ARCHIVES OF GENERAL PSYCHIATRY

Volume 53

January through December 1996

Editor
Jack D. Barchas, MD
New York, NY

Assistant to Editor
Peter M. Marzuk, MD
New York, NY

Editorial Administrator
Angela McGregor
New York, NY

Editorial Board

ARCHIVES
OF
GENERAL PSYCHIATRY

VOL 53 NO. 1, JANUARY 1996

Commentary

Neurodevelopmental Abnormalities and Schizophrenia: A Family Affair 11
Richard Jed Wyatt, MD

Original Articles

Rhesus Incompatibility as a Risk Factor for Schizophrenia in Male Adults 19
J. Meggin Hollister, PhD; Peter Laing, PhD; Sarnoff A. Mednick, PhD, DrMed

Schizophrenia After Prenatal Famine: Further Evidence 25
Ezra Susser, MD, DrPH; Richard Neugebauer, PhD; Hans W. Hoek, MD; Alan S. Brown, MD; Shang Lin, PhD; Daniel Labovitz, MD; Jack M. Gorman, MD

Search for Viral Nucleic Acid Sequences in Brain Tissues of Patients With Schizophrenia Using Nested Polymerase Chain Reaction 32
Alla M. Taller, MD; David M. Asher, MD; Kitty L. Pomeroy; Basil A. Eldadah; Mark S. Godec, MD; Peter G. Falkai, MD; Bernhard Bogert, MD; Joel E. Kleinman, MD, PhD; Janice R. Stevens, MD; E. Fuller Torrey, MD

Effects of Rapid Tryptophan Depletion in Patients With Seasonal Affective Disorder in Remission After Light Therapy 41
Raymond W. Lam, MD; Athanasios P. Zis, MD; Arvinder Grewal; Pedro L. Delgado, MD; Dennis S. Charney, MD; John H. Krystal, MD

American Medical Association
Physicians dedicated to the health of America

James S. Todd, MD
Executive Vice President
Kenneth E. Monroe
Deputy Executive Vice President
George D. Lundberg, MD
Editor in Chief, Scientific Information and Multimedia
James F. Rappel
Group Vice President, Business and Management Services
Robert L. Kennett
Vice President, Publishing
Michael D. Springer
Publisher
Mary C. Steermann
Director, Production and Distribution Division

Cheryl Iverson
Director, Editorial Processing Division
Peter L. Payerli
Director, Advertising Sales
Geoffrey A. Flick
Manager, Marketing Services

Advertising Office: J. P. Cahill & Associates, 341 S Waiola Ave, La Grange, IL 60525 (708) 352-1450. **AMA Physician Recruitment Advertising Department:** Carri Lynch, Supervisor, 800-262-2260.

Seasonal Changes in Mood and Behavior: The Role of Genetic Factors 47
Pamela A. F. Madden, PhD; Andrew C. Heath, DPhil; Norman E. Rosenthal, MD; Nicholas G. Martin, PhD

Anterior Paralimbic Mediation of Procaine-Induced Emotional and Psychosensory Experiences 59
Terence A. Ketter, MD; Paul J. Andreason, MD; Mark S. George, MD; Chulhee Lee, PhD; Debra S. Gill, MA; Priti I. Parekh; Mark W. Willis, MEng; Peter Herscovitch, MD; Robert M. Post, MD

High School Students Who Use Crack and Other Drugs 71
Denise B. Kandel, PhD, Mark Davies, MPH

Letters to the Editor

Response of Organic Catatonia to Risperidone 82
Edwin H. Cook, Jr, MD; Kerri Olson, PhD; Neil Pliskin, PhD

Panic Attacks: Klein's False Suffocation Alarm, Taylor and Rachman's Data, and Ley's Dyspneic-Fear Theory 83
Ronald Ley, PhD

In Reply 83
Donald F. Klein, MD

The Occurrence of Schizophrenia in Monozygotic Twins and Fractal Dendritic Development 85
Nicholas Pediaditakis, MD

Regular Departments

Index to Advertisers 5

This Month in *Archives of General Psychiatry* 10

Physician Recruitment Advertising 87

Instructions for Authors—See December 1995 issue, page 1083.

ARCHIVES OF GENERAL PSYCHIATRY

VOL 53 NO. 2, FEBRUARY 1996

ORIGINAL ARTICLES

Abnormal Electroencephalographic Sleep Profiles in Major Depression: Association With Response to Cognitive Behavior Therapy 99
Michael E. Thase, MD; Anne D. Simons, PhD; Charles F. Reynolds III, MD

Systematic Changes in Cerebral Glucose Metabolic Rate After Successful Behavior Modification Treatment of Obsessive-Compulsive Disorder 109
Jeffrey M. Schwartz, MD; Paula W. Stoessel, PhD; Lewis R. Baxter, Jr, MD; Karron M. Martin, RN; Michael E. Phelps, PhD

Clinical and Biochemical Effects of Catecholamine Depletion on Antidepressant-Induced Remission of Depression 117
Helen L. Miller, MD; Pedro L. Delgado, MD; Ronald M. Salomon, MD; Robert Berman, MD; John H. Krystal, MD; George R. Heninger, MD; Dennis S. Charney, MD

A Hospital-Based Twin Registry Study of the Heritability of *DSM-IV* Unipolar Depression 129
Peter McGuffin, MB, PhD, FRCP, FRCPsych; Randy Katz, PhD; Sarah Watkins, MB, MRCPsych; Joan Rutherford, MB, MRCPsych

American Medical Association
Physicians dedicated to the health of America

Increased Number of Vasopressin- and Oxytocin-Expressing Neurons in the Paraventricular Nucleus of the Hypothalamus in Depression 137
Jan S. Purba, MD, PhD; Witte J. G. Hoogendijk, MD; Michel A. Hofman, PhD; Dick F. Swaab, MD, PhD

Electroencephalographic Sleep Profiles During Depression: Effects of Episode Duration and Other Clinical and Psychosocial Factors in Older Adults 148
Mary Amanda Dew, PhD; Charles F. Reynolds III, MD; Daniel J. Buysse, MD; Patricia R. Houck, MS; Carolyn C. Hoch, PhD; Timothy H. Monk, PhD; David J. Kupfer, MD

Agoraphobia, Simple Phobia, and Social Phobia in the National Comorbidity Survey 159
William J. Magee, PhD; William W. Eaton, PhD; Hans-Ulrich Wittchen, PhD; Katherine A. McGonagle, PhD; Ronald C. Kessler, PhD

Public-Speaking Fears in a Community Sample: Prevalence, Impact on Functioning, and Diagnostic Classification 169
Murray B. Stein, MD; John R. Walker, PhD; David R. Forde, PhD

Depressed Mood and the Incidence of Alzheimer's Disease in the Elderly Living in the Community 175
D. P. Devanand, MD; Mary Sano, PhD; Ming-Xin Tang, PhD; Stuart Taylor, MD; Barry J. Gurland, MD; David Wilder, PhD; Yaakov Stern, PhD; Richard Mayeux, MD

REGULAR DEPARTMENTS

Index to Advertisers 93

This Month in *Archives of General Psychiatry* 98

Physician Recruitment Advertising 183

Instructions for Authors— See December 1995 issue, page 1083.

ARCHIVES OF GENERAL PSYCHIATRY

ARCHIVES OF GENERAL PSYCHIATRY

VOL 53 NO. 3, MARCH 1996

COMMENTARY

Alcohol Research: At the Cutting Edge 199
Enoch Gordis, MD

ORIGINAL ARTICLES

An 8-Year Follow-up of 450 Sons of Alcoholic and Control Subjects 202
Marc A. Schuckit, MD, Tom L. Smith, PhD

Early-Onset Alcoholics Have Lower Cerebrospinal Fluid 5-Hydroxyindoleacetic Acid Levels Than Late-Onset Alcoholics 211
Marie-Lourdes Fils-Aime, MD; Michael J. Eckardt, PhD; David T. George, MD; Gerald L. Brown, MD; Ivan Mefford, PhD; Markku Linnoila, MD, PhD

Six-Month Follow-up of Naltrexone and Psychotherapy for Alcohol Dependence 217
Stephanie S. O'Malley, PhD; Adam J. Jaffe, PhD; Grace Chang, MD; Sarah Rode, MA; Richard Schottenfeld, MD; Roger E. Meyer, MD; Bruce Rounsaville, MD

The Obsessive Compulsive Drinking Scale: A New Method of Assessing Outcome in Alcoholism Treatment Studies 225
Raymond F. Anton, MD; Darlene H. Moak, MD; Patricia K. Latham, PhD

Imipramine Treatment of Alcoholics With Primary Depression: A Placebo-Controlled Clinical Trial 232
Patrick J. McGrath, MD; Edward V. Nunes, MD; Jonathan W. Stewart, MD; Deberah Goldman, PhD; Vito Agosti, MSW; Katja Ocepek-Welikson, MPhil; Frederic M. Quitkin, MD

American Medical Association
Physicians dedicated to the health of America

A Long-term Follow-up of Male Alcohol Abuse 243
George E. Vaillant, MD

Enhanced Sensitivity of Pituitary β-Endorphin to Ethanol in Subjects at High Risk of Alcoholism 250
Christina Gianoulakis, PhD; Brinda Krishnan, MD; Joseph Thavundayil, MD

The Electroencephalogram After Alcohol Administration in High-Risk Men and the Development of Alcohol Use Disorders 10 Years Later: Preliminary Findings 258
Jan Volavka, MD, PhD; Pál Czobor, PhD; Donald W. Goodwin, MD; William F. Gabrielli, Jr, MD, PhD; Elizabeth C. Penick, PhD; Sarnoff A. Mednick, PhD, DrMed; Per Jensen, MD; Joachim Knop, MD; Fini Schulsinger, MD

The Effects of Alcohol Consumption on Laboratory-Induced Panic and State Anxiety 264
Matt G. Kushner, PhD; Thomas B. Mackenzie, MD; Joanna Fiszdon; David P. Valentiner, PhD; Edna Foa, PhD; Nicole Anderson; Douglas Wangensteen, PhD

REGULAR DEPARTMENTS

Index to Advertisers 189

Interactive Opportunities 189

This Month in *Archives of General Psychiatry* 194

Physician Recruitment Advertising 271

Instructions for Authors—See December 1995 issue, page 1083.

ARCHIVES OF GENERAL PSYCHIATRY

ARCHIVES
OF
GENERAL PSYCHIATRY

VOL 53 NO. 4, APRIL 1996

NEWS AND VIEWS

The Role of Psychotherapy in the Treatment of Depression: Review of Two Practice Guidelines 283
Jacqueline B. Persons, PhD; Michael E. Thase, MD; Paul Crits-Christoph, PhD

COMMENTARIES

The Role of Psychotherapy in the Treatment of Depression: Review of Two Practice Guidelines 291
John S. McIntyre, MD; Deborah A. Zarin, MD; Harold Alan Pincus, MD

The Role of Psychotherapy in the Treatment of Depression: Review of Two Practice Guidelines 298
A. John Rush, MD

The Role of Psychotherapy in the Treatment of Depression: Review of Two Practice Guidelines 301
Arnold E. Merriam, MD; T. Byram Karasu, MD

Practice Guidelines and Professional Challenges: What Psychotherapists Need to Do 303
James H. Kocsis, MD

ORIGINAL ARTICLES

Recovery in Geriatric Depression 305
George S. Alexopoulos, MD; Barnett S. Meyers, MD; Robert C. Young, MD; Tatsu Kakuma, PhD; Maria Feder, MD; Adam Einhorn, MBA; Eileen Rosendahl, PhD

Incidence and Correlates of Tardive Dyskinesia in First Episode of Schizophrenia 313
Miranda H. Chakos, MD; Jose Ma. J. Alvir, DrPH; Margaret G. Woerner, PhD; Amy Koreen, MD; Stephen Geisler, MD; David Mayerhoff, MD; Steven Sobel, MD; John M. Kane, MD; Michael Borenstein, PhD; Jeffrey A. Lieberman, MD

Hypothalamic-Pituitary-Adrenal Axis Activity in Panic Disorder: 24-Hour Secretion of Corticotropin and Cortisol 323
James L. Abelson, MD, PhD; George C. Curtis, MD

Mental Health Problems Among Homeless Mothers: Relationship to Service Use and Child Mental Health Problems 332
Bonnie T. Zima, MD, MPH; Kenneth B. Wells, MD, MPH; Bernadette Benjamin, MSc; Naihua Duan, PhD

Psychiatric Diagnosis in Child and Adolescent Suicide 339
David Shaffer, MB, BS, FRCP, FRCPsych; Madelyn S. Gould, PhD, MPH; Prudence Fisher, MS; Paul Trautman, MD; Donna Moreau, MD; Marjorie Kleinman, MA; Michael Flory, PhD, MPH

Personality Disorders Predict Onset of Axis I Disorders and Impaired Functioning Among Homosexual Men With and at Risk of HIV Infection 350
Jeffrey G. Johnson, PhD; Janet B. W. Williams, DSW; Raymond R. Goetz, PhD; Judith G. Rabkin, PhD; Robert H. Remien, PhD; Joshua D. Lipsitz, PhD; Jack M. Gorman, MD

Communication Disturbances in Schizophrenia and Mania 358
Nancy M. Docherty, PhD; Maddalena DeRosa; Nancy C. Andreasen, MD, PhD

REGULAR DEPARTMENTS

Index to Advertisers 277

This Month in *Archives of General Psychiatry* 282

Physician Recruitment Advertising 366

Instructions for Authors—See December 1995 issue, page 1083.

ARCHIVES OF GENERAL PSYCHIATRY

ARCHIVES OF GENERAL PSYCHIATRY

VOL 53 NO. 5, MAY 1996

ORIGINAL ARTICLES

A Symptom Provocation Study of Posttraumatic Stress Disorder Using Positron Emission Tomography and Script-Driven Imagery **380**
Scott L. Rauch, MD; Bessel A. van der Kolk, MD; Rita E. Fisler, EdM; Nathaniel M. Alpert, PhD; Scott P. Orr, PhD; Cary R. Savage, PhD; Alan J. Fischman, MD, PhD; Michael A. Jenike, MD; Roger K. Pitman, MD

The Identification and Validation of Distinct Depressive Syndromes in a Population-Based Sample of Female Twins **391**
Kenneth S. Kendler, MD; Lindon J. Eaves, PhD, DSc; Ellen E. Walters, MS; Michael C. Neale, PhD; Andrew C. Heath, DPhil; Ronald C. Kessler, PhD

A Controlled Trial Comparing Buprenorphine and Methadone Maintenance in Opioid Dependence **401**
Walter Ling, MD; Donald R. Wesson, MD; Charles Charuvastra, MD; C. James Klett, PhD

Sustained Cocaine Abstinence in Methadone Maintenance Patients Through Voucher-Based Reinforcement Therapy **409**
Kenneth Silverman, PhD; Stephen T. Higgins, PhD; Robert K. Brooner, PhD; Ivan D. Montoya, MD; Edward J. Cone, PhD; Charles R. Schuster, PhD; Kenzie L. Preston, PhD

Israeli Preschoolers Under Scud Missile Attacks: A Developmental Perspective on Risk-Modifying Factors **416**
Nathaniel Laor, MD, PhD; Leo Wolmer, MA; Linda C. Mayes, MD; Abigail Golomb, MD; Donald S. Silverberg, MD; Ronit Weizman, MD; Donald J. Cohen, MD

American Medical Association
Physicians dedicated to the health of America

All articles published, including editorials, letters, and book reviews, represent the opinions of the authors and do not reflect the policy of the American Medical Association, the Editorial Board, or the institution with which the author is affiliated, unless this is clearly specified.

James S. Todd, MD
Executive Vice President
Kenneth E. Monroe
Deputy Executive Vice President
George D. Lundberg, MD
Editor in Chief, Scientific Information and Multimedia
James F. Rappel
Group Vice President, Business and Management Services
Robert L. Kennett
Vice President, Publishing
Michael D. Springer
Publisher, New Media
Peter L. Payerli
Associate Publisher

Mary C. Steermann
Director, Production & Distribution Division
Cheryl Iverson
Director, Editorial Processing Division
Geoffrey A. Flick
Manager, Marketing Services

Advertising Office: J. P. Cahill & Associates, 341 S Waiola Ave, La Grange, IL 60525 (708) 352-0322. **AMA Physician Recruitment Advertising Department:** Carri Lynch, Supervisor, 800-262-2260.

Maldistribution of Interstitial Neurons in Prefrontal White Matter of the Brains of Schizophrenic Patients 425
Schahram Akbarian, MD, PhD; James J. Kim; Steven G. Potkin, MD; William P. Hetrick, PhD; William E. Bunney, Jr, MD; Edward G. Jones, MD, PhD

A Prospective 4-Year Follow-up Study of Attention-Deficit Hyperactivity and Related Disorders 437
Joseph Biederman, MD; Stephen Faraone, PhD; Sharon Milberger, DSc; Jessica Guite; Eric Mick; Lisa Chen; Douglas Mennin; Abbe Marrs; Cheryl Ouellette; Phoebe Moore; Thomas Spencer, MD; Dennis Norman, EdD; Timothy Wilens, MD; Ilana Kraus, MD; James Perrin, MD

NEWS AND VIEWS

The Contribution of α_2-Noradrenergic Mechanisms to Prefrontal Cortical Cognitive Function: Potential Significance for Attention-Deficit Hyperactivity Disorder 448
Amy F. T. Arnsten, PhD; Jenna C. Steere, MPH; Robert D. Hunt, MD

Catching up on Schizophrenia: The Fifth International Congress on Schizophrenia Research, Warm Springs, Va, April 8-12, 1995 456
Peter F. Buckley, MD; Robert W. Buchanan, MD (Rapporteurs); S. Charles Schulz, MD; Carol A. Tamminga, MD (Organizers)

CORRECTION

A Hospital-Based Twin Registry Study of the Heritability of *DSM-IV* Unipolar Depression 436
Peter McGuffin, MB, PhD, FRCP, FRCPsych; Randy Katz, PhD; Sarah Watkins, MB, MRCPsych; Joan Rutherford, MB, MRCPsych

REGULAR DEPARTMENTS

Index to Advertisers 373

This Month in *Archives of General Psychiatry* 378

Physician Recruitment Advertising 463

Instructions for Authors—See December 1995 issue, page 1083.

ARCHIVES OF GENERAL PSYCHIATRY

ARCHIVES OF GENERAL PSYCHIATRY

VOL 53 NO. 6, JUNE 1996

EDITORIAL

Violence, Crime, and Mental Illness: How Strong a Link? 481
Peter M. Marzuk, MD

ORIGINAL ARTICLES

Mental Disorder and Crime: Evidence From a Danish Birth Cohort 489
Sheilagh Hodgins, PhD; Sarnoff A. Mednick, DrMed, PhD; Patricia A. Brennan, PhD; Fini Schulsinger, MD; Marianne Engberg, MD, PhD

Mental Disorders and Homicidal Behavior in Finland 497
Markku Eronen, MD; Panu Hakola, MD, PhD; Jari Tiihonen, MD, PhD

Prevalence of Psychiatric Disorders Among Incarcerated Women: I. Pretrial Jail Detainees 505
Linda A. Teplin, PhD; Karen M. Abram, PhD; Gary M. McClelland, PhD

Prevalence of Psychiatric Disorders Among Incarcerated Women: II. Convicted Felons Entering Prison 513
B. Kathleen Jordan, PhD; William E. Schlenger, PhD; John A. Fairbank, PhD; Juesta M. Caddell, PhD

A Prospective Follow-up Study of Alcoholic Violent Offenders and Fire Setters 523
Matti Virkkunen, MD; Monika Eggert, MD; Robert Rawlings, MS; Markku Linnoila, MD, PhD

American Medical Association
Physicians dedicated to the health of America

Impulsive Aggression in Personality Disorder Correlates With Tritiated Paroxetine Binding in the Platelet 531
Emil F. Coccaro, MD; Richard J. Kavoussi, MD; Yvette I. Sheline, MD; Jennifer D. Lish, PhD; John G. Csernansky, MD

Excessive Mortality in Young Free-Ranging Male Nonhuman Primates With Low Cerebrospinal Fluid 5-Hydroxyindoleacetic Acid Concentrations 537
J. Dee Higley, PhD; Patrick T. Mehlman, PhD; David M. Taub, PhD; Sue B. Higley; Beth Fernald; James Vickers, DVM; Stephen G. Lindell; Stephen J. Suomi, PhD; Markku Linnoila, MD, PhD

High Rates of Violence, Crime, Academic Problems, and Behavioral Problems in Males With Both Early Neuromotor Deficits and Unstable Family Environments 544
Adrian Raine, PhD; Patricia Brennan, PhD; Birgitte Mednick, PhD; Sarnoff A. Mednick, PhD, DM

The Association of Sexual Assault and Attempted Suicide Within the Community 550
Jonathan R. T. Davidson, MD; Dana C. Hughes, RN, PhD; Linda K. George, PhD; Dan G. Blazer, MD, PhD

REGULAR DEPARTMENTS

Index to Advertisers 469

This Month in *Archives of General Psychiatry* 474

Instructions for Authors 556

Physician Recruitment Advertising 558

ARCHIVES OF GENERAL PSYCHIATRY

ARCHIVES OF GENERAL PSYCHIATRY

VOL 53 NO. 7, JULY 1996

COMMENTARY

Mapping Mental Illness: A New Era 574
John C. Mazziotta, MD, PhD

ORIGINAL ARTICLES

Normal Caudate Nucleus in Obsessive-compulsive Disorder Assessed by Quantitative Neuroimaging 577
Elizabeth H. Aylward, PhD; Gordon J. Harris, PhD; Rudolf Hoehn-Saric, MD; Patrick E. Barta, MD, PhD; Steven R. Machlin, MD; Godfrey D. Pearlson, MB, BS

Sex Differences in Human Brain Morphometry and Metabolism: An In Vivo Quantitative Magnetic Resonance Imaging and Positron Emission Tomography Study on the Effect of Aging 585
Declan G. M. Murphy, MD; Charles DeCarli, MD; Andrew R. McIntosh, PhD; Eileen Daly; Marc J. Mentis, MD; Pietro Pietrini, MD; Joanna Szczepanik, MA; Mark B. Schapiro, MD; Cheryl L. Grady, PhD; Barry Horwitz, PhD; Stanley I. Rapoport, MD

Functional Magnetic Resonance Imaging of Symptom Provocation in Obsessive-compulsive Disorder 595
Hans C. Breiter, MD; Scott L. Rauch, MD; Kenneth K. Kwong, PhD; John R. Baker, PhD; Robert M. Weisskoff, PhD; David N. Kennedy, PhD; Adair D. Kendrick; Timothy L. Davis, MS; Aiping Jiang, PhD; Mark S. Cohen, PhD; Chantal E. Stern, DPhil; John W. Belliveau, PhD; Lee Baer, PhD; Richard L. O'Sullivan, MD; Cary R. Savage, PhD; Michael A. Jenike, MD; Bruce R. Rosen, MD, PhD

Quantitative Brain Magnetic Resonance Imaging in Attention-Deficit Hyperactivity Disorder 607
F. Xavier Castellanos, MD; Jay N. Giedd, MD; Wendy L. Marsh; Susan D. Hamburger, MA, MS; A. Catherine Vaituzis; Daniel P. Dickstein; Stacey E. Sarfatti; Yolanda C. Vauss; John W. Snell, PhD; Nicholas Lange, PhD; Debra Kaysen; Amy L. Krain; Gail F. Ritchie, MSW; Jagath C. Rajapakse, PhD; Judith L. Rapoport, MD

American Medical Association
Physicians dedicated to the health of America

James S. Todd, MD
Executive Vice President
Kenneth E. Monroe
Deputy Executive Vice President
George D. Lundberg, MD
Editor in Chief, Scientific Information and Multimedia
James F. Rappel
Group Vice President, Business and Management Services
Robert L. Kennett
Vice President, Publishing
Michael D. Springer
Publisher, New Media
Peter L. Payerli
Associate Publisher

Mary C. Steermann
Director, Production & Distribution Division
Cheryl Iverson
Director, Editorial Processing Division
Geoffrey A. Flick
Manager, Marketing Services

Advertising Office: J. P. Cahill & Associates, 341 S Waiola Ave, La Grange, IL 60525 (708) 352-0322. **AMA Physician Recruitment Advertising Department:** Carri Lynch, Supervisor, 800-262-2260.

Brain Anatomic Magnetic Resonance Imaging in Childhood-Onset Schizophrenia 617
Jean A. Frazier, MD; Jay N. Giedd, MD; Susan D. Hamburger, MA, MS; Kathleen E. Albus; Debra Kaysen; A. Catherine Vaituzis; Jagath C. Rajapakse, PhD; Marge C. Lenane, MSW; Kathleen McKenna, MD; Leslie K. Jacobsen, MD; Charles T. Gordon, MD; Alan Breier, MD; Judith L. Rapoport, MD

Cerebral Structural Abnormalities in Obsessive-compulsive Disorder: A Quantitative Morphometric Magnetic Resonance Imaging Study 625
Michael A. Jenike, MD; Hans C. Breiter, MD; Lee Baer, PhD; David N. Kennedy, PhD; Cary R. Savage, PhD; Michael J. Olivares; Richard L. O'Sullivan, MD; David M. Shera, MS; Scott L. Rauch, MD; Nancy Keuthen, PhD; Bruce R. Rosen, MD, PhD; Verne S. Caviness, MD, PhD; Pauline A. Filipek, MD

Auditory Attentional Deficits in Patients With Schizophrenia: A Positron Emission Tomography Study 633
Daniel S. O'Leary, PhD; Nancy C. Andreasen, MD, PhD; Richard R. Hurtig, PhD; Marilyn L. Kesler; Margaret Rogers, PhD; Stephen Arndt, PhD; Ted Cizadlo; G. Leonard Watkins, PhD; Laura L. Boles Ponto, PhD; Peter T. Kirchner, MD; Richard D. Hichwa, PhD

Brain Glucose Metabolism During Non–Rapid Eye Movement Sleep in Major Depression: A Positron Emission Tomography Study 645
Andrew P. Ho, MD; J. Christian Gillin, MD; Monte S. Buchsbaum, MD; Joseph C. Wu, MD; Lennert Abel, MD; William E. Bunney, Jr, MD

LETTERS TO THE EDITOR

Retinoid Dysregulation May Result in Abnormal Expression of Glutamic Acid Decarboxylase in Schizophrenia 653
Ann B. Goodman

Venlafaxine in Obsessive-compulsive Disorder 653
Jose A. Yaryura-Tobias, MD; Fugen A. Neziroglu, PhD

In Reply 654
John H. Greist, MD

CORRECTION

The Obsessive-compulsive Drinking Scale: A New Method of Assessing Outcome in Alcoholism Treatment Studies 576
Raymond F. Anton, MD; Darlene H. Moak, MD; Patricia K. Latham, PhD

REGULAR DEPARTMENTS

Index to Advertisers 565

This Month in *Archives of General Psychiatry* 571

Physician Recruitment Advertising 656

Instructions for Authors— See June 1996 issue, page 556

ARCHIVES OF GENERAL PSYCHIATRY

ARCHIVES OF GENERAL PSYCHIATRY

VOL 53 NO. 8, AUGUST 1996

EDITORIAL

The Contribution of Psychotherapy and Pharmacotherapy Research to National Mental Health Care: Introduction to the Special Series 670
Larry E. Beutler, PhD; Jack D. Barchas, MD; Peter M. Marzuk, MD

ORIGINAL ARTICLES

Relapse Prevention by Acamprosate: Results From a Placebo-Controlled Study on Alcohol Dependence 673
Henning Sass, MD; Michael Soyka, MD; Karl Mann, MD; Walter Zieglgänsberger, MD

Replication of the Stockholm Adoption Study of Alcoholism: Confirmatory Cross-Fostering Analysis 681
Sören Sigvardsson, PhD; Michael Bohman, MD; C. Robert Cloninger, MD

Does Brief Dynamic Psychotherapy Reduce the Relapse Rate of Panic Disorder? 689
Ida M. Wiborg, PhD; Alv A. Dahl, MD, PhD

SPECIAL ARTICLES

Patterns of Mental Health Service Utilization 696
Kenneth I. Howard, PhD; Thomas A. Cornille, PhD; John S. Lyons, PhD; John T. Vessey, PhD; Robert J. Lueger, PhD; Stephen M. Saunders, PhD

Psychotherapy Research in Historical Perspective: Implications for Mental Health Care Policy 708
Robert L. Russell, PhD; David E. Orlinsky, PhD

American Medical Association
Physicians dedicated to the health of America

Psychotherapy of Depression: Implications for Reform of the Health Care System 717
John F. Clarkin, PhD; Paul A. Pilkonis, PhD; Kathryn M. Magruder, PhD

Advances in the Psychosocial Treatment of Anxiety Disorders: Implications for National Health Care 727
David H. Barlow, PhD; Cassandra L. Lehman

Alcohol Treatment and Health Care System Reform 737
Barbara S. McCrady, PhD; James W. Langenbucher, PhD

Psychosocial Treatment for Drug Abuse: Selected Review and Recommendations for National Health Care 749
Paul Crits-Christoph, PhD; Lynne Siqueland, PhD

CORRECTION

Prevalence of Psychiatric Disorders Among Incarcerated Women: I. Pretrial Jail Detainees 664
Linda A. Teplin, PhD; Karen M. Abram, PhD; Gary M. McClelland, PhD

REGULAR DEPARTMENTS

This Month in *Archives of General Psychiatry* 663

Index to Advertisers 665

Physician Recruitment Advertising 759

Instructions for Authors— See June 1996 issue, page 556

ARCHIVES OF GENERAL PSYCHIATRY

ARCHIVES OF GENERAL PSYCHIATRY

VOL 53 NO. 9, SEPTEMBER 1996

ORIGINAL ARTICLE

Maintenance Therapy for Chronic Depression: A Controlled Clinical Trial of Desipramine 769
James H. Kocsis, MD; Richard A. Friedman, MD; John C. Markowitz, MD; Andrew C. Leon, PhD; Nina L. Miller, MA; Leah Gniwesch, MA; Michael Parides, MS

COMMENTARY

Maintenance Therapy for Chronic Depression: A Controlled Clinical Trial of Desipramine 775
David J. Kupfer, MD; Ellen Frank, PhD

ORIGINAL ARTICLES

A Placebo-Controlled, Randomized Clinical Trial Comparing Sertraline and Imipramine for the Treatment of Dysthymia 777
Michael E. Thase, MD; Maurizio Fava, MD; Uriel Halbreich, MD; James H. Kocsis, MD; Lorrin Koran, MD; Jonathan Davidson, MD; Jerrold Rosenbaum, MD; Wilma Harrison, MD

Chronological Milestones to Guide Drug Change: When Should Clinicians Switch Antidepressants? 785
Frederic M. Quitkin, MD; Patrick J. McGrath, MD; Jonathan W. Stewart, MD; Katja Ocepek-Welikson, MPhil; Bonnie P. Taylor, MA; Edward Nunes, MD; Deborah Deliyannides, MD; Vito Agosti, MSW; Steven J. Donovan, MD; Eva Petkova, PhD; Donald F. Klein, MD

American Medical Association
Physicians dedicated to the health of America

All articles published, including editorials, letters, and book reviews, represent the opinions of the authors and do not reflect the policy of the American Medical Association, the Editorial Board, or the institution with which the author is affiliated, unless this is clearly specified.

Advertising Office: J. P. Cahill & Associates, 341 S Waiola Ave, La Grange, IL 60525 (708) 352-0322. **AMA Physician Recruitment Advertising Department:** Robert Lake, Supervisor, 800-262-2260.

Recovery After 5 Years of Unremitting Major Depressive Disorder 794
Timothy I. Mueller, MD; Martin B. Keller, MD; Andrew C. Leon, PhD; David A. Solomon, MD; M. Tracie Shea, PhD; William Coryell, MD; Jean Endicott, PhD

Immunodetection and Quantitation of Imidazoline Receptor Proteins in Platelets of Patients With Major Depression and in Brains of Suicide Victims 803
Jesús A. García-Sevilla, MD; Pablo V. Escribá, PhD; Magdalena Sastre, PhD; Claude Walzer, PhD; Xavier Busquets, PhD; Galina Jaquet, MD; Donald J. Reis, MD; José Guimón, MD

The Effects of Electroconvulsive Therapy on Quantitative Electroencephalograms: Relationship to Clinical Outcome 814
Harold A. Sackeim, PhD; Bruce Luber, PhD; Gary P. Katzman; James R. Moeller, PhD; Joan Prudic, MD; D. P. Devanand, MD; Mitchell S. Nobler, MD

COMMENTARY

Interictal Electroencephalographic Effects of Electroconvulsive Therapy: Can They Elucidate the Mechanism of Action? 826
Jan Volavka, MD, PhD; Pal Czobor, PhD

ORIGINAL ARTICLES

Effect of Antidepressant Medication on Morning and Evening Thyroid Function Tests During a Major Depressive Episode 833
Fabrice Duval, MD; Marie-Claude Mokrani, PhD; Marc-Antoine Crocq, MD; Martine Jautz, MAPsych; Paul Bailey, MRCPsych; Than-Son Diep, MD; Jean-Paul Macher, MD

Triiodothyronine Augmentation in the Treatment of Refractory Depression: A Meta-analysis 842
Ronnie Aronson, MD; Hilary J. Offman, MD; Russel T. Joffe, MD; C. David Naylor, MD, DPhil

REGULAR DEPARTMENTS

This Month in *Archives of General Psychiatry* 768

Instructions for Authors 850

Index to Advertisers 853

Physician Recruitment Advertising 854

ARCHIVES OF GENERAL PSYCHIATRY

ARCHIVES OF GENERAL PSYCHIATRY

VOL 53 NO. 10, OCTOBER 1996

NEWS AND VIEWS

Peering Into the 'Black Box': Measuring Outcomes of Managed Care 870
Harold Alan Pincus, MD; Deborah A. Zarin, MD; Joyce C. West, MPP

ORIGINAL ARTICLES

Subthreshold Psychiatric Symptoms in a Primary Care Group Practice 880
Mark Olfson, MD, MPH; W. Eugene Broadhead, MD, PhD; Myrna M. Weissman, PhD; Andrew C. Leon, PhD; Leslie Farber, PhD; Christina Hoven, PhD; Roger Kathol, MD

Comorbid Anxiety Disorder and the Functioning and Well-being of Chronically Ill Patients of General Medical Providers 889
Cathy Donald Sherbourne, PhD; Kenneth B. Wells, MD; Lisa S. Meredith, PhD; Catherine A. Jackson, PhD; Patti Camp, MA

Medical Costs Attributed to Depression Among Patients With a History of High Medical Expenses in a Health Maintenance Organization 899
Henry J. Henk, MS; David J. Katzelnick, MD; Kenneth A. Kobak, PhD; John H. Greist, MD; James W. Jefferson, MD

Counseling Typically Provided for Depression: Role of Clinician Specialty and Payment System 905
Lisa S. Meredith, PhD; Kenneth B. Wells, MD, MPH; Sherrie H. Kaplan, PhD, MPH; Rebecca M. Mazel, MA

Treating Major Depression in Primary Care Practice: Eight-Month Clinical Outcomes 913
Herbert C. Schulberg, PhD; Marian R. Block, MD; Michael J. Madonia, MSW; C. Paul Scott, MD; Eric Rodriguez, MD; Stanley D. Imber, PhD; James Perel, PhD; Judith Lave, PhD; Patricia R. Houck, MS; John L. Coulehan, MD

A Multifaceted Intervention to Improve Treatment of Depression in Primary Care 924
Wayne Katon, MD; Patricia Robinson, PhD; Michael Von Korff, ScD; Elizabeth Lin, MD, MPH; Terry Bush, PhD; Evette Ludman, PhD; Gregory Simon, MD, MPH; Edward Walker, MD

NEWS AND VIEWS

Some Economics of Mental Health 'Carve-Outs' 933
Richard G. Frank, PhD; Haiden A. Huskamp; Thomas G. McGuire, PhD; Joseph P. Newhouse, PhD

ORIGINAL ARTICLES

Enrollment Duration, Service Use, and Costs of Care for Severely Mentally Ill Members of a Health Maintenance Organization 938
Bentson H. McFarland, MD, PhD; Richard E. Johnson, PhD; Mark C. Hornbrook, PhD

Managing the Care of Schizophrenia: Lessons From a 4-Year Massachusetts Medicaid Study 945
Barbara Dickey, PhD; Sharon-Lise T. Normand, PhD; Edward C. Norton, PhD; Hocine Azeni, MA; William Fisher, PhD; Frederic Altaffer, PhD

Cost-effectiveness of Clozapine Monitoring After the First 6 Months 954
Mingliang Zhang, PhD; Richard R. Owen, MD; Sandra K. Pope, MPH; G. Richard Smith, MD

COMMENTARY

A Funny Thing Happened on the Way to Reform 959
Gary L. Tischler, MD; Boris M. Astrachan, MD

LETTER TO THE EDITOR

***TPH* Replication Study: Not!** 964
David A. Nielsen, PhD; David Goldman, MD; Matti Virkkunen, MD; Riitta Tokola, MD; Robert Rawlings, MS; Markku Linnoila, MD, PhD

REGULAR DEPARTMENTS

This Month in *Archives of General Psychiatry* 864

Index to Advertisers 865

Physician Recruitment Advertising 966

Instructions for Authors—See September 1996 issue, page 850

ARCHIVES OF GENERAL PSYCHIATRY

ARCHIVES OF GENERAL PSYCHIATRY

VOL 53 NO. 11, NOVEMBER 1996

COMMENTARY

Autism Research: Bringing Together Approaches to Pull Apart the Disorder 980
P. Anne McBride, MD; George M. Anderson, PhD; Theodore Shapiro, MD

ORIGINAL ARTICLES

Autism and the X Chromosome: Multipoint Sib-Pair Analysis 985
Joachim Hallmayer, MD; Joan M. Hebert, MA; Donna Spiker, PhD; Linda Lotspeich, MD; William M. McMahon, MD; P. Brent Petersen, MD; Peter Nicholas, LCSW; Carmen Pingree, MS; Alice A. Lin, MS; Luca L. Cavalli-Sforza, MD; Neil Risch, PhD; Roland D. Ciaranello, MD

Effects of Tryptophan Depletion in Drug-Free Adults With Autistic Disorder 993
Christopher J. McDougle, MD; Susan T. Naylor, RN, MSN; Donald J. Cohen, MD; George K. Aghajanian, MD; George R. Heninger, MD; Lawrence H. Price, MD

A Double-blind, Placebo-Controlled Study of Fluvoxamine in Adults With Autistic Disorder 1001
Christopher J. McDougle, MD; Susan T. Naylor, RN, MSN; Donald J. Cohen, MD; Fred R. Volkmar, MD; George R. Heninger, MD; Lawrence H. Price, MD

Nocturnal Serum Melatonin Profile in Major Depression in Children and Adolescents 1009
Mohammad Shafii, MD; Duncan R. MacMillan, MD; Mary P. Key, MS, MT; Ann McCue Derrick, RN, MS; Nancy Kaufman, MS; Irwin D. Nahinsky, PhD

Lifetime Prevalence, Demographic Risk Factors, and Diagnostic Validity of Nonaffective Psychosis as Assessed in a US Community Sample: The National Comorbidity Survey 1022
Kenneth S. Kendler, MD; Timothy J. Gallagher, PhD; Jamie M. Abelson, MSW; Ronald C. Kessler, PhD

American Medical Association
Physicians dedicated to the health of America

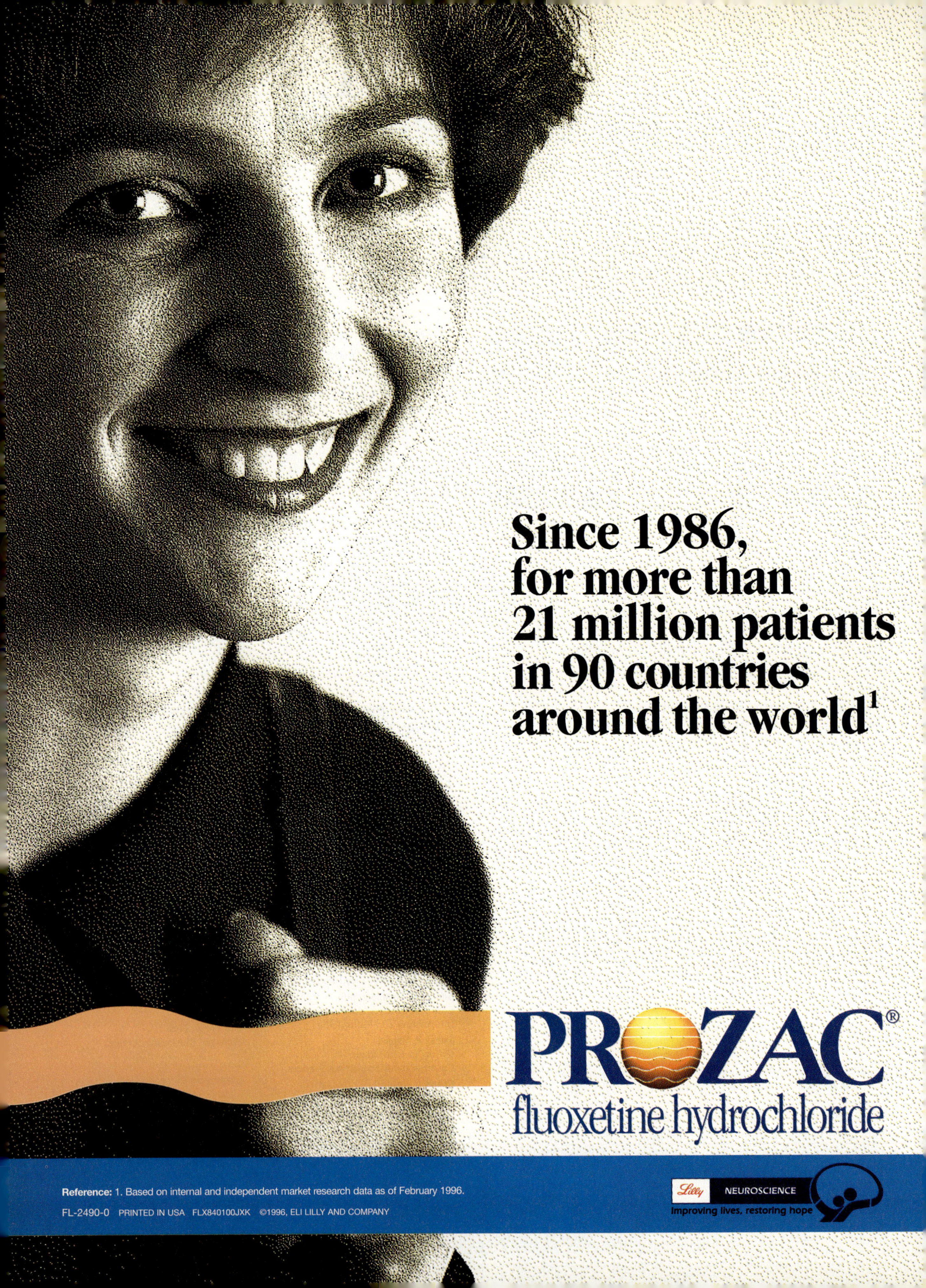
Since 1986, for more than 21 million patients in 90 countries around the world[1]
PROZAC®
fluoxetine hydrochloride
Reference: 1. Based on internal and independent market research data as of February 1996.
FL-2490-0 PRINTED IN USA FLX840100JXK ©1996, ELI LILLY AND COMPANY
Lilly NEUROSCIENCE
improving lives, restoring hope

Behavioral Observations at Age 3 Years Predict Adult Psychiatric Disorders: Longitudinal Evidence From a Birth Cohort 1033
Avshalom Caspi, PhD; Terrie E. Moffitt, PhD; Denise L. Newman, PhD; Phil A. Silva, PhD

Comorbidity Between Depressive Disorders and Nicotine Dependence in a Cohort of 16-Year-Olds 1043
David M. Fergusson, PhD; Michael T. Lynskey, MSc; L. John Horwood, MSc

Cognitive Correlates of Long-term Cannabis Use in Costa Rican Men 1051
Jack M. Fletcher, PhD; J. Bryan Page, PhD; David J. Francis, PhD; Kimberly Copeland, MA; Mary J. Naus, PhD; Chester M. Davis, PhD; Robin Morris, PhD; Dina Krauskopf, MA; Paul Satz, PhD

LETTERS TO THE EDITOR

Is Research in Normal and Ill Children Involving Radiation Exposure Ethical? 1059
Lt Col Charles T. Morton, MC, USAF

In Reply 1059
B. J. Casey, PhD; Jonathan D. Cohen, MD, PhD

In Reply 1060
Alan J. Zametkin, MD; David J. Schwartz; Monique Ernst, MD, PhD; Robert M. Cohen, MD, PhD

Parenthood, Completed Suicide, and Mental Disorders 1061
Erkki T. Isometsä, MD; Martti E. Heikkinen, MD; Markus M. Henriksson, MD; Hillevi M. Aro, MD, PhD; Mauri J. Marttunen, MD; Jouko K. Lönnqvist, MD, PhD

Schizophrenia and Temporal Lobe Epilepsy 1062
Amit Anand, MD

Alexander J. Mitchell, MB, BS 1063

In Reply 1063
James M. Gold, PhD; Bruce P. Hermann, PhD; Daniel R. Weinberger, MD

Alterations of Membrane Phospholipid Metabolism in Patients With Schizophrenia Assessed by Phosphorus Magnetic Resonance Spectroscopy 1065
Tony P. George, MD; Matthew W. Spence, MD, PhD

Rapid Eye Movement Density Among Adolescents With Major Depressive Disorder Revisited 1066
Raymond R. Goetz, PhD; Susan I. Wolk, MD; Jeremy D. Coplan, MD; Myrna M. Weissman, PhD; Ronald E. Dahl, MD; Neal D. Ryan, MD

REGULAR DEPARTMENTS

This Month in *Archives of General Psychiatry* 977

Index to Advertisers 984

Physician Recruitment Advertising 1071

Instructions for Authors— See September 1996 issue, page 850.

ARCHIVES OF GENERAL PSYCHIATRY

ARCHIVES
OF
GENERAL PSYCHIATRY

VOL 53 NO. 12, DECEMBER 1996

EDITORIAL

Quality of Care: A Call for Papers for the Annual Coordinated Theme Issues of the AMA Journals 1085
George D. Lundberg, MD; John E. Wennberg, MD

ORIGINAL ARTICLES

Childhood-Onset Schizophrenia: A Double-blind Clozapine-Haloperidol Comparison 1090
Sanjiv Kumra, MD; Jean A. Frazier, MD; Leslie K. Jacobsen, MD; Kathleen McKenna, MD; Charles T. Gordon, MD; Marge C. Lenane, MSW; Susan D. Hamburger, MA, MS; Amy K. Smith; Kathleen E. Albus; Javad Alaghband-Rad, MD; Judith L. Rapoport, MD

The Influence of Expressed Emotion, Family Dynamics, and Symptom Type on the Social Adjustment of Schizophrenic Young Adults 1098
Suzanne King, PhD; Mike J. Dixon, PhD

Schizophrenic Deficits in the Processing of Context: A Test of a Theoretical Model 1105
David Servan-Schreiber, MD, PhD; Jonathan D. Cohen, MD, PhD; Sandra Steingard, MD

Inhibitory Gating of an Evoked Response to Repeated Auditory Stimuli in Schizophrenic and Normal Subjects: Human Recordings, Computer Simulation, and an Animal Model 1114
Robert Freedman, MD; Lawrence E. Adler, MD; Marina Myles-Worsley, PhD; Herbert T. Nagamoto, MD; Christine Miller, PhD; Michael Kisley, MS; Kara McRae, BA; Ellen Cawthra, RN; Merilyne Waldo, PhD

Psychopathological and Behavioral Correlates of Dopaminergic Sensitivity in Alcohol-Dependent Patients 1123
Andreas Heinz, MD; Peter Dufeu, Dipl Psych; Silke Kuhn, Dipl Psych; Michael Dettling, MD; Klaus Gräf, MD; Irene Kürten, MTA; Hans Rommelspacher, MD; Lutz G. Schmidt, MD

American Medical Association
Physicians dedicated to the health of America

All articles published, including editorials, letters, and book reviews, represent the opinions of the authors and do not reflect the policy of the American Medical Association, the Editorial Board, or the institution with which the author is affiliated, unless this is clearly specified.

The Great Smoky Mountains Study of Youth: Goals, Design, Methods, and the Prevalence of *DSM-III-R* Disorders 1129
E. Jane Costello, PhD; Adrian Angold, MRCPsych; Barbara J. Burns, PhD; Dalene K. Stangl, PhD; Dan L. Tweed, PhD; Alaattin Erkanli, PhD; Carol M. Worthman, PhD

The Great Smoky Mountains Study of Youth: Functional Impairment and Serious Emotional Disturbance 1137
E. Jane Costello, PhD; Adrian Angold, MRCPsych; Barbara J. Burns, PhD; Alaattin Erkanli, PhD; Dalene K. Stangl, PhD; Dan L. Tweed, PhD

Suicidal Behavior Runs in Families: A Controlled Family Study of Adolescent Suicide Victims 1145
David A. Brent, MD; Jeff Bridge; Barbara A. Johnson, MD; John Connolly, MA

Psychosocial Risk Factors of Child and Adolescent Completed Suicide 1155
Madelyn S. Gould, PhD, MPH; Prudence Fisher, MS; Michael Parides, PhD; Michael Flory, PhD; David Shaffer, MD

LETTERS TO THE EDITOR

Studies of Ventricular Enlargement 1165
Rajendra Persaud, MSc, MPhil, MD, MRCPsych

In Reply 1166
Lee Friedman, PhD; John A. Jesberger; Herbert Y. Meltzer, MD; Helio Elkis, MD, PhD

The Relationship Between Plasma Haloperidol Concentrations and Clinical Results 1167
Diego J. Palao, MD; Alberte Araúxo, MD; Josep M. Haro, MD; Mercé Brunet, MD; Miguel Bernardo, PhD

In Reply 1168
Jan Volavka, MD, PhD; Thomas B. Cooper, MA; Pal Czobor, PhD; Morris Meisner, PhD

CORRECTION

Relapse Prevention by Acamprosate: Results From a Placebo-Controlled Study on Alcohol Dependence 1097
Henning Sass, MD; Michael Soyka, MD; Karl Mann, MD; Walter Zieglgänsberger, MD

REGULAR DEPARTMENTS

Reviewers for 1996 1081

This Month in *Archives of General Psychiatry* 1088

Index to Advertisers 1122

Index to Volume 53 1170

Physician Recruitment Advertising 1175

Instructions for Authors—See September 1996 issue, page 850.

ARCHIVES OF GENERAL PSYCHIATRY

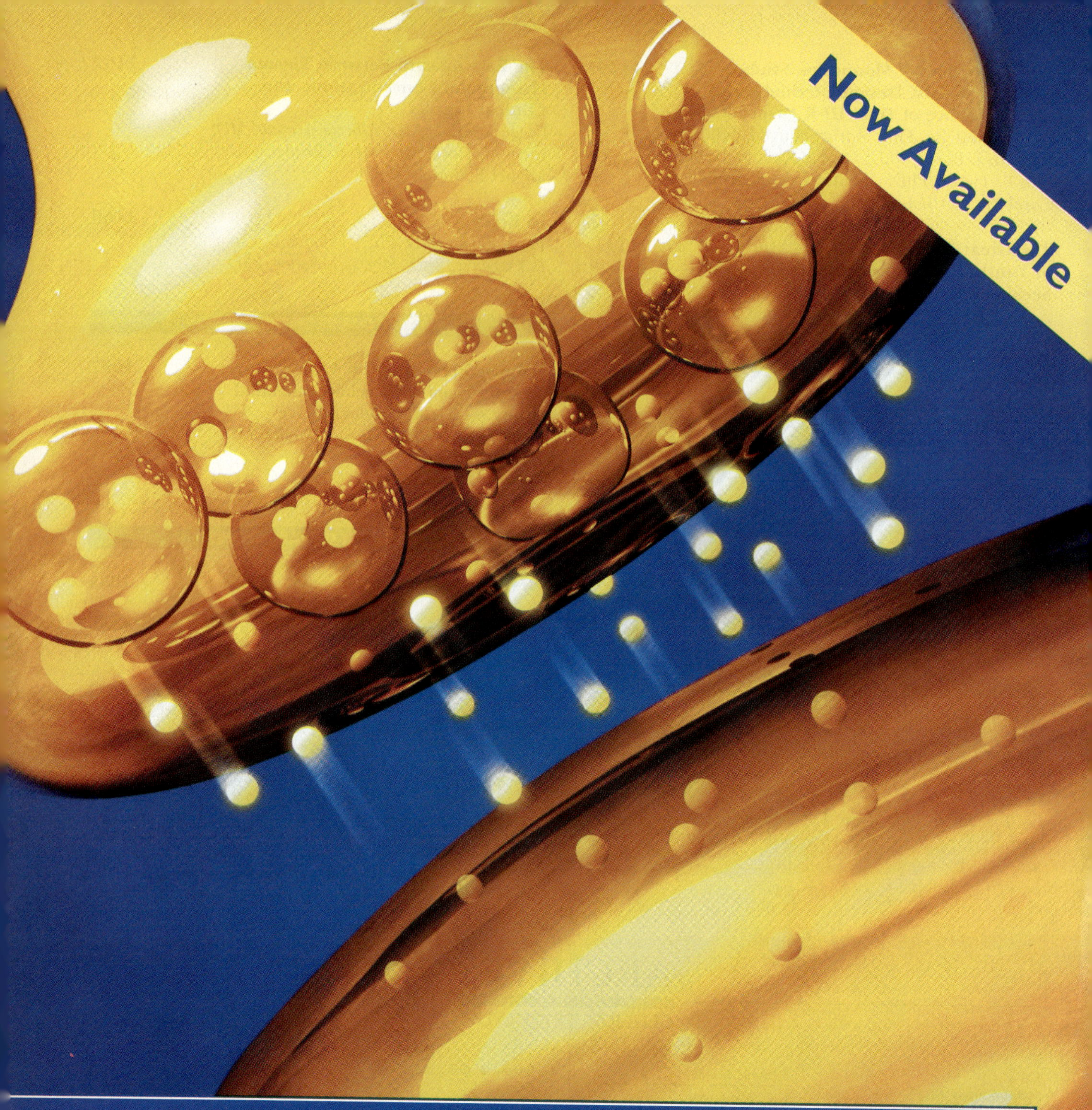
Now Available

THIS MONTH IN

ARCHIVES OF GENERAL PSYCHIATRY

Schizophrenia is regarded by some as a neurodevelopmental disorder that results from fetal exposure to environmental toxins such as influenza, heavy metals, famine, or obstetric complications. **Hollister et al** (page 19) present the first evidence that maternal/fetal rhesus incompatibility may increase the risk for schizophrenia. As was predicted, the rate of schizophrenia was greater with increasing birth order as the risk for maternal isoimmunization increases. The observations presented may provide supportive evidence that maternal antibodies can perturb fetal neurodevelopment either through secondary obstetric complications or some other unknown mechanism, resulting in schizophrenia.

Prenatal exposures that affect brain development might increase the risk of schizophrenia. With this in mind, **Susser et al** (page 25) examined whether exposure during early gestation to the famine of the Dutch Hunger Winter increased the risk of schizophrenia. The exposed birth cohorts were born in the cities of western Holland from October 15 to December 31 of 1945; these were compared with unexposed birth cohorts born in the same cities of Holland before and after those dates. The exposed birth cohorts had a twofold increase in schizophrenia, which suggests that prenatal nutrition could be related to the risk of schizophrenia.

Several authorities have hypothesized that schizophrenia may be caused by a persistent infection of the nervous system with a virus. **Taller et al** (page 32) extracted nucleic acids from selected areas of the brains of 31 patients with schizophrenia and 23 control subjects and used the sensitive method of "nested" polymerase chain reaction in an attempt to amplify nucleic acids of 12 viruses, most of them previously suspected of involvement in schizophrenia. None of the viruses was detected. Other causes including nonpersistent infections and infections with less common agents, should be considered for schizophrenia.

The biological effects of light therapy for seasonal affective disorder (SAD) were explored by **Lam et al** (page 41). Ten SAD patients in remission with light therapy underwent a double-blind, placebo-controlled study of rapid depletion of tryptophan, the amino acid precursor of serotonin. During the depletion session, which reduced plasma tryptophan levels by approximately 80%, but not during the placebo session, patients experienced a significant temporary relapse of their depressive symptoms. This study shows that the antidepressant effects of light therapy are tryptophan-dependent and suggests that light therapy may act through serotonergic mechanisms.

Recurrent seasonal depressive syndromes have been more completely described in recent years, including recurrent winter depression, also known as seasonal affective disorder (SAD), summer depression, and subsyndromal depression. **Madden et al** (page 47) performed a genetic analysis on self-report survey data on seasonal changes in mood and behavior obtained from Australian adult twins. They conclude that sensitivity to changes associated with the winter months (or the winter form of "seasonality") tends to run in families and this is largely due to biological predisposition. Their findings support continuing efforts to understand the role of seasonality in the development of mood disorders.

Midline (limbic) brain regions have been proposed to mediate emotional experiences. **Ketter et al** (page 59), using positron emission tomography scanning to determine brain blood flow, found that in healthy volunteers, intravenous doses of the local anesthetic procaine induced vivid emotional and sensory experiences while increasing anterior limbic activity. The left amygdala, a brain structure deep beneath the left temple, activated in subjects who experienced fear and deactivated in those who had euphoria. Visual areas in the back of the brain activated in those who had visual experiences. This study suggests that anterior limbic structures have important relationships to emotional experiences.

Crack cocaine represents the highest stage in the developmental sequence of drug involvement. **Kandel and Davies** (page 71) compared the psychosocial functioning of six groups of high school students, at different stages of drug involvement, with respect to family, peers, deviance, health, psychological symptoms, and drug-related problems. The sharpest differences in functioning occurred between alcohol and/or cigarettes and marijuana use. Delinquency and perceived peer drug use consistently increased with each higher stage of involvement. Students who used crack are the most maladjusted. That these youths started using alcohol and cigarettes two years earlier than their peers highlights the importance of early prevention and education efforts.

Neurodevelopmental Abnormalities and Schizophrenia

A Family Affair

DURING THE last decade, there has been a resurgence of interest in the relationship between prenatal and perinatal adversity and schizophrenia. Driving this interest is the notion that a physically traumatic event happening either in utero or during delivery disrupts the normal development of the central nervous system (CNS). In time, the altered CNS causes the individual to develop schizophrenia. This has become known as the neurodevelopmental hypothesis.[1-4] While a number of in utero events have been linked with schizophrenia, the one that has received the most scrutiny is maternal influenza during the second trimester of pregnancy. In this issue of the ARCHIVES, two other toxic events that occur during pregnancy and that may also lead to schizophrenia are described: RhD incompatibility[5] and severe nutritional deficiencies.[6] In their most severe form, the disorders produced by these events lead to death or to clearly observable neurological abnormalities; however, it is possible that some forms of schizophrenia are formes frustes of severe neurological disorders. A third study found no evidence of viral infection as a potential cause of schizophrenia.[7]

RhD INCOMPATIBILITY

The Rh (Rhesus) blood group system consists of over 40 antigens located on the surface of human erythrocytes. Of the five major antigens, the highly immunogenic RhD is the most clinically important because of its potential to cause hemolytic disease of the fetus and newborn in RhD-incompatible pregnancies (RhD-negative mother/RhD-positive offspring). RhD incompatibility occurs in about 10% of pregnancies of Caucasian women and in about 5% of pregnancies of African-American women; it is extremely rare in pregnancies of Oriental women, very few of whom are RhD-negative.[8]

The RhD-negative mother develops RhD antibodies to the fetus' erythrocytes in two stages. Unless the primigravid woman has had a previous transfusion, her risk of developing antibodies is negligible until her first delivery. At that point, if there is fetomaternal hemorrhaging, from tearing of the placenta, for example, and a substantial amount of fetal blood is released into the mother's bloodstream, the mother mounts a primary immune response that produces specific IgM antibodies. Fortunately, IgM antibodies are unable to cross the placenta, and even if the mother produces the IgM antibodies before giving birth, the fetus remains protected. During this first exposure to the fetal RhD antigen, the mother's population of B cells expands. These B cells remember the RhD antigen; when the woman is again exposed to RhD-positive erythrocytes during a subsequent pregnancy, these lymphocytes quickly mount a secondary immunological response. Specific IgG antibodies, which readily cross the placenta, are now made in high titers and attach themselves to the fetal erythrocytes, participating in their destruction. There is excessive breakdown of hemoglobin, and hyperbilirubinemia develops in untreated neonates. Since even small numbers of erythrocytes can trigger this reaction, the response may occur as early as the second trimester of a second or later pregnancy. The fetus becomes anemic and hypoxic, and a variety of symptoms develop.

See also pages 19, 25, and 32

During pregnancy, the fetus is usually protected against small excesses of bilirubin both by the placenta and by the mother's liver, which conjugates bilirubin with UDP-glucuronyltransferase. Conjugated bilirubin is water-soluble and easily cleared by the kidney. The liver of the newborn, however, particularly the premature newborn, has little reserve conjugating capability. Unconjugated bilirubin diffuses into cell membranes, and, most importantly, into the membranes of the CNS. Infants with bilirubin encephalopathy caused by hemolytic disease are spastic and have choreoathetosis and deafness to high-pitched frequencies.[9] Lesions are found in the globus pallidum, putamen, thalamus, hippocampus, and dentate nucleus of the cerebellum as well as in other brain regions.[10,11] Within the first week, death occurs in 70% of untreated cases.

During the mid-1950s, exchange transfusions were used to "wash out" the excess bilirubin in infants' blood, saving many lives and greatly decreasing morbidity[12]; in the early 1960s, intrauterine transfusions further improved the outcome for affected fetuses.[13] In the late

1960s, anti–D–γ-globulin began to be used after RhD-incompatible pregnancies to destroy RhD-positive erythrocytes as they entered the mother's bloodstream, before she could become sensitized. With rare exceptions, hyperbilirubinemia from RhD incompatibility should be a thing of the past. Nevertheless, it continues to contribute significantly to infant morbidity and mortality in the United States.[14]

RhD incompatibility, however, is not the only way a fetus can develop hyperbilirubinemia. ABO blood group incompatibility (an O mother and a fetus with A- or B-coated erythrocytes), which does not require sensitization, can affect first pregnancies. Although the jaundice is milder and less common than with RhD incompatibility, it occurs in 20% of all pregnancies.[15] When ABO incompatibility does occur, it does so within the first 24 hours of birth.[16] Gilbert's syndrome, which is still not fully understood, causes an apparently genetic reduction in hepatic UDP-glucuronyltransferase activity and can also increase indirect bilirubin concentrations in the fetus. It is also noteworthy that excessive vitamin K (menadione), as well as some antibiotics, increases indirect bilirubin concentrations.

Although exchange and intrauterine transfusions introduced prior to the use of anti–D–γ-globulin were lifesaving, several follow-up studies were done to determine whether smaller increases in bilirubin than occur with hemolytic disease of the fetus and newborn might have more subtle effects on the CNS. The follow-up studies were generally performed relatively early in life and found little to suggest adverse effects on the CNS. Some children, however, were reported to have mild athetosis and perhaps slight impairment on intelligence tests.[17] Nevertheless, a study using modern neuropsychological tests to evaluate cognitive function and schizophrenia spectrum symptoms is necessary to establish what if any effects persist for populations with a much more limited exposure to high prenatal and perinatal bilirubin concentrations than occurs in recognized hemolytic disease of the fetus and newborn.

Dr Hollister's landmark study of RhD incompatibility[5] had personal origins. Her sister has schizophrenia, and some readers will be familiar with her parents' involvement in the National Association for Research in Schizophrenia and Affective Disorder (NARSAD) and their development of NARSAD Artworks, a program that sells cards featuring the art of individuals with psychiatric illnesses to raise funds for research. Dr Hollister made the observation that her mother is RhD-negative and that her schizophrenic sister is RhD-positive and second-born and suffered birth complications; in contrast, both Dr Hollister and her psychiatrically healthy brother are RhD-negative and had no birth complications. From these observations, Dr Hollister speculated that RhD incompatibility and its concomitant complications may constitute a risk factor for schizophrenia. Having the good fortune to be working with Dr Sarnoff Mednick, who had previously discovered the association between second-trimester infection with the influenza virus and schizophrenia, Dr Hollister took advantage of the excellent Danish psychiatric registers to examine possible associations between RhD incompatibility and *International Classification of Diseases, Eighth Revision* (*ICD-8*)–diagnosed schizophrenia.

Dr Hollister and colleagues studied 1867 men born between 1959 and 1961 at University Hospital in Copenhagen, Denmark. In 1994, the male subjects were between 32 and 35 years old and had passed the maximum age of risk for developing schizophrenia. Twenty-one schizophrenic subjects and their mothers had their Rh phenotype determined. In those pregnancies with RhD incompatibility—the mother was RhD-negative and the fetus RhD-positive—the rate of schizophrenia was 2.1%. In RhD-compatible pregnancies, the rate of schizophrenia was 0.8%. Individuals with RhD-incompatible births were almost three times (relative risk, 2.78) more likely to develop schizophrenia than those with RhD-compatible births. Consistent with sensitivity developing after the first pregnancy, Hollister and colleagues found that the risk for developing schizophrenia was greater only in the second-born or later-born offspring.[5]

In addition to indicating how we might further diminish one form of schizophrenia, the study by Hollister and colleagues provides further evidence for the heterogeneity of schizophrenia, as did our previous understanding of the etiology of syphilis, the encephalopathies, vitamin deficiencies, and metabolic disorders, all of which at times produced symptoms similar to those of schizophrenia.

The putative relationship between RhD incompatibility and schizophrenia may also tell us something about other searches for the causes of schizophrenia, particularly those that are genetic. Clearly, RhD incompatibility is genetically determined, yet it is the interaction between the gene and the environment that causes the disorder. Most current genetic strategies look for gene linkages, or "fellow travelers." Genes that are close to one another on a chromosome tend to travel together through meiosis and can be tracked by identifying their fellow travelers. The general assumption in linkage studies is that all members of a family with a relatively rare disease, such as schizophrenia, will have similar alleles at the critical locus. Current genetic techniques are very powerful and have enjoyed considerable success. Nevertheless, while these techniques are certain to become even more powerful, it is unlikely that they could identify RhD incompatibility as a potential cause of schizophrenia, given that it is the interaction of common genes in two people at a specific time in their lives that produces the illness. Thus, despite the importance of molecular genetics, observation, intuition, and reflective synthesis remain principal tools in the science of psychiatry.[18]

Certainly, the study by Hollister and colleagues must be replicated. More importantly, there is ample material available to attempt such replications; a number of studies taking place in this country, including the Prenatal Determinants of Schizophrenia Study, provide the opportunity for such evaluations. This study is based on the cohort from the Child Health and Development Study, an investigation designed to examine the effects of prenatal exposures on early childhood disorders. Detailed records were kept from each prenatal care visit as well as from deliveries; furthermore, maternal blood was saved from each trimester, as was blood from the cord in some cases. Information is available for about 19 000 live births from 1959 through 1966 from the Oakland, Calif, hospital of the Kaiser Foundation Health Plan,[19] and for perhaps as many as 80 000 pregnancies from other centers with similar populations.[20]

NUTRITIONAL DEFICIENCIES

An important body of work about nutritional deficiencies and their relationship to neurological and neuropsychiatric disorders stems from tragic historical circumstances. Near the end of World War II, the Allies invaded France. They pushed north to the Netherlands in September 1944, crossing two branches of the Rhine River to advance on the main German industrial centers in the Ruhr Valley. Paratroopers dropped behind enemy lines attempting to capture and hold key bridges that cross the Rhine and connect the Netherlands to Germany. Their failure was the subject of a popular movie, *A Bridge Too Far* (1977). Meanwhile, Dutch railroad workers went on strike to aid the Allies, and the Nazis retaliated by embargoing and attempting to starve the inhabitants of Dutch cities; thus developed the Dutch Hunger Winter of 1944-1945. The famine was worst in the large cities of the western Netherlands; small towns were better off, as were communities in the east and north, which the Allied armies had occupied.[21] Many pregnant mothers and their fetuses were exposed to conditions of extreme famine. Unfortunately, this is not an uncommon occurrence during natural disasters and war. While looking back in anger, the world nevertheless gained invaluable knowledge.

Several features of the Dutch Hunger Winter made it possible to obtain this knowledge: (1) The famine was sharply delimited in time and place. Malnutrition increased from November 1944 but stopped abruptly in May 1945, when the Allies crossed the Rhine River and broke the blockade. (2) The type and extent of the nutritional deficiencies are well documented. (3) The Dutch kept excellent records on the medical and psychiatric outcomes of the individuals who lived through that experience.[21] In addition to birth records and a system of registers that are a consequence of Napoleon's conquest and administration, military records (including the Raven Progressive Matrices Test) and records from psychiatric contacts have been kept. Dr Ezra Susser's parents, Drs Zena Stein and Mervyn Susser, together with Drs Gerhart Saenger and Francis Marola, put together the database Dr Susser has been using to study the effects of the Dutch Hunger Winter on subsequent psychiatric illness. Thus, it appears that Dr Susser inherited not only his parents' inquisitiveness but his family's small business as well.

In an earlier publication, Susser and Lin[22] (1992) found that women but not men whose mothers were in the first trimester of pregnancy during the Dutch Hunger Winter had an elevated risk of developing schizophrenia. The present study[6] both expands and refines the findings of that earlier study. The exposed population was narrowed to include only those individuals who were conceived at the height of the famine and whose mothers had therefore carried them under conditions of extreme famine in the first trimester of pregnancy. Populations who received less than 42 kJ/d (1000 calories per day) for the longest period—toward the end of the Hunger Winter—were said to have suffered extreme famine. At the height of the famine, individuals were often receiving as little as 2.1 kJ/d (500 calories/d), much of it consisting of bread and potatoes (E. Susser, MD, DrPH, E-mail, November 10, 1995).

An increase in congenital neural tube defects, such as spina bifida and anencephaly, has previously been found in this population.[21] In the present study, Susser and colleagues found that, for both men and women, infants conceived at the height of the famine had an approximately twofold increased risk of developing schizophrenia. Notably, the effect was greater for narrowly defined schizophrenia than in the more broadly defined group, which might have included patients with affective disorders. Interestingly, there is also an increased risk of developing affective disorders from prenatal exposure to famine, but the risk period appears to be the second trimester.[23] It is now necessary to determine whether the lack of a specific nutritional factor in pregnancy is responsible for schizophrenia, similar to folic acid deficiency in pregnancy causing neural tube defects.

VIRUSES AND SCHIZOPHRENIA

There are several generic viral hypotheses of schizophrenia. The first suggests that an individual had a viral illness at roughly the same time as the onset of schizophrenia, that this illness precipitated the symptoms of schizophrenia, and that the schizophrenia remained despite the end of that original viral illness. In Boston, Mass, during the roughly 3 months of the 1918 influenza pandemic, 35 of 100 patients with influenza-associated psychiatric admissions to Boston Psychopathic Hospital (Massachusetts Mental Health Center) were believed to have schizophrenia.[24,25] It was noteworthy that no patients with a diagnosis of schizophrenia were below 18 years of age and few were above 30 years of age. In all cases, the psychosis began after the fever abated. In some cases, the influenza seemed to precipitate a latent psychosis, while for others it was not associated with any premorbid indicators.

A second hypothesis suggests that latent viruses may become active and precipitate psychosis. For example, the activation of a latent herpes simplex virus produces an encephalitis that, in its early stages, can resemble an acute form of schizophrenia.[26] Another hypothesis suggests that viruses may subtly attack the CNS, for instance, by taking over a "luxury function." Such a virus would not lyse the cells it infects but would interfere with the cells' ability to produce neurohormones, neurotransmitters, or cytokines.[27,28]

Another notion about viruses that fits the general theme of the other articles in this issue of the ARCHIVES is that, during fetal development, the pregnant mother may be exposed to a virus. That virus or perhaps the mother's or fetus' reaction to that virus damages the CNS. The first study hinting at such an association came from Mednick and colleagues[29] (1988), who found that pregnant women exposed to the type A2/Singapore influenza virus during their second trimester in greater Helsinki, Finland, had a greater-than-expected risk of having offspring who developed schizophrenia. There have now been almost 20 studies examining whether maternal infection with influenza or other viruses might subsequently cause schizophrenia in the offspring; the results of these studies are mixed.[30]

The study by Taller and colleagues[7] in this issue of the ARCHIVES explores the relationship between viruses and schizophrenia. Like Dr Hollister, Dr Torrey, who is a coauthor of that article, became interested in schizophrenia because of a sister's illness; he is perhaps best known as an advocate for the mentally ill. When I first met Dr Torrey in the early 1970s, he was already interested in a possible viral cause for schizophrenia. Much of his work has been epidemiological, and at least on this side of the Atlantic, he was one of a very small group looking at the epidemiology of schizophrenia. This led him to raise the fascinating and still-unanswered question[31,32] of whether schizophrenia is a new disorder, originating only about 200 years ago.[33] Dr Torrey's ability to ask intriguing questions and to obtain high-quality answers is evident in the work of Taller and colleagues. They used a direct approach to determine if there is evidence of viruses in the brains of deceased schizophrenics. Polymerase chain reaction (PCR) is one of those magical techniques, perhaps like the first x-ray films or computed tomography, that permit the seemingly impossible. Minute quantities of DNA or RNA—even one copy—can be amplified, allowing manipulation and identification. Polymerase chain reaction has already shown great promise in other areas of medicine. Nested polymerase chain reaction is a refinement that provides greater specificity.

Taller and colleagues did not find evidence of virus residues in the brains of schizophrenics. Specifically, there was no evidence of the DNA herpesviruses: herpes simplex virus type 1 (HSV-1), cytomegalovirus (CMV), Epstein-Barr virus (EBV), varicella-zoster virus (VZV), or human herpesvirus type 6 (HHV-6). Similarly, there was no evidence of the RNA viruses: influenza virus type A, the picornavirus group (enteroviruses, rhinoviruses), measles virus, mumps virus, rubella virus, human T-cell leukemia–associated virus type I (HTLV-I), or St Louis encephalitis virus. Although it is possible that one of these common viruses came and went without leaving its molecular fingerprint, if indeed a schizophrenia-causing virus persists in the brain, it is not likely to be one of those searched for here.

CONCLUSION

In addition to raising important etiologic questions, perhaps the most important clinical implication of the RhD incompatibility and nutritional deficiency studies is that some forms of schizophrenia may be preventable. Indeed, we may already have unknowingly begun preventing one form of schizophrenia. Because of the introduction of immunization with anti–D–γ-globulin, fewer individuals now develop the devastating CNS destruction produced by RhD incompatibility. Similar fetomaternal associations between immunological incompatibilities[34] and schizophrenia can be looked for and, if found, probably prevented. Preventing famine of the nature that occurred during the Dutch Hunger Winter is more of a social and political issue than a medical one, but some awareness of nutritional factors could ensure that pregnant women receive specific nutritional supplements even when sufficient calories are not available. For the medical sciences, however, further efforts are necessary to determine whether a specific dietary component is responsible for some forms of schizophrenia, much as folic acid deficiency during pregnancy is responsible for neural-tube defects. Finally, the article by Taller and colleagues does not directly address the issue of influenza infection during pregnancy; however, if influenza or other viral infections during the second trimester are found to contribute to schizophrenia, efforts could be made to immunize women of child-bearing age, as is currently done for other high-risk populations.

Much of our current research and care for schizophrenia focuses on improving treatment and rehabilitation. While we cannot overemphasize the importance of this for those who already suffer from the ravages of this disorder, it may be time to determine whether some forms of schizophrenia are preventable. As the RhD incompatibility and nutritional deficiency studies have so elegantly shown, it may not be necessary to wait until the gene or genes responsible for the genetic portion of schizophrenia are discovered to begin reorienting our approach to this extremely devastating and costly problem.[35]

Richard Jed Wyatt, MD
Neuropsychiatry Branch
NIH-NIMH Neuroscience Center at St Elizabeths
2700 Martin Luther King Jr Ave
Washington, DC 20032

Dr Wyatt is grateful to Ioline Henter for her excellent editorial assistance.

REFERENCES

1. Weinberger D. Implications of normal brain development for the pathogenesis of schizophrenia. *Arch Gen Psychiatry.* 1987;44:660-669.
2. Murray R, Lewis S. Is schizophrenia a neurodevelopmental disorder? *BMJ.* 1987;295:681-682.
3. Crow TJ, Ball J, Bloom SR, Brown R, Bruton CJ, Colter N, Frith CD, Johnstone EC, Owens DG, Roberts GW. Schizophrenia as an anomaly of development of cerebral asymmetry: a postmortem study and a proposal concerning the genetic basis of the disease. *Arch Gen Psychiatry.* 1989;46:1145-1150.
4. Waddington J. Schizophrenia: developmental neuroscience and pathobiology. *Lancet.* 1993;341:531-536.
5. Hollister JM, Laing P, Mednick SA. Rhesus incompatibility as a risk factor for schizophrenia in male adults. *Arch Gen Psychiatry.* 1996;53:19-24.
6. Susser E, Neugebauer R, Hoek HW, Brown AS,

Lin S, Labovitz D, Gorman JM. Schizophrenia after prenatal famine: further evidence. *Arch Gen Psychiatry.* 1996;53:25-31.
7. Taller AM, Asher DM, Pomeroy KL, Eldadah BA, Godec MS, Falkai PG, Bogert B, Kleinman JE, Stevens JR, Torrey EF. Search for viral nucleic acid sequences in brain tissues of patients with schizophrenia using nested polymerase chain reaction. *Arch Gen Psychiatry.* 1996;53:32-40.
8. Ose T, Tsuruhara T, Araki M, Hanaoka T, Bush OJ. Follow-up study of exchange transfusion for hyperbilirubinemia in infants in Japan. *Pediatrics.* 1967;40:196-201.
9. Larroche J-C, ed. *Perinatal Brain Damage.* New York, NY: John Wiley & Sons Inc; 1984.
10. Turkel S. Autopsy findings associated with neonatal hyperbilirubinemia. *Clin Perinatol.* 1990; 17:381-396.
11. Blackwood W, McMenemey WH, Meyer A, Norman RM, Russell DS. *Greenfield's Neuropathology.* Baltimore, Md: Williams & Wilkins; 1963.
12. Crome L, Stern J. *Pathology of Mental Retardation.* Baltimore, Md: Williams & Wilkins; 1972.
13. Mollison P. Haemolytic disease of the fetus and newborn. In: Mollison P, Engelfriet C, Conteras M, eds. *Blood Transfusion in Clinical Medicine.* Oxford, England: Blackwell Scientific Publications; 1993:543-591.
14. Chavez GF, Mulinare J, Edmonds LD. Epidemiology of Rh hemolytic disease of the newborn in the United States. *JAMA.* 1991;265:3270-3274.
15. Blanchette V, Zipursky A. Neonatal hematology. In: Avery G, ed. *Neonatology: Pathophysiology and Management of the Newborn.* Philadelphia, Pa: JB Lippincott; 1987:653-654.
16. Madlon-Kay D. The clinical significance of ABO blood group incompatibility. *Arch Fam Med.* 1993; 2:285-287.
17. Gerver J, Day R. Intelligence quotient of children who have recovered from erythroblastosis fetalis. *J Pediatr.* 1950;36:342-350.
18. Wyatt R. Science and psychiatry. In: Kaplan H, Sadock B, eds. *Comprehensive Textbook of Psychiatry IV.* Baltimore, Md: Williams & Wilkins; 1985:2016-2027.
19. van den Berg B. The California child health and development studies. In: Mednick S, Harway M, Finello K, eds. *Handbook of Longitudinal Research.* New York, NY: Praeger Publishers; 1984: 166-179.
20. Buka S, Tsuang M, Lipsitt L. Pregnancy/delivery complications and psychiatric diagnosis: a prospective study. *Arch Gen Psychiatry.* 1993;50: 151-156.
21. Stein Z, Susser M, Saenger G, Marolla F. *Famine and Human Development: The Dutch Hunger Winter of 1944-1945.* New York, NY: Oxford University Press; 1975.
22. Susser ES, Lin SP. Schizophrenia after prenatal exposure to the Dutch Hunger Winter of 1944-1945. *Arch Gen Psychiatry.* 1992;49:983-988.
23. Brown A, Susser E, Lin S, Neugebauer R, Gorman J. Increased risk of affective disorders in males after second trimester prenatal exposure to the Dutch Hunger Winter of 1944-45. *Br J Psychiatry.* 1995;166:601-606.
24. Menninger K. Psychosis associated with influenza. *JAMA.* 1919;72:235-241.
25. Menninger K. Influenza and schizophrenia. *Am J Psychiatry.* 1926;82:469-529.
26. Raskin D, Frank S. Herpes encephalitis with catatonic stupor. *Arch Gen Psychiatry.* 1974;31:544-546.
27. Oldstone M. Viral alteration of cell function: viruses can cause disease in the absence of morphological evidence of cell injury: implication for uncovering new diseases in the future. *Sci Am.* August 1989;261:42-48.
28. de la Torre J, Borrow P, Oldstone M. Viral persistence and disease: cytophathology in the absence of cytolysis. *Br Med Bull.* 1991;47:838-851.
29. Mednick SA, Machon RA, Huttunen MO, Bonett D. Adult schizophrenia following prenatal exposure to an influenza epidemic. *Arch Gen Psychiatry.* 1988;45:189-192.
30. Wyatt R, Apud J, Potkin S. New directions in the prevention and treatment of schizophrenia: a biological perspective. *Psychiatry.* In press.
31. Jeste D, del Carmen R, Lohr J, Wyatt R. Did schizophrenia exist before the 18th century? *Comp Psychiatry.* 1985;26:493-503.
32. Howells J, ed. *The Concept of Schizophrenia: Historical Perspectives.* Washington, DC: American Psychiatric Press; 1991.
33. Torrey E. *Schizophrenia and Civilization.* New York, NY: Jason Aronson Inc; 1980.
34. Wegman TG, Lin H, Guilbert L, Mosmann TR. Bidirectional cytokine interactions in the maternal-fetal relationship: is successful pregnancy a T_H2 phenomenon? *Immunol Today.* 1993;14:353-356.
35. Wyatt R, Henter I, Leary M, Taylor E. An economic evaluation of schizophrenia—1991. *Soc Psychiatry Psychiatr Epidemiol.* 1995;30:196-205.

Rhesus Incompatibility as a Risk Factor for Schizophrenia in Male Adults

J. Megginson Hollister, PhD; Peter Laing, PhD; Sarnoff A. Mednick, PhD, DrMed

Background: Rhesus (Rh) incompatibility is a cause of hemolytic disease of the fetus and newborn. Hemolytic disease results from the transplacentally transmitted maternal antibodies against Rh factor D and can cause permanent neurological damage in the affected newborn. This study examines the hypothesis that Rh incompatibility may be a risk factor for schizophrenia.

Methods: A sample of 1867 male subjects was divided into two groups, 535 Rh incompatible and 1332 Rh compatible, and compared on rate of schizophrenia.

Results: The rate of schizophrenia was significantly higher in the Rh-incompatible group (2.1%) compared with the Rh-compatible group (0.8%) ($P<.03$). In addition, since the risk for Rh hemolytic disease increases with second and later Rh incompatible pregnancies, it is noteworthy that the second- and later-born incompatible offspring exhibited a significantly higher rate of schizophrenia than second- and later-born compatible offspring ($P<.05$). Also, as predicted, the rate of schizophrenia among firstborn incompatible subjects was not significantly different from that of firstborn compatible subjects (1.1% vs 0.7%).

Conclusion: Rh incompatibility may be a risk factor for schizophrenia.

(Arch Gen Psychiatry. 1996;53:19-24)

Maternal infection with influenza during the second trimester of gestation is associated with an increased risk for schizophrenia in the offspring.[1,2] Several independent investigators worldwide have replicated these findings,[3-8] while others have not.[9-12] Influenza viruses elicit autoantibody production in humans and animals.[13-16] Certain autoantibodies of the IgG class cross the placenta and have adverse effects on the developing fetus,[17-19] leading us to consider whether maternal antibodies might cause perturbations in fetal neurodevelopment, in some cases resulting in schizophrenia.

Maternal alloantibodies against the Rhesus (Rh) D antigen are known to result in brain damage in humans secondary to hemolytic disease of the fetus and newborn (HDN). Transplacentally acquired maternal erythrocyte alloantibodies cause fetal erythrolysis in the liver and spleen of the fetus and newborn. In severe cases, death may occur in utero as early as week 18 of gestation as a consequence of hydrops fetalis secondary to profound anemia and associated hypoxia.[20] Post partum, HDN results in an accumulation of bilirubin in the neonate's circulation, which may result in kernicterus (yellow staining of neuronal elements of the brain, including the basal ganglia and hippocampus).[21] Infants who survive kernicterus often suffer from lasting brain damage, manifesting as choreoathetosis, sensorineural hearing deficits, and/or mental retardation.[22]

Rh incompatibility is the most serious cause of HDN. An Rh-negative (d) woman can become immunized to Rh-positive (D) blood through transfusion of D blood, or through miscarriage, abortion, or delivery of an Rh-positive fetus or infant. Hemolytic disease of the fetus and newborn rarely affects firstborn Rh-positive infants, and the incidence and severity of HDN is greater in second- and later-affected neonates.[20,23] In addition, several studies indicate that male fetuses are more likely than female fetuses to initiate maternal Rh D immunization.[24-26]

The neuroanatomical abnormalities

See Methods on next page

From the University of Pennsylvania, Philadelphia (Dr Hollister); the Social Science Research Institute, University of Southern California, Los Angeles (Drs Hollister and Mednick); Department of Immunology, University Hospital, Queens Medical Centre, Nottingham (England) University (Dr Laing); and the Institute of Preventive Medicine, Copenhagen, Denmark (Dr Mednick).

METHODS

SAMPLE SELECTION

The Danish Perinatal Project consists of data on the births of 9182 infants born to 9006 women between 1959 and 1961 at University Hospital in Copenhagen, Denmark. The births of almost all 9182 offspring were observed by senior obstetricians. Extensive data were recorded concerning the pregnancy, including ABO and Rh blood types of 8798 mothers and 3758 infants. A disproportionate amount of serological data from children of Rh-negative mothers was represented (40% vs 17% expected in the Danish population). The selective sampling biased toward offspring of Rh-negative mothers would be expected since these infants were at greatest risk for HDN. One hundred eighty-seven of the 3758 infants with complete serological data died before schizophrenia could develop and an additional 53 subjects were missing data for diagnosis or sex, reducing the sample to 3518 subjects. Other information that was collected included early neurobehavioral and physical examination results, psychiatric diagnoses of both parents, and socioeconomic status.[35]

In 1992 to 1993, the National Psychiatric Register of the Institute for Psychiatric Demography in Risskov, Denmark, was accessed to obtain psychiatric hospital diagnoses of the mothers, fathers, and children in this cohort. This register had its origin in 1938 when systematic registration of patients admitted to mental hospitals in Denmark was begun. It was computerized in 1969 and includes information from all 86 psychiatric institutions in Denmark. The diagnostic system in place at this time was the *International Classification of Diseases, Eighth Revision* (*ICD-8*). As of 1994, 50 of the male and 18 of the female offspring were registered as having *ICD-8* diagnoses of schizophrenia. The Rh phenotype is available for 26 of these 68 individuals (21 males and five females). Analyses were limited to male offspring owing to the small number of female offspring with schizophrenia, so the final sample consisted of 1867 male offspring. **Table 1** presents data for the female offspring for the readers' interest.

RISK GROUP CLASSIFICATION

Subjects were divided into Rh-In and Rh-Co groups. The Rh-In group consisted of subjects who were incompatible (Rh-negative mother/Rh-positive offspring—configuration 'd/D') and 110 Rh-positive subjects whose mothers were coded as "mother with known Rh, ABO, or other immunization (configuration imm/D)." In these instances, there was no way to know with certainty the type of immunization. Schizophrenia subsequently developed in two offspring in this category. The reported findings were statistically significant with or without including these two subjects. In addition, since Rh HDN and other types of fetal HDN are fundamentally similar, it is appropriate to include these subjects in the Rh-In group. Therefore, the Rh-In group represents virtually all pregnancies that could give rise to cases of HDN. The Rh-Co group consisted of all pregnancies (d/d, D/D, D/d, imm/d) that could not have given rise to Rh HDN.

STATISTICAL PROCEDURES

χ^2 Tests with continuity correction and two-tailed Fisher's exact test were conducted[36] for hypothesis 1 and hypothesis 2, respectively. Five χ^2 tests with continuity correction and two Fisher's exact tests were conducted for non–hypothesis-driven comparisons of the Rh-In and Rh-Co groups on demographic variables. Logistic regression was conducted to control for differences between the two groups. Three χ^2 tests with continuity correction were conducted comparing the two groups on variables associated with Rh HDN. Since these analyses were hypothesis driven, Bonferroni correction was utilized with a corrected P value of .02.

observed in schizophrenia have been ascribed to perturbations of fetal neurodevelopment, occurring especially during the second trimester.[1,27,28] Consistent with this view, HDN can impair fetal neurodevelopment at this time and may increase the risk for schizophrenia. Furthermore, since *some* of the neuropathological and clinical manifestations of kernicterus parallel those observed for *some* individuals with schizophrenia (ie, disturbed cytoarchitecture of the hippocampus,[29,30] choreoathetosis, and other neuromotor disturbances in infancy and childhood;[31,32] spontaneous abnormal movements in adults;[33] and mental retardation[34]), the postpartum hyperbilirubinemic phase of HDN may also be related to increased risk for schizophrenia.

See also pages 11, 25, and 32

The characteristic features of Rh HDN, which include occurrence only in Rh-incompatible (Rh-In) pregnancies, the tendency for males to initiate maternal Rh D immunization, sparing of firstborn individuals, and greatly increased incidence and severity in second- and later-affected offspring, suggest two hypotheses: (1) the rate of schizophrenia among male offspring from Rh-In pregnancies should be higher than the rate of schizophrenia among male offspring from Rh-compatible (Rh-Co) pregnancies; (2) the rate of schizophrenia among second- or later-born Rh-In offspring should be higher than the rate of schizophrenia among second- or later-born Rh-Co offspring. However, the rate of schizophrenia among firstborn Rh-In offspring should be similar to that among firstborn Rh-Co offspring.

We compared the rate of schizophrenia among offspring from Rh-In and Rh-Co pregnancies in the context of the Danish Perinatal Cohort.[35]

RESULTS

HYPOTHESIS 1

The rate of schizophrenia was found to be 2.1% in the Rh-In group compared with 0.8% in the Rh-Co group (χ^2 [1]=4.73, P=.03; relative risk=2.78, 95% confidence interval=1.2 to 6.6) (Table 1).

Table 1. Rate of Schizophrenia in Adulthood in Rhesus (Rh)-Incompatible and Rh-Compatible Groups

	Total No. of Schizophrenics/Total Sample Size (% With Schizophrenia)			
	Rh Incompatible	Rh Compatible	Total	Significance
Males	11/535 (2.1)	10/1332 (0.8)	**21/1867** (1.1)	.03*
All subjects	12/1062 (1.1)	14/2456 (0.6)	**26/3518** (0.7)	.12*
Females	1/527 (0.2)	4/1124 (0.4)	**5/1651** (0.3)	1.0†

*P value for χ^2.
†P value for Fisher's exact test.

Table 2. Rate of Schizophrenia in Rhesus (Rh)-Incompatible and Rh-Compatible Adult Males by Birth Order

	Total No. of Schizophrenics/Total Sample Size (% With Schizophrenia)			
Birth Order	Rh Incompatible	Rh Compatible	Total	Significance*
Firstborn	2/178 (1.1)	5/672 (0.7)	**7/850** (0.8)	.64
Second born	3/134 (2.2)	2/328 (0.6)	**5/462** (1.1)	.15
Third and later born	4/138 (2.9)	3/306 (0.9)	**7/444** (1.6)	.21
Second and later born	7/272 (2.6)	5/634 (0.8)	**12/906** (1.3)	.05

*P value for Fisher's exact test.

HYPOTHESIS 2

The rate of schizophrenia among second- and later-born Rh-In male offspring was significantly greater (2.6% vs 0.8%) than that of second- and later-born Rh-Co male offspring (Fisher's exact test [two-tailed]: *P*=.05, relative risk=3.32, 95% confidence interval=1.0 to 10.6). In addition, the rate of schizophrenia in firstborn Rh-In and Rh-Co male offspring was 1.1% and 0.7%, respectively. This difference was not significant (Fisher's exact test [two-tailed], *P*=.64) (**Table 2**).

OTHER ANALYSES

Possible confounding influences on our findings include parental diagnosis, age, marital status, number of previous pregnancies, length of gestation, and offspring mortality. No significant differences were observed between the two groups for paternal or maternal diagnosis of schizophrenia. Significant differences were observed in the age, marital status, and number of pregnancies of Rh-In and Rh-Co mothers. Significant differences between the Rh-In and Rh-Co groups were observed for length of gestation and death rate of neonates before the age of 1 year. The significant group differences can be explained as a recruitment bias affecting the subgroup for whom Rh blood group data were available for both mother and offspring. We found that Rh-In mothers were significantly older ($\chi^2[1]=7.73$, *P*=.005), more likely to be married ($\chi^2[1]=7.35$, *P*=.007), and to have more previous pregnancies ($\chi^2[1]=23.69$, *P*<.001) than Rh-Co mothers. Because HDN is confined almost exclusively to second and later pregnancies, mothers at risk of giving birth to offspring with Rh HDN are more likely to be older and married. Rh-Co mothers were more likely than Rh-In mothers to deliver prematurely ($\chi^2[1]=16.78$, *P*<.001) and to have newborns who died in the first year of life ($\chi^2[1]=9.60$, *P*=.002) (**Table 3**).

Logistic regression was conducted to control for the possible confounding influence of these sample differences on the reported findings. The rate of schizophrenia among the Rh-In group remained significantly higher than that of the Rh-Co group when marital status, age, number of pregnancies, and length of gestation were controlled for ($\chi^2[1]=5.90$, *P*=.02).

Since no direct measure of Rh HDN (ie, direct antiglobulin test) in offspring was available for this sample, we examined variables that may be indicative of Rh HDN. These variables included exchange transfusion, bilirubin levels, and jaundice. Exchange transfusions occurred significantly more often for Rh-In than for Rh-Co offspring, 21% and 3.5%, respectively ($\chi^2[1]=258.0$, *P*<.001). Bilirubin levels were available for a subsample, including 319 and 881 subjects in the Rh-In and Rh-Co groups, respectively. Rhesus incompatible subjects were more likely to have critically elevated bilirubin levels (>20 mg/100 mL) than the Rh-Co subjects, 27% vs 19%, respectively ($\chi^2[1]=7.48$, *P*=.006). A subsample of subjects had data reported on the presence of jaundice at the first clinical examination (Rh-In group, n=240; Rh-Co group, n=524). Subjects in the Rh-In subsample were more likely to be reported as having jaundice at the first clinical examination ($\chi^2[1]=20.25$, *P*<.001) than subjects in the Rh-Co subsample (63% vs 45%). The occurrence of exchange transfusions in one fifth of Rh-In subjects, the significantly elevated levels of bilirubin, and the reports of jaundice in a large proportion of Rh-In subjects support our contention that some subjects in the Rh-In group suffered from Rh HDN. Unfortunately, the sample sizes were too small to ascertain whether any of these variables were related to rate of schizophrenia.

COMMENT

Our findings demonstrate that the rate of schizophrenia is increased to 2.1% in male subjects who are Rh-In with their mothers. In contrast, the rate of schizophrenia is 0.8% among those without these characteristics. Also, the rate of schizophrenia is found to be greater in second- and later-born Rh-In offspring than in parity-matched Rh-Co male offspring. Moreover, the rate of schizophrenia is higher in third- or later-born than in second-born Rh-In male offspring (2.9% and 2.2%, respectively) in accordance with the fivefold increase of stillbirths attributed to HDN among second-affected infants. These findings should be considered preliminary as there are several limitations to this study, which will be discussed. We will then speculate on the teratogenic effects of Rh incompatibility that might lead to schizophrenia and conclude with suggestions for future research.

Table 3. Comparison of Rhesus (Rh)-Incompatible and Rh-Compatible Groups on Demographic Variables

Variable, %	Rh Incompatible	Rh Compatible	Significance
Maternal diagnosis of schizophrenia	0.4	0.5	1.0*
Paternal diagnosis of schizophrenia	0.4	0.2	.32*
Maternal age >23 y†	59	52	.005‡
Maternal marital status§	75	68	.007
Parity‖			
Firstborn	39	51	<.001‡
Second born	30	25	
Third born	31	24	
Gestation <38 wk	23	34	<.001‡
Infant mortality	2.9	6.6	.002‡

**P value for Fisher's exact test.*
†Median split of total sample.
‡P value for χ^2.
§Percentage who are currently married or were at one time.
‖Offspring included in study by birth order.

LIMITATIONS AND POSSIBLE CONFOUNDS

Limitations of this study include the use of hospital diagnoses, an Rh-Co sample that may be at high risk for other pregnancy and birth complications (PBCs), and a small number of schizophrenic subjects.

The reliability and validity of hospital diagnoses has been questioned. We argue that Danish hospital diagnoses tend to be conservative relative to experienced clinicians' interview diagnoses. Therefore, subjects given a hospital diagnosis of schizophrenia would almost always be diagnosed as schizophrenic during a more detailed clinical interview.[37,38] Furthermore, if errors in diagnostic typing occurred, it is unlikely that they would be more prevalent among Rh-In than among Rh-Co offspring.

The data for subjects in this sample were gathered for research purposes. However, certain medical procedures (such as taking a blood sample from the neonate) were not routine. As a result, this study consisted of a somewhat biased sample toward pregnancies that warranted serological examination.

In future studies, the rate of schizophrenia among female Rh-In offspring must be examined. The disproportionate number of male schizophrenic subjects in our sample is explained by differences in the age at onset between males and females and the age of the subjects when they were checked in the psychiatric register (32 years).[39-41] In addition to age-at-onset differences, the sexes may be differentially susceptible to gestational environmental factors. Therefore, analyzing the sexes separately may provide important information regarding Rh incompatibility as a risk factor for schizophrenia.

HOW MIGHT Rh INCOMPATIBILITY INCREASE THE RISK FOR SCHIZOPHRENIA?

Again, Rh incompatibility is the most serious cause of HDN. We suggest that the fetal hypoxia resulting from hemolysis in Rh HDN may have deleterious effects on fetal neurodevelopment, increasing the vulnerability for schizophrenia later in life. McNeil[42] suggests that prenatal, perinatal, and neonatal oxygen deprivation may increase the risk for schizophrenia. One brain region particularly vulnerable to hypoxia is the hippocampus.[21,43] Neuropathological studies have implicated the hippocampus as a brain region frequently found to be abnormal among schizophrenics.[44] The migration of neurons into the hippocampus is reaching a peak during the second trimester,[45] at which time the transfer of maternal antibodies to the fetus is under way.[46] Furthermore, a study from our laboratory,[1] which has been replicated several times, implicates the second trimester of gestation as critical in the development of schizophrenia.

Second, we proposed earlier that kernicterus at birth may be related to risk for schizophrenia in adulthood. The hyperbilirubinemic phase of postpartum Rh HDN can cause damage to the basal ganglia and hippocampus, brain areas associated with schizophrenia. In addition, some of the clinical manifestations of kernicterus are also observed in preschizophrenics and in adults with schizophrenia. However, given the mounting evidence of second-trimester perturbation in schizophrenia, we suggest that the *fetal* phase of Rh HDN rather than the neonatal phase may be the more critical period of insult. Furthermore, in this study, 19% of the Rh-Co group evidenced critically elevated bilirubin levels. Although the percentage was significantly less than in the Rh-In group (27%), the disparity is not all that great.

Both neuropathology studies and the second-trimester findings are consistent with the hypothesis that the maternal transfer of anti-D antibodies into a Rh-positive fetus, causing HDN (and the concomitant hypoxia and hyperbilirubinemia), may damage brain tissues associated with an increased risk for schizophrenia. Our findings of an increased rate of schizophrenia among Rh-In offspring, those who are at highest risk for Rh HDN, support this hypothesis.

SUGGESTIONS FOR FUTURE RESEARCH

Population prevalence of the d phenotype, information on the heterozygosity or homozygosity of the father's blood type, effects of parity, and the administration of anti-D prophylaxis must be considered in replication attempts. In addition, the presence of PBCs secondary to Rh HDN and their relationship to schizophrenia in adulthood must be further explored.

- The prevalence of the d phenotype ranges from 0% in a Thai population[47] to 20% to 40% in the Basque people.[48] The variance observed in the prevalence of D and d phenotypes worldwide raises the question as to whether populations with increased incidence of Rh incompatibility will also evidence an increased incidence of schizophrenia? To our knowledge, unusual rates of schizophrenia have not been observed in the above-mentioned regions.
- The homozygosity or heterozygosity of the paternal D factor may influence results. All offspring of homozygous D (DD) fathers and d (dd) mothers will be D (Dd), which will increase the probability of anti-D antibody production by the mother's immune system, thereby increasing the probability of HDN.[20]

- Replications must also consider the effect of parity. Nonfirstborn children will have the greatest probability of suffering from HDN,[20] and according to our hypothesis these trends will be evident as a correspondingly increased risk for schizophrenia throughout second and later Rh-In pregnancies.
- Rh HDN has been significantly reduced since the development of anti-D prophylaxis in the late 1960s.[29] Schizophrenia has also been reported to be on the decline. However, the decline has mainly been attributed to changes in both diagnostic practices and economic and social forces.[49] Replication attempts must include samples that predate the administration of anti-D prophylaxis.
- A relationship between PBCs and schizophrenia has been reported.[42,50] A relationship has also been observed for certain PBCs and HDN, such as asphyxia at delivery, pulmonary edema, and other respiratory difficulties.[51] The question arises as to whether PBCs themselves increase the risk for schizophrenia, whether the PBCs merely reflect manifestations of pathological processes occurring earlier in pregnancy that increase the risk for schizophrenia, or a combination of the two.
- These findings may also be relevant to the genetics of schizophrenia. The d genotype is inheritable and will cluster in families; therefore, so, too, will Rh-In pregnancies. If Rh incompatibility is a risk factor for schizophrenia, then schizophrenia would also tend to cluster in these families. These families might mistakenly be identified as having a genetic predisposition for schizophrenia, when in fact they may simply have a genetic predisposition for HDN.

CONCLUSION

This study implicates Rh incompatibility as a risk factor for schizophrenia, a risk factor that involves genetics, maternal immune functioning, PBCs, and fetal neurodevelopment. There are numerous ways in which the hypotheses discussed in this study can be tested. Attempts at replications using other perinatal cohorts are already under way. In addition, retrospective studies examining the psychiatric outcomes of adult survivors of HDN and kernicterus can be designed. Studies examining the rate of Rh incompatibility in large samples of schizophrenic subjects is another possible design. Other forms of fetal/maternal incompatibilities (ie, ABO incompatibility—maternal blood type O, offspring A, B, or AB) and their relationship to schizophrenia can be examined. Studies can be conducted that examine other human hemolytic conditions such as autoimmune hemolytic anemia. Research using animal models can explore the role of hemolysis, consequent hypoxia, and hyperbilirubinemia on fetal neurodevelopment and aberrant behavior. In future studies, the limitations discussed earlier can certainly be overcome through research design. Finally, the observations presented in this study may provide supportive evidence that maternal antibodies can perturb fetal neurodevelopment either through secondary obstetric complications or some other unknown mechanism, causing schizophrenia later in life. Therefore, a wider consideration of the possible role of maternal antibodies and other immune factors in the pathogenesis of schizophrenia is indicated.

Accepted for publication July 27, 1995.

This research was supported by National Institute of Mental Health grant MH46014; National Institute Mental Health Research Award MH00619 (Dr Mednick); and grants from the Medical Research Council, the Stanley Foundation.

The authors appreciate the editorial advice of Richard Wyatt, MD, and statistical suggestions of Patricia Brennan, PhD.

Reprint requests to University of Pennsylvania, Neuropsychiatry Section, 10th Floor, Gates Building, Philadelphia, PA 19104-4283 or E-mail: meggin@hirisk.psych.upenn.edu (Dr Hollister).

REFERENCES

1. Mednick SA, Machon RA, Huttunen MO, Bonnet D. Adult schizophrenia following prenatal exposure to an influenza epidemic. *Arch Gen Psychiatry.* 1988; 45:189-192.
2. Mednick SA, Huttunen MO, Machon RA. Prenatal influenza infections and adult schizophrenia. *Schizophr Bull.* 1994;20:263-267.
3. Kendell RE, Kemp IW. Maternal influenza in the etiology of schizophrenia. *Arch Gen Psychiatry.* 1989;46:878-882.
4. O'Callaghan E, Sham P, Takei N, Glover G, Murray R. Schizophrenia after prenatal exposure to the 1957 A2 influenza epidemic. *Lancet.* 1991;337:1248-1250.
5. Kunugi H, Nanko S, Takei N. Influenza and schizophrenia in Japan. *Br J Psychiatry.* 1992;161:274-275.
6. Fahy TA, Jones PB, Sham PC. Schizophrenia in Afro-Caribbean's in the UK following prenatal exposure to the 1957 A2 influenza epidemic. *Schizophr Res.* 1992;6:98-99.
7. Welham JL, McGrath JJ, Pemberton MR. Schizophrenia: birthrates and three Australian epidemics. *Schizophr Res.* 1993;9:142.
8. Adams W, Kendell RE, Hare EH, Munk-Jorgensen P. Epidemiological evidence that maternal influenza contributes to the aetiology of schizophrenia: an analysis of Scottish, English, and Danish data. *Br J Psychiatry.* 1993;163:522-534.
9. Bowler AE, Torrey EF. Influenza and schizophrenia: Helsinki vs Edinburgh. *Arch Gen Psychiatry.* 1990;47:876-877.
10. Crow TJ, Done DJ. Prenatal exposure to influenza does not cause schizophrenia. *Br J Psychiatry.* 1992;161:390-393.
11. Cannon M, Cotter D, Sham PC, Larkin C, Murray RM, Coffey VP, O'Callaghan E. Schizophrenia in an Irish sample following prenatal exposure to the 1957 influenza epidemic: a case-controlled, prospective follow-up study. *Schizophr Res.* 1994;11:95.
12. Selten J-PCJ, Slaets JPJ. Evidence against maternal influenza as a risk factor for schizophrenia. *Br J Psychiatry.* 1994;164:674-676.
13. Loza-Tulimowska M, Semkow R, Michalak T, Nowoslawski A. Autoantibodies in sera of influenza patients. *Acta Virol.* 1976;20:202-207.
14. Fox AE, Plescia OJ. An experimental model of autoimmune hemolytic anemia in mice. *Immunol Comm.* 1973;2:241-256.
15. Laing P, Knight JG, Hill JM, Harris AG, Oxford JS, Webster RG, Markwell MAK, Paul SM, Pert CB. Influenza viruses induce autoantibodies to a 37 kDa brain-specific protein in rabbit. *Proc Natl Acad Sci U S A.* 1989;86:1998-2002.
16. Guldner HH, Netler HJ, Szostecki C, Jaeger E, Will H. Human P68 autoantibodies recognize a common epitope of U1-RNA containing small nuclear ribonucleoprotein and influenza-B virus. *J Exp Med.* 1990;171:819-829.
17. Munro DS, Dirmikis SM, Humphries H, Smith T, Broadhead GD. The role of thyroid stimulating immunoglobulins of Graves' disease on neonatal thyrotoxicosis. *Br J Obstet Gynaecol.* 1978;85:849-857.
18. Papazian O. Transient neonatal myasthenia gravis. *J Child Neurol.* 1992;7:135-141.
19. Harley JB, Scofield RH, Reichlin M. Anti-Ro in Sjogren's syndrome and systemic lupus erythematosus. *Rheum Dis Clin North Am.* 1992;18:337-358.
20. Mollison PL. Haemolytic disease of the fetus and newborn. In: Mollison PL, Engelfriet CP, Contreras M, eds. *Blood Transfusion in Clinical Medicine.* Oxford, England: Blackwell Scientific Publications; 1993:543-591.

21. Rorke LB. Perinatal brain damage. In: Adams JH, Duchen LW, eds. *Greenfield's Neuropathology.* 5th ed. New York, NY: Oxford University Press; 1992: 639-708.
22. Watchko JF, Oski FA. Kernicterus in preterm newborns: past, present and future. *Pediatrics.* 1992;90:707-715.
23. Walker W, Murray S, Russell JK. Stillbirth due to haemolytic disease of the newborn. *J Obstet Gynaecol Br Empire.* 1957;44:573.
24. Scott JR. Immunologic risks to fetuses from maternal to fetal transfer of erythrocytes. In: *Proceedings of the Symposium on Rh Antibody Mediated Immunosuppression.* Raritan, NJ: Ortho Research Institute; 1976.
25. Renkonen KO, Seppala M. The sex of the sensitizing Rh-positive child. *Ann Med Exp Fenn.* 1962;40:108.
26. Renkonen KO, Timonen S. Factors influencing the immunization of Rh-negative mothers. *J Med Genet.* 1967;4:166-168.
27. Bogerts B. The neuropathology of schizophrenia: pathophysiological and neurodevelopmental implications. In: Mednick SA, Cannon TD, Barr CE, Lyon M, eds. *Fetal Neural Development and Adult Schizophrenia.* Cambridge, England: Cambridge University Press; 1991:153-173.
28. Beckman H, Jakob H. Prenatal disturbances of nerve cell migration in the entorhinal region: a common vulnerability factor in functional psychoses? *J Neural Transm.* 1991;84:155-164.
29. Kovelman JA, Scheibel AB. A neurohistological correlate of schizophrenia. *Biol Psychiatry.* 1984;19:1601-1621.
30. Altschuler L, Conrad A, Kovelman JA, Scheibel A. Hippocampal pyramidal cell orientation in schizophrenia. *Arch Gen Psychiatry.* 1987;44:1094-1098.
31. Walker EF, Savoie T, Davis D. Neuromotor precursors of schizophrenia. *Schizophr Bull.* 1994;20:441-451.
32. Mednick SA, Silverton L. High-risk studies of the etiology of schizophrenia. In: Tsuang M, Simpson JC, eds. *Handbook of Schizophrenia: Nosology, Epidemiology and Genetics.* Amsterdam, the Netherlands: Elsevier Science Publishers; 1988;3:543-562.
33. Fenton WS, Wyatt RJ, McGlashan TH. Risk factors for spontaneous dyskinesia in schizophrenia. *Arch Gen Psychiatry.* 1994;51:643-650.
34. Jones P, Murray R, Rodgers B. Childhood risk factors for adult schizophrenia in a general population birth cohort at age 43 years. In: Mednick SA, Hollister JM, eds. *Neural Development in Schizophrenia: Theory and Research.* New York, NY: Plenum Press. 1995:151-176.
35. Mednick SA, Mura E, Schulsinger F, Mednick B. Perinatal conditions and infant development in children with schizophrenic parents. *Soc Biol.* 1971;18 (suppl):S103-S113.
36. Siegel S. The case of two independent samples. *Nonparametric Statistics.* New York, NY: McGraw-Hill International Book Co; 1956:109.
37. Munk-Jorgensen P, Mortensen PB. Schizophrenia: a 13-year followup. *Acta Psychiatr Scand.* 1989;79:391-399.
38. Jorgensen A, Teasdale TW, Parnas J, Mednick SA, Schulsinger F. The Copenhagen High Risk Project: the diagnosis of maternal schizophrenia and its relation to offspring diagnosis. *Br J Psychiatry.* 1987;151:753-757.
39. Hafner H, Riecher-Rossler A, Maurer K, Fatkenheurer B, Loffler W. First onset and early symptomatology of schizophrenia: a chapter of epidemiological and neurobiological research into age and sex differences. *Eur Arch Psychiatry Clin Neurosci.* 1992;242:109-118.
40. Riecher-Rossler A, Fatkenheuer B, Loffler W, Maurer K, Hafner H. Is age of onset in schizophrenia influenced by marital status? some remarks on the difficulties and pitfalls in the systematic testing of a 'simple' question. *Soc Psychiatry Psychiatr Epidemiol.* 1992;27:122-128.
41. Gureje O. Gender and schizophrenia: age at onset and sociodemographic attributes. *Acta Psychiatr Scand.* 1991;83:402-405.
42. McNeil TF. Obstetric factors and perinatal injuries. In: Tsuang MT, Simpson JC, eds. *Handbook of Schizophrenia: Nosology, Epidemiology and Genetics.* Amsterdam, the Netherlands: Elsevier Science Publishers; 1988:319-344.
43. Ben Ari Y. Effects of anoxia and aglycemia on the adult and immature hippocampus. *Biol Neonate.* 1992;62:225-230.
44. Jeste DV, Lohr JB. Hippocampal pathologic findings in schizophrenia. *Arch Gen Psychiatry.* 1989;46:1019-1024.
45. Conrad AJ, Scheibel AB. Schizophrenia and the hippocampus: the embryological hypothesis extended. *Schizophr Bull.* 1987;13:577-587.
46. Adinolphi M. The development of the human blood-CSF-brain barrier. *Dev Med Child Neurol.* 1985;27:532-537.
47. Singh TS, Phookan MN. A note on the frequency of ABO and Rhesus blood groups in four Thai populations of Assam (India) and their position among Mongoloids of this region. *Anthropol Anz.* 1990;48:29-35.
48. Mourant AE, Kopec AC, Domaniewska-Sobczak K. *The Distribution of the Human Blood Groups and Other Biochemical Polymorphisms.* Oxford, England: Oxford University Press; 1976.
49. Stoll AL, Tohen M, Baldessarini RJ, Goodwin DC, Stein S, Katz S, Geenens D, Swinson RP, Goethe JW, McGlashan T. Shifts in diagnostic frequencies of schizophrenia and major affective disorders at six North American psychiatric hospitals, 1972-1988. *Am J Psychiatry.* 1993;150:1668-1673.
50. McNeil TF, Kaij L. Obstetric factors in the development of schizophrenia: complication in the births of preschizophrenics and in reproduction by schizophrenics. In: Wynne LC, Cromwell RL, Matthysse S, eds. *The Nature of Schizophrenia: New Approaches to Research and Treatment.* New York, NY: John Wiley & Sons; 1978:401-429.
51. Halitsky V. Sequelae in children who survived in utero fetal transfusion: a comparison with those who underwent postpartum exchange transfusion. In: Tegami N, ed. *Obstetrical Events and Developmental Sequelae.* Boca Raton, Fla: CRC Press Inc; 1990:111-126.

Announcement

Free Patient Record Forms Available

Patient record forms are available free of charge to ARCHIVES readers by calling or writing FORMEDIC, 12D Worlds Fair Dr, Somerset, NJ 08873-9863, telephone (908) 469-7031.

ORIGINAL ARTICLE

Schizophrenia After Prenatal Famine

Further Evidence

Ezra Susser, MD, DrPH; Richard Neugebauer, PhD; Hans W. Hoek, MD; Alan S. Brown, MD; Shang Lin, PhD; Daniel Labovitz, MD; Jack M. Gorman, MD

Background: Suggestive findings of an earlier study that prenatal nutritional deficiency was a determinant of schizophrenia prompted us to undertake a second test of the hypothesis using more precise data on both exposure and outcome.

Methods: Among persons born in the cities of western Netherlands during 1944 through 1946, we compared the risk for schizophrenia in those exposed and unexposed during early gestation to the Dutch Hunger Winter of 1944/1945. The frequency of hospitalized patients with schizophrenia at age 24 to 48 years in the exposed and unexposed birth cohorts was ascertained from a national psychiatric registry.

Results: The most exposed birth cohort, conceived at the height of the famine, showed a twofold and statistically significant increase in the risk for schizophrenia (relative risk [RR] = 2.0; 95% confidence interval [CI] = 1.2 to 3.4; $P<.01$) in both men (RR = 1.9; 95% CI = 1.0 to 3.7; P=.05) and women (RR = 2.2; 95% CI = 1.0 to 4.7; P= .04). Among all birth cohorts of 1944 through 1946, the risk for schizophrenia clearly peaked in this exposed cohort.

Conclusion: Prenatal nutritional deficiency may play a role in the origin of some cases of schizophrenia.

(Arch Gen Psychiatry. 1996;53:25-31)

WE TESTED the hypothesis that early prenatal nutritional deficiency is associated with an increased risk for schizophrenia.[1-3] The evidence grows that schizophrenia is, in some cases, a neurodevelopmental disorder.[4-9] For instance, numerous studies have now demonstrated that schizophrenia can be associated with abnormalities in brain structure[9,10] and in cognitive and behavioral development.[11-13] Prenatal nutritional deficiencies are important causes of other neurodevelopmental defects.[14-16] Therefore, their possible contribution to schizophrenic illness warrants investigation.

Birth cohorts exposed to early prenatal nutritional deficiency during the Dutch Hunger Winter of 1944/1945[17-20] were compared with those unexposed, with regard to the risk of hospitalization for schizophrenia in adulthood. In an earlier, more limited study,[1-3] we found a significant increase in schizophrenia in exposed women but not in men. Because this association could have important implications for the origin of schizophrenia, these suggestive findings prompted us to undertake a larger and more systematic investigation using new data on exposure and outcome. The present study was not an independent replication, but it was designed to extend and refine our earlier work.

See also pages 11, 19, and 32

Toward the end of World War II, a Nazi blockade precipitated a severe famine in western Netherlands. The Dutch Hunger Winter began in October 1944, gradually increased in intensity over the ensuing months, and ended abruptly on liberation in early May 1945.[17-19] The cities of western Netherlands were affected more than rural areas. At the height of the famine from February to April 1945, the population of these cities suffered severe adverse effects including high mortality from malnutrition.[17-19] The Dutch Hunger Winter was unique in that a famine of brief and clearly defined duration afflicted a population that

See Methods on next page

From the Department of Psychiatry (Drs Susser, Brown, Labovitz, and Gorman) and Gertrude H. Sergievsky Center (Dr Neugebauer), Columbia University, New York, NY; New York State Psychiatric Institute, New York (Drs Susser, Neugebauer, Brown, Labovitz, and Gorman); University Hospital Department of Psychiatry, Utrecht, the Netherlands (Dr Hoek); and Nathan Kline Institute for Psychiatric Research, New York (Dr Lin).

METHODS

We report on birth cohorts of 1944 through 1946 in the six cities in the famine region of the Netherlands with populations larger than 40 000 (Amsterdam, The Hague, Haarlem, Leiden, Rotterdam, and Utrecht). Obviously, the exact date of conception of the birth cohorts was not known. In a full-term pregnancy, conception would be 8 to 9 months prior to birth. For instance, full-term births in November 1945 would have been conceived in February and March 1945; full-term births in December 1945, in March and April 1945.

The cities of other regions of the Netherlands were not included in this analysis. These regions did experience periods of moderately low rations and were included in our earlier study.[1-3] However, because they were not exposed to severe famine and did not show a significant increase in congenital neural defects, a comparable refinement in the analysis was infeasible.

EXPOSURE

As stated above, three criteria were used to define the exposed birth cohorts: (1) low food rations during the first trimester, (2) conception at the height of the famine, and (3) increased congenital neural defects. To establish the first criterion, we used the average food ration during each trimester of gestation, previously documented for all monthly birth cohorts of 1944 through 1946.[17] For the birth cohorts of August through December 1945, average food rations during the first trimester were below 1000 kcal daily (4200 kJ).[1] These cohorts were defined as *exposed to low rations*. All other birth cohorts of 1944 through 1946 (born in 1944, in January through July 1945, and in 1946) were defined as *unexposed*.

For the second criterion, we relied on the documented health outcomes of the famine period. These data indicate that the height of the famine was toward the end of the Hunger Winter (during February through April 1945). The population was nutritionally depleted, and the effects on morbidity and mortality were most severe.[17-19] The early months of the Hunger Winter were not as harsh.

Among the cohorts of August through December 1945, only the later born (born October 15 through December 31, 1945) were conceived during the height of the famine and, therefore, met our second criterion for exposure. We shall refer to these later born as the EX2 cohort. Owing to the timing of their conception, the EX2 cohort was marked by fertility below 50% of previous levels.[17-19] The earlier born (born August 1 through October 14, 1945) were conceived in the early months of the Hunger Winter and did not meet our second criterion for exposure. We refer to these earlier born as the EX1 cohort. In accord with the lesser exposure, the EX1 cohort suffered a smaller decline in fertility.[17]

With regard to the third exposure criterion, increased risk for congenital neural defects, we examined the *International Classification of Diseases (ICD)* categories with established or strongly suspected links with early prenatal nutritional deficiency, including neural tube defects (*ICD-5*[22] spina bifida 731 and anencephaly 733; *ICD-6*[23] spina bifida 751 and other central nervous system anomalies including microcephaly 753.4). We reanalyzed the data of Stein et al[17] that were available only for male subjects. Data on deaths caused by these defects from birth to age 17 years were obtained from national mortality data of the Netherlands Central Bureau of Statistics.[17] Data on those surviving to age 18 years were obtained from military records.[17] Military induction was compulsory for all male individuals of these birth cohorts, and inductees were administered standardized medical examinations. The risk for congenital neural defects in the EX2, EX1, and unexposed

maintained excellent records on food rations during the famine and on health outcomes during the famine and in subsequent decades.[17-20]

With regard to exposure, our a priori hypothesis[1(p 983)] was that an increased risk for schizophrenia would be found among the birth cohorts conceived at the height of the famine and exhibiting an excess of congenital neural defects. Accordingly, in the present study, three criteria were used to define the exposed birth cohorts: (1) low food rations during the first trimester of gestation, (2) conception at the height of the famine as indicated by adverse health effects in the general population, and (3) a detectable excess of congenital neural defects. Whereas our prior study[1] relied on the first criterion alone, this current study obtained data that enabled us to differentiate between exposed birth cohorts satisfying only this first criterion and those satisfying all three criteria.

With regard to outcome, the data of the Dutch national psychiatric registry afforded comprehensive ascertainment of hospitalized patients with schizophrenia at 24 years of age and older in the exposed and unexposed birth cohorts. The registry data of our earlier study were restricted to schizophrenic patients hospitalized at age 32 years and older. This expansion of the outcome data was crucial because the first hospitalization for schizophrenia is most often before age 30 years, especially in men.[21] Taken together, the new data yielded, on the one hand, a considerably more precise definition of the exposed birth cohorts and, on the other, a larger number of cases that are more representative in terms of age at onset and course of illness. The sample size now ensured adequate statistical power to detect a meaningful association between a precisely defined prenatal famine exposure and the risk for narrowly defined schizophrenia.

RESULTS

Our a priori data analysis used the narrow definition of schizophrenia and the most recent discharge diagnosis. The risk for schizophrenia was significantly higher in the EX2 cohort than in the unexposed cohort (**Table 2**) (RR=2.0; 95% CI = 1.2 to 3.4; $P<.01$). The RR did not vary by gender; among men, the RR=1.9 (95% CI = 1.0 to 3.7; $P=.05$), and among women, the RR = 2.2 (95% CI = 1.0 to 4.7; $P=.04$). The risk for schizophrenia was not increased in the EX1 cohort.

Figure 2 shows the risk for schizophrenia in 17 successive birth cohorts of 1944 through 1946. The risk for schizophrenia peaked in the EX2 cohort and was otherwise stable.

We reanalyzed the finding for the EX2 cohort under a broad definition of schizophrenia and using other cohorts was computed as the total number of cases (deaths plus survivors to age 18 years) divided by the number of births (stillbirths were not included because causes of mortality were not available for stillbirths). The EX2 cohort had a detectable excess of congenital neural defects (relative risk [RR] = 2.5; 95% confidence interval [CI] = 1.3 to 4.9; $P<.01$), while the EX1 cohort did not (RR = 1.1, not significant) (**Table 1**).

For further confirmation, we examined secular trends in congenital neural defects. The birth cohorts of the years 1944 through 1946 were divided into 2-month periods. However, to maintain the integrity of the EX1 and EX2 cohorts, the period of May through December 1945 was divided into May through July, August 1 through October 14 (EX1), and October 15 through December 31 (EX2). For each of the 17 successive birth cohorts so defined, the risk for congenital neural defects (in male subjects) was computed as the number of cases divided by the number of births. The risk clearly peaked in the EX2 cohort (**Figure 1**).

Thus, the exposed birth cohorts comprised two distinct groups. The EX2 cohort met all three exposure criteria. The EX1 cohort met only one of the three criteria.

OUTCOME

Cases of schizophrenia were ascertained from the Dutch national psychiatric registry. Registry data were available for 1970 through 1992, comprising persons 24 to 48 years of age for the birth cohorts of 1944 through 1946. Data on cases were derived from psychiatric and university hospitals, which account for more than 90% of psychiatric admissions in the Netherlands. Data on each case included *ICD-8–ICD-9*[24] diagnosis, place of birth, and week of birth.

We used *narrow* and *broad* definitions of schizophrenia as in our previous study. Narrowly defined schizophrenia included only those cases in which the *ICD-8–ICD-9* diagnosis was that of paranoid, hebephrenic, residual, or catatonic schizophrenia,[1] in accordance with the modern criteria for schizophrenia.[25] While severely restricting the number of cases, this definition also minimized the risk of misclassification of affective psychoses as schizophrenia. Broadly defined schizophrenia included all cases with an *ICD-9* diagnosis of schizophrenia, irrespective of the subtype.

DATA ANALYSIS

We analyzed the data under the a priori narrow definition of schizophrenia, using the most recent discharge diagnosis. The risks for schizophrenia in the EX2 cohort, the EX1 cohort, and the unexposed cohort were computed by dividing the number of cases by the number of births minus deaths up to age 18 years. Risk was multiplied by 1000 to derive the risk (ie, cumulative incidence) per 1000 persons. The RRs in the exposed compared with the unexposed were calculated, and 95% CIs for these RRs were derived using the Taylor series.[26]

The χ^2 statistic was used to test the null hypothesis of no association between exposure and disease.[26] Owing to the large numbers of births in both the unexposed (136 691) and the exposed (EX1 = 5466; EX2 = 4190) cohorts, statistical power was sufficient even with the smaller number of cases under a narrow definition of schizophrenia and a refined definition of exposure. For example, for a "true" RR of 2.2, the probability that the null hypothesis would be rejected at $\alpha=.05$ was greater than 80%.

Seasonal and other fluctuations in the rate of schizophrenia were examined by dividing the birth cohorts of 1944 through 1946 into 17 successive cohorts, as described above for congenital neural defects in male subjects.

procedures for selecting the diagnosis. The association between early prenatal exposure to famine and schizophrenia was consistent under six approaches (**Table 3**).

COMMENT

This study offers evidence of a relation between early prenatal nutritional deficiency and the risk for hospitalized schizophrenia in adulthood. The EX2 birth cohort, conceived at the height of the Dutch Hunger Winter, had a significant, twofold increase in the risk for schizophrenia. The increased risk for schizophrenia in the EX2 cohort was evident in men as well as in women and occurred in the context of an otherwise stable incidence of schizophrenia. The EX1 cohort exhibited no increased risk for schizophrenia.

The exposure of the EX2 cohort to early prenatal nutritional deficiency is well established. This birth cohort (although born after the famine) was conceived in the worst months of the Hunger Winter when supplementary food supplies were virtually exhausted. Extensive evidence documents the nutritionally depleted state of the population.[17-19] Women conceiving during this period were nutritionally depleted prior to conception and, in addition, were poorly nourished after conception.

On several counts, the findings possess a high degree of specificity regarding both the prenatal famine exposure and the psychiatric outcomes. First, the EX2 cohort, conceived in the last months of the famine, were exposed only during early gestation because food was plentiful immediately on liberation. Second, the EX1 cohort showed no increased risk for schizophrenia after a lesser exposure during early gestation. Third, birth cohorts exposed to the famine in later stages of gestation exhibited no increased risk for schizophrenia. Fourth, the increased risk for schizophrenia in the EX2 cohort did not extend to other neuropsychiatric disorders. Affective disorders may have been increased in cohorts exposed to the famine later in gestation but were not increased in the EX2 cohort.[17,18,27] Fifth, while the increased risk was evident under all definitions of schizophrenia, it was most marked under a narrow definition consistent with modern criteria. Taken together, the notable specificity in these domains enhances the credibility of these findings as a whole and of the proposed nutritional explanation in particular.

Nonetheless, it is also important to consider alternative explanations that may be consistent with our findings. Selection processes could have led to an artifactual association between prenatal famine exposure and schizophrenia. In addition, other factors may have mediated or confounded the effects of prenatal famine exposure.

Table 1. Congenital Neural Defects* in Males of Birth Cohorts Exposed† and Unexposed† to Early Prenatal Nutritional Deficiency During the Dutch Hunger Winter of 1944 Through 1945: Prevalence Data

	Cohort		
	Exposed		
Prevalence Data	EX2 (n=2327)	EX1 (n=2993)	Unexposed (n=74 245)
Prevalence, per 1000 live births (No. of cases)	3.9 (9‡)	1.7 (5‡)	1.5 (115)
Relative risk (95% confidence interval)	2.5 (1.3-4.9)	1.1 (0.4-2.6)	...
P	<.01	.7	...

*Deaths from birth to age 17 years plus survivors at age 18 years (ICD [International Classification of Diseases]-5 *731, 733;* ICD-6 *751, 753.4).*

†*EX2 indicates exposed birth cohort of October 15 through December 31, 1945; EX1, exposed birth cohort of August 1 through October 14, 1945; and unexposed, all other births of 1944 through 1946 in the famine cities.*

‡*One case of October 1945 excluded because day of birth was missing.*

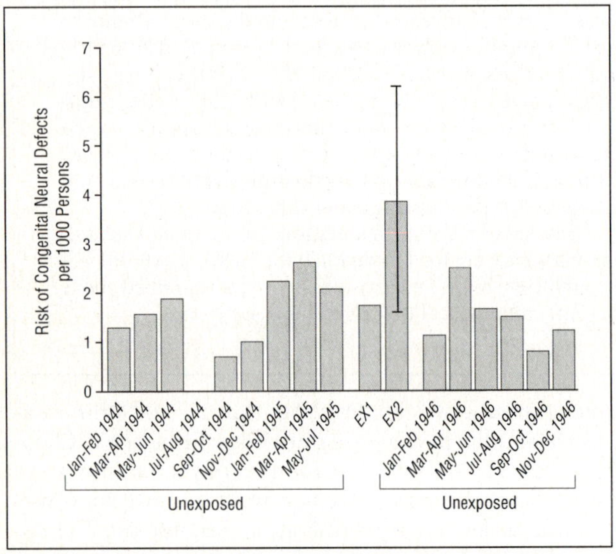

Figure 1. *Congenital neural defects in male individuals (death plus surviving subjects to age 18 years) in Dutch birth cohorts of 1944 through 1946. EX1 and EX2 indicate cohorts born August 1 through October 14, 1995, and October 15 through December 31, 1945, respectively; bar, 95% confidence limits.*

SELECTION BIAS

One possibility is selective conception. Persons conceiving during the famine, when fertility was low, may have had unusual characteristics. Hypothetically, women genetically predisposed to schizophrenia might be more inclined than others to attempt conception at such times. However, poor nutrition was probably the most critical factor in conception;[17] hence, the decline in fertility was more marked in the lower compared with the upper classes.[17,18] In this light, one might expect women predisposed to schizophrenia to have had especially *low* rates of conception during the famine period, as they may have been less successful than others in competing for black market and other extra ration food.

A second possibility is selective survival. The live births of the EX2 cohort represent conceptions that survived difficult circumstances. It has been suggested that the persistence of schizophrenia, despite reduced fertility and survival among cases, may be explained if genes that increase the risk for schizophrenia also confer a selective advantage in some other area.[28] Possibly EX2 births were selected for some genetic factor that is associated with better survival from conception to birth but that is also associated with an increased risk for schizophrenia.

OTHER FACTORS

Prenatal nutritional deficiency may have exerted an effect on the risk for schizophrenia only indirectly, via some other factor. Owing in part to their prenatal exposure to the famine, the EX2 cohort suffered a high perinatal mortality. Perinatal complications have been associated with an increased risk for schizophrenia.[7] However, some of the unexposed birth cohorts of 1944 through 1946 were also afflicted by high perinatal mortality, albeit for different reasons. The unexposed cohorts with high perinatal mortality did not experience increased rates of schizophrenia.

Prenatal nutritional deficiency could lead to maternal ingestion of food substitutes such as tulip bulbs,[1,17] could be a severe stressor that affects prenatal maternal hormones,[29] or could be followed by a rapid nutritional repletion.[20] These exposures could, in turn, have a toxic effect on fetal brain development. However, while there is extensive evidence that prenatal nutritional deficiency can directly affect brain development, there is no strong evidence to support these other exposures.

Finally, a thorough search was conducted for evidence of nonnutritional exposures that were specifically coincident with the height of the famine in the Netherlands and that could account for our findings.[17] None were identified. Moreover, there was no increased risk for schizophrenia among contemporaneous birth cohorts in the cities of other regions of the Netherlands unaffected by the famine (**Table 4**). Therefore, the increased risk cannot be caused by an exposure such as a viral epidemic coinciding in time with the famine, unless this exposure was also confined to the famine cities.

RELATION TO OUR PREVIOUS STUDY

Our earlier study of schizophrenia after prenatal exposure to the Dutch Hunger Winter[1] found an association in women but not in men. Three factors, the number of available patients, the age distribution of the patients, and the definition of the exposed cohort, probably all contributed to the difference in the present results. First, the smaller number of patients, 195 vs 284 in this study, allowed for more random fluctuation.[2,3] Second, in the previous study, patients hospitalized under the age of 32 years but not hospitalized after that age were omitted; therefore, we could not detect patients having an early onset of disease unless they were rehospitalized after age 32 years. The loss of early-onset cases may have weakened the results disproportionately in men because the average age at onset of schizophrenia is younger in men than

Table 2. Schizophrenia* in Birth Cohorts Exposed† and Unexposed† to Early Prenatal Nutritional Deficiency During the Dutch Hunger Winter of 1944 Through 1945: Cumulative Incidence Data

	All			Men‡			Women‡		
	Exposed			Exposed			Exposed		
Incidence Data	EX2 (n=4190)	EX1 (n=5466)	Unexposed (n=136 691)	EX2 (n=2184)	EX1 (n=2800)	Unexposed (n=69 943)	EX2 (n=2006)	EX1 (n=2666)	Unexposed (n=66 748)
Cumulative incidence per 1000 persons‡ (n cases)	3.8 (16)	2.0 (11)	1.9 (257)	4.1 (9)	2.5 (7)	2.2 (151)	3.5 (7)	1.5 (4)	1.6 (106)
Relative risk at age 24-48 y (95% confidence interval)	2.0 (1.2-3.4)	1.1 (0.6-2.0)	...	1.9 (1.0-3.7)	1.2 (0.5-2.5)	...	2.2 (1.0-4.7)	0.9 (0.4-2.6)	...
P	<.01	.82	...	.05	.70	...	.04	.91	...

Schizophrenia narrowly defined, ie, ICD-9 (International Classification of Diseases, Ninth Revision) *295.1,2,3,6.*
†*EX2 indicates exposed birth cohort of October 15 through December 31, 1945; EX1, exposed birth cohort of August 1 through October 14, 1945; and unexposed, all other births of 1944 through 1946 in the famine cities.*
‡*Denominators are live births minus deaths up to age 18 years. (Note that in men, denominators differ between Tables 1 and 2, being only live births in Table 1.)*

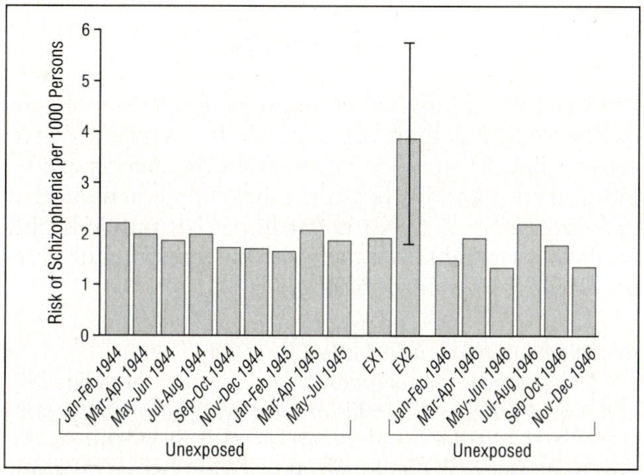

Figure 2. *Schizophrenia in adulthood (hospitalized subjects of 24 to 48 years of age) in Dutch birth cohorts of 1944 through 1946. EX1 and EX2 indicate cohorts born August 1 through October 14, 1995, and October 15 through December 31, 1945, respectively; bar, 95% confidence limits.*

Table 3. Schizophrenia in Birth Cohorts Exposed* and Unexposed to Early Prenatal Nutritional Deficiency During the Dutch Hunger Winter of 1944 Through 1945: Incidence Data Under Narrow and Broad Definitions of Schizophrenia

	Cumulative Incidence per 1000 Persons (No. of Cases)			
Approach	Exposed, EX2	Unexposed	Relative Risk (95% Confidence Interval)	*P*
Under Narrow Definition of Schizophrenia (*ICD-9* 295.1,2,3,6)				
Most recent discharge	3.8 (16)	1.9 (257)	2.0 (1.2-3.4)	<.01
Any discharge	4.5 (19)	2.4 (333)	1.9 (1.2-3.0)	<.01
Any discharge or admission	4.8 (20)	2.8 (385)	1.7 (1.1-2.7)	.02
Under Broad Definition of Schizophrenia (*ICD-9* 295, Any Subtype)				
Most recent discharge	5.3 (22)	3.6 (486)	1.5 (1.0-2.3)	.07
Any discharge	6.0 (25)	3.7 (510)	1.6 (1.1-2.4)	.02
Any discharge or admission	6.4 (27)	4.3 (584)	1.5 (1.0-2.2)	.04

EX2 indicates exposed birth cohort of October 15 through December 31, 1945; unexposed, see Tables 1 and 2; and ICD-9, International Classification of Diseases, Ninth Revision.

in women.[2,3] Third, the definition of the exposed birth cohort, based on official food rations alone, was relatively imprecise and did not take into account nutritional depletion over time, the precise timing of the exposure in gestation, and extra ration foods that could affect neurodevelopmental outcomes.

The RR under the broader classification of exposure (EX1+EX2) used in our previous study can be calculated from the data in Table 2. The overall RR was 1.5 (95% CI = 1.0 to 2.2; *P* =.048) and did not differ between men (RR=1.5) and women (RR=1.5). Thus, the effect of the new data was to remove the suggestion that the results varied by gender, as well as to reveal that the association is confined solely to the EX2 cohort.

IMPLICATIONS

Early prenatal nutritional deficiency, the most likely causative factor in the increased rate of schizophrenia among the EX2 cohort, could produce effects because of either general malnutrition or a specific micronutrient deficiency. Severe prenatal protein-calorie malnutrition is a rare exposure that occurs mainly in developing countries and, in developed countries, could account only for a small number of cases in special circumstances. A specific prenatal micronutrient deficiency, on the other hand, might play an important role in developed as well as in developing countries.[14,30,31]

The findings for neural tube defects such as spina bifida and anencephaly exemplify this point. Early prenatal folate deficiency has remained an important causative factor for neural tube defects in wealthy societies.[14,30,31] The incidence appears to depend on the specific micronutrient composition of the diet, and on the genetic background of the population, rather than on overall food intake, and it follows no simple gradient across rich and poor societies.

Table 4. Schizophrenia in Birth Cohorts of Nonfamine Cities of the Netherlands*: Incidence Among EX2 vs All Other Born in 1944 Through 1946

Diagnosis	Cumulative Incidence per 1000 Persons (No. of Cases) EX2 (n=3841)	All Other Births (n=57 138)	Relative Risk (95% Confidence Interval)	P
Schizophrenia under narrow definition	1.6 (6)	1.4 (81)	1.1 (.5-2.5)	.82

*Includes all nonfamine cities of population >40 000: Groningen, Leeuwarden, Zwolle, Enschede, Hengelo, Breda, Tilburgh, Eindhoven, Heerlen, and Maastricht. EX2 indicates exposed birth cohort of October 15 through December 15, 1945.

Prenatal nutritional deficiency could act in conjunction with either genetic factors or other prenatal exposures.[1,5-7,32-34] In this regard too, neural tube defects may serve as a useful paradigm. These defects are influenced by genetic factors, as well as by prenatal nutrition, and comprise several types that may be genetically distinct.[31] Recent findings suggest that in the presence of an impairment in homocysteine metabolism, which may be genetically determined, a higher than average periconceptional intake of vitamin B_{12} or of folate may compensate by overcoming the metabolic defect and, thereby, reduce the risk for neural tube defects in offspring.[35]

LIMITATIONS

First, this study used group data to define individuals as exposed. In contrast with most ecologic studies, however, the exposure was documented in detail and known to be pervasive in the population.[36]

Second, unconfounded estimates of deficiencies of particular nutrients cannot be determined from the available data. Caloric deficiency, protein deficiency, and deficiencies of specific micronutrients occurred simultaneously in the Dutch Hunger Winter, and each of these has been shown to be capable of affecting brain development in animal experiments.[37,38] To obtain individual exposure data and specify the relevant exposure, we are presently conducting a study of a large birth cohort in the United States; stored prenatal maternal serum samples are available to measure prenatal nutritional exposures in schizophrenic patients and matched controls.

Third, the time of birth was known, but the time of conception had to be inferred. The time of conception was estimated on the assumption of a full-term pregnancy. The great majority of births, including schizophrenic births and births after prenatal famine exposure, occur at full term.[17,39] However, if short gestations were more frequent among schizophrenic births compared with other births, the effect of this misclassification would be to deflate the estimates of the true RR for the EX2 cohort.

Fourth, complete data on congenital neural defects were available only for male patients. The morbidity data from military induction examinations, the basis for our a priori specification regarding timing of exposure, were lacking for female patients.

Fifth, data on social class of origin were not available in the psychiatric registry. No relation has been found in the Netherlands between schizophrenia and low social class of origin.[40] Moreover, since the exposed birth cohort was weighted toward the upper classes, any such association would tend to reduce the estimated RR in this study.

Other limitations of this study included the use of registry diagnoses, the absence of patients younger than 24 years of age, and the loss to emigration of a small number of the members of these birth cohorts. Because each of these factors would affect the exposed and unexposed cohorts in the same way, they cannot account for the association between prenatal nutritional deficiency and schizophrenia in this study.[1] Rather, they would tend to diminish the observed association owing to nondifferential misclassification.

CONCLUSION

The findings of this study link prenatal nutritional deficiency to the risk for schizophrenia. It has recently been shown that the incidence of neural tube defects can be reduced substantially by nutritional supplementation in early pregnancy.[14,30,31] It is our hope that public health implications might eventually also emerge from the present findings on schizophrenia.

Accepted for publication July 28, 1995.

This study was supported in part by the Theodore and Vada Stanley Foundation and by grant 1 P20-MH-50727 NYSPI from the National Institute of Mental Health for Developing Schizophrenia Research Center (Epidemiology Research Core), Washington, DC.

We thank the three original authors of the Dutch Famine Study: Zena Stein, MD, Mervyn Susser, MD, and Gerhart Saenger, PhD, for consultation on this manuscript. We also thank Peter Bosch and Constance van Rooijen of the Dutch Psychiatric Registry for their contribution to this work.

Reprint requests to New York State Psychiatric Institute, Box 24, 722 W 168th St, New York, NY 10032 (Dr Susser).

REFERENCES

1. Susser E, Lin SP. Schizophrenia after prenatal exposure to the Dutch Hunger Winter of 1944-1945. *Arch Gen Psychiatry.* 1992;49:983-988.
2. Jones P. Schizophrenia after prenatal exposure to the Dutch Hunger Winter of 1944-1945. *Arch Gen Psychiatry.* 1994;51:333. Letter.
3. Brown S, Susser E, Butler P, Richardson Andrews R, Kaufmann C, Gorman J. Neurobiological plausibility of prenatal nutritional deprivation as a risk factor for schizophrenia. *J Nerv Ment Dis.* In press.
4. Carpenter WT Jr, Buchanan RW. Medical progress schizophrenia. *N Engl J Med.* 1994;330:10:681-690.
5. Weinberger DR. Implications of normal brain development for the pathogenesis of schizophrenia. *Arch Gen Psychiatry.* 1987;44:660-669.
6. Murray RM. Is schizophrenia a neurodevelopmental disorder. *BMJ.* 1987;295: 681-682.
7. Waddington JL. Schizophrenia: developmental neuroscience and pathobiology. *Lancet.* 1993;341:531-538.
8. Bloom FE. Advancing a neurodevelopmental origin for schizophrenia. *Arch Gen*

Psychiatry. 1993;50:224-227.
9. Suddath RL, Christison GW, Torrey EF, Casanova MF, Weinberger DR. Anatomical abnormalities in the brain of monozygotic twins discordant for schizophrenia. *N Engl J Med.* 1990;322:789-794.
10. Andreasen NC, Arndt S, Swayze V II, Cizadlo T, Flaum M, O'Leary D, Erhardt JC, Yuh WT. Thalamic abnormalities in schizophrenia visualized through magnetic resonance image averaging. *Science.* 1994;266:294-298.
11. Fish B, Marcus J, Hans SL, Auerbach JG, Purdue S. Infants at risk for schizophrenia. *Arch Gen Psychiatry.* 1992;49:221-235.
12. Done DJ, Crow TJ, Johnstone EV, Sacker A. Childhood antecedents of schizophrenia and affective illness: social adjustment at ages 7 and 11. *BMJ.* 1994; 309:699-703.
13. Jones P, Rodgers B, Murray R, Marmot M. Child developmental risk factors for adult schizophrenia in the British 1946 birth cohort. *Lancet.* 1994;344: 1398-1402.
14. Medical Research Council Vitamin Study Research Group. Prevention of neural tube defects: results of the Medical Research Council Vitamin Study. *Lancet.* 1991;338:131-137.
15. Rosso PR. Prenatal nutrition and brain growth. In: van Gelder NM, Butterworth RF, Drujan BD, eds. *(Mal)nutrition and the Infant Brain.* New York, NY: Wiley-Liss Inc; 1990;25-40.
16. DeLong GR. Effects of nutrition on brain development in humans. *Am J Clin Nutr (Suppl).* 1993;57:286-290.
17. Stein Z, Susser M, Saenger G, Marolla F, eds. *Famine and Human Development: The Dutch Hunger Winter of 1944-45.* New York, NY: Oxford University Press; 1975.
18. Stein Z, Susser M, Saenger G, Marolla F. Nutrition and mental performance. *Science.* 1973;178:708-713.
19. Burger GCE, Drummond JC, Sandstead HR, eds. *Malnutriton and Starvation in Western Netherlands: September 1944-July 1945.* Hague, the Netherlands: General State Printing Office; 1948.
20. Ravelli GP, Stein ZA, Susser MW. Obesity in young men after exposure in utero and early infancy. *N Engl J Med.* 1976;295:349-353.
21. Jablensky A, Sartorious N, Ernberg G, Anker M, Korten A, Cooper JE, Day R, Bertelsen A. Schizophrenia: manifestations, incidence and course in different cultures: a World Helath Organization Ten Country Study. *Psychol Med Monogr Suppl.* 1992;20.
22. World Health Organization. *Manual of the International Statistical Classification of Diseases, Injuries, and Causes of Death.* Geneva, Switzerland: World Health Organization; 1938.
23. World Health Organization. *Manual of the International Statistical Classification of Diseases, Injuries, and Causes of Death.* Geneva, Switzerland: World Health Organization; 1948.
24. World Health Organization. *Mental Disorders: Glossary and Guide to Their Classification in Accordance With the Ninth Revision of the International Classification of Diseases.* Geneva, Switzerland: World Health Organization; 1978.
25. American Psychiatric Association. *Diagnostic and Statistical Manual of Mental Disorders.* 4th ed. Washington, DC: American Psychiatric Association; 1994.
26. Fleiss JL. *Statistical Methods for Rates and Proportions.* 2nd ed. New York, NY: John Wiley & Sons; 1981.
27. Brown AS, Susser ES, Lin SP, Neugebauer R, Gorman J. Increased risk of affective disorders in males after second trimester prenatal exposure to the Dutch Hunger Winter of 1944-45. *Br J Psychiatry.* 1995:166;606-606.
28. Crow TJ. Integrated viral genes as potential pathogens in the functional psychoses. *J Psychiatr Res.* 1987;21:479-485.
29. Huttenen M, Niskanen P. Prenatal loss of father and psychiatric disorders. *Arch Gen Psychiatry.* 1978;35:429-431.
30. Czeisel AE, Dudas I. Prevention of the first occurrence of neural-tube defects by periconceptional vitamin supplementation. *N Engl J Med.* 1992;327:1832-1835.
31. Elwood JM, Little J, Elwood JH. *Epidemiology and Control of Neural Tube Defects.* New York, NY: Oxford University Press; 1992.
32. Susser E, Susser M. Genetic epidemiology of psychiatric disorders: examples from schizophrenia. In: Michels R, ed. *Psychiatry.* Philadelphia, Pa: JB Lippincott Co; 1993.
33. Mednick SA, Machon RA, Huttunen MO, Bonett D. Adult schizophrenia following prenatal exposure to an influenza epidemic. *Arch Gen Psychiatry.* 1988; 45:189-192.
34. O'Callaghan E, Sham P, Takei N, Glover G, Murray RM. Schizophrenia after prenatal exposure to 1957 A2 influenza epidemic. *Lancet.* 1991;337:1248-1250.
35. Mills JL, McPartlin JM, Kirke PN, Lee YJ, Conley MR, Weir DG, Scott JM. Homocysteine metabolism in pregnancies complicated by neural-tube defects. *Lancet.* 1995;345:149-151.
36. Susser M. The logic in ecological, I. *Am J Publ Health.* 1994;84:825-829.
37. Morgane PJ, Austin-LaFrance R, Bronzino J, Tonkiss J, Diaz-Cintra S, Cintra L, Kemper T, Galler JR. Prenatal malnutrition and development of the brain. *Neurosci Biobehav Rev.* 1993;17:91-128.
38. Butler PD, Susser ES, Brown AS, Kaufmann CA, Gorman JM. Prenatal nutritional deprivation as a risk factor in schizophrenia: preclinical evidence. *Neuropsychopharmacology.* 1994;11:227-235.
39. Done DJ, Johnstone EC, Frith CD, Golding J, Shepherd PM, Crow TJ. Complications of pregnancy and delivery in relation to psychosis in adult life: data from the British Perinatal Mortality Survey Sample. *BMJ.* 1991;302:1576-1580.
40. Wiersma D, Giel R, DeJong A, Slooff CJ. Social class and schizophrenia in a Dutch cohort. *Psychol Med.* 1983;13:141-150.

ARCHIVES Circulation

The ARCHIVES is available by request to nonfederal physicians in the United States (50 states and Washington, DC) whose official American Medical Association masterfile record shows a primary specialty of psychiatry or child psychiatry in an office- or hospital-based practice as a staff physician, resident in training beyond the first year, or clinical fellow.

If you meet the above qualification criteria and are not currently receiving the ARCHIVES and would like to receive it each month, you must complete a free subscription request card. To receive a request card, please write to Kathryn Osten, American Medical Association, Circulation Processing Department, 515 N State St, Chicago, IL 60610 (fax 312-464-5831). A subscription request card will be sent to you in response. If you are a resident or fellow, please include verification of your training program and a complete mailing address.

ORIGINAL ARTICLE

Search for Viral Nucleic Acid Sequences in Brain Tissues of Patients With Schizophrenia Using Nested Polymerase Chain Reaction

Alla M. Taller, MD; David M. Asher, MD; Kitty L. Pomeroy; Basil A. Eldadah; Mark S. Godec, MD; Peter G. Falkai, MD; Bernhard Bogert, MD; Joel E. Kleinman, MD, PhD; Janice R. Stevens, MD; E. Fuller Torrey, MD

Background: We used polymerase chain reaction to search for nucleic acid sequences of several viruses in DNA and RNA extracted from brain tissues of schizophrenic and control subjects.

Methods: We extracted DNA and RNA templates from frozen brain specimens of 31 patients with schizophrenia and 23 nonschizophrenic control patients with other diseases. The extracts were subjected to polymerase chain reaction with oligonucleotide primers for 12 different viruses (cytomegalovirus, Epstein-Barr virus, herpes simplex virus type 1, human herpesvirus type 6, varicella-zoster virus, measles virus, mumps virus, rubella virus, the picornavirus group, influenza A virus, human T-cell lymphotropic virus type I, and St Louis encephalitis virus), several of which have been suspected of involvement in schizophrenia. Nested primers were used to increase the sensitivity of the method.

Results: No amplified nucleic acid sequences encoded by the selected viral genomes were detected in extracts of any brain specimens from either schizophrenic or control patients.

Conclusions: These data agree with previous studies that failed to find sequences of a number of viruses in the cerebrospinal fluid or selected areas of the brains of schizophrenic patients. Additional efforts should be undertaken to identify other known and unknown pathogens in schizophrenia, sampling more areas of the brain from subjects with a variety of clinical types of schizophrenia.

(Arch Gen Psychiatry. 1996;53:32-40)

From the Laboratory of Central Nervous System Studies, National Institute of Neurological Disorders and Stroke, National Institutes of Health, Bethesda, Md (Drs Taller, Asher, and Godec, Ms Pomeroy, and Mr Eldadah); Department of Psychiatry, University of Düsseldorf, Düsseldorf, Germany (Dr Falkai); Department of Psychiatry, Otto von Guericke University, Magdeburg, Germany (Dr Bogert); and Clinical Brain Disorders Branch, National Institute of Mental Health Neuroscience Center at St Elizabeths Hospital, Washington, DC (Drs Kleinman, Stevens, and Torrey).

CHRONIC schizophrenia is a common illness (estimated 1-month point prevalence rate in the United States, 0.7%; overall lifetime rate for schizophrenia/schizophreniform disorder, 1.5%)[1] with long duration and relatively poor response to therapy. Although its cause remains unknown, one hypothesis holds that a virus may be responsible. Factors suggesting possible viral involvement in the development of the schizophrenic process have been thoroughly reviewed.[2-10] We used polymerase chain reaction (PCR)[11,12] to examine nucleic acids extracted from brain tissues of schizophrenics, attempting to detect a variety of viral DNA or RNA sequences. We selected several viruses known to infect the central nervous system in childhood, as well as other viruses hypothesized to be involved in schizophrenia or of special interest to us.

The introduction of PCR to virology made it possible to detect extremely small amounts of viral nucleic acids in tissues and body fluids. The principles of PCR have been well explained in the popular scientific literature by its originator[13] and in the medical literature by others[14] and are summarized schematically in the **Figure**. Polymerase chain reaction can amplify any DNA for which the nucleotide sequence is known, by repeated cycles of denaturation (separation of the two DNA strands by heating), hybridization of two synthetic oligonucleotide primers selected to be complementary to selected sites on the separated DNA strands, followed by extension of a new DNA strand from the 3′ end of each primer catalyzed by a DNA polymerase enzyme. If the DNA polymerase is resistant to inactivation at high temperatures, it can be added to the reaction mixture at the start and remains active even after many cycles of heat denaturation of the DNA. The resulting

See Materials and Methods on next page

MATERIALS AND METHODS

PATIENTS

Postmortem brain tissue was obtained from autopsies conducted by the medical examiners of Washington, DC, and Düsseldorf, Germany. Tissues of 29 schizophrenic patients and 17 nonschizophrenic control patients were from the collection of the Neuropathology Section, Clinical Brain Disorders Branch, Intramural Research Program, National Institute of Mental Health at St Elizabeths Hospital, Washington, DC. Tissues of two schizophrenic patients and seven nonschizophrenic control patients were from the collection of the Department of Psychiatry, University of Düsseldorf. Specimens were collected randomly between 1978 and 1990. Preliminary diagnosis of psychiatric disorder was made by review of answers to a special screening questionnaire prepared by a psychiatrist and administered by a police officer to surviving friends or relatives of the subjects. Hospital records and outpatient records of psychiatric patients were then reviewed independently by two psychiatrists, who both agreed with the premortem diagnosis of schizophrenia. General medical records for control subjects, determined by review of the questionnaires not to have had psychiatric disorders, were unavailable; however, because the control subjects were from the same locations and socioeconomic groups as the schizophrenic subjects, it seems likely that if they had schizophrenia they would have had records in our institutions, the main providers of psychiatric care in the areas, and none did.

There were 31 patients with definite or probable schizophrenia and 23 patients without psychiatric diagnoses. Clinical and demographic characteristics are summarized in **Table 1**. Twenty-eight patients met the *DSM-III-R* criteria for schizophrenia. One patient had probable schizophrenia but also had a history of temporal lobectomy for epilepsy. Two patients appeared to have had typical schizophrenia but died 3 and 6 months after onset; to detect viral agents that might be present only early in illness, we included those patients with short durations of probable schizophrenia, even though strict *DSM-III-R* criteria require illness to last 6 months before a diagnosis of schizophrenia can be made. Schizophrenic patients tended to be younger than controls, and many more died of suicide.

As an additional control to validate that our technique was adequate to detect small amounts of a latent virus, we attempted to detect DNA sequences of herpes simplex virus (HSV) in trigeminal ganglia—known to harbor that virus in a majority of adults.[16] Trigeminal ganglia were obtained at the autopsies of three patients in the Clinical Center, National Institutes of Health, Bethesda, Md. (Those patients are not included in Table 1.) All were men aged 50 to 60 years with malignant diseases. Postmortem intervals for two subjects were 4.5 and 9.5 hours. The time of death of the third patient was not known.

SPECIMENS

Autopsies of schizophrenic and nonschizophrenic patients were performed at comparable intervals after death (Table 1)—a mean of 24 hours for control subjects and 18 hours for schizophrenics, with the longest postmortem interval 72 hours. (Studies with human brains removed at various intervals after death found RNA to be surprisingly stable, at least up to 84 hours post mortem[17]; DNA is thought to be even more stable.) Specimens of hippocampus, when available, and of hypothalamus (Washington, DC) or thalamus (Düsseldorf) were frozen promptly at −70°C and stored at that temperature for 3 to 15 years until extraction of nucleic acids. (Those areas were selected because they are thought to be affected by schizophrenia.[8]) Specimens from schizophrenic patients and controls were held in storage for comparable times.

NUCLEIC ACID EXTRACTS

Where necessary, the weight of each specimen was brought to 1.0 g by adding normal mouse brain tissue to increase the total yield of carrier nucleic acid. (Nucleic acid extracts of the same normal mouse tissue were included in each PCR as negative controls.) We obtained DNA and total RNA from brain tissues, trigeminal ganglia, control mouse brain, and cultured cells by extraction in guanidine isothiocyanate and centrifugation through cesium chloride, as previously described,[18-21] and these extracts were stored in aliquots of 20 μL at −70°C.

SELECTION AND PREPARATION OF VIRAL PRIMER SEQUENCES

Viruses of the herpes group—especially HSV and cytomegalovirus (CMV)—have been implicated in several studies of schizophrenia. We selected primers for HSV type 1(HSV-1), CMV, Epstein-Barr virus (EBV), varicella-zoster virus (VZV), and human herpesvirus type 6 (HHV-6) for screening. Primers for a number of RNA viruses (influenza virus type A, picornavirus group, and measles, mumps, and rubella viruses) postulated to be associated with schizophrenia[4,7,22-25] were also selected. Because of increasing interest in the neurotropic retrovirus human T-cell lymphotropic virus type I (HTLV-I),[26-28] we selected primers for that agent as well. (We assayed for HTLV-I proviral DNA transcript[29] rather than for viral RNA.) We also prepared primers for St Louis encephalitis virus,[21] not implicated in schizophrenia, as an additional control. The specific oligonucleotide primer pairs designed to amplify regions of viral sequences from 126 to 732 base pairs (bp) long are presented in **Table 2**,[30-50] which describes primer sequences, their identification codes, locations in the genome when known, predicted sizes of the target PCR-amplified cDNA products, and published sources of sequence information. Primers were synthesized on a PCR Mate 391 DNA synthesizer (Applied Biosystems, Foster City, Calif).

PREPARATION OF CONTROL VIRAL TEMPLATES

Control positive viral DNA or RNA templates were prepared for each virus. Most viral nucleic acids were extracted from cultured cells infected with standard strains of virus, as previously described[19,20]; strains were originally obtained from the American Type Culture Collection (ATCC), Rockville, Md, except as indicated. The HSV-1/KOS strain, measles virus/Edmonston strain, mumps virus/Enders strain, rubella virus/To 336 strain, and poliovirus type 1/Brunhilde and type 2/Lansing strains were grown in Vero E6 C1008 cells (ATCC) by adsorbing 1.0 mL of diluted virus stock on 75-cm² confluent monolayers of cells for 1 hour at 37°C. The virus was then aspirated and the fluid replaced with 15 mL of Eagle's minimum essential medium supplemented with 5% fetal bovine serum. The VZV/Ellen and CMV/AD-169 strains were propagated in WI-38

Continued on next page

cells (Viromed Inc, Minneapolis, Minn) as described, except that the inoculated cultures were first centrifuged at 150g for 30 minutes at 20°C[51] and then further adsorbed for 30 minutes at 37°C. The EBV was provided as a culture of persistently infected Raji cells (ATCC). The HHV-6/GS strain was provided as infected HSB-2 cells by the National Institute of Allergy and Infectious Diseases Acquired Immunodeficiency Syndrome Research and Reference Reagent Program (HSB-2/HHV-6GS; Ogden Bioservices Corp, Rockville, Md) and propagated by periodic addition of uninfected HSB-2 cells (CCRF-HSB-2) in RPMI medium supplemented with glutamine and 10% fetal bovine serum.[52] The St Louis encephalitis virus/Parton strain was propagated in C6/36 mosquito cells.[21] At appropriate intervals after infection, nucleic acids were extracted from the cells.[18-21] Influenza A virus/NWS/33 (hemagglutinin 1 and neuraminidase 1 [H1N1]) strain (ATCC) was propagated in the chorioallantoic sacs of embryonated hens' eggs and in brain tissue of suckling mice inoculated intracerebrally, and RNA was extracted from fluids and tissue, as above. We extracted HTLV-I proviral DNA from the brain tissue of an infected patient with mycosis fungoides and spastic paraparesis, as previously described.[53]

Nucleic acid extracts from uninfected Vero E6, WI-38, and HSB-2 cell cultures and from brain tissues of normal mice and humans served as negative controls. Only those experimental extracts in which sufficient nucleic acid was present for amplification, as confirmed by PCR using primers flanking a 437-bp region of the human β-globin (HBG) DNA sequence on chromosome 11,[30] were tested with viral primers. (Unfortunately, the HBG primers do not distinguish between RNA and contaminating genomic DNA.)

POLYMERASE CHAIN REACTIONS

The DNA templates were subjected to PCR[54] and RNA templates to reverse transcriptase PCR,[19-21] as previously described. Control templates of DNA or RNA from normal human brain, normal mouse brain, and cell cultures, as well as controls to which only water was added in place of template, were included in each set of PCRs with experimental samples to detect false-positive results.[55]

Nested PCR

To increase the sensitivity of the PCR, a second pair of inner primers was selected internal to the first pair, amplifying regions 50 to 70 bp smaller than the initial cDNA products, and these served as templates for nested PCR.[20]

Identification of PCR Products

The PCR products were visualized by electrophoresis in 1.2% agarose gels with ethidium bromide staining; identity of positively amplified fragments was confirmed by enzymatic cleavage with *Alu* I or *Ava* II.[19-21] In those few cases in which the original primers amplified products of questionable specificity, additional primer pairs from different parts of the viral gene were selected, and PCR was repeated to confirm the results.

SAFEGUARDS AGAINST CONTAMINATION

All viral controls were prepared and extracted in a laminar flow biosafety cabinet separate from the area used to extract the patient material. Recommended precautions for PCR[55] were observed to reduce the likelihood of contamination of nucleic acid extracts by accidental carryover of PCR products. Nested PCRs were set up in an area of the laboratory adjacent to the PCR thermal cycler, separate from the area in which the original nucleic acids were extracted. Identification of the PCR products by gel electrophoresis was performed only after the second round of amplification with inner primers was complete. The PCR products were never introduced into the viral or human nucleic acid template preparation areas.

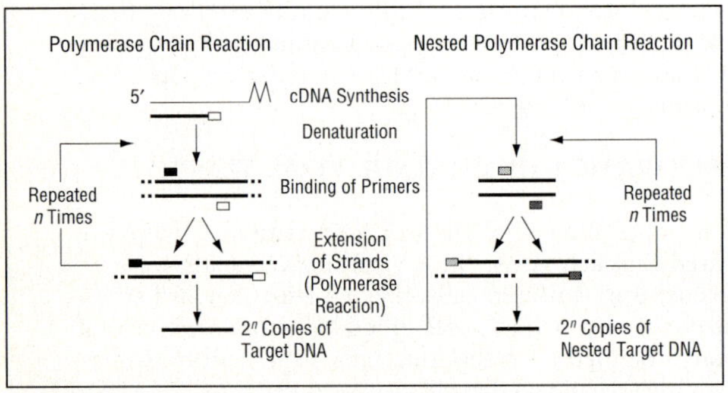

Detection of viral nucleic acids by polymerase chain reaction (PCR) (modified from Hyypiä et al[15]). Double-stranded complementary DNA (cDNA) is generated using a synthetic oligonucleotide primer complementary to a selected area of the viral nucleic acid and reverse transcriptase for RNA viruses or DNA polymerase for single-stranded DNA viruses. A short, double-stranded DNA product is then amplified by PCR—repeated cycles of the following three steps: (1) denaturation (separation of DNA strands by heating), (2) hybridization of each DNA strand with one of a pair of oligonucleotide primers, and (3) extension of new DNA strands from the 3′ end of each primer, catalyzed by a heat-stable DNA polymerase. To increase the sensitivity and specificity of PCR, a second series of amplification cycles can be conducted, using the initial short DNA product as the template with a nested pair of primers[12] that hybridize further in (3′) from the ends of the DNA strands, generating larger amounts of an even shorter DNA product. Specificity of PCR products is confirmed as described in the text.

amplified product or "amplicon" is a short, double-stranded DNA, the ends of which are defined by the 5′ ends of the synthetic primers. The identity of the DNA product can be confirmed by determining that it has the predicted size (estimated by measuring its electrophoretic mobility in gel compared with DNA of standard sizes) and sequence (by hybridization of the product to a complementary oligonucleotide probe, by cleavage with restriction endonuclease enzymes at predicted sites, or by more laborious direct analysis of the nucleotide sequence). The nucleic acids of DNA viruses are readily amplified and identified as described. As indicated in the Figure, RNA extracted from viruses can also be detected[15] by first transcribing it to complementary DNA (cDNA) using a reverse transcriptase enzyme and an appropriate oligonucleotide primer, which can be one of those used for PCR. The DNA or RNA selected for amplification by PCR (often called the nucleic acid template) need not be highly purified. The sensitivity and specificity of PCR can be increased by taking the double-stranded DNA product as a new template for a second series of amplification reactions, selecting "nested" primers internal to those used for the first series.[12]

Table 1. Clinical and Demographic Characteristics of Subjects

	Schizophrenic Subjects	Nonschizophrenic Subjects
No.	31	23
No. from Washington, DC/Düsseldorf, Germany	29/2	16/7
Age, y* (range)	41.0±14.1 (20-68)	54.0±21.4 (19-86)
Gender, No. F/M	11/20	8/15
Race, No. B/H/W†	19/0/12	10/1/12
Duration of schizophrenia, y* (range)	17.2±12.3 (0.3-42)	...
Cause of death, No.		
Accident	5	6
Homicide	0	3
Suicide	12‡	2
Cardiovascular§	5	6
Other‖	5	4
Unknown¶	4	2
Postmortem interval, h* (range)	18.3±10.9 (3.5-49.0)	24.2±16.4 (3.8-72.0)
Brain area tested, No.		
Hippocampus	11	7
Hypothalamus or thalamus	9	5
Both	11	11

*Values are mean±SD.
†H indicates Hispanic.
‡Includes one case in which an accident was not ruled out.
§Includes atherosclerotic coronary artery disease and myocardial infarction, and some patients had other diseases as well.
‖Includes malignant tumor, pneumonia, seizures, pulmonary embolus, subarachnoid hemorrhage, and possible myxedema/cardiomyopathy.
¶Includes "collapse," cardiac arrest, and hyponatremia.

RESULTS

All the target sequences of control viral nucleic acids extracted from infected cells were successfully amplified by the selected primers. More than one primer pair was used to amplify several different gene regions of CMV (including an early transcribed region), HHV-6, VZV, HTLV-I, and influenza virus type A (Table 2). The DNA from two of three normal trigeminal ganglia, subjected to PCR as an additional positive control, yielded the products predicted for HSV-1, and the specificity of those PCR products was confirmed by cleavage with *Alu* I, giving fragments of predicted sizes.

See also pages 11, 19, and 25

We successfully extracted DNA templates from the brains of all patients included in this report except for one schizophrenic patient. When amplified by the HBG primers, they produced fragments of 437 and 337 bp with outer and inner primers, respectively (Table 2); those few outer PCR products that did not produce clear bands in gel nonetheless gave definite bands with inner primers. The outer HBG primers were not amplified from cDNA transcripts of RNA extracted from any human brain tissue, but the nested inner HBG primers amplified products of predicted sizes from cDNA templates prepared from all subjects.

None of the DNA or RNA templates from brains of schizophrenic subjects yielded products of predicted target sizes in PCR with any viral primer pairs. Products giving prominent nonspecific bands (not usually of the sizes predicted for viruses) were amplified in some reactions, but they were consistently eliminated by nested PCR, and when tested with additional pairs of primers chosen from different genomic regions of the same virus, no specific amplification was confirmed. Two DNA specimens extracted from brains of control subjects yielded products of a size close to that predicted, using outer primers for HTLV-I (SK 110, SK 111), and one of those was digested by incubation with a restriction enzyme (*Alu* I), yielding fragments of the approximate sizes predicted for HTLV-I. However, using those products as templates, nested PCR with an inner pair of primers (SK 110-IN-1, SK 111-IN-2) did not yield the predicted smaller products, nor did an additional pair of primers from a different site in the HTLV-I genome (SK 54, SK 55) amplify products from the original templates, so the presence of HTLV-I in those brains was not confirmed.

In addition to the single specimen of a schizophrenic patient from which satisfactory DNA was not obtained, a few other specimens from schizophrenic patients (as indicated below) yielded too little nucleic acid to perform PCR with every primer pair. (All 23 control specimens yielded ample nucleic acid for successful PCR with all primer pairs.) In all, 30 specimens from schizophrenic patients were successfully tested for the DNA viruses CMV, EBV, HSV-1, and VZV and for the HTLV-I provirus, and 29 were tested for HHV-6. Brains of 23 schizophrenic patients were successfully tested for mumps virus and 22 for measles and rubella viruses. Brains of all 31 schizophrenic patients were tested for the other viruses. In short, except for the trigeminal ganglia of controls, in none of the human tissues tested were viral nucleic acids detected.

Table 2. Viral Oligonucleotide Primer Sequences Selected and cDNA Products Generated*

Target Genome	Amplified Region of Genome	Location in Genome (Nucleotide Nos.)	Primer Identification Code	Primer Sequence 5′-3′
				Control
Human genome	Human β-globin gene (chromosome 11)	62333-62353	HBG 1	CAA TAG AAA CTG GGC ATG TGG
		62769-62749	HBG 2	TGC AAT CAT TCG TCT GTT TCC
		62364-62384	HBG 3	GAC TCT TGG GTT TCT GAT AGG
		62740-62720	HBG 4	ACT GTA CCC TGT TAC TTC TCC
				DNA Viruses
CMV	Glycoprotein B gene	368-387	GB 5	TCT ACA ACA CTA CCC TCA AG
		780-760	GB 6	GTT TTG ATA ACT GTC CCT ATG
		401-420	GB 7	TGG GAG TCA ACA CTA CCA AG
		746-727	GB 8	ACC GTG CCT CCT ATA ACG CG
	Transforming region	1027-1046	Adtran 1	TGT ACT TAT GCT ACA TGA TG
		1491-1472	Adtran 2	ATG ATG ATA ATA ATG ATG AC
		1054-1073	Adtran 3	CTT TGA TTC ATC GTT CCT CC
		1464-1445	Adtran 4	CCA CCA CAC GAT ATA TAC AG
	Early transcribed gene	453-472	ET 1	GCG AGT GTT CCA TAA AAG CC
		917-898	ET 2	TCG TGG TCG ATG AAA CTG TG
		479-498	ET 3	TCC GCG AGA CCA TGC CAT CC
		891-872	ET 4	CAA GTG ACG TCC ATT TCT TG
EBV	5′ terminus	66-85	EBV 1	AGT ATG CCT GCC TGT AAT TG
		436-417	EBV 2	AGC TGC GGC CAG CAA TGC AA
		101-120	EBV 3	TTT GGC TGG CGG CTA TTG CC
		400-381	EBV 4	AGG TGG GTC CTC AAT CCT CC
HSV-1	Glycoprotein B gene	1066-1085	HSV 1	GTG GTT CGG CCA CCG CTA CT
		1465-1446	HSV 2	CCC CTC CCG GTA GCC GTA AA
		1127-1147	HSV 3	TTC GAG GAG GTG ATC GAC AAG
		1430-1411	HSV 4	CAA AGT CGC CAG TCG CCA GC
HHV-6	Unmarked gene	215-234	HHV-6 out #1	AGC CCA ACA TTC ATA TTC TA
		876-857	HHV-6 out #2	AGA TCG TAT GCG TCA TTA CG
		180-199	HHV-6 1	ACC GCG CAC GTG TTT TTT AT
		911-892	HHV-6 2	TAG AAT GCT TAC GAG AAG GT
		250-269	HHV-6 3	CAT ACT AGA ACA ACA GAG AG
		841-824	HHV-6 4	ATT TTA AAG ATT ACG GAC TT
VZV	70-kd membrane protein gene	480-499	VZ MP 1	TGC ACA GGA GGA TCT TGG GG
		929-910	VZ MP 2	AAC AGT GTG CTC GTG TTT AC
		510-529	VZ MP 3A	CAT CCA CGT TAT CCC TAC GT
		893-874	VZ MP 4A	TCC GCT TCC TTC TTA CCT TG
	Inverted repeat	5-24	VZ-REP-1	CGG GAT GGA CTC CAT GAC GG
		454-435	VZ-REP-2	CAC CTC GGG CCC TGT GGT GG
	Glycoprotein gpII gene	1837-1856	VZ-GP-1	ATT ATG TCC AGA GAT CTG TT
		2286-2267	VZ-GP-2	GTT AGA TAA AAA CGT GGT AA
	5′ terminus	967-986	VZ-1	GCT TAT ATA AAT TTA TGT GC
		1416-1397	VZ-2	CAC CTC CAG GCG TCA TTG CA
				RNA Viruses
Measles virus	Nucleocapsid protein gene	428-448	MNP 1	GGT TCG GAT GGT TCG AGA ACA
		904-884	MNP 2	GGT TCA TCA AGG ACT CAA GTG
		465-485	MNP 3	TGA AGT GCA AGA CCC TGA GGG
		864-844	MNP 4	TTC ATG CAG TCC AAG AGC AGG
Mumps virus	Hemagglutinin-neuraminidase gene	611-631	MHN 1	CAC CCA ATG GTT GCA CAA GAA
		1242-1222	MHN 2	CCA GGC ACA GAC AAG AAA TGC
		643-663	MHN 3	TCT CTA GGT AAG ACA CAC TGG
		1188-1168	MHN 4	GAA GTA TGA TCT CAA AGC ACG
Rubella virus	E1 protein region of polyprotein gene	657-677	RE1P 1	CTA CTA CAA GCA GTA CCA CCC
		1171-1151	RE1P 2	GGC GTG ACC CAC ACC TCA CCG
		687-707	RE1P 3	CGA GGT TGA ACC TGC CTT CGG
		1142-1122	RE1P 4	GCA GCG CAG CAA GCA GCA GGG
Picornaviruses (enteroviruses, rhinoviruses)	Capsid protein gene	165-180	OL 26	GCA CTT CTG TTT CCC C
		556-541	OL 27	CGG ACA CCC AAA GTA G
		187-208	OL 28	ATT GCA TAG ACT GCT CAC GCG
		532-512	OL 29	GCC ACA GAC TTG CGC GTT ACG

cDNA Product Size, Base Pairs	Restriction Enzyme	Cleavage Product Sizes, Base Pairs	Source
437	. . .	. . .	Lawn et al[30]
377			
413	*Alu* I	244/169	Cranage et al[31]
346			
465	*Ava* II	189/276	Nelson et al[32]
411			
465	*Ava* II	290/175	Greenaway and Wilkinson[33]
413			
371	*Alu* I	151/218/2	Baer et al[34]
300			
400	*Alu* I	181/219	Bzik et al[35]
304			
662	*Alu* I	303/359	Josephs et al[36]
732	*Alu* I	338/394	
592			
450	*Alu* I	240/210	Davidson[37]
384			
450	*Alu* I	240/210	Davidson and Scot[38]
450	*Alu* I	210/240	Keller et al[39]
450	*Alu* I	133/317	Davidson and Scot[40]
477	*Alu* I	138/11/328	Rozenblatt et al[41]
400			
632	*Alu* I	208/424	Waxham et al[42]
546			
515	*Alu* I	117/398	Nakhasi et al[43]
456			
391	*Alu* I	267/125	Toyoda et al,[44] Gama et al[45]
345			

(continued)

COMMENT

Particular interest in the study of schizophrenia as a disease with a possible viral cause has focused on the herpes group of viruses (CMV, EBV, HSV-1, and VZV), particularly CMV and HSV.[22,23,56-72] Cytomegalovirus was implicated by the finding of elevated levels of antibodies to that virus in the cerebrospinal fluid of schizophrenic patients.[60,61] The idea that HSV might play some role in the disease was suggested by the virologic and anatomic features of known latent infections with that virus[8]; it was postulated that HSV, remaining latent in the trigeminal ganglion from infancy, might travel up the nerve to the medial temporal cortex, considered to be the area most involved in schizophrenia.

Alexander and others[71] recently summarized studies attempting to find CMV in the cerebrospinal fluid and brain specimens of schizophrenics during the previous 10 years. Sensitive nucleic acid hybridization studies failed to detect CMV sequences in several areas of brains from schizophrenics,[57,65,66] although a CMV probe hybridized with DNA from the brain of one young schizophrenic patient described by Moises and coworkers.[68] However, using the same hybridization technique, others[57,65] failed to detect CMV, HSV-1, and VZV as well as the nonherpes JC and BK papovaviruses in the brains of schizophrenics. In the present study, PCR with nested primers—probably the most sensitive assay available for detecting viral nucleic acids in clinical material[73]—failed to detect sequences of six viruses of the herpes group, including CMV and HSV, in DNA extracted from the brains of schizophrenic patients. Our results with CMV are in accordance with previous failures of others to amplify CMV DNA by PCR from eight brains of schizophrenic patients.[71] (We selected primer pairs from three regions of the CMV genome different from those described by Alexander et al, and we increased the sensitivity of the method with nested primers.)

Because of other studies suggesting possible roles of enteroviruses in the development of schizophrenia,[7,25,74] we looked without success for RNA sequences well conserved in that group of viruses.[45,46]

An association between maternal infection with influenza virus during pregnancy and the later development of schizophrenia in offspring has been noted[24,75-82]; we tested RNA templates from schizophrenic and control brains against outer and inner primers selected from three genes that code for different proteins of influenza virus type A, again without success. Controversial data on fluctuations of the antibody titers to measles, mumps, and rubella viruses in cerebrospinal fluid or serum of schizophrenics,[22,83] together with the epidemiological finding of a significant relationship between some reportable viral diseases (measles among them) and the pattern of schizophrenic births in different parts of the world,[7] stimulated us to select sequences for those RNA viruses to test in our PCR survey. No amplification of any of those sequences from RNA templates extracted from schizophrenic brains or from control brains was obtained.

Table 2. Viral Oligonucleotide Primer Sequences Selected and cDNA Products Generated (cont)*

Target Genome	Amplified Region of Genome	Location in Genome (Nucleotide Nos.)	Primer Identification Code	Primer Sequence 5'-3'
Influenza virus type A	Hemagglutinin gene	1020-1039	FLU-HM-OUT-1	ATG GTT ACA GGA CTA AGA AA
		1439-1420	FLU-HM-OUT-2	TAA TTG GCT TTT TAC TTT CT
		1055-1074	FLU-HM-IN-1	ATA CAG AGG TCT ATT TGG AG
		1404-1385	FLU-HM-IN-2	CAT TTA AGT CAT GGA AAT CC
	Matrix protein gene	115-134	FLU-M1-OUT-1	TCT TTG CAG GGA AGA ACA CC
		584-565	FLU-M1-OUT-2	CTT GGG TGT AGT GCT GGC TA
		150-169	FLU-M1-IN-1	ATG GAA TGG CTA AAG ACA AG
		549-530	FLU-M1-IN-2	CAT GTC TGA TTA GTG GAT TG
	Polymerase 1 gene	470-489	FLU-POL-OUT-1	TGT TCA GAT CAA ATG GCC TC
		1039-1020	FLU-POL-OUT-2	TAC TTA GAA CAT TTC TGA AC
		505-524	FLU-POL-IN-1	GGA AGG CTC ATA GAC TTC CT
		1004-985	FLU-POL-IN-2	CTG GTT ATA TAT GTG ATC AT
HTLV-I	Polymerase gene	4738-4759	SK 110	CCC TAC AAT CCA ACC AGC TCA
		4923-4900	SK 111	GTG GTG AAG CTG CCA TCG GGT TTT
		4765-4786	SK 110-IN-1	GTA GAA CGC TCT AAT GGC ATT
		4890-4869	SK 111-IN-2	GGT TAA CAC ATT CAG GTG GTT G
		3365-3384	SK54	CTT CAC AGT CTC TAC TGT GC
		3483-3465	SK55	CGG CAG TTC TGT GAC AGG G
St Louis encephalitis virus	Capsid protein gene	87-106	SLE-CAP 1	GGG AAT TAC CCA ATG TCT AA
		468-449	SLE-CAP 2	ACT GCA ATG AAC TCG CCA GT
		127-146	SLE-CAP 3	GAA ACC GGG TTG TCA ATA TG
		428-409	SLE-CAP 4	GAG CAA CGA TCT GGT CCC TC

**cDNA indicates complementary DNA; CMV, cytomegalovirus; EBV, Epstein-Barr virus; HSV-1, herpes simplex virus type 1; HHV-6, human herpesvirus type 6; VZV, varicella-zoster virus; and HTLV-I, human T-cell lymphotropic virus type I.*

Because of increasing interest in the neurotropic properties of the oncogenic retrovirus HTLV-I (associated with myelopathy, meningoencephalitis, and myositis), also proposed to be a possible cause of schizophrenia,[28] we selected primers for the provirus of that agent. Our attempts to amplify sequences of HTLV-I were negative, consistent with earlier negative serological and immunological studies.[26,27]

The sensitivity of PCR in detecting viruses in peripheral blood and urine of infected patients has been documented,[73] but we attempted no independent confirmation of that demonstration. We did confirm that our PCR was adequate to detect latent infections with HSV-1 by examining extracts of DNA from trigeminal ganglia (often latently infected with HSV-1)[16] of three nonschizophrenic patients. We successfully amplified products of the size predicted for HSV-1 amplicons from two of those ganglia and confirmed their identity by endonuclease digestion. Using the same techniques described here, we previously detected measles viral sequences in brains of patients with subacute sclerosing panencephalitis[19] and JC papovavirus in subjects with progressive multifocal leukoencephalopathy.[54] Had any of the 12 viruses that we selected been present with any regularity in the brain specimens available for our study, it seems probable that we would have detected them as well. Our consistent failure to do so implies that the areas of the brains studied were unlikely to have been persistently infected with any of those 12 viruses. Of course, it remains possible that persistent infection with some other virus is involved in schizophrenia or that a causal agent present earlier in illness had either disappeared (leaving sequelae but not persisting) or was present in an amount too small to detect. Recently improved molecular biological methods to detect minute amounts of unique nucleic acids in complex mixtures[84,85] merit application to the study of schizophrenia. The importance of schizophrenia justifies intensified efforts to determine its etiology, including continued search for infectious pathogens[86] in more areas of the brain from patients with a wider spectrum of clinical variants.

Accepted for publication August 29, 1995.

David A. Katz, MD, National Institute of Neurological Disorders and Stroke, generously provided several specimens of trigeminal ganglion and cerebral cortex. Kendall O. Smith, PhD, formerly with the Division of Biologics Standards, provided the HSV-1/KOS strain. Maneth Gravell, PhD, National Institute of Neurological Disorders and Stroke, provided the EBV strain.

The Figure was adapted with the permission of the authors[15] and the Journal of General Virology.

Reprint requests to Laboratory of Method Development, Center for Biologics Evaluation and Research, Food and Drug Administration, HPM-255, 1401 Rockville Pike, Rockville, MD 20852-1448 (Dr Asher).

REFERENCES

1. Keith SJ, Regier DA, Rae DS. Schizophrenic disorders. In: Robins LN, Regier DA, eds. *Psychiatric Disorders in America: The Epidemiologic Catchment Area Study.* New York, NY: Free Press; 1991:33-52.
2. Crow TJ. Integrated viral genes as potential pathogens in the functional psychoses. *J Psychiatr Res.* 1987;21:479-485.
3. Crow TJ. The viral theory of schizophrenia. *Br J Psychiatry.* 1988;153:564-566.
4. Eaves L, Schulz SC, Sharp M, Asher DM, Bromet E, Cloninger CR, Gershon ES,

cDNA Product Size, Base Pairs	Restriction Enzyme	Cleavage Product Sizes, Base Pairs	Source
420	*Alu* I	235/185	Hiti et al[46]
350			
470	*Alu* I	215/255	Baylor et al[47]
400			
570	*Alu* I	260/310	Sivasubramanian and Nayak[48]
500			
186	*Alu* I	17/160/9	Evangelista et al[49]
126			
118	*Alu* I	90/29	
382	*Alu* I	184/198	Trent et al[50]
302			

Hall JC, Kaufmann C, Kendler K, McFarlin DE, Pert CB, Stevens J. Genetics, immunology, and virology. *Schizophr Bull.* 1988;14:365-382.

5. Pert CB, Knight JG, Laing P, Markwell MA. Scenarios for a viral etiology of schizophrenia. *Schizophr Bull.* 1988;14:243-247.
6. Torrey EF, Kaufmann CA. Schizophrenia and neuroviruses. In: Nasrallah HA, Weinberger DR, eds. *The Neurology of Schizophrenia.* Amsterdam, the Netherlands: Elsevier Science Publishers; 1986:361-376.
7. Torrey EF, Rawlings R, Waldman IN. Schizophrenic births and viral diseases in two states. *Schizophr Res.* 1988;1:73-77.
8. Torrey EF. A viral-anatomical explanation of schizophrenia. *Schizophr Bull.* 1991;17:15-18.
9. Waltrip RW II, Carrigan DR, Carpenter WJ Jr. Immunopathology and viral reactivation: a general theory of schizophrenia. *J Nerv Ment Dis.* 1990;178:729-738.
10. Yolken RH, Torrey EF. Viruses, schizophrenia, and bipolar disorder. *Clin Microbiol Rev.* 1995;8:131-145.
11. Saiki RK, Gelfand GH, Stoffel S, Scharf SJ, Higuchi R, Horn GT, Mullis KB, Erlich HA. Primer-directed enzymatic amplification of DNA with a thermostable DNA polymerase. *Science.* 1988;239:487-491.
12. Mullis K, Faloona F, Scharf S, Saiki R, Horn G, Erlich H. Specific enzymatic amplification of DNA in vitro: the polymerase chain reaction. *Cold Spring Harb Symp Quant Biol.* 1986;51:263-273.
13. Mullis KB. The unusual origin of the polymerase chain reaction. *Sci Am.* April 1990;262:56-61, 64-65.
14. Rosenthal N. Tools of the trade: recombinant DNA. *N Engl J Med.* 1994;331:315-317.
15. Hyypiä T, Auvinen P, Maaronen M. Polymerase chain reaction for human picornaviruses. *J Gen Virol.* 1989;70:3261-3268.
16. Warren KG, Devlin M, Gilden DH, Wrobleska Z, Brown SM, Subak-Sharp J, Koprowski H. Isolation of herpes simplex virus from human trigeminal ganglia, including ganglia from one patient with multiple sclerosis. *Lancet.* 1977;2:637-639.
17. Harrison PJ, Pearson RC. In situ hybridization histochemistry and the study of gene expression in the human brain. *Prog Neurobiol.* 1990;34:271-312.
18. Chirgwin JM, Przybala AE, MacDonald RJ, Rutter WJ. Isolation of biologically active ribonucleic acid from sources enriched in ribonuclease. *Biochemistry.* 1979;18:5294-5299.
19. Godec MS, Asher DM, Swoveland PT, Eldadah ZA, Feinstone SM, Goldfarb LG, Gibbs CJ Jr, Gajdusek DC. Detection of measles virus genomic sequences in SSPE brain tissue by the polymerase chain reaction. *J Med Virol.* 1990;30:237-244.
20. Godec MS, Asher DM, Murray RS, Shin ML, Greenham LW, Gibbs JC Jr, Gajdusek DC. Absence of measles, mumps and rubella viral genomic sequences from multiple sclerosis brain tissue by polymerase chain reaction. *Ann Neurol.* 1992;32:401-404.
21. Eldadah ZA, Asher DM, Godec MS, Pomeroy KL, Goldfarb LG, Feinstone SG, Levitan H, Gibbs CJ Jr, Gajdusek DC. Detection of flaviviruses by reverse-transcriprase polymerase chain reaction. *J Med Virol.* 1991;33:260-267.
22. King DJ, Cooper SJ, Earle JA, Martin SJ, McFerran NV, Wisdom GB. Serum and CSF antibody titres to seven common viruses in schizophrenic patients. *Br J Psychiatry.* 1985;147:145-149.
23. King DJ, Cooper SJ, Earle JA, Martin SJ, McFerran NV, Rima BK, Wisdom GB. A survey of serum antibodies to eight common viruses in psychiatric patients. *Br J Psychiatry.* 1985;147:137-144.
24. Mednick SA, Machon RA, Huttunen MO, Bonett D. Adult schizophrenia following prenatal exposure to an influenza epidemic. *Arch Gen Psychiatry.* 1988;45:189-192.
25. Squires RF, Saederup E. A review of evidence for GABergic predominance/glutamatergic deficit as a common etiological factor in both schizophrenia and affective psychoses: more support for a continuum hypothesis of functional psychosis. *Neurochem Res.* 1991;16:1099-1111.
26. Feenstra A, Kirch DG, Bracha HS, Wyatt RJ. Lack of evidence for a role of T-cell-associated retroviruses as an etiology of schizophrenia. *Biol Psychiatry.* 1989;25:421-430.
27. DeLisi LE, Sarin PS. Lack of evidence for retrovirus infection in schizophrenic patients. *Br J Psychiatry.* 1985;146:674-675.
28. Mattock C, Parker NE. HTLV-I infection and schizophrenia. *Lancet.* 1985;2:945.
29. Rodriguez M, Prayoonwiwat N, Pease LR. PCR detection of human T-cell lymphotrophic virus type I. In: Persing DH, Smith TF, Tenover FC, White TJ, eds. *Diagnostic Molecular Microbiology: Principles and Applications.* Washington, DC: American Society for Microbiology; 1993:316-321.
30. Lawn RM, Efstratiadis A, O'Connell C, Maniatis T. The nucleotide sequence of the human beta-globin gene. *Cell.* 1980;21:647-651.
31. Cranage MP, Kouzarides T, Bankier AT, Satchwell S, Weston K, Tomlinson P, Barrell B, Hart H, Bell SE, Minson AC, Smith GL. Identification of the human cytomegalovirus glycoprotein B gene and induction of neutralizing antibodies via its expression in recombinant vaccinia virus. *EMBO J.* 1986;5:3057-3063.
32. Nelson JA, Fleckenstein B, Jahn G, Galloway DA, McDougall JK. Structure of the transforming region of human cytomegalovirus AD 169. *J Virol.* 1984;49:109-115.
33. Greenaway PJ, Wilkinson GWG. Nucleotide sequence of the most abundantly transcribed early gene of human cytomegalovirus strain AD169. *Virus Res.* 1987;7:17-31.
34. Baer RJ, Bankier AT, Biggin MD, Deininger PL, Farrell PJ, Gibson TJ, Hatfull TF, Hudson GS, Sathwell SC, Seguin C, Tuffnell PS, Barrell BG. DNA sequence and expression of the B95-8 Epstein-Barr virus genome. *Nature.* 1984;310:207-211.
35. Bzik DJ, Fox BA, DeLuca NA, Person S. Nucleotide sequence specifying the glycoprotein gene, gB, of herpes simplex virus type 1. *Virology.* 1984;133:301-314.
36. Josephs SF, Salahuddin SZ, Ablashi DV, Schachter F, Wong-Staal F, Gallo RC. Genomic analysis of the human B-lymphotropic virus (HBLV). *Science.* 1986;234:601-603.
37. Davidson AJ. DNA sequence of the U_S component of the varicella-zoster virus genome. *EMBO J.* 1983;2:2203-2209.
38. Davidson AJ, Scot JE. DNA sequence of the major inverted repeat in the varicella-zoster virus genome. *J Gen Virol.* 1985;66:207-220.
39. Keller PM, Davidson AJ, Lowe RS, Bennett CD, Ellis RW. Identification and structure of the gene encoding gpII, a major glycoprotein of varicella-zoster virus. *Virology.* 1986;152:181-191.
40. Davidson AJ, Scot JE. The complete DNA sequence of varicella-zoster virus. *J Gen Virol.* 1986;67:1759-1816.
41. Rozenblatt S, Eizenberg O, Ben-Levy R, Lavie V, Bellini WJ. Sequence homology within the morbilliviruses. *J Virol.* 1985;53:684-690.
42. Waxham MN, Aronowski J, Server AC, Wolinsky JS, Smith JA, Goodman HM. Sequence determination of the mumps virus HN gene. *Virology.* 1988;164:318-325.
43. Nakhasi HL, Meyers BC, Liu T-Y. Rubella virus cDNA: sequence and expression of E1. *J Biol Chem.* 1986;261:16616-16621.
44. Toyoda H, Kohara Y, Suganuma T, Omata T, Imura N, Nomoto A. Complete nucleotide sequence of all three poliovirus serotype genomes: implication for genetic relationship, gene function and antigenic determinants. *J Mol Biol.* 1984;174:561-585.
45. Gama RE, Horsnell PR, Hughes PJ, North C, Bruce CB, Al-Nakib W, Stanway G. Amplification of rhinovirus specific nucleic acids from clinical samples using the

polymerase chain reaction. *J Med Virol.* 1989;28:73-77.
46. Hiti AL, Davis AR, Nayak DP. Complete sequence analysis shows that the hemagglutinins of the H0 and H2 subtypes of human influenza virus are closely related. *Virology.* 1981;111:113-124.
47. Baylor NW, Zhiping YL, Wagner RR. Transient expression and sequence of the matrix (M1) gene of WSN influenza A virus in a vaccinia vector. *Virology.* 1988; 163:618-621.
48. Sivasubramanian N, Nayak DP. Sequence analysis of the polymerase 1 gene and the secondary structure prediction of polymerase 1 protein of human influenza virus A/WSN/33. *J Virol.* 1982;44:321-329.
49. Evangelista A, Maroushek S, Minnigan H, Larson A, Retzel E, Haase A, Gonzalez-Dunia D, McFarlin D, Mingioli E, Jacobson S. Nucleotide sequence analysis of a provirus derived from an individual with tropical spastic paraparesis. *Microb Pathog.* 1990;8:259-278.
50. Trent DW, Kinney RM, Johnson BJB, Vorndam AV, Grant JA, Deubel V, Rice CM, Hahn C. Partial nucleotide sequence of St. Louis encephalitis virus RNA: structural proteins, NS1, ns2a, and ns2b. *Virology.* 1987;156:293-304.
51. Thiele GM, Bicak MS, Young A, Kinsey J, White RJ, Purtillo DT. Rapid detection of cytomegalovirus by tissue culture, centrifugation, and immunofluorescence with a monoclonal antibody to an early nuclear antigen. *J Virol Methods.* 1987;16:327-338.
52. Ablashi DV. Human B-lymphotropic virus (human herpesvirus-6). *J Virol Methods.* 1988;21:29-48.
53. Iannone R, Sherman MP, Rodgers-Johnson PEB, Beilke MA, Mora CA, Amin RM, Tinsley SR, Papsidero LD, Poiesz BJ, Gibbs CJ Jr. HTLV-I DNA sequences in CNS tissues of a patient with tropical spastic paraparesis and HTLV-I-associated myelopathy. *J Acquir Immune Defic Syndr.* 1992;5:810-816.
54. Buckle GJ, Godec MS, Rubi JU, Tornatore C, Major EO, Gibbs CJ Jr, Gajdusek DC, Asher DM. Lack of JC viral genomic sequences in multiple sclerosis brain tissue by polymerase chain reaction. *Ann Neurol.* 1992;32:829-831.
55. Kwok S, Higuchi R. Avoiding false positives with PCR. *Nature.* 1989;339:293-304.
56. Shrikhande S, Hirsch SR, Coleman JC, Reveley MA, Dayton R. Cytomegalovirus and schizophrenia: a test of a viral hypothesis. *Br J Psychiatry.* 1985; 146:503-506.
57. Stevens JR, Langloss JM, Albrecht P, Yolken R, Wang YN. A search for cytomegalovirus and herpes viral antigens in brains of schizophrenic patients. *Arch Gen Psychiatry.* 1984;41:795.
58. Taylor GR, Crow TJ, Higgins T, Reynolds G. Search for cytomegalovirus in postmortem brain tissue from patients with Huntington's chorea and other psychiatric disease by molecular hybridization using cloned DNA. *J Neuropathol Exp Neurol.* 1985;44:176-184.
59. Taylor GR, Crow TJ. Viruses in human brains: a search for cytomegalovirus and herpes virus 1 DNA in necropsy tissue from normal and neuropsychiatric cases. *Psychol Med.* 1986;16:289-295.
60. Torrey EF, Yolken RH. Cytomegalovirus antibody in cerebrospinal fluid of schizophrenic patients detected by enzyme immunoassay. *Science.* 1982;216:892-894.
61. Torrey EF, Yolken RH, Albrecht P. Cytomegalovirus as a possible etiological agent in schizophrenia. In: Morozov PV, ed. *Research in Viral Hypothesis of Mental Disorder.* Basel, Switzerland: Karger; 1983:150-160.
62. DeLisi LE, Smith SB, Hamovit JR, Maxwell ME, Goldin LR, Dingman CW, Gershon ES. Herpes simplex virus, cytomegalovirus and Epstein-Barr virus antibody titres in sera from schizophrenic patients. *Psychol Med.* 1986;16:757-763.
63. DeLisi LE, Goldin LR, Nurnberger JI, Simmons-Alling S, Hamovit J, Dingman CW. Failure to alleviate symptoms of schizophrenia with the novel use of an antiviral agent, acyclovir (Zovirax). *Biol Psychiatry.* 1987;22:216-220.
64. Bartova L, Rajcani J, Pogady J. Herpes simplex virus antibodies in the cerebrospinal fluid of schizophrenic patients. *Acta Virol.* 1987;31:443-446.
65. Carter GI, Taylor GR, Crow TJ. Search for viral nucleic acid sequences in the post mortem brains of patients with schizophrenia and individuals who have committed suicide. *J Neurol Neurosurg Psychiatry.* 1987;50:247-251.
66. Kudelova M, Rajcani J, Pogady J, Sramka M. Herpes simplex virus DNA in the brain of psychotic patients. *Acta Virol.* 1988;32:455-460.
67. Ebstein RP, Bennett ER, Hadjez J, Silver H, Yedgar S, Lerer B. Cyclic AMP second messenger signal generation in EBV-transformed lymphoblastoid cells from schizophrenic patients. *J Psychiatr Res.* 1990;24:121-127.
68. Moises HW, Ruger R, Reynolds GP, Fleckenstein B. Human cytomegalovirus DNA in the temporal cortex of a schizophrenic patient. *Eur Arch Psychiatry Neurol Sci.* 1988;238:110-113.
69. Pelonero AL, Pandurangi AK, Calabrese VP. Serum IgG antibody to herpes viruses in schizophrenia. *Psychiatry Res.* 1990;33:11-17.
70. Bennett ER, Yedgar S, Lerer B, Ebstein RP. Phospholipase A2 activity in Epstein-Barr virus-transformed lymphoblast cells from schizophrenic patients. *Biol Psychiatry.* 1991;29:1058-1062.
71. Alexander RC, Spector SA, Casanova M, Kleinman J, Wyatt RJ, Kirch DG. Search for cytomegalovirus in the postmortem brains of schizophrenic patients using the polymerase chain reaction. *Arch Gen Psychiatry.* 1992;49:47-53.
72. Fux M, Sarov I, Ginot Y, Sarov B. Herpes simplex virus and cytomegalovirus in the serum of schizophrenic patients versus other psychosis and normal controls. *Isr J Psychiatry Relat Sci.* 1992;29:33-35.
73. Hsia K, Spector DH, Lawrie J, Spector SA. Enzymatic amplification of human cytomegalovirus sequence by polymerase chain reaction. *J Clin Microbiol.* 1989; 27:1802-1809.
74. Eagles JM. Are polioviruses a cause of schizophrenia? *Br J Psychiatry.* 1992; 160:598-600.
75. Mednick SA, Machón RA, Huttunen MO, Barr CE. Influenza and schizophrenia: Helsinki vs Edinburgh. *Arch Gen Psychiatry.* 1990;47:875-876.
76. Maurizi CP. Why was the 1918 influenza pandemic so lethal? the possible role of a neurovirulent neuraminidase. *Med Hypotheses.* 1985;16:1-5.
77. Barr CE, Mednick SA, Munk-Jorgensen P. Exposure to influenza epidemics during gestation and adult schizophrenia: 40-year study. *Arch Gen Psychiatry.* 1990; 47:869-874.
78. Bowler AE, Torrey EF. Influenza and schizophrenia: Helsinki vs Edinburgh. *Arch Gen Psychiatry.* 1990;47:876-877.
79. Coggiano MA, Alexander RC, Kirch DG, Wyatt RJ, Kulaga H. The continued search for evidence of retroviral infection in schizophrenic patients. *Schizophr Res.* 1991;5:243-247.
80. Crow TJ, Done DJ, Johnstone EC. Schizophrenia and influenza. *Lancet.* 1991; 338:116-117.
81. Kendell RE, Kemp IW. Influenza and schizophrenia: Helsinki vs Edinburgh. *Arch Gen Psychiatry.* 1990;47:877-878.
82. Sham PC, O'Callaghan E, Takei N, Murray GK, Hare EH, Murray RM. Schizophrenia following pre-natal exposure to influenza epidemics between 1939 and 1960. *Br J Psychiatry.* 1992;160:461-466.
83. Vasil'eva OA, Kriukova LK, Podoplekina LE. Antibodies to measles, smallpox, influenza and arenaviruses in schizophrenic patients [in Russian]. *Zh Nevropatol Psikhiatr Im S S Korsakova.* 1986;86:106-108.
84. Lisitsyn N, Lisitsyn N, Wigler M. Cloning the differences between two complex genomes. *Science.* 1993;259:946-951.
85. Chang Y, Cesarman E, Pessin MS, Lee F, Culpepper J, Knowles DM, Moore PS. Identification of herpesvirus-like DNA sequences in AIDS-associated Kaposi's sarcoma. *Science.* 1994;266:1865-1869.
86. Kaufmann CA, Weinberger DR, Stevens JR, Asher DM, Kleinman JE, Sulima MP, Gibbs CJ Jr, Gajdusek DC. Intracerebral inoculation of animals with brain tissue from patients with schizophrenia: failure to observe consistent or specific behavioral and neuropathological effects. *Arch Gen Psychiatry.* 1988;45: 648-652.

Effects of Rapid Tryptophan Depletion in Patients With Seasonal Affective Disorder in Remission After Light Therapy

Raymond W. Lam, MD; Athanasios P. Zis, MD; Arvinder Grewal; Pedro L. Delgado, MD; Dennis S. Charney, MD; John H. Krystal, MD

Background: Previous studies show that rapid tryptophan depletion reverses the effects of therapy with serotonergic, but not noradrenergic, antidepressant drugs in patients with remitted nonseasonal depression. The objective of this study was to investigate the effects of rapid tryptophan depletion in patients with seasonal affective disorder (SAD) that was in clinical remission after light therapy.

Methods: Patients who met *DSM-III-R* criteria for recurrent major depressive episodes, seasonal (winter) pattern (equivalent to SAD), were treated with a standard course of light therapy. Ten patients with SAD in clinical remission after light therapy underwent rapid tryptophan depletion in a placebo-controlled, double-blind crossover study. Behavioral ratings and plasma tryptophan levels were obtained before and after rapid tryptophan depletion.

Results: Plasma total and free tryptophan levels were significantly reduced to 20% of normal levels by the rapid tryptophan depletion. The depletion session resulted in significant increases in depression scores compared with the sham control session. Six of 10 patients had a clinically significant relapse of their depression following the tryptophan depletion session.

Conclusions: Rapid tryptophan depletion appears to reverse the antidepressant effect of bright light therapy in patients with SAD. This suggests that the therapeutic effects of bright light in SAD may involve a serotonergic mechanism.

(Arch Gen Psychiatry. 1996;53:41-44)

From the Division of Mood Disorders, Department of Psychiatry, University of British Columbia, and Vancouver Hospital & Health Sciences Centre, Vancouver, BC (Drs Lam and Zis and Ms Grewal); University of Arizona, Tucson (Dr Delgado); and Yale University and Veterans Affairs Medical Center, West Haven, Conn (Drs Charney and Krystal).

SEASONAL AFFECTIVE disorder (SAD), or winter depression, is a subtype of mood disorder characterized by recurrent major depressive episodes that occur regularly in the fall and winter months, with spontaneous remission in the spring and summer.[1] The common symptoms of SAD include depressed mood and so-called atypical depressive symptoms such as hypersomnia, increased appetite, carbohydrate craving, and weight gain. Seasonal affective disorder appears to respond to exposure to bright light, termed *light therapy*.[1-4]

The pathophysiology of SAD and the mechanism of action of light therapy are still poorly understood,[5] but several lines of research suggest that serotonin mechanisms may be important.[6] Postmortem studies in normal humans have demonstrated marked seasonal fluctuations in serotonin concentration in the hypothalamus, with highest levels in autumn and lowest in winter.[7] Similarly, levels of serotonin metabolites such as 5-hydroxyindoleacetic acid (5-HIAA) in cerebrospinal fluid are highest in summer and autumn and lowest in winter and spring.[8-10] Studies on patients with SAD who were administered *m*-chlorophenylpiperazine found elevated euphoric-activation responses[11] and exaggerated prolactin and cortisol responses[12] compared with those in controls. These abnormalities were partially reversed after treatment with bright light. Finally, serotonergic medications such as D-fenfluramine,[13,14] tryptophan,[15] and fluoxetine[16,17] appear to be effective in the treatment of SAD.

Recent studies[18-20] suggested that rapid depletion of tryptophan, the dietary amino acid precursor of serotonin, can provide insights into the mechanism of antidepressant medications. In animals, brain serotonin function is correlated with plasma tryptophan level, which, in turn, is dependent on dietary trypto-

See Methods on next page

METHODS

This study was approved by the Human Ethics Committee of the University of British Columbia at Vancouver. Patients were administered the Structured Clinical Interview for *DSM-III-R*[27] (SCID)[28] by experienced psychiatrists. Patients met *DSM-III-R* criteria for recurrent major depressive episodes with a seasonal pattern (equivalent to SAD) and were studied in winter. Severity of symptoms was evaluated by psychiatrists using the Structured Interview Guide for the Hamilton Depression Rating Scale (HAM-D), Seasonal Affective Disorders Version (SIGH-SAD).[29] The SIGH-SAD generates the 21-item HAM-D[30] and a 29-item modified HAM-D that includes eight additional items for atypical depressive symptoms. Entry criteria prior to treatment included being medication free for at least 2 weeks (5 weeks if previously taking fluoxetine) and having a score greater than 15 on the 21-item HAM-D. Eligible patients then underwent a standard treatment regimen of 10 000-lux cool-white fluorescent light for 30 minutes daily between 7 AM and 8 AM. A light box fitted with a UV filter was used by patients at home. *Remission* was defined as a score of less than 8 on the 21-item HAM-D and a score of less than 12 on the 29-item modified HAM-D for at least 2 weeks.

After giving written informed consent, the patients with remitted SAD underwent a randomized, double-blind, counterbalanced protocol with two test sessions separated by at least a 5-day period. The experimental session (rapid tryptophan depletion) consisted of a 24-hour low-tryptophan diet (160 mg/d), with a blue placebo capsule given three times a day (on day 1), followed the next morning (day 2) by a tryptophan-free 15-amino acid drink. The control session (normal daily tryptophan intake) consisted of the low-tryptophan diet (160 mg/d) supplemented by identical blue capsules, each containing 500 mg of tryptophan on day 1, followed the next morning (day 2) by a 16-amino acid drink that included 2.3 g of tryptophan. Composition of the amino acid drink has been described elsewhere.[25] The mixture was flavored with chocolate syrup, and the most unpalatable ingredients were given in capsule form. Food prepared for the diet was given to patients to take with them, and patients continued with their morning light treatment during the test session days. Patients remained indoors and received less than 200-lux light exposure from 9 AM to 5 PM on day 2.

Behavioral ratings were obtained by raters who were blind to experimental session at 9 AM on day 1 prior to starting the diet, at 9 AM on day 2 prior to ingestion of the amino acid drink, and at 5 hours after ingestion (approximately 2 PM). Ratings included the Hamilton Anxiety Scale and the 29-item HAM-D modified to exclude the nine items that could not be rated within the same day, including sleep, eating (since patients were fasting), weight, and diurnal variation. The blind was successfully maintained in both patients and raters.

Blood samples were also drawn at behavioral rating times and immediately centrifuged at room temperature. Total tryptophan concentration was assayed from plasma, while free tryptophan concentration was assayed from an ultrafiltrate of plasma obtained by additional centrifuge (2000*g*) at room temperature for 30 minutes through a cellulose ultrafiltration membrane system (Amicon Co, Beverley, Mass). Both the plasma and the ultrafiltrate samples were frozen at $-70°$ for later assay using high-performance liquid chromatography with fluorometric detection.[31]

Behavioral and laboratory data were analyzed using repeated measures analysis of variance (ANOVA) with order of sessions as a grouping variable and with time and session (depletion, control) as repeated measures. Using this analysis, differences in responses between the depletion and control sessions would show up as significant main effects of session or time × session interaction effects. Analyses were performed on a personal computer using a statistical package.[32]

phan. Plasma tryptophan level can also be rapidly reduced by 80% within 3 to 5 hours by administering an oral tryptophan-free mixture containing large amounts of other amino acids.[21,22] This mixture induces hepatic protein synthesis that depletes available plasma tryptophan. In animals, and presumably in humans, this degree of tryptophan depletion reduces serotonin concentration in the brain to approximately 20% of normal levels.[20,23] Normal subjects who undergo rapid tryptophan depletion have transient mild, negative mood changes.[22,24] Patients with depression in remission after treatment with serotonergic antidepressant drugs have

See also page 47

transient depressive relapses when they undergo rapid tryptophan depletion,[25] but these relapses are infrequent in patients treated with noradrenergic antidepressant drugs.[26] The tryptophan dependence of serotonergic antidepressant response suggests that these drugs work by enhancing serotonin function.

In this study, we examined the effects of rapid tryptophan depletion in patients with SAD that was in remission with light therapy. We hypothesized that rapid tryptophan depletion, but not a sham control treatment, would reverse the antidepressant effects of light therapy in these patients.

RESULTS

Twelve patients entered the study, but two of them could not continue because of nausea and vomiting. One patient could not tolerate ingesting the 25 capsules, while the other became extremely nauseated and vomited after ingesting the amino acid mixture. Seven women and three men, ages 21 to 49 years, completed the study. Their mean age±SD was 33.0±8.8 years, and the mean±SD number of past depressive episodes was 10.0±7.0. Three of the patients had a history of mild hypomanic episodes during the summer. Most of the patients had experienced atypical depressive symptoms such as hypersomnia (n=10) and weight gain (n=6) during their winter depressions. At the time of testing, patients had their SAD

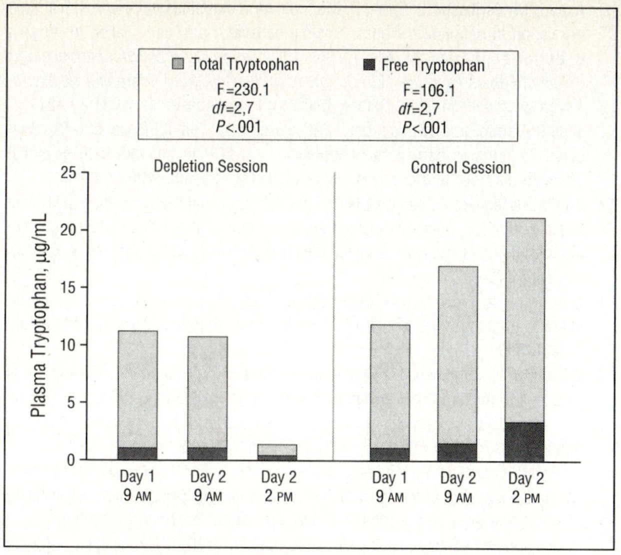

Figure 1. *Plasma total and free tryptophan levels during control and tryptophan depletion sessions in patients with seasonal affective disorder treated with light therapy (n=10). Significant time × session effects by repeated measures analysis of variance.*

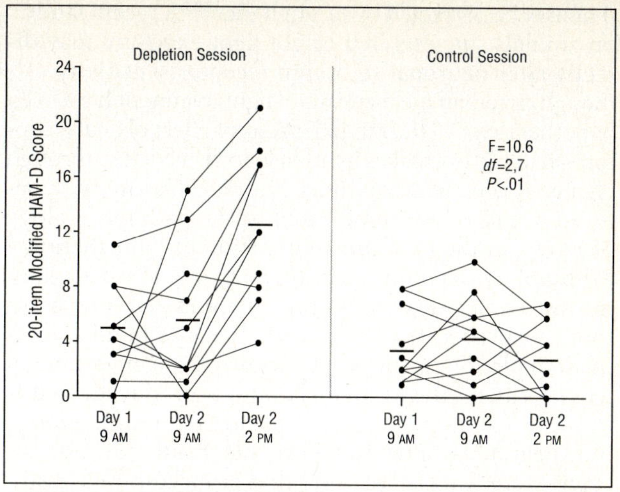

Figure 2. *Depression scores (on 20-item modified Hamilton Depression Rating Scale [HAM-D]) during control and tryptophan depletion sessions in patients with seasonal affective disorder treated with light therapy (n=10). Bars indicate mean scores; significant time × session effects by repeated measures analysis of variance.*

in remission for a mean±SD of 3.9±1.3 weeks (range, 3 to 7 weeks).

Figure 1 shows the plasma tryptophan concentrations, both total and free, during the depletion and control sessions. The baseline levels of total and free tryptophan in plasma were not significantly different between the depletion (total tryptophan level, 10.1±1.2 μg/mL; free tryptophan level, 1.1±0.1 μg/mL) and control sessions (total tryptophan level, 10.6±2.0 μg/mL; free tryptophan level, 1.2±0.2 μg/mL). The depletion session significantly lowered the levels of total and free tryptophan in plasma by a mean of 89% and 72%, respectively, whereas the control session led, as expected, to increases in plasma total and free tryptophan levels after tryptophan ingestion. This effect was statistically significant for plasma total tryptophan (session × time interaction, F=230.1; *df*=2,7; *P*<.001) and plasma free tryptophan (session × time interaction, F=106.1; *df*=2,7; *P*<.001) levels.

Figure 2 shows the modified HAM-D scores between depletion and control sessions. The repeated measures ANOVA found no main or interaction effects of order. There was no main effect of session, but there was a significant time × session interaction effect, with the depletion session showing significantly higher depression scores at 5 hours after ingestion (F=10.6; *df*=2,7; *P*<.01). Post hoc paired *t* tests found no significant differences between depletion and control sessions at baseline (day 1, 9 AM) or before the amino acid drink (day 2, 9 AM). A significant difference between sessions was found after the amino acid drink (day 2, 2 PM) (*t*=6.1, *df*=9, *P*<.001). Similarly, there was a significant time × session interaction for the HAM-A scores (F=7.2; *df*=2,7; *P*<.02), with higher scores after the depletion session. Six of the 10 patients experienced clinically significant depressive symptoms (defined as a score of 12 or greater) during the depletion session compared with none during the control session. Two other patients had marked increases in depression and anxiety ratings. By 5 PM, the patients' moods were improving and all patients recovered from the effects of the tryptophan depletion to baseline levels by the next day on resumption of normal dietary intake.

For the tryptophan depletion session, the correlations between changes in plasma total and free tryptophan levels and the change in HAM-D score before and after depletion were examined using one-tailed Pearson correlations. There were trends for significant negative correlations between changes in HAM-D score and changes in plasma total tryptophan levels (*r*=-.44, *df*=9, *P*<.10) and plasma free tryptophan levels (*r*=-.55, *df*=9, *P*<.07).

COMMENT

In this study, we demonstrated that rapid tryptophan depletion reversed the antidepressant effects of a standard course of bright light therapy in patients with SAD. Eight of the 10 patients showed significant depressive and anxiety symptoms after the depletion session. There was little clinical effect after the sham control session. The clinical symptoms experienced by patients during relapse were similar to their depressive symptoms prior to treatment with light therapy. There was also a trend to a significant negative correlation between the changes in plasma tryptophan levels and the change in depression scores during the tryptophan depletion session, although these were not statistically significant. The magnitude of the correlations (*r*=-.44, *r*=-.55) was similar to significant correlations reported in other studies of tryptophan depletion in patients with antidepressant-remitted nonseasonal depression,[25] and our results may well have reached statistical significance had we studied a larger number of subjects.

Our results suggest that the antidepressant effect of light therapy may be mediated through serotonergic mechanisms. These results are consistent with preliminary studies showing serotonergic dysfunction in SAD that may be corrected by bright light.[12,33] A recent study[34] on animals suggests that bright light exposure may directly alter neuronal serotonin receptor sensitivity. Although circadian mechanisms of light treatment have been hypothesized,[35,36] the rapid depressant effect of acute tryptophan depletion makes it unlikely to be mediated through changes in circadian rhythms. The pineal hormone melatonin has also been implicated in the pathophysiology of SAD and the mechanism of action of light therapy.[5] Tryptophan depletion may theoretically affect melatonin secretion since melatonin is synthesized from serotonin. However, the behavioral effects of rapid tryptophan depletion in this study occurred during a time of day in which little or no melatonin is produced, so it is unlikely that these effects were mediated through changes in pineal melatonin. However, our results do not entirely exclude a circadian rhythm or melatonin hypothesis for SAD, since different mechanisms may account for the tryptophan dependence of light-remitted depression in patients.

In summary, acute tryptophan depletion produces rapid and robust, but transient, reversal of antidepressant effects of bright light therapy. This suggests that serotonergic mechanisms may be involved in the mechanism of action of light treatment and, possibly, in the pathophysiology of SAD.

Accepted for publication July 28, 1995.

Supported in part by grants from the Medical Research Council of Canada (Drs Lam and Zis).

A modified version of this article was presented at the 33rd Annual Meeting of the American College of Neuropsychopharmacology, San Juan, Puerto Rico, December 12, 1994.

Reprint requests to Department of Psychiatry, University of British Columbia, 2255 Wesbrook Mall, Vancouver, BC V6T 2A1 (Dr Lam).

REFERENCES

1. Rosenthal NE, Sack DA, Gillin JC, Lewy AJ, Goodwin FK, Davenport Y, Mueller PS, Newsome DA, Wehr TA. Seasonal affective disorder. *Arch Gen Psychiatry.* 1984;41:72-80.
2. Rosenthal NE, Sack DA, Carpenter CJ, Parry BL, Mendelson WB, Wehr TA. Antidepressant effects of light in seasonal affective disorder. *Am J Psychiatry.* 1985;142:163-170.
3. Terman M, Terman JS, Quitkin FM, McGrath PJ, Stewart JW, Rafferty B. Light therapy for seasonal affective disorder. *Neuropsychopharmacology.* 1989;2:1-22.
4. Wehr TA, Rosenthal NE. Seasonality and affective illness. *Am J Psychiatry.* 1989;146:829-839.
5. Blehar MC, Lewy AJ. Seasonal mood disorders: consensus and controversy. *Psychopharmacol Bull.* 1990;26:465-494.
6. Jacobsen FM, Murphy DL, Rosenthal NE. The role of serotonin in seasonal affective disorder and the antidepressant response to phototherapy. In: Rosenthal NE, Blehar MC, eds. *Seasonal Affective Disorders and Phototherapy.* New York, NY: Guilford Press; 1989:333-341.
7. Carlsson A, Svennerhorn L, Winblad B. Seasonal and circadian monoamine variations in human brain examined post mortem. *Acta Psychiatr Scand (Suppl).* 1980;280:75-83.
8. Brewerton TD, Berrettini WH, Nurnberger JI Jr, Linnoila M. Analysis of seasonal fluctuations of CSF monoamine metabolites and neuropeptides in normal controls. *Psychiatry Res.* 1988;23:257-265.
9. Lacoste V, Wirz-Justice A. Seasonal variation in normal subjects. In: Rosenthal NE, Blehar MC, eds. *Seasonal Affective Disorders and Phototherapy.* New York, NY: Guilford Press; 1989:167-229.
10. Asberg M, Bertlisson L, Rydin E. Monoamine metabolites in cerebrospinal fluid in relation to depressive illness, suicidal behaviour and personality. In: Angrist B, Burrows GD, Lader M, eds. *Recent Advances in Neuropsychopharmacology: Selected Papers from the 12th Congress of the Collegium Internationale Neuro-Psychopharmacologicum.* Oxford, England: Pergamon Press; 1981:257-271.
11. Joseph-Vanderpool JR, Jacobsen FM, Murphy DL, Hill JL, Rosenthal NE. Seasonal variation in behavioral responses to m-CPP in patients with seasonal affective disorder and controls. *Biol Psychiatry.* 1993;33:496-504.
12. Garcia-Borreguero D, Jacobsen FM, Murphy DL, Joseph-Vanderpool JR, Chiara A, Rosenthal NE. Hormonal responses to the administration of *m*-chlorophenylpiperazine in patients with seasonal affective disorder and controls. *Biol Psychiatry.* 1995;37:740-749.
13. O'Rourke DA, Wurtman JJ, Brzezinski A, Nader TA, Chew B. Serotonin implicated in etiology of seasonal affective disorder. *Psychopharmacol Bull.* 1987;23:358-359.
14. O'Rourke D, Wurtman JJ, Wurtman RJ, Chebli R, Gleason R. Treatment of seasonal depression with D-fenfluramine. *J Clin Psychiatry.* 1989;50:343-347.
15. McGrath RE, Buckwald B, Resnick EV. The effect of L-tryptophan on seasonal affective disorder. *J Clin Psychiatry.* 1990;51:162-163.
16. Lam RW, Gorman CP, Michalon M, Steiner M, Levitt AJ, Corral MR, Watson GD, Morehouse RL, Tam W, Joff RT. A multi-center, placebo-controlled study of fluoxetine in seasonal affective disorder. *Am J Psychiatry.* In press.
17. Ruhrmann S, Kasper S, Hawellek B, Martinez B, Hoflich G, Nickelsen T, Moller H-J. Fluoxetine vs light therapy in the treatment of SAD. *Biol Psychiatry.* 1993;33:83A. Abstract.
18. Fernstrom JD. Effects of the diet on brain neurotransmitters. *Metabolism.* 1977;26:207-223.
19. Curzon G. Relationships between plasma, CSF and brain tryptophan. *J Neural Transm.* 1979;15:93-105.
20. Young SN, Ervin FR, Pihl RO, Finn P. Biochemical aspects of tryptophan depletion in primates. *Psychopharmacology.* 1989;98:508-511.
21. Harper AE, Benevenga NJ, Wohlhueter RM. Effects of ingestion of disproportionate amounts of amino acids. *Physiol Rev.* 1970;50:428-548.
22. Young SN, Smith SE, Pihl R, Ervin FR. Tryptophan depletion causes a rapid lowering of mood in normal males. *Psychopharmacology.* 1985;87:173-177.
23. Moja EA, Cipolla P, Castoda D, Tofanetti O. Dose-responsive decrease in plasma tryptophan and in brain tryptophan and serotonin after tryptophan-free amino acid mixtures in rats. *Life Sci.* 1989;44:971-976.
24. Delgado PL, Charney DS, Price LH, Landis H, Heninger GR. Neuroendocrine and behavioral effects of dietary tryptophan restriction in healthy subjects. *Life Sci.* 1989;45:2323-2332.
25. Delgado PL, Charney DS, Price LH, Aghajanian GK, Landis H, Heninger GR. Serotonin function and the mechanism of antidepressant action. *Arch Gen Psychiatry.* 1990;47:411-418.
26. Delgado PL, Price LH, Miller HL, Licinio J, Krystal JH, Heninger GR, Charney DS. Rapid serotonin depletion as a provocative challenge test for patients with major depression. *Psychopharmacol Bull.* 1991;27:321-330.
27. American Psychiatric Association. *Diagnostic and Statistical Manual of Mental Disorders, Revised Third Edition.* Washington, DC: American Psychiatric Association; 1987.
28. Williams JBW, Gibbon M, First MB. The Structured Clinical Interview for *DSM-III-R* (SCID), I: history, rationale, and description. *Arch Gen Psychiatry.* 1992;49:624-629.
29. Williams JBW, Link MJ, Rosenthal NE, Terman M. *Structured Interview Guide for the Hamilton Depression Rating Scale, Seasonal Affective Disorders Version (SIGH-SAD).* New York, NY: New York Psychiatric Institute; 1988.
30. Hamilton M. Development of a rating scale for primary depressive illness. *Br J Soc Clin Psychol.* 1967;6:278-296.
31. Anderson GM, Young JG, Cohen DJ, Schlicht KR, Patel N. Liquid-chromatographic determination of serotonin and tryptophan in whole blood and plasma. *Clin Chem.* 1981;27:775-776.
32. SPSS Inc. *SPSS for Windows, v.6.01.* Chicago, Ill: SPSS Inc; 1994.
33. Jacobsen FM, Mueller EA, Rosenthal NE, Rogers S, Hill JL, Murphy DL. Behavioral responses to intravenous meta-chlorophenylpiperazine in patients with seasonal affective disorder and control subjects before and after phototherapy. *Psychiatry Res.* 1994;52:181-197.
34. Mason R. The effect of light on neuronal sensitivity to noradrenaline and serotonin (5-HT). In: Thompson C, Silverstone T, eds. *Seasonal Affective Disorder.* London, England: CNS (Clinical Neuroscience); 1989:243-258.
35. Lewy AJ, Sack RL, Singer CM, White DM. The phase shift hypothesis for bright light's therapeutic mechanism of action: theoretical considerations and experimental evidence. *Psychopharmacol Bull.* 1987;23:349-353.
36. Sack RL, Lewy AJ, White DM, Singer CM, Fireman MJ, Vandiver R. Morning vs evening light treatment for winter depression. 1992;49:650]. *Arch Gen Psychiatry.* 1990;47:343-351.

Seasonal Changes in Mood and Behavior

The Role of Genetic Factors

Pamela A. F. Madden, PhD; Andrew C. Heath, DPhil; Norman E. Rosenthal, MD; Nicholas G. Martin, PhD

Background: Seasonal rhythms in mood and behavior (seasonality) have been reported to occur in the general population. Seasonal affective disorder, a clinically diagnosed syndrome, is believed to represent the morbid extreme of a spectrum of seasonality. Two types of seasonality have been clinically described: one characterized by a winter pattern and a second by a summer pattern of depressive mood disturbance.

Methods: By using methods of univariate and multivariate genetic analysis, we examined the relative contribution of genetic and environmental factors to the risk of seasonality symptoms that were assessed by a mailed questionnaire of 4639 adult twins from a volunteer-based registry in Australia.

Results: Seasonality was associated with a winter rather than a summer pattern of mood and behavioral change. In each behavioral domain (ie, mood, energy, social activity, sleep, appetite, and weight), a significant genetic influence on the reporting of seasonal changes was found. Consistent with the hypothesis of a seasonal syndrome, genetic effects were found to exert a global influence across all behavioral changes, accounting for at least 29% of the variance in seasonality in men and women.

Conclusions: There is a tendency for seasonal changes in mood and behavior to run in families, especially seasonality of the winter type, and this is largely due to a biological predisposition. These findings support continuing efforts to understand the role of seasonality in the development of mood disorders.

(Arch Gen Psychiatry. 1996;53:47-55)

SEASONAL INFLUENCE on the incidence of mood disorders has been recognized for centuries, and individual cases of seasonally recurring depressions and manias have been documented since classical times.[1-3] In recent years, syndromes of recurrent seasonal depression have been more completely described, including recurrent winter depression (which is also known as seasonal affective disorder [SAD]),[4] summer depression,[5] and subsyndromal winter depression.[6] The term "seasonal pattern" was incorporated into *DSM-III-R*[7] and *DSM-IV*[8] to describe any forms of recurrent mood disorders that show regular seasonal variations.

Patients with winter-SAD typically report that they oversleep, overeat, and gain weight during their depressive periods,[4,9-11] while patients with summer depression are more likely to report that they lose sleep and weight and have a decreased appetite.[12] Both patient groups report that they experience decreased energy, decreased socialization, and sadness during their depressions. There is evidence to suggest that winter-SAD is induced in vulnerable individuals by the decreased ambient light that occurs during the winter,[4] whereas summer-SAD may be induced by high temperatures. These associations have led researchers to treat patients who have winter-SAD with enhanced environmental lighting with some success.[4,13-15] Less is known about the therapeutic potential of decreasing environmental temperature or environmental light in patients with summer-SAD.

Clinical researchers who have worked on seasonality independently and in separate geographical regions have documented similar symptoms in patients who were recruited for SAD.[15-23] Boyce and Parker[24] found evidence of summer and winter forms of SAD in the southern hemisphere that corresponded to the symptom profiles described by clinical researchers who worked in the northern hemisphere.

See Patients and Methods on next page

From the Department of Psychiatry, Washington University School of Medicine, St Louis, Mo (Drs Madden and Heath), the Clinical Psychobiology Branch, National Institute of Mental Health, Bethesda, Md (Dr Rosenthal), and the Queensland Institute of Medical Research, Brisbane, Australia (Dr Martin).

PATIENTS AND METHODS

SAMPLE

The sample was drawn from an adult twin registry maintained by the Australian National Health and Medical Research Council, Brisbane. The Australian National Health and Medical Research Council Twin Registry is a volunteer twin panel that was first surveyed in 1980-1981.[28-30] In spring 1988 (November in Australia), a mailed questionnaire was sent to the 3808 twin pairs who had both responded to the original 1980-1981 mailing, with remailings and telephone follow-up of nonrespondents. Twins who did not return a mailed questionnaire were asked to complete an abbreviated telephone interview. Mailed questionnaire or telephone interview data were obtained from both members of 2997 twin pairs (79% pairwise response rate) and from one twin only from 334 pairs (83% individual response rate). However, since the abbreviated telephone interview did not include the Seasonal Pattern Assessment Questionnaire (SPAQ),[31] the final sample for the purposes of this article included 2487 twin pairs in which both members participated and 687 twin pairs in which only one twin responded to the questionnaire items on seasonality (65% pairwise response rate and 74% individual response rate). The zygosity assigned to the twin pairs was that determined by questionnaire in the original 1980-1981 study.[28,29] The same questionnaire was remailed in 1990 to a subsample of 500 female and 500 male respondents to the 1988 mailing, yielding 2-year test-retest data from 430 female and 410 male respondents. The mean (±SD) age for the 1988 sample was 41.3±12.7 years, and the age range of the twins was 25 to 89 years.

MEASUREMENTS

The SPAQ is a self-administered, retrospective questionnaire.[31] Based on behaviors determined to be abnormal in patients with SAD, this inventory inquires about the pattern and degree of seasonal changes in behavior, and the extent to which such seasonal changes are experienced as a problem by the respondent. This instrument has been widely used in epidemiological studies that were designed to determine the prevalence of SAD and of subclinical levels of seasonality in the general population.[6,14,17,32,33] Two sections from the SPAQ were used to answer the questions addressed in this study: six seasonal "change" items and 120 "calendar" items. By using five-point scales (range, 0 to 4), the SPAQ change section asks respondents to rate the degree of seasonal change that they experience across six behaviors: sleep length, social activity, mood, weight, appetite, and energy level. The calendar items ask the respondent to denote the months that are typically affected for each of five of the above-mentioned behaviors (excluding changes in energy level) and the direction of the changes (ie, best or most vs worst or least).

DATA ANALYSIS

Before attempting a genetic analysis, the data set was evaluated for the representativeness of the sampling. The assumption of equal environments between monozygotic (MZ) and dizygotic (DZ) twins was tested; the effects of age[34,35] and the effects of twins who were living in dissimilar seasonal environments[36] were examined. Important violations of the assumptions of the twin method were not found (data available on request).

Factor Analysis

Traditional factor analyses were performed separately for each sex, ignoring the twin structure of the data, to explore whether a seasonality construct (phenotype) could be observed in these data. More specifically, we examined the following issues: (1) whether sensitivity to changes in season, as measured by responses to the six change items on the SPAQ, could be explained by a single seasonality factor; (2) whether there is evidence for different seasonal patterns (eg, summer or winter), as indicated by relatively separate patterns of seasonal changes in mood and behavior on the 120 calendar items; and if so, (3) whether such patterns show differential associations with the degree of sensitivity to seasonal changes (as measured by the six change items on the SPAQ).

Three matrices of product-moment correlations among the six change and the 120 calendar variables were factor-analyzed[37]: (1) a 6×6 correlation matrix of the change items, (2) a 120×120 correlation matrix of the calendar items, and (3) a 126×126 correlation matrix of the full set of variables from both categories of data. An oblique rotation (Promax) was used to examine the degree of correlation among factors. In each analysis, the number of factors retained was determined by the number with eigenvalues greater than unity and the consistency of the solution across sexes. When too few factors are extracted, sex differences in the ordering of factors by magnitude may misleadingly result in very different factor solutions for males and females.[38]

Genetic Item Analysis

Vulnerability to seasonality was evaluated by performing genetic analyses using responses to the six seasonal change questions. The genetic analysis was begun at the level of the individual item.[29] Polychoric correlations for each item were estimated by the method of maximum likelihood[39] separately for each of the five zygosity groups. Polychoric correlations were also estimated for the test-retest data separately for men and women: these provide estimates of the proportion of variation in each seasonality item that is stable

Their findings are consistent with the hypothesis that seasonal changes in mood and behavior are related to changes in the physical environment and inconsistent with the argument that temporal patterns in symptoms can be explained as anniversary or adjustment reactions to the holiday season.

As with any finding, the clinical description of SAD is sensitive to limitations in the representativeness of the sample. Subjects for SAD research have been predominantly recruited by referral; hence, their reports are subject to bias owing to information on SAD that is disseminated through public

See also page 41

over time (for a comparison, see the study by Kendler et al[29]). Estimation of a polychoric correlation implies the assumption that a normal distribution of liability to seasonality underlies the observed categorical response distribution (a plausible assumption for a behavior that may be influenced by multiple genetic and environmental factors) and that the joint distribution of twin pair members for liability to seasonality is bivariate normal.

Univariate genetic analyses of the symptom scores were carried out under a multiple threshold model by the method of maximum likelihood.[29,40] Thresholds were allowed to vary as a function of sex, but were constrained to be the same in twins of the same sex from MZ, DZ like-sex, and DZ opposite-sex pairs. A series of standard genetic and environmental models were fitted to the data: models that tested for additive and nonadditive genetic effects and environmental effects (either shared or unshared with other family members) and models that allowed for gender differences in the relative magnitude of genetic and environmental effects. Environmental and additive genetic submodels were compared with the full model by the likelihood-ratio χ^2 test.[29,35]

Multivariate Genetic Analyses

Multivariate genetic factor analyses[35,36] were performed to test hypotheses about the number of genetic or environmental factors that were needed to explain the correlations observed between the seasonality symptoms. Multivariate genetic analysis is a generalization of factor analysis that permits estimation of separate genetic and shared and nonshared environmental common and specific factors. Common-factor effects influence two or more symptoms and will give rise to symptom clustering. Specific-factor effects influence only one particular symptom. We tested whether the genetic contribution to vulnerability to seasonal changes reflects a single dimension of genetic variation (or a single "genetic factor"), affecting a broad range of symptoms, or two or more genetic factors, perhaps associated with different symptom constellations.

We also examined whether the genetic factor structure closely paralleled the environmental factor structure (ie, the "common-pathway" model), or whether it was necessary to allow for different genetic vs environmental factor structures (ie, the "independent-pathway" model).[30,41] The independent-pathway models attribute the spectrum of seasonality symptoms to one or more underlying liability factors in which environmental and genetic factors are assumed to affect each symptom in qualitatively different ways. Statistically (see diagram of a one-factor model in the **Figure**, top), separate sets of environmental factor loadings and genetic factor loadings are estimated for the seasonality symptoms. This allows for the possibility that there may be distinct "genetic" and "environmental" clusters of symptoms, with certain symptoms occurring together because of a genetic predisposition, and other symptoms occurring because of environmental effects on behavior (eg, colder temperatures and shorter days leading to changes in sleep patterns, as well as providing fewer opportunities to socialize with friends, neighbors, and relatives).

Compared with the independent-pathway model, a common-pathway model hypothesizes that genetic and environmental effects on symptoms are mediated through one or more intervening biological final common pathways, and it is therefore more supportive of a biological explanation for symptom development. This is illustrated in the one-factor model in the Figure, bottom. The genetic factor loadings for each item are estimated as a scalar multiple ("h") of the corresponding environmental loadings with the heritability of the latent factor (ie, the proportion of the variance in the factor attributable to genetic effects) estimated as $h^2/(1+h^2)$.[35] We also examined the effects of estimating a mixed "common-pathway+independent-pathway" model, where genetic and environmental loadings on the first factor only were constrained to follow the common-pathway model. We might expect this mixed model to fit the data if the SPAQ is indeed providing a valid measure of seasonality, but additional genetic or environmental influences, unrelated to seasonality, are also contributing to correlations between the items of the SPAQ. The common-pathway model is a submodel of the independent-pathway model; hence, models of each type that estimated the same number of common factors were directly compared by using the likelihood-ratio χ^2 test.

The same genetic and environmental risk factors were assumed to affect the vulnerability to seasonal changes in men and women, but the magnitude of their effects were allowed to vary by gender in all models, except where indicated otherwise. Thus, correlations between additive genetic effects in unlike-sex pairs were fixed to .5, and correlations between shared environmental effects were fixed to unity.[35]

The multivariate genetic analyses were performed by using a structural equation–modeling package (LISREL7).[35,36,42] The raw data were summarized by polychoric correlations that were estimated by using a commercially available software package (PRELIS).[39] One- and two-factor models were fitted by asymptotic weighted least squares.[39,43] Beginning with simple one-factor environmental and genetic factor models, we systematically added genetic or environmental factors in an effort to select the simplest model, consistent with the observed data, to explain the determinants of seasonality. All models also allowed for environmental and additive and nonadditive genetic influences that were symptom-specific. Models that gave a poor fit to the data ($P<.05$) were rejected by the χ^2 goodness-of-fit test. Models that gave an adequate fit to the data by the goodness-of-fit test were compared by using the likelihood-ratio χ^2 test.

and professional channels, to traits associated with clinical research volunteerism (eg, severity of illness[25] or help-seeking behavior), and to criteria imposed by the researchers. Consequently, diagnostic criteria for seasonal mood disorders, based on such clinical descriptions, may be too broad or too narrow. Patients who are defined as suffering from SAD may actually constitute a heterogeneous group with different conditions[26]; or alternatively, the two types of SAD that have already been defined may merely represent a subset of a variety of pathological seasonal disorders that are present in the general population. This issue can be addressed by turning from clinical to community samples, which have not been selected for problem behavior or illness.

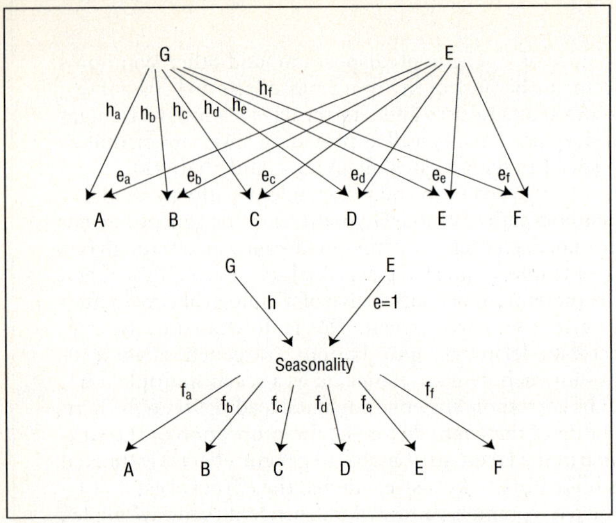

Latent genetic (G) and environmental (E) common factors that contribute to the variance and covariance of six seasonality symptoms (A through F). Top, Independent-pathway model in which genetic factor loadings of symptoms on the latent genetic factors are denoted by paths $h_a \ldots h_f$ and environmental factor loadings by paths $e_a \ldots e_f$. Bottom, Common-pathway model in which the contribution of G and E to the six seasonality items (h and e, respectively) are mediated through the latent factor seasonality, on which the items have loadings $f_a \ldots f_f$. Theoretically, separate genetic and environmental factors (E and H) both act on the intervening "seasonality" variable. Under this model, we can only estimate the relative *magnitude of the genetic influence (h) compared with the environmental (e) influence; hence, we follow the standard practice of fitting one parameter to unity[30,35,36] (e=1 in this case). Item genetic-specific and within-family environmental-specific factors have been omitted from the diagrams.*

Seasonality has been reported as a problem by a substantial proportion of the general population. When surveyed by mailed questionnaires, 25% of a randomly selected sample in New York City[27] and 27% of a Maryland sample[6] complained that seasonally experienced changes were a problem. Some 5% of the Maryland respondents[6] reported a degree of change and impairment that resembled the questionnaire response of patients who were clinically diagnosed as having SAD. Consistent with findings in clinical research, many fewer individuals report a summer vs a winter pattern of seasonal changes by mailed questionnaire. Only about 10% to 12% of the adults who participated in these surveys[6,27] reported that they felt worst during the summer compared with 43% to 50% of respondents who reported a winter pattern of behavioral changes.

This project was designed to evaluate the validity of the seasonality construct through the analysis of data from a volunteer sample of twin pairs who were not selected for problem behavior or illness. Our present approach differs from those of previous survey studies in that we formulate a description for symptoms of seasonality based on patterns of family resemblance that were observed in the data. If there are genetic influences on seasonality, we would expect to observe different degrees of similarity between identical vs fraternal twin pairs; hence, we have been able to differentiate combinations of symptoms that may share a biological (or environmental) predisposition without replicating the bias of self-selection that has confounded many laboratory and treatment studies on seasonality.

The literature suggests that the relatives of patients with SAD may have a higher prevalence of mood disorders in general and SAD in particular than the general population.[4,14] To date, however, no formal family studies of SAD have been conducted. It would be useful to know whether SAD as a disorder and seasonality as a trait are familially transmitted, and whether any such familial transmission has a biological basis. In the present study, we have set out to address two key hypotheses: (1) genetic vulnerability to seasonality is manifested by a seasonal change in a broad spectrum of behaviors that include mood, sleep pattern, social activity, weight, appetite, and energy; and (2) there exist genetic differences in vulnerability to seasonality that are manifested by summer and winter patterns of disturbance.

RESULTS

The twins in this survey were located throughout the Australian continent: about 40% of the sample were from the state of Victoria (the region most similar in seasonal change in sunlight exposure to Montgomery County, Maryland, where research on SAD has been pioneered[4-6]); 30% were from New South Wales; 10% were from Queensland; 5% were from South Australia; 5% were from Tasmania; 5% were from Western Australia; 3% were from Australian Capital Territory; and 2% were from the Northern Territory or overseas. Thirteen percent of our sample complained that seasonality was a personal problem, 17% reported that they felt worst during the winter, and 8% reported that they experienced a summer pattern of worsening in mood. Only 2% of our sample reported a degree of seasonality that resembled the response of patients who were clinically diagnosed as having SAD.[6] Of individual twins who reported behavioral changes during the winter, 28% to 33% reported increases in sleep, food intake, and weight (at most, 5% of winter-affected individuals reported decreases in these behaviors); by contrast, 26% to 31% reported decreases in weight, food intake, and sleep during the summer (9% to 12% reported increases in these behaviors).

FACTOR STRUCTURE

When a conventional factor analysis was performed, a one-factor solution was found to describe adequately the pattern of covariation of the six seasonal change items. All six items (sleep length, social activity, mood, weight, appetite, and energy level change) exhibited high loadings (in the range of .55 to .78), and a similar factor pattern was defined for both sexes. The analysis was consistent with the assumption of a single global seasonality factor.

Factor analysis of the 120 calendar items identified four oblique seasonal factors (two winter and two summer factors) that replicated across sexes. One factor had high loadings on items that specified a worsening of mood and a decrease in social activity during the winter; a second winter factor had high loadings on items that indicated an increase in weight, appetite, and sleep. The interfactor correlation between these two winter factors was .4 in both sexes. A third factor had high loadings on items that indicated a decrease in mood and social activity dur-

Table 1. Sample Sizes and Twin Pair and Test-Retest Polychoric Correlations for Seasonality Items*

Group	No.†	Correlations for Seasonality Change Items					
		Sleep Length	Social Activity	Mood	Weight	Appetite	Energy
Twins							
MZ females	854	.23	.29	.34	.34	.35	.31
DZ females	492	.15	.13	.04	.10	.21	.15
MZ males	390	.18	.26	.38	.31	.23	.26
DZ males	215	.15	.27	.14	.10	.12	.06
DZ opposite-sex	536	.09	.07	.10	.10	.08	.16
Retest sample							
Females	430	.45	.53	.48	.60	.51	.57
Males	410	.53	.52	.58	.61	.61	.54

*MZ indicates monozygotic; DZ, dizygotic

†Number of pairs for twin groups, but number of individuals for retest sample.

ing the summer; a fourth factor had high loadings on items that specified a summer increase in weight, appetite, and sleep. The interfactor correlations between the two summer factors was .4 in men and .2 in women, with only modest correlations between the summer and winter pairs of seasonal factors (−.05 to .19).

In the joint-factor analysis of the six seasonal change items and 120 calendar items, in women, the change items had positive loadings only on the winter factors, with no item loading higher than .04 on either summer factor. A similar trend was observed in the men (highest-loading item, .25). Sensitivity to changes in season, as measured by the six change items, seemed to be associated with winter rather than summer patterns of mood and behavioral changes, especially in women.

GENETIC ANALYSIS: INDIVIDUAL SEASONALITY ITEMS

Table 1 summarizes twin correlations for each zygosity group, separately for each seasonal change item. Two-year test-retest correlations are shown in the last two rows of Table 1. The MZ correlations are about one half of the reliability estimates, suggesting that about one half of the longitudinally stable variance is owing to factors responsible for family resemblance (ie, either genetic or environmental influences that are shared between a twin and co-twin). For most items, the DZ correlation was no more than one half the MZ correlation, implying an influence of genetic effects, especially for women. An analysis of variance[37] was performed to test the effect of season of return for the mailed questionnaire on the report of seasonal changes in behavior (summarized by the sum of the respondent's answers to the seasonal change items). No significant differences in the total score as a function of the season when the questionnaire was completed were found (men: F=0.21, *df*=3, 1979, and *P*=.89; women: F=1.17, *df*=3, 3673, and *P*=.31).

Table 2 summarizes the results of fitting genetic models to the data for each seasonal change item. The left-hand column on Table 2 shows, for each item, the χ^2 test of goodness of fit for the full model (ACE), allowing for both genetic and shared and unshared environmental effects. For two items, namely, sleep length and appetite, the goodness of fit of the best-fitting model was somewhat marginal (*P*=.02 and *P*=.04, respectively), and for the mood change item, the goodness of fit was poor (*P*=.002). Relaxing the constraint that threshold values be the same in MZ and DZ pairs led to an adequate fit for the latter item (χ^2=54.46, *df*=40, *P*=.06), but not for the former two items (sleep length: χ^2=57.56, *df*=40, *P*=.04; appetite: χ^2=56.96, *df*=40, *P*=.04). Allowing threshold values to differ between zygosity groups produced a negligible change in the estimate of the twin polychoric correlations and, hence, did not have any appreciable effect in the model-fitting analyses.

The next two columns give the likelihood-ratio χ^2 tests of submodels that assume either no shared environmental effects (AE) or no genetic effects (CE). The three right-hand-most columns of Table 2 give the parameter estimates under the best-fitting model. Parameter estimates have not been corrected for measurement error. There was no evidence of heterogeneity of genetic parameters across sex (ie, no genotype×sex interaction) for any symptom, except appetite, where models allowing for sex dependence of parameters are reported. In all cases, the environmental model gave a worse fit than the full model. This indicated a genetic influence on the vulnerability to seasonal changes. For the mood item only, the data were best explained by a model that incorporated nonadditive genetic as well as additive genetic effects, and the maximum likelihood estimate of the additive genetic variance was negative. (In twin studies, estimates of the additive and nonadditive genetic variances are strongly negatively correlated,[44] making it difficult to obtain accurate simultaneous estimates of additive and nonadditive genetic components.) Estimates of the broad heritability of the seasonal change items (ie, the proportion of the variance in liability accounted for by additive genetic plus nonadditive genetic factors) were in the range of 20% to 35%, uncorrected for reliability of measurement. This range increases to 39% to 73% if we take into account test-retest reliability and consider instead the proportion of the temporally stable variation explained by genetic factors.

Table 2. Univariate Genetic Analyses of Seasonality Items

'Change' Item	Goodness-of-Fit Full Model (ACE), χ^2 (*df*=67)	Likelihood-Ratio Tests Against Full Model: Genetic, (AE), χ^2 (*df*=1)	Environmental (CE), χ^2 (*df*=1)	Parameter Estimates Under Best-Fitting Model*: Additive Genetic Variance (a^2)	Dominance Genetic Variance (d^2)	Within-Family Environmental Variance (e^2)
Sleep length	92.00†	1.50	5.30†	22	...	78
Social activity	85.95	2.35	13.73‡	28	...	72
Mood§	105.89‖	1.55	36.35‡	−03	38	65
Weight	74.92	3.73	25.10‡	31	...	70
Appetite¶	87.06†	1.83	20.66‡	20,#35**	...	80,#65**
Energy level	77.79	1.61	13.98‡	29	...	71

*Parameter estimates are uncorrected for reliability of measurement.
†$P<.05$.
‡$P<.001$
§For "Mood," the full model estimated additive genetic plus dominance genetic effects (ADE).
‖$P<.01$.
¶For "Appetite," models reported allow for sex-dependent genetic or environmental effects (A_f, A_m, C_f, C_m, E_f, E_m, and a correlation for between shared environmental effects in males and females, r_c). Degrees of freedom for these models were 3 (environmental, genetic models) and 64 (full model).
#For males.
**For females.

Table 3. Goodness of Fit of Multivariate Genetic Models*

	No. of Common Factors										
	Independence Pathway				Common Pathway				Goodness of Fit		
Model	AG	NAG	SE	NSE	AG	NAG	SE	NSE	*df*	χ^2	*P*
1	1	0	0	2	...	...	...	...	282	289.90	.36
2	2	0	0	2	...	...	...	...	270	260.30	.65
3	1	1	0	2	...	...	...	...	270	264.68	.58
4	1	0	1	2	...	...	...	...	270	252.72	.77
5	2	0	1	2	...	...	...	...	258	230.02	.89
6	1	1	1	2	...	...	...	...	258	231.04	.89
7	1	0	2	2	...	...	...	...	258	233.34	.86
8	2	0	2	2	...	...	...	...	246	221.06	.87
9	2	1	1	2	...	...	...	...	246	219.57	.87
10	...	...	...	...	2	0	1	2	288	275.13	.70
11	...	...	...	...	1	1	1	2	288	285.81	.53
12	...	...	...	...	2_a	0	1	2	290	275.97	.71
13	1	0	1_a	1_a	1_a	0	0	1	281	248.87	.92

*AG represents additive genetic factors; NAG, nonadditive genetic factors; SE, shared environmental factors; NSE, nonshared environmental effects; and subscript a, sex-independent parameter(s), parameter estimate(s) constrained to be equal across sex.

MULTIVARIATE GENETIC ANALYSIS

Results of fitting multivariate genetic analyses are presented in **Table 3**. Each model tested a different hypothesis about common-factor effects, that is, about the number of genetic or environmental common factors that contribute to the correlations between the six seasonal change measures of seasonality in the SPAQ. Two hypotheses were rejected by an overall χ^2 test of goodness of fit ($P<.05$, results not shown): (1) the hypothesis that the SPAQ measures only a single dimension of liability to seasonality (ie, all models that estimated only one common factor [genetic or environmental] were rejected); and (2) the hypothesis that sensitivity to changes in season can be explained entirely by environmental (ie, shared and nonshared environmental) influences.

Of all the independent-pathway models, models with two nonshared environmental common factors, one shared environmental common factor, and either two additive genetic (model 5) or one additive genetic and one nonadditive genetic factor (model 6) were the simplest models consistent with the observed data.

The common-pathway models 10 and 11 gave a significantly worse fit than the more general independent-pathway models by the likelihood-ratio test (models 11 vs 6, $P<.004$; models 10 vs 5, $P=.04$). The simplest model to explain the observed data was a mixed model (model 13), with a common-pathway structure specified for the first factor and an independent-pathway structure specified for the second genetic and environmental factors. Under this model, additive genetic estimates were constrained to be the same across sex for the common-pathway factor. For the independent-pathway factors, the magnitude of the genetic estimates were allowed to dif-

Table 4. Factor Loadings and Heritability Estimates Under Best-Fitting Multivariate Genetic Model*

	Females					Males				
	'Common'-Pathway Factor		'Independent'-Pathway Factor			Common-Pathway Factor		Independent-Pathway Factor		
'Change' Item	Additive Genetic	Nonshared Environment	Additive Genetic	Shared Environment	Nonshared Environment	Additive Genetic	Nonshared Environment	Additive Genetic	Shared Environment	Nonshared Environment
Sleep length	.30	.47	.11	.28	.10	.29	.46	−.09	.28	.10
Social activity	.32	.50	.17	.23	.00	.31	.48	−.40	.23	.00
Mood	.44	.70	.30	.04	−.09	.45	.71	−.14	.04	−.10
Weight	.24	.38	.36	.16	.46	.26	.41	−.07	.16	.46
Appetite	.25	.40	.50	.24	.66	.32	.50	.01	.24	.66
Energy level	.40	.63	.23	.13	.18	.43	.68	.00	.13	.18

Table 4 does not include specific-factor loadings; hence, percentage of phenotypic variance that is explained by these common-factor effects will be less than 100%. The percentage of explained phenotypic variance was as follows: for females—common-pathway factor, 39%; independent-pathway factor, 9% (additive genetic), 4% (shared environment), and 12% (nonshared environment); for males—common-pathway factor, 43%; independent-pathway factor, 3% (additive genetic), 4% (shared environment), and 12% (nonshared environment).

fer by sex, but the shared and nonshared environmental estimates were constrained to be equal in men and women. This model gave an excellent fit to the data (*P*=.92), and there was no worsening of fit over the independent-pathway model by the likelihood-ratio test (models 13 vs 5, *P*=.71). Model 13 explained simply the genetic and environmental factors that predispose an individual to seasonality, and it was favored over all other models that were tested against the data.

Genetic and environmental factor loadings under this simplest model are summarized in **Table 4**. Loadings for the common-pathway factor follow a pattern consistent with the hypothesis that the genetic vulnerability to seasonality is manifested by changes in mood, sleep pattern, social activity, weight, appetite, and energy (ie, genetic effects exert a global influence across all six changes in behavior). The strongest genetic effects are on changes in mood and energy level. This seasonality factor has a heritability of 29% in both sexes, and it accounts for about 40% of the phenotypic variance in the individual seasonality symptoms in both sexes. The independent-pathway genetic, shared environmental, and nonshared environmental factors each account for a relatively small proportion of the phenotypic variation. The independent-pathway genetic factor in females appears to be an appetite and a weight factor with more modest loadings on changes in mood and energy. The corresponding genetic factor in males accounts for a trivial proportion of the total variation and is less amenable to interpretation.

COMMENT

Seasonal variations in mood and behavior, which we shall call seasonality, have been documented in reports on epidemiological research to occur along a spectrum of severity,[6,27,32,45-51] with patients who have SAD representing the extreme on that spectrum. The rest of that spectrum consists of subsyndromal-SAD: individuals who express asymptomatic seasonal behavioral changes and those who report no seasonal changes whatsoever.

Our results suggest that seasonality is heritable, with at least 29% of the variance in risk of seasonality due to genetic influences in men and women. Supportive of the hypothesis of a seasonal syndrome, we found genetic effects to exert a global influence across seasonal changes in eating, sleeping, weight change, socializing, energy level, and mood. Interestingly, genetic and environmental determinants of seasonality appeared to be mediated through a single biological pathway. Consequently, one would predict individuals who present with seasonality to include complaints on changes in mood, sleep length, social activity, weight, appetite, and energy level with a high degree of consistency across cases. These findings are inconsistent with those of Young et al,[18] that atypical symptoms of depression (ie, fatigue, hypersomnia, and increased weight and appetite) in patients with winter-SAD demonstrate a pattern of onset and course that is substantially different from patterns observed for other complaints that are commonly reported by these patients (ie, decreases in self-esteem, mood, interest, ability to concentrate, and problems with social withdrawal).

Consistent with problems that are commonly reported by individuals with winter-SAD, genetic predisposition to seasonality (as measured by the SPAQ) appears to be manifested by complaints associated with the atypical vegetative symptoms of depression (ie, increases in sleep, eating, and weight gain) and decreases in socialization, energy, and mood. This finding is compatible with the results from treatment outcome studies, which also have found that complaints of hypersomnia, overeating, and weight gain are predictors of a good response to phototherapy in patients who are diagnosed as having winter-SAD.[52,53]

Consistent with the results of Rosen and Rosenthal,[54] who used data collected in the northern hemisphere, we found patterns of response in our data to support the presence of summer and winter patterns of behavioral changes. However, our results indicate that genetic susceptibility for sensitivity to changes in season is only associated with winter forms of mood and behavioral changes. If a genetic predisposition to a summer form of seasonality exists, the prevalence of this condition must be too low in the general population of Australia to be detectable by using the sample sizes of the present study.

In interpreting our findings, several important limitations should be borne in mind. First, assessments of seasonality in the present study were carried out by a retrospective self-report questionnaire, and our findings were limited by the ability of the SPAQ to discriminate those individuals who were affected with seasonality from the unaffected persons in the general population. Our demonstration of significant familial aggregation of seasonality, and the fact that this familial aggregation is genetically determined, is another step in the ongoing evaluation of the validity and specificity of this questionnaire.

Second, our ability to detect a contribution to the risk of seasonality of environmental factor(s) shared by family members (eg, seasonal changes in the surrounding environment) may have been limited by characteristics of our sample. There is an overrepresentation of twins from southeastern Australia (40% of twins live in the state of Victoria). Assuming that latitude is a reasonable indicator of exposure to seasonal changes, an evaluation of the significance of the shared environmental contribution to the risk of seasonality ideally would require a more balanced sample in the distribution by geographical location. Sample sizes significantly larger than those used to test the hypotheses of this project are required to detect modest shared environmental influences against a background of genetic effects when MZ twin correlations are as low as those observed in the present study.[44]

Last, the low prevalence of clinical levels of seasonality (only 2%) limits the interpretation of our results to seasonality within the subclinical or normal range, and it precludes statements about genetic influences on SAD per se.

To conclude, there is a tendency for seasonality to run in families, and this is largely owing to a biological predisposition. These findings support continuing efforts to determine the role of seasonality in the development of affective disorder. Two questions remain: (1) Do the same genetic and environmental risk factors that determine the risk of seasonality, as we have found here, also predispose to clinically significant seasonal changes in mood? (2) Is the tendency to experience seasonal changes in mood and behavior transmitted along with a vulnerability to a mood disorder, or are these separate heritable factors?

Accepted for publication August 2, 1995.

This study was supported in part by grant AA07535 from the National Institutes of Health, Bethesda, Md, by a grant from the the Australian National Health and Medical Research Council, by postdoctoral training grant DA07261 from the National Institute on Drug Abuse, Bethesda, and by funds from the Clinical Psychobiology Branch, National Institute of Mental Health, Bethesda.

The authors acknowledge the contribution of Thomas A. Wehr, MD, for his helpful comments.

Reprint requests to Department of Psychiatry, Washington University School of Medicine, Box 8134, 4940 Children's Pl, St Louis, MO 63110 (Dr Madden).

REFERENCES

1. Castiglione A. *A History of Medicine.* New York, NY: Alfred A Knopf Inc; 1941.
2. Roccatagliata G. *A History of Ancient Psychiatry.* New York, NY: Greenwood Press Inc; 1986.
3. Wehr TA, Rosenthal NE. Seasonality and affective illness. *Am J Psychiatry.* 1989;146:829-839.
4. Rosenthal NE, Sack DA, Gillin C, Lewy AJ, Goodwin FK, Davenport Y, Mueller PS, Newsome DA, Wehr TA. Seasonal affective disorder: a description of the syndrome and preliminary findings with light therapy. *Arch Gen Psychiatry.* 1984;41:72-80.
5. Wehr TA, Sack DA, Rosenthal NE. Seasonal affective disorder with summer depression and winter hypomania. *Am J Psychiatry.* 1987;144:1602-1603.
6. Kasper S, Wehr TA, Bartko JJ, Gaist PA, Rosenthal NE. Epidemiological findings of seasonal changes in mood and behavior: a telephone survey of Montgomery County, Maryland. *Arch Gen Psychiatry.* 1989;46:823-833.
7. American Psychiatric Association, Committee on Nomenclature and Statistics. *Diagnostic and Statistical Manual of Mental Disorders, Revised Third Edition.* Washington, DC: American Psychiatric Association; 1987.
8. American Psychiatric Association, Committee on Nomenclature and Statistics. *Diagnostic and Statistical Manual of Mental Disorders, Fourth Edition.* Washington, DC: American Psychiatric Association; 1994.
9. Rosenthal NE, Sack DA, James SP, Parry BL, Mendelson WB, Tamarkin L, Wehr, TA. Seasonal affective disorder and phototherapy. *Ann N Y Acad Sci.* 1985;453:260-269.
10. Rosenthal NE, Rotter A, Jacobsen FM, Skewer RG. No mood-altering effects found following treatment of normal subjects with bright light in the morning. *Psychiatry Res.* 1987;22:1-9.
11. Oren D, Rosenthal NE. Seasonal affective disorders. In: Paykel ES, ed. *Handbook of Affective Disorders.* 2nd ed. New York, NY: Churchill Livingstone Inc; 1992:551-567.
12. Wehr TA, Giesen HA, Schulz PM, Anderson JL, Joseph-Vanderpool JR, Kelly K, Kasper S, Rosenthal NE. Contrasts between symptoms of summer depression and winter depression. *J Affect Disord.* 1991;23:173-183.
13. Lewy AJ, Sack RL, Miller LS, Hoban TM. Antidepressant and circadian phase-shifting effects of light. *Science.* 1987;235:352-353.
14. Terman M, Terman JS, Quitkin FM, McGrath PJ, Stewart JW, Rafferty AB. Light therapy for seasonal affective disorder: a review of efficacy. *Neuropsychopharmacology.* 1989;2:1-22.
15. Wirz-Justice A, Bucheli C, Graw P, Kielholz P, Fisch H-U, Woggon B. Light treatment of seasonal affective disorder in Switzerland. *Acta Psychiatr Scand.* 1986;74:193-204.
16. Garvey MJ, Wesner R, Godes M. Comparison of seasonal and non-seasonal affective disorders. *Am J Psychiatry.* 1988;145:100-102.
17. Thompson C, Isaacs G. Seasonal affective disorder—a British sample: symptomatology in relation to mode of referral and diagnostic subtype. *J Affect Disord.* 1988;14:1-11.
18. Young MA, Watel LG, Lahmeyer HW, Eastman CI. The temporal onset of individual symptoms in winter depression: differentiating underlying mechanisms. *J Affect Disord.* 1991;22:191-197.
19. Avery DH, Khan A, Dager SR, Cohen S, Cox GB, Dunner DL. Morning or evening bright light treatment of winter depression? the significance of hypersomnia. *Biol Psychiatry.* 1991;29:117-129.
20. Hellekson CJ, Kline JA, Rosenthal NE. Phototherapy for seasonal affective disorder in Alaska. *Am J Psychiatry.* 1986;8:1035-1037.
21. Takahashi K, Asano Y, Kohsaka M, Okawa M, Saski M, Honda Y, Higuchi T, Yamazaki J, Ishizuka Y, Kawaguchi K, Ohto T, Hanada K, Sugita Y, Maeda K, Nagayama H, Kotorii T, Egashira K, Takahashi S. Multi-center study of seasonal affective disorders in Japan. *J Affect Disord.* 1991;21:57-65.
22. Faedda GL, Tondo L, Teicher MH, Baldessarini RJ, Gelbard HA, Floris GF. Seasonal mood disorders: patterns of seasonal recurrence in mania and depression. *Arch Gen Psychiatry.* 1993;50:17-23.
23. Lingjaerde O, Reichborn-Kjennerud T. Characteristics of winter depression in the Oslo area (60°N). *Acta Psychiatr Scand.* 1993;88:111-120.
24. Boyce P, Parker G. Seasonal affective disorder in the southern hemisphere. *Am J Psychiatry.* 1988;145:96-99.
25. Wilhelmsen L, Ljungberg S, Wedel H, Werko L. A comparison between participants and non-participants in a primary preventive trial. *J Chronic Dis.* 1976; 29:331-339.
26. Berkson J. Limitations of the application of fourfold table analysis to hospital data. *Biometrics.* 1946;2:47-53.
27. Terman M. On the question of mechanism in phototherapy: considerations of clinical efficacy and epidemiology. *J Biol Rhythms.* 1988;3:155-172.
28. Jardine R, Martin NG, Henderson AS. Genetic covariation between neuroticism and the symptoms of anxiety and depression. *Genet Epidemiol.* 1984;1: 89-107.
29. Kendler KS, Heath A, Martin NG, Eaves LJ. Symptoms of anxiety and depression in a volunteer twin population: the etiologic role of genetic and environmental factors. *Arch Gen Psychiatry.* 1986;43:213-221.
30. Kendler KS, Heath A, Martin NG, Eaves LJ. Symptoms of anxiety and

symptoms of depression: same genes, different environments? *Arch Gen Psychiatry.* 1987;5:451-457.
31. Rosenthal NE, Genhart MJ, Sack DA, Skwerer RG, Wehr TA. Seasonal affective disorder and its relevance for the understanding and treatment of bulimia. In: Hudson JI, Pope HG Jr, eds. *The Psychology of Bulimia.* Washington, DC: American Psychiatric Press Inc; 1987:205-228.
32. Rosen LN, Targum SD, Terman M, Bryant MJ, Hoffman H, Kasper SF, Hamovit JR, Docherty JP, Welch B, Rosenthal NE. Prevalence of seasonal affective disorder at four latitudes. *Psychiatry Res.* 1990;31:131-144.
33. Thompson C, Stinson D, Fernandez M, Fine J, Isaacs G. A comparison of normal, bipolar and seasonal affective disorder subjects using the Seasonal Pattern Assessment Questionnaire. *J Affect Disord.* 1988;14:257-264.
34. Neale MC, Martin NG. The effects of age, sex and genotype on self-report drunkenness following a challenge dose of alcohol. *Behav Genet.* 1989;19:63-78.
35. Neale MC, Cardon LR. Multivariate analysis. In: Neale MC, Cardon LR, eds. *Methodology for Genetic Studies of Twins and Families.* Boston, Mass: Kluwer Academic Publishers; 1992:231-259.
36. Heath AC, Neale MC, Hewitt JK, Eaves LJ, Fulker DW. Testing structural equation models for twin data using LISREL. *Behav Genet.* 1989;19:9-35.
37. SAS Institute. *SAS/STAT User's Guide, Version 6.* 4th ed. Cary, NC: SAS Institute Inc; 1990:2.
38. Heath AC, Jardine R, Eaves LJ. The genetic structure of personality, I: phenotype factor structure of the EPQ in an Australian sample. *Personal Individ Diff. 1988;9:59-67.*
39. Joreskog KG, Sorbom D. *PRELIS: A Preprocessor for LISREL.* 2nd ed. Mooresville, Ind: Scientific Software; 1988.
40. Eaves LJ, Last KA, Young PA, Martin NG. Model-fitting approaches to the analysis of human behavior. *Heredity.* 1978;41:249-320.
41. Martin NG, Eaves LJ. The genetical analysis of covariance structure. *Heredity.* 1977;38:79-95.
42. Joreskog KG, Sorbom D. *LISREL7: A Guide to the Program and Applications.* 2nd ed. Chicago, Ill: SPSS Inc; 1989.
43. Browne MW. Asymptotically distribution-free methods for the analysis of covariance structures. *Br J Math Stat Psychol.* 1984;37:62-83.
44. Martin NG, Eaves LJ, Kearsey MJ, Davies P. The power of the classical twin study. *Heredity.* 1978;40:97-116.
45. Lingjaerde O, Bratlid T, Hansen T, Gotestam KG. Seasonal affective disorder and midwinter insomnia in the far north: studies on two related chronobiological disorders in Norway. *Clin Neuropharmacol.* 1986;9(suppl):187-189.
46. Potkin SG, Zetin M, Stamenkovic V, Kripke D, Bunney WE Jr. Seasonal affective disorder: prevalence varies with latitude and climate. *Clin Neuropharmacol.* 1986;9(suppl):181-183.
47. Booker JM, Hellekson CJ. Prevalence of seasonal affective disorder in Alaska. *Am J Psychiatry.* 1992;149:1176-1182.
48. Muscettola G, Barbato G, Ficca G, Beatrice M, Puca M, Aguglia E, Amati A. Seasonality of mood in Italy: role of latitude and sociocultural factors. *J Affect Disord.* 1995;33:135-139.
49. Armstrong C, McIntyre I. The winter of our discontent. *Today's Life Sci.* 1989; 1:10-17.
50. Haggag A, Eklund B, Linaker O, Gotestam KG. Seasonal mood variation: an epidemiological study in northern Norway. *Acta Psychiatr Scand.* 1990;81: 141-145.
51. Spoont MR, Depue RA, Krauss SS. Dimensional measurement of seasonal variation in mood and behavior. *Psychiatry Res.* 1991;39:269-284.
52. Oren DA, Jacobsen FM, Wehr TA, Cameron CL, Rosenthal NE. Predictors of response to phototherapy in seasonal affective disorder. *Compr Psychiatry.* 1992;33:111-114.
53. Stinson D, Thompson C. Clinical experience with phototherapy. *J Affect Disord.* 1990;18:129-135.
54. Rosen LN, Rosenthal NE. Seasonal variations in mood and behavior in the general population. *Psychiatry Res.* 1991;38:271-283.

ORIGINAL ARTICLE

Anterior Paralimbic Mediation of Procaine-Induced Emotional and Psychosensory Experiences

Terence A. Ketter, MD; Paul J. Andreason, MD; Mark S. George, MD; Chulhee Lee, PhD; Debra S. Gill, MA; Priti I. Parekh; Mark W. Willis, MEng; Peter Herscovitch, MD; Robert M. Post, MD

Background: Procaine activates limbic structures in animals. In humans, acute intravenous administration of procaine yields emotional and psychosensory experiences and temporal lobe fast activity. We studied procaine's acute effects on cerebral blood flow (CBF) in relationship to clinical responses.

Methods: Cerebral blood flow was assessed by positron emission tomography with oxygen-15–labeled water in 32 healthy volunteers. Data were analyzed with statistical parametric mapping and magnetic resonance imaging–directed regions of interest.

Results: Procaine increased global CBF and, to a greater extent, anterior paralimbic CBF. Subjects with intense procaine-induced fear compared with those with euphoria had greater increases in left amygdalar CBF. Absolute and normalized left amygdalar CBF changes tended to correlate positively with fear and negatively with euphoria intensity. Procaine-induced visual hallucinations appeared associated with greater global and occipital CBF increases. Absolute occipital CBF increases appeared to correlate positively with visual hallucination intensity.

Conclusions: Procaine increased anterior paralimbic CBF, and different clinical responses appeared to be associated with different patterns of CBF changes.

(Arch Gen Psychiatry. 1996;53:59-69)

From the Biological Psychiatry Branch, National Institute of Mental Health (Drs Ketter, George, and Post, Mss Gill and Parekh and Mr Willis), National Institute on Alcohol Abuse and Alcoholism (Dr Andreason), Biomedical Engineering and Implementation Branch (Dr Lee), and National Institutes of Health Clinical Center (Dr Herscovitch), Bethesda, Md. Dr Ketter is now affiliated with the Department of Psychiatry and Behavioral Sciences, Stanford (Calif) University School of Medicine.

SEVERAL LINES of evidence suggest that the limbic system plays a crucial role in mood regulation.[1-3] This system is strategically arranged to receive complex sensory information, process it by integrating information from past experiences, and thus imbue it with affective significance that would lead to appropriate behavioral and hormonal responses.[4] This view is consistent with literature demonstrating that patients with temporal lobe epilepsy frequently have secondary mood disorders that resemble primary affective illnesses,[5] and that temporal lobe depth electrode stimulation can yield emotional and psychosensory responses.[6,7]

Procaine and related local anesthetics selectively activate limbic structures in rats,[8,9] rabbits,[10] cats,[10] and monkeys.[11] In patients with mood disorders and healthy controls, intravenous administration of procaine yielded consistent emotional (from dysphoria and fear to euphoria and acute relief of chronic refractory depression), psychosensory (auditory and visual hallucinations), and hormonal (increased plasma corticotropin, cortisol, and prolactin, but not growth hormone, levels) responses as well as increased temporal lobe fast activity on quantitative electroencephalograms.[12] Although these data suggested that procaine had selective temporal lobe effects in humans,[12] temporalis muscle artifact could have confounded the electroencephalographic findings. Mapping of regional cerebral blood flow (rCBF) by positron emission tomography (PET) with oxygen-15–labeled water has less potential for surface artifacts, enhanced sensitivity in deep structures, and temporal resolution well matched to the plasma half-life and clinical duration of procaine, all of which are about 2 minutes. Based on the results of animal experiments and human clinical, hormonal, and electroencephalographic effects, we hypothesized that acute intravenous procaine would yield temporal lobe and related limbic rCBF changes, in concert with emotional and psychosensory ex-

See Subjects and Methods on next page

SUBJECTS AND METHODS

SUBJECTS

The nature and possible consequences of the study were explained and verbal and written informed consent was obtained from 32 volunteers (17 men and 15 women; mean±SD age, 30.1±7.5 years; range, 18 to 45 years) determined to be physically healthy by history, physical and neurologic examinations, electrocardiogram, routine serum chemistry studies (including human immunodeficiency virus test), comprehensive drug screen (and cerebral magnetic resonance [MR] imaging in 27), and never mentally ill by the Schedule for Affective Disorders and Schizophrenia–Lifetime Anxiety Version.[13]

PROCAINE CHALLENGE AND SCAN ACQUISITION

Regional cerebral blood flow (CBF) was determined after serial single-blind intravenous injections of procaine vs saline. We used a scanner (PC2048-15B, Scanditronix Inc, Uppsala, Sweden), with 6.9-mm in-plane and 5- to 6-mm axial full-width half-maximum resolution, 1110-MBq bolus intravenous injections of oxygen-15–labeled water, 4-minute scan acquisitions, and a 20-minute interscan duration. Individually molded Polyform (Smith and Nephew, Madison, Wis) thermoplastic masks restricted head motion, and postacquisition scan coregistration allowed voxel-by-voxel within-subject comparisons of rCBF after injections of procaine vs saline. A germanium 68/gallium-68 rotating pin source was used to obtain transmission scans, to allow correction of the emission scans for photon attenuation by the tissues of the head. Emission data were collected in 15 planes spaced 6.5 mm apart starting 10 mm above the canthomeatal line. Radial arterial blood sampling allowed blood gas and absolute rCBF determinations in all subjects. Regional CBF was calculated by means of a rapid least-squares method,[14] from dynamic PET scan data collected for 4 minutes and from the arterial time-activity curve.

Subjects were informed that procaine had various transient emotional and sensory effects, ranging from minimal to intense and from pleasant to unpleasant. They were instructed to lie quietly with eyes closed and monitor their sensory and emotional experiences during scans. Such experiences were self-rated with scales ranging from 0 (none) to 6 (very intense) (**Figure 1**, vertical axes). After an initial sham scan with single-blind intravenous saline and no tracer, to habituate subjects to the scanning environment, we obtained single-blind baseline (saline), low-dose procaine (0.46 mg/kg), high-dose procaine (1.84 mg/kg), and recovery (saline) PET studies. Experiential self-ratings and blood for hormonal studies were obtained at baseline and immediately after each scan. The serial single-blind intravenous doses of procaine or saline were each followed 15 seconds later by a 1110-MBq intravenous bolus injection of oxygen-15–labeled water. Tomographic image acquisition started when the radiotracer bolus reached the head and continued for 4 minutes. In 21 subjects, 5 minutes after the high-dose procaine injection, arterial blood was collected into tubes containing echothiophate (a pseudocholinesterase inhibitor to prevent procaine metabolism) for procaine concentration determination by a commercial laboratory. In 27 subjects, sagittally acquired MR images with slices 2.5 mm apart were obtained on a superconducting MR imaging system (Picker International, Cleveland, Ohio), using a magnetic field strength of 0.5-T for coregistration with PET images.

DATA ANALYSIS

Absolute, P_{CO_2}-adjusted absolute, and normalized rCBF data were analyzed by means of statistical parametric mapping (SPM). Image processing was performed on a workstation (SUN SPARCstation 2, Sun Microsystems Inc, Mountain View, Calif) with the use of ANALYZE imaging software (Biomedical Imaging Resource, Mayo Foundation, Rochester, Minn), PROMATLAB statistical software (Mathworks, Sherborn, Mass), and SPM software (MRC Cyclotron Unit, Hammersmith Hospital, London, England).[15] Scans were individually inspected for image quality and artifacts.

For the SPM analyses, scans were interpolated to 43 slices, and roll and yaw corrections were individually assessed and applied. Baseline (saline) and procaine images were coregistered to one another[16] and then individually reoriented parallel to the intercommissural plane,[17] and resized, rescaled, and resliced to yield stereotactically

periences. Not only was a specific pattern of anterior paralimbic activation demonstrated but different affective and psychosensory experiences were associated with different changes in rCBF.

RESULTS

Procaine yielded prominent psychosensory and emotional experiences (Figure 1) and distinctive rCBF changes (**Figure 2** through **Figure 5**). Experiential effects were maximal during the first 2 minutes of the procaine scans, the period with the greatest weighting in the image acquisition. Mean self-rated visual and auditory hallucinations, fear, and euphoria increased substantially with procaine (Figure 1, top). Although subjects consistently (29 of 32 subjects) reported procaine-induced auditory hallucinations (unformed buzzing, ringing, or electronic sounds), there was considerable heterogeneity of other clinical responses. To explore the rCBF concomitants of these experiences, the sample was divided into more homogeneous subgroups: (1) visual hallucinations: nine subjects with intense procaine-induced unformed visual hallucinations (lights or colors self-rated as intense or very intense); (2) no visual hallucinations: nine other subjects with no such hallucinations (Figure 1, center); the remaining 14 subjects had mild to moderate visual hallucinations; (3) fear: nine subjects with intense procaine-induced fear (self-rated as intense or very intense, with symptoms meeting criteria for clinical panic attacks[20]); and (4) euphoria: nine other subjects with intense or very intense euphoria (Figure 1, bottom). The remaining 14 subjects had mild to moderate or mixed emotional responses. Subgroups 1 and 2 did not overlap, and subgroups 3 and 4 did not overlap. The main experiential difference between groups 1 and 2 was visual hallucinations (Figure 1, center), and that between groups 3 and 4 was affective response (Figure 1, bottom).

In the 21 subjects in whom arterial blood procaine

normalized images corresponding to the human brain atlas of Talairach and Tournoux.[18] Images were smoothed with gaussian filters (10-mm transaxial and 6-mm axial) to increase spatial extents of focal activations and thus the probability that such activations would overlap across subjects. The coregistration, smoothing, and stereotactic normalization thus minimized the effects of any possible interscan spatial displacements. Global CBF was calculated from mean rCBF values in stereotactically normalized images after application of masks to exclude voxels with values less than one third of the maximum voxel for each image. For the normalized SPM analysis, a voxel-based analysis of covariance over the different baseline and activation conditions yielded four rCBF maps for each subject (baseline saline, low-dose procaine, high-dose procaine, and recovery saline) normalized to a mean global rCBF of 50 mL per 100 g of brain tissue per minute, and each with an associated error variance.[19] Statistically significant focal interscan changes in blood flow, assumed to be independent of global blood flow changes, were then calculated. Also, absolute and PCO_2-adjusted absolute SPM analyses were performed, in which focal interscan changes in blood flow were calculated, without any adjustment to normalize global blood flow.

As high-dose procaine yielded the most robust clinical and rCBF changes, this report describes comparisons of high-dose procaine and baseline (saline) rCBF. The rather complex relationships between procaine doses and experiential and rCBF effects will be described in a future article. Results were displayed as SPMs on transverse, coronal, and sagittal slices. The SPMs displayed voxels exceeding ascending color-coded z-thresholds (starting at $z=2.33$) corresponding to exponentially decreasing P values (starting at $P=10^{-2}$, not corrected for multiple comparisons). A strict Bonferroni-type correction requires a z-threshold of 3.75 (corresponds to about $P=10^{-4}$, not corrected for multiple comparisons), which was coded as yellow or above, while a more liberal correction in the setting of a priori hypotheses allows a z-threshold of 3.0 (corresponds to about $P=10^{-3}$, not corrected for multiple comparisons), which was coded as green or above. In addition, for experiential subgroups, mean increases and differences in mean increases in rCBF were calculated to examine heterogeneity of rCBF responses. To aid in visualization, SPM figures were displayed masked with cartoons of the cardinal axes and crucial cerebral structures in Talairach space.

In addition, in 27 subjects with available MR images, we performed a coregistered MR imaging–directed region of interest (ROI) analysis of changes in absolute, PCO_2-adjusted absolute, and normalized rCBF with high-dose procaine compared with saline (**Table 1** through **Table 3**). The original 15 slices of PET data for the saline and procaine conditions were coregistered to one another and to MR images by means of the ANALYZE surface matching subroutine. This yielded MR images resliced in planes identical to the PET images. The ROIs were defined on the MR images for the left and right amygdala (in the plane of its maximum diameter, corresponding to about 16 mm below the intercommissural plane in Talairach space) and then applied to the *unfiltered* saline and procaine PET images to provide analysis of changes in absolute, PCO_2-adjusted absolute, and normalized amygdalar rCBF. The two amygdalar ROIs were defined a priori on theoretical grounds as primary outcome measures in relationship to CBF activation and affective responses. Ten additional ROIs were defined to allow preliminary comparison of amygdalar changes with those in other structures as well as comparison of the findings of the ROI analysis with those of the SPM analysis. These additional ROIs included bilateral anterior and posterior cingulate and mesial occipital cortex (in a plane corresponding to about 20 mm above the intercommissural plane in Talairach space) and bilateral hippocampus and lateral frontal cortex (in a plane corresponding to the intercommissural plane in Talairach space).

Data were analyzed by two-tailed Student's t tests and Pearson correlation coefficients. Means (±SDs) are reported. For assessment of CBF effects of procaine in ROIs for the entire sample, a Bonferroni correction ($P<.004$) was applied to account for all 12 ROIs (Table 1). For assessment of CBF effects of procaine in the amygdala for experiential subgroups and correlations between affective responses and changes in amygdalar CBF, a Bonferroni correction ($P<.01$) was applied to account for the left and right amygdala ROIs and fear and euphoria responses (Tables 2 and 3). For other ROIs in Tables 2 and 3, no correction of P for multiple comparisons was applied.

concentrations were determined 5 minutes after high-dose procaine injection, levels were uniformly low to undetectable (mean, 0.11±0.17 μg/mL), indicating that no subject had remarkable abnormalities in procaine pharmacokinetics. Also, procaine concentrations did not significantly differ between experiential subgroups, or correlate with experiential measures, global CBF, or normalized and absolute rCBF, except for an inverse relationship with normalized (but not absolute) left lateral frontal lobe rCBF ($r=-.50$, $df=19$, $P<.04$).

GLOBAL CBF EFFECTS

Mean global CBF increased 13.1% from a baseline of 42.6±6.9 mL/100 g per minute to 48.2±11.2 mL/100 g per minute with high-dose procaine ($t=3.04$, $df=31$, $P<.005$). Mean PCO_2 decreased from 39.2±4.1 mm Hg at baseline to 36.6±4.8 mm Hg with procaine ($t=3.42$, $df=31$, $P<.002$), so that global CBF adjusted for PCO_2 (with an adjustment of $1.8\times[40-PCO_2]$ mL/100 g per minute) increased 23.3% from a baseline of 44.1±11.7 mL/100 g per minute to 54.4±13.7 mL/100 g per minute with procaine ($t=4.46$, $df=31$, $P<.001$) (Table 1, bottom). Subjects with intense procaine-induced visual hallucinations had greater increases in PCO_2-adjusted global CBF than those without ($t=2.92$, $df=14$, $P=.01$) (Table 2, bottom). There was a trend toward a positive correlation between increases (ie, procaine-saline) in PCO_2-adjusted global CBF and visual hallucination intensity ($r=.34$, $df=30$, $P<.06$), but not auditory hallucination, fear, or euphoria intensity ($|r|<.16$, $df=30$, $P>.39$).

SPM ANALYSIS OF rCBF EFFECTS

In the SPM analysis, procaine increased both PCO_2-adjusted absolute and normalized rCBF in anterior paralimbic structures, including the amygdala, anterior cingulate, hypothalamus, basal forebrain, insula, and or-

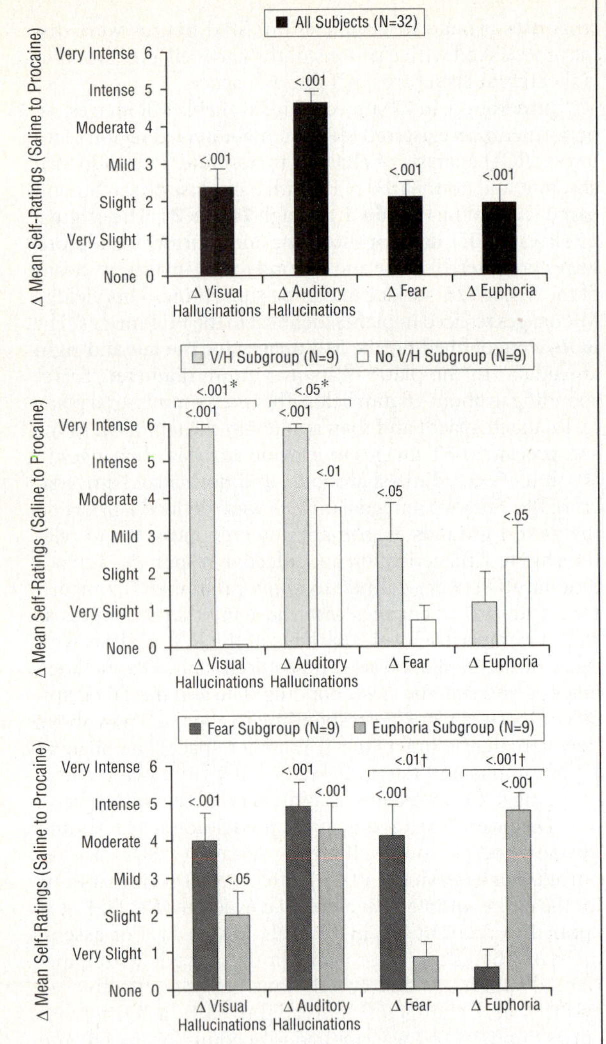

Figure 1. *Procaine experiential effects. Changes in self-rated sensory (visual and auditory hallucinations) and emotional (fear and euphoria) experiences from saline to procaine. Means and SEs are depicted. Top, All 32 subjects. Center, Nine subjects with intense procaine-induced visual hallucinations vs nine others without them. Bottom, Nine subjects with intense procaine-induced fear vs nine others with intense euphoria. Δ indicates changes in experiential measures from saline to procaine.* $P<.0125=.05/4$, *Bonferroni-type correction limits overall type I error to .05 for four comparisons.* P *values given above bars are by paired* t *test for saline vs procaine, except as otherwise specified. Asterisk indicates unpaired* t *test, visual hallucination (V/H) vs no V/H subgroup; dagger, unpaired* t *test, fear vs euphoria subgroup.*

bitofrontal cortex (Figure 2 and Figure 3, left and top right). Hereafter, for the sake of brevity, we will use the term *absolute* to indicate "P_{CO_2}-adjusted absolute." Maximal activation was at the same anterior cingulate voxel (Talairach coordinates −2, 20, and 24; Brodmann area 24) for both absolute (37.6% increase, z=5.48) and normalized (15.2% increase, z=5.31) analyses. Voxels with the second greatest local maximum were in the region of the hypothalamus for both the absolute (38.6% increase, z=5.47 at Talairach coordinates −4, −2, and −4) and normalized (15.1% increase, z=5.01 at Talairach coordinates 0, 0, and −8) analyses. Procaine decreased nor-

Table 1. Changes in Mean P_{CO_2}: Adjusted Absolute and Normalized CBF With Procaine*

	% Change in CBF With Procaine	
	Absolute	Normalized
Anterior limbic ROIs		
Right anterior cingulate	41.7†‡	16.7†‡
Left anterior cingulate	38.5†‡	14.4§‖
Right amygdala	33.9§	7.3
Left amygdala	23.2	0.1
Posterior limbic ROIs		
Right hippocampus	24.5§	0.6
Left hippocampus	17.7	−3.7
Right posterior cingulate	18.2	−3.1
Left posterior cingulate	17.8	−2.7
Neocortical ROIs		
Right mesial occipital lobe	18.6	−1.7
Left mesial occipital lobe	15.2	−5.2
Right lateral frontal lobe	16.1	−5.3
Left lateral frontal lobe	19.6§	−1.6
Global CBF (N=32)	23.3†	...

**CBF indicates cerebral blood flow; ROI, region of interest. N=27 for ROI analysis.* $P<.004=.05/12$, *limits overall type I error to .05 for 12 (ROI) comparisons.*
†*P<.001 vs baseline.*
‡*P<.004 versus posterior limbic and neocortical ROIs.*
§*P<.004 vs baseline.*
‖*P<.004 vs posterior limbic and neocortical ROIs (except* P=.009 *vs left posterior cingulate).*

malized (but not P_{CO_2}-adjusted absolute) rCBF in other (non–anterior paralimbic) structures, including cerebellum and neocortex (Figure 3, bottom right). As a confirmation, we repeated the absolute and normalized SPM analyses with two age- and gender-matched subgroups of 15 subjects each. In both subgroups, procaine yielded anterior paralimbic activation patterns remarkably similar to the whole group analysis and to one another (not illustrated).

Procaine-induced auditory hallucinations were the most common experiential effects, and superior temporal activation was evident in the entire group of 32 subjects (Figure 2 and Figure 3, left). There was considerable heterogeneity of rCBF responses to procaine (Figure 4). Nine subjects with intense procaine-induced visual hallucinations compared with nine without them had more prominent increases in mesial occipital, anterior paralimbic, and diffuse cortical rCBF (Figure 4, top two rows). However, in the statistical analysis (not illustrated), the visual hallucination compared with no visual hallucination subgroup had greater occipital (and other regional) rCBF increases that only exceeded the $P<.01$ threshold (absolute and normalized, not corrected for multiple comparisons).

There was less difference between the patterns of mean rCBF increases in nine subjects with intense procaine-induced fear and nine with intense procaine-induced euphoria (Figure 4, bottom two rows). In the statistical analyses (not illustrated), for the fear compared with the euphoria subgroup, rCBF changes only differed in a few scattered voxels and only exceeded the $P<.05$ threshold in the absolute and the $P<.01$ thresh-

Table 2. Changes in Mean P_{CO_2}: Adjusted Absolute and Normalized CBF With Procaine in Experiential Subgroups*

	% Change in CBF With Procaine							
	Fear vs Euphoria				With vs Without Visual Hallucinations			
	Absolute		Normalized		Absolute		Normalized	
	Fear (n=9)	Euphoria (n=9)	Fear (n=9)	Euphoria (n=9)	Visual Hallucinations (n=9)	No Visual Hallucinations (n=7)	Visual Hallucinations (n=9)	No Visual Hallucinations (n=7)
Anterior limbic ROIs								
Right anterior cingulate	54.8†‡	37.8†	26.2‡§	12.4	**70.6**‡§	**23.2**	24.0‡§	14.8
Left anterior cingulate	39.5†	47.5†	16.7	18.7†	51.4§	31.3	8.6	24.6†
Right amygdala	31.6	41.1	5.4	8.0	43.9†	30.1	1.3	18.4
Left amygdala	**52.8** (.04)	**−4.4**	**25.1** (.008)	**−26.3**	**75.6**§ (.004)	**−3.8**	23.8	−10.4
Posterior limbic ROIs								
Right hippocampus	25.9	30.2†	2.9	1.8	41.3†	15.5	−2.2	9.4
Left hippocampus	15.7	26.1	−3.1	0.3	35.8†	4.4	−4.9	−2.3
Right posterior cingulate	15.1	22.1	−6.8	−1.9	36.2†	−2.6	−3.7	−8.3
Left posterior cingulate	26.2	8.0	5.7	−14.9	41.2	3.9	−0.3	3.7
Neocortical ROIs								
Right mesial occipital lobe	26.8	14.8	**5.7**	**−8.6**	**43.8**§	**−4.5**	**3.5**	**−8.9**
Left mesial occipital lobe	11.8	20.8	−8.9	−4.5	**37.3**†	**2.8**	−2.6	−3.6
Right lateral frontal lobe	11.5	22.9	−8.4	−2.9	30.5†	7.3	−9.0	0.9
Left lateral frontal lobe	18.9	23.7	−2.2	−0.9	**35.4**†	**8.4**	−3.4	4.2
Global CBF (*P* vs baseline)	23.2 (.08)	26.2 (.02)	...	...	**44.6**§ (.0014)	**6.2** (.49)	...	...

**CBF indicates cerebral blood flow; ROI, region of interest. Left and right amygdala ROIs are primary outcome measures.* P<*.0125=.05/4 limits overall type I error to .05 for four (left and right amygdala for fear and euphoria) comparisons. For left amygdala,* P *values for comparison of size of CBF increase between subgroups are given in parentheses between columns. Correction of* P *for multiple comparisons not applied for other ROIs. Boldface values indicate* P<*.05 for euphoria vs fear or visual hallucinations vs no visual hallucinations.*

†P<*.01 vs baseline.*

‡P<*.01 vs posterior limbic and neocortical ROIs.*

§P<*.001 vs baseline.*

old in the normalized analysis (not corrected for multiple comparisons).

MR IMAGING–DIRECTED ROI ANALYSIS OF rCBF EFFECTS

In 27 subjects with MR images, visual inspection of individual PET baseline, high-dose procaine, and subtraction (procaine minus baseline) absolute CBF images coregistered with MR images qualitatively confirmed the activation pattern seen with the SPM analysis (Figure 5) and the absence of interscan spatial displacement. In general, the findings of the MR imaging–directed ROI analysis of the unfiltered PET images agreed with those of the SPM analysis of smoothed PET images with the important exception that the ROI analysis provided additional information regarding relationships between clinical responses and differential rCBF activation in the left and right amygdala, which was presumably absent from the SPM analysis because of smoothing and the small size of the amygdala.

Mean absolute and normalized amygdalar rCBF tended to rise more consistently in the right (24 of 27 subjects) than left (18 of 27 subjects) amygdala (χ^2=3.86, *df*=1, Fisher's exact *P*=.10). Absolute and normalized increases in bilateral anterior cingulate rCBF were particularly robust and exceeded rCBF increases in posterior limbic and cortical ROIs (Table 1).

Nine subjects with intense procaine-induced visual hallucinations, compared with seven without them, tended to have greater increases in absolute (*t*=3.9, *df*=14, *P*=.002, not corrected for multiple comparisons) and normalized (*t*=2.5, *df*=14, *P*=.02, not corrected for multiple comparisons) rCBF in right mesial occipital lobe (as well as left mesial occipital lobe and amygdala, and right anterior cingulate and lateral frontal lobe) (Table 2). In addition, visual hallucination intensities tended to correlate positively with increases in absolute (but not normalized) rCBF in mesial occipital, left amygdala, and right anterior cingulate ROIs (Table 3). However, the (trend) correlation between visual hallucinations and global CBF increases mentioned above may have contributed importantly, as these regional correlations were evident in the absolute but not normalized analysis.

Nine subjects with intense procaine-induced fear (dysphoria) compared with nine with euphoria tended to have greater increases in absolute (*t*=2.2, *df*=16, *P*=.04, significance threshold *P*<.01) and normalized (*t*=3.1, *df*=16, *P*=.01, significance threshold *P*<.01) left amygdalar rCBF (Table 2). In addition, changes in absolute and normalized left amygdalar rCBF tended to correlate positively with fear intensity (for normalized rCBF, *r*=.48, *df*=25, *P*<.01, significance threshold *P*<.01) and negatively with euphoria intensity (for normalized rCBF, *r*=−.47, *df*=25, *P*<.02, significance threshold *P*<.01) (Table 3). Similar correlations were also observed between fear and right mesial occipital rCBF, possibly be-

Table 3. Correlations Between Experiential Changes and Changes in CBF* (n=27)

	Δ Left Amygdala				Δ Right Mesial Occipital			
	Pco_2-Adjusted Absolute CBF		Normalized CBF		Pco_2-Adjusted Absolute CBF		Normalized CBF	
	r	*P*	*r*	*P*	*r*	*P*	*r*	*P*
Δ Fear†	**.350**	**.08**	**.481**	**.01**	.120	.56	.451	.02
Δ Euphoria‡	**−.467**	**.02**	−.466	.02	−.369	.06	**−.574**	**.002**
Δ Visual hallucinations§	.432	.03	.244	.22	**.502**	**.01**	.224	.27

*Δ indicates procaine-baseline changes for experiential ratings and cerebral blood flow (CBF). Boldface values indicate correlations with maximal |r| compared with all other regions of interest (ROIs). Δ Left amygdala vs Δ right mesial occipital CBF: r=.676, P<.001 absolute; r=.357, P<.07 normalized. Left and right amygdala ROIs are primary outcome measures. P<.0125=.05/4 limits overall type I error to .05 for four (left and right amygdala for anxiety and euphoria) comparisons. Correction of P for multiple comparisons was not applied for other ROIs.

†P>.12 for all 10 other ROIs.

‡P>.07 for all 10 other ROIs.

§P>.06 for all 10 other ROIs except r=.467, P<.02 for Δ visual hallucinations vs Δ right anterior cingulate absolute CBF; r=.388, P<.05 for Δ visual hallucinations vs Δ left mesial occipital absolute CBF; and r=−.422, P<.03 for Δ visual hallucinations vs Δ right lateral frontal normalized CBF.

cause of the correlation between rCBF changes in these two regions (Table 3). Changes in experiential measures generally correlated with changes in rCBF in the left amygdala and right mesial occipital cortex to a greater extent than other regions.

COMMENT

Procaine increased global CBF and both absolute and normalized rCBF in anterior paralimbic structures, including amygdala, anterior cingulate, hypothalamus, basal forebrain, insula, and orbitofrontal cortex. Different rCBF activation patterns were associated with different sensory and emotional experiences. Procaine yielded robust (24%) global and even more dramatic anterior paralimbic activation, which persisted even when the global effect was removed by normalization. This confirms the view derived from preclinical studies that procaine and related local anesthetics are selective limbic probes.

The procaine anterior paralimbic activation pattern resembles the distribution of the amygdala and its efferents[4] and, to some extent, that of basal forebrain cholinergic cell bodies and their efferents.[21-23] The anterior (amygdalocentric) portion of the limbic system has been hypothesized to mediate affective, motivational, and endocrine functions, in contrast to the posterior (hippocampocentric) portion, which may be more closely associated with learning and memory.[24] This view is consistent with the selective anterior paralimbic activation noted during procaine-induced emotional experiences.

Reciprocal connections between anterior cingulate and amygdala, insula, basal forebrain, anterior temporal lobe, and other anterior paralimbic structures[25] also mirror the procaine activation pattern. The anterior and posterior cingulate differ in cytoarchitecture[26] and connections with other brain regions.[25] Animal studies suggest that the anterior (executive) cingulate may mediate higher functions, such as affect, attention, semantic processing, and vocalization, while the posterior (evaluative) cingulate may mediate motor and sensory functions.[27] Concomitant procaine-induced affective arousal and anterior (greater than posterior) cingulate activation is consistent with this functional subdivision.

Procaine also yielded decreased normalized (but not absolute) neocortical and cerebellar rCBF, probably because these regions had more modest absolute rCBF increases than limbic structures. However, relative neocortical deactivation might yield limbic activation by release of neocortical modulation. In animals, procaine deactivates cortical[8,28] yet activates limbic[8,29-31] structures, and various anesthetics can cause agitation before sedation, perhaps because of deactivation of inhibitory (possibly neocortical) before excitatory (possibly paralimbic) centers.[32,33] Inhibitory structure deactivation has been proposed to explain preferential limbic activation by anesthetics.[34] However, the observed procaine-induced relative neocortical deactivation need not be causally related to limbic activation, and could even represent a mere artifact of the normalization process.

Subjects with intense procaine-induced visual hallucinations (compared with those without) tended to have greater right occipital cortical (absolute and normalized) and left amygdalar (absolute but not normalized) activation, while absolute (but not normalized) activations in these structures correlated with visual hallucination intensities. In addition, there tended to be positive correlations between the degree of rCBF activation in these structures that were greater in the absolute than in the normalized analyses. Excitatory amygdalar efferents[4] might allow limbic activation to drive visual cortex, yielding visual hallucinations. However, it is also possible that a substantial component of the observed relationships between absolute rCBF activations and visual hallucinations resulted from the (trend) correlation between procaine-induced changes in global CBF and visual hallucinations. This notion is further supported by the greatly attenuated correlations in the normalized analysis. Also, visual phenomena may even occur primarily because of limbic activity.[6] Patients with mood and anxiety disorders report diverse spontaneous paroxysmal psychosensory and emotional phenomena similar to those of patients with complex partial seizures and in excess of those of healthy and medical controls.[35] Limbic dysfunction (with or without associated neocortical changes) might contribute to mediation of such experiences.

The anterior limbic activation observed in subjects with intense fear and the correlation between fear and left amygdalar activation are consistent with evidence that this portion of the limbic system may contribute to the mediation of fear.[36] Indeed, fear is the most common affective response to limbic depth electrode stimulation in patients with epilepsy being evaluated for surgery.[6] Hence, endogenous or spontaneous anxiety and panic could be in part mediated by amygdalar dysfunction. This is consistent with the high levels of γ-aminobutyric $acid_A$–benzodiazepine receptors found in the amygdala,[4] the specific antianxiety effects of benzodiazepines injected in this region,[37] and the ability of γ-aminobutyric $acid_A$ and benzodiazepine antagonists injected into the amygdala to block anxiolytic effects of peripherally administered benzodiazepine.[38]

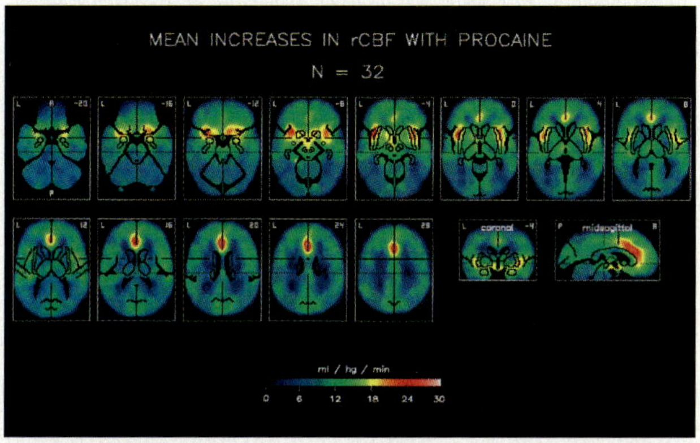

Figure 2. *Procaine increases anterior paralimbic regional cerebral blood flow (rCBF) (mean images). Images are transaxial, coronal, and midsagittal maps of mean increases in Pco_2-adjusted absolute rCBF from baseline (saline) to high-dose procaine in 32 healthy volunteers. Numbers in upper right corners indicate distance from the intercommissural plane in transaxial slices and distance from the anterior commissural plane in coronal slice. L indicates left; A, anterior; and P, posterior. Legend gives rCBF values in milliliters per 100 g of brain tissue per minute.*

The significant inverse relationship observed between left amygdalar rCBF and euphoria suggests a role for deactivation of this structure in procaine-induced euphoria. London et al[39] noted that global cerebral hypometabolism occurred in cocaine- and other drug-induced euphorias. However, our subjects with euphoria had global CBF increases as well as activation of mesial paralimbic structures (hypothalamus, basal forebrain, and anterior cingulate) related to pleasure and reward.[40] Differences between our findings and those of London et al could result from differences in drugs (cocaine vs procaine), subject groups (substance abusers vs healthy controls), or methods (cerebral glucose metabolism by fluorine-18–labeled deoxyglucose vs CBF by oxygen-15–labeled water.

The left amygdalar activation associated with procaine-induced fear and deactivation with euphoria suggests that this structure may contribute to the mediation of different emotional experiences, and that this function could be lateralized as right amygdalar rCBF increased independent of affective responses. Lateralized amygdalar relationships to affect may occur in rodents, as left amygdala electrical kindling decreases and right increases anxiety.[41]

The cingulate gyrus has also been linked to affective experience.[42] Electrical cingulate stimulation yielded various prominent affective experiences in some[43-45] but not all[46-48] studies, and cingulotomy can relieve affective symptoms in some patients.[49-51] In our study, procaine induced particularly robust anterior cingulate activation that was related to visual hallucination intensity in the absolute (but not normalized) analysis. However, in contrast to the left amygdala, anterior cingulate activa-

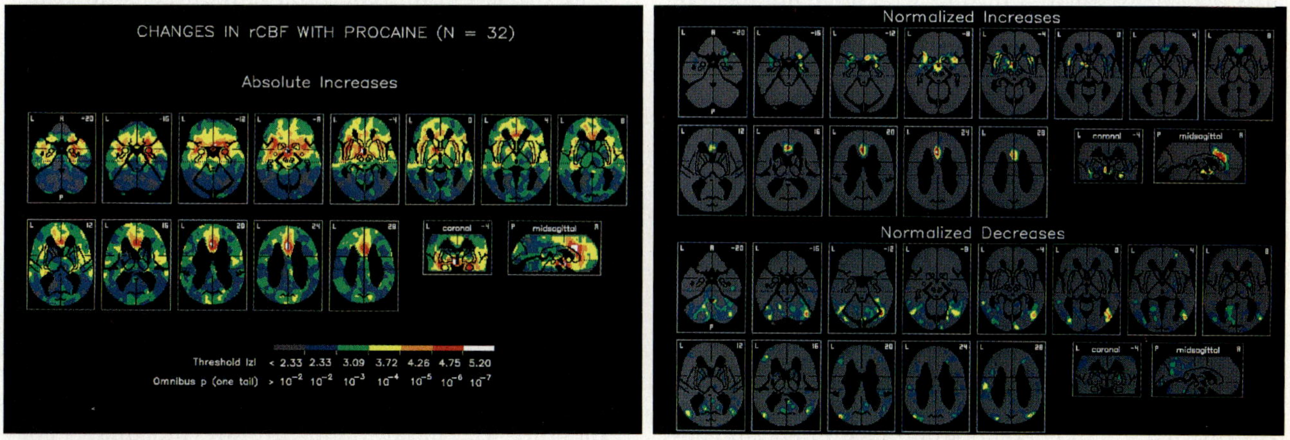

Figure 3. *Procaine increases anterior paralimbic regional cerebral blood flow (rCBF) (statistical parametric map images). Images are transaxial, coronal, and midsagittal* z*-maps of changes in rCBF from baseline (saline) to high-dose procaine in 32 healthy volunteers. Left, Increases in Pco_2-adjusted absolute rCBF. Right, top, Increases in normalized rCBF. Right, bottom, Decreases in normalized rCBF. Numbers in upper right corners indicate distance from the intercommissural plane in transaxial slices and distance from the anterior commissural plane in coronal slices. L indicates left; A, anterior; and P, posterior. Legend gives* z*-values and omnibus one-tailed* P *values (not corrected for multiple comparisons). A strict Bonferroni-type correction requires a threshold of about* $P=10^{-4}$*, coded as yellow or above. A more liberal correction in the setting of a priori hypotheses allows a threshold of about* $P=10^{-3}$*, coded as green or above. Note the similarities of anterior paralimbic increases in the corresponding absolute (left) and normalized (right, top) analyses. There were no voxels with decreases in the absolute analysis (not illustrated). Note the similarity of the pattern of neocortical and cerebellar decreases in the normalized analysis (right, bottom) to regions with minimal increases in the absolute analysis (left).*

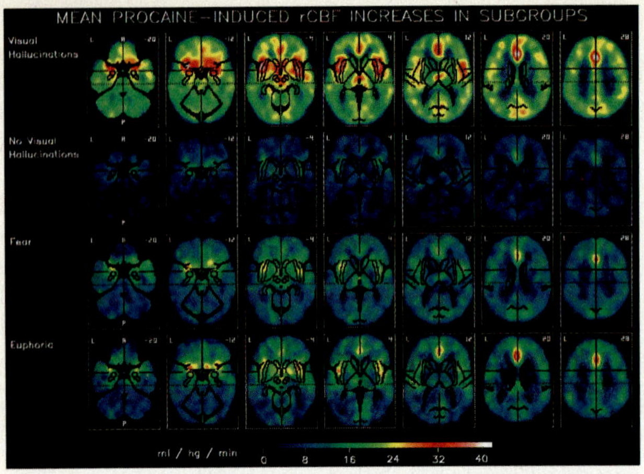

Figure 4. *Heterogeneity of clinical and regional cerebral blood flow (rCBF) responses to procaine. Images are transaxial maps of mean increases in Pco_2-adjusted absolute rCBF from baseline (saline) to high-dose procaine. First row, Nine subjects with intense procaine-induced visual hallucinations; second row, nine with no procaine-induced visual hallucinations; third row, nine with intense procaine-induced fear; and fourth row, nine with intense procaine-induced euphoria. Numbers in upper right corners indicate distance from the intercommissural plane in transaxial slices and distance from the anterior commissural plane in coronal slices. L indicates left; A, anterior; and P, posterior. Legend gives rCBF values in milliliters per 100 g of brain tissue per minute. Note the difference in diffuse activation between subjects with visual hallucinations and those without them, and the occipital flow in the visual hallucinations group, paralleling the findings of the region of interest analysis (Table 2). Mean differences between subjects with fear and those with euphoria were less pronounced. Differential left amygdalar responses in these two subgroups noted in the unfiltered region of interest analysis (Table 2) were not evident in these images, possibly because of the smoothing and the small size of the amygdala.*

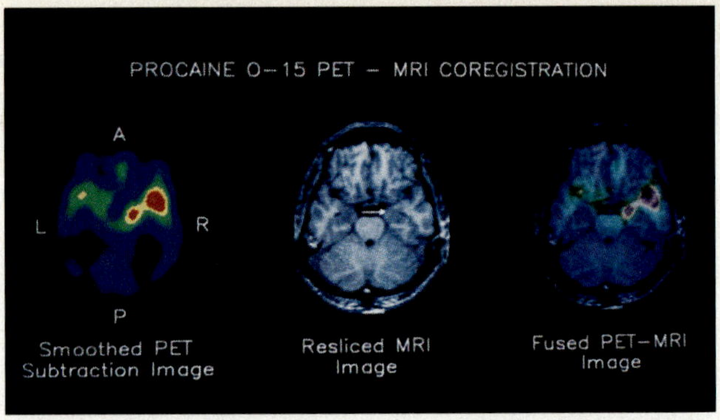

Figure 5. *Procaine-induced regional cerebral blood flow (rCBF) increases coregistered with magnetic resonance imaging (MRI) in an individual subject. Flame scale (blue<green<yellow<red) depicts absolute rCBF increases. Left, Positron emission tomographic (PET) subtraction (high-dose procaine minus saline) image, smoothed to aid visualization. The region of interest analysis (described in the text) did not involve the use of such smoothed subtraction images, but involved drawing regions on the coregistered magnetic resonance images and then transferring them to the* unfiltered *PET saline and procaine images for assessment of mean rCBF within regions. Center, Magnetic resonance image resliced in plane PET slice (corresponding to about 16 mm below the intercommissural plane in Talairach space), with an arrow indicating the right amygdala. Right, Fused PET-magnetic resonance image showing activation of right more than left anterior paralimbic rCBF in this individual.*

tion failed to correlate with affective responses to procaine.

A full discussion of possible mechanisms of procaine's selective anterior paralimbic activation is beyond the scope of this report, although we will briefly consider two important candidates. Like cocaine, procaine is a potent sodium-channel blocker. Sodium channels appear maximal in regions with large numbers of synapses in a widespread pattern consistent with procaine's ability to increase global rCBF, but quite different from the procaine anterior paralimbic activation pattern.[52] However, a sodium-channel mechanism for procaine's specific limbic activation cannot be categorically excluded, as it is possible that procaine could bind with enhanced affinity to an as yet uncharacterized sodium-channel subtype particularly abundant in anterior paralimbic structures.

Cholinergic mechanisms are of particular interest as high levels of choline acetyltransferase occur in the primate amygdala and related paralimbic structures,[4] and this system appears disrupted in mood disorders.[53] The procaine activation pattern somewhat resembles the distribution of efferents from basal forebrain cholinergic cell bodies (Ch1 to Ch4).[21-23] The nucleus basalis of Meynert (Ch4) has particularly dense limbic and paralimbic reciprocal connections and cortical efferents that might allow it to be a cholinergic relay between the limbic system and neocortex to allow affective states to modulate complex behaviors.[23,54,55] Procaine binds to muscarinic M2 receptors,[56] inhibits quinuclidinylbenzilate binding,[57] and is a noncompetitive (negative allosteric) modulator of nicotinic acetylcholine receptor-gated cation channels.[58-60] Muscarinic antagonists retard amygdaloid electrical kindling,[61-64] while direct amygdalar administration of the cholinomimetic carbachol yields amygdalar depolarization and repetitive firing,[65] and development of kindled seizures similar to amygdalar electrical kindling.[66,67] Recent work in our branch suggests that atropine inhibits and physostigmine weakly facilitates procaine seizure kindling in rodents (Terri Heynen and Susan Weiss, PhD, unpublished data, May 1995). Procaine derivatives have even shown promise as cholinergic receptor ligands.[57,68] Positron emission tomography and single-photon-emission computed tomography radiotracers with affinity for muscarinic receptor subtypes[69,70] may eventually aid in exploring whether cholinergic mechanisms account for procaine's specific anterior paralimbic activation pattern.

LIMITATIONS AND CAUTIONS IN INTERPRETATION

Procaine and related local anesthetics have complex direct vascular actions that could confound assessments of cerebral effects based on inferring neuronal activation from rCBF changes. In animals, lidocaine constricts pulmonary and mesenteric[71] but dilates pial[72] and nasal[73] vessels, while procaine constricts mesenteric,[71] nasal,[73] and carotid[74] but dilates coronary[75] vasculature. In humans, procaine may constrict umbilical vessels[76] and increase cerebrovascular resistance[77] but dilate intradermal vessels.[78] Possible impacts of procaine's vascular properties on our study include not affecting, attenuating (through vasoconstriction), or enhancing (through vasodilation) the apparent degree of activation. In view of the observed dramatic procaine-induced rCBF increases, only the latter entails a possible methodologic confounder. In addition, flow changes in large vessels (interior carotid and anterior and middle cerebral arteries) close to anterior paralimbic structures could be a confounding factor.

Several facts suggest it is unlikely that our findings are confounded in a major way by such vascular considerations. First, previous animal and human studies provide substantial evidence that procaine and related local anesthetics dramatically influence anterior paralimbic function as assessed by methods (cerebral glucose metabolism in rats and electrical activity in rats, cats, and humans) independent of major vascular confounders.[8,12,30,31,79,80] Second, we have observed correlations between procaine-induced rCBF and electroencephalographic changes.[81] Third, procaine-induced rCBF changes correlated with experiential measures. Fourth, it is unlikely that vascular effects could cause the observed left vs right amygdala ROI rCBF differences. Fifth, the procaine rCBF activation pattern, although bearing some resemblance to the major anterior cerebral vessels, has important differences, including more robust increases in the dorsal ("downstream") compared with ventral ("upstream") anterior cingulate and the abrupt cutoff of activation in the middle cingulate. Sixth, if there was a major vascular artifact caused by the anterior great vessels, then there ought to be a similar artifact caused by the posterior great vessels, and this was not observed. Seventh, one depressed patient who responded positively to intravenous procaine received a 30-minute continuous procaine infusion, and the same anterior paralimbic activation pattern was observed in cerebral glucose metabolism as assessed by the serial ("split") fluorine-18–labeled deoxyglucose method (unpublished data, T.A.K., M.S.G., and R.M.P., June 1993). Studies of cerebral function with fluorine-18–labeled deoxyglucose or biochemically specific (eg, muscarinic receptor or labeled procaine itself) radioligands could help further confirm that the vascular effects of procaine and the proximity of major arteries are not substantially confounding our findings.

Although the spatial and temporal resolution of our PET method appeared adequate to suggest procaine activation of anterior paralimbic rCBF, methods with greater resolution, such as functional MR imaging, may yield more detailed information. This technique could also allow intraindividual determinations of significant activations, which would be of considerable utility in exploring relationships between experiential and rCBF responses in view of the substantial interindividual differences in these measures. Recently developed methods using contrast agents with functional MR imaging might even allow quantitative (absolute) assessment of procaine's rCBF effects.[82] Also, more detailed pharmacokinetic data, such as blood procaine concentrations every 15 seconds, could aid in exploring relationships between procaine levels and experiential and rCBF responses, and would be particularly useful combined with methods with superior temporal resolution, such as functional MR imaging.

In the ROI analysis, right and left amygdala rCBF were primary outcome measures and a correction for multiple comparisons was applied. However, findings for other ROIs (in particular, occipital lobe ROIs and their relationships to visual hallucinations) must be considered with caution and require replication, as a correction for multiple comparisons was not applied. Similarly, in the SPM analysis, although mean images suggested differences between experiential subgroups, these findings did not exceed thresholds set to account for multiple comparisons. Assessment of these differences requires larger experiential subgroups.

CONCLUSION

This study suggests that procaine is a selective anterior paralimbic activator. Along with reports that paralimbic electrical stimulation yields pleomorphic affective and sensory responses,[6,7] our data suggest that functional changes in the same brain regions may be associated with highly divergent affective responses. In preliminary data from our group, patients with mood disorder had lower anterior paralimbic rCBF at rest than healthy controls[83] and markedly blunted procaine rCBF responses.[84] Taken together, these observations suggest that anterior paralimbic structures could contribute to the mediation of emotional experiences in health, and that dysfunction of these structures could underlie some of the affective and perceptual symptoms seen in mood disorders.

Accepted for publication July 28, 1995.

We thank the staff of the National Institutes of Health cyclotron facility for isotope production; Paul Baldwin; Gerard Jacobs; Stacey Stein; Shielah Green; Margaret Der, BScPharm; Melvin Packer, RT; Kimberly Robles, RT; and Brian Murry, RT, for data acquisition and processing; Joe Maisog, MD; Barry Horwitz, PhD; and James Haxby, PhD, for assistance with the data analysis; and Karen Berman, MD; William Theodore, MD; and James Haxby, PhD, for reviewing the manuscript.

Presented in part at the 48th Annual Meeting of the Society of Biological Psychiatry, San Francisco, Calif, May 22, 1993.

Reprint requests to Biological Psychiatry Branch, National Institute of Mental Health, Bldg 10, Room 3N212, 9000 Rockville Pike, Bethesda, MD 20892 (Dr Ketter).

REFERENCES

1. Papez JW. A proposed mechanism of emotion. *Arch Neurol Psychiatry.* 1937; 38:725-743.
2. Post RM. Does limbic system dysfunction play a role in affective illness? In: Doane BK, Livingston KE, eds. *The Limbic System: Functional Organization and Clinical Disorders.* New York, NY: Raven Press; 1986:229-249.
3. Stevens JR. Interictal clinical manifestations of complex partial seizures and their treatment. *Adv Neurol.* 1975;2:85-112.
4. Amaral DG, Price JL, Pitkanen A, Carmichael ST. Anatomical organization of the primate amygdaloid complex. In: Aggleton JP, ed. *The Amygdala: Neurobiological Aspects of Emotion, Memory, and Mental Dysfunction.* New York, NY: Wiley-Liss Inc; 1992:1-66.
5. Post RM, Uhde TW, Joffe RT, Bierer L. Psychiatric manifestations and implications of seizure disorders. In: Extein I, Gold MS, eds. *Medical Mimics of*

Psychiatric Disorders. Washington, DC: American Psychiatric Press; 1986:33-91.
6. Gloor P, Olivier A, Quesney LF, Andermann F, Horowitz S. The role of the limbic system in experiential phenomena of temporal lobe epilepsy. *Ann Neurol.* 1982;12:129-144.
7. Halgren E, Walter RD, Cherlow DG, Crandall PH. Mental phenomena evoked by electrical stimulation of the human hippocampal formation and amygdala. *Brain.* 1978;101:83-117.
8. Racine R, Livingston K, Joaquin A. Effects of procaine hydrochloride, diazepam, and diphenylhydantoin on seizure development in cortical and subcortical structures in rats. *Electroencephalogr Clin Neurophysiol.* 1975;38:355-365.
9. Post RM, Kennedy C, Shinohara M, Squillace K, Miyaoka M, Suda S, Ingvar DH, Sokoloff L. Metabolic and behavioral consequences of lidocaine-kindled seizures. *Brain Res.* 1984;324:295-303.
10. Wagman IH, De Jong RH, Prince DA. Effects of lidocaine on the central nervous system. *Anesthesiology.* 1967;28:155-172.
11. Munson ES, Gutnick MJ, Wagman IH. Local anesthetic drug-induced seizures in rhesus monkeys. *Anesth Analg.* 1970;49:986-997.
12. Kellner CH, Post RM, Putnam F, Cowdry R, Gardner D, Kling MA, Minichiello MD, Trettau JR, Coppola R. Intravenous procaine as a probe of limbic system activity in psychiatric patients and normal controls. *Biol Psychiatry.* 1987;22:1107-1126.
13. Endicott J, Spitzer RL. A diagnostic interview: the Schedule for Affective Disorders and Schizophrenia. *Arch Gen Psychiatry.* 1978;35:837-844.
14. Koeppe RA, Holden JE, Ip WR. Performance comparison of parameter estimation techniques for the quantitation of local cerebral blood flow by dynamic positron computed tomography. *J Cereb Blood Flow Metab.* 1985;5:224-234.
15. Friston KJ, Frith CD, Liddle PF, Frackowiak RS. Comparing functional (PET) images: the assessment of significant change. *J Cereb Blood Flow Metab.* 1991;11:690-699.
16. Woods RP, Cherry SR, Mazziotta JC. Rapid automated algorithm for aligning and reslicing PET images. *J Comput Assist Tomogr.* 1992;16:620-633.
17. Friston KJ, Passingham RE, Nutt JG, Heather JD, Sawle GV, Frackowiak RS. Localisation in PET images: direct fitting of the intercommissural (AC-PC) line. *J Cereb Blood Flow Metab.* 1989;9:690-695.
18. Talairach J, Tournoux P; Rayport M, trans. *Co-Planar Stereotactic Atlas of the Human Brain.* New York, NY: Thieme Medical Publishers Inc; 1988.
19. Friston KJ, Frith CD, Liddle PF, Dolan RJ, Lammertsma AA, Frackowiak RS. The relationship between global and local changes in PET scans. *J Cereb Blood Flow Metab.* 1990;10:458-466.
20. American Psychiatric Association, Committee on Nomenclature and Statistics. *Diagnostic and Statistical Manual of Mental Disorders, Revised Third Edition.* Washington, DC: American Psychiatric Association; 1987.
21. Gaykema RP, Gaal G, Traber J, Hersh LB, Luiten PG. The basal forebrain cholinergic system: efferent and afferent connectivity and long-term effects of lesions. *Acta Psychiatr Scand Suppl.* 1991;366:14-26.
22. Nieuwenhuys R. Survey of chemically defined cell groups and pathways: acetylcholine. In: Nieuwenhuys R, ed. *Chemoarchitecture of the Brain.* New York, NY: Springer-Verlag; 1985:7-11.
23. Mesulam MM. Structure and function of cholinergic pathways in the cerebral cortex, limbic system, basal ganglia and thalamus of the human brain. In: Bloom FE, Kupfer DJ, eds. *Psychopharmacology: The Fourth Generation of Progress.* New York, NY: Raven Press; 1995:135-146.
24. Mesulam MM. Neural substrates of behavior: the effects of brain lesions upon mental state. In: Nicholi AM, ed. *The New Harvard Guide to Psychiatry.* Cambridge, Mass: Harvard University Press; 1988:91-128.
25. Van Hoesen GW, Morecraft RJ, Vogt BA. Connections of the monkey cingulate cortex. In: Vogt BA, Gabriel M, eds. *Neurobiology of Cingulate Cortex and Limbic Thalamus: A Comprehensive Handbook.* Boston, Mass: Birkhauser; 1993:249-284.
26. Vogt BA. Structural organization of cingulate cortex: areas, neurons, and somatodendritic transmitter receptors. In: Vogt BA, Gabriel M, eds. *Neurobiology of Cingulate Cortex and Limbic Thalamus: A Comprehensive Handbook.* Boston, Mass: Birkhauser; 1993:19-70.
27. Vogt BA, Finch DM, Olson CR. Functional heterogeneity in cingulate cortex: the anterior executive and posterior evaluative regions. *Cereb Cortex.* 1992;2:435-443.
28. Elliot HW, Quilici GC, Elison C. Central effects of local anesthetics. *Fed Proc.* 1960;19:274.
29. Babb TL, Perryman KM, Lieb JP, Finch DM, Crandall PH. Procaine-induced seizures in epileptic monkeys with bilateral hippocampal foci. *Electroencephalogr Clin Neurophysiol.* 1979;47:725-737.
30. Adamec RE, Stark-Adamec C, Saint-Hilaire JM, Livingston KE. Basic science and clinical aspects of procaine HCl as a limbic system excitant. *Prog Neuropsychopharmacol Biol Psychiatry.* 1985;9:109-119.
31. Adamec RE, Stark-Adamec C. The effects of procaine HCl on population cellular and evoked response activity within the limbic system of the cat: evidence for differential excitatory action of procaine in a variety of limbic circuits. *Prog Neuropsychopharmacol Biol Psychiatry.* 1987;11:345-364.
32. Tanaka K, Yamasaki M. Blocking of cortical inhibitory synapses by intravenous lidocaine. *Nature.* 1966;209:207-208.
33. Scott DB. Toxic effects of local anaesthetic agents on the central nervous system. *Br J Anaesth.* 1986;58:732-735.
34. De Jong RH. Central nervous system effects. In: de Jong RH, ed. *Local Anesthetics.* St Louis, Mo: Mosby-Year Book Inc; 1994:264-303.
35. Silberman EK, Post RM, Nurnberger J, Theodore W, Boulenger JP. Transient sensory, cognitive and affective phenomena in affective illness: a comparison with complex partial epilepsy. *Br J Psychiatry.* 1985;146:81-89.
36. Rauch SL, Savage CR, Alpert NM, Miguel E, Baer L, Breiter HC, Fischman AJ, Manzo PA, Moretti C, Jenike MA. A positron emission tomographic study of simple phobic symptom provocation. *Arch Gen Psychiatry.* 1995;52:20-28.
37. Thomas SR, Lewis ME, Iversen SD. Correlation of [3H]diazepam binding density with anxiolytic locus in the amygdaloid complex of the rat. *Brain Res.* 1985;342:85-90.
38. Sanders SK, Shekhar A. Anxiolytic effects of chlordiazepoxide blocked by injection of GABA-A and benzodiazepine receptor antagonists in the region of the anterior basolateral amygdala of rats. *Biol Psychiatry.* 1995;37:473-476.
39. London ED, Cascella NG, Wong DF, Phillips RL, Dannals RF, Links JM, Herning R, Grayson R, Jaffe JH, Wagner HN. Cocaine-induced reduction of glucose utilization in human brain: a study using positron emission tomography and [fluorine 18]-fluorodeoxyglucose. *Arch Gen Psychiatry.* 1990;47:567-574.
40. Porrino LJ. Cortical mechanisms of reinforcement. In: Vogt BA, Gabriel M, eds. *Neurobiology of Cingulate Cortex and Limbic Thalamus: A Comprehensive Handbook.* Boston, Mass: Birkhauser; 1993:445-460.
41. Adamec RE, Morgan HD. The effect of kindling of different nuclei in the left and right amygdala on anxiety in the rat. *Physiology Behav.* 1994;55:1-12.
42. Devinsky O, Luciano D. The contributions of cingulate cortex to human behavior. In: Vogt BA, Gabriel M, eds. *Neurobiology of Cingulate Cortex and Limbic Thalamus: A Comprehensive Handbook.* Boston, Mass: Birkhauser; 1993:528-556.
43. Laitinen LV, Vilkki J. Observations on the transcallosal emotional connections. In: Laitinen LV, Livingston KE, eds. *Surgical Approaches in Psychiatry.* Baltimore, Md: University Park Press; 1973:74-80.
44. Meyer G, McElhaney M, Martin W, McGraw CP. Stereotactic cingulotomy with results of acute stimulation and serial psychological testing. In: Laitinen LV, Livingston KE, eds. *Surgical Approaches in Psychiatry.* Baltimore, Md: University Park Press; 1973:39-58.
45. Talairach J, Bancaud J, Geier S, Bordas FM, Bonis A, Szikla G, Rusu M. The cingulate gyrus and human behaviour. *Electroencephalogr Clin Neurophysiol.* 1973;34:45-52.
46. Lewin W, Whitty CWM. Effects of anterior cingulate stimulation in conscious human subjects. *J Neurophysiol.* 1960;23:445-447.
47. Escobedo F, Fernandez-Guardiola A, Solis G. Chronic stimulation of the cingulum in humans with behavioral disorders. In: Laitinen LV, Livingston KE, eds. *Surgical Approaches in Psychiatry.* Baltimore, Md: University Park Press; 1973:65-68.
48. Van Buren JM, Fedio P. Functional representation on the medial aspect of the frontal lobes in man. *J Neurosurg.* 1976;44:275-289.
49. Bailey HR, Dowling JL, Davies E. Cingulotractotomy and related procedures for severe depressive illness. In: Sweet WH, Obrador S, Martin-Rodriguez JG, eds. *Neurosurgical Treatment in Psychiatry, Pain, and Epilepsy.* Baltimore, Md: University Park Press; 1977:229-251.
50. Ballantine HT Jr, Levy BS, Dagi TF, Giriunas IB. Cingulotomy for psychiatric illness: report of 13 years' experience. In: Sweet WH, Obrador S, Martin-Rodriguez JG, eds. *Neurosurgical Treatment in Psychiatry, Pain, and Epilepsy.* Baltimore, Md: University Park Press; 1977:333-353.
51. Winston F. Treatment of depression after cingulotomy. In: Hitchcock ER, Ballantine HT Jr, Meyerson BA, eds. *Modern Concepts in Psychiatric Surgery.* New York, NY: Elsevier Science Publishing Co Inc; 1979:273-282.
52. Worley PF, Baraban JM. Site of anticonvulsant action on sodium channels: autoradiographic and electrophysiological studies in rat brain. *Proc Natl Acad Sci U S A.* 1987;84:3051-3055.
53. Janowsky DS, Risch SR. Role of acetylcholine mechanisms in the affective disorders. In: Meltzer HY, ed. *Psychopharmacology: The Third Generation of Progress.* New York, NY: Raven Press; 1987:527-533.
54. Mesulam MM, Geula C. Nucleus basalis (Ch4) and cortical cholinergic innervation in the human brain: observations based on the distribution of acetylcholinesterase and choline acetyltransferase. *J Comp Neurol.* 1988;275:216-240.

55. Mesulam MM, Hersh LB, Mash DC, Geula C. Differential cholinergic innervation within functional subdivisions of the human cerebral cortex: a choline acetyltransferase study. *J Comp Neurol.* 1992;318:316-328.
56. Hisayama T, Takayanagi I, Kumagai N, Kubo H. Interaction of 8-(N,N-diethylamino) octyl 3,4,5-trimethoxybenzoate hydrochloride, ryanodine and procaine with muscarinic cholinergic M2 receptor sites in smooth muscle. *J Pharmacol Exp Ther.* 1989;249:646-651.
57. Saraswati M, Hashmi M, Abood LG. 4-Bromoacetamidoprocaine: an affinity ligand for brain muscarinic and nicotinic cholinergic receptors. *Neurochem Res.* 1992;17:247-252.
58. Léna C, Changeux JP. Allosteric modulations of the nicotinic acetylcholine receptor. *Trends Neurosci.* 1993;16:181-186.
59. Yost CS, Dodson BA. Inhibition of the nicotinic acetylcholine receptor by barbiturates and by procaine: do they act at different sites? *Cell Mol Neurobiol.* 1993;13:159-172.
60. Arneric SP, Sullivan JP, Williams M. Neuronal nicotinic acetylcholine receptors: novel targets for central nervous system therapeutics. In: Bloom FE, Kupfer DJ, eds. *Psychopharmacology: The Fourth Generation of Progress.* New York, NY: Raven Press; 1995:95-110.
61. Arnold PS, Racine RJ, Wise RA. Effects of atropine, reserpine, 6-hydroxydopamine, and handling on seizure development in the rat. *Exp Neurol.* 1973; 40:457-470.
62. Cain DP, McKitrick DJ, Desborough KA. Effects of treatment with scopolamine and naloxone, singly and in combination, on amygdala kindling. *Exp Neurol.* 1987;96:97-103.
63. Westerberg V, Corcoran ME. Antagonism of central but not peripheral cholinergic receptors retards amygdala kindling in rats. *Exp Neurol.* 1987;95:194-206.
64. Cain DP, Desborough KA, McKitrick DJ. Retardation of amygdala kindling by antagonism of NMD-aspartate and muscarinic cholinergic receptors: evidence for the summation of excitatory mechanisms in kindling. *Exp Neurol.* 1988; 100:179-187.
65. Washburn MS, Moises HC. Muscarinic responses of rat basolateral amygdaloid neurons recorded in vitro. *J Physiol.* 1992;449:121-154.
66. Goddard GV. Analysis of avoidance conditioning following cholinergic stimulation of amygdala in rats. *J Comp Physiol Psychol.* 1969;68:1-18.
67. Cain DP. Bidirectional transfer of electrical and carbachol kindling. *Brain Res.* 1983;260:135-138.
68. Abood LG, Saraswati M, Lerner-Marmarosh N, Hashmi M. Affinity ligands and related agents for brain muscarinic and nicotinic cholinergic receptors. *Biochem Pharmacol.* 1993;45:2143-2148.
69. Wilson AA, Scheffel UA, Dannals RF, Stathis M, Ravert HT, Wagner HN Jr. In vivo biodistribution of two [18F]-labelled muscarinic cholinergic receptor ligands: 2-[18F]- and 4-[18F]-fluorodexetimide. *Life Sci.* 1991;48:1385-1394.
70. McPherson DW, DeHaven-Hudkins DL, Callahan AP, Knapp FF Jr. Synthesis and biodistribution of iodine-125-labeled 1-azabicyclo[2.2.2]oct-3-yl alpha-hydroxy-alpha-(1-iodo-1-propen-3-yl)-alpha-phenylacetate: a new ligand for the potential imaging of muscarinic receptors by single photon emission computed tomography. *J Med Chem.* 1993;36:848-854.
71. Altura BM, Altura BT. Effects of local anesthetics, antihistamines, and glucocorticoids on peripheral blood flow and vascular smooth muscle. *Anesthesiology.* 1974;41:197-214.
72. Altura BM, Lassoff S. Perivascular action of the local anaesthetic, lidocaine, on pial terminal arterioles: direct observations on the microcirculation. *Br J Pharmacol.* 1981;73:577-579.
73. Wang HW, Jackson RT. Effects of lidocaine and procaine on canine nasal blood vessels. *Ann Otol Rhinol Laryngol.* 1988;97:409-413.
74. Jacobs A, Keatinge WR. Effects of procaine and lignocaine on electrical and mechanical activity of smooth muscle of sheep carotid arteries. *Br J Pharmacol.* 1974;51:405-411.
75. Imai S, Nakazawa M, Imai H, Nabata H. Effects of procaine on the isolated dog coronary artery. *Arch Int Pharmacodyn Ther.* 1984;271:98-105.
76. Silva de Sa MF, Meirelles RS, Franco J Jr, Rodrigues R. Constriction of human umbilical artery induced by local anesthetics. *Gynecol Obstet Invest.* 1981; 12:123-131.
77. Scheinberg P, Jayne HW, Blackburn LI. Studies of cerebral circulatory functions following intravenous administration of procaine hydrochloride. *Arch Neurol Psychiatry.* 1952;68:815-818.
78. Willatts DG, Reynolds F. Comparison of the vasoactivity of amide and ester local anesthetics: an intradermal study. *Br J Anaesth.* 1985;57:1006-1011.
79. Adamec RE, Stark-Adamec C, Burnham WM, Bruun-Meyer S, Perrin R, Livingston KE. Power spectral analysis of EEG drug response in the kindled rat brain. *Electroencephalogr Clin Neurophysiol.* 1981;52:451-460.
80. Racine R, Burnham WM, Livingston K. The effect of procaine hydrochloride and diazepam, separately or in combination, on cortico-generalized kindled seizures. *Electroencephalogr Clin Neurophysiol.* 1979;47:204-212.
81. Parekh PI, Spencer JW, George MS, Gill DS, Ketter TA, Andreason PJ, Herscovitch P, Post RM. Procaine-induced increases in limbic rCBF correlate positively with increases in occipital and temporal EEG fast activity. *Brain Topography.* 1995;7:209-216.
82. Levin JM, Kaufman MJ, Mendelson JH, Cohen BM, Renshaw PF. Functional MR measurement of drug effect on the human brain. In: Program and abstracts of the Annual Meeting of the American College of Neuropsychopharmacology; December 12-16, 1994; San Juan, Puerto Rico. Abstract.
83. Ketter TA, Andreason PJ, George MS, Marangell LB, Pazzaglia PJ, Post RM. Reduced resting frontal lobe CBF in mood disorders. In: Program and abstracts of the 146th Annual Meeting of the American Psychiatric Association; May 22-27, 1993; San Francisco, Calif. Abstract NR298.
84. Ketter TA, Andreason PJ, George MS, Pazzaglia PJ, Marangell LB, Post RM. Blunted CBF response to procaine in mood disorders. In: Program and abstracts of the 146th Annual Meeting of the American Psychiatric Association; May 22-27, 1993; San Francisco, Calif. Abstract NR297.

ORIGINAL ARTICLE

High School Students Who Use Crack and Other Drugs

Denise B. Kandel, PhD, Mark Davies, MPH

Background: When it appeared in the 1980s, crack was thought to represent a completely new pathway of entry into drug use. Our objective was to identify the distinguishing characteristics of adolescents who have reached different stages of drug use, in particular the highest state represented by crack.

Methods: Adolescents (N=7611) representative of students in grades 7 to 12 from 53 New York state schools were classified in the following six mutually exclusive, cumulative categories of drug use: nonusers; alcohol and/or cigarette users only; marijuana users only; users of illicit drugs other than marijuana but neither cocaine nor crack; cocaine but not crack users; and crack users. The groups were compared in level of psychosocial functioning.

Results: Students who use illicit drugs show deficits in school performance, quality of family relationships, and health and increased psychological symptoms. Compared with nonusers, they are more delinquent and more actively involved with their peers and live in social environments in which the perceived use of drugs by other adolescents and parents is more extensive. Delinquency and extent of perceived drug use consistently increase with each higher stage of use. Crack users exhibit the lowest level of psychosocial functioning of any drug-using group.

Conclusions: There are stage-specific characteristics and common characteristics (delinquent participation, peer drug use) throughout the developmental sequence of drug use. Despite declines over the last two decades in the prevalence of the use of different drugs, young people who use drugs display characteristics over historical time similar to those of young drug users 20 years ago.

(Arch Gen Psychiatry. 1996;53:71-80)

MORE IS known about the extent of the use of crack by adolescents and young adults than about the characteristics of crack users compared with those of users of other types of drugs. Prevalence estimates of the use of crack have been released annually for national samples of high school seniors in the United States since 1987 and for eighth and 10th graders since 1990.[1] Several Canadian epidemiological reports are also available.[2-4] Fagan,[5] Fagan and Chin,[6,7] and Johnston and associates[8] have carried out studies of the spread of crack in low-income neighborhoods, and in particular of the relationship among crack, violence, and drug selling. One publication contrasts the characteristics of cocaine and crack users.[9]

Crack, which appeared suddenly in urban centers in the mid 1980s, was thought to represent a completely new pathway of entry into drug use, disrupting the normal social processes attending drug initiation and progression to use of various other forms of drugs (*New York Times*. March 28, 1989:A20). Although it was commonly believed that young people initiate drug use with crack, we have found that crack is the last drug in the sequence of drug use.[10] Except for the addition of crack, the developmental pattern identified in the early 1970s still characterizes adolescent pathways of drug use. The sequence involves at the earliest stage the use of at least one drug that is licit for adults, ie, alcohol or cigarettes. Among the illicit drugs, the use of marijuana precedes the use of cocaine other than crack; crack is the last drug used. We observed this pattern in a sample representative of junior and senior high school students in public

From the Department of Psychiatry and School of Public Health, Columbia University (Dr Kandel), and the New York State Office of Mental Health (Dr Kandel and Mr Davies), New York, NY.

See Subjects and Methods on next page

SUBJECTS AND METHODS

SAMPLE AND FIELD PROCEDURES

A school survey of the use of alcoholic beverages, cigarettes, marijuana, cocaine, crack, and other illicit drugs was conducted in a representative sample of 7611 students in grades 7 through 12 in New York state in spring 1988. The two-stage random sample is representative of junior and senior high school students attending public and private schools in New York state. A stratified sample of 54 schools was drawn, and two homerooms from each grade within each school were randomly selected. The four stratification criteria for school selection were (1) geographical area (New York City, other large cities with over 50 000 population, New York City suburbs, other metropolitan areas, and nonmetropolitan areas); (2) proportion of white enrollment (more or less than 50%); (3) public vs private schools; and (4) size of school enrollment in grades 7 and above. Thus, the schools were selected from 20 strata. Active or passive parental consent for the child's participation in the study was obtained, as required by individual schools. Active consent was required for all schools in New York City, where one school was dropped because only 10% of the parents returned the consent form. The completion rate for the target sample of 54 schools in the survey was 83.8%, and varied little by grade in school. Response rates varied from 88.0% in the seventh grade to 82.1% in the 11th grade and 82.4% in the 12th grade. The sample was weighted to reflect the variable probabilities of selection of schools and homerooms and the absentee factor in each school. Relative weights were constructed by using the reciprocals of the probability of selection and the school absentee rate. Final relative weights were obtained by scaling the sum of the weights to equal the number of students who participated in the survey. The logistic regressions included the stratification variables (geography, ethnicity, and funding status) to adjust for strata differences.

Students answered anonymous self-administered structured questionnaires in their classrooms. The closed-end questions covered drug use behaviors as well as domains of life and functioning important in adolescence. In particular, the students were asked how often they had used each of 10 classes of drugs in their lives and in the last month and at what age they initiated the use of each drug class. The specific field conditions, namely school setting, self-administration, and anonymity, maximize the validity and reliability of self-reports of drug use by young people.[13] There was internal consistency of drug reports. Only 1.7% of self-acknowledged lifetime cigarette users reported never to have smoked in answer to a question asking about age at first use of cigarettes. The parallel proportion among marijuana users was 1.3%.

DEFINITION OF VARIABLES

School performance was scored as the mean of the following four items: (1) grades in the fall term (1 indicates below D; 2, mostly Ds; 3, about half Cs and half Ds; 4, mostly Cs; 5, about half Bs and half Cs; 6, mostly Bs; 7, about half As and half Bs; and 8, mostly As); (2) time spent doing homework (1 indicates none; 2, about half an hour a day; 3, about 1 hour a day; 4, about 1½ hours a day; 5, about 2 hours a day; and 6, more than 2 hours a day); (3) how good a student the respondent was (1 indicates not too good; 2, about average; 3, good; 4, very good, and 5, extremely good); and (4) how far the student intended to go in school (1 indicates less than high school; 2, finish high school only; 3, technical, nursing, or business school; 4, some college but less than 4 years; 5, 4 years of college; 6, master's degree or some graduate school; and 7, doctorate or other professional degree) (Cronbach's α=.69, as a measure of internal consistency).

School nonattendance was scored as the sum of the number of school absences in the last year and the number of classes cut in the last month. School absences were coded as follows: 1, none or almost none; 2, 1 to 2 days; 3, 3 to 6 days; 4, 7 to 15 days; and 5, 16 or more days. Number of classes cut were coded as follows: 1, not at all; 2, 1 to 2 days; 3, 3 to 5 days; 4, 6 to 10 days; 5, 11 to 20 days; and 6, more than 20 days (Cronbach's α=.36).

Delinquency was scored as the sum of the number of delinquent acts committed over the past 12 months, from a list of the following 16 items: serious fight at school or work, taken something worth under $50, broken into house or business, set fire to property purposely, argued or had fight with parent, trouble with police, hurt someone badly enough to need bandages or doctor, damaged property at school or work on purpose, taken something from store without paying, hit a teacher or supervisor, taken or used car without permission, argued or had fight with friends, taken part in gang fight, taken something worth more than $50, used weapon to get something from person, and forged or passed bad checks (Cronbach's α=.76).

The Closeness to Parent Scale was the mean of the mother's and father's scores if both parents were in the household; the scale was scored for one parent if the family was not intact. Scales consist of the means of the following three items: how often parent praises child (1 indicates never; 2, one to three times a month; 3, about once a week; 4, several times a week; and 5, everyday); how close youth feels to parent (1 indicates not close; 2, not particularly close; 3, moderately close; 4, quite close; and 5, extremely close); and how dependent student is on parent for advice (1 indicates not at all; 2, a little; 3, quite a bit; 4, very much; and 5, completely) (Cronbach's α=.84).

and private schools in New York state.[10] Similarly, in a snowball sample of minority crack-using young adults in New York City composed of drug arrestees, community residents, and clients in drug treatment programs, crack was found to have been used after marijuana by four of five crack users.[7] Thus, crack appears to be the last drug to be tried both by adolescent drug users who are still in school as well as youths sampled from institutions. The latter group is usually more heavily involved in drug use than students in school.

A stage conceptualization provides a better understanding of the natural history of drug use and a framework within which to investigate more accurately the correlates, risk factors, and consequences of the use of various classes of drugs.[11] The notion of stages allows one to define clearly groups with specific patterns of use, to describe their attributes, and, in a longitudinal design, to isolate systematically within each group those individuals who progress to the next stage within a specific time interval.[12]

The number of parental rules was scored as the sum of the number of items checked on a list of the following 11: time for being in at night, about homework, amount of dating, time spent watching television, against going around with certain boys or girls, eating dinner with family, helping around the house, against smoking, against drinking alcohol, against using drugs, and concerning dress and hair (Cronbach's α=.67).

Extent of involvement in peer activities was scored as the mean frequency of participation in the following six activities: date, listen to records with friends, attend parties, hang out with a group of kids, drive around with friends, and get together with friends after school. Each activity was coded as follows: 1, rarely; 2, less than once a month; 3, one to three times a month; 4, once a week; 5, several times a week; and 6, everyday (Cronbach's α=.76).

Extent of close friends' drug use was scored as the mean of close friends' use of cigarettes, alcohol, marijuana, cocaine and/or crack, and pills (nonmedical use). Each item was coded as follows: 1, none; 2, few; 3, some; 4, most; and 5, all (Cronbach's α=.83).

The Thrill-Seeking Scale consisted of the mean of scores for the following two items: get a kick from things a little dangerous and like to test myself. Each item was coded as follows: 1, disagree strongly; 2, disagree somewhat; 3, agree somewhat; and 4, agree strongly (Cronbach's α=.71).

The Depressive Symptoms Scale score consisted of the mean of the following six items (with each item multiplied by 10): feeling too tired to do things; trouble going to sleep and/or staying asleep; feeling unhappy, sad, or depressed; feeling hopeless about the future; feeling nervous or tense; and worrying too much about things. Each item was coded as follows: 1, not at all; 2, somewhat; or 3, much (Cronbach's α=.79).

The Anxiety Scale score consisted of the mean of the following six items (with each item multiplied by 10): feeling afraid to be alone, being tense with strangers, feeling nervous speaking to group, worried about what people think of me, nervous about doing or saying wrong thing, and worried about making fool of myself. Each item was coded as follows: 1, not at all; 2, somewhat; or 3, much (Cronbach's α=.82).

The Depressive-Anxiety Combined Scale score consisted of the mean results of the Depressive Symptoms Scale and the Anxiety Scale.

Alcohol-related problems were scored as the sum of any of the following seven problems experienced as the result of drinking: becoming depressed; getting into trouble with teachers or the principal; getting into difficulties with friends, getting into trouble with family, getting into trouble with the police; being criticized by someone they were dating; and driving when high (Cronbach's α=.73). Cocaine-related problems were scored as the sum of any of the same seven problems experienced as the result of using cocaine (Cronbach's α=.79).

DATA ANALYSIS

We report results of two analyses. In a first step, descriptive analyses were implemented to present the attributes of students classified as nonusers or five mutually exclusive groups of drug users, representing successively higher stages of drug use. This classification is based on the documentation of stages of drug use in this[12] and other samples.[14] These analyses were restricted to 11th and 12th graders, since there is a relationship among age, patterns of drug use, and mean level of several of the characteristics being examined. In a second step, logistic regressions[15] were conducted on the total sample, with factors from major domains entered simultaneously in the equations to identify stage-specific attributes of drug use. Although the multiple regressions cannot establish causal sequences, they provide a succinct way of summarizing the relative additional importance of specific factors at the different stages.

Five logistic regression models were estimated, one each for the five hierarchical drug-using groups. In each regression model, the dependent variable (logit) was constructed by dividing the probability of being in the particular stage by the probability of being in the prior stage. For example, the probability of alcohol and/or cigarette use was compared with the probability of no use; the probability of marijuana use was compared with the probability of alcohol and/or cigarette use; and so on. The independent variables in each regression were identical and covered the domains of demographics, school commitment, family characteristics, peer group interaction, and health and /or psychological characteristics. The logistic regressions included the stratification variables (geography, ethnicity, and funding status) to adjust for strata differences. Exponentiated logistic regression coefficients (adjusted odds ratios) are given. For example, crack users are compared with cocaine-only users at different levels of delinquent acts, controlling for other covariates. When individuals with four delinquent acts are compared with those with three delinquent acts, the odds of using crack are multiplied by 1.2.

Because the number of respondents differs among the six user categories of the dependent variable, tests of significance for regression coefficients are executed with varying statistical power. There is more power to detect small regression coefficients when no use is compared with alcohol and/or cigarette use than when the use of illicit drugs other than marijuana is compared with cocaine use. Relative effects for specific independent variables should be compared using the absolute value of the odds ratios rather than the level of statistical significance.

In this report, we use the stage framework to inform our understanding of the distinguishing characteristics of young people who have reached different stages of drug use, in particular those who have reached the highest stage represented by crack. We examine functioning in the important domains of a young person's life, including family, peers, deviance, health, psychological symptoms, and drug-related problems. We document that young people still in school who use crack constitute the most maladapted group of youngsters.

We stress at the outset that the data we used for this investigation are cross-sectional and, in many instances, limit the causal inferences that can be made, since a causal order among most factors cannot be determined. For example, drug use could lead to increased delinquency as well as the reverse. However, very little systematic data have appeared in the literature describing the characteristics of crack users drawn from a representative sample of young people. None, to our knowledge, have relied on a developmental stage framework in their analyses.

Table 1. Recent and Daily Use of Drugs Among Students Who Ever Used Each Drug by Cumulative Pattern of Drug Use*

	Cumulative Pattern of Lifetime Drug Use					
Recent Drug Use	Alcohol Only	Cigarettes Only	Marijuana	OID but Not Cocaine	Cocaine but Not Crack	Crack
Last month						
Alcohol	40	...	69	80	85	86†‡
Cigarettes	...	26	55	62	81	83†‡§
Marijuana	...	...	32	48	64	75‡§‖
OID but neither cocaine nor crack	...	...	...	28	24	61‖
Cocaine and/or crack	...	...	...	...	25	56‖
Daily within last month						
Alcohol	1	...	3	7	9	29†‡‖
Cigarettes	...	5	27	35	60	54†‡§
Marijuana	...	...	1	4	11	28‡§‖
OID but neither cocaine nor crack	...	...	...	2	2	16‖
Cocaine and/or crack	...	...	...	...	1	9‖
Total No. of users	3392	2181	995	544	282	121

*Students include seventh to 12th graders. Unless indicated otherwise, data are presented as percentage of students. OID indicates illicit drugs other than marijuana.
†Differences were significant ($P<.05$) between alcohol and/or cigarette and marijuana users.
‡Differences were significant ($P<.05$) between marijuana and OID users.
§Differences were significant ($P<.05$) between OID and cocaine users.
‖Differences were significant ($P<.05$) between cocaine and crack users.

RESULTS

PREVALENCE OF DRUG USE AMONG JUNIOR AND SENIOR HIGH SCHOOL STUDENTS

Our interest is not in prevalence rates of drug use per se, but in the attributes of students who use different classes of drugs. Prevalence levels are only presented as background to the analyses. The rank order of the prevalences of use in this sample is typical of that reported in other epidemiological studies.[1] Alcohol (84%) and cigarettes (52%) were the most frequently used drugs. Less than one third of students (32%) reported having ever used any illicit drug, and less than one fifth (18%) reported having ever used an illicit drug other than marijuana. Marijuana was the most commonly used illicit drug (28%). Stimulants were next in prevalence (11%), followed by inhalants and cocaine in any form (6% each), psychedelics (5%), and crack (2%). Only a small minority of students (1%) reported having ever used heroin.

WHO ARE THE YOUNG PEOPLE WHO USE DRUGS?

A Classification of Drug Users

To understand what distinguishes young people who get involved in different patterns of drug use, the following six groups reflecting cumulative and hierarchical patterns of lifetime drug use were identified and compared: (1) never used any drugs; (2) used only alcohol and/or cigarettes; (3) used marijuana but no other illicit drugs; (4) used illicit drugs other than marijuana but neither cocaine nor crack; (5) used cocaine but not crack; and (6) used crack. The classification is based on results from analyses in which the specific position of crack was examined when marijuana, cocaine, and crack were the only illicit drugs included[10] and analyses in which marijuana, cocaine, and other illicit drugs, but not crack, were considered.[14,16] These analyses have documented that marijuana use precedes the use of other illicit drugs. While a strict order between these other illicit drugs and cocaine has not been systematically investigated, data presented in **Table 1** and **Table 2** support the suggested order of cocaine use between illicit drugs other than marijuana and crack. Cocaine and crack were specifically kept separate because of our interest in identifying the differentiating characteristics of crack users.

The classification reflects the developmental pathway of drug use characteristic of young people and captures their increasingly serious drug use in each succeeding category. Most users in a category have used drug(s) in the lower categories (data not presented). For example, 94.4% of those who have used cocaine have also used marijuana. Furthermore, the higher the drug class, the greater the persistence of use is, as reflected in the prevalence of current use among those who ever used the drug in their lives; the more frequent the use is, as reflected in the proportion of users who reported using the drug daily within the last month (Table 1); and the earlier the age is of first experimentation with all classes of drugs (Table 2). Adolescents who have experimented with crack are much more likely than any other group of youngsters to have experimented with other illicit drugs and to remain current and frequent users. For instance, more than twice as many marijuana users (75%) who also used crack reported using marijuana within the last 30 days preceding the survey, compared with those who had used only marijuana but no other illicit drugs (32%) (Table 1). Twice as many crack users reported using cocaine within the last 30 days, compared with cocaine users who did not use crack, and nine times as many used cocaine daily. Those who have used cocaine, but

Table 2. Age at Onset of Drug Use Among 11th and 12th Grade Students Who Ever Used Specific Drugs by Cumulative Pattern of Drug Use*

	Cumulative Pattern of Lifetime Drug Use				
Drug	Alcohol or Cigarettes Only	Marijuana	OID but Not Cocaine	Cocaine but Not Crack	Crack
Alcohol	12.8±2.7 (1086)	12.3±2.3 (604)	11.7±2.1 (348)	11.4±2.1 (214)	10.7±2.1 (66)†‡§
Cigarettes	13.2±2.5 (568)	13.0±2.2 (553)	12.4±2.2 (314)	11.8±2.2 (201)	11.1±2.2 (59)‡§‖
Marijuana	...	15.0±1.6 (598)	14.4±1.7 (271)	13.4±1.9 (207)	12.7±2.5 (65)‡§‖
Cocaine	...	...	...	15.8±1.3 (205)	14.9±2.4 (61)§
Crack	...	...	...	...	15.6±1.9 (59)

*Data are presented as mean±SD years of age (No. of students). OID indicates illicit drugs other than marijuana.
†Differences were significant ($P<.05$) between alcohol and/or cigarette and marijuana users.
‡Differences were significant ($P<.05$) between marijuana and OID users.
§Differences were significant ($P<.05$) between cocaine and crack users.
‖Differences were significant ($P<.05$) between OID and cocaine users.

not crack, are more likely to use cigarettes and marijuana than those who used illicit drugs other than marijuana but not cocaine.

In considering the age at onset of drug use among different types of drug users, we restricted the analysis to students in the 11th and 12th grades to give all youths an equal opportunity for experimenting with different classes of drugs (Table 2). Students who progressed to using illicit drugs other than marijuana, but neither cocaine nor crack, started smoking cigarettes or drinking alcohol 1 year earlier on average and started using marijuana about 7 months earlier than those who remained exclusive marijuana users. Cocaine users who did not progress to crack use started using all drug classes about 1½ years earlier than any other group, except crack users. Crack users initiated the use of all classes of drugs at least 2 years earlier than any other group. Their mean age at onset of marijuana use was 12.7 years, compared with 15.0 years for those who remained exclusive marijuana users.

Sociodemographic Background Characteristics

Because adolescents at the higher stages are older than those at the lower stages of drug use and because many of the criteria variables are related to age, **Table 3** through **Table 5** are also restricted to 11th and 12th graders.

By and large, the drug-using groups do not differ greatly from each other on sociodemographic characteristics (Table 3). White youths are more likely than minorities to report the use of any class of drug, especially illicit drugs other than cocaine and crack. Family intactness has a curvilinear relationship with position on the sequence of drug use. Income is positively associated with using any class of drugs, compared with not using any. Parental education is related to the use of any drug, rather than to specific drug classes.

Psychosocial Functioning

Much larger differences appear on indicators of psychosocial functioning than on sociodemographic characteristics. The following four areas of functioning, which cover the important dimensions of an adolescent's life, were examined as a function of the student's lifetime cumulative pattern of drug use: commitment to school, quality of relationship with parents and interactions with peers, conformity and participation in deviant activities, and health and psychological functioning. Selected results are presented in Table 3. In addition, we examined extent of drug use in the student's social environment (Table 5). In every arena, drug users, and especially users of illicit drugs, perform at a lower level and conform less than nonusers; users are also more likely than nonusers to live in environments in which the use of drugs is prevalent. There is a monotonic relationship with pattern of drug use, such that for each criterion, students at each successive stage of drug use show greater decrements in adjustment and greater involvement with drug-using peers. Youths who have used crack show the lowest level of psychosocial adjustment of any group. On some characteristics, cocaine users who have not used crack are most similar to those who have used illicit drugs other than marijuana but have not used cocaine. On some other characteristics, cocaine users who have not used crack are more similar to crack users than to any other group.

School Performance. As compared with nonusers, users of illicit drugs report lower school performance and lower interest in academic matters (Table 3). Users obtain lower grades, spend less time on their homework, and are absent from school much more frequently than those who have not used any drugs or have used alcohol or cigarettes exclusively. All crack users who cut classes in school within the past month did so at least 20 times (data not presented).

Family Relationships. Drug users have less satisfactory relationships with their parents than nonusers. Drug users are much less likely than nonusers to report that they are close to their parents (Table 3). Their parents are reported to be also less likely to set rules and standards for their children. Illicit drug users mention a smaller number of rules than nonusers or exclusive users of alcohol or cigarettes.

Peer Relationships. Drug users are much more oriented toward their peers and participate in many more

Table 3. Student Characteristics in Major Domains Among 11th and 12th Graders by Cumulative Pattern of Drug Use*

	Cumulative Pattern of Lifetime Drug Use					
Domains	None	Alcohol or Cigarettes Only	Marijuana	OID but Not Cocaine	Cocaine but Not Crack	Crack
Sociodemographic, % of students						
Male	47	49	49	42	48	70†‡
Ethnicity						
White	42	74	77	91	78	67†§‖
Black	32	11	12	2	5	8†§
Hispanic	12	8	6	3	13	8†‖
Other	14	7	3	4	4	17
Lives with both biological parents	55	72	64	62	54	47§¶
Household income ≥$20 000	68	78	84	82	79	82§¶
Parent is 4-year college graduate	52	34	40	32	27	32†§¶
Commitment to school, % of students						
Fall term grades of A	20	20	11	11	8	5¶
Does homework ≥1 hour per day	68	62	44	41	25	19‖¶
Absent ≥16 days in last year	11	8	16	16	41	51‖¶
Parent and peer relationship, mean±SD score#						
Closeness to Parents Index	3.4±0.9	3.2±0.9	3.1±0.9	2.9±0.9	2.8±0.9	2.4±1.0†‡¶
Parental rules	5.0±2.4	4.7±2.2	4.3±2.0	4.4±2.0	3.8±2.1	4.2±2.7‖¶
Peer activities	2.8±1.2	3.3±1.1	3.9±1.0	4.0±1.0	4.3±1.0	4.4±0.9§‖¶
Conformity and deviance						
Delinquency last year, mean±SD score¶	1.7±1.2	2.7±1.8	3.6±2.2	4.1±2.2	4.5±2.6	6.8±4.5†‡§¶
Attends religious services rarely or never, % of students	37	40	51	53	62	64‖¶
Health, % of students						
Self-reported health excellent	57	45	35	27	17	33†‡§‖¶
Seen physician more than twice in last year						
For physical illness	28	39	44	49	47	40§¶
For psychological problem	4	4	6	12	13	32†‡¶
Psychological characteristics, mean±SD score#						
Thrill seeking	1.9±0.9	2.4±0.9	2.6±0.8	2.8±0.8	2.9±0.9	3.1±0.9†§¶
Depressive symptoms	1.5±4.8	17.3±4.5	17.2±4.6	18.7±4.9	17.8±5.1	17.8±5.9†§‖
Total**	107	1056	575	334	194	60

*OID indicates illicit drugs other than marijuana.
†Differences were significant (P<.05) between marijuana and OID users.
‡Differences were significant (P<.05) between cocaine and crack users.
§Differences were significant (P<.05) between nonusers and alcohol and/or cigarette users.
‖Differences were significant (P<.05) between OID and cocaine users.
¶Differences were significant (P<.05) between alcohol and/or cigarette and marijuana users.
#Scoring is described in the "Definition of Variables" subsection of the "Subjects and Methods" section of the text.
**Totals represent smallest number of persons who answered any question.

activities with their peers than nonusers (Table 3).

Commitment to Conventional Institutions. Drug-using students are less religious and more involved in delinquent activities than nonusers (Table 3). The differences among the five drug-using groups on the mean summary scores of delinquent acts committed within the last year are striking. The higher the stage of drug use, the greater the delinquent participation was.

Health, Psychological Symptoms, and Drug-Related Problems. Drug-using youths report poorer health than nonusers, as reflected both in the subjective assessment of their health status and in the reported number of contacts with health professionals during the prior year. The differences are large for number of visits with a physician for a psychological problem (Table 3).

Except for thrill-seeking, which increases monotonically with increasing drug use, there are no systematic relationships between stage of drug use and scores on two scales of psychological symptoms, anxiety and powerlessness (data not presented). Depression is higher among those who have used any class of drugs than among nonusers; however, no systematic differences appear among users of the various classes of drugs.

The higher the stage of drug use, the greater the proportions are of students experiencing a drug-related problem, and the greater the number is of problems associated with the use of drugs (Table 4). Becoming depressed, driving after having a good bit to drink or after being high, and getting into trouble with one's family are the problems most often mentioned in relation to alcohol. Driving after being high is the most frequent problem associated with the use of cocaine.

The Social Context of Drug Use. Young people who use drugs live in social environments in which they perceive the use of drugs to be prevalent. The higher the stage of drug use, the more extensive the reported use of drugs by peers and parents is (Table 5). Of the students who

Table 4. Problems Experienced With the Use of Alcohol and Cocaine Among Alcohol and Cocaine Users by Cumulative Pattern of Drug Use, 11th and 12th Graders*

	Cumulative Pattern of Lifetime Drug Use						
	Alcohol-Related Problems					Cocaine-Related Problems	
	Alcohol or Cigarettes Only	Marijuana	OID but Not Cocaine	Cocaine but Not Crack	Crack	Cocaine but Not Crack	Crack
Students experiencing each problem two or more times in last year							
Becoming depressed	5	11	15	21	30†	8	16
Driving after having a good bit to drink or being high	1	5	8	18	27†‡	10	33§
Gotten into trouble with family	3	7	11	12	25†§‖	2	9
Gotten into trouble with teacher or principal	0.6	1.0	4	4	16§‖	2	14§
Gotten into difficulties with friends	4	7	10	11	16†	7	12
Criticized by dates	2	6	7	12	14†‡	10	14
Gotten into trouble with police	0.3	0.9	2	4	11	1	3
Students experiencing at least one problem two or more times	9	22	31	47	62†‡§‖	22	53§
No. of problems, mean±SD score	0.5±1.0	1.1±1.3	1.6±1.6	1.8±1.7	2.3±2.2†‖	0.8±1.3	2.0±2.0§
Total¶	1082	591	341	207	65	190	60

**Unless otherwise indicated, data are presented as percentage of students. OID indicates illicit drugs other than marijuana.*
*†Differences were significant (*P<.05*) between alcohol and/or cigarette and marijuana users.*
*‡Differences were significant (*P<.05*) between OID and cocaine users.*
*§Differences were significant (*P<.05*) between cocaine and crack users.*
*‖Differences were significant (*P<.05*) between marijuana and OID users.*
¶Totals represent smallest number of persons who answered any question.

ever used crack, 66% report that all or most of their close friends have used marijuana and 38% have used cocaine and/or crack, compared with only 8% and 0%, respectively, of the students who used no drugs.

The drug users' parents are also reported to smoke cigarettes, drink alcohol, and use medically prescribed tranquilizers within the last year more extensively than the nonusers' parents. The proportion of students who report that their parents drink alcohol daily or smoke cigarettes heavily is more than twice as high among all users of illicit drugs other than marijuana as among students who have never used any drugs. The largest differences appear for the use of tranquilizers. Sex-specific analyses indicate that the differences with respect to mothers' drug consumption are even greater than those for fathers (data not presented).

MULTIVARIATE ANALYSES

The data that we have presented provide a striking portrait of adolescents according to the different stages of drug use to which they have progressed. As we noted earlier, because these are cross-sectional data, the time order between the various covariates and the drug use patterns cannot be clearly established. We carried out logistic regressions on the total sample of students to identify more precisely than can be done from descriptive data, by controlling for age and other potentially confounding factors, the stage-specific correlates of the use of different substances along the developmental pathway of drug use. These analyses allow us to identify the common and unique factors that characterize those who are at one stage of use compared with those at the next adjacent stage. In several instances, we substituted a multi-item scale for individual items presented in Tables 3 to 5 to reduce the number of coefficients to be estimated. Thus, we combined four items into a school performance index and similarly combined the five separate items about number of friends using cigarettes, alcohol, marijuana, cocaine and/or crack, and pills (nonmedical use) into an "extent of peer drug use" scale.

Factors vary in their importance. Certain factors differentiate users at a higher stage from users at the preceding stage at all stages of drug use. Other factors are stage specific (**Table 6**). The two factors that underlie progression to almost every stage are degree of perceived drug use in the peer group and extent of delinquent participation. At every stage along the continuum of drug use, except for crack, students who have progressed to the next highest level compared with those at the adjacent lower level perceive increasingly more extensive use of drugs among their friends. Controlling for all other covariates, however, extent of drug use in the peer group does not differentiate cocaine from crack users. (The data presented in Table 5 suggest that for these youths there is an increase in the number of their friends using cocaine, which is obscured when the combined measure of friends' drug use is used in the multivariate model.) Except for the contrast between illicit drugs other than cocaine and cocaine, increasing delinquency is associated with increasingly higher position in the developmental sequence of drug use.

Other factors are stage specific. Minority students are relatively less likely to start using one of the legal drugs, but among those who have done so the proportions who use marijuana are higher than among nonminorities. The proportions who have progressed to illicit drug use other than cocaine among black youths are lower than among

Table 5. Perceived Friends' and Parents' Drug Use by Cumulative Pattern of Drug Use Among 11th and 12th Graders*

Reported Drug Use of Family and Friends	Cumulative Pattern of Lifetime Drug Use: None	Alcohol or Cigarettes Only	Marijuana	OID but Not Cocaine	Cocaine but Not Crack	Crack
Used by most or all of friends						
Cigarettes	6	18	43	58	72	75†‡§‖
Alcohol	16	46	71	82	88	82†‡§‖
Marijuana	8	6	31	39	66	66‡§‖
Cocaine and/or crack	0	1	1	1	22	38†‖¶
Used by mother and/or father						
Pack or more of cigarettes	22	25	30	38	44	50‡§
Alcohol every day	11	13	14	20	20	28§
Tranquilizers in last year	2	6	9	17	15	25†‡§
Total#	112	1093	586	344	202	62

**Unless otherwise indicated, data are presented as percentage of students. OID indicates illicit drugs other than marijuana.*
†Differences were significant (P<.05) between nonusers and alcohol and/or cigarette users.
‡Differences were significant (P<.05) between alcohol and/or cigarettes and marijuana users.
§Differences were significant (P<.05) between marijuana and OID users.
‖Differences were significant (P<.05) between OID and cocaine users.
¶Differences were significant (P<.05) between cocaine and crack users.
#Totals represent smallest number of persons who answered any question.

white youths, whereas the proportions who have progressed to cocaine and crack use are higher. Parental education level is negatively related to progression to the use of most substances, except for marijuana, for which the relationship is positive. Once an adolescent has experimented with alcohol and/or cigarettes, the higher the parents' education, the higher the probability is that the adolescent will use marijuana. For all other drug classes, the higher the parental education, the lower the rate is of use. Family intactness is important for marijuana use, the illicit drug that provides an initial point of entry to the use of all other illicit drugs. Once having taken that step, family intactness is not associated with any further change in drug use pattern.

School-related factors, such as level of academic achievement and school attendance, are especially important at the first two stages of use. High academic performance is related to lower rates of alcohol or cigarette use and lower rates of marijuana use among those who already experimented with a legal drug. However, these academic factors appear to be relatively unimportant for higher stages of use, except for nonattendance at school, which differentiates those who have progressed to using crack, once having used cocaine, from those who have not.

Lack of commitment to conventional values, as reflected in religious participation, is associated with marijuana use.

Of the family-related variables, lack of closeness to parents and a strong orientation toward peers and away from parents are associated with progression to cocaine use, once the adolescent has experimented with other illicit drugs. Perceived parental use of certain drugs is related to specific stages of drug use. Perceived parental alcohol and/or cigarette use is related to the child's use of these same drugs; parental use of medically prescribed tranquilizers is related to the child's use of marijuana and other illicit drugs.

Psychological symptoms play a specific role in the stage of illicit drug use. Thrill-seeking is positively related to initial experimentation with legal drugs and also differentiates those who have only used marijuana from those who have used other illicit drugs other than cocaine; thrill-seeking is negatively related to using crack compared with other forms of cocaine. Those who have used crack have experienced psychological problems severe enough to require professional help.

COMMENT

In most areas of their lives, students who use drugs perform at a lower level than their peers who are nonusers. Crack users are the most maladjusted of all the drug users. On most characteristics, crack users are more maladjusted or more involved in drug-using peer groups than youths who have used cocaine but not in the form of crack. Two major conclusions can be drawn from the findings. First, after controlling for all other factors, drug use by peers and delinquent participation emerge as the two most important factors that differentiate drug users from nonusers of particular classes of drugs at each stage of the developmental sequence of drug use. At each higher stage of drug use, users are more actively involved with peers whom they perceive to be heavily involved in drug use. At each higher stage, users also are more delinquent. Second, the sharpest differences between drug use patterns occur between alcohol and/or cigarettes and marijuana.

Other than perceived drug use by peers and self-reported delinquency, most other factors are stage specific. Young people who become involved in drug use are alienated from two of the most important institutions in their lives, school and family, but differentially so at different phases. Lowered academic commitment is important in the early stages preceding experimentation with an illicit drug. Detachment from parents is important at later stages in the progression from use of illicit drugs other than marijuana to cocaine. Health deficits increase, especially among students who have progressed to marijuana use and those who have progressed to co-

Table 6. Predictors of Different Stages of Drug Involvement Among Seventh Through 12th Graders by Cumulative Pattern of Drug Use*

	Cumulative Pattern of Lifetime Drug Use				
Predictors†	None vs Alcohol or Cigarettes Only	Alcohol or Cigarettes vs Marijuana	Marijuana vs OID	OID vs Cocaine but Not Crack	Cocaine vs Crack
Sociodemographic					
Male	1.0	1.0	0.7‡	2.0§	1.5
Grade in school (age)	1.2§	1.4§	0.9‖	1.3§	0.7§
Ethnicity					
Black (vs white)	0.6‡	1.6‡	0.2§	3.7‡	3.8‖
Hispanic	0.7	1.3	1.0	3.1‡	1.2
Family not intact	0.9	1.4‡	1.0	1.5‖	0.9
Parental educational level	0.9§	1.1‡	1.0	0.9	0.9
Commitments					
School performance index	0.9	0.7§	1.0	0.8	1.2
School nonattendance	1.2‡	1.3§	1.0	1.3‡	1.2
Frequency of attending religious services	1.0	0.9§	1.1	1.0	1.0
No. of delinquent acts in last 12 mo	1.3§	1.1§	1.1§	1.0	1.2§
Family characteristics					
Closeness to Parents Scale	0.8§	0.9‖	0.9	0.9	0.9
Combined parental cigarette and alcohol use¶	1.2§	1.0	1.1	1.0	1.0
Parental use of tranquilizers¶	1.1	1.1‖	1.1‖	0.9	1.2
Peer group interactions					
Extent of involvement in peer activities	1.3§	1.3§	1.0	1.2	1.1
Extent of peer drug use	4.1§	2.9§	1.9§	2.4§	1.3
Health and/or psychological characteristics					
Visits to doctor for emotional problems¶	1.2	1.1	1.1	1.1	1.2‖
Thrill-Seeking Scale¶	1.3§	1.1	1.2‡	0.9	0.7
Depression-Anxiety Scale	1.1	0.5§	1.6‖	0.7	0.8
Constant	−3.6§	−6.6§	−2.7‡	−4.7§	−0.4
Total No. of students	4434	4840	1890	1071	429

*Unless otherwise indicated, data are shown as exponentiated logistic regression coefficients (adjusted odds ratio). OID indicates illicit drugs other than marijuana.
†Other variables included in the models, but not shown, are sampling strata variables (ie, region of state, public vs private school), ethnicity (other and missing), parental rules, and Powerlessness Scale.
‡P<.01.
§P<.001.
‖P<.05.
¶Dummy for missing value is included in model, but coefficient is not shown.

caine use. Parental alcohol and cigarette use are important for initial experimentation with a legal drug; parental use of a medically prescribed tranquilizer is important for experimentation with illicit drugs. One possibility is that through their use of medically prescribed psychotropic drugs, parents may indicate by example to their children that drugs can be used to handle psychological problems. The children, in turn, may use illicit drugs to handle their own feelings of psychological distress. These analyses suggest that, for some youngsters, the use of illicit drugs may represent a form of self-medication.

We mentioned earlier that characteristics of drug users are rarely investigated within a hierarchical developmental stage framework. We had carried out a similar analysis in the mid 1970s. In contrast to the cross-sectional data presented herein, the earlier report was based on prospective longitudinal data from a sample of New York State students whom we followed up over a 6-month interval. The stage-specific factors identified in that earlier analysis[17,18] are similar to those identified in this sample, almost 20 years later. Perceived drug use in the peer group was the most important factor related to progression at all stages of drug use. Lack of closeness to parents and psychological problems, reflected in depressive symptoms, were found in the earlier study to be particularly strong predictors of progressing from use of marijuana to use of other illicit drugs. Parental alcohol use predicted initiation into legal drug use; parental use of prescribed psychotropic drugs predicted initiation into illicit drug use. Thus, there are regularities in the relevance of stage-specific factors for drug use over historical time, even though prevalence levels might differ over the same period. Similarly, Bachman and collaborators[19] concluded that despite historical fluctuations in overall levels of use, the characteristics of high school seniors who get involved in use of different classes of drugs do not appear to change much over time. Although collected in 1988, the present data still have relevance for our understanding of factors related to adolescent drug use today.

Several limitations of the data need to be highlighted. As we have noted, since these data are cross-sectional, it is not possible to determine whether the declining levels of functioning observed among these youths are determinants or consequences of drug use. Probably both processes are involved. Poorer adjustment tends to precede experimentation with illicit drugs.[17-24] Lowered adjustment is further exacerbated by drug use.[24-27] In addition, this is a school sample. The conclusions characterize young people who are still attending school and cannot necessarily be generalizable to all adolescents. School dropouts have higher rates of drug use than regular students.[28] Whether or not the correlates and risk factors of drug use differ as well between students and dropouts is not known. Finally, the self-reported drug use reports suffer from limitations in validity inherent in such reports. However, the strong differences observed between self-acknowledged users and nonusers argue against a high degree of unreliability and low validity of reports.

Youths who use drugs have many needs. Strengthening both their commitment to schooling and education and their ties to their families might contribute to a reduction in the risk of initiating and persisting in the use of drugs. Age at onset of drug use is continuing to emerge as a crucial risk factor for progression into the most severe forms of drug use. This finding highlights the importance of developing early prevention and education efforts, especially since the postponement of drug experimentation may in itself have positive public health consequences for a young person's well-being, over and beyond that of reducing progression to use of more serious classes of drugs.

Accepted for publication July 19, 1995.

Partially supported by an award from the New York State Department of Mental Hygiene, Albany, NY; a grant from the William T. Grant Foundation, New York, NY; and Research Scientist Award KO5 DA00081 from the National Institute on Drug Abuse, Rockville, Md (Dr Kandel). Partial support for computer costs was provided by Mental Health Clinical Research Center Grant MH30906 from the National Institute of Mental Health, Rockville, Md (New York State Psychiatric Institute).

The research assistance of Christine Schaffran is gratefully acknowledged.

Correspondence to Columbia University, 722 W 168th St, Box 20, New York, NY 10032 (Dr Kandel).

REFERENCES

1. Johnston LD, Bachman JG, O'Malley PM. *Smoking, Drinking, and Illicit Drug Use Among American Secondary School Students, College Students, and Young Adults, 1975-1991.* Rockville, Md: National Institute on Drug Abuse; 1992.
2. Smart RG. 'Crack' cocaine use in Canada: a new epidemic? *Am J Epidemiol.* 1988;127:1315-1317.
3. Smart RG. Crack cocaine use: a review of prevalence and adverse effects. *Am J Drug Alcohol Abuse.* 1991;17:13-26.
4. Smart RG, Adlaf EM. Alcohol, cannabis, cocaine and other substance use among Ontario adults 1977-1987. *Can J Public Health.* 1988;79:206-207.
5. Fagan J. Editor's introduction: myths and realities about crack. *Contemp Drug Probl.* 1990;17:1-7.
6. Fagan J, Chin K. Initiation into crack and cocaine: a tale of two epidemics. *Contemp Drug Probl.* 1989;16:579-618.
7. Fagan J, Chin K. Social processes of initiation into crack. *J Drug Issues.* 1991; 21:313-342.
8. Johnson BD, Hamid A, Sanabria H. Emerging models of crack distribution. In: Mieczkowksi T, ed. *Drugs and Crime: A Reader.* Boston, Mass: Allyn-Bacon; 1991:56-78.
9. Ringwalt CL, Palmer JH. Cocaine and crack users compared. *Adolescence.* 1989; 24:851-859.
10. Kandel DB, Yamaguchi K. From beer to crack: developmental patterns of involvement in drugs. *Am J Public Health.* 1993;83:851-855.
11. Kandel DB. Issues of sequencing of adolescent drug use and other problem behaviors. *Drugs Soc.* 1989;3:55-76.
12. Robins LN, Davis DH, Wish E. Detecting predictors of rare events: demographic, family and personal deviance as predictors of stages in the progression toward narcotic addiction. In: Straus JS, Haroutun B, Roff M, eds. *The Origins and Course of Psychopathology.* New York, NY: Plenum Press; 1977: 379-406.
13. Turner CF, Lessler JT, Gfroerer JC, eds. *Survey Measurement of Drug Use: Methodological Studies.* Rockville, Md: US Dept of Health and Human Services, Alcohol, Drug Abuse, and Mental Health Administration; 1992.
14. Kandel DB, Yamaguchi K, Chen K. Stages of progression in drug involvement from adolescence to adulthood: further evidence for the gateway theory. *J Stud Alcohol.* 1992;53:447-457.
15. Agresti A. *Categorical Data Analysis.* New York, NY: John Wiley & Sons Inc; 1990.
16. Kandel DB, Faust R. Sequences and stages in patterns of adolescent drug use. *Arch Gen Psychiatry.* 1975;32:923-932.
17. Kandel DB, Kessler R, Margulies R. Antecedents of adolescent initiation into stages of drug use. In: Kandel D, ed. *Longitudinal Research on Drug Use.* Washington, DC: Hemisphere-Wiley; 1978:73-99.
18. Kandel DB. Developmental stages in adolescent drug involvement. In: Lettieri D, Sayers M, Pearson HW, eds. *Theories on Drug Abuse.* Rockville, Md: National Institute on Drug Abuse; 1980:120-127.
19. Bachman JG, O'Malley PM, Johnston LD. Smoking, drinking and drug use among American high school students: correlates and trends, 1975-1979. *Am J Public Health.* 1981;71:59-69.
20. Block J, Block JH, Keyes S. Longitudinally foretelling drug usage. *Child Dev.* 1988;59:336-355.
21. Brook JS, Whiteman M, Nomura C, Gordon AS, Cohen P. Personality, family, and ecological influences on adolescent drug use. *J Chem Depend Treatment.* 1988;1:123-162.
22. Jessor R, Jessor SL. *Probl Behav Psychosoc Dev.* Orlando, Fla: Academic Press Inc; 1977.
23. Kaplan HB. *Deviant Behavior in Defense of Self.* Orlando, Fla: Academic Press Inc; 1980.
24. Pandina RJ, Labouvie EW, Johnson V, White HR. The relationship between alcohol and marijuana use and competence. *J Health Soc Policy.* 1990;3:89-108.
25. Hansell S, White HR. Adolecent drug use, psychological distress, and physical symptoms. *J Health Social Behav.* 1991;32:288-301.
26. Kandel D, Davies M, Karus D, Yamaguchi K. The consequences in young adulthood of adolescent drug involvement: an overview. *Arch Gen Psychiatry.* 1986; 43:746-754.
27. Newcomb MD, Bentler PM. *Consequences of Adolescent Drug Use.* Newbury Park, Calif: Sage Publications; 1988.
28. Mensch B, Kandel D. Dropping out of high school and drug involvement. *Sociol Educ.* 1988;61:95-113.

Take The Next Logical Step.

Easy Access To The Information You Need

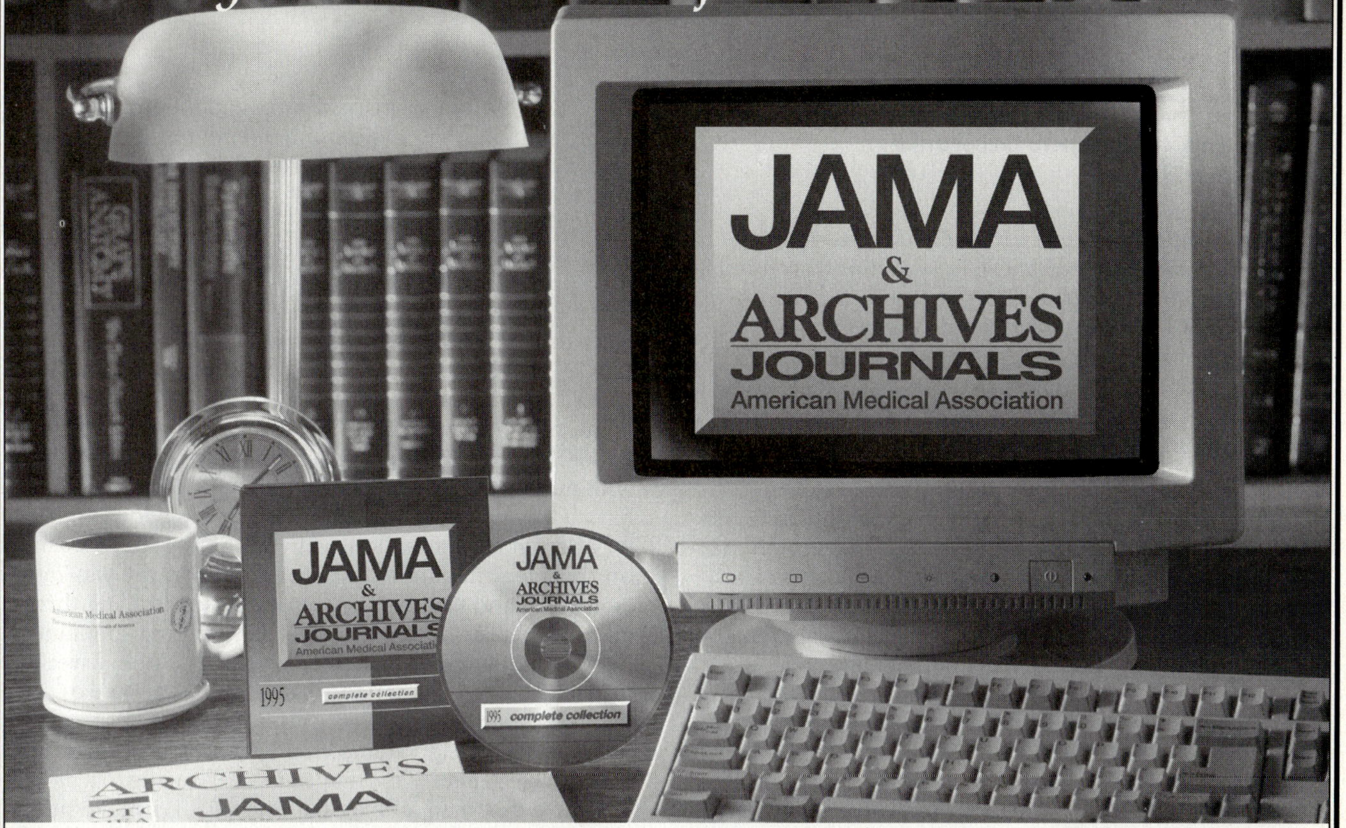

Introducing the complete JAMA & Archives Journals on CD-ROM. Superb reference materials have traditionally played a critical role in the practice of medicine. However, with the body of knowledge expanding so rapidly, along with increased pressures to maintain a broader base of expertise, conventional formats alone are no longer enough.

Now, with JAMA & Archives Journals on CD-ROM, you can easily search, cross-reference, print and save medical information from 10 of the world's most respected journals – right on your own computer. Plus, you have instant links to complete MEDLINE® references associated with the journal articles, along with a five-year JAMA & Archives Journals index.

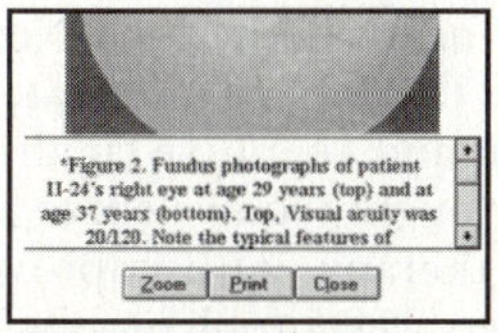

Zoom in on graphics and print complete articles.

An easy-to-use format, based on the journals themselves, makes the act of browsing the material very familiar. The powerful access capabilities quickly retrieve exactly the information you need.

Whether you're just beginning, or already well along in recognizing the ease of computer-based medical reference materials, JAMA & Archives Journals on CD-ROM is your next logical addition.

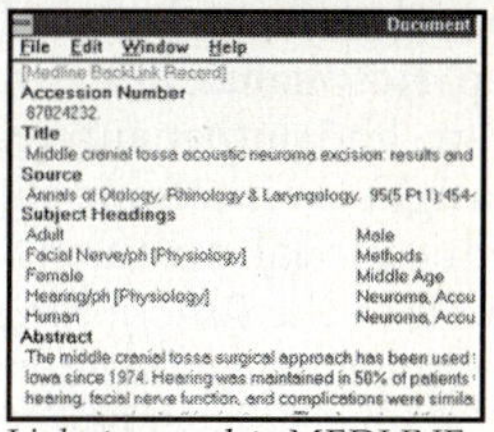

Links to complete MEDLINE references and 5-year abstracts.

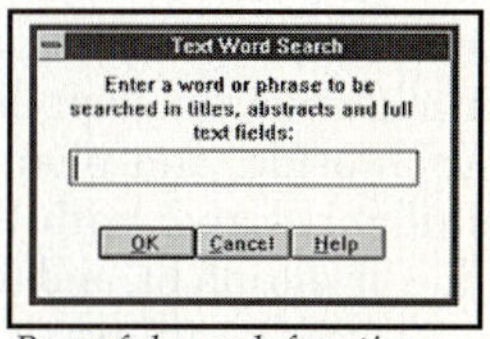

Powerful search functions can be performed by anyone.

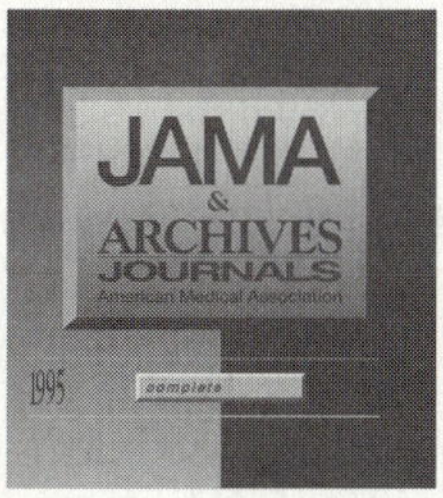

Minimum Windows System Requirements: 386-SX, 540 KB hard disk space, 4 MB RAM, VGA monitor. **Macintosh format not yet available.** OVID Software from OVID Technologies, Inc.

☐ **Yes, please send me**

JAMA & Archives Journals on CD-ROM

☐ 1995 Archival Disk **$150***
One disk includes editorial content from January-December 1995 for JAMA and all nine Archives Journals. 1995 Archival Disk will be shipped in February 1996.

☐ 1996 Quarterly Subscription **$250***
The first disk, containing editorial content for January through March 1996, will be shipped in April 1996. Each subsequent quarterly disk will be cumulative with the final disk in the subscription term containing the entire editorial content for 1996.

To order by phone, call
1-800-AMA-2350
Or, fax to **312-464-5831**
Mail coupon to: AMA Subscription Dept. CD, P.O. 10946, Chicago, IL 60610-0946

Please complete and return with your order:

Name
❑ MD/DO ❑ Other (please specify)________
Address
City State
Country
Zip/Postal Code
Phone ________ Fax ________
❑ Check made payable to AMA ❑ VISA ❑ MC ❑ AmEx ❑ Optima
Card # ________
Exp. Date ______ Signature ________

*Residents in AZ, CA, CT, DC, IL, IA, MN, NJ, NY, NC, WI, add required sales tax. In Canada, add GST. Contact AMA Subscription Dept for institution and foreign rates. Rates subject to change.
Payment must accompany order. Nonrefundable.

P6FAB

Response of Organic Catatonia to Risperidone

Although cases of catatonia have been shown to be acutely responsive to several interventions, including benzodiazepines and electroconvulsive therapy,[1,2] some individuals do not respond to these interventions. A review of the literature does not reveal previous reports of catatonia treated with risperidone. Therefore, we report the response to risperidone of a patient with persistent organic catatonia.

Report of a Case. Mr A's initial symptoms occurred during graduate school after the death of a close friend. He had a severe flulike illness for which he required residence for several weeks in the college infirmary. However, he was able to complete his PhD program in mathematics. When he was 31 years old, he had an apparent episode of catatonic excitement, followed by catatonic stupor. The initial course of catatonic stupor was episodic, but catatonic stupor became constant by the time he was 45 years old. His initial computed tomographic scan revealed discrete bilateral orbitofrontal atrophy, which did not change after more than a decade of follow-up. Hospitalization, partial hospitalization, nursing home care, and outpatient treatment including family therapy, insight-oriented and supportive psychotherapy, psychoeducational treatment, and group therapy all contributed to the functioning of his family. He required lifesaving medical treatment owing to complications, which included a severe episode of pulmonary embolism. In addition, he was treated with several antidepressants for at least 12 weeks at therapeutic dosages, including imipramine hydrochloride (up to 400 mg/d), desipramine hydrochloride, amitriptyline hydrochloride, fluoxetine hydrochloride, and phenelzine sulfate. Augmentation of antidepressants with lithium carbonate, triiodothyronine, tryptophan, and trifluoperazine hydrochloride (up to 70 mg/d) was unsuccessful. In addition, he was treated with trifluoperazine alone, clozapine (limited, by orthostatic hypotension and sedation, to 450 mg/d for 6 weeks, but with only 50% to 90% compliance caused by the failure of nursing home personnel during that time to provide adequate supervision of medication administration; their expectation of self-administration was not possible during that phase of his illness), haloperidol decanoate, thiothixene hydrochloride, chlorpromazine hydrochloride, and thioridazine hydrochloride. Because of marked improvement with intravenous amobarbital, he was treated with oral amobarbital, which was ineffective. He did not respond to intramuscular or oral lorazepam, alprazolam, clonazepam, or propanolol. He developed a syndrome of inappropriate antidiuretic hormone while taking carbamazepine and did not respond to phenytoin. In addition, he did not respond to pergolide mesylate, bromocriptine mesylate, or levodopa/carbidopa.

When Mr A was 47 years old, he had been mute and akinetic for over 18 months since electroconvulsive therapy was discontinued because of the onset of partial complex seizures and tolerance to the effects of electroconvulsive therapy three times weekly at maximal current levels. Because of his catatonic stupor, he had received tube feedings and anticoagulant prophylaxis for 18 months before initiation of risperidone. One hour of 2500-lux phototherapy was administered each morning with minimal improvement of akinetic mutism. One milligram of risperidone two times a day was added and he began speaking and walking with prompting after 5 weeks on this combination treatment. Phototherapy was discontinued and risperidone was increased to 2 mg three times a day. Six days later, he began walking spontaneously, initiating conversations, and eating. Within 2 weeks of increasing risperidone to 2 mg three times a day, he had only slight psychomotor retardation and expressed insights never before demonstrated about his illness and need for treatment. This may have been owing to a more complete treatment of his catatonic negativism. Risperidone was reduced to 1.5 mg two times a day because of a resting tremor and bradykinesia. However, within 4 weeks of this reduction, he became mute and abulic. His catatonic symptoms improved within 2 weeks of increasing his risperidone dose back to 3 mg two times a day. Four months later, his dose was reduced to 4.5 mg/d, and he was hospitalized because he stopped eating and moving completely. He responded several weeks after risperidone was increased to 4 mg two times a day. After several months, he spontaneously expressed a wish to return to work, while understanding his limitations. Neuropsychological testing revealed that he had moderately severe psychomotor retardation and cognitive rigidity. His response to risperidone was roughly equivalent to his response to electroconvulsive therapy, with improvement in his memory and Category Test problem solving scores. The Wisconsin Card Sort Test was not sensitive to his neuropsychological impairment.

After 13 years of follow-up by the same clinician, the patient never reported definite hallucinations, but had pathologic guilt about his friend's death. His recollection of his catatonic episodes was that he felt fatigued and abulic but alert.

Risperidone is an atypical neuroleptic that is an antagonist with high affinity for 5-HT_7, 5-HT_{2A}, D_2, D_3, D_4, H_1, α_{1B}, and α_2 receptors.[3-6] Future US availability of medications that potently inhibit 5-HT_{2A} and/or 5-HT_7 receptors, but not D_2 receptors,[2] may allow treatment of the residual psychomotor retardation and cognitive inflexibility in this patient. This case demonstrates that patients who are not responsive to treatment currently should be considered to be potentially responsive to treatment as research leads to the development of new therapeutic interventions.

Edwin H. Cook, Jr, MD
Kerri Olson, PhD
Neil Pliskin, PhD
University of Chicago
MC 3077
5841 S Maryland Ave
Chicago, IL 60637

1. Menza M, Harris D. Benzodiazepines and catatonia: an overview. *Biol Psychiatry.* 1989;26:842-846.
2. Rogers D. Catatonia: a contemporary approach. *J Neuropsychiatry Clin Neurosci.* 1991;3:334-340.
3. Roth B, Craigo S, Choudhary S, Uluer A, Monsma F Jr, Hen Y, Meltzer H, Sibley D. Binding of typical and atypical antipsychotic drugs to 5-hydroxytryptamine-6 and 5-hydroxytryptamine-7 receptors. *J Pharmacol Exp Ther.* 1994;268:1403-1410.
4. Leysen JE, Janssen PM, Gommeren W, Wynants J, Pauwels PJ, Janssen PA. In vitro and in vivo receptor binding and effects on monoamine turnover in rat brain regions of the novel antipsychotics risperidone and ocaperidone. *Mol Pharmacol.* 1992;41:494-508.
5. Seeman P, Van Tol H. Dopamine receptor pharmacology. *Trends Pharmacol Sci.* 1994;15:264-270.
6. Sleight AJ, Koek W, Bigg DC. Binding of antipsychotic drugs at alpha 1A- and alpha 1B-adrenoceptors: risperidone is selective for the alpha 1B-adrenoceptors. *Eur J Pharmacol.* 1993;238:407-410.

Panic Attacks: Klein's False Suffocation Alarm, Taylor and Rachman's Data, and Ley's Dyspneic-Fear Theory

In a recent letter on Klein's[1] false suffocation alarm theory of panic attacks, Taylor and Rachman[2] reported two sets of data that purportedly support predictions derived from the theory. One set supports the validity of their measure of suffocation fear[3] as an index of the sensitivity of the putative suffocation alarm: "As predicted, subjects with high suffocation fear reported significantly more panic attacks than subjects with low suffocation fear . . . "[2] The other set gave the results of a brief structured interview,[2] in which subjects with high suffocation fears reported a significantly greater incidence of panic in enclosed spaces and in other situations and a greater incidence of spontaneous panic than did subjects with low suffocation fears.

The primary point to be made here is that Taylor and Rachman's results also support Ley's[4] theory of panic, a theory predicated on the assumption that the classic "panic attack is marked by uncontrollable high intensity dyspnea (sense of impending suffocation) . . ., "[5] a feature that characterizes Klein's subsequent false suffocation alarm theory. Differences between Ley's theory and Klein's later theory can be found in Klein's ad hoc invention of a relatively complex network of loosely connected hypothetical mechanisms based on a shaky foundation of "natural experiments," conditions to which Taylor and Rachman allude in their letter.[2]

The secondary point to be made underscores Taylor and Rachman's caution that "Further progress in elucidating and evaluating Klein's theory will require precise definitions of the postulated suffocation alarm mechanism and the validation of acceptable means of measuring its operation."[3] In a critical commentary on the suffocation alarm theory, Ley[6] concludes that (1) there is no physiological evidence for a suffocation alarm and no theoretical advantage for postulating such an alarm, (2) there are clear examples of suffocation in which an alarm has never been reported or observed (eg, carbon monoxide poisoning, heroin overdoses, inhalation of 100% nitrogen), and (3) the results of an experiment by Fowler[7] demonstrate that the breaking point of breath holding can be doubled if subjects are given several inhalations of 8.2% oxygen and 7.5% carbon dioxide, gases that do not increase PO_2, but that increase PCO_2 significantly beyond the level obtained during prolonged inhalation of 5% carbon dioxide in air, the challenge test that Klein uses to induce his variety of "panic attacks."

In summary, the results by Taylor and Rachman point clearly to the significance of a sense of uncontrollable dyspnea/suffocation in panic attacks but provide no direct evidence for the hypothetical mechanisms that constitute Klein's false suffocation alarm theory. Do the assumptions that the brain has a "suffocation detector" that, if "deranged," erroneously triggers an "evolved suffocation alarm system" add anything to our common understanding that a sense of *uncontrollable* suffocation is frightening?

Ronald Ley, PhD
University at Albany
State University of New York
1400 Washington Ave
Albany, NY 12222

1. Klein DF. False suffocation alarms, spontaneous panics, and related conditions: an integrative hypothesis. *Arch Gen Psychiatry.* 1993;50:306-317.
2. Taylor S, Rachman S. Klein's suffocation theory of panic. *Arch Gen Psychiatry.* 1994;51:505-506.
3. Rachman S, Taylor S. Analyses of claustrophobia. *J Anxiety Disord.* 1993;7:281-291.
4. Ley R. Dyspneic-fear and catastrophic cognitions in hyperventilatory panic attacks. *Behav Res Ther.* 1989;27:549-554.
5. Ley R. The many faces of Pan: psychological and physiological differences among three types of panic attacks. *Behav Res Ther.* 1992;30:347-357.
6. Ley R. The 'suffocation alarm' theory of panic attacks: a critical commentary. *J Behav Ther Exp Psychiatry.* 1994;24:269-273.
7. Fowler W. Breaking point of breath holding. *J Appl Physiol.* 1954;6:536-545.

In reply

Ley claims that the findings of Taylor and Rachman[1] support his theory as well as mine. However, I do not believe this is substantiated by Ley's article[2] in which he states that a classic "panic attack" is marked by "uncontrollable high intensity dyspnea (sense of impending suffocation)." However, this has nothing to do with chronic suffocation fear, which Taylor and Rachman address. Nowhere in Ley's (clinical rather than data-based) presentation of a variety of panics does he make any specific prediction that chronic suffocation fear predicts any sort of panic. If anything, Ley's "anticipatory panic attack" or "cognitive panic attack," both marked by anticipatory anxiety, might better be predicted by chronic fear of suffocation than the "classic panic attack" heralded by acute dyspnea. However, since Ley did not address this issue, his claim for substantive support from Taylor and Rachman is unwarranted.

As we have pointed out,[3] carbon monoxide asphyxiation does challenge the false suffocation alarm theory of panic since such unfortunates asphyxiate but do not panic. One possibility is that carbon monoxide and similar agents disable the suffocation monitor or alarm system. This apparently ad hoc hypothesis finds support in the discovery by Prabhakar et al[4] and Snyder (personal communication, April 18, 1994) that carbon monoxide is an inhibitory neurotransmitter within the carotid body, since we had hypothesized[5] that the carotid body is a suffocation monitor. This strategically placed organ assays the blood level of oxygen and carbon dioxide and directly incites a central nervous system–driven respiratory response when hypoxic or hypercapnic signals of putative suffocation are detected.

Therefore, we are currently determining if carbon monoxide has antipanic effects as shown by blocking carbon dioxide panicogenesis. Fortunately, there is an extensive literature on the safe experimental administration of carbon monoxide to humans.[6] Prabhakar is currently investigating an animal model (personal communication, July 12, 1995).

Ley also

> *questions the plausibility of a 'suffocation alarm' [by] . . . death from an overdose of heroin. Why does an excessive amount of heroin relax the respiratory muscles to the point that breathing stops, thus producing suffocation to the point of lethal asphyxiation, but not activate the 'suffocation alarm'?*

Ley incorrectly states that heroin produces suffocation "by relaxation of the respiratory muscles." Rather it is by direct suppression of central respiratory centers.

We have cited[7] the extensive literature on respiratory control, which indicates that endorphines and endorphinomimetic drugs, such as morphine and heroin, profoundly depress the sensitivity of central nervous system to the stimulating effects of carbon dioxide, thus disabling the suffocation alarm system.

This too is open to experimental test. Two possibilities arise. One is the placebo-controlled, double-blind pretreatment with morphine of panic patients prior to a panic challenge. This may demonstrate that the potency and severity of challenge-produced panics are markedly decreased. However, it is open to the objection that this may be a nonspecific anxiolytic effect of morphine. Therefore, this design does not definitively address the question.

Instead, we induce an acute endorphinergic deficit via the antiopiate naloxone in normal subjects. The hypothesis is that, by sharply increasing suffocation sensitivity, naloxone may permit panic attacks in normal subjects who are almost always refractory to lactate and carbon dioxide panicogenesis. This study is under way. Facchinetti,[8] who independently replicated the findings of our group that lactate induces panic attacks in patients with severe premenstrual syndrome, has suggested that premenstrual syndrome may be caused by a phasic endorphinergic deficit. This may also be true of panic disorder, and we have suggested that this may provide a bridge between the suffocation alarm and separation anxiety.[7]

Ley's third counterexample is that the inhalation of pure nitrogen gives rise to dizziness and feelings of faintness that result from cerebral hypoxia but does not incur a suffocation alarm, despite the fact that asphyxia would occur if inhalation of nitrogen were continued. No data are given or reference is cited concerning the degree of asphyxia incurred. He also neglects the well-known phenomenon of nitrogen narcosis, which may also subvert the alarm systems. This too is open to experimentation.

As further counterevidence, Ley presents the study by Fowler[9] who indicates that the mean breath-holding breaking point of 52.3 seconds could be extended to a mean of 102.5 seconds if the subject were allowed to take several deep breaths of a gas containing 8.2% oxygen and 7.5% carbon dioxide, a mixture that did not increase their PO_2 but did increase their end tidal carbon dioxide to 52.3 mm Hg. Ley[10] states:

> *While it is a remarkable finding in itself that the breaking point of breath holding could be almost doubled during a period of steadily rising PCO_2 . . . an equally relevant finding, for the purpose of this commentary, was that 'suffocation alarms' were not reported by any of the subjects during the breath-holding suffocation induction or rising PCO_2.[10]*

Why is this experiment relevant? On exposure to 5% carbon dioxide, panic patients experience panic in approximately 13 minutes. Fowler described a period of exposure to carbon dioxide of less than 2 minutes. We agree with Ley that the increment in blood carbon dioxide is fairly moderate in our studies, averaging 50.5 mm Hg. It seems probable that when you have fairly minor but progressive increments in PCO_2, the monitor integrates this over time. A few breaths of carbon dioxide at a concentration only slightly above lung concentrations is not too alarming. However, a maintained increment would indicate a putatively suffocating circumstance.

Ley quotes Fowler as describing how repeated rebreathing periods eventually get the patients very uncomfortable, perspiring, with feelings of "not enough air."[9] One wonders what would have happened if they had been maintained in this hypercapnic condition for periods similar to those we used. That the distress of forced breath holding by self-induced laryngeal closure is temporarily alleviated by breathing activity is also irrelevant. Ley's attempt to use Fowler's data to discredit the false suffocation alarm theory is unwarranted.

Ley states that "one must ask where in the world outside a laboratory would one find that it contains 5% carbon dioxide." The obvious answer is wherever one would be forced to breathe his or her own exhalations, as occurs during smothering.

Ley concludes that a sense of uncontrollable suffocation is frightening, as if that is sufficient to deal with the facts. However, Ley inexplicably ignores my discussion of Ondine's Curse. These children, when grown up, are completely insensitive to carbon dioxide and have no sense of suffocation under asphyxiating circumstances. Can there be any clearer proof of the existence of a suffocation detector than the demonstration of subjects who do not have one?

To sum up, Ley raises a number of objections to the false suffocation alarm theory of panic disorder. He makes several irrelevant and immaterial claims and ignores relevant facts. His claim that the data of Taylor and Rachman support his theory is erroneous. His citation of the suffocating but nonpanicking effects of carbon monoxide, nitrogen, and opiates is challenging and, indeed, suggests experiments to further our understanding of this complex situation. However, his refutation is premature, at best.

Donald F. Klein, MD
Depatment of Therapeutics, Unit 22
New York State Psychiatric Institute
722 W 168th St
New York, NY 10032

1. Taylor S, Rachman S. Klein's suffocation theory of panic. *Arch Gen Psychiatry.* 1994;51:505-506.
2. Ley R. The many faces of Pan: psychological and physiological differences among three types of panic attacks. *Behav Res Ther.* 1992;30:347-357.
3. Klein DF. Testing the suffocation alarm theory of panic disorder. *Psychiatr Times.* 1995;12:14.
4. Prabhakar, NR, Dinerman JL, Agani FH, Snyder, SH. Carbon monoxide: a role in carotid body chemoreception. *Proc Natl Acad Sci U S A.* 1995;92: 1994-1997.
5. Klein DF. The suffocation false alarm hypothesis: panic disorder as the smothering response gone awry. *Currents.* 1994;13:5-13. Interview.
6. Benignus VA, Petrovick MK, Newlin-Clapp L, Prah JD. Carboxyhemoglobin and brain blood flow in humans. *Neurotoxicol Teratol.* 1992;14:285-290.
7. Klein DF. False suffocation alarms, spontaneous panics, and related conditions: an integrative hypothesis. *Arch Gen Psychiatry.* 1993;50:306-317.
8. Facchinetti F, Romano G, Fava M, Gennazzani AR. Lactate infusion induces panic attacks in patients with premenstrual syndrome. *Psychosom Med.* 1992;54:228-296.
9. Fowler W. Breaking point of breath holding. *J Appl Physiol.* 1954;6:536-545.
10. Ley R. The 'suffocation alarm' theory of panic attacks: a critical commentary. *J Behav Ther Exp Psychiatry.* 1994;25:269-273.

The Occurrence of Schizophrenia in Monozygotic Twins and Fractal Dendritic Development

The reduced (48%) incidence of schizophrenia in monozygotic twins when the co-twin develops schizophrenia[1] has long remained a puzzle and a challenge. Attempts have been made to explain the phenomenon by the use of the concept of incomplete penetrance and a possible postzygotic, mitotic crossover that could account for the discordance. A study conducted by Polymeropoulos et al[2] claims "no genetic marker discordances were identified between the co-twins, still leaving the possibility that a tissue-specific, mitotic crossover may have occurred in one of the discordant twins."

A more promising explanation is suggested by experimental observations of neuronal dendritic development in the sea slugs *Aplesias* (similar development also is known to occur in the daphnid and the fruit fly). In identical twins of such slugs, their giant neurons are located initially in spatial configurations identical to each other in their respective ganglia. Furthermore, it has been observed that this identical initial configuration of the developing dendrites in twin cohorts of *Aplesias* soon diverges into different fractal patterns (ie, similar in branching ratios on any scale but not identical in spatial coordinates).[3] Such divergence can only be due to random, environmental, perturbing influences after birth. The final outcome of the fractal deployment of dendrites within the boundaries and constraints of the initial genetic algorithm thus can be considered to be the result of the sum of such random influences in each twin.

It is plausible to assume that this phenomenon occurs in the developing neuronal systems of all higher organisms, including humans. This implies a different final dendritic structural arrangement for each human co-twin and hence a different functional reality, even though they began with identical genetic programming.

If such randomized dendritic deployment expresses itself as a sufficiently faulty functional abnormality, schizophrenia occurs in at least one co-twin. The probability is that the other co-twin will be protected approximately 50% of the time from also expressing a full-blown, clinically identifiable schizophrenia. Nevertheless, as any experienced clinician will attest, subtle signs of peculiar thought and behavioral patterns will still be found in the other co-twin (ie, a kind of "background noise" reflecting their common genetic origin).

It is our belief that this phenomenon may shed some light on the influences of detailed dendritic structure on brain function. The gross dendritic structure is no doubt genetically programmed. The peculiar thought and behavioral patterns identifiable in both twins reflect a common heritage close to the threshold of instability and, hence, schizophrenia. The "toss-of-the-coin" associated with the occurrence or lack of occurrence of schizophrenia in nearly 50% of the co-twins of twins with schizophrenia proves that twins reflect a final level of sensitivity to "faulty wiring" of genetic origin.

Structural defects in the brains of schizophrenics, shown by magnetic resonance imaging, have been well established. In a study by Weinberger et al,[4] the affected twin had a smaller anterior pes hippocampus and less regional cerebral blood flow in the dorsolateral prefrontal cortex during performance of a particular task (Wisconsin card sorting test). The detected abnormalities on magnetic resonance imaging may be the macroscopic consequence of such fractal divergence of the dendrite patterns as they unfold differently (similarly but not identically) for each of the co-twins, as I have outlined.

Nicholas Pediadiatakis, MD
Glenwood Professional Village
3123 Essex Circ
Raleigh, NC 27608

1. Onstad S, Skre I, Torgensen S, Kringlen E. Twin concordance for *DSM-III-R* schizophrenia. *Acta Psychiatr Scand.* May 1991:395-401.
2. Polymeropoulos MH, Xiao H, Torrey EF, Crow T, DeLisi LE, Merril CR. Search for a genetic event in monozygotic twins discordant for schizophrenia. *Psychiatry Res.* July 1993:27-36.
3. Changeux J-P. *Neuronal Man.* 7th ed. New York, NY: Pantheon Books; 1983: 209.
4. Weinberger DR, Berman KF, Suddath R, Torrey EF. Evidence of dysfunction of a prefrontal-limbic network in schizophrenia: a magnetic resonance imaging and regional cerebral blood flow study of discordant monozygotic twins. *Am J Psychiatry.* 1992;149:890-897.

ARCHIVES OF GENERAL PSYCHIATRY

The traditional clinical dictum that more neurobiologically disturbed, depressed patients should be treated preferentially with pharmacotherapy instead of psychotherapy remains unproven. **Thase et al** (page 99) compared response to cognitive behavior therapy (CBT) in 50 outpatients with normal all-night polysomnograms (PSGs) and 40 outpatients defined by a constellation of PSG abnormalities. The abnormal PSG group showed poor responses to CBT on several analyses, a lower recovery rate, and a higher recurrence rate during follow-up. Depressed patients with abnormal PSG profiles may suffer from a state of central nervous system dysfunction that interferes with the therapeutic strategies used in CBT.

Shwarz et al (page 109) used to study regional brain glucose metabolic rates in nine drug-free patients with OCD both before and after 10 weeks of behavioral therapy facilitated by cognitive techniques. Findings replicated their previous report of decreased caudate nucleus metabolism in treatment-responders vs poor responders. When data were combined with previous findings, they observed that pretreatment pathological correlations of brain activity among the right caudate nucleus, orbital cortex, and thalamus decreased significantly after successful behavior treatment.

Miller et al (page 117) have shown that remitted depressed subjects, who were treated with serotonin (ie, fluoxetine and setraline) reuptake inhibitors, demonstrated a depressive relapse when catecholamine function was reduced by administration of the tyrosine hydroxylase inhibitor, α-methylparatyrosine. Considered with previous studies that assessed the effects of reduced serotonin function in antidepressant-remitted depressed patients, these findings suggest that antidepressants may not work through a single monoamine-related mechanism.

Major depression tends to run in families. To examine whether this phenomenon is best explained by genetic factors or shared family environment, **McGuffin et al** (page 129) studied identical and fraternal twins in which at least one of each pair had received treatment for depression. The results of biometric model fitting suggest that genetic factors have a powerful effect, and these are probably individual specific with no contribution from the environment shared by the twin pairs. The findings suggest that major depression has a biological basis and that its etiology might be elucidated using molecular genetic strategies.

Various hypothalamic systems may be involved in depression. In a postmortem study **Swaab et al** (page 137) found that compared with controls, the number of vasopressin- and oxytocin-expressing neurons in the paraventricular nucleus in major and bipolar depressed patients was increased by 56% and 23%, respectively. This group also reported recently on an activation of corticotropin-releasing hormone producing neurons in the same brain area in depressed patients. All three peptides might contribute to the symptoms of depression.

Sleep disturbances in adults aged 60 years or older, especially during depressive illness, have gained recognition as major public health and quality-of-life issues. **Dew et al** (page 148) report that EEG sleep alterations were significantly more pronounced in elders who were early in their depressive episodes (4 months or less), compared with elders depressed for longer periods and with nondepressed elders. In addition, psyhosocial stressors and supports and clinical and demographic characteristics were each associated with EEG sleep profiles during depression.

Magee et al (page 159) present data from the National Comorbidity Survey on the prevalence, impairment, comorbidities, and help-seeking for phobias. They find that phobias are increasingly prevalent, often associated with serious role impairment, usually go untreated, and are risk factors for many other disorders. It is not clear that persons with phobias recognize that they have a mental illness, or that help is available.

Fears about public speaking are believed to be common, but whether such fears constitute a serious problem is unknown. **Stein et al** (page 169) conducted a randomized community survey and found that nearly 10% of persons reported severe public speaking anxiety that resulted in marked distress and/or interference with their work, social life, or education.

The relationship between depression and Alzheimer's disease has been poorly understood. Over a 5-year period **Devanand et al** (page 175) found the incidence of Alzheimer's disease among healthy elderly individuals to be three times higher for those with depression compared with those without depression. Because depressed mood also increased in frequency with worsening cognitive performance in both the cross-sectional and longitudinal components of the study, the authors conclude that depression may be a prodrome or an early manifestation of Alzheimer's disease rather than a risk factor.

ORIGINAL ARTICLE

Abnormal Electroencephalographic Sleep Profiles in Major Depression

Association With Response to Cognitive Behavior Therapy

Michael E. Thase, MD; Anne D. Simons, PhD; Charles F. Reynolds III, MD

Background: To test the hypothesis that depressed patients with selected neurobiologic disturbances are less responsive to psychotherapy, we examined responses to cognitive behavior therapy in relation to electroencephalographic sleep profiles.

Methods: Under a prospective, case-control design, 90 outpatients with probable or definite endogenous major depression (Schedule for Affective Disorders and Schizophrenia and Research Diagnostic Criteria) were stratified into abnormal and normal sleep subgroups (on the basis of an empirically validated electroencephalographic sleep profile) and more severe and less severe depression subgroups (on the basis of pretreatment Hamilton scores). Response to 16 weeks of treatment was analyzed for both intention-to-treat and completers (n=82) samples. Outcomes during a 36-month prospective follow-up were assessed with survival analyses.

Results: Abnormal sleep profiles and higher pretreatment depression severity were independently associated with poorer outcomes on several analyses. The association between sleep abnormality and cognitive behavior therapy response was not significant in the completers analyses, however, largely because of differential attrition. During follow-up, pretreatment depression severity was predictive of relapse and a lower recovery rate, whereas sleep abnormality was predictive of a lower recovery rate and a higher risk of recurrence.

Conclusions: Depressed patients characterized by higher severity and/or an abnormal electroencephalographic sleep profile were relatively less responsive to cognitive behavior therapy. These associations are hypothesized to result from a constellation of neurophysiologic disturbances that interfere with the acquisition, application, and implementation of the skills emphasized in cognitive behavior therapy.

(Arch Gen Psychiatry. 1996;53:99-108)

ELECTROENCEPHALOGRAPHIC (EEG) sleep recordings have been widely used to study the neurobiologic characteristics of depression.[1-3] One line of research has focused on the ability of EEG sleep recordings to predict treatment response. While most of this research has examined response to pharmacotherapy, EEG sleep studies also might be useful predictors of response or nonresponse to psychotherapy.[4] For example, identification of an EEG sleep profile associated with poor response to psychotherapy could reveal a specific pattern of biologic dysfunction that warrants somatic forms of therapy.[4,5]

In 1987, we began a series of studies in which depressed patients were evaluated with EEG sleep studies before and after treatment with cognitive behavior therapy (CBT).[4,6,7] In previous articles,[4,6] we reported that reduced rapid eye movement (REM) latency, a well-replicated correlate of depression,[1-3] was not associated with response to CBT. During the course of this study, several other groups failed to find any relationship between REM latency and response to individual CBT,[8] group CBT,[9] or interpersonal psychotherapy.[10] Our group subsequently replicated this finding in independent samples of depressed men[11] and hospitalized patients.[12]

While such a confluence of findings is compelling, several methodological issues warrant consideration. First, because 50% to 80% of depressed outpatients enrolled in clinical trials of psychotherapy typically respond, a neurobiologic correlate of poor response could occur in as few as 20% to 50% of outpa-

See Methods on next page

From the Department of Psychiatry, Western Psychiatric Institute and Clinic, University of Pittsburgh (Pa) School of Medicine. Dr Simons is now with the Department of Psychology, University of Oregon, Eugene.

METHODS

PATIENTS

The procedures used for recruitment, assessment, and treatment have been described in detail in earlier reports.[4,6,20,21] To summarize briefly, outpatients were initially evaluated by a clinician-psychiatrist team. Patients meeting *DSM-III-R* criteria for major depressive disorder were referred to our research team for secondary evaluation, including medical history, physical examination, laboratory screening studies, and an interview using both the Schedule for Affective Disorders and Schizophrenia (SADS)[22] and the 17-item Hamilton Rating Scale for Depression (HRSD).[23]

Patients were eligible for the study if they (1) met Research Diagnostic Criteria[24] for a diagnosis of primary major depression (unipolar, nonpsychotic, and probable or definite endogenous subtypes), (2) had HRSD scores of 14 or greater, and (3) did not suffer from conditions that might cause depression (eg, hypothyroidism), invalidate EEG sleep studies (eg, sleep apnea), and/or require medication that might cause either of these confounding factors (eg, corticosteroids or β-blockers). Patients with antecedent dysthymia or index episodes of major depression of at least 18 months' duration were excluded, as were those with recent histories of drug or alcohol abuse. Individuals with well-established diagnoses of borderline and/or antisocial personality disorder also were excluded.

About 200 outpatients were evaluated by our team, of whom 99 met entry criteria and 93 provided written informed consent. The major reasons for exclusion were dysthymia, insufficient severity, and/or Research Diagnostic Criteria nonendogenous subtype. One patient had a spontaneous remission and two others dropped out after completing EEG sleep assessment. Patients were enrolled in two waves: the first wave (1987-1989) was predominantly female (45 women and 17 men). The second wave (1989-1991) was predominantly male (six women and 25 men), largely because of the simultaneous participation of 20 subjects in the Men's Depression Study.[11] Demographic and clinical characteristics for the 90 patients are summarized in **Table 1**.

EEG SLEEP STUDIES

On completion of a 14-day medication- and alcohol-free observation period, patients underwent reassessment with the HRSD, Beck Depression Inventory (BDI),[25] and Global Assessment Scale (GAS)[26] before beginning either 3 (n=70) or 4 (n=20) consecutive nights of study in our Sleep Evaluation Center. The methods used for EEG sleep studies have been described elsewhere.[4,11]

Analyses of EEG sleep records focused on 16 visually scored variables describing different aspects of sleep continuity, sleep architecture, and REM sleep.[27] Excellent interrater reliability of visual scoring has been achieved and maintained in our laboratory for most measures, with only minutes (and percentage) of stage 3 sleep showing intraclass correlation coefficients less than .8. Accordingly, we used the more reliable measure of percentage of slow wave sleep instead of reporting stage 3 and stage 4 separately. In earlier reports,[4,6,7] data from nights 2 and 3 of study were used, allowing night 1 for accommodation. Results from the first 2 nights were used in the current report so that patients from the men's study and control groups of healthy normals and depressed inpatients (studied in 2-night protocols) could be compared. Preliminary analysis revealed that the polygraphic measurement of nocturnal penile tumescence in the men's study did not alter EEG sleep recordings on nights 1 and 2.[28]

PRELIMINARY SLEEP ANALYSES

The EEG sleep variables from our sample were compared with those of an age- and sex-equated normal control group (n=25) and a group of depressed inpatients (n=20).[12] The controls (15 women, 10 men; mean age, 36.5 years) had no personal history of psychopathologic conditions according to the lifetime version of the SADS,[29] although they were not screened with respect to family history of affective disorder.

Using a series of 1×3 analyses of covariance (covariate: age), significant differences were found on six of 16 comparisons (see **Table 2**). Inpatients differed from controls on six measures, whereas outpatients differed from controls on only two measures. Inpatients had more severe disturbances than outpatients on four measures.

EEG SLEEP CLASSIFICATION

As it was apparent that our outpatient sample did not have particularly disturbed EEG sleep, a multivariate analysis was conducted to identify a subgroup with more markedly abnormal profiles.[30-32] The methods employed for this classification are summarized below. First, the inpatients were used as the "abnormal" criterion group compared with age-matched (±5 years) normal controls. The sleep variables of the inpatients and controls were entered into a stepwise discriminant analysis, which yielded a discriminant index score derived from three variables (REM latency, sleep efficiency, and REM density). A score was computed for each subject by subtracting a score derived from the controls [−116.2+0.0049 (REM latency) + 4.51 (REM density) + 2.40 (sleep efficiency)] from one derived from depressed inpatients [−95.7 − 0.047 (REM latency) + 6.12 (REM density) + 2.18 (sleep efficiency)]; discriminant index scores of zero or lower were considered abnormal. The classification accurately discriminated between inpatients (15 [75%] of 20) and controls (19 [95%] of 20) (χ^2=20.4, *df*=1, *P*<.001). The construct validity of this classification was supported by the fact that each of the variables had been

tients. Second, it is likely that such an abnormality would be associated with a relatively poorer response rather than with absolute resistance. Samples of at least 80 subjects would be necessary to have the statistical power to detect a moderate effect in a biologically disturbed subgroup. Third, factors such as symptomatic severity, chronicity, diagnostic comorbidity, high levels of dysfunctional attitudes, and/or complicating medical conditions also are related to poor therapy outcomes.[7,12-15] To control for the impact of such factors, investigators would need to shown to be disturbed in previous studies of endogenous depression.[1-3,30-32] Second, cross-validation was performed on new, age-equated groups of depressed inpatients (n=24) and age- and sex-matched controls (n=24); 20 inpatients (83%) and 20 controls (83%) were identified correctly (χ^2=21.3, *df*=1, *P*<.001). Next, the stability of the classification was estimated in 20 unmedicated inpatients who were restudied after 2 to 4 weeks. The classification was found to have a test-retest concordance of 80% (κ=0.6, *P*<.01).

When our outpatient sample was classified using this method, 40 cases (44%) met criteria for an "abnormal" sleep profile and 50 cases (56%) were classified as "normal." Demographic and baseline clinical characteristics were compared for the two groups using a series of *t* tests and χ^2 tests (see Table 1). Although the groups were generally similar, patients with abnormal sleep profiles were significantly older (*P*=.002) and were more likely to have HRSD scores greater than 20 (*P*=.04).

COGNITIVE BEHAVIOR THERAPY

The 16-week, 20-session acute-phase therapy protocol (twice-weekly sessions for 4 weeks, weekly thereafter)[33] began following completion of EEG sleep studies. Patients were not permitted to take any form of psychotropic medication during CBT. All therapists had completed 2 or more years of supervised training and had received external certification according to the standards established by Shaw[34] for use in the NIMH Treatment of Depression Collaborative Research Program.[35] Therapists received ongoing weekly supervision from one of the authors (A.D.S. or M.E.T.).

MEASUREMENT OF OUTCOME

During treatment, the BDI, HRSD, and GAS were measured biweekly. All ratings and therapy sessions were conducted without knowledge of EEG sleep results. *Remission* was defined as termination from treatment with at least two consecutive HRSD scores of 6 or less. *Treatment failure* was defined by a final HRSD score greater than 10 *and* a reduction from baseline of less than 50%. Patients with intermediate outcomes were considered to be in *partial remission*.

Following treatment, patients with remissions and partial remissions entered a controlled 3-year follow-up protocol. Patients agreed not to immediately seek further treatment, in return for prompt evaluation of potential relapses and renewed treatment. Semistructured evaluations using the HRSD and Life II interview[36] were performed at 1, 3, 6, 9, 12, 18, 24, 30, and 36 months posttreatment. Patients who maintained remissions for 6 months or more were classified as *recovered*.[37] *Relapse* was defined by an increase in HRSD score of 14 or greater for 2 or more weeks *and DSM-III-R* criteria for major depression prior to recovery.[37] A *recurrence* was defined as an episode meeting criteria for relapse after a period of recovery.[37]

STATISTICAL ANALYSIS

The abnormal/normal sleep classification was used as the principal grouping factor. Because increased severity also may predict poorer CBT response,[20,21,35] the sample was divided into less severe (HRSD score ≤20) and more severe (HRSD score ≥21) depression subgroups, using a median split. Significantly greater proportions of cases were aggregated within the abnormal sleep/more severe (n=23) and normal sleep/less severe (n=32) cells than in the abnormal sleep/less severe (n=17) and normal sleep/more severe (n=18) cells (see Table 1).

Our principal hypothesis was that the abnormal sleep group would have a less favorable outcome than the normal sleep group. We also predicted an additive interaction, so that patients with higher HRSD scores and abnormal sleep profiles would have the worst outcomes. For the treatment phase, these hypotheses were tested using two series of analyses of variance (ANOVAs) with repeated measures. The first set of ANOVAs followed the intention-to-treat principle,[38] with the last observation carried forward method used to account for the missing observations of dropouts. This method's shortcomings[38] were partly offset by our study's low attrition rate and by frequent measurement of the dependent variables. In the absence of prospective ratings of all dropouts (the ideal strategy for an intention-to-treat analysis), the last observation carried forward method is the most widely used alternative to take into account the clinical status of noncompleters. The second series of ANOVAs used only the data from the patients who completed the treatment protocol (completers). A power analysis documented that effect sizes as small as d=0.30 (ie, a 3-point difference in HRSD scores) could be detected with a power of 81% for the intention-to-treat sample and 75% for the completers, assuming 10% attrition.[39]

We initially did not covary age because it may be an inextricable correlate of both endogenous depression[3,31,32] and depressive EEG sleep abnormality.[1-3,32] However, concerns that the age difference between the normal and abnormal sleep groups might confound results led us to repeat the ANOVAs after stratifying the sample into older (≥38 years) and younger (<38 years) subgroups, using a median split. This post hoc analysis addressed both the independent and interactive effects of age with respect to depression severity and sleep abnormality.

Categorical outcomes were compared with χ^2 tests, Fisher's exact probability tests, or survival analyses of life-table data,[40] as appropriate for either cross-sectional or longitudinal data. Follow-up data were analyzed with the Cox proportional hazards model[40] so that the relative effects of sleep abnormality, pretreatment depression severity (HRSD scores), the sleep group×severity interaction, and history of depression could be compared. For all survival analyses, dropouts were censored at the point of attrition. All categorical comparisons were performed with one-sided tests, as justified by their use to test specific a priori hypotheses.[39]

either exclude patients with more complicated conditions or enroll a sample large enough to permit stratification or multivariate analyses. Fourth, the EEG sleep profiles of depressed outpatients are typically much less disturbed than those of inpatients.[3,16] This point is particularly important because the predictive value of an abnormal biologic test result is severely compromised when the proportions of true-positive and false-positive cases do not differ greatly.[17] The use of composite EEG sleep profiles may yield more robust predictors than individual EEG sleep variables,[16,18,19] although this method has not been evaluated in studies of psychotherapy.

With these issues in mind, reexamination of the studies reviewed above revealed that (1) all had samples of less than 60 subjects,[6,8-12] (2) four included patients with chronic major depression, dysthymia, and/or significant comorbidity,[8,9,11,12] (3) none prescreened patients to ensure enrollment of a sufficient number with EEG sleep abnormalities, and (4) all examined single EEG sleep variables. We were able to address each of these shortcomings in our completed outpatient study, and we now report on the relationship between EEG sleep and CBT response in 90 depressed outpatients, including 40 with abnormal pretreatment profiles.

RESULTS

The abnormal sleep group received 18.6 (5.1) sessions of therapy (values are mean [SD]), whereas the normal sleep group received 19.3 (3.4) sessions ($t_{88}=-0.74$, $P=.46$). Attrition rates were comparable in the more severe (7% [n=3]) and less severe (10% [n=5]) depression subgroups ($\chi^2=0.2$, $df=1$, $P=.63$). Attrition rates for the abnormal and normal sleep groups were 15% (n=6) and 4% (n=2), respectively ($\chi^2=3.3$, $df=1$, $P=.04$). Reasons for early termination included noncompliance (abnormal sleep, n=1), dissatisfaction with therapy (abnormal sleep, n=5), moved out of state (normal sleep, n=1), and hospitalization following a suicide attempt (normal sleep, n=1).

SYMPTOMATIC IMPROVEMENT

For the intention-to-treat sample, the ANOVA main effects for time were highly significant, reflecting the fact that most patients improved considerably (see **Table 3** and **Figure 1** and **Figure 2**). Both the main effects for severity and the severity group×time interactions were significant on the HRSD and BDI. The interactions reflected the fact that the more and less severe depression groups became more similar over time (see Figure 1). Significant effects for both sleep group and the sleep group×time interaction were found on the HRSD and GAS. Figure 2 illustrates that these interaction effects were caused by the abnormal sleep group's poorer outcome after week 6. Neither the severity group×sleep group interaction effects nor the three-way interaction terms (time×sleep group×severity group) were significant. The results for the completers sample are reported in the bottom half of Table 3. Although the results were generally similar to those of the intention-to-treat analyses, neither the main effects for sleep group nor the sleep group×time interactions were significant.

The ANOVAs assessing the effects of age revealed little evidence of confounding factors: only two of the 42 relevant F ratios (six main effects, 18 two-way interactions, and 18 three-way interactions) were statistically significant. In both the intention-to-treat and completers samples, there were significant age×time interactions on the BDI. These interactions reflected the tendency for younger patients to start with higher BDI scores and show relatively greater change over the course of therapy. Controlling for age did not influence the significance of the previously reported main effects and interactions involving the severity group and sleep group.

Table 1. Pretreatment Demographic and Clinical Descriptors for the Total Patient Sample and Subgroups With Abnormal or Normal Electroencephalographic Sleep Profiles*†

	Total (N=90)	Abnormal (n=40)	Normal (n=50)
Age, y			
Current	38.4 (9.7)	42.9 (10.2)	34.9 (7.7)‡
At onset	31.8 (11.0)	34.6 (12.2)	29.7 (9.6)§
Sex, No. (%)			
M	40 (44)	22 (55)	18 (36)
F	50 (56)	18 (45)	32 (64)
Marital status, No. (%)			
Single, never married	28 (31)	10 (25)	18 (36)
Married	50 (56)	24 (60)	26 (52)
Other	12 (13)	6 (15)	6 (12)
Employment status, No. (%)			
Employed	62 (69)	25 (62)	37 (74)
Homemaker	8 (9)	5 (12)	3 (6)
Student	6 (7)	2 (6)	4 (8)
Other	14 (15)	8 (20)	6 (12)
Education, y	14.6 (2.5)	14.5 (2.5)	14.6 (2.6)
High school, No. (%)	18 (20)	9 (22)	9 (18)
Some college, No. (%)	34 (38)	14 (35)	20 (40)
College graduate, No. (%)	20 (22)	9 (22)	11 (22)
Postgraduate, No. (%)	18 (20)	8 (21)	10 (20)
Endogenous, No. (%)			
Probable	19 (21)	7 (18)	12 (24)
Definite	71 (79)	33 (82)	38 (76)
Previous episodes of depression			
No.	1.6 (2.2)	1.8 (2.1)	1.5 (2.3)
Single episode, No. (%)	40 (44)	15 (38)	25 (50)
Recurrent, No. (%)	50 (56)	25 (62)	25 (50)
Episode duration, wk	41.7 (28.1)	39.0 (27.9)	43.7 (28.3)
HRSD score	20.3 (4.1)	20.9 (4.6)	19.9 (3.7)
Score >20, No. (%)	41 (46)	23 (58)	18 (36)∥
GAS score	53.3 (8.1)	52.6 (8.7)	53.7 (7.5)
BDI score	27.2 (8.4)	28.6 (9.0)	26.0 (7.7)

*HRSD indicates Hamilton Rating Scale for Depression; GAS, Global Assessment Scale; and BDI, Beck Depression Inventory.
†Values are mean (SD) unless otherwise specified.
‡$t_{88}=4.2$, $P<.001$.
§$t_{88}=2.2$, $P=.03$.
∥$\chi^2=4.1$, $df=1$, two-tailed $P=.02$.

RESPONSE AT TERMINATION

For the intention-to-treat sample, end-point scores on the BDI, HRSD, and GAS were significantly higher in the abnormal sleep group (see **Table 4**). Similar albeit nonsignificant trends were seen among the completers ($P=.09$, .10, and .10 for the BDI, HRSD, and GAS, respectively). There were no significant effects by severity group or the sleep group×severity group interaction in either the intention-to-treat or completers analyses.

The categorical outcomes of the more and less severe depression groups were as follows: remission, 46% (n=19) vs 65% (n=32); partial remission, 32% (n=13) vs 16% (n=8); and treatment failure, 22% (n=9) vs 18% (n=9) ($\chi^2=3.8$, $df=2$, $P=.08$). Survival analysis revealed a similar trend for the more severe group to have a slower time

Table 2. Pretreatment Electroencephalographic Sleep Measures in Depressed Outpatients Compared With Normal Controls and Depressed Inpatients*

	Controls (n=25)	Depressed Outpatients (n=90)	Depressed Inpatients (n=20)	Group Effect ANCOVA, F†	Between-Group Comparisons‡
Sleep Continuity					
Time spent asleep, min	410.6 (46.5)	381.8 (51.5)	354.1 (39.0)	8.23§	C OP IP
Sleep latency, min‖	17.4 (12.9)	19.7 (14.9)	34.9 (29.6)	3.69¶	$\overline{\text{C OP}}$ IP
Awake, min	20.1 (21.3)	31.9 (32.1)	30.7 (35.9)	1.39	
No. of awakenings	4.9 (2.6)	5.9 (3.0)	3.5 (2.0)	5.40#	$\overline{\text{OP C}}$ IP; OP $\overline{\text{C IP}}$
Awake last 2 hours, min**	7.2 (8.6)	15.6 (15.1)	20.1 (28.2)	4.51#	C $\overline{\text{OP IP}}$
Sleep efficiency, %	91.6 (6.2)	88.2 (8.2)	84.3 (8.3)	6.24§	$\overline{\text{C OP}}$ IP
NREM Sleep					
Stage 1, %	4.7 (2.4)	4.6 (2.6)	3.6 (2.5)	1.01	
Stage 2, %	60.9 (9.7)	60.0 (8.8)	60.2 (8.8)	0.45	
Slow wave sleep, %**	11.2 (7.1)	12.4 (8.6)	10.6 (7.1)	1.30	
REM Measures					
REM, %	23.0 (5.4)	23.0 (5.3)	25.5 (6.7)	1.66	
REM, min**	96.0 (28.4)	88.5 (25.0)	91.8 (27.6)	0.54	
REM activity, U**	139.0 (57.7)	133.1 (64.1)	141.2 (59.8)	0.17	
REM density, U/min	1.43 (0.36)	1.48 (0.44)	1.53 (0.51)	0.91	
REM latency, min**	86.5 (35.2)	73.2 (24.2)	52.4 (21.1)	12.81§	$\overline{\text{C OP}}$ IP
REM periods, No.	3.8 (0.9)	3.8 (0.8)	3.8 (0.7)	0.05	
REM intensity	0.33 (0.12)	0.35 (0.15)	0.39 (0.15)	1.01	

*ANCOVA indicates analysis of covariance; NREM, non–rapid eye movement; and REM, rapid eye movement. Values are mean (SD).
†Covariate: age, df=2, 132.
‡Student-Newman-Keuls test; groups joined by a line (for example, $\overline{\text{C OP}}$) do not differ significantly. C indicates controls; OP, depressed outpatients; and IP, depressed inpatients.
§P<.003 (critical P following Bonferroni correction: P=.05/16).
‖Logarithmic transformations were done for analyses because of nonnormal distributions.
¶P<.05.
#P<.01.
**Square root transformations were done for analyses because of nonnormal distributions.

Table 3. Analyses of Variance of Continuous Outcome Measures (F Ratios)*

	Time	Severity Group	Sleep Group	Time × Sleep	Time × Severity	Sleep × Severity	Time × Sleep × Severity
Intention-to-treat analyses†							
df	8, 688	1, 86	1, 86	8, 688	8, 688	1, 86	8, 79
HRSD	113.98‡	4.27§	4.33§	2.39§	5.58‡	1.86	0.82
GAS	88.71‡	3.15	5.13§	3.27‡	1.49	1.31	0.92
BDI	110.89‡	3.88‖	2.89	1.45	3.07§	0.84	0.70
Completers analyses							
df	8, 624	1, 78	1, 78	8, 624	8, 624	1, 78	8, 624
HRSD	115.24‡	8.37‡	1.46	1.49	3.83§	0.64	0.51
GAS	91.08‡	6.68§	1.27	1.70	1.23	0.27	0.62
BDI	119.43‡	6.08‖	1.21	0.82	2.35‖	0.15	0.52

*HRSD indicates Hamilton Rating Scale for Depression; GAS, Global Assessment Scale; and BDI, Beck Depression Inventory.
†Last observation carried forward.
‡P<.001.
§P<.01.
‖P<.05.

to remission (Mantel-Cox χ^2=2.1, *df*=1, *P*=.07). Among completers, remission rates were 50% (19/38) and 67% (32/48) for the more and less severe groups, respectively (χ^2=2.4, *df*=1, *P*=.06).

The abnormal and normal sleep groups had the following categorical outcomes: remission, 45% (n=18) vs 66% (n=33); partial remission, 25% (n=10) vs 22% (n=11); and treatment failure, 30% (n=12) vs 12% (n=6) (χ^2=5.4, *df*=2, *P*=.04). All five patients who dropped out of the abnormal sleep group because of dissatisfaction with therapy were classified as treatment failures. The abnormal sleep group also had a significantly slower onset of remission (Mantel-Cox χ^2=4.8, *df*=1, *P*=.02). Among completers, remission rates were 53% (18/34) and 69% (33/48) for the abnormal and normal sleep groups, respectively (χ^2=2.1, *df*=1, *P*=.07).

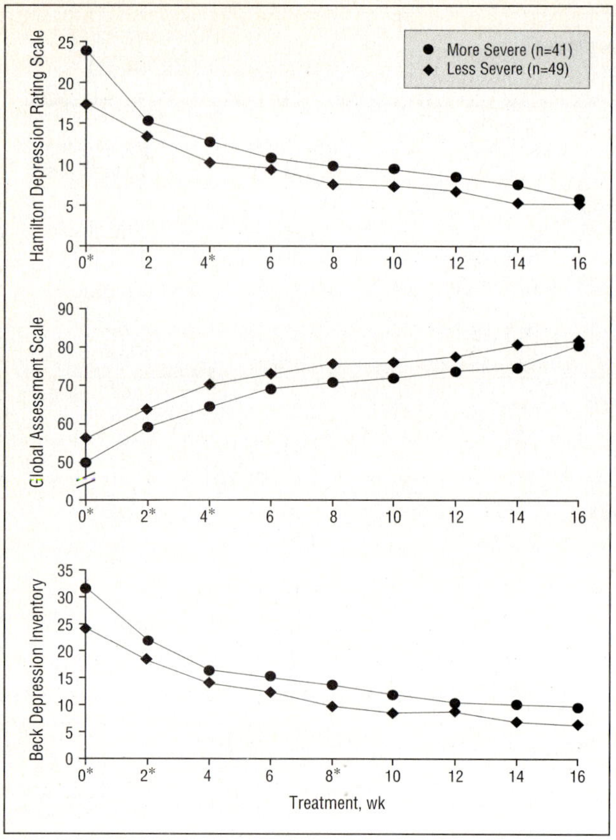

Figure 1. *Changes in symptomatic measures over time in patients with less severe and more severe pretreatment depression levels. Results are from intention-to-treat analyses. Asterisks indicate significant between-group differences (Student-Newman-Keuls tests).*

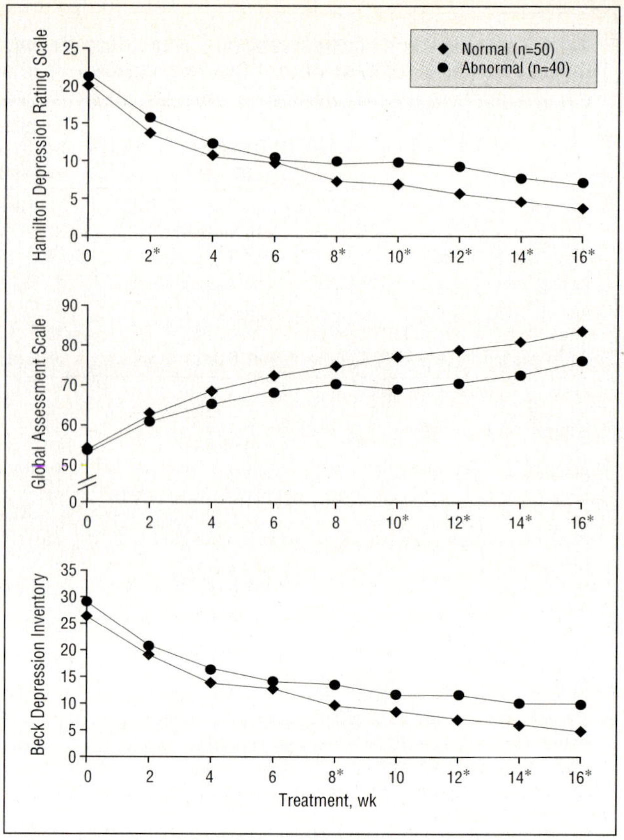

Figure 2. *Changes in symptomatic measures over time in patients with normal and abnormal pretreatment sleep profiles. Results are from intention-to-treat analyses. Asterisks indicate significant between-group differences (Student-Newman-Keuls tests).*

RATES OF RELAPSE, RECOVERY, AND RECURRENCE

Sixteen (23%) of the 71 patients entering follow-up relapsed. Sleep group was not significantly associated with relapse risk (abnormal sleep, 4/28; normal sleep, 12/43; Mantel-Cox χ^2=1.5, *df*=1, *P*=.22). The proportional hazard of relapse was significantly related to pretreatment HRSD score (*P*=.006) (see **Table 5**). In addition, patients in partial remission were nearly five times more likely to relapse than those in full remission (Mantel-Cox χ^2=35.6, *df*=1, *P*<.001).

Among the 55 patients who did not relapse, 42 (76%) recovered. The recovery rate was significantly lower in the abnormal sleep group (67% [16/24]) than in the normal sleep group (84% [26/31]) (Mantel-Cox χ^2=4.6, *df*=1, *P*=.02). Pretreatment HRSD scores (*P*=.04) and the interaction of sleep group×severity group (*P*=.01) also contributed to the likelihood of recovery (see Table 5). Median (SD) time to recovery was 40.3 (10.9) weeks for the abnormal sleep group and 35.9 (5.5) weeks for the normal sleep group. Although the abnormal sleep group had significantly greater variability in speed of recovery ($F_{15,25}$=3.89, *P*<.001), the mean values did not differ significantly after adjustment for unequal variances ($t_{19.8}$=1.47, two-tailed *P*=.16).

Seventeen (40%) of the 42 patients who recovered subsequently suffered recurrences. Recurrence rates were 56% (9/16) and 31% (8/26) for the abnormal and normal sleep groups, respectively (Mantel-Cox χ^2=2.7, *df*=1, *P*=.05). However, only a history of prior episodes of depression was significantly related to the proportional hazard of recurrence (see Table 5; Mantel-Cox χ^2=3.9, *df*=1, *P*=.03). Further inspection of these data revealed an interaction between sleep group and history of depressive episodes. Specifically, 75% (12/16) of patients in the abnormal sleep group had recurrent depression (compared with 38% [10/26] of patients in the normal sleep group; Fisher's exact probability test, *P*=.02); nine of the 12 in the former group suffered recurrences. By contrast, none of four first episode/abnormal sleep patients, four of 10 recurrent depression/normal sleep patients, and four of 16 first episode/normal sleep patients suffered recurrences (see **Figure 3**; Mantel-Cox χ^2=4.5, *df*=1, *P*=.02).

Five patients withdrew from follow-up, including four with abnormal sleep profiles (Fisher's exact probability test, *P*=.04). Thus, only 10% (4/40) of patients in the abnormal sleep group responded to treatment (ie, complete or partial remission), did not relapse, recovered, and were known not to have suffered a recurrence, compared with 30% (15/50) of patients in the normal sleep group (χ^2=5.3, *df*=1, *P*=.01).

Table 4. End-of-Treatment Symptom Ratings and Analyses of Variance (F Ratios)*

	Mean (SD) End-of-Treatment Symptom Ratings				Analyses of Variance (F Ratios)†		
	Abnormal Sleep		Normal Sleep				
	More Severe Depression	Less Severe Depression	More Severe Depression	Less Severe Depression	Severity Group	Sleep Group	Sleep × Severity
Intention-to-treat analyses							
No. of patients	23	17	18	32	...	...	...
HRSD	6.4 (5.9)	8.6 (6.7)	5.3 (5.6)	3.8 (4.1)	0.07	6.41‡	2.57
GAS	80.4 (13.8)	73.4 (15.7)	82.1 (17.4)	86.8 (9.6)	0.15	6.44‡	3.92§
BDI	11.4 (10.9)	10.5 (9.0)	8.2 (9.2)	4.7 (4.6)	1.49	6.21‡	0.56
Completers analyses							
No. of patients	20	14	18	30	...	...	...
HRSD	5.9 (5.9)	6.5 (5.0)	5.3 (5.6)	3.4 (3.6)	0.27	2.60	1.33
GAS	81.5 (14.2)	77.9 (11.7)	82.1 (17.4)	87.2 (9.2)	0.08	2.76	2.12
BDI	10.7 (11.5)	7.8 (6.3)	8.2 (9.2)	4.2 (4.5)	3.72	2.68	0.09

*HRSD indicates Hamilton Rating Scale for Depression; GAS, Global Assessment Scale; and BDI, Beck Depression Inventory.
†For the intention-to-treat analyses, df=1, 86; for the completers analyses, df=1, 78.
‡$P<.01$.
§$P<.05$.

Table 5. Summary of Cox Proportional Hazard Model Analyses for Risks of Relapse, Recovery, and Recurrence*

	Relapse (n=71)	Recovery (n=55)	Recurrence (n=42)
No. of events	16	42	17
Overall model, χ^2†	13.98‡	10.36§	7.90∥
Sleep group	0.64 (1.57)	−2.21 (0.96)§	0.60 (1.56)
Severity	0.18 (0.06)§	−0.08 (0.05)∥	0.06 (0.07)
Sleep × severity	−0.05 (0.07)	0.11 (0.05)§	−0.02 (0.07)
Past episodes	−0.15 (0.27)	−0.07 (0.18)	−0.55 (0.30)∥

*Values are β weights, with SEs in parentheses.
†df=4.
‡$P\leq.001$.
§$P\leq.01$.
∥$P\leq.05$.

COMMENT

The major goal of this study was to determine if there is a psychobiologic boundary to CBT response in depression. In contrast to six earlier reports using less powerful methods,[6-11] we found that patients with abnormal sleep profiles generally had less favorable outcomes than patients with normal sleep profiles. Consistent with earlier reports from this project,[12,20,21] we found that patients with higher pretreatment HRSD scores tended to have poorer outcomes. However, there was little evidence of an additive interaction between severity of depression and sleep abnormality. The failure to confirm a hypothesized interaction invokes the possibility of a type II error, although the posttreatment symptom scores revealed no trends in the expected direction. It is possible that our outpatient sample did not have enough markedly severe cases, ie, patients with pretreatment HRSD scores of 25 or greater,[12] to permit detection of an additive effect. In any event, it does not appear that assessment of symptom severity can serve as a proxy for the information provided by the polysomnogram.

It is interesting that the relationship between sleep abnormality and treatment response was not significant in the completers analysis, nor was it apparent in the intention-to-treat sample during the first 4 weeks of treatment, ie, when patients were seen twice weekly. In fact, 53% (18/34) of the completers in the abnormal sleep group achieved a full remission. In a similar vein, severity was not related to outcome by week 16 in either the intention-to-treat or completers sample. Treatment intensity and/or therapeutic tenacity thus may help to offset the negative impact of symptom severity or EEG sleep disturbance.

The discrepancy between the results of the intention-to-treat and completers analyses was relatively small (<10% difference in remission rates) but, nonetheless, it was large enough to determine statistical significance. This difference was largely attributable to the statistical methods used to account for the dropouts. On one hand, the last observation carried forward method assumes that patients who drop out would have remained at the same level of symptoms, and because the abnormal sleep group had greater attrition, the intention-to-treat analyses probably overestimated the impact of the sleep abnormality. On the other hand, attrition from the abnormal sleep group was greater because of dissatisfaction with therapy (nonresponse), suggesting that the completers analysis probably underestimated the "true" difference between groups. Which approach gives the more valid estimate of the significance of an abnormal EEG sleep profile? We favor the intention-to-treat analysis on the basis of four findings "untainted" by a last observation carried forward artifact: (1) There was differential attrition, which in and of itself is an important finding. (2) There was a significant difference between the abnormal and normal sleep groups on the survival analysis of remission rates, which censored the data of dropouts. (3) The abnormal sleep group had a significantly lower recovery rate. (4) Patients in the abnormal sleep group with recurrent depression had a markedly increased recurrence rate despite the presumed prophylactic effect of CBT.[41,42] The

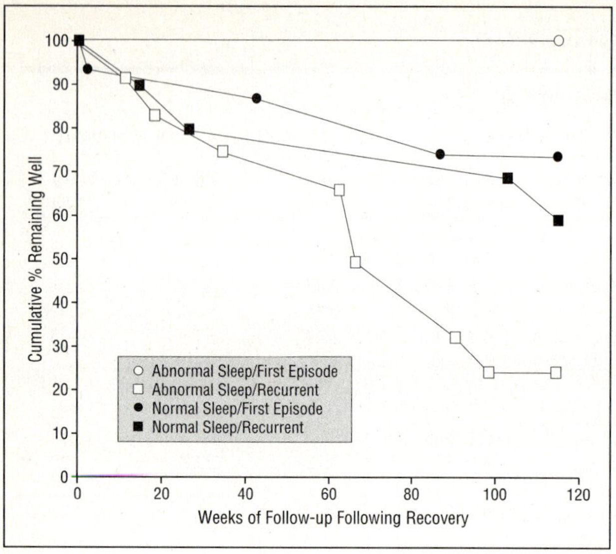

Figure 3. *Recurrence rates following recovery stratified by sleep group and history (Wilcoxon* χ^2*=4.5,* df=*1,* P=*.02).*

latter two findings are particularly informative because only patients who completed the therapy protocol entered the follow-up.

We propose that sleep abnormality may impair CBT response via a series of interrelated neurobiologic processes. For example, an abnormal sleep profile often is associated with increased hypothalamic-pituitary-adrenocortical activity,[43-46] which also may predict a poorer response to psychotherapy.[5,9,12,47,48] Hypercortisolism is implicated in the genesis of depressive cognitive disturbances[49,50] and may ultimately cause neurotoxicity[51] and cortical atrophy.[52] Hypercortisolemia and poor sleep efficiency are also associated with increased sympathoadrenal activity,[3,53,54] probably initiated by the effect of corticotropin-releasing hormone on the pituitary and locus ceruleus.[55-58] Such increased arousal may worsen neuropsychological capabilities, both directly[59] and via the cumulative effects of sleep loss.[60] Furthermore, increased corticotropin-releasing hormone levels[61] and elevated indices of sympathoadrenal activity[62] are associated with higher levels of dysphoric cognition. Increased REM density is similarly correlated with more intensely negative cognitions and affects.[63,64] In this regard, high levels of dysfunctional attitudes and hopelessness have been associated with poorer responses to CBT.[13,21,65] Prolonged activation of the hypothalamic-pituitary-adrenocortical and sympathomedullary systems mediates stress responses and may deplete mesocortical biogenic amines,[66] reducing volitional psychomotor activity, hedonic capacity, and appetitive behavior.[67] Thus, patients manifesting one or more of these neurobiologic disturbances may be functionally handicapped in a learning-based therapy such as CBT.[68,69] Affected individuals may have difficulty concentrating, grasping abstract concepts, generalizing from one topic to another, and/or recalling material. Patients with more marked disturbances also may be less capable of using therapeutic interventions to suppress dysphorogenic cognitions or effect improvements in mood, undercutting the therapeutic value of CBT methods in vivo. It remains to be seen if patients with abnormal sleep profiles might be more responsive to psychotherapies emphasizing interpersonal or psychodynamic strategies.

An important limitation of this study is the lack of randomized comparison groups. Without a pharmacotherapy group, it cannot be definitively concluded that more severely depressed patients or those with abnormal sleep profiles would have done better with antidepressant treatment. Conversely, we cannot conclude that the more favorable outcome of the normal sleep group observed would have exceeded the effect of a credible attention-placebo approach. A controlled clinical trial directly comparing these treatment options in patient groups defined by EEG sleep profiles is now warranted. Other potential limitations center around the generalizability and applicability of our findings. For example, it is likely that the relatively high treatment response rates are caused by our exclusion of more complicated and chronic cases. The expense and inconvenience of all-night sleep studies, coupled with their relatively modest predictive power vis-à-vis CBT response, also limit the practical application of these findings. In future studies it will be important to determine if selected clinical assessments (eg, assessment of mood reactivity, abstract concept formation, or attention span) might provide a more efficient way to measure the psychobiologic processes proposed to impair CBT response.

Over the years, the relative merits of psychotherapy and pharmacotherapy as treatments of endogenous and reactive forms of nonpsychotic depression have been debated extensively.[5,70,71] Furthermore, comparative treatment outcome studies using clinical classifications of endogeneity have not resolved this debate.[70,72] We have found that two psychobiologic indicators, clinical severity and an abnormal EEG sleep profile, are associated with a poorer response to CBT. While it would be overzealous to conclude that CBT is contraindicated for treatment of patients characterized by such disturbances, a significant minority of depressed outpatients may require pharmacotherapy to correct or control underlying neurophysiologic abnormalities.

Accepted for publication September 13, 1995.

This work was supported in part by Mental Health Clinical Research Center grants MH-41884, MH-40023, and MH-30915 from the National Institute of Mental Health, Bethesda, Md, as well as a grant from the Depression Network of the John D. and Catherine T. MacArthur Foundation, Chicago, Ill.

We acknowledge the contributions of the staff and faculty of the Cognitive Therapy Clinic and the Sleep Evaluation Center at the Western Psychiatric Institute and Clinic, including our principal therapists (Joseph Howell, PhD, Lisa Keller, MSN, Carol Hughes, MSW, and Jean Smith, MSN) and research staff (Janice McGeary, RN, Jack Cahalane, MSW, Gregory Garamoni, PhD, Tim Harden, Marilyn Kraus, Amy Fasiczka, Susan Berman, and Lisa Stupar). We also thank David J. Kupfer, MD, Ellen Frank, PhD, Joel Greenhouse, PhD, and Larry Muenz, PhD, for their helpful comments.

Reprint requests to the Department of Psychiatry, Western Psychiatric Institute and Clinic, University of Pittsburgh School of Medicine, 3811 O'Hara St, Pittsburgh, PA 15213 (Dr Thase).

REFERENCES

1. Benca RM, Obermeyer WH, Thisted RA, Gillin JC. Sleep and psychiatric disorders: a meta-analysis. *Arch Gen Psychiatry.* 1992;4:651-668.
2. Buysse DJ, Kupfer DJ. Sleep disorders in depressive disorders. In: Mann JJ, Kupfer DJ, eds. *Biology of Depressive Disorders Part A: A Systems Perspective.* New York, NY: Plenum Press; 1993:123-154.
3. Thase ME, Kupfer DJ. Current status of EEG sleep in the assessment and treatment of depression. In: Burrows GD, Werry JS, eds. *Advances in Human Psychopharmacology.* Greenwich, Conn: JAI Press Inc; 1987;4:93-148.
4. Thase ME, Simons AD. The applied use of psychotherapy in the study of the psychobiology of depression. *J Psychother Pract Res.* 1992;1:72-80.
5. Rush AJ. A phase III study of cognitive therapy of depression. In: Williams JBW, Spitzer RL, eds. *Psychotherapy Research: Where Are We and Where Should We Go?* New York, NY: Guilford Press; 1984:216-233.
6. Simons AD, Thase ME. Biological markers, treatment outcome, and 1 year follow-up of endogenous depression: electroencephalographic sleep studies and cognitive therapy. *J Consult Clin Psychol.* 1992;60:392-401.
7. Simons AD, Gordon J, Monroe SM, Thase ME. Toward an integration of cognitive factors, life events, and sleep EEG in depression: effects on course and outcome of cognitive therapy. *J Consult Clin Psychol.* In press.
8. Jarrett RB, Rush AJ, Khatami M, Roffwarg HP. Does the pretreatment polysomnogram predict response to cognitive therapy in depression outpatients? a preliminary report. *Psychiatry Res.* 1990;33:285-299.
9. Corbishley M, Beutler L, Quan S, Bamford C, Meredith K, Scogin F. Rapid eye movement density and latency and dexamethasone suppression as predictors of treatment response in depressed older adults. *Curr Ther Res.* 1990;47:846-859.
10. Buysse D, Kupfer DJ, Frank E, Monk T, Rittenour A, Ehlers CL. Electroencephalographic sleep studies in depressed patients treated with psychotherapy, I: baseline studies in responders and nonresponders. *Psychiatry Res.* 1992;42:13-26.
11. Thase ME, Reynolds CF III, Frank E, Jennings JR, Nofzinger E, Fasiczka AL, Garamoni GL, Kupfer DJ. Polysomnographic studies of unmedicated depressed men before and after treatment with cognitive behavior therapy. *Am J Psychiatry.* 1994;151:1615-1621.
12. Thase ME, Simons AD, Reynolds CF III. Psychobiological correlates of poor response to cognitive behavior therapy. *Psychopharmacol Bull.* 1993;29:293-301.
13. Sotsky SM, Glass DR, Shea MT, Pilkonis PA, Collins JF, Elkin I, Watkins JT, Imber SD, Leber WR, Moyer J, Oliveri ME. Patient predictors of response to psychotherapy and pharmacotherapy: findings in the NIMH Treatment of Depression Collaborative Research Program. *Am J Psychiatry.* 1991;148:997-1008.
14. Shea MT, Pilkonis PA, Beckham E, Collins JF, Elkin I, Sotsky SM, Docherty JP. Personality disorders and treatment outcome in the NIMH Treatment of Depression Collaborative Research Program. *Am J Psychiatry.* 1990;147:711-718.
15. Hoberman HM, Lewinsohn PM, Tilson M. Group treatment of depression: individual predictors of outcome. *J Consult Clin Psychol.* 1988;56:393-398.
16. Buysse DJ, Kupfer DJ. Diagnostic and research applications of electroencephalographic sleep studies in depression: conceptual and methodological issues. *J Nerv Ment Dis.* 1990;178:405-414.
17. Arana GW, Baldessarini RJ, Ornsteen M. The dexamethasone suppression test for diagnosis and prognosis in psychiatry. *Arch Gen Psychiatry.* 1985;42:1193-1204.
18. Kupfer DJ, Spiker DG, Coble PA, Neil JF, Ulrich RF, Shaw DH. Sleep and treatment prediction in endogenous depression. *Am J Psychiatry.* 1981;138:429-434.
19. Mendlewicz J, Kempenaers C, de Maertelaer V. Sleep EEG and amitriptyline treatment in depressed inpatients. *Biol Psychiatry.* 1991;30:691-702.
20. Thase ME, Simons AD, Cahalane J, McGeary J, Harden T. Severity of depression and response to cognitive behavior therapy. *Am J Psychiatry.* 1991;148:784-789.
21. Thase ME, Simons AD, McGeary J, Hughes C, Harden T, Friedman E. Relapse after cognitive behavior therapy of depression: potential implications for longer courses of treatment? *Am J Psychiatry.* 1992;149:1046-1052.
22. Endicott J, Spitzer RL. A diagnostic interview: the Schedule for Affective Disorders and Schizophrenia. *Arch Gen Psychiatry.* 1978;35:837-848.
23. Hamilton M. A rating scale for depression. *J Neurol Neurosurg Psychiatry.* 1960;23:56-62.
24. Spitzer RL, Endicott J, Robins E. Research Diagnostic Criteria: rationale and reliability. *Arch Gen Psychiatry.* 1978;35:773-782.
25. Beck AT, Ward CH, Mendelson M, Mock J, Erbaugh J. An inventory for measuring depression. *Arch Gen Psychiatry.* 1961;4:561-571.
26. Endicott J, Spitzer RL, Fleiss JL, Cohen J. The Global Assessment Scale: a procedure for measuring the overall severity of psychiatric disturbance. *Arch Gen Psychiatry.* 1976;33:766-771.
27. Rechtschaffen A, Kales AA. *A Manual of Standardized Terminology, Techniques, and Scoring for Sleep Stages of Human Subjects.* Washington, DC: US Dept of Health, Education, and Welfare; 1968.
28. Thase ME, Reynolds CF III, Jennings JR, Frank E, Howell J, Houck PR, Kupfer DJ. Technical note: do nocturnal penile tumescence recordings alter electroencephalographic sleep? *Sleep.* 1987;10:486-490.
29. Spitzer RL, Endicott J. *Schedule for Affective Disorders and Schizophrenia–Lifetime Version.* New York: New York State Psychiatric Institute Biometrics Research; 1975.
30. Gillin JC, Duncan W, Pettegrew KD, Frankel BL, Snyder F. Successful separation of depression, normal, and insomniac subjects by EEG sleep data. *Arch Gen Psychiatry.* 1979;36:85-90.
31. Feinberg M, Gillin JC, Carroll BJ, Greden JF, Zis AP. EEG studies of sleep in the diagnosis of depression. *Biol Psychiatry.* 1982;17:305-316.
32. Thase ME, Kupfer DJ, Ulrich RF. Electroencephalographic sleep in psychotic depression: a valid subtype? *Arch Gen Psychiatry.* 1986;43:886-893.
33. Beck AT, Rush AJ, Shaw BF, Emery G. *Cognitive Therapy of Depression.* New York, NY: Guilford Press; 1979.
34. Shaw BF. Specification of the training and evaluation of cognitive therapists for outcome studies. In: Williams JBW, Spitzer RL, eds. *Psychotherapy Research: Where Are We and Where We Should Go?* New York, NY: Guilford Press; 1984:173-189.
35. Elkin I, Shea MT, Watkins JT, Imber SD, Sotsky SM, Collins JF, Glass DR, Pilkonis PA, Leber WR, Docherty JP, Fiester SJ, Parloff MB. National Institute of Mental Health Treatment of Depression Collaborative Research Program: general effectiveness treatments. *Arch Gen Psychiatry.* 1989;46:971-982.
36. Keller MB, Lavori PW, Friedman B, Nielsen E, Endicott J, McDonald-Scott P, Andreasen NC. The longitudinal interval follow-up evaluation. *Arch Gen Psychiatry.* 1987;44:540-548.
37. Frank E, Prien RF, Jarrett RB, Keller MD, Kupfer DJ, Lavori P, Rush AJ, Weissman MM. Conceptualization and rationale to consensus definitions of terms in major depressive disorder: response, remission, recovery, relapse, and recurrence. *Arch Gen Psychiatry.* 1991;48:851-855.
38. Lavori PW. Clinical trials in psychiatry: should protocol deviation censor patient data? *Neuropsychopharmacology.* 1992;6:39-63.
39. Kraemer HC, Thiemann S. *How Many Subjects? Statistical Power Analysis in Research.* Newbury Park, Calif: Sage Publications Inc; 1987.
40. Cox DR, Oakes D. *Analysis of Survival Data.* London, England: Chapman & Hall; 1984.
41. Simons AD, Murphy GE, Levine JI, Wetzel RD. Cognitive therapy and pharmacotherapy for depression: sustained improvement over 1 year. *Arch Gen Psychiatry.* 1986;43:43-48.
42. Evans MD, Hollon SD, DeRubeis RJ, Piasecki JM, Grove WM, Garvey MJ, Tuason VB. Differential relapse following cognitive therapy and pharmacotherapy for depression. *Arch Gen Psychiatry.* 1992;49:802-809.
43. Poland RE, McCracken JT, Lutchmansingh P, Tondo L. Relationship between REM sleep latency and nocturnal cortisol concentrations in depressed patients. *J Sleep Res.* 1992;1:54-57.
44. Giles DE, Schlesser MA, Rush AJ, Orsulak PJ, Fulton CL, Roffwarg HP. Polysomnographic findings and dexamethasone nonsuppression in depression: a replication and extension. *Biol Psychiatry.* 1987;22:872-882.
45. Mendlewicz J, Kerhofs M, Hoffman G, Linkowski P. Dexamethasone suppression test and REM sleep in patients with major depressive disorder. *Br J Psychiatry.* 1984;145:383-388.
46. Feinberg M, Carroll BJ. Biological 'markers' for endogenous depression: effect of age, severity of illness, weight loss, and polarity. *Arch Gen Psychiatry.* 1984;41:1080-1085.
47. Robbins DR, Alessi NE, Colfer MV. Treatment of adolescents with major depression: implications of the DST and melancholia clinical subtype. *J Affect Disord.* 1989;17:99-104.
48. McKnight DL, Nelson-Gray RO, Barnhill J. Dexamethasone suppression test and response to cognitive therapy and antidepressant medications. *Behav Ther.* 1992;1:99-111.
49. Rubinow DR, Post RM, Savard R, Gold PW. Cortisol hypersecretion and cog-

nitive impairment in depression. *Arch Gen Psychiatry.* 1984;41:279-283.
50. Reus VI. Hormonal medication of the memory disorder in depression. *Drug Dev Res.* 1985;4:489-500.
51. McEwen BS, Angulo J, Cameron H, Chao HM, Daniels D, Gannon MN, Gould E, Mendelson S, Sakai R, Spencer R, Woolley C. Paradoxical effects of adrenal steroids on the brain: protection versus degeneration. *Biol Psychiatry.* 1992; 31:177-199.
52. Kellner CH, Rubinow DR, Gold PW, Post RM. Relationship of cortisol hypersecretion to brain CT scan alterations in depression patients. *Psychiatry Res.* 1983;8:191-197.
53. Jimerson DC, Insel TR, Reus VI, Kopin I. Increased plasma MHPG in dexamethasone-resistant depressed patients. *Arch Gen Psychiatry.* 1983;40:173-176.
54. Rosenbaum AH, Maruta T, Schatzberg AF, Orsulak PJ, Jiang NS, Cole JO, Schildkraut JJ. Toward a biochemical classification of depressive disorders, VII: urinary-free cortisol and urinary MHPG in depression. *Am J Psychiatry.* 1983;140:314-318.
55. Gold PW, Goodwin FK, Chrousos GP. Clinical and biochemical manifestations of depression: relation to the neurobiology of stress. *N Engl J Med.* 1988;319: 413-420.
56. Nemeroff CB. New vistas in neuropeptide research in neuropsychiatry: focus on corticotropin-releasing factor. *Neuropsychopharmacology.* 1992;6:69-75.
57. Dunn AJ, Berridge CW. Physiological and behavioral responses to corticotropin-releasing factor administration: is CRF a mediator of anxiety or stress response? *Brain Res Rev.* 1990;15:71-100.
58. Ehlers CL, Reed TK, Henriksen SJ. Effects of corticotropin-releasing factor and growth hormone-releasing factor on sleep and activity in rats. *Neuroendocrinology.* 1986;42:467-474.
59. Hartlage S, Alloy LB, Vazquez C, Dykman B. Automatic and effortful processing in depression. *Psychol Bull.* 1993;113:247-278.
60. Horne JA. Human sleep, sleep loss and behavior implications for the prefrontal cortex and psychiatric disorder. *Br J Psychiatry.* 1993;162:413-419.
61. DeJong JA, Roy A. Relationship of cognitive factors to CSF corticotropin-releasing hormone in depression. *Am J Psychiatry.* 1990;147:350-352.
62. Sampson JA, Mirin SM, Hauser ST, Fenton BT, Schildkraut JJ. Learned helplessness and urinary MHPG levels in unipolar depression. *Am J Psychiatry.* 1992;149:806-809.
63. Kramer M. The selective mood regulatory function of dreaming: an update and revision. In: Moffitt AR, Kramer M, Hoffman RF, eds. *The Function of Dreaming.* Albany: State University of New York Press; 1993:139-195.
64. Nofzinger EA, Schwartz RM, Reynolds CF III, Thase ME, Jennings RJ, Frank E, Fasiczka AL, Garamoni GI, Kupfer DJ. Affect intensity and phasic REM sleep in depressed men before and after treatment with cognitive behavior therapy. *J Consult Clin Psychol.* 1994;62:83-91.
65. Stewart JW, Mercier MA, Quitkin FM, McGrath PJ, Nunes E, Young J, Ocepek-Welikson K, Tricamo E. Demoralization predicts nonresponse to cognitive therapy in depressed outpatients. *J Cogn Psychother.* 1993;7:105-116.
66. Weiss JM. Stress-induced depression: critical neurochemical and electrophysiological changes. In: Madden J, ed. *Neurobiology of Learning, Emotion, and Affect.* New York, NY: Raven Press; 1991:123-154.
67. Wilner P, Golembiowski K, Klimer V, Muscat R. Changes in mesolimbic dopamine may explain stress-induced anhedonia. *Psychobiology.* 1991;19:79-84.
68. Thase ME. Cognitive-behavioral therapy of severe unipolar depression. In: Grunhaus L, Greden JF, eds. *Severe Depressive Disorders.* Washington, DC: American Psychiatric Press; 1994:269-296.
69. Fennell MJV, Teasdale JD, Jones S, Damle A. Distraction in neurotic and endogenous depression. *Psychol Med.* 1987;17:441-452.
70. American Psychiatric Association. Practice guideline for major depressive disorder in adults. *Am J Psychiatry.* 193;150(suppl 4):1-26.
71. Free ML, Oei TPS. Biological and psychological processes in the treatment and maintenance of depression. *Clin Psychol Rev.* 1989;9:653-688.
72. Thase ME. Reeducative psychotherapy. In: Gabbard GO, ed. *Treatments of Psychiatric Disorders: The DSM-IV Edition.* Washington, DC: American Psychiatric Press; 1995:1169-1204.

ORIGINAL ARTICLE

Systematic Changes in Cerebral Glucose Metabolic Rate After Successful Behavior Modification Treatment of Obsessive-Compulsive Disorder

Jeffrey M. Schwartz, MD; Paula W. Stoessel, PhD; Lewis R. Baxter, Jr, MD; Karron M. Martin, RN; Michael E. Phelps, PhD

Background: We sought to determine in a new patient sample whether symptomatic improvement in obsessive-compulsive disorder treated with behavior modification is accompanied by significant changes in glucose metabolic rates in the caudate nucleus, measured with positron emission tomography, as seen in a previous study. Second, by combining samples from this and the previous study, we also examined whether there were pathologic correlational relationships among brain activity in the orbital cortex, caudate nucleus, and thalamus that obtained before behavioral treatment of obsessive-compulsive disorder, but that decreased significantly with symptom improvement.

Methods: Nine patients with obsessive-compulsive disorder were studied with positron emission tomography before and after 10 weeks of structured exposure and response prevention behavioral and cognitive treatment. Results were analyzed both alone and combined with those from nine similar subjects from the previous study.

Results: Behavior therapy responders had significant ($P<.05$) bilateral decreases in caudate glucose metabolic rates that were greater than those seen in poor responders to treatment. Before treatment, there were significant correlations of brain activity between the orbital gyri and the head of the caudate nucleus and the orbital gyri and the thalamus on the right. These correlations decreased significantly after effective treatment.

Conclusions: These results replicate and extend previous findings of changes in caudate nucleus function with behavior therapy for obsessive-compulsive disorder. A prefrontal cortico-striato-thalamic brain system is implicated in mediation of symptoms of obsessive-compulsive disorder.

(Arch Gen Psychiatry. 1996;53:109-113)

OBSESSIVE-COMPULSIVE disorder[1] (OCD) is a common, debilitating psychiatric illness characterized by recurrent, unwanted thoughts (obsessions) and conscious, ritualized acts (compulsions), usually attributed to attempts to deal with anxiety generated by the obsessions. Medications that are strong serotonin reuptake inhibitors[2] and specific behavioral therapies that use the principles of exposure and response prevention (deconditioning)[3] are effective in reducing the symptoms of OCD in many patients. Although the cause is uncertain, recently many investigators[4-12] have postulated a role for a cortico-striato-thalamic brain system in the mediation of OCD symptoms.

Cerebral glucose metabolic rates are a sensitive indicator of brain functional demands and can be measured accurately and noninvasively in humans with positron emission tomography (PET) and the fludeoxyglucose F 18 method.[13] We have reported a study[12] that demonstrated statistically significant decreases in glucose metabolic rates in the right head of the caudate nucleus (a part of the neostriatum in the basal ganglia) after effective treatment of OCD with either medication alone (fluoxetine hydrochloride) or behavior modification using exposure and response prevention techniques without medication. Although subject numbers were too small to examine patients treated with drug vs behavior therapy separately in that first investigation, we also reported then that when responders to either treatment were combined for analyses, there were significant pretreatment correlations among elements in an orbital prefrontal cortex to caudate nucleus to thalamus circuit, and that such correlations decreased significantly after effective treatment. We believe that these pretreatment correlations in functional activity

See Patients and Methods on next page

From the Departments of Psychiatry (Drs Schwartz, Stoessel, and Baxter and Ms Martin) and Pharmacology (Drs Baxter and Phelps), The Brain Research Institute (Dr Baxter), and the Laboratory of Nuclear Medicine (Drs Baxter and Phelps), UCLA School of Medicine, Los Angeles, Calif.

PATIENTS AND METHODS

This study was carried out under guidelines established by the UCLA Human Subjects' Protection Committee, Los Angeles, Calif.

PATIENTS

In our original study,[12] nine patients with OCD were treated with behavior modification alone. We initially planned to have 11 new subjects in this study, but PET difficulties led to loss of data for the second scan in two subjects. Results from the nine remaining new subjects, analyzed with and without the nine from the previous publication,[12] are reported. All subjects were outpatients in the UCLA Neuropsychiatric Hospital OCD Treatment Program. Patients were asked to undergo fludeoxyglucose PET scanning before and after behavior therapy, which they chose after a careful discussion of all treatment options. All had a current primary diagnosis of *DSM-III-R* OCD that had been present for at least 1 year. All patients were in good physical health. All denied substance abuse. We did not perform urine drug screens. All patients were drug free by history for at least 2 weeks (4 weeks for medications with a long half-life, such as fluoxetine) before their initial PET scan, and remained drug free throughout the study.

In the previously reported behavior treatment group, there were diagnoses of cyclothymic disorder, panic disorder, and acrophobia in one subject each.[12] In this new subject group, no patient currently met criteria for other *DSM-III-R* Axis I psychiatric disorders. Two subjects in the new group of nine, and five in the previous group, had had major depression in the past, but all were euthymic at the time of study; none met *DSM-III-R* criteria for major depression, and the score for item 1 on the Hamilton Depression Rating Scale was less than 2.

Patient demographics and rating scale scores are given in **Table 1**.

SYMPTOM SEVERITY RATINGS

Subject behaviors were rated with the Yale-Brown Obsessive-Compulsive Scale[15,16] (YB-OCS), the 17-item Hamilton Depression Rating Scale,[17] the Hamilton Anxiety Rating Scale,[18] and the Global Assessment Scale[19] at the time of each PET scan. Responders to treatment were defined, a priori, as those who were rated as either "much improved" or "very much improved" on item 18 of the YB-OCS (which is taken from the Clinical Global Impression Scale) at the time of the second PET scan. Nonresponders were those who scored "no change" or "minimally improved" on the same item.

TREATMENT

Patients met one to two times a week with their therapist (J.M.S., P.W.S., or K.M.M.) for approximately 1 hour for review of assignments for individualized exposure and response-prevention exercises, which they did as homework, and self-monitored with diaries and/or graphs. Completion of exposure and response-prevention assignments was facilitated by cognitive techniques.[20] Homework was reviewed and evaluated with therapists at the next meeting. Some patients had occasional therapist-aided exposure and response-prevention sessions. Many also attended a cognitive-behavioral therapy group for patients with OCD.[20] None took any psychoactive medications during the study. All had supportive advice from their individual treaters, in addition to formal behavior therapy. All patients had 8 to 12 (mean, 10) weeks of therapy before undergoing a second PET scan.

among these brain regions in OCD are pathologic, since they were not seen in normal controls or in patients with unipolar major depression in a subsequent study.[14]

We interpreted the results of that previous study[12] as supporting the idea that a pathologic activity "capture" of this cortico-striato-thalamic circuit could be responsible for the brain's mediation of the fixed, repetitive thoughts and behaviors seen in OCD. Similarly, we proposed that effective OCD treatments restore the normal ability of functions in the head of the caudate nucleus to determine, or "gate," whether a given stimulus captures this circuit, and thus the individual's behavior.[12]

We report here a new study of patients with OCD in which fludeoxyglucose PET scanning was done before and after behavior therapy alone for OCD treatment. The purpose of this study was twofold: (1) to attempt to replicate our previous findings with an independent sample and (2) to provide additional subjects whose results could be combined with those from behavior therapy–treated subjects from the first study, which was performed with identical methods. This would allow sufficient subject numbers to examine whether the previously observed treatment-sensitive correlational relationships among elements of this orbital prefrontal cortico-striato-thalamic brain circuit would be observed in a population of patients treated successfully with behavior therapy alone.

RESULTS

Six of the new behavior-treated patients were judged to be responders by the preestablished criterion; three were nonresponders or poor responders. Rating scale scores before and after treatment are presented in **Table 2**, along with those of subjects from the previous study.

We replicated our previous finding of a greater decrease in right Cd/hem in those judged treatment responders than in nonresponders from the pretreatment to posttreatment scans (responders: pretreatment, 1.27 ± 0.06; posttreatment, 1.19 ± 0.13; poor responders: 1.23 ± 0.05 and 1.24 ± 0.04, respectively; Kruskal-Wallis test statistic=2.4; $P=.06$) in our new sample of nine subjects. (The **Figure** illustrates the right caudate nucleus findings from before to after treatment.) With patients from the new and old studies combined, even when good and poor responders were pooled, right Cd/hem showed a statistically significant decrease after treatment (1.27 ± 0.10 vs 1.20 ± 0.12; $t=3.16$, $df=17$, $P=.003$). When data for patients from the new and old studies were combined, left Cd/hem also changed significantly more after effective treatment, with responders showing a significantly greater change than nonresponders (1.21 ± 0.11 to 1.18 ± 0.16 vs 1.14 ± 0.12 to 1.21 ± 0.09, respectively; Kruskal-Wallis test statistic=5.1, $P=.02$). (In our previous study with a sample half this size,

PET METHODS

The PET methods were exactly those of our previous study.[12] For these nine new patients, neuroanatomic regions of interest were determined by one of us (L.R.B., who had reviewed all scans in the previous study for neuroanatomic accuracy after regions of interest were determined by a student) who was unaware of subject identity, diagnosis, and scan sequence. Since "normalized" metabolic rates gave the same results in our previous study when calculated from raw radiation counts without a blood input function, and we had concerns about the accuracy of blood sampling data in some subjects, we decided to use raw radiation counts from each region of interest, normalized by dividing the local cerebral metabolic rate for glucose of that region by that of the ipsilateral cerebral hemisphere, which yielded a dimensionless ratio, to generate data for each of the two patient samples analyzed. (This is analogous to the method used to calculate region of interest values in single photon emission computed tomography.)

STATISTICAL ANALYSES

Results are presented as mean±SD, as in our previous report.[12] From the results of our previous study, we made a clear, a priori prediction that normalized metabolic rates in the right caudate nucleus, normalized to the ipsilateral hemisphere (Cd/hem), would decrease significantly from before to after treatment in responders to behavior therapy in this new group of nine subjects. Furthermore, the degree of Cd/hem change in those judged to be "responders" would be significantly greater than in those judged to be "nonresponders."

We also postulated for the total group of 18 patients (nine from this study plus nine from the previous study) that there might be a significant decrease in both left and right normalized caudate metabolic rates. In addition, we postulated that treatment responders would show significant pretreatment correlations among the orbital gyri, heads of the caudate nuclei, and thalami, likewise as seen previously[12]; such correlations would show a significant decrease in strength after symptomatic improvement.

Group statistical comparisons for parametric measures with normal distributions (eg, region of interest/ipsilateral hemisphere values) were made with the paired *t* test for data from the same individual at the two times of scanning. When there were concerns about low subject numbers, normal distributions, or equality of intergroup variances, we performed the nonparametric Wilcoxon signed rank test or the nonparametric Kruskal-Wallis analysis of variance for intrasubject and intersubject evaluations, respectively. The nonparametric Kendall's τ, with a correction for tied values, was used for rank-order correlations between percentage change in the nonparametric behavioral rating scale scores and percentage change in normalized regional metabolic rates. (Kendall's τ is valid with $n>8$.[21]) For correlations of region of interest/ipsilateral hemisphere values among brain regions of interest, Pearson's *r* was used, since the numbers of patients were sufficiently large (n=12) and normal distributions obtained, as determined by visual inspection of frequency histograms. Fisher's *z* transformation was used to evaluate the significance of differences between correlations.

Based on the results of our previous report,[12] from which we had clear expectations as to direction of change, we used one-tailed statistical tests, looking for differences in a specified direction in Cd/hem (decreases) from before to after successful treatment in this new sample of nine subjects. No corrections were made for multiple tests, since this was an attempt to replicate previous findings. When data obtained by combining results from this and the previous study were examined, however, two-tailed probability estimates were used.

left Cd/hem did not show a significant difference between responders and nonresponders.) None of the above methods of comparison gave significant changes in the orbital gyri or thalami, bilaterally, for this new group of nine subjects, or for the group of 18 subjects from this and the previous study ($P>.10$).

There was a trend for a positive rank-order correlation between percentage change in total YB-OCS score before and after treatment and the percentage change in right Cd/hem ($\tau=.32$, $P=.07$) and left Cd/hem ($\tau=.26$, $P=.1$). The correlation of left orbital cortex/ipsilateral hemisphere to YB-OCS score was significant ($\tau=.51$, $P=.003$), but that of the right orbital cortex/ipsilateral hemisphere was not ($\tau=.07$, $P=.70$) when all 18 subjects were considered.

We examined correlations among the head of the caudate nucleus, thalamus, and orbital gyri (**Table 3**) before and after successful treatment by combining treatment responders from both studies (n=12). (Numbers of nonresponders were too small for valid correlation coefficients.) The right orbital cortex/hemisphere value was correlated significantly with ipsilateral Cd/hem and thalamus/hemisphere before treatment, but not after, and the differences before and after treatment were significant ($P<.05$), as seen in our previous study for responders to drug or behavior therapy, combined. In this study, however, results were not impressive on the left, as in the previous study[12] (see Table 3).

Table 1. OCD Behavior Treatment Populations*

	New Sample	Previous Sample
No. of subjects	9	9
Drug-free, No.	9	9
Age, y	33.4±6.6	34.7±6.0
Sex, No. M/F	2/7	4/5
Right handed, No.	9	8
YB-OCS		
Total	25.7±4.0	23.9±5.5
Obsessive (items 1-5)	13.4±2.1	12.0±3.8
Compulsive (items 6-10)	12.2±2.5	11.9±2.9
HAM-D	3.9±2.6	7.8±5.7
HAM-A	7.4±6.6	22.8±7.4
GAS	62.8±7.2	59.1±8.6

**OCD indicates obsessive-compulsive disorder; YB-OCS, Yale-Brown Obsessive-Compulsive Scale; HAM-D, Hamilton Depression Rating Scale; HAM-A, Hamilton Anxiety Rating Scale; and GAS, Global Assessment Scale. Data are given as mean±SD unless otherwise specified.*

COMMENT

The results of this study replicate those of our previous report in showing significant changes in right caudate glucose metabolic activity, normalized to the ipsilateral hemi-

Table 2. Treatment Response*

	New Sample (N=9)			Previous Sample (N=9)		
	Score			Score		
	Pretreatment	Posttreatment	P	Pretreatment	Posttreatment	P
Responders (n=6)						
YB-OCS						
Total	24.3±2.7	12.5±2.0	<.05	22.3±4.1	13.5±4.0	<.05
Obsessive (items 1-5)	12.3±0.9	6.8±1.5	<.05	11.3±3.6	7.0±2.3	≥.05
Compulsive (items 6-10)	12.0±2.0	5.7±1.1	<.05	11.0±2.4	6.5±2.7	<.05
HAM-D	3.5±2.5	2.0±1.4	≥.05	5.5±3.3	5.2±3.1	≥.05
HAM-A	6.8±7.3	4.7±4.9	≥.05	20.2±4.3	18.3±4.4	≥.05
GAS	66.1±3.4	81.0±5.5	<.05	60.0±9.6	71.8±4.8	≥.05
Poor Responders (n=3)						
YB-OCS						
Total	28.3±4.7	20.0±5.0	<.05	27.0±5.7	22.0±4.9	≥.05
Obsessive (items 1-5)	15.7±2.1	11.7±3.1	≥.05	13.3±3.1	11.3±2.6	≥.05
Compulsive (items 6-10)	12.7±3.3	8.3±1.9	≥.05	13.7±2.6	10.7±2.6	≥.05
HAM-D	4.7±2.5	4.7±0.9	≥.05	12.3±5.8	5.3±4.1	≥.05
HAM-A	8.7±4.6	7.0±0.0	≥.05	28.0±8.2	21.7±4.6	≥.05
GAS	56.5±7.7	65.7±4.0	≥.05	57.3±3.3	58.7±6.3	≥.05

YB-OCS indicates Yale-Brown Obsessive-Compulsive Scale; HAM-D, Hamilton Depression Rating Scale; HAM-A, Hamilton Anxiety Rating Scale; and GAS, Global Assessment Scale.

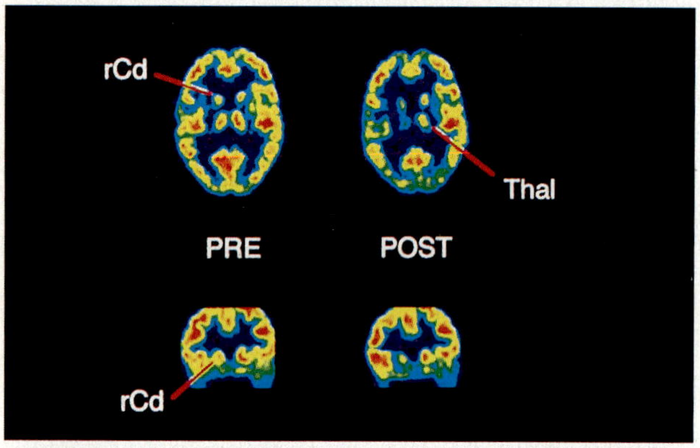

Fludeoxyglucose F 18 positron emission tomographic scans of a patient with obsessive-compulsive disorder who responded to behavior modification treatment, before and after 2 months of therapy. Horizontal and coronal sections (both 7 mm thick) are shown at the same brain levels for scans obtained before and after treatment. Decreases in glucose metabolic rates are particularly striking on the right. rCd indicates head of the right caudate nucleus; Thal, thalamus.

Table 3. Normalized Region of Interest Correlations Before and After Treatment for Behavior Treatment Responders*

	r	
	Before Treatment	After Treatment
L caudate to L orbit	.46	−.01
R caudate to R orbit	.74†	.28‡
L orbit to L thalamus	.34	.05
R orbit to R thalamus	.81§	.14‡
L caudate to L thalamus	.66‖	.36
R caudate to R thalamus	.69‖	.41

*Combined from both studies (N=12).
†Individual pretreatment correlation, P<.01 (one tailed).
‡Pretreatment to posttreatment correlation, P<.05.
§Individual pretreatment correlation, P<.001 (one tailed).
‖Individual pretreatment correlation, P<.05 (one tailed).

sphere, after effective behavior modification treatment of OCD; such changes are not seen when treatment is not effective. Our previous study[12] also demonstrated that normal controls showed significantly less change on rescanning after 10 weeks than did patients with OCD who responded to behavior or drug treatment.

By combining data from this new sample of patients with results from our nine patients with OCD from the previous, similar study, we were able to demonstrate statistically significant pretreatment correlations among the right orbital gyri, head of the caudate nucleus, and thalamus that decreased after effective behavioral treatment. Previously, we found similar results in a mixed OCD population treated with either behavior modification or fluoxetine. The fact that such effects can be demonstrated after behavior therapy alone—and that the correlations among these brain regions are not seen in normal controls or patients with unipolar major depression[14]—suggests that "coupling" of activity among elements in this cortico-striato-thalamic circuit may be related to the expression of OCD symptoms.[12,22]

Although there was a suggestion of similar effects on the left side of the brain, most results were not as impressive as on the right. This hint of asymmetry is similar to that observed in our previous report.[12] Although there are other possibilities,[22] it is noteworthy that Hollander et al[23] found increased right compared with left cortical neurologic soft signs in their patients with OCD, perhaps implying that right cortex function is more disordered than that on the left in OCD. Although the orbital gyri did not show a significant change in glucose metabolic activity from pretreatment to posttreatment, the significant correlation of change in left orbital cortex rates with change in YB-OCS score is similar to that reported by Swedo et al[24] after medication treatment of OCD.

Rauch et al[25] reported increases in cerebral blood flow in similar orbital gyrus, striatum, and thalamus brain regions, as well as several limbic structures, after acutely increasing OCD symptoms with stimulus provocation. McGuire et al[26] also reported positive PET-measured blood-flow correlations with OCD symptoms in brain regions that included the inferior frontal cortex, the striatum, and the thalamus—though, again, changes were observed in other brain regions as well. Both these groups of investigators noted that their experimental methods acutely increased anxiety as well as more specific OCD behaviors. Nevertheless, it is interesting to note that brain regions reported to correlate with OCD symptoms by both of these groups of investigators include the ones in which we see changes in activity and intercorrelations after effective drug or behavior treatment.[12]

As pointed out previously,[4-12] known functions of the caudate nucleus, and the orbital prefrontal cortico-striato-thalamic system of which it is a key element, do seem to fit the symptoms of OCD and may be the brain basis for its mediation. Further, specifically in regard to the localization of this brain change after behavior therapy for OCD, there is now a wealth of data implicating the caudate nucleus in "implicit memory," as well as "procedural" or "process learning"—including the ability to acquire new habits and skills necessary for the successful initiation of approach or avoidance behaviors.[27-30] In light of these and other findings, it should not be surprising that the deconditioning (or "extinguishing") of OCD symptoms accomplished through cognitive-behavioral therapy might be accompanied by a change in function in the head of the caudate nucleus, and in the cortico-striato-thalmic system of which it is a key element.[12,20,31]

Accepted for publication June 1, 1995.

This study was supported in part by a National Alliance for Research on Schizophrenia and Depression Established Investigator Award (Dr Baxter); contract AM03-76-SF00012 from the US Department of Energy, grant MH37916, and Research Scientist Development Award KO1-MH00752 (Dr Baxter) from the National Institute of Mental Health; donations from the Charles and Lelah Hilton Family, Mr and Mrs Brian Harvey, Mr and Mrs A. L., the Jennifer Jones Simon Foundation, and the Judson Braun Chair in Psychiatry, UCLA.

We are indebted to N. Satyamurthy, PhD, and his cyclotron staff, and Jorge Barrio, PhD, and his chemistry staff for synthesis of fludeoxyglucose; also to Ron Sumida, Lawrence Pang, Francine Aguilar, Der-Jen Liu, Mike Raghian, and Mark Hulgan for technical assistance with scanning. Sanjaya Saxena, MD, Arthur Brody, MD, Mark Colgan, MS, and Jay Carlyle provided other technical assistance.

We would also like to acknowledge the late Daniel X. Freedman, MD, whose constant encouragement and constructive criticisms contributed greatly to the experiment presented here.

Reprint requests to University of Alabama at Birmingham, 1001 Sparks Research Bldg, 1720 Seventh Ave S, Birmingham, AL 35294-0017 (Dr Baxter).

REFERENCES

1. Jenike MA, Baer L, Minichiello WE, eds. *Obsessive-Compulsive Disorders: Theory and Management.* 2nd ed. Chicago, Ill: Year Book Medical Publishers; 1990.
2. DeVeaugh-Geiss J. Pharmacologic treatment of obsessive-compulsive disorder. In: Zohar J, Insel T, Rasmussen S, eds. *The Psychobiology of Obsessive-Compulsive Disorder.* New York, NY: Springer Publishing Co; 1991:187-207.
3. Baer L, Minichiello WE. Behavior therapy for obsessive-compulsive disorder. In: Jenike MA, Baer L, Minichiello WE, eds. *Obsessive-Compulsive Disorders: Theory and Management.* 2nd ed. Chicago, Ill: Year Book Medical Publishers; 1990:203-232.
4. Cummings JL, Frankel M. Gilles de la Tourette's syndrome and the neurological basis of obsessions and compulsions. *Biol Psychiatry.* 1985;20:1117-1126.
5. Baxter LR, Phelps ME, Mazziotta JC, Guze BH, Schwartz JM, Selin CE. Local cerebral glucose metabolic rates in obsessive-compulsive disorder: a comparison with rates in unipolar depression and normal controls. *Arch Gen Psychiatry.* 1987;44:211-218.
6. Rapoport JL, Wise SP. Obsessive-compulsive disorder: is it a basal ganglia dysfunction? *Psychopharmacol Bull.* 1988;24:380-384.
7. Modell JG, Mountx JM, Curtis GC, Greden JF. Neurophysiologic dysfunction in basal ganglia/limbic striatal and thalamocortical circuits as a pathogenetic mechanism of obsessive-compulsive disorder. *J Neuropsychiatry.* 1989;1:27-36.
8. Baxter LR, Schwartz JM, Guze BH, Bergman K, Szuba MP. Neuroimaging in obsessive-compulsive disorder: seeking the mediating neuroanatomy. In: Jenike MA, Baer L, Minichiello WE, eds. *Obsessive-Compulsive Disorders: Theory and Management.* 2nd ed. Chicago, Ill: Year Book Medical Publishers; 1990:167-188.
9. Insel TR. Obsessive-compulsive disorder: a neuroethological perspective. *Psychopharmacol Bull.* 1988;24:365-369.
10. Insel TR, Winslow JT. Neurobiology of obsessive-compulsive disorder. In: Jenike MA, Baer L, Minichiello WE, eds. *Obsessive-Compulsive Disorders: Theory and Management.* 2nd ed. Chicago, Ill: Year Book Medical Publishers; 1990:116-131.
11. Rapoport JL. Recent advances in obsessive-compulsive disorder. *Neuropsychopharmacology.* 1991;5:1-10.
12. Baxter LR, Schwartz JM, Bergman KS, Szuba MP, Guze BH, Mazziotta JC, Akazraju A, Selin CE, Ferng H-K, Munford P, Phelps ME. Caudate glucose metabolic rate changes with both drug and behavior therapy for obsessive-compulsive disorder. *Arch Gen Psychiatry.* 1992;49:681-689.
13. Phelps ME, Mazziotta JC. Positron emission tomography: human brain function and biochemistry. *Science.* 1985;228:799-809.
14. Baxter LR. Neuroimaging studies of obsessive compulsive disorder. *Psychiatr Clin North Am.* 1992;15:871-884.
15. Goodman WK, Price LH, Rasmussen SA, Mazure C, Fleischmann RL, Hill CL, Heninger GR, Charney DS. The Yale-Brown Obsessive-Compulsive Scale, I: development, use, and reliability. *Arch Gen Psychiatry.* 1989;46:1006-1011.
16. Goodman WK, Price LH, Rasmussen SA, Mazure C, Delgado P, Heninger GR, Charney DS. The Yale-Brown Obsessive Compulsive Scale, II: validity. *Arch Gen Psychiatry.* 1989;46:1012-1016.
17. Hamilton M. Development of a rating scale for primary depressive illness. *Br J Soc Psychol.* 1967;6:278-296.
18. Hamilton M. Diagnosis and rating of anxiety. *Br J Psychiatry.* 1969;3(special issue):76-79.
19. Spitzer RL, Endicott J. *Schedule for Affective Disorders and Schizophrenia.* New York, NY: New York State Psychiatric Institute; 1978.
20. Schwartz JM, Martin K, Baxter LR. Neuroimaging and cognitive-behavioral self-treatment in obsessive-compulsive disorder: practical and philosophical considerations. In: Hand I, Goodman W, eds. *Obsessive-Compulsive Disorder: Recent Research.* Berlin, Germany: Springer-Verlag; 1992:82-101.
21. Hayes WL. *Statistics.* New York, NY: Holt Rinehart & Winston; 1963.
22. Baxter LR. Neuroimaging studies of human anxiety disorders. In: Bloom FE, Kupfer DJ, eds. *Neuropsychopharmacology: The 4th Generation of Progress.* New York, NY: Raven Press; 1994:1287-1299.
23. Hollander E, Schiffman E, Cohen B, Rivera-Stein MA, Rosen W, Gorman JM, Fyer AJ, Papp L, Liebowitz MR. Signs of central nervous system dysfunction in obsessive-compulsive disorder. *Arch Gen Psychiatry.* 1990;47:27-32.
24. Swedo SE, Pietrini P, Leonard HL, Schapiro MB, Rettew DC, Goldberger EL, Rapoport SI, Rapoport JL. Cerebral glucose metabolism in childhood-onset obsessive-compulsive disorder: revisualization during pharmacotherapy. *Arch Gen Psychiatry.* 1992;49:690-694.
25. Rauch SL, Jenike MJ, Alpert NA, Baer L, Breiter HCR, Savage CR, Fischman AJ. Regional cerebral blood flow measured during symptom provocation in obsessive-compulsive disorder using oxygen 15–labeled CO_2 and positron emission tomography. *Arch Gen Psychiatry.* 1994;51:62-70.
26. McGuire PK, Bench CJ, Frith CD, Marks IM, Frackowiak RSJ, Dolan RJ. Functional anatomy of obsessive-compulsive phenomena. *Br J Psychiatry.* 1994;164:459-468.
27. Phillips AG, Carr GD. Cognition and the basal ganglia: a possible substrate for procedural knowledge. *Can J Neurol Sci.* 1987;14:381-385.
28. Packard MG, Hirsh R, White NM. Differential effects of fornix and caudate nucleus lesions on two radial maze tasks: evidence for multiple memory systems. *J Neurosci.* 1989;9:1465-1472.
29. Mittleman G, Whishaw IQ, Jones GH, Koch M, Robbins TW. Cortical, hippocampal and striatal mediation of schedule-induced behaviors. *Behav Neurosci.* 1990;104:399-409.
30. Packard MG, White NM. Lesions of the caudate nucleus selectively impair 'reference memory' acquisitions in the radial maze. *Behav Neural Biol.* 1990;53:39-50.
31. Schwartz JM. Cognitive-behavioral self-treatment for obsessive-compulsive disorder systematically alters cerebral metabolism: a mind-brain interaction paradigm for psychotherapists. In: Hollander E, Stein DJ, eds. *Obsessive-Compulsive Disorders: Diagnosis, Etiology, Treatment.* New York, NY: Marcel Dekker Inc. In press.

Clinical and Biochemical Effects of Catecholamine Depletion on Antidepressant-Induced Remission of Depression

Helen L. Miller, MD; Pedro L. Delgado, MD; Ronald M. Salomon, MD; Robert Berman, MD; John H. Krystal, MD; George R. Heninger, MD; Dennis S. Charney, MD

Background: Most hypotheses of the therapeutic mechanism of action of antidepressant drugs have focused on the role of the monoamines. We examined the effect of catecholamine depletion on antidepressant-induced remission.

Method: The tyrosine hydroxylase inhibitor α-methylparatyrosine and the antihistamine diphenhydramine hydrochloride were administered, during separate test sessions, to depressed patients in remission maintained with either norepinephrine reuptake inhibitors (desipramine [n=7] or mazindol [n=2]) or serotonin reuptake inhibitors (fluoxetine hydrochloride [n=9] or sertraline hydrochloride [n=1]). Because of considerable sedation associated with α-methylparatyrosine testing, diphenhydramine was used as an active control rather than an inactive placebo. The effects of α-methylparatyrosine and diphenhydramine on depression, anxiety, and plasma catecholamine metabolites were assessed.

Results: α-Methylparatyrosine produced similar significant decreases in plasma 3-methoxy-4-hydroxyphenylethyleneglycol and homovanillic acid levels in the treatment groups. α-Methylparatyrosine produced a robust increase in depressive symptoms on the Hamilton Depression Rating Scale, including depressed mood, decreased concentration, anhedonia, loss of interest, and feelings of worthlessness, helplessness, and hopelessness, in the desipramine-mazindol but not in the fluoxetine-sertraline group. Diphenhydramine had no effects on mood in either treatment group.

Conclusions: The therapeutic effects of norepinephrine reuptake inhibitors, but not serotonin reuptake inhibitors, are reversed by catecholamine depletion. Considered with previous reports that serotonin depletion produces depressive relapses in patients in remission maintained with serotonin reuptake inhibitors, but not norepinephrine reuptake inhibitors, these findings suggest that antidepressants may not work via a single monoamine-related mechanism.

(Arch Gen Psychiatry. 1996;53:117-128)

THE ROLE of brain norepinephrine and dopamine function in the mechanism of action of antidepressant drugs has been the subject of intensive research during the past three decades.[1-5] Initially, the catecholamine hypotheses of depression postulated that a deficiency of norepinephrine was responsible for depression. The early hypotheses were based on the clinical observations of the mood-lowering effect of such drugs as reserpine, which depletes catecholamines, as well as the clinical efficacy of the monoamine oxidase inhibitors and tricyclic antidepressants, which increase the synaptic availability of catecholamines.[1,2]

Subsequently, preclinical investigations of the mechanisms of antidepressant action have characterized the effects of antidepressant drugs on noradrenergic and dopaminergic receptor function. Long-term treatment with some, but not all, antidepressant drugs has been demonstrated to decrease the function of presynaptic α_2-adrenergic autoreceptors.[6-15] A more consistent observation is that most antidepressant drugs decrease β-adrenergic receptor density and function.[16-23] Conversely, long-term antidepressant administration generally enhances the behaviorally and electrophysiologically assessed α_1-adrenergic receptor responsiveness.[24-30]

Antidepressant administration does not consistently alter dopamine D_2 receptor density[31-33] but may decrease dopamine D_1 receptor binding in limbic areas.[32-34] Antidepressant effects on the limbic

From the Department of Psychiatry, Yale University School of Medicine, New Haven, Conn, and the Department of Veterans Affairs Medical Center, West Haven, Conn.

See Patients and Methods on next page

PATIENTS AND METHODS

PATIENTS

Nineteen previously depressed patients in clinical remission for at least 2 weeks while receiving antidepressant treatment gave written informed consent to participate in a research study of the behavioral effects of catecholamine depletion. The patients were informed that acute reduction of catecholamine levels by α-methylparatyrosine might lead to a change in their mood, possibly causing a return of their depressive symptoms.

Diagnoses were made by consensus of two research psychiatrists (before antidepressant treatment) with the use of *DSM-III-R* criteria. Diagnoses were based on direct interview with the Structured Clinical Interview for *DSM-III-R*, Yale Depression Inventory,[64] and medical records. Each of the 19 patients met *DSM-III-R* criteria for major depressive episode. One patient also met criteria for major depressive episode with melancholia. Approximately 50% of the patients also met criteria for another Axis I or Axis II diagnosis, although in every case major depression was believed to be the primary reason for presentation for treatment. Demographic and diagnostic data for the patient groups are listed in **Table 1**.

The patients studied had therapeutic responses (as defined below) and were currently receiving treatment with a selective norepinephrine or dopamine reuptake inhibitor (desipramine hydrochloride [n=7] or mazindol [n=2]) or selective serotonin reuptake inhibitors (fluoxetine hydrochloride [n=9] or sertraline hydrochloride [n=1]).[65-67] Antidepressant treatment was provided by a research psychiatrist (P.L.D. or H.L.M.) in the Mood Disorders Outpatient Clinic (n=18) or the Affective Disorders Inpatient Unit (n=1) of the West Haven (Conn) Department of Veterans Affairs Medical Center. The antidepressant medication assignment to desipramine, mazindol, fluoxetine, or sertraline was not random and was based on several factors, including the patient's previous response to antidepressant drugs and participation in other research protocols. In addition, the patients in the study had been in remission for varying lengths of time (Table 1). Testing was performed after the patient had remained clinically stable for at least 2 weeks.

Before testing, each patient was judged by the investigator to have had a marked therapeutic response to the antidepressant, no longer to meet criteria for a current episode of major depression, and to have a total 25-item Hamilton Depression Rating Scale (HDRS) score of 15 or less.

PROCEDURE

α-Methylparatyrosine and Diphenhydramine Testing

Subjects underwent α-methylparatyrosine and diphenhydramine hydrochloride control testing approximately 1 week apart. Assignment to initial test conditions was random and double-blind. Approximately one half of subjects had α-methylparatyrosine testing first (n=9); the other half had diphenhydramine control testing first (n=10). Because of considerable sedation associated with α-methylparatyrosine testing, diphenhydramine was used as an active control rather than an inactive placebo. The patients continued to receive their antidepressant medication daily throughout α-methylparatyrosine and diphenhydramine testing.

Each test sequence consisted of 4 consecutive days: a baseline test day during which no medication was given (baseline); 2 days of treatment with either α-methylparatyrosine, 1 g three times daily, or diphenhydramine hydrochloride, 50 mg three times daily (day 1), and α-methylparatyrosine, 1 g twice daily, or diphenhydramine hydrochloride, 50 mg twice daily (day 2); and a posttest evaluation (follow-up day). Subjects were given a low-monoamine diet for the 4 days of testing to minimize variability in catecholamine turnover. Serum was collected each morning (at 9 AM) for determination of 3-methoxy-4-hydroxyphenylethyleneglycol (MHPG) and HVA levels. Be-

and cortical dopamine D_3, D_4, and D_5 receptors have not yet been studied. Mesolimbic dopamine function, as assessed by amphetamine- and apomorphine-induced spontaneous locomotor activity, is enhanced by tricyclic antidepressants and electroconvulsive therapy, possibly via increased postsynaptic dopamine receptor responsiveness.[35] Nigrostriatal dopamine function, as assessed by dopamine agonist–stimulated stereotypy, shows less consistent results.[33] Biochemical and behavioral investigations indicate that long-term treatment with some, but not all, antidepressant drugs reduces dopamine autoreceptor function.[33,36-38]

Studies of repeated antidepressant dosing have shown inconsistent results on norepinephrine uptake site density, as measured by tritiated desipramine.[39-43] A recent study[44] that used radiolabeled nisoxetine, a potent and relatively specific ligand for the norepinephrine uptake site, demonstrated significantly decreased binding in multiple brain regions, including the hippocampus, thalamus, and amygdala, after long-term administration of desipramine or electroconvulsive therapy.

More recently, the effects of antidepressant drugs on tyrosine hydroxylase, the rate-limiting enzyme in the biosynthesis of norepinephrine and dopamine, have been examined. Long-term administration of several types of antidepressants reduces the expression of this protein, as measured by immunoblot assays, and decreases tyrosine hydroxylase activity, as measured by norepinephrine precursor accumulation in response to tyrosine hydroxylase inhibition.[45-47] Studies of tyrosine hydroxylase messenger RNA levels in response to long-term administration of antidepressants have shown variable results.[45-49]

Clinical investigations of the mechanism of antidepressant action suggest that long-term antidepressant treatment frequently, but not invariably, results in decreased responsiveness of presynaptic α_2-adrenergic function.[50-53] To our knowledge, no studies have been conducted of central α_1- or β-adrenergic function in depressed patients. One investigation[54] that used the heart rate and blood pressure responses to isoproterenol as an index of β_1-adrenergic receptor function found reduced effects after antidepressant treatment.

Although these data are not the primary subject of this report, extensive preclinical and clinical data strongly implicate serotonin in the mechanism of action of antihaviorial ratings were obtained once on the baseline day (at 9 AM), twice a day during medication administration (at 9 AM and 4:30 PM, days 1 and 2), and once on the follow-up day (at 9 AM) (see **Table 2** for the schedule of α-methylparatyrosine and diphenhydramine test sessions).

Behavioral ratings consisted of the 25-item, modified HDRS,[64] the Hamilton Anxiety Scale,[68] and the Side Effect Symptom Checklist.[69] The Symptom Checklist is a self-rated scale consisting of 23 items, each scored from 0 (not at all) to 3 (severe). Items included headache, constipation, poor memory, nausea or vomiting, feeling drowsy or sleepy, blurred vision, increased appetite, difficulty starting urination, trouble concentrating, nightmares, difficulty sitting still, irregular or pounding heartbeat, diarrhea, frequent need to urinate, dry mouth, decreased appetite, tremors or shakiness, rash, ringing in the ears, sweating, faintness or light-headedness, poor coordination, and stiffness in muscles.

Biochemical Assays

Plasma free levels of HVA[70] and MHPG[71] were measured by gas chromatography and mass spectrometry, with the use of deuterated internal standards.

Data Analysis

The effects of α-methylparatyrosine and diphenhydramine on the two patient groups (desipramine-mazindol and fluoxetine-sertraline) and on the biochemical and behavioral measures were initially evaluated by means of an analysis of variance with repeated measures (ANOVA). This allowed an assessment of the statistical significance of the main effects of patient group (desipramine-mazindol vs fluoxetine-sertraline), drug (α-methylparatyrosine vs diphenhydramine), and time of measurement (changes during the periods sampled). The central question of the data analysis was focused on whether the patients in the desipramine-mazindol group reacted differently to α-methylparatyrosine than the patients in the fluoxetine-sertraline group. In the ANOVA involving the entire patient sample, this was manifested primarily in the interaction of group with drug and time. In the ANOVA calculated in the groups separately, the interaction of drug and time demonstrated the significance of the α-methylparatyrosine effects within each group.

The significant interactions were further evaluated with paired and nonpaired *t* tests to assess how and when the patients differed in their response to α-methylparatyrosine. This was primarily done by subtracting the baseline value from the value at each time point on the variable of interest. This resulted in a change score at each time point after administration of α-methylparatyrosine or diphenhydramine. By subtracting the change after diphenhydramine treatment from the change after α-methylparatyrosine treatment, an estimate of the net α-methylparatyrosine effect could be obtained. Pearson correlations were calculated to evaluate the relationships among the net α-methylparatyrosine effects on depressive symptoms and catecholamine metabolites and the clinical characteristics listed in Table 1. Results are reported as significant when $P<.05$, with a two-tailed test.

Another analysis of behavioral data used the concept of depressive relapse as previously defined (P.L.D, H.L.M., R.M.S., Julio Licinio, MD, J.H.K., G.R.H., D.S.C., unpublished data, January 1995).[57,58] Relapse was defined as an increase in depressive symptoms such that the total HDRS score had increased by 50% or more from before testing and was now 17 or more. Patients were categorized as having had relapses or not, and Fisher's exact test was applied.

The effects of α-methylparatyrosine and diphenhydramine on total HDRS scores in five of the patients in the desipramine-mazindol group and five of those in the fluoxetine-sertraline group have been described in a short preliminary report.[72]

depressant drugs.[55,56] Considered with the evidence cited above regarding norepinephrine and dopamine, a crucial research and clinical question is whether the different classes of antidepressant drugs work via a common neurobiologic mechanism or whether distinct neuronal effects can lead to similar therapeutic properties.

A clinical research strategy recently used by our group to study the role of the different monoamine systems in the mechanism of action of antidepressant drugs has been the use of monoamine depletion paradigms to determine the effect of reduced monoamine availability on the maintenance of antidepressant-induced remission. In a series of investigations (P.L.D, H.L.M., R.M.S., Julio Licinio, MD, J.H.K., G.R.H., D.S.C., unpublished data, January 1995)[57,58] we demonstrated that rapid plasma tryptophan depletion temporarily reverses antidepressant responses in many antidepressant-treated patients in remission. Furthermore, recent findings indicate that patients who have responded to selective serotonin reuptake inhibitors frequently experience a transient depressive relapse during rapid tryptophan depletion, but patients whose conditions have improved with norepinephrine reuptake inhibitors (such as desipramine) rarely experience such a relapse (P.L.D, H.L.M., R.M.S., Julio Licinio, MD, J.H.K., G.R.H., D.S.C., unpublished data, January 1995). These data suggested that enhancement of the serotonin function may not represent a common mechanism of antidepressant action, and that the therapeutic responses of some antidepressants may be more primarily related to effects on other monoamine systems.

The purpose of the present investigation was to determine if rapid reduction in the brain catecholamines, norepinephrine and dopamine, induces a transient depressive relapse in depressed patients with an antidepressant-maintained recent remission. A reduction in brain catecholamine levels is produced by administration of α-methylparatyrosine via inhibition of tyrosine hydroxylase.[59] In clinical investigations, α-methylparatyrosine (in dosages ranging from 1 to 4 g/d) produces substantial decreases in urinary excretion of catecholamine metabolites and cerebrospinal fluid levels of the dopamine metabolite homovanillic acid (HVA) with no change in the 5-hydroxytryptophan metabolite 5-hydroxyindoleacetic acid.[60-62] A maximal reduction of catecholamine metabolites during α-methylparatyrosine treatment occurs

Table 1. Patient Characteristics*

Patient No./ Gender/Age, y	Diagnosis*	Current Antidepressant Medication/Dose, mg/d	No. of Previous Unsuccessful Antidepressant Trials	No. of Previous Major Depressive Episodes	Hamilton Depression Scale Score† Medication Initiation	Hamilton Depression Scale Score† Baseline	Weeks of Remission at Time of AMPT Testing
Selective Serotonin Reuptake Inhibitor Responders							
1/M/47	MD, ALCe	Fluoxetine hydrochloride/20	0	0	30	0	11
2/F/21	MD, Bul, BoPD	Fluoxetine hydrochloride/60	0	2	30	0	90
3/M/59	MD, ALCe	Fluoxetine hydrochloride/20	1	0	28	9	15
4/F/53	MD, ALCe, OCD	Fluoxetine hydrochloride/20	1	>3	28	6	4
5/F/26	MD, Bul	Fluoxetine hydrochloride/20	0	0	28	7	7
6/F/34	MD	Fluoxetine hydrochloride/20	0	0	34	0	60
7/M/42	MD, PD	Fluoxetine hydrochloride/60	2	>3	32	4	5
8/M/35	MD, DPD	Fluoxetine hydrochloride/60	0	0	42	5	32
9/M/35	MD, PSAe	Fluoxetine hydrochloride/80	3	0	31	8	7
10/F/44	MD	Sertraline hydrochloride/75	5	0	30	10	8
Norepinephrine Reuptake Inhibitor Responders							
1/M/59	MD	Desipramine hydrochloride/200	0	>3	35	15	2
2/F/34	MD	Desipramine hydrochloride/200	0	0	32	3	12
3/M/57	MDM, ALCe	Desipramine hydrochloride/300	2	2	59	15	2
4/M/32	MD, MJe	Desipramine hydrochloride/250	3	1	37	7	10
5/M/46	MD, APD	Desipramine hydrochloride/250	0	>3	23	4	12
6/M/42	MD	Desipramine hydrochloride//300	1	0	31	13	11
7/M/46	MD	Desipramine hydrochloride/300	0	0	38	10	17
8/M/48	MD	Mazindol/4	0	0	30	14	12
9/M/57	MD, ALCe	Mazindol/4	...	...	42	2	30

*ALCe indicates alcohol abuse in remission; APD, avoidant personality disorder; BoPD, borderline personality disorder; Bul, bulimia; DPD, dependent personality disorder; MD, major depression; MDM, major depression with melancholia; MJe, marijuana abuse in remission; OCD, obsessive-compulsive disorder; PD, panic disorder; PSAe, polysubstance abuse in remission; and AMPT, α-methylparatyrosine.

†Hamilton Depression Scale scores shown reflect those obtained just before the start of the current antidepressant treatment (medication initiation) and just before the start of AMPT or diphenhydramine hydrochloride testing (baseline).

Table 2. Schedule for AMPT and Diphenhydramine Test Sessions*

Test Day	Time	Procedure
Baseline day	9 AM	Vital signs (BP, pulse, temperature, urinalysis); ratings of mood, plasma MHPG, HVA
Drug day 1	9 AM	Vital signs; ratings of mood, plasma MHPG, HVA; diphenhydramine hydrochloride, 50 mg, or AMPT, 1 g
	Noon	Diphenhydramine hydrochloride, 50 mg, or AMPT, 1 g
	3 PM	Diphenhydramine hydrochloride, 50 mg, or AMPT, 1 g
	4:30 PM	Ratings of mood, vital signs
Drug day 2	9 AM	Vital signs; ratings of mood, plasma MHPG, HVA; diphenhydramine hydrochloride, 50 mg, or AMPT, 1 g
	Noon	Diphenhydramine hydrochloride, 50 mg, or AMPT, 1 g
	4:30 PM	Ratings of mood, vital signs
Follow-up day	9 AM	Vital signs; ratings of mood, plasma MHPG, HVA

*AMPT indicates α-methylparatyrosine; BP, blood pressure; MHPG, 3-methoxy-4-hydroxyphenylethyleneglycol; and HVA, homovanillic acid.

after 2 to 3 days of treatment.[61,63] We predicted that depressed patients who experienced remissions during treatment with norepinephrine reuptake inhibitor drugs, but not those who had remissions with serotonin reuptake inhibitors, would experience a return of depressive symptoms while receiving α-methylparatyrosine.

RESULTS

α-METHYLPARATYROSINE–INDUCED CHANGES IN PLASMA MHPG AND HVA LEVELS

As predicted, α-methylparatyrosine produced robust and significant decreases in plasma HVA levels in both antidepressant groups.[73] The ANOVA in the desipramine-mazindol and fluoxetine-sertraline groups, respectively, for plasma HVA level showed a drug and time interaction ($F=18.9$, $df=3,18$, $P<.001$; and $F=7.34$, $df=3,15$, $P=.003$). α-Methylparatyrosine significantly decreased plasma HVA levels from baseline on day 2 in the desipramine-mazindol group and on day 2 and the follow-up day in the fluoxetine-sertraline group (**Figure 1**).

α-Methylparatyrosine produced robust decreases in plasma MHPG levels in both antidepressant drug groups. The effect was slightly greater in the fluoxetine-sertraline group, probably because of the reduced baseline MHPG levels produced by desipramine treatment.[74] The drug and time interaction was highly significant ($F=14.2$, $df=3,21$, $P<.001$), and plasma MHPG level was significantly decreased from baseline on day 2 and the follow-up day in the fluoxetine-sertraline group. In the desipramine-mazindol group, the drug and time interaction was

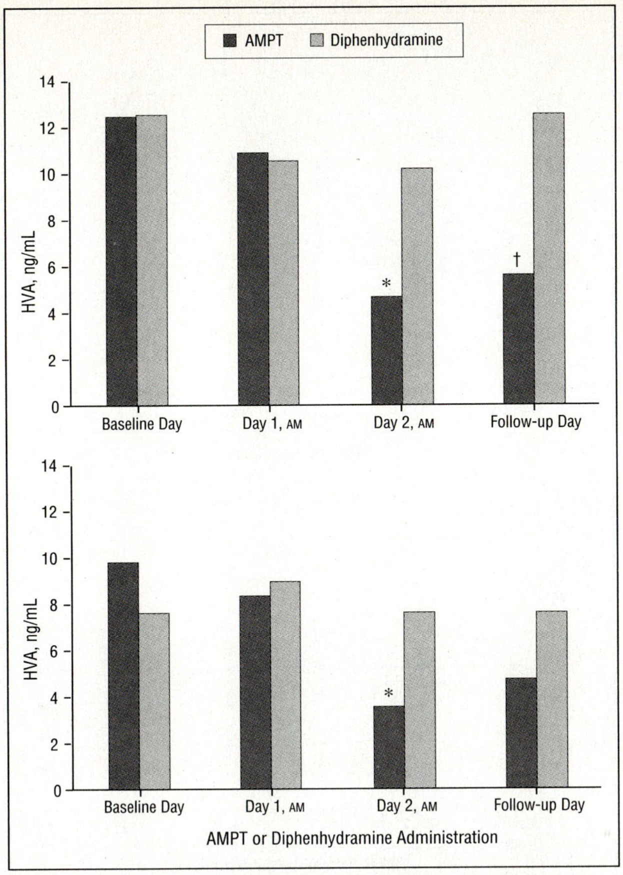

Figure 1. *The effect of α-methylparatyrosine (AMPT) and diphenhydramine hydrochloride on plasma homovanillic acid (HVA) levels in patients who responded to fluoxetine hydrochloride (n=9) or sertraline hydrochloride (n=1) (top) and to desipramine hydrochloride (n=7) or mazindol (n=2) (bottom). There were significant decreases (asterisk,* $P<.001$*; dagger,* $P<.01$*) during and just after AMPT administration. There were no significant decreases in plasma HVA level during diphenhydramine administration. Values for baseline and day 1 reflect measurements before drug administration. Follow-up day values reflect measurements after discontinuation of drug administration.*

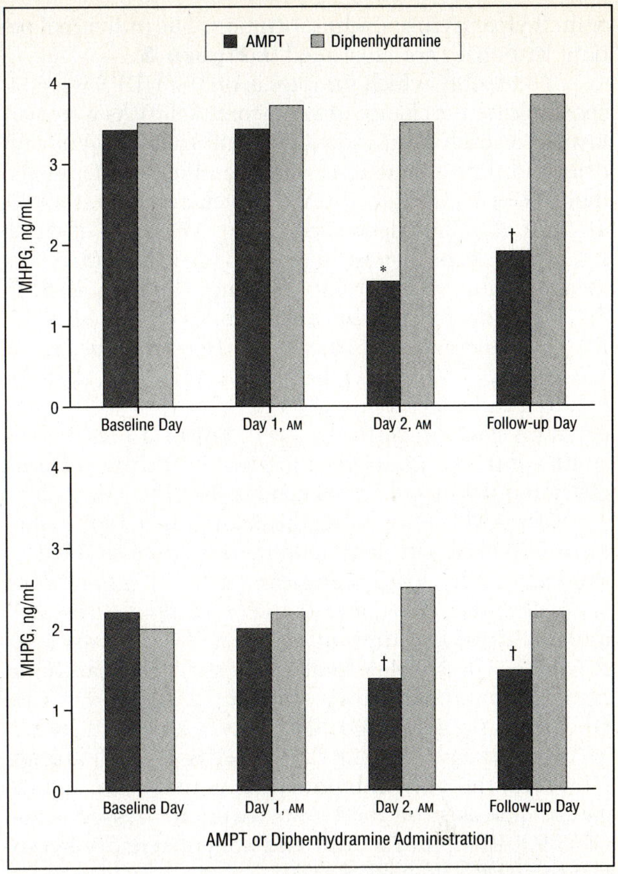

Figure 2. *The effect of α-methylparatyrosine (AMPT) and diphenhydramine hydrochloride on plasma 3-methoxy-4-hydroxyphenylethyleneglycol (MHPG) levels in patients who responded to fluoxetine hydrochloride (n=9) or sertraline hydrochloride (n=1) (top) and to desipramine hydrochloride (n=7) or mazindol (n=2) (bottom). There were significant decreases (asterisk,* $P<.01$*; dagger,* $P<.05$*) in plasma MHPG levels during AMPT administration. There were no significant decreases in plasma MHPG level during diphenhydramine administration. Values for baseline and day 1 reflect measurements before drug administration. Follow-up day values reflect measurements after discontinuation of drug administration.*

also significant ($F=7.02$, $df=3,21$, $P=.002$), and plasma MHPG level was significantly decreased from baseline on day 2 and the follow-up day (**Figure 2**).

The effects of α-methylparatyrosine and diphenhydramine on plasma MHPG and HVA levels did not differ in the desipramine-mazindol and fluoxetine-sertraline groups. The group, drug, and time interaction was not significant ($F=0.66$, $df=3,33$, $P=.58$), and at no time point were the changes in MHPG and HVA levels significantly different between the two patient groups.

BEHAVIORAL EFFECTS OF α-METHYLPARATYROSINE IN PATIENTS IN REMISSION TAKING ANTIDEPRESSANTS

Norepinephrine Reuptake Inhibitors

The ANOVA assessing the change in depressive symptoms (reflected in the HDRS total score) during α-methylparatyrosine and diphenhydramine administration in depressed patients in remission who were receiving either desipramine (n=7) or mazindol (n=2) showed significant main effects of drug ($F=22.42$, $df=1,8$, $P=.001$) and time ($F=8.22$, $df=5,40$, $P<.001$). The interaction of drug (α-methylparatyrosine vs diphenhydramine) and time of sampling was also significant ($F=13.70$, $df=5,40$, $P<.001$). This interaction reflects the significant increase in depressive symptoms elicited by α-methylparatyrosine compared with diphenhydramine administration during the time points sampled. Paired *t* tests showed significant increases from total HDRS scores obtained before α-methylparatyrosine administration (day 1 AM measurement) compared with HDRS scores in the evening of the first day of α-methylparatyrosine administration (day 1 PM; 8.9 ± 5.2 vs 16.4 ± 9.2, $t=3.25$, $P=.001$) and the morning (day 2 AM; 8.9 ± 5.2 vs 23.1 ± 9.1, $t=4.86$, $P=.001$) and evening (day 2 PM; 8.9 ± 5.2 vs 17.8 ± 8.6, $t=3.63$, $P=.007$) of the second day of α-methylparatyrosine administration. No significant changes from the baseline HDRS scores were found after diphenhydramine administration. Eight of the nine patients (six of seven treated with desipramine and two of two treated with mazindol) met relapse criteria during α-methylparatyrosine administration. One of the nine patients (receiving desipramine) met criteria for relapse during diphenhydramine administration. This patient also had a relapse during α-methylparatyrosine administration. The individual patient responses are illustrated in **Figure 3**.

To identify which symptoms on the HDRS were responsible for the change in total score, ANOVAs were performed on each of the individual HDRS items. Significant drug and time interactions were identified for depressed mood (F=4.15, *df*=5,40, *P*=.004); psychic anxiety (F=3.89, *df*=5,40, *P*=.006); decreased energy (F=8.64, *df*=5,40, *P*<.001); loss of interest (F=5.07, *df*=5,40, *P*<.001); decreased ability to experience pleasure (F=5.23, *df*=5,40, *P*<.001); decreased concentration (F=8.81, *df*=5,40, *P*<.001); increased feelings of worthlessness or failure (F=3.40, *df*=5,40, *P*=.01), helplessness (F=4.50, *df*=5,40, *P*=.002), and hopelessness (F=6.06, *df*=5,40, *P*<.001); and agitation (F=2.49, *df*=5,40, *P*=.05). **Table 3** presents the results of paired *t* tests used to identify the time of peak effect and the magnitude of change for these effects.

The ANOVA assessing the change in anxiety symptoms, as reflected in the Hamilton Anxiety Scale (HAM-A) total score, disclosed significant main effects of drug (F=6.45, *df*=1,8, *P*=.04) and time (F=4.76, *df*=5,40, *P*=.002) and the drug and time interaction (F=7.62, *df*=5,40, *P*<.001). The HAM-A total score was significantly increased from the day 1 AM score (6.7±3.0) at day 1 PM (9.6±4.5, *t*=2.7, *P*=.03), day 2 AM (14.2±8.3, *t*=2.7, *P*=.02), and day 2 PM (11.7±5.8, *t*=2.8, *P*<.05) ratings. However, the only individual items that were significantly increased on the HAM-A were depressed mood (F=3.93, *df*=5,40, *P*=.005) and somatosensory symptoms (F=2.83, *df*=5,40, *P*=.03).

Assessment of side effects associated with α-methylparatyrosine compared with diphenhydramine administration showed a significant drug and time interaction only for constipation (F=2.54, *df*=5,40, *P*=.04), with α-methylparatyrosine leading to a slight increase. Both α-methylparatyrosine and diphenhydramine induced drowsiness, as indicated by a significant main effect of time (F=4.42, *df*=5,40, *P*=.003). The drowsiness caused by α-methylparatyrosine (day 1 AM, 1.7±0.9, to maximal effect at day 1 PM, 2.6±0.7) and diphenhydramine (day 1 AM, 1.6±0.9, to maximal effect at day 1 PM, 2.3±0.7) was similar in degree and duration.

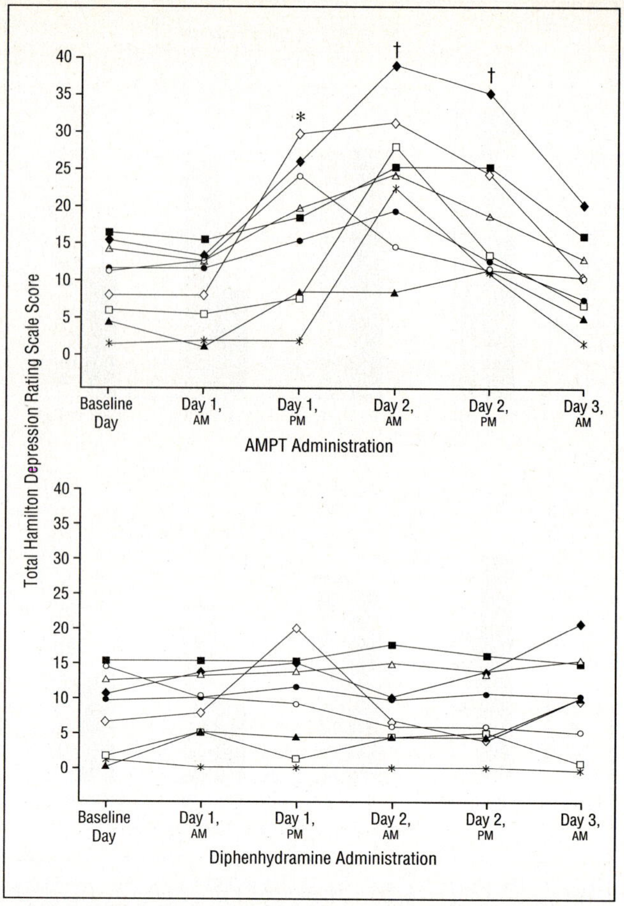

Figure 3. *Scores on the 25-item Hamilton Depression Rating Scale for each of nine depressed patients in remission who were taking either desipramine hydrochloride (n=7) or mazindol (n=2) before (baseline and day 1 AM ratings), during administration of either α-methylparatyrosine (AMPT) (1 g at 9 AM, 1 PM, and 4 PM on day 1; 1 g at 9 AM and 1 PM on day 2) or diphenhydramine hydrochloride (50 mg at 9 AM, 1 PM, and 4 PM on day 1; 50 mg at 9 AM and 1 PM on day 2), and at follow-up (day 3). Asterisk indicates* P<.05 *compared with day 1 AM, paired* t *test, two tailed; dagger,* P<.01 *compared with day 1 AM, paired* t *test, two tailed. Each of the nine patients is represented by a different symbol.*

Serotonin Reuptake Inhibitors

In contrast to effects observed in patients treated with desipramine or mazindol, α-methylparatyrosine did not produce an exacerbation of depressive symptoms in patients treated with fluoxetine (n=9) or sertraline (n=1). The ANOVA examining the change in the HDRS total score showed a nonsignificant main effect of drug (F=0.04, *df*=1,9, *P*=.84) and a significant main effect of time (F=3.69, *df*=5,45, *P*=.007). However, the interaction of drug and time was not significant (F=1.22, *df*=5,45, *P*=.32). Paired *t* tests indicated that at no time point was there a significant change from baseline in HDRS scores after either α-methylparatyrosine or diphenhydramine administration (**Figure 4**).

None of the 10 patients who were receiving fluoxetine or sertraline for maintenance met relapse criteria during either α-methylparatyrosine or diphenhydramine administration.

To determine if any individual symptom on the HDRS was changed by α-methylparatyrosine compared with diphenhydramine, ANOVAs were calculated for each of the individual HDRS items. The only symptom for which there was a significant drug and time interaction was terminal insomnia (F=2.85, *df*=5,45, *P*=.03). However, at no time point was the change in the report of terminal insomnia from baseline significantly different after α-methylparatyrosine compared with diphenhydramine administration. For comparison with the effects of α-methylparatyrosine in the patients who received desipramine and mazindol for maintenance, **Table 4** lists the effects of α-methylparatyrosine on individual HDRS items in the patients who received fluoxetine and sertraline.

In contrast to effects identified in the patients who received desipramine and mazindol, α-methylparatyrosine did not produce an increase in the HAM-A score. The ANOVA showed nonsignificant main effects of drug (F=0.42, *df*=1,9, *P*=.53) and time (F=1.2, *df*=5,45, *P*=.33) and a nonsignificant drug and time interaction (F=0.67,

Table 3. Individual Hamilton Depression Rating Scale Items Found Significant on Analysis of Variance During AMPT Administration in Patients Responding to Desipramine (n=7) or Mazindol (n=2)

Item	Baseline Day*	Day 1, AM*	Day 1, PM	Day 2, AM	Day 2, PM	Follow-up Day
Depressed mood	1.0±0.5	0.9±0.6	1.4±1.1	1.7±1.1†	1.4±0.9	0.9±0.8
Psychic anxiety	0.9±0.8	0.4±0.5	0.9±1.3	1.6±1.2†	1.2±1.1†	0.8±0.8
Loss of energy	0.8±0.7	0.9±0.8	2.2±1.0‡	2.8±0.4‡	2.1±0.8§	1.1±0.6
Loss of interest	0.7±0.5	0.8±0.7	1.6±1.1†	2.1±0.6§	1.6±0.9†	1.0±0.7
Loss of pleasure	0.7±0.5	0.7±0.5	1.2±1.2	1.8±0.8§	1.6±0.9§	1.0±0.9†
Decreased concentration	0.7±0.9	0.6±0.5	1.8±1.2§	2.6±0.7‡	1.8±1.0§	0.7±0.5
Agitation	0.1±0.3	0.1±0.3	0.3±0.7	0.9±1.1§	0.4±0.7	0.1±0.3
Helplessness	0.6±0.5	0.4±0.5	1.1±1.1	1.8±1.0§	0.9±0.8	0.6±0.7
Hopelessness	0.4±0.5	0.6±0.5	1.1±1.3	1.3±1.0§	1.0±1.1	0.7±1.0
Worthlessness/failure	0.4±0.5	0.4±0.5	1.0±1.1†	0.9±1.0†	0.6±0.7	0.6±0.7

*These ratings were obtained before α-methylparatyrosine (AMPT) administration (see Table 2).
†P<.05 vs day 1 AM, paired t test, two tailed.
‡P<.001 vs day 1 AM, paired t test, two tailed.
§P<.01 vs day 1 AM, paired t test, two tailed.

df=5,45, *P*=.65). Furthermore, none of the individual items on the HAM-A were significantly increased by α-methylparatyrosine.

Assessment of side effects associated with α-methylparatyrosine compared with diphenhydramine administration showed a significant drug and time interaction only for decreased concentration (F=2.59, *df*=5,40, *P*=.04), with diphenhydramine producing a slight increase. Both α-methylparatyrosine and diphenhydramine induced drowsiness, as indicated by a significant main effect of time (F=6.12, *df*=5,40, *P*<.001). The drowsiness resulting from α-methylparatyrosine (day 1 AM, 1.6±0.5, to maximal effect at day 1 PM, 2.5±1.1) and diphenhydramine (day 1 AM, 1.4±0.5, to maximal effect at day 1 PM, 2.3±1.2) was similar in degree and duration.

Comparison of Effects in Patients Treated With Norepinephrine and Serotonin Reuptake Inhibitors for Maintenance

As detailed above, α-methylparatyrosine produced clinically and statistically significant increase in depressive symptoms in patients maintained with desipramine or mazindol. In marked contrast, α-methylparatyrosine had essentially no effect on these symptoms in patients receiving fluoxetine or sertraline.

The ANOVA comparing the effects of α-methylparatyrosine and diphenhydramine on total HDRS score in all of the patients demonstrated a highly significant group (desipramine-mazindol vs fluoxetine-sertraline) and drug (α-methylparatyrosine vs diphenhydramine) and time interaction (F=9.71, *df*=5,85, *P*<.001). This indicates that α-methylparatyrosine and diphenhydramine had statistically significantly different effects in the two patient groups during the period sampled. Specifically, α-methylparatyrosine, compared with diphenhydramine, produced significantly greater increases in the HDRS total score from the day 1 AM score in desipramine-mazindol–treated patients compared with the fluoxetine-sertraline–treated patients at the day 2 AM (14.6±9.4 vs 1.1±5.6, *t*=4.5, *P*<.001) and day 2 PM (9.1±7.0 vs 0.3±5.9, *t*=3.1, *P*=.006) ratings. Further reinforcing the observation that the magnitude of the effect of α-methylparatyrosine on HDRS score was different for the two groups are the differences in the rate of depressive relapse. None of the 10 fluoxetine-sertraline–treated patients met criteria for relapse, while eight of nine desipramine-mazindol–treated patients had relapses after administration of α-methylparatyrosine (*P*<.001, Fisher's exact test).

The ANOVA assessing specific items on the HDRS also showed greater α-methylparatyrosine effects in the desipramine-mazindol group. Significant group and drug and time interactions were found for depression (F=3.2, *df*=5,85, *P*=.01), psychic anxiety (F=3.6, *df*=5,85, *P*=.005), loss of interest (F=3.32, *df*=5,85, *P*=.009), decreased ability to experience pleasure (F=2.73, *df*=5,85, *P*=.02), decreased concentration (F=4.24, *df*=5,85, *P*=.002), and increased feelings of worthlessness or failure (F=2.90, *df*=5,85, *P*=.02), helplessness (F=4.58, *df*=5,85, *P*<.001), and hopelessness (F=3.66, *df*=5,85, *P*=.005). For each of these items, the α-methylparatyrosine–induced increases were significantly greater in the desipramine-mazindol–treated patients at multiple time points.

α-Methylparatyrosine also produced larger increases in the total HAM-A score in the desipramine-mazindol group. The ANOVA found a significant group and drug and time interaction (F=6.90, *df*=5,85, *P*<.001). The increase in the HAM-A from day 1 AM after α-methylparatyrosine administration compared with diphenhydramine was significantly greater at the day 2 AM (7.8±9.1 vs −1.5±4.5, *t*=2.8, *P*=.02) and day 2 PM (5.3±5.1 vs −1.4±4.9, *t*=2.9, *P*=.02) ratings in the desipramine-mazindol group compared with the fluoxetine-sertraline group.

The effect of α-methylparatyrosine and diphenhydramine on side effects was not different for the two patient groups for any item.

FACTORS ASSOCIATED WITH RETURN OF DEPRESSION

Since the patients were not randomly assigned to each treatment group, it is possible that specific clinical characteristics were related to the response to α-methylparatyrosine. Given the relatively small number of patients in each subgroup, the findings must be interpreted with caution. Inspection of the clinical characteristics of the patients studied, shown in Table 1, suggests that diagnosis, number of previous depressive episodes or unsuccessful antidepressant trials, and weeks in remission cannot account for the differential response to α-methylparatyrosine since the two patient groups were similar in regard to these factors. It is possible that the severity of depressive symptoms, as reflected by the HDRS scores at baseline, may be related to α-methylparatyrosine responsiveness because the desipramine- and mazindol-maintained patients had higher HDRS scores at this time. However, there was no correlation between baseline HDRS score and α-methylparatyrosine–induced increases in the HDRS score (r=.20, P=.41), and ANOVA covarying for baseline HDRS did not change the significance of the reported findings. There also was no apparent relationship between the effect of α-methylparatyrosine on plasma HVA (r=.18, P=.68) or MHPG levels and changes in the HDRS in the desipramine-mazindol–treated patients (r=.10, P=.79).

COMMENT

The primary finding of this investigation is that administration of α-methylparatyrosine to depressed patients in remission led to a clinically significant return of depressive symptoms in patients whose remissions were maintained with the norepinephrine reuptake inhibitors desipramine and mazindol, but not in patients whose remissions were maintained with the serotonin reuptake inhibitors fluoxetine and sertraline. Diphenhydramine proved to be a successful control in that it produced a degree of drowsiness and anergy similar to that from α-methylparatyrosine, but did not significantly alter depressive symptoms in either patient group.

The α-methylparatyrosine evoked the core symptoms of depression, such as depressed mood, loss of interest, anhedonia, decreased concentration, and sense of worthlessness and failure. Moreover, the symptom complex and depressive cognitive content induced by α-methylparatyrosine often closely resembled the unique features manifested by the patient before successful treatment.

Interpretation of these findings is contingent on the extent to which α-methylparatyrosine reduced brain norepinephrine and dopamine synthesis. As noted, α-methylparatyrosine is an inhibitor of the first and rate-limiting step in catecholamine synthesis, the enzyme tyrosine hydroxylase. In the present study, administration of α-methylparatyrosine rapidly reduced plasma metabolites of norepinephrine and dopamine. The magnitude of reduction in catecholamine metabolites was similar to that reported previously in healthy human subjects[61] and psychiatric patients.[63] Since α-methylparatyrosine easily passes the blood-brain barrier and tyrosine hydroxylase is present in brain catecholamine-containing neurons,[73] it is likely that substantial brain catecholamine depletion occurred during α-methylparatyrosine testing.

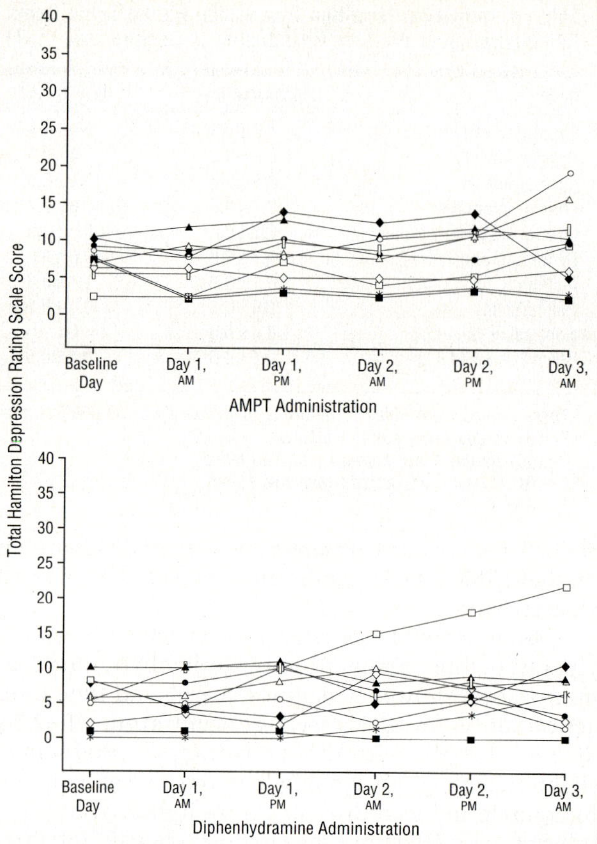

Figure 4. *Scores on the 25-item Hamilton Depression Rating Scale for each of 10 depressed patients in remission who were taking either fluoxetine hydrochloride (n=9) or sertraline hydrochloride (n=1) before (baseline and day 1 AM ratings), during administration of either α-methylparatyrosine (AMPT) (1 g at 9 AM, 1 PM, and 4 PM on day 1; 1 g at 9 AM and 1 PM on day 2) or diphenhydramine hydrochloride (50 mg at 9 AM, 1 PM, and 4 PM on day 1; 50 mg at 9 AM and 1 PM on day 2), and at follow-up (day 3). There were no significant changes in scores as a result of AMPT or diphenhydramine administration. Each of the 10 patients is represented by a different symbol.*

The α-methylparatyrosine–induced decreases in plasma HVA and MHPG levels were similar in the patients who received desipramine-mazindol and fluoxetine-sertraline for maintenance. This suggests that the differential effects of α-methylparatyrosine on depressive symptoms are related to the therapeutic mechanism of action of the antidepressant drugs used.

It is possible, however, that specific clinical characteristics of the depressed patients studied may be related to α-methylparatyrosine responsiveness. The therapeutic effects of desipramine and mazindol, as reflected by higher HDRS scores before α-methylparatyrosine testing, appear to have been less than those of fluoxetine or sertraline. Although, as noted, there was no correlation between baseline HDRS score and α-methylparatyrosine–induced increases in the HDRS score, it is possible that incomplete antidepressant effects are a factor in the observed findings. Other factors that need further study and may be relevant to the α-methylparatyrosine effects could

Table 4. Individual Hamilton Depression Rating Scale Items During AMPT Administration in Patients Responding to Fluoxetine (n=9) or Sertraline (n=1)

Item	Baseline Day*	Day 1, AM*	Day 1, PM	Day 2, AM	Day 2, PM	Follow-up Day
Depressed mood	0.1±0.3	0.0±0.0	0.0±0.0	0.1±0.3	0.0±0.0	0.3±0.7
Psychic anxiety	0.6±0.5	0.7±0.7	0.4±0.5	0.2±0.4	0.4±0.5	1.0±1.2
Loss of energy	0.4±0.5	0.4±0.5	2.1±0.9†	1.5±1.3‡	2.0±1.2‡	1.3±1.0§
Loss of interest	0.5±0.7	0.5±0.7	0.6±0.7	0.6±0.8	0.6±0.8	0.8±1.1
Loss of pleasure	0.4±0.7	0.5±0.7	0.5±0.7	0.6±0.8	0.6±0.8	0.7±1.0
Decreased concentration	0.6±0.7	0.6±0.7	1.2±1.2	0.9±1.0	1.1±1.0	0.7±0.8
Agitation	0.1±0.3	0.1±0.3	0.1±0.3	0.1±0.3	0.3±0.5	0.3±0.5
Helplessness	0.1±0.3	0.2±0.4	0.1±0.3	0.1±0.3	0.0±0.0	0.3±0.5
Hopelessness	0.1±0.3	0.1±0.3	0.1±0.3	0.2±0.4	0.2±0.4	0.1±0.3
Worthlessness/failure	0.1±0.3	0.1±0.3	0.2±0.4	0.1±0.3	0.1±0.3	0.1±0.3

**These ratings were obtained before α-methylparatyrosine (AMPT) administration (see Table 2).*
†P<.001 vs day 1 AM, paired t test, two tailed.
‡P<.01 vs day 1 AM, paired t test, two tailed.
§P<.05 vs day 1 AM, paired t test, two tailed.

be melancholic diagnosis, history of refractoriness to antidepressant drugs, gender, and duration of antidepressant-induced remission. Additional studies using random drug assignment will be helpful in determining whether other factors besides antidepressant drug type are related to α-methylparatyrosine effects.

COMPARISON WITH PREVIOUS STUDIES WITH α-METHYLPARATYROSINE

One previous investigation assessed the behavioral effects of α-methylparatyrosine in antidepressant-treated depressed patients. In three depressed patients who had a therapeutic response to imipramine, α-methylparatyrosine had no significant effect on the antidepressant response.[75] In one of these patients, α-methylparatyrosine administration was started before initiation of antidepressant treatment, and that patient went on to have a therapeutic response to imipramine. Although these data are provocative, strong inferences cannot be drawn from this study because the number of patients was small, there was no placebo control, and imipramine is a potent serotonin reuptake inhibitor as well as norepinephrine reuptake inhibitor.

In general, α-methylparatyrosine has not been reported to produce major alterations in mood in medical patients.[60,61] In a recent study by our group,[76] drug-free depressed patients were uniformly unable to distinguish α-methylparatyrosine from diphenhydramine and did not experience significant increases in HDRS score with either condition. This contrasts with the early reports of Brodie et al[62] and Bunney et al.[63,77] They found that α-methylparatyrosine worsened the symptoms of three of four psychotically depressed patients. This exacerbation was reversed by discontinuation of the α-methylparatyrosine. The discrepancy between the two sets of studies may result from differences in patient characteristics, since patients in one study were psychotic and in the other they were not. Alternatively, as noted by others,[78] these reported effects of α-methylparatyrosine may simply have been a sedative effect rather than a primary action on depressed mood.

COMPARISON WITH PREVIOUS STUDIES USING TRYPTOPHAN DEPLETION

In the initial investigation, approximately 70% of depressed patients who had recently improved with antidepressant medications experienced a transient relapse of depressive symptoms when tryptophan was depleted. In this study, patients successfully treated with the selective norepinephrine reuptake inhibitor desipramine were less likely to have relapses (only 20% relapse rate) than those treated with a selective serotonin reuptake inhibitor or monoamine oxidase inhibitor (90% relapse rate). However, we were not able to ascertain whether the observed relapse rates with different antidepressant drugs resulted from the neuropharmacologic properties of the drugs or specific patient characteristics. Patients with a history of previous antidepressant drug nonresponse and those with a subdiagnosis of melancholia were more likely to be treated with a serotonin reuptake inhibitor or monoamine oxidase inhibitor.[57]

To extend this work, treatment-naive depressed patients who were primarily nonmelancholic were randomly assigned to receive either fluoxetine or desipramine. Antidepressant drug responders were then subjected to tryptophan depletion. Depressed patients who achieved therapeutic responses to fluoxetine were significantly more likely to experience a transient depressive relapse during tryptophan depletion than those patients who responded to desipramine. The data from these investigations suggest that maintenance of an antidepressant response to fluoxetine is much more acutely dependent on brain serotonin content than maintenance of the response to desipramine (P.L.D, H.L.M., R.M.S., Julio Licinio, MD, J.H.K., G.R.H., D.S.C., unpublished data, January 1995).

The effects of tryptophan depletion also have been evaluated in drug-free depressed patients.[79] Depressed mood in these patients did not worsen during tryptophan depletion. This contrasts sharply with the dramatic and rapid return of depression in patients tested after therapeutic antidepressant treatment (P.L.D, H.L.M., R.M.S., Julio Licinio, MD, J.H.K., G.R.H., D.S.C., unpublished data, January 1995).[57,58] In fact, of patients tested with tryptophan depletion before and after antidepressant treatment, none had a depressive relapse during the drug-free state but 60% had relapses after successful antidepressant treatment.

IMPLICATIONS FOR THE PATHOGENESIS OF DEPRESSION AND THE MECHANISM OF ACTION OF ANTIDEPRESSANT TREATMENTS

The results of these and other studies provide an opportunity to reexamine critically the role of brain monoamine function in the pathogenesis of depression and the mechanism of action of antidepressant drugs. The findings of the investigations with tryptophan depletion and α-methylparatyrosine suggest that the efficacy of antidepressant drugs may not be the result of a common mechanism involving a single monoamine system. Serotonin and norepinephrine reuptake inhibitors may work via primary actions on serotonin and norepinephrine function, respectively. Alternatively, these two classes of antidepressant drugs may exert their therapeutic properties by affecting the function of as yet unidentified neuronal systems that are regulated by these monoamine systems.

In both drug-free depressed patients and healthy subjects, tryptophan depletion and α-methylparatyrosine do not produce marked alterations in depressed mood. These results raise the possibility that alterations in serotonin, dopamine, and norepinephrine systems do not reflect the primary abnormality causing depressive illness. An alternative explanation is that in depressed patients these systems are maximally dysfunctional such that further manipulations do not worsen depressive systems.[76,79] The recent report that healthy subjects with a family history of depression experienced a lowering of mood after tryptophan depletion indicates that additional studies of tryptophan depletion are needed, particularly in depressed patients who are drug free and in remission.[80]

Clinical experience and the results of several controlled studies indicate that the efficacy of serotonin reuptake inhibitors and norepinephrine-inhibiting drugs are approximately equal. Furthermore, while most depressed patients respond to the first trial of either antidepressant class, patients who do not respond to one class of antidepressant, in general, do not respond to the second class[81,82] (but see also Delgado et al[83] and Beasley et al[84]). These investigations, and others,[85] argue against the proposition that specific subtypes of depressive illness exist based on alterations in monoamine function and against the suggestion that these drugs work solely by distinct monoamine-related mechanisms. The findings may be viewed as consistent with the idea, noted above, that the primary abnormality of depression, like the mechanism of action of antidepressant treatments, may result from an abnormality in a neuronal system, which remains to be discovered, that is highly regulated by the brain's monoamine systems.

In this regard, there are several neuropeptide systems, the most salient being corticotropin-releasing hormone and neuropeptide Y, that are regulated by the monoamines and have been hypothesized to be involved in the pathogenesis of depression and the mechanism of action of antidepressant drugs. In fact, corticotropin-releasing hormone and neuropeptide Y may exert a reciprocal regulation of emotional responsiveness, possibly via an interaction of these two systems in the amygdala.[86-88]

The complexity and interdependency in neurotransmitter, neuropeptide, receptor, and intracellular messenger systems in brain suggest that antidepressant action may not lie in the modification of a single neurotransmitter or neuropeptide, but involves the upregulation or down-regulation of the expression of multiple proteins in multiple neuronal cell types.[89,90] The key brain structures involved in antidepressant action need to be identified. In conjunction with further understanding of the effects of antidepressant drug action at sites distal to receptor recognition sites, the development of new classes of antidepressant drugs will be facilitated.

Accepted for publication September 6, 1995.

This study was funded by grants from the Department of Veterans Affairs (Drs Miller, Delgado, and Charney). Plasma HVA and MHPG assays were performed by Harold Landis and Robert Reynolds at the Yale Mental Health Clinical Research Center, Gas Chromatography–Mass Spectroscopy Laboratory (grant MH-30929).

We thank Lowell Goodman, MD, and Wyeth Laboratories, Philadelphia, Pa, for providing mazindol.

The assistance of Kathleen Colonese, Lisa Roach, and Melissa Giunti in conducting this study is gratefully acknowledged. Pedro Mendia and Evelyn Testa provided excellent statistical and technical assistance.

Reprint requests to Department of Veterans Affairs Medical Center, 950 Campbell Ave, West Haven, CT 06516 (Dr Charney).

REFERENCES

1. Schildkraut JJ. The catecholamine hypothesis of affective disorders: a review of supporting evidence. *Am J Psychiatry.* 1965;122:509-522.
2. Bunney WE Jr, Davis JM. Norepinephrine in depressive reactions. *Arch Gen Psychiatry.* 1965;13:483-494.
3. Siever LJ, Davis KL. Overview: toward a dysregulation hypothesis of depression. *Am J Psychiatry.* 1985;142:1017-1031.
4. Delgado PL, Price LH, Heninger GR, Charney DS. Neurochemistry of affective disorders. In: Paykel ES, ed. *Handbook of Affective Disorders.* New York, NY: Churchill Livingstone; 1992:219-253.
5. Kapur S, Mann JJ. Role of the dopaminergic system in depression. *Biol Psychiatry.* 1992;32:1-17.
6. Lacroix D, Blier P, Curet O, deMontigny C. Effects of long-term desipramine administration on noradrenergic neurotransmission: electrophysiological studies in the rat brain. *J Pharmacol Exp Ther.* 1991;257:1081-1090.
7. Cohen RM, Aulakh CS, Campbell IC, Murphy DL. Functional subsensitivity of $alpha_2$ adrenoceptors accompanies reductions in yohimbine binding after clorgyline treatment. *Eur J Pharmacol.* 1982;81:145-148.
8. Sugrue MF. A study of the sensitivity of rat brain $alpha_2$-adrenoceptors during chronic antidepressant treatments. *Naunyn Schmiedebergs Arch Pharmacol.* 1982;320:90-96.
9. Scuvee-Moreau JJ, Svensson TH. Sensitivity in vivo of central α_2- and opiate receptors after chronic treatment with various antidepressants. *J Neural Transm.* 1982;54:51-63.
10. Spyraki C, Fibiger HC. Functional evidence for subsensitivity of noradrenergic $alpha_2$-receptors after chronic desipramine treatment. *Life Sci.* 1980;27:1863-1876.
11. Heal DJ, Lister S, Smith SL, Davies CL, Molyneux SG, Green AR. The effects of acute and repeated administration of various antidepressant drugs on clonidine-

induced hypoactivity in rats and mice. *Neuropharmacology.* 1983;22:983-992.
12. Heal DJ, Akagi A, Bowdler JM, Green AR. Repeated electroconvulsive shock attenuates clonidine-induced hypoactivity in rodents. *Eur J Pharmacol.* 1981; 75:231-237.
13. Kostowski W, Obersztyn M. Chronic administration of desipramine and imipramine but not zimelidine attenuates clonidine induced depression of avoidance behavior in rats. *Pol J Pharmacol Pharm.* 1988;40:341-349.
14. McKenna KF, Baker GB, Coutts RT, Greenshaw AJ. Chronic administration of the antidepressant-antipanic drug phenelzine and its *N*-acetylated analogue: effects on monoamine oxidase, biogenic amines, and α_2-adrenoreceptor. *J Pharmacol Sci.* 1992;81:832-835.
15. Davis M, Menkes DB. Tricyclic antidepressants vary in decreasing alpha$_2$-adrenoceptor sensitivity with chronic treatment: assessment with clonidine inhibition of acoustic startle. *Br J Pharmacol.* 1982;77:217-222.
16. Duman RS, Strada SJ, Enna SJ. Effect of imipramine and adrenocorticotropin administration on the rat brain norepinephrine-coupled cyclic nucleotide generating system: alterations in alpha and beta adrenergic components. *J Pharmacol Exp Ther.* 1985;234:409-414.
17. Garcha G, Smokcum RW, Stephenson JD, Weeramathri TB. Effect of some atypical antidepressants on beta adrenoceptor binding and adenylate cyclase activity in the rat forebrain. *Eur J Pharmacol.* 1985;108:1-7.
18. Sulser F. New perspectives on the molecular pharmacology of affective disorders. *Eur Arch Psychiatr Neurol Sci.* 1989;238:231-239.
19. Gillespie DD, Manier DH, Sanders-Bush E, Sulser F. The serotonin norepinephrine link in brain, II: the role of serotonin in the regulation of beta adrenoceptors in the low agonist affinity conformation. *J Pharmacol Exp Ther.* 1988; 244:154-159.
20. Olpe HR, Schellenberg A. Reduced sensitivity of neurons to noradrenaline after chronic treatment with antidepressant drugs. *Eur J Pharmacol.* 1980;63: 7-13.
21. Schultz JE, Siggins GR, Schocker FW. Effects of prolonged treatment with lithium and tricyclic antidepressants on discharge frequency, norepinephrine responses and beta receptor binding in rat cerebellum: electrophysiological and biochemical comparison. *J Pharmacol Exp Ther.* 1981;216:28-38.
22. McManus DJ, Greenshaw AJ. Differential effects of chronic antidepressants in behavioural tests of β-adrenergic and GABA3 receptor function. *Psychopharmacology.* 1991;103:204-208.
23. Przegalinski E, Baran L, Siwanowicz J, Bigajska K. Repeated treatment with antidepressant drugs prevents salbutamol-induced hypoactivity in rats. *Pharmacol Biochem Behav.* 1984;21:695-698.
24. Menkes DB, Kehne JH, Gallager DW, Aghajanian GK, Davis M. Functional supersensitivity of CNS alpha$_1$ adrenoceptors following chronic antidepressant treatment. *Life Sci.* 1983;33:181-188.
25. Hong KW, Rhim BY, Lee WS. Enhancement of central and peripheral alpha$_1$ adrenoceptor sensitivity and reduction of alpha$_2$ adrenoceptor sensitivity following chronic imipramine treatment in rats. *Eur J Pharmacol.* 1986;120:275-283.
26. Maj J, Rogoz Z, Skuza G, Sowinska H. Repeated treatment with antidepressant drugs potentiates the locomotor response to (+)-amphetamine. *J Pharm Pharmacol.* 1984;36:127-130.
27. Maj J, Klimek V, Nowak G. Antidepressant drugs given repeatedly increase binding to alpha$_1$ adrenoceptors in the rat cortex. *Eur J Pharmacol.* 1985;119: 113-116.
28. Menkes DB, Aghajanian GK. α_2-Adrenoceptor-mediated responses in the lateral geniculate nucleus are enhanced by chronic antidepressant treatment. *Eur J Pharmacol.* 1981;74:27-35.
29. Menkes DB, Aghajanian GK, McCall RB. Chronic antidepressant treatment enhances α-adrenergic and serotonergic responses in the facial nucleus. *Life Sci.* 1980;27:45-55.
30. Sapena R, Morin D, Zini R, Tillement JP. Evaluation of central adrenergic receptor signal transmissions after an antidepressant administration to the rat. *Biochem Pharmacol.* 1992;44:1067-1072.
31. Antkiewicz-Michaluk L, Rokosz-Pelc A, Vetulani J. Increased low-affinity 3H-spiroperidol binding to rat cortical membranes after chronic antidepressant treatments. *Pol J Pharmacol Pharm.* 1985;37:317-323.
32. Martin KF, Needham PL, Atkinson J, Cowen A, Neal DJ, Buckett WR. Rat striatal and mesolimbic D-1 receptor binding is not altered by antidepressant treatments including ECS and sibutramine HCl. *Br J Pharmacol.* 1988;95:896P. Abstract.
33. Willner P. Dopamine and depression: a review of recent evidence, III: the effects of antidepressant treatments. *Brain Res Rev.* 1983;6:237-246.
34. Klimek V, Nielsen M. Chronic treatment with antidepressants decreases the number of [^{3}H]SCH 23390 binding sites in the rat striatum and limbic system. *Eur J Pharmacol.* 1987;139:163-169.
35. Serra G, Cully M, D'Augulia PS, Demontis MG, Gessa GL. On the mechanisms involved in the behavioral supersensitivity to DA-agonists induced by chronic antidepressants. In: Gessa GL, Serra G, eds. *Dopamine in Mental Depression.* Oxford, England: Pergamon Press; 1990:121-138.
36. Chiodo LA, Antelman SM. Repeated tricyclics induce a progressive dopamine autoreceptor subsensitivity independent of daily drug treatment. *Nature.* 1980; 287:451-454.
37. MacNeill DA, Gower M. Do antidepressants induce dopamine autoreceptor subsensitivity? *Nature.* 1982;298:302-303.
38. Diggory GL, Buckett WR. Chronic antidepressant administration fails to attenuate apomorphine-induced decreases in rat striatal dopamine metabolites. *Eur J Pharmacol.* 1984;105:257-263.
39. Racagni G, Mocchetti I, Calderini G, Battistella A, Brunello N. Temporal sequence of changes in central noradrenergic system of rat after prolonged antidepressant treatment: receptor desensitization and neurotransmitter interactions. *Neuropharmacology.* 1983;22:415-424.
40. Biegon A. Effect of chronic desipramine treatment on dihydro-alprenolol, imipramine, and desipramine binding sites: a quantitative autoradiographic study in the rat brain. *J Neurochem.* 1986;47:77-80.
41. Modigh K. Long term effects of electroconvulsive shock therapy on synthesis, turnover and uptake of brain monoamines. *Psychopharmacology.* 1976;49: 170-185.
42. Minchin MCW, Williams J, Bowdler JM, Green AR. Effect of electroconvulsive shock on the uptake and release of noradrenaline and 5-hydroxytryptamine in rat brain slices. *J Neurochem.* 1983;40:765-768.
43. Gleiter CH, Nutt DJ. Repeated electroconvulsive shock increases the number of [^{3}H]desipramine binding sites in rat cerebral cortex. *Psychopharmacology.* 1988;96:426-427.
44. Bauer ME, Tejani-Butt SM. Effects of repeated administration of desipramine or electroconvulsive shock on norepinephrine uptake sites measured by [^{3}H]nisoxetine autoradiography. *Brain Res.* 1992;582:208-214.
45. Melia KR, Nestler EJ, Duman RS. Chronic imipramine treatment normalizes levels of tyrosine hydroxylase in the locus coeruleus of chronically stressed rats. *Psychopharmacology.* 1992;108:23-26.
46. Nestler EJ, McMahon A, Sabban EL, Tallman JF, Duman RS. Chronic antidepressant administration decreases the expression of tyrosine hydroxylase in the rat locus coeruleus. *Proc Natl Acad Sci U S A.* 1990;87:7522-7526.
47. Moret C, Briley M. Effect of antidepressant drugs on monoamine synthesis in brain in vivo. *Neuropharmacology.* 1992;31:679-684.
48. Melia KR, Rasmussen K, Terwilliger RZ, Haycock JW, Nestler EJ, Duman RS. Coordinate regulation of the cyclic AMP system with firing rate and expression of tyrosine hydroxylase in the rat locus coeruleus: effects of chronic stress and drug treatments. *J Neurochem.* 1992;58:494-502.
49. Brady LS, Gold PW, Herkenham M, Lynn AB, Whitfield HJ Jr. The antidepressants fluoxetine, idazoxan and phenelzine alter corticotropin-releasing hormone and tyrosine hydroxylase mRNA levels in rat brain: therapeutic implications. *Brain Res.* 1992;55:121-133.
50. Charney DS, Heninger GR, Sternberg DE, Redmond DE, Leckman JF, Maas JW, Roth RH. Presynaptic adrenergic receptor sensitivity in depression: the effect of long-term desipramine treatment. *Arch Gen Psychiatry.* 1981;38:1334-1340.
51. Charney DS, Heninger GR, Sternberg DE. Alpha$_2$ adrenergic receptor sensitivity and the mechanism of action of antidepressant therapy: the effect of long-term amitriptyline treatment. *Br J Psychiatry.* 1983;142:265-275.
52. Charney DS, Heninger GR, Sternberg DE. The effect of mianserin on alpha-2 adrenergic receptor function in depressed patients. *Br J Psychiatry.* 1984;144: 407-416.
53. Price LH, Charney DS, Heninger GR. Effects of trazodone treatment on alpha-2 adrenoreceptor function in depressed patients. *Psychopharmacology.* 1986; 89:38-44.
54. Pohl R, Yeragani VK, Balon R. Effects of isoproterenol in panic disorder patients after antidepressant treatment. *Biol Psychiatry.* 1990;28:203-214.
55. Charney DS, Delgado PL. Current concepts of serotonin neuronal function and the pathophysiology of depression. In: Elliott M, Heal DJ, Marsden CA, eds. *Experimental Approaches to Anxiety and Depression.* London, England: John Wiley & Sons Ltd; 1992:197-218.
56. Blier P, deMontigny C. Current advances and in the treatment of depression. *Trends Pharmacol Sci.* 1994;15:220-226.
57. Delgado PL, Charney DS, Price LH, Aghajanian GK, Lanais H, Heninger GR. Serotonin function and the mechanism of antidepressant action: reversal of antidepressant induced remission by rapid depletion of plasma tryptophan. *Arch Gen Psychiatry.* 1990;47:411-418.
58. Delgado PL, Price LH, Miller HL, Salomon RM, Licinio J, Krystal JH, Heninger GR, Charney DS. Rapid serotonin depletion as a provocative challenge test for patients with major depression: relevance to antidepressant action and the neurobiology of depression. *Psychopharmacol Bull.* 1991;27:321-330.

59. Widerlov E, Lewander T. Inhibition of the in vivo biosynthesis and changes of catecholamine levels in rat brain after α-methyl-*p*-tyrosine: time- and dose-response relationships. *Naunyn Schmiedebergs Arch Pharmacol.* 1978;304: 111-123.
60. Sjoerdsma A, Engelman K, Spector S. Inhibition of catecholamine synthesis in man with alpha methyl tyrosine, an inhibitor of tyrosine hydroxylase. *Lancet.* 1965;2:1092-1094.
61. Engelman K, Horwitz D, Jequier E. Biochemical and pharmacologic effects of alpha-methyltyrosine in man. *J Clin Invest.* 1968;47:577-594.
62. Brodie HKH, Murphy DL, Goodwin FK, Bunney WE Jr. Catecholamines and mania: the effect of alpha-methyl-para-tyrosine on manic behavior and catecholamine metabolism. *Clin Pharmacol Ther.* 1971;12:218-224.
63. Bunney WE Jr, Brodie HKH, Murphy DL, Goodwin FK. Studies of alpha-methyl-para-tyrosine, L-dopa, and L-tryptophan in depression and mania. *Am J Psychiatry.* 1971;127:872-881.
64. Mazure C, Nelson C, Price LH. Reliability and validity of the symptoms of major depressive illness. *Arch Gen Psychiatry.* 1986;43:451-456.
65. Richelson E. Antidepressants: pharmacology and clinical use. In: Karasu T, ed. *Treatments of Psychiatric Disorders.* Washington, DC: American Psychiatric Association Press; 1989;3:1773-1787.
66. Hyttel J. Citalopram: pharmacological profile of a specific serotonin uptake inhibitor with antidepressant activity. *Prog Neuropsychopharmacol Biol Psychiatry.* 1982;6:277-295.
67. Cusack B, Nelson A, Richelson E. Binding of antidepressants to human brain receptors: focus on newer generation compounds. *Psychopharmacology.* 1994; 114:559-565.
68. Hamilton M. The assessment of anxiety states by rating. *Br J Med Psychol.* 1959;32:50.
69. Woods SW, Charney DS, Goodman WK, Heninger GR. Carbon dioxide–induced anxiety. *Arch Gen Psychiatry.* 1988;45:43-52.
70. Bacopoulos NG, Redmond DE, Roth RH. Serotonin and dopamine metabolites in brain regions and cerebrospinal fluid of a primate species: effects of ketamine and fluphenazine. *J Neurochem.* 1979;32:1215-1218.
71. Maas JW, Hattox SE, Landis DH. The determination of a brain arteriovenous difference for 3-methoxy-4-hydroxyphenylethylene glycol (MHPG). *Brain Res.* 1976;118:167-173.
72. Delgado PL, Miller HL, Salomon RM, Licinio J, Heninger GR, Gelenberg AJ, Charney DS. Monoamines and the mechanism of antidepressant action: effects of catecholamine depletion on mood of patients treated with antidepressants. *Psychopharmacol Bull.* 1994;29:389-396.
73. Cooper JR, Bloom FE, Roth RH. *The Biochemical Basis of Neuropharmacology.* New York, NY: Oxford University Press; 1991:220-284.
74. Charney DS, Heninger GR, Steinberg DE, Roth RH. Plasma MPHG in depression: effects of acute and chronic desipramine treatment. *Psychiatry Res.* 1981; 5:217-229.
75. Shopsin B, Gershon S, Goldstein M, Friedman E, Wilk S. Use of synthesis inhibitors in defining a role for biogenic amines during imipramine treatment in depressed patients. *Psychopharmacol Commun.* 1975;2:239-249.
76. Miller HL, Delgado PL, Salomon RM, Heninger GR, Charney DS. Effects of AMPT in drug free depressed patients. *Neuropsychopharmacology.* In press.
77. Bunney WE Jr, Gershon ES, Murphy DL, Goodwin FK. Psychobiological and pharmacological studies of manic-depressive illness. *J Psychiatry Res.* 1972; 9:207-226.
78. Mendels J, Frazer A. Brain biogenic amine depletion and mood. *Arch Gen Psychiatry.* 1974;30:447-451.
79. Delgado PL, Price LH, Miller HL, Salomon RM, Aghajanian GK, Heninger GR, Charney DS. Serotonin and the neurobiology of depression: effects of tryptophan depletion in drug-free depressed patients. *Arch Gen Psychiatry.* 1994; 51:865-874.
80. Benkelfat C, Ellenbogen MA, Dean P, Palmour RM, Young SN. Mood lowering effect of tryptophan depletion: enhanced susceptibility in young men at genetic risk for major affective disorders. *Arch Gen Psychiatry.* 1994;51:687-700.
81. Nolen WA, van de Putte JJ, Dijken WA, Kamp JS, Blansjaar BA, Kramer HJ, Haffmans J. Treatment strategy in depression, I: non-tricyclic and selective reuptake inhibitors in resistant depression: a double-blind partial crossover study on the effects of oxaprotiline and fluvoxamine. *Acta Psychiatr Scand.* 1988;78:668-675.
82. Charney DS, Miller HL, Licinio J, Salomon RS. Treatment of depression. In: Nemeroff CB, Schatzberg AF, eds. *The American Psychiatric Press Textbook of Psychopharmacology.* Washington, DC: American Psychiatric Press Inc; 1995: 575-601.
83. Delgado PL, Price LH, Charney DS, Heninger GR. Efficacy of fluvoxamine in treatment-refractory depression. *J Affect Disord.* 1988;15:55-60.
84. Beasley CM Jr, Sayler ME, Cunningham GE, Weiss AM, Masica DN. Fluoxetine in tricyclic refractory major depressive disorder. *J Affect Disord.* 1990;20:193-200.
85. Joyce PR, Paykel ES. Predictors of drug response in depression. *Arch Gen Psychiatry.* 1989;46:89-99.
86. Heilig M, Kook GF, Edoman R, Britton KT. Corticotropin-releasing factor and neuropeptide's role in emotional integration. *Trends Neurol Sci.* 1994;17:80-85.
87. Owens MJ, Nemeroff CB. The role of corticotropin-releasing factor in the pathophysiology of affective and anxiety disorders: laboratory and clinical studies. *Ciba Found Symp.* 1993;172:296-316.
88. Owens MJ, Nemeroff CB. Physiology and pharmacology of corticotropin releasing factor. *Pharmacol Rev.* 1991;43:425-473.
89. Hudson CJ, Young LT, Li PP, Warsh JJ. CNS signal transduction in the pathophysiology and pharmacology of affective disorders and schizophrenia. *Synapse.* 1993;13:278-293.
90. Nestler EJ, Duman RS. Intracellular messenger pathways as mediators of neural plasticity. In: Bloom F, Kupfer D, eds. *Psychopharmacology: The Fourth Generation of Progress.* New York, NY: Raven Press; 1995:695-704.

ORIGINAL ARTICLE

A Hospital-Based Twin Register of the Heritability of *DSM-IV* Unipolar Depression

Peter McGuffin, MB, PhD, FRCP, FRCPsych; Randy Katz, PhD; Sarah Watkins, MB, MRCPsych; Joan Rutherford, MB, MRCPsych

Objectives: To estimate the contribution of genes and shared family environment to the liability to *DSM-IV* major depression and to examine the influence of certain proband characteristics on twin concordance.

Methods: We studied 177 probands with major depressive disorder ascertained via the Maudsley Hospital Twin Register (London, England) and their same-sex co-twins. Diagnostic assessments were carried out blind to zygosity and information on the other member of the twin pair. Probandwise concordances were used to compute correlations in liability, and model fitting was performed using maximum likelihood procedures.

Results: The probandwise concordance was 46% in monozygotic (n=68) and 20% in dizygotic (n=109) twins, a statistically highly significant difference. There was no evidence of a sex difference in heritability or of shared environmental effects. Depending on the assumed population risks for *DSM-IV*, major depression estimates of heritability were between 48% and 75%. A duration of longest episode of less than 13 months, multiple episodes, and an endogenous rather than neurotic pattern of symptoms, as established by the *International Classification of Diseases, Ninth Revision*, in the proband were associated with a trend toward a higher monozygotic-dizygotic concordance ratio. Using log-linear analysis, only the association between duration of episodes and monozygotic-dizygotic concordance ratio was significant.

Conclusions: Liability to *DSM-IV* major depression has a substantial heritable component, and there is no evidence of an effect of shared family environment. Some proband characteristics, especially shorter duration of episodes, may be associated with a larger degree of genetic determination.

(Arch Gen Psychiatry. 1996;53:129-136)

From the Department of Psychological Medicine, University of Wales College of Medicine, Cardiff (Drs McGuffin and Watkins); the Department of Psychology, Toronto General Hospital, Toronto, Ontario (Dr Katz); and The Ridgewood Centre, Surrey, England (Dr Rutherford).

ALTHOUGH THERE is consistent evidence from many studies that unipolar depressive disorders are familial,[1,2] the role of genetic factors has seemed less certain. At least some of the ambiguities and apparent contradictions have resulted from differences in the approaches to diagnosis and classification used in twin studies. For example, investigators before the 1970s invariably lumped unipolar and bipolar disorders together in a broad neo-Kraepelinian category of manic-depressive disorder. Such studies overall showed a pattern of higher monozygotic (MZ) than dizygotic (DZ) concordance.[3] The first twin study to clearly differentiate between unipolar and bipolar disorders was a careful register-based investigation by Bertelsen and colleagues.[4] Although there was a suggestion of a stronger genetic effect in bipolar disorder, there was significantly higher MZ than DZ concordance, irrespective of whether the twins were ascertained via unipolar or bipolar probands.

Other early studies, explicitly confined to subjects with episodes of depression and no history of mania, focused on nonendogenous or neurotic forms of disorder. Slater and Shields[5] found zero concordance in both MZ and DZ twins in a small study based on probands with neurotic depression ascertained via the Maudsley Hospital Twin Register, London, England; but, in a Danish study, Shapiro[6] found MZ-DZ differences in concordance suggestive of a modest genetic effect for nonendogenous depression. Subsequently, Torgersen[7] reported no differences in the concordance for neurotic depression in MZ and DZ twins but did find evidence of a moderate genetic effect for *DSM-III*[8] major depression.

See Methods on next page

METHODS

ASCERTAINMENT OF PROBANDS

As described elsewhere,[15] we screened all available written material on probands having a first contact diagnosis of "depression" or "depression?" listed on the Maudsley Hospital Twin Register since its inception in 1948 until the beginning of 1986. (The register consists entirely of same-sex pairs.) This yielded a total of 408 probands on whom a checklist, based on *DSM-III* criteria[8] for affective disorders, was scored and the syndrome checklist of the Present State Examination[16] was completed. Subjects fulfilling *DSM-III* criteria for major affective disorder, all of whom also had one or more recognizable affective disorder syndromes based on the Present State Examination, were retained for study.

This left a total of 215 probands, of whom 34 turned out to have had one or more episodes of mania (in most cases, this had followed the index episode of first contact with the hospital). For the purposes of this report, this subsample is, therefore, set aside. There were no other additional or "comorbid" diagnoses requiring the exclusion of probands.

In the remaining sample, consisting of 181 probands and their co-twins, three pairs of twins appear on the register both as probands *and* as co-twins. As we have discussed elsewhere,[15] the complications of ascertainment when only twin pairs with at least one affected can possibly be included in the sample are best dealt with by considering individuals rather than twin pairs. Thus, we adopt probandwise concordance rate as the simplest and most appropriate measure and assume that each proband is ascertained independently. Each twin pair is then counted once for each member independently ascertained, and the approach becomes equivalent to the usual proband method of ascertainment in segregation analysis.

ZYGOSITY TESTING

Assignment to zygosity was carried out as previously described.[15] This was based on red blood cell typing, which was available on 55 pairs, and, in other pairs, on a combination of photographs, information from case notes, and a zygosity questionnaire. This combined information was found to be superior to questionnaires alone and gave 94% agreement with red blood cell typing. In only one proband–co-twin pair were zygosity questionnaire data missing, and there was insufficient other information to make a confident assignment of zygosity; they were excluded from subsequent analyses. This left 180 proband–co-twin pairs, on which the blindfold diagnostic assessment was carried out, and, as a result of which, a further three probands were excluded (see below), leaving a total of 177.

DIAGNOSTIC ASSESSMENT

We aimed to interview personally as many of the probands and co-twins as possible. Complete blindness was not possible, but, where feasible, the proband and co-twin had different interviewers. Inevitably, because we were dealing with a sample based on the register that accumulated over nearly four decades, a substantial proportion were nonsurvivors, not traced, or those who refused to be interviewed.[15] A total of 144 subjects (40% of the entire sample) were interviewed using the Present State Examination[16] augmented with the Past History schedule[17] and extra questions, so that classification could be obtained according to *DSM-III*,[8] *DSM-III-R*,[18] and other alternative operational criteria.[19] The interviewed subjects consisted of 69 probands and 75 co-twins.

In addition, whether or not an interview was possible, all available information was gleaned from hospital charts, which in the main were detailed and of high quality; from other written sources, such as letters or reports from general practitioners; and, where possible, from an interview with another informant. Hospital charts were available on all probands and 26 co-twins. Case note information from general practitioners was obtained for 48 co-twins. In addition, some limited information was available from twin register records, including clinical findings from earlier smaller studies that had been carried out before the era of standardized interviews and operationalized diagnostic criteria.[5,20]

In all, new information was obtained on a total of 129 co-twins and the sources are summarized in **Table 1**. This left 13 co-twins who refused interview, 13 who could not be traced, and 22 who were dead. In none of these 48 co-twins (18 MZ and 30 DZ) was there evidence from the original twin register files or from subsequent inquiry to National Health Service records that they had ever received treatment for psychiatric disorder within the United Kingdom. Based on all of this material, one of us (J.R.) compiled typewritten abstracts in which all information about zygosity and personal identity other than a code number were deleted.

Two of us (S.W. and P.McG.), aided by a symptom checklist, independently assessed 20 randomly selected abstracts of co-twins and then compared our diagnoses, using both *DSM-III-R* and *International Classification of Diseases, Ninth Revision* (*ICD-9*).[21] By *DSM-III-R* criteria, co-twins were assigned to three categories: major affective disorder, other psychiatric disorder, or unaffected. By *ICD-9* criteria, the categories were manic depressive disorder, neurotic depression, other psychiatric disorder, or unaffected.

We obtained very good agreement for *DSM-III-R* categories (weighted $\kappa = 0.92 \pm 0.07$, Pearson's $r = .96 \pm .04$, $P < .001$) and for *ICD-9* (weighted $\kappa = 0.86 \pm 0.09$, Pearson's $r = .95 \pm .03$, $P < .001$). Consequently, the remainder of the abstracts were assessed by a single rater. In this article, we will only use the *ICD-9* criteria to separate subjects into endogenous (manic-depressive disorder, *ICD-9* 296) and neurotic (depressive neurosis, *ICD-9* 300.4) categories. Since carrying out our assessments, *DSM-IV* criteria have been published.[22] For the category of major depression, the main difference from *DSM-III-R* is the

Adoption study evidence has also been conflicting. A major adoptee family study[9] supported the importance of genetic factors in depression, but two other studies[10,11] suggested that environmental factors are of greater relevance.

More recently, two studies taking, as their starting point, twins unselected for psychiatric disorder have also produced apparently conflicting results. An Australian study[12] of 446 volunteer twin pairs investigated a variety of common psychiatric disorders, including depression for which the MZ concordance rate was actually slightly lower than that in DZ pairs. Kendler and colleagues[13] carried out a population-based twin study of major depression in women, using a sample of 1033 additional requirement of an "impairment" criterion. All subjects classified by us as fulfilling criteria for *DSM-III-R* major depression also fulfilled this impairment criterion and, indeed, all but two had sought treatment at some time. They will, therefore, be described as cases of *DSM-IV* major depression in the rest of this article.

PROBAND CHARACTERISTICS

We sought to divide up the sample according to presence or absence of clinical features that might be expected to affect the degree of genetic determination of unipolar depression such as an endogenous vs neurotic pattern of symptoms. As the latter is not included in *DSM-III-R* or *DSM-IV*, their separation was made as described above, using *ICD-9* criteria. We also considered that age at onset of disease, duration of the longest episode, and number of episodes might be relevant, since all have been suggested as having a bearing on the familiality of affective disorder.[2]

The effects of proband characteristics were assessed by examining the significance of MZ-DZ differences, using a Pearson χ^2, and the size of MZ-DZ differences, as reflected in the concordance ratio. The MZ-DZ concordance ratio is a crude measure of degree of genetic determination compared with estimating heritability (see below) and, as such, has been the subject of criticism.[23] However, we have argued that it is a useful measure when population-based rates cannot be estimated and it has been shown[24] that the MZ-DZ concordance ratio generally is directly proportional to heritability.

Whether MZ-DZ concordance ratios differed significantly was examined using log-linear analysis, as implemented in SPSS/PC+ testing (SPSS Inc, Chicago, Ill)[25] for significant interactions between concordance, zygosity, and each of the proband factors in turn.

MEASURES OF SHARED ENVIRONMENT

We questioned the interviewed probands and their co-twins about whether they were still in regular contact, for how long they had lived together, and whether they had shared a bedroom and, if so, for how long. We also asked a standard set of questions, following Loehlin and Nichols[26] on the degree to which, as children, the twins were treated alike by friends and parents. The aim here was to examine the equal environments assumption[27] that MZ and DZ twins share the environment to an approximately similar extent.

GENETIC MODEL

The data were analyzed under the assumption that depression is a threshold trait and that, within the population, liability to develop depression is a continuous variable that receives contributions from environmental and genetic effects acting in a mainly additive fashion. It is assumed that the distribution of liability is normal or can be readily transformed to normality and only those individuals whose liability at some stage exceeds a certain threshold manifest the disorder. Knowing the population frequency or the disorder and the frequency in a certain class of relatives such as MZ or DZ twins, we can compute a correlation in liability, which is effectively a tetrachoric correlation.[28,29]

We assume that liability has a mean of zero and variance $V_p = 1$. Assuming also that the combination of genetic and environmental sources of variation is additive, then

$$V_p = h^2 + c^2 + s^2,$$

where h^2 is the heritability or proportion of variance in liability contributed by additive genetic effects; c^2, the proportion of variance contributed by environment shared by siblings; and s^2, the proportion of variance attributable to environmental factors not shared by siblings. Error variance is also included in this term. We apply a simple model where, in women, the expected correlation between MZ twins,

$$r_{MZ} = h^2 + c^2$$

and the correlation between DZ twins,

$$r_{DZ} = 1/2\, h^2 + c^2.$$

We allow for the possibility that heritability and the proportion of variance contributed by shared environment differ between the sexes by introducing coefficients *a* and *b*, so that, for men

$$r_{MZ}=ah^2+ bc^2$$

and

$$r_{DZ}=1/2\, ah^2 + bc^2.$$

We incorporate this model into a FORTRAN computer program TWIN, which uses the GEMINI subroutine[30] to maximize a log likelihood of the form

$$\ln L = \sum_{i=1}^{N} A_i \ln P_i + U_i \ln (1 - P_i),$$

where P_i is the proportion of relatives predicted by the model as affected and A_i and U_i are the observed numbers of affected and unaffected relatives in the *i*th category. We have four categories of relatives consisting of MZ and DZ same-sex co-twins of male and female probands.

A full model, where there are both additive genetic and shared environmental factors, is compared with reduced models with either c^2 fixed at zero (ie, additive genetic effects only), h^2 fixed at zero (ie, only shared environmental effects account for twin similarity), or both h^2 and c^2 fixed at zero (ie, no familial affect). Sex differences in heritability or shared environmental effects are tested for by examining the effects of fixing the coefficients *a* and *b* at 1. These comparisons between nested models are made using a likelihood ratio test that depends on the fact that minus twice the difference in log likelihoods is asymptotically a χ^2, with degrees of freedom equal to the difference in the number of parameters between the two models being compared. We can also assess goodness-of-fit of each model using a Pearson χ^2, where degrees of freedom equal the number of observed correlations minus the number of estimated parameters.

same-sex pairs from the Virginia Twin Registry. Their best fitting model using *DSM-III-R* criteria provided an estimate of heritability of 42% for major depression. Although a structured interview was used with good interrater reliability, the interpretation of *DSM-III-R* criteria was very broad, resulting in a lifetime prevalence of major depression in women of 31%. Nevertheless, all of the familiality of major depression was accounted for by additive genetic effects, with no evidence of shared environmental factors. This pattern was borne out in a subsequent analysis of the Virginia twin sample,[14] where the subjects were followed up and model fitting was applied, taking into account reliability of the lifetime diagnosis of major depression. It was found that more than half of what had previously been attributed to environmental variance was probably explained by measurement error, increasing the estimate of heritability to about 70%. Again, there was evidence only of individual-specific environmental effects.

The only other twin study of depression on which biometric model fitting has been published was our previous report[15] that suggested a heritability similar to that in the earlier Virginia twin study report[13] (of about 51%). However, we also found a significant familial environmental effect accounting for about 31% of the variance in liability.[15] We pointed out that these results were preliminary, based on still incomplete data, and that a more definitive set of conclusions would depend on the application of a rigorously blindfold assessment of all the available information. This has now been completed and represents by far the largest systematically ascertained clinical sample of twins with unipolar depression to be reported to date. In this article, we report the findings and results of model fitting and compare and contrast the results with other studies.

RESULTS

DIAGNOSTIC CONCORDANCE

As noted earlier, on blind diagnostic assessment, three of the 180 probands did not fulfill *DSM-III-R/DSM-IV* criteria for major depression and these were excluded from the analysis, leaving a total of 177 probands and their co-twins. The frequency of affective disorder in co-twins is summarized in **Table 2** together with the correlations in liability. The mean age at onset was similar for MZ (39.9 years) and DZ (39.6 years) twins. Among the MZ co-twins, one of the men had had episodes of both mania and depression and, therefore, fulfilled criteria for bipolar disorder; otherwise, conditions of all of the co-twins were classed as concordant and unipolar depression only. In both sexes, MZ concordance is significantly greater than DZ concordance.

It is possible that biases could have been introduced by the varying sources of information used to arrive at the diagnoses in the probands and co-twins. Although the rate of major depression was slightly higher, at 36%, in the co-twins of interviewed probands than in co-twins of noninterviewed probands (perhaps reflecting differences in quality of information), this was not statistically significant (χ^2= 2.13, *df*=1, *P*=.14). Furthermore, there was no significant difference (χ^2= 1.31, *df*=1, *P*=.26) in the proportion of MZ probands who were interviewed (34%) compared with DZ probands (42%). Neither was there any difference with respect to zygosity in terms of the period of time between age at onset in the proband and age at which last information was available on proband or co-twin. This had a mean (±SE) of 14.68 (±0.668) years for MZ pairs and 14.50 (±1.0) years for DZ pairs.

To assess further whether the differences in sources of information on co-twins introduced any biases in calculating concordance rates, or in subsequent model fitting, we can divide the co-twin data into three groups: co-twins who were interviewed, co-twins who were not interviewed but on whom there was some other new source of information, and co-twins on whom there was no additional data other than that contained in the twin register files. All of the last group of missing co-twins were assumed to be unaffected in the twin register files and, at the time of our follow-up, had no contacts that we were able to detect either with psychiatric services in the United Kingdom or with their general practitioner for treatment of psychiatric symptoms. All were classified in the blind rating as unaffected by major depression.

Hence, although there was overall a much higher rate of major depression in co-twins who were interviewed (44%) compared with those who were not (18%) (χ^2=12.8, *df*=1, *P*<.001), this was almost entirely accounted for by the missing co-twins. There was no significant difference in the blindly assessed rate of de-

Table 1. Sources of Co-twin Information

Source	No. of Co-twins	% of Total
Interview (interview and charts*)	76 (51)	43 (29)
Hospital charts only	13	7
General practitioner information only	13	7
Death certificate/coroner only†	5	3
Mailed questionnaire only	2	1
Proband interview only	20	11
No additional information, ie, original twin register files and probands' hospital charts only	48	27
Total	**177**	**100**

**Subjects who had interviews plus information from hospital and/or general practitioner.*
†Includes four suicides.

Table 2. Affective Disorder in the Co-twins of Proband With *DSM-IV* Major Depression

	DSM-IV Major Depression							
	Monozygotic			Dizygotic				
Sex	n	Concordance, %	r* (SE)	n	Concordance, %	r* (SE)	χ^2†	P
Men	24	45.8**	.79 (0.08)	27	14.8	.38 (0.18)	5.81	.02
Women	44	45.5	.70 (0.09)	82	22.0	.35 (0.09)	7.51	.01
Combined	68	45.6**	. . .	109	20.2	. . .	9.63	.00

**Correlation in liability (r) assuming population risk of .035 in men and .084 in women.*
†Pearson χ^2 (1 df) cross-tabulating zygosity by probandwise concordance.
‡Includes one co-twin with bipolar affective disorder.

Table 3. Model Fitting Results for *DSM-IV* Major Depression*

Model	Parameter Estimates h^2 (SE)	c^2 (SE)	*a*	*b*	−2 ln *L* +Constant	χ^2	*df*	*P*
1	0.76 (0.23)	0.03 (0.19)	1.07	0.77	202.98	0.0	0	
2	0.77 (0.19)	0.04 (0.16)	[1.0]	0.23	103.00	0.028	1	.86
3	0.75 (0.21)	0.03 (0.17)	1.08	[1.0]	202.98	0.001	1	.99
4	0.75 (0.06)	[0.0] (. . .)	[1.0]	[1.0]	203.31	0.34	3	.95
5	[0.0] (. . .)	0.55 (0.05)	[1.0]	[1.0]	218.75	16.27	3	.001
6	[0.0] (. . .)	[0.0] (. . .)	[1.0]	[1.0]	311.95	146.57	4	<.001

*h^2 *Indicates heritability of liability;* c^2, *variance in liability explained by shared environment;* a *and* b, *coefficients that allow for sex differences in heritability and shared environment, respectively; L, maximum likelihood; and data in brackets, fixed parameters.*

pression, in the noninterviewed twins on whom we had other sources of new information (35%), and in the interviewed co-twins (χ^2=1.05, *df*=1, *P*=.3). Neither was there a significant difference in the number of interviewed MZ co-twins (27/68 [40%]) compared with DZ co-twins (50/109 [46%]) (χ^2=0.77, *df*=1, *P*=.38). Furthermore, the proportion of the sample on which no new information was available was nearly exactly the same for MZ (26%) compared with that for DZ (28%) co-twins (χ^2=0.0, *df*=1, *P*= 1.0).

One approach might, therefore, be to simply ignore the missing co-twins, which would give us a sex averaged MZ probandwise concordance of 31 (62%) of 50 and a DZ concordance of 22 (28%) of 78. However, it seems likely that our success in follow-up was biased in favor of co-twins who were, or who had become, affected by psychiatric disorder and, therefore, a more conservative approach is to accept the blind rating of unaffected at face value and to include the missing co-twins in the denominator when calculating concordance rates.

ENVIRONMENTAL MEASURES

We found that there was no difference between MZ and DZ twins in the length of time they had lived together or shared a bedroom. Monozygotic twins more often than DZ twins reported dressing alike as children, being treated alike by parents, having joint friends, or being in the same class at school. All of these differences were significant at *P*<.05. However, there was no significant relationship between concordance for depression and any of these measures. Similarly, reporting being in current contact vs not in current contact had no significant relationship with concordance. We, therefore, proceeded with model fitting under the assumption that environments of relevance to the development of depression are shared to the same extent by MZ and DZ twins.

MODEL FITTING

The results of model fitting are summarized in **Table 3**. We assumed a population risk figure to age 65 years for hospital-treated depression of 16.6% for women and 8.5% for men.[31] This was derived from the Camberwell case register (Camberwell is the old borough of London, in which the Maudsley Hospital is situated). We have no precise estimate of the lifetime risk of *DSM-IV* depression in a British population. However, our probands can be taken as a representative sample of patients referred to hospital for depression, of whom 50.4% of the female and 41.1% of the male unipolar cases were found to fulfill the criteria for major depression. This allows us to obtain an approximate risk for *DSM-IV* major depression of 16.6%×50.4%=8.4% for women and 8.5%×41.1%=3.5% for men. Using a method described elsewhere,[32] we calculate that the SEs of these estimate are 0.1% and 0.2%, respectively.

Fixing the sex difference coefficients at values of *a*=1 or *b*=1 resulted in negligible changes in the likelihood (models 2 and 3) as did fixing *a*=1 and *b*=1 (not shown). This suggests that the size of genetic and shared environmental effects is the same in men and women and, therefore, subsequent model fitting was carried out under the assumption of no sex differences for these familial effects. When we fitted a reduced model with additive genetic effects only (model 4), this resulted in little change in the likelihood compared with the general model (model 1) and produced a good fit (Pearson's χ^2=0.34, *df*=3, *P*=.95). However, a shared environment model with h^2 fixed at zero produced a substantial drop in likelihood and a poor fit (likelihood ratio χ^2=15.77, *df*=3, *P*=.001; Pearson χ^2=16.27, *df*=3, *P*=.001). Finally a no-transmission model with h^2 and c^2 both fixed zero resulted in an extremely poor fit (likelihood ratio χ^2=108.97, *df*=4, *P*<.001; Pearson χ^2=146.57, *df*=4, *P*<.001).

We also carried out model fitting, assuming the higher concordances obtained when missing co-twins are excluded from the analysis. This again suggested no sex differences in the components of variance in liability and resulted in the most satisfactory model on grounds of parsimony and goodness-of-fit being h^2=0.80, c^2=0 (Pearson's χ^2=0.12, *df*=3, *P*=.8). Finally, as estimates of h^2 and c^2 depend on the population frequency of the disorder, we explored the effect of model fitting using the much higher lifetime prevalences of major depression of 21% in women and 13% in men reported in a recent survey in the United States.[33] This resulted in a similar overall pattern with, once again, no sex differences in the familial variance components and no evidence of shared environment since c^2 became fixed at the boundary value of zero during iteration. The most acceptable model therefore provided estimates of h^2=0.48 and c^2=0.0 (likelihood ratio χ^2=6.03, *df*=3, *P*=.11; Pearson's χ^2=5.77, *df*=3, *P*=.12).

Table 4. Concordance for *DSM-IV* Major Affective Disorder According to Proband Characteristics

Proband Characteristics	Monozygotic (MZ) n	Monozygotic (MZ) Concordance, %	Dizygotic (DZ) n	Dizygotic (DZ) Concordance, %	χ^2†	MZ-DZ Concordance Ratio
No. of episodes						
>2	47	49	59	20	9.67	2.45
≤2	21	38	50	20	2.60	1.90
Age at onset, y						
<36, early	36	42	50	20	4.77	2.5
≥36, late	25	52	42	19	7.91	2.21
Illness subtype						
Neurotic, *ICD-9** 300.4	27	33	36	22	0.97	1.50
Endogenous, *ICD-9* 296.X	41	54	73	19	14.45	2.84
Episode duration, mo						
≤13	31	61	47	17	16.2	3.59
>13	26	31	49	22	0.6	1.41

*ICD-9 *indicates* International Classification of Diseases, Ninth Revision.[21]
†*Pearson* χ^2 *(1* df*) cross-tabulating zygosity by probandwise concordance.*

PROBAND EFFECTS

Concordance by zygosity is presented in **Table 4**, according to the presence or absence of certain proband characteristics. The mean number of episodes reported by probands was two, and they were, therefore, divided into those having had one or two episodes and those having had more than two episodes. Similarly, the mean age at onset was 36 years and this was used to divide the sample into an early- and late-onset group. The mean for the duration of longest episode was 13 months, and this was used as another way of dichotomizing the sample. *ICD-9* neurotic/endogenous and dichotomy patterns were applied as described earlier.

Age at onset had no effect on MZ-DZ differences. However, having an endogenous pattern of symptoms, having a longest episode of 13 months or less, and having had more than two episodes were all associated with higher MZ than DZ concordance. To test whether each of these dichotomous proband factors had a significant effect on the MZ-DZ concordance ratio, we applied log-linear models testing for a three-way interaction among proband factor, concordance, and zygosity. Only the proband factor relating to duration of longest episode proved to have a significant effect (likelihood ratio χ^2=4.59, *df*=1, *P*=.03).

COMMENT

Our results suggest that liability to *DSM-IV* unipolar depression is highly heritable. Our estimate of heritability of liability, when we use population risk figures derived from a study of hospital-treated depression,[31] is considerably larger than that obtained in our previous report[15] based on less complete and nonblind diagnostic assessments. At over 70%, this estimate is similar to that obtained in a recent report of the Virginia twin study of depression in women.[14]

In another respect, our new findings increase the similarities with the results of the Virginia twin study of depression in women. We no longer have evidence of family environment that is shared by twins having an influence on liability to major depression. We, thus, agree with Kendler and coworkers[13,14] who found that genetic factors were the sole source of similarity for major depression in female twins, as well as with the only other study[7] to have used a modern operational definition of major depression. This produced results suggestive of absent shared environmental effects but moderate heritability.[13]

Where our results show disagreements with the Virginia study is in population risks for depression. We obtained population estimates (albeit indirect) of 8.4% in women and 3.5% in men. Kendler and colleagues, in their initial report,[13] found that major depression is extremely common in women with a lifetime risk of over 30%. Part of the difference in the breadth of case definition must arise from differences in the designs of the studies. Our study was based on a hospital twin register, and our series was ascertained through probands who, by definition, are hospital patients and so presumably have been sufficiently impaired to either seek treatment or be referred by others. Furthermore, all but two of the co-twins in our study who were diagnosed as having *DSM-IV* depression had sought medical help at some time. By contrast, the Virginia twin series is population based and so the studies of depression used subjects who were unselected for psychiatric disorder and presumably included "cases" who had not previously come to medical attention.

This pattern is in keeping with epidemiological studies in general,[34] where the identification of a proportion of subjects who have never received hospital treatment is the rule rather than the exception. Nevertheless, most recent epidemiological surveys[34] have produced lifetime prevalences of *DSM-III* or *DSM-III-R* major depression of between 6% and 16% in women and between 3% and 9% in men. Thus, our own estimates are toward the lower end of the usual range, but that of Kendler and colleagues is considerably higher. This suggests that differences between our study and that of the Virginia group also depend on the way that diagnostic criteria were applied. To explore the effects of broader population estimates on model fitting to our own data, we used figures from the US National Comorbidity Survey,[33] where lifetime prevalences of 21% in women and 13% in men were found. This produced a pattern of results that was unchanged, ie, there was no evidence of shared environmental effects or of sex differences in heritability. However, the estimate of heritability of liability to major depression was lowered at 48%.

Although it is probably meaningless to argue that either a broad or a narrow interpretation of similar diagnostic criteria is more correct, it is important to realize that such differences in interpretation can result in differences in estimates of heritability, if not in the overall pattern of results. There are obvious advantages in the population-based approach, as adopted by the Virginia group, in that an estimate of the population prevalence of the disorder is directly built into the study, overcoming the need to rely on indirect estimate derived from external source. There is, however, one way that we can obtain an estimate of the population rate of depression using our own data alone, and this is to assume that it is safe to fix c^2 at zero (and both a and b at 1) and then find the maximum likelihood estimate of h^2 and the population rate simultaneously. This results in a population rates of 8.9% (±2.9%) for women and 5.7% (±3.4%) for men, which (although the SEs are large) is fairly close to the estimates of 8.4% and 3.5% that we derived from the Camberwell Case Register figures of Sturt et al[31] and is comfortably within the range of lifetime prevalences from (pre–National Comorbidity Survey findings) in the review by Smith and Weissman.[34] The estimate of heritability associated with these population rates was 70%, and the model fitted well (Pearson's χ^2=0.48, *df*=1, *P*=.99).

As we have noted, the main difference between *DSM-III-R* and *DSM-IV* criteria for major depression is the introduction of an impairment criterion in *DSM-IV*. This might be expected to stabilize the population estimates of the frequency of major depression and resolve some of the discrepancies between studies. In this respect, it is of interest that Kendler and colleagues[14] found that, although the lifetime diagnosis of depression in a population-based sample had only moderate reliability, among the factors predicting reliability were treatment seeking and being impaired by the disorder.

An obvious advantage of using a hospital-based register to ascertain probands for our twin study is that the probands have, by definition, sought treatment and are likely to have been impaired. However, one of the problems is that, to obtain a sufficient sample size for our statistical analyses, we included subjects listed over a period of time stretching back over more almost four decades. This inevitably meant that a substantial proportion of co-twins, more than half, could not be interviewed because of death, difficulties in tracing, or refusal. We obtained other information from written sources on most of the noninterviewed co-twins, but this still left 27% on whom we had no new information in addition to that in the twin register files. The blind rating of abstracts based on this, in some cases fairly scant, information classified all of the missing co-twins as unaffected. We can be reasonably confident that there were no cases of hospital-treated depression in the missing co-twins. Untreated disorder cannot, of course, be ruled out. We might, therefore, have simply ignored the missing cases, which would give us an MZ concordance of 62% and a DZ concordance of 28%, resulting in an estimate of heritability of approximately 80%. The argument against accepting these higher concordances is that our sources of new information were almost certainly biased in the direction of co-twins who had themselves suffered from psychiatric symptoms. This, in turn, probably reflects the fact that co-twins who had psychiatric disorder were the most readily traced and possibly the most cooperative subjects. Some support for our preferentially accepting the lower and more conservative concordances comes from the only other hospital-based study to use modern explicit diagnostic criteria,[7] which yielded an MZ concordance of 37% and a DZ concordance of 20%, as well as from the preliminary findings of a Swedish twin study containing subjects both from the general population and ascertained via hospitals. This gave concordances for narrowly defined affective disorder of 48% in MZ and 23% in DZ twins.[35]

When we explored our own data further, dividing the sample according to certain proband characteristics, an interesting, if inconclusive, pattern of results emerged. When probands had an endogenous subtype of depression, we found significantly higher MZ than DZ concordance, but when the probands had an *ICD-9* neurotic subtype, the MZ-DZ concordance difference was small and nonsignificant. Although fitting log-linear models failed to show a significant interaction among subtype, zygosity, and concordance, the overall pattern of results were in keeping with the findings of Torgersen[7] and, more generally, with the suggestion of Slater and Shields[5] in their earlier study that neurotic depression has low heritability. The only study that disagrees is that of Shapiro,[6] which found that MZ concordance was substantially higher than DZ concordance for nonendogenous depression. Again, some of the differences may be owing both to different diagnostic practice and use of terms.[36]

Other proband characteristics that were of interest are the number of episodes and the duration of the longest episode.[37,38] Where the proband had a longest episode of 13 months or less or had more than two episodes, the MZ concordance was significantly higher than the DZ concordance. By contrast, the proband having longer episodes or only having one or two episodes were each associated with nonsignificant differences between MZ and DZ concordances. Log-linear analysis showed that the MZ-DZ concordance ratios differed significantly only when probands were split according to duration of longest episode. Nevertheless, the results at least suggest that multiple episodes, with durations of 13 months or less, may characterize those forms of depression with a more marked degree of genetic determination.

Although it has been suggested that early onset is associated with greater familiality of affective disorder than late onset,[39] we have not been able to show this in our family studies.[40] Similarly, an earlier vs later age at onset in the proband in the present study appeared to have no influence on the rate of the disorder in co-twins.

Our findings suggest that liability to unipolar depression, as defined by *DSM-IV* criteria, is substantially heritable with no sex difference in heritability and no evidence of a shared family environmental component. Our results also suggest that having episodes lasting 13 months or less, multiple episodes, or an endogenous pattern of symptoms may characterize those forms of depressive disorder where genetic factors are most prominent.

Accepted for publication August 29, 1995.

This study was supported by a grant from the Medical Research Council (United Kingdom).

Reprint requests to Department of Psychological Medicine, College of Medicine, University of Wales, Heath Park, Cardiff, Wales CF4 4XN (Dr McGuffin).

REFERENCES

1. McGuffin P, Katz R. Nature, nurture and affective disorders. In: Deakin JWK, ed. *The Biology of Depression.* London, England: Gaskell Press; 1986:26-51.
2. Tsuang MT, Faraone SV. *The Genetics of Mood Disorders.* Baltimore, Md: John Hopkins University Press; 1990.
3. Gershon ES, Bunney WF, Leckman J F, Van Eerdewegh M, DeBauche BA. The inheritance of affective disorders: a review of data and hypotheses. *Behav Genet.* 1976;6:227-261.
4. Bertelsen A, Harvard B, Gauge M. A Danish twin study of manic-depressive disorders. *Br J Psychiatry.* 1977;130:330-351.
5. Slater E, Shields J. Genetical aspects of anxiety. *Br J Psychiatry.* 1969:62-71. Special Publication No. 3.
6. Shapiro RW. A twin study of non-endogenous depression. *Acta Jutland.* 1971; 49:273-281.
7. Torgersen S. Genetic factors in moderately severe and mild affective disorders. *Arch Gen Psychiatry.* 1986;43:222-226.
8. American Psychiatric Association. *Diagnostic and Statistical Manual of Mental Disorders, Third Edition.* Washington, DC: American Psychiatric Association; 1980.
9. Wender PH, Kety SS, Rosethal D, Schulsinger F, Ortmann J, Lunde L. Psychological disorders in the biological and adoptive relatives of individuals with affective disorders. *Arch Gen Psychiatry.* 1986;43:923-929.
10. Cadoret RJ, O'Gorman TW, Heywood E, Troughton E. Genetic and environmental factors in major depression. *J Affect Disord.* 1985;9:155-164.
11. Von Knorring AL, Cloninger CR, Bodman N, Sigvardsson S. An adoption study of depressive disorders and substance abuse. *Arch Gen Psychiatry.* 1983;40: 943-950.
12. Andrews G, Stewart G, Allen R, Henderson AS. The genetics of six neurotic disorders: a twin study. *J Affect Disord.* 1990;19:23-29.
13. Kendler KS, Neale MC, Kessler RC, Heath AC, Eaves LJ. A population based twin study of major depression in women: the impact of varying definitions of illness. *Arch Gen Psychiatry.* 1992;49:273-281.
14. Kendler KS, Neale MC, Kessler RC, Heath AC, Eaves LJ. The lifetime history of major depression in women: reliability of diagnosis and heriability. *Arch Gen Psychiatry.* 1993;50,863-870.
15. McGuffin P, Katz R, Rutherford J. Nature, nurture and depression: a twin study. *Psychol Med.* 1991;20:329-335.
16. Wing JK, Cooper JE, Sartorius N. *The Measurement and Classification of Psychiatric Symptoms.* Cambridge, England: Cambridge University Press; 1974.
17. McGuffin P, Katz R, Aldrich J. Past and present state examination: the assessment of lifetime ever psychopatholgy. *Psychol Med.* 1986;16:461-465.
18. American Psychiatric Association. *Diagnostic and Statistical Manual of Mental Disorders, Revised Third Edition.* Washington DC: American Psychiatric Association; 1987.
19. McGuffin P, Farmer AE, Harvey I. A polydiagnostic application of operational criteria in studies of psychotic illness: development and reliability of the OPCRIT system. *Arch Gen Psychiatry.* 1991;48:764-770.
20. Da Fonseca AF. Affective equivalents. *Br J Psychiatry.* 1963;109:464-469.
21. World Health Organisation. *The ICD-9 Classification of Mental and Behavioural Disorders: Clinical Descriptions and Diagnostic Guidelines.* Geneva, Switzerland; 1992.
22. American Psychiatric Association. *Diagnostic and Statistical Manual, Fourth Edition.* Washington, DC: American Psychiatric Association; 1994.
23. Kendler KS. Limitations of the ratio of concordance rates in monozygotic and dizygotic twins. *Arch Gen Psychiatry.* 1989;46:477-478.
24. Farmer AE, McGuffin P, Bebbington P. The phenomena of schizophrenia. In: Bebbington P, McGuffin P, eds. *Schizophrenia: The Major Issues.* London, England: Heinemann Medical Books; 1988:36-50.
25. Norusis MJ. *SPSS/PC+ Advanced Statistics.* Chicago, Ill: SPSS Inc; 1990.
26. Loehlin JC, Nichols RC. *Heredity, Environment and Personality.* Austin, Tex: University of Texas Press; 1976.
27. Plomin R, DeFries JL, McLean JE. *Behavioral Genetics: A Primer.* San Francisco, Calif: WH Freeman Co; 1980.
28. Falconer DS. The inheritance of liability to certain diseases, estimated from the incidence among relatives. *Ann Hum Genet.* 1965;29:51-76.
29. Reich T, James JW, Morris CA. The use of multiple thresholds in determining the mode of transmission of semi-continuous traits. *Ann Hum Genet London.* 1972;36:163-184.
30. Lalouel JM. Optimisation of functions. In: Morton NE, Rao DC, Lalouel JM, eds. *Methods of Genetic Epidemiology.* New York, NJ: S Karger AG; 1983: 235-259.
31. Sturt E, Kumakura N, Der G. Life-long morbidity risk for depressive disorder in the general population. *J Affect Disord.* 1984;7:109-122.
32. McGuffin P, Farmer AE, Gottesman II, Murray RM, Reveley A. Twin concordance for operationally defined schizophrenia: confirmation of familiality and heritability. *Arch Gen Psychiatry.* 1984;41:541-545.
33. Kessler RC, McGonagle KA, Zhao S, Nelson CB, Hughes M, Eshleman S, Wittchen HU, Kendler KS. Lifetime and 12-month prevalence of *DSM-III-R* psychiatric disorders in the United States: results from the National Comorbidity Survey. *Arch Gen Psychiatry.* 1994;51:8-19.
34. Smith AL, Wiessman MM. Epidemiology. In: Paykel ES, ed. *Handbook of Affective Disorders.* New York, NY: Churchill Livingstone Inc; 1992:111-130.
35. Kendler KS, Pedersen N, Johnson L, Neale MC, Aleksander AA. Pilot Swedish twin study: affective illness, including hospital and population ascertained subsamples. *Arch Gen Psychiatry.* 1993;50:699-705.
36. Farmer A E, McGuffin P. Classification of the depressions: contemporary confusion revisited. *Br J Psychiatry.* 1989;155:437-443.
37. Bland C, Newman SC, Orn H. Recurrent and non recurrent depression. *Arch Gen Psychiatry.* 1986;43:1085-1089.
38. Gershon ES, Weissman MM, Guroff JJ, Prusoff BA, Leckman JF. Validation criteria for major depression through controlled family study. *J Affect Disord.* 1986;11:125-131.
39. Weissman MM, Merikangas K, Wickramaratne P, Kidd LL, Prusoff B, Leckman JF, Pauls D. Understanding the clinical heterogeneity of major depression using family data. *Arch Gen Psychiatry.* 1986;43:431-434.
40. McGuffin P, Katz R, Bebbington P. Hazard, heredity and affective disorder: a family study. *J Psychiatr Res.* 1987;31:365-375.

ORIGINAL ARTICLE

Increased Number of Vasopressin- and Oxytocin-Expressing Neurons in the Paraventricular Nucleus of the Hypothalamus in Depression

Jan S. Purba, MD, PhD; Witte J. G. Hoogendijk, MD; Michel A. Hofman, PhD; Dick F. Swaab, MD, PhD

Background: Cerebrospinal fluid levels of arginine vasopressin (AVP) and oxytocin (OXT) have been found to change in mood disorders. In the present study, the numbers of AVP-immunoreactive (IR) and OXT-IR neurons were determined in the paraventricular nucleus (PVN) of the human hypothalamus.

Methods: Postmortem brain tissue was fixed in formalin, embedded in paraffin, and stained for AVP and OXT using immunocytochemical techniques. The number of IR neurons in the PVN was estimated by morphometry in eight depressed patients ranging in age from 21 to 85 years and eight age-matched controls ranging in age from 23 to 88 years.

Results: The numbers of AVP-IR and OXT-IR neurons in the PVN of patients with mood disorder were increased by 56% and 23%, respectively. No differences were found in AVP-IR or OXT-IR cell numbers between three patients with major depression and three patients with bipolar depression. The numbers of AVP-IR and OXT-IR neurons in two patients with depression not otherwise specified were within the same range as in the six other patients with a mood disorder.

Conclusions: The AVP and OXT neurons were activated in the PVN in patients with major depression or bipolar disorder. This activation may be associated with activation of the hypothalamic-pituitary-adrenal axis in these patients, since both AVP and OXT are known to potentiate the effects of corticotropin-releasing hormone. Because of their central effects, activation of AVP and OXT neurons may also be related to symptoms of major depression or bipolar disorder.

(Arch Gen Psychiatry. 1996;53:137-143)

THREE HYPOTHALAMIC systems are currently considered to be involved in depression: (1) The suprachiasmatic nucleus (SCN), the clock of the hypothalamus, shows strong annual variations in neuronal activity[1-3] that may be related to annual fluctuations in mood.[4,5] (2) The corticotropin-releasing hormone (CRH) neurons of the paraventricular nucleus (PVN), which regulate the hypothalamic-pituitary-adrenal (HPA) axis, have recently been found to be strongly activated in depression.[6,7] This finding is of particular interest since there are similarities between signs and symptoms of major depression and the behavioral effects of centrally administered CRH in laboratory animals[8] and of transgenic mice with CRH overproduction.[9] (3) The hormone levels of arginine vasopressin (AVP) and oxytocin (OXT) were found to be changed in the cerebrospinal fluid (CSF) in mood disorders.[10,11] These CSF levels are influenced by the synthesizing activity of the AVP and OXT neurons of the PVN.[12]

The present report deals with changes in AVP and OXT neurons in the PVN in patients with depression. Arginine vasopressin– and OXT-producing neurons from the PVN and supraoptic nucleus in the hypothalamus project to the neurohypophysis, where they are released into the general circulation. In the periphery, these peptides are involved in the regulation of diuresis and reproductive processes.[13-15] In addition, nerve fibers containing AVP and OXT innervate a large number of brain areas,[16,17] where AVP and OXT act as neurotransmitters or neuromodulators.[18,19] These extrahypothalamic projections are thought to be implicated in the regulation of body temperature, blood pressure, and osmolality, as well as in cognition, attention, and mood.[10,11,20]

From the Netherlands Institute for Brain Research (Drs Purba, Hoogendijk, Hofman, and Swaab) and the Valerius Clinic, Department of Psychiatry, Free University (Dr Hoogendijk), Graduate School Neurosciences Amsterdam (the Netherlands).

See Materials and Methods on next page

MATERIALS AND METHODS

Eight patients, four men and four women aged 21 through 85 years (mean±SEM, 61±8 years) with a clinical diagnosis of mood disorder according to *DSM-III-R*,[28] were entered in this study. The patients were selected using the clinical records and, if necessary, an interview with the clinician who treated the patients. Three patients fulfilled *DSM-III-R* criteria for major depression (patients 1, 3, and 5), three had bipolar disorders (patients 2, 4, and 7), one had an organic syndrome with depressed mood following a cardiac arrest and resuscitation (patient 6), and one had an unspecified depressive disorder, ie, not fulfilling *DSM-III-R* criteria for major depression (patient 8). Control brains were obtained from subjects without any evidence of a psychiatric disorder and were matched for age and sex (**Table 1**). The controls consisted of four men and four women aged 23 through 88 years (mean±SEM, 60±9 years).

The neuropathological diagnosis of depressed patients and controls was performed at the Free University of Amsterdam (Wouter Kamphorst, MD, PhD), the Academic Medical Center of the University of Amsterdam (Dirk Troost, MD, PhD), or the Netherlands Brain Bank, Amsterdam (Frans C. Stam, MD, PhD). For clinicopathological information see Table 1. Brains were weighed, and the hypothalamus was dissected and fixed in 4% formaldehyde for about 1 month. The hypothalamic area containing the PVN was dehydrated in graded ethanol and embedded in paraffin. Serial 6-μm frontal sections were cut on a Leitz microtome (Leica Instruments GmbH, Nussloch, Germany). Every 50th section was mounted on a chrome-alum–coated object slide, deparaffinized, hydrated, and stained with thionine to locate the PVN before immunocytochemical staining and to determine neuropathological alterations in the hypothalamus. Two series of sections taken at regular 300-μm intervals throughout the region in which the PVN could be discerned by thionine staining were stained immunocytochemically for AVP or OXT.

IMMUNOCYTOCHEMICAL PROCEDURES

To remove cross-reactivity from anti-AVP (obtained from rabbit Truus, January 29, 1989) or anti-OXT (obtained from rabbit 02-T, January 29, 1989), the antisera were preadsorbed twice with OXT or AVP glutaraldehyde-coupled sepharose beads.[29] The second incubation resulted in complete removal of cross-reactivity in the assay.[30] In addition, similarly purified antisera had been checked for cross-reactivity in alternating 6-μm sections of the PVN and had revealed no cells staining with both antisera.[30] Mounted sections were hydrated and stained using the following procedure: (1) incubation with purified AVP antiserum (Truus OXT), 1:1000, or purified OXT antiserum (02-T AVP), 1:1000, in 0.05-mol/L TRIS containing 0.9% sodium chloride (TRIS-buffered saline [TBS], pH 7.6) with 0.5% Triton X-100 (All incubations were performed for 1 hour at room temperature and subsequently overnight at 4°C in plastic boxes to prevent evaporation.); (2) washing in TBS (twice for 10 minutes each time); (3) incubation with goat anti–rabbit IgG serum (obtained from goat Betsie), 1:1000, in TBS at room temperature for 30 minutes; (4) washing in TBS (twice for 10 minutes each time); (5) incubation with peroxidase antiperoxidase, 1:500, in TBS at room temperature for 30 minutes; (6) washing in TBS (twice for 10 minutes each time); (7) rinsing in 0.05-mol/L TRIS hydrochloride (pH 7.6); (8) incubation with 0.5-mg/mL 3-3′-diaminobenzidine (Sigma Chemical Co, St Louis, Mo) in 0.05-mol/L TRIS hydrochloride containing 0.01% hydrogen peroxide at room temperature for 10 minutes; (9) rinsing in distilled water followed by dehydration in graded ethanol at room temperature; and (10) coverslipping with Entellan (a rapid-mounting medium for microscopy) (Merck, Darmstadt, Germany).

MORPHOMETRY

Cross-sectional areas of the PVN in AVP- and OXT-stained sections were measured with a digitizer connected to an HP 9000/835 computer (Hewlett-Packard Co, Palo Alto, Calif) using a Zeiss microscope (Carl Zeiss Inc, Thornwood, NY) with a PLAN ×2.5 objective and PLAN ×12.5 eyepieces. If the cross-sectional area of the PVN extended beyond the field of vision in a particular section, this area was measured stepwise. A quadrangular grid in one of the eyepieces was then used as a reference. The sections containing three or more stained neurons were included in the measurements. The PVN was measured on the right side of the brain, except for two cases in which the nucleus was not entirely present within the dissected tissue on that side.

The volume of the AVP and OXT cell groups in the PVN was determined by integrating area measurements from the most rostral to the most caudal sections of each population of cells.[31]

Numerical AVP and OXT cell densities in the PVN were estimated by counting the total number of nuclear profiles of immunoreactive neurons per unit area, followed by a discrete unfolding procedure[32] with the modification proposed by Cruz-Orive[33] and a correction for section thickness. For this purpose, nuclear profile areas of AVP or OXT cells were measured using the equipment described above, with a PLAN ×40 objective. To take fluctuations in cell density into account, AVP and OXT cell nuclei in the PVN were sampled in a random, systematic way[34] by measuring all nuclear profiles in every 200th section throughout the PVN (ie, at 1200-μm intervals).

The total numbers of AVP and OXT cells in the PVN were computed by multiplying the average numerical cell density times the volume of the population.

STATISTICS

Differences among the groups were assessed using the Mann-Whitney *U* two-tailed test. Values are expressed as mean±SEM. The critical level for statistical significance was $P \leq .05$.

There are at least two opposite lines of evidence for the possible changes in activity of AVP- and OXT-producing neurons in mood disorders. First, patients with depression often manifest hyperactivity of the HPA axis.[6,7,21] In addition, AVP is involved in the modulation of the activity of the HPA axis, eg, by potentiating a CRH-induced corticotropin release from the pituitary.[22,23] Moreover, CRH and AVP are colocalized in an increased number of PVN neurons in depressed patients.[6] On the basis of these two findings one would expect increased activ-

Table 1. Clinicopathological Information and OXT-IR and AVP-IR Cell Numbers in the Paraventricular Nucleus*

Patient No./ Age, y/Sex	Brain Weight, g	Postmortem Delay, h	Fixation Time, d	Cause of Death	Clinical Diagnosis (*DSM-III-R*)	Medication in Last Month	No. of Cells OXT-IR	No. of Cells AVP-IR
Patients With Depression								
1/21/M	1492	24	33	Overdose of opiate	Major depression	Amytriptyline	27 190	34 856
2/39/M	1220	48	30	Respiratory insufficiency	Bipolar disorder	Moclobemide, 450 mg/d, clorazepam, 2.5 mg/d, fluphenazine, lithium carbonate	25 470	34 431
3/55/F	1320	7	30	Cardiac failure	Major depression with mood-congruent, psychotic features	Maprotiline, 150 mg/d, oxazepam, 100 mg/d, flupentixol, 5 mg/d	36 794	34 964
4/63/M	1210	24	33	Cardiac failure	Bipolar disorder	Haloperidol, 15 mg/d, temazepam, 20 mg/d, diazepam, 40 mg/d, promethazine, 100 mg/d	37 940	32 003
5/70/M	NA	48	28	Cardiac failure	Major depression with mood-congruent, psychotic features	Fluvoxamine, 250 mg/d, lorazepam, sulpiride, 800 mg/d, lisinopril, 5 mg/d	26 436	26 222
6/73/F	1032	96	28	Cardiac failure	Organic mood syndrome, depressed	Tranylcypramine, 70 mg/d	33 922	38 657
7/80/F	1300	24	69	Bronchopneumonia	Bipolar disorder	Lithium carbonate, haloperidol amantadine	32 052	39 549
8/85/F	1260	72	49	Bronchopneumonia	Depressive disorder not otherwise specified	Trazodone	28 395	29 015
Mean±SEM/ 61±8/...	1262 ±52	43±10	38±5	...	...	...	31 025 ±1711†	33 712 ±1598‡
Controls								
1/23/M	1310	13	11	Acute death, brain-stem encephalitis	...	Antibiotics	20 546	10 461
2/30/F	1330	24	39	Acute death, intramural dissecting hematoma of coronary artery, cardiac failure	...	No medication	27 958	11 481
3/42/F	1370	5	33	Metastatic carcinoma of mamma, multiple cerebral and meningeal metastases, radiation, bronchopneumonia	...	Nicomorphine	20 390	21 683
4/63/M	1420	33	35	Myocardial infarction, cardiac failure	...	No medication	25 632	28 400
5/68/M	1366	7	58	Myocardial infarction, cardiac failure following bypass thrombosis	...	Streptokinase and trinitroglycerine	26 505	20 692
6/83/M	1280	26	42	Perforated diverticulitis of colon, sepsis, myocardial infarction	...	Antibiotics, heparin infusion	25 504	21 645
7/81/F	1210	30	NA	Liver cirrhosis, liver carcinoma, alcohol intoxication, pneumonia	...	Vitamin B (Neurobion), antibiotics	31 116	27 604
8/88/F	1030	11	11	Basal cell carcinoma of ear, cardiac failure, urine infection	...	Digitalis, antibiotics	24 743	30 881
Mean±SEM/ 60±9/...	1290 ±43	19±4	33±6	...	...	...	25 299 ±1264†	21 606 ±2658‡

**OXT-IR indicates oxytocin-immunoreactive; AVP-IR, arginine vasopressin–immunoreactive; and NA, not available.*
†*P*=.03.
‡*P*=.003.

ity, especially of parvocellular AVP neurons, in depression. Concerning blood and CSF levels of AVP, OXT, and their neurophysins, changes in different directions have been reported that may depend, at least partly, on the type of depression. Increased CSF levels of neurophysins were found in patients who had bipolar affective disorder compared with patients who had unipolar depression and controls.[24] However, the basal levels of AVP neurophysin in plasma and CSF were found to be lower in a group of patients with major depression.[10,25-27]

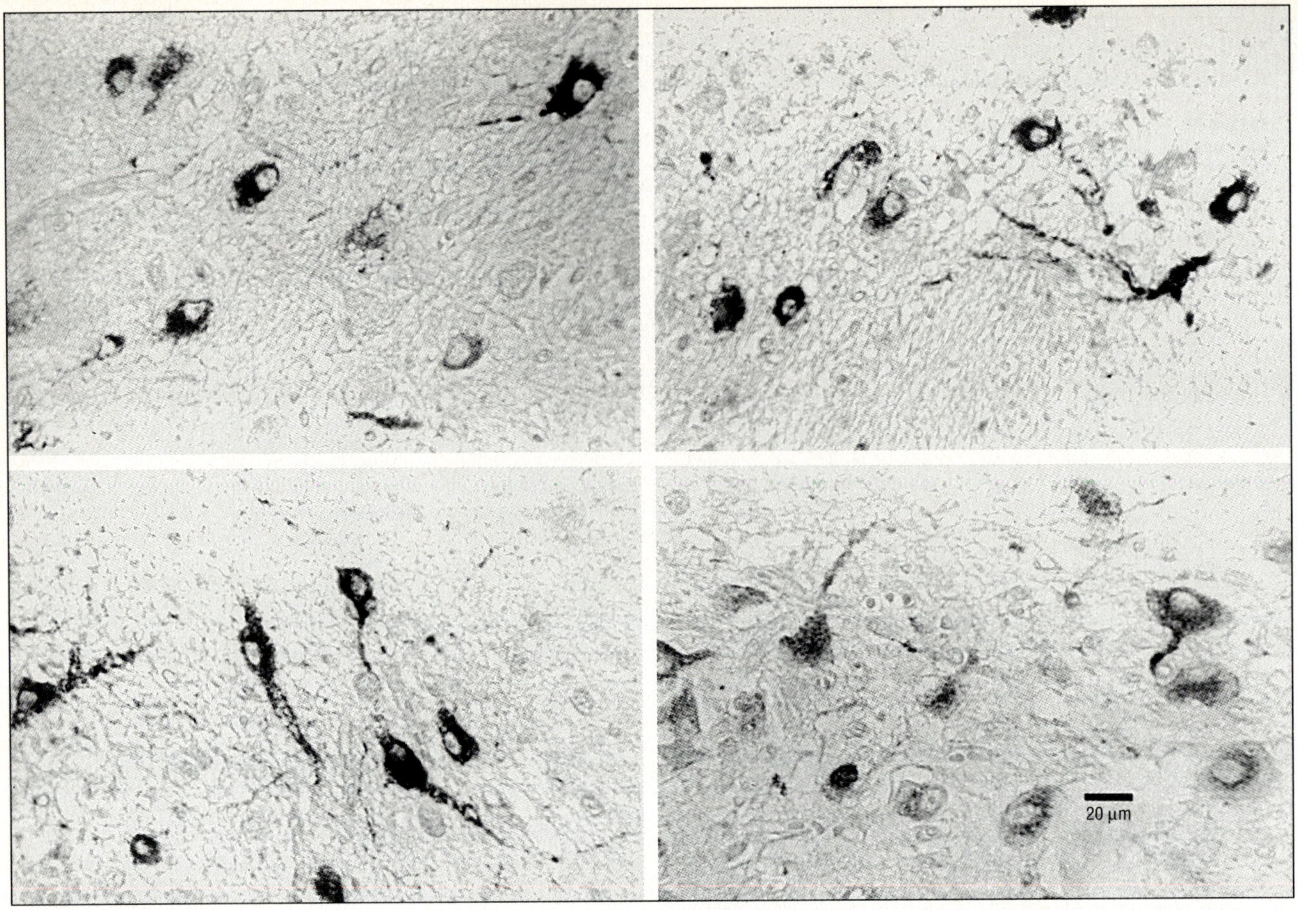

Frontal section (6 µm) of paraventricular nucleus of human hypothalamus. Top left, Control subject (patient 6) (antioxytocin). Top right, Patient with mood disorder (patient 2) (antioxytocin). Bottom left, Control subject (patient 6) (antivasopressin). Bottom right, Patient with mood disorder (patient 2) (antivasopressin).

To obtain direct information on possible changes in PVN neurons in mood disorders, in the present study, numbers of AVP-IR and OXT-IR neurons in the PVN were determined in depressed patients.

RESULTS

Age, brain weight, postmortem delay, and fixation time did not differ between patients with a mood disorder and controls (*P*=.87, *P*=.45, *P*=.11, and *P*=.82, respectively). Although there was no significant difference in postmortem time between controls and patients with a mood disorder and earlier studies had shown that postmortem interval does not affect AVP and OXT staining,[30,35,36] the potential effect of postmortem interval on the number of peptidergic neurons was investigated by applying linear regression analysis. No significant relationship was found between postmortem interval and the number of OXT-IR neurons (*r*=.63, *P*>.1) or AVP-IR neurons (*r*=.20, *P*>.6) in the PVN.

The intensity of the OXT staining was found to be similar in controls and patients with a mood disorder, but the intensity of the AVP staining was only slightly diminished in the latter group (**Figure**).

The number of OXT-IR neurons in the PVN was 23% higher in patients with a mood disorder than in controls (*P*=.03), and the mean nuclear diameter of the OXT-IR neurons was greater in patients with a mood disorder than in controls (*P*=.03) (**Table 2**).

The number of AVP-IR neurons in the PVN was 56% higher in patients with a mood disorder than in controls (*P*=.003), whereas the nuclear diameter of the AVP-IR neurons did not differ significantly between the two groups (Table 2). There were no differences between the three patients with major depression and the three patients with bipolar disorder in either OXT or AVP cell numbers (*P*=.82 for each). The AVP-IR and OXT-IR neuron numbers of the two patients with a depressive disorder not otherwise specified (Table 1, patients 6 and 8) were within the same range as in the six patients with major depression or bipolar disorder.

COMMENT

Mood disorders are characterized by persistent disturbances of mood, cognitive, psychomotor, and biological functions.[37] The symptoms of depression in older patients are basically not different from those in younger patients: depressed mood, apathy and anhedonia, insomnia, weight loss, feelings of worthlessness or inappropriate guilt, psychomotor agitation and retardation, concentration problems, loss of memory, and suicidal ideation or thoughts of death.[38]

Table 2. OXT-IR and AVP-IR Cell Populations in the Paraventricular Nucleus*

	OXT-IR Neurons			AVP-IR Neurons		
	Volume, mm^3	Neuron No., $\times 10^3$	Cell Nuclear Diameter, μm	Volume, mm^3	Neuron No., $\times 10^3$	Cell Nuclear Diameter, μm
Controls (n=8)	3.89±0.49	25.30±1.26	8.83±0.20	2.74±0.38	21.60±2.66	9.35±0.45
Depressed patients (n=8)	3.57±0.27	31.02±1.71	9.64±0.35	3.29±0.35	33.71±1.59	10.18±0.41
P†	.67	.03	.03	.29	.003	.17

*Values are mean±SEM. OXT-IR indicates oxytocin-immunoreactive; AVP-IR, arginine vasopressin–immunoreactive.
†Differences were assessed using the two-tailed Mann-Whitney U test.*

Various centrally active neuropeptides have been suggested to play a role in the pathophysiologic processes of affective disorders.[39] In this respect, it should be noted that in humans the SCN shows very strong annual fluctuations in neuronal activity. The number of AVP-expressing neurons in the SCN is about twice as high in the autumn as in the summer.[1-3] October and November, when the number of AVP-expressing neurons in the SCN is highest, is also when the frequency of depression is highest.[4,40] Since, in addition, light therapy is an effective treatment of seasonal depression and directly stimulates the SCN,[4,40-42] the annual fluctuation in the SCN might be causally related to this type of depression. As a seasonal fluctuation does not occur in the number of AVP neurons in the PVN,[1] annual changes should not have influenced the present data.

A second hypothalamic peptidergic system that has been shown to be related to depression is the HPA axis. This system is known to be hyperactive in depressed patients on the basis of hormone assays.[8] Recently, our group has shown that CRH neurons were strongly activated both in the three patients with bipolar disorder and in the three patients with major depression; ie, the number of CRH neurons had increased threefold to fourfold,[6] and the amount of CRH messenger RNA had doubled[7]; in the patients with major depression, the number of AVP-coexpressing CRH neurons had increased as well.[6] It was remarkable that in the two patients with a depressive disorder not otherwise specified, the CRH neurons were not activated,[6] whereas the OXT and AVP neurons were found to be activated in these two patients in the present report. Whether this means that different types of depression go together with different types of neuropeptidergic responses needs to be studied in more detail.

A third hypothalamic peptidergic system that might be involved in depression is formed by the AVP and OXT neurons of the supraoptic nucleus and PVN.[10] We found an increased number of neurons expressing AVP or OXT associated with depression. This is an indication of increased neuropeptide production and release, as shown, for example, for AVP in the course of aging, where a gradual increase in the number of neurons expressing AVP[36] goes together with other signs of increased peptide production, such as increased nucleolar size[43] and Golgi apparatus[44] and increased plasma levels of AVP.[45] With respect to the fact that we observed activation of AVP, OXT (in the present report), and CRH neurons[6,7] in depression, it is of interest to note that both AVP and OXT potentiate the CRH-mediated corticotropin release.[46-51] The AVP nerve terminals found in the external zone of the rat median eminence originate from the hypothalamic PVN.[52] The PVN also contains the CRH neurons in the human hypothalamus that project to the median eminence.[53] The CRH neurons in the PVN coexpress AVP in increasing numbers during the course of aging.[53] In the rat, OXT neurons that also contain CRH are present in both magnocellular and parvocellular subnuclei of the PVN,[54,55] but in the human PVN this coexistence has not yet been studied.

Increased corticosterone levels have been found in animals treated with OXT,[56] indicating that not only AVP but also OXT may potentiate the effects of CRH release. Our results showed an increase of 56% in AVP-IR neuron numbers and an increase of 23% in OXT-IR neuron numbers in depressed patients. Animal experiments have shown that CRH and AVP also act in a synergistic manner centrally, ie, on behavior.[57] Thus, the increased corticotropin release caused by increased activity of CRH-IR neurons, as observed recently in depressed patients,[6] might be potentiated by increased release of AVP and OXT. Our results show changes that might contribute to the hyperactivity of the HPA axis in depression,[8] confirming the postulation of Bardeleben and Holsboer[58] that the action of CRH in depression is enhanced by AVP. It is also interesting to note that OXT had an effect similar to that of antidepressants in two animal experimental tests that are considered relevant as animal models of depression.[59]

We did not find any difference in AVP-IR or OXT-IR cell numbers between patients with major depression and patients with bipolar disorder. This is in agreement with the similar increase in CRH activity found in both groups.[6,7] We do not know which of the two types of OXT and AVP neurons are activated: (1) neuroendocrine neurons that release their peptides into the capillary loops of the pituitary portal system or the neurohypophysis[13-15] or (2) neurons that transport their peptides to other parts of the brain, where they act as neurotransmitters or neuromodulators.[18,35] Currently, we cannot distinguish between these two cell types in the human PVN. In the human PVN, in contrast to that of the rat, these different types of neurons are not localized in particularly well-developed subnuclei.[60] In addition, suitable tracing procedures to solve this problem are not yet available for the postmortem brain.

There is little information in the literature on the possible effects of antidepressant drugs on the AVP or OXT system in the PVN. Although the clinical use of the serotonin transporter inhibitor fluoxetine was recently found to be associated with the occurrence of an inappropriate antidiuretic hormone syndrome in some patients, no evidence was found that this compound had an effect on osmoregulated AVP release or on the ability of a normal person to excrete a water load.[61] The diabetes insipidus of manic-depressive patients treated with lithium salts seems to be caused by activation of the collecting ducts of the kidney.[62] Although such an effect might lead to a compensating increase in AVP production by the PVN, the similar AVP and OXT changes in major depression and bipolar disorder, the strongly variable amount and kind of medication the patients had received, and the lack of effect of fluoxetine on AVP release indicate that it is more likely that the observed activation of OXT and AVP neurons is related to depression than that it is caused by the drug treatment. The idea that activation of OXT and AVP neurons is related to depression is reinforced by the observation of De Bellis et al,[63] who found significant decreases in CSF CRH and AVP levels and in Hamilton Depression Scale ratings following fluoxetine treatment. The overdose of opiates taken by patient 1 did not influence our conclusions, since opiates inhibit AVP and OXT secretion.[64]

As described above, increased AVP and OXT activity might contribute to the activation of the neuroendocrine HPA axis. Furthermore, increased AVP and OXT activity might affect other parts of the brain as neurotransmitters or neuromodulators. At present, one can only speculate about the possible central effects of OXT and AVP activation in depressed patients. Increased AVP and OXT cell activity might contribute to mood changes and cognitive impairment,[10] eg, by also potentiating the central CRH effects. Indeed, together with a decrease in Hamilton Depression Scale ratings, CSF AVP levels decrease following fluoxetine treatment of depressed patients.[63] Moreover, hypomanic episodes have been observed following administration of AVP.[10] One can also speculate about possible AVP- or OXT-potentiated central CRH effects on stress-related phenomena such as anxiety or sleep disturbances. These phenomena may in turn contribute to the diagnosis of major depression. Another interesting speculation is that the possible amnesiac effect of OXT might have an adaptive value in minimizing the emotional trauma of certain forms of stress, including depression.[65] The activation of OXT neurons may also play a role in the metabolic changes that are disturbed in depression. Various studies have shown that OXT is an important inhibitory factor in the modulation of food intake[66,67] and that it modifies fat and glucose metabolism.[14,67] One might therefore speculate that the weight loss, inhibition of food intake, and decreased motivation to eat seen in depressed patients are based not only on increased CRH activity[21,68,69] but also on the activation of OXT neurons, as observed in the present study.

One future research strategy might be to measure the individual symptoms of depression quantitatively, preferably prospectively. In this way, stronger and more specific correlations between particular symptoms and changes in hypothalamic systems might be detected, eg, between weight loss and the activation of OXT-IR cells in the PVN.

In conclusion, we found increased activity in the OXT and AVP neurons in the PVN of patients with mood disorder, regardless of the type of depression. Confirmation of these findings using quantitative in situ hybridization[70] and determining the exact central and peripheral consequences of this activation require further study.

Accepted for publication July 10, 1995.

This study was supported by the Deventer-Maas Foundation, The Hague, the Netherlands, by E. J. M. Stevens, and by grant 900557007 from the Netherlands Research Council, The Hague.

The authors thank Arja A. Sluiter and Bart Fisser for technical assistance; Gerben van der Meulen for photographic work; and Hans L. G. Blauwgeers, MD, Ernst J. Colon, MD, PhD, Pieternel Kölling, MD, Max Kross, MD, PhD, Margaret E. I. Schipper, MD, Ernst W. H. Jansen Steun, MD, PhD, and Rob A. I. de Vos, MD, for well-documented brain material. Human brain tissue was obtained from the Netherlands Brain Bank, Amsterdam (coordinator, Rivka Ravid, PhD).

Reprint requests to Netherlands Institute for Brain Research, Meibergdreef 33, 1105 AZ Amsterdam, the Netherlands (Dr Swaab).

REFERENCES

1. Hofman MA, Swaab DF. Seasonal changes in the suprachiasmatic nucleus of man. *Neurosci Lett.* 1992;139:257-260.
2. Hofman MA, Swaab DF. Diurnal and seasonal rhythms of neuronal activity in the suprachiasmatic nucleus of humans. *J Biol Rhythms.* 1993;38:163-171.
3. Hofman MA, Purba JS, Swaab DF. Annual variation in the vasopressin neuron population of the human suprachiasmatic nucleus. *Neuroscience.* 1993;53:1103-1112.
4. Rosenthal NE, Sack DA, Skwerer RG, Jacobsen FM, Wehr TA. Phototherapy for seasonal affective disorder. *J Biol Rhythms.* 1988;3:101-120.
5. Wehr TA, Rosenthal NE. Seasonality and affective illness. *Am J Psychiatry.* 1989;146:829-839.
6. Raadsheer FC, Hoogendijk WJG, Stam FC, Tilders FJH, Swaab DF. Increased number of corticotropin-releasing hormone neurons in the hypothalamic paraventricular nuclei of depressed patients. *Neuroendocrinology.* 1994;60:436-444.
7. Raadsheer FC, Van Heerikhuize JJ, Lucassen PJ, Tilders FJH, Swaab DF. Increased corticotropin-releasing hormone (CRH) mRNA in paraventricular nucleus of patients with Alzheimer's disease or depression. *Am J Psychiatry.* 1995;152:1372-1376.
8. Holsboer F, Sprengler D, Heuser I. The role of corticotropin-releasing hormone in the pathogenesis of Cushing's disease, anorexia nervosa, alcoholism, affective disorders and dementia. *Prog Brain Res.* 1992;93:385-417.
9. Stenzel-Poore MP, Heinrichs SC, Rivest S, Koob GF, Vale WW. Overproduction of coticotropin-releasing factor in transgenic mice: a genetic model of anxiogenic behavior. *J Neurosci.* 1994;14:2579-2584.
10. Legros JJ, Ansseau M. Neurohypophyseal peptides and psychopathology. *Prog Brain Res.* 1992;93:455-461.
11. Legros JJ, Ansseau M, Timsit-Berthier M. Neurohypophyseal peptides and psychiatric disease. *Regul Pept.* 1993;45:133-138.
12. Jolkkonen J, Tuomisto L, Van Wimersma Greidanus TjB, Riekkinen PJ. Vasopressin levels in the cerebrospinal fluid of rats with lesions of the paraventricular and suprachiasmatic nuclei. *Neurosci Lett.* 1988;86:184-188.
13. Gash DM, Boer GJ, eds. *Vasopressin: Principles and Properties.* New York, NY: Plenum Press; 1987.
14. Cunningham ET Jr, Sawchenko PE. Reflex control of magnocellular vasopressin and oxytocin secretion. *Trends Neurosci.* 1991;14:406-411.
15. Swaab DF, Hofman MA, Lucassen PJ, Purba JS, Raadsheer CF, Van de Nes JAP. Functional neuroanatomy and neuropathology of the hypothalamus. *Anat Embryol.* 1993;187:317-330.
16. Buijs RM, Swaab DF, Dogterom J, Van Leeuwen FW. Intra- and extrahypothalamic vasopressin and oxytocin pathways in the rat. *Cell Tissue Res.* 1978;186:423-433.
17. Fliers E, Swaab DF, Pool CW, Verwer RWH. The vasopressin and oxytocin neurons in the human supraoptic nucleus and paraventricular nucleus with aging and in senile dementia. *Brain Res.* 1985;342:45-53.

18. Buijs RM. The ultra structural localization of amines, amino acids and peptides in the brain. *Prog Brain Res.* 1982;55:167-183.
19. Swanson LW. The hypothalamus. In: Björklund A, Hokfelt T, Swanson LW, eds. *Handbook of Chemical Neuroanatomy.* Amsterdam, the Netherlands: Elsevier Science Publishers; 1987;5:1-124.
20. De Wied D, Versteeg V. Neurohypophyseal principles and memory. *Fed Proc.* 1979;38:2348-2354.
21. Holsboer-Trachsler E, Stochler R, Hatzinger M. Repeated administration of combined dexamethasone-human corticotropin releasing hormone stimulating test during treatment of depression. *Psychiatry Res.* 1991;38:163-171.
22. Callahan MF, Thore CR, Sundberg DK, Gruber KA, O'Steen K, Morris M. Excitotoxin paraventricular nucleus lesions: stress and endocrine reactivity and oxytocin mRNA levels. *Brain Res.* 1992;597:8-15.
23. Bartanusz V, Jezova D, Bertini LT, Tilders FJH, Aubry JM, Kiss J. Stress-induced increase in vasopressin and corticotropin-releasing factor expression in hypophysiotropic paraventricular nucleus. *Endocrinology.* 1993;132:895-902.
24. Legros JJ, Genen V, Linkowski P, Mendelwicz J. Increased neurophysins I and II cerebrospinal fluid concentration from bipolar versus unipolar depressed patients. *Neuroendocrinol Lett.* 1983;5:201-205.
25. Gjerris A, Hummer M, Vendsborg P, Christiensen NJ, Rafaelson DJ. Cerebrospinal fluid vasopressin changes in depression. *Br J Psychiatry.* 1985;147: 696-701.
26. Laruelle M, Seghers A, Goffinet S, Bonchez S, Legros JJ. Plasmatic vasopressin neurophysin in depression: basic levels and relations with HPA axis. *Biol Psychiatry.* 1990;27:1249-1261.
27. Linkowski P, Genen V, Kerkhofs M, Mendlewicz J, Legros JJ. Cerebrospinal fluid neurophysins in affective illness and schizophrenia. *Eur Arch Psychiatry Neurol Sci.* 1984;234:162-165.
28. American Psychiatric Association. *Diagnostic and Statistical Manual of Mental Disorders, Revised Third Edition.* Washington, DC: American Psychiatric Association; 1987.
29. Pool CW, Madlener S, Diegenbach PC, Sluiter AA, Van der Sluis P. Quantification of antiserum reactivity in immunocytochemistry. *J Histochem Cytochem.* 1984;32:921-928.
30. Wierda M, Goudsmit E, Van der Woude PF, Purba JS, Hofman MA, Swaab DF. Oxytocin cell number in the human paraventricular nucleus remains constant with aging and in Alzheimer's disease. *Neurobiol Aging.* 1991;12:511-516.
31. Van Eden CG, Uylings HBM, Van Pelt J. Sex-difference and left-right asymmetries in the prefrontal cortex during postnatal development in the rat. *Dev Brain Res.* 1984;12:146-153.
32. Weibel ER. *Stereological Methods: Practical Methods for Biological Morphometry.* Orlando, Fla: Academic Press Inc; 1979;1:186-196.
33. Cruz-Orive LM. Particle shape-size distributions, the general spheroid problem, II: stochastic model and practical guide. *J Microsc.* 1978;112:153-167.
34. Uylings HBM, Van Eden CG, Hofman MA. Morphometry of size/volume variables and comparison of their bivariate relations in the nervous system under different conditions. *J Neurosci Methods.* 1986;18:19-37.
35. Fliers E, Guldenaar SEF, Van der Waal N, Swaab DF. Extrahypothalamic vasopressin and oxytocin in the human brain: presence of vasopressin cells in the bed nucleus of the stria terminalis. *Brain Res.* 1986;375:363-367.
36. Van der Woude PF, Goudsmit E, Wierda M, Purba JS, Hofman MA, Swaab DF. No vasopressin cell loss in the human paraventricular and supraoptic nucleus during aging and in Alzheimer's disease. *Neurobiol Aging.* 1995;16:11-18.
37. Kalin NH, Dawson G. Neuroendocrine dysfunction in depression: hypothalamic-anterior pituitary systems. *Trends Neurosci.* 1986;9:261-266.
38. Mendels J. Clinical management of the depressed geriatric patient: current therapeutic options. *Am J Med.* 1993;94:12-18.
39. Judd LL, Craig RS, Parker DC, Janowsky DS, Segal DS, Huey LY. Blunted prolactin response. *Arch Gen Psychiatry.* 1982;39:1413-1416.
40. Rosenthal NE, Levendosky AA, Skwerer RG, Joseph-Vanderpool JR, Kelly KA, Hardin T, Kaspar S, DellaBella P, Wehr TA. Effects of light treatment on core body temperature in seasonal affective disorders. *Biol Psychiatry.* 1990;27:39-50.
41. Lewy AJ. Treating chronobiologic sleep and mood disorders with bright light. *Psychiatry Annu.* 1987;17:664-669.
42. Van Someren EJW, Mirmiran M, Swaab DF. Non-pharmacological treatment of sleep and wake disturbances in aging and Alzheimer's disease: chronobiological perspectives. *Behav Brain Res.* 1993;57:235-253.
43. Hoogendijk JE, Fliers E, Swaab DF, Verwer RWH. Activation of vasopressin neurons in the human supraoptic and paraventricular nucleus in senescence and senile dementia. *J Neurol Sci.* 1985;69:291-299.
44. Lucassen PJ, Salehi A, Pool CW, Gonatas NK, Swaab DF. Activation of vasopressin neurons in aging and Alzheimer's disease. *J Neuroendocrinol.* 1994; 6:673-680.
45. Frolkis VV, Golovchenko SF, Medved VI, Frolkis RA. Vasopressin and cardiovascular system in aging. *Gerontology.* 1982;28:290-302.
46. Yates FE, Maran JW. Stimulation and inhibition of adrenocorticotropin release. In: Knobil E, Sawyer WH, eds. *Handbook of Physiology.* Washington, DC: American Physiology Society; 1974;4(pt 2):367-404.
47. Gillies G, Lowry P. Corticotropin releasing factor may be modulated by vasopressin. *Nature.* 1979;278:463-464.
48. Gillies GE, Linton EA, Lowry PJ. Corticotropin releasing activity of the new CRF is potentiated several times by vasopressin. *Nature.* 1982;299:355-357.
49. Carlson DE, Dornhorst A, Seif SM, Robinson AG, Gann DS. Vasopressin-dependent and -independent control of the release of adrenocorticotropin. *Endocrinology.* 1982;110:680-682.
50. Vale WJ, Vaughan J, Yamamoto G, Bruhn T, Douglas C, Dalton D, Rivier C, Rivier J. Assay of corticotropin releasing factor. *Methods Enzymol.* 1983;103: 565-577.
51. Makara GB. The relative importance of hypothalamic neurons containing corticotropin-releasing factor or vasopressin in the regulation of adrenocorticotropic, hormone secretion. In: *Functional Anatomy of the Neuroendocrine Hypothalamus.* New York, NY: John Wiley & Sons Inc; 1992:43-53.
52. Vandesande F, Dierickx K. Identification of the vasopressin producing and of oxytocin producing neurons in the hypothalamic magnocellular neurosecretory system of the rat. *Cell Tissue Res.* 1975;164:153-162.
53. Raadsheer FC, Sluiter AA, Ravid R, Tilders FJH, Swaab DF. Localization of corticotropin-releasing hormone (CRH) neuron in the paraventricular nucleus of the human hypothalamus: age dependent colocalization with vasopressin. *Brain Res.* 1993;615:50-62.
54. Sawchenko PE, Swanson LW, Vale WW. Corticotropin-releasing factor: co-expression within distinct subsets of oxytocin-, vasopressin-, and neurotensin-immunoreactive neurons in the hypothalamus of male rat. *J Neurosci.* 1984; 4:1118-1129.
55. Pretel S, Piekut DT. Coexistence of CRF peptide and oxytocin mRNA in the paraventricular nucleus. *Peptides.* 1990;11:621-624.
56. Muir JL, Pfister HP. Influence of exogenously administered oxytocin on the corticosterone and prolactin response to psychological stress. *Pharmacol Biochem Behav.* 1988;29:699-703.
57. Elkabir DR, Wyatt ME, Vellucci SV, Herbert J. The effects of separate or combined infusions of corticotropin-releasing factor and vasopressin either intraventricularly or into the amygdala on aggressive and investigative behaviour in the rat. *Regul Pept.* 1990;28:199-214.
58. Bardeleben U, Holsboer F. Cortisol response to a combined dexamethasone-human corticotropin-releasing hormone challenge in patients with depression. *J Neuroendocrinol.* 1989;1:485-488.
59. Arletti R, Bertolini A. Oxytocin acts as an antidepressant in two animal models of depression. *Life Sci.* 1987;41:1725-1730.
60. Swaab DF, Purba JS, Hofman MA. Alterations in the hypothalamic paraventricular nucleus and its oxytocin neurons (putative satiety cells) in Prader-Willi syndrome: a study of five cases. *J Clin Endocrinol Metab.* 1995;80:573-579.
61. Faull CM, Rooke P, Baylis PH. The effect of a highly specific serotonine agonist on osmoregulated vasopressin secretion in healthy man. *Clin Endocrinol.* 1991;35:423-430.
62. Singer I, Rotenberg D, Puschet JB, Franko EA. Lithium-induced nephrogenic diabetes insipidus: in vivo and in vitro studies. *J Clin Invest.* 1972;51:1081-1091.
63. De Bellis MD, Gold PW, Geracioti Jr TD, Listwak SJ, Kling MA. Association of fluoxetine treatment with reductions in CSF concentrations of corticotropin-releasing hormone and arginine vasopressin in patients with major depression. *Am J Psychiatry.* 1993;150:656-657.
64. Lutz-Bucher B, Koch B. Evidence for a direct inhibitory effect of morphine on the secretion of posterior pituitary hormones. *Eur J Pharmacol.* 1980;66:375-378.
65. Gibbs DM. Dissociation of oxytocin, vasopressin and corticotropin secretion during different types of stress. *Life Sci.* 1984;35:487-491.
66. Olson BR, Drutarosky MD, Stricker EM, Verbalis J. Brain oxytocin receptors mediate corticotropin-releasing hormone-induced anorexia. *Am Physiol Soc.* 1991;260:R448-R452.
67. Altzuler N, Rosenberg CR, Winkler B, Fuchs AR, Hill PS, Hruby VJ. The metabolic effects of oxytocin are mediated by a uterine type of receptor and are inhibited by oxytocin antagonist and by arginine vasopressin in the dog. *Life Sci.* 1992;50:739-746.
68. Britton DR, Koob GF, River J, Vale W. Intraventricular corticotropin-releasing hormone enhances behavioral effects of novelty. *Life Sci.* 1982;31:363-367.
69. Morley JE, Levine AS. Corticotropin-releasing factor in grooming and ingestive behavior. *Life Sci.* 1982;31:1459-1464.
70. Lucassen PJ, Goudsmit E, Pool CW, Mengod G, Palacios JM, Raadsheer FC, Guldenaar SEF, Swaab DF. In situ hybridization for vasopressin mRNA in the human supraoptic and paraventricular nucleus: quantitative aspects of formalin-fixed paraffin-embedded tissue sections as compared to cryostat sections. *J Neurosci Methods.* 1995;57:221-230.

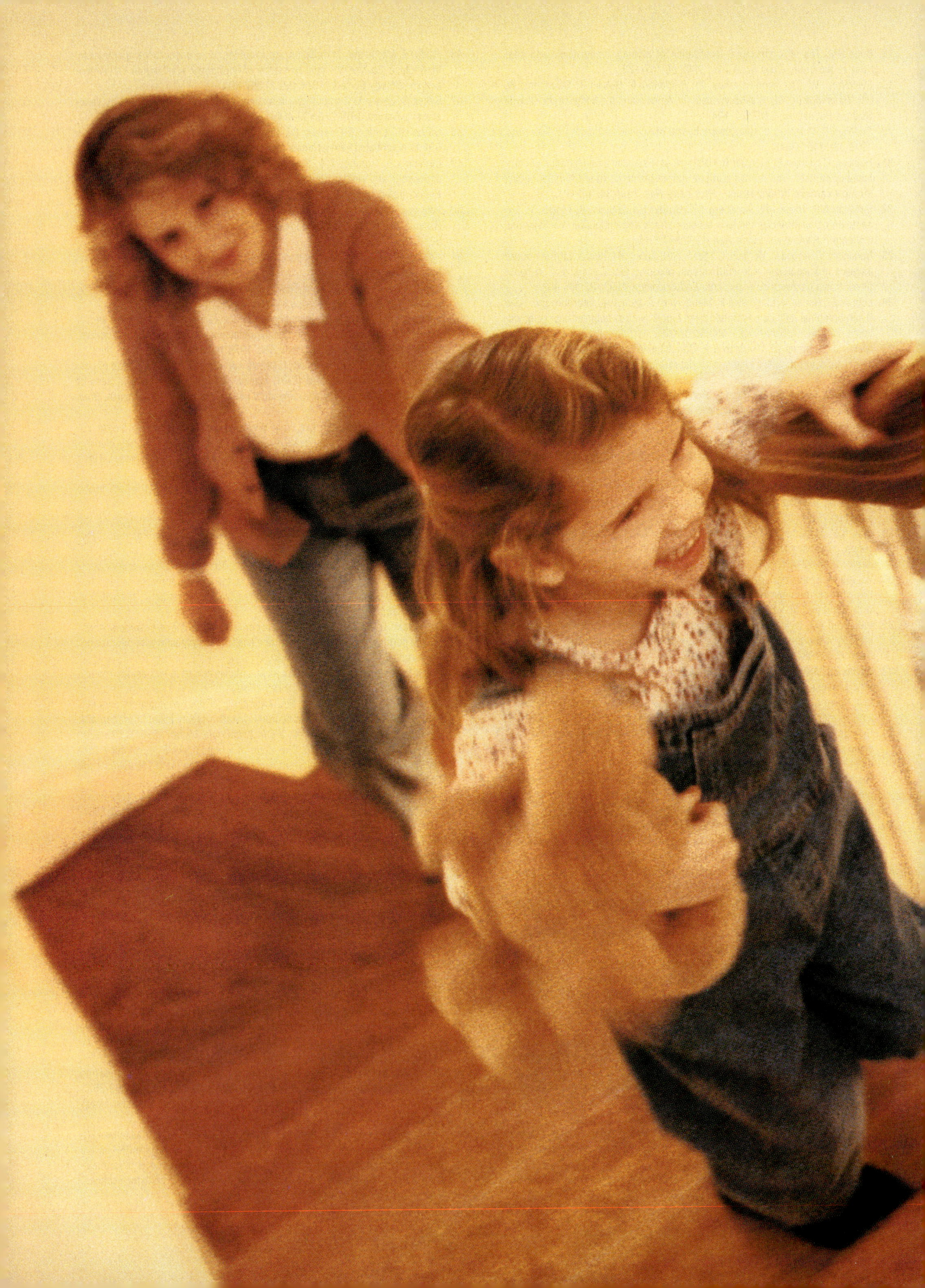

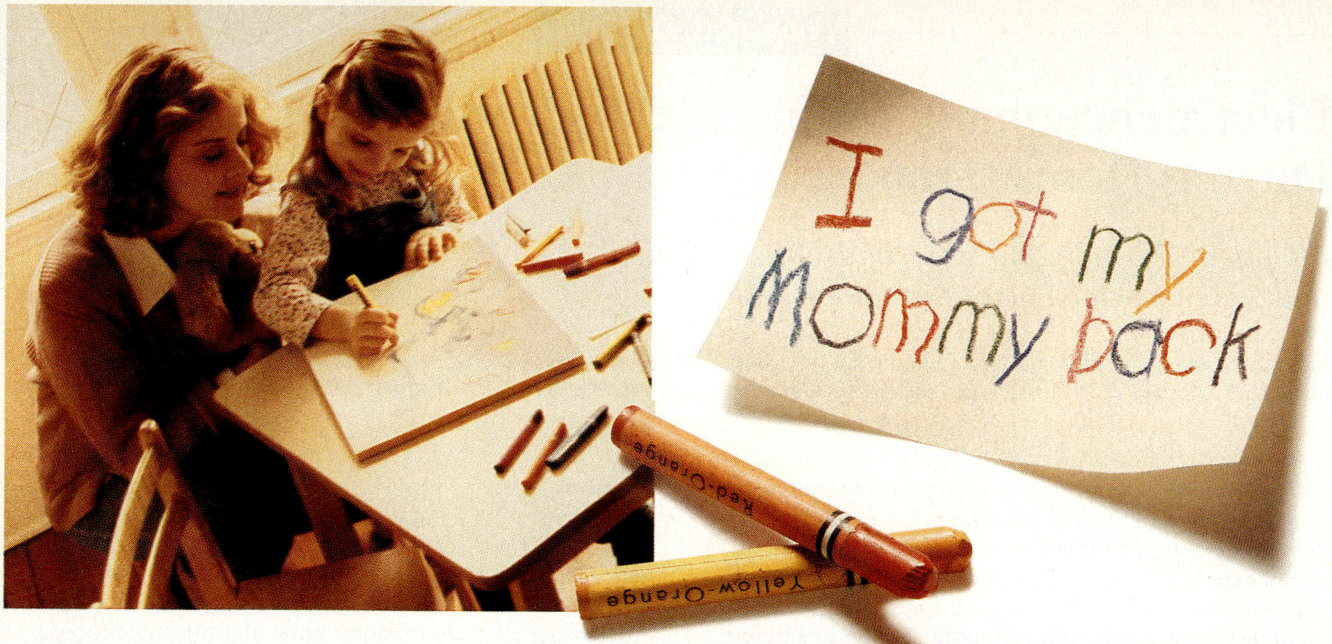

- Efficacy clearly demonstrated in depressed outpatients[1]
- Effective treatment in hospitalized depressed patients with major depressive disorder and melancholia meeting DSM-III-R™ criteria[2]
- No differential response in patients suffering from the symptoms of psychomotor agitation or psychomotor retardation that may accompany depression, based on subgroup analysis of effects on outcome[1]
- EFFEXOR should be taken in two or three divided doses with food

The most common adverse events reported in EFFEXOR clinical trials (incidence >10% and ≥ 2X that of placebo) were nausea, somnolence, dry mouth, dizziness, constipation, nervousness, sweating, asthenia, abnormal ejaculation/orgasm, and anorexia.

Counsel patients that nausea diminishes in most patients.

The effectiveness of EFFEXOR in long-term use (>6 weeks) has not been systematically evaluated in controlled trials.

EFFEXOR is contraindicated in patients taking monoamine oxidase inhibitors (MAOIs). EFFEXOR should not be used in combination with an MAOI or within at least 14 days of discontinuing treatment with an MAOI because of potential for serious adverse reactions. Based on the half-life of EFFEXOR, at least 7 days should be allowed after stopping EFFEXOR before starting an MAOI.

Treatment with EFFEXOR is associated with sustained increases in blood pressure in some patients. The incidence was seen at >5% at dosages above 200 mg/day and appears to be dose dependent. Regular monitoring of blood pressure is recommended.

As with any psychotropic drug, EFFEXOR may impair judgment, thinking, or motor skills; patients should be advised to exercise caution until they have adapted to therapy.

Please see brief summary of Prescribing Information on previous page of this advertisement.

Tablets: 25 mg, 37.5 mg, 50 mg, 75 mg, and 100 mg

VENLAFAXINE HCl

EFFEXOR® MEANS EFFECTIVE

ORIGINAL ARTICLE

Electroencephalographic Sleep Profiles During Depression

Effects of Episode Duration and Other Clinical and Psychosocial Factors in Older Adults

Mary Amanda Dew, PhD; Charles F. Reynolds III, MD; Daniel J. Buysse, MD; Patricia R. Houck, MS; Carolyn C. Hoch, PhD; Timothy H. Monk, PhD; David J. Kupfer, MD

Background: Limited evidence suggests that polysomnographic alterations may be more prominent early in a depressive episode. Whether the effects of episode duration extend beyond middle age and appear in late-life depression as well has important implications for treatment decisions and for understanding depressive illness across the life span. Furthermore, the impact of episode duration on sleep has not been examined in the context of other factors related to clinical history and psychosocial status.

Methods: Eighty-three persons aged 60 years or older with recurrent depression were studied: 34 had been depressed for 2 to 16 weeks and 49 for longer periods. An age- and gender-matched group of 48 persons with no history of major depression served as controls. Initial univariate analyses examined duration effects on electroencephalographic (EEG) sleep measurements. Multivariate analyses considered the combined effects of episode duration, clinical variables, and psychosocial variables on EEG sleep profile.

Results: Episode duration was strongly associated with sleep continuity, architecture, and rapid eye movement: subjects who were earlier in their depressive episodes had their sleep impaired more than those later in their episodes, who, in turn, were more impaired than controls. Moreover, clinical characteristics of subjects' depressive illness, demographic variables, and psychosocial stressors and supports had unique effects on the EEG sleep profile.

Conclusion: Episode duration appears to be a potent factor to consider when evaluating sleep during depression. The additional contribution of clinical and psychosocial characteristics to the prediction of the EEG sleep profile demonstrates the importance of incorporating these variables into models of the psychobiologic characteristics of depression. The results are relevant to the timing and focus of therapeutic interventions.

(Arch Gen Psychiatry. 1996;53:148-156)

A GROWING body of evidence indicates that depression is associated with both qualitative[1-4] and quantitative[5-8] sleep alterations and that these associations grow stronger across the life span.[5,9] Indeed, sleep disturbances in adults aged 60 years or older, especially in the context of depressive illness, have gained recognition as major public health and quality-of-life issues.[10,11] These issues are likely to become more prominent as the mean age of the US population continues to increase.

While subjective sleep disturbance is a hallmark of depression, constituting a cardinal symptom for diagnosis and implicated in the disorder's pathogenesis,[1] alterations in electroencephalographic (EEG) sleep measurements have been less reliable "markers" for depression, especially in older adults. Such changes occur during normal aging[10,12] as well as in other psychiatric illnesses.[13] Furthermore, as observed in younger populations,[7] not all older adults who meet diagnostic criteria for depression display the full profile of "classic" sleep stigmata.[7,9,14,15] It has been suggested that the lack of sensitivity of the EEG sleep profile to depressive illness per se may be largely because of heterogeneity in depression severity, physical health status, or clinical history.[15-19] Such factors have rarely been examined in their own right as correlates of EEG sleep measurements. However, even when these factors are controlled by study design to limit their possible influence, variability in the level

From the Departments of Psychiatry (Drs Dew, Reynolds, Buysse, Hoch, Monk, and Kupfer and Ms Houck), Epidemiology (Dr Dew), and Psychology (Dr Dew), University of Pittsburgh School of Medicine and Western Psychiatric Institute and Clinic, Pittsburgh, Pa.

See Methods on next page

METHODS

SUBJECTS

Data were collected from 131 persons aged 60 years or older enrolled in ongoing studies of sleep in late life.[32,33] Eighty-three of these subjects were recruited for an investigation of maintenance therapies in late-life depression; data presented here were gathered prior to treatment. To enter the investigation, these subjects were required (1) to meet Research Diagnostic Criteria (RDC)[34] for nondelusional unipolar major depression, as determined by the Schedule for Affective Disorders and Schizophrenia–Lifetime Version (SADS-L),[35] (2) to have scores exceeding 16 on the 17-item Hamilton Rating Scale for Depression (HAM-D),[36] and (3) to be in at least their second lifetime episode of depression, with one or more episodes occurring within the 3 years before onset of the current episode. None had suffered the death of a loved one within the past 6 months. Because depressed persons who had already sought care would not constitute a representative sample,[15] subjects were recruited from multiple sources, including public information efforts (eg, radio advertisements, resulting in 45% of the sample [n=37]) and traditional clinical referrals (55% of the sample [n=46]).[37] Subjects recruited from these sources showed no systematic differences on any measures in the present study.

The remaining 48 subjects, who serve as controls, were age- and gender-matched to the 83 depressed subjects. They were recruited through the same public information efforts noted above to participate in investigations of sleep in healthy, nondepressed individuals and were required (1) to demonstrate no evidence of lifetime psychiatric disorder, as determined with the SADS-L, (2) to have HAM-D scores below 8, and (3) to have no subjective sleep/wake complaint.

All 131 subjects met other stringent health criteria for study inclusion.[32,33,37] They had no evidence of dementia (Mini-Mental State Examination[38] score ≥27) or current substance abuse. Physical examinations, electrocardiograms, and laboratory studies screened out persons with serious or uncontrolled physical problems.[37] Chronic medical conditions (eg, heart disease) did not exclude subjects, provided the condition was stable either without medication or with medications (listed below) not known to have significant sleep or mood effects. These conditions were not associated with self-reported sleep disturbance, daytime sleepiness, or EEG sleep variables.

Subjects' mean age was 67.5 years (SD, 6.0 years; range, 60 to 91 years), 26% were men, most had at least a high school education (83%; mean, 13 years of education), and most were white (92%). Fifty-seven percent (n=75) took at least one prescribed medication (including analgesics, diuretics, calcium channel-blocking agents, estrogen, β-blockers, digoxin, cimetidine/ranitidine, β-agonists, antihistamines as needed, and/or oral hypoglycemics).

PROCEDURE

Subjects kept a daily sleep-wake log for a 14-day period free of psychotropic drugs.[39] They were asked to refrain from alcohol use during this time. They then had 3 consecutive nights of polysomnography performed using standard procedures[32] at the Sleep and Chronobiology Center, Western Psychiatric Institute and Clinic, Pittsburgh, Pa. Bedtime and wake-up time was at subjects' habitual times as determined by their sleep/wake logs. Polysomnographic technologists used standard criteria for scoring sleep,[40] with periodic checks of interrater reliability.[41] Automated delta-wave and REM activity analyses were conducted using standard methods of period and amplitude analysis.[42] Psychosocial data were collected by trained personnel while subjects were at the center. Informed consent was obtained after study procedures were fully explained.

MEASURES

Polysomnography

Measures represent averages over nights 2 and 3, with night 1 considered an adaptation night. They include indices of sleep continuity, sleep architecture, and REM sleep, listed in **Table 1**.

Depression History Characteristics

Duration of current depressive episode was ascertained using the SADS-L and was based on subjects' reports as well as collateral information from medical records and relatives. The 83 depressed subjects were classified into those who were (1) relatively early in their current episode (≤4 months [n=34]; median duration, 2.25 months [9 weeks]; range, 2 weeks to 4 months) or (2) depressed for a longer time (>4 months [n=49]; median duration, 7.5 months [30 weeks]; range, 5 to 48 months).

The classification was achieved by dichotomizing the distribution of months of illness at the median. A histo-

Continued on next page

of EEG sleep disturbance among depressed individuals is still observed.[17,20,21]

Of interest, then, are hints from laboratory studies of EEG sleep variables and from depression treatment studies that another factor may be critical, namely, the duration of an individual's depressive episode at the time of evaluation. To our knowledge, the only investigation of the effects of episode duration on EEG sleep characteristics is earlier work from our laboratory on a small middle-aged cohort. This work suggested that sleep alterations, particularly in rapid eye movement (REM) indices, are more pronounced during the earliest weeks of depressive episodes than later on.[17,20] However, because these early-episode observations were made during a recurrence of depression, while the late-episode observations had been made previously during individuals' most recent episode, the unique effects of episode duration could not be disentangled from the cumulative history of depressive illness.

There are other compelling reasons to investigate this parameter further. Episode duration is already recognized as a potent factor to consider when initiating treatment for depression,[22] with early treatment often leading to more advantageous outcomes, especially during recurrent episodes.[23,24] Efficacious outcomes may be linked in part to the ability of somatic treatments to produce gram of this skewed distribution is shown in the **Figure**, which also includes a box plot summarizing key features of the distribution.[43] The median duration was 5 months, with a mean of 7 months. The interquartile range (the middlemost 50% of the distribution) lay between 3 and 9 months' duration. Although we considered, for conceptual reasons, cutting the distribution at an earlier point than the median, so that persons with earlier-episode depression would have been ill for less than 2 months,[17] we could not do so because there would have been too few cases in the early-episode group for adequate statistical power.

Additional information regarding current and previous depressive episodes was also obtained and is given in the top half of **Table 2**.[34-36,44]

Psychosocial Characteristics

In addition to demographic characteristics, indices of stress and social support were assessed among depressed subjects (bottom half of Table 2).[45-47] With respect to stress, severity of chronic medical (nonpsychiatric) burden was determined from trained nurses' evaluations using the Cumulative Illness Rating Scale,[45] modified for older adults[31] (ratio of severity across all organ systems to number of systems affected, higher score=greater burden). Whether subjects had experienced a recent acute life event or stressor that had directly contributed to the onset of current depression was ascertained using the SADS-L (ie, determination using RDC that the episode was caused by situational factors). Third, the Perceived Stress Scale[46] assessed the degree to which subjects appraised their daily lives as chronically stressful during the past month. Because this measure was highly skewed, it was dichotomized into high chronic stress (top third of the sample) vs low chronic stress.

The degree to which subjects felt they had available emotional and practical support from others was determined using the Interpersonal Support Evaluation List,[47] adapted for older adults.[48] This measure was also dichotomized into low (bottom third of the sample) vs high support because of skewness.

ANALYSES

Univariate analyses were initially performed to examine polysomnographic differences across the three study groups: early-episode depressed subjects, later-episode depressed subjects, and nondepressed controls. Planned contrasts to evaluate the hypothesized pattern of group differences were computed using one-way analyses of variance.[49]

Although some EEG measures were partially redundant by virtue of their definition and computation (ie, sleep efficiency with sleep maintenance and REM density with REM intensity), we report descriptive analyses for each to allow complete comparison with other cohorts for which such data have routinely been presented.[17,32] However, only one index from each pair of redundant variables could be included in subsequent multivariate analyses to prevent multicollinearity and singularity problems.[50] (The requirement to eliminate redundancy does not imply that EEG measures had to be uncorrelated for multivariate analyses; those included did tend to be intercorrelated [median r=.19; interquartile range, .07 to .32].)

Multivariate analyses examined (1) whether the duration of the current episode was associated with an overall profile of sleep differences among depressed subjects, (2) whether this association was maintained even when other clinical and psychosocial factors were considered, and (3) the relationship to the EEG sleep profile of each of these other factors in its own right. Canonical correlation analysis was employed to address these issues.

This analysis enabled us to examine possible dimensions along which a diverse constellation of sleep indices might be related to episode duration and the other potential predictors in depressed subjects. The goal of the procedure is to analyze relationships between two sets of variables (here, a set of sleep indices and a set of potential predictors).[50,51] The analysis derives a linear combination (a canonical variate) of the sleep variables and a linear combination of the predictors so that the correlation between this pair of linear combinations (the canonical R) is maximized. Each canonical variate represents an underlying dimension describing a given set of variables, and the variate is conceptually interpreted in a manner identical to factor interpretation in factor analysis. The analysis is mathematically identical to, for example, discriminant function or regression analysis, in which a string of predictors is examined relative to an outcome. In the present situation, however, we have not only a string of potential predictors but also a complete set of outcomes (ie, the sleep indices). Canonical correlation analysis is thus a generalization of more familiar multivariate techniques to more complex situations.

The relatively small sample of depressed persons precluded use of a single analysis to simultaneously consider the effects on sleep of all the predictors. Thus, two separate canonical analyses were performed to examine the effects of episode duration on sleep in the context of (1) other clinical factors and then (2) psychosocial characteristics.

biological responses in the form of marked, immediate changes in REM sleep.[25-27] Could episode duration itself, then, independent of clinical history and other personal factors, be associated with important differences in EEG sleep profile? If so, these differences might, in turn, aid in making both the targeting of therapies and the judgment of their likely success even more precise.

In the present study we evaluate the role of episode duration on older adults' sleep profiles during depression, unconfounded by cumulative depressive history or by illness severity. Moreover, we determine whether episode duration remains important even after other clinical and psychosocial factors are considered. Examining the contribution of these other factors is a second critical study goal because there is increasing evidence that sleep changes during depression may be influenced by multiple biological and psychosocial characteristics of the ill individual.[28-30] In particular, the effects of factors such as acute life stressors, ongoing strains, and social supports on sleep and depressive symptoms are often profound.[3,28,31] Full understanding of any unique effects of episode duration on EEG sleep profiles in depression can only be achieved by examining such effects in studies that consider the impact of these other environmental factors as well.

Table 1. EEG Sleep Measures in Three Study Groups*

	Duration of Major Depressive Episode ≤4 mo (n=34)	Duration of Major Depressive Episode >4 mo (n=49)	No Depression (n=48)	ANOVA, F†
Sleep continuity				
Total recording period, min	465.4 (63.4)	451.7 (55.2)	459.4 (44.1)	0.26
Sleep latency, min	36.2 (38.9)	25.5 (23.2)	17.8 (10.4)	13.43‡
Time spent awake, min	83.7 (42.5)	64.9 (42.2)	51.7 (31.4)	13.55‡
Time spent asleep, min	343.3 (59.8)	359.0 (55.8)	390.6 (36.4)	18.41‡
Sleep efficiency, % §‖	73.2 (12.0)	79.3 (10.4)	83.6 (6.1)	23.62‡
Sleep maintenance, % §¶	79.3 (9.2)	88.4 (8.9)	87.0 (6.1)	18.69‡
Sleep architecture				
Stage 1, % #	8.5 (9.3)	6.1 (4.2)	5.7 (3.9)	4.47**
Stage 2, %	59.9 (9.5)	60.3 (8.5)	61.0 (8.0)	0.35
REM, %	23.8 (6.4)	24.4 (5.0)	21.9 (4.8)	2.80
Delta, %	7.0 (7.5)	8.4 (8.3)	10.8 (9.1)	3.59††
Delta ratio ‡‡	1.16 (0.3)	1.25 (0.3)	1.27 (0.4)	2.18
REM measures				
Latency, min #	45.6 (24.4)	54.5 (27.1)	63.0 (24.3)	12.24‡
Activity #§§	133.7 (57.8)	128.9 (64.7)	124.7 (53.0)	0.50
Density ‖‖	1.7 (0.6)	1.5 (0.5)	1.5 (0.5)	4.32**
Intensity ¶¶	0.40 (0.2)	0.37 (0.2)	0.32 (0.1)	5.23**
No. of REM periods	3.7 (1.1)	3.6 (0.9)	3.9 (0.8)	1.22
REM counts/min, period 1	8.0 (4.3)	6.5 (4.2)	5.4 (3.9)	8.33##
REM ratio §***	1.71 (1.4)	1.54 (1.5)	1.22 (1.0)	4.09**

*Values are mean (SD). Measures were derived from visual scoring, except for delta ratio, REM counts per minute, and REM ratio, which were derived from automated analysis.[42] EEG indicates electroencephalographic; ANOVA, analysis of variance; and REM, rapid eye movement.

†Test for linear trend. Except for delta ratio, REM counts per minute, and REM ratio, df=1, 128 for F tests. For the delta ratio, data were missing for 15 persons with no depression, so that df=1, 113 for F tests. For REM counts per minute and REM ratio, data were missing for one person with a major depressive episode greater than 4 months in duration, so that df=1, 127 for F tests.

‡$P<.001$.

§Transformation used prior to F tests: ln (x+1).

‖Percentage of total recording period spent asleep.

¶Percentage of total recording period spent asleep, adjusted for sleep latency.

#Transformation used prior to F tests: $\sqrt{x}$.

**$P<.05$.

††$P=.06$.

‡‡Ratio of delta wave counts per minute in non-REM period 1 to delta wave counts per minute in non-REM period 2.[42]

§§REM frequency per minutes of REM sleep.

‖‖REM activity per REM time.

¶¶REM activity per time spent asleep.

##$P<.01$.

***Ratio of REM counts per minute in REM period 1 to REM counts per minute in REM period 2.

RESULTS

RELATIONSHIP OF EPISODE DURATION TO POLYSOMNOGRAPHY

Table 1 presents data relevant to the association of EEG sleep measures with the occurrence and duration of depression. We hypothesized not only that depressed persons' sleep would be adversely affected relative to nondepressed controls but also that persons with early-episode depression would score most poorly of all. Results of planned contrasts testing this linear hypothesis are shown in the last column of Table 1: not only was REM latency progressively shorter across the three study groups but there was also a strong and significant linear decline for other sleep continuity, architecture, and REM measures. The decline in sleep continuity indices was particularly pronounced. In addition, stage 1 sleep percentage increased across the groups, and a marginally significant ($P<.06$) reduction in delta sleep percentage was evident. In addition, REM density and intensity were relatively increased in subjects with early-episode depression, as were automated measures of REM activity.

UNIQUE EFFECTS OF DEPRESSION DURATION AND OTHER CHARACTERISTICS

The univariate analyses reveal differences on individual sleep indices but do not evaluate (1) whether, among depressed subjects, episode duration was reliably related to a complete profile of interrelated sleep deficiencies or (2) whether the impact of episode duration on sleep was maintained even when other aspects of clinical and psychosocial status were considered. Canonical correlation analysis addressed these issues.

The set of sleep indices used in the canonical analyses included the variables found in the initial univariate analyses (Table 1) to have at least modest relationships (ie, $r>.15$ for effect size, from planned contrast)[52] to episode duration. Additionally, for variables that overlapped conceptually and computationally (sleep efficiency with maintenance and REM density with intensity), only one index from each pair was included in the canonical analyses, as specified above.

With respect to the predictors, Table 2 shows that there were no sizable or significant differences in these variables as a function of episode duration. This provides preliminary evidence that the observed relationships between episode duration and the EEG sleep measures (Table 1) cannot be explained solely by study group differences in these other characteristics.

Analysis 1: Effects of Episode Duration and Other Depressive History Variables

A single canonical correlation was sufficient to explain the linkage between the set of sleep variables and the set of duration and clinical variables. This correlation of .63 accounted for 39.9% of the shared variability between variable sets ($F[90, 417]=1.31$, $P=.04$); after removal of the first pair of canonical variates, insignificant shared variability remained ($F[72, 379]=1.12$, $P=.24$). The first pair of canonical variates, therefore, accounted for the significant relationships between the two sets of variables.

The first column of **Table 3** provides additional information from this analysis. The loadings of the sleep variables on their canonical variate are shown at the top of the first column, and the loadings of the predictor set of clinical variables on their canonical variate are shown at the bottom of the first column. These values are analogous to factor loadings in factor analysis; the larger the loadings, the stronger the relationships of variables to their respective canonical variates.

Considering the sleep variables first, and using a cutoff of ±.20 for loading interpretation,[53] the sizes of their loadings indicate that all of the sleep indices (except time spent asleep) are important for their canonical variate. This suggests that there was only a single underlying dimension, representing a continuum from poor to good sleep, across the indices; ie, depressed subjects' sleep could not be further differentiated using additional unique dimensions, such as a continuity dimension vs an REM dimension. Instead, at the poor end of the sleep continuum, for example, subjects' sleep reflected a complete constellation of longer sleep latency (indicated by a positive loading of .47), reduced sleep efficiency (negative loading of −.61), heightened stage 1 sleep percentage (.45), reduced delta sleep (−.31), shortened REM latency (−.35), increased REM density (.44), more REM counts per minute in REM period 1 (.20), and a larger REM ratio (.32).

The variables in the clinical predictor set that were important relative to this sleep profile are those with loadings of at least .20 at the bottom of the first column in Table 3. These included, notably, episode duration: the loading of .50 indicates a strong relationship between relatively early status in the current episode and having a poorer sleep profile, even after including the effects of other predictors. Several of the other clinical variables, however, were important correlates of sleep profile in their own right: subjects with poorer sleep during their current episode had been younger at their first lifetime episode (−.33), had more previous hospitalizations (.50), and had more prior episodes (.26). Concerning current episode characteristics, subjects with poorer sleep had greater symptom severity (.25), had greater functional severity (.27), and were more likely to have episodes characterized as RDC endogenous (.35) and RDC agitated (.33).

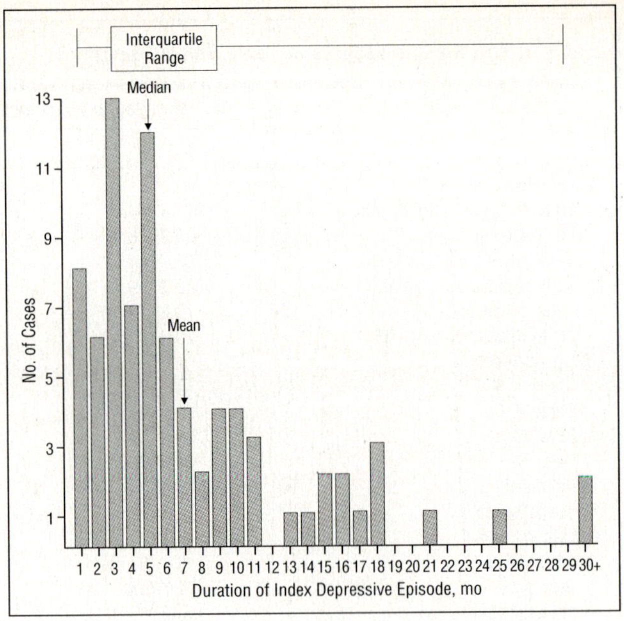

Histogram and box plot of the duration of the depressive episodes of 83 subjects.

Although the number of cases was too small for analysis, it is noteworthy that seven of the 83 persons were hospitalized at the time of study. Recomputing analysis 1 omitting these persons did not produce any appreciable change in the findings. Moreover, since hospitalized individuals scored at the poor end of the HAM-D and Global Assessment Scale (GAS), hospitalization per se reflected severity of illness, and multiple measures of illness severity were included in the multivariate analyses.

In sum, among the 83 depressed subjects, a unidimensional sleep profile emerged in which the quality of subjects' sleep ranged from poor (across multiple indices) to better. This continuum of sleep was, in turn, significantly associated with a set of predictors that included episode duration as well as other characteristics of subjects' depressive history and current status.

Analysis 2: Effects of Episode Duration in the Context of Psychosocial Characteristics

A single canonical correlation accounted for the linkage between the set of sleep variables and the set of episode duration plus psychosocial variables. This correlation of .62 explained 38.5% of the variability between variable sets ($F[72, 403]=1.35$, $P=.04$). After removal of the first pair of canonical variates, insignificant shared variability remained ($F[56, 361]=1.07$, $P=.36$). The first pair of canonical variates, therefore, accounted for the significant relationships between the two sets of variables.

The second column of Table 3 lists loadings of the

Table 2. Depressive History and Psychosocial Characteristics of Depressed Subjects as a Function of Duration of Current Depressive Episode*

	Duration of Major Depressive Episode		
	≤4 mo (n=34)	>4 mo (n=49)	Test Statistic†
Depression History Variables‡			
Age at first episode, y §	47.3 (16.6)	45.9 (18.1)	0.36
No. of past episodes §‖	4.7 (2.4)	5.2 (4.5)	0.09
≥3 past hospitalizations, % (No.)	15 (5)	10 (5)	0.39
Lifetime comorbidity with any other RDC disorder, % (No.) ¶	26 (9)	12 (6)	2.74
Remission prior to current episode, wk §‖	63.3 (46.4)	53.8 (43.9)	1.01
Symptom severity, current episode §#	21.9 (3.8)	22.4 (3.8)	0.57
Functional severity, current episode §‖#	56.3 (4.9)	57.2 (5.0)	0.86
Current episode RDC endogenous, % (No.)	47 (16)	61 (30)	1.63
Current episode RDC agitated, % (No.)	12 (4)	10 (5)	0.50
Current episode RDC retarded, % (No.)	12 (4)	16 (8)	0.34
Psychosocial Variables‡			
Current age, y §	67.7 (5.6)	66.0 (6.3)	1.27
Male, % (No.)	26 (9)	27 (13)	0.02
Level of education, y §	12.1 (2.3)	12.5 (2.2)	0.98
Chronic medical burden severity index §#	1.6 (0.4)	1.6 (0.4)	0.00
Occurrence of major life stressor prior to episode onset, % (No.)	32 (11)	41 (20)	0.61
High perceived chronic stress, % (No.) #	38 (13)	27 (13)	1.28
High level of social support, % (No.) #	62 (21)	67 (33)	0.28

**RDC indicates Research Diagnostic Criteria.*

†t test for continuous variables, χ^2 test for dichotomous variables. None of the test statistic values was significant, and all reflected small to modest effect sizes (point biserial r or ϕ value <.20).

‡Determined using the Schedule for Affective Disorders and Schizophrenia–Lifetime Version, unless otherwise indicated.

§Values are mean (SD).

‖Logarithmic transformation was performed before the t test was computed.

¶Lifetime disorders in the sample included panic disorder (n=1), generalized anxiety disorder (n=5), phobia (n=3), alcoholism (n=7), and other substance abuse (n=2). Cases in these categories are not mutually exclusive. Diagnoses concurrent with the present episode of depression were panic disorder (n=1), phobia (n=2), and intermittent depression (n=5). The small numbers of cases of specific past or current RDC diagnoses precluded consideration of individual diagnoses in the analyses.

#Symptom severity was assessed with the Hamilton Rating Scale for Depression,[36] functional severity with the Global Assessment Scale,[44] chronic medical burden with the Cumulative Illness Rating Scale,[45] perceived chronic stress with the Perceived Stress Scale,[46] and social support with the Interpersonal Support Evaluation List.[47] See the "Methods" section for further details.

sleep variables on their canonical variate from analysis 2 and loadings of the psychosocial variable set on their canonical variate. Similar to analysis 1, the majority of the sleep indices load on a single underlying dimension, and that dimension is best described as representing a continuum of poor to better sleep.

The predictors that were most strongly related to their canonical variate (indicating their relative importance to sleep) included, again, episode duration (loading=.39). Several psychosocial variables were also important correlates of sleep profile: depressed persons with poorer sleep were currently older (.40), more likely to be male (.63), and less educated (−.40). They also had higher chronic medical burden (.32), had lower social support (−.23), and were more likely to have experienced a major life stressor that contributed to episode onset (.30).

In sum, a unidimensional sleep profile, representing a continuum of poor to better sleep, emerged relative to the set of psychosocial variables (plus episode duration) included in analysis 2. Episode duration remained associated with poorer sleep. Several psychosocial variables themselves were also related to sleep among the depressed subjects.

COMMENT

The present study explored the contributions of multiple clinical and psychosocial variables to the EEG sleep profile in depressed elders, focusing on the role played by duration of depressive episode. Episode duration was strongly associated with diverse sleep measures: persons who were relatively early in their episode evinced the poorest sleep profile, followed by later-episode subjects, who in turn showed greater sleep impairment than nondepressed controls. This pattern was pronounced not only for REM measures but also for non-REM sleep and sleep continuity measures. The pattern held for both visual and computer-derived (automated) measures.

These findings are important on two counts. First, from a methodologic perspective, we documented these effects beyond a piecemeal, univariate examination of episode duration–sleep variable differences by performing multivariate analyses of the impact of duration on a complete ensemble of EEG measures. Second, the very fact that a constellation of sleep measures—extending well beyond REM latency—was associated with duration provides direct evidence that REM latency, particularly dur-

Table 3. Relationships Between Sleep Variables and Predictor Variables Among Depressed Subjects*

	First Canonical Variate Loading	
	Analysis 1	Analysis 2
Sleep Variable Set		
Sleep latency	.47	.05
Time spent asleep	−.06	−.06
Sleep efficiency	−.61	−.32
Stage 1 sleep %	.45	.66
Delta sleep %	−.31	−.69
REM latency	−.35	−.26
REM density	.44	.30
REM counts/min, period 1	.20	.07
REM ratio	.32	.20
Analysis 1: Predictor Set		
Shorter duration of current episode	.50	
Depression history		
Age at first episode	−.33	
No. of past episodes	.26	
No. of past hospitalizations	.50	
Lifetime comorbidity with other RDC disorder	−.18	
Duration of remission prior to current episode	.19	
HAM-D, current episode	.25	
GAS, current episode	.27	
Current endogenous depression	.35	
Current agitated depression†	.33	
Canonical correlation, analysis 1	.63‡	
Analysis 2: Predictor Set		
Shorter duration of current episode		.39
Psychosocial characteristics		
Current age		.40
Male		.63
Level of education		−.40
Chronic medical burden		.32
Occurrence of major life stressor		.30
Perceived chronic stress		.03
Level of social support		−.23
Canonical correlation, analysis 2		.62‡

*REM indicates rapid eye movement; HAM-D, Hamilton Rating Scale for Depression; and GAS, Global Assessment Scale.

†Because Research Diagnostic Criteria agitated major depression and retarded major depression are mutually exclusive, they were combined to create an ordinal variable with three levels (agitated, neither, or retarded) for these analyses.

‡$P<.05$.

ing depression, should not be conceptually divorced or studied in isolation from other aspects of sleep physiology.[8,54,55] Evidence that these elements reflected a single underlying continuum ranging from "good" to "poor" sleep also empirically supports others' conclusions regarding a basic unidimensionality underlying diverse sleep indices that appears to hold across the life span.[56]

To our knowledge, ours is the first analysis of the effects of duration of depression on sleep in older adults. In earlier work in a middle-aged cohort, similar effects on REM sleep were found,[17,20] but the possibility could not be eliminated that these effects were caused by greater cumulative depressive illness rather than by episode duration per se. We disentangled these effects, although our cross-sectional between-subjects study design leaves open the possibility that the observed episode duration–sleep relationship could be caused by other unmeasured differences between early- and late-episode subjects. For example, individuals who enroll in a treatment study later in their depression may be in some way less severely ill or may have more psychosocial supports available than individuals who enroll earlier in their depression; both categories of variables are known to influence treatment seeking.[57,58] However, the fact that earlier- and later-episode subjects in the present study did not differ on a wide array of such clinical and psychosocial variables helps to limit the impact of this possibility. Clearly, the strongest design for addressing the episode duration–EEG sleep relationship would be to longitudinally study a cohort of persons with untreated depression to examine the EEG sleep profile across a single episode of illness. This would also allow examination of intraepisode changes—eg, individuals' habituation to or compensation for symptoms—that might contribute to duration-related patterns of EEG sleep. However, application of this design would be difficult, given the ethical priority to offer treatment as soon as an episode is recognized.

It is also noteworthy that our findings regarding duration effects, like those obtained previously,[17,20] pertain to individuals with recurrent unipolar, nondelusional disease. It is not known whether such effects can be generalized to incident cases of unipolar depression or other forms of depressive illness.

Given these caveats, what mechanism might be responsible for greater perturbations of EEG sleep earlier in an elder's depressive episode? Concerning the effects on REM sleep, it has been suggested that REM changes reflect or covary with other biological abnormalities that may be more pronounced early in an episode.[17] Such abnormalities include corticotropin-releasing factor/hypothalamic-pituitary-adrenal axis alterations as well as core body temperature and motor activity rhythms.[30,59,60] Concerning non-REM and sleep continuity alterations, the effects we observed were not evident in the middle-aged cohort studied previously.[17] However, in the same way that aging appears to magnify the strength of the association of depressive illness with these components of sleep,[1,10,61,62] perhaps aging ultimately reveals the effects of episode duration on these components—effects that are less visible earlier in the life span.

Beyond the impact of episode duration, we found that both clinical and psychosocial factors were associated with EEG sleep profiles. Subjects who were more severely ill during their current episode and who met criteria for endogenous and/or agitated depression showed a more impaired sleep profile. Moreover, subjects who had a longer, more severe history of depressive illness had poorer sleep during their episode. Since persons with recurrent depression often manifest EEG abnormalities even during remission from acute illness,[7] these associations with current sleep profile may reflect permanent biological scarring, ie, residual impairment in sleep physiologic characteristics produced by illness chronicity. Alternatively, EEG sleep may itself represent a premorbid vulnerability factor for recurrent depression.[63,64]

Regarding psychosocial factors, depressed subjects

with the poorest sleep were older and more likely to be male—correlates observed previously in healthy, nondepressed samples.[3,32] Of particular significance, those with poorer sleep profiles had fewer psychosocial assets: they were less educated, carried a greater chronic medical burden, and experienced less social support. Finally, while perceived chronic stress was not highly related to sleep profile (perhaps because of the inadequacy of only a brief self-report measure of such strain[65]), the occurrence of acute life stressors prior to episode onset was strongly related to poorer sleep. These findings provide further evidence of the pathogenic role of certain environmental factors in the EEG sleep profile.[3]

In sum, our findings of the effects of not only episode duration but also a variety of other clinical and psychosocial variables on the EEG sleep profile suggest the importance of building multifactorial models of sleep disturbance, particularly in the context of depression.[28,30] The strength of the observed effects demands more extended consideration and replication in other cohorts. Determination of why episode duration influences sleep requires particular attention. At the very least, however, our data suggest issues important for interventions with older adults who are depressed. For example, should persons whose depression is identified relatively early receive treatment with a heavier focus on alleviating sleep abnormalities, compared with the treatment offered to—or most beneficial for—individuals who have been depressed for more extended periods? In addition, to what extent can improvements in sleep be achieved by targeting interventions not only to the depression per se but also to other characteristics of individuals' personal and psychosocial environments?

Accepted for publication July 19, 1995.

This research was supported in part by grant AG-06836 from the National Institute on Aging, Bethesda, Md; by grants MH37869, MH00295, MH30915, and MH43832 from the National Institute of Mental Health, Rockville, Md; and by a grant from the John D. and Catherine T. MacArthur Foundation Mental Health Research Network on the Psychobiology of Depression and Other Affective Disorders, Chicago, Ill.

Correspondence to Department of Psychiatry, University of Pittsburgh School of Medicine, 3811 O'Hara St, Pittsburgh, PA 15213 (Dr Dew).

REFERENCES

1. Ford DE, Kamerow DB. Epidemiologic study of sleep disturbances and psychiatric disorders: an opportunity for prevention? *JAMA.* 1989;262:1479-1488.
2. Buysse DJ, Reynolds CF, Monk TH, Hoch CC, Yeager AL, Kupfer DJ. Quantification of subjective sleep quality in healthy elderly men and women using the Pittsburgh Sleep Quality Index (PSQI). *Sleep.* 1991;14:331-338.
3. Dew MA, Reynolds CF, Monk TH, Buysse DJ, Hoch CC, Jennings JR, Kupfer DJ. Psychosocial correlates and sequelae of electroencephalographic sleep in healthy elders. *J Gerontol.* 1994;49:8-18.
4. Rodin J, McAvay G, Timko C. A longitudinal study of depressed mood and sleep disturbances in elderly adults. *J Gerontol.* 1988;43:45-53.
5. Reynolds CF, Kupfer DJ. Sleep research in affective illness: state of the art circa 1987. *Sleep.* 1987;10:199-215.
6. Hoch CC, Buysse DJ, Reynolds CF. Sleep and depression in late life. *Clin Geriatr Med.* 1989;5:259-274.
7. Kupfer DJ, Ehlers CL. Two roads to rapid eye movement latency. *Arch Gen Psychiatry.* 1989;46:945-948.
8. Gillin JC, Borbely AA. Sleep: a neurobiological window in affective disorders. *Trends Neurosci.* 1985;8:537-542.
9. Knowles JB, MacLean AW. Age-related changes in sleep in depressed and healthy subjects: a meta-analysis. *Neuropsychopharmacology.* 1990;3:251-259.
10. National Institutes of Health. *Consensus Development Conference on the Treatment of Sleep Disorders in Older People.* Bethesda, Md: National Institutes of Health; 1990;8. No. 3.
11. National Institutes of Health Consensus Development Panel on Depression in Late Life. Diagnosis and treatment of depression in late life. *JAMA.* 1992;268:1018-1024.
12. Webb WB. Age-related changes in sleep. *Clin Geriatr Med.* 1989;5:275-287.
13. Benca RM, Obermeyer WH, Thisted RA, Gillin JC. Sleep and psychiatric disorders: a meta-analysis. *Arch Gen Psychiatry.* 1992;49:651-668.
14. Buysse DJ, Kupfer DJ. Diagnostic and research applications of electroencephalographic sleep studies in depression: conceptual and methodologic issues. *J Nerv Ment Dis.* 1990;178:405-414.
15. Vitiello MV, Prinz PN, Avery DH, Williams DE, Ries RK, Bokan JA, Khan A. Sleep is undisturbed in elderly, depressed individuals who have not sought health care. *Biol Psychiatry.* 1990;27:431-440.
16. Kupfer DJ, Reynolds CF, Grochocinski VJ, Ulrich RF, McEachran AB. Aspects of short REM latency in affective states: a revisit. *Psychiatry Res.* 1986;17:49-59.
17. Kupfer DJ, Ehlers CL Frank E, Grochocinski VJ, McEachran AB. EEG sleep profiles and recurrent depression. *Biol Psychiatry.* 1991;30:641-655.
18. Ansseau M, Kupfer DJ, Reynolds CF, McEachran AB. REM latency distribution in major depression: clinical characteristics associated with sleep onset REM periods. *Biol Psychiatry.* 1984;19:1651-1666.
19. Spiker DG, Coble P, Cofsky J, Foster FG, Kupfer DJ. EEG sleep and severity of depression. *Biol Psychiatry.* 1978;13:485-488.
20. Kupfer DJ, Frank E, Grochocinski VJ, Gregor M, McEachran AB. Electroencephalographic sleep profiles in recurrent depression. *Arch Gen Psychiatry.* 1988;45:678-681.
21. Reynolds CF, Kupfer DJ, Houck PR, Hoch CC, Stack JA, Berman SR, Zimmer B. Reliable discrimination of elderly depressed and demented patients by electroencephalographic sleep data. *Arch Gen Psychiatry.* 1988;45:258-264.
22. Regier DA, Hirschfeld R, Goodwin FK, Burke J, Lazar J, Judd LL. The NIMH Depression/Awareness, Recognition, and Treatment Program: structure, aims and scientific basis. *Am J Psychiatry.* 1988;145:1351-1357.
23. Kupfer DJ, Frank E, Perel JM. The advantage of early treatment intervention in recurrent depression. *Arch Gen Psychiatry.* 1989;46:771-775.
24. Reynolds CF, Frank E, Perel JM, Miller MD, Cornes C, Rifai AH, Pollock BG, Mazumdar S, George CJ, Houck PR, Kupfer DJ. Treatment of consecutive episodes of major depression in the elderly. *Am J Psychiatry.* 1994;151:1740-1743.
25. Hochli D, Riemann D, Zulley J, Berger M. Initial REM sleep suppression by clomipramine: a prognostic tool for treatment response in patients with a major depressive disorder. *Biol Psychiatry.* 1986;21:1217-1220.
26. Gillin JC, Wyatt RJ, Fram D, Snyder F. The relationship between changes in REM sleep and clinical improvement in depressed patients treated with amitriptyline. *Psychopharmacology.* 1978;59:267-272.
27. Kupfer DJ, Shipley JE, Perel JM, Pollack B, Coble PA, Spiker DG. Antidepressants and EEG sleep: search for specificity. In: Dahl SG, Gram LF, Paul SM, Potter WZ, eds. *Clinical Pharmacology in Psychiatry: Selectivity in Psychotropic Drug Action: Promises or Problems?* New York, NY: Springer-Verlag NY Inc; 1987:167-173.
28. Reynolds CF, Dew MA, Monk TH, Hoch CC. Sleep disorders in late life: a biopsychosocial model for understanding pathogenesis and intervention. In: Coffey CE, Cummings JL, eds. *Textbook of Geriatric Psychiatry.* Washington, DC: American Psychiatric Association Press; 1994:323-331.
29. Reynolds CF, Hoch CC, Buysse DJ, Houck PR, Schlernitzauer M, Pasternak RE, Frank E, Mazumdar S, Kupfer DJ. Sleep after spousal bereavement: a study of recovery from stress. *Biol Psychiatry.* 1993;34:791-797.
30. Kupfer DJ. Maintenance treatment in recurrent depression: current and future directions. *Br J Psychiatry.* 1992;161:309-316.
31. Miller MD, Paradis CF, Houck PR, Mazumdar S, Stack JA, Rifai AH, Mulsant B, Reynolds CF. Rating chronic medical illness burden in geropsychiatric practice and research: application of the Cumulative Illness Rating Scale. *Psychiatry Res.* 1992;41:237-248.
32. Reynolds CF, Monk TH, Hoch CC, Jennings JR, Buysse DJ, Houck PR, Jarrett DB, Kupfer DJ. Electroencephalographic sleep in the healthy 'old old': a comparison with the 'young old' in visually scored and automated measures. *J Gerontol.* 1991;46:39-46.

33. Reynolds CF, Frank E, Perel JM, Imber SD, Cornes C, Morycz RK, Mazumdar S, Miller MD, Pollock BG, Rifai AH, Stack JA, George CJ, Houck PR, Kupfer DJ. Combined pharmacotherapy and psychotherapy in the acute and continuation treatment of elderly patients with recurrent major depression: a preliminary report. *Am J Psychiatry.* 1992;149:1687-1692.
34. Spitzer RL Endicott J, Robins E. Research Diagnostic Criteria: rationale and reliability. *Arch Gen Psychiatry.* 1978;35:773-782.
35. Endicott J, Spitzer RL. A diagnostic interview: the Schedule for Affective Disorders and Schizophrenia. *Arch Gen Psychiatry.* 1978;35:837-844.
36. Hamilton M. Development of a rating scale for primary depressive illness. *Br J Soc Clin Psychol.* 1967;6:278-296.
37. Stack JA, Paradis CF, Reynolds CF, Houck PR, Frank E, Anderson B, Mayo AL, Miller MD, Rifai AH, Perel JM, Kupfer DJ. Does recruitment method make a difference? effects on protocol retention and treatment outcome in elderly depressed patients. *Psychiatry Res.* 1995;56:17-24.
38. Folstein MF, Folstein SE, McHugh PR. Mini-Mental State: a practical method for grading the cognitive state of patients for the clinician. *J Psychiatr Res.* 1975;12:189-198.
39. Reynolds CF, Grochocinski VJ, Monk TH, Buysse DJ, Giles DE, Coble PA, Matzzie JV, Doman J, Monahan J, Kupfer DJ. Concordance between habitual sleep times and laboratory recording schedules. *Sleep.* 1992;15:571-575.
40. Rechtschaffen A, Kales A. *A Manual of Standardized Terminology, Techniques, and Scoring System for Sleep Stages of Human Subjects.* Washington, DC: US Dept of Health, Education, and Welfare; 1965. National Institutes of Health publication 204.
41. Campbell PI, Reynolds CF, Berman SR, Hoch CC, Stack JA, Houck PR. Assessment of sleep fragmentation in the elderly: a reliability study. *Sleep Res.* 1987;16:547.
42. Kupfer DJ, Frank E, McEachran AB, Grochocinski VJ. Delta sleep ratio: a biological correlate of early recurrence in unipolar affective disorder. *Arch Gen Psychiatry.* 1990;47:1100-1105.
43. Tukey JW. *Exploratory Data Analysis.* Reading, Mass: Addison-Wesley Publishing Co; 1977.
44. Endicott J, Spitzer RL, Fleiss JL, Cohen J. The Global Assessment Scale: a procedure for measuring overall severity of psychiatric disturbance. *Arch Gen Psychiatry.* 1976;33:766-771.
45. Linn BS, Linn BW, Gurel L. Cumulative Illness Rating Scale. *J Am Geriatr Soc.* 1968;16:622-626.
46. Cohen S, Kamarck T, Mermelstein R. A global measure of perceived stress. *J Health Soc Behav.* 1983;24:385-396.
47. Cohen S, Mermelstein R, Kamarck T, Hoberman HM. Measuring the functional components of social support. In: Sarason IG, Sarason B, eds. *Social Support: Theory, Research and Applications.* The Hague, the Netherlands: Martinus Nijhoff Publishers; 1985:73-94.
48. Williamson GM, Schulz R. Relationship orientation, quality of prior relationship, and distress among caregivers of Alzheimer's patients. *Psychol Aging.* 1990;5:502-510.
49. Rosenthal R, Rosnow RL *Contrast Analysis: Focused Comparisons in the Analysis of Variance.* New York, NY: Cambridge University Press; 1985.
50. Tabachnick BG, Fidell LS. *Using Multivanate Statistics.* 2nd ed. New York, NY: Harper & Row; 1989.
51. Levine MS. *Canonical Analysis and Factor Comparison.* Beverly Hills, Calif: Sage Publications Inc; 1977.
52. Cohen J. *Statistical Power Analysis for the Behavioral Sciences.* 2nd ed. Hillsdale, NJ: Lawrence Erlbaum Associates Inc Publishers; 1983.
53. Gorsuch RL. *Factor Analysis.* 2nd ed. Hillsdale, NJ: Lawrence Erlbaum Associates Inc Publishers; 1983.
54. Feinberg I, Floyd TC. The regulation of human sleep: clues from its phenomenology. *Hum Neurobiol.* 1982;1:185-194.
55. Kupfer DJ, Reynolds CF. Sleep and psychiatric disorder: a meta-analysis. *Arch Gen Psychiatry.* 1992;49:669-670.
56. Hudson JI, Pope HG, Sullivan LE, Waternaux CM, Keck PE, Broughton RJ. Good sleep, bad sleep: a meta-analysis of polysomnographic measures in insomnia, depression, and narcolepsy. *Biol Psychiatry.* 1992;32:958-975.
57. Dew MA, Bromet EJ, Schulberg HC, Parkinson DK, Curtis EC. Factors affecting service utilization for depression in a white collar population. *Soc Psychiatry Psychiatr Epidemiol.* 1991;26:230-237.
58. Dew MA, Dunn LO, Bromet EJ, Schulberg HC. Factors affecting help-seeking during depression in a community sample. *J Affect Disord.* 1988;14:223-234.
59. Borbely AA. The S-deficiency hypothesis of depression and the two-process model of sleep regulation. *Pharmacopsychiatria.* 1987;20:23-29.
60. Ehlers CL Kupfer DJ. Hypothalamic peptide modulation of EEG sleep in depression: a further application of the S-process hypothesis. *Biol Psychiatry.* 1987;22:513-517.
61. Borbely AA. A two-process model of sleep regulation. *Hum Neurobiol.* 1982; 1:195-204.
62. Reynolds CF, Hoch CC, Buysse DJ, George CJ, Houck PR, Mazumdar S, Miller M, Pollock BG, Rifai AH, Frank E, Cornes C, Morycz RK, Kupfer DJ. Sleep in late-life recurrent depression: changes during early continuation therapy with nortriptyline. *Neuropsychopharmacology.* 1991;5:85-96.
63. Giles DE, Biggs MM, Ruch AJ, Roffwarg HP. Risk factors in families of unipolar depression, I: incidence of illness and reduced REM latency. *J Affect Disord.* 1988;14:51-59.
64. Giles DE, Etzel BA, Reynolds CF, Kupfer DJ. Stability of polysomnographic parameters in unipolar depression: a cross-sectional report. *Biol Psychiatry.* 1989; 25:807-810.
65. Turner RJ, Wheaton B, Lloyd DA. The epidemiology of social stress. *Am Sociol Rev.* 1995:60:104-125.

Agoraphobia, Simple Phobia, and Social Phobia in the National Comorbidity Survey

William J. Magee, PhD; William W. Eaton, PhD; Hans-Ulrich Wittchen, PhD; Katherine A. McGonagle, PhD; Ronald C. Kessler, PhD

Background: Data are presented on the general population prevalences, correlates, comorbidities, and impairments associated with *DSM-III-R* phobias.

Methods: Analysis is based on the National Comorbidity Survey. Phobias were assessed with a revised version of the Composite International Diagnostic Interview.

Results: Lifetime (and 30-day) prevalence estimates are 6.7% (and 2.3%) for agoraphobia, 11.3% (and 5.5%) for simple phobia, and 13.3% (and 4.5%) for social phobia. Increasing lifetime prevalences are found in recent cohorts. Earlier median ages at illness onset are found for simple (15 years of age) and social (16 years of age) phobias than for agoraphobia (29 years of age). Phobias are highly comorbid. Most comorbid simple and social phobias are temporally primary, while most comorbid agoraphobia is temporally secondary. Comorbid phobias are generally more severe than pure phobias. Despite evidence of role impairment in phobia, only a minority of individuals with phobia ever seek professional treatment.

Conclusions: Phobias are common, increasingly prevalent, often associated with serious role impairment, and usually go untreated. Focused research is needed to investigate barriers to help seeking.

(Arch Gen Psychiatry. 1996;53:159-168)

THIS ARTICLE presents nationally representative data on the general population descriptive epidemiology of *DSM-III-R* agoraphobia (with or without panic), social phobia, and simple phobia from the National Comorbidity Survey (NCS).[1] The focus is on prevalence, sociodemographic correlates, comorbidity, impairment, and professional help seeking.

RESULTS

PREVALENCE

Lifetime and 30-day prevalence estimates are presented in **Table 1**. As reported previously,[1] lifetime prevalence estimates are 6.7% for agoraphobia, 11.3% for simple phobia, and 13.3% for social phobia. The prevalence estimates for agoraphobia and simple phobia are over twice as high among women as among men, with female-male prevalence ratios of 2.2:1.0 for agoraphobia ($z = 5.7$, $P<.05$) and 2.3:1.0 for simple phobia ($z = 7.4$, $P<.05$). The female-male prevalence ratio for social phobia is considerably lower (1.4:1.0), although still statistically significant ($z = 3.4$, $P<.05$).

Lifetime prevalence estimates generally decline with age, as shown in Table 1, suggesting the possible existence of cohort effects. Analysis of age-at-onset curves, shown in **Figure 1**, **Figure 2**, and **Figure 3**, documents that these cohort differences are significant for all three phobias and most pronounced for agoraphobia. Despite the apparent sex difference in the age effect in Table 1, none of the cohort effects in the Figures 1 through 3 differs significantly by sex. Intercohort differences emerge quite early in life for agoraphobia and, while most pronounced for the difference between the most recent (ages 15 to 24 years at interview) vs earlier (ages 25 to 54 years at interview) cohorts, are also shown in Figure 1 to be statistically significant within the three later cohorts. Intercohort differences in simple and social phobias are con-

See Methods on next page

From the Department of Psychiatry, The University of Wisconsin, Madison (Dr Magee); the Department of Mental Hygiene, The Johns Hopkins University, Baltimore, Md (Dr Eaton); the Department of Clinical Psychology, The Max Planck Institute of Psychiatry–Clinical Institute, Munich, Germany (Dr Wittchen); and the Institute for Social Research (Drs McGonagle and Kessler) and the Department of Sociology (Dr Kessler), The University of Michigan, Ann Arbor.

METHODS

SAMPLE

As described in more detail in previous articles published in the ARCHIVES,[1-3] the NCS was administered to a stratified, multistage area probability sample of 8098 respondents (age range, 15 to 54 years) selected from the noninstitutionalized household population of the coterminous United States and to a supplemental sample of students in campus group housing. The survey was fielded between September 1990 and March 1992. The response rate was 82.4%. The data were weighted for differential probabilities of selection and differential nonresponse and to adjust the sample to approximate the cross-classification of the population distribution on a range of sociodemographic characteristics. These weights are described in more detail elsewhere.[1]

DIAGNOSTIC ASSESSMENT

The NCS diagnoses are based on a modified version of the World Health Organization's Composite International Diagnostic Interview (WHO-CIDI),[4] a structured interview designed to be administered by trained interviewers who are not clinicians. Phobias were assessed by asking respondents whether there was ever a time in their life when any of 19 potentially phobic situations always made them so afraid that they either tried to avoid it or felt very uncomfortable in the situation. These situational descriptors were presented in three lists (five situations for agoraphobia, eight for simple phobia, and six for social phobia). The main change in the version of the CIDI developed at The University of Michigan, Ann Arbor, for the NCS (UM-CIDI) was that respondents were asked to review these lists visually as the interviewer read the stem questions in an effort to focus memory search and reduce chances of inducing the "no" response set that has been documented to occur when "yes-no" questions are presented in lists of this sort.[5]

Respondents who endorsed one or more situational descriptors were then administered the structured CIDI questions that assessed *DSM-III-R* criteria for agoraphobia (with or without panic), simple phobia, or social phobia. Short-term test-retest reliabilities of the diagnoses generated from these structured questions were assessed in the WHO-CIDI Field Trials. Values of κ were .68 for agoraphobia, .59 for simple phobia, and .64 for social phobia.[6] Although disorder-specific validity estimates have not been reported, a comparison of CIDI diagnoses and clinical diagnoses made by one of two psychiatrists in the CIDI Field Trials documented good concordance ($\kappa = .76$) for the anxiety and phobic disorders as a whole.[6] The psychiatrists in this concordance study were either observers of the CIDI interviews or, on a small number of occasions, administered the CIDI. The psychiatrists were then allowed to ask whatever additional questions they wished to complete a *DSM-III-R* criteria checklist as the basis for clinical diagnoses.

ANALYSIS PROCEDURES

Estimates of disorder prevalences, professional help seeking, and proportions of cases with impairment were obtained by calculating means for dichotomous outcomes using the PSRATIO program in the OSIRIS software package.[7] Age-at-onset curves were calculated using the SURVIVAL procedure in the SPSS software package.[8] Cross-sectional estimates of sociodemographic correlates and bivariate comorbidities were obtained by estimating odds ratios (ORs) based on logistic regression models with dichotomous predictor variables using the LOGISTIC procedure in the SAS software package.[9]

Owing to the complex sample design and weighting of the NCS, special analysis procedures were required to obtain unbiased estimates of SEs of parameter estimates. The Taylor series linearization method[10] was used to adjust SEMs. The method of Balanced Repeated Replications,[11] operationalized in a SAS MACRO,[9] was used to adjust SEs of ORs. Odds ratios for bivariate models are reported below, with 95% confidence intervals (CIs) adjusted for design effects (ie, the effects of weighting and clustering of observations). All statistical tests were evaluated at the .05 level of significance, using two-tailed tests and design-based SEs.

fined to cases with disease onsets after age 16 years. While the cohort effect for social phobia in Figure 3 is largely owing to relatively early age at onset among the most recent cohort, intercohort differences are statistically significant both between the most recent and earlier cohorts and within the earlier cohorts. It is also noteworthy that simple and social phobias generally have earlier estimated ages at onset than agoraphobia, based on retrospective self-reports. Median ages at onset in the oldest cohort, where years of risk are greatest, are 15 years for simple phobia, 16 years for social phobia, and 29 years for agoraphobia.

Thirty-day prevalence estimates are 2.3% for agoraphobia, 5.5% for simple phobia, and 4.5% for social phobia. The estimates for agoraphobia and simple phobia are substantially higher among women than among men, with prevalence ratios of 2.2:1.0 for agoraphobia ($z = 3.4$, $P < .05$) and 3.8:1.0 for simple phobia ($z = 7.2$, $P < .05$). The female-male prevalence ratio for social phobia is much smaller (1.4:1.0), but still statistically significant ($z = 2.2$, $P < .05$). Age differences (which could also be interpreted as cohort differences) are generally not significant, although there is a fairly consistent trend for 30-day prevalence estimates to be highest in the youngest cohort.

SOCIODEMOGRAPHIC CORRELATES

Bivariate associations between sociodemographic variables and 30-day phobias are presented in **Table 2** as a way of providing descriptive information on the social distribution of phobias. Thirty-day agoraphobia is negatively related to income and education and is significantly elevated among blacks; homemakers; persons who are neither working, nor students, nor homemakers; and those who live with someone other than a spouse. Thirty-day simple phobia is negatively related to education but not income, and it is significantly elevated among Hispanics, all persons who are not employed (including stu-

Table 1. Lifetime and 30-Day Prevalences of Agoraphobia (With or Without Panic), Simple Phobia, and Social Phobia in the United States by Age and Sex

	Prevelance, % (SE)					
	Agoraphobia		Simple Phobia		Social Phobia	
Age Group, y	Lifetime	30-Day	Lifetime	30-Day	Lifetime	30-Day
Total sample						
15-24	7.7 (0.7)	3.0 (0.6)	10.8 (1.1)	6.2 (0.9)	14.9 (1.1)	7.3 (0.7)
25-34	6.3 (0.7)	2.3 (0.5)	11.9 (0.9)	5.2 (0.8)	13.8 (1.1)	4.4 (0.7)
35-44	5.3 (0.7)	1.9 (0.4)	11.9 (1.2)	5.4 (0.6)	12.1 (1.1)	3.2 (0.5)
45-54	5.8 (1.1)	1.7 (0.7)	10.0 (1.2)	5.1 (0.7)	12.2 (1.1)	2.9 (0.6)
Total	6.7 (0.4)	2.3 (0.3)	11.3 (0.6)	5.5 (0.5)	13.3 (0.7)	4.5 (0.4)
Men						
15-24	5.4 (1.0)	2.4 (0.7)	7.0 (1.3)	2.5 (0.9)	12.7 (1.4)	6.6 (1.1)
25-34	2.2 (0.6)	0.6 (0.3)	7.0 (0.7)	1.9 (0.5)	11.3 (1.4)	3.5 (0.6)
35-44	4.9 (1.0)	1.1 (0.2)	7.6 (1.2)	2.5 (0.5)	10.7 (1.6)	2.9 (0.6)
45-54	3.7 (1.1)	1.8 (0.9)	4.6 (1.0)	2.2 (0.7)	9.2 (1.2)	1.8 (0.5)
Total	4.1 (0.5)	1.4 (0.3)	6.7 (0.5)	2.3 (0.4)	11.1 (0.8)	3.8 (0.4)
Women						
15-24	10.2 (1.3)	3.7 (0.9)	14.9 (1.9)	10.3 (1.5)	17.3 (2.0)	8.1 (1.1)
25-34	9.8 (1.3)	3.8 (0.9)	16.0 (1.7)	8.1 (1.5)	16.0 (1.6)	5.2 (1.2)
35-44	7.7 (1.1)	2.7 (0.7)	16.3 (1.8)	8.4 (1.0)	13.6 (1.4)	3.4 (0.7)
45-54	8.0 (1.7)	1.6 (0.8)	15.7 (2.0)	8.1 (1.4)	15.3 (1.8)	4.0 (1.1)
Total	9.0 (0.7)	3.1 (0.4)	15.7 (1.1)	8.7 (0.8)	15.5 (1.0)	5.2 (0.5)

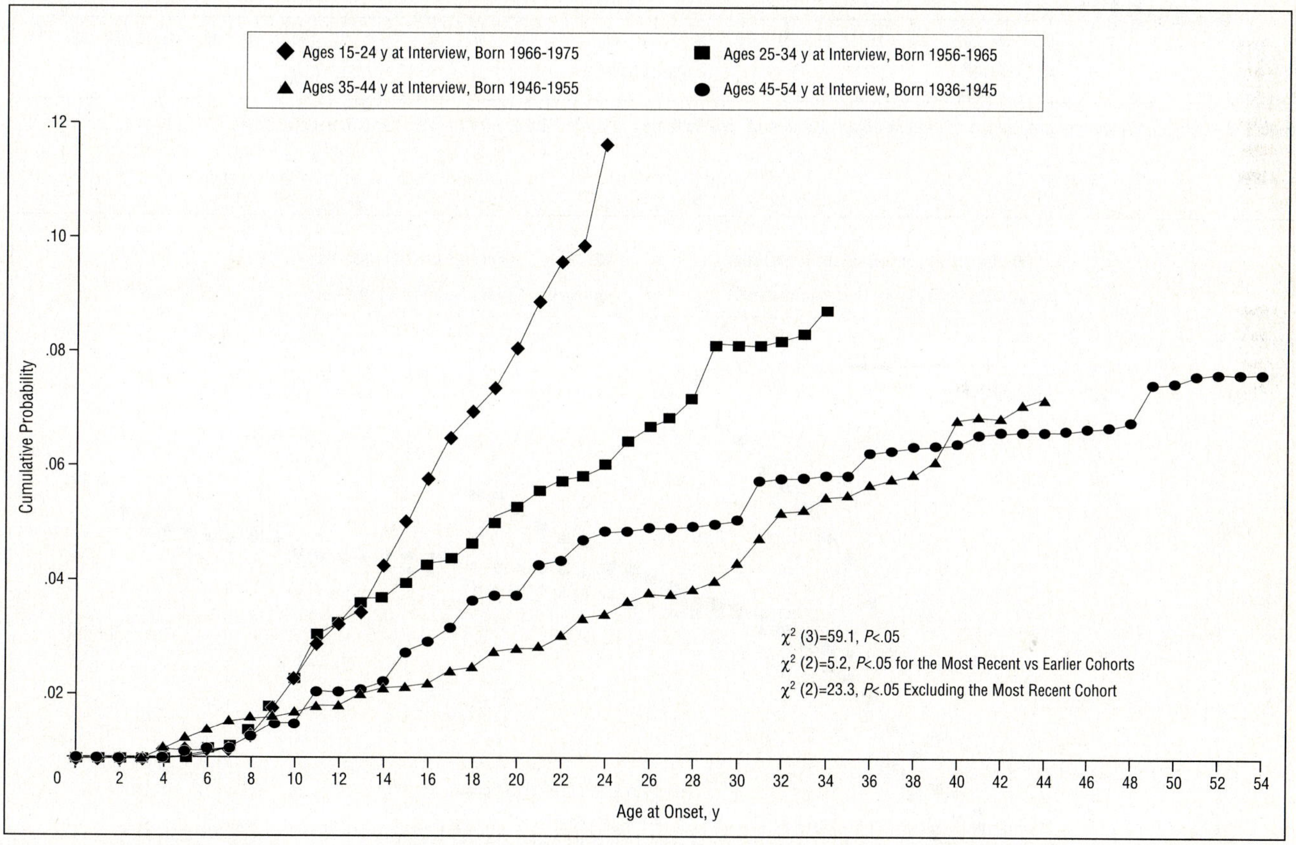

Figure 1. *Cumulative lifetime prevalence of agoraphobia by cohort. Numbers in parentheses indicate degrees of freedom.*

dents, homemakers, and others), and those who live with their parents. Thirty-day social phobia is negatively related to education and income and significantly elevated among the never married; students; persons who are neither working, nor students, nor homemakers; and those who live with their parents. None of the phobias is meaningfully associated with either region of the country or urbanicity. Multivariate relationships were also examined and found to be quite similar to those reported in Table 2. (The results of these and other analyses that

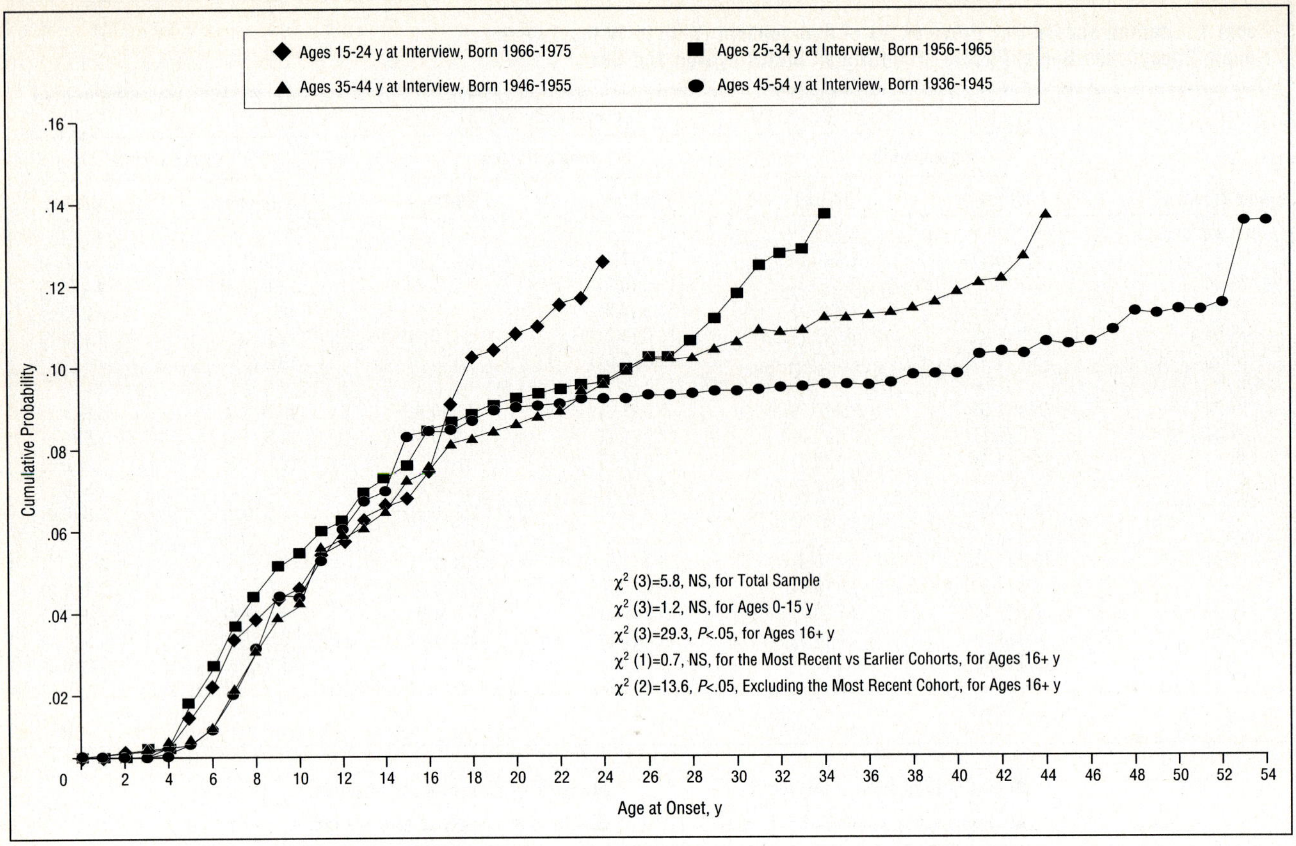

Figure 2. *Cumulative lifetime prevalence of simple phobia by cohort. NS indicates not significant; numbers in parentheses, degrees of freedom.*

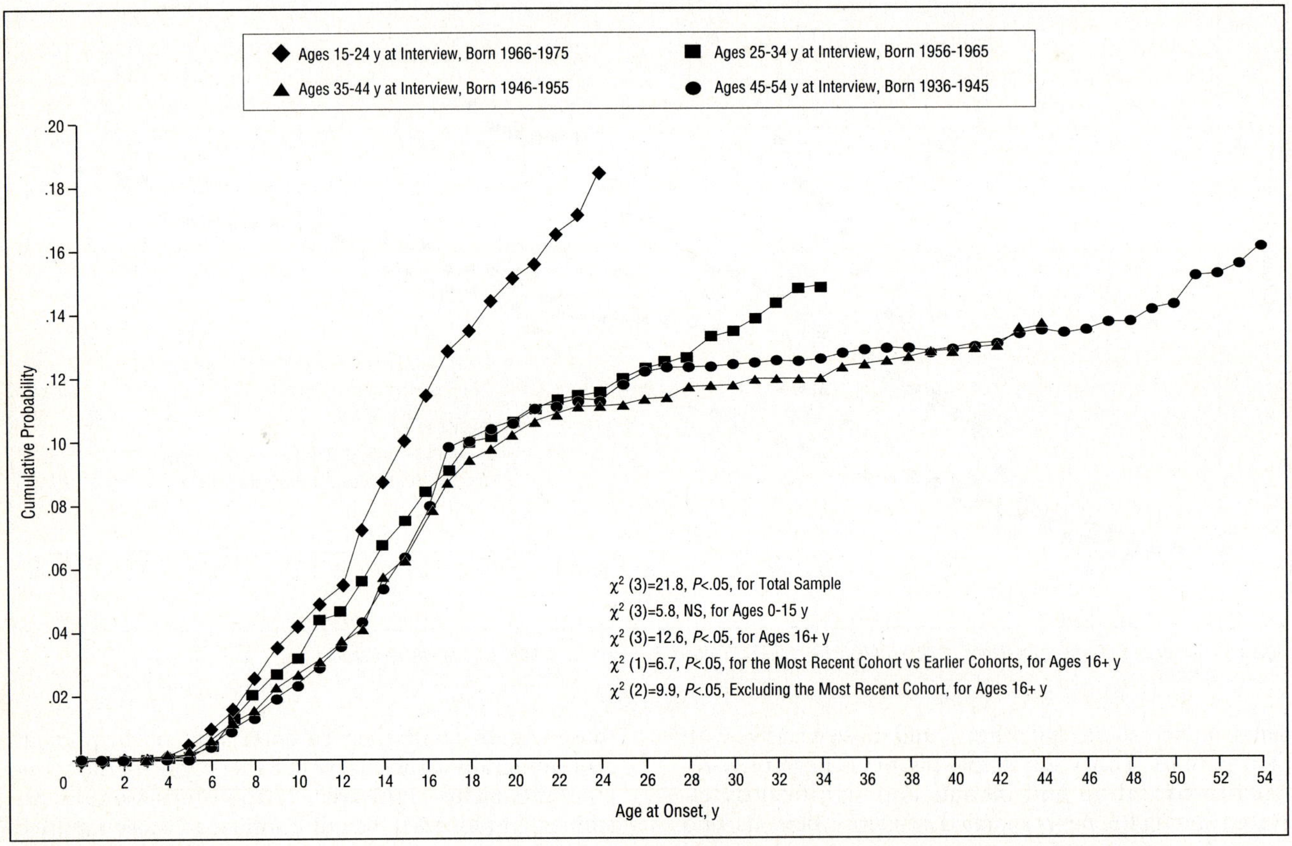

Figure 3. *Cumulative lifetime prevalence of social phobia by cohort. NS indicates not significant; numbers in parentheses, degrees of freedom.*

Table 2. Bivariate Associations of Sociodemographic Factors With Past-Month Phobias

Characteristics	OR (95% CI)*		
	Agoraphobia	Simple Phobia	Social Phobia
Race			
White	1.00 . . .	1.00 . . .	1.00 . . .
Black	1.97† (1.02-3.84)	1.33 (0.80-2.22)	0.79 (0.37-1.66)
Hispanic	1.35 (0.41-4.46)	1.83† (1.24-2.71)	1.04 (0.55-1.96)
Other	1.20 (0.00-99)	1.20 (0.54-2.67)	0.67 (0.19-2.42)
Education,‡ y			
0-11	8.99† (3.74-21.60)	3.14† (2.07-4.76)	3.03† (1.84-4.99)
12	4.94† (2.24-10.87)	2.06† (1.97-4.15)	1.71† (1.11-2.64)
13-15	2.70 (0.95-7.65)	1.87† (1.12-3.13)	1.90 (0.84-2.31)
16+	1.00 . . .	1.00 . . .	1.00 . . .
Income‡ ×$1000			
0-19	7.74† (3.70-16.19)	2.02† (1.16-3.50)	2.19† (1.40-3.43)
20-34	3.48† (1.54-7.91)	1.66 (0.93-2.96)	1.64† (1.01-2.66)
35-69	2.31† (1.20-4.43)	1.75 (0.97-3.16)	1.42 (0.91-2.21)
70+	1.00 . . .	1.00 . . .	1.00 . . .
Marital status			
Married/cohabiting	1.00 . . .	1.00 . . .	1.00 . . .
Separated/divorced/widowed	1.21 (0.56-2.65)	1.38 (0.86-2.22)	1.49 (0.92-2.42)
Never married	1.23 (0.71-2.16)	1.07 (0.72-1.58)	1.97† (1.50-2.69)
Employment			
Working	1.00 . . .	1.00 . . .	1.00 . . .
Student	1.93 (0.90-4.13)	1.49† (1.01-2.21)	2.48† (1.78-3.44)
Homemaker	2.90† (1.14-7.33)	2.48† (1.44-4.26)	1.32 (0.77-2.25)
Other	7.38† (3.42-15.91)	2.91† (1.66-5.07)	2.79† (1.80-4.32)
Household composition			
Live alone	1.00 . . .	1.00 . . .	1.00 . . .
Live with spouse	2.10 (0.93-4.74)	1.42† (1.01-2.00)	0.83 (0.45-1.52)
Live with other	2.58† (1.13-5.89)	1.30 (0.85-2.01)	1.15 (0.58-2.26)
Live with parents	3.08† (1.09-8.72)	2.41 (1.46-3.98)	1.88† (1.06-3.36)
Region			
Northeast	1.33 (0.59-3.04)	1.25 (0.83-1.91)	0.90 (0.55-1.47)
Midwest	1.06 (0.60-1.87)	0.95 (0.62-1.45)	0.79 (0.48-1.29)
South	1.00 . . .	1.00 . . .	1.00 . . .
West	0.82 (0.36-1.84)	1.06 (0.53-2.14)	0.84 (0.59-1.60)
Urbanicity			
Metropolitan	1.08 (0.65-1.81)	1.07 (0.66-1.72)	1.06 (0.68-1.64)
Other urban	1.01 (0.61-1.67)	1.16 (0.77-1.73)	1.00 (0.65-1.49)
Nonurban	1.00 . . .	1.00 . . .	1.00 . . .

**OR indicates odds ratio; CI, confidence interval.*
†Significant at the .05 level, two-tailed test.
‡Students excluded from education and income analyses.

are described in the text without the presentation of results can be obtained from the public-access Internet file described in the acknowledgments.) Correlates of 30-day prevalence among lifetime cases controlling for age at onset and time since onset were also examined and found to be largely nonsignificant, suggesting indirectly that the persistence of phobias is unrelated to these sociodemographic variables.

COMORBIDITY

As shown in **Table 3**, the vast majority of persons with phobia (87.6% of persons with agoraphobia, 83.4% of persons with simple phobia, and 81.0% of persons with social phobia) reported at least one other lifetime *DSM-III-R*/NCS disorder. These proportions are significantly higher than those found among the subsample of NCS respondents who reported never having a phobia, with bivariate ORs of 6.8 (agoraphobia), 5.3 (simple phobia), and 4.8 (social phobia). Disorder-specific ORs show that lifetime phobias are strongly comorbid with each other (OR range, 7.1 to 8.7), with other anxiety disorders (OR range, 2.7 to 11.9), and with affective disorders (OR range, 3.1 to 10.0). Phobias are more weakly comorbid with alcohol and drug dependence (OR range, 1.7 to 2.9), and they are not significantly comorbid with either alcohol or drug abuse without dependence (OR range, 0.9 to 1.2). The single largest OR in the data is between panic disorder and agoraphobia (11.9), a result observed because agoraphobia with panic and agoraphobia without panic were not distinguished in defining agoraphobia. There is also a very large OR between mania and simple phobia (10.0). It is noteworthy that only a minority (35.8%) of the respondents diagnosed in the UM-CIDI as having lifetime agoraphobia reported ever having an unexpected panic attack (including 21.6% with panic disorder and an additional 14.6% with panic attacks but not panic disorder) despite the high panic-agoraphobia OR.

Table 3. Percent of Subjects With Lifetime Phobia With Other Lifetime NCS/*DSM-III-R* Disorders and Bivariate ORs of Lifetime Comorbidity*

Other Disorder	Agoraphobia %	Agoraphobia OR (95% CI)	Simple Phobia %	Simple Phobia OR (95% CI)	Social Phobia %	Social Phobia OR (95% CI)
Affective						
Major depression	45.9	4.81† (3.65-6.35)	42.3	4.55† (3.63-5.70)	37.2	3.65† (2.98-4.46)
Dysthymia	16.0	3.14† (2.25-4.40)	15.8	3.42† (2.66-4.39)	14.6	3.15† (2.37-4.19)
Mania	8.6	7.89† (5.44-11.45)	8.0	10.05† (5.62-17.95)	5.1	4.60† (2.55-8.30)
Any affective	50.9	5.03† (3.90-6.50)	46.8	4.66† (3.79-5.73)	41.4	3.74† (3.14-4.45)
Anxiety						
Generalized anxiety disorder	19.8	5.80† (4.39-7.66)	16.0	4.87† (3.45-6.89)	13.3	3.77† (2.83-5.03)
Agoraphobia	...	...	27.0	8.67† (6.77-11.11)	23.3	7.06† (5.65-8.83)
Simple phobia	45.6	8.67† (6.77-11.11)	...	...	37.6	7.75† (6.35-9.48)
Social phobia	46.5	7.07† (5.65-8.83)	44.5	7.75† (6.35-9.48)	...	...
Panic disorder	21.6	11.88† (8.04-17.55)	14.8	7.87† (5.23-11.83)	10.9	4.83† (3.54-6.61)
Panic attacks‡	35.8	10.01† (7.55-13.28)	27.0	7.25† (5.29-9.95)	20.7	4.67† (3.73-5.85)
PTSD	22.6	4.08† (2.73-6.08)	19.7	3.68† (2.68-5.06)	15.8	2.69† (2.05-3.55)
Any anxiety§	74.1	8.79† (6.13-12.61)	68.7	8.50† (6.82-10.58)	56.9	5.80† (4.89-6.88)
Substance abuse						
Alcohol abuse without dependence	9.3	0.98 (0.60-1.59)	11.3	1.25 (0.96-1.63)	10.9	1.20 (0.93-1.54)
Alcohol dependence	21.2	1.70† (1.25-2.32)	23.6	2.08† (1.65-2.62)	23.9	2.17† (1.78-2.64)
Drug abuse without dependence	4.2	0.93 (0.55-1.57)	5.0	1.15 (0.69-1.90)	5.3	1.24† (0.85-1.81)
Drug dependence	17.3	2.86† (2.09-3.92)	14.8	2.47† (1.83-3.34)	14.8	2.56† (1.93-3.40)
Any substance	36.3	1.63† (1.23-2.15)	39.4	1.95† (1.58-2.41)	39.6	2.01† (1.69-2.38)
Aggregate						
Any other disorder	87.6	6.80† (4.87-11.37)	83.4	5.34† (4.18-6.81)	81.0	4.77† (3.80-5.98)
One other	15.1	0.75 (0.56-0.97)	17.1	0.88 (0.71-1.11)	18.9	1.02 (0.81-1.29)
Two others	18.5	1.69† (1.30-2.21)	13.7	1.24 (0.96-1.58)	14.1	1.33† (1.08-1.63)
Three others	54.0	4.68† (3.52-6.24)	52.5	5.00† (3.95-6.33)	48.0	4.32† (3.60-5.18)

**NSC indicates National Comorbidity Survey; ORs, odds ratios; CI, confidence interval; and PTSD, posttraumatic stress disorder.*
†Significant at the .05 level, two-tailed test.
‡With or without panic disorder.
§Excluding the relevant phobia(s).

As shown in **Table 4**, comorbid agoraphobia is usually secondary (55.4% of comorbid cases) in the sense of agoraphobia onset occurring at a later age than at least one other comorbid condition. Comorbid simple phobia and social phobia, in comparison, are usually temporally primary (56.8% for simple phobia and 52.6% for social phobia). These results are consistent with the earlier observation that the retrospectively reported median ages at onset of simple and social phobias are during the adolescent years (15 to 16 years) compared with a median age at onset of 29 years for agoraphobia.

IMPAIRMENT AND PROFESSIONAL HELP SEEKING

The proportions of persons with lifetime phobia who perceived themselves to ever have significant role impairment (as operationalized by a report that the phobia interfered "a lot," rather than "some," "a little," or "not at all," with their life and activities), who sought professional help, or who took medication more than once for their phobias are presented in **Table 5**. All three of these severity indicators are consistently more prevalent among comorbid than pure cases and, within the subsample of comorbid cases, more prevalent among those with a lifetime history of panic.

Perceived role impairment is significantly less prevalent overall among persons with agoraphobia (26.5%) than among persons with either simple (34.2%, $z=2.4$, $P<.05$) or social (33.5%, $z=2.4$, $P<.05$) phobias. However, there is no significant difference across types of phobia in the prevalence of perceived role impairment in the subsample of those with panic attacks. A higher proportion of persons with agoraphobia (41.0%) sought professional help for their phobias at some time in their life than those with either simple (30.2%, $z=3.1$, $P<.05$) or social (19.0%, $z=4$, $P<.05$) phobias. Furthermore, a higher proportion of persons with agoraphobia reported lifetime use of medications for their phobias (21.6%) than those with either simple (8.0%, $z=5.9$, $P.05$) or social (6.2%, $z=7.5$, $P<.05$) phobias. Overall, approximately half of persons with agoraphobia, simple phobia, and social phobia reported at least one outcome indicative of severity at some time in their life (either a lot of interference, professional help seeking, or use of medications more than once).

The opposite-sign pattern seen in Table 5, ie, a lower proportion of persons with agoraphobia who reported impairment but higher proportions of those who reported help seeking and use of medication, implies that the relationship between perceived impairment and treatment differs by type of phobia. This is examined directly in **Table 6**, where it is shown that the probabilities of professional help seeking and use of medication among the persons with agoraphobia at a given level of perceived role impairment are generally higher than among the persons with simple or social phobias who reported the same levels of role impairment.

Table 4. Temporal Ordering of Comorbid Phobias

	% (SE) Among Persons With a History of Each Phobia		
Disorder	Agoraphobia	Simple Phobia	Social Phobia
Pure*	12.4 (2.7)	16.6 (1.5)	19.0 (1.5)
Temporally primary†	20.3 (2.2)	40.2 (1.9)	33.6 (2.1)
Same year‡	12.0 (2.0)	10.0 (1.7)	9.5 (1.3)
Temporally secondary§			
Any affective disorder	17.3 (2.5)	9.8 (1.8)	9.4 (1.2)
Some other phobia	23.9 (2.2)	17.0 (2.2)	21.1 (1.6)
Some other anxiety disorder	6.3 (1.1)	3.0 (0.4)	4.3 (1.0)
Alcohol abuse or dependence	10.8 (2.1)	6.2 (1.2)	6.4 (0.9)
Drug abuse or dependence	10.3 (2.2)	3.5 (0.9)	3.8 (0.8)
Conduct disorder	10.6 (2.3)	9.4 (1.9)	8.9 (1.1)
Any of the above	55.4 (3.9)	33.1 (2.7)	37.8 (2.0)

**This phobia is the respondent's only lifetime National Comorbidity Survey (NCS)* DSM-III-R *disorder.*

†*This phobia was at an earlier age of onset (based on retrospective self-reports) than any other disorder and was followed by the onset of at least one other NCS/*DSM-III-R *disorder.*

‡*This phobia and at least one other NCS/*DSM-III-R *disorder were at the same ages of onset, which were earlier than those of any other disorder.*

§*At least one other NCS/*DSM-III-R *disorder occurred at an earlier age than this phobia.*

Table 5. Lifetime Perceived Role Impairment, Help Seeking, and Use of Medication for Pure and Comorbid Phobias

	% (SE) Among Persons With Each Subtype of Phobia			
Disorder	Perceived Role Impairment	Sought Help	Medication	Any
Agoraphobia				
Pure	2.8 (2.1)	22.3 (9.4)	4.7 (2.8)	23.6 (9.5)
Comorbid, no panic attacks	22.0 (3.2)	25.6 (4.2)	13.2 (3.3)	38.9 (5.1)
Comorbid with panic attacks	40.7 (4.1)	69.4 (4.8)	39.2 (4.0)	78.0 (3.4)
Total	26.5 (2.2)	41.0 (2.9)	21.6 (1.9)	51.2 (3.0)
Simple phobia				
Pure	24.5 (4.4)	30.3 (4.9)	6.3 (4.0)	52.2 (5.5)
Comorbid, no panic attacks	33.2 (3.4)	22.5 (2.1)	4.7 (1.2)	46.1 (2.9)
Comorbid with panic attacks	41.8 (4.9)	46.6 (4.1)	16.1 (3.2)	66.7 (4.2)
Total	34.2 (2.4)	30.2 (1.9)	8.0 (1.3)	52.6 (2.3)
Social phobia				
Pure	14.4 (3.3)	4.0 (1.5)	0.3 (0.3)	17.3 (3.3)
Comorbid, no panic attacks	34.9 (2.8)	19.1 (2.0)	5.3 (1.1)	46.8 (2.8)
Comorbid with panic attacks	46.3 (5.7)	31.8 (4.3)	13.9 (2.8)	60.0 (5.5)
Total	33.5 (2.0)	19.0 (1.8)	6.2 (0.8)	44.1 (2.3)

Given that the finding of less role impairment among persons with agoraphobia than among those with other phobias is inconsistent with prior research,[12-17] an analysis of more objective role impairment was conducted. This was done by estimating logistic regression equations, in which measures of 30-day agoraphobia, simple phobia, and social phobia were used to predict various measures of current role impairment, controlling for sociodemographic variables (age, sex, education, marital status, number of preschool-aged children in the home, and interactions between sex and marital status and between sex and preschoolers), and comorbid disorders. The analyses showed that agoraphobia and simple phobia, but not social phobia, are associated with significantly increased work absence among employed men (equivalent to 1.1 days per month for persons with agoraphobia and 0.7 day per month for persons with simple phobias [$z = 6.7$ and 6.1, respectively], compared with a nonsignificant 0.05 days per month for persons with social phobia [$z = 0.1$]) but not among employed women. In addition, simple and social phobias, but not agoraphobia, are associated with low social support (defined as the lowest decile in the sample), with ORs of 1.92 (95% CI, 1.11 to 3.35) for simple phobia and 1.74 (95% CI, 1.03 to 2.95) for social phobia, compared with a nonsignificant OR of 1.08 (95% CI, 0.23 to 5.04) for agoraphobia. None of the phobias was significantly related to financial adversity, as defined by either low family income in the total sample or low earnings in the subsample of the employed.

COMMENT

PREVALENCE

Previous studies of phobias in North American community samples have largely been based on *DSM-III* criteria, as defined in the Diagnostic Interview Schedule.[18] The NCS agoraphobia lifetime prevalence estimate of 6.7% is at the upper end of the range of these earlier surveys (2.9% to 6.9%),[19,20] while the NCS simple phobia lifetime prevalence estimate of 11.3% is in the middle of the range in earlier surveys (6.5% to 21.6%).[21] The NCS social phobia lifetime prevalence estimate of 13.3%, in comparison, is far above the range in earlier surveys (1.6% to 3.2%),[20,22] although lower than in a recent European community epidemiologic survey (16.0%) that used *DSM-III-R* criteria and made diagnoses with the CIDI.[23] Furthermore, a recent epidemiologic survey of a Canadian community, based on *DSM-III-R* criteria, reported a period prevalence of social phobia (7.1%)[24] that is quite similar to the NCS 12-month prevalence estimate of 7.9%.[1]

A blind clinical reappraisal of a subsample of NCS respondents who endorsed the stem question for social phobia found that 100% of CIDI cases were confirmed as cases and 84% of noncases were confirmed as noncases,[25] documenting that the higher prevalence in the NCS than in earlier surveys is not owing to invalidity. But how can this high prevalence be explained? At least three factors appear to be involved.

First, the phobia stem questions in the NCS are based on *DSM-III-R*, which requires either avoidance or distress on exposure, rather than the narrower *DSM-III* requirement of avoidance. This has a much larger effect on the prevalence of social phobia than other phobias, because it is much more difficult to avoid social situations than the situations associated with simple phobia or agoraphobia.

Second, while the NCS descriptors for simple phobia and agoraphobia were similar in number and word-

Table 6. Lifetime Help Seeking and Use of Medication by Level of Perceived Role Impairment

Perceived Role Impairment	% (SE) Among Persons With Each Level of Perceived Impairment Caused by Phobia		
	Agoraphobia	Simple Phobia	Social Phobia
A lot			
Help seeking*	70.5‡ (6.4)	40.3 (4.3)	28.2 (2.9)
Medications†	42.1 (5.6)	11.4 (2.4)	11.4 (2.3)
Some			
Any help	39.6 (4.7)	27.2 (3.1)	15.3 (2.3)
Medications	18.5 (3.6)	6.3 (2.2)	5.9 (1.1)
A little			
Any help	30.4 (4.2)	21.0 (3.2)	13.0 (2.3)
Medications	14.0 (4.4)	6.2 (2.9)	1.1 (0.8)
None			
Any help	13.2 (7.9)	26.6 (6.6)	21.6 (10.1)
Medications	8.1 (5.8)	6.6 (3.8)	0.0 ...

*Seeking help for the fear from a nonpsychiatric medical doctor, a mental health specialist, or any other professional (eg, priest, minister, rabbi, counselor, or nurse).

†Taking medication more than once because of the fear.

‡Percentage of subjects with lifetime agoraphobia who sought any help in the subsample of those who reported "a lot" of role impairment due to the phobia.

ing to those used in the Epidemiologic Catchment Area (ECA) there was an expansion from three social phobia descriptors in the earlier surveys to six in the NCS. The ECA asked about low-prevalence social-phobic fears: of eating in public (endorsed by 2.7% of ECA respondents and 2.7% of NCS respondents), of speaking to new acquaintances (endorsed by 4.7% of ECA respondents and not included in the NCS), and of speaking in front of a small group of people you know (endorsed by 6.5% of ECA respondents). The third of these questions was modified in the NCS to delete the words "you know," with an increase in the prevalence of endorsement to 14.6%. The new questions added to the NCS all tapped high-prevalence social-phobic fears: of having to use the toilet when away from home (endorsed by 6.3%), of writing when someone watches (endorsed by 6.1%), of talking to people and not having anything to say or sounding foolish (endorsed by 13.5%), and of speaking in public (endorsed by 29.1%).

Third, the estimated prevalence of social phobia is more sensitive than those of simple phobia or agoraphobia to changes in diagnostic criteria, as documented by the fact that the prevalence estimates for agoraphobia and simple phobia did not change very much when the diagnostic criteria were changed from *DSM-III-R* to *DSM-III* (from 6.7% to 5.5% for agoraphobia and from 11.3% to 10.9% for simple phobia). The prevalence estimate for social phobia, in comparison, changes substantially, from 13.3% to 8.3%, with this change in diagnostic criteria. When diagnosis was further restricted to the NCS respondents who endorsed one of the situational descriptors most comparable to those used in the *Diagnostic Interview Schedule–DSM-III* surveys, the lifetime social phobia prevalence dropped to 4.8%, which is close to the estimates in the earlier surveys.

AGE AT ONSET

A limitation of the age-at-onset analysis is that the NCS asked respondents to date their age at first onset of their unrealistic fear, not the age when they first developed a full phobic syndrome. Nonetheless, the estimated median ages at onset of 15 years for simple phobia, 16 years for social phobia, and 29 years for agoraphobia are quite similar to those obtained by Ost[26] in a review of clinical studies (between 7 and 20 years for separate simple phobias, 16 years for social phobia, and 28 years for agoraphobia).

COHORT EFFECTS

The significant intercohort difference in lifetime phobia prevalence was found to be more pronounced for agoraphobia than for the other phobias and only to appear for later-onset cases of simple and social phobias. These specifications could explain why Burke et al,[27] who examined cohort differences in onset distributions of total phobia in the ECA (not distinguishing among agoraphobia, simple phobia, and social phobia) up to age 29 years, failed to document consistent evidence for increasing prevalences in more recent cohorts.

Although it is conceivable that evidence for increasing prevalences of phobias in more recent cohorts could be owing to a methodological artifact involving either greater recall failure among older respondents or greater exclusion from the sample of older phobics, neither of these possibilities can explain the fact that the significant cohort differences in lifetime simple and social phobias are confined to later-onset cases. This specification raises the possibility that there is heterogeneity in the causes of simple and social phobias depending on age at onset. More precise assessment of this possibility, however, will require analysis of longitudinal data to distinguish a true cohort effect from a methodological artifact.

SOCIODEMOGRAPHIC CORRELATES

The finding that agoraphobia and simple phobia are approximately twice as prevalent among women as among men while there is a much smaller sex difference in social phobia is consistent with the results of several previous studies.[19,20,28-32] The strong and negative association of at least one indicator of socioeconomic status (education or income) with all three phobias is also consistent with previous research.[33,34] The inconsistency of the associations between phobias and other sociodemographic correlates mirrors inconsistencies found in earlier epidemiologic studies.[14,20,21,23,26-28,35,36]

COMORBIDITY

The NCS finding of significant comorbidities between phobias and other disorders are consistent with prior clinical studies[37-39] and community epidemiologic surveys.[12,22,40] The strongest of the NCS comorbidities is that between panic and agoraphobia (OR = 11.9), a result consistent with prior research[41-43] and owing to the fact that we did not distinguish agoraphobia with panic from agoraphobia without panic in the definition of agoraphobia. Despite this very high OR, however, only about one third of NCS agoraphobic respondents reported ever having an unexpected panic attack, a result also found in the ECA Study.[44] Subsequent clinical reanalysis of ECA cases found that many of those classified as agoraphobic without panic had, in fact, misdiagnosed simple or social phobias,[45] a result that is consistent with the fact that agoraphobia without a history of panic is very rare in clinical samples.[46,47] More detailed analysis of the NCS data is currently under way to discriminate persons with agoraphobia who deny ever having simple or social phobic fears from those with such fears (who could have misdiagnosed simple or social phobias) in an effort to evaluate the possibility that a similar diagnostic confusion underlies the appearance that agoraphobia without panic is more common than agoraphobia with panic in the NCS.

Another important result concerning comorbidity is that all the phobias were found to be more weakly comorbid with substance use disorders than with other anxiety disorders or affective disorders. This result is consistent with a comprehensive review of the literature by Schuckit and Hesselbrock, who concluded that "the available data, while imperfect, do not prove a close relationship between lifelong anxiety disorders and alcohol dependence."[48]

Finally, the NCS result that comorbid simple and social phobias are usually temporally primary while comorbid agoraphobia is usually temporally secondary is consistent with previous results of both clinical and epidemiologic studies.[14,22,49,50] However, it is important to remember that both the NCS and many of the previous studies that examined temporal priority between phobias and other disorders dated the age at onset of the first fear of phobic situations rather than of first meeting full diagnostic criteria. It is possible that an assessment of the latter would lead to different conclusions concerning temporal priorities between phobias and comorbid disorders. Although clinical studies might be expected to provide valid data of this sort, such studies often rely on retrospective patient reports that are subject to the same sort of bias.[35] The only rigorous way to obtain unequivocal data on this issue is to use longitudinal general population data. Data of this sort document that anxiety disorders generally occur before comorbid affective disorders, but are less clear that anxiety disorders predict the subsequent onset of substance use disorders.[51-53]

IMPAIRMENT

The NCS results concerning perceived role impairments are at odds with most other clinical and community studies in finding that a somewhat smaller proportion of persons with agoraphobia (26.5%) than those with either simple (34.2%) or social (33.5%) phobias reported that their phobia "interfered a lot" with their "life and activities." This might be caused by imprecision in the single self-reported question used to assess perceived role impairment, which could miss the fact that avoidance of public places impairs ability to work much more than does avoidance of harmless animals or avoidance of social situations. More detailed and objective assessments of role functioning have generally found that the rank ordering of the different phobias in terms of impairment varies depending on the way impairment is assessed,[14,15] a result that is consistent with our analysis of the impairments associated with current phobias. More detailed assessment of functional impairments is needed in future epidemiologic research on this issue.

PROFESSIONAL HELP SEEKING

The NCS results are consistent with earlier community surveys in finding that only a minority of individuals with phobia ever seek professional help,[15,24,54] as well as in finding that persons with agoraphobia are more likely than are those with other phobias to obtain treatment.[54] While it has previously been assumed that the higher prevalence of help seeking among persons with agoraphobia is an effect of their greater impairment, the NCS results suggest that this might not be the case, as this association persists after controlling for perceived impairment. One plausible interpretation of this result is that subjects with agoraphobia are more likely than are those with other phobias to interpret their symptoms in mental health terms. This could occur because the symptoms of agoraphobia first occur much later than the symptoms of other phobias and, because of this, are more readily seen as deviations from some prior standard of behavior, rather than the way things have always been. Or it could be that fears of agoraphobic situations are more readily interpreted as pathological than fears of simple phobic situations (which might be interpreted as caused by cautiousness rather than mental disorder) or social phobic situations (which might be interpreted as caused by shyness rather than mental disorder). Whatever the case may be, the objective role impairments, barriers associated with problem recognition, and subsequent help seeking among individuals with simple and social phobias need to be studied more seriously in future research.

Accepted for publication September 7, 1995.

The National Comorbidity Survey (NCS) is a collaborative epidemiologic investigation of the prevalence, causes, and consequences of psychiatric morbidity and comorbidity in the United States, supported by the National Institute of Mental Health (grants R01 MH/DA46376 and R01 MH49098) and the National Institute of Drug Abuse (through a supplement to R01 MH/DA46376), Rockville, Md, and the W. T. Grant Foundation, New York, NY (grant 90135190; Dr Kessler, Principal Investigator). Preparation of this report was also supported by Research Scientist Award K05 MH00507 and by Training grants T32 MH14641 and T32 MH16806 from the National Institute of Mental Health. Collaborating NCS sites and investigators are The Addiction Research Foundation, Toronto, Ontario (Robin Room, PhD); Duke University Medical Center, Durham, NC (Dan Blazer, MD, PhD, and Marvin Swartz, MD); The Johns Hopkins University, Baltimore, Md (James Anthony, MD, William Eaton, PhD, and Philip Leaf, PhD); the Max Planck Institute of Psychiatry-Clinical Institute, Munich, Germany (Hans-Ulrich Wittchen, PhD); the Medical College of Virginia, Richmond (Kenneth Kendler, MD); The University of Michigan, Ann Arbor (Lloyd Johnston, PhD, and Ronald Kessler, PhD); New

York University, New York (Patrick Shrout, PhD); SUNY Stony Brook (Evelyn Bromet, PhD); the University of Miami, Miami, Fla (R. Jay Turner, PhD); and Washington University School of Medicine, St Louis, Mo (Linda Cottler, PhD).

A complete list of NCS publications can be obtained from the NCS Study Coordinator, Room 1006, Institute for Social Research, The University of Michigan, Box 1248, Ann Arbor, MI 48106-1248. The text of this and other NCS publications, working papers, and the raw data from the NCS can also be obtained from the NCS home page by using the URL: http://www.umich.edu/~ncsum/.

We appreciate the thoughtful comments of Murray Stein and the anonymous reviewers.

Reprint requests to Survey Research Center, The University of Michigan, 426 Thompson St, PO Box 1248, Ann Arbor, MI 48106-1248 (Dr Kessler).

REFERENCES

1. Kessler RC, McGonagle KA, Zhao S, Nelson CB, Hughes M, Eshleman S, Wittchen H-U, Kendler KS. Lifetime and 12-month prevalence of *DSM-III-R* psychiatric disorders in the United States: results from the National Comorbidity Survey. *Arch Gen Psychiatry.* 1994;51:8-19.
2. Wittchen H-U, Zhao S, Kessler RC, Eaton WW. *DSM-III-R* generalized anxiety disorder in the National Comorbidity Survey. *Arch Gen Psychiatry.* 1994;51: 355-364.
3. Warner LA, Kessler RC, Hughes M, Anthony JC, Nelson CB. Prevalence and correlates of drug use and dependence in the United States: results from the National Comorbidity Survey. *Arch Gen Psychiatry.* 1995;52:219-229.
4. World Health Organization. *Composite International Diagnostic Interview (Version 1.0).* Geneva, Switzerland: WHO; 1990.
5. Kessler RC, Wethington E. The reliability of life events reports in a community survey. *Psychol Med.* 1991;21:1-16.
6. Wittchen, H-U. Reliability and validity studies of the WHO-Composite International Diagnostic Interview (CIDI): a critical review. *J Psychiatr Res.* 1994;28:57-84.
7. University of Michigan. *OSIRIS VII.* Ann Arbor, Mich: Institute for Social Research, The University of Michigan; 1981.
8. Norusis MJ. *SPSS Advanced Statistics User's Guide.* Chicago, Ill: SPSS Inc; 1990.
9. SAS Institute. *SAS 6.03.* Cary, NC: SAS Institute; 1988.
10. Woodruff RS, Causey BD. Computerized method for approximating the variance of a complicated estimate. *J Am Stat Assoc.* 1976;71:315-321.
11. Koch GG, Lemeshow S. An application of multivariate analysis to complex sample survey data. *J Am Stat Assoc.* 1972;67:780-782.
12. Davidson JRT, Hughes DL, George LK, Blazer DG. The boundary of social phobia: exploring the threshold. *Arch Gen Psychiatry.* 1994;51:975-983.
13. Agras S, Sylvester D, Oliveau D. The epidemiology of common fears and phobias. *Compr Psychiatry.* 1969;10:151-156.
14. Wittchen H-U, Essau CA, von Zerssen D, Krieg CJ, Hecht H. Lifetime and six-month prevalence of mental disorders in the Munich follow-up study. *Eur Arch Psychiatry Clin Neurosci.* 1992;241:247-258.
15. Angst J, Dobler-Mikola A. The Zurich Study, V: anxiety and phobia in young adults. *Eur Arch Psychiatry Clin Neurol Sci.* 1985;235:171-178.
16. Costello CG. Fears and phobia in women: a community study. *J Abnorm Psychol.* 1982;91:280-286.
17. Uhlenhuth EH, Balter MB, Mellinger GG, Cisin IH, Clinthorpe J. Symptom checklist syndromes in the general population: correlations with psychotherapeutic drug use. *Arch Gen Psychiatry.* 1983;40:1167-1173.
18. Robins LN, Helzer JE, Croughan JL, Ratcliff KS. National Institute of Mental Health Diagnostic Interview Schedule: its history, characteristics and validity. *Arch Gen Psychiatry.* 1981;38:381-389.
19. Bland RC, Orn H, Newman SC. Lifetime prevalence of psychiatric disorders in Edmonton. *Acta Psychiatr Scand.* 1988;77:24-32.
20. Dagonda M, Angst J. The Zurich Study, XX: social phobia and agoraphobia. *Eur Arch Psychiatry Clin Neurosci.* 1993;243:95-102.
21. Robins LN, Helzer J, Weissman MM, Orvaschel H, Gruenberg E, Burke JD Jr, Regier DA. Lifetime prevalence of specific psychiatric disorders in three sites. *Arch Gen Psychiatry.* 1984;41:949-958.
22. Schneier FR, Johnson J, Hornig C, Liebowitz M, Weissman M. Social phobia: comorbidity and morbidity in an epidemiologic sample. *Arch Gen Psychiatry.* 1992;49:282-288.
23. Wacker HR, Mullejans R, Klein KH, Battegay R. Identification of cases of anxiety disorders and affective disorders in the community according to *ICD-10* and *DSM-III-R* using the Composite International Diagnostic Interview (CIDI). *Int J Meth Psychiatr Res.* 1992;2:91-100.
24. Stein MB, Walker JR, Forde DR. Setting diagnostic thresholds for social phobia: considerations from a community survey of social anxiety. *Am J Psychiatry.* 1994;151:408-412.
25. Wittchen, H-U, Zhao, S, Abelson, JM, Abelson, JL, Kessler, RC. Reliability and procedural validity of UM-CIDI *DSM-III-R* phobic disorders. *Psychol Med.* In press.
26. Ost L-G. Age of onset of different phobias. *J Abnorm Psychol.* 1987;96:223-229.
27. Burke KC, Burke JD, Rae DS, Regier DA. Comparing age at onset of major depression and other psychiatric disorders by birth cohorts in five US community populations. *Arch Gen Psychiatry.* 1991;48:789-795.
28. Boyd JH, Rea DS, Thompson JW, Burns BJ, Bourdon K, Locke BZ, Regier DA. Phobia: prevalence and risk factors. *Soc Psychiatry Psychiatr Epidemiol.* 1990; 25:314-323.
29. Chen C, Wong J, Lee N, Chan-Ho M, Lau JT, Fung M. The Shatin Community Mental Health Survey in Hong Kong, II: major findings. *Arch Gen Psychiatry.* 1993;50:125-133.
30. Hwu HG, Yeh EK, Chang LY. Prevalence of psychiatric disorders in Taiwan as defined by the Chinese Diagnostic Interview Schedule. *Acta Psychiatr Scand.* 1989;79:136-147.
31. Joyce PR, Bushnell JA, Oakley-Browne MA, Wells JE, Hornblow AR. The epidemiology of panic symptomatology and agoraphobic avoidance. *Compr Psychiatry.* 1989;30:303-312.
32. Bourdon KH, Boyd JH, Rae DS, Burns BJ, Thompson JW, Locke BZ. Gender differences in phobias: results of the ECA community survey. *J Anxiety Disord.* 1988;2:227-241.
33. Canino GJ, Bird HR, Shrout PE, Rubio-Stipec M, Bravo M, Marinez R, Sesman M, Guevara LM. The prevalence of specific psychiatric disorders in Puerto Rico. *Arch Gen Psychiatry.* 1987;44:727-735.
34. Eaton WW, Dryman A, Weissman MM. Panic and phobia. In: Robins LN, Regier DA, eds. *Psychiatric Disorders in America: The ECA Study.* New York, NY: The Free Press; 1991:155-179.
35. Brown DR, Eaton WW, Sussman L. Racial differences in prevalence of phobic disorders. *J Nerv Ment Dis.* 1990;178:434-441.
36. Escobar JI, Karno M, Burnam AH, RL, Golding J. Distribution on major mental disorders in an US metropolis. *Acta Psychiatr Scand.* 1988;78(suppl):45-53.
37. Wittchen H-U, Essau CA, Kreig J-C. Anxiety disorders: similarities and differences of comorbidity in treated and untreated groups. *Br J Psychiatry.* 1991; 159(suppl):23-33.
38. De Ruiter C, Rijken H, Garssen B, van Schaik A, Kraaimaat F. Comorbidity among the anxiety disorders. *J Anxiety Disord.* 1989;3:57-68.
39. Sanderson WC, DiNardo PA, Rapee RM, Barlow DH. Syndrome comorbidity in patients diagnosed with a *DSM-III-R* anxiety disorder. *J Abnorm Psychol.* 1990; 99:308-312.
40. Dick CL, Sowa B, Bland RC, Newman SC. Phobic disorders. *Acta Psychiatr Scand.* 1994;89(suppl):36-44.
41. Weissman MM, Myers JK, Harding PS. Psychiatric disorders in a US urban community. *Am J Psychiatry.* 1978;135:459-462.
42. Weissman MM, Merikangas KR. The epidemiology of anxiety and panic disorders: an update. *J Clin Psychiatry.* 1986;47:11-17.
43. Wittchen H-U. Zum Spontanverlauf unbehandelter Falle mit Angst-storungen und Depressionen. In: Wittchen H-U, von Zerssen D, eds. *Verlaufe Behandelter und Unbehandelter Depressionen und Angst-storungen.* Heidelberg, Germany: Springer Verlag; 1988.
44. Weissman MM, Leaf PJ, Blazer DG, Boyd JH, Florio L. The relationship between panic disorder and agoraphobia: an epidemiologic perspective. *Psychopharmacol Bull.* 1986;22:787-791.
45. Horwarth E, Lish JD, Johnson J, Hornig CD, Weissman M. Agoraphobia without panic: clinical reappraisal of an epidemiologic finding. *Am J Psychiatry.* 1993;150:1496-1501.
46. Klein DF, Gorman JM. A model of panic and agoraphobia development. *Acta Psychiatr Scand.* 1987;76(suppl):87-95.
47. Klein DF, Klein HM. The nosology, genetics, and theory of spontaneous panic and phobias. In: Tyrer PJ, ed. *Psychopharmacology of Anxiety.* New York, NY: Oxford University Press; 1989.
48. Schuckit MA, Hesselbrock V. Alcohol dependence and anxiety disorders: what is the relationship? *Am J Psychiatry.* 1994;151:1723-1734.
49. Angst J, Vollrath M, Merikangas KR, Ernst C. Comorbidity of anxiety and depression in the Zurich cohort study of young adults. In: Maser JD, Cloninger CR, eds. *Comorbidity of Mood and Anxiety Disorders.* Washington, DC: American Psychiatric Press; 1990:123-138.
50. Lesser IM, Rubin RT, Pecknold JC, Rifkin A, Swinson RP, Lydiard RB, Burrows GD, Noyes R Jr, DuPont RL Jr. Secondary depression in panic disorder and agoraphobia. *Arch Gen Psychiatry.* 1988;45:437-443.
51. Murphy JM. Diagnostic comorbidity and symptom co-occurrence: The Stirling County Study. In: Maser JD, Cloninger CR, eds. *Comorbidity of Mood and Anxiety Disorders.* Washington, DC: American Psychiatric Press; 1990:153-176.
52. Hagnell O, Tunvia K. Prevalence and nature of alcoholism in a total population. *Soc Psychiatry.* 1972;7:190-201.
53. Vaillant G. *The Natural History of Alcoholism.* Cambridge, Mass: Harvard University Press; 1983.
54. Thompson JW, Burns BJ, Bartko J, Boyd JH, Taube CA, Bourdon KH. The use of ambulatory service by persons with and without phobia. *Med Care.* 1988; 26:183-198.

Public-Speaking Fears in a Community Sample

Prevalence, Impact on Functioning, and Diagnostic Classification

Murray B. Stein, MD; John R. Walker, PhD; David R. Forde, PhD

Background: Recent epidemiologic studies have revealed that social phobia is more prevalent than has been previously believed. An unresolved issue is the extent to which public-speaking fears constitute a recognizable form of social phobia in a community sample and, moreover, to what extent these fears are associated with functional morbidity.

Methods: To examine the prevalence and impact of public-speaking fears and their relationship to social phobia in a community sample, we conducted a randomized telephone survey of 499 residents of Winnipeg, Manitoba, a medium-sized midwestern metropolitan area.

Results: One third of the respondents reported that they had excessive anxiety when they spoke to a large audience. The onset of fears was early (ie, 50%, 75%, and 90% by the ages of 13, 17, and 20 years, respectively). Anxious cognitions about public speaking included the following fears: doing or saying something embarrassing (64%), one's mind going blank (74%), being unable to continue talking (63%), saying foolish things or not making sense (59%), and trembling, shaking, or showing other signs of anxiety (80%). In total, 10% (n=49) of the respondents reported that public-speaking anxiety had resulted in a marked interference with their work (2%), social life (1%), or education (4%), or had caused them marked distress (8%). Twenty-three persons (5%) had public-speaking anxiety in isolation (ie, without evidence of additional kinds of social fears).

Conclusions: These data support the inclusion of severe forms of public-speaking fears within the social phobia construct and, furthermore, suggest that public-speaking anxiety may have a detrimental impact on the lives of many individuals in the community.

(Arch Gen Psychiatry. 1996;53:169-174)

SOCIAL PHOBIA has been the focus of several recent community surveys.[1] Studies that have used *DSM-III* criteria have found current rates of 2% to 3% for social phobia in the general population[2-5]; however, studies that have used *DSM-III-R* or *DSM-IV* criteria have found much higher rates for social phobia (7% to 8%).[6,7] In large part, these discrepant findings can be accounted for by differences in the assessment approaches that were used by the diagnostic instruments particular to each study.[7,8] For example, the version of the Diagnostic Interview Schedule used in the Epidemiologic Catchment Area Study[4,5] assessed three social situations (*not* including public speaking), whereas the version of the Comprehensive International Diagnostic Interview used in the National Comorbidity Survey[6] assessed six situations (including public speaking).

Clinicians have come to realize that social phobia may be subclassified on the basis of the extent and specific nature of the social fears.[9-12] Among the possible subtyping schemata for social phobia, a "specific" or "performance" subtype has been recognized that consists primarily (although not exclusively) of persons with public-speaking fears. In clinical samples, patients with performance-only fears are considerably *less* impaired by their symptoms than patients with the more "generalized" form of the disorder. Although this seems to be true for *clinical samples*, it is not known to what extent public-speaking (ie, in front of a large group of unfamiliar people) fears—the most common form of social anxiety in nonclinical samples[12]—carry a sufficient burden of disability and distress that they become "clinically significant." In other words, what pro-

From the Anxiety Disorders Research Program, Department of Psychiatry (Drs Stein and Walker) and the Winnipeg Area Study, Department of Sociology (Dr Forde), University of Manitoba, Winnipeg. Dr Stein is now with the Department of Psychiatry, University of California–San Diego, La Jolla. Dr Forde is now with the Department of Criminology and Criminal Justice, University of Memphis, Memphis, Tenn.

See Subjects and Methods on next page

SUBJECTS AND METHODS

SUBJECT SAMPLE

The data reported were collected as part of the 1993 Winnipeg (Manitoba) Area Study, which is an annual community survey that has been carried out since 1981. Winnipeg is a city of 650 000 inhabitants with a stable economy and population base, located in the Canadian midwest. Following two pilot tests, 10 professional interviewers, all of whom had previous experience with population surveys, spent 9 hours practicing for this project with the help of an instruction handbook that was written specifically for this version of the Winnipeg Area Study.

The goal of the study was to interview approximately 500 respondents during 1 month. We used a two-stage sampling frame in which we used (1) a random sample of 3000 telephone numbers, with approximately one in three being active, excluding out-of-service and business telephone numbers, to obtain a probability sample of households, and (2) a random predesignation of a male or female respondent within each household to ensure an equal representation of male and female participants. Past experience on the Winnipeg Area Study indicated that women were more likely than men to answer the telephone. If the person who answered was of the specified gender, only that person could be interviewed. If the person was not of the specified gender, that person was asked if someone of the appropriate gender was in the household. If there was no one of the specified gender who lived there, the respondent could only be the person who answered the telephone. If a person of the designated gender was living there, the interviewer was to ask for this person or the oldest if there was more than one. If the eligible respondent was not at home or for some other reason was not available, every effort was made to set up another interview appointment. No substitution was permitted if the eligible respondent refused. Addition selection criteria were respondents who were 18 years of age or older and the dwelling unit that was their usual place of residence.

Each interviewer was to complete up to 10 telephone call attempts to a household and to vary the time of the call and date. All interviews were conducted over the telephone, either at the respondent's residence or occasionally at another telephone number (location) that was convenient to the respondent. Our items about public speaking came near the beginning of the interview, which also included questions about the respondent's sociodemographic status and opinions about a variety of social issues (as part of another study). The median length of the interview was 34 minutes (range, 15 to 127 minutes).

QUESTIONNAIRE DESIGN

The questionnaire, available in its entirety from the authors, is summarized here. After an introduction that described the nature of the survey, the interviewer asked, "How nervous or uncomfortable would you be speaking in front of a small group of people you know?" This was followed by the question: "How nervous or uncomfortable would you be speaking in front of a large audience" (ie, "public speaking")? Response categories were as follows: "Much more nervous (uncomfortable) than other people," "Somewhat more nervous than other people," or "No more nervous than other people." Respondents who answered much or somewhat more nervous than other people to this probe were questioned further about public-speaking anxiety. They were asked whether they felt nervous about public speaking because "you are afraid that you might say or do something embarrassing," "you are afraid that your mind will go blank," "you are afraid that you will be unable to continue talking," "you are afraid that you will say foolish things or not make sense," or "you are afraid that you will tremble, shake, or show other signs of anxiety." Response categories here were "yes," "no," or "don't know." The respondent was then asked, "How old were you when you first had difficulty with public speaking?" Finally, the respondent was asked whether discomfort about public speaking "has made it difficult for you to find a job, change jobs, or get a better job"; "has interfered with your normal social activities with family, friends, or neighbors"; "has interfered with your education"; or "has bothered you personally." Response categories for this series of queries were along a one- to seven-point scale, where a response rating of 1 indicated "not at all," a response rating of 4 indicated "somewhat," and a response rating of 7 indicated "a great deal." For the purpose of these analyses, only persons who gave a response rating of 6 or 7 were considered to have met the criterion for a positive response. This very conservative criterion was set to include only severe levels of disability or distress.

DATA ANALYSIS AND STATISTICAL PROCEDURES

We generated frequency tables for respondent characteristics in the relevant response categories. Sample sizes varied for different questions because of differences in the number of evaluable responses. The statistical association between certain dependent variables and subject classification was analyzed by multiway frequency tables using the χ^2 test; the odds ratios (ORs) with 95% confidence intervals (CIs) are reported, where indicated. Logistic regressions that controlled for relevant demographic characteristics (eg, age, gender) were used in select instances. All tests were two-tailed, and $P<.05$ was considered statistically significant.

portion of people with public-speaking fears in the community are adversely affected by these fears to a degree that warrants a "diagnosis"?

This is an important, heretofore unanswered question, given that the *International Classification of Diseases, 10th Revision*, seems to *exclude* explicitly from the social phobia category persons whose fear is of speaking in front of a large crowd,[13] presumably because such fears are thought to be so common (or so trivial) as to not merit a diagnosis. On the other hand, *DSM-IV* criteria permit the application of the social phobia diagnosis to persons whose fear is of speaking in front of large crowds.[14] In neither case, however, did the respective diagnostic committees have access to empiric data with regard to the prevalence and importance of public-speaking anxiety in the community. The purpose of the present study was to make such data available.

In our previous survey,[7] we found that approxi-

Table 1. Sociodemographic Profile of Respondents in the 1993 Winnipeg (Manitoba) Area Study (N=499)*

Characteristic	Frequency, No. (%)
Gender	
M	216 (43.3)
F	283 (56.7)
Age, y	
18-29	122 (24.5)
30-44	191 (38.2)
45-64	103 (20.7)
≥65	83 (16.6)
Marital status	
Married	285 (57.5)
Divorced or separated	61 (12.2)
Widowed	42 (8.5)
Never married	108 (21.8)
Current employment	
Full-time	232 (46.5)
Part-time	87 (17.4)
Retired	98 (19.6)
Unemployed	38 (7.6)
Other	44 (8.8)
Annual personal income, $	
0-19 999	183 (46.6)
20 000-39 999	134 (34.1)
40 000-69 999	65 (16.5)
≥70 000	11 (2.8)
Education level, y	
0-11	123 (24.7)
12	137 (27.6)
13-15	218 (43.9)
≥16	19 (3.8)

**Subject numbers vary owing to differential response rates for various questions.*

mately one third of respondents judged themselves much more nervous than other people with regard to public speaking (defined as formal speaking in front of a large group of unfamiliar people). However, the design of that study—wherein respondents were asked to identify their *worst* source of social anxiety, and then to restrict subsequent answers to *that* particular situation—did not enable us to determine how many persons had substantial public-speaking fears accompanied by "social phobia–like" cognitions, or to examine the extent to which public-speaking fears resulted in social, occupational, or educational impairment. To our knowledge, these issues—which the present study was designed to explore—have not previously been addressed in an epidemiologic sample.

RESULTS

CHARACTERISTICS OF THE SURVEY SAMPLE

Demographic characteristics of the survey sample are summarized in **Table 1**. The sociodemographic profile of the respondents and persons in the household was similar to that of the city's population as determined by the 1986 census. This representation was achieved through a rigorous process of callbacks that continued until the interviewer made contact for an interview or refusal. Many interviews were completed on the initial telephone call (28%), and half (50%) of the interviews were completed on the first or second telephone call to a household. The mean number of callbacks was 2.2, with 2% of interviews taking more than 10 callbacks.

Analysis of the designated gender in the household indicates that 16% of the households had three or more adults, but in 94% of the households, only one person met the criteria for the designated respondent. Thus, the sample faces a 6% chance of households having more than one potential respondent where the respondent would be the first adult to answer the telephone or the oldest adult if the other gender answered. The effects of the potential bias of callbacks and availability to answer the telephone will be tested later in this article. Overall, the response rate for the survey was 76% of the eligible households.

PREVALENCE OF PUBLIC-SPEAKING FEARS

One hundred sixty-seven persons (34%) reported that they were "much more nervous than other people" when they were speaking to a large audience; these individuals will be referred to here as those with "substantial public-speaking fears" (SPSFs). One hundred fourteen persons (23%) judged themselves as "somewhat more nervous than other people" in this situation. These rates are comparable with those found in our previous survey (ie, 31% and 24%, respectively),[7] suggesting that these rates are stable within the community.

A mean (±SD) of 1.99±2.21 callbacks was required to complete the interview with persons with SPSFs, compared with 2.26±2.30 callbacks for persons without SPSFs (t=1.25, df=489, P=.21). Approximately equal proportions of SPSFs (11%) and non-SPSFs (16%) required greater than two callbacks to complete the interview (χ^2=2.34, df=1, P=.13). These data demonstrate that persons with SPSFs were not inadvertently oversampled by virtue of their being more likely to be at home when they were telephoned.

Among persons with SPSFs, the age at onset was early, with 50% of persons reporting an onset by the age of 13 years, 75% by the age of 17 years, and 90% by the age of 20 years. This early age at onset is consistent with the early age at onset of social phobia in clinical samples.[12,15-17]

Of those persons with SPSFs (n=167), less than one third (n=59 or 12% of the respondents) rated themselves as much more nervous than other people when they were speaking to a small group of familiar people. This finding, consistent with that of our previous survey,[7] confirms that fears about speaking in front of large vs small groups are not equivalent phenomena. If public speaking is considered to refer only to small groups—an approach apparently adopted by the *International Classification of Diseases, 10th Revision*—then it is to be expected that reports of public-speaking fears will be only about one third as prevalent as they would be if the whole range of public-speaking experiences (ie, including large groups) is included.

SOCIODEMOGRAPHIC FACTORS ASSOCIATED WITH PUBLIC-SPEAKING FEARS

Persons with SPSFs (**Table 2**) were significantly more likely to be female (OR=2.62 [CI, 1.75 to 3.94]), significantly less likely to have more than a high school education (OR=0.42 [CI, 0.29 to 0.63]), and significantly less likely to have a personal income of $40 000 or more per year (OR=0.42 [CI, 0.22 to 0.80) compared with persons without SPSFs. Persons with SPSFs were no more likely than persons without SPSFs to have been never married (OR=1.29 [CI, 0.81 to 2.10]) or unemployed (OR=1.90 [CI, 0.96 to 3.75]).

To determine whether public-speaking fears were *independently* associated with a lower level of educational attainment, lower personal income, and lower likelihood of being currently employed, we conducted separate logistic regression analyses for these three dependent variables, by covarying for the potential confounding effects of gender and age. When age and gender were controlled for, persons with SPSFs were found to be less likely to have personal incomes of $40 000 or more per year (OR=0.51 [CI, 0.26 to 0.995]), less likely to have a postsecondary education (OR=0.43 [CI, 0.29 to 0.64]), and more likely to be unemployed (OR=2.60 [CI, 1.27 to 5.30]) than persons without SPSFs.

Table 2. Demographic Contrast of Persons Who Reported That They Had SPSFs (n=167) vs Those Persons Without SPSFs (n=324)*

	No. (%) of Persons	
Characteristic	**SPSFs**	**Without SPSFs**
Gender†		
M	47 (28.1)	164 (50.6)
F	120 (71.9)	160 (49.4)
Age, y		
18-29	32 (19.2)	86 (26.5)
30-44	67 (40.1)	116 (35.8)
45-64	39 (23.4)	60 (18.5)
≥65	29 (17.4)	62 (19.1)
Marital status		
Married	104 (62.7)	174 (54.0)
Divorced or separated	14 (8.4)	47 (14.6)
Widowed	16 (9.6)	25 (7.8)
Never married	32 (19.3)	76 (23.6)
Current employment		
Full- or part-time	92 (64.3)	223 (73.1)
Unemployed	17 (11.9)	21 (6.9)
Retired	34 (23.8)	61 (20.0)
Annual personal income, $‡		
0-19 999	70 (56.0)	110 (42.1)
20 000-39 999	41 (32.8)	91 (34.9)
40 000-69 999	12 (9.6)	51 (19.5)
≥70 000	2 (1.6)	9 (3.4)
Education level, y§		
0-11	49 (29.3)	70 (21.7)
12	61 (36.5)	75 (23.3)
13-15	55 (32.9)	160 (49.7)
≥16	2 (1.2)	17 (5.3)

**Subject numbers vary owing to differential response rates for various questions. SPSFs indicates substantial public-speaking fears.*
†Odds ratio (OR) =2.62 (confidence interval [CI], 1.75 to 3.94).
‡OR=0.42 (CI, 0.23 to 0.78) for having a personal annual income of $40 000 or more.
§OR=0.42 (CI, 0.29 to 0.62) for having more than a high school education.

ANXIOUS COGNITIONS PERTAINING TO PUBLIC-SPEAKING FEARS

To assist us further in determining whether persons with SPSFs were similar to patients with other recognized forms of social phobia, we thought that it would be interesting to ascertain whether they had typical social phobic cognitions with regard to public speaking. We elected to inquire specifically about each of the cognitions and concerns that are included in the *DSM-IV* criteria for social phobia.[14] Among the respondents with SPSFs (n=167), the percentages of those who responded affirmatively to fearful cognitions associated with public speaking were as follows: "afraid you might say or do something that will be embarrassing," 64%; "afraid that your mind will go blank," 74%; "afraid that you will be unable to continue talking," 63%; "afraid that you will say foolish things or not make sense," 58%; and "afraid that you will tremble, shake, or show other signs of anxiety," 80%. Nearly all (96%) of the respondents with SPSFs reported that they had at least one of these cognitions and concerns that are considered to be characteristic of social phobia.

IMPACT OF PUBLIC-SPEAKING FEARS

Although many persons in the community reported that they had substantial public-speaking fears in association with social phobia–like cognitions, an overriding question is how many of these individuals were *adversely affected* by their fears? The *DSM-IV* explicitly states that for a diagnosis of social phobia to be applied, the fears must be associated with significant impairment or distress, whereas a requirement for impairment is an implicit requirement in the *International Classification of Diseases, 10th Revision*. Impairment and distress were rated along a seven-point scale (response ratings: 1="not at all," 4="somewhat," and 7="a great deal"); the range of responses of persons with SPSFs is shown in the **Figure**. If one adopts a very high threshold for severity by insisting on a rating of at least 6 to satisfy a requirement for interference, then the number of persons with SPSFs who would meet or exceed this criterion is as follows: 12 persons (7%) reported that their public-speaking fears made it markedly difficult for them to find a job, change jobs, or get a better job; six persons (4%) reported a marked interference with normal social activities; and 22 persons (14%) reported a definite interference with their education. In total, 29 persons (17% of the persons with SPSFs, or 6% of the respondents) reported an adverse impact on one or more important aspects of their lives that they attributed to public-speaking fears. Arguably, these persons would fit within the diagnostic guidelines for social phobia according to the *International Classification of Diseases, 10th Revision*, if the category was broadened to permit the inclusion of persons with "large-group" public-speaking fears. Thirty-one respondents (19% of the persons with SPSFs) reported that public-speaking fears

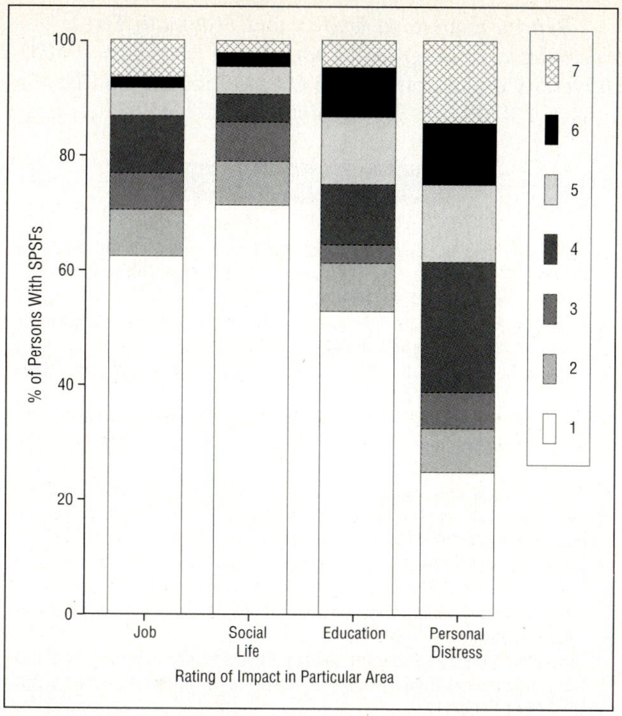

Proportion (percentage) of persons with substantial public-speaking fears (SPSFs) who reported impairment (in three domains) or distress (one- to seven-point scale, where ratings of 1 and 7 indicate "none" and "a great deal," respectively).

had caused them marked (ie, a rating of at least 6 on the scale of 7) distress. When *either* disability *or* distress were considered conjointly (as per the *DSM-IV* criteria), a total of 49 persons (29% of persons with SPSFs, or 10% of the respondents) would fulfill *DSM-IV* syndromal criteria (without considering possible medical or psychiatric exclusionary criteria)[12] for social phobia. This rate would nearly double (to 16% of the respondents) merely by including persons who rated their disability or distress as a response rating of 5 on the seven-point scale.

PUBLIC-SPEAKING FEARS IN ISOLATION

An important question to ask is, "How many of these people have public-speaking fears in isolation, as opposed to those who are likely suffering from a more generalized form[18] of social phobia in which public-speaking fears are just one manifestation thereof?" We are able to ascertain the number of people with substantial fears that are *exclusive* to public speaking by eliminating people who also endorse problems with speaking in front of a small group of familiar people. When this distinction is applied, we find that approximately one half (47% [23/49]) of persons in the community who meet *DSM-IV* syndromal criteria for social phobia—ie, 5% of respondents—do so *solely on the basis of public-speaking fears.*

COMMENT

In light of recent evidence that social phobia is more common than previously supposed,[1] we conducted this study to determine expressly the prevalence of public-speaking fears in the community. Unlike most previous surveys,[3-8] which focused on a respondent's "worst" phobia and rated disability in reference to that particular phobia, we designed the present survey to assess disability and distress that were specific to public-speaking fears. To our knowledge, this has not been previously attempted in a community sample.

We found that 5% to 10% of the people (depending on the impairment severity threshold that was selected) with substantial public-speaking fears and associated disability or distress do indeed strongly resemble persons with other types of social anxiety in the community.[5-8] Specifically, they have an early age at onset, they are overrepresented by females, and they tend to have less education and lower incomes than persons without substantial public-speaking fears. Furthermore, they have negative cognitions about public speaking that are prototypical of those experienced by patients with social phobia. For these reasons, it would seem reasonable to conclude tentatively that severe public-speaking fears (ie, those associated with substantial disability or distress) belong in the social phobia diagnostic spectrum.

We confirmed previous findings of a high rate of public-speaking fears among the general population.[1] In interpreting this finding, it should be kept in mind that we asked people "How nervous *would* you be . . . ?" not "How nervous have you been . . . ?" Consequently, it is likely that the respondents included some people who *hypothesized* that they *would* be extremely nervous when they were in a public-speaking situation, even though they may not have actually had the opportunity to test this hypothesis (eg, they may not actually have had a public-speaking engagement). Nevertheless, when these persons were asked to assess the *actual*—not imagined—impact of public-speaking fears on their lives, a substantial subsection of the community (5% to 10%, depending on the criteria used) reported that these fears had affected them adversely. These data underscore the point that even though a particular fear may be "common," it did not necessarily follow that commonality should be equated with triviality. For most persons, it was indeed the case that their public-speaking fears were inconsequential. For a sizable minority, however, it was their judgment that their public-speaking phobia had hindered them significantly in one or more meaningful psychosocial domains. It will be important in future studies to document objectively the extent to which public-speaking fears lead to functional disability and, moreover, the pathways through which this occurs.

We found a tendency for persons with substantial public-speaking anxiety to be less gainfully employed and to have lower educational attainment than persons without substantial public-speaking anxiety. Thus, the demographics of public-speaking anxiety associated with social phobia in this nonclinical sample parallels that experienced by patients with social phobia in clinical settings.[17,19] Our data are complementary to those of Davidson et al,[4,8] who found that social phobia in a North Carolina community—even in a form that was *subthreshold* in terms of strict *DSM-III* criteria—was associated with more frequent school performance and attendance problems, as well as increased rates of work problems. It is important to highlight, however, that their data and our own do not, of course, demonstrate a causal relationship (ie, that public-speaking anxiety *resulted in* employment and academic underperformance).

Although we can infer from our data that approximately half the people with substantial public-speaking fears experience those fears in isolation, it is likely that the other half experience difficulty with public speaking as merely one manifestation of a more global condition (eg, generalized social phobia).[18] This remains to be clarified with additional research through which the links between SPSFs and functional disability will be delineated. This research effort would be greatly abetted if ensuing revisions to the *International Classification of Diseases* and the *DSM* were to sanction a special social phobia subtype designation for those persons who suffer *exclusively* from public-speaking fears (ie, in the absence of other kinds of social fears). In the interim, we would encourage researchers to begin to subtype their patients with social phobia in this manner.

Finally, on a more treatment-oriented note, we wish to comment on the public health issues that are raised by this study. Our data suggest that public-speaking fears are associated with disability in a large sector (5% to 10%) of the population. In particular, we were surprised to see that so many respondents reported that public-speaking fears had interfered with their education (a finding that was echoed by the reports of Davidson et al[4,8] of high rates of impaired school performance during adolescence in persons with social phobia). This raises the possibility that the problem could be ameliorated by focusing preventative and early interventional efforts on educational services at the elementary or junior high school levels. This would be appropriate because many of the interventions that are used to help people with public-speaking anxiety (eg, self-help and skills-oriented programs such as Toastmasters) are educational in nature. Perhaps a greater emphasis could be placed on public speaking and formal presentations as part of the regular curriculum, with specialized referral services then reserved for and made available to children with more extensive difficulties. Future studies that test the utility and cost-effectiveness of such measures will significantly advance our knowledge in this area.

Accepted for publication September 13, 1995.

This work was supported in part by a Scholarship Award from the Medical Research Council of Canada, Ottawa, Ontario (Dr Stein).

Reprint requests to Anxiety and Traumatic Stress Disorders Research Program, Department of Psychiatry (0603), University of California–San Diego, 9500 Gilman Dr, La Jolla, CA 92093-0603 (Dr Stein).

REFERENCES

1. Walker JR, Stein MB. Epidemiology of social phobia. In: Stein MB, ed. *Social Phobia: Clinical and Research Perspectives.* Washington, DC: American Psychiatric Press Inc; 1995:43-75.
2. Pollard CA, Henderson JG. Four types of social phobia in a community sample. *J Nerv Ment Dis.* 1988;176:440-445.
3. Degonda M, Angst J. The Zurich Study, XX: social phobia and agoraphobia. *Eur Arch Psychiatry Clin Neurosci.* 1993;243:95-102.
4. Davidson JT, Hughes DL, George LK, Blazer DG. The epidemiology of social phobia: findings from the Duke Epidemiological Catchment Area Study. *Psychol Med.* 1993;23:709-718.
5. Schneier FR, Johnson J, Hornig CD, Liebowitz MR, Weissman MM. Social phobia: comorbidity and morbidity in an epidemiologic sample. *Arch Gen Psychiatry.* 1992;49:282-288.
6. Kessler RG, McGonagle KA, Zhao S, Nelson CB, Hughes M, Eshleman S, Wittchen H-U, Kendler KS. Lifetime and 12-month prevalence of *DSM-III-R* psychiatric disorders in the United States: results from the National Comorbidity Survey. *Arch Gen Psychiatry.* 1994;51:8-19.
7. Stein MB, Walker JR, Forde DR. Setting diagnostic thresholds for social phobia: considerations from a community survey of social anxiety. *Am J Psychiatry.* 1994;51:408-412.
8. Davidson JRT, Hughes DC, George LK, Blazer DG. The boundary of social phobia: exploring the threshold. *Arch Gen Psychiatry.* 1994;51:975-983.
9. Gelernter CS, Stein MB, Tancer ME, Uhde TW. An examination of syndromal validity and diagnostic subtypes in social phobia and panic disorder. *J Clin Psychiatry.* 1992;53:23-27.
10. Heimberg RG, Hope DA, Dodge CS, Becker RE. *DSM-III-R* subtypes of social phobia: comparison of generalized social phobics and public-speaking phobes. *J Nerv Ment Dis.* 1990;178:172-179.
11. Heimberg RG, Holt CS, Schneier FR, Spitzer RL, Liebowitz MR. The issue of subtypes in the diagnosis of social phobia. *J Anxiety Disord.* 1993;7:249-269.
12. Hazen AL, Stein MB. Differential diagnosis and comorbidity of social phobia. In: Stein MB, ed. *Social Phobia: Clinical and Research Perspectives.* Washington, DC: American Psychiatric Press Inc; 1995:3-41.
13. World Health Organization. *The ICD-10 Classification of Mental and Behavioural Disorders: Clinical Descriptions and Diagnostic Guidelines.* Geneva, Switzerland: World Health Organization; 1992.
14. American Psychiatric Association. *Diagnostic and Statistical Manual of Mental Disorders, Fourth Edition.* Washington, DC: American Psychiatric Press Inc; 1994.
15. Amies PL, Gelder MG, Shaw PM. Social phobia: a comparative clinical study. *Br J Psychiatry.* 1983;142:174-179.
16. Solyom L, Ledwidge B, Solyom C. Delineating social phobia. *Br J Psychiatry.* 1986;149:464-470.
17. Liebowitz MR, Fyer J, Gorman JM, Klein DF. Social phobia: review of a neglected anxiety disorder. *Arch Gen Psychiatry.* 1985;42:729-736.
18. Mannuzza S, Schneier F, Chapman TF, Liebowitz MR, Klein DF, Fyer AJ. Generalized social phobia: reliability and validity. *Arch Gen Psychiatry.* 1995;52:230-237.
19. Schneier FR, Heckelman LR, Garfinkel R, Campeas R, Fallon BA, Gitow A, Street L, Del Bene D, Liebowitz MR. Functional impairment in social phobia. *J Clin Psychiatry.* 1994;55:322-331.

ORIGINAL ARTICLE

Depressed Mood and the Incidence of Alzheimer's Disease in the Elderly Living in the Community

D. P. Devanand, MD; Mary Sano, PhD; Ming-Xin Tang, PhD; Stuart Taylor, MD; Barry J. Gurland, MD; David Wilder, PhD; Yaakov Stern, PhD; Richard Mayeux, MD

Background: It remains unclear whether depression increases the risk for dementia in the elderly. We evaluated the relationship between depressed mood at baseline and the incidence of dementia, particularly Alzheimer's disease, in the elderly living in the community.

Methods: A total of 1070 elderly individuals, aged 60 years or older, were identified as part of a registry for dementia in the Washington Heights community of North Manhattan, NY. In a prospective, longitudinal design with follow-up for 1 to 5 years, annual physician evaluation and neuropsychological testing were used to assess levels of cognitive impairment and to diagnose dementia. Depressive symptoms were evaluated with the 17-item Hamilton Rating Scale for Depression. Based on clinical considerations and a validity study, a positive score for the depressed mood item was used in statistical analyses. To confirm the results, the total Hamilton Rating Scale for Depression score was also evaluated as the "depression" variable.

Results: Of the 1070 subjects, 218 met criteria for dementia at baseline evaluation. In the 852 subjects without dementia, depressed mood was more common in individuals with greater cognitive impairment. In a follow-up study of 478 of these subjects without dementia (mean±SD, 2.54±1.12 years of follow-up), the effect of baseline depressed mood on the end-point diagnosis of dementia (93% had possible or probable Alzheimer's disease) was evaluated in a Cox proportional hazards model. Depressed mood at baseline was associated with an increased risk of incident dementia (relative risk, 2.94; 95% confidence interval, 1.76 to 4.91; $P<.001$). This effect remained after adjustment for age, gender, education, language of assessment, Blessed Memory Information and Concentration test scores, and Blessed Functional Activity Scale scores (relative risk, 2.05; 95% confidence interval, 1.16 to 3.62; $P<.02$). Similar results were obtained when the total Hamilton Rating Scale for Depression score was used as the depression variable, with the use of the same covariates (relative risk, 1.07 per point interval; 95% confidence interval, 1.02 to 1.11; $P<.01$).

Conclusions: Depressed mood moderately increased the risk of developing dementia, primarily Alzheimer's disease. Whether depressed mood is a very early manifestation of Alzheimer's disease, or increases susceptibility through another mechanism, remains to be determined.

(Arch Gen Psychiatry. 1996;53:175-182)

From the Gertrude H. Sergievsky Center and the Center for Alzheimer's Disease Research in New York City (Drs Devanand, Sano, Tang, Taylor, Gurland, Wilder, Stern, and Mayeux), the Center for Geriatrics at Columbia University (Drs Gurland and Wilder), the Department of Biological Psychiatry, New York State Psychiatric Institute (Drs Devanand, Stern, and Mayeux), and the Departments of Psychiatry (Drs Devanand, Taylor, Gurland, and Wilder) and Neurology (Drs Sano, Tang, Stern, and Mayeux), College of Physicians and Surgeons of Columbia University, New York, NY.

IN THE ELDERLY, it remains unclear whether depression increases the risk of dementia. Depression may be associated with cognitive deficits, and some patients with dementia manifest depressive symptoms.[1-6] Approximately 10% to 30% of patients with Alzheimer's disease (AD) meet criteria for major depression.[7-10] However, some symptoms used to diagnose depressive disorders, including psychomotor change, apathy or lack of interest, sleep difficulties, and disturbances in thinking or concentration, frequently occur in demented patients who are not depressed.[11-13] These nonspecific symptoms may artificially raise the reported prevalence of depression in demented patients.

In the clinically depressed elderly, mild cognitive impairment is not uncommon.[14,15] This cognitive dysfunction improves to varying degrees once the depressive symptoms subside.[16,17] However, there is growing evidence that some of these clinically depressed patients with cognitive impairment develop irreversible dementia in 2 or more years,[16,18,19] although there are some dissenting reports.[20,21] In clinical samples, follow-up studies indicate that cognitively intact elderly patients with depression have only a slightly higher probability of developing dementia than the general population.[22,23]

See Subjects and Methods on next page

SUBJECTS AND METHODS

SUBJECTS

All subjects provided written informed consent to participate in the Washington Heights–Inwood and Columbia Aging Project, a prospective investigation of AD and dementias associated with Parkinson's disease and stroke. Informed consent was obtained from subjects and appropriate advocates, as defined by the Columbia University (New York, NY) institutional review board that approved this project. Sources of potential subjects included referrals by community-based health care providers, random samples from a commercial list and a list obtained from the Health Care Financing Agency, a state agency list of home care recipients, self-referred volunteers, and solicitation by news media. Other details of subject recruitment to this community registry have been described elsewhere.[34,35] Recruitment was limited to a geographically defined area of northern Manhattan.

The present study sample was selected by excluding all subjects identified by a physician to have stroke (by history or by focal neurologic signs or by radiologic evidence consistent with stroke), Parkinson's disease, Huntington's disease, multiple sclerosis, brain tumor, schizophrenia, or mental retardation. Major depression was not an exclusion criterion. Subjects were examined at their residence (home or nursing home), senior citizen center, other community facility, or in a research clinic. Follow-up was conducted with an identical set of evaluation procedures at 1-year intervals for a maximum of 5 years.

DIAGNOSTIC EVALUATION

All evaluations were conducted in either English or Spanish, based on the subjects' primary language and their opinion of which language would yield better performance. A physician obtained a semistructured medical history, conducted a physical and neurologic examination, completed the modified short Blessed Memory Information and Concentration test (BMIC),[36] reviewed the Blessed Functional Activity Scale (BFAS parts 1 and 2),[34,36] and completed the Clinical Dementia Rating.[37] Prescribed medications were reviewed and recorded. The physician, usually a neurologist or internist, also obtained a history of psychotropic medication use and electroconvulsive therapy and made the diagnosis of major depression based on clinical impression. The physician used *DSM-III-R* criteria[38] as a guideline, but there was no attempt to establish reliability of the physician's diagnosis of major depression.

A research technician administered a standardized neuropsychological test battery that assessed memory (verbal and nonverbal), orientation, abstract reasoning, language, and visuospatial abilities. These procedures have been described elsewhere.[34]

The initial diagnosis of dementia was based on a fixed paradigm that used a priori cutoff scores on the neuropsychological tests and evidence of impairment in social or occupational function.[34,35] These cutoff scores on neuropsychological tests were established after the cognitive effects of depression, stroke, and Parkinson's disease were taken into account.[34] As a result, the cutoff scores were conservative enough to avoid misclassification of these three conditions as dementia. The final diagnosis was based on a consensus conference between physicians and neuropsychologists. The diagnosis of dementia was based on the *DSM-III-R* criteria and required evidence of memory impairment and other cognitive deficits based on a neuropsychological test paradigm, as well as evidence of impairment in social or occupational function based on the formal functional assessment, elicited history, or both. After this final consensus diagnosis, subjects who were rated as demented were classified according to cause, based on the available medical and neurologic information. The criteria of the National Institute of Neurological and Communicative Disorders and Stroke–Alzheimer's Disease and Related Disorders Association[39] were used to make the diagnosis of possible or probable AD. In this consensus diagnostic conference, there was no attempt to classify depressive diagnoses according to *DSM-III-R*.

Nondemented subjects were classified into one of three categories: (1) no cognitive impairment (no more than one neuropsychological test score below cutoffs, no functional impairment, and Clinical Dementia Rating of 0); (2) mild cognitive impairment (two or more test scores below cutoffs, no functional impairment, and Clinical Dementia Rating of 0); and (3) moderate cognitive impairment (two or more test scores below cutoffs, no functional impairment, and Clinical Dementia Rating of 0.5).

Follow-up evaluations were conducted at annual in-

Few epidemiologic studies have directly assessed depression as a risk factor for dementia, and many have excluded depressed individuals during sample selection.[24] These studies, mostly of the case-control type, suggest that a history of medically treated depression is more common in cases of dementia than in controls,[25-31] with limited contrary evidence.[32] Overall, these studies suggest that a history of depression slightly increases the risk of dementia.[24]

Major limitations of many of these epidemiologic studies include the use of a case-control design, reliance on history of depression obtained primarily from medical records and informant interviews, absence of direct evaluation of depression, and low statistical power.[33] To our knowledge, there are no published longitudinal epidemiologic studies that have used systematic assessments of depression and cognition to determine whether depression is a risk factor for dementia. In a prospective, longitudinal, population-based study that used direct clinical evaluation of elderly subjects identified from a community registry in a circumscribed geographic area, we evaluated the relationship between the presence of depression and the incidence of dementia, particularly AD.

RESULTS

BASELINE SAMPLE

Baseline information was collected for 1070 subjects. Their demographic and clinical features are described in **Table 1**. The ethnic breakdown was 30% non-Latino white, 41% Latino, and 27% African American, with 1% in other categories. For some clinical variables, eg, psytervals, with the use of the same diagnostic consensus conference procedures. Follow-up diagnoses were made without knowledge of any baseline information. At the diagnostic consensus conference, staff were aware of whether the subject was depressed at that time. However, this did not influence the diagnosis of dementia because the primary dementia criterion, cognitive deficit, was based on a fixed neuropsychological test score paradigm. In addition, subjects were studied as part of a larger study with goals unrelated to those of this report.

DEPRESSION

Two senior researchers formally trained and supervised the interviewers in the use of the HRSD, with the aid of didactic sessions, videotapes, and in-person interviews. The trained interviewer used a semistructured interview guide to administer the 17-item HRSD to the patient.[40] In demented subjects, additional information was obtained from an informant.

To establish reliability, in a series of 52 elderly subjects (32 patients with stroke and 20 normal controls; mean age, 71.5 years), three trained raters and one clinical psychologist conducted interviews in pairs in which one rater administered the scale and the other rater observed the interview. Both raters made independent ratings. Intraclass correlation coefficients were .86 for the depressed mood item and .96 for the total HRSD score.

In a separate validity study of 36 elderly subjects (13 patients with Parkinson's disease and 23 normal controls; mean age, 73.4 years), a trained interviewer administered the HRSD and a psychiatrist (S.T.) independently conducted the Structured Clinical Interview for *DSM-III-R*[38] to diagnose major depressive disorder. In these 36 subjects, the mean (±SD) HRSD score was 4.4±2.8. Six (17%) of these 36 subjects met criteria for major depressive disorder. For the single HRSD item of depressed mood relative to the Structured Clinical Interview for *DSM-III-R* diagnosis of major depressive disorder, sensitivity was 83% and specificity was 70%. Sensitivity and specificity were not improved further by the inclusion of any other HRSD item, or by the total HRSD score (dichotomized as ≥10 or <10).

The symptoms of lack of interest, agitation, insomnia, and weight loss are not uncommon in AD, and the diagnosis of major depression and the total HRSD score can be misleading in such cases. Given these considerations, and the results of the validity study, the HRSD depressed mood item alone (dichotomized as present or absent) was the main variable used for "depression" in statistical analyses. To confirm the results obtained with the depressed mood item, the total HRSD score was also evaluated as the depression variable.

Recent evidence[41,42] suggests a strong association between the presence of the apolipoprotein E-ε4 allele and AD. During the last year of the study, blood was drawn from a subset of available subjects who consented to assessment of the apolipoprotein E genotype.

STATISTICAL ANALYSIS

Baseline Evaluation

Analyses by χ^2 or two-tailed Student's *t* tests were conducted to compare the demographic and clinical features in subjects with and without dementia. Analyses of variance and χ^2 analyses were used to compare relevant demographic and clinical variables in the three subgroups with no, mild, and moderate cognitive impairment. A logistic regression model was used to assess the independent effects of age, education, language, and depression on the diagnosis of dementia.

Follow-up

Cox proportional hazards models[43] were used to assess the relative risk (RR) of incident dementia associated with depression. The timing variable was the duration from the initial visit to the first follow-up time point at which the diagnosis of dementia was made. Follow-up Cox analyses were recalculated with adjustment for age, gender, education, language of assessment (English or Spanish), BMIC scores (range, 0 to 28), and BFAS scores (range, 0 to 17).

In the sample subset in which apolipoprotein E genotypes were determined, subjects with the apolipoprotein E-ε4 allele (homozygous or heterozygous) were classified into one group, and the remaining subjects formed the other group. The Cox proportional hazards model was used to determine if the association of depression with incident dementia remained after accounting for the effect of apolipoprotein E-ε4 on disease risk.

chiatric history, information was not obtained, or could not be obtained reliably, in 1% to 7% of subjects. Compared with the 852 subjects rated as not demented, the 218 demented patients were older, had less education, and were more impaired on tests of cognition (BMIC) and functional ability (BFAS). Of the demented subjects, 89% were given a diagnosis of possible or probable AD with or without concomitant contributory conditions.

Compared with subjects without dementia, the subjects with dementia more frequently scored positively on the HRSD depressed mood item and had significantly higher HRSD total scores (Table 1). Patients with dementia were more likely to be prescribed anxiolytic medications. The two groups did not differ with respect to a history of psychiatric disorder or current or past treatment with antidepressant medications or electroconvulsive therapy (Table 1). The specific type of past psychiatric disorder was not ascertained.

A logistic regression model was used to identify the independent effects of median age (≤74 years vs >74 years), education (≤8 years vs >8 years), language (English or Spanish), and depression on the diagnosis of dementia at baseline evaluation. Median age (RR, 6.22; 95% confidence interval [CI], 4.17 to 9.13; $P<.001$) and education (RR, 2.27; 95% CI, 1.53 to 3.36; $P<.001$) were strongly associated, but depressed mood (RR, 1.34; 95% CI, 0.96 to 1.87; $P<.1$) and language (RR, 1.38; 95% CI, 0.93 to 2.04; $P=.11$) were not associated with the diagnosis of dementia at baseline evaluation.

The degree of cognitive impairment was rated in 849 of the 852 subjects who were not demented at baseline evaluation. Of the 849 subjects, 452 (53%) had no cognitive impairment, 243 (29%) had mild cognitive impairment, and 112 (13%) had moderate cognitive impairment. In these three subgroups, the demographic and clinical features were compared (**Table 2**). There were no differences in gender, history of psychiatric disorder, or current psychotropic medication usage. Greater cognitive impairment was associated with increased age, lower education, and Spanish as the language of assessment. The presence of major depression as determined by the physician's clinical impression, as well as positive scores for the depressed mood item and the total HRSD score, increased significantly with greater cognitive impairment.

In the 849 subjects without dementia, the subgroups with and without a positive score for the HRSD depressed mood item were compared on cognitive performance and functional ability. The depressed group performed more poorly on the BMIC (mean±SD, 4.9±4.4 vs 4.0±4.2; t=2.9, P<.005) and showed greater functional impairment on the BFAS (2.7±3.3 vs 1.5±2.6; t=6.8, P<.001).

Table 1. Baseline Demographic and Clinical Features of the Sample*

Variable	Dementia	No Dementia	P†
Baseline sample, No.	218	852	...
Age, y (mean±SD)	81.9±8.1	73.4±7.3	<.001
Gender, % F	78.4	69.4	<.01
Education, y (mean±SD)	6.8±4.3	9.7±4.8	<.001
Language of assessment, %			
English	47.9	61.9	<.001
Spanish	52.1	38.1	...
BMIC (mean±SD)	16.4±7.1	4.3±4.3	<.001
BFAS (mean±SD)	5.3±4.2	1.1±1.7	<.001
Total HRSD score (mean±SD)	6.1±5.6	4.5±4.6	<.001
HRSD depressed mood item, % positive score	49.1	37.4	<.01
Current antidepressant use, %	2.4	2.2	.86
Current anxiolytic use, %	8.5	3.1	<.001
History of psychiatric disorder, %	10.5	7.9	.23
Ever took antidepressants, %	4.0	6.8	.16
Ever received ECT, %	2.2	1.8	.70

*BMIC indicates Blessed Memory Information and Concentration Test (range, 0 to 28); BFAS, Blessed Functional Activity Scale (parts 1 and 2; range, 0 to 17); HRSD, Hamilton Rating Scale for Depression; and ECT, electroconvulsive therapy.

†A test of significance for χ^2 (categorical variables) or two-tailed t test (continuous variables), as appropriate.

FOLLOW-UP SAMPLE

Of the 849 subjects rated not demented at baseline evaluation, at least one follow-up evaluation was conducted in 478 subjects during a 1- to 5-year period (mean±SD follow-up, 2.54±1.12 years). The number of subjects followed up at each time point was as follows: 391 at year 1, 346 at year 2, 216 at year 3, and 105 at year 4. Of the 353 subjects who were not followed up, 165 subjects were recruited in the last year of the study, which has ended. Reasons for failure to reexamine the others were death (n=15), unavailability for follow-up or relocation (n=125), and refusal (n=48). There were no significant differences in gender, age, language, and depression scores between subjects who were and were not followed up. Duration of follow-up was greater in subjects with a high level of education compared with those with a low level of education (χ^2=9.2, P<.01). The mean (±SD) number of years of education was 10.4±4.8 for subjects who were followed up and 8.9±4.7 for subjects who were not followed up.

The persistence of depressed mood over time was evaluated in the subjects who were followed up. One hundred seven (62%) of the 173 subjects with depressed mood at baseline had depressed mood at 1-year follow-up, and 75% of the 283 subjects without depressed mood at baseline did not have depressed mood at 1-year follow-up (χ^2=62.1, P<.001). Similarly, 63% of subjects with depressed mood at baseline had depressed mood at 2-year follow-up, and 73% of subjects without depressed mood at baseline did not have depressed mood at 2-year follow-up (χ^2=42.8, P<.001). These findings suggested that depressed mood was often an enduring symptom and provided indirect evidence that the interviewers made consistent ratings during the study.

Of the 478 subjects who were followed up, 61 reached the end-point diagnosis of dementia. These 61 subjects comprised 36 (21%) of 173 subjects who were depressed and 25 (9%) of 283 subjects who were not depressed at baseline evaluation (χ^2=13.3, P<.001). At baseline evaluation, these 36 depressed subjects had higher depression (HRSD) and functional impairment (BFAS) scores and were more likely to be Latino (Spanish-speaking) than the 25 nondepressed subjects who developed dementia on follow-up (**Table 3**). However, these two groups did not differ in age, gender, duration from the baseline visit to the final diagnosis of dementia, and BMIC scores. The mean (±SD) HRSD score in the depressed group (9.0±6.1) indicated that the depressive syndromes experienced by these subjects were often mild. On the HRSD depressed mood item (scored 0 [absent] to 4 [severely depressed]), 22 (61%) of these 36 depressed subjects received a score of 1, 11 subjects (31%) received a score of 2, three subjects (8%) received a score of 3, and none received a score of 4. The 36 depressed subjects who developed dementia on follow-up did not differ significantly in baseline total HRSD scores (mean±SD, 9.0±6.1) from the 137 depressed subjects (7.5±4.9; t=1.56) who did not develop dementia on follow-up.

Fifty-seven (93%) of these 61 incident dementia cases were classified as possible (n=9) or probable (n=48) AD. Of the remaining four incident dementia cases, one had progressive supranuclear palsy. The other three incident dementia cases had a progressive clinical course consistent with AD but had other conditions (head injury, alcohol dependence with motor vehicle accident, and multiple sclerosis that developed after the initial evaluation) that were deemed contributing factors. Regardless of dementia subtype, data for all subjects were retained in the main analyses. A Cox proportional hazards model evaluated the effect of baseline depressed mood on the end-point diagnosis of dementia. The RR for reaching this end point was significantly greater in subjects with depressed mood at baseline (RR, 2.94; 95% CI, 1.76 to 4.91; P<.001). The **Figure** presents the survival curves for

Table 2. Baseline Features of Subgroups With No, Mild, and Moderate Cognitive Impairment*

Variable	No Cognitive Impairment	Mild Impairment	Moderate impairment	P†
Total No.	452	279	118	...
Gender, % F	70.1	66.7	73.7	.34
Age, y (mean±SD)	71.6±6.6	74.5±7.5	77.7±7.8	<.001
Education, y (mean±SD)	11.8±4.2	7.8±4.3	6.7±4.2	<.001
Language, % Spanish	25.7	48.6	50.8	<.001
BMIC (mean±SD)	2.5±2.8	5.5±4.1	8.6±5.2	<.001
BFAS (mean±SD)	0.7±1.3	1.3±1.5	2.4±2.4	<.001
Past psychiatric disorder, %	8.5	6.9	8.5	.72
Current antidepressant use, %	1.4	3.3	2.6	.21
Current anxiolytic use, %	2.5	4.5	2.6	.33
Ever took antidepressants, %	8.7	3.6	6.0	.06
Ever received ECT, %	2.4	1.0	1.2	.46
Major depression, current %‡	1.5	2.9	6.8	<.01
Total HRSD score (mean±SD)	3.8±3.9	4.9±4.6	6.6±6.3	<.001
Depressed mood, %	30.3	42.9	52.5	<.001

*BMIC indicates Blessed Memory Information and Concentration Test; BFAS, Blessed Functional Activity Scale (parts 1 and 2); ECT, electroconvulsive therapy; and HRSD, Hamilton Rating Scale for Depression.

†Level of significance in analysis of variance or χ^2, as appropriate.

‡Diagnosis of major depression was based on the clinical impression of the physician, usually a neurologist or internist.

Table 3. Comparison of Depressed and Nondepressed Subjects With Incident Dementia*

Variable	Depressed	Not Depressed	P†
No. (%)	36 (20.8)	25 (8.8)	<.001
Gender, % F	72.0	75.0	.79
Language, % Spanish	66.7	32.0	<.01
Age, y (mean±SD)	78.75±8.14	80.16±9.42	.54
Duration to dementia, y (mean±SD)	1.79±1.02	1.88±0.65	.67
Total HRSD score (mean±SD)	9.0±6.1	2.4±2.3	<.001
BMIC (mean±SD)	7.72±4.71	7.72±5.9	.99
BFAS (mean±SD)	2.89±2.8	1.74±1.69	.05

*HRSD indicates Hamilton Rating Scale for Depression; BMIC, Blessed Memory Information and Concentration Test; and BFAS, Blessed Functional Activity Scale (parts 1 and 2).

†A test of significance for χ^2 (categorical variables) or two-tailed *t* test (continuous variables), as appropriate.

reaching dementia in subjects with and without depression at baseline. The Cox proportional hazards model was then recalculated with age, gender, education, language, and BMIC and BFAS scores included as covariates. Baseline depressed mood remained significantly associated with the end-point diagnosis of dementia (RR, 2.05; 95% CI, 1.16 to 3.62; $P<.02$). The covariates of age (RR, 1.11 per year interval; 95% CI, 1.07 to 1.15; $P<.001$), education (RR, 1.97; 95% CI, 1.05 to 3.68; $P<.05$), BMIC scores (RR, 1.14 per point interval; 95% CI, 1.08 to 1.20; $P<.001$), and BFAS scores (RR, 1.14 per point interval; 95% CI, 1.02 to 1.28; $P<.02$) were significantly associated with an increased risk of developing dementia on follow-up; gender and language showed no significant effects. Similar results were obtained when the four non-AD cases were excluded, with depressed mood significantly associated with the diagnosis of AD on follow-up (RR, 1.91; 95% CI, 1.07 to 3.42; $P=.03$), and the covariates of age, education, BMIC scores, and BFAS scores showed significant effects.

With the use of the same covariates, the Cox analyses were repeated with the total HRSD score as the depression variable. The results were unchanged, with the total HRSD score significantly associated with the endpoint diagnosis of dementia (RR, 1.07 per point interval; 95% CI, 1.02 to 1.11; $P<.01$), and the covariates of age, education, BMIC scores, and BFAS scores showed significant effects. Similar results were obtained with the HRSD score dichotomized into high ($\geq$10) or low (<10) scores (RR, 2.16; 95% CI, 1.14 to 4.08; $P<.02$), and the same covariates remained significantly associated with an increased risk of developing dementia on follow-up.

Of the 48 nondemented subjects with moderate cognitive impairment at baseline evaluation, 30 (62%) met criteria for dementia on follow-up. One possibility is that nearly all these subjects with moderate cognitive impairment would have met criteria for dementia if followed up long enough. To control for the possibility that the definition of moderate cognitive impairment in this study was synonymous with very early dementia, the Cox proportional hazards model was recalculated after exclusion of these 48 subjects with moderate cognitive impairment. The results were unchanged, with the exception that BFAS scores no longer showed a significant effect. Baseline depression (RR, 2.31; 95% CI, 1.04 to 5.15; $P=.04$), age (RR, 1.07 per year interval; 95% CI, 1.07 to 1.19; $P<.001$), education (RR, 3.85; 95% CI, 1.62 to 9.13; $P<.05$), and BMIC scores (RR, 1.13 per point interval; 95% CI, 1.04 to 1.22; $P<.01$) were significantly associated with an increased risk of developing dementia on follow-up; gender, language, and BFAS scores showed no significant effects.

In the subset of 121 subjects who were assessed for the apolipoprotein E genotype, a Cox proportional hazards model evaluated the effect of age, baseline depressed mood, and the presence of the apolipoprotein E-ϵ4

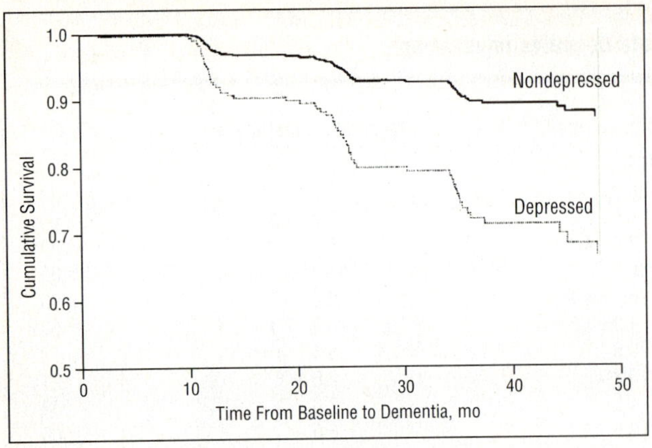

Cumulative survival for subjects with depressed mood at baseline evaluation (dotted line) and for subjects without depressed mood at baseline evaluation (solid line), as a function of time from baseline evaluation to the diagnosis of dementia during follow-up.

allele on the end-point diagnosis of dementia. In this analysis, the magnitude of the RR for reaching this end point was unchanged in subjects with depressed mood at baseline (RR, 2.82; 95% CI, 0.93 to 8.6; *P*=.07). The 33 subjects with the apolipoprotein E-ϵ4 allele manifested a significantly higher relative risk for incident dementia than the 88 subjects without the apolipoprotein E-ϵ4 allele (RR, 4.79; 95% CI, 1.25 to 18.32; *P*=.02), and age showed a significant effect (RR, 1.12 per year interval; 95% CI, 1.05 to 1.20; *P*<.001).

COMMENT

In community-residing elderly subjects without dementia, the presence of depressed mood was associated with a moderately increased risk of dementia on follow-up. This increased risk applied primarily to the development of AD, because at baseline evaluation (89%) and during follow-up (93%) most subjects with dementia met National Institute of Neurological and Communicative Disorders and Stroke–Alzheimer's Disease and Related Disorders Association criteria for possible or probable AD. The presence of depressed mood conferred a RR of 2.05 after controlling for all the major clinical risk factors for dementia that were evaluated, and remained significant after the non-AD dementia cases were excluded. These results were confirmed when similar results were obtained with the HRSD total score as the depression variable. In addition, in the subset in which the apolipoprotein E genotype was assessed, factoring in the effect of the apolipoprotein E-ϵ4 allele did not attenuate the strength of the association between depressed mood and incident dementia. Overall, the RR obtained in this prospective, longitudinal study is at the upper end of the range of the RRs observed in other epidemiologic studies that used case-control designs.[24]

In this study, the subjects were identified and recruited specifically for a community registry that examined risk factors for dementia, and were not randomly sampled from the general elderly population. As a result, the proportion of subjects with dementia, and of subjects with cognitive impairment but without dementia, was high. At the baseline examination of subjects without dementia, the prevalence of depressed mood was higher in subjects with greater cognitive impairment, as has been observed by others.[31] This finding suggests that depressed mood may be more a prodromal or early sign than a risk factor for dementia.[26,29,44] However, in the longitudinal data set, when the Cox analyses were conducted after removal of the subgroup with moderate cognitive impairment at baseline evaluation, depressed mood remained a risk factor for dementia. This argues against the notion that depressed mood is more a prodromal or early sign than a risk factor for dementia. Careful prospective assessment of the onset of depression and of cognitive decline would be necessary to address this issue in future research.

Another possibility is that depression-induced cognitive dysfunction led subjects to meet criteria for dementia at an earlier time point without affecting the total incidence. Several features of our study suggest that this was unlikely. Depressive symptoms were predominantly very mild to mild and therefore were unlikely to result in cognitive impairment of a magnitude sufficient to lead to the diagnosis of dementia. Of note, the cutoff scores on the neuropsychological test paradigm for the diagnosis of dementia were established after the cognitive effects of depression were taken into account and were conservative enough to avoid misclassification. Incident dementia was diagnosed only when there was measurable deterioration in cognitive performance and functional ability compared with baseline evaluation. Therefore, it is unlikely that subjects had "depressive pseudodementia" at baseline evaluation and later worsened to meet criteria for dementia during follow-up.[1,19]

Other epidemiologic data, obtained primarily from cross-sectional studies, have suggested a weak association between depression and cognitive impairment. In North Carolina, 2% of a community sample had a depressive disorder and some cognitive impairment.[45] In the United Kingdom–United States cross-national diagnostic project, Gurland et al[44] reported no association between depressive and cognitive symptoms in New York (*r*=.14) and in London (*r*=−.01). In an Australian community study,[46] eight of 274 met diagnostic criteria for depression and dementia, a finding no different from that expected by chance. However, there was a significant association between depressive and cognitive symptoms (*r*=.30). A recent study[31] from Sweden found a complex relationship between mood disturbance and cognitive impairment in 1304 community-residing subjects who were aged 75 years or older. Depressive symptoms increased as cognitive function declined, but a further cognitive decline was associated with a decrease in depressive symptoms.

Some of these discrepancies in the epidemiologic literature may result from sample size and selection and methods of ascertainment. In this study, the strengths included the large sample size, the prospective design with systematic follow-up, the direct evaluation of community-residing subjects by physicians, detailed neuropsychological assessment to evaluate cognitive impairment and dementia, and the use of trained research personnel to assess depressive symptoms with a standard rating instrument. The use of these methods might have increased the sensitivity to detect the associations observed, in contrast to previous studies that used cross-sectional designs and screening instruments to assess cognitive status.

Most of the depressed subjects had mild symptoms, a finding consistent with other epidemiologic data in the elderly.[24,47] In these mildly depressed subjects, there was an increased RR for incident dementia. One limitation was that diagnostic subtype classification of the depressive illness, eg, major depression, dysthymic disorder, or minor depression, was not attempted. It remains unclear whether the 17-item HRSD is optimal to assess depression in these subjects, and other instruments also need to be evaluated in future research.[48,49] Another limitation, inherent to all community studies of this type, is that the most severely depressed subjects may have refused study participation. There was indirect evidence that this did not occur, because at baseline evaluation there was no difference in the severity of depression between those subjects who subsequently did and did not participate in the follow-up phase. The follow-up rate was less than ideal but was fairly good for a community study with large minority representation.

Although exposure to minor tranquilizers and antidepressants might be expected to be associated with cognitive impairment and an increased likelihood of a diagnosis of dementia, the few case-control studies that have examined this issue failed to find any association.[26,27,32] In this study, the low frequency of antidepressant use limited statistical power and precluded any definitive conclusions.

The common occurrence of depression early during the course of intellectual deterioration has been postulated to be secondary to awareness of eroding cognitive capacities.[7] Depressed patients with AD have degenerative changes in the noradrenergic nucleus locus ceruleus and the substantia nigra,[50] and this points to catecholaminergic deficit as a possible mechanism for the depression observed in some patients with AD. In addition, there is evidence of degeneration of serotoninergic neurons early in the course of AD.[51] The onset of these early degenerative changes may be associated with depression being a prodromal or early sign in a subgroup of patients with AD. Other recent evidence indicates that elderly patients with major depression, particularly those with late onset, have elevated rates of baseline white matter lesions and other structural abnormalities on magnetic resonance images.[52-55] However, whether this subgroup of depressed patients with subcortical lesions has an increased risk of developing dementia remains to be established. In our study, patients with historical or clinical or radiologic evidence of stroke were excluded. However, computed tomographic scans and magnetic resonance images were not available in most of these community-residing subjects, and the contribution of cerebrovascular disease to the clinical picture could not be ascertained.

In conclusion, using a prospective, longitudinal design with detailed clinical assessment in a large sample and controlling for a range of known risk factors, we found depressed mood to be associated with a moderately increased risk of dementia, predominantly AD. Depression is known to worsen the prognosis in other illnesses in the elderly, eg, stroke[56] and myocardial infarction.[57] However, it remains unclear whether successful treatment of depression delays the time point at which the individual at risk meets clinical diagnostic criteria for AD. Another unresolved question is whether depression is a prodromal sign of AD or represents an intermediary factor related in some way to another risk factor that has yet to be identified. These issues need clarification in future research.

Accepted for publication July 28, 1995.

This work was supported by federal grants AG07232, AG08702, and AG10963 from the National Institute of Aging; MH44176 and MH50038 from the National Institute of Mental Health; and the Charles S. Robertson Memorial Gift for Research in Alzheimer's Disease.

Reprint requests to Sergievsky Center, 630 W 168th St, New York, NY 10032 (Dr Mayeux).

REFERENCES

1. Devanand DP, Nelson JC. Concurrent depression and dementia: implications for diagnosis and treatment. *J Clin Psychiatry.* 1985;46:389-392.
2. O'Connor DW, Pollitt PA, Roth M. Coexisting depression and dementia in a community survey of the elderly. *Int Psychogeriatr.* 1990;2:45-53.
3. Emery VO, Oxman TE. Update on the dementia spectrum of depression. *Am J Psychiatry.* 1992;149:305-317.
4. Roth M. The natural history of mental disorder in old age. *J Ment Sci.* 1955; 101:281-301.
5. Kral VA. The relationship between senile dementia (Alzheimer type) and depression. *Can J Psychiatry.* 1983;28:304-306.
6. La Rue A, Spar J, Hill CD. Cognitive impairment in late-life depression: clinical correlates and treatment implications. *J Affective Disord.* 1986;11:179-184.
7. Reifler BV, Larson E, Hanley R. Coexistence of cognitive impairment and depression in geriatric outpatients. *Am J Psychiatry.* 1982;139:623-626.
8. Greenwald BS, Kramer-Ginsberg E, Marin DB, Laitman LB, Hermann CK, Mohs RC, Davis KL. Dementia with coexistent major depression. *Am J Psychiatry.* 1989;146:1472-1478.
9. Wragg RE, Jeste DV. Overview of depression and psychosis in Alzheimer's disease. *Am J Psychiatry.* 1989;146:577-587.
10. Rovner BW, Broadhead J, Spencer M, Carson K, Folstein MF. Depression and Alzheimer's disease. *Am J Psychiatry.* 1989;146:350-353.
11. Burke WJ, Rubin EH, Morris JC. Symptoms of 'depression' in dementia of the Alzheimer type. *Alzheimer Dis Assoc Disord J.* 1988;2:356-362.
12. Cummings JL. Dementia and depression: an evolving enigma. *J Neuropsychiatry.* 1989;1:236-242.
13. Forsell Y, Jorm AF, Fratiglioni L, Grut M, Winblad B. Application of *DSM-III-R* criteria for major depressive episode to elderly subjects with and without dementia. *Am J Psychiatry.* 1993;150:1199-1202.
14. Alexopoulos GS. Heterogeneity and comorbidity in dementia-depression syndromes. *Int J Geriatr Psychiatry.* 1991;6:125-127.
15. Sackeim HA, Steif BL. The neuropsychology of depression and mania. In: Georgotas AC, Cancro R, eds. *Depression and Mania.* New York, NY: Elsevier Science Publishing Co Inc; 1988:265-289.
16. Reynolds CF, Kupfer DJ, Hoch CC, Stack JA, Houck PR, Sewitch DE. Two year follow-up of elderly patients with mixed depression and dementia: clinical and electroencephalographic findings. *J Am Geriatr Soc.* 1986;34:793-799.
17. Stoudemire A, Hill CD, Morris R, Lewison BJ. Long-term outcome of treatment resistant depression in older adults. *Am J Psychiatry.* 1993;150:1539-1540.
18. Reding M, Haycox J, Blass J. Depression in patients referred to a dementia clinic. *Arch Neurol.* 1985;42:894-896.
19. Alexopoulos GS, Meyers BS, Young RC, Mattis S, Kakuma T. The course of geriatric depression with 'reversible dementia': a controlled study. *Am J Psychiatry.* 1993;150:1693-1699.
20. Rabins PV, Merchant A, Nestadt G. Criteria for diagnosing reversible dementia caused by depression: validation by 2-year follow-up. *Br J Psychiatry.* 1984; 144:488-492.
21. Pearlson GD, Rabins PV, Kim WS, Speedic LJ, Moberg PJ, Burns A, Bascom

MJ. Structural brain CT changes and cognitive deficits in elderly depressives with and without reversible dementia ('pseudodementia'). *Psychol Med.* 1989; 19:573-584.

22. Murphy E. The prognosis of depression in old age. *Br J Psychiatry.* 1983;142: 111-119.
23. Baldwin RC, Jolley DJ. The prognosis of depression in old age. *Br J Psychiatry.* 1986;149:574-583.
24. Jorm AF, Van Duijn CM, Chandra V, Fratiglioni L, Graves AB, Heyman A, Kokmen E, Kondo K, Mortimer JA, Rocca WA, Shalat SL, Soininen H, Hofman A, for the EURODEM Risk Factors Research Group. Psychiatric history and related exposures as risk factors for Alzheimer's disease: a collaborative re-analysis of case-control studies. *Int J Epidemiol.* 1991;20:S43-S47.
25. Barclay LL, Zemcov A, Blass JP, McDowell FH. Factors associated with duration of survival in Alzheimer's disease. *Biol Psychiatry.* 1985;20:86-93.
26. Broe GA, Henderson AS, Creasey H, McCusker E, Korten AE, Jorm AF, Longley W, Anthony JC. A case-control study of Alzheimer's disease in Australia. *Neurology.* 1990;40:1698-1707.
27. French LR, Schuman LM, Mortimer JA, Hutton JT, Boatman RA, Christians B. A case-control study of dementia of the Alzheimer type. *Am J Epidemiol.* 1985; 121:414-421.
28. Shalat SL, Seltzer B, Pidcock C, Baker EL. Risk factors for Alzheimer's disease: a case-control study. *Neurology.* 1987;37:1630-1633.
29. Heyman A, Wilkinson WE, Stafford JA, Helms MJ, Sigmon AH, Weinberg T. Alzheimer's disease: a study of epidemiological aspects. *Ann Neurol.* 1984; 15:335-341.
30. Kokmen E, Beard CM, Chandra V, Offord KP, Schoenberg BS. Clinical risk factors for Alzheimer's disease: a population based case-control study. *Neurology.* 1991;41:1393-1397.
31. Forsell Y, Jorm AF, Winblad B. Association of age, sex, cognitive dysfunction, and disability with major depressive symptoms in an elderly sample. *Am J Psychiatry.* 1994;151:1600-1604.
32. Soininen H, Heinonen OP. Clinical and etiological aspects of senile dementia. *Eur Neurol.* 1982;21:401-410.
33. Van Djuin CM, Stijnen T, Hofman A. Risk factors for Alzheimer's disease: overview of the EURODEM collaborative re-analysis of case-control studies. *Int J Epidemiol.* 1991;20:S4-S11.
34. Stern Y, Andrews H, Pittman J, Sano M, Tatemichi TK, Lantigua R, Mayeux R. Diagnosis of dementia in a heterogeneous population: development of a neuropsychological paradigm-based diagnosis of dementia and quantified correction for the effects of education. *Arch Neurol.* 1992;49:453-460.
35. Stern Y, Gurland B, Tatemichi TK, Tang M-X, Wilder D, Mayeux R. Influence of education and occupation on the incidence of Alzheimer's disease. *JAMA.* 1994; 271:1004-1010.
36. Blessed G, Tomlinson BE, Roth M. The association between quantitative measures of dementia and of senile change in the cerebral grey matter of elderly subjects. *Br J Psychiatry.* 1968;114:797-811.
37. Hughes CP, Berg L, Danzinger WL, Coben LA, Martin RL. A new clinical scale for the staging of dementia. *Br J Psychiatry.* 1982;140:566-572.
38. American Psychiatric Association, Committee on Nomenclature and Statistics. *Diagnostic and Statistical Manual of Mental Disorders, Revised Third Edition.* Washington, DC: American Psychiatric Press Inc; 1987.
39. McKhann G, Drachman D, Folstein M. Clinical diagnosis of Alzheimer's disease: report of the NINCDS-ADRDA Work Group under the auspices of Department of Health and Human Services Task Force on Alzheimer's Disease. *Neurology.* 1984;34:939-944.
40. Williams J. A structured interview guide for the Hamilton Depression Scale. *Arch Gen Psychiatry.* 1988;45:742-747.
41. Saunders AM, Strittmatter WJ, Schmechel D, St Goerge-Hyslop PH, Pericak-Vance MA, Joo SH, Roses AD. Association of apolipoprotein E allele e4 with late-onset familial and sporadic Alzheimer's disease. *Neurology.* 1993;43:1467-1472.
42. Mayeux R, Stern Y, Ottman R, Tatemichi TK, Tang M-X, Maestre G, Ngai C, Tycko B, Ginsberg H. The apolipoprotein e4 allele in patients with Alzheimer's disease. *Ann Neurol.* 1993;34:752-754.
43. Lawless JF. *Statistical Model and Methods for Lifetime Data.* New York, NY: John Wiley & Sons Inc; 1982.
44. Gurland B, Copeland J, Kuriansky J, Kelleher M, Sharpe L, Dean L. *The Mind and Mood of Aging.* London, England: Croom Helm; 1983.
45. Blazer D, Williams CD. Epidemiology of dysphoria and depression in an elderly population. *Am J Psychiatry.* 1980;137:439-444.
46. Kay DWK, Henderson AS, Scott R, Wilson J, Rickwood D, Grayson DA. Dementia and depression among the elderly living in the Hobart community: the effect of the diagnostic criteria on the prevalence rates. *Psychol Med.* 1985; 15:771-788.
47. Blazer D, Swartz M, Woodbury M, Manton K, Hughes D, George LK. Depressive symptoms and depressive diagnoses in a community population. *Arch Gen Psychiatry.* 1988;45:1078-1084.
48. Yesavage JA, Brink TL, Rose TL, Adey M. The Geriatric Depression Rating Scale: comparison with other self-report and psychiatric rating scales. In: Crook T, Ferris S, Bartus R, eds. *Assessment in Geriatric Psychopharmacology.* New Canaan, Conn: Mark Powley; 1983:153-167.
49. Alexopoulos GS, Abrams RC, Young RC, Shamoian CA. Cornell Scale for Depression in Dementia. *Biol Psychiatry.* 1988;23:271-284.
50. Zubenko GS, Moossy J. Major depression in primary dementia: clinical and neuropathological correlates. *Arch Neurol.* 1988;45:1182-1186.
51. Nordberg A. Neuroreceptor changes in Alzheimer disease. *Cerebrovasc Brain Metab Rev.* 1992;4:303-328.
52. Coffey CE, Figiel GS, Djang WT, Weiner RD. Subcortical hyperintensity on magnetic resonance imaging: a comparison of normal and depressed elderly subjects. *Am J Psychiatry.* 1990;147:187-189.
53. Baldwin RC, Benbow SM, Marriott A, Tomensen B. Depression in old age: a reconsideration of cerebral disease in relation to outcome. *Br J Psychiatry.* 1993;163:82-90.
54. Lesser IM, Miller BL, Boone KB, Hill-Guttierez E, Mehringer CM, Wang K, Mena I. Brain injury and cognitive function in late-onset psychotic depression. *J Neuropsychiatry Clin Neurosci.* 1991;3:33-40.
55. Krishnan KR, McDonald WM, Escalona PR, Doraiswamy PM, Na C, Figiel GS, Ellinwood EH Jr. Neuroanatomical substrates of depression in the elderly. *Eur Arch Psychiatry Clin Neurosci.* 1993;243:41-46.
56. Morris PLP, Robinson RG, Andrzejewski P, Samuels J, Price TR. Association of depression with 10-year poststroke mortality. *Am J Psychiatry.* 1993;150: 124-129.
57. Frasure-Smith N, Lesperance F, Talajic M. Depression following myocardial infarction: impact on 6-month survival. *JAMA.* 1993;270:1819-1825.

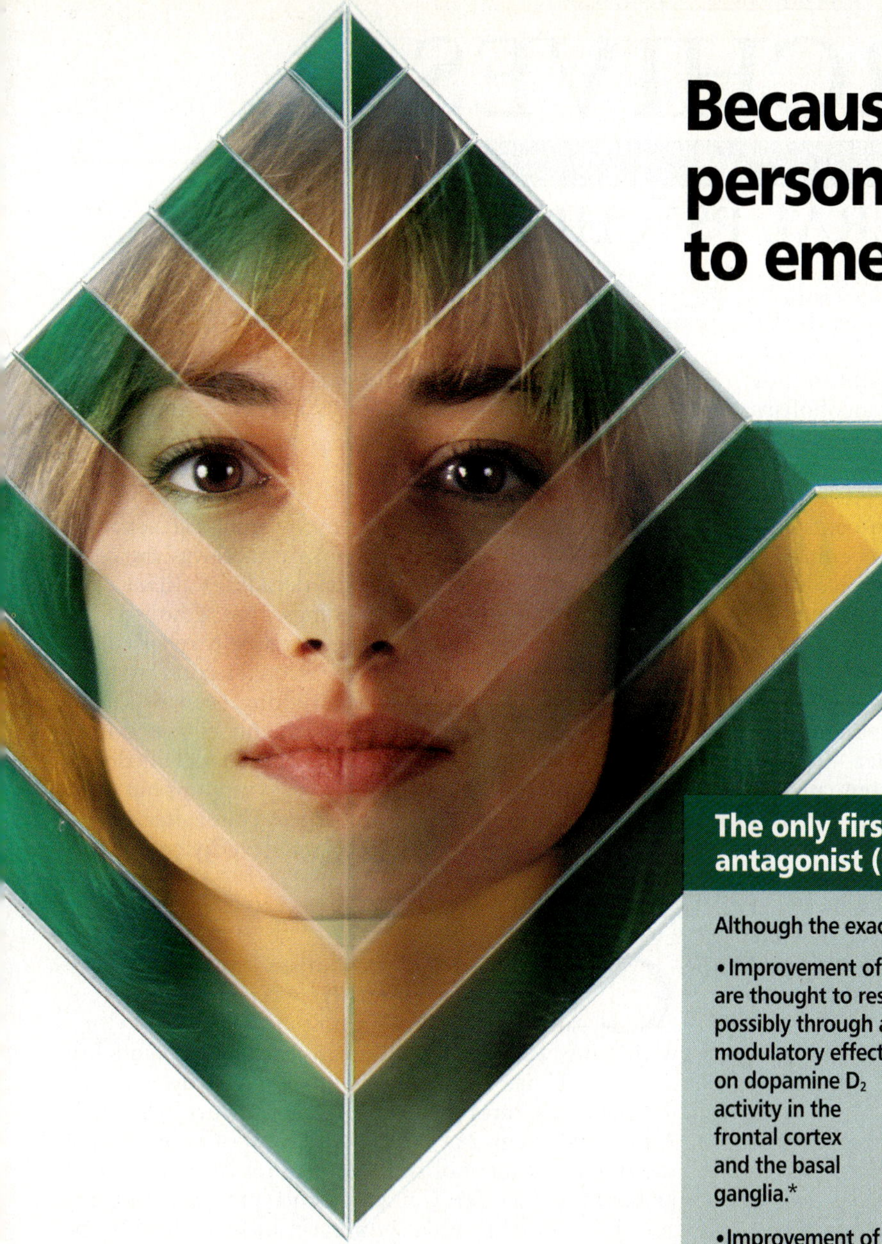

Because a whole person is waiting to emerge.

The only first-choice serotonin/dopamine antagonist (SDA).

Although the exact mechanism of action is unknown:

- Improvement of negative symptoms and lessened risk of EPS are thought to result from blockade of serotonin 5-HT_2 receptors, possibly through a modulatory effect on dopamine D_2 activity in the frontal cortex and the basal ganglia.*
- Improvement of positive symptoms is thought to result from blockade of dopamine D_2 receptors in the limbic system.*

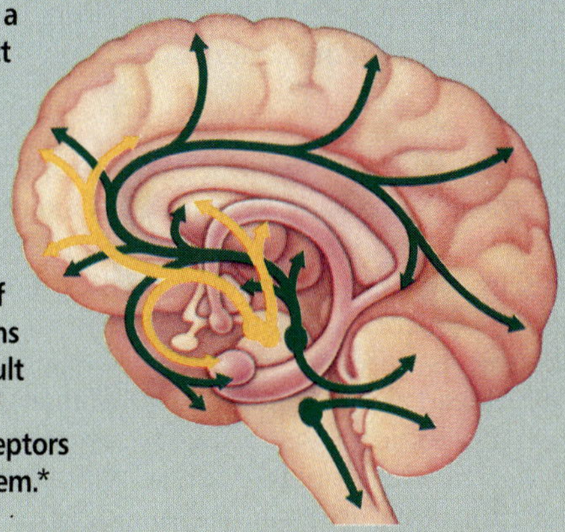

Dopaminergic system   Serotoninergic system

*Ereshefsky L, Lacombe S. Pharmacological profile of risperidone. *Can J Psychiatry.* 1993;38(Suppl 3):S80-S88.

Please see the brief summary of Prescribing Information adjacent to this ad.

JANSSEN · PHARMACEUTICA · RESEARCH FOUNDATION ·   SB SmithKline Beecham Pharmaceuticals

1-, 2-, 3-, 4-mg tablets

Risperdal®
RISPERIDONE

A first choice in psychosis.

Gianoulakis et al (page 250) investigated the basal activity and the response of the pituitary β-endorphin system to alcohol in individuals at high and low risk of developing alcoholism. Compared with low-risk subjects, high-risk subjects presented with lower basal levels of plasma β-endorphin. Alcohol ingestion induced a dose-dependent increase of plasma β-endorphin content in the high-risk but not low-risk subjects. This enhanced sensitivity of the pituitary β-endorphin to alcohol in high-risk subjects may be important in controlling alcohol consumption.

It is unclear why the risk for alcohol problems is elevated among those with panic disorder. **Kushner et al** (page 264) found that alcohol attenuated responses during a panic provocation procedure in subjects with panic disorder. These findings suggest that drinking aimed at obtaining these short-term anxiety-reducing effects may contribute to the high rate at which alcohol problems co-occur with panic disorder. Paradoxically, in the long term, drinking is considered a poor anxiety management strategy, since research shows that chronic alcohol use leads to a worsening of anxiety and other undesirable consequences.

To explore the genetic predisposition to alcoholism, **Volavka et al** (page 258) examined electroencephalographic (EEG) response to a dose of alcohol in 19-year-old sons of alcoholics and sons of nonalcoholic controls in 1979 or 1980. In the early 1990s, these subjects were interviewed to ascertain whether they had developed alcohol and other substance use disorders. The results indicate that a family history of alcoholism predicts the development of substance dependence. Lower EEG response to a dose of alcohol was associated with the later development of alcohol dependence. Thus, lower sensitivity to alcohol effects may predispose to alcoholism.

Naltrexone has been shown to improve abstinence rates and to reduce the risk of relapse in individuals with alcohol dependence, but whether these improvements are sustained following cessation of treatment is unknown. In a 6-month follow-up of alcohol-dependent subjects who had participated in a 12-week controlled trial of naltrexone and psychotherapy, **O'Malley et al** (page 217) found that naltrexone was associated with lower rates of heavy drinking and alcohol-related diagnoses. Differences in level of drinking between naltrexone use and placebo, however, diminished over time, which suggests that continued treatment may benefit some patients.

The course of alcoholism in two groups of men from very different social backgrounds was prospectively charted for several decades. **Vaillant et al** (page 243) noted three major findings. First, although 40% of men with 2 years of abstinence eventually relapsed, after 5 years of abstinence, relapse was rare. In contrast, most men who maintained controlled drinking, even for 3 to 10 years, eventually relapsed. Second, highly educated men began alcohol abuse significantly later than socially disadvantaged men and experienced fewer symptoms but were less likely to achieve stable abstinence. Third, after 5 to 15 years of increasing symptomatology, severity of alcoholism did not continue to progress.

Characteristics of alcoholism in men may vary with age of at onset. Men with an early onset of alcoholism often exhibit antisocial behaviors, with many fulfilling criteria for antisocial personality disorder. Those with antisocial personality disorder often have low rates of central serotonin turnover. **Fils-Aime et al** (page 211) studied a group of men seeking treatment for alcoholism who did not have antisocial personality disorder. Compared with men with late onset of alcoholism, men with early onset had reduced central serotonergic turnover and a history of fighting. Serotonergic treatment strategies in men with alcoholism might best be targeted toward the early-onset group.

Multiple genetic factors interact with the environment to produce a risk for alcoholism. This 8-year follow-up by **Schuckit et al** (page 202) of 450 of 453 subjects demonstrates one biological and genetically influenced factor that predicted future alcoholism. For this relatively highly functional group of men, a low level of response to alcohol was a significant predictor of severe alcohol problems over the subsequent decade and explained much of the relation between a family history and the future development of alcoholism. The data provide evidence about one possibly important risk factor for severe drinking problems, a finding that might lead to more effective prevention strategies.

A Commentary by Dr Enoch Gordis, director of the National Institute on Alcohol Abuse and Alcoholism, is included in this issue (page 199).

Alcoholism in patients seeking treatment is often accompanied by depression. The appropriate treatment of alcoholics with primary depression, which either preceded their alcoholism or continued during long periods of sobriety, has not been well studied. In a double-blind placebo-controlled study, **McGrath et al** (page 232) report that imipramine combined with individual relapse prevention counseling is effective for the treatment of primary depression in alcoholic outpatients. Among subjects whose depression responded to treatment, there was evidence of decreased alcohol abuse with imipramine treatment. These data support antidepressant treatment of primary depression in carefully selected alcoholics.

Alcohol craving has been an illusive concept to accurately quantify during alcoholism treatment studies. **Anton et al** (page 225) have developed and validated a self-rated instrument, the Obsessive-Compulsive Drinking Scale (OCDS), which measures obsessive thinking about alcohol and its compulsive use. The OCDS is correlated with analogue craving scales. The scores of the OCDS change over time in relation to drinking outcome. Early treatment OCDS scores correlated with future drinking. This instrument could prove useful to measure the change in a dimension of craving during alcoholism treatment studies.

Notice to Authors

Length of Text. Ideally, the text of manuscripts (not including abstract, tables, figures, and references) should be under 5000 words. Include a word count on the title page.

Title. The title should be short, specific, and descriptive, emphasizing the main point of the article. Avoid two-part titles, if at all possible. Do not number titles, eg, "I" or "Part I." Title length, including punctuation and spaces, ideally should be under 100 characters and must not exceed 200 characters.

Abstract. The abstract should be structured into four parts and be no longer than 250 words.

Tables and Figures. Material should provide substantive data and not merely illustrate the text. While the main finding of a table or figure may be discussed in the narrative, the table or figure should not duplicate the text. Although no specific guideline applies to all articles, the number and length of tables and figures should be considered carefully and kept to a minimum.

References. All references should be selected carefully to acknowledge previous work or to document a specific point. They should not be exhaustive.

Please consult the "Instructions for Authors" on page 1083 of the December 1995 issue for other details regarding manuscript preparation.

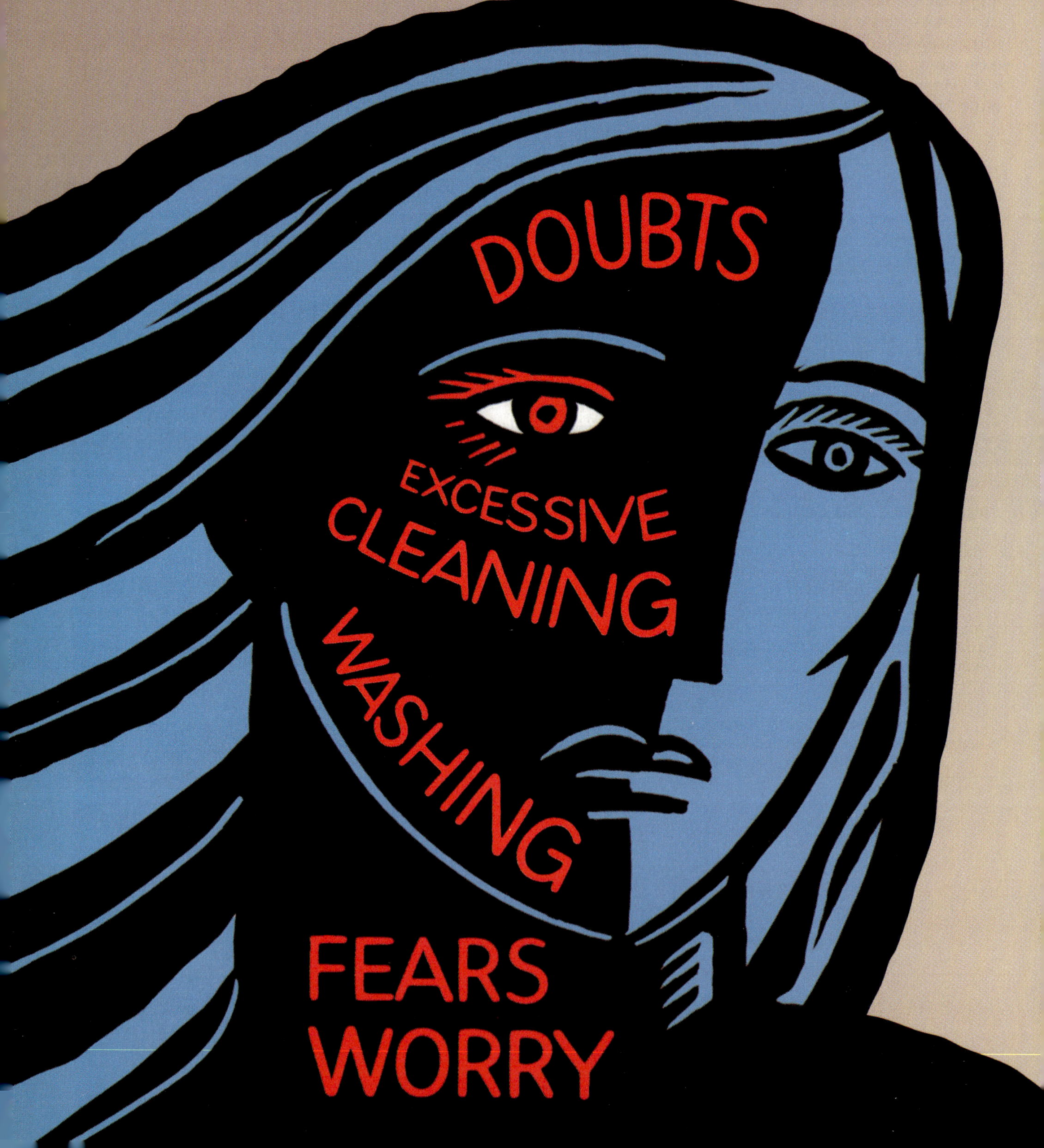
DOUBTS
EXCESSIVE
CLEANING
WASHING
FEARS
WORRY

Alcohol Research

At the Cutting Edge

IT IS a happy coincidence that the *Archives of General Psychiatry* is presenting a superb group of articles on alcoholism in this issue. The National Institute on Alcohol Abuse and Alcoholism (NIAAA) is celebrating its 25th anniversary during this academic year, and much of the research described in these articles was supported by the NIAAA. The Editorial Board has kindly invited me to introduce this issue. I think the best way of doing that is to comment on major conceptual advances made during the last decades, with some illustrations from current research.

A SIGNIFICANT FRACTION OF VULNERABILITY TO ALCOHOLISM IS INHERITED

That alcoholism runs in families has long been known, but only since the 1970s has a mix of twin and adoption studies demonstrated that much of this vulnerability is inherited. The important Swedish adoption study of Cloninger et al[1] has recently been replicated.[2] What is inherited is not yet known, nor is it known whether what is inherited is specific to alcohol. Among many reasonable possibilities are differences in temperament, different initial sensitivity to the rewarding or aversive qualities of alcohol, different abilities to develop tolerance after repeated exposure, different rates and routes of alcohol metabolism, different taste preferences, different signaling from peripheral sites to the brain after drinking alcohol, and different abilities to relate memories of drinking experiences to their consequences.

The search for the relevant genes is now being actively pursued in several settings. It is difficult because alcoholism is likely to be polygenic, with each gene contributing only a portion of the vulnerability. The NIAAA-supported Cooperative Study on the Genetics of Alcoholism (COGA) is a multisite study at six centers. Extensive diagnostic instruments were created for this project, hundreds of probands and families have been interviewed, a complex computerized pedigree database has been incorporated, and all the techniques of statistical genetics and molecular biology are being applied to "informative" families. Phenotypic markers shown previously to be relevant to alcohol are incorporated in the study, including biochemical markers, evoked potential responses, and tests of initial sensitivity to alcohol (the latter being a strong predictor of later alcoholism).[3] The project is moving rapidly ahead, using both candidate genes and microsatellite markers that span the whole genome. The intramural program of the NIAAA is studying with similar techniques the inheritance of alcoholism, specifically, that type of alcoholism marked by early onset[4] or sociopathy. Research with animals is helping to understand the neurochemistry and inheritance of alcohol preference and alcohol effects. Scientists have bred strains of rats over many generations that reliably demonstrate strong or absent alcohol preference. Other investigators are applying the techniques of identifying quantitative trait loci (QTL) to mice and rats to identify the genes responsible for a variety of responses to alcohol, including preference. Similarities between the mouse and human genome give hope that the animal work will provide clues that will accelerate the search of the human genome for alcohol-related genes.

See also pages 202, 211, 217, 225, 232, and 243 and JAMA, *March 13, 1996*

It is important to keep in mind the expected payoff if the search for genes is successful. When the functions of the protein products of these genes are identified, this information will help lead to the development of new treatments and better-focused prevention efforts for those individuals identified as most vulnerable to maladaptive responses. If history is any guide, the study of the abnormal will again shed light on normal physiology. Finally, only with precision in genetic understanding can we define clearly the role of the environment (during development and via current stressors) in increasing the risk for alcoholism.

In alcoholism, genes are not destiny; they only indicate risk. Many genetic discoveries have the potential for misuse: discrimination in employment, insurance, and health care, and stigmatization. Our field is no exception. Our goal will be to bring to people the benefits of genetics research and to avoid its hazards.

APPLICATION OF NEUROSCIENCE TO DRINKING AND THE PHENOMENON OF ADDICTION

All the new techniques of neuroscience (for example, patch clamping, imaging, expression of isolated receptor messenger RNA in in vitro expression systems, electrophysiology, neurochemistry, microdialysis, and cognitive neuroscience) are now being applied to fundamental phenomena of alcohol use and abuse. How alcohol influences the variable expression of receptor subunits and how the initial pattern of subunits affects sensitivity to alcohol are both under study. The role of the reinforcing neural reward circuits and their essential neurotransmitters is being elucidated. The hypothalamic-pituitary-adrenal axis and stress are being studied as one route to abnormal drinking. The toxic effects of alcohol on the structure and function of the nervous system are being explained. Subtle aspects of cognitive impairment are being studied using sophisticated cognitive testing combined with imaging. Important insights into the specificity of ethanol action at various receptors (using clinically realistic concentrations) have revolutionized thinking. No specific receptor for ethanol is known, but the "cutoff phenomenon" observed at several receptors[5] (alcohols of increasing chain length function up to a certain chain length but then lose their effect) suggests that it is not correct to see the actions of alcohol simply as a solvent effect on membrane lipids: alcohols appear to fit into hydrophobic pockets on proteins with steric limitations that vary among receptors.

Clearly, the hope for our neuroscience research is the development of new medications for treatment. The recent approval by the Food and Drug Administration of naltrexone for the early management of alcoholism following withdrawal is the result of work inspired by both clinical observation and neuroscience.[6,7] The clinical clue was the report of some heroin addicts who reacted less to alcohol after they had been treated with naltrexone for their heroin addiction. The neuroscience background was the older demonstration in animals that opiate antagonists reduced a variety of ingestive behaviors, including alcohol intake. Naltrexone in combination with counseling had two main effects: it delayed the time to the first drink and reduced the proportion of "slips" that became full-blown binges. The article in this issue on naltrexone is an important continuation of this work.[8] Meanwhile, European investigators have conducted large controlled clinical trials with acamprosate (calcium acetyl homotaurinate) in newly detoxified alcoholics and have found that this drug is also effective in maintaining abstinence.[9]

ACCEPTANCE OF THE STUDY OF MENTAL PROCESSES IN ALCOHOL ACTION

Certain prior experiences with alcohol, some of which can only be ascertained by asking about mental processes, affect the reaction to alcohol. For example, under certain dosing conditions, the development of tolerance to alcohol measured with specific behaviors can be accelerated if the test behavior is rewarded[10] or practiced while the subject is intoxicated.[11] Certain responses to alcohol can be produced with placebo beverages that simulate alcoholic beverages in individuals who expect certain effects from drinking. Different definitions of *craving* have been offered, largely in response to criticism that the term has been used loosely. More precise definitions are permitting more targeted research on this important construct.[12]

NEW INSIGHTS INTO HOW ALCOHOL DAMAGES ORGANS

Novel mechanisms of toxicity are under intense study. In withdrawal, the potential for excitatory neurotransmitter and glucocorticoid damage to the hippocampus is leading to reconsideration of the safety of nonmedical detoxification. Areas of investigation in liver damage include the role of autoantibodies to adducts of liver protein with acetaldehyde, the role of different dietary fats together with alcohol in causing damage, and the role of intestinal endotoxin and a network of inflammatory cytokines that are stimulated by endotoxin following alcohol ingestion.[13] Different possible mechanisms of fetal damage from alcohol are being studied. Finally, the coronary protective effect of moderate alcohol use is being investigated: mechanisms of protection as well as the risk-benefit tradeoffs of moderate drinking at different stages of life.[14]

NEW APPROACHES TO TREATMENT

Two major trends have evolved. First, methods of clinical trials long standard in most areas of medicine have now become essential in alcoholism research: randomization, appropriate controls, blinding, power calculations, and defined and objectively measured outcomes. The older approaches, which were the equivalent of "deep in my heart I know our program works," can no longer be funded and are (slowly) disappearing from discourse, even in nonresearch settings. Excellent trials that have produced decisive evidence include the Veterans Administration Cooperative Studies on disulfiram[15] (no effect on total abstinence, modest effect on number of drinking days) and lithium[16] (no effect), as well as the work with naltrexone referred to above. Other trials with a variety of receptor-related agents are in progress, all with good design. Subgroups of alcoholics with psychiatric comorbidity may benefit from pharmacotherapies that do not work well with alcoholism alone.[17] The impression that alcoholism is heterogeneous has led to important matching studies (such as the NIAAA cooperative study, Project MATCH [Matching Alcoholism Treatment to Client Heterogeneity]) to determine whether matching carefully typed patients to clearly differentiated manual-driven verbal treatments can improve outcome.[18] The second trend, of course, is the application of neuroscience to the development of new pharmacologic agents. This trend is likely to become stronger with time and is our best current hope for new therapy.

PREVENTION CAN BE STUDIED RIGOROUSLY

Interventions can generally be divided into two categories: those aimed at individuals or small groups (such as school-based programs) and those that affect the whole population through regulatory and legal controls (such as age limits for drinking or beverage price policy). Prevention research is difficult: investigators have little control over activities in the community that frequently change and can affect outcomes. Nevertheless, important results have been obtained in well-designed studies.

Young lives have been saved by two measures: increasing the legal drinking age to 21 years[19,20] and setting the maximum blood alcohol limit in young drivers at 0.02% (so-called zero tolerance).[21] School-based programs closely linked to other community activities can reduce drinking in preadolescents. It is now evident that measures that affect the whole population also affect heavy drinkers. Historical analysis[22] and computer modeling[23] indicate that highway deaths and cirrhosis deaths have varied inversely with the price of beverage alcohol and that even heavy drinkers drink less in response to increased price.

To assess the long-term effects of prevention interventions, it is important to know how alcohol problems change with time, both in individuals and in society. The remarkable longitudinal study of several hundred individuals over decades reported in this issue of the ARCHIVES[24] demonstrates not only the high mortality of alcohol abuse and dependence but also the wide fluctuations in alcohol use and abuse during the lives of individuals. National long-term trends can be studied only with excellent epidemiology. One major advance has been the recent NIAAA National Longitudinal Alcohol Epidemiologic Study (NLAES),[25] a nationwide household survey that involved a careful national sample of 42 862 people. The survey was designed to analyze not merely by separate symptoms of alcoholism and other psychiatric conditions, as previous studies have done, but also by the presence of total syndromes, as defined by *DSM-III-R*, *DSM-IV*, and *ICD-10* (*International Statistical Classification of Diseases, 10th Revision*).

Final Note: It is clear that we are closer to answering the fundamental questions regarding alcohol abuse and alcoholism: Why is it that millions of otherwise intelligent and dependable people cannot stop abusive drinking even though they know they are killing themselves? How can we better prevent alcohol problems, and if they occur, treat them better and reverse their consequences? The articles in this issue of the ARCHIVES are examples of why we can look to the future with confidence. Young investigators about to choose a field of research should consider alcoholism as a topic whose importance, scientific interest, and intellectual challenge are extraordinary.

Enoch Gordis, MD
Director
National Institute
on Alcohol Abuse
and Alcoholism
Suite 400
6000 Executive Blvd
Bethesda, MD 20892-7003

More information concerning the points covered in this article can be found in the following two fully referenced publications of the NIAAA: Special Reports to the US Congress on Alcohol and Health, *triennial reports that describe progress in developing knowledge on alcohol abuse and alcoholism, and* Alcohol Alert, *a quarterly bulletin for clinicians and other health professionals. Information on these publications may be obtained by writing to the National Institute on Alcohol Abuse and Alcoholism Scientific Communications Branch, Suite 409, Willco Bldg, MSC 7003, 6000 Executive Blvd, Bethesda, MD 20892-7003, or by calling 301-443-3860.*

REFERENCES

1. Cloninger CR, Bohman M, Sigvardsson S. Inheritance of alcohol abuse. *Arch Gen Psychiatry.* 1981;38:861-868.
2. Sigvardsson S, Bohman M, Cloninger CR. Replication of the Stockholm Adoption Study of Alcoholism. *Arch Gen Psychiatry.* In press.
3. Schuckit MA, Smith TL. An 8-year follow-up of 450 sons of alcoholics and control subjects. *Arch Gen Psychiatry.* 1996;53:202-210.
4. Fils-Aime M-L, Eckardt MJ, George DT, Brown GL, Mefford I, Linnoila M. Early-onset alcoholics have lower cerebrospinal fluid 5-hydroxyindoleacetic acid levels than late-onset alcoholics. *Arch Gen Psychiatry.* 1996;53:211-216.
5. Chaoying L, Peoples RW, Weight FF. Alcohol action on a neuronal membrane receptor: evidence for a direct interaction with the receptor protein. *Proc Natl Acad Sci U S A.* 1994;91:1-5.
6. Volpicelli JR, Alterman AI, Hayashida M, O'Brien CP. Naltrexone in the treatment of alcohol dependence. *Arch Gen Psychiatry.* 1992;49:876-880.
7. O'Malley SS, Jaffe AJ, Chang G, Schottenfeld RS, Meyer RE, Rounsaville B. Naltrexone and coping skills therapy for alcohol dependence: a controlled study. *Arch Gen Psychiatry.* 1992;49:881-887.
8. O'Malley SS, Jaffe AJ, Chang G, Rode S, Schottenfeld R, Meyer RE, Rounsaville B. Six-month follow-up of naltrexone and psychotherapy for alcohol dependence. *Arch Gen Psychiatry.* 1996;53:217-224.
9. Sass H, Soyka M, Mann K, Zieglgänsberger W. Relapse prevention by acamprosate: results from a placebo-controlled study in alcohol dependence. *Arch Gen Psychiatry.* In press.
10. Haubenreisser T, Vogel-Sproft M. Reinforcement reduces behavioural impairment under an acute dose of alcohol. *Biochem Behav.* 1987;26:29-33.
11. Le AD, Kalant H. Influence of intoxicated practice on the development of acute tolerance to the motor impairment effect of ethanol. *Psychopharmacology.* 1992;106:572-576.
12. Anton RF, Moak DH, Latham PK. The Obsessive-Compulsive Drinking Scale: a new method of assessing outcome in alcoholism treatment studies. *Arch Gen Psychiatry.* 1996;53:225-231.
13. Lands WEM. Cellular signals in alcohol-induced liver injury: a review. *Alcohol Clin Exp Res.* 1995;19:928-938.
14. National Institute on Alcohol Abuse and Alcoholism. *Moderate Drinking.* Washington, DC: Public Health Service; 1992. Alcohol Alert No. 16. Publication PH315.
15. Fuller RK, Branchey L, Brightwell DR, Derman RM, Emrick CD, Iber FL, James KE, Lacoursiere RB, Lee KK, Lowenstam I, Maany I, Neiderhiser D, Nocks JJ, Shaw S. Disulfiram treatment of alcoholism: a Veterans Administration Cooperative Study. *JAMA.* 1986;256:1449-1455.
16. Dorus W, Ostrow DG, Anton R, Cushman P, Collins JF, Schaefer M, Charles HL, Hayashida M, Malkerneker U, Willenbring M, Fiscella R, Sather MR. Lithium treatment of depressed and nondepressed alcoholics. *JAMA.* 1989;262:1646-1652.
17. McGrath PJ, Nunes EV, Stewart JW, Goldman D, Agosti V, Ocepek-Welikson K, Quitkin FM. Imipramine treatment of alcoholics with primary depression: a placebo-controlled clinical trial. *Arch Gen Psychiatry.* 1996;53:232-240.
18. Project MATCH Research Group. Project MATCH: rationale and methods for a multisite clinical trial matching patients to alcoholism treatment. *Alcohol Clin Exp Res.* 1993;17:1130-1145.
19. O'Malley PM, Wagenaar AC. Effects of minimum drinking age laws on alcohol use, related behaviors, and traffic crash involvement among American youth: 1976-1987. *J Stud Alcohol.* 1991;52:478-491.
20. Wagenaar AC. Preventing highway crashes by raising the legal minimum age for drinking: the Michigan experience 6 years later. *J Safety Res.* 1986;17:101-109.
21. Hingson R, Heeren T, Winter M. Lower legal blood alcohol limits for young drivers. *Public Health Rep.* 1994;109:736-744.
22. Cook PJ. The effect of liquor taxes on drinking, cirrhosis, and auto accidents. In: Moore MH, Gerstein DR, eds. *Alcohol and Public Policy: Beyond the Shadow of Prohibition.* Washington, DC: National Academy of Sciences; 1981:255-285.
23. Chaloupka FJ. Effects of price on alcohol-related problems. *Alcohol Health Res World.* 1993;17:46-53.
24. Vaillant GE. A long-term follow-up of male alcohol abuse. *Arch Gen Psychiatry.* 1996;53:243-249.
25. Grant BF. Alcohol consumption, alcohol abuse and alcohol dependence: the United States as an example. *Addiction.* 1994;89:1357-1365.

An 8-Year Follow-up of 450 Sons of Alcoholic and Control Subjects

Marc A. Schuckit, MD, Tom L. Smith, PhD

Background: Between 1978 and 1988, 453 sons (age range, 18 to 29 years) of alcoholic and control subjects were evaluated for their level of reaction (LR) to alcohol. This article presents the results of the 8.2-year follow-up of 450 of these men. The three goals were (1) to attempt to replicate results of the follow-up of the first 223 subjects, (2) to evaluate the potential impact of the quantity and frequency of drinking at the time of the original study on the relationship between LR and alcoholic outcome (ALC), and, most importantly, (3) to test if the relationship between family history (FH) and ALC might be mediated by LR in a subset of the sample.

Methods: Face-to-face structured follow-up interviews were carried out with the subjects and separately with an additional informant, and blood samples, as well as urine specimens, were obtained for determination of state markers of heavy drinking and drug toxicology screens.

Results: First, the rate of development of *DSM-III-R* abuse and dependence on alcohol was 14.1% and 28.6%, respectively, for family history positive (FHP) subjects, compared with 6.6% and 10.8%, respectively, for family history negative (FHN) men. Second, neither consideration of the quantity nor the frequency of drinking at the time of the original study, nor their combination, effectively diminished the relationships between LR and ALC. Third, among men who drank and demonstrated the 15% highest and lowest scores on LR at about the age of 20 years (ie, 30% of the relevant population), the correlation between FH and ALC was greatly reduced when LR was considered, but the correlation between LR and ALC was not greatly diminished when the impact of FH was evaluated.

Conclusions: In this sample of moderately functional white men, the development of alcoholism occurred in relationship to an FH of alcoholism, but alcohol abuse or dependence was unrelated to prior psychiatric disorders. For this group, LR at the age of 20 years was associated with future alcoholism in a manner that was independent of the drinking practices at the time of the original study. At least among those men with clearly high and low LR scores, these data are consistent with the conclusion that LR might be a mediator of the alcoholism risk.

(Arch Gen Psychiatry. 1996;53:202-210)

Family, twin, and adoption studies have documented the importance of genetic influences in alcoholism, and these studies have revealed several indications about how complex these factors are likely to be.[1-7] Among the complicating factors is evidence of genetic heterogeneity[8] where there are likely to be multiple genetic factors that increase the risk for alcohol-related problems through different mechanisms. For example, a number of genetically influenced conditions (eg, schizophrenia, antisocial personality disorder [ASPD], and mania) each carry an elevated risk for alcoholism[9-11]; however, the majority of alcohol-dependent men and women do not demonstrate any of these preexisting major psychiatric conditions.[12] It is likely that there are still important subgroups among these more straightforward alcoholic individuals.

In recognition of the multifactorial and possibly polygenic nature of these influences in alcoholism, along with the likelihood of genetic heterogeneity, in 1978, we began a prospective investigation of individuals from a large number of families of alcoholics. It was hoped that these subjects might help to identify a "theme" of characteristics, or even a phenotype associated with the increased alcoholism risk observed in some alcoholic families. In structuring the investigation, the effects of genetic heterogeneity were partially controlled by excluding individuals who demonstrated major preexisting psychiatric disorders (eg, ASPD, schizophrenia, and mania) in themselves or a first-degree relative. The potential impact of a fetal alcohol syndrome[13] was minimized by placing an emphasis on offspring of alcoholic fathers, with no alcohol dependence in the mother antedating the birth of the subject.

Thus, the sample that formed the basis for the major analyses presented be-

See Subjects and Methods on next page

From the Department of Psychiatry, School of Medicine, University of California–San Diego, and the Alcohol Research Center, Veterans Affairs Medical Center, San Diego.

SUBJECTS AND METHODS

All 453 men, originally tested between the ages of 18 and 29 years, had been located and contacted.[26,27] They represented 454 initial evaluations, but one subject had been tested twice a number of years apart; thus, there were 453 individuals involved. Follow-up evaluations were all carried out between 1989 and 1994, with the 1989 interviews focusing on men who were originally tested in 1978 or 1979 and so on. During follow-up, three men had died: one died of heart disease, one died of acquired immunodeficiency syndrome (AIDS) associated with sexual transmission, and one committed suicide during an alcoholic binge (follow-up data were available on all three men). Three of the subjects refused a personal interview, with the result that face-to-face evaluations were carried out regarding 450 (99.3%) of the 453 men. The structured interview used *DSM-III-R* diagnostic criteria[28] to review abuse and dependence on alcohol and all illicit substances and to evaluate the development of any major anxiety disorders, major affective disorders, and schizophrenia. The interview was a modification of an interview developed from the Schedule for Affective Disorders and Schizophrenia[29] by the Alcohol Research Center, Veterans Affairs Medical Center, San Diego.

The subject's self-reports on substance use patterns, substance use disorders, and psychiatric conditions were corroborated through an identical face-to-face interview that was administered to the additional informant, usually the spouse, but with questions altered to address the subject's history. In addition, a blood sample was obtained from each subject for evaluation of state markers of heavy drinking (eg, γ-glutamyltransferase[14]), and a urine sample was used for a drug toxicology screening.

The final period of the follow-up sessions with the subject and the additional informant reviewed the history of substance use disorders and major psychiatric conditions in the subject's first- and second-degree relatives by using *DSM-III-R* criteria. This procedure was used to check the accuracy of the initial FH diagnosis and to determine whether any relatives had experienced a substance use disorder during follow-up.

The first step in the analyses reported herein was to determine the FH status by using data from all the intake and follow-up interviews with the subjects and the information supplied by the additional informant at follow-up. For all the data presented in **Table 1** and **Table 2**, a man was classified as having an FHP if he had a father with alcohol abuse or dependence, and 59.9% of these men had at least one additional alcoholic first- or second-degree relative. The FHN status was established if no first- or second-degree relative had alcohol abuse or dependence. By using these rules, two of the 450 subjects were excluded from the analyses because, during follow-up, one had discovered that he was adopted, and the other had learned from his mother that she was not sure of the identity of his father. With these exclusions, there were 448 men left in the analyses. To limit the data in this report to the most homogeneous samples possible, 58 FHP men were also excluded because, while they did have an alcoholic relative, this did not include the father; this left 390 subjects eligible for these analyses. In addition, 32 men who were originally classified as having an FHN were found to have an alcoholic second-degree relative; therefore, they were excluded because they could not clearly be labeled as having full FHN nor full FHP status. Thus, the final sample for the first set of analyses comparing the two FH groups in Table 1 included 358 subjects (ie, 192 FHPs and 166 FHNs).

Continued on next page

low is composed of individuals who were family history positive (FHP)—at higher risk for future alcoholism based on alcohol abuse or dependence in the father. For each subject who was at higher risk, a family history negative (FHN) control was selected, matched on the quantity and frequency of drinking, smoking, and drug use histories, as well as on demography. Because of the desire to incorporate an alcohol challenge component into the work, all FHP and FHN pairs had some experience with alcohol. Between 1978 and 1988, subjects were originally studied between the ages of 18 and approximately 29 years, with the upper limit chosen for fear that individuals who had not experienced alcohol dependence by their late 20s might be those who did not carry the biological risk for this disorder, and the lower age reflecting the need for informed consent and the desire to evaluate reactions to alcohol in subjects with adult physical development and the need for informed consent.

To select FHP- and FHN-matched pairs, each year between 1978 and 1988, a questionnaire was distributed to about 700 individuals who were selected at random from lists of students and nonacademic staff at the University of California–San Diego. Repetitive mailings were used to generate a 50% to 70% response rate, depending on the financial resources. Then, all available higher-risk FHP subjects who were drinkers but not alcohol-dependent were identified, and specific subjects were contacted at random, with an estimated 80% of those approached agreeing to participate. The purpose of the large mailing was to generate a large enough pool of FHNs to allow for matching with FHPs on age, race, religion, education, and height-weight ratio, as well as smoking and drug and alcohol use histories. Appropriate higher-risk FHP individuals and lower-risk FHN controls were invited to the laboratory for face-to-face evaluations, by using subsections of the Schedule for Affective Disorder and Schizophrenia (SADS) for a more detailed alcohol and drug use history and for the collection of blood samples to evaluate state markers of heavy drinking as a verification of the recent alcohol use patterns.[14] When family histories of alcoholism and other psychiatric disorders were unclear, subjects were asked for permission for research staff to gather additional information from at least one first-degree relative.

During the years, 453 separate subjects were evaluated for short-term challenges with alcohol, with most sessions involving placebo, 0.75 mL/kg, or ethanol, 1.1 mL/kg. The theory to be tested grew out of anecdotal reports from alcohol-dependent patients who from an early age were able to consume large amounts of alcohol with relatively little effects. Thus, as described in more detail elsewhere,[1] the need for more alcohol to get the effects achieved

For several of the analyses, a single score that related to the LR to alcohol at approximately the age of 20 years was required. This measure was based on the change from baseline to 1 hour (the time of the peak blood alcohol concentration) after the consumption of ethanol, 0.75 mL/kg, focusing on the three measures available on the largest number of subjects. These included the high and drug subscale scores for the Subjective High Assessment Scale, the total change in body sway following alcohol, and the alcohol-related change in the cortisol level.[16,18,19,24] Because not all men had all measures at the key time point, and to address changes in protocols during the years (eg, the subset of 126 men who also received a diazepam challenge), a *z* score approach was used. To accomplish this, *z* scores were generated separately within each of the protocol subgroups, as the research method changed slightly every 5 years when new funding was sought for continuation of the project. These *z* scores were selected for an individual based on the number that was most deviant from that group mean for that measure. In protocols in which multiple doses of alcohol had been used, *z* scores for the 0.75-mL/kg dose were generated separately based on subgroups in a manner that controlled for order effects. To produce the *z* score within each relevant subgroup, the mean value for the measure was determined for the group, each individual's score was subtracted from that mean, and the resulting figure was divided by the SD for the variable within that subgroup. The final LR variable for an individual was derived across the Subjective High Assessment Scale, body sway, and cortisol level by using the lowest *z* score that was generated as an indication of that subject's lowest intensity of response. Because of the possible racial differences on the LR, seven subjects who were not fully white were excluded, while, for 16 men, data on the LR were missing at the key time point; thus, the analyses on the reaction to alcohol focused on 335 individuals.

For the analyses reported in Table 2 and **Table 3**, alcoholism at outcome was defined as an individual who met *DSM-III-R* criteria for alcohol abuse or dependence during follow-up. However, because alcoholism at outcome is a dichotomous variable, a second outcome measure was used, namely, the number of the nine *DSM-III-R* diagnostic items or alcohol problems that was fulfilled by the individual during follow-up.

Having determined the FH, LR, and outcome scores, the next step in the analyses was to explore the relationships between the LR and outcome, controlling for the pattern of alcohol intake at time 1 (ie, approximately the age of 20 years), when the men were originally tested with alcohol. Included in these analyses in Table 3 was a measure of the average quantity of alcohol consumed per occasion during the 6 months before original testing analyzed as the number of 10 gram units of alcohol consumed. The frequency of alcohol intake at time 1 was measured as the average number of days per month on which drinking occurred in the 6 months before testing. Pearson correlation coefficients were determined with regard to the relationships among the variables (continuous and dichotomous); then, partial correlations were generated to control for the impact of specific variables (eg, the relationship between LR and alcoholism at outcome, controlling for the measures of alcohol intake at time 1). Similar correlation and partial correlation approaches were used in Table 2 to evaluate the relationships between the characteristics of subjects at time 1 (eg, FH and LR) and the two versions of the alcohol outcomes at follow-up.

by others with less alcohol consumption could contribute to escalating intake and a higher risk for problems.

During test sessions, the time-to-peak blood alcohol concentration (BAC) and the rate of disappearance of ethanol from the blood following challenges was identical in the two family groups.[15] Despite these similarities, approximately 40% of the FHP subjects but less than 10% of the FHN subjects demonstrated low levels of subjective feelings of intoxication, as measured on the Subjective High Assessment Scale following the alcohol challenges.[16] A recent meta-analysis has corroborated that basic conclusion.[17] Subsets of the 453 subjects were also evaluated for alcohol-related changes in a motor performance task (body sway), for alterations in prolactin, cortisol, and corticotropin (adrenocorticotropic hormone) levels, and for electrophysiological changes following drinking.[16,18-24] Each of these measures has revealed less intense responses to alcohol in FHP subjects than in FHN controls. A subgroup of 126 men (63 FHP and FHN pairs) were included in this sample who were tested for their intensity of response to a comparison brain depressant (ie, diazepam) with no evidence that the same men who showed the decreased reaction to alcohol demonstrated a decreased response to the benzodiazepine.[25]

However, a difference between FHP and FHN groups at approximately the age of 20 years does not indicate whether the diminished response relates to the future risk for alcohol use disorders or other syndromes. Several years ago, the data from the follow-up evaluations of the first 223 of the 453 men were analyzed.[26] These data indicated that a low level of response to alcohol at the age of 20 years was a relatively potent predictor of alcohol abuse or dependence almost 10 years later. That sample was not large enough to carry out more sophisticated analyses, and, without replication, the results were considered preliminary.

To date, the data support the theory that, in a society of heavy drinkers where alcohol is readily available and intoxication is often encouraged, some people who drink ad libitum might be at a disadvantage in learning to control their alcohol intake. One mechanism that might impair the ability to regulate intake carefully is the need for relatively large amounts of alcohol to have an effect from early on in the drinking career. This might serve to maximize the chances of consumption of large doses of alcohol that, in turn, could cause body damage and produce both pharmacokinetic and pharmacodynamic tolerance, the need for even higher doses of alcohol, the subsequent association with heavier drinking coevals, and so on. This low level of response to alcohol would not, of course, be relevant to everyone, but it is one possible factor among other influences in producing the alcoholism risk. Thus, people who do not choose to drink ad libitum but who severely limit their alcohol intake would not be at a high risk for alcoholism, regardless of the in-

Table 1. Demography, Substance Use Patterns, and Follow-up Diagnoses for 358 Men*

Variable	FHP (n=192)	FHN (n=166)	Statistic†	P
Time 1: intake				
Alcohol use, mean (SD)				
Average quantity, drinks/d	2.9 (1.50)	2.7 (1.39)	1.59	.12
Average frequency, d/mo	8.5 (6.05)	9.2 (6.28)	−1.10	.28
Time 2: follow-up				
Mean (SD)				
Age	31.1 (2.92)	31.4 (2.96)	−1.16	.25
Follow-up, y	8.1 (1.56)	8.3 (1.72)	−0.63	.53
Level of education, y	15.7 (1.53)	16.2 (1.66)	−3.26	.001
Alcohol use				
Maximum quantity, drinks/d	10.4 (5.89)	8.8 (4.89)	2.71	.007
Maximum frequency, d/mo	17.6 (9.14)	17.6 (8.95)	0.02	.99
DSM-III-R dependence items	1.5 (1.84)	0.8 (1.36)	4.27	.001
Interval substance use, %				
Alcohol	100	100	...	...
Cannabinol	71.9	58.4	7.13	.007
Stimulant	38.0	30.7	2.09	.15
Other drugs	34.9	28.3	1.78	.19
Interval diagnosis, %‡				
Any diagnosis	51.0	28.3	19.08	<.001
Alcohol				
Abuse	14.1	6.6	5.19	.03
Dependence	28.6	10.8	17.38	<.001
Cannabinol				
Abuse	1.8	2.9	<1	.57
Dependence	3.6	2.2	1.45	.57
Stimulant				
Abuse	0.9	0.7	<1	.89
Dependence	2.7	0.7	1.50	.22
Anxiety or depressive diagnosis	3.6	3.6	<1	.99
Other diagnoses	2.7	3.6	<1	.63

FHP indicates family history positive; FHN, family history negative.
†t Test values for means; χ^2 test values for percentages.
‡Subjects may have more than one diagnosis so percentages of "Any diagnosis" will not equal the sum of the individual diagnoses percentages.

tensity of their alcohol reaction when they are young. Also, people who have, for whatever reason, fallen into a pattern of relatively high-alcohol intake before evaluation for their response to alcohol might be difficult to study because of the impact of their recent drinking histories on their level of reaction (LR), which make the interpretation of the LR unclear. Finally, it is hypothesized that the LR to alcohol might be accurately measured only at the extremes, and that smaller differences in the intensities of this measure that fluctuate around the median might be less meaningful.

The present article describes the most recent analyses that include the remaining 227 subjects; thus, this generated a complete sample of 450 men who were successfully followed up. The goals were (1) to determine if data from the full sample replicated the relationship between FH and the subsequent risks for alcoholism and other disorders, (2) to probe further the possible impact of the drinking practices early in life on the relationship between the LR and alcoholic outcome, and (3) to evaluate if individuals who demonstrated very low or high levels of response to alcohol differed on their risk for alcoholism in the full sample. The number of subjects is now large enough to test whether the low response to alcohol might be a mechanism through which FH operates in increasing the risk for alcoholism in a subset of alcoholic families.

RESULTS

Sufficient data were available for the average quantity of alcohol consumed per occasion and the frequency of alcohol intake at time 1 on all 450 subjects, but, for reasons described earlier, clear FH categories could only be established for the 358 men in Table 1. At original testing, the two FH groups were similar on demography and drinking history. At follow-up, the two groups were similar on age (mean±SD, 31.2±2.94 years), an average of 8.19±1.64 years had elapsed since initial testing, and 59% were married or living as married, 4% were separated or divorced, and 37% were single. The FHP subjects had a mean±SD of 15.7±1.53 years of education compared with 16.21±1.66 years for FHN subjects ($t=-3.26$, $P<.001$).

Table 1 first demonstrates that, despite the exclusion of some subjects from the analyses because of an unclear FH, the men in the two FH groups were still similar on drinking patterns at the age of 20 years. While all men had consumed alcohol at follow-up and the two groups remained similar on the highest number of drinking days per month, during the interval since original testing, FHP subjects as a group consumed a higher number of maximum drinks per day and endorsed a higher number of *DSM-III-R* dependence items. The FHN and FHP individuals had been matched on their exposure to drugs other than alcohol at the age of 20 years, but, during follow-up, a significantly higher proportion of FHP subjects had used marijuana, although the two FH groups did not differ significantly on the proportion exposed to stimulants (amphetamines or cocaine) or other drugs (hallucinogens, opiates, solvents, etc).

Table 1 also outlines the proportion of FHP and FHN individuals who met criteria for a substance use disorder or a major psychiatric disorder during follow-up. Significantly more of the FHP subjects fulfilled criteria for a diagnosis. The two FH groups were most different for their levels of alcoholism (alcohol abuse or dependence), a *DSM-III-R* diagnosis noted for 42.7% of the FHP subjects and 17.4% of the FHN men (χ^2=21.55, $P<.001$). The groups were especially different for their rates of alcohol dependence, with an almost threefold FH difference. In the absence of alcohol abuse or dependence, approximately 5% of each FH group fulfilled criteria for cannabinol abuse or dependence, and 3.6% of the FHP men vs 1.4% of the FHN subjects met criteria for dependence on amphetamines or cocaine—a difference that was not statistically significant (χ^2=1.19, P=.28). While not shown in Table 1, when the rates of other drug prob-

Table 2. Relationships Among FH, LR, and Outcome Measures*

Variable	FH+LR	ALC Dx	ALC PROB
Full sample (n=335)	.14 (<.01 [.23])	...	...
FH	...	−.27 (<.001 [−.25])	−.20 (<.001 [−.66])
Control for LR	...	−.24 (<.001 [−.22])	−.18 (<.001 [−.58])
LR	...	−.25 (<.001 [−.14])	−.19 (<.001 [.37])
Control for FH	...	−.22 (<.001 [−.12])	−.16 (<.001 [−.32])
Middle 70% (n=171)	.08 (.31 [.07])	...	...
FH	...	−.23 (<.01 [−.21])	−.16 (<.05 [−.64])
Control for LR	...	−.23 (<.01 [−.20])	−.15 (<.05 [−.62])
LR	...	−.20 (<.01 [−.17])	−.07 (.40 [−.23])
Control for FH	...	−.20 (<.01 [−.15])	−.05 (.51 [−.18])
Delete extreme QF and limit to extreme 20% LR (n=96)	.36 (<.001 [.86])	...	...
FH	...	−.27 (<.01 [−.25])	−.30 (<.01 [−.99])
Control for LR	...	−.15 (<.14 [−.14])	−.20 (<.05 [−.67])
LR	...	−.37 (<.001 [−.15])	−.35 (<.001 [−.48])
Control for FH	...	−.31 (<.001 [−.12])	−.26 (<.001 [−.37])
Delete extreme QF and limit to extreme 15% LR (n=72)	.41 (<.001 [1.07])	...	...
FH	...	−.31 (<.01 [−.28])	−.30 (<.01 [−.93])
Control for LR	...	−.16 (.18 [−.15])	−.14 (.24 [−.43])
LR	...	−.43 (<.001 [−.15])	−.46 (<.001 [−.54])
Control for FH	...	−.35 (<.01 [−.13])	−.38 (<.001 [−.47])
Delete extreme QF and limit to extreme 10% LR (n=47)	.46 (<.001 [1.38])	...	...
FH	...	−.23 (.13 [−.22])	−.25 (.09 [−.85])
Control for LR	...	.01 (.94 [.01])	−.01 (.99 [−.003])
LR	...	−.51 (<.001 [−.16])	−.54 (<.001 [−.62])
Control for FH	...	−.47 (<.001 [−.17])	−.50 (<.001 [−.62])

**FH refers to the presence or absence of a family history of alcoholism; LR refers to the level of reaction to alcohol; ALC Dx, a diagnosis of alcohol abuse or dependence during the follow-up; ALC PROB, the number of the nine* DSM-III-R *alcohol dependence items observed during the interval since testing; and QF, quantity and frequency. Data are given as standardized coefficients, correlations, and partials, and* P *values [nonstandardized coefficients] are cited in parentheses (note that the maximal coefficient is established by the matrix of the variables and is not 1.0).*

lems in individuals with alcohol abuse or dependence were included in the analyses, 10.4% of the FHP subjects and 7.2% of the FHNs fulfilled criteria for cannabinol abuse or dependence (χ^2=1.11, P=.30), while the same was true with regard to stimulants for 12% of the FHP subjects and 5% of the FHN men (χ^2=5.77, P<.05). The two FH groups did not differ on the incidence of major anxiety or depressive disorders during follow-up.

Table 3 relates information on the 335 white men for whom the LR variable could be clearly established. The major goal of Table 3 is to explore the relationship between the LR variable at the age of about 20 years and the two major outcome variables at approximately the age of 30 years, after controlling for the measures of alcohol intake at the age of about 20 years. The first line of Table 3 describes the overall relationship between the LR and outcome, while the final three lines indicate whether this correlation is merely a reflection of either the quantity or frequency of drinking at the age of 20 years. The negative correlation between the LR and the outcome measures indicates that the lower the reaction to alcohol, the higher the risk for problems. It can be seen that neither the number of occasions per month on which drinking occurred during the 6 months before initial testing, nor the average number of drinks consumed per occasion at the age of 20 years greatly diminished the relationship between the LR and the outcome variables. These data are consistent with the conclusion that the intensity of response to alcohol at the time of initial testing was not merely a reflection of the quantity and frequency of alcohol intake at that age, at least in the manner in which the LR correlates with the outcomes.

Table 2 presents a series of analyses that looked at the full sample on which the LR was available (n=335) and then offers information on predefined subgroups. Each set of analyses describes the correlation between the two predictors (FH and LR), the relationship between each of these and the two outcome variables (the development of alcoholism and the number of alcohol problems), and the partial correlation coefficient between each of the two predictors (FH and LR) and the two outcomes while controlling for the second predictor. In each column, the first number is the standardized coefficient. However, because this table technically compares across subsamples, nonstandardized coefficients are also presented in parentheses. In interpreting the latter results, it is important to remember nonstandardized coefficient values are affected by the metrics of the variables, and the largest maximal coefficient is not 1.00. Because the same general conclusions apply to standardized and nonstandardized approaches, and because the same levels of statistical significance apply to both, for the sake of clarity, only the more commonly used standardized approaches are discussed in the text.

For the full sample of 335 men on whom clear FHs and clear LR values are available, the correlation between

Table 3. Impact of the Drinking Pattern at Time 1 on the Relationship of LR to Outcomes (n=335)*

Variable	ALC Dx	ALC PROB
LR	−.25†	−.19†
Controlling for		
FRQ_{T1}	−.23†	−.16†
QNT_{T1}	−.21†	−.15‡
Both	−.19†	−.13‡

**LR refers to the level of reaction to alcohol; ALC Dx, a diagnosis of alcohol abuse or dependence during the follow-up; ALC PROB, the number of the nine DSM-III-R alcohol dependence items observed during the interval since testing; FRQ_{T1}, the average number of days per week on which alcohol was consumed; and QNT_{T1}, the number of drinks per occasion at the time of original testing.*

†$P<.001$.

‡$P<.01$.

FH and LR was .14, indicating that FHP subjects had a lower LR score. If the entire range of reactions to alcohol was considered (ie, the high and low extremes of the LR were not highlighted), FH correlated with the future development of alcoholism and with the number of alcohol problems during the interval at a level of −.27 and −.20, respectively—values that decreased only slightly when the LR was used as a covariate. At the same time, the correlation coefficients between the full range of LR scores and the two outcome variables almost a decade later were −.25 and −.19, respectively—values that also showed little diminution when FH was used as a covariate. Thus, for the full sample of 335 men, FH and LR predicted outcome, but appeared to do so relatively independently.

However, as discussed in the introduction, it was hypothesized a priori that the LR was not likely to relate to an outcome if at the age of 20 years the individual was a very infrequent drinker (with a subsequent lack of exposure to alcohol and thus no ability of the intensity of reaction to alcohol to impact on the alcoholism risk among infrequent imbibers). Also, because of the previously noted difficulties in clearly interpreting the LR in the presence of heavy drinking, those subjects who were the heaviest drinkers at the age of 20 years were excluded a priori. Thus, in the remaining analyses in Table 2, 22 of the 335 men who at the age of 20 years drank one or less times per month and the 70 who consumed alcohol 12 or more times each month (ie, drank half again as often as weekend drinkers) were excluded, so that 73% of these subjects were included in the final analyses.

Evaluating these same relationships among FH, LR, and outcomes but focusing on those men whose LR scores at the age of 20 years were near the mean (ie, the middle 70% on the LR), FH (at −.23) and LR (at −.20) predicted alcoholism at outcome, but, as in the full sample, appeared to do so independently of each other, since controlling for either did not affect the relationship between the other and outcome. However, as discussed in the introduction, as a predictor of alcohol problems, the major impact of the LR on outcome would be expected to occur when the values of this variable were either fairly high (indicating a high level of intensity of reaction to alcohol and a probable low risk for alcoholism), or when they were very low (indicating a low level of reaction to alcohol and a probable high risk for future alcoholism or alcohol problems).

Thus, the series of results offered toward the bottom of Table 2 best captures the potential impact of the LR by focusing on the relevant individuals who fell into the highest and lowest 15% on the LR (ie, 30% of the group). Here, the LR now correlated with FH at .41. In this subset, FH related to alcoholism and alcohol problem outcomes at −.31 and −.30, respectively, and the correlation coefficients between the LR and the two outcomes were −.43 and −.46, respectively. Of even greater importance in this subsample chosen for an optimal theoretic impact of the LR, the partial correlation coefficients between the LR and the outcomes controlling for the impact of FH did not diminish greatly. In distinction from this, the correlation coefficients between FH and the two outcomes dropped to nonsignificant correlation coefficients of −.16 and −.14, respectively. For this subgroup representing the 15% upper and lower extremes on the LR, therefore, FH and LR related to the two outcomes, but the LR appears to be carrying most of the effect of FH in its ability to predict severe alcohol problems in the future.

Table 2 also explores the impact of focusing on the upper 10% and lower 10% on the LR (ie, 20% of the sample), revealing a correlation coefficient between FH and LR of .46, and an apparent greater impact of LR when used as a covariate in the correlation coefficients between FH and outcome when compared with the potential impact of FH in diminishing the relationship between the LR and outcomes. The picture observed with the upper and lower 20% (ie, 40% of the sample) reflected a similar pattern, but, because the incorporation of individuals whose LR score was closer to the mean, the findings are not as striking.

While not shown in the table, analyses similar to those offered in Table 2 were carried out for the FHP and FHN groups separately. These resulted in relatively small numbers of subjects in each relevant cell. However, both FHP and FHN subgroups demonstrated the same pattern of an increasing association between diagnoses of alcoholism and extreme LR scores as shown in Table 2 for the entire sample, showing an absence of an interaction between FH and LR. That is, FH did not moderate the relation between the LR and outcome. In addition, using hierarchic multiple regression within any of the extreme samples (ie, upper and lower 15% or 10%), an FH by the LR interaction term contributed nothing when it was entered following the main effect entries for FH and LR.

It is also important to look at possible interactions between the level of response to alcohol and FH as predictors of outcome for the larger sample, not just the extremes. Focusing on the sample most relevant to the original hypotheses, for these 223 men, there were no significant LR-by-FH interactions for the diagnosis of alcoholism ($\beta=.27$, the nonstandardized weight or $b=.10$, $P=.07$) or for alcohol problems ($\beta=.22$, $b=.27$, $P=.14$). Of course, it is possible that a significant interaction might be observed in a larger sample. An alternate approach is to take the full range of the LR and divide it into six levels of equal numbers of subjects to evaluate the relationship between FH and outcome across the LR levels. An evaluation of these results suggested a nonsignificant trend for FH having a closer relationship to outcome at low to middle levels of the LR than at higher levels of the LR.

An additional potential interaction of interest is between the LR and alcohol consumption at time 1. While no formal prediction of such an interaction was made a priori, the relationship is implied by the decision to exclude the subjects who drank the heaviest and the lightest from the analyses. Thus, the relationships between the LR and the two outcomes were evaluated within the 22 men who drank lightly at time 1, with a nonsignificant trend for alcoholism ($r=-.40$, b=−.12, $P=.07$) but none for alcohol problems ($r=-.20$, b=.25, $P=.35$). For the 70 men who drank the heaviest from time 1, the LR did not significantly predict alcoholism ($r=-.08$, b=−.05, $P=.51$) nor alcohol problems ($r=.03$, b=.08, $P=.79$). In the full sample of 335 men that included these light and heavy drinkers, there were nonsignificant interactions for the LR by drinking status at time 1 in predicting alcoholism ($\beta=-.07$, b=−.004, $P=.36$) and alcohol problems ($\beta=-.03$, b=−.005, $P=.73$).

Finally, for the sake of completeness, the assumption of linearity between the LR and outcomes was evaluated by using both residual plots and the entering of LR polynomials (up to quartic). There was no evidence for nonlinearity between the LR and the two outcomes for either the full sample or the extreme subsamples.

COMMENT

This article describes data from a longitudinal evaluation of 450 healthy young men. The first major goal of the work was to determine if information from this complete sample replicated the relationship between FH and the subsequent risk for alcoholism, drug abuse or dependence, and psychiatric disorders that was initially reported in the first 223 subjects.[26] Indeed, a positive FH of alcoholism was associated with an almost threefold increased risk for alcohol abuse or dependence in the sons of alcoholic fathers, even though the original sample was composed of relatively high-functioning blue- and white-collar men. Consistent with the prior results, at follow-up, nonalcoholic subjects did not have significantly higher risks for abuse or dependence on any other substance, although, if alcoholic individuals were considered, the risk for dependence on stimulants was slightly but significantly enhanced as well. There was no indication that an FH of alcoholism was associated with a higher risk for major psychiatric disorders—a finding that was likely related to the selection of men whose alcoholic fathers had no evidence of antisocial personality disorder, schizophrenia, or manic-depressive disease. These findings are consistent with additional studies from our group that indicated that, for at least a substantial proportion of alcohol-dependent individuals, the substance use disorder was not likely to have developed as a consequence of a preexisting psychiatric syndrome.[1,12,26,30,31]

With regard to the second goal, Table 3 demonstrates that the relationship between the LR and the two outcome measures remained robust even after covarying the results for the impact of the quantity and frequency of alcohol intake at the age of 20 years. These data complement the findings from earlier analyses that demonstrated that the initial FHP and FHN differences on the reaction to alcohol were observed despite close matching on their quantity and frequency of alcohol intake. Thus, in earlier reports, despite differences on the LR, the two FH groups were similar on state markers of heavy drinking (eg, γ-glutamyltransferase) and on the rate of disappearance of ethanol from the blood.[14-16,18-24] With regard to the importance of having demonstrated equal rates of disappearance of ethanol for subjects with FHP and FHN backgrounds, a recent publication has shown that the rate of metabolism of alcohol is relatively sensitive to even modest changes in the alcohol-intake pattern.[32] Also supporting the probable independence of the LR measure from the pattern of drinking at the age of 20 years is the demonstration through our own evaluations, as well as those of Porjesz and Begleiter,[33] that the differences between the FH groups on the LR remained robust even when relatively low-level drinking pairs were considered; for these individuals, gross underreporting of alcohol-intake patterns might be less likely.[33]

In considering the methods used to evaluate the quantity and frequency of alcohol intake at the age of about 20 years, it is important to recognize that there were no alternative, more appropriate approaches. For example, subjects might have been placed in a hospital environment for 1 or 2 weeks before laboratory testing to ensure abstinence, but such procedures would have been prohibitively expensive and would have severely limited the number of subjects who could be tested. Alternatively, subjects who had never consumed alcohol could have been initially selected for study, but this represented 2% or less of the young male sample surveyed in San Diego, raising the probability that the sample would be unique. It might also have been possible to test prepubertal children of alcoholic individuals to ensure that the subjects had no prior experience with alcohol, but this would have raised ethical problems with regard to the administration of intoxicating doses of alcohol to such young individuals, as well as similar concerns with regard to exposure of alcohol to otherwise abstinent subjects who were at high risk for alcoholism.

The major goal of these analyses, presented in Table 2, was to evaluate the relationship between the LR and an alcoholic outcome, and to take advantage of the larger sample to explore whether this relationship might account for the mechanism through which FH operates in a subsample of alcoholic families. It was hypothesized that the intensity of reaction to alcohol as a potential mediator of an alcoholism outcome would only be relevant to individuals who demonstrated relatively high or low levels of response to alcohol. This potential risk factor was not thought to apply to individuals who did not expose themselves to drinking situations, and the LR was hypothesized to operate even after excluding the subjects who had relatively high levels of alcohol intake at the age of 20 years. Testing this theory required a large number of subjects to focus on appropriate subgroups. The bottom portion of Table 2 reveals that, at least among the individuals at the extreme high and low 10% to 15% of the LR (ie, 20% to 30% of the population), FH correlated with the LR at a value of greater than .40, and the LR related to the outcomes with correlation coefficients of between .43 and .54. These latter correlation coefficients were not diminished to any great extent when the impact of covarying for FH was evaluated. However, consistent with the possibility that the LR acts as a potential mediating variable between FH and alcoholism in some people, covarying for the LR resulted in a relationship between FH and outcomes that was no longer statistically significant (Table 2). Interestingly, within the men who scored in the middle range on the LR, it appeared as if both the LR and FH predicted future alcoholism and did so independently.

The important question with regard to interaction effects was also evaluated. Neither the LR by drinking status at time 1 nor the LR by FH interactions yielded significant results. Still, some suggestive evidence of the effect of interactions was found, and the presence of such interactions should be tested in any future research in this area. For example, it may not have been necessary to exclude subjects who drank lightly at time 1 from the general analyses.

The paradigm used in this study cannot directly evaluate whether the LR is itself genetically influenced. However, this question has been addressed in two studies of twins in Australia and Indiana. These laboratories used an alcohol challenge to compare levels of concordance on the response to alcohol in monozygotic and dizygotic twin pairs.[34] The studies indicated a likelihood that genetic factors contributed to the subjective responses to alcohol, hormonal changes following alcohol challenges, and the alcohol-induced alterations in body sway, although the contribution of environmental factors could not be excluded.[35] Additional support for the importance of genetic factors for determining the level of response to alcohol comes from comparisons of lines of rodents that were selectively bred to consume voluntarily higher and lower amounts of alcohol in a free-choice situation with water available.[36] A common theme apparent in these studies was that a lower level response to alcohol was associated with high levels of alcohol consumption.[36-38]

In interpreting these results, it is important to recognize the limitations of the data. First, while FH was assigned based on all available information, an optimal study would have interviewed all available first- and second-degree relatives of the subjects. Unfortunately, this step would have been prohibitively expensive for a sample this large, especially because family members were geographically widely dispersed. However, other research has revealed that the major informants used here (ie, sons of alcoholics) are likely to be among the most reliable sources of information with regard to alcohol problems in their parents.[39] In addition, the practice of gathering information from multiple informants, as was done in this study, has been demonstrated to be superior to obtaining data from only one source.[40] Finally, any errors in FH assignment in this study would have served to diminish (not magnify) the relationships among the variables that were evaluated here.

A second caveat is that even a sample of 450 men who were successfully followed up during almost a decade is barely large enough to test adequately the third question raised in the introduction. Among the 450 individuals, 92 were excluded from the key analyses to focus only on men with an alcoholic father as compared with clearly FHN control subjects. Because some of the analyses were limited to only those individuals for whom clear information on the LR were available (excluding those with missing data at key time points), the sample decreased further to 335 individuals. When one recognizes that the LR is a potential mediator of the alcoholism risk that is only likely to apply to those individuals with high and low levels of responses, the exclusion of subjects whose LR measures fell near the mean resulted in final samples in the cells at the bottom of Table 2 of between 72 and 47 individuals. Thus, while the data are consistent with the possibility that the LR operates as a mediator of the FH risk associated with future alcoholism, the relatively small-sample size in these cells requires caution with regard to any definitive conclusions.

Another qualification is the need to emphasize that the data focused on males. When the study began in the 1970s, children of alcohol-dependent mothers were excluded for fear that any FHP vs FHN differences might reflect a fetal alcohol effect. The population was restricted to sons because of the possibility that men and women might carry different types of predispositions toward alcoholism, with a subsequent risk that a large-scale longitudinal study would result in two smaller subgroups that could not be combined into one large sample. If this had been the case, many of the analyses reported in Table 2 could not have been carried out. Faced with the choice between male and female subjects, the former were selected because of their higher probability of experiencing alcoholism in the future. However, while the present study cannot relate adequate information on women, as part of the Collaborative Study of the Genetics of Alcoholism, investigative data are currently being gathered on 18- to 29-year-old sons *and daughters* of alcohol-dependent men and women. Future work in the present study will also gather data on the daughters of our present subjects.

There are additional problems inherent in this type of work. No sample can be selected fully at random. For example, FHP subjects and FHN controls were selected from the approximately 70% of the respondents to a yearly mailed questionnaire. Also, the subjects selected for study were relatively highly functional men who were old enough to give informed consent and who already had experience with alcohol. Thus, the subjects were not necessarily representative of males in the general population in San Diego. Also, potential subjects with antisocial personality disorder, those with other causes of early-onset alcoholism, and those with preexisting severe cognitive deficits were not likely to be included in the sample. However, the present group of 450 individuals is relatively large, and data from the alcohol challenge component of the Collaborative Study of the Genetics of Alcoholism have basically replicated the FHP and FHN differences in a blue-collar, less highly functional, more racially heterogenous group.[41] In addition, a meta-analysis of alcohol challenge results has replicated some of the FH findings reported here.[17] The present work also suffers from the lack of a perfect, standardized mechanism for measuring the LR, as well as imperfections in determining alcoholic outcomes.

Despite all of these caveats, the results have generated a response to each of the three questions posed in the introduction, and they have a number of implications with regard to future directions for this research. First, while the relationship between the LR to alcohol and the future development of alcoholism is significant and appears to be powerful enough to have a possible clinical relevance, the specific marker of potential risk, namely, a relatively low level of responsivity to alcohol, is likely to act in concert with other moderating and mediating variables. Thus, the next stage in the follow-up of these 450 men to be carried out from 1994 to 1999 is focusing on those individuals who did not experience alcohol abuse and dependence despite low levels of response to alcohol. Of equal interest will be subjects who experienced alcoholism despite relatively high sensitivities to the alcohol challenge. Such evaluations might help to identify psychologic and environmental influences that interact with FH and responsivity to alcohol to produce the risk for alcoholism. These factors to be studied include more detailed evaluations of the expectations of the effects of alcohol, styles of coping with stress, levels of life stress, social support systems, and several personality attributes.

Another important next step for this work is a response to the fact that, for the reasons described earlier, the original sample was limited to 18- to 29-year-old men. However, even at the first stage of follow-up, 54% of the subjects had children, with a likelihood that this proportion will increase over time; these sons and daughters of the original subjects will now offer the opportunity to observe prospectively from an early age a population of both males and females at a future high risk for alcoholism. Evaluations will be carried out via interviews with the parent and, once the children are old enough, with the sons and daughters themselves.

Accepted for publication August 2, 1995.

This research was supported by the Veterans Affairs Research Service of the San Diego (Calif) Veterans Affairs Medical Center, and by grants 05526, 08401, and 08403 from the National Institute on Alcohol Abuse and Alcoholism, Washington, DC.

The authors thank Jeff Klein, who has been involved in all stages of this research.

Correspondence to Department of Psychiatry (116A), 3350 La Jolla Village Dr, San Diego, CA 92161-2002 (Dr Schuckit).

REFERENCES

1. Schuckit MA. A clinical model of genetic influences in alcohol dependence. *J Stud Alcohol.* 1994;55:5-17.
2. Cotton NS. The familial incidence of alcoholism. *J Stud Alcohol.* 1979;40:89-116.
3. Cadoret RJ. Development of alcoholism in adoptees raised apart from alcoholic biologic relatives. *Arch Gen Psychiatry.* 1980;37:561-563.
4. Kendler KS, Heath AC, Neale MC, Kessler RC, Eaves LJ. A population-based twin study of alcoholism in women. *JAMA.* 1992;268:1877-1882.
5. Goodwin DW, Schulsinger F, Mollen N, Hermansen L, Winokur G, Guze SB. Drinking problems in adopted and nonadopted sons of alcoholics. *Arch Gen Psychiatry.* 1974;31:164-169.
6. Devor EJ, Cloninger CR. Genetics of alcoholism. *Annu Rev Genet.* 1989;23:19-36.
7. Chakravarti A, Lander ES. Genetic approaches to the dissection of complex diseases. *Banbury Rep.* 1990;33:307-315.
8. Greenberg DA. There is more than one way to collect data for linkage analysis. *Arch Gen Psychiatry.* 1992;49:745-750.
9. Mueser KT, Yarnold PR, Bellack AS. Diagnostic and demographic correlates of substance abuse in schizophrenia and major affective disorder. *Acta Psychiatr Scand.* 1992;85:48-55.
10. Hesselbrock MN. Gender comparison of antisocial personality disorder and depression in alcoholism. *J Subst Abuse.* 1991;3:205-219.
11. Tohen M, Waternaux CCM, Tsuang MT. Outcome in mania: a 4-year prospective follow-up of 75 patients utilizing survival analysis. *Arch Gen Psychiatry.* 1990;47:1106-1111.
12. Schuckit MA. The clinical implications of primary diagnostic groups among alcoholics. *Arch Gen Psychiatry.* 1985a;42:1043-1049.
13. Streissguth AP, Landesman-Dwyer S, Martin JC, Smith DW. Teratogenic effects of alcohol in humans and laboratory animals. *Science.* 1980;209:353-361.
14. Irwin M, Baird S, Smith TL, Schuckit M. Use of laboratory tests to monitor heavy drinking by alcoholic men discharged from a treatment program. *Am J Psychiatry.* 1988;145:595-599.
15. Schuckit MA. Peak blood alcohol levels in men at high risk for the future development of alcoholism. *Alcohol Clin Exp Res.* 1981;5:64-66.
16. Schuckit MA, Gold EO. A simultaneous evaluation of multiple markers of ethanol/placebo challenges in sons of alcoholics and controls. *Arch Gen Psychiatry.* 1988;45:211-216.
17. Pollock VE. Meta-analysis of subjective sensitivity to alcohol in sons of alcoholics. *Am J Psychiatry.* 1992;149:1534-1538.
18. Schuckit MA. Body sway: differences after drinking in sons of alcoholics and controls. In: Pichot P, Berner P, Folf R, Thau K, eds. *Psychiatry: the State of the Art.* London, England: Plenum Publishing Co Ltd; 1985;5:138-161.
19. Schuckit MA. Ethanol-induced changes in body sway in men at high alcoholism risk. *Arch Gen Psychiatry.* 1985;42:375-379.
20. Schuckit MA, Risch SC, Gold EO. Alcohol consumption, ACTH level, and family history of alcoholism. *Am J Psychiatry.* 1988;145:1391-1395.
21. Schuckit MA, Polich J, Gold EO, Croot K, Finn P. P3 latency after ethanol in sons of alcoholics and controls. *Biol Psychiatry.* 1988;24:310-315.
22. Schuckit MA, Parker DC, Rossman LR. Prolactin responses to ethanol in men at elevated risk for alcoholism and controls. *Biol Psychiatry.* 1983;18:1153-1159.
23. Schuckit MA, Gold EO, Risch SC. Serum prolactin levels in sons of alcoholics and control subjects. *Am J Psychiatry.* 1987;144:854-859.
24. Schuckit MA, Gold EO, Risch SC. Plasma cortisol levels following ethanol in sons of alcoholics and controls. *Arch Gen Psychiatry.* 1987;44:942 945.
25. Schuckit MA, Duthie LA, Mahler HIM, Irwin M, Monteiro MG. Subjective feelings and changes in body sway following diazepam in sons of alcoholics and control subjects. *J Stud Alcohol.* 1991;52:601-608.
26. Schuckit MA. Low level of response to alcohol as a predictor of future alcoholism. *Am J Psychiatry.* 1994;151:184-189.
27. Twitchell GR, Hertzog CA, Klein JK, Schuckit MA. The anatomy of a follow-up. *Br J Addict.* 1992;87:251-257.
28. American Psychiatric Association. *Diagnostic and Statistical Manual of Mental Disorders, Revised Third Edition.* Washington, DC: American Psychiatric Press; 1987.
29. Schuckit MA, Irwin M, Howard T, Smith T. A structured diagnostic interview for identification of primary alcoholism: a preliminary evaluation. *J Stud Alcohol.* 1988;49:93-99.
30. Brown SA, Schuckit MA. Changes in depression among abstinent alcoholics. *J Stud Alcohol.* 1988;49:412-417.
31. Schuckit MA, Hesselbrock VM. Alcohol dependence and anxiety disorders: what is the relationship? *Am J Psychiatry.* 1994;151:1723-1734.
32. Whitfield JB, Martin NG. Alcohol consumption and alcohol pharmacokinetics: interactions within the normal population. *Alcohol Clin Exp Res.* 1994;18:238-243.
33. Porjesz B, Begleiter H. Reactions to alcohol in sons of alcoholics. Presented at the International Society for the Biomedical Research on Alcoholism Satellite Symposium on Genetics and Alcohol-Related Diseases; June 19, 1992; Bordeaux, France.
34. Martin NG, Oakeshott JG, Gibson JB, Starmer GA, Perl J, Wilks AV. A twin study of psychomotor and physiological responses to an acute dose of alcohol. *Behav Genet.* 1985;15:305-347.
35. Heath AC, Martin NG. Genetic differences in psychomotor performance decrement after alcohol: a multivariate analysis. *J Stud Alcohol.* 1992;53:262-271.
36. Li T, Lumeng L, Doolittle DP. Selective breeding for alcohol preference and associated responses. *Behav Genet.* 1993;23:163-170.
37. Lumeng L, Waller MB, McBride WJ, Li TK. Different sensitivities to ethanol in alcohol-preferring and nonpreferring rats. *Pharmacol Biochem Behav.* 1982;16:125-130.
38. Stewart RB, Kurtz DI, Zweifel M, Li TK, Froehlich JC. Differences in the hypothermic response to ethanol in rats selectively bred for oral ethanol preference and nonpreference. *Psychopharmacology.* 1992;106:169-174.
39. Sher KJ, Descutner C. Reports of paternal alcoholism: reliability across siblings. *Addict Behav.* 1986;11:25-30.
40. Andreasen NC, Rice J, Endicott J, Reich T, Coryell W. The family history approach to diagnosis: how useful is it? *Arch Gen Psychiatry.* 1986;43:421-429.
41. Schuckit MA, Tsuang JW, Anthenelli RA, Tipp JE, Nurnberger JI. Alcohol challenges in young men from alcoholic pedigrees and control families: a report from the COGA project. *J Stud Alcohol.* In press.

Early-Onset Alcoholics Have Lower Cerebrospinal Fluid 5-Hydroxyindoleacetic Acid Levels Than Late-Onset Alcoholics

Marie-Lourdes Fils-Aime, MD; Michael J. Eckardt, PhD; David T. George, MD; Gerald L. Brown, MD; Ivan Mefford, PhD; Markku Linnoila, MD, PhD

Background: We investigated the interrelationships of age at onset of excessive alcohol consumption, family history of alcoholism, psychiatric comorbidity, and cerebrospinal fluid monoamine metabolite concentrations in abstinent, treatment-seeking alcoholics.

Methods: We studied 131 recently abstinent alcoholics. Supervised abstinence was maintained on a research ward at the National Institutes of Health Clinical Center for a minimum of 3 weeks. All alcoholics received a low-monoamine diet for a minimum of 3 days before lumbar puncture. Lumbar punctures were performed in the morning after an overnight fast. Monoamine metabolites and tryptophan in cerebrospinal fluid were quantified with liquid chromatography by means of electrochemical detection. Psychiatric diagnoses were established from blind-rated Schedule for Affective Disorders and Schizophrenia–Lifetime version interviews administered by a research social worker. Severity and age at onset of excessive alcohol consumption were documented with a structured lifetime drinking history questionnaire and with selected alcoholism screening questionnaires (CAGE and Michigan Alcoholism Screening Test). Family history of alcoholism was obtained from the probands.

Results: A majority of the treatment-seeking, primarily white male alcoholics had a lifetime history of psychiatric disorders other than alcoholism. None fulfilled criteria for antisocial personality disorder. Early-onset alcoholics (onset of excessive consumption before 25 years of age) had a more severe course of alcoholism and lower mean cerebrospinal fluid 5-hydroxyindoleacetic acid concentration than late-onset alcoholics. Patients who reported both parents to be alcoholics had particularly low mean cerebrospinal fluid 5-hydroxyindoleacetic acid, homovanillic acid, and tryptophan concentrations.

Conclusion: Among treatment-seeking alcoholics, early age at onset is generally associated with a more severe course of alcoholism and lower cerebrospinal fluid 5-hydroxyindoleacetic acid concentration.

(Arch Gen Psychiatry. 1996;53:211-216)

EPIDEMIOLOGIC surveys have found that alcoholism is the most common mental or substance abuse disorder among men in the United States.[1] Like most mental disorders, alcoholism is heterogeneous and tends to occur in families. To facilitate psychobiologic and molecular genetic studies on alcoholism, criteria have been proposed to define relatively homogeneous subgroups.

Cloninger et al[2] developed a classification scheme for alcoholism, based on a large-scale adoption study conducted in Stockholm, Sweden, that has had great heuristic value. Two subtypes of alcoholism were defined, types 1 and 2. Seventy-five percent of men and all women in the Stockholm sample fulfilled criteria for type 1 alcoholism. These patients were characterized by a relatively late age at onset of heavy drinking, anxious personality traits, and adverse environmental conditions during development. The type 2 alcoholics were all men, had alcoholic fathers with antisocial traits, began heavy drinking at an early age, exhibited antisocial personality traits, and a functional adoptive family did not reduce the risk of expression of the inherited vulnerability.[2] Irwin et al[3] and Lamparski et al[4] were only partially successful in validating the findings of Cloninger et al.[2] Irwin et al[3] found that, regardless of family history, the main factor defining the course and characteristics of an alcoholic seeking treatment was the age at onset. Lamparski et

From the Laboratory of Clinical Studies, Division of Intramural Clinical and Biological Research, National Institute on Alcohol Abuse and Alcoholism (Drs Fils-Aime, Eckardt, George, Brown, and Linnoila), and the Laboratory of Clinical Science, National Institute of Mental Health (Dr Mefford), Bethesda, Md.

See Patients and Methods on next page

PATIENTS AND METHODS

PATIENTS

All participants (n=131) were selected from recently abstinent alcoholics undergoing research and treatment on the inpatient research ward of the National Institute on Alcohol Abuse and Alcoholism at the National Institutes of Health Clinical Center in Bethesda, Md. Most participants resided in the Washington, DC, metropolitan area and became aware of the program by physician referral, word of mouth, or weekly advertisements in a major metropolitan newspaper. All patients met Research Diagnostic Criteria[11] for alcoholism and had negative results of urine drug screens at the time of admission. Written informed consent was obtained before the start of the study.

PROCEDURES

The standard procedure for obtaining CSF samples consisted of at least 3 weeks of supervised abstinence from alcohol on a locked research ward and a minimum of 3 days on a low-monoamine diet.[12] The low-monoamine diet excluded certain beverages (eg, chocolate drinks), fruits (eg, bananas), nuts (eg, walnuts), vegetables (eg, tomatoes), meats (eg, chicken livers), dairy products (eg, aged cheese), fish (eg, smoked fish), and soft drinks sweetened with aspartame. Lumbar punctures were performed between 9 and 10 AM, after overnight bed rest and fast. Approximately 32 mL of CSF was collected while the patient was in the left lateral decubitus position. The first 12 mL of CSF was collected as a single aliquot into a tube on wet ice, mixed thoroughly, aliquoted to 1-mL test tubes, and stored immediately at −70°C. None of the samples was ever thawed before analysis.

Concentrations of the major CSF metabolites of norepinephrine (3-methoxy-4-hydroxyphenylglycol [MHPG]), dopamine (homovanillic acid [HVA]), serotonin (5-HIAA), and the serotonin precursor tryptophan were determined with high-pressure liquid chromatography by means of a slight modification of the method of Scheinin et al.[13] Analyses were conducted in a single run. The within-run coefficient of variation for all of the analytes was less than 10%.

All alcoholics were administered a structured psychiatric instrument, the Schedule for Affective Disorders and Schizophrenia–Lifetime version,[14] by a social worker. The resulting diagnoses were based on a subsequent blind rating by another social worker and a psychiatrist. Diagnoses were reviewed and any inconsistencies were resolved by a senior psychiatrist (G.L.B.). Diagnoses were categorized as current, past, and lifetime (current and/or past). Alcoholism screening instruments (ie, the Michigan Alcoholism Screening Test[15] and the CAGE[16]) were administered, and information on recent and chronic alcohol consumption and alcohol-related behavior was obtained from structured research questionnaires completed by the patients.[17] Information on current and past use of other drugs, including cigarettes and caffeine, and parental history of alcoholism was collected from the patients, and selected laboratory variables (aspartate aminotransferase, alanine aminotransferase, and γ-glutamyltransferase) were quantified.

All statistics were computed by means of the BMDP statistical software package.[18]

al[4] reported difficulty in applying the Cloninger classification scheme because a majority of alcoholics could not be confidently assigned to either type.

von Knorring et al[5] operationalized a two-group classification scheme based primarily on age at onset and secondarily on complications thought to be consequences of antisocial behavioral traits. This scheme results in every alcoholic being assigned to one of the subgroups. Similar to the Cloninger et al[2] criteria, von Knorring et al[5] called late-onset alcoholics type 1 and early-onset type 2. Unlike Cloninger et al,[2] von Knorring et al[5] did not require a paternal family history of alcoholism for type 2. The classification scheme of von Knorring et al[5] has proved useful in psychobiologic studies. Type 2 alcoholics have lower mean platelet monoamine oxidase activity than type 1 alcoholics and healthy volunteers[6]; this biochemical trait has been associated with the personality trait of sensation seeking. Approximately half of type 2 alcoholics have also been reported to experience a strong urge to consume alcohol in response to an intravenous infusion of the serotonin 2C receptor agonist meta-chlorophenylpiperazine.[7] Studies of early-onset, violent Finnish alcoholics have demonstrated that their impaired impulse control is associated with a low mean concentration of 5-hydroxyindoleacetic acid (5-HIAA), the major metabolite of serotonin, in the cerebrospinal fluid (CSF).[8,9]

Based on the above findings, we postulated that alcoholics who engage in excessive alcohol consumption by 25 years of age (type 2) have reduced central serotonin turnover.[10] In the present study, we tested this hypothesis as well as determined the effects of (1) family history of alcoholism, (2) degree of antisocial behavioral traits, and (3) depression concurrent with alcoholism on CSF 5-HIAA concentrations in a large group of carefully characterized alcoholics after a minimum of 3 weeks of supervised abstinence. Levels of CSF monoamine metabolites were determined after at least 3 days on a low-monoamine diet and were quantified in a single large assay to exclude interassay variability.

RESULTS

The average (±SD) age of the alcoholics was 39.2±9.8 years. The sample was composed of 122 men and nine women, consisting of 112 whites, 17 African Americans, and two Hispanics.

The age at onset of excessive alcohol consumption was calculated by subtracting the years of excessive consumption (more than three drinks per 24 hours, on the average) from the current age. The 90 alcoholics who had an onset of excessive consumption by 25 years of age had lower levels of 5-HIAA than the alcoholics with an onset after 25 years of age (*P*=.01; **Figure 1**). There were

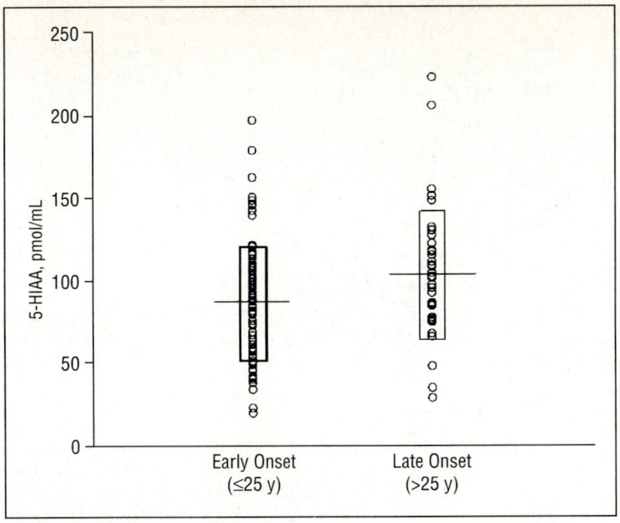

Figure 1. *Mean±SD cerebrospinal fluid levels of 5-hydroxyindoleacetic acid (5-HIAA) in alcoholics as a function of age at onset of excessive alcohol consumption* (P=.01).

Table 1. Concentrations of CSF Variables*

	Mean±SD		
	Early Onset (n=90)	Late Onset (n=41)	*P*
5-HIAA, pmol/mL	85.6±34.7	103.6±38.9	.01
HVA, pmol/mL	149.5±62.3	163.4±58.5	.24
MHPG, pmol/mL	43.4±12.1	43.4±13.4	.99
Tryptophan, pmol/mL	3515±989	3437±692	.65

**CSF indicates cerebrospinal fluid; 5-HIAA, 5-hydroxyindoleacetic acid; HVA, homovanillic acid; and MHPG, 3-methoxy-4-hydroxyphenylglycol.*

no differences in CSF HVA, MHPG, or tryptophan concentrations between the groups (**Table 1**).

Early-onset alcoholics were younger (36.3±8.8 years) than late-onset alcoholics (46.1±8.7 years) (*P*<.001). They consumed more alcohol per drinking occasion during the preceding 6 months, had more years of excessive alcohol consumption, and had higher CAGE and Michigan Alcoholism Screening Test scores (**Table 2**). There were no group differences in frequency of drinking during the past 6 months or in time between the last drink and the lumbar puncture.

There were no differences in CSF 5-HIAA, HVA, MHPG, or tryptophan levels between alcoholics with only paternal alcoholism, only maternal alcoholism, or either parent exhibiting alcoholic behavior and the rest of the sample. The 12 alcoholics with paternal *and* maternal alcoholism had significantly lower levels of 5-HIAA (79±5 vs 92±38 pmol/mL; *P*=.03), HVA (132±30 vs 156±63 pmol/mL; *P*=.03), and tryptophan (2976±655 vs 3536±912 pmol/mL; *P*=.04) than the rest of the sample.

Relationships among various predictor variables and CSF 5-HIAA, HVA, MHPG, and tryptophan concentrations were determined by means of multiple regression techniques wherein each dependent variable, one at a time, was predicted by those independent variables with which it was significantly correlated (*r*≥.17; *P*≤.05). Fifty-five percent of the variance in 5-HIAA level was explained by levels of HVA, tryptophan, and MHPG and the CAGE score (*P*<.001). Higher levels of HVA predicted higher levels of 5-HIAA (*P*<.001), and lower levels of tryptophan tended to predict higher levels of 5-HIAA (*P*=.06). Neither MHPG level (*P*=.40) nor the CAGE score (*P*=.81) was significant when the other variables were considered.

Fifty-six percent of the variance in HVA level was explained by levels of 5-HIAA and MHPG, years of excessive alcohol consumption, and CAGE score (*P*<.001). Increasing levels of 5-HIAA and MHPG predicted higher levels of HVA (*P*<.001 and *P*=.03, respectively), and increasing years of excessive alcohol consumption tended to predict lower levels of HVA (*P*=.08). The CAGE did not explain significant amounts of variance (*P*=.78) when the other variables were considered.

Fourteen percent of the variance in MHPG level was explained by age and levels of HVA and 5-HIAA (*P*<.001). Increasing age predicted higher MHPG levels (*P*=.01), and increasing HVA levels predicted higher MHPG levels (*P*=.02). The level of 5-HIAA did not explain significant amounts of variance (*P*=.87) when the other variables were considered.

Seventeen percent of the variance in tryptophan was explained by levels of 5-HIAA, aspartate aminotransferase (45±47 U/L), γ-glutamyltransferase (127±188 U/L), and alanine aminotransferase (52±62 U/L) (*P*<.001). Decreasing levels of 5-HIAA predicted higher levels of tryptophan (*P*=.004; **Figure 2**), and increasing levels of aspartate aminotransferase predicted higher levels of tryptophan (*P*=.04); there was a trend for higher levels of γ-glutamyltransferase to predict higher levels of tryptophan (*P*=.08). Levels of alanine aminotransferase did not predict (*P*=.26) tryptophan levels when the other variables were considered.

In addition to satisfying Research Diagnostic Criteria for a lifetime (current and/or past) diagnosis of alcoholism, 90 alcoholics (69%) also satisfied criteria for other lifetime psychiatric disorders. Thirty-six alcoholics (27%) had diagnoses that coexisted with alcoholic behavior, while 54 (41%) had psychiatric disorders that were separable from alcoholic behavior, ie, current diagnosis of alcoholism and past psychiatric diagnosis or past diagnosis of alcoholism and current psychiatric diagnosis.

In the 54 alcoholics who satisfied criteria for other lifetime psychiatric disorder(s) that were separable from alcoholic behavior, most frequent were drug use, mood, and anxiety disorders (**Table 3**). Thirty-one had one other diagnosis, 13 had two, five had three, and five had four or more diagnoses.

Sixty-eight alcoholics (52%) had other lifetime psychiatric disorders that were *not* separable from alcoholic behavior, with the most frequent being mood and anxiety disorders (Table 3). Of these 68, 32 (47%) had some psychiatric disorders that were distinct from alcoholic behavior and some that were not separable.

Alcoholics with a lifetime diagnosis of some form of depression (major, minor or intermittent, or depres-

Table 2. Alcoholism-Related Variables*

	Mean±SD		
	Early Onset (n=90)	Late Onset (n=41)	*P*
CAGE (4 items)	3.8±0.5	3.5±0.8	.02
MAST (25 weighted items)	43.8±22.3	35.2±6.9	.02
Days between last drink and lumbar puncture	38.0±22.1	34.8±22.4	.44
No. of drinking occasions in last 6 mo	126.9±55.2	127.6±53.9	.94
Alcohol consumed per occasion in last 6 mo, g†	221.4±115.4	170.6±154.8	.04
Years of excessive alcohol consumption (yearly average, >3 drinks/d)	18.2±9.0	9.7±7.8	<.001

*CAGE is an alcoholism screening questionnaire that contains four structured research questions. MAST indicates Michigan Alcoholism Screening Test.

†A standard drink contains 11.2 to 14.0 g of alcohol, depending on beverage.

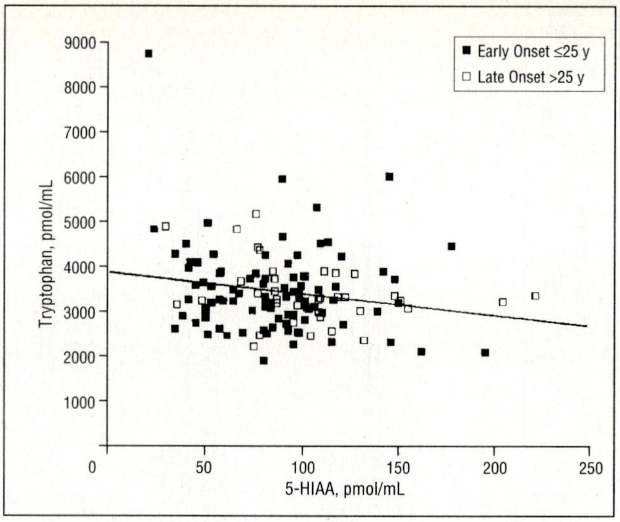

Figure 2. *Relationship between 5-hydroxyindoleacetic acid (5-HIAA) and tryptophan (*r=−.19; P=.03*).*

sion not otherwise specified) did not have low CSF 5-HIAA levels. Moreover, there were no differences in 5-HIAA levels between alcoholics with no diagnosis of depression and those with major depression; major depression or depression not otherwise specified; minor or intermittent depression; or minor, intermittent, or depression not otherwise specified.

Nineteen alcoholics reported attempting suicide, and they did not differ from the others in 5-HIAA, HVA, MHPG, or tryptophan levels. Early- and late-onset (n=14 and 5, respectively) alcoholics were equally likely to have attempted suicide (15.6% and 15.2%, respectively). Moreover, there were no differences in the seriousness of intent scores according to the Schedule for Affective Disorders and Schizophrenia–Lifetime version for the most serious attempt.

Comparisons among prevalence of psychiatric diagnoses in early- and late-onset alcoholics showed that individuals with early onset were also more likely to have a lifetime diagnosis of drug use disorder (*P*<.03).

Although no alcoholics satisfied Schedule for Affective Disorders and Schizophrenia–Lifetime version criteria for antisocial personality disorder, summed scores across the four criteria disclosed higher values for early- than for late-onset alcoholics (*P*=.001). The early-onset alcoholics exhibited poorer occupational performance (*P*<.001) and more childhood (*P*=.001) and adult (*P*=.001) behaviors defined as antisocial than the late-onset alcoholics. Occupational, childhood, adult, and summed antisocial behavior scores were not significantly correlated with 5-HIAA levels for early- or late-onset alcoholics or for the entire sample. Also, there was no relationship between a father's alcoholic status and degree of antisocial traits in the alcoholic offspring.

COMMENT

The present study was designed to determine relationships among levels of various CSF monoamine metabolites, alcohol-related behavior, psychiatric comorbidity, and parental alcoholism. Quantification of alcohol-related behavior and determination of parental alcoholism was based on self-report. Psychiatric comorbidity was determined by administration of the Schedule for Affective Disorders and Schizophrenia–Lifetime version, with subsequent blind rating of responses by clinicians who used Research Diagnostic Criteria. The levels of CSF monoamine metabolites were determined in a single large assay after at least 3 days of low-monoamine diet and 3 weeks of supervised abstinence.

Alcoholics who began excessive alcohol consumption by 25 years of age (early onset) had significantly lower CSF 5-HIAA concentrations than alcoholics with a late onset (Figure 1). The HVA, MHPG, and tryptophan concentrations were similar among the early- and late-onset alcoholics (Table 1). Even though early-onset alcoholics had a more extensive alcohol history than late-onset alcoholics (Table 2), alcohol-related behaviors or alcohol consumption did not correlate with CSF 5-HIAA concentrations in either the total sample or the two subsamples.

In addition to exhibiting more severe alcoholism, early-onset alcoholics also exhibited more antisocial behavioral traits. Similar findings have been reported by Irwin et al.[3] Neither study, however, included patients who met criteria for antisocial personality disorder. These findings differ from those of Cloninger,[19] who suggested that late-onset alcoholics exhibit a more severe alcoholism and have a poorer prognosis.

An earlier study from our program[20] also reported lower CSF 5-HIAA concentrations in early- vs late-onset alcoholics. This finding did not, however, achieve statistical significance. The major differences between the two studies are the larger sample size and the elimination of between-assay variability in the present study and a different age at onset criterion. The present age at onset criterion was selected to test directly the hypotheses of Cloninger et al[2] and Irwin et al.[3] Although other investigators have reported reduced CSF 5-HIAA concentrations in abstinent alcoholics, they have not addressed

Table 3. Lifetime Psychiatric Disorders in Diagnosed Alcoholics (N=131)

Diagnosis*	No. of Patients: Separable From Alcoholic Behavior	Coexistent With Alcoholic Behavior
Mood disorders		
Hypomania	1	0
Major depression	7	0
Minor and intermittent depression	14	0
Depression NOS	0	61
Anxiety disorders		
Panic	6	0
Phobia	4	0
Obsessive compulsive	2	0
Generalized anxiety	10	0
Anxiety NOS	9	0
Posttraumatic stress	2	0
Drug use disorder	29	1
Psychotic disorders NOS	0	3
Organic disorder NOS	0	2
Attention deficit disorder	0	2

More than one diagnosis per individual is possible. NOS indicates not otherwise specified.

the issue of subgrouping. Ballenger et al[21] studied abstinent, young male alcoholics and reported one of the largest differences between alcoholics and controls. The demographics of their sample suggest that a large proportion of the patients were early-onset alcoholics. Banki[22] reported low CSF 5-HIAA levels in recently abstinent alcoholic men and women, and Takahashi et al[23] found low CSF 5-HIAA concentrations in alcoholics who had undergone severe withdrawal.

Parental alcoholism had little effect on levels of monoamine metabolites, except that lower concentrations of 5-HIAA, HVA, and tryptophan were observed in the 12 alcoholics who reported that both of their parents were alcoholic. Determination of family history of alcoholism by structured questioning of the alcoholics rather than having additional verification by relatives or significant others is a less-than-optimal practice,[24] even though it yields more accurate results for the family history of alcoholism than for most other mental disorders.[25]

The observed interrelationships among CSF monoamine metabolite concentrations are generally compatible with the existing literature.[26] Higher levels of HVA and lower levels of tryptophan predicted higher levels of 5-HIAA. Higher levels of 5-HIAA and MHPG predicted higher levels of HVA, whereas increasing years of excessive alcohol consumption tended to predict lower levels of HVA. Increasing age and HVA levels predicted higher levels of MHPG, as previously reported.[27] Decreasing levels of 5-HIAA and increasing levels of aspartate and alanine aminotransferase predicted higher levels of tryptophan. The negative relationship between CSF tryptophan and 5-HIAA concentration (Figure 2) is seemingly contrary to the suggestion that free tryptophan crossing the blood-brain barrier drives the rate of serotonin synthesis.[28] Virkkunen and Narvanen[29] found, however, that Finnish violent alcoholics with low CSF 5-HIAA concentrations had high ratios of plasma tryptophan to large neutral amino acids. These data are in accordance with a recent suggestion that in humans, under certain circumstances, the activity of tryptophan hydroxylase per se, rather than the free extracellular tryptophan concentration, may be rate limiting for central serotonin turnover.[30]

In addition to satisfying Research Diagnostic Criteria for a lifetime diagnosis of alcoholism, 90 individuals also satisfied criteria for other lifetime psychiatric disorders. This relatively high prevalence of comorbidity has been reported by others[31,32] and consisted of disorders that were separable from alcoholic behavior as well as those that were not separable. In the 54 alcoholics with past or present psychiatric disorders that were separable from alcoholic behavior, the most frequent were drug use, mood, and anxiety disorders (Table 3). Mood and anxiety disorders were the most frequent psychiatric disorders observed (Table 3) in the 68 alcoholics for whom the psychiatric disorders were not separable from alcohol-related behavior.

In studies on violent, antisocial alcoholics in Finland, the patients with a family history of paternal alcoholism had the lowest CSF 5-HIAA concentration.[33] The Finnish patients, as a group, had much lower CSF 5-HIAA concentrations than the present sample. Because CSF 5-HIAA is influenced by genetic and environmental variables, it may be that the genetic variation is more apparent at the extremes of the distribution, such as was observed among the Finnish patients. A history of suicide attempts was also related to extremely low CSF 5-HIAA levels among alcoholic violent Finns,[8,34] but the present study replicates our previous finding[35] of a lack of a relationship between CSF 5-HIAA and suicide attempts among American treatment-seeking alcoholics, free of personality disorders and with 5-HIAA levels in the normal range.

Rosenthal et al[36] reported that depressed patients, who themselves did not have a drinking problem but had a family history of alcoholism, had a lower mean CSF 5-HIAA concentration than equally depressed patients free of a family history of alcoholism. Although family history of depression was not determined in the present study, a personal history of depressive episodes was not associated with a low CSF 5-HIAA concentration.

In conclusion, we found that early-onset alcoholics had a lower mean CSF 5-HIAA concentration than late-onset alcoholics. Early-onset alcoholics also had a more severe course of illness than late-onset alcoholics. Psychiatric comorbidity and family history positive for paternal alcoholism did not correlate with CSF 5-HIAA, but a history of alcoholism in both parents was correlated with low CSF 5-HIAA concentration.

Accepted for publication May 4, 1995.

Reprint requests to National Institute on Alcohol Abuse and Alcoholism, 10/3C103, 10 Center Dr MSC-1256, Bethesda, MD 20892-1256 (Dr Linnoila).

REFERENCES

1. Robins LN, Helzer JE, Weissman MM, Orvaschel H, Gruenberg E, Burke JD, Regier DA. Lifetime prevalence of specific psychiatric disorders in three sites. *Arch Gen Psychiatry.* 1984;41:949-958.
2. Cloninger R, Bohman M, Sigvardsson S. Inheritance of alcohol abuse: cross fostering analysis of adopted men. *Arch Gen Psychiatry.* 1981;38:861-868.
3. Irwin M, Schuckit M, Smith T. Clinical importance of age of onset in type 1 and type 2 primary alcoholics. *Arch Gen Psychiatry.* 1990;47:320-324.
4. Lamparski DM, Roy A, Nutt DJ, Linnoila M. The criteria of Cloninger et al. and von Knorring et al. for subgrouping of alcoholics: a comparison in a clinical population. *Acta Psychiatr Scand.* 1991;84:497-502.
5. von Knorring AL, Bohman M, von Knorring L, Oreland L. Platelet MAO activity as a biological marker in subgroups of alcoholism. *Acta Psychiatr Scand.* 1985; 72:51-58.
6. von Knorring L, Oreland L, von Knorring AL. Personality traits and platelet MAO activity in alcohol and drug abusing teenage boys. *Acta Psychiatr Scand.* 1987;75:307-314.
7. Benkelfat C, Murphy DL, Hill JL, George DT, Nutt D, Linnoila M. Ethanollike properties of the serotonergic partial agonist m-chlorophenylpiperazine in chronic alcoholic patients. *Arch Gen Psychiatry.* 1991;48:383.
8. Linnoila M, Virkkunen M, Scheinin M, Nuutila A, Rimon R, Goodwin FK. Low cerebrospinal fluid 5-hydroxyindoleacetic acid concentration differentiates impulsive from nonimpulsive violent behavior. *Life Sci.* 1983;33:2609-2614.
9. Virkkunen M, Nuutila A, Goodwin FK, Linnoila M. Cerebrospinal fluid monoamine metabolites in male arsonists. *Arch Gen Psychiatry.* 1987;44:241-247.
10. Roy A, Virkkunen M, Linnoila M. Reduced central serotonin turnover in a subgroup of alcoholics? *Prog Neuropsychopharmacol Biol Psychiatry.* 1987;11: 173-177.
11. Spitzer R, Endicott J, Robins E. Research diagnostic criteria: rationale and reliability. *Arch Gen Psychiatry.* 1978;35:773-782.
12. Muscettola G, Wehr T, Goodwin FK. Effect of diet on urinary MHPG excretion in depressed patients and normal control subjects. *Am J Psychiatry.* 1977; 134:914-916.
13. Scheinin M, Chang W, Kirk K, Linnoila M. Simultaneous determination of 3-methoxy-4-hydroxyphenylglycol, 5-hydroxyindoleacetic acid and homovanillic acid in cerebrospinal fluid with high performance liquid chromatography using electrochemical detection. *Anal Biochem.* 1983;131:246-253.
14. Endicott J, Spitzer R. A diagnostic interview: the Schedule for Affective Disorders and Schizophrenia. *Arch Gen Psychiatry.* 1978;35:837-844.
15. Selzer ML. The Michigan Alcoholism Screening Test: the quest for a new diagnostic instrument. *Am J Psychiatry.* 1971;127:1653-1658.
16. Mayfield DG, McLeod G, Hall P. The CAGE questionnaire: validation of a new alcoholism screening instrument. *Am J Psychiatry.* 1974;131:1121-1123.
17. Eckardt MJ, Parker ES, Noble EP, Feldman DJ, Gottschalk LA. Relationship between neuropsychological performance and alcohol consumption in alcoholics. *Biol Psychiatry.* 1978;13:551-564.
18. Dixon WJ. *BMDP Statistical Software Manual.* Berkeley, Calif: University of California Press; 1990.
19. Cloninger R. Neurogenetic mechanisms in alcoholism. *Science.* 1987;236:410-416.
20. Roy A, DeJong J, Lamparski D, Adinoff B, George T, Moore V, Garnett D, Kerich M, Linnoila M. Mental disorders among alcoholics. *Arch Gen Psychiatry.* 1991; 48:423-427.
21. Ballenger J, Goodwin F, Major L, Brown G. Alcohol and central serotonin metabolism in man. *Arch Gen Psychiatry.* 1979;36:224-227.
22. Banki C. Factors influencing monoamine metabolites and tryptophan in patients with alcohol dependence. *J Neural Transm.* 1981;50:98-101.
23. Takahashi S, Yamane H, Kondo H, Tani M. CSF monoamine metabolites in alcoholism, a comparative study with depression. *Folia Psychiatr Neurol Jpn.* 1974;28:347-354.
24. Andreasen NC, Rice J, Endicott J, Reich T, Coryell W. The family history approach to diagnosis: how useful is it? *Arch Gen Psychiatry.* 1986;43:421-429.
25. Roy M-A, Walsh D, Prescott CA, Kendler K. Biases in the diagnosis of alcoholism by the family history method. *Alcohol Clin Exp Res.* 1994;18:845-851.
26. Agren H, Mefford IN, Rudorfer MV, Linnoila M, Potter WZ. Interacting neurotransmitter systems: a non-experimental approach to the 5HIAA-HVA correlation in human CSF. *Psychiatry Res.* 1986;20:175-193.
27. Cutler NR, Kay AD, Agren H, Linnoila M, Potter WZ. Cerebrospinal fluid monoamine metabolites in 32 healthy men aged 19-77 years. *Brain Dysfunct.* 1988; 1:192-196.
28. Fernstrom JD, Wurtman RJ. Brain serotonin content: physiological regulation by plasma neutral amino acids. *Science.* 1972;178:414-416.
29. Virkkunen M, Narvanen S. Plasma insulin, tryptophan and serotonin levels during the glucose tolerance test among habitually violent and impulsive offenders. *Neuropsychobiology.* 1987;17:19-23.
30. Nielsen D, Goldman D, Virkkunen M, Tokola R, Rawlings R, Linnoila M. Suicidality and 5-hydroxyindoleacetic acid concentration associated with a tryptophan hydroxylase polymorphism. *Arch Gen Psychiatry.* 1994;51:34-38.
31. Schuckit M. The clinical implications of primary diagnostic groups among alcoholics. *Arch Gen Psychiatry.* 1985;42:1043-1049.
32. Hesselbrock M, Meyer R, Keener J. Psychopathology in hospitalized alcoholics. *Arch Gen Psychiatry.* 1985;42:1050-1055.
33. Linnoila M, DeJong J, Virkkunen M. Family history of alcoholism in violent offenders and impulsive fire setters. *Arch Gen Psychiatry.* 1989;46:613-616.
34. Virkkunen M, DeJong J, Bartko J, Linnoila M. Psychobiological concomitants of a history of suicide attempts among violent offenders and impulsive fire setters. *Arch Gen Psychiatry.* 1989;42:604-606.
35. Roy A, Lamparski D, DeJong J, Moore V, Linnoila M. Characteristics of alcoholics who attempt suicide. *Am J Psychiatry.* 1990;147:761-765.
36. Rosenthal N, Davenport Y, Cowdry R, Webster M, Goodwin F. Monoamine metabolites in cerebrospinal fluid of depressive subgroups. *Psychiatry Res.* 1980;2:113-119.

ORIGINAL ARTICLE

Six-Month Follow-up of Naltrexone and Psychotherapy for Alcohol Dependence

Stephanie S. O'Malley, PhD; Adam J. Jaffe, PhD; Grace Chang, MD; Sarah Rode, MA; Richard Schottenfeld, MD; Roger E. Meyer, MD; Bruce Rounsaville, MD

Background: The goal of this study was to examine the persistence of naltrexone's effects on drinking outcomes among alcoholics following discontinuation of treatment and to determine whether coping skills therapy improves long-term outcomes compared with supportive therapy.

Methods: Eighty of 97 alcohol-dependent subjects randomized to receive naltrexone or placebo and either coping skills therapy or supportive therapy for 12 weeks were assessed at a 6-month off-treatment follow-up.

Results: Subjects who received naltrexone were less likely to drink heavily or to meet criteria for alcohol abuse or dependence than subjects who received placebo. The effect of naltrexone therapy on abstinence rates persisted only through the first month of follow-up. Coping skills therapy was associated with decreased levels of drinking among subjects who received placebo. Psychotherapy condition, however, did not predict alcohol diagnosis at follow-up.

Conclusions: Some but not all of the benefits resulting from short-term naltrexone treatment persist after discontinuation of treatment. The findings suggest that continued treatment with naltrexone may be beneficial for some patients.

(Arch Gen Psychiatry. 1996;53:217-224)

THE IMPORTANCE of follow-up studies of initial clinical trials of pharmacotherapy and psychotherapy has been emphasized but not always pursued in practice.[1] Pharmacological interventions that are beneficial initially may exhibit rebound effects caused by receptor changes resulting from long-term administration. In addition, information about the durability of improvement following discontinuation of pharmacotherapy may suggest the need for extended drug treatment. With regard to psychotherapy interventions, the follow-up period can be used to evaluate the possibility that alternative treatments differentially influence the subject's ability to function after treatment termination. In cognitive behavioral interventions, for example, patients are taught new skills that they can apply to new problems, thereby acting as their own therapist.

In an earlier report,[2] we examined the effectiveness of naltrexone in combination with two different forms of psychotherapy in the treatment of alcohol dependence. Subjects were randomly assigned to one of four groups for 12 weeks: (1) naltrexone and coping skills therapy, (2) naltrexone and supportive therapy, (3) placebo and coping skills therapy, and (4) placebo and supportive therapy. The major findings were that naltrexone treatment reduced the number of days in which alcohol was consumed and increased the time to relapse to heavy drinking. In addition, we found that rates of continuous abstinence were highest for subjects receiving naltrexone and supportive psychotherapy. Among those subjects who had an initial drink, however, those receiving naltrexone and coping skills therapy had the lowest rate of relapse. Reduction in relapse rates with naltrexone treatment has also been reported by Volpicelli and colleagues,[3] who studied 70 alcohol-dependent outpatients at the Philadelphia (Pa) Veterans Affairs Medical Center. Naltrexone appeared to differentially prevent

From the Department of Psychiatry, Yale University School of Medicine, New Haven, Conn (Drs O'Malley, Jaffe, Schottenfeld, and Rounsaville and Ms Rode); Division of Psychiatry, Department of Medicine, Harvard Medical School and Brigham and Women's Hospital, Boston, Mass (Dr Chang); and Association of Academic Health Centers, Washington, DC (Dr Meyer).

See Subjects and Methods on next page

SUBJECTS AND METHODS

SUBJECTS

Subjects were recruited through advertisements in New Haven (Conn) area newspapers and from among patients seeking treatment at the outpatient Alcohol Treatment Unit of the Connecticut Mental Health Center. Individuals were eligible to participate if they (1) met the *DSM-III-R* criteria for alcohol dependence,[6] (2) had achieved 7 to 30 days of abstinence just prior to the first therapy session, and (3) were 18 to 65 years old. Criteria for exclusion were (1) a current *DSM-III-R* diagnosis of dependence on other substances, except nicotine; (2) a history of opioid abuse; (3) a history of psychosis; (4) current suicidality, homicidality, or psychiatric symptoms that required other medications; (5) current disulfiram use; (6) significant cerebral, renal, thyroid, or cardiac disease; (7) a history of cirrhosis or laboratory evidence of significant hepatocellular injury; and (8) in women, pregnancy, nursing, or refusal to use a reliable method of birth control.

A total of 104 subjects were randomized in a 2×2 factorial design into one of four treatment conditions: naltrexone and coping skills therapy, naltrexone and supportive therapy, placebo and coping skills therapy, and placebo and supportive therapy. Treatment was provided for 12 weeks. The treatment groups did not differ significantly in rates of study completion. The final sample on which the analyses are based consists of 97 subjects who received therapy and medication for at least 1 week.

The sample was primarily male (74% [n=72]), white (93% [n=90]), employed full-time (73% [n=71]), and unmarried (66% [n=64]). Their mean (SD) age was 40.5 (9.7) years. On average, they drank on 60% of the days (36 days) during the 60-day pretreatment baseline period and consumed a mean of 11.2 (9.2) standard drinks per drinking occasion.

STUDY CONDITIONS AND PROCEDURES

In each of the study conditions, subjects were seen weekly by therapists with MA or PhD degrees in individual treatment sessions that were guided by a manual.

Pharmacotherapy

Subjects were prescribed 50 mg of naltrexone or a matching placebo to be taken daily. Riboflavin, 25 mg, was incorporated into all capsules as a compliance marker.[2,7]

Coping Skills/Relapse Prevention Therapy

This therapy is based on Marlatt and Gordon's[8] model of relapse prevention and uses didactic presentations, cognitive and behavioral rehearsal within sessions, and homework exercises to foster the acquisition of coping skills.[9,10] The main components include (1) self-monitoring and a functional analysis of drinking behavior; (2) teaching, modeling, and role-playing of coping skills, such as stress and anger management; (3) cognitive and behavioral strategies for handling problems, urges, and cravings; (4) development of problem-solving skills; and (5) development of leisure activities that do not involve alcohol. In addition, patients are informed about the abstinence violation effect,[7] involving negative self-evaluations that typically follow a drinking lapse. Patients are taught to keep a lapse from turning into a relapse by anticipating the abstinence violation effect, monitoring and changing their thoughts and feelings following a slip, and using new behaviors, such as leaving the situation or calling a friend.

Supportive Therapy

Patients were encouraged by their therapist to remain abstinent without being taught specific coping skills. Therapist references to content relevant to coping skills or relapse prevention were prohibited. Instead, the therapist inquired about how the patient was doing in more general terms as well as inquiring specifically about drinking behavior. In addition, the therapist encouraged and supported the patient's efforts at abstinence and self-derived strategies. This approach was primarily nondirective, but the therapist could give advice if asked by the patient.

A detailed description of study conditions and procedures can be found in the original report of the initial 12-week treatment outcomes.[2]

DATA COLLECTION AND MEASURES

Subjects were assessed prior to treatment (baseline), weekly during treatment, at termination from treatment, and at

relapse among those subjects who "sampled" an initial alcoholic drink.

These data suggest that naltrexone, an opioid receptor antagonist, may modify some of the effects of alcohol that are reinforcing and that "prime" further drinking. Similarly, naltrexone may improve abstinence rates by blocking conditioned neuroendocrine changes that occur in response to environmental cues previously paired with alcohol consumption.[4,5]

The durability of naltrexone's effects on abstinence and heavy drinking following discontinuation of treatment has yet to be evaluated. As a result, this investigation examines clinical outcomes over the 6-month period following treatment termination for the patients who participated in our 12-week controlled clinical trial of naltrexone and psychotherapy in the treatment of alcohol dependence.[2] Three main questions are addressed:

1. After naltrexone treatment is discontinued, do subjects who received naltrexone continue to have higher abstinence rates and lower rates of heavy drinking over time than subjects who received placebo? A related question is whether there are differences in the long-term outcome of naltrexone and placebo subjects as measured by *DSM-III-R* criteria for alcohol abuse and dependence. Specifically, are subjects who received naltrexone less likely to be classified at follow-up as having an alcohol diagnosis than subjects who received placebo?

2. What is the relationship between the success-

6-month follow-up. Patients were evaluated before, during, and after treatment by a research assistant with a bachelor's degree. In addition, the study psychiatrist met with the patient prior to treatment to discuss the study medication, which was begun on the day of the first therapy session. Weekly ratings (eg, medication side effects, global functioning, and completion of session therapy tasks) were also made by the therapist.

FOLLOW-UP PROCEDURES

At the end of the initial 12-week treatment trial, the study medication was discontinued for all subjects. Subjects requesting additional counseling were referred to the outpatient Alcohol Treatment Unit of the Connecticut Mental Health Center or to private therapists.

Six months after completion of the treatment phase, subjects were invited by telephone and/or letter to participate in a 1-hour follow-up interview with a research assistant. The research assistant used the time-line follow-back technique[11] to elicit information about the number of drinks consumed each day for the 6 months following treatment termination. The time-line follow-back interview has been demonstrated to provide reliable and valid retrospective assessments of drinking for up to 360 days.[12] The subject was also interviewed using the alcohol section of the Structured Clinical Interview for *DSM-III-R* (SCID)[13] to determine whether the subject had experienced symptoms of alcohol abuse or dependence during the 6-month follow-up period. The research assistant and the subject remained blind to the pharmacotherapy condition until the end of the interview, at which time an envelope was opened, revealing whether the subject had been taking naltrexone or placebo. The research assistant was also blind to the psychotherapy condition.

DATA ANALYSIS PLAN

Our primary outcome variables included measures of drinking status derived from the time-line follow-back assessment and diagnoses of alcohol abuse or dependence ascertained with the SCID at follow-up. Initially, several continuous variables were considered, including percentage of days drinking and percentage of days of heavy drinking. The distributions of these variables, however, did not meet the assumption of approximate normality and were highly skewed. Attempts to transform the data failed to resolve this problem. As a result, data from the time-line assessment were used to categorize the subject's drinking status during each month of the follow-up into three ordered categories: (1) no drinking, (2) light-moderate drinking, and (3) heavy drinking. No drinking was coded if the subject abstained throughout the 30-day period. Light-moderate drinking was used to indicate a day or more of drinking one to four drinks for men and one to three drinks for women. Heavy drinking was coded based on five or more drinks on an occasion for men or four or more drinks on an occasion for women on 1 or more days of the month. Thus, six time points were established for this ordinal-dependent variable (ie, months 1 to 6 of follow-up).

To analyze the repeated ordinal classifications of drinking status during the six monthly follow-up periods, a random-effects ordinal logistic regression model[14] was used, as implemented in the MIXOR software program.[15] The random-effects ordinal regression model is an ordinal analogue of the random-effects regression models[16,17] that have been used for repeated-outcome variables measured on a continuous scale. This model was used to characterize the repeated ordinal responses in terms of time-related changes in drinking level across the follow-up period. In these analyses, linear trends across time were considered in addition to effects averaged over time. Specific tests were conducted to determine the effect of medication and psychotherapy as well as the medication-by-psychotherapy interaction on overall drinking levels during the follow-up period (overall condition effects) and on time-related changes in drinking during the follow-up period (condition-by-time interactions).

As a follow-up to the longitudinal analysis, rates of any drinking (nonabstention) and rates of heavy drinking for each of the six monthly time points were analyzed separately using logistic regression analyses. We also examined drinking and heavy drinking rates during the 12-week treatment period for the subjects comprising the follow-up sample. The dependent measures of drinking and heavy drinking are similar to the two major outcomes in our initial trial, time to first drink and time to first relapse. In the survival analyses described in the original report of the treatment-phase results,[2] subjects who dropped out of treatment were assumed to have failed in addition to those subjects who were observed to have drunk or relapsed during the period in which they were observed. Finally, subjects were characterized based on whether they had ever drunk and based on whether they had at least 1 day of heavy drinking during the 6-month period.

ful maintenance of abstinence during treatment and clinical status at the end of the follow-up as measured by *DSM-III-R* criteria for alcohol abuse or dependence? The answer to this question provides information needed to evaluate whether the goal of naltrexone treatment should be abstinence or reduced use.

3. Does coping skills therapy result in more enduring changes in drinking behavior than supportive therapy? In coping skills/relapse prevention therapy, the patient is taught concrete coping strategies to use once treatment has ended. In contrast, specific coping skills were not taught to patients receiving supportive therapy. As a result, we hypothesized that subjects who received coping skills therapy would be better equipped to cope with high-risk situations once treatment ended and thus would have better drinking-related outcomes than subjects who received supportive therapy.

RESULTS

FOLLOW-UP SAMPLE

Rates of Follow-up

Eighty of the original 97 subjects treated with study medication for at least 1 week participated in the follow-up interview, for a follow-up rate of 82%. The interview rate did not differ by randomized treatment condition ($\chi^2 < 1.03$ for all): naltrexone/coping skills, 21 (88%) of 24; naltrexone/supportive, 19 (86%) of 22; placebo/coping skills, 20 (83%)

Table 1. Demographic and Baseline Characteristics of the Follow-up Sample by Treatment Assignment

	Naltrexone		Placebo	
	Coping Skills (n=21)	Supportive (n=19)	Coping Skills (n=20)	Supportive (n=20)
Mean (±SD) age, y	44.0±10.4	41.2±11.6	39.7±9.2	37.0±8.0
Male, No. (%)	15 (71)	18 (95)	13 (65)	15 (75)
White, No. (%)	17 (81)	18 (95)	19 (95)	19 (95)
Married, No. (%)	9 (43)	8 (42)	5 (25)	5 (25)
Employed, No. (%)	17 (81)	15 (79)	14 (70)	14 (70)
Mean (±SD) pretreatment drinking*				
Drinking days, %	63.2±29.2	61.9±21.0	59.3±23.5	61.8±28.0
Heavy drinking days, %†	41.4±26.1	50.2±26.3	44.7±25.7	54.1±28.5

*Measures of drinking during the 90 days prior to study participation.
†Five or more drinks per day for men and four or more drinks per day for women.

of 24; and placebo/supportive, 20 (74%) of 27. All subjects were interviewed in a face-to-face session, with the exception of two subjects who were interviewed by telephone.

Follow-up interviews were completed within 6 months of their due date for 71 subjects and beyond the 6-month window for nine subjects. There were no significant differences in timeliness of follow-up associated with treatment group.

Interviewed vs Noninterviewed Subjects

There were no statistically significant differences between interviewed subjects and those unavailable for follow-up on the following demographic variables: age, gender, marital status, educational level, and employment status. All of the minority subjects (n=7) were reached for follow-up; therefore, all the noninterviewed subjects were white.

Compared with the 80 subjects who were interviewed, subjects who were unavailable for follow-up were less likely to have completed 10 or more weeks of treatment (78% [62/80] vs 35% [6/17]; χ^2=11.92, *df*=1, *P*=.001). Mean treatment participation was longer for subjects who completed the follow-up (11.5 [3.0] weeks) than for subjects who did not (7.3 [4.3] weeks; *t*=−3.76, Satterthwaite *df*=19.1, *P*=.001). Subjects who were and were not reached for follow-up were similar on the percentage of drinking days and heavy drinking days at baseline.

BASELINE CHARACTERISTICS

The demographic and baseline drinking characteristics of subjects who participated in the follow-up are presented in **Table 1** by randomized treatment group. The groups did not differ significantly on race, marital status, education, employment, or measures of drinking at baseline. Men were slightly overrepresented in the supportive therapy condition (χ^2=3.39, *P*=.07). Patients who received naltrexone tended to be older (mean age, 42.7 [10.9] years) than subjects who received placebo (mean age, 38.4 [9.1] years) (F[1, 76]=3.52, *P*=.07).

TREATMENT RECEIVED DURING FOLLOW-UP

As described above, naltrexone treatment was discontinued at the end of the trial. Subjects were free, however, to seek additional psychotherapy with providers other than study staff. Forty-six percent of the subjects (n=37) reported attending at least one session of additional treatment (eg, individual, group, or family therapy, self-help groups). There were no significant differences in rates of participation in additional treatment for the four treatment groups: naltrexone/coping skills, 43% (9/21); naltrexone/supportive, 53% (10/19); placebo/coping skills, 50% (10/20); and placebo/supportive, 40% (8/20).

DRINKING STATUS DURING TREATMENT

As can be seen in **Table 2**, subjects in the follow-up sample who initially received naltrexone were less likely to drink (45% [18/40]) while in treatment than subjects who received placebo (78% [31/40]) (*P*<.01). Supportive therapy also tended to be associated with lower rates of nonabstention during treatment than coping skills therapy (51% [20/39] vs 71% [29/41], *P*<.10). When heavy drinking was considered (**Table 3**), subjects who had received naltrexone were less likely to have a day of heavy drinking during treatment than subjects who had received placebo (25% [10/40] vs 60% [24/40], *P*<.01). No differences were found for psychotherapy or for the interaction of medication and psychotherapy.

DRINKING BEHAVIOR DURING FOLLOW-UP

Table 4 presents the results of the random-effects ordinal logistic regression analysis for the six monthly follow-up periods. Note that the direction of the estimates is such that positive values indicate a positive association with increased levels of drinking (ie, from abstinent to light-moderate to heavy). As can be seen in Table 4, there was a significant main effect of time, suggesting that levels of drinking increased over the 6-month follow-up period (*P*<.05). The main effect of medication condition was of marginal significance (*P*=.06), favoring naltrexone over placebo. The data, however, show strong condition-by-time interaction effects. The significant positive medication-by-time interaction (*P*<.001) indicates that the effect of medication condition diminishes over time. For purposes of interpreting this time-by-condition interaction, Tables 2 and 3 present rates of any drinking (light-moderate and heavy) and rates of heavy drinking across time by randomized treatment condition. As can be seen, naltrex-

Table 2. Rates of Drinking During Treatment and Follow-up by Treatment Assignment

	Drinking, No. (%)*					
	Naltrexone		Placebo		χ^2	
	Coping Skills (n=21)	Supportive (n=19)	Coping Skills (n=20)	Supportive (n=20)	Medication	Therapy
Treatment	12 (57)	6 (32)	17 (85)	14 (70)	8.81†	3.55‡
Follow-up						
Month 1	8 (38)	5 (26)	14 (74)§	10 (53)§	7.35†	2.26
Month 2	12 (57)	6 (32)	14 (70)	11 (55)	2.68	3.32‖
Month 3	12 (57)	9 (47)	14 (70)	13 (65)	1.91	0.45
Month 4	12 (57)	10 (53)	14 (70)	12 (60)	<1	<1
Month 5	15 (71)	11 (58)	12 (60)	13 (65)	<1	<1
Month 6	14 (67)	11 (58)	11 (55)	13 (65)	<1	<1
Overall	16 (76)	15 (79)	19 (95)	15 (75)	1.3	1.5

*These data reflect subjects who reported drinking on 1 or more days in each of the specified periods and are not cumulative.
†$P<.01$.
‡$P<.05$.
§Sample reduced by one subject because of missing data.
‖$P<.10$.

Table 3. Rates of Heavy Drinking During Treatment and Follow-up by Treatment Assignment

	Heavy Drinking, No. (%)*					
	Naltrexone		Placebo		χ^2	
	Coping Skills (n=21)	Supportive (n=19)	Coping Skills (n=20)	Supportive (n=20)	Medication	Therapy
Treatment	5 (24)	5 (26)	13 (65)	11 (55)	9.50†	<1
Follow-up						
Month 1	2 (10)	4 (21)	12 (63)‡	10 (53)‡	13.24§	<1
Month 2	5 (24)	6 (32)	14 (70)	10 (50)	8.21†	<1
Month 3	5 (24)	8 (42)	12 (60)	12 (60)	5.87‖	<1
Month 4	6 (29)	8 (42)	11 (55)	12 (60)	3.90‖	<1
Month 5	7 (33)	8 (42)	8 (40)	12 (60)	1.21‖	1.66
Month 6	6 (29)	7 (37)	7 (35)	12 (60)	1.74	2.21
Overall	9 (43)	13 (68)	16 (80)	15 (75)	3.93‖	<1

*These data reflect subjects who reported heavy drinking (five or more drinks per day for men and four or more drinks per day for women) on 1 or more days in each of the specified periods and are not cumulative.
†$P<.01$.
‡Sample reduced by one subject because of missing data.
§$P<.001$.
‖$P<.05$.

one was associated with a strong positive effect in the early follow-up period that diminished over time. During the first month of follow-up (Table 2), logistic regression analyses indicate that subjects who had received naltrexone during treatment remained significantly less likely to slip and consume some alcohol than subjects who had received placebo (33% [13/40] vs 63% [24/38], $P<.01$). At month 2, this difference was no longer statistically significant. When heavy drinking was considered (Table 3), naltrexone-treated subjects were significantly less likely to drink heavily than subjects who had received placebo through month 4, with no differences associated with medication condition in months 5 and 6.

The main effect of psychotherapy was nonsignificant; however, there was a negative psychotherapy-by-month interaction ($P<.002$), indicating that coping skills therapy had a slight negative effect initially that improved across time. However, a significant three-way interaction of medication, psychotherapy, and time was also found ($P<.05$). An examination of Tables 2 and 3 suggests that while the changes in rates of drinking and heavy drinking across the follow-up times were relatively similar for the two groups that received naltrexone, the changes in rates across time for the two placebo groups were quite dissimilar. The naltrexone coping skills group and the naltrexone supportive group each exhibited approximately a 30% increase in drinking and a 20% increase in heavy drinking across time during the follow-up. The placebo supportive group showed approximately a 10% increase in drinking and heavy drinking rates over time, whereas the placebo coping skills group showed a pronounced decrease in both any drinking and heavy drinking rates over time (19% and 28%, respectively). By the sixth month of follow-up, subjects who received placebo and coping skills therapy had rates of drinking and heavy drinking that were similar to those of the two groups originally treated with naltrexone.

Table 4. Random-Effects Ordinal Logistic Regression Analysis of the Effects of Time and Treatment Condition Across 6 Months of Follow-up (n=80)*

Effect†	Parameter Estimate, Mean (SE)	z	P
Overall time	0.147 (0.061)	2.4	.02
Overall condition			
Medication	−0.673 (0.355)	−1.298	.06
Psychotherapy	−0.142 (0.363)	−0.392	.70
Medication×psychotherapy	0.056 (0.357)	0.158	.87
Condition×time			
Medication×time	0.240 (0.061)	3.909	.001
Psychotherapy×time	−0.192 (0.061)	−3.133	.002
Medication×psychotherapy× time	0.133 (0.065)	2.042	.04

Ordinal outcome variables were 0, no drinking; 1, one to four drinks for men or one to three drinks for women on any day (light-moderate drinking); and 2, more than four drinks for men and more than four drinks for women on 1 or more days in a 30-day period.

†All effects were centered for this analysis. The codes for the effects are, for medication: naltrexone, 1; placebo, −1; for psychotherapy: coping skills, 1; supportive therapy, −1; and for time: months 1 through 6, −2.5, −1.5, −0.5, 0.5, 1.5, and 2.5, respectively.

When the entire follow-up period was considered, the percentage of subjects who drank at least once during the 6-month follow-up did not differ significantly as a function of either the psychotherapy type or medication condition. The percentage of subjects who had at least 1 day of heavy drinking over the 6-month follow-up period was significantly higher for placebo-treated subjects than for naltrexone-treated subjects (78% [31/40] vs 55% [22/40], $P<.05$).

ALCOHOL-RELATED DIAGNOSES AT FOLLOW-UP

At the follow-up interview, subjects were reinterviewed with the alcohol section of the SCID. In responding to these questions, subjects were asked to consider the 6 months following treatment termination. Positive responses were used to assign a diagnosis of alcohol abuse or dependence using the criteria specified in *DSM-III-R*, except that the time frame was restricted to the follow-up period. Diagnosis (no diagnosis, abuse, or dependence) was related to medication, psychotherapy, and their interaction as independent variables using logistic regression analysis. Since SCID data were not obtained for three subjects, the sample size for this analysis was 77. The results indicated that naltrexone was superior to placebo in preventing another episode of alcohol abuse or dependence ($\chi^2=7.66$, $P<.01$). Of the subjects who had received placebo, 24% (9/38) met the criteria for alcohol abuse and 39% (15/38) met the criteria for dependence. In contrast, only 13% (5/39) of naltrexone-treated subjects met the criteria for alcohol abuse and 18% (7/39) met the criteria for alcohol dependence. Diagnosis at follow-up was unrelated to the type of psychotherapy received during treatment or to the interaction of medication condition and psychotherapy ($\chi^2<1$ for both).

RELATIONSHIP BETWEEN DRINKING DURING TREATMENT AND ALCOHOL-RELATED DIAGNOSES AT FOLLOW-UP

Given evidence from the initial treatment trial that naltrexone may prevent uncontrolled drinking once drinking is initiated, we were interested in examining the relationship between alcohol consumption during treatment and the probability of receiving an alcohol diagnosis at the 6-month follow-up. The logistic regression analysis predicting diagnosis from drinking during treatment, medication, and the interaction of medication and drinking during treatment revealed a significant effect of drinking during treatment ($\chi^2=7.57$, $P<.01$). Subjects who abstained during treatment were less likely to receive a diagnosis of alcohol abuse (10% [3/31]) or dependence (13% [4/31]) at follow-up than subjects who drank (abuse, 24% [11/46]; dependence, 39% [18/46]). Medication condition and the interaction of medication with abstinence during treatment did not predict diagnosis in this analysis, which simultaneously considered abstinence during treatment.

COMMENT

The results of this naturalistic follow-up study suggest that some but not all of the benefits resulting from short-term treatment with naltrexone persist after discontinuation of treatment. Although naltrexone resulted in higher abstinence rates during treatment, this effect was no longer apparent by the second month of follow-up. The effect of naltrexone on relapse rates was more durable and persisted in a diminished fashion through month 4 of follow-up. In addition, the percentage of subjects who avoided relapse over the entire follow-up period was higher for naltrexone than for placebo. Finally, subjects who had received naltrexone were significantly less likely to meet the criteria for a diagnosis of alcohol abuse or dependence over the course of the follow-up period than subjects who had received placebo.

In understanding naltrexone's ability to support abstinence, one hypothesis is that cues associated with drinking may act like a "priming dose" of alcohol and elicit an appetitive motivational response, perhaps through conditioned endogenous opioid release. For those patients receiving placebo, this response may lead to drinking. If naltrexone blocks this response to drinking-related stimuli, these alcohol-related cues may lose their ability to elicit craving, alcohol-related thoughts, and drinking behavior. This hypothesis derives from work by Stewart and colleagues,[5] who have argued that conditioned stimuli associated with drug use can elicit neural states that are similar to those produced by the drug itself, thereby increasing the probability of drug-related thoughts and behaviors. Using a conditioned place preference paradigm in mice, Cunningham and colleagues[18] have demonstrated that opioid antagonists can facilitate the extinction of the conditioned reinforcing effects of alcohol in the absence of alcohol ingestion. The longitudinal analysis in our sample, however, suggests that the ability of naltrexone to support abstinence does not persist for long after medication discontinuation.

Although the effect of the medication condition diminished over time, there was no evidence of rebound effects following discontinuation of naltrexone. In particular, for several months into follow-up, patients who received naltrexone continued to have lower relapse rates than patients who received placebo. The diminution of differences between naltrexone and placebo observed over time following medication discontinuation adds credence to the conclusion that the medication effects observed during treatment result from naltrexone and not from some other, unknown baseline patient characteristic.

It is noteworthy that only one third of the naltrexone subjects had resumed drinking to the point that they had the full syndrome of alcohol abuse or dependence by the end of the follow-up period, compared with almost two thirds of the placebo subjects. The interpretation of this finding requires consideration of the method used to obtain the diagnostic information. Subjects were asked whether they had experienced any of the problems/symptoms that constitute the *DSM-III-R* criteria for alcohol abuse and dependence across the 6-month follow-up period without reference to prior symptoms that might have remitted during treatment. Naltrexone patients entered the follow-up period with substantially better functioning than placebo patients, as reflected by differences in abstinence and heavy-drinking rates for the treatment period. In addition, the naltrexone group continued to have lower rates of heavy drinking through month 4 of follow-up. Hence, the period in which to accrue the consequences of heavy drinking that contribute to the diagnosis of alcohol abuse or dependence was limited. With a longer follow-up period, it is conceivable that the differences in diagnosis rates might diminish over time.

Based on these findings, we believe that continued naltrexone therapy beyond 12 weeks may be beneficial for some patients, although this hypothesis will need to be empirically tested. The period of treatment could be extended to allow for greater stabilization and integration of psychosocial changes that could help maintain abstinence once naltrexone was discontinued. As an alternative, naltrexone could be used on a short-term basis, with the possibility of resuming naltrexone during high-risk periods or following initial resumption of drinking. Peachy and Annis[19,20] have used a similar treatment strategy, integrating the use of calcium carbamide, an alcohol-sensitizing agent, and relapse-prevention techniques. Continuous calcium carbamide coverage is provided to initiate a stable abstinence period. Subsequently, the medication is used in high-risk situations that are identified by the patient, and this use is gradually discontinued as the patient develops alternative coping strategies for dealing with high-risk situations.[19]

The findings also have implications for the alcohol-related goals of short-term naltrexone treatment. In both of the published clinical trials of naltrexone for alcohol dependence,[2,3] the goal of treatment was abstinence. Nonetheless, many subjects sampled alcohol. Of those who drank, the majority receiving placebo met the criteria for heavy drinking, whereas subjects receiving naltrexone relapsed to heavy drinking at a lower rate. To relate this initial treatment effect of naltrexone to long-term functioning, we examined the relationship between abstinence during treatment and the presence of an alcohol diagnosis at follow-up. Abstinence during treatment significantly predicted whether subjects met the criteria for a diagnosis of alcohol abuse or dependence. The interaction between medication condition and abstention during treatment was nonsignificant, suggesting that subjects who abstained during treatment had significantly better 6-month outcomes than subjects who did not abstain, irrespective of medication condition. It should be remembered, however, that subjects initially treated with naltrexone were much more successful in maintaining abstinence during treatment than subjects who received placebo. Given that abstinence has been found to be a strong predictor of long-term outcome in other studies[21] as well as in this investigation, we continue to recommend abstinence as the goal of naltrexone therapy for alcohol dependence. Unless naltrexone is to be taken indefinitely, we predict that patients who drink, albeit moderately, while supported pharmacologically by naltrexone will increase their drinking over time once the medication is discontinued. The question of whether naltrexone can be used to promote moderation training in nonalcoholic heavy drinkers, however, is currently being investigated by others.[22]

Our hypothesis that subjects who received coping skills/relapse prevention training would have better clinical outcomes than subjects who received supportive therapy was partially supported by the data. The results of the random-effects ordinal regression analyses revealed a significant interaction between medication condition, psychotherapy condition, and time. The advantage of coping skills therapy was apparent primarily among subjects who had been randomized to placebo. At the outset of the follow-up period, the two placebo groups had higher rates of drinking and of heavy drinking than the two naltrexone groups. Over the 6-month period, these rates worsened slightly for patients who had received placebo and supportive therapy. In contrast, rates of drinking and heavy drinking declined substantially over time for placebo-treated subjects who had received coping skills therapy. Among the patients who had received naltrexone, there was no additional advantage conferred by participation in coping skills therapy. Naltrexone-treated subjects who received either form of psychotherapy showed similar increases in drinking and heavy drinking over the follow-up period.

Since the groups were equivalent in the use of other treatment during the follow-up, we hypothesize that the improvement of the placebo/coping skills group may have been caused by a delayed emergence of treatment efficacy associated with coping skills therapy. Carroll et al[21] also observed greater improvement during follow-up for cocaine abusers who received coping skills therapy vs clinical management and discussed the possible mechanisms of the effect, many of which also apply to the current study. Specifically, subjects in all treatment conditions received a number of nonspecific interventions during treatment, including weekly monitoring by research staff, support and encouragement from the therapist and research staff, and positive expectations for treatment and medication. Following treatment termination, however, subjects had to rely on their own resources. Coping skills therapy, which sought to teach generalizable coping skills, may have provided patients with more tools for addressing their drinking problem during follow-up. In contrast, the supportive therapy specifically precluded the teaching of coping skills, and as a result, these patients may not have had as many personal resources available to them. The failure to find differential efficacy between the two psychotherapies provided in conjunction with naltrexone may have been caused by the fact that these subjects were doing very well when they began the follow-up period.

A number of limitations must be considered in evaluating the results of this study. First, we relied exclusively on self-reports of drinking and alcohol-related problems during follow-up. Although self-reports of drinking obtained with the time-line follow-back method have been found to be reliable and valid,[12] information from other, corroborating measures, such as liver enzyme levels or collateral reports, would have been useful. While there is no reason to expect differences in the accuracy of reporting by patients who received naltrexone and patients who received placebo, the availability of such corroborating information would increase our confidence in the findings.

The small sample size represents another limitation. The issue of sample size is particularly problematic for assessment of psychotherapy effects, which tend to involve small to medium effect sizes.[23] Finally, our follow-up rate of 82% was only modest, limiting our ability to characterize the long-term course of the entire sample. In particular, it can be assumed that individuals with poorer outcomes were more likely to have been unavailable for follow-up.

CONCLUSIONS

The results of this study suggest that, compared with patients treated with placebo, patients initially treated with naltrexone continue to experience lower relapse rates and fewer alcohol-related consequences following discontinuation of treatment. At the same time, the advantage of naltrexone vs placebo appears to diminish over the follow-up period, suggesting that continued treatment with naltrexone beyond 12 weeks may be beneficial for some patients. Given that abstinence during treatment is a strong predictor of alcohol-related diagnoses at the end of the follow-up period, those patients who have not been able to attain a sustained period of abstinence may be candidates for longer-term naltrexone treatment. In addition, the finding that placebo patients who had received coping skills therapy improved over the course of follow-up suggests that teaching generalizable coping skills may contribute to better long-term outcomes.

Accepted for publication December 10, 1995.

This research was supported in part by grants P50-03-510, K02-AA00171, and RO1-AA09538 from the National Institute on Alcohol Abuse and Alcoholism, Bethesda, Md.

Preliminary results from this study were presented at the annual meeting of the Research Society on Alcoholism, San Antonio, Tex, June 22, 1993, and the annual meeting of the American Psychiatric Association, Philadelphia, Pa, May 24, 1994.

The authors thank Donald Hedeker, PhD, Kevin Lynch, MA, and Victor Golubchikov, MA, for their assistance in conducting the data analyses. DuPont-Merck, Wilmington, Del, generously provided the naltrexone and placebo used in this study.

Reprint requests to Substance Abuse Treatment Unit, Yale University School of Medicine, Box 18, 1 Long Wharf, New Haven, CT 06511 (Dr O'Malley).

REFERENCES

1. Nicholson RA, Berman JS. Is follow-up necessary in evaluating psychotherapy? *Psychol Bull.* 1980;93:261-278.
2. O'Malley SS, Jaffe AJ, Chang G, Schottenfeld RS, Meyer RE, Rounsaville BJ. Naltrexone and coping skills therapy for alcohol dependence: a controlled study. *Arch Gen Psychiatry.* 1992;49:881-887.
3. Volpicelli JR, Alterman AI, Hayashida M. Naltrexone in the treatment of alcohol dependence. *Arch Gen Psychiatry.* 1992;49:876-880.
4. O'Malley SS. Strategies to maximize the efficacy of naltrexone for alcohol dependence. In: Onken LS, Blaine JD, Boren JJ, eds. *Potentiating the Efficacy of Medications: Integrating Psychosocial Therapies With Pharmacotherapies in the Treatment of Drug Dependence.* Washington, DC: National Institute of Drug Abuse; 1995. Publication NIH 95-3899.
5. Stewart J, de Wit H, Eikelboom R. Role of unconditioned and conditioned drug effects in the self-administration of opiates and stimulants. *Psychol Rev.* 1984; 91:251-268.
6. American Psychiatric Association. *Diagnostic and Statistical Manual of Mental Disorders, Revised Third Edition.* Washington, DC: American Psychiatric Association; 1987.
7. Fuller RK, Williford WO, Lee KK, Derman R. Veterans Administration Cooperative Study of Disulfiram in the Treatment of Alcoholism: study design and methodological considerations. *Control Clin Trials.* 1984;5:263-273.
8. Marlatt GA, Gordon JR, eds. *Relapse Prevention.* New York, NY: Guilford Press; 1985.
9. Carroll K, Schottenfeld R. *A Therapist's Manual for Relapse Prevention in the Treatment of Alcoholism.* New Haven, Conn: Yale University School of Medicine; 1988.
10. Jaffe AJ, Korner P, Witte G, Brown J. *Relapse Prevention for the Treatment of Problem Drinking: A Manual for Therapists and Patients.* New Haven, Conn: Yale University School of Medicine; Farmington: University of Connecticut Health Center; 1989.
11. Sobell MB, Maisto SA, Sobell LC, Cooper AM, Cooper T, Sanders B. Developing a prototype for evaluating alcohol treatment effectiveness. In: Sobell LC, Sobell MB, Ward E, eds. *Evaluating Alcohol and Drug Abuse Treatment Effectiveness: Recent Advances.* New York, NY: Pergamon Press; 1980:129-150.
12. Sobell LC, Sobell MB. Timeline follow-back: a technique for assessing self-reported ethanol consumption. In: Allen J, Litten R, eds. *Measuring Alcohol Consumption: Psychosocial and Biochemical Methods.* Totowa, NJ: Humana Press Inc; 1992:41-72.
13. Spitzer RL, Williams JBW. *Structured Clinical Interview for DSM-III-R.* New York, NY: Biometrics Research Division, New York State Psychiatric Institute; 1985.
14. Hedeker D, Gibbons RD. A random-effects ordinal regression model for multilevel data. *Biometrics.* 1994;50:933-944.
15. Hedeker D. *MIXOR, A Fortran Program for Mixed-Effects Ordinal Probit and Logistic Regression.* Chicago: University of Illinois at Chicago Prevention Research Center, School of Public Health; 1993.
16. Laird NM, Ware JH. Random effects models for longitudinal data. *Biometrics.* 1982;38:963-974.
17. Gibbons RD, Hedeker D, Elkin I, Waternaux C, Kraemer HC, Greenhouse JB, Shea MT, Imber ST, Sotksy SM, Watkins JT. Some conceptual and statistical issues in analyses of longitudinal psychiatric data. *Arch Gen Psychiatry.* 1993; 50:739-750.
18. Cunningham CL, Okorn DM, Dickinson SD. Naloxone interferes with expression of ethanol-induced conditioned place preference. *Alcohol Clin Exp Res.* 1994;18:518.
19. Annis HM. A cognitive-social learning approach to relapse: pharmacotherapy and relapse prevention counseling. *Alcohol Alcohol.* 1991;1(suppl 1):527-530.
20. Peachy JE, Annis HM. New strategies for using the alcohol-sensitizing drugs. In: Naranjo CA, Sellers EM, eds. *Recent Advances in New Psychopharmacological Treatments for Alcoholism.* Amsterdam, the Netherlands: Elsevier Science Publishers; 1985:199-216.
21. Carroll KM, Rounsaville BJ, Nich C, Gordon LT, Wirtz PW, Gawin F. One-year follow-up of psychotherapy and pharmacotherapy for cocaine dependence: delayed emergence of psychotherapy effects. *Arch Gen Psychiatry.* 1994;51:989-997.
22. Bohn MJ, Kranzler HR, Beazoglou D, Staehler BA. Naltrexone and brief counseling to reduce heavy drinking: results of a small clinical trial. *Am J Addict.* 1994;3:91-99.
23. Kazdin RM, Bass E. Power to detect differences between alternate treatments in comparative psychotherapy outcome research. *J Consult Clin Psychol.* 1989; 57:138-147.

ORIGINAL ARTICLE

The Obsessive Compulsive Drinking Scale

A New Method of Assessing Outcome in Alcoholism Treatment Studies

Raymond F. Anton, MD; Darlene H. Moak, MD; Patricia K. Latham, PhD

Background: The 14-item Obsessive Compulsive Drinking Scale (OCDS) is a quick and reliable self-rating instrument that provides a total and two subscale scores that measure some cognitive aspects of alcohol "craving." This study validated further its utility as an alcoholism severity and treatment outcome instrument.

Methods: Alcoholism severity and analogue craving scales were administered at baseline, and the OCDS was given at baseline and weekly to 41 alcohol-dependent individuals who participated in a 12-week pharmacologic and cognitive-behavioral treatment trial. Repeated-measures analysis of variance was used to examine group differences in the OCDS scores of those individuals who remained abstinent or drank during the trial.

Results: At baseline, the OCDS was correlated with the alcohol composite score of the addiction severity index (r=.48), the alcohol dependence scale (r=.42), the analogue craving measures (range r=.40 to .57), and prestudy alcohol consumption (r=.60). Most importantly, the OCDS total and subscale scores were significantly different between individuals who had relapse drinking, who had "slip" drinking, and who remained abstinent, with relapsers showing the highest scores.

Conclusions: The OCDS scores appear to be sensitive to alcoholism severity and change during abstinence and relapse drinking. Since the shared variance with analogue craving measures is only about 20% to 30%, it appears to be measuring a largely independent dimension of alcohol dependence. Its ease of use (5 minutes per self-rating), reliability, validity, and analytic capabilities support its utility as a tool to measure severity and improvement during alcoholism treatment trials.

(Arch Gen Psychiatry. 1996;53:225-231)

MANY CLINICIANS and researchers believe that "craving" an abusable substance is a central phenomenon related to addiction. Craving alcohol appears to be intimately related to the loss of control over consumption and to compulsive alcohol use.[1] Although craving is taken into account in the *International Classification of Disease, Tenth Revision* classification of alcohol dependence, it is not explicitly mentioned in *DSM-IV*, which does consider the inability to cut down or control alcohol consumption a core feature of the alcohol dependence syndrome.

Despite wide clinical recognition and mention in the literature, craving remains ill defined and its measurement nonspecific. For instance, although it is recognized that craving and its broad manifestations should be measured in alcoholism pharmacotherapy trials,[2] most studies use a simple analogue scale to quantify craving, which leaves the interpretation to the patient. Several studies have indicated that the meaning of craving differs among substance-dependent individuals and professional caregivers.[3,4] The multidimensionality of craving could explain this discrepancy.

Although craving has been defined in behavioral and physiologic terms, the most widely used assessments in substance abuse research have been subjective. Tiffany[5] suggested that craving for alcohol might best be viewed as an automatic behavior. Implicit in this concept is that craving exists at a noncognitive or subcortical neuropsychologic level, an idea consistent with clinical observation and supported by clinical and basic research.[6] However, the accurate measurement of the cognitive elements associ-

See Patients and Methods on next page

From the Institute of Psychiatry, Medical University of South Carolina, Charleston.

PATIENTS AND METHODS

The items numbered 1, 6, 7, and 10 on the YBOCS-hd were conceptually divided into two separate items on the OCDS (**Figure 1**) but scaled from 0 to 4 in a similar fashion to the other items on the scale. These split items, although rated separately by the individual, were combined into one score for that item by using the higher score of the split items, thereby allowing the maximum OCDS total score to be 40, which is the same as the YBOCS and the YBOCS-hd.

Subjects for this study were 41 patients (29 men and 12 women; 37 whites and four African Americans) who signed informed consent to participate in an ongoing, randomized, double-blind 12-week trial of naltrexone or placebo for the treatment of alcohol dependence and who were recruited through direct outpatient referral either from clinicians or personal response to advertisements. All patients received weekly sessions of cognitive behavioral therapy in addition to the double-blind medication. The data analysis used total study group data without partitioning into treatment cells. Inclusion criteria included meeting *DSM-III-R* criteria for alcohol dependence, drinking an average of at least five standard drinks per day in the month before study entry, living within an hour's travel of the study site, having a stable living situation and a person acting as a collateral informant of drinking behavior, and a negative urine drug screen for substances of abuse. Exclusion criteria included a history of inpatient alcohol detoxification, the presence of a current *DSM-III-R* axis 1 diagnosis including substance abuse other than alcohol, notable medical illness requiring medication, results of liver function tests greater than 2.5 times normal, pregnancy, and current legal charges other than driving under the influence. All patients were required to abstain from alcohol for 5 days before study entry and were monitored frequently during the baseline evaluation period to ensure compliance.

Baseline assessment measures of alcoholism severity included the Addiction Severity Index[12] and the Alcohol Dependence Scale (ADS).[13] At baseline, subjects were instructed to rate the OCDS for the last week of drinking before entry into the study. Three 10-cm analogue craving scales were given at the same time as the OCDS. The global analogue scale, which stated "the amount of my craving for alcohol," was anchored at one end "very little" and at the other "a great deal." The frequency analogue scale, which stated "my craving for alcohol happened," was anchored at one end "rarely" and at the other "almost all the time." The intensity analogue scale, which stated "the intensity of my craving for alcohol," was anchored at one end "none" and at the other "irresistible." Analogue lines were divided by 1-cm hatch marks, and patients were asked to place a mark anywhere on the line that best described their craving in the past week. The distance from the lower anchored end to the patient's mark was measured in millimeters and used for scoring.

Alcohol consumption for the 90 days before study entry was obtained by a timeline followback method.[14] During the treatment trial the patients were seen weekly to ascertain alcohol ingestion by means of the timeline followback method and to assess their level of "craving for alcohol." The OCDS was given along with the analogue craving scales, and the patients were instructed to rate these on the basis of a composite experience of the previous week.

Of the 41 subjects who entered the active phase of the treatment trial, five patients dropped out before the final week 12 assessment. Two patients in the relapse group, two in the slip group, and one in the abstinent group terminated early. Of the patients who completed the trial, 21 had data available on all 12 assessment weeks, while 91% of the overall weekly assessments were completed by the total study population. Alcohol consumption data were obtained on all patients for all missing visits, even after study dropout, by applying the timeline followback method at the next visit after the visit missed or at week 12 for those patients who dropped out early. For the purposes of the present study, the subjects' responses to treatment were categorized into three distinct outcomes: group 1 included those subjects who remained abstinent throughout the 12-week treatment trial (n=20), group 2 had an alcohol "slip" during the trial but did not meet the criterion for relapse (n=13), and group 3 met the criterion for alcohol relapse, which was defined as having five or more drinks on two consecutive days some time during the study period (n=8). The number (mean±SD) of standard drinks consumed during the 12-week study was zero for group 1, 37±31 for group 2, and 172±73 for group 3. The OCDS total and subscale scores (obsessive thoughts about alcohol subscale and compulsive drinking subscale) were also compared.

Descriptive statistics summarized the population characteristics. Pearson's Product-Moment Correlation coefficients were obtained between the OCDS total score and the subscale scores, the ADS, the Alcohol Composite Score of the Addiction Severity Index, and each analogue craving scale.

A multivariate approach to repeated-measures analysis of variance was conducted for the OCDS total and subscale scores with the use of the baseline and all 12 treatment weeks. Since only 21 subjects had complete data for each of the 13 time points, the data were reanalyzed with substitution of the following for the missing data points: (1) the mean of the specific time point calculated for the total population, (2) the mean of the specific time point for the drinking category, and (3) carrying forward the last available data point for each subject. The results of all three methods of analysis were similar. The last-point-carried-forward method was used for further examination of group, time, and group by time interaction effects.

To decompose further the interaction between drinking category and time (weeks in the study), a post hoc analysis at each time point with the Student-Newman-Keuls multiple range test was completed.

ated with alcohol craving, such as thoughts of alcohol, conditioned automatic behaviors, and cognitive mechanisms that resist action-provoking images and behaviors, may be possible, as is done in other putative subcortical psychiatric disorders, such as obsessive-compulsive disorder.

Some time ago Edwards and Gross[1] and more recently Modell et al[7,8] suggested that many aspects of craving (eg, the compulsive drive to consume alcohol, recurrent and persistent thoughts about alcohol, and the struggle to control these drives and thoughts) are similar to the thought patterns and behaviors of patients with

Directions: The questions below ask you about your drinking alcohol and your attempts to control your drinking. Please circle the number next to the statement that best applies to you.

1. How much of your time when you're not drinking is occupied by ideas, thoughts, impulses, or images related to drinking?
(0) None
(1) Less than 1 hour a day
(2) 1-3 hours a day
(3) 4-8 hours a day
(4) Greater than 8 hours a day

2. How frequently do these thoughts occur?
(0) Never
(1) No more than 8 times a day
(2) More than 8 times a day, but most hours of the day are free of those thoughts
(3) More than 8 times a day and during most hours of the day
(4) Thoughts are too numerous to count and an hour rarely passes without several such thoughts occurring.

Insert the Higher Score of Questions 1 or 2 here_____

3. How much do these ideas, thoughts, impulses, or images related to drinking interfere with your social or work (or role) functioning? Is there anything you don't or can't do because of them? [If you are not currently working, how much of your performance would be affected if you were working?]
(0) Thoughts of drinking never interfere—I can function normally.
(1) Thoughts of drinking slightly interfere with my social or occupational activities, but my overall performance is not impaired.
(2) Thoughts of drinking definitely interfere with my social or occupational performance, but I can still manage.
(3) Thoughts of drinking cause substantial impairment in my social or occupational performance.
(4) Thoughts of drinking interfere completely with my social or work performance.

4. How much distress or disturbance do these ideas, thoughts, impulses, or images related to drinking cause you when you're not drinking?
(0) None
(1) Mild, infrequent, and not too disturbing
(2) Moderate, frequent, and disturbing, but still manageable
(3) Severe, very frequent, and very disturbing
(4) Extreme, nearly constant, and disabling distress

5. How much of an effort do you make to resist these thoughts or try to disregard or turn your attention away from these thoughts as they enter your mind when you're not drinking? (Rate *your efforts made to resist these thoughts*, not your success or failure in actually controlling them.)
(0) My thoughts are so minimal, I don't need to actively resist. If I have thoughts, I make an effort to *always* resist.
(1) I try to resist most of the time.
(2) I make some effort to resist.
(3) I give in to all such thoughts without attempting to control them, but I do so with some reluctance.
(4) I completely and willingly give in to all such thoughts.

6. How successful are you in stopping or diverting these thoughts when you're not drinking?
(0) I am completely successful in stopping or diverting such thoughts.
(1) I am usually able to stop or divert such thoughts with some effort and concentration.
(2) I am sometimes able to stop or divert such thoughts.
(3) I am rarely successful in stopping such thoughts and can only divert such thoughts with difficulty.
(4) I am rarely able to divert such thoughts even momentarily.

7. How many drinks do you drink each day?
(0) None
(1) Less than 1 drink per day
(2) 1-2 drinks per day
(3) 3-7 drinks per day
(4) 8 or more drinks per day

8. How many days each week do you drink?
(0) None
(1) No more than 1 day per week
(2) 2-3 days per week
(3) 4-5 days per week
(4) 6-7 days per week

Insert the Higher Score of Questions 7 or 8 here_____

9. How much does your drinking interfere with your work functioning? Is there anything that you don't or can't do because of your drinking? [If you are not currently working, how much of your performance would be affected if you were working?]
(0) Drinking never interferes—I can function normally.
(1) Drinking slightly interferes with my occupational activities, but my overall performance is not impaired.
(2) Drinking definitely interferes with my occupational performance, but I can still manage.
(3) Drinking causes substantial impairment in my occupational performance.
(4) Drinking problems interfere completely with my work performance.

10. How much does your drinking interfere with your social functioning? Is there anything that you don't or can't do because of your drinking?
(0) Drinking never interferes—I can function normally.
(1) Drinking slightly interferes with my social activities, but my overall performance is not impaired.
(2) Drinking definitely interferes with my social performance, but I can still manage.
(3) Drinking causes substantial impairment in my social performance.
(4) Drinking problems interfere completely with my social performance.

Insert the Higher Score of Questions 9 or 10 here_____

11. If you were prevented from drinking alcohol when you desired a drink, how anxious or upset would you become?
(0) I would not experience any anxiety or irritation.
(1) I would become only slightly anxious or irritated.
(2) The anxiety or irritation would mount, but remain manageable.
(3) I would experience a prominent and very disturbing increase in anxiety or irritation.
(4) I would experience incapacitating anxiety or irritation.

12. How much of an effort do you make to resist consumption of alcoholic beverages? (Only *rate your effort to resist*, not your success or failure in actually controlling the drinking.)
(0) My drinking is so minimal, I don't need to actively resist. If I drink, I make an effort to always resist.
(1) I try to resist most of the time.
(2) I make some effort to resist.
(3) I give in to almost all drinking without attempting to control it, but I do so with some reluctance.
(4) I completely and willingly give in to all drinking.

13. How strong is the drive to consume alcoholic beverages?
(0) No drive
(1) Some pressure to drink
(2) Strong pressure to drink
(3) Very strong drive to drink
(4) The drive to drink is completely involuntary and overpowering.

14. How much control do you have over the drinking?
(0) I have complete control.
(1) I am usually able to exercise voluntary control over it.
(2) I can control it only with difficulty.
(3) I must drink and can only delay drinking with difficulty.
(4) I am rarely able to delay drinking even momentarily.

Insert the Higher Score of Questions 13 or 14 here_____

Figure 1. *The Obsessive Compulsive Drinking Scale (reproduced with permission from Anton et al[11]).*

obsessive-compulsive illness. Modell et al[7,8] modified the Yale-Brown Obsessive Compulsive Scale (YBOCS)[9,10] to measure these aspects in heavy drinkers (the YBOCS-hd). The YBOCS-hd was found to differentiate alcoholics from normal drinkers reliably[7] and to be related to an analogue measure of subjective craving in alcoholics.[8] We modified the original 10-item interview scale into a 14-item self-rated questionnaire, the Obsessive Compulsive Drinking Scale (OCDS), which is easily administered, has excellent concurrent validity with the YBOCS-hd (r=.83), exhibits excellent test-retest reliability (r=.96) and internal consistency (Cronbach's α=.86), and, in a preliminary fashion, was sensitive to change during the course of a 12-week treatment trial.[11]

To validate further the OCDS and provide an indication for its use in prospective alcoholism treatment re-

Table 1. Baseline Characteristics of Subjects by Drinking Status During Treatment*

	Abstinent (n=20)	'Slip' Drinking (n=13)	Relapse Drinking (n=8)
Age, y	45±9.3	44.2±8.7	38.2±10.8
Race, No. (%)			
White	17 (85)	12 (92.3)	8 (100)
African American	3 (15)	1 (7.7)	0 (0)
Gender, No. (%)			
M	14 (70)	8 (61.5)	7 (87.5)
F	6 (30)	5 (38.5)	1 (12.5)
Education, y	14.3±2.6	14.3±2.9	15.5±5.2
Marital status, No. (%)			
Married	13 (65)	10 (76.9)	5 (62.5)
Remarried	1 (5)	1 (7.7)	1 (12.5)
Divorced	3 (15)	1 (7.7)	0 (0)
Never married	3 (15)	1 (7.7)	2 (25)
Addiction Severity Index			
Alcohol Composite Score	0.6847±0.16	0.6889±0.17	0.8162±0.11
Alcohol Dependence Scale	16.2±5.7	18.5±7.3	18.0±7.0
Alcohol intake in week before study entry, g/d	107±93	96±56	98±74

**There were no statistically significant differences between the groups at study entry. Unless otherwise indicated, values are expressed as mean ±SD.*

search, it was administered to a group of well-characterized alcohol-dependent individuals before the start of a double-blind pharmacotherapy trial of the opiate antagonist naltrexone, combined with cognitive behavioral therapy, and given weekly during the 12-week trial period. To substantiate construct validity, the relationship of the OCDS scores to baseline alcoholism severity measures, alcohol consumption, and craving was examined. As a measure of criterion-related validity and sensitivity to change, OCDS scores were examined in individuals who either remained abstinent, had an alcohol slip, or relapsed during the 12-week rating period.

RESULTS

The baseline characteristics of the patient sample as they were distributed into the three outcome groups (ie, abstinent, alcohol slip, and alcohol relapse) are detailed in **Table 1**. The patients were mostly middle-aged, white married men who had, on average, several years of post-secondary education.

These demographic variables did not differ significantly between the drinking outcome groups. The baseline ADS score for the study population was 17.27±6.43, and the Alcohol Composite Score on the Addiction Severity Index was 0.71±0.16. Study patients drank on average 102±78 g of alcohol per day in the 7 days before entry into the study.

Table 2 gives the correlations at study entry between the OCDS total and subscale scores, other independent measures of alcohol severity, and analogue craving scales. Although the total OCDS score and both subscales were significantly correlated with the Alcohol Composite Score and the ADS scores, the total score and the obsessive thoughts of drinking subscale were more highly correlated than the compulsive drinking subscale with these measures. The correlation of the OCDS scores with the alcohol composite score from the Addiction Severity Index was higher than the correlation of the OCDS scores with the ADS scores, which may reflect the time period the Alcohol Composite Score evaluates (the 30 days before study), in contrast to the ADS, which is not limited to these 30 days.

Table 2. Relationship of the OCDS With Measures of Alcoholism Severity and Analogue Measures of Alcohol Craving at Baseline*

	Severity		Craving		
OCDS Score	ALCOMP	ADS	Global	Frequency	Intensity
Total	.48†	.42‡	.40‡	.52†	.57†
Obsessive	.46‡	.39§	.31§	.40‡	.49†
Compulsive	.36§	.32§	.38§	.52†	.49†

**Values are Pearson's Product-Moment Correlation coefficients. OCDS indicates Obsessive-Compulsive Drinking Scale; ALCOMP, Alcohol Composite Score from the Addiction Severity Index; and ADS, Alcohol Dependence Scale.*
†*P<.001.*
‡*P<.01.*
§*P<.05.*

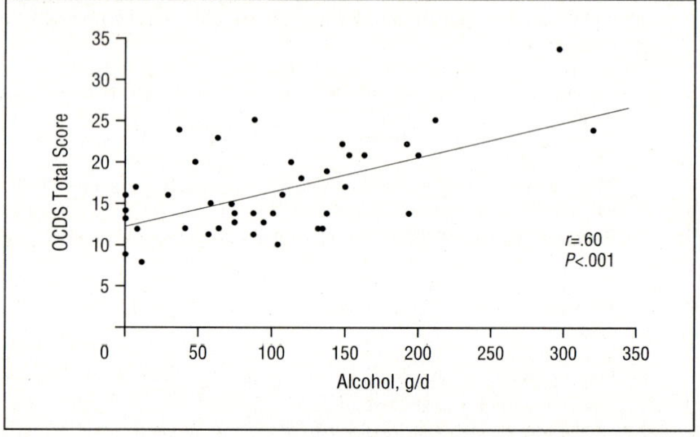

Figure 2. *Relationship of Obsessive-Compulsive Drinking Scale (OCDS) scores at baseline to the quantity of alcohol consumed in the week before study entry.*

See also pages 199, 202, 211, 217, 232, and 243

The highly significant positive relationship between the OCDS total score and the three analogue scales of craving is especially evident for the measurements of frequency and intensity of craving. Even though both subscales exhibit significant correlations with all analogue craving measures, the compulsive drinking subscale appears to be more closely related to the frequency of craving than the obsessive thoughts of alcohol subscale.

Figure 2 shows the significant positive relationship between the amount of alcohol consumed in the week before study entry and the OCDS total score at study entry. Despite being significant, the correlation is not strong, and the amount of alcohol consumed accounts for only

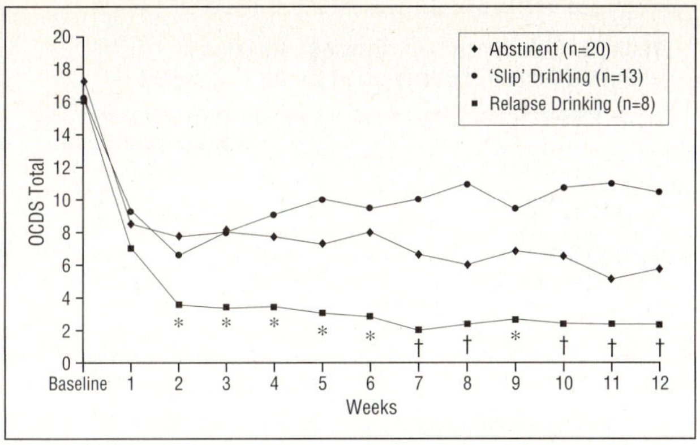

Figure 3. *Obsessive-Compulsive Drinking Scale (OCDS) total scores in three drinking outcome groups during a 12-week treatment period. The data are plotted with the use of the last point carry forward substitution for missing data. Asterisk indicates* P<.05 *for the abstinent group vs the slip and relapse groups (Student-Newman-Keuls multiple-group comparisons); dagger, all groups differ from each other at* P<.05.

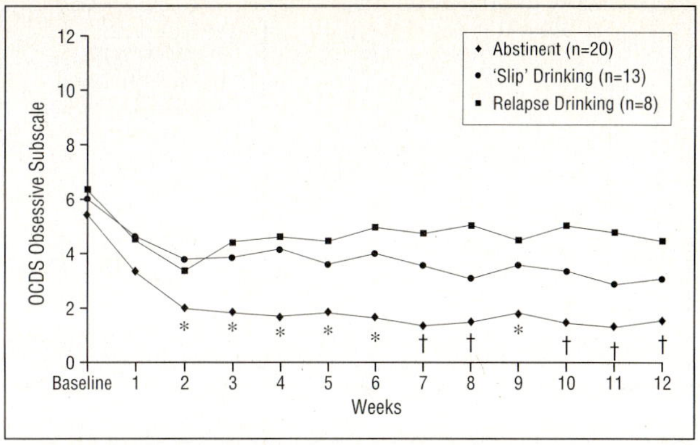

Figure 4. *Obsessive-Compulsive Drinking Scale (OCDS) obsessive subscale score in three drinking outcome groups during a 12-week treatment period. The data are plotted with the use of the last point carry forward substitution for missing data. Asterisk indicates* P<.05 *for the abstinent group vs the slip and relapse groups (Student-Newman-Keuls multiple-group comparisons); dagger, all groups differ from each other at* P<.05.

36% of the variance in the total OCDS score. The correlation of the amount of alcohol consumed and the obsessive subscale score was r=.47 (P=.002), while the correlation of the baseline amount of alcohol consumed and the compulsive subscale score was r=.57 (P<.001).

The total OCDS scores during the 12-week study for the three patient groups stratified by their intake of alcohol during the study (abstinent, alcohol slip, and alcohol relapse) are shown in **Figure 3**. There was a main effect of time on the total OCDS score (F=40.67, df=12, P<.001) such that all groups had a reduction in score during the course of treatment. Importantly, there was a main effect of drinking group (F=24.49, df=2, P<.001) as well as an interaction between drinking group and time (F=3.62, df=24, P<.001). Decomposition of this interaction term by means of weekly group comparisons showed that at baseline and in week 1 there was no difference between patient groups (Figure 3). However, in weeks 2 through 12, there was a significant difference in the total OCDS score between abstinent patients and the groups who slipped or relapsed. In general, after week 7 the slip and relapse drinking groups also significantly differed from each other. As shown in Figure 3, patients who relapsed had higher OCDS total scores than those who only slipped, and both drinking groups had higher scores than those who maintained continual abstinence. For example, at week 2 of treatment, the abstainer group had a 75% decrease in the total OCDS score from study entry compared with only a 56% decrease exhibited by the relapse drinking group (t=3.9 df=39, P<.001).

The obsessive thoughts about drinking subscale (**Figure 4**) and the compulsive drinking behavior subscale (**Figure 5**) showed longitudinal characteristics similar to those of total OCDS scores. For the obsessive subscale, there was a main effect of time (F=11.21, df=12, P<.001), a main effect of drinking group (F=17.09, df=2, P<.001), and an interaction between time and drinking group (F=1.83, df=24, P=.01). For the compulsive drinking behavior subscale (Figure 5), there was a main effect of time (F=57.70, df=12, P<.001), a main effect of drinking group (F=25.37, df=2, P<.001), and an interaction between time and drinking group (F=4.11, df=24, P<.001). For both subscales, the abstinent group had lower scores than the two drinking groups from week 2 through the end of the study. However, the slip drinking group differed from the relapse drinking group only after week 7 of the study.

The relationship between OCDS and analogue craving scores at week 3, the point at which scores stabilized during the initial phase of treatment, and alcohol consumption during the remainder of the study was examined. **Table 3** indicates that the OCDS scores in general, and the obsessive subscale in particular, were more highly correlated with future alcohol consumption than was the analogue craving scale score.

COMMENT

These data further substantiate the validity of the OCDS as an instrument capable of quantifying craving for alcohol in alcohol-dependent individuals. Although the OCDS and its two subscales were significantly correlated with the amount of alcohol consumed and with other independent measures of craving, the shared variance between these crucial alcohol consumption–related measures was not large. This suggests that the OCDS is measuring a largely independent domain of the alcohol-dependence syndrome. The positive relationship of the OCDS total and subscale scores to independent measures of alcoholism severity implies that as the severity of this illness progresses, so does the intensity of the obsessive thoughts about alcohol and the compulsive behaviors to use alcohol. This provides support for the construct validity of the alcohol-related thoughts and behaviors rated on the OCDS.

Criterion-related validity of the OCDS is provided by the longitudinal data presented for treatment study subjects. The OCDS total and subscale scores fall during the acquisition of sobriety and remain low in abstaining patients. Patients who drink alcohol, but who do not relapse, have higher OCDS scores than those who remain abstinent. Finally, those patients who eventually relapse have even higher OCDS scores that remain el-

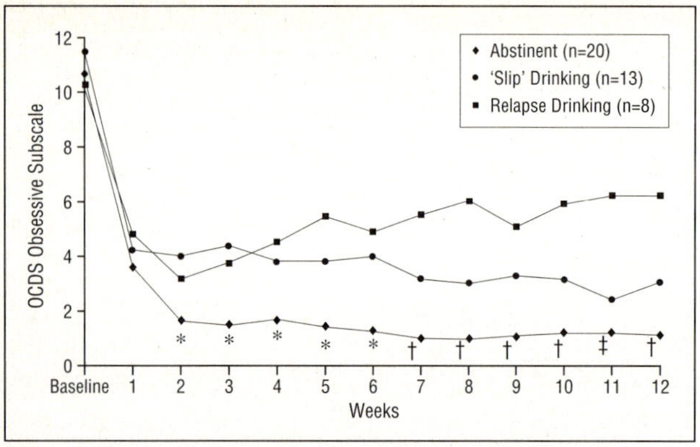

Figure 5. *Obsessive-Compulsive Drinking Scale (OCDS) compulsive subscale score in three drinking outcome groups during a 12-week treatment period. The data are plotted with the use of the last point carry forward substitution for missing data. Asterisk indicates* P<.05 *for the abstinent group vs the slip and relapse groups (Student-Newman-Keuls multiple-group comparisons); dagger, all groups differ from each other at* P<.05*; and double dagger,* P<.05 *for the relapse group vs the abstinent and slip groups, but the slip and abstinent groups were not significantly different from each other.*

Table 3. Relationship of 'Craving' Measures to Future Alcohol Consumption During Treatment

	Total Standard Drinks, Weeks 4-12	
Week 3 Score	***r****	***P***
OCDS† total	.30	.05
Obsessive subscale	.36	.02
Compulsive subscale	.22	.17
Analogue craving	.24	.13

**Values are Pearson's Product-Moment Correlation coefficients.*
†OCDS indicates Obsessive-Compulsive Drinking Scale.

evated. Abstaining patients exhibit about a 75% drop in OCDS total score during the first 2 weeks of treatment. In contrast, those subjects who drink at least some alcohol during the study have only a less than 50% drop in the OCDS total during this period.

After the initial period of "improvement," the patients who relapse have a steady increase in the OCDS scores but never appear to return to baseline prestudy levels, which could be a function of study dropout and the last score being carried forward in the analysis. Alternatively, treatment may have allowed these patients to stabilize at a lower level of alcohol craving and consumption than before treatment at least for the brief period studied (12 weeks). Scores on the OCDS obtained for these patients after the termination of treatment would be useful in addressing this issue. In any case, the longitudinal data clearly show that the OCDS is capable of measuring changes in craving for alcohol and that changes in the dimension(s) quantified by the scale vary in relationship to alcohol consumption. We have previously illustrated that for certain patients the total OCDS score in general, and the obsessive thoughts of alcohol subscale in particular, may increase before relapse drinking.[11] The scale, therefore, may be useful in monitoring patients during treatment to identify individuals who may be at risk for imminent uncontrolled drinking, since individuals with higher OCDS scores early in treatment (between weeks 2 and 3) had greater alcohol consumption in future weeks.

The relationship of the amount of alcohol consumption to the OCDS score has been previously described[11] in an inpatient population of alcoholics and is similar to the relationship obtained in the present sample of less severely alcohol-dependent outpatients. The amount of alcohol consumption predicts only about 20% of the variance in OCDS scores. There are several explanations for this finding. For instance, alcoholics may think frequently about alcohol and also spend a fair amount of time resisting these thoughts in a semisuccessful effort to control or reduce their alcohol intake, especially in the period immediately before treatment seeking. To the extent that patients are able not to drink or that external contingencies prevent them from consuming alcohol in an amount commensurate with their thoughts of drinking, then the variability between thoughts, resistance, and alcohol consumption will increase. Alternatively, if alcohol consumption is largely automatic, that is, not under conscious control, as postulated by Tiffany,[5] then individuals may consume varying amounts of alcohol without having awareness of the thoughts before drinking. Consequently, individuals will be unable to resist the thoughts and impulses about alcohol before treatment because they are unaware of them. In fact, the goal of cognitive behavioral therapy is to allow individuals to identify these thoughts and impulses and to provide nonautomatic cognitive coping strategies that will enhance resistance to them until the automatic nature of their generation becomes unconditioned.[5] By means of this theoretical framework, the items that make up the OCDS have face validity, and this instrument might be especially suited to measure change during treatment trials where cognitively oriented coping skills techniques are used. Additionally, medications,[15,16] some of which are used to treat both obsessive-compulsive disorder and alcohol dependence, may enhance the individual's ability to resist these thoughts by decreasing the automatic nature of a cue-induced drinking situation, and by enhancing cognitive awareness of alcohol-related thoughts and motivation to resist, such as when comorbid depression is treated. Again, the face validity of the items of the OCDS and their sensitivity to change would make it a suitable instrument to quantify improvement during pharmacologic treatment trials.

The OCDS may be especially suited to outpatient comparative treatment trials in which improvement between two treatments is being examined and analyzed. In the most recent alcoholism treatment trials, the primary dependent variables related to alcohol consumption used a relapse end-point model that is most suited to time series analysis.[17-19] In this type of analysis, a return to alcohol consumption is measured, usually starting from an abstinent, or zero, consumption state. Therefore, one can only measure a worsening in status or a time to a specific event (ie, alcohol relapse). It is not possible to gauge incremental improvement from a baseline dysfunctional state. However, a higher score on the OCDS implies greater dysfunction, with improvement indicated by a drop in the score. As such, the OCDS performs in a psychometric fashion during change assessment similar to that of the YBOCS,[9,10] from which it was originally derived, and to other traditional psychiatric rating scales, such as the Hamilton Rating Scales for Depression[20] and Anxiety,[21] the Brief Psychiatric Rating Scale,[22] and the Beck Depression Inventory.[23]

In summary, the OCDS appears to be a reliable and valid self-rating instrument for the measurement of a dimension of alcohol dependence that might be best described as the cognitive correlate of craving. While it shares measurement variance with the amount of alcohol consumption and analogue measures of craving, it appears to be capturing a dimension of alcoholism that is to a great extent independent of these measures. The OCDS is sensitive to both the severity of alcohol dependence and acute change during treatment for this condition. The change in OCDS scores is associated with changes in drinking behavior and can be used to establish group means and variance, such that classic analysis of variance techniques can be applied for quantification of group differences. The ease of use (5 minutes per self-rating), excellent patient acceptance, reliability, validity, and psychometric and analytic properties suggest its usefulness as a tool to measure improvement in alcohol dependence both in clinical treatment programs and during treatment trials.

Accepted for publication November 7, 1995.

This work was supported by grant RO1-AA09568 from the National Institute on Alcohol Abuse and Alcoholism.

We acknowledge the statistical assistance of James Dias, PhD, and the assistance of Mary Radin and Daphne Thompson in the preparation of the manuscript.

Reprint requests to Institute of Psychiatry, Medical University of South Carolina, 171 Ashley Ave, Charleston, SC 29425 (Dr Anton).

REFERENCES

1. Edwards G, Gross MM. Alcohol dependence: provisional description of a clinical syndrome. *BMJ.* 1976;1:1058-1061.
2. Linnoila M, Fawcett J, Fuller RK, Harford TC, Martin PB, Meyer RE, Romach MK, Sellers EM. Evaluation of pharmacologic treatments for alcohol abuse, dependence, and their complications. In: Prien RF, Robinson DS, eds. *Clinical Evaluation of Psychotropic Drugs: Principles and Guidelines.* New York, NY: Raven Press; 1994:625-649.
3. Kozlowski LT, Mann RE, Wilkinson DA, Poulos CX. 'Cravings' are ambiguous: ask about urges or desires. *Addict Behav.* 1989;14:443-445.
4. Sitharthan T, McGrath D, Sitharthaan G, Saunders JB. Meaning of craving in research on addiction. *Psychol Rep.* 1992;71:823-826.
5. Tiffany ST. A cognitive model of drug urges and drug-use behavior: role of automatic and nonautomatic processes. *Psychol Rev.* 1990;97:147-168.
6. Robinson TE, Berridge KC. The neural basis of drug craving: an incentive-sensitization theory of addiction. *Brain Res Rev.* 1993;18:247-291.
7. Modell JG, Glaser FB, Mountz JM, Schmaltz S, Cyr L. Obsessive and compulsive characteristics of alcohol abuse and dependence: quantification by a newly developed questionnaire. *Alcohol Clin Exp Res.* 1992a;16:266-271.
8. Modell JG, Glaser FB, Cyr L, Mountz JM. Obsessive and compulsive characteristics of craving for alcohol in alcohol abuse and dependence. *Alcohol Clin Exp Res.* 1992b;16:272-274.
9. Goodman WK, Price LH, Rasmussen SA, Mazure C, Delgado P, Heninger GR, Charney DS. The Yale-Brown Obsessive Compulsive Scale, I: development, use, and reliability. *Arch Gen Psychiatry.* 1989a;46:1006-1011.
10. Goodman WK, Price LH, Rasmussen SA, Mazure C, Delgado P, Heninger GR, Charney DS. The Yale-Brown Obsessive Compulsive Scale, II: validity. *Arch Gen Psychiatry.* 1989b;46:1012-1016.
11. Anton RF, Moak DH, Latham P. The Obsessive Compulsive Drinking Scale: a self-rated instrument for the quanitification of thoughts about alcohol and drinking behavior. *Alcohol Clin Exp Res.* 1995;19:92-99.
12. McLellan AT, Luborsky L, Woody GE, O'Brien CP. An improved diagnostic evaluation instrument for substance abuse patients: the Addiction Severity Index. *J Nerv Ment Dis.* 1980;168:26-33.
13. Skinner HA, Allen BA. Alcohol dependence syndrome: measurement and validation. *J Abnorm Psychol.* 1982;91:199-209.
14. Sobell LC, Sobell MB, Leo CI, Cancilla A. Reliability of a timeline method: assessing normal drinkers' reports of recent drinking and a comparative evaluation across several populations. *Br J Addict.* 1988;83:393-402.
15. Kranzler HR, Burleson J, Korner P, DelBoca F, Bohn M, Brown J, Liebowitz N. Placebo-controlled trial of fluoxetine as an adjunct to relapse prevention in alcoholics. *Am J Psychiatry.* 1995;152:391-397.
16. Naranjo CA, Bremner KE. Evaluation of the effects of serotonin uptake inhibitors in alcoholics: a review. In: Naranjo CA, Sellers EM, eds. *Novel Pharmacological Interventions for Alcoholism.* New York, NY: Springer-Verlag; 1992; 105-117.
17. Dorus W, Ostrow DG, Anton RF, Cushman P, Collins JF, Schaefer M, Charles HL, Desai P, Hayashida M, Malkerneker U, Willenbring M, Fiscella R, Sather MR. Lithium treatment of depressed and nondepressed alcoholics. *JAMA.* 1989; 262:1646-1652.
18. Volpicelli JR, Alterman AI, Hayashida M, O'Brien CP. Naltrexone in the treatment of alcohol dependence. *Arch Gen Psychiatry.* 1992;49:876-880.
19. O'Malley SS, Jaffe AJ, Chang G, Schottenfeld RS, Meyer RE, Rounsaville B. Naltrexone and coping skills therapy for alcohol dependence. *Arch Gen Psychiatry.* 1992;49:881-887.
20. Hamilton MA. A rating scale for depression. *J Neurol Neurosurg Psychiatry.* 1960;23:56-62.
21. Hamilton M. The assessment of anxiety states by rating. *Br J Med Psychol.* 1959;32:50-55.
22. Overall JE, Gorham DR. The Brief Psychiatric Rating Scale. *Psychol Rep.* 1962; 10:799-812.
23. Beck AT, Ward CH, Mendelsohn M, Mock J, Erbaugh J. An inventory for measuring depression. *Arch Gen Psychiatry.* 1961;4:561-571.

ORIGINAL ARTICLE

Imipramine Treatment of Alcoholics With Primary Depression

A Placebo-Controlled Clinical Trial

Patrick J. McGrath, MD; Edward V. Nunes, MD; Jonathan W. Stewart, MD; Deberah Goldman, PhD; Vito Agosti, MSW; Katja Ocepek-Welikson, MPhil; Frederic M. Quitkin, MD

Background: Depressive disorders are commonly comorbid with alcoholism, particularly in treatment-seeking samples. If antidepressant treatment were safe and improved the treatment outcome in the subset of actively drinking alcoholics with depression, this would be of clinical importance.

Methods: We conducted a randomized, 12-week placebo-controlled trial of imipramine hydrochloride combined with weekly relapse prevention psychotherapy. The subjects were 69 actively drinking alcoholic outpatients with current depressive disorders. The first onset of depression was either antecedent to the abuse of alcohol or occurred during prolonged periods of sobriety. Depression and drinking outcomes at 12 weeks, as well as their relationship, were measured.

Results: Imipramine treatment was safe and associated with improvement in depression in both adequately treated and intention-to-treat samples. While there was no overall effect on drinking outcome, patients whose mood improved showed decreased alcohol consumption that was more marked in those treated with imipramine.

Conclusions: Imipramine treatment is effective for primary depression among actively drinking alcoholic outpatients, and may improve alcoholic outcome for those whose depression responds to treatment.

(Arch Gen Psychiatry. 1996;53:232-240)

If contributions to physical illnesses, suicide, homicide, and accidental death are considered, alcoholism is the fourth leading cause of death in the United States.[1] Data from multiple epidemiologic samples show that depression is commonly comorbid with alcoholism.[2-7] Data from the Epidemiologic Catchment Area study,[5] for example, show that 5% of male alcoholics and 19% of female alcoholics have a lifetime history of major depression. As would be expected, even higher rates of comorbid major depression ranging from 8% to 53% are seen in treatment-seeking subjects[8] and in primary care settings.[9] If antidepressant treatment of comorbid depression could improve outcome for this subset of alcoholics, this could have a significant public health impact.

The nature of the relationship between depression and alcoholism is complex and controversial. Comorbidity could be a coincidence, one disorder could cause or influence the course of the other, they could both be caused by an underlying condition, or alcohol intoxication and withdrawal could cause depressive symptoms that mimic primary depression.[10,11] While it is the consensus of several comprehensive reviews[8,12,13] that the two disorders are not simply manifestations of a single underlying illness, subsequently reported data call this into question.[14-17] It is clear from careful prospective studies[18-20] that transient depressive symptoms, chronologically secondary to alcoholism, are common among alcoholics and remit rapidly with abstinence. This suggests that comorbid depression, at least in males hospitalized for alcoholism, is probably most often a manifestation of alcohol's toxic effects. The frequency of such secondary major depression has been documented by prospective follow-up data from the Collaborative Study on the Psychobiology of Depression which show that 28% of alcoholics without affective disorder at intake developed major depression

From the New York State Psychiatric Institute and the College of Physicians and Surgeons, Columbia University, New York, NY.

See Subjects and Methods on next page

SUBJECTS AND METHODS

SUBJECTS

Subjects were recruited to a university-based depression research clinic through advertisements and referrals. They were between the ages of 18 and 65 years, met the *DSM III-R* criteria for either current alcohol dependence or abuse *and* for current major depression, dysthymia, or depressive disorder not otherwise specified. Depressive disorder was required to be primary, defined as either having had its onset prior to the onset of alcohol abuse or having continued during at least 6 months of sobriety. Subjects were excluded because of a history of mania, psychosis, seizure disorder, severe current physical dependence on alcohol requiring inpatient detoxification, abstinence of 2 weeks' duration at baseline, or for current serious and unstable physical illnesses. Also excluded were subjects meeting criteria for dependence on another substance, apart from nicotine, within the last 6 months and women not using adequate contraception. A history of hypomania or of current abuse of other substances was not exclusionary, provided that alcohol was clearly the main substance of abuse.

PROCEDURES

The *DSM III-R* diagnoses were made by a research psychiatrist using the structured clinical interview for *DSM III-R*, patient version.[34] The temporal sequence of addictive and nonaddictive disorders was determined by dating the age of onset of each structured clinical interview depressive and addictive disorder and by dating any periods of abstinence of 6 months or longer by a procedure that has subsequently been refined and tested for reliability.[35] Each diagnosis was reviewed for presence prior to a depressive disorder or during an abstinent period. The presence of any structured clinical interview depressive disorder during an abstinent period or prior to the onset of alcoholism or alcohol abuse defined *primary* depression. This assumes that 6 months of abstinence is adequate to exclude depression induced by intoxication or withdrawal, a reasonable but undocumented assumption. All other comorbid subjects were considered secondary and excluded from our study. Atypical depression was diagnosed according to Columbia University's criteria for atypical depression, using a structured diagnostic scale.[36] Physical evaluation consisted of medical history, physical examination, electrocardiogram, chemistry screening, urinalysis, and urine screen for drugs of abuse.

Eligible patients who signed informed consent were given single-blind placebo for 1 week. Patients whose depression was not rated "much improved" or "very much improved" on the improvement item of the Clinical Global Impressions Scale (CGI)[37] for depression were randomized to receive placebo or imipramine hydrochloride in a single daily dose given at bedtime for 12 weeks under double-blind conditions. A 12-week trial was planned to allow adequate time for antidepressant response and subsequent work toward abstinence in counseling and Alcoholics Anonymous (AA).

MEDICATION TREATMENT AND ASSESSMENT

Patients randomized to imipramine hydrochloride began at 50 mg and increased by 50 mg every 3 to 5 days until a maximum dose of 300 mg was reached, there was significant improvement, or side effects became dose limiting. Medication was given in a single evening dose using identical tablets of imipramine or placebo. An adequate trial of imipramine was prospectively defined as 4 weeks of double-blind medication with a minimum dose of at least

Continued on next page

by 6 years later compared with 12% of never-ill subjects.[21] A controlled trial of desipramine in the treatment of secondary depression in abstinent alcoholics has documented efficacy in this group.[22]

The prevalence of primary depression among alcoholics is much less clear. The "self-medication hypothesis" proposes that some patients with primary depression or anxiety disorders drink to alleviate dysphoric affect and may become secondarily alcoholic as a result.[23,24] While studies of male subjects tend not to find significant rates of primary depression,[25] studies that include women do.[5,26] For example, in a reanalysis of the Epidemiologic Catchment Area data, Helzer and Pryzbeck[5] found that while male alcoholics had only a slightly increased risk of major depression compared with the total sample (5% vs 3%), female alcoholics were more likely to have depression than females in the total population (19% vs 7%). Further, in women depression was antecedent in the majority of cases (66%), while alcohol abuse was antecedent in the majority of men (78%).

Taken together, these studies suggest that while most depression among alcoholics is a secondary consequence of their alcoholism, a small but significant minority of alcoholics, particularly women, has primary depression that may either contribute to the development of alcoholism or exacerbate its course once developed.

Clinical trials of antidepressant treatment of alcoholics have generally not supported efficacy.[27-30] These older studies have substantial shortcomings in that most employed low dosage, short duration of treatment, and ascertained depression only by cross-sectional scales, which are likely to detect transient substance-induced mood syndromes unlikely to benefit from antidepressant treatment. Newer preliminary open trials of antidepressant treatment of alcoholics with primary depression[31] and in severe comorbid suicidal depression in inpatients[32] have shown promising results. Among alcoholics not selected for depression, preliminary evidence suggests decreased depression among subjects with major depression using fluoxetine treatment.[33] Controlled studies are needed to confirm these preliminary observations.

Our study enrolled alcohol-abusing subjects who gave a history of clear primary depression in a placebo-controlled antidepressant trial using a vigorous antidepressant treatment regimen to address three main questions: (1) Does primary depression identified in actively drinking alcoholics respond to tricyclic antidepres-

150 mg of imipramine hydrochloride for 2 consecutive weeks or the equivalent number of placebo capsules.

Patients were seen weekly and assessed for depression and alcohol consumption using the TimeLine Follow-Back,[38] the CGI,[39] and the Hamilton Depression Scale (HAM-D).[40] Plasma levels of imipramine and desipramine were measured at weeks 6 and 12. Attendance at AA was rated for the previous 7 days as percentage of days attending of 7 days. Saliva samples were screened for alcohol at each visit using an enzymatic dipstick method.[40] Urine samples for alcohol and drugs of abuse were obtained at baseline and end of treatment. Whenever possible, a collateral informant was interviewed at baseline and the end of the trial to confirm the patient's report. While data from collateral informants were not systematically collected, about two thirds of our subjects had such informants and almost all were contacted at the end of treatment. Any discrepancies between subject report and informant report were resolved conservatively and all available data were considered in ratings prior to any unblinding.

Patient response was rated for depression and for alcohol consumption in the last week of the study using the CGI criterion of much improved or better as described above. Patients who were abstinent or whose amount of alcohol use declined by at least 50%, supported by any available significant other report, were considered responders if they also met the response criterion for depression.

COUNSELING

Patients were seen for weekly individual relapse prevention counseling sessions by a therapist who had been trained in the method of Marlatt and Gordon[41] and received weekly individual supervision by a psychologist experienced in the treatment of substance abuse. The focus of the counseling was identifying individual high-risk situations for drinking and developing cognitive and behavioral coping strategies to avoid alcohol use in those situations. Attendance at AA was strongly encouraged.

STATISTICAL ANALYSIS

For purposes of efficacy analysis, the adequately treated sample was defined prospectively as including those who had a minimum of 4 weeks of randomized medication treatment with at least 2 consecutive weeks receiving 150 mg or more of imipramine hydrochloride daily, or an equivalent number of placebo capsules. Ratings from the last observation were carried forward for those subjects who did not complete all 12 weeks of treatment. Intention-to-treat analyses included all randomized patients and carried last observation forward for dropouts and those who completed less than 12 weeks.

Categorical measures were compared by χ^2 analysis, corrected for continuity. The Fisher's exact test was used for contingency tables with any expected frequency of five or less. Confidence intervals for relative risk were calculated by the method of Cornfield[42] and included the Yates' correction.

Continuous baseline measures were compared by analysis of variance and outcome measures by analysis of covariance, using the baseline score as the covariate, after testing for homogeneity of slope. Variance estimates are SDs except for measures of relative risk where SE is used. Tests with a prospective hypothesis are reported one tailed and indicated in the text as such; all others are reported two tailed. Baseline variables were examined as predictors of outcome by comparing means or contingency tables for responders and nonresponders.

sants? (2) Is a tricyclic antidepressant safe to administer to actively drinking alcoholic outpatients without physical dependency on alcohol? (3) Do patients whose depression responds to an antidepressant and concurrent alcohol counseling decrease their drinking?

RESULTS

PATIENT FLOW AND SAMPLE DESCRIPTION

Of approximately 480 telephone inquiries from potential subjects, 123 who were interested and possibly eligible were screened in person. Twenty-three (19%) subjects did not meet inclusion criteria for either alcohol abuse or a depressive disorder or both, eight (6%) were excluded because of a physical illness, and seven (6%) were uninterested in study participation. Of the remaining 85 patients who began the single-blind placebo washout week, 11 (13%) responded to placebo with much improved depression, five (6%) were excluded because they were abstinent at both baseline and randomization visits, and 69 (81%) were randomized, with 36 to imipramine and 33 to placebo.

Demographic, diagnostic, and severity characteristics of randomized subjects are presented in **Table 1**. Although groups were comparable on almost all measures, significantly more subjects randomized to imipramine were currently married. According to *DSM III-R* criteria, patients largely were alcohol dependent with histories of early-onset chronic depressive illness of moderate severity and atypical subtype. To assess depressive severity, HAM-D scores were compared for these subjects with a sample of 926 depressed outpatients treated in our clinic who had no current substance abuse or dependence. The depressed sample had a mean (±SD) HAM-D score at baseline of 13.4±5.5, which was slightly but statistically significantly lower than the subjects in this study ($F=4.9$ [1,993], $P<.03$). The relatively low HAM-D scores for both groups may be a result of the large proportion of subjects meeting criteria for atypical depression, since overeating and oversleeping are not scored on this version. The scores also indicate that these subjects are at least as depressed as many subjects in outpatient clinical trials of uncomplicated depression. They had high prevalences of panic disorder and past dysthymia and modest histories of dependence on other substances. Their drinking was moderately heavy with a moderate severity of alcoholism on the Michigan Alcoholism Screening Test[43] (mean [±SD] score, 13.8±6.5), a standard alcoholism severity measure. At baseline, sub-

Table 1. Demographic and Diagnostic Characteristics of Randomized Subjects*

Variable	Treatment Group: Imipramine Hydrochloride (n=36)	Treatment Group: Placebo (n=33)	Difference Between Groups: Test Statistic	Difference Between Groups: P
Female, %	48.5	53.3	χ^2=0.12	.72
Mean (±SD) age, y	37.4 (6.7)	10.6 (9.1)	F=1.64	.11
White, %	83.3	78.8	χ^2=2.66	.45
Currently married, %	30.6	9.1	χ^2=4.34	.04
Mean (±SD) education, y	14.5 (2.3)	14.5 (3.2)	F=0.02	.99
Employed, %	42.9	59.4	χ^2=1.22	.27
Alcohol dependence	94.4	96.9	...	1
Major depression	72.2	71.0	.00	1
Bipolar depression, NOS	11.1	12.1	...	1
Atypical depression†	70.4	72.4	.00	.50
Past dysthymia	48.1	44.8	.00	1
Mean (SD)				
Hamilton Depression Scale, 21 items	15.4 (5.2)	14.3 (5.2)	.85	.34
HSCL-90, summary	20.0 (4.9)	21.6 (5.6)	.46	.65
Age at onset of alcohol disorder, y	28.6 (15.2)	25.7 (9.2)	.94	.33
Proportion of days drinking‡	63.8 (33.5)	68.0 (31.8)	.65	.52
Proportion of days drinking heavily (≥6 oz/d), %‡	38.3 (34.4)	51.5 (39.3)	1.48	.14
Drinks per drinking day, mean§	9.1 (6.5)	11.4 (13.7)	.90	.37

*All diagnoses definite plus probable by DSM-III-R unless otherwise indicated. NOS indicates not otherwise specified; HSCL-90, Hopkins Symptom Checklist, 90-item self-rated version.
†Atypical depression, definite and probable, by Columbia criteria.[36]
‡Drinking measures from the TimeLine Follow Back for the week before beginning the study.[38]
§Two-tailed Fischer's exact test employed for expected call frequencies 5 or less.

jects had attended meetings (mean±SD) of AA on 3.8±7.8 days of the last 30 days.

Urine drug screens at baseline were positive for other substances of abuse in 16% of cases: tetrahydrocannabinol, four; benzodiazepine, four; and cocaine on two occasions, one. There was no difference in positive urine drug screens by treatment. Patients receiving active imipramine attended a comparable number of counseling sessions (mean±SD, 7.8±5.0) as those receiving placebo (mean±SD, 6.9±3.0; t [63] = 0.9; P, not significant).

Thirteen patients dropped out after randomization: nine (13%) because of side effects from imipramine and four who were receiving placebo; three (4%) placebo-treated patients dropped out because of noncompliance; and one (1%) because of elective hospitalization for alcohol detoxification (χ^2 [1]=1.1; P, not significant). The most common side effect resulting in discontinuation was severe sedation experienced by four patients; other side effects included dizziness, constipation, gastrointestinal distress, urinary retention, and a single case of drug rash. No patient discontinued medication because of a clear adverse interaction between imipramine and alcohol and no seizures or hepatotoxicity occurred.

There were trends for dropouts to differ from the adequately treated group by being less likely to have had panic attacks (0% vs 25%; χ^2 [1]=3.8, $P<.06$) and more likely to be from an ethnic minority (41% vs 14%; χ^2 [1]=3.3; $P<.07$). Panic attacks may not be representative of panic disorder here as the possible relationship of panic attacks to alcohol withdrawal was not ascertained in our study. Dropouts attended AA significantly less frequently at baseline (mean±SD, 0.8%±1.5 of days vs 11.0%±23% of days in the previous month, $P<.02$). Other demographic, diagnostic, and severity of illness variables did not differ between adequately treated subjects and dropouts. Family history showed high levels of both depressive disorder (86%) and alcohol use disorders (86%) among first-degree relatives.

Because baseline of marital status differed between groups, analyses of covariance were run including this as a covariate. No significant effects of this were found, although the small number of subjects in some cells made full assessment of interactions impossible. For simplicity, the results are reported without the covariate.

Fifty-six patients (81% of those randomized) met criteria for adequate medication treatment. Thirty-five (51%) of those randomized completed the entire 12 weeks of the trial.

GLOBAL AND DEPRESSION TREATMENT OUTCOME FOR ADEQUATELY TREATED SUBJECTS

Measures of overall treatment outcome are presented in **Table 2**. Global response was rated on the CGI scale where patients rated much improved or very much improved on *both* depression and on alcohol ratings were considered to be responders. By this definition, response to imipramine (52%; confidence interval, 33% to 70%) was significantly better than response to placebo (21%; confidence interval, 9% to 38%). Expressed as a relative risk, the probability of response to imipramine was 2.51±0.41 (mean±SEM) compared with placebo (confidence interval, 1.07 to 6.45). Using HAM-D as a measure of depression outcome, patients receiving imipramine were significantly less depressed at end point than patients taking

Table 2. Treatment Outcome at End Point for Completers*

	Treatment Group		Difference Between Groups	
	Imipramine Hydrochloride (n=27)	Placebo (n=29)	χ^2 or F†	*P*‡
Global response rate, %	52	21	4.6	<.05
HAM-D Scale, 21 items, mean (±SD)	9.4 (7.7)	12.4 (9.7)	0.6	<.03
HAM-D Scale decreased ≥50%§	48	31	1.1	NS
HAM-D Scale decreased ≥50% and final HAM-D Scale ≤6	37	28	0.1	NS
Abstinent, last week, %	44	22	1.1	NS
Abstinent, last 4 wk, %	31	21	1.1	NS

*NS indicates not significant.
†χ^2, df=1; F [1, 53].
‡One tailed.
§Hamilton Depression (HAM-D) Scale score decreased from baseline by 50% or more.

placebo, although the magnitude of change was modest. Using more stringent definitions of response including the proportion attaining a decrease in HAM-D score of 50% or more as well as the proportion attaining both a decrease in HAM-D score of 50% or more and a final score of 6 or less, there were no differences between imipramine and placebo. There were no differences between treatments in rates of abstinence from alcohol in either the last week or the last 4 weeks of the trial.

Summary and subscale scores of the self-rated 90-item Hopkins Symptom Checklist[44] were examined by two-way analysis of covariance for evidence of treatment effect by drug and by categorization of depression response. There were no mean differences between treatments for the summary or any of the subscale scores. Patients categorized as depression responders, however, did rate themselves significantly better on the summary and on all but one of the subscales (paranoia) than did nonresponders. There were no significant interactions between depression response and treatment. These self-rating results support the clinician ratings of depression response.

INTENTION-TO-TREAT ANALYSES

When the sample of all randomized patients was considered in an intent-to-treat analysis using last observation in an end-point analysis, 15 (42%) of 36 patients randomized to imipramine were rated to be responders on both depression and alcohol abuse and six (18%) of 33 patients randomized to placebo (χ^2 [1]=3.4, *P*<.05, one tailed). For the intention-to-treat sample of all 69 randomized subjects, mean (±SD) HAM-D scores at the end of treatment, corrected for baseline, were 10.3±7.2 for imipramine-treated patients and 12.7±6.9 for placebo-treated patients (F [1,66]=2.69). This corresponds to a *P* value of .05 for the directional hypothesis tested.

CONTINUOUS MEASURES OF TREATMENT OUTCOME FOR DRINKING

Drinking outcome was measured by comparing patients treated with imipramine with those treated with placebo on measures derived from the TimeLine Follow Back for the final week in the study for each patient. Placebo-treated patients drank on 30.8%±32.9% (mean±SD) of the drinking days compared with 28.3%±33.1% for imipramine-treated patients (F [1,58]=.09; *P*, not significant); placebo patients drank heavily (defined as ≥6 oz per drinking day) on 9.0%±16.2% of days compared with 13.5%±24.2% of the drinkingdays for imipramine-treated patients (F [1,58]=1.02; *P*, not significant). The mean (±SD) number of standard drinks per drinking day was 4.1±4.1 for placebo-treated patients and 3.7±4.8 for imipramine-treated patients (F [1,58]=1.0; *P*, not significant). While these results indicate no overall improvement in drinking because of imipramine treatment, testing the hypothesis requires examining drinking in patients whose depression has responded to treatment, as this is proposed to be the mediating factor.

MEASURES OF ALCOHOL RESPONSE WITHIN DEPRESSION RESPONDERS

The results of two-way analyses of covariance of alcohol consumption among depression responders and nonresponders, using baseline score as the covariate, are presented in **Table 3**. Depression response, medication treatment, and the interaction of depression response and medication treatment were tested in the model. There was a significant main effect for depression response on mean number of standard drinks daily, proportion of days drinking, and on days drinking heavily (≥6 oz per day). There was no main effect for drug treatment. Significant interactions were found for mean number of daily drinks and for percentage of days drinking heavily, in the direction of less pathological drinking for patients taking imipramine.

SUBGROUP ANALYSIS

The principal subgroup of interest with sufficient sample size to analyze usefully is patients with major depression. Among the 41 adequately treated subjects with current major depression, the global response rates were 55% (11/20) for imipramine, and 29% (6/21) for placebo. This is essentially identical to the response rates for the whole

Table 3. Drinking Outcome Measures by Depression Response and by Drug for Study Completers*

Outcome Variable Mean (SD)	Depression Responders IMI	Depression Responders PBO	Depression Nonresponders IMI	Depression Nonresponders PBO	Depression Response F	Depression Response P	Drug Effect F	Drug Effect P	Interaction F	Interaction P
Mean drinks per drinking day (n=56)	1.5 (2.5)	4.0 (5.1)	6.4 (5.6)	4.1 (3.6)	4.8	<.05	.01	NS	4.5	<.05
No. (%) of days drinking (n=56)	17 (30)	25 (35)	42 (33)	33 (32)	4.2	<.05	.00	NS	1.2	NS
No. (%) of days drinking heavily (≥6 oz, n=56)	1 (4)	5 (6)	29 (30)	11 (19)	11.1	<.01	2.3	NS	4.4	<.05
No. (%) of days drinking lightly (≤6 oz, n=56)	25 (38)	21 (33)	19 (34)	31 (35)	0.1	NS	0.3	NS	0.8	NS
No. (%) of days AA attendance (n=33)	3 (6)	8 (11)	20 (33)	16 (30)	2.4	NS	0.1	NS	0.8	NS

**IMI indicates imipramine hydrochloride; PBO, placebo; and NS, not significant.*

sample, although with the small sample size the difference between drug and placebo fails to reach statistical significance ($\chi^2[1]=1.96$, *P*=.08, one tailed). As in the whole sample, there were no overall changes in drinking between treatment groups but there were significant effects of depression response. Depression responders to either treatment had significantly fewer heavy drinking days at end point, although among this smaller sample the interaction of treatment by depression response was not significant. While this indicates similarity to the whole sample, the sample size is simply insufficient to draw definite conclusions.

DOSES AND BLOOD LEVELS

The mean (±SD) dose of imipramine received by adequately treated subjects was 262±43 mg daily, with placebo patients receiving a comparable number of pills. The mean (±SD) plasma level of imipramine plus desipramine at the end of treatment was 1148±927 nmol/L (322±260 ng/mL) (n=23). There was a trend for subjects whose depression responded to have a higher plasma level (1455±1136 nmol/L [408±319 ng/mL]; n=12) than nonresponders (817±429 nmol/L [229±138 ng/mL]; n=11; *t* [21]=1.8, *P*<.10) and also greater variability in level (F=5.3, *P*<.02). Using a cutoff level at the end, treatment of 802 nmol/L [225 ng/mL] or more to define adequate treatment, three (80%) of 15 responders with depression met this criterion vs three (75%) of 12 nonresponders (Fisher's exact test, 0.30), a nonsignificant difference. A similar result was obtained for alcohol response, considered by itself. However, responders also tended to have been prescribed a higher daily dose (275±40 mg for responders and 232±64 mg for nonresponders; *t*=1.95 [21]; *P*<.07). When a ratio between blood level and prescribed dose was calculated, the difference between responders and nonresponders (5.7±5.7 nmol/L [1.6±1.6 ng/mL] per mg daily dose for responders) and 3.9±2.9 nmol/L [1.1±0.8 ng/mL per mg] for nonresponders (*t* [21]=1.0; *P*, not significant) was not significant, although again the variability was greater in the responders (F=4.0, *P*<.05). Since dosage escalation was curtailed in nonresponders mainly because of side effects, this may suggest that responders were better able or more willing to tolerate imipramine's side effects. The greater variability in level among responders does not suggest that nonresponse was strongly related to noncompliance in our patients, but rather perhaps that doses tended to be increased to toleration in nonresponders and not increased in responders, leading to more variability in the latter group.

COURSE OF RESPONSE

Patients in the study were categorized based on ratings from the weekly CGI improvement scores for alcohol abuse and depression as to whether depression improved first, alcohol improved first, or both improved simultaneously. This was done for the first manifestation of any improvement ("minimal improvement" or better) and for improvement to the criteria of significant response for the study. Rating the onset of at least minimal improvement for the 20 adequately treated subjects who responded, 13 (65%) improved first in alcohol abuse, four (20%) improved first in depression, and three (15%) improved simultaneously on both. A similar pattern of alcohol abuse improving first was obtained when rating the onset of much improved or better was considered. There were no significant differences between imipramine and placebo with regard to which disorder improved first.

AA ATTENDANCE

The possible effect of attendance at AA during the study on drinking measures from the TimeLine Follow Back was examined as an independent variable in a multivariate analysis of variance with baseline drinking, treatment, and depression response as the other independent variables. Neither effect of AA attendance nor interaction with the other independent variables was found for any of the dependent measures. This is consistent with the evidence on AA where uncontrolled studies generally report a modest benefit of AA attendance on drinking outcomes, but where controlled studies have not found this effect.[45]

PREDICTORS OF RESPONSE

Responders to treatment did not differ from nonresponders on demographic, *DSM III-R* diagnoses, or severity variables at baseline. However, the relatively small sample size gives limited power. There may be subgroups who have a better prognosis but analysis of this issue requires larger samples.

COMMENT

These data support the hypothesis that imipramine treatment of moderately ill, actively drinking alcoholic outpatients with current depression of a primary type, ascertained by history, results in statistically significant, albeit modest, improvement in depression in patients who receive an adequate trial. This treatment did not cause serious adverse events in our subjects, even those few who drank heavily while receiving active imipramine therapy. However, our subjects were not physically dependent to the degree that they required detoxification, they were relatively physically healthy, and our sample size was relatively small. This does not establish safety for more seriously ill patients, and imipramine treatment should be given cautiously to actively drinking alcoholics. Furthermore, the reduction of occasions of heavy drinking is correlated with depression response in those whose depression responded to treatment. While this is consistent with the hypothesis that an improvement in depression also improves the outcome of comorbid alcoholism, at least in the near term, it is not definitive. The course of response analysis suggests that improvement in drinking was antecedent to improvement in depression, which might indicate that the causality was reversed and decreased drinking caused decreased depression. The large proportion of subjects with atypical depression may have limited the benefit from imipramine therapy, consistent with a large body of data suggesting a poorer response to imipramine than to other treatments in depressed patients with atypical depression.[46]

Unfortunately, while imipramine-treated subjects decreased pathological drinking, they did not attain sobriety any more frequently than placebo-treated patients. Since sobriety is the most widely accepted long-term treatment goal for alcoholic patients, this is an unsatisfactory outcome. Certainly, reduction of harm by decreased pathological drinking would be worthwhile but there are as yet insufficient data to show that return to social drinking by alcoholic subjects as a result of treatment is often sustained. Other treatment with either enhanced psychosocial treatments or possibly other pharmacologic treatments may be indicated for these patients and antidepressants must be viewed as adjunctive. This conclusion must be tempered with the knowledge that imipramine has been shown to be a marginally effective treatment for atypical depression, which was the subtype of most of our subjects. Other agents such as selective serotonin reuptake inhibitors, buproprion, or monoamine oxidase inhibitors might be more effective. While our sample was not selected for atypical depression, it may be that this is common among alcoholics but to our knowledge that has not been studied systematically.

Other treatment possibilities to improve on these outcomes worthy of further research include pharmacologic strategies such as naltrexone coadministration,[47,48] should safety data support this. The lack of imipramine effect on drinking, independent of depression response, is in accord with previous studies. Available studies suggest either clinically modest or no attenuation of drinking in alcoholics not selected for depression, even by selective serotonin reuptake antidepressants for which preclinical data indicate suppression of alcohol consumption.[33,49,50]

The hypothesis of our study was that improvement in depression may be associated with improvement in drinking behavior, not that antidepressants per se reduce drinking. To address this issue, analyses were conducted within the subgroup of patients whose depression has responded to treatment. These showed that mood improvement while receiving either treatment was associated with significant decreases in both average drinking and particularly in heavy drinking, which supports the hypothesis. That result would be compatible with mood improvement consequently, rather than a cause of decreased drinking. When drinking response was measured in relation to drug treatment and depression response, however, there was also a treatment interaction indicating that patients overall drank less when taking imipramine only when their depression responded to treatment.

The course of response analysis on the other hand gives no support for the idea that it is improvement in depression that drives decreases in drinking. It is possible that minor degrees of symptomatic change in depression, which were not detectible by global ratings, did precede significant changes in alcohol consumption. The overall improvements in drinking in both treatment groups might have obscured differential effects between medication and placebo that might be seen with a larger sample.

Overall, these data do not support a pure self-medication model of the relationship between alcoholism and primary depression because of the modest effect of treating depression on drinking outcomes. They are more consistent with a model whereby depression, even when it is primary as far as can be determined in nonabstinent patients, is an independent factor that interacts with alcoholism and worsens its course. These data do support the value of identifying primary depression by history in actively drinking outpatients without physiologic dependence on alcohol and the treatment of those patients with a tricyclic antidepressant. The treatment of secondary depression was not addressed in this trial; a controlled study of treating secondary depression in abstinent alcoholics has been reported showing good results with desipramine treatment.[22]

STUDY LIMITATIONS

Since treatment effects appeared to be more robust in the adequately treated subsample, it is possible that differential attrition of subjects with regard to some significant variable could have enhanced the outcome for the adequately treated sample. An equally plausible explanation is that an adequate exposure in both dose and duration is necessary for antidepressant effects to be manifested,[51] making an analysis of the adequately treated sample analysis more powerful. Intention-to-treat analyses sacrifice power by including subjects who are not exposed to adequate treatment and therefore require larger sample sizes to show significant differences. The sample size in our study limited the power to find robust differences in the intention-to-treat sample. Because of the substantial dropout rate, clinical application of these data must be cautious. Only replications of the present study with larger sample sizes can definitively resolve this question.

We solicited comorbid subjects who were not seriously physically dependent on alcohol and who were generally seeking treatment for depression, which limits its generalizability. While these subjects are not representative of patients seen in usual alcoholism treatment settings, they may be more representative of patients seen in other mental health settings or in primary care, where alcoholism is not the presenting problem but where the clinician identifies it during evaluation of another disorder.

The period of observation in our trial was short in terms of the natural history of alcohol-use disorders. Studies employing longer periods of follow-up would be necessary to determine if these benefits are sustained. The low completion rate for the 12-week trial (51%), while typical of substance-abusing populations, increases the risk of undetected differential attrition and limits the generalizability to those who completed the trial. Studies diagnosing and treating such patients from well-defined populations would be necessary to determine this.

Ratings of both depression and drinking were made by the treating psychiatrist. Although the clinician was blinded to treatment assignment, possible knowledge of side effects may have influenced the ratings, especially given imipramine's distinctive side-effect profile. However, patient self-ratings of depression were concordant with clinician ratings, suggesting that this was not a major source of bias. Ideally, an independent evaluator blinded to possible side effects would have been used.

Assessment of drinking was primarily by self-report with input from weekly measures of salivary alcohol and input from significant others when available. Generally, available laboratory measures have been of limited use in subjects not severely physically dependent on alcohol because they are frequently normal at baseline. Nonetheless, serial measures of γ-glutamyl transferase and mean corpuscular volume would have been preferable to provide more objective measures of drinking behavior. Also, newer measures, like the level of carbohydrate-deficient transferrin, have become available although they also have significant limitations of sensitivity and specificity.[52] Even in the absence of rater bias, the presence of side effects perceived by the patient could have influenced the reports of drinking behavior, since the patients were not blinded to the hypothesis.

Future studies of this group of patients appear to be warranted by these findings. Such studies should characterize patients with regard to atypical subtype of depression, as these data suggest that alcoholic patients not meeting criteria for atypical depression respond best to a tricyclic antidepressant, as do nonalcoholic depressed subjects. The use of other antidepressants, like the selective serotonin uptake inhibitors, may be advantageous since some data suggest that they may be more effective than the tricyclics in atypical depression.[53] The data suggesting that selective serotonin uptake inhibitors have some modest effects in suppressing alcohol consumption in both animals[54] and human subjects[49,50] make these possibly more attractive than the tricyclics as they may have some effect independent of their antidepressant effects. Some preliminary data also suggest that selective serotonin uptake inhibitors are effective in depressed alcoholics.[33]

Accepted for publication December 10, 1995.

This study was supported by grant AA9539 from the National Institute on Alcohol Abuse and Alcoholism, Rockville, Md; by the state of New York; and by grant NIMH 30906 from the Mental Health Clinical Research Center, New York, NY.

We thank Thomas F. Babor, PhD, and Roger Meyer, MD, for design and measurement consultation; Deborah Deliyannides, MD, Stephen Donovan, MD, Jerry Finkel, MD, Ron Goldman, MD, Ilisse Perlmutter, MD, Lawrence Peters, MD, Margaret Spinelli, MD, and Steven Wager, MD, for treating patients in the study; Naomi Quart, MSW, for counseling the subjects; Donald E. Klein, MD, for helpful comments on the manuscript; Eva Petkova, PhD, for statistical consultation, Ellen Jimenez for manuscript preparation; and the clinic staff of the Depression Evaluation Service and the Staten Island Research Clinic for patient recruitment and support services. Medication and matching placebo were supplied by Ciba-Geigy Corp, Summit, NJ.

Reprint requests to the Depression Evaluation Service, Unit 35, New York State Psychiatric Institute, 722 W 168th St, New York, NY 10032 (Dr McGrath).

REFERENCES

1. Institute of Medicine. *Causes and Consequences of Alcohol Problems.* Washington, DC: National Academy Press; 1987.
2. Weissman MM, Myers JK. Clinical depression in alcoholism. *Am J Psychiatry.* 1980;137:372-373.
3. Boyd JH, Burke JD, Gruenberg E, Holzer CE, Rae DS, George LK, Karuo M, Stoltzman R, McEvoy L. Exclusion criteria of *DSM-III*: a study of co-occurrence of hierarchy-free syndromes. *Arch Gen Psychiatry.* 1984;41:983-989.
4. Helzer JE, Canino GJ, Hwu HG, Bland RC, Newman S, Yeh EK. Alcoholism: a cross-national comparison of population survey with the Diagnostic Interview Schedule. In: Rose RM, Barrett JE, eds. *Alcoholism: Origins and Outcome.* New York, NY: Raven Press; 1988:31-47.
5. Helzer JE, Pryzbeck TR. The co-occurrence of alcoholism and other psychiatric disorders in the general population and its impact on treatment. *J Stud Alcohol.* 1988;49:219-224.
6. Regier DA, Farmer ME, Rae DS, Locke BZ, Keith SJ, Judd LL, Goodwin FK. Comorbidity of mental disorders with alcohol and other drug abuse: results from the Epidemiologic Catchment Area (ECA) Study. *JAMA.* 1990;264:2511-2518.
7. Rohde P, Lewinsohn PM, Seeley JR. Comorbidity of unipolar depression, II: comorbidity with other mental disorders in adolescents and adults. *J Abnorm Psychol.* 1991;100:214-222.
8. Merikangas KR, Gelernter CS. Comorbidity for alcoholism and depression. *Psychiatr Clin North Am.* 1990;13:613-632.
9. Coulehan JL, Zettler-Segal M, Block M, McClelland M, Schulberg HC. Recognition of alcoholism and substance abuse in primary care patients. *Arch Intern Med.* 1987;147:349-352.
10. Schuckit MA. Genetic and clinical implications of alcoholism and affective disorder. *Am J Psychiatry.* 1986;143:140-147.

11. Meyer RE. Prospects for a rational pharmacotherapy of alcoholism. *J Clin Psychiatry.* 1989;50:403-412.
12. Cloninger CR, Reich T, Wetzel R. Alcoholism and affective disorders: familial association and genetic models. In: Goodwin DW, Erickson CK, eds. *Alcoholism and Affective Disorders: Clinical, Genetic, and Biochemical Studies.* New York, NY: SP Medical & Scientific Books; 1979:57-86.
13. Schuckit MA. Genetic and clinical implications of alcoholism and affective disorder. *Am J Psychiatry.* 1986;143:140-147.
14. Finn PR, Kleinman I, Pihl RO. The lifetime prevalence of psychopathology in men with multigenerational family histories of alcoholism. *J Nerv Ment Dis.* 1990;178:500-504.
15. Winokur G, Coryell W. Familial alcoholism in primary unipolar major depressive disorder. *Am J Psychiatry.* 1991;148:184-188.
16. Ingraham LJ, Wender PH. Risk for affective disorder and alcohol and other drug abuse in the relatives of affectively ill adoptees. *J Affect Disord.* 1992; 26:45-52.
17. Kendler KS, Heath AC, Neale MC, Kessler RC, Eaves LJ. Alcoholism and major depression in women. *Arch Gen Psychiatry.* 1993;50:690-698.
18. Schuckit MA, Winokur G. A short term follow-up of women alcoholics. *Dis Nerv Sys.* 1972;33:672-678.
19. Schuckit MA. The clinical implications of primary diagnostic groups among alcoholics. *Arch Gen Psychiatry.* 1985;42:1043-1049.
20. Brown SA, Schuckit MA. Changes in depression among abstinent alcoholics. *J Stud Alcohol.* 1988;49:412-417.
21. Coryell W, Endicottt J, Keller M. Major depression in a nonclinical sample. *Arch Gen Psychiatry.* 1992;49:117-125.
22. Mason BJ, Kocsis JH. Desipramine treatment of alcoholism. *Psychopharm Bull.* 1991;27:155-161.
23. Quitkin FM, Rifkin A, Kaplan J, Klein DF. Phobic anxiety syndrome complicated by drug dependence and addiction: a treatable form of drug abuse. *Arch Gen Psychiatry.* 1972;27:159-162.
24. Khantzian EJ. The self-medication hypothesis of addictive disorders: focus on heroin and cocaine dependence. *Am J Psychiatry.* 1985;142:1259-1264.
25. Powell BJ, Penick EC, Othmer E, Bingham SF, Rice AS. Prevalence of additional psychiatric syndromes among male alcoholics. *J Clin Psychiatry.* 1982; 43:404-407.
26. Hesselbrock M, Meyer RE, Keener JJ. Psychopathology in hospitalized alcoholics. *Arch Gen Psychiatry.* 1985;42:1050-1055.
27. O'Sullivan K. Depression and its treatment in alcoholics: a review. *Can J Psychiatry.* 1984;29:379-384.
28. Shaw JA, Donley P, Morgan DW, Robinson JA. Treatment of depression in alcoholics. *Am J Psychiatry.* 1975;132:641-644.
29. Ciraulo DA, Jaffe JH. Tricyclic antidepressants in the treatment of depression associated with alcoholism. *J Clin Psychopharm.* 1981;1:146-150.
30. Liskow BI, Goodwin DW. Pharmacological treatment of alcohol intoxication, withdrawal and dependence: a critical review. *J Stud Alcohol.* 1987;48:356-370.
31. Nunes EV, McGrath PJ, Quitkin FM, Stewart JW, Harrison W, Tricamo E, Ocepete-Welikson K. Imipramine treatment of alcoholism with comorbid depression. *Am J Psychiatry.* 1993;150:963-965.
32. Cornelius J, Salloum IM, Cornelius MD, Perel JM, Thase ME, Ehler JG; Mann JJ. Fluoxetine trial in suicidal depressed alcoholics. *Psychopharm Bull.* 1993; 29:195-199.
33. Kranzler HR, Burleson JA, Korner P, Del Boca FK, Bohn MJ, Brown J, Liebowitz N. Placebo-controlled trial of fluoxetine as an adjunct to relapse prevention in alcoholics. *Am J Psychiatry.* 1995;152:391-397.
34. Spitzer RL, Williams JBW, Gibbon M, First MB. The structured clinical interview for *DSM-III-R* (SCID), I: history, rationale, and description. *Arch Gen Psychiatry.* 1992;49:624-629.
35. Nunes EV, Goehl L, Seracini A, Deliyannides D, Donovan S, Koenig T, Quitkin FM, Williams J. Evaluation of depression and panic disorder in methadone patients using a modification of the structured clinical interview for *DSM III-R*: test-retest reliability. *Am J Addict.* In press.
36. Stewart JW, Rabkin JG, Quitkin FM, McGrath PJ, Klein DF. Atypical depression. In: Dunner DL, ed. *Current Psychiatric Therapy.* Philadelphia, Pa: WB Saunders Co; 1992:215-220.
37. Guy W, ed. *ECDEU Assessment Manual for Psychopharmacology, Revised Edition.* Rockville, Md: National Institute of Mental Health; 1976. US Dept of Health, Education, and Welfare publication (ADM) 76-338.
38. Sobell MB, Maisto SA, Sobell LC, Cooper AM, Cooper TC, Sanders M. Developing a prototype for evaluating alcohol treatment effectiveness. In: Sobell LC, Sobell MB, Ward E, eds. *Evaluating Alcohol and Drug Abuse Treatment Effectiveness: Recent Advances.* Elmsford, NY: Pergamon Press Inc; 1980.
39. Hamilton M. A rating scale for depression. *J Neurol Neurosurg Psychiatry.* 1960;23:56-62.
40. Kapur BM, Israel Y. Alcohol dipstick: a rapid method for analysis of ethanol in body fluids. In: Chang NC, Chao HM, eds. *Early Identification of Alcohol Abuse.* Rockville, Md: US Dept of Health and Human Services; 1985:1-30. Research Monograph No. 17.
41. Marlatt GA, Gordon JR. *Relapse Prevention.* New York, NY: Guilford; 1985.
42. Cornfield J. A statistical problem arising from retrospective studies. In: Neyman J, ed. *Proceedings of the Third Berkeley Symposium on Mathematical Statistics and Probability.* Berkeley, Calif: University of California Press; 1956;4:135-148.
43. Selzer M. The Michigan alcoholism screening test: the quest for a new diagnostic instrument. *Am J Psychiatry.* 1971;127:1653-1658.
44. Derogatis LR. *SCL-90 Administration, Scoring, and Procedures Manual.* Baltimore, Md: Clinical Psychiatry Research; 1977.
45. Montgomery HA, Miller WR, Tonigan JS. Does alcoholics anonymous involvement predict treatment outcome? *J Subst Abuse Treat.* 1995;12:241-246.
46. Quitkin FM, Stewart JW, McGrath PJ, Tricamio E, Rabkim JG, Ocepele-Welikson K, Nunes E, Harrison W, Klein DF. Columbia atypical depression: a subgroup of depressives with better response to MAOI than to tricyclic antidepressants or placebo. *Br J Psychiatry.* 1993;163(suppl 21):30-34.
47. Omalley SS, Jaffe AJ, Chang G, Schottenfeld RS, Meyer RE, Rounsaville B. Naltrexone and coping skills therapy for alcohol dependence: a controlled study. *Arch Gen Psychiatry.* 1992;49:894-898.
48. Volpicelli JR, Alterman AI, Hayashida M, O'Brien CP. Naltrexone in the treatment of alcohol dependence. *Arch Gen Psychiatry.* 1992;49:876-880.
49. Naranjo CA, Kadlec KE, Sanhueza P, Woodley-Remus D, Sellers EM. Fluoxetine differentially alters alcohol intake and other consummatory behaviors. *Clin Pharmacol Ther.* 1990;47:490-498.
50. Gorelick DA, Paredes A. Effect of fluoxetine on alcohol consumption in male alcoholics. *Alcohol Clin Exp Res.* 1992;16:261-265.
51. Quitkin FM. The importance of dose in prescribing antidepressants. *Br J Psychiatry.* 1985;147:593-597.
52. Stibler S. Carbohydrate-deficient transferrin in serum: a new marker of potentially harmful alcohol consumption reviewed. *Clin Chem.* 1991;37:2029-2037.
53. Reimherr FW, Wood DR, Byerley B, Brainard J, Grosser BI. Characteristics of responders to fluoxetine. *Psychopharm Bull.* 1987;30:70-72.
54. Naranjo CA, Sellers EM, Lawrin MO. Modulation of ethanol intake by serotonin uptake inhibitors. *J Clin Psychiatry.* 1986;47(suppl):16-22.

A Long-term Follow-up of Male Alcohol Abuse

George E. Vaillant, MD

Background: This study attempted to determine the course of male alcohol abuse from the age of 40 years to 60 or 70 years, to estimate the duration of abstinence required for stable remission and to study the hypothesis of progression of symptoms in chronic alcohol abuse.

Methods: The subjects were 268 former Harvard University (Cambridge, Mass) undergraduates (college sample) and 456 nondelinquent inner-city adolescents (core city sample) who had been repeatedly studied in multidisciplinary fashion since 1940. Since 47 years of age, these men have been followed up biennially by questionnaire and every 5 years by physical examination. At some point during their lives, 55 (21%) of the college and 150 (33%) of the core city men met *DSM-III* criteria for alcohol abuse. The college cohort has been followed until the age of 70 years, the core city cohort until age 60 years. The dependent variables were mortality and alcohol abuse status every 5 years.

Results: By 60 years of age, 18% of the college alcohol abusers had died, 11% were abstinent, 11% were controlled drinkers, and 59% were known to be still abusing alcohol. By 60 years of age, 28% of the core city alcohol abusers had died, 30% were abstinent, 11% were controlled drinkers, and only 28% were known to be still abusing alcohol.

Conclusions: In three respects the two socially divergent samples resembled each other. After abstinence had been maintained for 5 years, relapse was rare. In contrast, return to controlled drinking without eventual relapse was unlikely. Alcohol abuse could continue for decades without remission or progression of symptoms. The samples differed in that the core city men began to abuse alcohol when younger and, although they were more likely than the college men to become alcohol dependent, the core city men were twice as likely to achieve stable abstinence.

(Arch Gen Psychiatry. 1996;53:243-249)

Approximately 100 000[1] deaths in the United States each year can be attributed directly or indirectly to alcohol; thus, alcohol abuse vies with strokes and accidents as the third most important cause of death in this country. Nevertheless, we know far more about the natural course of most cancers than we do of alcohol abuse. A major reason for our ignorance is the scarcity of long-term prospective follow-up studies.

Indeed, there are three unanswered questions regarding the clinical course of alcoholism that can be answered only by prolonged follow-up. First, why does the prevalence of alcohol abuse decline sharply with age?[2] Is the explanation for this decline stable abstinence, or return to asymptomatic drinking, or high mortality, or poor case finding among the elderly? Second, if alcohol abuse persists over the life course, does it really progress inexorably, as investigators such as Jellinek[3] believed? Or, over time, do some individuals without remission remain chronic alcohol abusers without progressing to dependence? Third, how long must abstinence or return to controlled drinking persist before an individual's recovery can be considered secure? In cancer, remission must often last for 5 years before relapse is considered unlikely. In alcohol treatment studies, however, investigators often speak of recovery after the alcohol abuser has been symptom-free for 6 months or 1 year.

To the extent that the natural course of alcoholism can be addressed from a 50-year study confined to white

See Subjects and Methods on next page

From Harvard Medical School and Brigham and Women's Hospital, Boston, Mass.

SUBJECTS AND METHODS

A prospective cohort study of two socially contrasting samples of men has been conducted since 1940.

STUDY PARTICIPANTS

The core city sample (mean±SD date of birth, 1929±2) included 456 men first studied from early adolescence until age 31 years as a nondelinquent control group for Glueck and Glueck's well-known studies of juvenile delinquents.[5,6] Ninety percent of these men came from working-class or welfare families; 61% of their parents were foreign-born. They resided in high-crime inner-city Boston, Mass, neighborhoods. Their mean IQ was 95±12; 48% graduated from high school and 7% from college. Their 1976 mean income was approximately $15 000. The sample included no African Americans.

At the time of original study, the men, their parents, and their teachers were interviewed individually. More than 90% of the surviving participants were reinterviewed at 25 and 31 years of age.[6] At these interviews alcohol abuse or its absence was specifically recorded. When the men reached age 47 years, a 2-hour semistructured interview with a detailed 23-item section on lifetime problem drinking was used to reinterview 87% of the surviving men.[4]

The college sample (mean±SD date of birth, 1921±2) included 268 Harvard University sophomores selected for a study of "normal" development from 1938 to 1942. Selection criteria required the absence of known physical or mental illness and a freshman grade average above C.[7] Although half of the sample worked during college to help pay tuition and/or were on scholarships, most of their parents were upper or middle class and were born in this country. Their estimated mean IQ was 130; 76% attended graduate school; and their 1976 mean income was approximately $50 000. Up to 47 years of age, the college sample was studied in roughly the same fashion as the core city sample; after age 47 years the college sample was studied in an identical manner to the core city sample.[4,8]

DATA COLLECTION

From age 47 years until the present, both groups were followed up by biennial questionnaires and by obtaining reports of physical examinations every 5 years. Besides gathering information regarding health, work, and relationships, the biennial questionnaires inquired about alcohol use. In addition to describing quantity and frequency of alcohol use, the men were asked five questions: whether (1) they, (2) their friends, (3) their families, or (4) their physicians had been concerned about their drinking, and (5) whether and for how long they had stopped drinking.

MEASUREMENT OF ALCOHOL ABUSE

Presence or Absence of Alcohol Abuse by Age 47 Years

For both samples, 2-hour interviews at age 48±3 years were performed by clinicians, most with two or more years of experience in alcohol clinics. Interviews at age 31 years and recent psychiatric, medical, and arrest records also were reviewed. These records confirmed the participants' self-reports and documented alcohol-related problems. On the basis of all of the available data, clinicians rated the men on two scales of alcohol abuse. (The core city men were also rated on an 11-point scale, developed by Cahalan,[9] to assess alcohol-related social deviance.)

The first scale from the American Psychiatric Association's *DSM-III*[10] reflected a three-category medical model for diagnosing alcoholism, where 1 represents no alcohol abuse; 2, alcohol abuse; and 3, alcohol dependence (tolerance or withdrawal symptoms from alcohol *in addition* to alcohol abuse). Diagnosis was made by consensus of two clinicians; the extensive evidence for convergent validity of diagnosis is discussed elsewhere.[4,8]

The second scale used was the Problem Drinking Scale, an equally weighted 16-point scale (similar to the Michigan Alcoholism Screening Test)[11] devised to combine the emphasis of the *DSM-III* on physiologic dependence and the emphasis of the Cahalan scale on social deviance. The scale assigned points for social, legal, medical, and employment problems caused by alcohol abuse and points for blackouts, going on the wagon, seeking treatment, and admitting to problems with control and withdrawal symptoms. Measurement of alcohol in a breath sample and laboratory drug screens were not performed.

Presence or Absence of Alcohol Abuse After Age 47 Years

Since age 47 years, if any man who was not previously classified as an alcohol abuser reported two or more of the four alcohol-related problems (eg, wife or physician complains, participant feeling guilty, etc) on the biennial questionnaire for two consecutive questionnaires (see the "Data Collection" section), he was reclassified as an alcohol abuser. Because the follow-up depended largely on questionnaires, after age 47 years no further attempt was made to distinguish alcohol abuse from dependence. Progression

men, this report will attempt to provide answers to the three questions posed above. The report prospectively builds on a 1976 follow-up study[4] of two contrasting community samples: 456 underprivileged inner-city adolescents and 268 Harvard University (Cambridge, Mass) sophomores. In the current study, all the alcohol abusers identified in those samples were followed up until 60 years of age (the core city men) and 70 years of age (the college men).

RESULTS

AGE AT ONSET OF ALCOHOL ABUSE

By age 70 years, 52 (21%) of the 249 college men who remained in the study at age 47 years had met *DSM-III* criteria for alcohol abuse (as had three of the 13 who dropped out of the study). At some point, 21 (38%) of the 55 men also met *DSM-III* criteria for dependence. By of symptoms, however, could be determined from the serial physical exams and assessments of social functioning.

Age at Onset of Alcohol Abuse

The age at which each participant first met criteria for alcohol abuse was estimated from the repeated interviews and questionnaires. Age at development of dependence was not determined.

SMOKING

Pack-years of cigarette smoking were estimated by review of all information at age 47 years and at age 60 years. Age at stable smoking cessation was estimated.

OUTCOME DEFINITIONS

Quinquennial alcohol use status was determined by estimating the use or abuse status of each alcohol abuser every 5 years. This status estimate was based on the questionnaires administered every 2 years and physical examinations obtained every 5 years.

Alcohol use or abuse status was categorized as follows: (1) *abstinent:* less than one drink (0.5 oz of alcohol) per month for more than a year; (2) *social drinker:* not yet an abuser, or follow-up suggests that original diagnosis of *DSM-III* alcohol abuse could be challenged because of brief duration (<5 years) *and* minimal symptoms (Problem Drinking Scale score <5) *and* subsequent problem-free drinking for 10 years or more; (3) *return to controlled drinking:* a former alcohol abuser consuming more than one drink per month for at least 2 years but with no reported problems; (4) *continued alcohol abuse:* clear history of sustained alcohol abuse and one or more acknowledged problems caused by drinking in the past 2 years; relapse to *alcohol abuse* from a status of *stable abstinence* or of *stable return to controlled drinking* required reporting at least *two* or more problems caused by alcohol use; and (5) *dead:* death certificates were obtained for all alcohol abusers (and nonabusers) categorized as deceased.

Complete physical examinations were sought for all subjects every 5 years. Data from physical examinations and death certificates were used to determine presence or absence of *cancer* and *heart disease*.

Final outcome status was determined as follows. At the most recent follow-up or at the time of death or long-term institutionalization, each alcohol abuser was assigned to one of four categories: (1) *stable abstinence* in the community (3 years or more); (2) *stable return to controlled drinking* (3 years or more); (3) *reclassified social drinker* (original diagnosis of previous alcohol abuse open to question because of brevity, minimal symptoms (Problem Drinking Scale score <5), and 10 to 40 years of return to social drinking; and (4) *chronic alcohol abuse,* which was alcohol abuse, usually chronic, during the last 3 years of follow-up or during the 3 years before death or institutionalization. (Although this broad definition theoretically could include men who had abused alcohol for only 1 year, 83 of the 86 men assigned to this outcome category had abused alcohol for 6 to 40 years. The three exceptions died after 1, 3, and 5 years of alcohol abuse, respectively.)

ATTRITION

Before age 47 years, 19 (7%) of the 268 men from the college sample could not be classified for presence or absence of alcohol abuse because of nonparticipation or death in World War II. Before age 47 years, 23 (5%) of the 456 core city men could not be classified because of early death, nonparticipation, or difficulty in location.

Since age 47 years, the alcohol-abusing subjects in both samples were less likely than nonabusers to return questionnaires, but not significantly so. In an average mailing, 61% of non–alcohol abusers and 53% of abusers returned questionnaires. Questionnaire nonresponders were interviewed by telephone or in person. Subjects with whom contact was lost and nonresponding subjects were traced through credit agencies and departments of motor vehicles. During any given 5-year period, no more than 2% to 3% of participants were unavailable, and only 1% of the sample appeared permanently unavailable. Alcohol-abusing participants were somewhat more likely to withdraw from the study. As of 1992, 21 of the known 150 alcohol-abusing core city men and two of the known 52 alcohol-abusing college men had dropped out. The mortality of nonresponders and dropouts was monitored through the National Death Index.

STATISTICAL ANALYSIS

The significance of differences between groups was determined by the χ^2 test for categoric predictors or Student's *t* test for continuous predictors. All tests were two tailed, with a *P* value of .05 considered significant. The log-rank test was used to contrast age at onset of alcohol abuse between the two groups. Logistic regression was employed to determine whether alcohol abuse was a risk factor for mortality even after controlling for multiple hypothesized risk factors (obesity, blood cholesterol level, blood pressure, and smoking). Results are presented as odds ratios and are accompanied by 95% confidence intervals.

age 60 years, 150 (35%) of the 433 core city men who remained in the study at age 47 years whose alcohol abuse status was known had met *DSM-III* criteria for alcohol abuse. At some point, 77 (51%) of the core city alcohol abusers also met criteria for alcohol dependence. The average age at onset of alcohol abuse was a decade later for the 51 college men who developed alcohol abuse by age 60 years (mean, 40.2±9.9 years) than it was for the 149 core city men (mean, 29.2±9.5 years). **Figure 1** illustrates graphically the differing age at onset between the two groups. The difference was highly significant (log-rank statistic=38.5, *df*=1, *P*<.01).

OUTCOME STATUS OF ALCOHOL ABUSERS

Table 1 summarizes the outcome status for the two cohorts at age 60 years. As noted, 21 of the 150 core city alcohol abusers dropped out of the study after age 47 years.

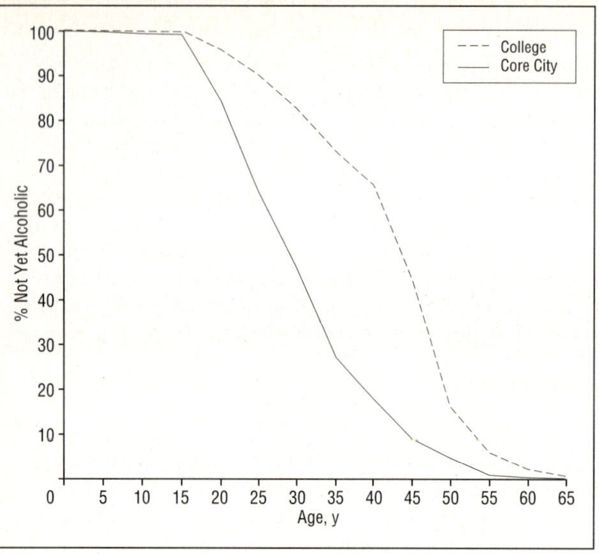

Figure 1. *Approximate age at which each of the 150 core city and the 52 college alcohol abusers with complete data sets first met the* DSM-III *criteria for alcohol abuse. Age at onset before age 45 years was based in part on retrospective data.*

Table 1. Final Outcome Status for the Two Cohorts of Alcohol Abusers at Last Contact or Time of Death

	No. (%)	
	College (n=52)*	**Core City (n=129)†**
Stable abstinence (≥3 y)	10 (19)	48 (37)‡
Return to controlled drinking (≥3 y)	5 (10)	18 (14)
Reclassified as social drinker	6 (11.5)	8 (6)
Chronic alcohol abuse	31 (59.5)	55 (43)
Total	**52 (100)**	**129 (100)**
Dead by age 60 y	8 (15)	38 (25)
Dead by age 70 y	22 (40)§	. . .

**N=52 because data sets for three alcohol abusers are incomplete.*
†*N=129 because data sets for 21 core city alcohol abusers are incomplete.*
‡χ^2=5.5, df=2, P=.02.
§*The death rate for 55 college alcohol abusers was significantly greater than the 16% of 194 college nonalcoholics who had died by age 70 years* (χ^2=15.6, df=1, P<.01).

Roughly half of the men in both samples achieved stable remission, but stable abstinence was significantly more common in the core city cohort. Of the 129 core city men whose alcoholic careers were known, only 31% (n=19) of the 62 core city men who met criteria for alcohol abuse achieved stable abstinence, in contrast to 43% (n=29) of the 67 core city men classified as dependent. However, this difference did not reach statistical significance (χ^2=2.2, *df*=1, *P*=.14). Of the 18 core city men who returned to controlled drinking, nine (50%) had met criteria for alcohol dependence. An equal proportion, 28 (51%), of the 55 men who continued to abuse alcohol until age 60 years or death were alcohol dependent.

Table 1 also shows that by age 60 years, 38 (25%) of the 150 core city alcohol abusers had died. In contrast, only 37 (14%) of the 264 core city non–alcohol abusers had died (χ^2=8.3, *df*=1, *P*<.01). For the same period (20 to 60 years of age), the comparable mortality for white men living in the United States was also 14%.[12] Of the 78 core city men who met criteria for alcohol dependence, 25 (32%) died; this was significantly more than the 13 (18%) of the 72 alcohol abusers who died by age 60 years (χ^2=3.9, *df*=1, *P*<.05).

At age 60 years, the comparable mortality for the 194 nonalcoholic college men was only 5%—much lower than the national rate and only a third of the 15% mortality noted for alcohol-abusing college men. By age 70 years, 13 (62%) of the 21 alcohol-dependent college men were dead, contrasted to 17% of the 228 non–alcohol-dependent college men (χ^2=23.4, *df*=1, *P*<.01). For comparison, 40% of 20-year-old white men living in the United States would be dead by age 70 years.[12]

In both samples, the risk of heart disease and cancer was roughly two times the risk for alcohol abusers as for non–alcohol abusers. Heavy smoking greatly increased the mortality of alcohol abusers in both groups. Thirty (31%) of the 97 core city alcohol abusers with sustained one-pack-per-day smoking habits died before age 60 years; 24 (22%) of the 111 similarly heavy-smoking but non–alcohol-abusing core city participants died before age 60 years. Only 16 (11%) of the 146 non–heavy-smoking, non–alcohol-abusing core city men were dead. Among the 52 college alcohol abusers, 15 of the 22 deaths by age 70 years occurred among the 23 alcohol abusers with the heaviest (≥50 pack-year) smoking habits. When the effect of smoking was controlled by logistic regression, the odds ratio for mortality among the alcohol abusers remained clinically and statistically significant in the college sample (odds ratio, 3.32 [95% confidence interval, 1.40 to 7.91]) and in the core city sample (odds ratio, 2.71 [95% confidence interval, 1.30 to 5.63]).

Alcohol abuse appeared associated with failure to stop smoking. For example, by age 65 years, 54 (84%) of the 64 heavy-smoking but nonalcoholic college men had stopped smoking. In contrast, only 15 (37%) of the 41 heavy-smoking *and* alcohol-abusing college men had stopped smoking. This difference between the two groups in smoking cessation was significant (χ^2=25.6, *df*=1, *P*<.01).

PROGRESSION OF SYMPTOMS

Figure 2 depicts the life course of alcohol abuse among the core city alcohol abusers who have continued to participate in the study. The number of subjects is 121 and not 129 because the eight core city alcohol abusers who were reclassified as social drinkers in Table 1 were excluded. At age 60 years, data were missing for nine of these 121 core city alcohol abusers. Only 30 (27%) of the remaining 112 men were still classified as alcohol abusers at age 60 years. This reduction in prevalence of alcohol abuse resulted more from high mortality (n=31 [28%]) and stable abstinence (n=34 [30%]) than from return to controlled drinking (n=12 [11%]).

Figure 3 demonstrates that the life course of alcohol abuse for the college men was similar to that for the core city men, except that the core city men began abusing alcohol at a younger age and appeared more likely to achieve stable abstinence. At age 60 years, excluding

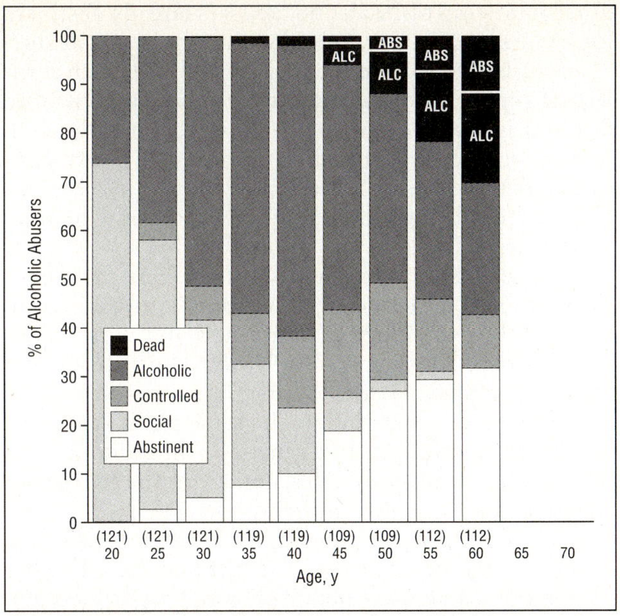

Figure 2. *Quinquennial alcohol use status of the 121 core city men who remained active in the study and met the criteria for* DSM-III *alcohol abuse. (The eight men who were reclassified as social drinkers because of brief duration of alcohol abuse and minimal symptoms have been excluded.) ALC indicates the proportion of deaths that occurred among alcohol abusers; ABS, the proportion among stably abstinent men.*

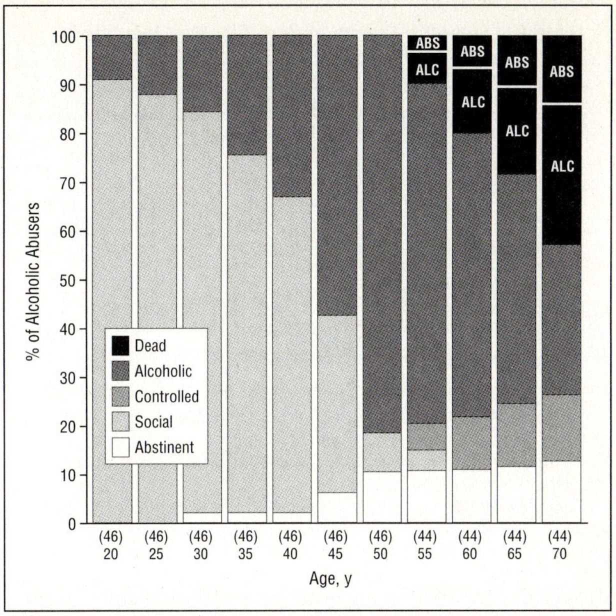

Figure 3. *Quinquennial alcohol use status of the 46 college men who met* DSM-III *criteria for alcohol abuse. (The six alcohol abusers reclassified as social drinkers and the three alcohol abusers with incomplete data sets have been excluded.) ALC indicates the proportion of deaths that occurred among alcohol abusers; ABS, the proportion among stably abstinent men.*

six men reclassified as social drinkers and two men with missing data, eight (18%) of the remaining 44 college men were dead, five (11%) were classified as abstinent, and five (11%) were classified as controlled drinkers. At age 60 years, 26 (59%), and at age 70 years, only 14 (32%), of the college men were still abusing alcohol. Just as the mean age of alcohol abuse onset was a decade later for the college sample, their mean age of peak prevalence and then their steady decline in alcohol abuse appeared to occur a decade later.

Many members of the surviving college sample spent the last 20 years (ages 50 to 70 years) alternating between periods of controlled drinking and periods of alcohol abuse. They reported continued alcohol-related problems with their health, self-esteem, and families. Yet, despite decades of observation, their sustained patterns of alcohol abuse seldom progressed to job loss, dependence, or the need for detoxification.

It is possible that alcohol dependence contributes to the likelihood of stable abstinence. None of the 34 college men who met criteria only for alcohol abuse achieved five or more years of abstinence, in contrast to 10 (48%) of the 21 college men classified dependent (χ^2=11.0, df=1, P<.01). As noted previously, the alcohol-dependent core city men were also more likely to become abstinent, but the difference was not statistically significant. About 40% of men with stable abstinence in each cohort attended Alcoholics Anonymous for a year or more.

DURATION OF ABSTINENCE REQUIRED FOR STABLE REMISSION

The association between length of abstinence and probability of relapse was examined for the 10 college and 46 core city alcohol abusers who reported at least 2 years of abstinence and who subsequently survived for at least 8 years. Eventual relapse to alcohol abuse occurred in 23 (41%) of the 56 men who reported 2 years of abstinence. Nine relapses occurred in year 3, five relapses in year 4, six relapses during years 5 through 7, and three relapses during years 8 through 13. After 6 years of abstinence, subsequent relapse to abuse of alcohol seemed unlikely. The mean length of recorded abstinence among the 33 men not reporting relapse was 18 years (range, 9 to 33 years).

Table 2 shows that if 5 to 6 years of abstinence was adequate to predict stable future abstinence, return to controlled drinking was a much less stable state. In 1977, at the end of the age 20 to 47 years follow-up period, 21 of the core city men had been classified as having achieved stable abstinence of 3 years or more, and 22 men had been classified as returned to controlled drinking for 3 years or more.[4] Of the 21 core city men with 3 or more years of abstinence in 1977, 18 (86%) were still abstinent in 1992 or at death. The mean length of known abstinence for these 18 men was 20 years (range, 3 to 37 years). Of the 22 men with 3 or more years of controlled drinking, only eight men (including three who were reclassified as social drinkers) were *still* known to be drinking in a controlled fashion in 1992 or at death. Three others became stably abstinent and four withdrew from the study. For the seven controlled drinkers who relapsed to sustained alcohol abuse, the mean duration of alleged controlled drinking before relapse was 12 years (range, 5 to 28 years).

COMMENT

Longitudinal studies appear necessary to understand alcohol abuse. First, some studies have suggested that in-

Table 2. Long-term Course of Core City Men Identified in 1977 as Practicing Stable Abstinence or Return to Controlled Drinking

	1977 Status	
1992 Status	≥3 y of Abstinence (<1974-1977) (n=21)	≥3 y of Controlled Drinking (<1974-1977) (n=22)
Abstinent	18	3
Controlled drinking	1	8*
Relapse	1†	7
Dropped out or contact lost	1†	4‡

**Three of these eight men abused alcohol only briefly, with minimal symptoms, and were reclassified as social drinkers.*

†Before relapse or loss of contact, both these men were abstinent for 13 years.

‡The mean length of controlled drinking before loss of contact was 8 years.

dividual alcohol abuse is unstable and fluctuates greatly over time.[4] Such a picture is derived from cross-sectional "snapshots" obtained over too short a time frame. In the present study of men's lives examined in 5-year blocks rather than in 1-month blocks, alcohol abuse appeared relatively stable. Men identified as alcohol abusers, when contrasted to social drinkers, appeared to continue to experience far more alcohol-related problems, not the least of which was a twofold increase in mortality. In part, the increased mortality may be mediated by the failure of alcohol abusers to stop smoking.[13]

Nevertheless, as the alcohol abusers aged, the prevalence of alcohol abuse steadily declined. At age 60 years, only 28% of the surviving core city abusers whose status was known were still symptomatic. At age 70 years, only 32% of the surviving college abusers were still symptomatic. The reasons for this decline were both stable abstinence *and* high mortality.

By studying only the severely alcohol-dependent clients of detoxification centers, clinicians often believe that Jellinek[3] was right in asserting that alcoholism is a "progressive disease." However, the long-term evidence from a community sample such as the present one suggests that, rather than progressing, chronic alcohol abuse often appears merely to fluctuate in severity. Analogous to the reported eating habits of the chronically obese, the reported daily alcohol consumption of many of the college alcohol abusers fell within normal limits. However, analogous to the obese, alcohol abusers in concert with their friends, relatives, and physicians continue to perceive their alcohol use as problematic.

Since systematic follow-ups of abstinent alcohol abusers are seldom undertaken, the long-term stability of abstinence has been unclear. However, data from the few existing follow-up studies support the finding from this study that 2 years of abstinence is inadequate to provide a basis for long-term prognosis. Reanalysis of data from a previously reported 8-year follow-up[14] noted that, when followed up from 4 to 14 years (mean, 8 years), 45% of 33 alcohol-dependent men and women relapsed after 2 years of abstinence. However, after 5 years of follow-up, only 9% relapsed, and none relapsed after 6 years. In another follow-up of 29 alcohol abusers already abstinent for 2 years, six (21%) relapsed within the next 2 years.[15]

Finally, short-term epidemiologic studies such as the RAND report have suggested that return to controlled drinking is relatively common.[16] However, long-term follow-up studies of controlled drinking[17-19] have confirmed the findings in Table 2 that return to a stable pattern of trouble-free drinking among chronic alcohol abusers is unlikely.

Since these contrasting cohorts of white men born between 1917 and 1932 are small and hardly representative of the general population, the above conclusions may not be broadly applicable. However, controlling for birth cohort and sex, the lifetime rate of alcohol abuse in the two cohorts is roughly the same as that observed for United States population samples.[2,4] In addition, most findings from the study were similar for the two socioeconomically very different samples.

The findings are limited by the absence of information from significant others. The fact that the follow-up data in this article were obtained by self-report does not control for heavy drinkers who manifested but failed to acknowledge alcohol-related problems. Such men would have been incorrectly classified as having returned to controlled drinking. Three factors mitigate this limitation. First, some men undoubtedly were alcohol abusers who denied problems, but their total number cannot be large. Of the 181 alcohol abusers in the study who were assigned final outcome status in Table 1, only 23 (13%) were actually classified as having returned to controlled drinking. Second, the self-reports of sustained abstinence (mean duration, 19 years) and of active alcohol abuse can be considered relatively reliable. Third, the study depended on "CAGE"-type questions[20] to identify alcohol-related problems on the biennial questionnaire. (CAGE is an acronym for questions about cutting down on drinking, annoyance at others' concern about drinking, feeling guilty about drinking, and using alcohol as an eye-opener in the morning.) Although the present data and data from other studies suggest that alcohol abusers underreport daily alcohol consumption by about 50%,[21] studies that have used the CAGE-type questions yield relatively reliable data that are superior to biochemical tests and roughly comparable with data obtained from significant others.[22,23]

Because of their highly selective nature, the samples enjoyed two serendipitous advantages that may actually help to elucidate the course of alcoholism for the general population. First, both samples were selected as normal nondelinquent adolescents in subcultures and during historical epochs in which alcohol was the principal drug of abuse. Thus, the confounding problems of dual diagnosis (eg, sociopathy, polydrug abuse, and schizophrenia) that obscure the natural course of alcohol abuse were minimized. Second, since the men shared the same contemporary culture and historical epoch, they experienced similar federal controls, alcohol cost structure, and drinking mores. Recovery from alcohol abuse could be viewed as a function of the natural course of the disorder rather than the result of changes in social mores.

The significant differences in age at onset of alcohol abuse between the college and core city samples were probably a result of the fact that familial disorganization, late adolescent delinquency, and dropping out of school—far more common among the core city sample—all lead to increased risk for early onset of drug abuse of all kinds and to rapid progression of alcohol abuse to dependence.[24]

This report has not discussed predictors of recovery nor reviewed other long-term studies of the natural course of alcohol abuse. However, these topics are reviewed at length in a recently published book.[25] As in the long-term follow-up by Edwards et al,[26] variables as promising as alcoholic heredity, family disorganization, number and severity of alcohol problems, and alcohol clinic treatment fail to predict long-term outcome. In part, this failure of prediction is because alcohol abusers with the best prognosis come from two divergent groups. On the one hand, socially disadvantaged men, in part as a function of the early onset of severe alcohol dependence, often become stably abstinent. However, because of poor health habits (especially smoking and diet), they are also more likely to die. On the other hand, alcohol abusers with excellent social supports, high education, good health habits, and late onset of minimal alcohol abuse are more likely to survive and resume problem-free drinking, but such men also appeared more likely to maintain a pattern of lifelong intermittent alcohol abuse. Thus, as Figure 3 illustrates, the college sample despite their educational and social advantages were less likely to abstain from their alcohol abuse than were the disadvantaged core city sample.

Accepted for publication July 10, 1995.

This work was supported by research grants KO5-MH00364 and MH42248 from the National Institute of Mental Health, Bethesda, Md.

I am indebted to John Orav, PhD, for helpful advice. As is evident in my coauthored articles, the bibliography, and the acknowledgments in my cited books, at least a score of individuals, living and dead, could be included as coauthors in this 50-year study.

Reprint requests to Division of Psychiatry, Brigham and Women's Hospital, 75 Francis St, Boston, MA 02115 (Dr Vaillant).

REFERENCES

1. McGinnis JM, Foege WH. Actual causes of death in the United States. *JAMA.* 1993;270:2207-2212.
2. Robins LN, Regier DA. *Psychiatric Disorders in America.* New York, NY: Free Press; 1991.
3. Jellinek EM. *The Disease Concept of Alcoholism.* New Haven, Conn: Hillhouse Press; 1960.
4. Vaillant GE. *The Natural History of Alcoholism: Paths to Recovery.* Cambridge, Mass: Harvard University Press; 1983.
5. Glueck S, Glueck E. *Unraveling Juvenile Delinquency.* New York, NY: Commonwealth Fund; 1950.
6. Glueck S, Glueck E. *Delinquents and Nondelinquents in Perspective.* Cambridge, Mass: Harvard University Press; 1968.
7. Heath CW. *What People Are.* Cambridge, Mass: Harvard University Press; 1945.
8. Vaillant GE, Schnurr PP, Baron JA, Gerber PD. A prospective study of the effects of cigarette smoking and alcohol abuse on mortality. *J Gen Intern Med.* 1991;6:299-304.
9. Cahalan D. *Problem Drinkers: A National Survey.* San Francisco, Calif: Jossey Bass Inc; 1970.
10. American Psychiatric Association, Committee on Nomenclature and Statistics. *Diagnostic and Statistical Manual of Mental Disorders, Third Edition.* Washington, DC: American Psychiatric Association Press; 1980.
11. Selzer ML. The Michigan alcoholism screening test: the quest for a new diagnostic instrument. *Am J Psychiatry.* 1971;127:1653-1658.
12. *Vital Statistics of the United States, Volume II—Mortality.* Washington, DC: US Dept of Health Statistics; 1988.
13. DiFranza J, Guerrera M. Alcoholism and smoking. *J Stud Alcohol.* 1990;51:130-135.
14. Vaillant GE, Clark W, Cyrus C, et al. Prospective study of alcoholism treatment: eight-year follow-up. *Am J Med.* 1983;75:455-463.
15. Loosen PT, Dew BW, Prange AJ. Long-term predictors of outcome in abstinent alcoholic men. *Am J Psychiatry.* 1990;147:1662-1666.
16. Armor DJ, Polich JM, Stanbul HB. *Alcoholism and Treatment.* New York, NY: John Wiley & Sons Inc; 1978.
17. Pendery ML, Maltzman IM, West LJ. Controlled drinking by alcoholics? New findings and a reevaluation of a major affirmative study. *Science.* 1982;217:169-175.
18. Edwards G. A later follow-up of a classic case series: D. L. Davies' 1962 report and its significance for the present. *J Stud Alcohol.* 1985;46:181-190.
19. Miller WR, Leckman AL, Delaney HD, Tinkcom M. Long-term follow-up of behavioral self-control training. *J Stud Alcohol.* 1992;53:249-261.
20. Ewing JA. Detecting alcoholism: the CAGE questionnaire. *JAMA.* 1984;252:1905-1907.
21. Smith PF, Remington PL, Williamson DF, Anda RF. A comparison of alcohol sales data with survey data on self-reported alcohol use in 21 states. *Am J Public Health.* 1990;80:309-312.
22. Moore RD, Bone LR, Geller G, Mamon JA, Stokes EJ, Levine DM. Prevalence, detection, and treatment of alcoholism in hospitalized patients. *JAMA.* 1989;261:403-407.
23. Cyr MG, Wortman SA. The effectiveness of routine screening questions in the detection of alcoholism. *JAMA.* 1988;259:51-54.
24. Vaillant GE. Evidence that the type 1/type 2 dichotomy in alcoholism must be re-examined. *Addiction.* 1994;89:1049-1057.
25. Vaillant GE. *The Natural History of Alcoholism Revisited.* Cambridge, Mass: Harvard University Press; 1995.
26. Edwards G, Brown D, Oppenheimer E, Sheehan M, Taylor C, Duckitt A. Long-term outcome for patients with drinking problems: the search for predictors. *Br J Addict.* 1988;83:917-927.

ORIGINAL ARTICLE

Enhanced Sensitivity of Pituitary β-Endorphin to Ethanol in Subjects at High Risk of Alcoholism

Christina Gianoulakis, PhD; Brinda Krishnan, MD; Joseph Thavundayil, MD

Background: Previous studies have demonstrated that a moderate dose of ethanol induced a significant increase in the plasma β-endorphin content of subjects from families with a history of alcoholism (high risk [HR]), but not of subjects from families without a history of alcoholism (low risk [LR]). The objective of this study was to examine the response of the pituitary β-endorphin and adrenal cortisol systems to various concentrations of ethanol in male and female subjects at high and low risk of the future development of alcoholism.

Methods: All subjects participated in four experimental sessions. In each session the subjects were given a drink containing one of the following doses of ethanol: 0, 0.25, 0.50, and 0.75 g of ethanol per kilogram of body weight (for a 60- to 70-kg individual). Blood samples were taken at 0 minutes and at 15, 45, 120, and 180 minutes after the drink for estimation of the blood alcohol, plasma β-endorphin, and plasma cortisol levels.

Results: The concentration of alcohol in the blood at various intervals after the drink was similar among the subjects, regardless of the risk group. Ethanol increased the plasma level of β-endorphin–related peptides of the HR but not of the LR subjects in a dose-dependent manner. All subjects showed a small decrease in plasma cortisol level with time, but ethanol ingestion did not significantly alter the plasma cortisol levels.

Conclusion: This study indicates that the pituitary β-endorphin system, but not the adrenal cortisol system, of the HR subjects shows an enhanced sensitivity to ethanol, which may be an important factor in controlling ethanol consumption.

(Arch Gen Psychiatry. 1996;53:250-257)

CONTROLLED STUDIES, such as twin, adoption, and cross-fostering studies and detailed pedigree analysis, support the concept of an inherited predisposition to alcoholism while simultaneously emphasizing the importance of social and environmental interactions in generating the clinical phenotype of alcoholism.[1,2] Selectively bred strains and lines of animals exhibiting either preference for or aversion to ethanol solutions[3,4] indicate the influence of genetic factors in excessive alcohol consumption.

Endogenous opioid peptides,[5-7] such as β-endorphin, have been implicated in the processes of reward and reinforcement.[8-11] The major sites of β-endorphin biosynthesis are the pituitary gland and the arcuate nucleus of the hypothalamus[9]; corticotropin-releasing hormone (CRH) increases the release of both hypothalamic and pituitary β-endorphin peptides.[12,13] Since an interaction of ethanol with the endogenous opioid system has been demonstrated at both the behavioral and biochemical levels,[8] the endogenous opioid system may mediate some of ethanol's reinforcing effects.

In vivo and in vitro exposure of the pituitary gland and hypothalamus to ethanol demonstrated a fast, transient increase of β-endorphin release, followed by an insensitivity of the tissues to subsequent ethanol exposure for a period of about 60 minutes.[12-14] Furthermore, differences were observed between the alcohol-preferring (C57BL/6) and alcohol-avoiding (DBA/2) mice on basal release, on the magnitude and duration of the ethanol-stimulated release of β-endorphin, which is more pronounced and longer lasting in the alcohol-preferring

See Subjects and Methods on next page

From the Department of Psychiatry, McGill University, and Douglas Hospital Research Centre, Verdun, Quebec.

SUBJECTS AND METHODS

SUBJECTS

High-risk and low-risk subjects were recruited as follows: 18 subjects through a newspaper article (45%); 11 through friends (27.5%); six through members of the alcohol research group at Douglas Hospital, Verdun, Quebec (15%); three through a family member participating in the study (7.5%); and two through a family member under treatment (5%). The risk factor was determined by a structured interview of the Michigan Alcoholism Screening Test (MAST)[33] and the *DSM-III-R*[34] administered by a specially trained research assistant. In brief, family histories were taken from as many family members as possible and a family pedigree was constructed. For family members who were available for interview, the diagnosis of alcoholism was based on a score greater than 10 on the MAST and the presence of alcohol dependence as determined by the *DSM-III-R*. For family members who were unavailable for interview (family members who were dead, living outside Montreal, or unwilling to participate in the study), the Family History Research Diagnostic Criteria was used.[35] Families were considered to have a strong positive history if they had a minimum of two generations with a history of alcoholism (eg, father and paternal grandfather being alcoholics). Although the presence of alcoholism in the family of the mother was not a necessary selection criterion, it was not excluded. Indeed, two male and three female HR subjects had an alcoholic maternal grandfather or grandmother or other close relatives. However, subjects whose mother had been or was an alcoholic were excluded from the study to avoid including subjects exposed to ethanol in utero; fetal ethanol exposure can alter the response of the offspring to stress.[36-38] Since genetic vulnerability to alcoholism is equally transmitted to daughters from either their fathers or mothers,[39] both daughters and sons of alcoholic fathers could have inherited the vulnerability to alcoholism and could be included in the HR group. Thus, sons and daughters of these selected families who were not alcoholic themselves were assumed to have a high familial risk for alcoholism and made up the HR group. Low-risk subjects were recruited from families with a strong negative history for alcoholism as determined from their family history using the same criteria as for the HR families. Sons and daughters of these families were assumed to have a low familial risk for alcoholism and made up the LR group.

All HR and LR subjects participating in the study were between 20 and 30 years of age. Subjects were screened for alcohol consumption using the MAST, *DSM-III-R*, and a Drinking Behavior Scale,[40] administered by a specially trained research assistant. In addition, all individuals underwent a complete medical examination. Exclusion criteria included heavy drinking; long-term use of prescribed medication for major psychiatric disorders; history of alcoholism; presence of diabetes mellitus, liver, brain, or kidney disease, or other chronic disease; use of other drugs; and heavy cigarette smoking (more than 10 cigarettes per day). Two HR subjects with antisocial personality disorder were included in the study. None of the LR subjects had antisocial personality disorder. Subjects with a MAST score equal to or less than 10 who did not meet the *DSM-III-R* criteria for alcohol dependence were included in the study. However, subjects with a MAST score between 8 and 10 who admitted to having a period in their life of heavy or problem drinking were excluded from the study even if they did not meet the *DSM-III-R* criteria for alcohol dependence.

The project was designed to include a sample size of 24 subjects in each group (12 men and 12 women, matched for sex, age, drinking behavior, and cigarette smoking). However, one HR male, one LR male, and two HR female subjects dropped out of the study—a dropout rate of 12.5% for the HR subjects and 4.2% for the LR subjects. None of the subjects dropped out of the study owing to nausea or vomiting caused by the alcohol drinks. When one subject dropped out, his or her matched pair was also withdrawn from the study. Thus, 20 HR (10 men and 10 women) and 20 LR (10 men and 10 women) subjects completed the study. The investigations were approved by the Research Ethics Board of the Douglas Hospital for Humans and were conducted in accordance with the guidelines proposed in the Declaration of Helsinki. Informed consent was obtained from all subjects and they could withdraw from the study at any time.

ADMINISTRATION OF THE PLACEBO OR ETHANOL DRINKS AND BLOOD SAMPLING

Matched pairs of subjects participated in four testing sessions, one placebo and three alcohol sessions. The minimum interval between sessions was 5 days. All subjects had to abstain from alcohol for 48 hours prior to testing. Female subjects were tested on days 3 or 4 and 8 or 9 of the reproductive cycle (follicular phase). All four sessions were

Continued on next page

mice, and on the length of the ethanol nonresponsive period, which is shorter in these mice.[12,14] Therefore, it is reasonable to suggest that individuals at high risk of alcoholism and animals exhibiting high ethanol consumption may have inherited an increased sensitivity of the endogenous opioid system to ethanol, presenting a more pronounced release of opioid peptides following ethanol consumption.

Currently, there are only a few reports on the effects of ethanol on plasma β-endorphin levels in humans. Studies using normal human volunteers demonstrated that ethanol ingestion induced an increase in the plasma cortisol, adrenal corticotropin (ACTH), and β-endorphin levels.[15] Ethanol administration to both human subjects and experimental animals has been reported to increase, decrease, or cause no significant change in the plasma cortisol levels.[16-25] Studies by Schuckit et al[22,26] demonstrated that ingestion of a high dose of ethanol (1.1 mL of ethanol per kilogram of body weight) but not of a lower dose of ethanol (0.75 mL of ethanol per kilogram of body weight) induced a significant increase in plasma ACTH and cortisol levels in the sons of nonalcoholics but not in the sons of alcoholics. Since ethanol stimulates the release of CRH and ACTH, which in turn stimulate the release of cortisol,[14,27-30] increased release of cortisol is often considered an indication of increased release of CRH and ACTH. Since ACTH and β-endorphin share the same precursor and are co-released from the pitucompleted within 2 months for the male subjects and within 3 months for the female subjects. The project was designed to include 12 subjects in each of the four groups. The four ethanol dosages (0, 0.25, 0.50, and 0.75 g) were administered in a 4×4 Latin square standard design, so that three subjects from each group would receive one of the four doses during their first experimental session. This design was chosen to allow us to distinguish between the effects of stress associated with the laboratory environment or the novelty of the experimental procedure and the specific effects of ethanol.

On the day of testing, subjects arrived at the research unit at 8 AM, a catheter was placed in the arm vein, and they were allowed to rest. At 8:30 AM subjects were given two slices of dry toast to avoid the feeling of nausea experienced when receiving alcohol on an empty stomach. Nausea could act as a stressor, increasing the plasma levels of β-endorphin, ACTH, and cortisol, thus making it difficult to distinguish between the effects of stress and the specific effects of ethanol. Subjects were allowed to drink water, but not coffee or tea, and were not allowed to smoke for the duration of the experiment. At 9 AM a blood sample was drawn and each subject was given either the placebo or one of the ethanol drinks, which they were instructed to drink within 2 to 5 minutes. To prepare the placebo drink, one part degassed tonic water was mixed with two parts unsweetened orange juice. The lip of the glass was dipped in alcohol to provide the taste and smell of alcohol. To prepare the ethanol drinks, one part 95% alcohol was mixed with two parts unsweetened orange juice. Additional blood samples were obtained at 15, 45, 120, and 180 minutes after the drink was taken for estimation of the blood alcohol and plasma β-endorphin and cortisol levels. The experiment was performed in a double-blind fashion, and neither the subject nor the attending physician or nurse knew the ethanol dose ingested in each session. In the consent form, the subjects were informed that they would consume four doses of ethanol in a random order. To test the success of the placebo drink, at about 15, 60, 90, and 180 minutes after the drink was taken, the subjects were asked in a casual manner how they felt in general, whether they felt dizzy, and how they thought the drink they had received compared in strength with a glass of wine or a beer, or a standard drink of whiskey, gin, or vodka. Immediately following the placebo drink, all subjects thought they had ingested alcohol. However, about 30 to 60 minutes later, owing to the absence of the physiological effects of alcohol, the subjects, particularly those who had received high alcohol doses in earlier sessions, concluded that they had received either the placebo or a low dose of alcohol.

ESTIMATION OF BLOOD ALCOHOL LEVEL

To estimate the blood alcohol level, 250 μL of freshly drawn blood was mixed with 1.0 mL of ice-cold 6% trichloroacetic acid and centrifuged at 4°C. The supernatant was kept frozen at −75°C. The alcohol dehydrogenase method was used (Sigma NAD-ADH Kit, Sigma Chemical Co, St Louis, Mo).[41]

ESTIMATION OF PLASMA CORTISOL AND β-ENDORPHIN LEVELS

Measurement of the plasma level of immunoreactive β-endorphin was performed by radioimmunoassay, using an antiserum specific to the C-terminus of β-endorphin 1-31 at a final dilution of 1:30 000 as described previously.[16,42] Prior to the radioimmunoassay, the β-endorphinlike peptides were extracted from the plasma using C-18 Sep-Pak cartridges (Waters Scientific, Mississauga, Ontario).[16,43] The intra-assay and interassay coefficients of variation were 3.5% and 12.4%, respectively. The molecular weight forms of β-endorphinlike peptides in the plasma were estimated using Sephadex G-75 (Pharmacia, Uppsala, Sweden) chromatography as described previously.[16,43] For estimation of total (bound plus free) plasma cortisol levels, plasma was extracted in absolute ethanol, and cortisol was determined by radioimmunoassay according to a previously published procedure[16,44] using cortisol antiserum (F3-314, Endocrine Sciences, Tarzana, Calif) at a final dilution of 1:1000. The intra-assay and interassay coefficients of variation were 9% and 11%, respectively.

STATISTICAL ANALYSIS

The results are presented as mean ± SD or SEM. The statistical significance of the differences among the various groups was estimated either by a one-way analysis of variance (ANOVA) or by a two-way repeated-measures ANOVA with risk as one of the independent variables and time as the other independent variable. The ANOVAs were followed by Newman-Keul's multiple comparison test or by Fisher's least significant difference test to determine the significance of the difference between the different risk groups, sexes, and sampling times after the placebo or ethanol drinks. A value of $P<.05$ was considered significant.

itary gland under various conditions,[31] it may be expected that an increase in plasma β-endorphin level would be associated with an increase in plasma ACTH and cortisol levels.

This study was designed to address the following questions: (1) Does the pituitary β-endorphin system of the subjects at high risk (HR) and low risk (LR) of the future development of alcoholism respond differently to high than to low concentrations of ethanol, as was shown for experimental animals?[12,14,32] (2) For the same dose of ethanol, is the response of the pituitary β-endorphin system of the HR subjects different from that of the LR subjects? and (3) What is the effect of various doses of ethanol on the plasma cortisol level in HR and LR subjects? To investigate these questions, the effect of 0, 0.25, 0.50, and 0.75 g of ethanol per kilogram of body weight on plasma β-endorphin and cortisol levels was estimated in LR and HR subjects. These doses of ethanol were chosen because when taken by a 60- to 70-kg individual they correspond to approximately none, 1, 2, and 3 standard drinks, respectively.

RESULTS

SUBJECT DESCRIPTION

Twenty HR subjects (10 men and 10 women) with an average MAST score of 1.54±4.29 and 20 LR subjects (10 men and 10 women) with an average MAST score of 0.33±1.35 participated in the present study. The HR sub-

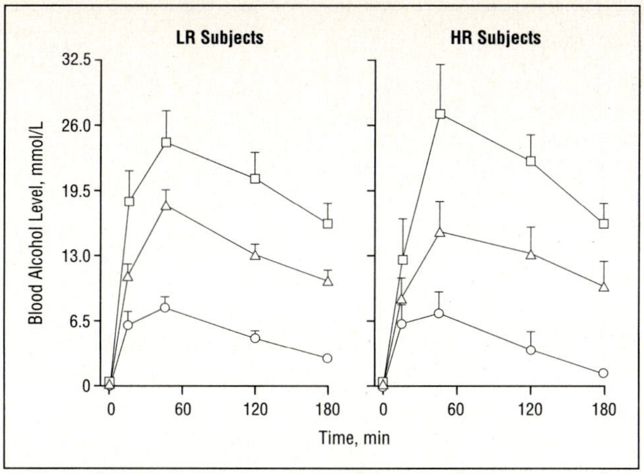

Figure 1. *Mean blood alcohol concentration at various intervals following ingestion of 0.25 (circles), 0.50 (triangles), and 0.75 (squares) g of ethanol for low-risk (LR) and high-risk (HR) subjects.*

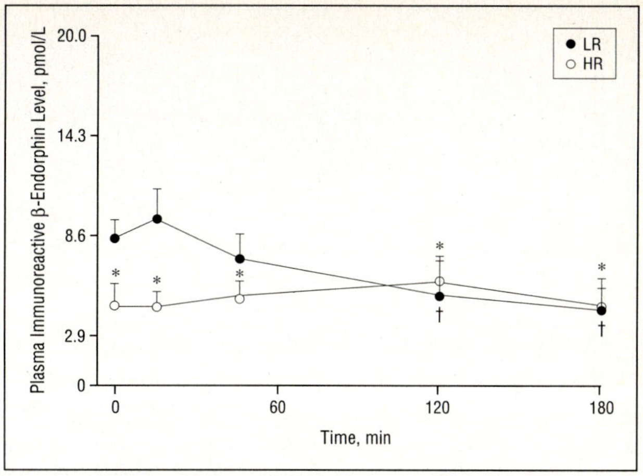

Figure 2. *Plasma levels of immunoreactive β-endorphin for the low-risk (LR) and high-risk (HR) subjects following ingestion of the placebo drink. Asterisk indicates a significant difference from the levels of the LR group at 0 and 15 minutes after the drink (*P*<.05; Fisher's least significant difference test); plus sign, significant difference from the levels of the LR group at 0 and 15 minutes after the drink (*P*<.05; Newman-Keul's multiple comparison test).*

jects had an average of 4.94±2.50 alcoholic relatives in the last two generations, while the LR subjects had none. High-risk and low-risk subjects were matched for sex, age, body weight, drinking behavior (quantity and frequency), and smoking behavior. All subjects were white. The average age was 27.32±2.47 years for the HR and 26.33±3.29 years for the LR subjects. The average age at the onset of regular drinking was 18.6±2.33 years and 19.5±2.70 years for the HR and LR subjects respectively. The HR subjects drank on an average of 7.64±4.20 days per month and had 5.21±2.37 drinks on each drinking day, while the LR subjects drank on an average of 7.35±4.33 days per month and had 4.71±2.71 drinks on each drinking day. Although none of the subjects were drinking excessively or were alcoholic at the time of testing, the HR subjects had a higher MAST score than the corresponding LR subjects. This was expected, since selection of HR subjects with very low MAST scores only would have favored the selection of members of the HR families who had not inherited the predisposition for alcoholism.

BLOOD ALCOHOL LEVEL

As shown in **Figure 1**, for each dose of ethanol administered, both HR and LR subjects exhibit similar blood alcohol concentrations. For each risk group and dose of ethanol, a two-way repeated-measures ANOVA with sex and time as the independent variables indicated that for both LR and HR subjects there was a significant main effect of time on blood alcohol level but no significant main effect of sex or the interaction of sex with time.

EFFECTS OF SEX ON PLASMA β-ENDORPHIN AND CORTISOL LEVELS

Since both male and female subjects were used in this study, sex differences in the responses of β-endorphin and cortisol to ethanol may exist. To investigate the presence of such differences for each risk and session group, a two-way repeated-measures ANOVA was performed with sex and time as the independent variables. For both LR and HR groups, there was no significant main effect of sex and no significant interaction between sex and time factors on the response of either pituitary β-endorphin or adrenal cortisol to the placebo or ethanol drinks. Since no differences were observed, the male and female data were combined for each risk group for subsequent statistical analysis.

BASAL LEVELS OF PLASMA β-ENDORPHIN AND CORTISOL

The basal levels of both plasma β-endorphin and cortisol at 0 minutes (9 AM) were lower in the HR than in the LR subjects. For each hormone, two-way ANOVAs were performed with session and risk factors as the independent variables. Results indicated a significant main effect of risk on the basal levels of both plasma β-endorphin ($F[1,38]=4.4$; $P<.04$) and cortisol ($F[1,38]=4.9$; $P<.03$), with no significant main effect of session and no significant interaction between risk and session factors. The absence of a significant effect of habituation to the laboratory environment and experimental procedure on basal plasma β-endorphin and cortisol levels may be due to previous participation of the subjects in studies conducted by other members of the Alcohol Research Program.

EFFECT OF THE PLACEBO AND ETHANOL DRINKS ON PLASMA β-ENDORPHIN LEVELS

As shown in **Figure 2**, following the placebo drink the LR but not the HR subjects showed a gradual decrease in the plasma level of β-endorphin, as would be expected from the β-endorphin circadian rhythm. A two-way repeated-measures ANOVA with risk and time as the independent variables indicated no significant main effect of risk, but a significant main effect of time ($F[4,152]=2.65$; $P<.03$) and a significant interaction of risk with time ($F[4,152]=2.45$; $P<.05$). Post hoc analy-

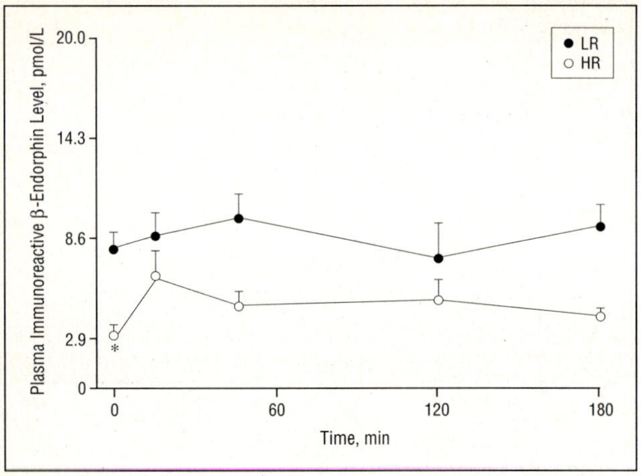

Figure 3. *Plasma levels of immunoreactive β-endorphin for the low-risk (LR) and the high-risk (HR) groups following ingestion of 0.25 g of ethanol. Asterisk indicates a significant difference from the levels of the LR group at 0, 15, 45, 120, and 180 minutes after the drink (*P<.05*; Fisher's least significant difference test).*

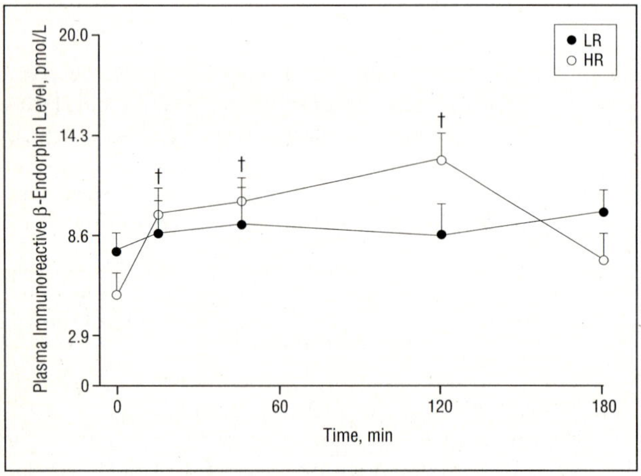

Figure 4. *Plasma levels of immunoreactive β-endorphin for the low-risk (LR) and the high-risk (HR) groups following ingestion of 0.50 g of ethanol. Plus sign indicates a significant difference from the levels of the HR group prior to drinking the alcohol solution (0 minutes) (*P<.05*; Newman-Keul's multiple comparison test).*

sis using Fisher's least significant difference test indicated a significant difference between the plasma β-endorphin level of HR subjects at 0, 15, 45, 120, and 180 minutes after the drink and the plasma β-endorphin level of LR subjects at 0 and 15 minutes after the drink. However, there was no significant difference in the plasma β-endorphin level between the HR and LR subjects at 45, 120, and 180 minutes after the drink.

Figure 3, **Figure 4**, and **Figure 5** demonstrate the effects of 0.25, 0.50, and 0.75 g of ethanol per kilogram of body weight, respectively, on plasma β-endorphin content. Ethanol ingestion increased the plasma level of β-endorphin of the HR but not the LR subjects in a dose-dependent manner. In the LR subjects, ethanol ingestion abolished the gradual decrease in plasma β-endorphin level that occurs with time, without inducing a significant increase above basal levels. Statistical analysis of the data indicated that in the HR but not the LR subjects, the plasma level of β-endorphin at 15, 45, and 120 minutes following

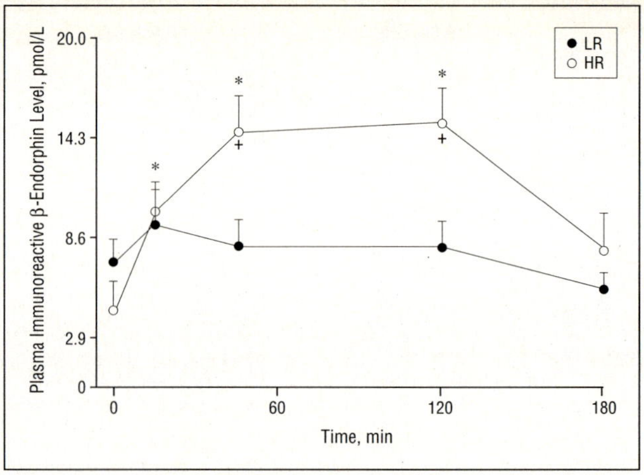

Figure 5. *Plasma levels of immunoreactive β-endorphin for the low-risk (LR) and high-risk (HR) groups following ingestion of 0.75 g of ethanol. Asterisk indicates a significant difference from the levels of the HR subjects prior to the ethanol drink (0 minutes) (*P<.05*; Newman-Keul's multiple comparison test); plus sign, a significant difference from the levels of the LR subjects at 0, 15, 45, 120, and 180 minutes after the drink (*P<.05*; Newman-Keul's multiple comparison test).*

ingestion of the 0.50- and the 0.75-g ethanol drinks (Figures 4 and 5) was significantly higher than the level at 0 minutes ($P<.05$; Newman-Keul's multiple comparison test). Furthermore, in contrast to the placebo drink, following the 0.25- and 0.50-g ethanol drinks, the level of β-endorphin in the plasma of the HR subjects was not significantly different from the level in the plasma of LR subjects (Figures 3 and 4). However, at 45 and 120 minutes following ingestion of the 0.75-g ethanol drink, the plasma β-endorphin level of the HR subjects was significantly higher than that of the LR subjects (Figure 5) ($P<.05$; Newman-Keul's multiple comparison test).

To compare the response of the β-endorphin system to ethanol between the HR and LR subjects for each of the doses of ethanol studied, a two-way repeated-measures ANOVA was performed with risk and time as the independent variables. Such analysis indicated that for all three doses of ethanol used, there was no significant main effect of risk but that there was a significant main effect of time for the 0.50-g ($F[4,152]=2.69$; $P<.03$) and 0.75-g ($F[4,152]=6.2$; $P<.01$) ethanol doses and a significant interaction between the risk and time factors for the 0.75-g ethanol dose ($F[4,152]=2.57$; $P<.04$). To further evaluate the differences between the two risk groups in the plasma β-endorphin level following ingestion of each of the various doses of ethanol, a three-way ANOVA with risk, dose, and time as the three independent variables and the plasma β-endorphin level as the dependent variable was performed. Results demonstrated that although there was no significant main effect of risk ($F[1,760]=2.76$; $P<.09$), there was a significant main effect of dose ($F[3,760]=2.68$; $P<.05$) and a significant main effect of time ($F[4,760]=2.45$; $P<.05$). There was also a significant interaction of risk with the dose of ethanol ($F[3,760]=6.95$; $P<.001$).

Using data from all three alcohol testing sessions, the plasma level of immunoreactive β-endorphin was corre-

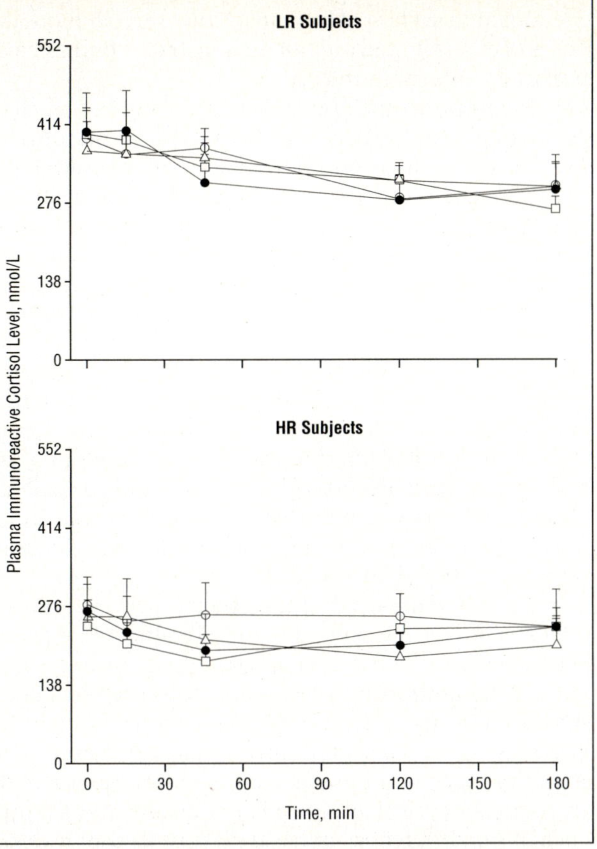

Figure 6. *Plasma content of immunoreactive cortisol of low-risk (LR) and high-risk (HR) subjects following ingestion of the placebo (solid circles); 0.25 g of ethanol (open circles); 0.50 g of ethanol (triangles); and 0.75 of g ethanol (squares).*

lated with the corresponding blood alcohol level. This linear regression analysis indicated that the changes in plasma immunoreactive β-endorphin level were positively correlated with the changes in blood alcohol level in HR (r=.91; $P<.001$), but not in LR (r=.26; $P<.35$) subjects.

In agreement with our previous findings,[16] gel filtration analysis of the β-endorphinlike peptides in the plasma of HR and LR individuals prior to and at 45 minutes after the drink indicated that the increase in the total level of immunoreactive β-endorphin in the plasma was associated with a significant increase of the β-lipotropin–sized peptides (data not shown).

EFFECT OF THE PLACEBO AND ETHANOL DRINKS ON PLASMA CORTISOL LEVELS

Figure 6 demonstrates that ethanol ingestion did not induce an increase above the basal levels in the plasma level of immunoreactive cortisol. For each dose of ethanol, the changes in the plasma level of immunoreactive cortisol were statistically evaluated using a two-way repeated-measures ANOVA with risk and time as the independent variables. There was a significant main effect of time with the placebo drink ($F[4,152]=2.75$; $P<.05$); the 0.50-g ethanol drink ($F[4,152]=2.81$; $P<.05$); and the 0.75-g ethanol drink ($F[4,152]=2.65$; $P<.05$); but not for the 0.25-g ethanol drink ($F[4,152]=1.52$; $P<.19$). There was a significant main effect of risk for the placebo drink ($F[1,152]=4.31$; $P<.05$); the 0.50-g ethanol drink ($F[1,152]=4.55$; $P<.05$); and the 0.75-g ethanol drink ($F[1,152]=3.85$; $P<.05$); but not for the 0.25-g ethanol drink ($F[1,152]=2.68$; $P<.10$). There was no significant interaction between risk and time factors.

COMMENT

This investigation indicated that the pituitary β-endorphin system of the HR subjects is more sensitive to ethanol than that of the LR subjects. Using the difference in the plasma β-endorphin level between the 0 and 120 minutes following ethanol ingestion and setting the level of significance at .05 and the power at .80, it was estimated that to detect a significant effect of ethanol on the plasma β-endorphin level, 80 HR subjects are needed for the 0.25-g ethanol dose, 15 for the 0.50-g ethanol dose, and 10 for the 0.75-g ethanol dose. Thus, the number of HR subjects used in this study was sufficient to detect significant effects of ethanol on the plasma β-endorphin level following ingestion of the 0.50- and 0.75-g ethanol doses but not following the 0.25-g ethanol dose. Although this number is small, it has been demonstrated that when the HR subjects are from families with an extensive history of alcoholism, a relatively low number of subjects may be sufficient to demonstrate significant differences between the LR and HR individuals in the responses of ACTH and cortisol levels to ethanol.[22]

Careful examination of the plasma β-endorphin levels following the placebo drink indicated that although HR subjects show lower plasma β-endorphin levels than LR subjects for the first 45 minutes, at 120 and 180 minutes the plasma β-endorphin levels between HR and LR subjects are indistinguishable. Thus, the deficiency of β-endorphin in the HR subjects may be limited to the early morning hours and may be due to an earlier occurrence of the peak in the circadian cycle of plasma β-endorphin in the HR compared with LR subjects. Studies using experimental animals have demonstrated that the plasma ACTH response to restraint stress was of greater magnitude in the trough compared with the peak of the circadian cycle for both intact and adrenalectomized rats.[45] Since ACTH and β-endorphin are co-released under a number of physiological conditions,[27,28,31] the response of the pituitary β-endorphin system to stress and ethanol may be stronger during the trough than during the peak of the circadian β-endorphin cycle. In future studies, the pattern of the circadian β-endorphin cycle in HR and LR individuals and the effect of ethanol ingestion during the trough (early afternoon) and peak (early morning) periods of the circadian β-endorphin cycle should be investigated. This approach will serve to determine whether the deficiency in the morning basal ACTH[46] and β-endorphin levels, as well as the higher ethanol-induced increase in the plasma β-endorphin level in the HR subjects, is due to different sensitivities of the pituitary β-endorphin systems or to different patterns of the β-endorphin circadian cycle between HR and LR subjects.

The significance of the enhanced plasma β-endorphin level in mediating ethanol's reinforcing effects is not clear since, owing to the blood-brain barrier, β-endorphin peptides from the peripheral circulation cannot reach and interact with the reward centers of the brain. However, β-endorphin and other small peptides have been shown to cross the blood-brain barrier[47,48] in small but sufficient quantities to induce effects on analgesia, electroencephalographic activity, and learning.[48,49] In addition, plasma β-endorphin may interact with regions of the brain outside the blood-brain barrier, pituitary β-endorphin may reach the level of the median eminence and hypothalamus via the retrograde transport mechanism,[50] and ethanol may alter the blood-brain barrier.[51] At present, there are no studies on the effect of peripheral β-endorphin on brain reward processes or on the comparison of the subjective effects of ethanol with the corresponding increases in peripheral β-endorphin level.

One of the hypotheses proposed for the implication of the endogenous opioid system in alcoholism is the "opioid deficiency hypothesis,"[52] which suggests that HR subjects have inherited a deficiency in the basal activity of the endogenous opioid system. Since ethanol enhances the activity of the opioid system, HR subjects consume high quantities of alcohol to compensate for this deficiency. Therefore, differences in the basal activity and response of the endogenous opioid system to alcohol among individuals may be important in determining their risk for excessive alcohol consumption, with low basal activity and a higher response of the endogenous opioid system to alcohol being associated with a higher risk for alcoholism. The lower basal levels of plasma β-endorphin (shown in this study), ACTH,[46] and cortisol[22] associated with higher β-endorphin response following ethanol ingestion support this hypothesis.

Administration of opioid antagonists such as naltrexone, naloxone, ICI-174864, and others decreases voluntary ethanol consumption in a number of experimental animals without altering water intake, supporting a role of the endogenous opioid system in controlling ethanol consumption.[53-58] Recently, clinical trials demonstrated that naltrexone, a nonspecific opioid antagonist, decreased the craving for alcohol and relapse to heavy drinking. However, according to the opioid deficiency hypothesis, opioid antagonists, by binding to the opioid receptors and blocking the effects of the endogenous opioid peptides, are creating an opioid deficiency and should increase the craving for alcohol instead of decreasing it. This apparent paradox may be explained by the high doses of opioid antagonists used, which were sufficient to occupy all opioid binding sites. Thus, even though drinking would increase the release of opioid peptides, they could not interact with their specific opioid receptors to mediate the reward mechanisms that eventually lead to a decreased craving for alcohol and decreased relapse to heavy drinking.[52,59,60]

Previous studies demonstrated that in rats and mice the release of β-endorphin peptides by both the pituitary gland and hypothalamus,[12,14,32] following exposure to various concentrations of ethanol, presents an inverse U-shaped dose-response curve, with low concentrations (10 to 25 mmol of ethanol per liter) inducing a more pronounced increase in the release of β-endorphin than high concentrations (30 to 120 mmol of ethanol per liter). Thus, one of the objectives of this investigation was to test the presence of a biphasic response to ethanol by the pituitary β-endorphin system of humans. However, the moderate doses of ethanol used did not demonstrate a biphasic pattern of β-endorphin release.

In our previous,[16] but not present, study, a small increase in plasma cortisol was observed at 15 minutes following ethanol ingestion. This discrepancy could be due to the longer resting period prior to ethanol ingestion in this study. The present data also demonstrate an apparent lack of concordance between the β-endorphin and cortisol responses to ethanol. Since the time course of stimulated cortisol secretion is different from that of β-endorphin, an increase in cortisol release may have occurred at a later time and was missed owing to infrequent blood sampling. Furthermore, ethanol may have altered the responsiveness of adrenal cortex to pituitary ACTH. In future studies, more frequent blood sampling and estimation of β-endorphin, ACTH, and cortisol levels may indicate whether this association occurs and, if it does, whether it is taking place at the level of the pituitary or adrenal cortex.

Sex differences in the plasma cortisol level during the follicular but not luteal phase of the reproductive cycle have been reported.[61,62] In the present study, significant sex differences in the morning plasma cortisol level were not observed, although the female subjects were tested in the follicular phase of the reproductive cycle. A larger number of subjects and more precise control for the phase of the reproductive cycle may be needed to demonstrate the presence of sex differences in basal plasma cortisol levels.

In summary, ingestion of moderate doses of ethanol induces a dose-dependent increase in the plasma β-endorphin level of HR but not LR subjects, suggesting an increased sensitivity of their pituitary β-endorphin system to ethanol, a factor that could be important in mediating ethanol's reinforcing effects.

Accepted for publication November 7, 1995.

This study was supported by the Alcohol Research Program at Douglas Hospital and the Alcoholic Beverage Medical Research Foundation, Baltimore, Md.

We are grateful to Sylvie Larocque and the nursing staff of the Research Unit of Douglas Hospital for their technical assistance in performing this investigation, as well as to Sharon Welner, PhD, for editorial assistance.

REFERENCES

1. Cloninger CR, Bohman M, Sigvardsson S, Von Knorring AL. Psychopathology in adopted-out children of alcoholics: the Stockholm adoption study. In: Galanter M, ed. *Recent Developments in Alcoholism.* New York, NY: Plenum Press; 1985:37-51.
2. Goldman D, Linnoila M. Genetic approaches to alcoholism. *Prog Neuropsychopharmacol Biol Psychiatry.* 1986;10:237-242.
3. Eriksson K, Rusi M. Finnish selection studies on alcohol-related behaviors: general outline. In: McClearn GE, Deitrich RA, Erwin G, eds. *Development of Animal Models as Pharmacogenetic Tools.* Boulder, Colo; 1978:87-117. National Institute of Alcohol Abuse and Alcoholism Research Monograph 6.
4. Keane B, Leonard BE. Rodent models of alcoholism: a review. *Alcohol Alcohol.* 1989;24:299-309.
5. Hughes J, Smith TW, Kosterlitz HW, Fathergill LA, Morgan BA, Morris HR. Identification of two related pentapeptides from the brain with potent opiate agonist activity. *Nature.* 1975;258:577-579.
6. Bradbury AF, Smyth DG, Snell CR, Birdsall NJM, Hulme EC. C-fragment of

lipotropin has a high affinity for brain opiate receptors. *Nature.* 1976;260:793.
7. Goldstein A, Tachibana S, Lowney LI, Hold L. Dynorphin (1-13): an extraordinarily potent opioid peptide. *Proc Natl Acad Sci U S A.* 1979;76:6666-6670.
8. Olson GA, Olson RD, Kastin AB. Endogenous opiates: 1989 review. *Peptides.* 1990;11:1277-1304.
9. Khachaturian H, Lewis ME, Schafer MKH, Watson SJ. Anatomy of the CNS opioid systems. *Trends Neurosci.* 1985;10:111-119.
10. Van Ree JM, De Wied D, Bradbury AF, Hulme EC, Smyth DG, Snell CR. Induction of tolerance to the analgesic action of lipotropin C-fragment. *Nature.* 1976;64:792-794.
11. Spanagel R, Herz A, Shippenberg T. Opposing tonically active endogenous opioid systems modulate the mesolimbic dopaminergic pathway. *Proc Natl Acad Sci U S A.* 1991;89:2046-2050.
12. De Waele JP, Papachristou DN, Gianoulakis C. The alcohol-preferring C57BL/6 mice present an enhanced sensitivity of the hypothalamic β-endorphin system to ethanol than the alcohol-avoiding DBA/2 mice. *J Pharmacol Exp Ther.* 1992; 261:788-794.
13. Keith LD, Crabbe JC, Robertson LM, Kendall JW. Ethanol-stimulated endorphin and corticotropin secretion in vitro. *Brain Res.* 1986;367:222-229.
14. De Waele JP, Gianoulakis C. Effects of single and repeated exposures to ethanol on the hypothalamic β-endorphin and CRH release by the C57BL/6 and DBA/2 strains of mice. *Neuroendocrinology.* 1993;57:700-709.
15. Naber D, Soble MG, Pickar D. Ethanol increases opioid activity in plasma of normal volunteers. *Pharmacopsychiatry.* 1981;14:160-161.
16. Gianoulakis C, Beliveau D, Angelogianni P, Meaney M, Thavundayil J, Tawar V, Dumas M. Different pituitary β-endorphin and adrenal cortisol response to ethanol in individuals with high and low risk for future development of alcoholism. *Life Sci.* 1989;45:1097-1109.
17. Valimaki MK, Harkonen M, Eriksson CJP, Ylikahri RH. Sex hormone and adrenocortical steroids in men acutely intoxicated with ethanol. *Alcohol.* 1984; 1:89-93.
18. Mendelson JH, Stein S. Serum cortisol levels in alcoholic and non-alcoholic subjects during experimentally induced ethanol intoxication. *Psychosom Med.* 1966;28:616-626.
19. Tabakoff B, Jaffe R, Ritzmann R. Corticosterone concentrations in mice during ethanol drinking and withdrawal. *J Pharm Pharmacol.* 1978;30:371-374.
20. Mendelson JH, Ogata M, Mello NK. Adrenal function and alcoholism, I: serum cortisol. *Psychosom Med.* 1971;33:145-157.
21. Seto A, Triconi S, Goodwin DW, Kolodney R, Sullivan T. Biochemical correlates of ethanol-induced flushing in Orientals. *J Stud Alcohol.* 1978;39:1-11.
22. Schuckit MA, Gold E, Risch C. Plasma cortisol levels following ethanol in sons of alcoholics and controls. *Arch Gen Psychiatry.* 1987;44:942-945.
23. Jenkins JS, Conolly J. Adrenocortical response to ethanol in man. *BMJ.* 1968; 2:804-805.
24. Merry J, Marks V. Plasma-hydrocortisone response to ethanol in chronic alcoholics. *Lancet.* 1969;1:921-923.
25. Schuckit MA. Differences in plasma cortisol after injection of ethanol in relatives of alcoholics and controls. *J Clin Psychiatry.* 1984;45:374-376.
26. Schuckit MA, Risch SC, Gold EO. Alcohol consumption, ACTH level, and family history of alcoholism. *Am J Psychiatry.* 1988;145:1391-1395.
27. Rivier C, Bruhn T, Vale W. Effect of ethanol on the hypothalamic-pituitary axis in the rat: role of corticotropin-releasing factor. *J Pharmacol Exp Ther.* 1984; 229:127-131.
28. Gambert SR, Pontzer CH, Barboriak JJ. Effect of ethanol consumption on central nervous system (CNS) β-endorphin and ACTH. *Horm Metab Res.* 1981; 13:242-243.
29. Noble EP, Kakihana R, Butte JC. Corticosterone metabolism in alcohol-adapted mice. In: Roach MK, McIssac WM, Creaven PJ, eds. *Biological Aspects of Alcohol.* Austin, Tex: The University of Texas Press; 1971:389.
30. Leppaluoto J, Rapeli M, Varis R, Ranta T. Secretion of anterior pituitary hormones in man: effects of ethyl alcohol. *Acta Physiol Scand.* 1975;95:400-406.
31. Guillemin R, Vargo T, Rossier J, Minick S, Ling N, Rivier C, Vale W, Bloom F. β-endorphin and adrenocorticotropin are secreted concomitantly by the pituitary gland. *Science.* 1977;197:1367-1369.
32. Gianoulakis C. Characterization of the effects of short-term ethanol administration on the release of β-endorphin peptides by the rat hypothalamus. *Eur J Pharmacol.* 1990;180:21-29.
33. Selzer ML. The Michigan Alcoholism Screening Test: the quest for a new diagnostic instrument. *Am J Psychiatry.* 1971;127:1653-1658.
34. American Psychiatric Association. *Diagnostic and Statistical Manual of Mental Disorders, Revised Third Edition.* Washington, DC: American Psychiatric Association; 1987.
35. Endicott J, Andreasen N, Spitzer RL. *Family History Research Diagnostic Criteria.* New York, NY; New York State Psychiatric Institute: 1975.
36. Angelogianni P, Gianoulakis C. Prenatal exposure to ethanol alters the ontogeny of the β-endorphin response to stress. *Alcohol Clin Exp Res.* 1989;13: 564-571.
37. Weinberg J, Nelson LR, Taylor AN. Hormonal effects of fetal alcohol exposure. In: West JR, ed. *Alcohol and Brain Development.* New York, NY: Oxford University Press; 1986:310-342.
38. Taylor AN, Branch BJ, Nelson LR, Lane LA, Poland RE. Prenatal ethanol and ontogeny of pituitary-adrenal responses to ethanol and morphine. *Alcohol.* 1986; 3:255-259.
39. Kendler KS, Neale MC, Heath AC, Kessler RC, Eaves LJ. A twin-family study of alcoholism in women. *Am J Psychiatry.* 1994;151:707-715.
40. Cahalan D, Cisin H. American drinking practices: summary from a national probability sample. *J Stud Alcohol.* 1968;29:130.
41. Hawkins RD, Kalant H, Khana JM. Effects of chronic intake of ethanol on rate of ethanol metabolism. *Can J Physiol Pharmacol.* 1966;44:241-257.
42. Gianoulakis C, Chan JCD, Kalant H, Chretien M. Chronic ethanol treatment alters the biosynthesis of β-endorphin by the rat intermediate lobe. *Can J Physiol Pharmacol.* 1983;61:967-976.
43. Bennett HPJ, Browne CA, Solomon S. Purification of the two major forms of rat pituitary corticotropin using only reverse phase liquid chromatography. *Biochemistry.* 1981;20:4530-4538.
44. Krey L, Lu K, Butler W, Hotchkis J, Piva F, Knoble E. Surgical disconnections of the medial basal hypothalamus and pituitary function in the rhesus monkey, II: GH and cortisol secretion. *Endocrinology.* 1975;96:1088-1093.
45. Bradbury MJ, Cascio CS, Scribner KA, Dallman MF. Stress-induced adrenocorticotropin secretion: diurnal responses and decreases during stress in the evening are not dependent on corticosterone. *Endocrinology.* 1991;128:680-688.
46. Waltman C, McCaul BE, Svikis D, Boyed G, Wand GS. oCRH-stimulated ACTH release is blunted in sons of alcoholic fathers. *Alcohol Clin Exp Res.* 1993;17: 443. Abstract.
47. Banks WA, Kastin AJ. Minireview: saturable transport of peptides across the blood-brain barrier. *Life Sci.* 1987;41:1319-1338.
48. Banks WA, Kastin AJ. Editorial review: peptide transport systems for opiates across the blood-brain barrier. *Am J Physiol.* 1990;259:E1-E10.
49. Banks WA, Kastin AJ, Barrera CM. Delivering peptides to the central nervous systems: dilemmas and strategies. *Pharm Res.* 1991;8:1345-1350.
50. Bergland RM, Page RB. Pituitary-brain vascular relations: a new paradigm. *Science.* 1979;204:18-24.
51. Banks WA, Kastin AJ. The potential for alcohol to affect the passage of peptide and protein hormones across the blood-brain barrier: a hypothesis for a disturbance in brain-body communication. In: Zakharis S, ed. *Alcohol and the Endocrine System.* Bethesda, Md; National Institute of Alcohol Abuse and Alcoholism: 1993. NIH publication 93-3533. Research Monograph 23.
52. Volpicelli JR, O'Brien CP, Alterman AI, Hayashida M. Naltrexone and the treatment of alcohol dependence: initial observations. In: Reid LD, ed. *Opioids, Bulimia and Alcohol Abuse & Alcoholism.* New York, NY: Springer-Verlag; 1990: 195-214.
53. Altshuler HL, Philips PE, Feinhandler DE. Alteration of ethanol self-administration by naltrexone. *Life Sci.* 1980;26:679-688.
54. Reid LD, Hunter GA. Morphine and naloxone modulate intake of ethanol. *Alcohol.* 1984;1:33-37.
55. Hubbell CL, Czirr SA, Hunter GA, Beaman CM, LeCann NC, Reid LD. Consumption of ethanol solution is potentiated by morphine and attenuated by naloxone persistently across repeated daily administrations. *Alcohol.* 1986;3: 39-54.
56. Kornet M, Goosen C, Van Ree JM. Effect of naltrexone on alcohol drinking and after a period of imposed abstinence in free-choice drinking rhesus monkeys. *Psychopharmacology.* 1991;104:367-376.
57. Froehlich JC, Harts J, Lumeng L, Li T-K. Naloxone attenuates voluntary ethanol intake in rats selectively bred for high ethanol preference. *Pharmacol Biochem Behav.* 1990;35:385-390.
58. Froehlich JC, Zweifel M, Hart J, Lumeng L, Li T-K. Importance of delta opioid receptors in maintaining high alcohol drinking. *Psychopharmacology.* 1991; 103:467-472.
59. Volpicelli JR, Alterman AI, Hayashida M, O'Brien CP. Naltrexone in the treatment of alcohol dependence. *Arch Gen Psychiatry.* 1992;49:876-880.
60. O'Malley SS, Jaffe AJ, Chang G, Schottenfeld RS, Meyer RE, Rounsaville B. Naltrexone and coping skills therapy for alcohol dependence: a controlled study. *Arch Gen Psychiatry.* 1992;49:881-887.
61. Zumoff B, Fukushima DK, Weitzman ED, Kream J, Hellman L. The sex difference in plasma cortisol concentration in man. *J Clin Endocrinol Metab.* 1974; 39:805-808.
62. Schoneshofer M, Harendt H, Vescei P. Simultaneous radioimmunoassay for corticosterone and deoxycortisol in human serum: sex differences in the mean serum concentrations. *J Clin Chem Clin Biochem.* 1977;15:69-75.

The Electroencephalogram After Alcohol Administration in High-Risk Men and the Development of Alcohol Use Disorders 10 Years Later

Preliminary Findings

Jan Volavka, MD, PhD; Pál Czobor, PhD; Donald W. Goodwin, MD; William F. Gabrielli, Jr, MD, PhD; Elizabeth C. Penick, PhD; Sarnoff A. Mednick, PhD, DrMed; Per Jensen, MD; Joachim Knop, MD; Fini Schulsinger, MD

Background: In 1979 through 1980, electroencephalographic (EEG) responses to an alcohol challenge in 19-year-old sons of alcoholics as well as in sons of nonalcoholic control subjects were examined. The familial risk status of the subjects and greater EEG sensitivity to alcohol were hypothesized to predict the development of alcoholism 10 years later.

Methods: In 1990 through 1992, diagnostic interviews were completed to ascertain alcohol and other substance use disorders in these subjects and to update their family history.

Results: Updated family history of alcoholism predicted the development of substance dependence. Density of alcoholic relatives (the number of alcoholic relatives divided by the number of known relatives) was positively related to the severity of alcohol use disorders in the probands. Contrary to expectation, a greater EEG response at age 19 years was not related to the later development of alcohol dependence. Instead, the opposite was observed: a *smaller* EEG alpha frequency response to alcohol at age 19 years was related to the development of alcohol dependence and high quantity and frequency of alcohol consumption 10 years later.

Conclusions: Lower EEG response to a small dose of alcohol may be associated with the later development of alcohol dependence. This result is based on a small number of subjects and should be interpreted with caution. Although this result is opposite to our 1980 hypothesis, it is consistent with much of the recent literature.

(Arch Gen Psychiatry. 1996;53:258-263)

GENETIC contribution to alcoholism exists.[1-3] Genetic predisposition to alcoholism may be mediated by a *low innate sensitivity* to the effects of alcohol.[4] According to this theory, prealcoholics "are at the lower end of a continuum of sensitivity to moderate doses of alcohol."[5(p 8)] The low innate sensitivity may ultimately lead to alcohol dependence if an individual possessing it chooses to drink. That individual will need more drinks to achieve the same level of intoxication as his more "normal-sensitive" drinking companions. Repeated exposure to large amounts of alcohol will lead to greater risk for developing dependence. Conversely, high innate sensitivity protects against alcoholism. Data indicate lower innate sensitivity to alcohol among subjects with positive family history for alcoholism (FHP), mostly among sons of alcoholic fathers, compared with control subjects with negative family history for alcoholism (FHN).[6,7]

An alternative theory states that individuals are at high risk for alcoholism if they perceive the effects of their initial doses of alcohol as normalizing their psychobiological functioning. One specific theory focused on the reduction of tension provided by small doses of alcohol. This *tension-reduction* theory postulates that prealcoholics are tense and that alcohol reduces tension; consequently, alcohol is particularly reinforcing to these individuals.[8,9] This theory would predict that the electroencephalograms (EEGs) of individuals at high risk for the development of alcoholism, compared with their normal-risk coun-

See Subjects and Methods on next page

From the Nathan S. Kline Institute for Psychiatric Research, Orangeburg, NY, and Department of Psychiatry, New York University, New York (Drs Volavka and Czobor); Department of Psychiatry, Kansas University Medical Center, Kansas City (Drs Goodwin, Gabrielli, and Penick); Social Science Research Institute, University of Southern California, Los Angeles (Dr Mednick); and Institute of Preventive Medicine, Copenhagen, Denmark (Drs Jensen, Knop, and Schulsinger).

SUBJECTS AND METHODS

SUBJECTS: THE 1979-1980 EEG STUDY

The subjects were selected from a cohort born in 1959 through 1961 in Copenhagen. In 1979, we searched the Central Psychiatric Register of Denmark and local Alcoholism Clinic records to determine which of the fathers had received the diagnosis of alcoholism. In this way, 448 fathers were identified as alcoholics. Their 255 sons were defined as high-risk subjects. Control subjects (n=125) were sons of men who did not have a diagnosis of alcoholism registered in the records mentioned above. The sons of alcoholic fathers and their control subjects have been followed up in a continuing multidisciplinary longitudinal prospective study.[16,17]

METHODS

Alcohol Challenge

As a part of the 1979-through-1980 examination of this sample, we gave an alcohol challenge with an EEG to 43 sons of alcoholic fathers and 28 control subjects.[12] All had used alcohol, and none was alcohol dependent. Furthermore, subjects were asked how much beer, wine, and hard liquor they had consumed during the previous week. At that time, the two groups did not differ in their current drinking practices.

The challenge consisted of 0.5-g/kg dose of alcohol diluted in currant juice. The subjects were told that the drink contained alcohol. No placebo session was done. Electroencephalographic records were obtained before and then repeatedly after alcohol administration. Arresting EEG with eyes closed was recorded in 71 subjects before and then at 30, 60, and 120 minutes after alcohol ingestion. We obtained measures of spectral energy for four frequency bands (theta, slow alpha, fast alpha, and beta) as well as the mean frequency within the alpha band. These measures were obtained for six scalp leads (C3, C4, P3, P4, O1, and O2). Additional details describing the methods of EEG recording and analysis have been published.[12] Some of the EEG data were incomplete; therefore, our original analyses[12] included only 48 subjects (31 sons of alcoholic fathers and 17 control subjects).

Quantitative measures of EEG alpha activity differentiated these two groups. After 0.5-g/kg dose of alcohol, the sons of alcoholic fathers exhibited a greater decrease of the average frequency of the EEG alpha activity, a greater increase of the slow alpha energy, and a greater decrease of the fast alpha energy than did the control subjects. Thus, the EEG findings obtained in 1979 through 1980 suggested that sons of alcoholic fathers were more sensitive to alcohol than were the controls. Similar EEG effects of alcohol were reported in men with a family history of alcoholism.[18]

One of the possible interpretations of these findings was that the greater EEG response to alcohol in the sons of alcoholic fathers reflected a greater reduction of tension and anxiety; at the time of the original data analysis in the early 1980s, some of us reasoned that this mechanism might account for the expected increase of vulnerability to alcohol abuse and dependence among the sons of alcoholic fathers.

Purpose of the Present Study

The results obtained in 1979 through 1980 involved young men who were at risk but who had not yet developed alcohol abuse or dependence.[12] Thus, we did not know whether the electrophysiological features that distinguished sons of alcoholics from control subjects were related to subsequent alcohol use disorders. We have now completed a follow-up of the men whose EEG response to a single dose of alcohol we described 10 years ago.[12] The main purpose of the present study is to describe relationships between the EEG response to a single dose of alcohol 10 years ago and the subsequent drinking behavior of these same men who are now approximately 30 years old. The principal hypothesis of this study was that the decrease of the average EEG alpha frequency after alcohol challenge would be related to the development of alcohol dependence. This hypothesis was based on the assumption that the EEG response to alcohol is a reflection of biological mechanisms that enhance the reinforcing effects of alcohol and, thus, render the subjects at risk more vulnerable to alcohol dependence. Alcohol dependence (rather than alcohol abuse) was the principal outcome variable among the results that we present in this study since the diagnosis of dependence is more consistent[19] and

Continued on next page

terparts, would show higher frequency and lower amplitude (with more beta activity) before alcohol consumption. After the administration of alcohol, the EEGs of high-risk persons, compared with their normal-risk counterparts, would show a pronounced increase of slow alpha activity, which, in general, is associated with relaxation.

As predicted by the theory, FHP subjects showed relatively high amounts of fast activity in the EEG[10] in the alcohol-free condition; this finding was partially consistent with another study.[11] Our previous results[12] are compatible with the tension-reduction theory. However, there exist EEG data that are not consistent with that theory.[13,14] The propensity to develop alcohol use disorders may be inherited jointly with the propensity for other substance use disorders.[15]

RESULTS

ALCOHOL USE AND FAMILY HISTORY

Among the 64 subjects included in this 1990-through-1992 follow-up study, there were 42 FHP and 22 FHN subjects according to family history data obtained during the 1990-through-1992 interviews. Seven of these subjects were diagnosed with alcohol dependence, 16 with alcohol abuse (but not alcohol dependence), and 41 with neither. **Table 2** shows that four (18%) of the 22 FHN subjects, but 19 (45%) of the 19 FHP subjects, developed an alcohol use disorder. The group difference was not statistically significant (Fisher's exact test).

genetic influences are more likely to be detected in the development of alcohol dependence than of alcohol abuse.[5]

Follow-up Interviews

In 1979 through 1980, 71 subjects received an alcohol challenge with EEG, as mentioned above (also see **Table 1**). In 1990 through 1992, a psychiatrist (P.J.) conducted structured follow-up interviews with the subjects in their homes. These interviews at the 1990-through-1992 follow-up and their preliminary results in the entire sample (including the subjects who did not have an alcohol challenge) have been described elsewhere.[16,17] The interview yielded the following data.

1. *DSM-III-R* diagnoses, including psychoactive substance use disorders,[20] were obtained by a structured comprehensive diagnostic interview.[21]

2. Data on the *drinking practices* in 1990 through 1992 were obtained. Similar to the interview conducted in 1979 through 1980, the subjects were asked how much beer, wine, and hard liquor they had consumed on each day during the previous week. The quantities reported by the subjects were converted to grams of ethyl alcohol[22] and averaged over the week for subsequent analyses. In addition to this measure of quantity, we derived a measure of drinking frequency; this was the number of days (in the week preceding the interview) during which the subject consumed any alcoholic beverage. Thus, the drinking frequency ranged between 0 and 7. Finally, problems and symptoms associated with abusive drinking were also reviewed.

3. Family history of psychiatric disorders (including substance use disorders) was also obtained during the interview. The interview included the family history review of psychiatric disorders, using the Andreasen's family history interview schedule.[23] On the basis of the family history obtained in this interview, the subjects with at least one alcoholic first- or second-degree relative were classified as FHP; the others were classified as FHN. The *density of alcoholic relatives* was calculated for each FHP subject by dividing the number of alcoholic first- and second-degree relatives by the number of known first- and second-degree relatives. For the purpose of the current study, we used the interview as the sole source of information on family history of alcoholism.

Data Analysis

The follow-up information was obtained in 64 of the 71 subjects. Seven of the 71 subjects were unavailable for follow-up: three failed to respond to our attempts at reaching them, one refused to cooperate, one left Denmark, one lived too far away (within Denmark), and one died. In 21 of the 64 subjects with 1990-through-1992 follow-up data available, the EEG from at least one scalp lead was distorted by artifacts at one (or more) of the four time points; therefore, none of their data could be used in a conventional repeated measures analysis of variance (ANOVA). Thus, unbalanced ANOVA for repeated measures was used to study relationship between drinking outcome and the EEG in the current study. This method uses cases with incomplete observations.[24,25] The empirical bayesian approach used in the unbalanced repeated measures ANOVA provides valid estimates of the true model parameters even if missing data occur systematically (eg, if the probability of missing data depends on symptom severity). Model parameter estimates yielded by the unbalanced repeated measures ANOVA were tested by Wald's χ^2 statistic.[24,26] This statistic, unlike the traditional F, is applicable for the maximum likelihood–based estimates of the unbalanced ANOVA model.[27,28]

Each of the five EEG variables (energy in four frequency bands and the mean alpha frequency) was used as the dependent variable in separate repeated measures ANOVAs. Although our primary hypothesis was not concerned with the theta or beta bands, we analyzed these bands for descriptive purposes. The analyses were performed for trichotomous classification (dependence, abuse, and absence), based on the diagnosis of alcohol use disorder. The outcome measure was used as a between-subjects factor in the analyses. The time (baseline and 30, 60, and 120 minutes), anteroposterior electrode location (central, parietal, and occipital), and lateral electrode location (right, left) served as within-subjects factors. Interactions between outcome and time were used to test whether differences in outcomes were associated with differences in the EEG response.

Relationship between the density of alcoholic relatives and alcohol use disorders in the probands (FHN and FHP) was examined using logistic regression analysis. The trichotomous classification (dependence, abuse, and absence) based on the diagnosis of alcohol use disorder served as the dependent variable. The density of alcoholic relatives was positively associated with greater severity of alcoholism in the probands (n=64, Wald's χ^2=4.15, *df*=1, $P<.05$).

The average densities of alcoholic relatives for the FHP subjects who evidenced alcohol dependence (n=6), alcohol abuse (n=13), and no alcohol use disorder (n=23) were 0.20±0.10, 0.18±0.11, and 0.17+0.09, respectively. There were no statistically significant differences in densities among these three groups. However, the density of alcoholic relatives was related to the mean frequency in the EEG after alcohol, ie, the higher density was associated with a greater decrease of the mean alpha frequency (n= 42, Wald's χ^2=19.7, *df*=3, $P<.001$). Updated family history status (FHP or FHN) was related to the change of the mean alpha frequency over time (for the interaction between family history and time, Wald's χ^2=15.06, *df*=3; $P<.002$), with a greater decrease of the mean alpha frequency in the FHP group. These results are consistent with our previous data.[12]

The self-reported drinking practices during the week preceding the 1979-through-1980 and 1990-through-1992 follow-up interviews are summarized in **Table 3**. As expected, the alcohol substance use disorders were associated with higher quantities and frequencies of current alcohol consumption.

USE OF OTHER SUBSTANCES

Abuse of or dependence on substances other than alcohol were diagnosed in 11 subjects (Table 2). Ten of the 11 individuals were ascertained among the FHP subjects; the number is too small to permit meaningful sta-

Table 1. Timing of Tests and Assessments Reported in This Article*

Test or Assessment	1979-1980	1990-1992
Fathers' records searched for diagnosis of alcoholism	Yes	No
EEG* and alcohol challenge	Yes	No
Current drinking practices	Yes	Yes
Diagnostic interview for alcohol use disorders	Yes	Yes
Diagnostic interview for other mental disorders	No	Yes
Systematic interview for family history, including alcoholism†	No	Yes

*Complete list of procedures was published elsewhere.[16] EEG indicates electroencephalography.

†For the purpose of the current report, we used the interview as the sole source of information on family history of alcoholism.

Table 2. Substance Dependence and Abuse: Alcohol Separated From Other Substances

Diagnosis in 1990-1992 at Age 30 y	Subject Group* FHN	FHP	Total
Alcohol dependence	1	6†	7
Alcohol abuse	3	13‡	16
No alcohol use disorder	18§	23‖	41
Total	**22**	**42**	**64**

*FHN indicates family history negative for alcoholism; FHP, family history positive.

†One case of polysubstance dependence.

‡Four cases of cannabis dependence and one case of polysubstance dependence.

§One case of cannabis dependence.

‖Two cases of cannabis dependence, one case of cannabis abuse, and one case of amphetamine dependence.

Table 3. Drinking Practices in 1979-1980 and in 1990-1992*

	1979-1980		1990-1992	
Diagnosis in 1990-1992	Quantity, g†	Frequency, d‡	Quantity, g†	Frequency, d‡
Alcohol dependence (n=7)	174±56	3.57±1.27	482±282§‖	5.29±2.29§¶
Alcohol abuse (n=16)	160±33	3.56±1.79	324±310	3.56±2.10
No alcohol use disorder (n=41)	150±53	3.32±2.27	143±125	2.63±2.17

*Values are mean±SD.

†Grams of ethyl alcohol consumed in various beverages during the week preceding the interview.

‡No. of days in the preceding week when any alcoholic beverage was consumed (range, 0 to 7).

§Statistically significant (analysis of variance, $P<.05$) diagnostic group effect.

‖Post hoc pairwise comparison showed that the alcohol-dependent and alcohol-abusing groups did not differ from each other, but both differed from the group with no alcohol disorder.

¶Post hoc pairwise comparison showed a significant difference between the alcohol-dependent group and the group with no alcohol disorder.

tistical evaluation. Nevertheless, it appears that the substance use disorders (other than alcohol) are overrepresented among the FHP subjects.

Our expanded hypothesis stated that FHP subjects would evidence a higher prevalence of psychoactive (alcohol and/or other substances) use disorders (**Table 4**). To test this expanded hypothesis, we compared the FHN with the FHP groups on the prevalence of substance dependence, substance abuse, and no substance use disorder. The groups differed significantly on the substance dependence vs no substance use disorder ($P<.027$). The group differences on substance dependence vs substance abuse and substance abuse vs no substance use disorder were not statistically significant (Fisher's exact test).

EEG RESPONSE TO ALCOHOL CHALLENGE

Diagnostic Categories (Alcohol Use Disorders)

To test the relationship between alcohol use disorders and the EEG response, we used the trichotomous classification: alcohol dependence (AD), alcohol abuse (AA), and no alcohol disorder (NA) (see Table 2). One analysis was performed for each of the five EEG variables. Significant interactions between outcome and time were detected for two EEG variables: mean alpha frequency (χ^2=23.31, *df*=6, $P<.001$) and beta energy (χ^2=20.67, *df*=6, $P<.002$). The interaction between outcome and time was independent of the EEG electrode locations.

Mean Alpha Frequency. Post hoc analyses of the interaction for the mean EEG alpha frequency (see the preceding paragraph) revealed that the AD group differed from the NA group (χ=15.3, *df*=3, $P<.002$) and from the AA group (χ=24.5, *df*=3, $P<.001$). The AA and NA groups did not differ from each other (χ=3.7, *df*=3, P=.302) (**Figure 1**). The examination of changes over time showed a significant time effect ($P<.001$) in each of the three groups (AD, AA, and NA). Thus, alcohol administration was followed by a decrease of the mean alpha frequency in all three groups; the decrease was *less pronounced* in the AD group than in the AA and NA groups. Thus, our hypothesis was not supported by data. The changes of the mean alpha frequency after alcohol (averaged over the three time points) in individual subjects are displayed in **Figure 2**.

To explore the possibility that the exclusion of the seven subjects who were unavailable for follow-up (see "Methods" subsection of "Subjects and Methods" section) has biased our principal results concerning alpha frequency, we compared the mean alpha frequency EEG response to alcohol in the seven subjects unavailable for follow-up with the response in the 64 subjects we did

Table 4. Substance Dependence and Abuse: Alcohol and Other Substances Combined*

	No. of Patients		
Diagnosis in 1990-1992	FHN	FHP	Total
Substance dependence†	2	14	**16**
Substance abuse	3	9	**12**
No substance use disorder	17	19	**36**
Total	**22**	**42**	**64**

**FHN* indicates family history negative for alcoholism; FHP, family history positive.*

†The likelihood of FHP was greater in subjects with substance dependence than in those with no substance use disorder (Fisher's exact test; $P<.027$*).*

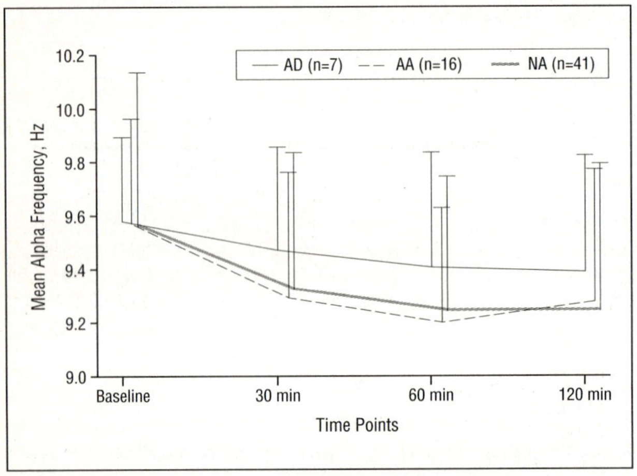

Figure 1. *Mean alpha frequency before and after a single dose of alcohol: group averages. Separately for each of the four time points, averages and SDs for the three outcome groups are displayed: alcohol dependence (AD), alcohol abuse (AA), and no alcohol use disorder (NA). The data were averaged over all scalp derivations available. The electroencephalography was performed in 1979 through 1980, and the outcomes of alcohol use were assessed in 1990 through 1992.*

follow up. An ANOVA procedure analogous to that described above was used. The interaction between time and unavailable for follow-up (yes or no) was not significant (χ^2=2.37, *df*=3, *P*=.499). Thus, the unavailability of seven subjects did not appear to bias the mean alpha frequency results.

Beta Energy. Post hoc analyses analogous to those performed for the alpha frequency (described above) were performed for the interaction involving beta energy. The AD group differed from the NA group (χ^2=18.00, *df*=3, $P<.001$) and the AA group (χ^2=14.5, *df*=3; $P<.002$). The AA and NA groups did not differ from each other (χ^2=1.6, *df*=3, *P*=.67). The beta energy increased over time in all three groups, but this effect reached the level of statistical significance only in the AA group (χ^2=11.2, *df*=3, $P<.01$).

Drinking Practices During the Week Preceding Interviews

Mean EEG alpha frequency was the dependent variable in Wald's tests examining the interaction between time

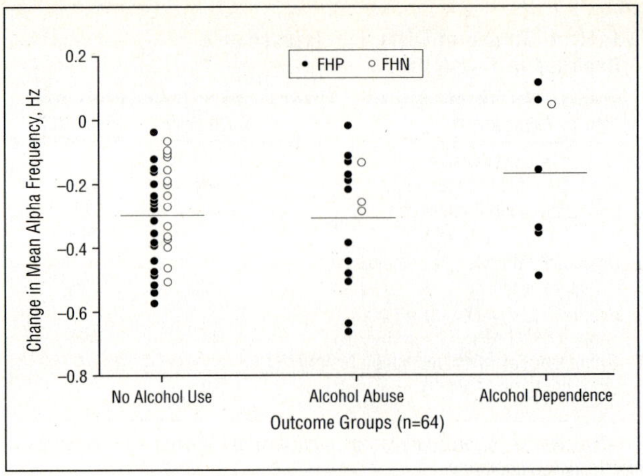

Figure 2. *Mean alpha frequency: change from baseline in individuals. For each of the 64 subjects from both groups, ie, the family history positive (FHP) and family history negative (FHN) for alcoholism, the mean alpha frequency was averaged over the three post–alcohol time points (30, 60, and 120 minutes). The difference between this average and the baseline is displayed for individual subjects in each of the outcome groups with group averages, based on the same data as in Figure 1.*

(minutes after alcohol administration) and a measure of drinking practices. A separate Wald test was performed for each of the four drinking practice variables: quantity and frequency of alcohol consumption in 1979 through 1980, and quantity and frequency in 1990 through 1992 (see Table 3 for descriptive data on drinking practices). Neither of the 1979-through-1980 variables yielded significant results. However, the 1990-through-1992 quantity and frequency of alcohol consumption showed significant interactions (χ^2=28.9, $P<.001$ and χ^2=9.21, $P<.027$, respectively, with *df*=3 for both tests). The sign of the interaction indicated that the smaller alpha mean frequency responses in 1979 through 1980 were associated with greater alcohol consumption in 1990 through 1992. These results are consistent with those obtained using alcohol use disorder diagnoses.

COMMENT

Our findings should be interpreted with caution in view of the small number of cases diagnosed with alcohol dependence so far; however, these results, based on diagnoses, are strengthened by consistent findings based on current drinking practices. Other limitations stem from the multiple tests performed and also from the fact that our hypothesis was not supported. No placebo session was included; this shortcoming makes it difficult to evaluate the EEG effects of alcohol in our study; thus, the observed response represents a composite of the effects of expectation and of actual pharmacological effects.

Although the differences between the alcohol-dependent group and the other groups in the mean alpha frequency after alcohol reached the level of statistical significance, there was a considerable overlap between the groups. It seems that a minority of the subjects with alcohol dependence (those who may be showing some EEG insensitivity) are responsible for this difference. The subjects have not yet passed through their age window of risk for the development of substance abuse disorders. Additional subjects are expected to develop these disorders by the time of the next follow-up approximately 10 years hence. At that time, the reliability of the current findings can be evaluated. Thus, given all these methodological problems, our results are best considered as hypothesis generating rather than conclusive.

With these limitations in mind, we report that a single dose of alcohol was followed by an average decrease of the mean EEG alpha frequency. Such decrease is a typical effect of moderate doses of alcohol.[29] Although this effect occurred in each of the three outcome groups, the average size of this effect was *smaller* in the group of subjects who would (10 years later) become dependent on alcohol. The direction of this group difference was opposite to our hypothesis and opposite to earlier findings comparing high-risk and low-risk groups. A similarly unexpected differentiation of the alcohol-dependent subjects from the other groups emerged in the analyses of beta energy. These results are in the opposite direction to our hypothesis, but they are consistent with the increasing evidence that low sensitivity to alcohol is a risk factor for the development of alcoholism.[7,13]

Accepted for publication December 10, 1995.

Supported in part by grant AA08176 from the National Institute on Alcohol Abuse and Alcoholism, Rockville, Md.

We thank V. E. Pollock, PhD, for the recording and computer analyses of electroencephalograms, and M. Galanter, MD, and H. Kalant, MD, PhD, for valuable comments.

Reprint requests to Nathan Kline Institute, Orangeburg, NY 10962 (Dr Volavka).

REFERENCES

1. Goodwin DW, Schulsinger F, Moller N, Hermansen L, Winokur G, Guze SB. Drinking problems in adopted and nonadopted sons of alcoholics. *Arch Gen Psychiatry.* 1974;31:164-169.
2. Cloninger CR, Bohman M, Sigvardsson S. Inheritance of alcohol abuse: cross-fostering analysis of adopted men. *Arch Gen Psychiatry.* 1981;38:861-868.
3. Goodwin DW. The genetics of alcoholism. In: McHugh PR, McKusick VA, eds. *Genes, Brain and Behavior.* New York, NY: Raven Press; 1990:219-226.
4. Goodwin DW. *Alcoholism: The Facts.* New York, NY: Oxford University Press; 1981.
5. Schuckit MA. A clinical model of genetic influences in alcohol dependence. *J Stud Alcohol.* 1994;55:5-17.
6. Pollock VE. Meta-analysis of subjective sensitivity to alcohol in sons of alcoholics. *Am J Psychiatry.* 1992;149:1534-1538.
7. Schuckit MA. Low level of response to alcohol as a predictor of future alcoholism. *Am J Psychiatry.* 1994;151:184-189.
8. Docter RF, Naitoh P, Smith JC. Electroencephalographic changes and vigilance behavior during experimentally induced intoxication with alcoholic subjects. *Psychosom Med.* 1966;28:605-615.
9. Volavka J, Pollock V, Gabrielli WF Jr, Mednick SA. The EEG in persons at risk for alcoholism. In: Galanter M, ed. *Recent Developments in Alcoholism.* New York, NY: Plenum Press; 1985:21-36.
10. Gabrielli WF, Mednick SA, Volavka J, Pollock VE, Schulsinger F, Itil TM. Electroencephalograms in children of alcoholic fathers. *Psychophysiology.* 1982; 19:404-407.
11. Ehlers CL, Schuckit MA. EEG fast frequency activity in the sons of alcoholics. *Biol Psychiatry.* 1990;27:631-641.
12. Pollock VE, Volavka J, Goodwin DW, Mednick SA, Gabrielli WF, Knop J, Schulsinger F. The EEG after alcohol administration in men at risk for alcoholism. *Arch Gen Psychiatry.* 1983;40:857-861.
13. Ehlers CL, Schuckit MA. Evaluation of EEG alpha activity in sons of alcoholics. *Neuropsychopharmacology.* 1991;4:199-205.
14. Kaplan RF, Hesselbrock VM, O'Connor S, DePalma N. Behavioral and EEG responses to alcohol in nonalcoholic men with a family history of alcoholism. *Prog Neuropsychopharmacol Biol Psychiatry.* 1988;12:873-885.
15. Mathew RJ, Wilson WH, Blazer DG, George LK. Psychiatric disorders in adult children of alcoholics: data from the Epidemiologic Catchment Area project. *Am J Psychiatry.* 1993;150:793-800.
16. Knop J, Goodwin DW, Jensen P, Penick E, Pollock V, Gabrielli W, Teasdale TW, Mednick SA. A 30-year follow-up study of the sons of alcoholic men. *Acta Psychiatr Scand Suppl.* 1993;370:48-53.
17. Goodwin DW, Knop J, Jensen P, Gabrielli WF Jr, Schulsinger F, Penick EC. Thirty-year follow-up of men at high risk for alcoholism. *Ann N Y Acad Sci.* 1994;708:97-101.
18. Bauer LO, Hesselbrock VM. EEG, autonomic and subjective correlates of the risk for alcoholism. *J Stud Alcohol.* 1993;54:577-589.
19. Rapaport MH, Tipp JE, Schuckit MA. A comparison of *ICD-10* and *DSM-III-R* criteria for substance abuse and dependence. *Am J Drug Alcohol Abuse.* 1993; 19:143-151.
20. American Psychiatric Association. *Diagnostic and Statistical Manual of Mental Disorders, Third Edition, Revised.* Washington, DC: American Psychiatric Association; 1987.
21. Othmer E, Penick EC, Powell BJ, Read MR, Othmer SC. *Psychiatric Diagnostic Interview, Revised (PDI-R): Manual.* Los Angeles, Calif: Western Psychological Services Publishers and Distributors; 1989.
22. Turner C. How much alcohol is in a 'standard drink'? an analysis of 125 studies. *Br J Addict.* 1990;85:1171-1175.
23. Andreasen NC, Endicott J, Spitzer RL, Winokur G. The family history method using diagnostic criteria: reliability and validity. *Arch Gen Psychiatry.* 1977; 34:1229-1235.
24. Schluchter MD. Unbalanced repeated measures models with structured covariance matrices. In: Dixon WJ, Brown MB, Engelman L, Jennrich RI, eds. *BMDP Statistical Software Manual.* Berkeley: University of California Press; 1990; 2:1207-1244.
25. Rubin DB. Inference and missing data. *Biometrika.* 1976;63:581-592.
26. Bollen KA. *Structural Equations With Latent Variables.* New York, NY: John Wiley & Sons Inc; 1989.
27. Gibbons RD, Hedeker D, Elkin I, Waternaux C, Kraemer HC, Greenhouse JB, Shea MT, Imber SD, Sotsky SM, Watkins JT. Some conceptual and statistical issues in analysis of longitudinal psychiatric data: application to the NIMH Treatment of Depression Collaborative Research Program dataset. *Arch Gen Psychiatry.* 1993;50:739-750.
28. Gibbons RD, Hedeker D, Waternaux C, Davis JM. Random regression models: a comprehensive approach to the analysis of longitudinal psychiatric data. *Psychopharmacol Bull.* 1988;24:438-443.
29. Ehlers CL, Wall TL, Schuckit MA. EEG spectral characteristics following ethanol administration in young men. *Electroencephalogr Clin Neurophysiol.* 1989; 73:179-187.

ORIGINAL ARTICLE

The Effects of Alcohol Consumption on Laboratory-Induced Panic and State Anxiety

Matt G. Kushner, PhD; Thomas B. Mackenzie, MD; Joanna Fiszdon; David P. Valentiner, PhD; Edna Foa, PhD; Nicole Anderson; Douglas Wangensteen, PhD

Background: This study tested whether alcohol consumption reduces anxiety and panic associated with a panic-challenge procedure.

Methods: Subjects with panic disorder were randomly assigned to consume either a moderate dose of alcohol or a nonalcoholic placebo. All subjects were told that they were drinking alcohol to control beverage expectancies. Following the beverage administration, subjects underwent a panic challenge (35% carbon dioxide) and a series of anxiety symptom assessments.

Results: Subjects who consumed alcohol reported significantly less state anxiety both before and after the challenge. In response to the challenge, subjects who consumed alcohol experienced significantly fewer panic attacks when applying liberal panic criteria; however, this effect only approached significance when applying conservative panic criteria.

Conclusions: These findings suggest that alcohol acts acutely to reduce both panic and the anxiety surrounding panic, and they lend support to the view that drinking behavior among those with panic disorder is reinforced by this effect. We suggest that this process may contribute to the high rate at which alcohol-use disorders co-occur with panic disorder.

(Arch Gen Psychiatry. 1996;53:264-270)

Alcohol-use disorders co-occur (are comorbid) with panic disorder at a rate that exceeds chance significantly.[1,2] It has been suggested that those with panic disorder are at an increased risk for the development of alcohol problems as they are prone to drink to relieve the symptoms of panic.[3,4] Conversely, "kindling" and hyperventilation are processes that have been posited to account for the emergence of panic-like symptoms in alcoholics by way of the chemical and cognitive effects of multiple alcohol withdrawals.[5,6] It has also been suggested that panic disorder and alcoholism are related by a shared familial factor.[7] Although each of these processes has received limited empirical support, it is generally agreed that the causes underlying high comorbidity rates remain speculative.[1]

Correlational and descriptive methods, although useful in identifying the extent of comorbidity, are less suited to studying the putative causes underlying comorbidity. Such studies do show that panic disorder typically precedes alcoholism among those who are comorbid[8,9] and that many comorbid patients report that they use alcohol to control anxiety and panic.[4,10] Although these studies would appear to imply a causal path from panic disorder to pathologic alcohol use, their methods preclude the drawing of firm conclusions regarding causal relationships.[1,11]

Experimental methodologies offer an underutilized approach to testing hypothesized causal connections between alcohol use and panic symptoms. In fact, recent reviews conclude that the bulk of experimental studies find a stress response–dampening effect for alcohol among normal subjects.[12] However, it cannot be assumed that alcohol's effect on contrived laboratory stressors among normal subjects would generalize to alcohol's effect on clinical anxiety phenomena among those with panic disorder.

In the present study, we tested directly the acute effects of alcohol on panic symptoms. We administered either alco-

See Subjects and Methods on next page

From the Departments of Psychiatry (Drs Kushner and Mackenzie and Ms Anderson), Psychology (Ms Fiszdon), and Physiology (Dr Wangensteen), University of Minnesota, Minneapolis; the Department of Psychology and Human Development, Vanderbilt University, Nashville, Tenn (Dr Valentiner); and the Department of Psychiatry, Medical College of Pennsylvania, Philadelphia (Dr Foa).

SUBJECTS AND METHODS

SUBJECTS

Screening

A trained research assistant prescreened newspaper ad respondents by telephone and scheduled those appearing to qualify for a final screen and study appointment. Inclusion required a *DSM III-R* diagnosis of current panic disorder (based on SCID-P version[15]) and a current age of 21 to 55 years. Exclusion criteria were (1) a history of alcoholism; (2) being a self-described nondrinker; (3) regular use of psychiatric medications (greater than three times per week); (4) currently pregnant or lactating; (5) current psychotic disorder; (6) current major depression; and (7) current respiratory or cardiovascular illness, including hypertension.

Final Sample

Thirty-four qualified subjects agreed to participate and attended the study appointment. Data from three of these subjects could not be used because of protocol violations (eg, unable or unwilling to inhale minimum amounts of the carbon dioxide as outlined below). The remaining 31 individuals made up the final subject sample (nine males and 22 females) and ranged in age from 21 to 51 years (mean age±SD=31±8 years).

Group Assignments

Group assignment slots were ordered randomly in blocks of 10 (five placebo slots and five alcohol slots) by the drawing of lots. As individuals were found to be qualified and agreed to be scheduled for a study appointment, they were placed in the next open slot in the randomized group assignment order.

Human Subjects Usage

This study was reviewed and approved by the University of Minnesota's Committee on the Use of Human Subjects in Research. All subjects provided informed consent to participate in this study, and each was paid $50.

MEASURES

Psychological Symptoms, Alcohol Use, and Integrity of Study Manipulations

Subjects responded to the Brief Symptom Inventory (BSI), the State-Trait Anxiety Inventory (STAI), and the Beck Depression Inventory (BDI).[16-18] With reference to the year preceding the study, subjects were asked to rate their typical quantity and frequency of alcohol consumption, as well as their episodes of heavy drinking (≥5 drinks).

Subjects also provided intensity ratings on a number of single-item scales, including (1) fearful anticipation of the challenge ("Challenge Fearfulness"), (2) subjective intoxication, (3) straightforwardness of the study, and (4) similarity of drinking in the study to drinking outside the study. Subjects responded to each of these items using a Visual Analog Scale format, in which they were asked to place a mark on a 100-mm line with a rating of 0 indicating not at all, and a rating of 100 indicating extremely so. Scores were determined by measuring (in millimeters) the distance from the left anchor of the scale (0) to the subject's mark.

Panic Symptoms and Panic Attacks

During the experiment, subjects responded to a modified version of the Acute Panic Inventory (API) that includes the original 17-item API,[19] as well as 10 items added more recently (J. Gorman, personal communication, April 1992). Items include *DSM-III-R* somatic and cognitive panic attack symptoms, as well as a number of other stress/anxiety symptoms. To increase the items' sensitivity to symptom variation, we modified the original four-point response format by having subjects rate each item, using the Visual Analog Scale format and scoring described above. A total API score was derived by averaging all API item responses.

In addition to the total API, a panic attack was counted as present if at least one API cognitive fear symptom *and* at least four API somatic panic symptoms were endorsed in response to the challenge. By adjusting the minimum API item intensity rating required to count a panic symptom as present, we identified panic attacks using two criteria. A lower symptom intensity panic criteria (*liberally defined panic*) counted cognitive fear symptoms as present when rated at an intensity of at least 50 (half of maximum). A higher symptom intensity panic criteria (*conservatively defined panic*) counted cognitive fear symptoms as present when rated at an intensity of at least 75 (three fourths of maximum). For both panic criteria, somatic symptoms were counted as present when relevant API items were rated at an intensity of at least 33 (one third of maximum). Both of these definitions meet *DSM-III-R* panic attack criteria and are largely consistent with past research assessing discrete panic attacks in response to a laboratory challenge.[20,21]

Biologic Measures

Measurement of blood pressure (millimeters of Hg) and heart rate (beats/minute) was accomplished using an automated recording system that produces a point measurement 45 to 60 seconds after activation. This system is attached to the subject by an arm-cuff. Blood alcohol levels (BAL) were measured using a pocket-sized breath alcohol testing device (Alco-Sensor III, ALCOPRO, Knoxville, Tenn), which estimates grams of alcohol per deciliter of blood, accurate to ±0.005 g/dL.

PROCEDURES

Study Appointment

All appointments were scheduled for the late afternoon,[22] and female subjects were scheduled exclusively during the first 2 weeks of their menstrual cycle.[23] Subjects had been instructed to (1) not take psychiatric medications for the 3 days preceding the study, (2) not drink alcohol for 24

Continued on next page

hours preceding the study, (3) not consume caffeinated products for 4 hours prior to the study, and (4) not eat for 4 hours preceding the study.

Alcohol Administration

All subjects were told that they would be given a moderate dose of alcohol; however, they were actually assigned randomly to receive either alcohol or a nonalcoholic placebo (see above). The experimenter mixed drinks from factory-labeled bottles of tonic water and 100-proof vodka (mixed 3:1) in front of the subject. The experimenter was blind to subjects' beverage group placement and was unaware of whether the vodka bottle actually contained vodka (alcohol group) or flat tonic water (placebo group). Subjects in the alcohol group were given an amount of alcohol that targeted a BAL of 0.085 g/dL[24] (approximately two standard drinks for a 55-kg [120-pound] woman and approximately 3.5 drinks for a 77-kg [170-pound] man). Subjects in the placebo group were given a matched volume of placebo with approximately 10 mL of a lime and vodka mixture (1:1) squirted on top of their drink to enhance the beverage deception. Following the 20-minute drinking period, subjects were asked to sit quietly for an additional 20 minutes, during which the alcohol they consumed was absorbed.

Carbon Dioxide Challenge and Vital Lung Capacity

A gas delivery system was constructed that delivered premixed 35% carbon dioxide and 65% oxygen through a standard gas mask held in place by the subject. The mask was attached to a 30-L bag that, in turn, was attached to a spirometer measuring the volume of gas inhaled. For the vital lung capacity (VC) determination, the bag was filled with 100% oxygen and subjects were instructed to inhale as much as possible after exhaling as much as possible. The greatest volume inhaled of two trials was recorded as the subject's VC.

For the panic challenge, subjects took a single inhalation of the 35% carbon dioxide, using the same method as described for the VC; however, subjects were told to inhale until the indicator on the spirometer reached a mark showing their VC volume (65% of the VC was established a priori as minimum for considering a challenge to be valid). Subjects were told: "You will be breathing a gas mixture containing carbon dioxide and oxygen. Although the gas mixture has no known health risks, it is possible that it will make you feel uncomfortable, anxious, or panicky for up to several minutes following the inhalation."

Assessments

A prestudy mailing assessment (BSI, BDI, STAI, alcohol use, and health-screen questionnaire) was completed by subjects at their homes. During the experiment, subjects completed a baseline assessment (API, STAI, heart rate, and blood pressure level) that was followed by the beverage administration (alcohol or placebo). After the beverage administration, subjects completed a prechallenge assessment 10 minutes before the carbon dioxide challenge and a postchallenge assessment 10 minutes after the carbon dioxide challenge (STAI, degree of subjective intoxication, heart rate/blood pressure, and a breath BAL read and recorded by a Clinical Research Center nurse). At the prechallenge assessment, subjects also provided a Challenge Fearfulness rating.

A challenge assessment was initiated 30 seconds following the carbon dioxide inhalation, where subjects responded to the API based on their "peak reaction" to the challenge. A single-point heart rate and blood pressure measurement was also completed from 1.0 to 1.5 minutes following the challenge. (However, we realized, after these data were collected, that this physiological measurement was likely to have missed a brief point-of-panic burst in these response domains. Therefore, to avoid the false impression that these data necessarily represented peak challenge responding, they are not analyzed herein.[25]) With the aim of providing pilot data for future studies, subjects were also asked to repeat the carbon dioxide challenge and assessments; however, these data are not analyzed herein. Finally, subjects completed an exit questionnaire assessing the integrity of the study manipulations and underwent a final breath BAL measurement. The final BAL measurement was taken by the experimenter, breaking the blind in anticipation of the poststudy debriefing.

Poststudy Debriefing and Exit

The experimenter completely debriefed subjects and provided information regarding local panic disorder treatment options. Information was provided both orally and in written form, which subjects took home. Subjects who consumed alcohol remained for approximately 2 hours following the conclusion of the study to allow the alcohol in their system to largely metabolize. Transportation home was arranged for all subjects.

STATISTICAL ANALYSIS

A two-tailed significance level of $P<.05$ was used for all analyses. We employed t tests to confirm the expected similarity of the two groups on measures taken at the mailed and study baseline assessments. The t test was also used to evaluate group differences on exit measures assessing the integrity of experimental manipulations. To evaluate hypothesized beverage effects on the prechallenge and postchallenge assessment measures, we employed analysis of covariance (ANCOVA), using beverage group as the independent variable and the relevant baseline effect as the covariate.

We had planned to use the same ANCOVA approach to analyze hypothesized beverage effects on challenge API scores; however, we recognized that three outlying baseline API scores discovered in the alcohol group (see the "Results" section) might violate assumptions associated with this parametric analytic approach.[26] Statisticians recommend the use of distribution-free nonparametric tests for such data.[27,28] Therefore, we calculated the degree of change from each subject's baseline API score to their challenge API score and then rank-transformed these data. We then applied the Wilcoxon rank sum test using the t approximation for the significance level.[28] Finally, χ^2 tests were used to evaluate the effect of beverage group status on panic attack frequency at the challenge assessment.

Table 1. Check of Experimental Manipulations by Beverage Group*

Variables	Beverage Group† Alcohol (n=16) Mean	SD	Placebo (n=15) Mean	SD	Group Difference *t* Value‡
Inhalation compliance, % of VC	96.97	12.64	92.97	9.92	NS
Subjective intoxication, 0-100 VAS score					
Prechallenge	58.56	18.85	26.87	22.83	4.22§
Postchallenge	50.81	23.44	17.27	20.14	4.26§
Blood alcohol level, g/dL					
Prechallenge	0.076	0.015	0.0	0.0	NA
Postchallenge	0.079	0.016	0.0	0.0	NA
Similarity to drinking outside of study, 0-100 VAS score	58.31	32.36	39.13	32.72	1.64‖
Straightforwardness of study, 0-100 VAS score	74.56	22.43	79.07	24.89	NS

*VC indicates vital lung capacity; VAS, Visual Analog Scale; NS, not significant; and NA, no test conducted.

†Subjective intoxication was significantly different from a mean population of 0 (ie, "no intoxication") for both groups at both assessment points, ie, prechallenge (alcohol group: $t[15]=12.42$, $P<.001$; placebo group: $t[14]=4.55$, $P<.001$) and postchallenge (alcohol group: $t[15]=8.67$, $P<.001$; placebo group: $t[14]=3.31$, $P<.01$).

‡*t* Tests were conducted with a df=29.

§$P<.001$.

‖$P<.10$.

hol or placebo to subjects with panic disorder prior to their undergoing a panic challenge (35% carbon dioxide). Because panic challenge responding is reduced by agents that block naturally occurring panic attacks,[13,14] this method should provide a valid test of alcohol's antipanic effects. We hypothesized that subjects consuming alcohol would respond less strongly to the panic challenge and would demonstrate less anxiety surrounding the challenge. Confirmation of this hypothesis would provide evidence of alcohol's capacity to reduce panic symptoms and would lend support to the view that this effect promotes drinking behavior among those with panic disorder.

RESULTS

STUDY MANIPULATION CHECKS

Table 1 shows beverage group comparisons on measures assessing the integrity of study manipulations. Suggesting good compliance with the inhalation instructions, both groups inhaled nearly the same volume of gas during the carbon dioxide challenge as during their VC assessment. Suggesting that the placebo deception was successful, subjects in both beverage groups reported a level of subjective intoxication that was significantly greater than 0 (ie, no intoxication) (Table 1, dagger footnote). However, subjects in the alcohol group reported a significantly greater degree of subjective intoxication than did those in the placebo group.

Also pointing to the success of the placebo deception, the groups did not differ on their ratings of the study's straightforwardness or on the similarity of drinking in the study to their typical drinking outside of the study (Table 1). However, group differences on the latter rating did approach significance, with the alcohol group reporting a greater similarity between drinking in the study and their typical drinking. As expected, only the alcohol group had a BAL level greater than zero, with the targeted BAL (0.085 g/dL) being reached with reasonable precision (Table 1).

MAILED QUESTIONNAIRES AND BASELINE ASSESSMENT

Suggesting the initial comparability of the study groups, no significant group differences were found on the mailed assessment measures (BDI, STAI [State and Trait], alcohol consumption measures, and BSI). In the laboratory, but prior to any experimental manipulations (baseline assessment), no significant group differences emerged on state anxiety, typical panic API, challenge fearfulness, interview ratings of agoraphobia, or heart rate and blood pressure. However, the mean baseline API score was significantly greater ($t[29]=2.58$, $P<.01$) in the alcohol group (mean±SD=21.3±18.1) than in the placebo group (mean±SD=8.2±7.8).

This finding was surprising, because group membership had been assigned randomly and no intervention had been introduced by the time this measure was taken. An examination of individual subject scores revealed three alcohol group subjects who had outlying baseline API scores (from 2 to 3 SDs above the sample mean [see the "Statistical Analysis" subsection under the "Methods" section for special consideration given the analysis of these data]).

PRECHALLENGE AND POSTCHALLENGE ASSESSMENTS

Table 2 shows prechallenge and postchallenge measures by beverage group. Baseline state anxiety was a significant covariate, demonstrating a positive association to both prechallenge and postchallenge state anxiety ($r=.40$ and $r=.29$, respectively). As predicted, state anxiety scores were significantly lower in the alcohol group at both the

Table 2. Prechallenge and Postchallenge by Beverage Group*

Variables	Alcohol (n=16) Raw Mean	Alcohol (n=16) Adjusted Mean	Alcohol (n=16) SD	Placebo (n=15) Raw Mean	Placebo (n=15) Adjusted Mean	Placebo (n=15) SD
Prechallenge Assessment						
State anxiety score†	26.94	24.90	13.76	36.13	38.30	18.84
Heart rate, beats/min	72.31	73.20	11.57	77.40	76.44	15.66
Blood pressure, mm Hg						
Systolic	116.06	116.72	9.85	120.93	120.23	11.03
Diastolic	74.44	74.89	9.86	78.07	77.57	14.10
Challenge fearfulness,‡ 0-100 VAS score	31.63	28.95	26.22	41.80	44.64	28.38
Postchallenge Assessment						
State anxiety score§	32.06	30.33	14.89	41.53	43.38	22.05
Heart rate, beats/min	79.44	80.24	10.51	82.67	81.80	14.54
Blood pressure, mm Hg						
Systolic	111.13	111.76	10.28	116.87	116.18	11.78
Diastolic	71.50	71.95	9.91	75.73	75.25	12.41

*VAS indicates Visual Analog Scale. Adjusted means control for prebeverage baseline effects. Significance tests based on covariate analysis.
†P<.01.
‡P<.08.
§P<.05.

prechallenge and postchallenge assessments (F[1,28]=6.32, *P*<.01; and F[1,28]=4.00, *P*<.05, respectively]).

Heart rate and blood pressure measures, while showing group differences in the predicted direction, did not reach statistical significance at either the prechallenge or postchallenge assessments. Those in the placebo group had greater challenge fearfulness by the Visual Analog Scale ratings (shown for the prechallenge assessment, Table 2); however, this effect did not quite reach conventional two-tailed statistical significance (F[1,28]=3.37, *P*<.08). Again, baseline challenge fearfulness was a significant covariate in this analysis (*r*=.48).

CHALLENGE ASSESSMENT

The API

As predicted, subjects in the placebo group showed more increase over baseline on the challenge API than did subjects in the alcohol group (alcohol group mean±SD rank =11.9±7.6; placebo group mean±SD rank=19.6±8.4) (*t*[28]=2.64, *P*<.01). (Note that one subject in the placebo group was not included in these or the panic attack comparisons as she reported being too upset by the challenge to respond accurately to the API measure. Also another subject in the placebo group failed to provide responses on two API items ["going crazy" and "feeling weak"], which were coded as missing in these analyses.) Because the API samples a heterogeneous set of symptoms, we repeated the above analysis for the separate API items. Significant group effects in the predicted direction were noted for the following: fear of dying (*t*[28]=3.50, *P*<.001), fear in general (*t*[28]=2.70, *P*<.01), difficulty swallowing (*t*[28]=2.27, *P*<.05), chest pain (*t*[28]=2.66, *P*<.01), and sweating (*t*[28]=2.10, *P*<.04). Additionally, the following API items showed group differences in the predicted direction that were nearly significant (*P*<.10): shakiness, dizziness, breathlessness, desire to flee, difficulty speaking, and difficulty working.

Panic Attacks

Using the liberally defined panic criteria (see the "Methods" section), a significantly greater proportion of subjects in the placebo group met criteria for a challenge-induced panic attack (85.7%) than was the case for subjects in the alcohol group (50%) (χ^2 [1, *N*=30]=4.28, *P*<.05). (Because one cell count was less than five, we determined that this group difference was also significant at the *P*<.05 level, using Fisher's exact test.) Finally, using the conservatively defined panic criteria, 50% of the placebo group met criteria for a panic attack vs 25% of the alcohol group, a difference that only approached statistical significance (χ^2[1, *N*=30]=2.01, *P*<.15).

COMMENT

Using subjects with panic disorder, we found that a moderate dose of alcohol decreased responding to a laboratory panic challenge and decreased anxiety before and after the challenge as well. These findings point to the potential for alcohol's anxiolytic properties to serve as a reinforcer of drinking behavior among those with panic disorder. This process may help to explain the high frequency with which alcohol problems co-occur with panic disorder. However, these findings and conclusions must be considered in light of the several caveats and limitations discussed below.

Unlike self-report measures, alcohol produced effects on psychophysiologic measures that, while in the predicted direction, failed to reach statistical significance. Although it is well known that fear manifestations (self-report, behavioral, physiological) may be desynchronous,[29] we speculate further that alcohol's complex effects on autonomic functioning may help explain the desynchrony found in this study. Alcohol was predicted to decrease autonomic responding by decreasing anxiety; however, alcohol has also been found to initially increase autonomic responding in nonstressed organisms.[30] These countervailing alcohol effects may have each partially masked the other.

Regarding methodology, because the blind was broken for each subject immediately following data collection, the experimenter could conceivably have begun to link certain behaviors occurring during the experiment to a specific group placement. Although this seems unlikely, given the highly routinized protocol (eg, subjects were seated and did not speak or move about during the experiment), data addressing this issue were, unfortunately, not collected. Nevertheless, we have no reason to believe that the experimenter's blind was compromised in this way. Also, our discovery of three alcohol group subjects with outlying baseline API scores raises questions about initial group comparability; however, a variety of well-validated measures (the BDI, STAI, and BSI) suggested that the groups were comparable initially.

Also germane to study findings was our use of an expectancy manipulation (EM) design vs a standard double-blind–placebo (DBP) design. In the EM design, subjects given a drink containing either alcohol or placebo are all told that they are drinking alcohol; in a DBP design, drink content is left ambiguous. Because it is rare that people drink a beverage of which the content or effect is ambiguous, EM designs mirror more closely the way people use alcohol in nonresearch settings.[31,32] Additionally, by telling all subjects that they have consumed alcohol, the EM design, unlike the DBP design, controls effects due to the belief that one has or has not consumed alcohol.[33]

However, the valid implementation of the EM design requires that placebo subjects *believe* that they are drinking alcohol. The present study met this requirement as indexed by the significant degree of subjective intoxication registered by the placebo group, as well as by the absence of group differences in ratings of the study's straightforwardness. However, the placebo group reported feeling less intoxicated than did the alcohol group. It is possible, therefore, that group differences in anxiety responding resulted, in part, from group differences in level of subjective intoxication. This alternative interpretation seems unlikely, however, as post hoc analyses that controlled for the effects of subjective intoxication did not alter the reported results.

The fact that placebo subjects are deceived about what they are drinking in the EM design also raises ethical issues. Therefore, we followed guidelines by the *Recommended Council Guidelines on Ethyl Alcohol Administration in Human Experimentation*[34] on the use of deception including (1) a full debriefing, (2) a consent form clearly indicating subjects may or may not receive alcohol and the amount of alcohol that they may receive, (3) a full disclosure of risk, and (4) truthful answers in response to direct questions. Also, those deceived were not given a psychoactive or dangerous drug and were paid volunteers recruited through advertisements, rather than from among hospital patients.

In interpreting our findings, it may be appropriate to view alcohol's general anxiolytic effects separately from its specific antipanic effects.[35,36] Although the stress-dampening properties of alcohol are well known,[12] this study demonstrates further that alcohol reduces anxiety in anticipation of exposure to a panicogenic situation (the carbon dioxide challenge). These findings are consistent with earlier suggestions that alcohol can attenuate the anticipatory anxiety underlying agoraphobia.[1,35]

Although alcohol reduced panic challenge responding, we cannot conclude firmly that alcohol acted directly on pathophysiology that is unique to panic. For example, it is possible that panic responding was reduced indirectly by alcohol's lowering of the anticipatory anxiety platform from which the carbon dioxide challenge was undertaken.[37] Also, although panic challenge responses are described as highly similar to natural panic,[37] challenge responding may confound panic with nonpanic anxiety distress.[38] Therefore, alcohol may have diminished nonpanic anxiety–distress elements of the challenge response but not panic elements of the challenge response. Studies that include a placebo-control challenge in addition to a panic challenge could potentially help to clarify these issues.

Regarding mechanisms of action, one possibility is that alcohol shares effects with the antipanic drug alprazolam on γ-aminobutyric acid (GABA)-ergic functioning.[39-41] Alcohol has also been shown to reduce responsiveness in locus ceruleus,[42] a brain system that has been linked to panic.[36] Alcohol may also interfere with cognitive processes potentially related to panic, such as self-focused attention.[43] As noted earlier, the possibility that alcohol affects generalized anxiety and panic through separate processes should also be considered.[35,36]

Although not addressed directly, our findings are consistent with the view that those with panic may seek alcohol to obtain symptom relief. If true, panic treatment should minimize an important motive to drink (ie, symptom reduction) among comorbid patients. Case histories[44,45] have reported decreased drinking in comorbid patients following panic treatment. A placebo-controlled study[46] found that imipramine reduced relapse to drinking among depressed alcoholics who also had panic disorder. As yet, however, definitive studies into the effects of panic on alcohol use have not been conducted.

We conjecture that a confluence of factors acts to either promote or inhibit drinking among those with panic. For example, drinking may be both promoted by the short-term anxiolytic effects of alcohol and inhibited by the long-term anxiogenic effects of alcohol.[47] Further, it seems likely that subgroups of those with panic disorder may be more or less prone to escalate drinking aimed at the control of anxiety and panic. Variations in sensitivity to the anxiolytic properties of alcohol,[42] personality dimensions,[48] beliefs about alcohol, and availability of effective coping responses[49] may all influence the likelihood that alcohol is used to control anxiety and panic.

Finally, we note that comorbidity is most likely a complex, multidetermined phenomenon. From this viewpoint, the idea that alcohol's anxiolytic properties contribute to the genesis of comorbidity is more likely to supplement than to supplant other putative comorbidity explanations. In any case, laboratory paradigms, such as those described herein, show promise as an approach to the further study of many questions related to comorbidity.

Accepted for publication November 1, 1995.

This research was supported, in part, by the following grants to the first author: R29-AA09871 from the National Institute on Alcohol Abuse and Alcoholism, Rockville, Md; 15228 from the Graduate School of the University of Minnesota, Minneapolis; and MRF-72-92 from the Minnesota Medical Foundation, Minneapolis, and from the University of Minnesota's General Clinical Research Center under grant MO1-RR00400 from the National Institutes of Health, Bethesda, Md.

We acknowledge and thank Mike Boyle of the Department of Cardiopulmonary Services, University of Minnesota, for support in the implementation of this research.

Reprint requests to Department of Psychiatry, Box 393, University of Minnesota, Mayo Memorial Bldg, 420 Delaware St SE, Minneapolis, MN 55455 (Dr Kushner).

REFERENCES

1. Kushner MG, Sher KJ, Beitman BD. The relation between alcohol problems and the anxiety disorders. *Am J Psychiatry.* 1990;147:685-695.
2. Himle JA, Hill EM. Alcohol abuse and the anxiety disorders: evidence from the Epidemiologic Catchment Area Survey. *J Anx Disord.* 1991;5:237-245.
3. Quitkin FM, Rifkin A, Kaplan J, Klein D. Phobic anxiety syndrome complicated by drug dependence and addiction. *Arch Gen Psychiatry.* 1972;27:159-162.
4. Norton GR, Malan J, Cairns SL, Wozney KA, Broughton R. Factors influencing drinking behavior in alcoholic panickers and non-panickers. *Behav Res Ther.* 1989;27:167-171.
5. George DT, Nutt DJ, Dwyer BA, Linnoila M. Alcoholism and panic disorder: is the comorbidity more than coincidence? *Acta Psychiatr Scand.* 1990;81:97-107.
6. Roelofs SM. Hyperventilation, anxiety, craving for alcohol: a subacute alcohol withdrawal syndrome. *Alcohol.* 1985;2:501-505.
7. Merikangas KR, Leckman JF, Prusoff BA, Pauls DL, Weissman MM. Familial transmission of depression and alcoholism. *Arch Gen Psychiatry.* 1985;42: 367-372.
8. Mullaney JA, Trippett CJ. Alcohol dependence and phobias: clinical description and relevance. *Br J Psychiatry.* 1979;135:565-573.
9. Stockwell T, Smail P, Hodgson R, Canter S. Alcohol dependence and phobic anxiety states, II: a retrospective study. *Br J Psychiatry.* 1984;144:58-63.
10. Bibb J, Chambless DL. Alcohol use and abuse among diagnosed agoraphobics. *Behav Res Ther.* 1986;24:49-58.
11. Schuckit MA, Hesselbrock V. Alcohol dependence and anxiety disorders: what is the relationship? *Am J Psychiatry.* 1994;151:1723-1734.
12. Cappell H, Greeley J. Alcohol and tension reduction: an update on research and theory. In: Blane HT, Leonard KE, eds. *Psychological Theories of Drinking and Alcoholism.* New York, NY: Guilford Press; 1987.
13. Sanderson WC, Wetzler S, Asnis GM. Alprazolam blockade of CO_2-provoked panic in patients with panic disorder. *Am J Psychiatry.* 1994;151:1220-1222.
14. Pols H, Zandbergen J, de Loof C, Griez E. Attenuation of carbon dioxide–induced panic after clonazepam treatment. *Acta Psychiatr Scand.* 1991;84: 585-586.
15. Spitzer RL, Williams JBW, Gibbon M, First MB. *Structured Clinical Interview for DSM-III-R-Patient Edition (SCID-P, 9/1/89 Version).* New York, NY: Biometrics Research Department; 1989.
16. Derogatis LR. *Brief Symptom Inventory,* Baltimore, Md: Clinical Psychometric Research; 1975.
17. Spielberger CD, Gorsuch RL, Lushene RE, Vagg P, Jacobs G. *Manual for the State-Trait Anxiety Inventory.* Palo Alto, Calif: Consulting Psychologist Press; 1983.
18. Beck AT, Ward CH, Mendelson M, Mock J, Erbaugh J. An Inventory for measuring depression. *Arch Gen Psychiatry.* 1961;4:561-571.
19. Dillon DJ, Gorman JM, Liebowitz MR, Fyer AJ, Klein DF. Measurement of lactate-induced panic and anxiety. *Psychiatry Res.* 1987;20:97-105.
20. Papp LA, Klein DF, Martinez J, Schneier F, Cole R, Liebowitz MR, Hollander E, Fyer AJ, Jordan F, Gorman JM. Diagnostic and substance specificity of carbon-dioxide–induced panic. *Am J Psychiatry.* 1983;150:250-257.
21. Rapee RM, Brown TA, Antony MM, Barlow DH. Response to hyperventilation and inhalation of 5.5% carbon dioxide enriched air across the *DSM-III-R* anxiety disorders. *J Abnorm Psychol.* 1992;101:538-552.
22. Jones BM. Circadian variation in the effects of alcohol on cognitive performance. *Q J Stud Alcohol.* 1974;35:1212-1219.
23. Jones BM, Jones MK. Alcohol effects in women during the menstrual cycle. *Ann N Y Acad Sci.* 1976;273:576-587.
24. Fisher HR, Simpson RI, Kapur BM. Calculation of blood alcohol concentration (BAC) by sex, weight, number of drinks and time. *Can J Publ Health.* 1987; 78:300-304.
25. Gorman JM, Fyer MR, Goetz R, Askanazi J, Liebowitz MR, Fyer AJ, Kinney J, Klein DF. Ventilatory physiology of patients with panic disorder. *Arch Gen Psychiatry.* 1988;45:31-39.
26. Cohen J, Cohen P. *Applied Multiple Regression/Correlation Analysis for the Behavioral Sciences.* Hillsdale, NJ: L Erlbaum Associates Inc; 1983.
27. Siegel S. *Nonparametric Statistics for the Behavioral Sciences.* New York, NY: McGraw-Hill International Book Co; 1956.
28. Conover WJ, Inman RL. Rank transformations as a bridge between parametric and nonparametric statistics. *Am Statist.* 1981;35:124-133.
29. Rachman SJ, Hodgson RS. Synchrony and desynchrony in fear and avoidance. *Behav Res Ther.* 1974;12:311-318.
30. Sayette MA. Heart rate as an index of stress response in alcohol administration research: a critical review. *Alcohol Clin Exp Res.* 1993;17:802-809.
31. Kirsch I, Rosadino MJ. Do double-blind studies with informed consent yield externally valid results? *Psychopharmacology.* 1993;110:437-442.
32. Kirsch I, Weixel, LJ. Double-blind versus deceptive administration of a placebo. *Behav Neurosci.* 1988;102:319-323.
33. Rohsenow DJ, Marlatt GA. The balanced placebo design: methodological considerations. *Addict Behav.* 1981;6:107-122.
34. National Advisory Council on Alcohol Abuse and Alcoholism. *Recommended Council Guidelines on Ethyl Alcohol Administration in Human Experimentation (Revised June 1989).* Rockville, Md: National Institute on Alcohol Abuse and Alcoholism; 1989.
35. Klein DF. Delineation of two drug-responsive anxiety syndromes. *Psychopharmacologia.* 1964;5:397-408.
36. Gorman JM, Liebowitz MR, Fyer AJ, Stein J. A neuroanatomical hypothesis for panic disorder. *Am J Psychiatry.* 1989;146:148-161.
37. Sanderson WC, Wetzler S. Five percent carbon dioxide challenge: valid analogue and marker of panic disorder? *Biol Psychiatry.* 1990;27:689-701.
38. Barlow DH, Brown TA, Craske MG. Definitions of panic attacks and panic disorder in the *DSM-IV:* implications for research. *J Abnorm Psychol.* 1994;103: 553-564.
39. Ballenger JC, Burrows GD, Dupont RL, Lesser I, Noyes R, Pecknold J, Riskin A, Swinson R. Alprazolam in panic disorder and agoraphobia: results from a multicenter trial. *Arch Gen Psychitry.* 1988;45:413-422.
40. Gray J. Drug effects on fear and frustration: possible limbic site of action of minor tranquilizers. In: Iverson LL, Snyder SD, eds. *Handbook of Psychopharmacology.* New York, NY: Plenum Press; 1977:433-529.
41. Noestoros J. Ethanol specifically potentiates GABA mediated neurotransmission in feline cerebral cortex. *Science.* 1980;209:708-710.
42. Levenson RW, Oyama ON, Meek PS. Greater reinforcement from alcohol for those at risk: parental risk, personality risk, and sex. *J Abnorm Psychol.* 1987; 96:242-253.
43. Hull JG. A self-awareness model of the causes and effects of alcohol consumption. *J Abnorm Psychol.* 1981;90:586-600.
44. Baron DH, Sands BF, Ciraulo DA, Shader RI. The diagnoses and treatment of panic disorder in alcoholics: three cases. *Am J Drug Alcohol Abuse.* 1990;16: 287-295.
45. Marks I. *Cure and Care of Neuroses: Theory and Practice of Behavioral Psychotherapy.* New York, NY: John Wiley & Sons Inc; 1981.
46. Nunes EV, McGrath PJ, Quitkin FM, Stewart JP, Harrison W, Tricamo E, Ocepek-Welikson K. Imipramine treatment of alcoholism with comorbid depression. *Am J Psychiatry.* 1993;150:963-965.
47. Stockwell T, Hodgson R, Rankin H. Tension reduction and the effects of prolonged alcohol consumption. *Br J Addict.* 1982;77:65-73.
48. Cloninger CR. Neurogenic adoptive mechanisms in alcoholism. *Science.* 1987; 236:410-416.
49. Cooper ML, Russel M, Skinner JB, Frone MR, Mudar P. Stress and alcohol use: moderating effects of gender coping, and alcohol expectancies. *J Abnorm Psychol.* 1992;101:139-152.

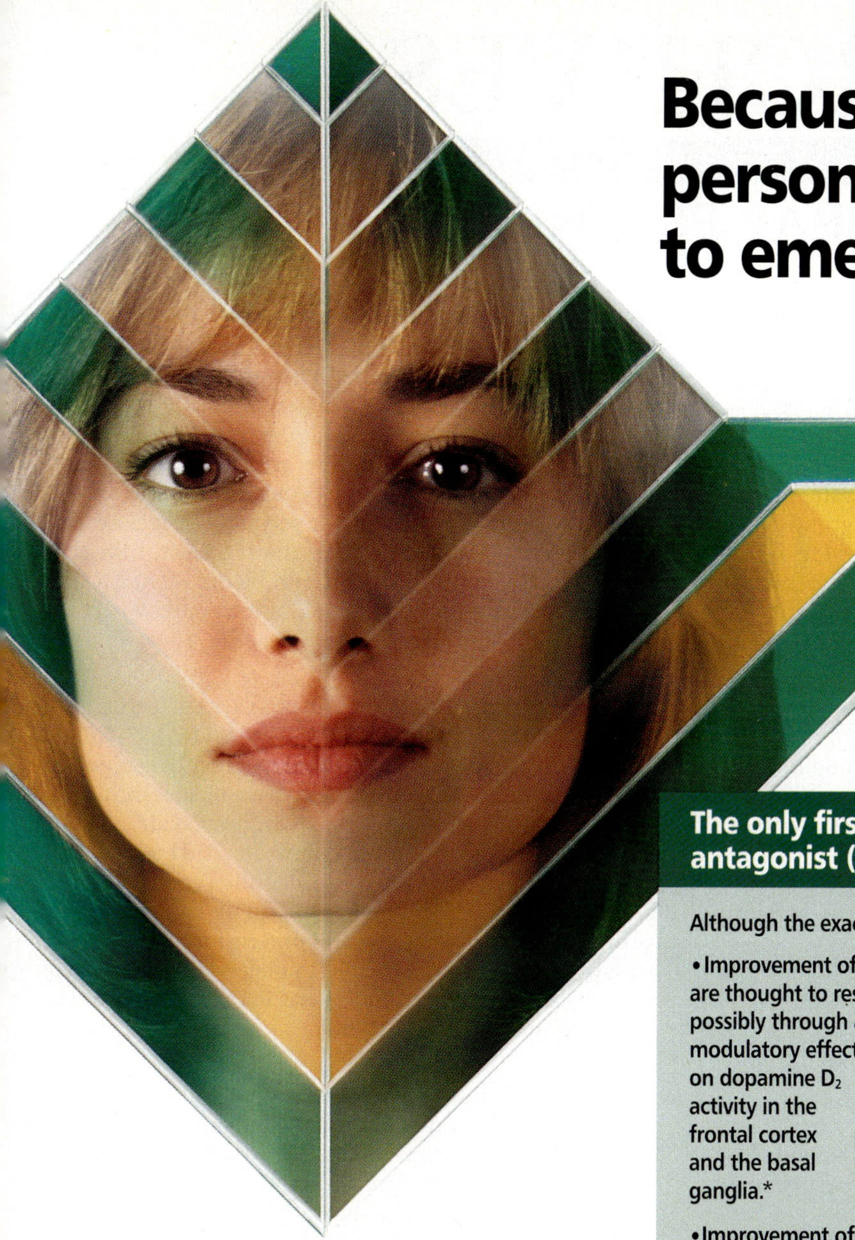

Because a whole person is waiting to emerge.

The only first-choice serotonin/dopamine antagonist (SDA).

Although the exact mechanism of action is unknown:

- Improvement of negative symptoms and lessened risk of EPS are thought to result from blockade of serotonin 5-HT_2 receptors, possibly through a modulatory effect on dopamine D_2 activity in the frontal cortex and the basal ganglia.*
- Improvement of positive symptoms is thought to result from blockade of dopamine D_2 receptors in the limbic system.*

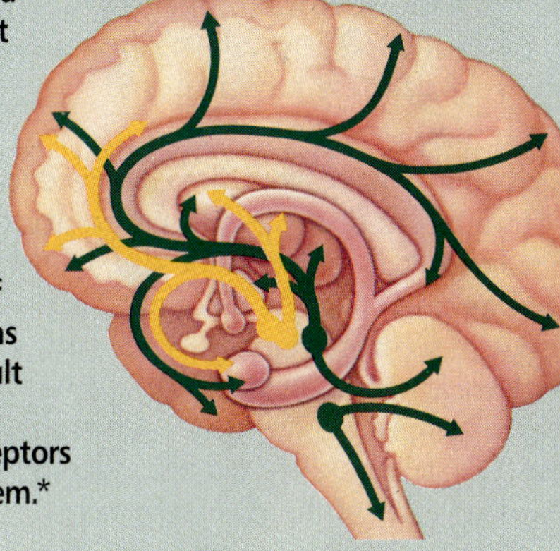

Dopaminergic system   Serotoninergic system

1-, 2-, 3-, 4-mg tablets

Risperdal®
RISPERIDONE

A first choice in psychosis.

*Ereshefsky L, Lacombe S. Pharmacological profile of risperidone. *Can J Psychiatry.* 1993;38(Suppl 3):S80-S88.

Please see the brief summary of Prescribing Information adjacent to this ad.

 JPI-RS-123D

JANSSEN · PHARMACEUTICA · RESEARCH FOUNDATION · SmithKline Beecham Pharmaceuticals

Persons et al (page 283) review recent practice guidelines' assessments of the role of psychotherapy in the treatment of major depression in adults. The guidelines were published by the American Psychiatric Association (APA) and by the Depression Guideline Panel of the Agency for Health Care Policy and Research (AHCPR). They argue that the APA guideline understates the value of cognitive, behavioral, brief psychodynamic, and group therapies and that both guidelines understate the value of psychotherapy alone in the treatment of more severely depressed outpatients.

Four commentaries on the two practice guidelines are included in this issue (pages 291, 298, 301, and 303).

Geriatric depression often occurs simultaneously with medical and neurological disorders, which may influence its outcome and complicate the prescription of antidepressant treatment. **Alexopoulos et al** (page 305) compared the recovery rates of elderly and younger patients with major depression. Their findings challenge the view that geriatric depression has a worse outcome than depression of younger adults. However, patients with depression whose first episode occurred in late life may be at higher risk of chronicity. Some clinicians prematurely reduce the amount of antidepressants prescribed prior to the complete recovery of these patients.

Tardive dyskinesia (TD) is believed to be caused by antipsychotic drugs. However, prior reports indicate that it may also be due to the disease process. **Chakos et al** (page 313) found that patients, in their first episode of schizophrenia who developed TD with drug treatment were more severely ill and had poorer prognoses than patients who did not develop TD. This suggests that TD vulnerability may be related to the particular form or severity of the disease process.

Dysregulation of the neuroendocrine "stress" hypothalamic-pituitary-adrenal (HPA) axis is observed in depression and may play a role in the pathophysiologic processes of panic disorder. **Abelson et al** (page 323) assessed corticotropin and cortisol secretion over 24 hours and found subtle abnormalities in HPA axis activity in patients with panic disorder. Patients had elevated overnight cortisol levels, but stress axis activity was modulated by illness severity and treatment seeking. Further research is needed to determine whether these abnormalities represent causes, consequences, or epiphenomena of the disorder.

Homeless families embody two generations at risk of mental health problems and limited access to care. **Zima et al** (page 332) found that 72% of homeless mothers reported having high psychological distress, a probable lifetime major mental illness, or a substance abuse disorder; yet only 15% had ever received mental health services. Compared with the general population, homeless mothers had a greater unmet need for services. Mothers with a probable mental disorder were also more likely to have children with depression or behavior problems. Mental health services for both generations should be integrated with housing services and primary care.

Mental illness is likely to be a cause of teen suicide and of recent increases in suicide rates among young men. **Shaffer et al** (page 339) interviewed parents and friends of more than 120 teen suicides and a similar number of controls. Long-standing psychiatric disturbance, most commonly a mood disorder, had been present in 90% of the suicides. In boys, it was often combined with substance or alcohol abuse. Screening for these disorders may provide an effective approach to prevention; the high rate of substance and alcohol abuse in male suicides may provide a clue to the cause of increases in that group over the past 3 decades.

Johnson et al (page 350) report that the presence of personality disorders predicted onset of axis I disorders and serious functional impairment in a community sample of homosexual men with and at risk of human immunodeficiency virus (HIV) infection, after HIV status and lifetime psychiatric history were controlled statistically. These findings indicate that homosexual men with personality disorders may be at risk for onset of Axis I disorders and serious impairment.

The speech of people with schizophrenia and mania is often difficult to understand. **Docherty et al** (page 358) developed a "natural language" measure to assess type and severity of communication disturbances in speech and applied it to speech samples from manic, schizophrenic, and nonpsychiatric subjects. The schizophrenic and manic subjects showed higher frequencies of six different types of communication failures than the controls. The proportions of different types of unclarity differed among the diagnostic groups. This new measure may be helpful in describing differences in communication disturbances among individuals and in elucidating cognitive weaknesses underlying psychotic communication failures.

The Role of Psychotherapy in the Treatment of Depression

Review of Two Practice Guidelines

Jacqueline B. Persons, PhD; Michael E. Thase, MD; Paul Crits-Christoph, PhD

We review two recent practice guidelines' assessments of the role of psychotherapy in the treatment of major depression in adults. We examine the practice guideline published by the American Psychiatric Association (APA) and that published by the Depression Guideline Panel of the Agency for Health Care Policy and Research. We focus on the guidelines' evaluations of psychotherapies, their statements about the role of psychotherapy in first-line treatment of depression, and the procedures they recommend for choosing among psychotherapies. We argue that the APA guideline understates the value of cognitive, behavioral, brief psychodynamic, and group therapies. Both guidelines understate the value of psychotherapy alone in the treatment of more severely depressed outpatients. The APA guideline overvalues the role of combined psychotherapy-pharmacotherapy regimens, particularly in view of the greater cost of this strategy. The APA guideline also makes recommendations about choosing among psychotherapies that are not well supported by empirical evidence. We conclude with some guidelines for guideline development.

(Arch Gen Psychiatry. 1996;53:283-290)

Practice guidelines have enormous potential. They are expected to directly affect the behavior of practicing clinicians. They are likely to be adopted by managed care and insurance companies and may be used in malpractice lawsuits and other litigation to establish standards of care. Therefore, it is essential that practice guidelines provide a balanced, up-to-date review of what is known about effective treatment.

In 1993, practice guidelines for the treatment of depression were published by the American Psychiatric Association (APA)[1] and by the Depression Guideline Panel of the Agency for Health Care Policy and Research (AHCPR).[2] The APA guideline addressed the treatment of depression by psychiatrists, and the AHCPR guideline addressed the treatment of depression in primary care.

From the Department of Psychiatry, University of California at San Francisco, and Center for Cognitive Therapy, Oakland, Calif (Dr Persons); Western Psychiatric Institute and Clinic, Department of Psychiatry, University of Pittsburgh School of Medicine, Pa (Dr Thase); and Department of Psychiatry, University of Pennsylvania, Philadelphia (Dr Crits-Christoph).

Both guidelines have many strengths. However, we argue that the APA guideline undervalues the efficacy of cognitive therapy (CT), behavior therapy (BT), brief psychodynamic psychotherapy, and group therapies. To support our thesis, we review both guidelines' assessments of these psychotherapies. We also examine both guidelines' statements about the role of psychotherapy in the first-line treatment of depression. We argue that both guidelines understate the value of psychotherapy alone in the treatment of more severely depressed outpatients. In addition, the APA guideline overvalues the use of combined psychotherapy-pharmacotherapy regimens. Finally, we argue that the APA guideline makes recommendations about choosing among pyschotherapies that are not well supported by the available empirical evidence. We preface our discussion with an examination of the methods of evaluation used to write the two guidelines, and we conclude with a brief discussion of the limitations of controlled trials and some guidelines for future guideline development.

METHODS OF EVALUATION

The AHCPR Clinical Practice Guideline was written by the Depression Guideline Panel, a 12-member multidisciplinary group chaired by A. John Rush, MD. Each section of the guideline was informed by a report prepared by an expert in the field. One of us (M.E.T.) wrote two reviews for the AHCPR document: on monoamine oxidase inhibitor therapy and on treatment-resistant depression. Each report provided a comprehensive literature review and, when possible, a quantitative meta-analysis of the relevant treatment outcome literature. To assist with the literature reviews and meta-analyses, the Depression Guideline Panel provided computerized literature searches and biostatistical consultation.

See also pages 291, 298, 301, and 303

The APA document was written by a work group of six psychiatrists chaired by T. Byram Karasu, MD. Most members of the work group were experts in at least one area pertaining to mood disorders, and Dr Karasu is a prominent figure in the area of psychotherapy. The work group conducted a literature search covering the period 1971 through 1991 but did not conduct meta-analyses. The work group also sought input from over 140 psychiatrists and from two nonpsychiatrist experts in psychotherapy research (Irene Elkin, PhD, and Myrna Weissman, PhD). Comments were also solicited from over 36 mental health organizations.

EVALUATIONS OF THE PSYCHOTHERAPIES

Cognitive Therapy

The AHCPR panel examined 22 acute-phase randomized controlled trials of CT in adult or geriatric patients and conducted a meta-analysis to estimate the effects of each treatment. When CT was compared with other acute-phase treatments, the panel concluded that

> Overall, cognitive therapy was similar in efficacy to all other psychotherapies taken together . . . Compared to medication alone, cognitive therapy had a slight advantage.[2(p 76)]

In contrast, the APA guideline states,

> There is some evidence that cognitive therapy reduces depressive symptoms during the acute phase of less severe, nonmelancholic forms of major depression,[3] but not significantly differently from pill placebo coupled with clinical management.[4]1(p 5)

(The references cited *within* quotes from both the AHCPR and APA guidelines are those that appear in the guidelines' reference lists; they are bracketed here and renumbered to follow the sequence of references in our article.)

When compared with the AHCPR guideline's meta-analytic evaluation, the APA guideline's review underestimates the efficacy of CT. The APA guideline's statement that "there is some evidence that cognitive therapy reduces depressive symptoms . . . , but not significantly differently from pill placebo . . . " does not, in our view, reflect a balanced assessment of the available empirical evidence. The statement that CT does not differ significantly from pill placebo coupled with clinical management is based on results from a single, albeit quite important, study (the Treatment of Depression Collaborative Research Program [TDCRP][4]) and ignores the results of a number of other studies. For example, controlled studies have found CT's efficacy to be comparable or superior to pharmacotherapy (as conducted by psychiatrists),[3-8] interpersonal therapy (IPT),[4] BT,[9-11] behavioral marital therapy,[12,13] and short-term psychodynamic psychotherapy.[9,10] (The study by Hollon et al[6] had not been published at the time the APA guideline was written, and it was apparently not included in the AHCPR review either, even though results from the follow-up phase of this study were cited in both practice guidelines.) In addition, four of five studies conducted in the United Kingdom showed that CT was statistically significantly more effective than treatment-as-usual or protocol pharmacotherapy provided by general practitioners.[14-17] Two meta-analyses have documented CT's efficacy when compared with waiting-list, alternate psychotherapeutic or pharmacotherapy control conditions.[18,19] The APA guideline's statement that CT "reduces depressive symptoms" does not convey clearly that empirical studies consistently document *remission* rates following CT that are comparable to those following pharmacotherapy.

Behavior Therapy

The AHCPR guideline states,

> In the panel's analysis, the overall efficacy of behavioral therapy was 55.3 percent. Compared to wait-list, behavioral therapy was 17.1 percent more effective; compared to all other forms of psychotherapy, behavioral therapy was 9.1 percent more effective. Compared to medication alone, it was 23.9 percent more effective. [This figure measures the proportion of patients assigned to the treatment who stayed in treatment and improved.][2(p 78)]

The APA guideline states,

> Behavior therapy has been reported to be effective in the acute treatment of patients with mild to moderately severe depressions, especially when combined with pharmacotherapy.[9,20-23]1(p 5)

The APA guideline states that BT is most effective when combined with medications. However, the research cited in the guideline does not support this assertion: none of the studies cited even included a combined BT and pharmacotherapy condition! We are aware of only three empirical studies that do examine this question directly.[24-26] Two[25,26] of the three trials did report more *rapid* improvement for patients receiving combined treatment, but there were no statistically significant differences between BT and combined treatment at posttreatment in any of the studies.

Brief Psychodynamic Psychotherapy

The AHCPR guideline states,

> The acute effects of brief dynamic psychotherapy were investigated in seven randomized controlled trials[9,10,20,24,27-29] of which six could be metaalyzed . . . The overall efficacy of brief dynamic psychotherapy in these six studies was 34.8 percent. Compared to other therapies, brief dynamic psychotherapy may be

slightly less effective. Compared to medication, it was 8.4 percent more effective.[2(p 81)]

The APA guideline states,

> Brief psychodynamic psychotherapy may be used in the acute-phase treatment of depression, especially as an adjunct to pharmacologic treatment. The efficacy of brief psychodynamic psychotherapy as a single modality in the treatment of major depression has not been conclusively demonstrated by controlled studies; although it has been shown to be more effective than a waiting list control,[9] the latter is considered a less than satisfactory control condition. Its effectiveness in comparison to other psychotherapeutic approaches requires further research. Research on combined pharmacotherapy and brief psychodynamic psychotherapy[30,31] is equally sparse and inconclusive.[1(p 5)]

We concur with the AHCPR guideline's statement that brief dynamic therapy may have a slightly weaker overall effect than other therapies and with the AHCPR's outline of the limitations of available studies of brief psychodynamic psychotherapy that may have weakened its effects in the research trials. These limitations include the fact that most studies were of group, not individual, treatment; therapy generally was not procedurally specified; and most of the investigators were aligned with another mode of psychotherapy.

We agree with the APA guideline's statement that the efficacy of brief psychodynamic psychotherapy has not been "conclusively demonstrated." Nevertheless, the APA guideline does not, in our view, present a full and balanced review of the evidence of the efficacy of brief psychodynamic psychotherapy. The APA guideline's evaluation of brief dynamic therapy is incomplete in its assessment of the efficacy data, and its recommendation that the therapy is best used in conjunction with medication is not supported by any empirical evidence.

The APA guideline cites the study[9] of depressed elders as showing that brief dynamic therapy is superior to a waiting-list control, but it fails to mention that, in this study, brief dynamic therapy did not differ significantly from cognitive and behavioral treatments for depression, two modalities that have received more extensive empirical support. Additional evidence supporting the efficacy of brief psychodynamic therapy is available from a study by Hersen et al,[24] in which brief dynamic therapy practiced by experienced clinicians (without the benefit of a treatment manual) produced significant improvements in the depressive symptoms of unipolar depression in women. In fact, outcome of brief dynamic therapy was not statistically significantly different from amitriptyline hydrochloride treatment, social skills training, or social skills training plus amitriptyline treatment. This study also included a 6-month continuation phase and showed that monthly sessions of dynamic therapy achieved the same outcome as continuation therapy with amitriptyline. Inferences from the study by Hersen et al are limited by the fact that patients in the dynamic therapy and social skills training conditions also received a pill placebo.

The statement in the APA guideline that brief dynamic therapy is especially useful as an adjunct to medication is not supported by *any* empirical evidence. Neither of the studies cited by the APA guideline (Daneman[30] and Covi et al[31]) found evidence of a significant additive effect for the combination of brief dynamic therapy and pharmacotherapy on reduction of depressive symptoms or remission rates.

Group Therapy

The AHCPR guideline did not specifically review group therapy. However, it did compare the efficacy of group and individual forms of BT and CT using meta-analysis and found that group and individual BT did not differ in effectiveness, whereas individual CT was slightly superior to group CT.

The APA guideline states,

> The role of group therapy in the treatment of depression is based on clinical experience rather than on systematic controlled studies.[1(p 6)]

This statement by the APA guideline ignores a very large body of published outcome studies of various forms of group therapy. Perhaps the APA guideline's conceptualization of group therapy was restricted to traditional "process"-oriented groups, which have not been studied extensively. If cognitive, behavioral, and other newer approaches to group therapy are included in the review, a large number of published empirical studies are available. While it is true that many are small studies of restricted samples (eg, women only) or use less rigorous methods (eg, patients were not required to meet *DSM-III*[32] criteria for major depression), the results of these studies are nevertheless fairly consistent.

Group behavior therapy and group CT have repeatedly been shown to produce statistically significant changes in depressive symptoms.[15,17,23,27,29,33-39] In two studies,[15,17] group CT was statistically significantly more effective than treatment as usual provided by general practitioners.

Other Psychotherapies

Although we are critical of the APA guideline's reviews of cognitive, behavioral, brief psychodynamic, and group therapies, we find that more balanced reviews are presented for IPT and marital and/or family therapy. The APA and AHCPR practice guidelines' conclusions for IPT and marital and/or family therapy are essentially in agreement. In fact, when compared with the APA guideline's assessments of the other time-limited therapies, APA's reviews of IPT and marital and/or family therapy are relatively positive. For example, the failure of IPT to surpass the placebo-clinical management condition in the TDCRP is not mentioned in the APA guideline. Similarly, the APA guideline notes, on the basis of a single study, that successful couples therapy may reduce the risk of depressive relapse; in contrast, the much more intensively studied long-term effects of CT and BT are described as inconclusive.

To their credit, both treatment guidelines clearly state that no data from controlled outcome studies support the efficacy of long-term psychodynamic psychotherapy or psychoanalysis in the treatment of depression in adults. In view of the fact that long-term psychodynamic theory was a dominant paradigm in psychiatry for decades, these are forthright and responsible statements. The AHCPR guideline extends this statement to point out that no data from controlled outcome studies support the efficacy of *any* form of long-term psychotherapy for depression.

The guidelines' reviews of supportive psychotherapy, a widely used modality, are unclear. The AHCPR acknowledges (correctly) that supportive psychotherapy has not been studied in randomized controlled trials but asserts that "a closely related therapy, IPT, has been specifically designed for depressed patients and formally tested."[1(p 87)] We doubt that most practitioners of interpersonal therapy would consider it to be "closely related" to supportive therapy. The APA provides a relatively lengthy description of supportive therapy but does not point out that its efficacy has not been demonstrated in controlled studies.

ROLE OF PSYCHOTHERAPY IN FIRST-LINE TREATMENT FOR DEPRESSION

The recommendations about first-line treatment made by both guidelines raise two issues: the issue of severity and the issue of combined pharmacotherapy-psychotherapy regimens. We discuss each in turn.

Severity

The AHCPR guideline makes the following recommendations about first-line treatment:

> Patients with moderate to severe major depressive disorder are appropriately treated with medication, whether or not formal psychotherapy is also used.[2(p 39)]

and

> Patients with mild to moderate major depression who prefer psychotherapy alone as the initial acute treatment choice may be treated with this option.[2(p 40)]

The APA guideline recommends,

> Most patients are best treated with antidepressant medication coupled with psychotherapeutic management or psychotherapy [II]. Some patients with mild to moderate degrees of impairment may be treated with psychotherapeutic management or psychotherapy alone . . .[1(pp 19-20)]

[Roman numeral II codes recommendations based on "moderate clinical confidence."[1(p 19)]]

The two guidelines concur in the recommendation that severely depressed patients should receive pharmacotherapy (with or without psychotherapy) and that only some mildly to moderately depressed patients ought to receive psychotherapy alone. Although some studies support the recommendation that only mildly to moderately depressed outpatients ought to receive psychotherapy alone, others do not. Thus, we believe that the empirical evidence on this question is more mixed than both practice guidelines' recommendations indicate.

Certainly, there is voluminous evidence that endogenously depressed outpatients or severely depressed inpatients benefit from pharmacotherapy.[2] By contrast, there is virtually no evidence that psychotherapy is an effective, principal treatment of psychotic depression or depression in inpatients. In a recent study of 30 unmedicated depressed inpatients who were treated for up to 4 weeks with daily CT, Thase[40] found a significantly poorer outcome in patients with Hamilton Rating Scale for Depression (HAM-D) scores of 25 or greater and/or patients with hypercortisolemia.

However, when depressed outpatients are examined, the evidence relating psychotherapy outcome to severity of depression is not so clearcut. Some data support the guidelines' assertions that more severely depressed patients benefit less from psychotherapy alone than do less severely depressed patients. In a recent analysis of the outcome of a large series of depressed outpatients treated with CT alone (n=129), IPT alone (n=112), or IPT plus pharmacotherapy (n=352), Thase et al[41] found a significant treatment type by severity interaction. Among patients with pretreatment HAM-D scores of 20 or greater, psychotherapy alone and combined IPT-pharmacotherapy regimens were equally effective. By contrast, in the more severe subgroup, combined IPT-pharmacotherapy regimens were statistically significantly more effective than CT or IPT alone. In their meta-analytic review, Robinson et al[19] found a modest, inverse relationship between pretreatment severity and response to a diverse group of time-limited psychotherapies.

However, other studies do not support the notion that more severely depressed patients benefit less from psychotherapy than do less severely depressed patients. Data from the TDCRP on this question are mixed. In the TDCRP,[4] a pretreatment HAM-D score of 20 or greater was used to identify a more severe subgroup. Consistent with the guidelines' recommendations, active drug treatment was statistically significantly more effective than both placebo plus clinical management and CT. However, contrary to both guidelines' conclusions, more severely depressed patients who received IPT did not differ in outcome from those who received active drug treatment.

Using the same definition of severity as the TDCRP, Hollon et al[6] found that CT and pharmacotherapy were equally effective treatments of severely depressed outpatients (this study was apparently published too late for review by the APA). McLean and Taylor[42] also failed to find a difference in response to BT or amitriptyline treatment associated with severity in a reanalysis of the 1979 report by McLean and Hakstian.[20]

The construct of endogeneity overlaps significantly with symptomatic severity.[43,44] Both practice guidelines recommend that melancholic (endogenous) depressions should be treated with pharmacotherapy instead of, or in combination with, psychotherapy.

Some studies support this recommendation. Using the more inclusive Research Diagnostic Criteria definition of endogenous depression, Prusoff et al[45] and Gallagher and Thompson[46] found poorer response to psychotherapy (IPT and a pooled grouping of dynamic, cognitive, and behavioral treatments, respectively) in patients with endogenous depression compared with patients with nonendogenous cases. In a reanalysis of the data from a clinical trial by Thase et al,[47] amitriptyline (either alone or with BT) was significantly more effective than a combined grouping of BT and dynamic therapy plus placebo. Melancholic patients were also significantly more likely to drop out of this study unless their treatment included active pharmacotherapy.[48] McKnight et al[7] similarly reported that melancholic patients had a poorer response to CT than nonmelancholics. However, these investigators also found poorer response to amitriptyline treatment in melancholics than in nonmelancholics.

We are not aware of any published prospective studies using the more restrictive diagnosis of melancholia that report a positive response to psychotherapy. However, other studies using the broader Research Diagnostic Criteria definition have not found a relationship between outcome and a clinical diagnosis of endogenous depression in studies of IPT,[49] CT,[5,6,49-52] or BT.[53]

In summary, while there is evidence in support of both practice guidelines' recommendation to limit use of psychotherapy alone to mild-to-moderate episodes of depression, empirical support for this recommendation is hardly uniform. We recommend that psychotherapy alone be considered a treatment option for more severely depressed outpatients who wish to pursue it and who are able to work productively in therapy. To restrict the use of CT, BT, or IPT to only "some outpatients with mild-to-moderate" depressions appears to overstate the relationship between severity and psychotherapy response. We fully agree with the AHCPR recommendation to reconsider use of pharmacotherapy if patients are not responding after 6 to 12 weeks of treatment with psychotherapy alone.

Combined Treatment

The APA guideline recommends that,

> Most patients are best treated with antidepressant medication coupled with psychotherapeutic management or psychotherapy [II].[1(pp 19-20)]

In this statement, the APA guideline seems to recommend combined pharmacotherapy-psychotherapy regimens for most patients. We use the term *seems* because there is some ambiguity in the APA's recommendation (this itself is a problem). Perhaps when the APA recommends coupling antidepressant medication with "psychotherapeutic management," it is referring to the standard monitoring and education that accompany any competently administered drug treatment. Our careful reading of the document, however, suggests that the APA is referring to a more intensive adjunct treatment. The term *psychotherapeutic management* refers, the guideline states, to a type of psychotherapy "sometimes referred to as 'supportive psychotherapy.'"[1(p 4)] The detailed description of the therapy indicates that it is more extensive than would ordinarily be provided by psychopharmacologists.

In contrast, the AHCPR guideline recommends combined pharmacotherapy-psychotherapy regimens only for certain cases, stating,

> Combined treatment may have an advantage for patients with partial responses to either treatment alone (if adequately administered) and for those with a more chronic history or poor interepisode recovery. However, combined treatment may provide no unique advantage for patients with uncomplicated, nonchronic major depressive disorder.[2(p 41)]

When the two guidelines' recommendations about the use of combined treatment are compared, we find the approach taken by the AHCPR to have firmer empirical support. In fact, the evidence comparing combined treatment (pharmacotherapy plus psychotherapy) to either modality alone provides little support for the APA's recommendation that most patients need combined treatment.

Several published studies support the APA guideline's assertion that combined pharmacotherapy-psychotherapy regimens are superior to treatment with a single modality. Blackburn et al[5] found that while CT and combined treatment (CT plus antidepressant medication) did not differ in efficacy for depressed patients treated in general practice settings, the combined treatment was more effective than CT alone in their more chronically ill psychiatric clinic subsample. Interpretation of this study is limited by the inefficacy of pharmacotherapy in the general practice setting. Weissman et al[54] found combined treatment to be superior to both amitriptyline alone and IPT alone at posttreatment. As reviewed earlier, two reports[25,26] found that depressed patients who received BT in combination with antidepressants improved more *rapidly* than those receiving BT alone, but combined treatment was not more effective by the completion of the therapy protocol. Finally, in a pooled analysis of six studies in which patients were treated with either psychotherapy alone (CT or IPT) or combined treatment (antidepressants plus IPT), Thase et al[41] found a trend in favor of the combined treatment condition, with a significant advantage for combined treatment in the more severely depressed subgroup of patients.

However, an even larger number of studies has found little or no benefit for combined psychotherapy-pharmacotherapy regimens compared with single modalities[6-8,24,27,30,31,52] For example, Hollon et al[6] found that CT plus imipramine was statistically significantly superior to imipramine alone on some measures (ie, the Depression Subscale of the Minnesota Multiphasic Personality Inventory and Raskin) but not others (ie, HAM-D or Beck Depression Inventory); CT plus imipramine was not statistically significantly different from cognitive behavior therapy alone on any outcome measure. Two longer-term studies also found no prophylactic advantage for the combination of IPT and pharmacotherapy compared with pharmacotherapy alone as either a continuation therapy[55] or maintenance-phase treatment.[56]

In meta-analyses, Conte et al[57] and the AHCPR[2] concluded that combined psychotherapy-pharmacotherapy regimens were only slightly superior to psychotherapy alone or pharmacotherapy alone. Hollon et al,[58] Persons,[59] and Manning and Frances[60] drew similar conclusions in qualitative reviews.

We conclude that although some empirical evidence supports the notion that combined treatment is more effective than single-modality treatment, the evidence is not strong enough to warrant the recommendation made by the APA guideline, particularly in view of the increased cost of this treatment strategy. The AHCPR came to essentially the same conclusion we did.

CHOOSING AMONG PSYCHOTHERAPIES

When psychotherapy alone is used as the first-line treatment, the AHCPR offers a single guideline for choosing among therapies:

> Since it has not been established that all forms of psychotherapy are equally effective in major depressive disorder, if one is chosen as the sole treatment, it should have been studied in randomized controlled trials.[2(p 84)]

Extrapolating from this principle, the AHCPR guideline states that

> Long-term therapies are not currently indicated as first-line acute phase treatments for patients with major depressive disorder.[2(p 84)]

The APA guideline points out that differential efficacy of the various psychotherapies has not been established, and it offers a detailed statement about how the clinician might choose among available psychotherapies, stating,

> The *psychosocial therapeutic program* may range from psychotherapeutic management [supportive psychotherapy] to one of a number of forms of systematic psychotherapy. The approach most congruent with the patient's needs should be chosen. The differential efficacies of and the indications for the various psychotherapies have not been fully established by formal studies. Interpersonal therapy may be suited for individuals who have experienced recent interpersonal conflicts or difficult role transitions [II]. Cognitive therapy may be used for those who desire and/or tolerate structured guidance to correct their distorted concepts of themselves and others [II]. The psychodynamic approach or psychoanalysis may be used in the presence of chronic self-underestimation, excessive self-expectations, chronic interpersonal conflicts, or unresolved early losses or separations, if the patient is inclined to be introspective, psychologically minded, and motivated and has a stable environment [II]. Marital, family, behavior, and group therapies may also be used [II].[1(p 20)]

In these statements, the APA guideline recommends with equal confidence therapies that have little or no empirical evidence of efficacy (eg, supportive psychotherapy and psychoanalysis) and therapies that are supported by significant amounts of efficacy data (eg, BT, CT, and IPT). The assertion by both guidelines that one type of psychotherapy has generally not been shown to be superior to another is empirically justified. However, psychotherapies differ considerably in the degree to which they are supported by empirical evidence, and it is disappointing that those differences are not reflected in the APA's recommendations about selecting psychotherapies.

Instead, the APA guideline seems to rely on what has been called the matching hypothesis, the notion that the most effective therapy for a patient is one that matches the patient's areas of difficulty and the areas of functioning emphasized by the therapy. Thus, patients with distorted attitudes and beliefs are proposed to benefit most from CT, and those with interpersonal difficulties are presumed to benefit most from IPT. However, little evidence supports the matching hypothesis, and several studies contradict it.[33,49,61-67] For example, patients with high levels of distorted cognitions and/or dysfunctional attitudes respond *less* favorably to CT than do patients with lower levels of cognitive distortion![49,61,64-66] Similarly, patients with marked interpersonal difficulties may be less responsive to IPT.[49]

SUMMARY AND CONCLUSIONS

The two practice guidelines reviewed here are laudable first efforts. However, like others,[68] we argue that psychotherapy deserves greater weight in the description of treatment options for major depression.

In the review of the two guidelines presented here, we agree more often with the AHCPR guideline than with the APA guideline. We believe that this is because the AHCPR took a more empirical approach to its task than did the APA. The AHCPR explicitly stated its intent to "focus on randomized controlled clinical trials as the highest level of credible evidence for treatment efficacy."[2(p 8)] It undertook a massive literature review and, when feasible, conducted meta-analyses that formed the basis for its recommendations. In fact, our major area of disagreement with the AHCPR guideline, namely, its recommendations about the use of psychotherapy in more severe depressions, deals with an issue for which a quantitative meta-anlysis was not completed. The APA also undertook a literature review but, as we argued above, did not rely consistently on the empirical literature in developing its guideline.

Limitations of Controlled Clinical Trials

Although our critique of the AHCPR and APA practice guidelines emphasizes the importance of controlled clinical trials, several limitations of controlled trials deserve mention. First, most clinical trials enroll only a minority of the patients who are screened for participation; patients are typically excluded if they have significant psychiatric or medical comorbid conditions, as do many, if not most, depressed patients. Clinical trials are limited, of course, to patients who will accept random assignment to treatment condition. Differential attrition and the fidelity with which treatments are administered can influence the results of a controlled trial. Even powerful statistical techniques, such as meta-analysis, can obscure the impact of systematic biases in patient selection.

Second, epidemiologic data indicate that most depressed people do not seek treatment in a psychiatric setting. Thus, clinical trials conducted in psychiatric research centers are skewed by their enrollment of "convenience" samples. Third, the findings of individual clinical trials must be interpreted cautiously. Even studies with 30 to 40 subjects per condition lack the statistical power to deter small, but clinically meaningful, differences between treatments, let alone interactions between treatment and patient characteristics, for example. Despite these weaknesses (and others), we view controlled clinical trials as the most objective means available for assessing treatment efficacy.

Guidelines for Guideline Development

Based on our review of the AHCPR and APA practice guidelines for treatment of depression, we offer several recommendations for future guideline development.

First, as we have emphasized throughout, we recommend that future practice guidelines give the highest priority to controlled clinical trials. More concretely, we recommend that the review of each treatment alternative include a comprehensive, quantitative review of the available empirical outcome evidence or a clear statement that no efficacy data are available.

Second, we recommend that practice guidelines be written by multidisciplinary panels. Input from several disciplines will reduce biases arising from intellectual or practice traditions in any one discipline. This is particularly important in view of the fact that most of the clinical trials examining efficacy of psychotherapy have been conducted by psychologists. The procedure used by the APA (professionals representing one discipline wrote the draft guideline and then asked for comments from reviewers from other disciplines) did not, in our view, adequately protect the guideline from bias.

Third, we recommend that future practice guidelines include some discussion of cost; an argument can be made that treatment quality cannot be evaluated independently of its cost.

Finally, we recommend that practice guidelines be revised periodically so that new research findings can be incorporated in a timely manner. The process of guideline development should be seen as continuing past the point of publication, so that comments, criticisms, and suggestions for revision are welcomed on an ongoing basis.

Accepted for publication August 25, 1995.

This work was supported in part by grants MH50367 (Dr Persons), MH-30915 (Clinical Research Center), and MH-41884 (Dr Thase) from the National Institute of Mental Health, Rockville, Md, and grants DA-07673 and DA-08541 from the National Institute on Drug Abuse, Rockville, Md (Dr Thase).

The authors thank Irene Elkin, PhD, Ellen Frank, PhD, David J. Kupfer, MD, Peter Lewinsohn, PhD, and K. Daniel O'Leary, PhD, for their helpful comments, and Andrew Bertagnolli for his assistance with library work.

Reprint requests to Center for Cognitive Therapy, 5435 College Ave, Suite 102, Oakland, CA 94618-1502 (Dr Persons).

REFERENCES

1. American Psychiatric Association. Practice guideline for major depressive disorder in adults. *Am J Psychiatry.* 1993;150(suppl4):1-26.
2. Depression Guideline Panel. *Clinical Practice Guideline Number 5: Depression in Primary Care, 2: Treatment of Major Depression.* Rockville, Md: US Dept of Health and Human Services, Agency for Health Care Policy and Research; 1993. AHCPR publication 93-0551.
3. Rush AJ, Beck AT, Kovacs M, Hollon S. Comparative efficacy of cognitive therapy and pharmacotherapy in the treatment of depressed outpatients. *Cognit Ther Res.* 1977;1:17-38.
4. Elkin I, Shea MT, Watkins JT, Imber SD, Sotsky SM, Collins JF, Glass DR, Pilkonis PA, Leber WR, Docherty JP, Fiester SJ, Parloff MB. National Institute of Mental Health Treatment of Depression Collaborative Research Program: general effectiveness of treatments. *Arch Gen Psychiatry.* 1989;46:971-982.
5. Blackburn IM, Bishop S, Glen AIM, Whalley LJ, Christie JE. The efficacy of cognitive therapy in depression: a treatment trial using cognitive therapy and pharmacotherapy, each alone and in combination. *Br J Psychiatry.* 1981;139:181-189.
6. Hollon SD, DeRubeis RJ, Evans MD, Wiemer JJ, Garvey JG, Grove WM, Tuason VB. Cognitive therapy and pharmacotherapy for depression: singly and in combination. *Arch Gen Psychiatry.* 1992;49:774-781.
7. McKnight DL, Nelson-Gray RO, Barnhill J. Dexamethasone suppression test and response to cognitive therapy and antidepressant medication. *Behav Ther.* 1992;1:99-111.
8. Murphy GE, Simons AD, Wetzel RD, Lustman PJ. Cognitive therapy and pharmacotherapy. *Arch Gen Psychiatry.* 1984;41:33-41.
9. Thompson LW, Gallagher D, Breckenridge JS. Comparative effectiveness of psychotherapies for depressed elders. *J Consult Clin Psychol.* 1987;55:385-390.
10. Gallagher DE, Thompson LW. Treatment of major depressive disorder in older adult outpatients with brief psychotherapies. *Psychotherapy.* 1982;19:482-490.
11. Shaw BF. Comparison of cognitive therapy and behavior therapy in the treatment of depression. *J Consult Clin Psychol.* 1977;45:543-551.
12. Jacobson NS, Dobson K, Fruzzetti AE, Schmaling KB, Salusky S. Marital therapy as a treatment for depression. *J Consult Clin Psychol.* 1991;59:547-557.
13. O'Leary KD, Beach SRH. Marital therapy: a viable treatment for depression and marital discord. *Am J Psychiatry.* 1990;147:183-186.
14. Scott AIF, Freeman CPL. Edinburgh primary care depression study: treatment outcome, patient satisfaction, and cost after 16 weeks. *BMJ.* 1992;304;883-887.
15. Ross M, Scott M. An evaluation of the effectiveness of individual and group cognitive therapy in the treatment of depressed patients in an inner city health centre. *J R Coll Gen Pract.* 1985;35:239-242.
16. Teasdale JD, Fennell MJV, Hibbert GA, Amies PL. Cognitive therapy for major depressive disorder in primary care. *Br J Psychiatry.* 1984;144:400-406.
17. Scott MJ, Stradling SG. Group cognitive therapy for depression produces clinically significant reliable change in community-based settings. *Behav Psychother.* 1990;18:1-19.
18. Dobson KS. A meta-analysis of the efficacy of cognitive therapy for depression. *J Consult Clin Psychol.* 1989;57:414-419.
19. Robinson LA, Berman JS, Neimeyer RA. Psychotherapy for the treatment of depression: a comprehensive review of controlled outcome research. *Psychol Bull.* 1990;108:30-49.
20. McLean PD, Hakstian AR. Clinical depression: comparative efficacy of outpatient treatments. *J Consult Clin Psychol.* 1979;47:818-836.
21. Brown RA, Lewinsohn PM. A psychoeducational approach to the treatment of depression: comparison of group, individual, and minimal contact procedures. *J Consult Clin Psychol.* 1984;52:774-783.
22. Usaf SO, Kavanaugh DJ. Mechanisms of improvement in treatment for depression: test of a self-efficacy and performance model. *J Cognit Psychother.* 1990;4:51-70.
23. Nezu AM, Perri MG. Social problem-solving therapy for unipolar depression: an initial dismantling investigation. *J Consult Clin Psychol.* 1989;57:408-413.
24. Hersen M, Bellack AS, Himmelhoch JM, Thase ME. Effects of social skill training, amitriptyline, and psychotherapy in unipolar depressed women. *Behav Ther.* 1984;15:21-40.
25. Roth D, Bielski R, Jones M, Parker W, Osborn G. A comparison of self-control therapy and combined self-control therapy and antidepressant medication in the treatment of depression. *Behav Ther.* 1982;13:133-144.
26. Wilson PH. Combined pharmacological and behavioural treatment of depression. *Behav Res Ther.* 1982;20:173-184.
27. Covi L, Lipman RS. Cognitive-behavioral group psychotherapy combined with imipramine in major depression. *Psychopharmacol Bull.* 1987;23:173.
28. Kornblith, SJ, Rehm, LP, O'Hara MW, Lamparski DM. The contribution of self-reinforcement training and behavioral assignments to the efficacy of self-control therapy for depression. *Cognit Ther Res.* 1983;7:499-528.
29. Steuer JL, Mintz J, Hammen CL, Hill MA, Jarvik LF, McCarley T, Motoike P, Rosen R. Cognitive-behavioral and psychodynamic group psychotherapy in treatment of geriatric depression. *J Consult Clin Psychol.* 1984;52:180-189.
30. Daneman EA. Imipramine in office management of depressive reactions: a double-blind study. *Dis Nerv Syst.* 1961;22:213-217.

31. Covi L, Lipman RS, Derogatis LR, Smith JE III, Pattison JH. Drugs and group psychotherapy in neurotic depression. *Am J Psychiatry.* 1974;131:191-198.
32. American Psychiatric Association, Committee on Nomenclature and Statistics. *Diagnostic and Statistical Manual of Mental Disorders, Third Edition.* Washington, DC: American Psychiatric Association; 1980.
33. Rehm LP, Kaslow NJ, Rabin AS. Cognitive and behavioral targets in a self-control therapy program for depression. *J Consult Clin Psychol.* 1987; 55:60-67.
34. Fleming BM, Thornton DW. Coping skills training as a component in the short-term treatment of depression. *J Consult Clin Psychol.* 1980;48:652-654.
35. Graff RW, Whitehead GI III, LeCompte M. Group treatment with divorced women using cognitive-behavioral and supportive-insight methods. *J Couns Psychol.* 1986;33:276-281.
36. Comas-Diaz L. Effects of cognitive and behavioral group treatment on the depressive symptomatology of Puerto Rican women. *J Consult Clin Psychol.* 1981;49:627-632.
37. Fuchs CZ, Rehm LP. A self-control behavior therapy program for depression. *J Consult Clin Psychol.* 1977;45:206-215.
38. Nezu AM. Efficacy of a social problem-solving therapy approach for unipolar depression. *J Consult Clin Psychol.* 1986;54:196-202.
39. Rude SS. Relative benefits of assertion or cognitive self-control treatment for depression as a function of proficiency in each domain. *J Consult Clin Psychol.* 1986;54:390-394.
40. Thase ME. Cognitive behavior therapy of severe unipolar depression. In: Grauhaus L, Greden JF, eds. *Severe Depressive Disorders.* Washington, DC: American Psychiatric Press Inc; 1994:269-296.
41. Thase ME, Greenhouse J, Frank E, Reynolds III, CF, Pilkonis PA, Hurley K, Grochocinski VJ, Kupfer DJ. Correlates of remission of major depression during standardized trials of psychotherapy, pharmacotherapy, or their combination: results from the Pittsburgh 600. *Psychopharmacol Bull.* 1994;30:642. Abstract.
42. McLean P, Taylor S. Severity of unipolar depression and choice of treatment. *Behav Res Ther.* 1992;30:443-451.
43. Zimmerman M, Spitzer RL. Melancholia: from *DSM-III* to *DSM-III-R. Am J Psychiatry.* 1989; 146:20-28.
44. Rush AJ, Weissenburger JE. Melancholic symptom features and *DSM-IV. Am J Psychiatry.* 1994; 151:489-498.
45. Prusoff BA, Weissman MM, Klerman GL, Rounsaville BJ. Research Diagnostic Criteria subtypes of depression: their role as predictors of differential response to psychotherapy and drug treatment. *Arch Gen Psychiatry.* 1980;37:796-803.
46. Gallagher DE, Thompson LW. Effectiveness of psychotherapy for both endogenous and nonendogenous depression in older adult outpatients. *J Gerontol.* 1983;38:707-712.
47. Thase ME, Himmelhoch JM, Hersen M, Bellack AS. Poor response to psychosocial treatments in melancholia. Presented at the annual meeting of the American Psychiatric Association; May 12, 1984; Los Angeles, Calif.
48. Last CG, Thase ME, Hersen M, Bellack AS, Himmelhoch JM. Patterns of attrition for psychosocial and pharmacological treatments of depression. *J Clin Psychiatry.* 1985;46:361-366.
49. Sotsky SM, Glass DR, Shea MT, Pilkonis PA, Collins JF, Elkin I, Watkins JT, Imber SD, Leber WR, Moyer J, Oliveri ME. Patient predictors of response to psychotherapy and pharmacotherapy: findings in the NIMH Treatment of Depression Collaborative Research Program. *Am J Psychiatry.* 1991;148:997-1008.
50. Simons AD, Thase ME. Biological markers, treatment outcome, and 1-year follow-up of endogenous depression: electroencephalographic sleep studies and response to cognitive therapy. *J Consult Clin Psychol.* 1992;60:392-401.
51. Kovacs M, Rush J, Beck AT, Hollon SD. Depressed outpatients treated with cognitive therapy or pharmacotherapy: a one-year follow-up. *Arch Gen Psychiatry.* 1981;38:33-39.
52. Beck AT, Hollon SD, Young JE, Bedrosian RC, Budenz D. Treatment of depression with cognitive therapy and amitriptyline. *Arch Gen Psychiatry.* 1985;42:142-148.
53. Thase ME. Cognitive and behavioral treatments for depression: a review of recent developments. In: Ayd FJ, Taylor IJ, Taylor BT, eds. *Affective Disorders Reassessed.* Baltimore, Md: Ayd Medical Communications; 1983.
54. Weissman MM, Prusoff BA, Dimascio A, Neu C, Goklaney M, Klerman GL. The efficacy of drugs and psychotherapy in the treatment of acute depressive episodes. *Am J Psychiatry.* 1979;136 (suppl 4B):555-558.
55. Klerman GL, DiMascio A, Weissman M, Prusoff B, Paykel ES. Treatment of depression by drugs and psychotherapy. *Am J Psychiatry.* 1974;131:186-191.
56. Frank E, Kupfer DJ, Perel JM, Cornes C, Jarrett DB, Mallinger AG, Thase ME, McEachran AB, Grochocinski VJ. Three-year outcomes for maintenance therapies in recurrent depression. *Arch Gen Psychiatry.* 1990;47:1093-1099.
57. Conte HR, Plutchik R, Wild KV, Karasu TB. Combined psychotherapy and pharmacotherapy for depression. *Arch Gen Psychiatry.* 1986;43:471-479.
58. Hollon SD, Shelton RC, Loosen PT. Cognitive therapy and pharmacotherapy for depression. *J Consult Clin Psychol.* 1991;59:88-99.
59. Persons JB. Outcome of psychotherapy for unipolar depression. In: Giles T, ed. *Effective Psychotherapy: A Handbook of Comparative Research.* New York, NY: Plenum Press; 1993.
60. Manning DW, Frances AJ. Combined therapy for depression: critical review of the literature. In: Manning DW, Frances AJ, eds. *Combined Pharmacotherapy and Psychotherapy for Depression.* Washington, DC: American Psychiatric Press; 1990:3-33.
61. Evans MD, Hollon SD, DeRubeis RJ, Piasecki JM, Grove WM, Garvey MJ, Tuason VB. Differential relapse following cognitive therapy and pharmacotherapy for depression. *Arch Gen Psychiatry.* 1992;49:802-808.
62. Imber SD, Pilkonis PA, Sotsky SM, Elkin I, Watkins JT, Collins JF, Shea MT, Leber WR, Glass DR. Mode-specific effects among three treatments for depression. *J Consult Clin Psychol.* 1990;58:352-359.
63. Zeiss AM, Lewinsohn PM, Muñoz RF. Nonspecific improvement effects in depression using interpersonal skills training, pleasant activity schedules, or cognitive training. *J Consult Clin Psychol.* 1979;47:427-439.
64. Keller KE. Dysfunctional attitudes and the cognitive therapy for depression. *Cognit Ther Res.* 1983;7:437-444.
65. Jarrett RB, Eaves GG, Grannenmann BD, Rush AJ. Clinical, cognitive, and demographic predictors of response to cognitive therapy for depression: a preliminary report. *Psychiatry Res.* 1991; 37:245-260.
66. Thase ME, Simons AD, McGeary J, Cahalane JF, Hughes C, Harden T, Friedman E. Relapse after cognitive behavior therapy of depression: potential implications for longer courses of treatment? *Am J Psychiatry.* 1992;149:1046-1052.
67. Diguer L, Barber JP, Luborsky L. Three concomitants: personality disorders, psychiatric severity, and outcome of dynamic psychotherapy of major depression. *Am J Psychiatry.* 1993; 150:1246-1248.
68. Muñoz RF, Hollon SD, McGrath E, Rehm LP, VandenBos GR. On the AHCPR Depression in Primary Care guidelines: further considerations for practitioners. *Am Psychol.* 1994;49:42-61.

The Role of Psychotherapy in the Treatment of Depression

Review of Two Practice Guidelines

Persons and colleagues[1] are to be commended for their detailed examination of two major practice guidelines on the care of patients with major depressive disorder. As they point out, practice guidelines have great potential, with important clinical, professional, and legal implications. In their article, they make a number of valuable and helpful suggestions. For example, their suggestion that practice guidelines undergo periodic revision is in agreement with the American Medical Association guide[2] and is consistent with the American Psychiatric Association (APA) practice guideline project[3] (which calls for revisions at 3- to 5-year intervals). However, in addition to such valuable suggestions, Persons et al also make some factual errors, underplay the limitations in the research literature (and thus ignore the role of clinical consensus in developing guidelines), and, most important, appear not to understand that the main purpose of practice guidelines is to assist clinicians (in this case psychiatrists) in making clinical decisions.

Persons et al argue that the APA guideline understates the value of psychotherapy in the treatment of this disorder. Actually, the APA guideline is crystal clear in its unequivocal support of the role of psychotherapy in the treatment of major depression. The "Summary of Recommendations" states, "Effective treatments for major depression include psychotherapy, antidepressant medications, and ECT [I]."[3] The bracketed [I] represents the strongest level of endorsement of recommendations and means "recommended with substantial clinical confidence." We are at a loss to understand how this key statement concerning the effectiveness of psychotherapy in the treatment of depressive disorder could be ignored or misunderstood.

Merriam and Karasu, in their commentary,[4] respond to the criticisms of Persons et al about the specific psychotherapies (cognitive therapy, behavior therapy, and brief psychodynamic psychotherapy). Since we are in agreement with comments by Merriam and Karasu, rather than repeat those arguments, we will focus instead on some broader issues raised by Persons et al in their article: the need to consider the target audience in developing and reviewing practice guidelines, the issue of incorporating cost into guideline recommendations, the concept of psychotherapeutic management and its role in the APA practice guideline, and the challenge of integrating empirical data with clinical wisdom in developing guidelines.

See also pages 283, 298, 301, and 303

THE TARGET AUDIENCE

The two practice guidelines under discussion were developed for different audiences: the Agency for Health Care Policy and Research (AHCPR) developed guidelines for primary care physicians,[5,6] and APA developed guidelines for psychiatrists.[3] Although Persons et al[1] focus on the differences in treatment recommendations between these two documents,[3,6] the remarkable (and encouraging) fact is that they are so consistent, with the few differences being easily attributable to different target audiences. For example, while a considerable portion of the AHCPR guideline addresses the diagnosis of major depressive disorder, the APA's does not, based on the assumption that psychiatrists have the expertise to make use of available documents (including *DSM-IV*[7]) and do not generally need additional guidance in this area. In the area of treatment recommendations, it is critical to understand the nature of the different patient populations likely to be seen by these different groups of clinicians. Compared with psychiatrists, primary care physicians are likely to see patients with depressive disorders that are less severe, less recurrent, and less likely to be complicated by psychiatric comorbidities but more likely to be complicated by general medical comorbidities.[8] In addition, psychiatrists are likely to see more patients who have had prior unsuccessful treatment experiences. The AHCPR guideline is based on certain assumptions about the knowledge and skills of primary care physicians, as well as the likely patient population. The APA guideline is similarly informed with regard to psychiatrists. Thus, it makes sense that the AHCPR guideline focuses on first-line treatments for patients with relatively uncomplicated disorders, and the APA guideline has an additional focus on patients with complicated disorders who may need combined and/or intensive treatments. As Rush[9] points out, it is this latter group that frequently requires moving beyond the available empirical data and considering clinical experience (the alternative being to tell such patients that you cannot care for them because they are dissimilar to patients in clinical trials).

THE ISSUE OF COST

Persons et al argue that treatment costs should be an important consideration in the development of practice guidelines. Here we have a fundamental disagreement. The APA Guideline Steering Committee decided that, at this time, costs will generally not be a factor in the formulation of guidelines. There are several reasons for this position. Although cost is certainly an important consideration for those who must allocate scarce resources among members of a population, we do not believe that the average psychiatrist plays this role, or that the average patient expects that his or her psychiatrist is doing this. The purpose of practice guidelines is to guide clinical decision making. Such decisions must first be informed by a synthesis of all available information of the likely consequences for the patient of different treatment strategies. The choice among these strategies would then be made by the patient and clinician in light of other relevant external considerations. Certainly, in many instances, cost would be such a consideration. But how could a national guideline incorporate this information? First, there would need to be a national consensus on whose cost (eg, the patient's, employer's, insurer's/managed care organization's, society's) and which costs (eg, direct treatment costs or also indirect costs, such as decreased work productivity, family burden) would be considered.[10] Second, reliable data about such costs would need to be analyzed. In our view, neither the consensus nor the data are available. Hence, the APA's current position is that, at this time, cost issues will not routinely be part of our guidelines. The professional association will make recommendations to psychiatrists about the likely effectiveness of the available treatment strategies, while the decision about the affordability of the different treatments will have to be made elsewhere.

PSYCHOTHERAPEUTIC MANAGEMENT

The concept of psychotherapeutic management is an essential component of the APA's practice guideline and is an excellent example of the necessity of including recommendations emanating from a consensus of clinicians. This concept arose from a synthesis of available literature (eg, regarding such interventions as "clinical management" and "supportive psychotherapy") and clinical experience regarding what good clinicians actually do for their depressed patients, above and beyond providing a specific treatment (whether it be a medication, electroconvulsive therapy, or a specific psychotherapy). The concept is fully explained and operationalized in the APA guideline.

While we agree with Persons et al that the efficacy of psychotherapeutic management has not been demonstrated in controlled studies, the system of coding for references and for key recommendations in the guideline makes the quality of the evidence underlying the recommendations clear.

Let us now look at Persons et al's discussion of "combined psychotherapy-pharmacotherapy regimens." Up until this section of the article, Persons et al were critical of the APA guideline, undervaluing the role of psychotherapy in the treatment of depression. However, in this section, the argument is now made that the APA guideline "overvalues the role of combined psychotherapy-pharmacotherapy regimens." Since, as noted by Persons et al, "There is voluminous evidence that endogenously depressed outpatients and severely depressed inpatients benefit from pharmacotherapy," the alternative to the combined therapies would seem to be pharmacotherapy alone. In the preparation of the APA guideline, there was a very strong clinical consensus that pharmacotherapy, if not combined with psychotherapy, should be practiced in a therapeutic relationship where attention is given to the issues included in the definition of "psychotherapeutic management." Hence, the recommendation, "*most* patients are best treated with antidepressant medication coupled with psychotherapeutic management *or* psychotherapy"[3] (italics added). Persons et al seemed to read "all" for "most" and to ignore the distinction between psychotherapeutic management and the specific psychotherapies. They also failed to understand that "most patients" applied to the target audience of psychiatrists, whose patients, as we noted, are more likely to have complications that require more intensive modalities of treatment.

In addition, for those patients treated with a combination of pharmacotherapy and psychotherapy, Persons et al make a strange argument. They identify several studies, meta-analyses, and qualitative reviews that conclude that combined psychotherapy-pharmacotherapy was only slightly superior to psychotherapy alone or pharmacotherapy alone. They then discount the value of "slightly superior" and simply declare "the evidence is not strong enough to warrant the recommendation made by the APA practice guideline." By whose decree is the evidence not strong enough? What do the authors think most patient would choose if they were told one approach was "slightly superior"?

THE CHALLENGE OF INTEGRATING EMPIRICAL AND CLINICAL DATA

Practice guidelines cannot simply be a compilation of research findings. To be useful, they must integrate available empirical data with all other relevant information to provide clinicians and their patients with the best possible guidance for making treatment decisions. The input of clinicians is essential to frame the issues to be covered and to fill in the gaps left by a research base of limited breadth and generalizability.

Controlled clinical trials do not represent the patient population of either primary care physicians or psychiatrists very well, owing to the effects of various inclusion and/or exclusion criteria as well as patient selection. In addition, controlled trials frequently focus on single, well-described treatments, which may not be representative of the dosage, intensity, or treatment modalities that are actually in widespread use (eg, combined treatments and nonmanualized psychotherapies are two types of treatments that are understudied in controlled trials). This partly explains the need for practice guidelines. If research data were directly applicable to all clinical care, then a systematic synthesis of available data, such as a meta-analysis, would suffice. Instead, data must be "translated" before application to patients.

Both the Institute of Medicine[11] and the American Medical Association[2] recognize the need for both clinical and empirical input into guidelines. In keeping with these principles, the APA guidelines are developed by a work group under the auspices of a Steering Committee. The members of the guideline work group are, by policy, psychiatrists in active clinical practice with diverse expertise and practice experiences relevant to the topic. Thus, we believe that every member of the depression work group was "an expert in the treatment of major depression," as contrasted with Persons et al's comment, "most members of the work group were experts in at least one area pertaining to mood disorders." The work group is guided by the policies established by the Steering Committee in "systematically reviewing data in the literature and forging consensus on the implications of that data as well as describing a clinical consensus."[12]

Although sound methods exist for integrating empirical data from similar studies (eg, meta-analysis), it is more difficult to systematically gather and integrate clinical data. The APA currently makes use of widespread, iterative reviews of drafts of its guidelines to gather the input of clinicians and other interested parties. For example, drafts of the depression guideline were sent to over 800 individuals as well as over 100 organizations (including most of the major mental health provider, patient, and advocacy organizations). Comments were collated by guideline page and carefully reviewed by the work group, the oversight committee, and the staff, and incorporated, as appropriate, into subsequent drafts. (Only individuals and organizations who made lengthy comments were listed in the published guidelines.) Although this is not as systematic a method as we would like, it is the best available to us at this time. However, the APA plans to improve on this process for future guidelines (including the revision of the depression guideline) by making use of its developing Practice Research Network to provide systematic data on practice patterns and outcomes by psychiatrists.

As indicated at the beginning of this article, we appreciate the efforts of Persons et al in increasing the attention to practice guidelines. We also commend the editorial staff of the ARCHIVES for allotting a significant portion of this issue to the topic of practice guidelines. We hope that the field as a whole will give increasing attention to practice guidelines, so that they can grow as vehicles for improving the care of patients.

John S. McIntyre, MD
Department of Psychiatry
St Mary's Hospital
Rochester, NY 14611

Deborah A. Zarin, MD
Harold Alan Pincus, MD
Washington, DC

REFERENCES

1. Persons JB, Thase ME, Crits-Christoph P. The role of psychotherapy in the treatment of depression: review of two practice guidelines. *Arch Gen Psychiatry.* 1996;53:283-290.
2. American Medical Association Practice Parameters Partnership. *Attributes to Guide the Development of Practice Parameters.* Chicago, Ill: American Medical Association; 1990.
3. American Psychiatric Association. Practice guideline for major depressive disorders in adults. *Am J Psychiatry.* 1993;150(suppl 4):1-26.
4. Merriam AE, Karasu TB. The role of psychotherapy in the treatment of depression: review of two practice guidelines. *Arch Gen Psychiatry.*1996;53:301-302.
5. Depression Guideline Panel. *Clinical Practice Guideline Number 5: Depression in Primary Care, 1: Detection and Diagnosis.* Rockville, Md: US Dept of Health and Human Services, Agency for Health Care Policy and Research; 1993. AHCPR publication 93-0550.
6. Depression Guideline Panel. *Clinical Practice Guideline Number 5: Depression in Primary Care, 2: Treatment of Major Depression.* Rockville, Md: US Dept of Health and Human Services, Agency for Health Care Policy and Research; 1993. AHCPR publication 93-0551.
7. American Psychiatric Association. *Diagnostic and Statistical Manual of Mental Disorders, Fourth Edition.* Washington, DC: American Psychiatric Association; 1994.
8. Rogers WH, Wells KB, Meredith LS, Sturm R, Burnam MA. Outcomes for adult outpatients with depression under prepaid of fee-for-service financing. *Arch Gen Psychiatry.* 1993;50:517-525.
9. Rush AJ. The role of psychotherapy in the treatment of depression: review of two practice guidelines. *Arch Gen Psychiatry.* 1996;53:298-300.
10. Krupnick J, Pincus HA. The cost-effectiveness of psychotherapy: a plan for research. *Am J Psychiatry.* 1992;149:1295-1305.
11. Field MJ, Lohr KN, eds, for Institute of Medicine. *Guidelines for Clinical Practice: From Development to Use.* Washington, DC: National Academy Press; 1992.
12. Zarin DA, Pincus HA, McIntyre JS. Practice guidelines. *Am J Psychiatry.* 1993;150:174-177.

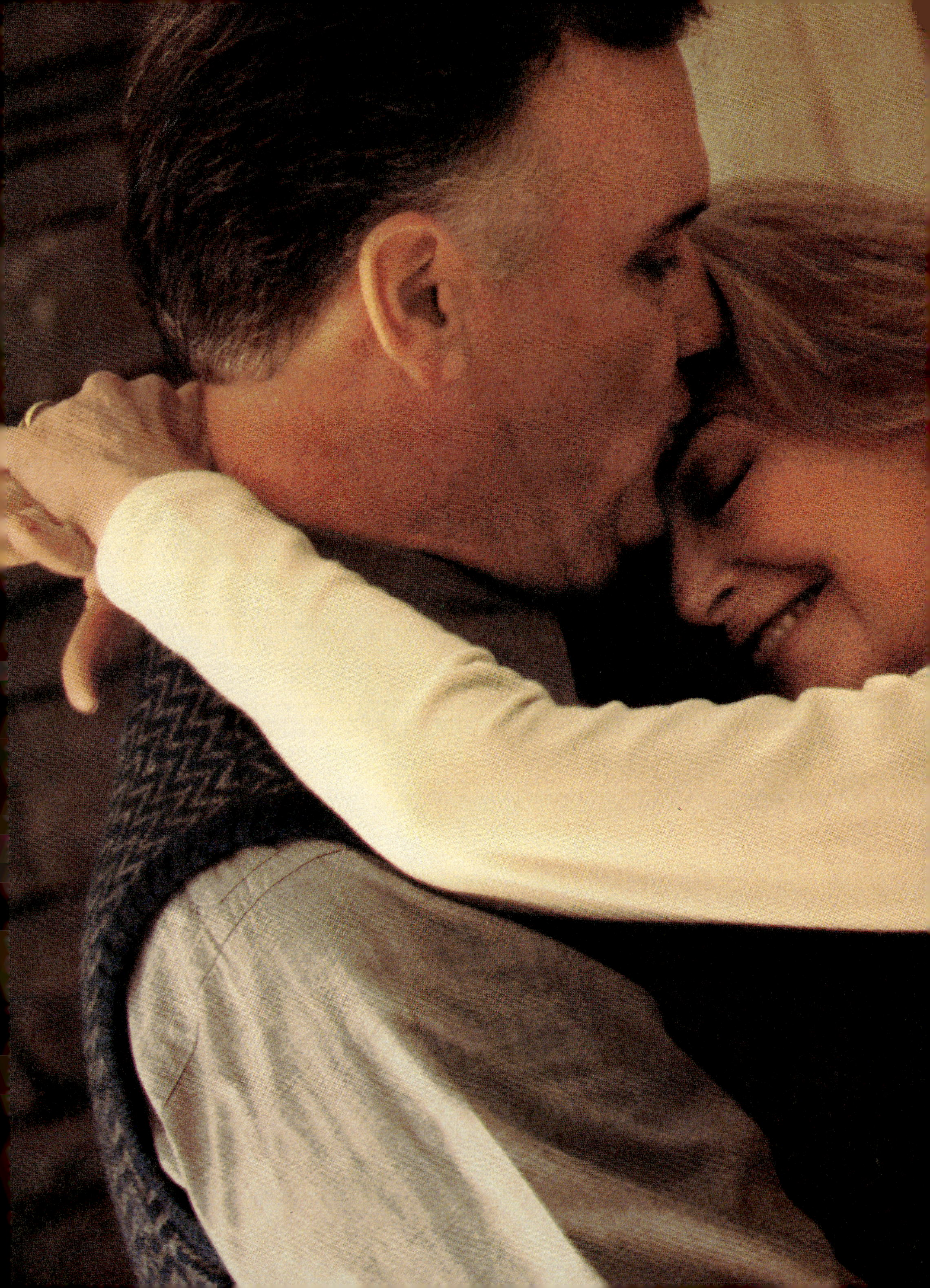

COMMENTARY

The Role of Psychotherapy in the Treatment of Depression

Review of Two Practice Guidelines

PERSONS AND colleagues[1] have raised some intriguing, provocative, and clinically important issues in their review and critique of two clinical practice guidelines: one by the Agency for Health Care Policy and Research (AHCPR),[2,3] aimed at primary care (PC) practitioners, and the second by the American Psychiatric Association (APA),[4] directed toward psychiatrists. In essence, Persons et al find a greater basis for recommending psychotherapy alone as a treatment for major depressive disorder, and they view the stronger call for combined treatment (medication and psychotherapy) by the APA as lacking empirical support. They make several recommendations for subsequent guideline development (eg, multidisciplinary panels, comments on cost, highest reliance on randomized controlled trials [RCTs], periodic revisions, etc).

The following comments, intended to be explanatory rather than in defense of, in particular, the AHCPR guidelines, focus on the philosophical basis underpinning the development and use of clinical practice guidelines. Assumptions made about guidelines bear directly on how guidelines are developed, the mix of reliance on empirical data (eg, controlled studies) vs clinical judgment, as well as on the final format of the guidelines (eg, very specific vs more general).

Debate about practice guidelines can generally be attributed to two major forces: (1) limitations in empirical knowledge and (2) attempts to address a wide range of presumed audiences. The latter often leads to "endorsement" or "recommendation" of treatments for which direct empirical data are lacking (eg, to ensure coverage), while the former often leads to a greater (or lesser) reliance on "clinical judgment." Taken together, these two forces logically lead to differences among practice guidelines of the type noted by Persons et al. Ultimately, such differences cannot be resolved without further scientific efforts, ie, guidelines relying more on clinical judgment need to be evaluated by scientific study.

The AHCPR guidelines were explicitly developed for PC providers, not for psychiatrists, psychologists, managed care administrators, or lawyers. Of course, we recognized that the guidelines would be used (and misused) by those needing to rationalize cost containment, deny care, or win lawsuits. Practice guidelines, in our view, should be written to ultimately provide physicians and their patients the best available information about diagnosis and treatment, regardless of the potential attacks or misuse by others.

Guidelines can only make recommendations based on group-based (nomothetic) data that may apply more, less, or not at all to selected individuals (ideographic decisions). We assumed that only the professional, in collaboration with his or her patient, can decide which recommendations should (or should not) be followed and to what degree, because group-based data must be factored in, but will not fully dictate, the tailoring of treatments to individuals. Consequently, malpractice lawsuits based on "guideline violations" should not be won if a reasonable case is made for divergences from guidelines in individual cases. We viewed practitioners as responsible for remaining up to date in the relevant areas and, in particular, to be trained and skilled in applying group-based scientific data to individual patients.

Those who reimburse health care cannot avoid the ethical problem of denying payment for treatments that have not yet been fully studied scientifically, but which are commonly used and anecdotally or consensually viewed as indicated. It means that a treatment that has not been fully studied is not necessarily effective or ineffective.

See also pages 283, 291, 301, and 303

In essence, scientific knowledge can never fully answer the complex questions that clinicians face on a daily basis.[5] The tailoring of group-based data to individual patients requires an in-depth understanding of the biological and psychological basis for the disorder and its relevant treatment, so that individual adjustments of guideline recommendations can be made for particular patients to optimize outcome, while minimizing harm and discomfort. In other words, guidelines cannot replace professional judgment by creating a "cookbook" to be followed by nonprofessionals because of the limitations inherent in applying group-based data to individual patients.

The AHCPR Guideline Panel viewed its role as furnishing PC providers with well-established scientific information that, while likely to evolve, was solid enough that guideline revisions would be called for less (every 4 to 6 years) rather than more (eg, yearly) frequently. Thus, we relied more heavily on scientifically established information.

Specialists, on the other hand, must go beyond well-established science to help those patients who do not respond to less-complex, but better-studied, treatments provided in PC settings. We also assumed that these patients would be more likely referred to specialty care. Consequently, we assumed that specialty practitioners would have to rely more heavily on clinical experience and on a suggestive, but often not yet definitive, scientific knowledge base,[5] given the unrepresentative nature of patients likely to be seen by psychiatrists. That is, specialty providers (eg, psychiatrists) would be more likely to deliver care and address problems that are less fully addressed by the available science than PC providers. Thus, a greater reliance on professional judgment is called for by guideline developers for specialty, as contrasted with PC, providers. For this reason, there is a greater reliance on RCTs by the AHCPR than the APA guidelines.

In fact, if we had been strictly empirical (eg, RCT data for all recommendations), the paucity of RCT studies actually conducted in PC settings would have precluded guideline development. Instead, we reasoned by analogy and evaluated the generalizability of published findings whenever possible; for example, by comparing studies in PC with those in psychiatric settings to develop the AHCPR guidelines. In addition, we provided levels of certainty (eg, less firmly supported recommendations were rated B or C, rather than A) for our recommendations.

Because guidelines are not standards of care,[6] they do not "dictate" what must be done (or not done) in individual cases. Most often, guidelines, as is the case with the AHCPR document, recommend (or suggest) more or less strongly based on (*a*) what is known and (*b*) the degree to which a particular patient "fits" the populations on which the knowledge has been developed.

The AHCPR guidelines, for example, do not "restrict the use of cognitive therapy, behavioral therapy, or interpersonal psychotherapy to only some outpatients with mild to moderate depressions."[1] Second, it is not feasible to reissue guidelines at a high enough frequency (eg, every 6 months) to fully inform nonmedical personnel (eg, managed care administrators, lawyers), as suggested by Persons et al in the introductory paragraph of their study. These individuals must still consult with experts.

The call by Persons et al for a mandate to require multidisciplinary panels for all guidelines is a bit naive and logically (if not politically) incorrect. For example, I doubt that a psychiatrist or psychologist would have much that is useful to say about guidelines for conducting retinal surgery. Rather, it seems most logical that the discipline mix of any guideline panel should be guided by the treatment called for and the people likely to deliver the treatment, as well as those experts in research on and actual provision of these treatments. Depending on the topic of the guideline, the panel, logically, would be more or less "multidisciplinary."

Persons et al suggest that future guidelines should also address cost issues. The AHCPR Panel looked at the available cost data and found it to be so lacking that cost was not addressed. By and large, cost issues are still not well resolved. It is my own judgment that cost issues are not germane to what is best for the patient. The science may strongly recommend a treatment (eg, excellent scientific evidence) that simply cannot be delivered for various practical reasons (lack of providers, treatment not available, not covered by insurance, or not affordable).

Another major problem is how to define cost (eg, Cost to whom? Pharmacy costs? Health care plan costs? Community costs?). Furthermore, how to cost out important clinical consequences is unresolved. What is the cost of a dry mouth to a radio talk show host as opposed to a forest ranger?—Are they the same? Is there any cost or is it only an inconvenience unless something costly to the system providing the service or payers happens as a consequence? How often does it happen? The cost of orthostatic hypotension to an elderly patient may be high (eg, falling that results in a hip fracture) but less costly to a 25-year-old. Thus, to increase the accuracy of cost estimates, one must define the population of interest far beyond the disorder definition.

Finally, the personal cost (pain, suffering, and inconvenience) cannot be easily assigned a dollar amount. These are value judgments: not convertible to dollars and cents. For example, one can forego anesthesia for minor surgery or many dental procedures, thereby reducing dollar costs to the system, while increasing discomfort to some patients. Is the dollar cost of anesthesia convertible to units of discomfort?

Let us now turn to the issue of weighing and interpreting empirical data. Persons et al take issue with a greater strength given to medication as opposed to psychotherapy alone for the more severely ill outpatients with major depressive disorder. There were three reasons for this recommendation by the AHCPR Panel: (1) The evidence for efficacy using a placebo, or nonspecific control was greater for medication than for psychotherapy alone (see AHCPR guideline[3(p6)]). (2) The symptom severity required to enter virtually all medication efficacy trials has been uniformly higher than the symptom severity required to enter psychotherapy trials in outpatients. Thus, we have more data on the efficacy of medication and less on psychotherapy alone for the more severely ill outpatients. (3) During 1992 and 1993, we realized that the length of stay in, and access to, inpatient treatment was being reduced and would likely become even more restricted by 1995; ie, yesterday's inpatients are today's outpatients. As Persons et al note, inpatient studies of psychotherapy alone were not available, yet medications have documented efficacy in this group. Combined with the principle that we adopted to recommend a studied treatment over an unstudied one, medication "trumped" psychotherapy in the treatment of today's more severely ill outpatients.

It is notable, however, that severity alone was not the sole factor in recommending psychotherapy vs medication (see AHCPR[3(pp39,43,90)]). Chronicity of illness, patient preference, prior response, general medical status, etc, all contribute to the strategic decision to select psychotherapy, medication, or the combination. We placed the burden of choice on the patients and their doctors, especially since the evidence to support a prescriptive predictor was not fully developed. (Prescriptive predictors are those pretreatment features that strongly recommend one treatment type [eg, fluoxetine vs amitriptyline] or strategy [eg, medication vs psychotherapy] over another.)

Other reasons to be less enthusiastic about psychotherapy alone as a first-line treatment *for the more severely depressed* was, at the time, the lack of any RCTs of medication vs psychotherapy in PC patients. However, recent studies[7,8] do suggest efficacy, although analyses of pretreatment severity as "predictors" were not conducted in either report. These issues cannot be fully settled without further study of targeted groups in PC settings.

It is notable that the APA and AHCPR guidelines are remarkably congruent, even when it comes to recommendations for combined treatment (ie, medication and psychotherapy). The AHCPR guideline recommends either treatment alone, given the evidence for acute-phase efficacy as measured by symptoms. However, based on logic and some circumstantial evidence (eg, by Weissman et al[9,10] and Blackburn et al[11,12]), the AHCPR document suggests that the combination of medication and psychotherapy may be particularly useful in the more complex situations (ie, depressions in the context of concurrent, chronic general-medical, or other psychiatric disorders, or in patients who fail to respond fully to either treatment alone). It is logical to expect that these kinds of patients are more likely to be seen by psychiatrists, who, in turn, are more likely to use combination treatment, ie, to follow the stronger recommendations for combined treatment found in the APA guidelines.

A comment about the language of this and other guideline debates seems appropriate. I believe that we must avoid language borrowed from the legal system and adversarial culture in which we live. For example, Persons et al recommend multidisciplinary panels to "protect from bias."[1] According to the *Webster's Collegiate Dictionary*, *bias* is "an indication of temperament or outlook—especially a highly personal and unreasoned distortion of judgment." The authors suggest that multidisciplinary panels reduce "biases," presumably by adding mutually contradictory biases together. Such a view is not empirically founded. Biases exist in all human endeavors. Multiple biases do not lead to a "bias-free" result.

Most important, a bias should not be assumed, simply because the message does not match the beliefs of the reader (ie, it is not necessary to shoot the messenger if one disagrees with the message). Rather, discussion and empirical evaluation of the content of the message itself is indicated.

Guidelines can be written by (1) stating the rules of evidence, (2) stating the types of evidence, (3) noting where inferences have been made, (4) noting the types of inferences made, and (5) providing a rationale for the inferences. Thus, full disclosure of the thinking processes (ie, evidence, assumptions, and inferences) should be an explicit part of all guidelines, which, in turn, allow further scientific evaluation of the evidence, the inferences, and the assumptions. Disagreements about conclusions, and the identified deficiencies in the scientific literature, provide a rational basis for further research and subsequent guideline revisions. In sum, let's avoid attributing motives (eg, "biases") to guideline developers and, rather, evaluate both the evidence and reasoning leading to the guidelines.

Finally, and perhaps most important of all, discussion and debate about specific practice guidelines should not lead payers to decide not to reimburse for reasonable treatments that are largely endorsed by both scientific evidence and most practitioners; limitations in our scientific knowledge or interprofessional differences should not become a rationale for arbitrary cost containment efforts.

A. John Rush, MD
Department of Psychiatry
University of Texas Southwestern Medical Center
5959 Harry Hines Blvd, Suite 600
Dallas, TX 75235

REFERENCES

1. Persons JB, Thase ME, Crits-Christoph P. The role of psychotherapy in the treatment of depression: review of two practice guidelines. *Arch Gen Psychiatry.* 1996;53:283-290.
2. Depression Guideline Panel. *Clinical Practice Guideline Number 5: Depression in Primary Care, 1: Detection and Diagnosis.* Rockville, Md: US Dept of Health and Human Services, Agency for Health Care Policy and Research; 1993. AHCPR publication 93-0550.
3. Depression Guideline Panel. *Clinical Practice Guideline Number 5: Depression in Primary Care, 2: Treatment of Major Depression.* Rockville, Md: US Dept of Health and Human Services, Agency for Health Care Policy and Research; 1993. AHCPR publication 93-0551.
4. American Psychiatric Association. Practice guidelines for major depressive disorder in adults. *Am J Psychiatry.* 1993;150(suppl 4):1-26.
5. Rush AJ, Prien R. From scientific knowledge to the clinical practice of psychopharmacology: can the gap be bridged? *Psychopharmacol Bull.* 1995; 31:7-20.
6. Field MJ, Lohr KN, eds, for the US Institute of Medicine, Division of Health Care Services, Committee on Clinical Practice Guidelines. *Guidelines for Clinical Practice: From Development to Use.* Washington, DC: National Academy Press; 1992.
7. Mynors-Wallis LM, Gath DH, Lloyd-Thomas AR, Tomlinson D. Randomised controlled trial comparing problem solving treatment with amitriptyline and placebo for major depression in primary care. *BMJ.* 1995;310:441-445.
8. Schulberg HC, Block MR, Madonia MJ, Rodriguez E, Scott CP, Lave J. Applicability of clinical pharmacotherapy guidelines for major depression in primary care settings. *Arch Fam Med.* 1995;4:106-112.
9. Weissman MM, Kasl SV, Klerman GL. Follow-up of depressed women after maintenance treatment. *Am J Psychiatry.* 1976;133:757-760.
10. Weissman MM, Klerman GL, Prusoff BA, Sholomskas D, Padian N. Depressed outpatients: results one year after treatment with drugs and/or interpersonal psychotherapy. *Arch Gen Psychiatry.* 1981;38:51-55.
11. Blackburn IM, Bishop S, Glen AIM, Whalley LJ, Christie JE. The efficacy of cognitive therapy in depression: a treatment trial using cognitive therapy and pharmacotherapy, each alone and in combination. *Br J Psychiatry.* 1981;139:181-189.
12. Blackburn IM, Eunson KM, Bishop S. A two-year naturalistic follow-up of depressed patients treated with cognitive therapy, pharmacotherapy and a combination of both. *J Affect Disord.* 1986;10: 67-75.

The Role of Psychotherapy in the Treatment of Depression

Review of Two Practice Guidelines

PERSONS ET AL,[1] in their critique in this issue of the ARCHIVES of the "Practice Guideline for Major Depressive Disorder in Adults"[2] by the American Psychiatric Association, raise a number of issues familiar to the members of the guideline work group from our deliberations in preparing this monograph.

Their main arguments are that we underestimated the values of various psychotherapies in general as treatments for major depression, we underestimated the value of psychotherapy as a solo treatment in severe depression, we overestimated the value of combined psychotherapy and pharmacotherapy, and we strayed from available empirical evidence in providing guidance as to the choice of psychotherapies.

Persons and colleagues argue that we understated the value of cognitive therapy. More precisely, in our monograph we commented on cognitive behavior therapy. We relied heavily on the findings of the Treatment of Depression Collaborative Research Program,[3] which we found well designed. We accurately reported the conclusions of this study, which indicated that cognitive behavior therapy reduces depressive symptoms, but not differentially from treatment consisting of pill placebo coupled with clinical management. The authors' cite studies comparing cognitive therapies with other psychotherapies[4-9] or with various forms of treatment by general practitioners,[10-12] but such comparisons are irrelevant to their argument against our recommendations.

The authors take issue with our statement that behavior therapy is more effective when coupled with medication treatment. However, they concede that there is good evidence that depression treated with a combination of the two modalities responds more rapidly. Isn't the rapid alleviation of symptoms the goal of treatment?

The authors criticize our recommendation that brief psychodynamic psychotherapy is best used in conjunction with medication. Since they clearly agree with our conclusion that the effectiveness of brief psychodynamic therapy has not been conclusively demonstrated as a solo treatment, the only two options available as recommendations would be to use it in conjunction with medication treatment as we did or to discourage its use altogether in the treatment of major depression. We felt that the latter alternative would have been unnecessarily restrictive in its interpretation of the sparse evidence that currently exists concerning this issue, given the wealth of clinical experience that supports the use of this form of treatment.

See also pages 283, 291, 298, and 303

In reference to the issue of group therapy, we are puzzled as to why the authors would criticize our statement that "the role of group therapy in the treatment of depression is based on clinical experience rather than on systematic controlled studies,"[2] when they acknowledge the evidence that they cite to the contrary that "many are small studies of unrestricted samples (eg, women only) or utilize less rigorous methods (eg, patients were not required to meet DSM-III criteria for major depression). . . ."[2] This statement would seem to support rather than undermine our conclusions.

Another criticism leveled against the APA guideline is that we inappropriately limited the recommendation of psychotherapy as a solo treatment to those afflicted with mild or moderate forms of the disorder. The authors also discuss "whether severely depressed patients benefit less from psychotherapy than do less severely depressed patients,"[1] an issue entirely extraneous to that of the acceptability of psychotherapy as a solo treatment. In regard to this issue, however, there simply is no convincing evidence that psychotherapy is an acceptable solo treatment for the most severely depressed. Even the best evidence the authors cite in support of their argument[13] pertains to outpatients, not severely depressed inpatients. We additionally note that this article (and 12 other of the 65 references cited by the authors exclusive of the references to the two guidelines themselves), was not published in time to be available to the work group as the APA guideline was drafted. We were surprised to have literature not available to us and that remains in press being used to upbraid us for our conclusions. Interpreted more broadly, this indicates the active state of investigation in this field and how incomplete our knowledge is of many of the issues. Awareness of this fact led us to place particular value on the opinion of our expert consultants. The clear indication for some form of somatic intervention in the treatment of severe depression was a vigorously held expert opinion. We continue to believe that our recommendation to this effect is clinically sound.

The authors additionally object to our statement that "most patients are best treated with antidepressant medication coupled with psychotherapeutic management or psychotherapy."[2] We gave a detailed explanation of what we meant by the term *psychotherapeutic management*. To briefly recapitulate, this treatment modality encompasses the establishment of a supportive relationship, the guarantee of availability in times of crisis, the maintenance of vigilance regarding dangerousness to self and others, the provision of education about the illness and the goals of treatment, the provision of encouragement and feedback concerning the patient's progress, the provision of guidance regarding the patient's interactions with his personal and work environment and any pending decisions that might be made or postponed, and the setting and monitoring of realistic goals on the way to remission. This recommendation stems from the guideline work group's conviction that if the prescription of antidepressant medications is not offered in the context of formal psychotherapy, it must at the very least be accompanied by such interventions. We were more than surprised to have this seemingly straightforward recommendation misinterpreted by Persons et al as indicating that "the APA practice guideline seems to recommend combined pharmacotherapy-psychotherapy for most patients."[1] We never made such a recommendation, and it was far from our intent to have our guideline so construed.

Persons et al also found problematic our comments regarding the choice of psychotherapy, if such is to be offered. We introduced this topic in our guideline with the statement that

> although various therapies are discussed here and in the literature as distinct entities, such separate categorizations are primarily useful for heuristic or research purposes. In practice, psychiatrists use a combination or synthesis or various approaches and strategies; these in turn are determined by and individually tailored to each patient on the basis of that person's particular conditions and coping capacities. Furthermore, in actual application the techniques and the therapist-patient relationship are powerfully intertwined.[2]

We also indicated that a particular psychotherapeutic approach might be chosen on the basis of a patient's particular needs. Persons et al criticize this recommendation on the basis that empirical evidence for such selection is lacking. While we agree that this is not an issue on which a great deal of evidence exists, we stand by our recommendation that all treatment should be offered in a manner that takes the patient's needs, aptitudes, and liabilities into account, rather than to be based on some other non–patient-centered variable, such as therapist inclination or theoretic background.

We take issue with the primacy that Persons et al place on the use of controlled clinical trials in the promulgation of practice guidelines. Patients seen in everyday clinical practice, with their medical and psychiatric comorbidities and their rational and irrational preferences, represent a population distinctly different from those enrolled in controlled clinical trials. While such trials shed light on certain specific issues, they cannot be used to determine many practical aspects of treatment. To do so in some cases would undermine rather than enhance the unique adaptation of the various principles of treatment that is specifically offered to each patient. We agree that guidelines benefit from a multidisciplinary perspective. Our text was sent for comment to hundreds of individuals and organizations representing the full array of mental health and general medical professionals, including those representing psychologists, nurses, social workers, marital and family therapists, and family practitioners.

In regard to the issue of cost, which Persons et al would like to see included in future guidelines, we must acknowledge that we are unable to meaningfully enter this factor into treatment recommendations at this time. We do not know what the true cost of an illness is to the patient, insurers, or employers; nor is there reliable information regarding the costs of treatment using various therapeutic approaches, factoring in the likelihood and degree and speed of recovery for each.

Finally, we agree that guidelines should be timely and therefore are to be revised at 3- to 5-year intervals as a matter of policy.

Arnold E. Merriam, MD
T. Byram Karasu, MD
Department of Psychiatry
Albert Einstein College of Medicine
Belfer 202
1300 Morris Park Ave
Bronx, NY 10461

REFERENCES

1. Persons JB, Thase ME, Crits-Cristoph P. The role of psychotherapy in the treatment of depression: review of two practice guidelines. *Arch Gen Psychiatry.* 1996;53:283-290.
2. American Psychiatric Association. Practice guideline for major depressive disorder in adults. *Am J Psychiatry.* 1993;150(suppl 4):1-26.
3. Elkin I, Shea MT, Watkins JT, Imber SD, Sotsky SM, Collins JF, Glass DR, Pilkonis PA, Leber WR, Docherty JP, Fiester SJ, Parloff MB. National Institute of Mental Health Treatment of Depression Collaborative Research Program: general effectiveness of treatments. *Arch Gen Psychiatry.* 1989;46:971-982.
4. Murphy GE, Simons AD, Wetzel RD, Lustman PJ. Cognitive therapy and pharmacotherapy. *Arch Gen Psychiatry.* 1984;41:33-41.
5. Thompson LW, Gallagher D, Breckenridge JS. Comparative effectiveness of psychotherapies for depressed elders. *J Consult Clin Psychol.* 1987; 55:385-390.
6. Gallagher DE, Thompson LW. Treatment of major depressive disorder in older adult outpatients with brief psychotherapies. *Psychotherapy.* 1982;19:482-490.
7. Shaw BF. Comparison of cognitive therapy and behavior therapy in the treatment of depression. *J Consult Clin Psychol.* 1977;45:543-551.
8. Jacobson NS, Dobson K, Fruzzetti AE, Schmaling KB, Salusky S. Marital therapy as a treatment for depression. *J Consult Clin Psychol.* 1991;59:547-557.
9. O'Leary KD, Beach SRH. Marital therapy: a viable treatment for depression and marital discord. *Am J Psychiatry.* 1990;147:183-186.
10. Scott AIF, Freeman CPL. Edinburgh primary care depression study: treatment outcome, patient satisfaction, and cost after 16 weeks. *BMJ.* 1992; 304;883-887.
11. Ross M, Scott M. An evaluation of the effectiveness of individual and group cognitive therapy in the treatment of depressed patients in an inner city health centre. *J R Coll Gen Pract.* 1985; 35:239-242.
12. Teasdale JD, Fennell MJV, Hibbert GA, Amies PL. Cognitive therapy for major depressive disorder in primary care. *Br J Psychiatry.* 1984;144:400-406.
13. Hollon SD, DeRubeis RJ, Evans MD, Wiemer MJ, Garvey MJ, Grove WM, Tuason VB. Cognitive-therapy and pharmacotherapy for depression: singly and in combination. *Arch Gen Psychiatry.* 1992; 49:774-781.

COMMENTARY

Practice Guidelines and Professional Challenges

What Psychotherapists Need to Do

Drs Persons, Thase, and Crits-Christoph[1] are to be congratulated for a concise, thorough, and well-executed review of the empirical basis supporting or contradicting the various recommendations for the psychotherapy of depression in the American Psychiatric Association and Agency for Health Care Policy and Research guidelines. The recommendations about guideline development given by the authors are eminently reasonable. What is most striking about the overall field of psychotherapy is the paucity of outcome research available. It behooves the mental health professions to understand this deficiency and to decide on a remedial course of action.

Psychotherapy does not have a major research tradition. Psychoanalytic psychotherapy, the most widely practiced technique, has developed as a professional service delivered by psychiatrists, psychologists, and social workers who have received training in graduate and postgraduate programs organized and operated by professional guilds. Therapeutic techniques have been taught by practicing professionals based on texts written by eminent psychoanalysts. Treatment principles have been derived primarily from recommendations based on anecdotal case material. This is not dissimilar to the average situation in medicine, surgery, and a variety of nonmedical professions, including law, teaching, and the clergy. In fact, it is anomalous that a profession is asked to defend the validity or value of its service based on the results of empirically conducted outcome research.

It may be helpful to understand some of the factors that led to the current predicament faced by psychotherapy. There has been an increasing trend in recent decades to put medical and surgical treatments on more scientifically sound foundations. Nowhere has this been more prominent than in the area of pharmaceuticals. The evolution of methods for the conduct of randomized clinical trials and a stringent set of standards for the testing of efficacy and safety (implemented and administered by the Food and Drug Administration and associated advisory committees in the United States) of new drug treatments had led to a burgeoning empirical database supporting drug treatments of various medical and psychiatric disorders. It is of interest that, despite large expenditures for research and development, the pharmaceutical industry thrives on and profits from psychiatric drugs and continues to attract some of the most eminent neuropsychopharmacology researchers into employment.

See also pages 283, 291, 298, and 301

In this context, the gauntlet was thrown down by clinical psychopharmacology researchers such as Gerald Klerman and Donald Klein et al[2-4] for comparable studies of the efficacy of psychotherapy and combined psychotherapy and drug treatment. With some notable exceptions (Aaron Beck and followers of cognitive behavioral therapy; Klerman and Weissman et al in the area of interpersonal psychotherapy), the challenge has been largely ignored. The bulk of total worldwide expenditures for psychotherapy research has been provided by the National Institute of Mental Health in the United States and has been minuscule in comparison with the research dollars the pharmaceutical industry devotes to studying psychotropic drugs. Yet, until recently, psychotherapy has thrived, clinics and practices have been filled, and the mental health professions have been continually expanding. This situation was facilitated by rather uncritical third-party insurance and government-supported programs of reimbursement for psychotherapy services.

The forces that have produced the current changes are well known. They include greater degrees of employer and third-party cost consciousness, increasingly conservative taxpayer and congressional fiscal postures toward government-funded medical/psychiatric reimbursement, and an ideological shift from an era of social and environmental determinism to biologically and genetically based theories.

Efficacy and safety demonstrated by empirical outcome research rather than expert clinical judgment may be an unusual and unfair standard to pose for a professional service. Outcome studies have not been required for reimbursement for legal, educational, or theological services. Nonetheless, psychotherapy has two major strategic disadvantages as a professional service: a history of being funded by governmental and private medical insurance, sources that are currently intensely focused on cost-cutting; and the fact that pharmaceuticals are the major alternative treatment. These factors tend to put psychotherapy in the position of needing to demonstrate safety and efficacy by stringent government-type standards, in addition to a new imperative to compete in comparisons of cost-effectiveness.

I believe that the technology exists for the conduct of methodologically sound psychotherapy research. Unfortunately, psychotherapy research is even more expensive and technically demanding than clinical psychopharmacology research. Only a handful of investigators are currently qualified to conduct high-quality psychotherapy research. Given these considerations, the psychotherapy professions (primarily psychiatry, clinical psychology, and social work) have two main alternative paths available. One route would be passivity and acceptance of the scaling back of reimbursement for these largely untested and unproven treatments for mental disorders. Such a road might result in smaller numbers of psychotherapy practitioners who would receive lower reimbursements for their services. A second possibility would be for the practicing professionals to fund research and development efforts to support the effectiveness and cost-benefit of the treatments they deliver. Presumably, mechanisms for taxing membership and solicitation of other potential revenue sources could be coordinated and implemented through the national professional associations for the purpose of funding outcome research. A great deal of active leadership would be required in these efforts. This would be the proactive position. Such a database would be enormously helpful in the future revision of practice guidelines, as suggested by Persons et al, for the treatment not only of depression, but for all mental disorders.

James H. Kocsis, MD
Professor of Psychiatry
Cornell University Medical Center
New York, NY 10021

The author would like to thank Theodore Shapiro, MD; George Makari, MD; and Randy Lehrer, MSW, for helpful critiques of an earlier version of this Commentary.

REFERENCES

1. Persons JB, Thase ME, Crits-Cristoph P. The role of psychotherapy in the treatment of depression: review of two practice guidelines. *Arch Gen Psychiatry.* 1996;53:283-290.
2. Klein DF, Zitrin CM, Woerner MG, Ross DC. Treatment of phobias, II: behavior therapy and supportive psychotherapy: are there any specific ingredients? *Arch Gen Psychiatry.* 1983;40:139-145.
3. Klein DF. The specificity of psychotherapy. *Biol Psychiatry.* 1983;18:1105.
4. Klerman GL. The psychiatric patient's right to effective treatment: implications of Osheroff v Chestnut Lodge. *Am J Psychiatry.* 1990;147:409-418.

Recovery in Geriatric Depression

George S. Alexopoulos, MD; Barnett S. Meyers, MD; Robert C. Young, MD; Tatsu Kakuma, PhD; Maria Feder, MD; Adam Einhorn, MBA; Eileen Rosendahl, PhD

Background: Clinical characteristics of depression, age at illness onset, medical burden, disability, cognitive impairment, lack of social support, and poor living conditions may influence the course of depression. This study investigates the timetable of recovery and the role of the above factors in predicting recovery in elderly patients with major depression.

Methods: Recovery was studied in 63 elderly (age >63 years) and 23 younger patients with depression who were followed up for an average of 18.2 months (SD, 13.1 months) under naturalistic treatment conditions. Diagnosis was assigned according to Research Diagnostic Criteria after administration of the Schedule for Affective Disorders and Schizophrenia. The Longitudinal Follow-up Interval Examination was used to identify recovery.

Results: The recovery rate of depressed elderly patients was similar to that of younger depressed patients. In the elderly patients, age, antidepressant treatment, age at onset, and chronicity of episode were significantly associated with time to recovery since entry. Among these parameters, late age at onset was the strongest predictor of slow recovery. In younger patients, long time to recovery was predicted by weak social support, younger age, cognitive impairment, and low intensity of antidepressant treatment. In the elderly, the intensity of antidepressant treatment began to decline within 16 weeks from entry and approximately 10 weeks prior to recovery.

Conclusions: These findings challenge the view that geriatric depression has a worse outcome than depression in younger adults. However, depressed patients with onset of first episode in late life may be at higher risk for chronicity. Antidepressant treatment prescribed by clinicians may decline prior to recovery despite evidence that high treatment intensity is effective in preventing relapse.

(Arch Gen Psychiatry. 1996;53:305-312)

A LONG-HELD clinical view is that depressive episodes are self-limited. However, the National Institute of Mental Health (NIMH) Collaborative Depression Study observed that 30% of mixed-age depressed patients had not recovered within 1 year and 12% were still depressed after over 5 years of follow-up.[1] Geriatric depression often occurs in the context of social impoverishment, disability, and medical and neurological disorders that may influence the course of depressive disorder. For this reason, the outcome of geriatric depression requires special consideration. Studies of geriatric depression using a naturalistic treatment design observed chronicity rates ranging from 18% to 35% over a period of 1 to 2 years,[2-7] although an Australian study observed a chronicity rate of 11% in 1 year.[8] Nonetheless, a recent geriatric study[5] that used methods similar to those of the NIMH Collaborative Depression Study observed that 28% of elderly patients with depression remained chronically depressed, a rate comparable to that reported in younger adults.[1]

Most studies of mixed-age populations agree that chronicity of depression is predicted by high severity of the depressive syndrome and long duration of the current or previous episodes.[1,9-11] The rate of recovery for a given depressive episode appears to decrease over time. The NIMH Collaborative Depression Study observed that 50% of subjects recovered within 6 months, 70% within 1 year, 81% within 2 years, and 88% within 5 years.[1] Therefore, the more chronic an episode, the more likely it is to remain chronic. In addition, there is some evidence that the length of the immediately preceding episode predicts the episode under investigation, suggesting that each depressed patient has a tendency to have episodes of approximately the same duration.[10]

Geriatric studies have reported that chronicity of depression may be predicted by long duration of the current episode, coexisting medical illness, high severity of depression, and nonmelancholic presentation.[2,3,12] Disagreements among studies of predictors of chronicity in ger-

See Methods on next page

From Cornell University Medical College, White Plains, NY (Drs Alexopoulos, Meyers, Young, and Kakuma); The New York (NY) Hospital (Dr Feder and Mr Einhorn); and the Long Island Jewish Hospital and the Albert Einstein College of Medicine, New Hyde Park, NY (Dr Rosendahl).

iatric depression may be owing to differences in samples and research methods.

The main goal of this study was to describe the timetable and predictors of recovery in elderly patients with major depression. Unlike studies of younger adults, this investigation focused on age at illness onset, medical burden, disability, cognitive impairment, lack of social support, and poor living conditions as factors that may interfere with recovery. This study adopted a design and data analysis approach similar to that of the NIMH Collaborative Depression Study.[1,9,10] This approach led to an investigation of special aspects of geriatric depression while it permitted comparisons of its findings with the large body of work contributed by the NIMH Collaborative Depression Study.

METHODS

The subjects were 86 patients who sought treatment at the inpatient or outpatient services of a freestanding psychiatric university hospital. They all arrived at the hospital through the usual referral mechanisms. Research advertisements were not used. All the patients were consecutively recruited and gave written informed consent, agreeing to participate in a longitudinal study that does not control antidepressant treatment. Twelve patients, four men and eight women, were invited to participate in the study but refused. All of these patients had received a *DSM-III-R* diagnosis of major depression by their physicians: nine were diagnosed as having recurrent major depression; three, moderate major depression; six, severe major depression without psychotic features; and three, major depression with psychotic features.

Inclusion criteria were (1) the presence of major depressive disorder diagnosed according to the Research Diagnostic Criteria (RDC)[13]; (2) a Geriatric Depression Scale (GDS)[14] score higher than 14 and a 24-item Hamilton Depression Rating Scale[15] score higher than 17; (3) the presence of an informant who has knowledge of the patient's history and has enough contact so that he or she can observe behavioral changes within 1 week; and (4) residence at a distance within a 45-minute drive from the research facilities.

Exclusion criteria were (1) a history of a psychiatric illness (except personality disorder) other than unipolar depressive disorder diagnosed prior to the onset of their first depressive episode; (2) severe or acute medical illness, ie, metastatic cancer, decompensated cardiac, liver, or renal failure, major surgery, and stroke or myocardial infarction 6 months prior to study entry; (3) delirium, spinocerebellar degeneration, Huntington's chorea, Parkinson's disease, or multi-infarct dementia; (4) cognitive dysfunction, ie, forgetfulness, restriction of activities such as driving, shopping, housekeeping, paying bills, and visiting friends, for longer than 6 months prior to the onset of depression, and a Mini-Mental State Examination[16] score lower than 15; and (5) severe behavioral disability defined as complete impairment in the performance of activities of daily living domain of the Philadelphia Multilevel Assessment Instrument (MAI).[17]

These criteria produced a sample of patients with major depressive disorder whose cognitive functions ranged from normal to mild dementia. Patients with major medical illness, severe dementia, and severe disability were excluded because these factors may interfere with rating of psychopathologic features, thus requiring specifically designed and validated clinical instruments.

Because the study focused on predictors of outcome of geriatric major depressive disorder, a rather large sample of elderly patients was necessary. A smaller comparison group that consisted of younger adults with major depressive disorder was also used. The younger comparison group was formed by recruiting one younger patient (aged <65 years) for every three elderly patients. Therefore, the sample of geriatric patients is approximately three times larger than that of younger patients.

All the subjects underwent assessment with the Schedule for Affective Disorders and Schizophrenia–Lifetime Version.[18] Severity of depression was quantified with the 24-item Hamilton Depression Rating Scale[15] and the GDS.[14] The GDS is a self-rated scale that was specifically designed and validated in geriatric populations. The GDS and other self-rated instruments in this study were rated by the patients in the presence of a research assistant who explained each item and sought to ensure that the scores provided by the patients accurately reflected the patients' views on the specific items. Because cognitive impairment may interfere with rating of depressive symptoms, the Cornell Scale for Depression in Dementia[19] was also used. The Cornell Scale is an interviewer-rated scale that is completed on the basis of information collected from both the depressed patient and an informant. The Cornell Scale has been validated in demented and nondemented elderly subjects.[20]

Overall cognitive impairment was evaluated using the Mini-Mental State Examination [16] and the Mattis Dementia Rating Scale.[21] The Mini-Mental State Examination is a widely used instrument that permits comparison of findings of this study with findings of others. The Mattis Dementia Rating Scale is sensitive in discriminating mildly demented patients from nondemented patients.[22]

Medical illness, lack of social support, and poor environment may all influence the course of depression. To study the potential effect of these factors on recovery, the MAI was used. The MAI was chosen because its item selection is comprehensive and permits global rating (five-grade scale) on a variety of domains, as well as the use of psychometrically validated indices. The medical health domain relies on assessment of self-rated health (by the patient), presence of health conditions, and health behavior.

RESULTS

Of the 86 subjects, 63 were older than 64 years and 23 were younger (**Table 1**). Elderly patients had demographic characteristics similar to the younger adults, except for education. Approximately 11% of the elderly subjects had less than 10 years of education, while all the younger subjects had more years of education. Similarly, 25% of the elderly group had graduated from college and/or had postgraduate studies, compared with 44% of younger patients. Psychotic depression was more frequent in the elderly group compared with the younger group ($\chi^2=5.74$, $df=1$, $P<.02$). There were no significant differences in severity of depression, cognitive impairment, medical health, social support, and physical environment between el-

Physical impairment was also rated with the Cumulative Illness Rating Scale-G.[23] This scale provides a format for rating impairment in 13 relatively independent organ areas. Ratings are made on a five-digit severity scale. In this study, the total Cumulative Illness Rating Scale-G score of 12 areas was used; scores for psychiatric impairment were not included in the total score. Social support was assessed using the social support domain of the MAI,[17] which depends on ratings of family interactions with friends. Finally, the physical environment domain was used. The subindices of this domain are subjective view of housing and subjective view of neighborhood.

Although antidepressant treatment may modify the course of depression, we did not control for treatment. However, the intensity of somatic treatment was classified according to a five-grade composite scale: 0, no treatment; 1, treatment with benzodiazepines; 2, treatment with cyclic antidepressants at daily doses lower than 75 mg of imipramine hydrochloride, desipramine hydrochloride, amitriptyline hydrochloride, doxepin hydrochloride, maprotiline hydrochloride, or amoxapine, 50 mg of nortriptyline hydrochloride, 30 mg of phenelzine sulfate, 20 mg of tranylcypromine sulfate, 100 mg of trazodone hydrochloride, or 100 mg of bupropion hydrochloride; 3, treatment with cyclic antidepressants at daily doses of 75 to 125 mg of imipramine hydrochloride or equivalent drugs, 50 to 60 mg of nortriptyline hydrochloride, 30 to 45 mg of phenelzine sulfate, 20 to 30 mg of tranylcypromine sulfate, 101 to 200 mg of trazodone hydrochloride, 6 to 10 mg of fluoxetine hydrochloride, or 101 to 200 mg of bupropion hydrochloride; 4, treatment with cyclic antidepressants at daily doses of 126 to 200 mg of imipramine hydrochloride or equivalent drugs, 61 to 80 mg of nortriptyline hydrochloride, 46 to 60 mg of phenelzine sulfate, 31 to 40 mg of tranylcypromine sulfate, 201 to 299 mg of trazodone hydrochloride, 11 to 20 mg of fluoxetine hydrochloride, or 200 to 300 mg of bupropion hydrochloride; and 5, treatment with cyclic antidepressants at daily doses greater than 200 mg of imipramine hydrochloride or equivalent drugs, 80 mg of nortriptyline hydrochloride, 60 mg of phenelzine sulfate, 40 mg of tranylcypromine hydrochloride, 300 mg of trazodone hydrochloride, 20 mg of fluoxetine hydrochloride, or 300 mg of bupropion hydrochloride. The composite treatment intensity scale was a modification of the scale used by Keller et al.[1,24] Elderly patients with depression often receive low doses of antidepressants. For this reason, the composite treatment was modified to include a broader range of lower doses, so that it can capture variability in the treatment of elderly patients.

After the initial evaluation, the patients and informants had in-person evaluations every 6 months. In addition, the subjects had telephone evaluations 3 months after each in-person session. Therefore, patients and informants had contact with the investigators every 3 months. Each patient-informant pair was assigned to the same assistant who visited the subjects at their homes if they were unable to come to the hospital. These follow-up procedures were intended to reduce attrition and allow accurate detection of outcome events during the follow-up period. The Longitudinal Interval Follow-Up Evaluation (LIFE)[25] was used to identify recovery of depression. The LIFE requires that the interviewer make retrospective weekly ratings of symptom levels for the diagnosis assigned during the initial interview. Anchor points, eg, patient's birthday and holidays, are used to facilitate recall. Ratings were assigned weekly using the following six-point scale of the LIFE Psychiatric Status Ratings (PSR): 1, usual self; 2, residual (one or more symptoms of no more than mild degree); 3, partial remission (meets considerably less symptoms than RDC criteria but still has obvious evidence of the disorder); 4, marked (does not meet RDC criteria but has obvious symptoms of major depression); 5, definite criteria (meets RDC criteria for major depression but no prominent psychotic symptoms or extreme impairment in functioning); and 6, definite criteria (meets RDC criteria for major depression with prominent psychotic symptoms or extreme impairment in functioning). Recovery was defined as beginning with the first week of 8 consecutive weeks with a PSR of 1 or 2.

Cumulative and instantaneous probabilities of recovery from the index episode of major depressive disorder were estimated using the Kaplan-Meier method.[26] The average follow-up was 18.2 months (SD, 13.1 months). The relationship of each "hypothesized predictor" to recovery was first examined using the life-table method for the categorical variables and a univariate Cox regression for the continuous variables. The hazard rates of potential predictors of recovery were then examined for proportionality after graphical representation of the estimated survival functions. Because the hypothesized predictors that initially appeared to have a significant relationship to recovery met the proportionality assumption, the semiparametric proportional hazards model was used for multivariate analysis. Variables that appeared significant were reexamined using forward and backward multiple Cox regression analyses. Interactions of the variables that appeared to predict recovery were later included in the model.

derly and younger patients. The younger group included a rather large number of middle-aged patients. This may have been in part a result of the requirement that major depression not be preceded by psychiatric disorders other than personality disorders. The rather small age difference between the elderly group and the younger group allows clinically interesting comparisons, since middle-aged patients with depression have more clinical and social similarities with elderly depressed patients than very young adults.

ATTRITION

Of the 86 patients, one was unavailable for follow-up prior to recovery and refused further participation. In addition, one patient died of suicide by hanging and five died of other causes prior to recovery. The causes of death were cardiovascular disease for three patients, cerebrovascular disease for one, and pneumonia for one. Estimation of the cumulative probability to recovery by the Kaplan-Meier method takes into consideration attrition of subjects due to withdrawal from the study or death. Estimates of cumulative probability are based on those who remained in the study and therefore were candidates for recovery. However, inherent in the Kaplan-Meier method is the assumption that patients who withdrew or died would have had a similar probability of recovery as patients who remained in the study. Review of the five patients who died prior to recovery showed that several of them had received high-intensity antidepressant treat-

Table 1. Characteristics at Entry for 63 Elderly and 23 Younger Patients With Major Depression*

Variable	Elderly Patients With Depression	Younger Patients With Depression
Gender, No. (%)		
Men	17 (27)	8 (35)
Women	46 (73)	15 (65)
Status at entry, No. (%)		
Inpatient	45 (71)	14 (61)
Outpatient	18 (29)	9 (39)
Previous episodes, No. (%)		
0	15 (24)	7 (30)
1	21 (33)	7 (30)
2	10 (16)	2 (9)
>2	17 (27)	7 (30)
RDC subtypes, No. (%)		
Endogenous	48 (76)	18 (78)
Psychotic	18 (28)	1 (4)
Age, y†	74.9/5.6/65/86	54.6/11/26/64
Severity of depression†		
24-HDRS	26.3/6.8/18/43	27.3/7.2/18/43
Cornell Scale for Depression in Dementia	18.4/5.9/10/30	19.6/4.9/12/29
Geriatric Depression Scale	19.9/3.9/15/29	23.0/4.0/15/29
Cognitive impairment†		
MMSE	27.5/2.7/18/30	29/1.5/25/30
DRS	133.3/9.2/103/144	140.3/3.8/131/144
Medical health†	5.4/2.9/0/12	5.0/3.8/0/16
Social support (MAI)†	52.7/12.5/28/82	56.0/16.9/21/82
Physical environment (MAI)†	74.9/5.6/65/86	56.6/7.8/42/68

*RDC indicates Research Diagnostic Criteria; 24-HDRS, 24-item Hamilton Depression Rating Scale; MMSE, Mini-Mental State Examination; DRS, Mattis Dementia Rating Scale; and MAI, Philadelphia Multilevel Assessment Instrument.

†Data are given as mean/SD/minimum/maximum score.

ment, ie, composite treatment scores of 5, 5, 4, 3, and 3. For this reason, their prognosis may have been worse than that of the patients who remained alive and continued in the study. Mortality, therefore, may have biased the sample toward a population with favorable prognosis, and the proportion of patients remaining ill during the follow-up period may be an underestimate.

CUMULATIVE PROBABILITY OF RECOVERY

Cumulative probabilities of recovery were estimated since entry to the study. In the elderly group (aged >64 years), the probability of recovering within 1 week since entry to the study was 8%; within 4 weeks, 14%; within 8 weeks, 24%; within 13 weeks, 35%; within 26 weeks, 59%; within 1 year, 74%; within 1.5 years, 77%; and within 2 years, 77%. Similar recovery rates were noted in the younger group (**Figure 1**). The probability of recovery since entry for the younger group (aged <65 years) was 9% within 1 week; 13% within 4 weeks; 26% within 8 weeks; 43% within 13 weeks; 61% within 26 weeks; 74% within 1 year; 79% within 1.5 years; and 86% within 2 years.

Estimation of time to recovery since the onset of the depressive episode showed that the cumulative probability of recovery in the elderly group was 5% within 4 weeks; 10% within 8 weeks; 13% within 13 weeks; 29% within 26 weeks; 56% within 1 year; 64% within 1.5 years; and 67% within

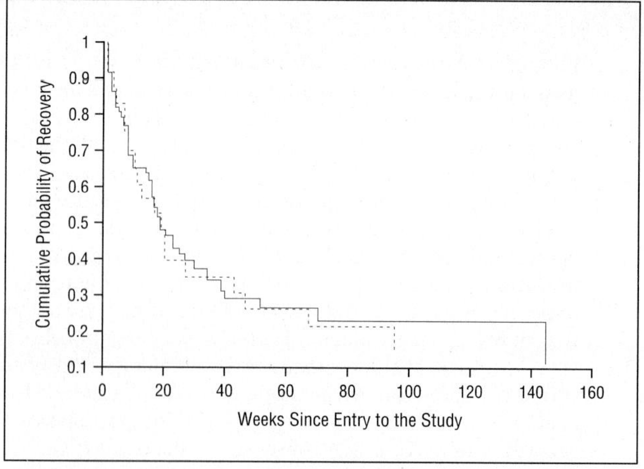

Figure 1. *Kaplan-Meier survival curves for the index episode of 63 elderly patients (aged >64 years) (solid line) and 23 younger patients (aged <65 years) (dotted line) with major depressive disorder. At entry, all subjects were experiencing an episode. Seven subjects were "censored," six died, and one was unavailable for follow-up.*

2 years. In the younger group, the cumulative probability to recovery since onset was 9% within 4 weeks; 9% within 8 weeks; 13% within 13 weeks; 35% within 26 weeks; 52% within 1 year; 65% within 1.5 years; and 78% within 2 years.

PREDICTION OF RECOVERY

Following the approach outlined in the "Methods" section, variables such as age, sex, marital status, maximum antidepressant treatment received during the depressive episode, chronicity of episode (from onset to study entry), age at onset, severity of depression, cognitive impairment, medical health, social support, and physical environment were examined for their ability to predict recovery since entry into the study. In the elderly group (n=63; 28.6% censored), a model including age, antidepressant treatment, age at onset, and chronicity of episode offered the highest prediction of time to recovery (**Table 2**). Among these parameters, age at onset was the strongest predictor, indicating an association between late onset of depression and slow recovery. Onset of depression was categorically divided into late (after age 64 years) and early (before age 65 years) onset. Survival curves were then calculated on the basis of the mean age, age at onset, intensity of antidepressant treatment, chronicity of depression, Mattis Dementia Rating Scale score, and MAI social support domain of this sample using the Cox proportional hazard model. The cumulative probability of recovery at 2 years was estimated to be 64% for the late-onset patients and 90% for the early-onset geriatric patients with depression (**Figure 2**). Chronicity of episode (onset to study entry) was also associated with slow recovery. Antidepressant treatment had both a linear and a quadratic relationship to recovery (Table 2), suggesting that the intensity of antidepressant treatment had an increasing effect on recovery but reached a ceiling. Because maximum antidepressant treatment received during the episode may not be the only treatment parameter relevant to recovery, the above analyses were repeated twice. Initially, a model identical to the above was used except that the treatment variable was replaced with the maximum treatment intensity offered during the first 4 weeks after

Table 2. Predictors of Recovery in 63 Elderly and 23 Younger Patients With Major Depression

Predictors*	Risk Ratio	Wald χ^2	*P*	Relative Risk (95% Confidence Interval)
Elderly Patients With Depression				
Since entry†				
Age	1.00	0.01	.91	1.00 (0.94-1.05)
Treatment	5.91	5.09	.02	5.91 (1.26-27.68)
Treatment × treatment	0.75	6.22	.01	0.75 (0.59-0.94)
Age at onset	0.97	8.57	.003	0.97 (0.95-0.99)
Onset to entry	1.00	3.74	.05	1.004 (1.00-1.009)
Since onset‡				
Age	0.97	0.74	.39	0.97 (0.92-1.03)
Treatment	0.89	0.90	.34	0.89 (0.69-1.13)
Age at onset	0.98	6.69	.01	0.97 (0.96-0.99)
Younger Patients With Depression				
Since entry§				
Age	0.78	6.33	.01	0.78 (0.64-0.95)
Treatment	0.04	4.55	.03	0.042 (0.002-0.773)
Age × treatment	1.067	4.65	.03	1.067 (1.006-1.131)
DRS total score	1.25	5.22	.02	1.26 (1.03-1.53)
Social support (MAI)	2.26	7.58	.006	2.26 (1.27-4.05)
Since onset‖				
Age	0.93	5.37	.02	0.93 (0.88-0.99)
Treatment	1.02	0.01	.93	1.02 (0.63-1.67)
DRS total score	1.21	5.46	.02	1.21 (0.03-1.42)
Social support (MAI)	1.91	6.53	.01	1.91 (1.16-3.13)

*Treatment refers to the intensity of somatic treatment classified according to a five-grade operationalized scale; the treatment × treatment interaction indicates a quadratic relationship between treatment intensity and time to recovery. DRS indicates Mattis Dementia Rating Scale; MAI, Philadelphia Multilevel Assessment Instrument.

†Likelihood ratio χ^2 for overall model=14.24; df=5, $P<.01$.

‡Likelihood ratio χ^2 for overall model=9.98; df=3, $P<.02$.

§Likelihood ratio χ^2 for overall model=27.56; df=5, $P<.001$.

‖Likelihood ratio χ^2 for overall model=16.03; df=4, $P<.003$.

entry to the study. Later, the same model was used but the treatment variable was the maximum treatment intensity offered during the 4 weeks prior to recovery or at the end of follow-up. In each of these analyses, age at onset was significantly associated with slow recovery (model including maximum treatment during the first 4 weeks: Wald χ^2 for age at onset=5.45, $P<.02$; model including maximum treatment during the 4 weeks preceding recovery or at the end of follow-up: Wald χ^2 for age at onset=5.57, $P<.02$). Age, treatment intensity, or chronicity of episode (from onset to entry) were not significantly associated with recovery in either model.

In the younger group (n=23; 17.4% censored) the strongest predictor of long time to recovery was poor social support, while older age, low intensity of antidepressant treatment (maximum level during the episode), age by treatment interaction, and cognitive impairment also were significantly associated with slow recovery (Table 2). As in the geriatric group, this analysis was repeated twice. First, a model with the above parameters was used except that the treatment variable was the maximum treatment during the first 4 weeks of the study. Then, the same model was used but the treatment variable was replaced with the maximum treatment intensity during the 4 weeks prior to recovery or prior to the end of the study. In each of these analyses, poor social support predicted slow recovery (analysis, Wald χ^2=4.82, $P<.03$; second analysis, Wald χ^2=7.01, $P<.008$). There was a significant association between cognitive impairment and time to recovery in the first analysis (Wald χ^2=3.71, $P<.05$) but only a nonsignificant trend (Wald χ^2=2.8, $P<.14$) in the second analysis.

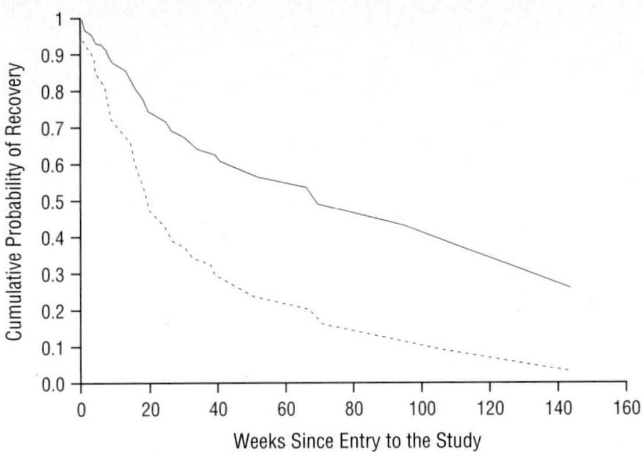

Figure 2. *Estimated mean survival curves for the index episode of 25 elderly patients (aged >64 years) with late-onset (after age 64 years) major depression (solid line) and 38 elderly patients with early-onset (prior to age 64 years) major depression (dotted line). At entry, all patients were experiencing an episode. The survival curves illustrate the probability of remaining depressed for the "average" elderly subject with late- or early-onset depression.*

Predictors of time to recovery since the onset of the depressive episode were studied using the approach employed to analyze predictors of time to recovery since entry. In the elderly group (n=63), the model including age, maximum antidepressant treatment intensity during the episode, and age at onset of illness was significant in predicting time to recovery since onset of depression. Late age at onset remained a significant predictor of slow recovery, while age and antidepressant treatment were no longer significant (Table 2). The cumulative probability of recovery within 2 years from onset was 48% for those with late-onset and 80% for those with early-onset depression. In the younger group (n=23), slow recovery since the onset of the depressive episode was predicted by weak social support, cognitive impairment, and young age, while antidepressant treatment was not significant (Table 2). The overall model was also significant (likelihood ratio χ^2=16.03, *df*=4, $P<.003$).

SYMPTOMS DURING THE EPISODE

The course of depressive episode was examined by reviewing the PSR scores obtained during the period starting from entry into the study and the beginning of recovery. Therefore, this analysis included the PSR scores until the first week (of 8 consecutive weeks) in which PSR scores of 1 or 2 were obtained and thus criteria for recovery were met.

At entry to the study, the modal PSR score for both the elderly and younger subjects was 5.0. The average PSR score dropped below 4.0 for the first time during the seventh week (mean PSR, 3.96; SD, 1.15) in the elderly group and during the fifth week (mean PSR, 3.73; SD, 0.80) in the younger subjects. During the rest of the episode, the PSR score fluctuated between an average of 3.25

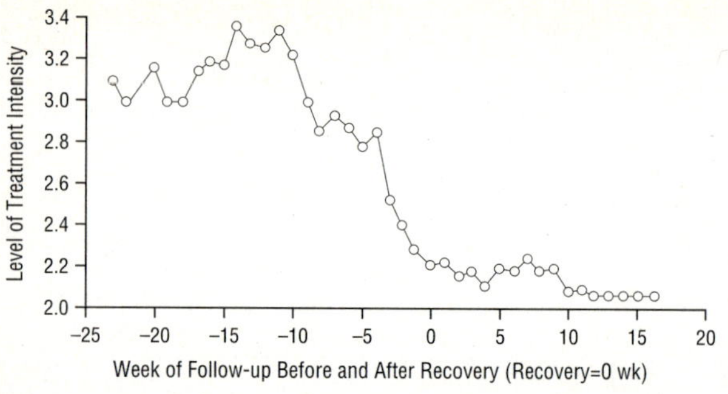

Figure 3. *Mean intensity of somatic antidepressant treatment classified according to a five-grade operationalized scale (see "Methods" section for details) during the follow-up period in 63 elderly patients with major depression. A drop in mean treatment intensity occurred 10 weeks prior to recovery and approximately 16 weeks since entry to the study.*

and 4.33 in the elderly group and between 2.87 and 4.00 in the younger group.

Severity of depression throughout the depressive episode was examined by identifying the percentage of time that the patients met full criteria (PSR score of 5 or 6) prior to recovery. The median proportion of time spent with full criteria (PSR score of 5 or 6) was 33.3% (mean, 34.5%; SD, 31.5) for the elderly group and 28.5% (mean, 19.7%; SD, 24.7) for the younger group.

CHRONICITY

At 2 years of follow-up, 26% (22/86) of the patients failed to meet criteria for recovery. The percentage of nonrecovery was 29% (18/63) for the elderly group and 17% (4/23) for the younger patients with depression. The criterion for recovery requires that patients receive PSR scores of 1 or 2 for 8 consecutive weeks. However, even in nonrecovered patients, depressive symptoms may fluctuate significantly from mild symptomatic states that do not meet RDC criteria for major depression (PSR score of 3 or 4) to extremely severe major depression (PSR score of 6). In this sample, of the 22 elderly patients with depression who did not recover, 18% (4/22) met full criteria for major depression (PSR score of 5 or 6) for more than 50% of the time in the study, and 82% (18/22) met less than full criteria for more than 50% of the time. Of the four younger patients who did not recover, 25% (1/4) met full criteria for major depression for more than half the follow-up period while 75% (3/4) had symptoms that did not meet RDC criteria for major depression for more than half of their follow-up time.

ANTIDEPRESSANT TREATMENT

The average intensity of antidepressant treatment received during the episode (prior to recovery) was calculated weekly. There was a precipitous decline in the intensity of antidepressant treatment as of the 16th week of the study and a plateau at an average treatment intensity of approximately 2.4 after the 40th week. The decline in antidepressant treatment intensity appeared to start approximately 10 weeks prior to recovery and was stabilized after recovery (**Figure 3**). There were no significant differences in treatment intensity between elderly and younger patients.

SUICIDE

Of the 86 subjects followed up during this study, one committed suicide by hanging. He was a 69-year-old white married businessman who was hospitalized for his second episode of major depression after a major business setback. A previous major depressive episode at 52 years of age, in which he responded favorably to electroconvulsive therapy (ECT), had followed the death of his first wife. During his second episode, the patient was hospitalized because of suicidal ideation and received 12 courses of bilateral ECT. He achieved partial improvement and was prescribed nortriptyline hydrochloride, 75 mg/d. He was discharged at his and his family's insistence after 9 weeks of hospitalization since he denied suicidal ideation. The patient hanged himself 1 week later, during the 10th week of the study.

Two patients attempted suicide during the study. The first patient was a 75-year-old white married woman who had her first episode of major depression at 40 years of age. This episode responded to ECT, but the patient had four more episodes of major depression at 41, 43, 68, and 75 years of age. Three of these episodes were treated with ECT. The patient improved after each episode, but during the interepisode intervals, depressed and irritable mood, hopelessness, and chronic suicidal ideation gradually developed. Eighteen weeks after she entered the study and while in her fifth episode of major depression (index episode), she attempted suicide by ingesting an unknown number of diazepam tablets. There was no distinct adverse life event; the patient attributed her suicide attempt to intensified feelings of hopelessness.

The second patient who attempted suicide scratched her wrists superficially 9 weeks after entry to the study while she was in her third episode of major depression (index episode). She was a 65-year-old white widowed retired nurse who had a history of two suicide attempts. She had her first episode of major depression at 63 years of age, approximately 1 year after receiving the diagnosis of breast cancer, which was treated with mastectomy and radiation. She responded to nortriptyline hydrochloride, 150 mg/d, but had two recurrences of depression within 2 years. During the interepisode periods, she maintained a hopeless outlook about her health and her future and had vague suicidal thoughts. The patient attributed her suicide attempt to increasing loneliness and concerns about caring for her own needs.

COMMENT

The principal findings of this study are that (1) elderly patients with major depression have approximately the same timetable of recovery as younger depressed patients; (2) late age at onset is a predictor of chronicity in geriatric depression; and (3) the intensity of antidepressant treatment prescribed by clinicians is reduced prior to the occurrence of recovery.

In this study, approximately 60% of either elderly or younger patients with depression recovered within 6 months from entry to the study and only an additional 20% of patients recovered during the following 1½ years. Therefore, both elderly and younger patients are more likely to remain depressed if they do not recover relatively early during the follow-up period. It should be pointed out that the younger sample included a large number of middle-aged patients. This factor might have contributed to the absence of differences in recovery between the elderly and the younger patients. The geriatric group had a significantly higher proportion of patients with major depression with psychotic features than the younger group. Psychotic depression has been found to respond poorly to antidepressants alone.[27,28] However, the geriatric patients did not have a worse recovery rate than the younger subjects. Comparable recovery rates in elderly and younger patients have been reported by studies that used methods similar to ours, including the NIMH Collaborative Study[1] and Hinrichsen's study[5] of an elderly sample. Even studies that used different methods have reported rates of recovery comparable to ours, ranging from 65% to 82% over a period of 1 to 2 years.[6-8,10,11]

It is clinically meaningful to study time to recovery since the onset of a depressive episode. The exact onset of an episode is often difficult to determine. However, in a subset of 20 elderly patients in our sample, we noted high interrater reliability (intraclass correlation r=.94) in identifying the duration of past depressive episodes when elderly patients and informants were interviewed by two raters using the LIFE[25]; this procedure was identical to the interview procedure of this study. Although no validity study was conducted, we believe interviewing of patients and informants resulted in reliable identification of the onset of the index episode. Using onset as the benchmark, about 55% of either elderly or younger depressed patients recovered within 1 year, but the rate of recovery was precipitously diminished after 1 year.

During episodes, depressive symptoms fluctuated. Both elderly and younger patients met RDC criteria for major depression for about 30% of the time, and they had milder symptoms the rest of the time. In elderly patients, depressive symptoms dropped below the level of major depression for the first time in 7 weeks after entry, while a similar drop occurred in younger patients after 5 weeks. The rather long time to improvement of the elderly group parallels the observation that elderly depressed patients require longer exposure to antidepressants than younger depressed patients[29]; nonetheless, focused studies are needed to evaluate the speed of response of geriatric depression.

In this study, nonrecovery of geriatric depression was predicted by late age at onset of depression even when maximum intensity of antidepressant treatment was taken into consideration. This observation is in accordance with findings of a retrospective study that noted that elderly patients with late-onset depression had longer hospital stays and more residual symptoms than patients with early-onset depression.[30] The reasons for the association between late onset of depressive disorder and chronicity are unclear. We have suggested that depression with onset during senescence is a heterogeneous condition and includes a large group of patients in whom medical and neurological disorders play an important role.[31] This view is supported by evidence of greater medical morbidity and mortality in late- compared with early-onset geriatric depression,[32,33] studies suggesting higher frequency of neuropsychological[34,35] and neuroradiological abnormalities[36-38] in late- compared with early-onset geriatric depression, and studies showing low frequency of affective disorders in the families of patients with late- compared with early-onset depression.[39] However, some studies failed to confirm the association between late depression onset and high medical and neurological morbidity.[30,40,41] Heterogeneity in the pathogenesis of late-life depressive disorders may be an important factor for these discrepancies. Impaired medical health and dementing disorders have been found to trigger depression[42] or worsen its course.[43] Moreover, it has been reported that neuroradiological[44] and cognitive abnormalities[43] are associated with poor response to treatment with antidepressants. It is possible that latent medical or neurological disorders contribute to the low recovery rate observed in late-onset depression. Nonetheless, studies of late-onset depression have limitations that include: (1) problems in the reliability of age at onset; (2) use of diverse categorical definitions of age at onset; (3) use of relatively small clinical samples from multiple sites; (4) lack of inclusion of subsyndromal depression, which limits the pathogenetic variability of late-onset depression; (5) difficulties in identifying appropriate control groups; and (6) the assumption that depression is homogeneous over time, although patients may experience episodes with different pathogenetic contributors during different episodes.

In a subset of 20 patients in the present study, the interrater reliability between two raters who interviewed subjects and informants at different times was high (intraclass correlation for age at first episode of major depression, .91). Moreover, age at onset was treated as a continuous variable. Despite methodological precautions, our findings are subject to limitations inherent in investigations of age at onset. Studies using longer follow-up will offer the opportunity to refute or validate the relationship between late age of depression onset, low recovery rate, and medical and dementing disorders, since most latent disorders will become apparent with aging and influence recovery directly.

In the younger group, weak social support was the strongest predictor of low recovery rate; this relationship was not observed in the elderly. This finding requires confirmation since the small number of younger adults does not allow definitive conclusions. However, similar findings have been reported by others,[45,46] who proposed that depression may become more autonomous and less responsive to psychosocial factors with increasing age.

Antidepressant treatment may influence the outcome of depression. Although the intensity of antidepressant treatment was taken into consideration, this approach cannot fully account for the heterogeneity of the currently available treatments or any specific interactions with predictors of recovery. Controlled treatment studies of long duration are needed to further examine the strength of predictors of recovery that were identified by this investigation.

In this study, the intensity of antidepressant treatment began to decline after 16 weeks since entry to the study. In the geriatric group, the drop in the intensity of antidepressant treatment began 10 weeks prior to recovery. Recovery was defined as a state of minimal or no symptoms or signs of depression. Therefore, improvement of depression may have started well prior to the occurrence of recovery. A possible explanation may be that physicians reduced the doses of antidepressants after the first signs of improvement because of concerns about side effects or at the request of patients who may have been more vociferous about side effects after improvement of depression. An alternative speculation may be that the clinicians lacked awareness of the importance of continuation treatment in prevention of relapse in geriatric depression.[47] This study cannot identify the reasons for early reduction in antidepressant treatment. Specifically designed studies with a focus on factors influencing the antidepressant prescription during the acute and continuation phases of treatment appears to be an appropriate next step. Therefore, our findings provide the background for effectiveness research studies on prophylactic treatment of geriatric depression.

Our results are limited by the relatively small sample for the number of comparisons attempted. This approach amply explores the data but generates findings that require confirmation through more focused studies. Another limitation is the lack of sampling from a broad community population. Because the subjects were patients of a large freestanding psychiatric hospital, patients with severe or persistent depression may be overrepresented. However, our findings may be applicable to the numerous geriatric patients who are treated for depression in similar settings. For this reason, we believe that they are clinically relevant.

Accepted for publication August 29, 1995.

This research was supported by grants R01 MH42819, T32 MH19132, and P20 MH49762, from the NIMH (Rockville, Md) and by a grant from the Xerox Foundation.

Reprint requests to Cornell University Medical College, Director, Cornell Institute of Geriatric Psychiatry, The New York Hospital–Cornell Medical Center, Westchester Division, 21 Bloomingdale Rd, White Plains, NY 10605 (Dr Alexopoulos).

REFERENCES

1. Keller MB, Lavori PV, Mueller TI, Endicott J, Coryell W, Hirschfeldt RMA, Shea T. Time to recovery, chronicity, and levels of psychopathology in major depression. *Arch Gen Psychiatry.* 1992;49:809-816.
2. Baldwin RC, Jolley DJ. The prognosis of depression in old age. *Br J Psychiatry.* 1986;149:574-583.
3. Murphy E. The prognosis of depression in old age. *Br J Psychiatry.* 1983;142:111-119.
4. Kennedy GJ, Kelman HR, Thomas C. Persistence and remission of depressive symptoms in late life. *Am J Psychiatry.* 1991;148:174-178.
5. Hinrichsen GA. Recovery and relapse from major depressive disorder in the elderly. *Am J Psychiatry.* 1992;149:1575-1579.
6. Stoudemire A, Hile CD, Morris R, Martino-Saltzman D, Lewison B. Long-term effective and cognitive outcome in depressed older adults. *Am J Psychiatry.* 1993;150:896-900.
7. Meats P, Timol M, Jolley D. Prognosis of depression in the elderly. *Br J Psychiatry.* 1991;159:659-663.
8. Burvill PW, Hall WD, Stampfer HG, Emmerson JP. The prognosis of depression in old age. *Br J Psychiatry.* 1991;158:64-71.
9. Keller MB. Chronic and recurrent affective disorders: incidence, course, and influencing factors. In: Racagnio G, ed. *Chronic Treatment in Neuropsychiatry.* New York, NY: Raven Press; 1985:111-120.
10. Keller MB, Lavori PW, Rice J, Coryell W, Hirschfeldt RMA. The persistent risk of chronicity in recurrent episodes of nonbipolar major depressive disorder: a prospective follow-up. *Am J Psychiatry.* 1986;143:24-28.
11. Alexopoulos GS, Chester JG. Outcomes of geriatric depression. *Clin Geriatr Med.* 1992;8:363-376.
12. Georgotas A, McCue RE, Cooper TB, Nogachandran N, Friedhoff A. Factors affecting the delay of antidepressant effect in responders to nortriptyline and phenelzine. *Psychiatry Res.* 1989;28:1-9.
13. Spitzer R, Endicott J, Robins E. Research diagnostic criteria. *Arch Gen Psychiatry.* 1978;35:773-782.
14. Yesavage JA, Brink TL, Rose TL, Adey M. The geriatric depression rating scale: comparison with other self-report and psychiatric rating scales. In: Crook T, Ferris S, Bartus R, eds. *Assessment in Geriatric Psychopharmacology.* New Canaan, Conn: Mark Powley Associates; 1983:153-165.
15. Hamilton M. A rating scale for depression. *J Neurol Neurosurg Psychiatry.* 1960;23:56-62.
16. Folstein MF, Folstein SF, McHugh PR. Mini-mental state: a practical method for grading the cognitive state of patients for the clinician. *J Psychiatr Res.* 1975;12:189-198.
17. Lawton MP, Moss M, Fulcomer M, Kleban MH. A research and service-oriented multilevel assessment instrument. *J Gerontol.* 1982;37:91-99.
18. Spitzer RL, Endicott J. *Schedule for Affective Disorders and Schizophrenia: Life-Time Version.* 3rd ed. New York, NY: Biometrics Research Division, New York State Psychiatric Institute; 1979.
19. Alexopoulos GS, Abrams RC, Young RC, Shamoian CA. Cornell scale for depression in dementia. *Biol Psychiatry.* 1988;23:271-284.
20. Alexopoulos GS, Abrams RC, Young RC, Shamoian CA. Use of the Cornell scale in non-demented patients. *J Am Geriatr Soc.* 1988;36:230-236.
21. Mattis S. *Dementia Rating Scale.* Odessa, Fla: Psychological Assessment Resources; 1989.
22. Shay KA, Duke LW, Conboy T, Harrell LE, Callaway R, Foles DG. The clinical validity of the MOHS Dementia Rating Scale in staging Alzheimer's dementia. *J Geriatr Psychiatry Neurol.* 1991;4:18-25.
23. Miller MD, Paradis CF, Houck PR, Mazumdar S, Stack JA, Rifai H, Mulsant B, Reynolds CF. Rating chronic medical illness burden in geropsychiatric practice and research: application of the Cumulative Illness Rating Scale. *Psychiatry Res.* 1991;41:237-248.
24. Keller MB, Klerman GL, Lavori PW, Fawcett JA, Coryell W, Endicott J. Treatment received by depressed patients. *JAMA.* 1982;248:1848-1855.
25. Keller MB, Lavori PW, Friedman B, Nielsen E, Endicott J, McDonald-Scott P, Andreasen NC. The longitudinal interval follow-up evaluation. *Arch Gen Psychiatry.* 1987;44:540-548.
26. Kalbfleisch J, Prentice RL. *The Statistical Analysis of Failure Time Data.* New York, NY: Wiley & Sons Inc; 1980.
27. Chan CH, Janisak PG, Davis JM, Altman E, Andriukaitis S, Hedeker D. Response of psychotic and non-psychotic depressed patients to tricyclic antidepressants. *J Clin Psychiatry.* 1987;48:197-200.
28. Kroessler D. Relative efficacy of rates for therapies of delusional depression. *Convuls Ther.* 1985;1:173-182.
29. Georgotas A, McCue RE. The additional benefit of extending an antidepressant trial past seven weeks in the depressed elderly. *Int J Geriatr Psychiatry.* 1989;4:191-195.
30. Conwell Y, Nelson JC, Kim KM, Majure CM. Depression in late life: age of onset as marker of a subtype. *J Affect Disord.* 1989;17:189-195.
31. Alexopoulos GS. Clinical and biological findings in late-onset depression. In: Tasman A, Goldfinger SM, Kaufman CA, eds. *Review of Psychiatry.* Washington, DC: American Psychiatric Press; 1990:9.
32. Roth M, Kay DWK. Affective disorders arising in the senium, II: physical disability as an etiological factor. *J Ment Sci.* 1956;102:141-150.
33. Jacoby RJ, Levy R, Bird JM. Computed tomography and the outcome of affective disorder: a follow-up study of elderly subjects. *Br J Psychiatry.* 1981;139:288-292.
34. Alexopoulos GS, Young RC, Meyers BS. Geriatric depression: age of onset and dementia. *Biol Psychiatry.* 1993;34:141-145.
35. Alexopoulos GS, Meyers BS, Young RC, Mattis S, Kakuma T. The course of geriatric depression with 'reversible dementia.' *Am J Psychiatry.* 1993;150:1693.
36. Alexopoulos GS, Young RC, Shindledecker R. Brain computed tomography in geriatric depression and primary degenerative dementia. *Biol Psychiatry.* 1992;31:591-599.
37. Jacoby RJ, Levy R. Computed tomography in the elderly, III: affective disorder. *Br J Psychiatry.* 1980;136:270-275.
38. Coffey CE, Figiel GS, Djang WT, Cress M, Saunders WB, Weiner RD. Leukoencephalopathy in elderly depressed patients referred for ECT. *Biol Psychiatry.* 1988;24:143-161.
39. Baron M, Mendlewicz J, Klotz J. Age-of-onset and genetic transmission in affective disorders. *Acta Psychiatr Scand.* 1981;64:373-380.
40. Greenwald BS, Kramer-Ginsberg E. Age of onset in geriatric depression: relationship to clinical variables. *J Affect Disord.* 1988;15:61-68.
41. Herrmann N, Lieff S, Silberfeld M. The effect of age of onset on depression in the elderly. *J Geriatr Psychiatry Neurol.* 1989;2:182-187.
42. Eastwood MR, Corbin SL. The relationship between physical illness and depression in old age. In: Murphy E, ed. *Affective Disorders in the Elderly.* New York, NY: Churchill Livingstone; 1986:177-186.
43. Young RC, Mattis S, Alexopoulos GS, Meyers BS, Shindledecer R, Dahr AK. Verbal memory and plasma drug concentrations in elderly depressives treated with nortriptyline. *Psychopharmacol Bull.* 1991;27:291-294.
44. Young RC, Nambudiri D, Alexopoulos GS, Roe R. Brain morphology and response to nortriptyline in elderly depressives. In: *Abstracts of the American Association for Geriatric Psychiatry.* Washington, DC: American Association for Geriatric Psychiatry; 1990.
45. Hughes DC, DeMalie D, Blazer DG. Does age make a difference in the effects of physical health and social support on the outcome of the major depressive episode? *Am J Psychiatry.* 1993;150:728-733.
46. Blazer DG, Hughes DC, George LK. Age and impaired subjective support: predictors of depressive symptoms at one year follow-up. *J Nerv Ment Dis.* 1992;180:172-178.
47. Georgotas A, McCue RE, Cooper TB. How effective and safe is continuation therapy in elderly depressed patients? *Arch Gen Psychiatry.* 1988;45:929-932.

ORIGINAL ARTICLE

Incidence and Correlates of Tardive Dyskinesia in First Episode of Schizophrenia

Miranda H. Chakos, MD; Jose Ma. J. Alvir, DrPH; Margaret G. Woerner, PhD; Amy Koreen, MD; Stephen Geisler, MD; David Mayerhoff, MD; Steven Sobel, MD; John M. Kane, MD; Michael Borenstein, PhD; Jeffrey A. Lieberman, MD

Background: There is controversy over whether tardive dyskinesia (TD) is solely a consequence of antipsychotic drug treatment or in part may reflect an intrinsic aspect of the disease process. Pathophysiologic factors could, independently or in concert with drug effects, lead to the development of dyskinetic signs.

Methods: We studied prospectively 118 patients in their first episode of psychosis who were treatment-naive or had less than 12 weeks of antipsychotic drug exposure at study entry. Patients received standardized antipsychotic drug treatment and were evaluated for up to 8½ years with regular assessments of psychopathologic signs and symptoms and side effects.

Results: The cumulative incidence of presumptive TD was 6.3% after 1 year of follow-up, 11.5% after 2 years, 13.7% after 3 years, and 17.5% after 4 years. Persistent TD had a cumulative incidence of 4.8% after 1 year, 7.2% after 2 years, and 15.6% after 4 years. Taken individually, both antipsychotic drug dose, entered as a time-dependent covariate, and poor response to treatment of the first psychotic episode were significant predicters of time to TD. When antipsychotic drug dose and treatment response were examined together, treatment responders had significantly lower hazards for presumptive TD than nonresponders (hazard ratio, 0.29; 95% confidence interval, 0.09 to 0.97). Dose was a trend-level predicter, with each 100-mg chlorpromazine equivalent unit increase in dose associated with a 5% increase in the hazard of presumptive TD (hazard ratio, 1.05; 95% confidence interval, 0.99 to 1.11).

Conclusion: Poor response to the treatment of a first episode of psychosis and, to a lesser extent, antipsychotic drug dose are important factors in the development of TD. This suggests that there may be a disease-related vulnerability to TD manifest with antipsychotic drug exposure. Potential pathophysiologic factors might include neurodevelopmentally induced structural neuropathologic characteristics, sensitization of nigrostriatal dopamine neurons, and the induction of glutamatergically mediated neurotoxic effects.

(Arch Gen Psychiatry. 1996;53:313-319)

SINCE THE mid-1960s there has been a progressive increase in case reports and epidemiologic studies of tardive dyskinesia (TD).[1] The prevalence of TD reported in a recent multicenter study of patients treated with antipsychotic drugs ranged from 13.3% among patients at a voluntary psychiatric hospital to 36.1% among patients at a state hospital.[2] With an increase in the number of patients exposed to long-term antipsychotic drug treatment with high-potency medications at higher doses, the apparent prevalence rate of TD increased from a mean of less than 5% before 1965 to approximately 25% in 1980.[3,4] The cumulative incidence of TD in treated patients is approximately 5% per year of antipsychotic drug treatment.[5] However, a recent study[6] reports higher persistent TD rates during the first 5 years of treatment in long-term outpatients receiving maintenance antipsychotic medications.

Several factors, including increased age,[2,4,7-9] gender,[2,4] and diagnosis (neuromedical and psychiatric),[4,7,10-12] may predispose to the development of TD. There is controversy as to whether TD is solely a consequence of antipsychotic drug treatment or in part reflects an intrinsic aspect of the disease process. Investigators have suggested that spontaneous involuntary movement disorders could be a feature of severe chronic schizophrenia unmodified by antipsychotic drugs.[13,14] Other

See Subjects and Methods on next page

From the Department of Psychiatry, Hillside Hospital, Long Island Jewish Medical Center, Albert Einstein College of Medicine, Glen Oaks, NY. Dr Lieberman is now with the Department of Psychiatry, University of North Carolina School of Medicine, Chapel Hill.

SUBJECTS AND METHODS

These data are from a prospective study of psychobiology in first-episode schizophrenia that is an ongoing cohort investigation of patients identified as treatment-naive or having less than 12 weeks of lifetime antipsychotic drug exposure. The first-episode sample has also been evaluated as a subgroup of the larger, ongoing Prospective Study of TD Development at our institution. The first-episode sample differed from the rest of the patient cohort on several factors. They had no or minimal antipsychotic drug treatment at study entry, while the larger sample was not limited to patients for whom antipsychotic drugs had been newly prescribed. Moreover, more comprehensive clinical information was available on the first-episode sample, including treatment response data, premorbid adjustment, ratings of psychopathologic signs and symptoms, and complete prospective antipsychotic drug histories.

We report on 118 subjects from the first-episode study. These subjects have been evalauted for up to 8½ years (median, 2.5 years), with TD examinations performed every 8 weeks. The follow-up duration varied mainly because of the continuing recruitment of first-episode patients into the prospective study, with later recruits contributing shorter durations. A detailed description of the design and methods has been reported previously.[18,19]

SUBJECT SELECTION

Patients admitted to the hospital for a first episode of psychosis were evaluated for the study with the Schedule for Affective Disorders and Schizophrenia (SADS).[20] The purpose and nature of the study were explained to eligible patients and their families, and informed consent was obtained. Eligible patients were in their first episode of psychosis; had a diagnosis of schizophrenia, schizophreniform disorder, or schizoaffective disorder by Research Diagnostic Criteria[21]; and were between the ages of 16 and 40 years. They had no or less than 12 weeks of antipsychotic drug exposure, no history of current substance abuse, and no neuromedical illness that could influence their diagnosis, such as endocrinopathy, hydrocephalus, or seizure disorder. Patients with prior antipsychotic drug exposure had a medication washout period of at least 2 weeks prior to beginning treatment. All patients were acutely psychotic with marked psychopathologic conditions at the time of study entry.

ASSESSMENTS

Measurement Instruments

Patients had baseline evaluations for psychopathologic conditions, extrapyramidal status, and involuntary movements using the SADS Change Version plus psychosis and disorganization items (SADS-C&PD),[22] Clinical Global Impressions (CGI) ratings,[23] Global Assessment Scale (GAS),[24] a modified Simpson Dyskinesia Scale (SDS),[25] a modified Simpson-Angus Extrapyramidal Scale (SAEPS),[26] and a modified Scale for the Assessment of Negative Symptoms (SANS).[27] Patients also received baseline ratings on the Premorbid Adjustment Scale (PAS)[28] for childhood, early and middle adolescence, and adulthood. This scale is designed to evaluate the degree of achievement of developmental goals and role performance in multiple areas of function at each of several periods of a subject's life prior to the onset of schizophrenia. After the initiation of treatment, patients were evaluated biweekly with the SADS-C&PD, SANS, SAEPS, and CGI for 12 weeks and every 4 weeks thereafter. Evaluations with the SDS were completed every 8 weeks. The SDS includes 28 items and a 6-point global score ranging from 0 (no TD) to 5 (severe TD). In addition, seven body-area items that correspond to the Abnormal Involuntary Movement Scale (AIMS)[29] were scored on a scale ranging from 0 to 5.

Antipsychotic Drug Treatment

Following baseline assessments, patients were treated in accordance with a standardized algorithm. They were initially treated with fluphenazine hydrochloride; the dosage was increased to 20 mg/d for 6 weeks. If extrapyramidal signs (EPS) developed, patients were given benztropine mesylate, 2 to 6 mg/d. If benztropine was ineffective for akathisia, lorazepam or propranolol hydrochloride could be added. For patients whose condition did not improve by week 6, the fluphenazine dosage was doubled to 40 mg/d by mouth for an additional 4 weeks. If there was still no improvement, patients were switched to haloperidol, 20 mg/d by mouth for 6 weeks, and if there was no improvement, 40 mg/d for 6 weeks. If there was still no improvement, a third antipsychotic drug from a different biochemical class was tried, usually molindone hydrochloride, up to 300 mg/d. Treatment-resistant patients were then considered for a trial of clozapine.

Remission was operationally defined as a rating no greater than 3 on any of the SADS-C&PD positive psy-

studies have suggested that exposure to antipsychotic drug treatment is the pathogenic factor in TD development[6] and that greater severity and persistence of TD is associated with greater antipsychotic drug exposure, that is, longer duration of treatment and a higher antipsychotic drug dose.[15,16] An alternative view is that TD vulnerability may be associated with disease-related pathophysiologic factors and that vulnerable individuals are most likely to show abnormal movements when exposed to antipsychotic drug treatment.

Most studies of TD rates and risk factors have been cross-sectional and have sampled primarily patients with chronic conditions and long treatment histories. For those found to have TD, the time of onset was usually not known. The major prospective studies of TD incidence have examined patients who were ill and treated for some time prior to study entry[5,6] or have dealt with elderly patients.[8,9] We have previously reported the incidence of extrapyramidal signs and idiopathic dyskinesia in treatment-naive patients with schizophrenia.[17] We now report the incidence and demographic and clinical correlates of TD in first-episode patients over the course of their long-term follow-up while receiving antipsychotic drug treatment.

chotic symptoms items, a rating of 3 (mild) or less on the CGI severity items, and a rating of 2 (much improved) or 1 (very much improved) on the CGI improvement items. This level of response was required to be sustained for 8 weeks (four consecutive biweekly ratings). Patients were classified as having full remission if they had no residual positive symptoms and a rating of 2 (mild) or less on each of the negative symptom global items of the SANS; partial remission was defined as persisting positive symptoms (eg, mild residual delusions, hallucinations, or thought disorganization below the levels required to meet remission criteria) or a global score of 3 (moderate) or greater on the SANS negative symptom items. Patients who failed to achieve criteria for full or partial remission were classified as nonresponders.

After patients reached remission, they entered the maintenance phase, during which the general treatment strategy was to gradually reduce the daily dose of antipsychotic medication to the lowest effective level. One year from the time of remission, the benefits and risks of continued treatment were explained to patients who had continued to be stable, and they were given the option of medication withdrawal. Patients who chose to discontinue medication were closely followed up for signs of relapse. Relapsing patients were re-treated with the medication to which they had initially responded.

Antipsychotic drug exposure history during the course of study participation was recorded prospectively, based on records of medications prescribed by the treating research psychiatrist, monthly patient evaluation interviews, and family reports on medication compliance. This allowed for accurate assessment of both the duration and dosage of antipsychotic drug treatment during the study period.

TD and EPS Diagnosis and Detection

Patients receiving a global score of 1 (questionable TD) or greater on the SDS as rated by the research psychiatrist were sent for rating confirmation by designated "expert raters" from the Prospective Study of TD Development.[7] These raters were blind to the patient's stage of illness and treatment. Cases of presumptive TD were defined as patients who received a global TD rating of at least 2 (mild TD) on the SDS according to each of the three expert raters independently at the same time. Cases of persistent TD were patients who met criteria for presumptive TD and whose TD symptoms persisted for at least 3 months in follow-up evaluations performed by the expert raters. (Interrater reliability was .91 on the SDS global items for the expert raters.)

Having EPS was operationally defined as having at least two scores of 2 (mild) *or* one score of 3 (moderate) on any of the modified SAEPS items for gait (item 1), rigidity (item 4), tremor (item 7), akinesia (item 9), or akathisia (item 10) *or* as having a "yes" response on the item for dystonia within the first episode of illness.

Data Analysis

Two sets of analyses were done, the first using presumptive TD and the second using persistent TD as the outcome variable. Survival analysis was used to estimate the cumulative incidence of presumptive and persistent TD and to assess the effects of risk factors. The risk factors assessed in the analyses of persistent TD were limited to antipsychotic drug dose and treatment responder status. Analyses involving persistent TD and the larger set of clinical and demographic variables (**Table 1**) are not included in this report because of the small number of persistent TD cases. Cox proportional hazards regression was used to estimate the effects, using hazard ratios, of single predicter variables as well as sets of predicter variables (**Table 2**). Antipsychotic drug dose, EPS, and type of antipsychotic drug (clozapine vs typical antipsychotic drugs) had values that varied over time. They were entered into the analyses as time-dependent covariates. Antipsychotic drug dose levels were converted in chlorpromazine equivalent units because of the different potency levels of the various antipsychotic drugs used. Ninety-five percent confidence intervals were generated for the hazard ratios, equivalent to setting the type I error level at .05.

We assessed whether treatment response during the first episode was a significant predicter of TD. Because of the unequal follow-up among patients, time to treatment response (or censoring date for nonresponders) was controlled for in these analyses. Treatment response and antipsychotic drug dose, with clozapine status and time to treatment response, were entered simultaneously in proportional hazards regression to try to unravel the independent effects of these variables.

We tested whether the proportional hazards assumption was valid by incorporating into the models terms measuring the interaction of the predicter with the logarithm of the time to outcome. Residual plots were also inspected to assess the fit of the proportional hazards model.

RESULTS

PATIENT CHARACTERISTICS

Sixty-one (52%) of the 118 patients in the sample were male. The mean (SD) age at study entry was 25.2 (6.6) years. Forty-one percent were white, 37% were black, 12% were Hispanic, 7% were Asian, and 3% were of mixed racial background. Seventy percent of patients in the sample had schizophrenia and 30% had schizoaffective disorder. Patients had high levels of psychopathologic symptoms at study entry. The mean (SD) score on the GAS[24] was 27.1 (9.0), and the mean severity of illness score on the CGI[23] was 5.5 (1.0).

Seventy-three percent of patients had no prior antipsychotic drug treatment at study entry. Eleven percent had between 2 and 12 weeks of prior treatment (mean, 5 weeks); 16% had less than 2 weeks of prior treatment (mean, 4 days). Fourteen patients failed to meet remission criteria with treatment during follow-up. The median time to remission for the sample was 9 weeks. Patients who ended study participation prior to 5 years of follow-up did not differ from other study patients in their treatment outcome. Thirteen patients received cloza-

Table 1. Demographic and Clinical Factors and Tardive Dyskinesia Risk*

	Hazard Ratio (95% Confidence Limits)
Female sex	0.79 (0.31, 2.02)
White vs nonwhite	0.45 (0.16, 1.26)
Black vs nonblack	1.37 (0.55, 3.41)
Age	0.98 (0.91, 1.05)
Diagnosis of schizoaffective disorder	0.56 (0.16, 1.94)
Baseline positive symptoms	1.26 (0.77, 2.06)
Baseline negative symptoms	1.27 (0.72, 2.25)
Childhood PAS score	1.67† (1.09, 2.58)
Early adolescent PAS score	1.41 (0.89, 2.22)
Late adolescent PAS score	1.24 (0.87, 1.77)
Adult PAS score	1.17 (0.80, 1.71)
EPS (time-dependent)	1.52 (0.55, 4.23)

*PAS indicates Premorbid Adjustment Scale; EPS, extrapyramidal signs.
†*P*<.05.

Table 2. Effects of Neuroleptic Dose and Treatment Response on Presumptive and Persistent TD*

	Hazard Ratio (95% Confidence Limits)	
	Presumptive TD	Persistent TD
Dose and clozapine use		
Dose†‡	1.06 (1.01, 1.12)	1.12 (1.03, 1.22)
Clozapine use‡	0.54 (0.07, 4.37)	2.56 (0.32, 20.5)
Treatment response§		
Treatment responder	0.07 (0.01, 0.39)	0.10 (0.01, 0.96)
Weeks to treatment response	0.99 (0.99, 1.00)	0.99 (0.98, 1.00)
Treatment response§ and dose		
Dose†‡	1.06 (1.00, 1.12)	1.05 (0.97, 1.13)
Clozapine use‡	0.50 (0.06, 4.08)	0.68 (0.07, 6.70)
Treatment responder	0.06 (0.01, 0.38)	0.09 (0.01, 0.98)
Weeks to treatment response	0.99 (0.98, 1.00)	0.99 (0.98, 1.01)

*TD indicates tardive dyskinesia.
†The hazard ratios for neuroleptic dose are in 100-mg chlorpromazine equivalent units.
‡Dose and clozapine use are time-dependent covariates.
§Treatment response is for the first episode of illness.

pine at some point during the study period. Ten of these patients received clozapine after nonresponse to treatment in their first episode; three received clozapine after nonresponse to treatment in a subsequent episode of illness.

OCCURRENCE OF TD

One of the 118 patients had involuntary movements prior to treatment (mild chewing and choreoathetoid finger movements). Of the 117 patients at risk for TD, 19 developed presumptive TD during the course of the study. Seventeen of these 19 cases received global severity ratings of mild TD at the time of confirmation and two received ratings of moderate TD. All cases had body area global ratings of at least 2 in an orofacial region, and 11 had ratings of at least 2 in both orofacial and extremity or trunk regions. At the time of initial case detection, 16 of the 19 patients who met the criteria for presumptive TD also met the Research Diagnosis for TD criteria for probable TD.[30] These criteria require ratings of mild involuntary movements in two or more body areas or of moderate movements in one body area.[30] The 19 cases were subsequently reexamined by the expert raters at regular intervals to determine the persistence of movements. Ten of these cases met the Research Diagnosis for TD criteria for persistent TD (movements persisted for at least 3 months); two cases never had movements persisting for 3 months but met the criteria for presumptive TD (as defined above) at their last rating; one case met the criteria for masked probable TD (had presumptive TD but movements diminished within 2 weeks following an increase in dosage); and six met the criteria for transient TD (movements never persisted for a 3-month period and were not present at the time of the last examination, and the dosage had not been increased).

Survival analysis was performed to estimate the cumulative incidence of TD in first-episode schizophrenia as a function of real calendar time since onset of treatment. The cumulative incidence of presumptive TD was 6.3% after 1 year of follow-up, 11.5% after 2 years, 13.7% after 3 years, and 17.5% after 4 years. Persistent TD had a cumulative incidence of 4.8% after 1 year, 7.2% after 2 years, and 15.6% after 4 years (see the **Figure**).

RISK FACTORS FOR PRESUMPTIVE TD

Demographic Factors

Table 1 summarizes the hazard ratios and their corresponding 95% confidence limits for risk factors for presumptive TD. Neither age, sex, diagnosis, nor race had significant effects on presumptive TD.

Clinical Factors

Baseline psychopathologic measures and EPS were not significant predicters of presumptive TD (Table 1). Presumptive TD development was predicted by greater impairment on childhood PAS score (hazard ratio, 1.67; 95% CI, 1.09 to 2.58). However, when dose, clozapine exposure, treatment response status, and time to response were controlled for, childhood PAS score did not significantly predict TD risk (hazard ratio, 1.38; 95% CI, 0.85 to 2.25).

Antipsychotic Drug Exposure and Treatment Response

Antipsychotic drug treatment and treatment outcome were associated with TD development (Table 2). Controlling for clozapine treatment, each 100-mg chlorpromazine equivalent increase in antipsychotic drug dose resulted in a 6% increase in the hazard of presumptive TD (hazard ratio, 1.06). The hazard ratio for clozapine status was not significantly different from zero. Controlling for time to treatment response (or censoring date), treatment responders had a significantly lower hazard for presump-

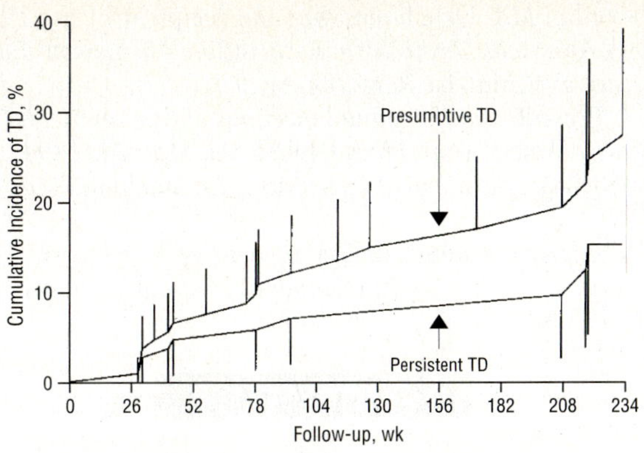

Cumulative incidence of presumptive and persistent tardive dyskinesia (TD). Error bars depict upper 95% confidence intervals for probable TD and lower 95% confidence intervals for persistent TD during weeks in which TD cases occurred.

tive TD (hazard ratio, 0.07). When antipsychotic drug dose and treatment response were considered together, along with clozapine status and time to treatment response, treatment responders continued to have lower hazards for presumptive TD (hazard ratio, 0.06), while dose was a trend-level predicter of presumptive TD (hazard ratio, 1.06; χ^2=3.83, *df*=1, *P*=.05). It should be noted, however, that the hazard ratios for antipsychotic drug dose were nearly identical whether or not treatment response was included in the model.

Persistent TD

The effects of treatment responder status and antipsychotic drug dose on persistent TD were similar to those for presumptive TD. When treatment response, antipsychotic drug dose, clozapine use, and weeks to treatment response were entered simultaneously, treatment responder status remained a strong predicter of TD (hazard ratio, 0.09).

COMMENT

The findings of this study indicate that the incidence of TD in patients with first-episode schizophrenia followed up from the start of treatment is comparable to incidence rates in larger studies of more heterogeneous patient samples.

The association of development of TD with antipsychotic medication dose has been reported in cross-sectional[31] and prospective[6,32] studies of patients with chronic schizophrenia. However, development of TD has also been associated with a poorer treatment response in patients with long-term treatment,[33,34] with a greater risk of relapse after medication discontinuation,[35] and with more severe forms of schizophrenia, including increased levels of negative symptoms, cognitive impairment, and "organic" features.[36-41] In the present study, TD was related to greater impairment on childhood PAS score, poor response to treatment of first episode of psychosis, and greater antipsychotic drug exposure. The association of TD development with impairment on childhood PAS score and poor treatment response suggests that medication exposure alone does not determine TD status. Rather, patients who are more severely ill and less responsive to treatment have increased vulnerability to TD. Higher doses of antipsychotic drugs received by sicker patients may constitute an accurate measure of the true severity of illness. Alternatively, patients who have a poor antipsychotic response may receive greater exposure to medication, developing TD as a result of higher doses and longer duration of treatment. We attempted to disentangle the association of treatment outcome and drug exposure with TD development by Cox regression analysis. Remission status from first psychotic episode remained a significant predicter of time to presumptive TD development, while antipsychotic drug dose was only a trend-level predicter. However, medication exposure and level of remission are inevitably confounded in any naturalistic treatment study. The only way to disentangle the effects of illness severity from antipsychotic drug dose would be to randomly assign good responders and poor responders to high- and low-dose treatment conditions and evaluate them longitudinally to determine TD outcome. This would be clearly unethical and thus unfeasible.

It is unclear what pathophysiologic factors may be responsible for the increased TD vulnerability in patients with more severe forms of schizophrenia. Crow et al[42] suggested that the structural neuropathologic conditions involving neuronal loss in their type 2 form of schizophrenia might underlie this effect. Consistent with this hypothesis is the proven association between increasing age (and, by extension, age-dependent decrease in neuronal number) and TD vulnerability.[4,8] We hypothesize that pathologic overactivity of mesolimbic and mesocortical dopamine neural systems, possibly the result of a process of endogenous neurochemical sensitization, may mediate persistence of psychotic symptoms despite adequate treatment of the first psychotic episode, while increased TD vulnerability may be caused by overactive nigrostriatal dopamine activity from this process that is enhanced by antipsychotic drug exposure.[35,43] Another possible pathophysiologic mechanism derives from the potential involvement of glutamatergic neuronal activity, which has been implicated in schizophrenia,[44] and how this activity might be affected by typical antipsychotic drugs. Coyle[45] suggested that dopamine receptor blockade may enhance cortical striatal glutamatergic activity, which may exceed levels required for excitatory or trophic functions, producing neurotoxic effects. Thus, there are existing hypotheses about primary pathophysiologic or disease-treatment interactive processes that could result in TD development.

The lack of an association between time to TD development and EPS in the first episode of young, essentially treatment-naive patients differs from the results of the larger, ongoing Prospective Study of TD Development.[5] We hypothesize that the EPS response of patients with little or no exposure to antipsychotic drugs may differ from the EPS response of chronically ill patients. Moreover, sustained treatment with antipsychotic medication may alter the neural substrates that underlie various forms of EPS and alter their expression.[46,47]

The lack of an association between age and TD development is in contrast to the positive association of age with TD development that has been previously reported,[2,5,8] but the lack of association is not surprising given the youth and limited age range of our first-episode patients. We also did not find a significant difference between men and women. However, the literature is not consistent with regard to gender effects (particularly in premenopausal women), and some results suggest that these effects vary with age.[2,6,48]

Unlike previous studies,[6,49] we found no association between race and TD risk. This may be because of the small number of TD cases in our study and the standardized treatment protocol. Since black patients may be treated with higher doses of antipsychotic drugs,[49] racial differences in TD risk may be found only at higher treatment doses.

There are some advantages in our ongoing prospective cohort study of essentially treatment-naive schizophrenics for the study of TD incidence and risk factors. First, to a greater extent than in previous prospective studies of TD,[5,6] we are confident that none of our patients had signs of TD in the past. In addition, rather than retrospective data on medication exposure, we had complete prospective medication records. Finally, the availability of treatment response and clinical data allowed us to examine the interrelationships of many variables that had not previously been studied prospectively in relation to TD development.

A limitation of the present study design is that, to an extent, medication dosage (in the context of the treatment algorithm) was influenced by treatment response. Thus, it is difficult to disentangle the independent effects on TD development of treatment outcome and medication exposure. Another limitation of the present analysis is the small number of cases of presumptive and persistent TD, which may have limited our ability to identify additional risk factors.

These factors notwithstanding, the incidence of TD in our sample of 118 patients with first-episode schizophrenia was comparable to the incidence rates prospectively determined in much larger samples.[5,6]

CONCLUSIONS

Our findings indicate that poor treatment outcome from first episode of psychosis, greater medication exposure, and greater impairment on childhood PAS score are associated with TD development. The findings suggest that there may be a disease-related vulnerability to TD that is manifest with drug exposure. They also suggest that the minimum effective dosage of antipsychotic medication should be used for schizophrenic patients who require long-term treatment.

Accepted for publication October 12, 1995.

This study was supported by grants MH411646 and MH32369, by Research Scientist Development Award MH00537 (Dr Lieberman), and by Mental Health Clinical Research Center grant MH41960 for the study of schizophrenia, all from the National Institute of Mental Health, Rockville, Md. Dr Chakos was the recipient of the 1993/1994 American Psychiatric Association Wisniewski Early Career Psychiatrist Research Award.

Presented at the annual meetings of the American Psychiatric Association, Philadelphia, Pa, May 23, 1994, and the Society of Biological Psychiatry, Philadelphia, May 20, 1994.

Reprint requests to Department of Psychiatry, University of North Carolina School of Medicine, Chapel Hill, NC 27599-7160 (Dr Lieberman).

REFERENCES

1. Jeste DV. Epidemiology. In: Jeste DV, Wyatt RJ, eds. *Understanding and Treating Tardive Dyskinesia.* New York, NY: Guilford Press; 1982:10-38.
2. Woerner, MG, Kane JM, Lieberman JA, Alvir JM, Bergmann KJ, Borenstein M, Schooler NR, Mukherjee S, Rotrosen J, Rubinstein M, Basavaraju N. The prevalence of tardive dyskinesia. *J Clin Psychopharmacol.* 1991;11:34-42.
3. Jeste DV, Wyatt RJ. Changing epidemiology of tardive dyskinesia: an overview. *Am J Psychiatry.* 1981;138:297-309.
4. Kane JM, Smith JM. Tardive dyskinesia: prevalence and risk factors, 1959 to 1979. *Arch Gen Psychiatry.* 1982;39:473-481.
5. Kane JM, Woerner M, Borenstein M, Wegner J, Lieberman J. Integrating incidence and prevalence of tardive dyskinesia. *Psychopharmacol Bull.* 1986;22:254-258.
6. Morgenstern H, Glazer WM. Identifying risk factors for tardive dyskinesia among long-term outpatients maintained with neuroleptic medications. *Arch Gen Psychiatry.* 1993;50:723-733.
7. Kane JM, Woerner M, Lieberman JA, Kinon BJ. Tardive dyskinesia: prevalence, incidence and risk factors. *J Clin Psychopharmacol.* 1988:8:259-262.
8. Saltz BL, Woerner MG, Kane JM, Lieberman JA, Alvir JMJ, Bergmann KJ, Blank K, Koblenzer J, Kahaner K. Prospective study of tardive dyskinesia incidence in the elderly. *JAMA.* 1991;266:2402-2406.
9. Jeste DV, Caligiuri MP, Paulsen JS, Heaton RK, Lacro JP, Harris MJ, Bailey A, Fell RL, McAdams LA. Risk of tardive dyskinesia in older patients: a prospective longitudinal study of 266 outpatients. *Arch Gen Psychiatry.* 1995;52:756-765.
10. Casey DE. Tardive dyskinesia and affective disorders. In: Casey DE, ed. *Tardive Dyskinesia and Neuroleptics: From Dogma to Reason.* Washington, DC: American Psychiatric Press; 1985:1-20.
11. Woerner MG, Saltz BL, Kane JM, Liebermann JA, Alvir JMJ. Diabetes and development of tardive dyskinesia. *Am J Psychiatry.* 1993;150:966-968.
12. Yassa R, Ghadirian AM, Schwartz G. Prevalence of tardive dyskinesia in affective disorder patients. *J Clin Psychiatry.* 1983;44:410-412.
13. Owens DG, Johnstone EC. The disabilities of chronic schizophrenia: their nature and the factors contributing to their development. *Br J Psychiatry.* 1980;136:384-395.
14. Owens DG, Johnstone EC, Frith CD. Spontaneous involuntary disorders of movement. *Arch Gen Psychiatry.* 1982;39:452-461.
15. Kane JM, Woerner M, Sarantakos S, Kinon B, Lieberman J. Do low dose neuroleptics prevent or ameliorate tardive dyskinesia? In: Casey DE, ed. *Tardive Dyskinesia and Neuroleptics: From Dogma to Reason.* Washington, DC: American Psychiatric Press; 1985:99-108.
16. Kane JM, Rifkin A, Woerner M. Low-dose neuroleptic treatment of outpatient schizophrenics. *Arch Gen Psychiatry.* 1983;40:893-896.
17. Chatterjee A, Chakos M, Koreen A, Geisler S, Sheitman B, Alvir J, Lieberman JA. Prevalence and clinical correlates of extrapyramidal signs and spontaneous dyskinesias in never medicated schizophrenic patients. *Am J Psychiatry.* 1995;152:1724-1729.
18. Lieberman JA, Jody D, Alvir JMJ, Ashtari M, Levy D, Bogerts B, Degreef G, Mayerhoff D, Cooper T. Brain morphology, dopamine and eye-tracking abnormalities in first-episode schizophrenia: prevalence and clinical correlates. *Arch Gen Psychiatry.* 1993;50:357-368.
19. Lieberman J, Jody D, Geisler S, Alvir J, Loebel A, Szymanski S, Woerner M, Borenstein M. Time course and biologic correlates of treatment response in first-episode schizophrenia. *Arch Gen Psychiatry.* 1993;50:369-376.
20. Endicott J, Spitzer RI. A diagnostic interview: the Schedule for Affective Disorders and Schizophrenia. *Arch Gen Psychiatry.* 1978;35:837-844.
21. Spitzer RL, Endicott J, Robins E. Research Diagnostic Criteria. *Arch Gen Psychiatry.* 1978;35:773-782.
22. Spitzer RL, Endicott J. *Schedule for Affective Disorders and Schizophrenia–*

Change Version. 3rd ed. New York: New York State Psychiatric Institute; 1978.
23. National Institute of Mental Health. Rating scales and assessment instruments for use in pediatric psychopharmacology research. *Psychopharmacol Bull*. 1985; 21:839-844.
24. Endicott J, Spitzer RI, Fleiss JD, Cohen J. The Global Assessment Scale: a procedure for measuring overall severity of psychiatric disturbance. *Arch Gen Psychiatry*. 1976;33:766-771.
25. Simpson GM, Lee JH, Zoubek B, Gardos G. A rating scale for tardive dyskinesia. *Psychopharmacology*. 1979;64:171-179.
26. Simpson GM, Angus JWS. A rating scale for extrapyramidal side effects. *Acta Psychiatr Scand Suppl*. 1970;212:1-58.
27. Andreasen NC, Olsen S. Negative vs positive schizophrenia: definition and validation. *Arch Gen Psychiatry*. 1982;39:789-794.
28. Cannon-Spoor HE, Potkin SG, Wyatt RJ. Measurement of premorbid adjustment in chronic schizophrenia. *Schizophr Bull*. 1982;8:470-484.
29. Guy W. Abnormal Involuntary Movement Scale. In: *ECDEU Assessment Manual for Psychopharmacology*. Washington, DC: US Public Health Service; 1976: 534-537.
30. Schooler NR, Kane JM. Research diagnoses for tardive dyskinesia. *Arch Gen Psychiatry*. 1982;39:486-487.
31. Muscettola G, Pampallona S, Barbato G, Casiello M, Bollini P. Persistent tardive dyskinesia: demographic and pharmacological risk factors. *Acta Psychiatr Scand*. 1993;87:29-36.
32. Cavallaro R, Regazzetti MG, Mundo E, Brancato V, Smeraldi E. Tardive dyskinesia outcomes: clinical and pharmacologic correlates of remission and persistence. *Neuropsychopharmacology*. 1993;8:233-239.
33. Thomas P, McGuire R. Orofacial dyskinesia, cognitive function and medication. *Br J Psychiatry*. 1986;149:216-220.
34. Chouinard B, Annable L, Ross-Chouinard A, Nestoros JN. Factors related to tardive dyskinesia. *Am J Psychiatry*. 1979;136:79-83.
35. Lieberman JA, Alvir J, Geisler S, Ramos-Lorenzi J, Woerner M, Novacenko H, Cooper T, Kane JM. Methylphenidate response, psychopathology and tardive dyskinesia as predictors of relapse in schizophrenia. *Neuropsychopharmacology*. 1994;11:107-118.
36. Richardson MA, Pass R, Bregman Z. Contrasts between patients' characteristics associated with tardive dyskinesia versus those associated with parkinsonism-like symptoms. In: Wolf ME, Mosnaim AD, eds. *Tardive Dyskinesia: Biological Mechanisms and Clinical Aspects*. Washington, DC: American Psychiatric Press; 1988:107-122.
37. Waddington JL, Hanafy AY, Dolhin C, Kinesella A. Cognitive dysfunction, negative symptoms, and tardive dyskinesia in schizophrenia. *Arch Gen Psychiatry*. 1987;44:907-912.
38. Waddington JL, O'Callaghan E, Larken D. Cognitive dysfunction in schizophrenia: organic vulnerability factor or state marker for tardive dyskinesia. *Brain Cogn*. 1993;23:56-70.
39. Wegner JT, Catalano F, Gibralter J, Kane JM. Schizophrenics with tardive dyskinesia-neuropsychological deficit and family psychopathology. *Arch Gen Psychiatry*. 1985;42:860-865.
40. Liddle PF, Barnes TRE, Speller J, Kibel D. Negative symptoms as a risk factor for tardive dyskinesia in schizophrenia. *Br J Psychiatry*. 1993;163:776-780.
41. Wegner JT, Kane JM, Weinhold P, Woerner M, Kinon B, Lieberman J. Cognitive impairment in tardive dyskinesia. *Psychiatry Res*. 1985;16:331-337.
42. Crow TJ, Owens DGC, Johnstone ED, Cross AJ, Owen F. Does tardive dyskinesia exist? In: Ban TA, Pichot P, Poldinger LW, St Gallen W, eds. *Modern Problems in Pharmacology*. Basel, Switzerland: Karger; 1983:206-219.
43. Lieberman JA, Kinon BJ, Loebel AD. Dopaminergic mechanisms of idiopathic and drug induced psychosis. *Schizophr Bull*. 1990;16:97-110.
44. Olney JW, Farber NB. Glutamate receptor dysfunction and schizophrenia. *Arch Gen Psychiatry*. 1995;52:998-1007.
45. Coyle J. Glutamate, oxidative stress and schizophrenia. Presented at the International Congress on Schizophrenia Research; April 10, 1995; Hot Springs, Va.
46. Chakos MH, Mayerhoff DI, Loebel AD, Alvir JM, Lieberman JA. Incidence and correlates of acute extrapyramidal symptoms in first episode schizophrenia. *Psychopharmacol Bull*. 1992;28:81-86.
47. Chakos MH, Lieberman JA, Bilder RM, Lerner G, Bogerts B, Degreef G, Wu H, Ashtari M. Increase in caudate nuclei volumes of first episode schizophrenic patients taking antipsychotic drugs. *Am J Psychiatry*. 1994;151:1430-1436.
48. Kowlakowska T, William AO, Ardern M, Reveley MA. Tardive dyskinesia in schizophrenics under 60 years of age. *Biol Psychiatry*. 1986;21:161-169.
49. Glazer WM, Morgenstern H, Doucette J. Race and tardive dyskinesia among outpatients at a CMHC. *Hosp Community Psychiatry*. 1994;45:38-42.

A selective serotonin
reuptake inhibitor for OCD

LUVOX™

fluvoxamine maleate 50 mg & 100 mg SCORED TABLETS

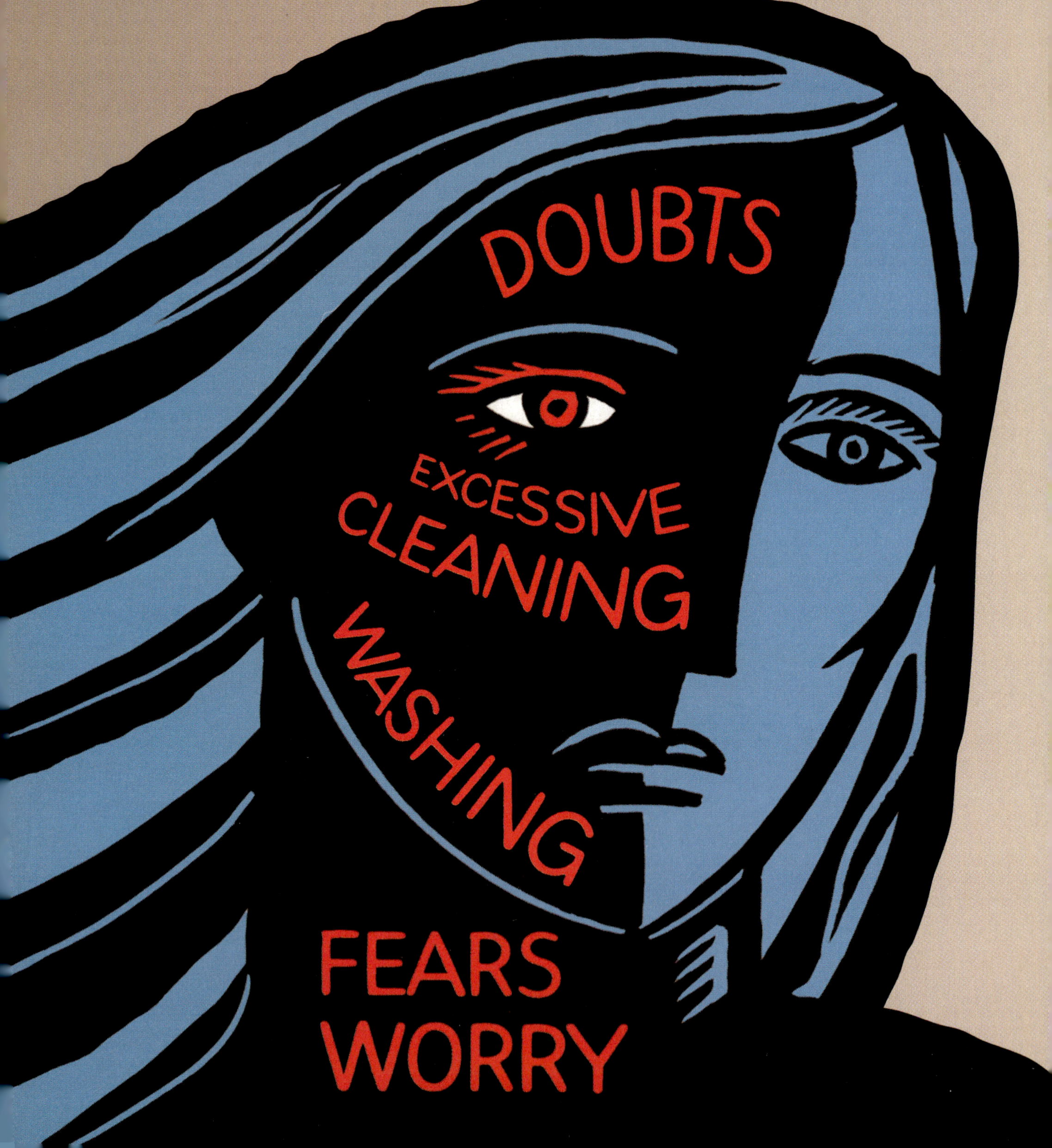

Hypothalamic-Pituitary-Adrenal Axis Activity in Panic Disorder

24-Hour Secretion of Corticotropin and Cortisol

James L. Abelson, MD, PhD; George C. Curtis, MD

Background: Oversecretion of corticotropin-releasing hormone and/or dysregulation of the hypothalamic-pituitary-adrenal (HPA) axis may contribute to pathophysiologic processes in panic disorder, but documentation of HPA axis disturbance in panic has been inconsistent. In the current study we examined HPA axis activity in panic disorder over a full circadian cycle, using frequent blood sampling to provide detailed assessment of corticotropin and cortisol secretion.

Methods: Twenty patients with panic disorder and 12 normal control subjects were studied. Blood samples were drawn every 15 minutes for 24 hours and assayed for corticotropin and cortisol levels.

Results: Patients with panic disorder had elevated overnight cortisol secretion and greater amplitude of ultradian secretory episodes. Patients who entered the study through clinical referral channels had greater cortisol secretion than those recruited by advertisements. Patients with panic disorder who had a low frequency of panic attacks had elevated daytime corticotropin levels and elevated corticotropin ultradian amplitude. Patients with a high frequency of attacks had shifted corticotropin circadian cycles.

Conclusions: Patients with panic disorder demonstrate subtle alterations in HPA axis activity, characterized by overnight hypercortisolemia and increased activity in ultradian secretory episodes, but HPA axis alterations in panic are modulated by illness severity and treatment seeking. It remains unclear whether HPA axis dysregulation in panic represents a pathogenic defect within the axis itself. Inconsistencies in prior work may reflect the subtlety of the abnormalities seen, differences in clinical characteristics of patients studied, and the use of different probes and measurement contexts.

(Arch Gen Psychiatry. 1996;53:323-331)

CONSIDERABLE interest has focused on the potential role of corticotropin-releasing hormone (CRH) and the hypothalamic-pituitary-adrenal (HPA) axis in pathophysiologic processes in panic disorder.[1] Supporting evidence, however, has been inconsistent. Blunted corticotropin responses to CRH have been reported in panic in some studies[2,3] but not in others.[4,5] Both normal and elevated rates of cortisol nonsuppression following dexamethasone have been reported.[6,7] Urinary free cortisol results have also been inconsistent.[8,9] Elevated plasma cortisol levels were reported in an "afternoon continuous test" setting,[10] but elevations were not reported during monitoring over a similar but more prolonged period in another context.[3] Potential explanations for these variable findings include (1) modulation of HPA activity by acute and chronic stress effects, resulting in complex and poorly understood mixtures of down-regulation and sensitization[11]; (2) separate regulation of stress effects and central drive/circadian rhythm,[12] with uncertainty as to which, if either, is altered in panic; (3) possible effects of clinical features, such as symptom severity (eg, panic frequency), functional impairment, or complications (eg, agoraphobia or depression)[13,14]; (4) distortion of results in brief studies caused by circadian and pulsatile characteristics of HPA activity[15]; and (5) possible subtlety of alterations in panic that results in detection difficulty.

In the present study we undertook a detailed examination of HPA axis activity in panic over a full circadian cycle, with (1) frequent sampling to allow characterization of both circadian rhythm and pulsatile/ultradian patterns, (2) examination of corticotropin and cortisol levels to allow some separation of adrenal and pituitary effects, and (3) attention to clinical variables, such as panic frequency, disability, and treatment seeking.

From the Anxiety Disorders Program, Department of Psychiatry, University of Michigan, Ann Arbor.

See Subjects and Methods on next page

SUBJECTS AND METHODS

PATIENTS AND CONTROLS

Twenty patients with panic disorder and 12 normal control subjects were studied. All were evaluated using a Structured Clinical Interview for *DSM-III-R*,[16] focusing on anxiety and affective disorders but including screens for substance use disorders and psychosis. Subjects were between 18 and 42 years of age; were medically healthy as confirmed by history, physical examination, and screening laboratory tests; reported no exposure to psychoactive medication for at least 2 weeks and passed a urine drug screen and plasma benzodiazepine screen at the time of study entry; and were taking no medication that might affect HPA axis activity. All sexually active women were using contraceptive precautions other than birth control pills, had regular menstrual cycles for the prior 6 months, had a negative result on a urine pregnancy screen, and were studied within 7 days of onset of menses.

Patients were recruited from among those applying for treatment to a university anxiety disorders program (n=6) and those who responded to advertisements in community newspapers (n=14). All patients met *DSM-III-R* criteria for panic disorder and had experienced at least one panic attack per week for the prior 3 weeks. Eleven had mild agoraphobia, three had moderate agoraphobia, and six had panic disorder alone. Two patients had histories of major depressive disorder and two had histories of substance abuse (all in remission for more than 6 months). In both cases with past depressive episodes, panic symptoms had occurred first and dominated the clinical picture. Four patients had current or past generalized anxiety disorder. One patient had social phobia and one had a simple phobia (heights). No other current or past Axis I disorders were detected.

Control subjects were recruited by advertisements in community newspapers. They had no history of Axis I disorder and reported no Axis I disorder in first-degree relatives.

DESIGN AND PROCEDURES

The full protocol included an initial detailed evaluation of HPA axis functioning, 10 weeks of treatment with alprazolam, and repeated evaluation of the HPA axis (reported separately). Subjects who met entry criteria and passed all screening tests provided written informed consent and were scheduled for admission to a clinical research center. Patients received free clinical care during the 10-week treatment protocol. One patient withdrew from the study during treatment, and her data were discarded. Control subjects were studied once and were paid $200.

On the day of study subjects had an intravenous catheter placed in a forearm vein and were admitted to the clinical research center by 5 PM. A constant, "keep open" drip of normal saline (with 3000 U per liter of heparin) was maintained throughout the monitoring period. Blood sampling began at 6 PM. Every 15 minutes for the next 24 hours, clinical research center nurses drew a 3-mL blood sample through the intravenous catheter into a syringe and placed it in a chilled tube containing ethylenediaminetetraacetic acid. Samples were placed on ice, separated in a refrigerated centrifuge within 2 hours, and frozen for later analysis. During the night (11 PM to approximately 7 AM), a small-bore extension line (183-cm arterial line tubing) was used to permit sampling from outside the subjects' bed curtains. Subjects remained at bed rest except for bathroom use throughout the monitoring period. They were served regular hospital meals, receiving dinner prior to initiation of blood sampling on day 1 and breakfast at approximately 8 AM and lunch at about noon on day 2. A CRH stimulation test (reported separately) was performed between 5:50 PM and 8 PM on day 2 (CRH given at 6 PM), after which subjects were fed dinner and discharged.

MEASURES

Assays were conducted at a commercial laboratory (Hazelton Inc, Washington, DC) using commercially available kits. Corticotropin levels were measured using the immunoradiometric assay kit from Nichols Institute (San Juan

RESULTS

The patients and controls did not differ significantly in age, weight, or sex ratios. Mean ages, sex distributions, and summary characteristics of the patients' panic disorder at entry into the study are presented in **Table 1**. Corticotropin and cortisol data are presented in **Figure 1** through **Figure 3**, which reveal that mean hormone values were higher for patients than for controls at almost every sampling point. The main exception was corticotropin from 6 PM to 10 PM, when patient values were slightly lower than control values. Analyses revealed that group differences were not consistently significant, but several specific and significant findings were embedded in the small overall elevations.

CORTISOL

Cortisol group means and comparisons for specific periods are presented in **Table 2**. Patients had significantly elevated overnight cortisol levels (evident in Figure 1), but patients' cortisol levels were not elevated during the day. There was a trend (P=.07) for patients to have elevated cortisol levels over the entire 24-hour period.

Cortisol secretion was more readily modeled by cosine curves in control subjects than in patients; the modeling produced significantly better "goodness-of-fit" correlations for controls ($P<.05$). Patients had elevated ultradian amplitudes compared with controls (P=.01) but did not differ in the mean frequency of these ultradian oscillations (5.1±1.8 cycles per 24 hours for patients, 5.2±1.9 cycles per 24 hours for controls; P=.90).

Pulse wave analyses confirm that patients' increased cortisol secretion was caused by increases in secretory burst amplitude but not in pulse frequency or background secretion. The mean pulse amplitude was significantly higher for patients than for controls (175±60 nmol/L vs 55±60 nmol/L , P=.03), but the algorithm detected similar numbers of pulses for the two groups (8.0±2.1 for patients and 6.9±2.0 for controls, P=.19) and similar basal cortisol levels.

Capistrano, Calif). Cortisol levels were measured using the Kallestead Quanticoat radioimmunassay from Sanofi Diagnostics (Chaska, Minn). Sensitivities were 14 nmol/L for the cortisol assay and 0.3 pmol/L for the corticotropin assay. All coefficients of variation were less than 17%.

Assessment of patients' clinical status included the Panic Attack and Anticipatory Anxiety Scale, the Marks/Sheehan Phobia Scale, the Sheehan Disability Scale, and the Hamilton Anxiety Scale.[17] Panic attack frequency was determined from the Panic Attack and Anticipatory Anxiety Scale and recorded as the average number of attacks per week over the month prior to evaluation for the study. Agoraphobic avoidance was recorded as the sum of the avoidance scores on the agoraphobia items of the Marks/Sheehan Phobia Scale. Disability was recorded as the sum of the scores on the four subscales of the Sheehan Disability Scale, which reflect the patient's subjective assessment of impairment in the arenas of work, social and leisure activities, and home and family responsibilities.

ANALYSES

Raw data were log-transformed prior to all analyses of means to improve their fit to a normal distribution curve. We first compared patients with controls using *t* tests, looking for differences in 24-hour, overnight (10 PM to 6 AM), and daytime (6 AM to 5:45 PM) means (the initial 4-hour epoch, 6 PM to 10 PM, was considered an accommodation period and was analyzed separately). We used similar comparisons to look for differences between patients who entered the study after responding to advertisements and those who entered through routine clinical referral channels and for differences between patients with frequent panic attacks (more than two per week) and patients with less frequent attacks (two or fewer per week).

Rhythm characteristics of hormone secretion were examined using a dual approach. First, we conducted repeated-measures analyses of variance comparing groups, using corticotropin and cortisol levels averaged over 2-hour blocks (to smooth curves by reducing the influence of sample timing relative to secretory bursts). Group differences in secretory profiles are reflected in significant group-by-time interactions. We report such differences as circadian rhythm shifts, however, only when they were confirmed by circadian timing differences detected by a commercially available modeling program (Cosifit, CirceSoft, Waltham, Mass).[18] This program applies multioscillator cosinor models to raw hormonal data. It finds a best-fitting 24-hour cosine curve for each subject and then adds additional oscillators and determines the best-fitting model. Our data were best fit by a three-oscillator model in which the first oscillator was fixed at 1 cycle per day (circadian), the second oscillator was fixed at 2 cycles per day (hemicircadian), and the program was allowed to determine the frequency of a third oscillator, thus identifying the ultradian rhythm producing the best-fitting curve. The hemicircadian oscillator appeared to partially adjust the circadian rhythm to its natural, nonsinusoidal shape. The third (ultradian) oscillator appeared to capture activity in transient bursts that were superimposed on the circadian rhythm. The program automatically applies the model to each subject's data and provides the mesor, the amplitudes, and times of acrophase of the circadian, hemicircadian, and ultradian rhythms, and goodness-of-fit correlation coefficients (measuring how well the data are fit by the model). Group differences for these variables were determined using *t* tests.

Corticotropin and cortisol are both secreted in a pulsatile fashion.[15,19] We used the Kushler-Brown pulse detection algorithm to examine the cortisol data.[20] This algorithm uses an exponential decay model based on the known half-life of a hormone and locates pulses with appropriate decay curves. It provides estimates of the number of pulses, average pulse amplitude, and background or basal levels. Because it requires three to five samples per half-life, we were not able to apply it to the corticotropin data.

Data are presented as means±SDs. We present raw-data means rather than the log-transformed values used in analyses since the raw values are more meaningful to most readers. All statistical tests were two-tailed and were considered significant at $P \leq .05$.

The bulk of the patients' cortisol elevation was accounted for by the six patients who entered the study through routine referral channels rather than through responses to advertisements. These clinic patients had significantly higher 24-hour mean cortisol levels than the advertisement patients ($t=2.3$, $P=.03$). The 24-hour and overnight mean cortisol levels of the clinic patients were also significantly elevated relative to controls (Table 2), whereas the advertisement patients differed from controls only in overnight mean cortisol levels and then only at a trend level ($P<.10$). These findings are presented in Figure 2.

A multiple regression analysis (all subjects combined) revealed that the bulk of the 24-hour secretion was accounted for by the circadian and ultradian amplitudes ($r=.8$), with both making significant contributions ($P<.001$), while the hemicircadian amplitude did not contribute significantly. This is consistent with the impression that the hemicircadian component of the cosinor analyses improved fit by adjusting the shape of the circadian rhythm to its natural, nonsinusoidal shape, but the hemicircadian component was not capturing additional secretory activity. The ultradian and circadian amplitudes were not related to each other ($r=.2$, $P=.39$). A very strong correlation ($r=.8$, $P<.001$) between ultradian amplitude (from the cosinor analysis) and pulse amplitude (from the pulse detection algorithm) indicates that these measures capture the same component of cortisol secretory activity. These findings suggest that most cortisol secretion is contained within two components, the major early morning activation impelled by the circadian clock and superimposed secretory episodes, occurring with an approximate frequency of six per 24 hours.

CORTICOTROPIN

Corticotropin group means and comparisons for specific periods are presented in Table 2. Patients and controls had similar corticotropin levels (Figure 3). There were no significant patient-control differences seen in the basic means analyses (24-hour, overnight, daytime).

Table 1. Demographic Characteristics and Illness Severity for All Patients, Patient Subgroups, and Controls*

	Patients					
	All (n=20)	Clinic (n=6)	Advertisement (n=14)	High PA (n=10)	Low PA (n=10)	Controls (n=12)
Age, y	30.6±6.1	30.8±6.2	30.6±6.3	32.4±4.9	28.9±7.0	28.1±4.4
No. of men/No. of women	8/12	4/2	4/10	3/7	5/5	3/9
Duration of illness, y	5.8±7.9	4.7±5.4	6.2±9.0	4.0±3.0	7.5±10.8	...
Age of onset, y	25.0±7.3	26.3±6.4	24.4±7.8	28.4±4.4†	21.5±8.1	...
Panic attacks per week	3.5±2.7	3.6±2.9	3.5±2.7	5.6±2.3‡	1.5±0.5	...
Agoraphobic avoidance score§	7.0±5.5	8.5±4.8	6.4±5.8	10.5±4.4‡	3.5±4.1	...
Sheehan Disability Scale score‖	16.3±8.4	23.2±7.5¶	13.4±7.1	21.0±7.7‡	11.6±6.3	...
Hamilton Anxiety Scale score#	15.6±8.0	17.5±7.3	14.7±8.4	21.3±7.1‡	9.8±3.5	...

*Values are mean±SD. Clinic patients were compared with advertisement patients, and high-frequency panic attack (high PA) patients were compared with low-frequency panic attack (low PA) patients. See the text for additional comparisons.
†$P<.05$ compared with low PA patients.
‡$P<.01$ compared with low PA patients.
§Sum of the avoidance scores on the agoraphobia items of the Marks/Sheehan Phobia Scale (range, 0 to 24).
‖Range, 0 to 35.
¶$P<.05$ compared with advertisement patients.
#Range, 0 to 56.

Cosinor analyses of corticotropin data detected an elevation in circadian amplitude in patients (patients' mean, 1.7±0.7 pmol/L; controls' mean, 1.1±0.5 pmol/L; t=2.2, P=.03), consistent with the higher peak in the early morning hours seen for patients in Figure 3. There were no other patient-control differences in the cosinor analyses.

In contrast to the cortisol results, there were no differences between clinic patients and advertisement patients or between clinic patients and controls on any measures of corticotropin activity.

CORTICOTROPIN-CORTISOL RATIO

The sensitivity of the adrenal cortex to stimulation by corticotropin was estimated by calculating the corticotropin-cortisol ratio. Group means were calculated for the entire 24-hour cycle, overnight, and for 4-hour epochs. No differences between patients and controls were seen at any time.

EFFECTS OF ILLNESS SEVERITY

Because prior work demonstrated modulation of a biological abnormality by attack frequency in patients with panic disorder,[13] we dichotomized patients by panic attack frequency and compared the two groups with each other and with controls. Corticotropin and cortisol levels for these patient subgroups are included in Table 2 and **Figure 4**. Cosinor analyses revealed that patients with low panic attack frequency (two or fewer per week) had significantly elevated corticotropin mesor, circadian amplitude, and ultradian amplitude relative to both patients with high panic attack frequency and controls ($P<.05$ for all comparisons). Patients with low panic attack frequency also had significantly higher daytime mean corticotropin levels relative to both patients with high panic attack frequency (t=2.3, P=.04) and controls (Table 2). Patients with high panic attack frequency did not differ from controls in mean corticotropin levels or in any derived amplitude variable.

Despite normal corticotropin levels, patients with high panic attack frequency did have an abnormal shift in their circadian rhythm, evidenced by a significant group-by-time interaction ($P<.001$) in the repeated-measures analysis of variance comparing them with controls (corticotropin levels averaged into 2-hour epochs over 24 hours) and by a significantly earlier circadian acrophase (P=.01) relative to controls in the cosinor analyses. As can be seen in Figure 4, compared with controls, patients with high panic attack frequency had corticotropin levels that started lower, rose faster and perhaps slightly higher, but ended up lower again by 6 PM on day 2. They had lower corticotropin levels during the initial 4-hour epoch than both controls and patients with low panic attack frequency (t=3.1, P=.006 for both); no other group differences for any hormone variable were seen for this epoch.

Patients with a high and low frequency of panic attacks did not differ from each other on any measure of cortisol secretion. Both groups tended to have elevated overnight cortisol levels compared with controls ($P<.10$), so both contributed to the patient-control difference in overnight cortisol secretion described above. Compared with controls, however, patients with low panic attack frequency did have elevated 24-hour cortisol levels (Table 2) and elevated daytime cortisol pulse amplitude (t=2.7, P=.01). Patients with high panic attack frequency did not differ from controls on these or other cortisol measures. The six clinic patients who accounted for the bulk of the cortisol elevation were evenly distributed between the high- and low-frequency panic attack groups (three in each group).

There is evidence that men have higher corticotropin levels than women despite comparable cortisol levels.[21] Because our low-frequency panic attack group had both the highest corticotropin levels and the highest proportion of men, we reexamined the effect of panic attack frequency on corticotropin levels using female subjects only. Although the resultant groups are small, the analyses show that the higher proportion of men in the low-frequency panic attack group does not account for

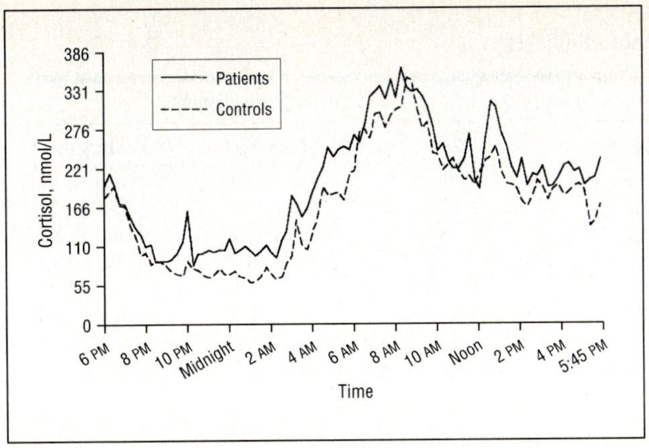

Figure 1. *Cortisol levels (measured every 15 minutes) in patients with panic disorder and control subjects over a 24-hour period. To avoid visual complexity, error bars are not included. Statistically meaningful differences are described in the text.*

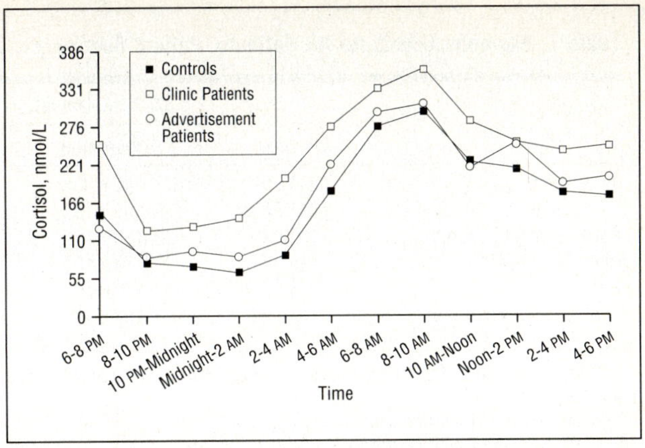

Figure 2. *Cortisol levels averaged over 2-hour epochs for 24 hours in patients with panic disorder recruited through routine referral channels (clinic patients), patients recruited through newspaper advertisements, and normal control subjects.*

their elevated corticotropin level. Group differences were even more pronounced with men excluded: Compared with patients who had high panic attack frequency (n=7), patients who had low panic attack frequency (n=5) had elevated corticotropin levels throughout the 24-hour cycle, with significantly elevated 24-hour and daytime means ($P<.009$ for both). Female patients with low panic attack frequency also had significantly elevated mean 24-hour and daytime corticotropin levels ($P<.05$) compared with female controls (n=9). Samples sizes were too small to allow separate analyses of men.

The lower corticotropin levels seen in patients with high panic attack frequency relative to patients with low panic attack frequency could reflect adrenal changes in response to chronic overdrive of the HPA axis in these more severely ill patients. If so, patients with high panic attack frequency should secrete more cortisol per unit of corticotropin (lower corticotropin-cortisol ratio). Because of potential sex effects (see above), we tested this prediction using female subjects only, excluding the period of intrinsic circadian activation (2 AM to 10 AM), when high ambient corticotropin levels could obscure subtle differences in adrenal sensitivity. We compared patients with high and low panic attack frequency and controls and found a significant group effect ($F=4.4$, $P<.03$). Patients with high panic attack frequency had the lowest corticotropin-cortisol ratio (mean, 1.3 ± 0.6), and post hoc analyses (Scheffe's) showed that patients with high panic attack frequency had a corticotropin-cortisol ratio that was significantly lower than the ratio in patients with low panic attack frequency (mean, 2.8 ± 0.8; $P<.05$) and that showed a trend to be lower than the ratio in controls (mean, 2.5 ± 1.2; $P<.08$).

Pearson product-moment correlations were used to further explore relationships between severity of illness (agoraphobic avoidance, panic attack frequency, Hamilton Anxiety Scale score, and total disability) and HPA axis activity. There were no significant correlations between any severity measure and any of the cortisol measures. Daytime corticotropin level was inversely related to severity of agoraphobic avoidance ($r=-.5$, $P=.04$). No other correlations between severity measures and corticotropin measures were significant. Neither age of illness onset nor duration of illness was correlated with any HPA axis measure.

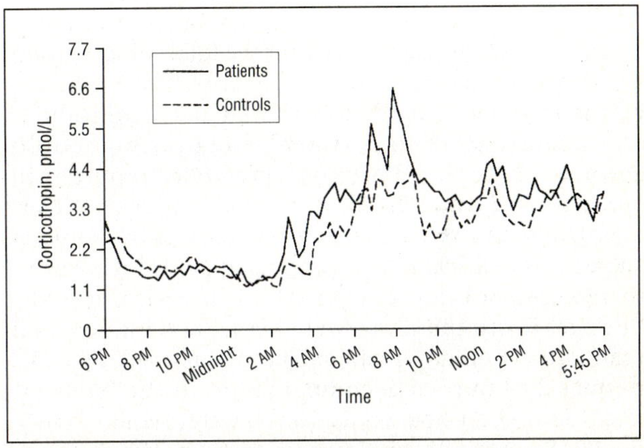

Figure 3. *Corticotropin levels (measured every 15 minutes) in patients with panic disorder and control subjects over a 24-hour period. To avoid visual complexity, error bars are not included. Statistically meaningful differences are described in the text.*

OTHER POTENTIAL CONFOUNDING FACTORS

The elevation in cortisol levels in clinic patients relative to advertisement patients could be caused by differences in severity of illness. However, the groups did not differ significantly on three of the four measures of illness severity and had essentially identical panic attack frequencies (Table 1). The clinic patients were significantly more disabled than the advertisement patients, but there was no direct relationship between total disability and overnight or 24-hour cortisol levels ($r<.3$, $P>.20$ for both). The clinic and advertisement patient groups did not differ in age of illness onset or duration of illness.

There were no significant correlations between age and any HPA axis variables. There were no differences in age between the patients and controls, between clinic patients and advertisement patients, or between patients with high- and low-frequency panic attacks.

Unfortunately, we did not use any quantitative measure of depressive symptoms. Two cases of secondary depression were noted at screening. Three patients devel-

Table 2. Hormone Levels for All Patients, Patient Subgroups, and Control Subjects*

	Cortisol, nmol/L			Corticotropin, pmol/L		
	24 h	Overnight	Daytime	24 h	Overnight	Daytime
All patients	200±50	145±80†	260±55	3.1±1.3	2.3±1.1	4.1±1.7
Clinic patients	235±65‡	190±130†	285±55	3.1±1.4	2.3±1.0	4.1±1.9
Advertisement patients	185±40	130±45	245±50	3.1±1.3	2.3±1.2	4.0±1.7
High PA patients	195±65	155±105	250±50	2.5±1.0	1.9±0.7	3.3±1.4
Low PA patients	205±40†	140±50	270±60	3.7±1.3	2.6±1.3	4.9±1.7†
Control subjects	170±35	102±40	230±45	2.6±0.9	1.8±0.8	3.4±1.1

*Values are mean±SD. Patient groups were compared with controls. See the text for additional comparisons. High PA indicates high-frequency panic attack; low PA, low-frequency panic attack.

†$P<.05$ compared with controls.

‡$P<.01$ compared with controls.

oped depressive episodes subsequent to completion of this study.[22] These five patients did not differ from the remaining patients on any HPA axis measure.

There were no differences between men and women on any cortisol measure, either for the total subject group or for patients alone. Men had higher corticotropin levels than women, but differences were not significant.

Reactivity to experimental conditions could account for some HPA axis overactivity reported in patients with panic disorder in other settings.[2] We attempted to minimize environmental factors by studying subjects at bed rest over a prolonged period. However, there was some evidence of reactivity effects in our study. First, corticotropin levels were higher at 6 PM on day 2 than at 6 PM on day 1 (all subjects combined, $P<.05$), despite 24 hours of accommodation to the environment. Second, 24-hour cortisol levels were predicted (r=.5, $P<.05$) by overnight restlessness, measured by the longest time during the night that subjects appeared to the nurse to be sleeping without disruption (monitored every 15 minutes; shorter durations suggested greater restlessness and were associated with higher cortisol levels).

COMMENT

Detailed examination over a full circadian cycle suggests that patients with panic disorder demonstrate subtle alterations in HPA axis activity that appear to vary with treatment seeking and illness severity. When detectable, these alterations are similar to those seen in depression,[23-26] characterized by hypercortisolemia (particularly overnight), increased activity in ultradian secretory episodes, and possibly some adrenal sensitization (reflected in decreased corticotropin-cortisol ratios in more severely ill patients). The HPA axis may be less tightly controlled in patients with panic disorder than in control subjects, reflected in poorer fit to multioscillator cosine curve modeling and in increased activity in episodic secretory bursts (greater ultradian and pulse amplitude). These findings are consistent with the suggestions of others that patients with panic disorder have less stable[3] or more acutely reactive[2] HPA axes.

Both basic science[12] and clinical evidence[24] suggest that the HPA axis is not controlled by a monolithic regulatory process. The circadian rhythm and stress response, for example, may be controlled by separate central nervous system mechanisms.[12] Our data support the concept of separable components within the HPA axis. We were able to apportion the bulk of 24-hour cortisol secretion into two primary components, one tied to the dominant circadian rhythm and the early morning activation of the HPA axis, the other reflecting higher-frequency, episodic secretory activity. Both our multioscillator cosinor analyses and our pulse detection algorithm seemed to identify the same higher-frequency (6 to 8 cycles per day) activity. These data are consistent with the findings of a depression study[24] that differentiated circadian timing fluctuations from abnormalities in ultradian rhythm and suggested that depressed patients may have separate abnormalities in these differing components. The ultradian rhythm identified in the depressed patients had the same frequency (6 cycles per day) as that seen in our patients with panic disorder. It is unclear whether the alterations in ultradian amplitude seen in our patients with panic disorder reflect sensitivity within the noncircadian, acute stress response component of HPA axis control. These alterations could also reflect an aspect of the system's adaptation to chronic stress or could constitute an intrinsic marker of illness. Follow-up work is needed to further delineate the neuroendocrine and possible clinical correlates of elevations in the amplitude of cortisol secretory episodes at a frequency of 6 cycles per day. Further use of analytic approaches, such as multioscillator cosinor analysis, that dissect the HPA axis into component parts may offer opportunities to identify disturbances with greater biological and clinical specificity.[24]

Abnormalities were less evident for corticotropin than cortisol secretion in our total patient group. The much shorter half-life of corticotropin relative to our sampling interval, resulting in less complete and therefore more variable capturing of corticotropin secretion, and greater variability within the corticotropin assay itself made it more difficult to detect group differences in corticotropin secretion. The differential impact of panic attack frequency on corticotropin secretion also contributed to this difficulty, in that differing types of corticotropin abnormalities in the two frequency subgroups were obscured in total group comparisons. The low-frequency panic attack group accounted entirely for the only detectable overall abnormality in corticotropin

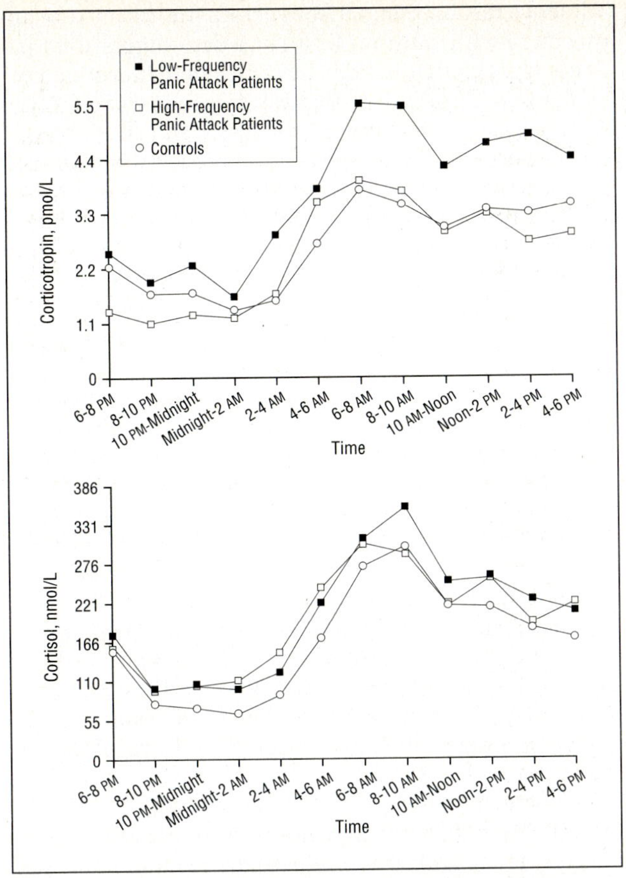

Figure 4. *Corticotropin and cortisol levels averaged over 2-hour epochs for 24 hours in patients with panic disorder who had two or fewer panic attacks per week, patients with more than two panic attacks per week, and normal control subjects.*

secretion, an elevated circadian amplitude in patients. This subgroup also had elevations in corticotropin ultradian amplitude and daytime corticotropin levels. The high-frequency panic attack group did not share these abnormalities and instead showed a shift in corticotropin circadian rhythm. Despite these corticotropin differences, both groups contributed to the overnight hypercortisolemia and elevated cortisol ultradian amplitude.

Further research is needed before abnormalities in HPA axis components, such as corticotropin ultradian amplitude or daytime corticotropin levels, can be accurately interpreted, but some speculative interpretation may be useful in shaping subsequent studies. The system's normal pulsatile pattern of activity may be entrained by environmental perturbations in such a way that heightened acute reactivity is reflected in the types of abnormalities seen in patients with low-frequency panic attacks—elevated corticotropin ultradian amplitude, corticotropin elevations that are particularly striking during waking hours, and elevated daytime cortisol pulse amplitude. If so, these findings may be less evident in patients with high-frequency panic attack because of greater levels of chronic activation, evidenced by adrenal sensitization (reduced corticotropin-cortisol ratio) that reduces corticotropin secretion by increased feedback inhibition and perhaps by a related enhancement of sensitivity to feedback inhibition.[27] Such factors could in fact produce the abnormal shift seen in the circadian corticotropin rhythm of the patients with high-frequency panic attack (lower levels in the evening but a steep rise in the early morning). Sensitivity to feedback inhibition normally fluctuates across the circadian cycle and is enhanced during the evening nadir,[28] which would magnify any abnormal enhancement of feedback inhibition and, coupled with increased cortisol secretion per unit of corticotropin, should drive corticotropin levels lower in the evening. Normal loss of sensitivity to cortisol feedback inhibition during the early morning HPA axis activation[28-30] would minimize the impact of cortisol feedback and still allow a rapid rise in corticotropin levels.

These speculations lead to testable hypotheses. Patients with high-frequency panic attacks should account for the elevation in glucocorticoid receptor binding seen in panic (thought to reflect negative feedback efficiency).[27] Patients with high-frequency panic attacks should be more likely than patients with low-frequency panic attacks to show enhanced cortisol response to corticotropin[25] and increased adrenal size.[26] Patients with low-frequency panic attacks should show greater corticotropin responses to environmental perturbations, such as meals or psychological stressors. Blockade of feedback inhibition (eg, by metyrapone) may unmask a similar acute reactivity in patients with high-frequency panic attacks. Follow-up studies addressing these hypotheses may be worthwhile.

The mechanisms producing the noted HPA axis changes in patients with high-frequency panic attack are not clear. They could reflect a biological defect (either genetic or developmental in origin) that produces increased hypothalamic drive and contributes in a causal way to greater illness severity. They could also reflect the compensatory responses of the HPA axis to more severe illness. These mechanisms are unlikely to be a direct consequence of frequent panic attacks because there is little evidence that attacks themselves produce significant HPA axis activity.[31,32] One other possibility must be addressed: they could be caused by associated depressive symptoms. Unfortunately, we do not have a quantitative assessment of depressive symptoms to examine. However, none of our patients was in a depressive episode at the time of study. Whether depressive symptoms in the absence of a full depressive episode can produce HPA axis dysregulation has not been empirically addressed, but in studies documenting dexamethasone nonsuppression in patients with panic disorder, HPA axis overactivity was not attributable to depressive symptoms.[33] Extremely high correlations (r>.90) between Hamilton Anxiety Scale and Hamilton Depression Scale scores in patients with panic disorder (O. G. Cameron, MD, PhD, unpublished data, 1994) and our failure to find any relationships between Hamilton Anxiety Scale scores and HPA axis activity further undermine the hypothesis that depressive symptoms account for the HPA axis dysregulation seen. We were able to document prior or subsequent episodes of major depression in five of our patients, and most of them (four of five) were in the high-frequency panic attack group. However, HPA axis dysregulation in depression appears to be a state marker,[34] and none of our patients was depressed at the time of study. These five patients did not differ from other patients in

HPA axis activity. These patients did not contribute to the increased cortisol secretion we saw in our cohort of clinic-referred patients (see below), since only one of them was in this group.

If patients with panic disorder have increased acute reactivity to environmental perturbations, as others[2] suggest, then the environmental context of HPA axis studies becomes very important. We attempted to minimize environmental perturbations in this study by keeping subjects at bed rest in a stable context for a prolonged period. However, impact of reactivity to environment on the HPA axis is still suggested by higher corticotropin levels at the end of 24-hour monitoring than at the beginning and by the relationship between overnight "restlessness" and 24-hour cortisol levels. We therefore cannot rule out the possibility that reactivity to study conditions explains the HPA axis dysregulation seen in patients with panic disorder, even in this setting. Replication of the urinary free cortisol studies,[8,9] with urine collected at home but with overnight samples separated from daytime samples, might clarify this matter.

The detection of the most robust hypercortisolemia in our six clinic patients raises interesting questions about the role of treatment seeking in HPA axis activity. Because this group is small, we must be cautious in drawing conclusions, but the potential implications of this source of patient effect on HPA axis measures are of sufficient importance that they must be contemplated and follow-up pursued. Clinic patients differed from advertisement patients in their spontaneous treatment seeking, which likely resulted from their greater levels of disability (subjective functional impairment). Others have reported an association in panic disorder between greater disability and increased HPA axis activity.[35] Patients with panic disorder complicated by secondary depression or agoraphobia are also more likely to have elevated cortisol secretion than patients with uncomplicated panic disorder.[8,36,37] In patients with panic disorder, then, treatment seeking, functional impairment, and a more complicated course of illness may be associated with greater HPA axis activity. If so, several important questions should be addressed. Does HPA axis overactivity in patients with panic disorder reflect some aspect of their distress, dysfunction, or ability to cope with their panic attack symptoms? Could HPA axis dysregulation more generally be linked to the degree of behavioral dysfunction created by a disorder? Could more consistent demonstration of HPA axis dysregulation in depression than in panic disorder reflect differential levels of functioning in populations studied[10] rather than illness-specific biologic characteristics? The roles of treatment seeking and functional disability in modulating neuroendocrine systems should be examined further. Because changes in health care systems are making it more difficult to find patients for research, and because advertising may be increasingly used to recruit patient participants, clear understanding of the impact of these factors may be critical in interpreting future data on the HPA axis in psychiatric disorders.

Because different probes of the HPA axis may tap different aspects of its regulation and because contextual and clinical factors may differ between studies and influence results, comparisons across studies must be approached with caution. Results to date suggest that patients with panic disorder have elevated afternoon cortisol levels,[10] normal corticotropin responses to CRH in the morning[4,5] but blunted responses in the evening,[2,3] elevated evening "basal" corticotropin levels when samples are drawn prior to an infusion[2] but normal morning levels when examined in a nonchallenge context,[38] possibly elevated urinary free cortisol secretion, but only if secondary depression or agoraphobia is also present,[8,9] and inconsistent responses to dexamethasone.[6,7] Our data bring some clarity to this inconsistent set of results by suggesting that there are some elements of HPA axis dysregulation in patients with panic disorder, but the abnormalities seen are not substantial, are modulated by illness severity, and may also be modulated by or entwined with non–disease-specific aspects of the behavioral consequences of the disorder for patients' functioning. A number of specific hypotheses emerge and require more direct study: The degree of HPA axis dysregulation is related to the impact of a disorder on functioning. More severely ill patients show more evidence of chronic, central overdrive in the stress axis, and this may be seen in adrenal changes. Tonic central drive and acute responsivity may be separately modulated, and patients with panic disorder may show evidence of dysregulation in one or the other or both.

Hypothalamic-pituitary-adrenal axis dysregulation in panic disorder may not be a simple reflection of diagnostic categorization. Others have made a similar suggestion based on HPA axis studies of depression.[24] The complexity is quite challenging but is not surprising, given the critical importance of the HPA axis to adaptation and survival.[39]

Accepted for publication October 4, 1995.

This research was supported in part by Clinical Research Center grant M01RR00042 from the National Institutes of Health, Bethesda, Md, and by a grant from the Upjohn Co, Kalamazoo, Mich.

Michael Bronzo, MD, and the Clinical Research Center nurses provided critical assistance in management and execution of the study. Sandy Ostrowski (University of Michigan Clinical Research Center, Ann Arbor), Brenda Benson (National Institute of Mental Health, Rockville, Md), and Sam Listwak (National Institute of Mental Health) managed the blood samples and facilitated completion of assays. Hedieh Haghighatgou, MSW, assisted in data management, and David Mauger, PhD (Department of Biostatistics, University of Michigan), helped with statistical analyses. Philip W. Gold, MD (National Institute of Mental Health), and Oliver G. Cameron, MD, PhD, helped in the development of the protocol. Dr Cameron also assisted in running the experiment, and Dr Gold oversaw completion of the corticotropin assays. Thomas Uhde, MD (Wayne State University, Detroit, Mich), oversaw completion of the cortisol assays. Elizabeth Young, MD, provided helpful review of earlier drafts of the manuscript.

Correspondence to Anxiety Disorders Program, Room C435, Med Inn Bldg/0840, 1500 E Medical Center Dr, Ann Arbor, MI 48109-0840 (Dr Abelson).

REFERENCES

1. Pihoker C, Nemeroff CB. The role of corticotropin-releasing factor in the pathophysiology of anxiety disorders. In: Hoehn-Saric R, McLeod DR, eds. *Biology of Anxiety Disorders.* Washington, DC: American Psychiatric Press; 1993:103-119. Progress in Psychiatry series.
2. Roy-Byrne PP, Uhde TW, Post RM, Gallucci W, Chrousos GP, Gold PW. The corticotropin-releasing hormone stimulation test in patients with panic disorder. *Am J Psychiatry.* 1986;143:896-899.
3. Holsboer F, von Bardeleben U, Buller R, Heuser I, Steiger A. Stimulation response to corticotropin-releasing hormone (CRH) in patients with depression, alcoholism and panic disorder. *Horm Metab Res.* 1987;16(suppl):80-88.
4. Brambilla F, Bellodi L, Perna G, Battaglia M, Sciuto G, Diaferia G, Petraglia F, Panerai A, Sacerdote P. Psychoimmunoendocrine aspects of panic disorder. *Neuropsychobiology.* 1992;26:12-22.
5. Rapaport MH, Risch SC, Golshan S, Gillin JC. Neuroendocrine effects of ovine corticotropin-releasing hormone in panic disorder patients. *Biol Psychiatry.* 1989; 26:344-348.
6. Coryell W, Noyes R. HPA axis disturbance and treatment outcome in panic disorder. *Biol Psychiatry.* 1988;24:762-766.
7. Curtis GC, Cameron OG, Nesse RM. The dexamethasone suppression test in panic disorder and agoraphobia. *Am J Psychiatry.* 1982;139:1043-1046.
8. Kathol RG, Anton R, Noyes R, Lopez AL, Reich JH. Relationship of urinary free cortisol levels in patients with panic disorder to symptoms of depression and agoraphobia. *Psychiatry Res.* 1988;24:211-221.
9. Uhde T, Joffe RT, Jimerson DC, Post RM. Normal urinary free cortisol and plasma MHPG in panic disorder: clinical and theoretical implications. *Biol Psychiatry.* 1988;23:575-585.
10. Goldstein S, Halbreich U, Asnis G, Endicott J, Alvir J. The hypothalamic-pituitary-adrenal system in panic disorder. *Am J Psychiatry.* 1987;144:1320-1323.
11. Lopez JF, Young EA, Herman JP, Akil H, Watson SJ. Regulatory biology of the HPA axis: an integrative approach. In: Risch SC, ed. *Central Nervous System Peptide Mechanisms in Stress and Depression.* Washington, DC: American Psychiatric Press; 1991:1-52.
12. Akil H, Morano MI. The biology of stress: from periphery to brain. In: Watson SJ, ed. *Biology of Schizophrenia and Affective Disease.* Washington, DC: American Psychiatric Press. In press.
13. Charney DS, Heninger GR, Breier A. Noradrenergic function in panic anxiety: effects of yohimbine in healthy subjects and patients with agoraphobia and panic disorder. *Arch Gen Psychiatry.* 1984;41:751-763.
14. Meador-Woodruff JH, Haskett RF, Grunhaus L, Akil H, Watson SJ, Greden JF. Postdexamethasone plasma cortisol and B-endorphin levels in depression: relationship to severity of illness. *Biol Psychiatry.* 1987;22:1137-1150.
15. Veldhuis JD, Iranmanesh A, Johnson ML, Lizarralde G. Twenty-four-hour rhythms in plasma concentrations of adenohypophyseal hormones are generated by distinct amplitude and/or fequency modulation of underlying pituitary secretory bursts. *J Clin Endocrinol Metab.* 1990;71:1616-1623.
16. Spitzer RL, Williams JBW. *Structured Clinical Interview for DSM-III-R: Upjohn Version–Revised.* New York, NY: Biometrics Research Dept, New York State Psychiatric Institute; 1986.
17. Ballenger J, Burrows G, DuPont RJ, Lesser I, Noyes RJ, Pecknold J, Rifkin A, Swinson R. Alprazolam in panic disorder and agoraphobia: results from a multicenter trial, I: efficacy in short-term treatment. *Arch Gen Psychiatry.* 1988; 45:413-422.
18. Teicher MH, Barber NI. COSIFIT: an interactive program for simultaneous multioscillator cosinor analysis of time-series data. *Comput Biomed Res.* 1990; 23:283-295.
19. Veldhuis JD, Iranmanesh A, Lizarralde G, Johnson ML. Amplitude modulation of a burstlike mode of cortisol secretion subserves the circadian glucocorticoid rhythm. *Am J Physiol.* 1989;257:E6-E14.
20. Kushler RH, Brown MB. A model for the identification of hormone pulses. *Stat Med.* 1991;10:329-340.
21. Roelfsema F, Van Den Berg G, Frölich M, Veldhuis JD, Van Eijk A, Buurman MM, Etman BHB. Sex-dependent alterations in cortisol response to endogenous adrenocorticotropin. *J Clin Endocrinol Metab.* 1993;77:234-240.
22. Abelson JL, Curtis GC. Discontinuation of alprazolam after successful treatment of panic disorder: a naturalistic follow-up study. *J Anxiety Disord.* 1993; 7:107-117.
23. Linkowski P, Medlewicz J, Leclercq R, Brasseur M, Hubain P, Golstein J, Copinschi G, Van Cauter E. The 24-hour profile of adrenocorticotropin and cortisol in major depressive illness. *J Clin Endocrinol Metab.* 1985;61:429-438.
24. Halbreich U, Asnis GM, Shindledecker R, Zumoff B, Nathan RS. Cortisol secretion in endogenous depression, II: time-related functions. *Arch Gen Psychiatry.* 1985;42:909-914.
25. Jaeckle RS, Kathol RG, Lopez JF, Meller WH, Krummel SJ. Enhanced adrenal sensitivity to exogenous cosyntropin (ACTH α^{1-24}) stimulation in major depression: relationship to dexamethasone suppression test results. *Arch Gen Psychiatry.* 1987;44:233-240.
26. Nemeroff CB, Krishnan KRR, Reed D, Leder R, Beam C, Dunnick NR. Adrenal gland enlargement in major depression: a computed tomographic study. *Arch Gen Psychiatry.* 1992;49:384-387.
27. Yehuda R, Boisoneau D, Mason JW, Giller EL. Glucocorticoid receptor number and cortisol excretion in mood, anxiety, and psychotic disorders. *Biol Psychiatry.* 1993;34:18-25.
28. Dallman MF, Akana SF, Scribner KA, Bradbury MJ, Walker C-D, Strack AM, Cascio CS. Stress, feedback, and facilitation in the hypothalamic-pituitary-adrenal axis. *J Neuroendocrinol.* 1991;4:517-526.
29. Späth-Schwalbe E, Gofferje M, Kern W, Born J, Fehm HL. Sleep disruption alters nocturnal ACTH and cortisol secretory patterns. *Biol Psychiatry.* 1991; 29:575-584.
30. Fehm HL, Späth-Schwalbe E, Pietrowsky R, Kern W, Born J. Entrainment of nocturnal pituitary-adrenocortical activity to sleep processes in man: a hypothesis. *Exp Clin Endocrinol.* 1993;101:267-276.
31. Cameron OG, Lee MA, Curtis GC, McCann DS. Endocrine and physiological changes during 'spontaneous' panic attacks. *Psychoneuroendocrinology.* 1987; 12:321-331.
32. Carr DB, Sheehan DV, Surman OS, Coleman JH, Greenblatt DJ, Heninger GR, Jones KJ, Levine PH, Watkins WD. Neuroendocrine correlates of lactate-induced anxiety and their response to chronic alprazolam therapy. *Am J Psychiatry.* 1986;143:483-494.
33. Coryell W, Noyes R, Schlechte J. The significance of HPA axis disturbance in panic disorder. *Biol Psychiatry.* 1989;25:989-1002.
34. Linkowski P, Medlewicz J, Kerkhofs M, Leclercq R, Golstein J, Brasseur M, Copinschi G, Van Cauter E. 24-Hour profiles of adrenocorticotropin, cortisol, and growth hormone in major depressive illness: effect of antidepressant treatment. *J Clin Endocrinol Metab.* 1987;65:141-152.
35. Coryell W, Noyes R, Reich J. The prognostic significance of HPA-axis disturbance in panic disorder: a 3-year follow-up. *Biol Psychiatry.* 1991;29:96-102.
36. Kathol RG, Anton R, Noyes R, Gehris T. Direct comparison of urinary free cortisol excretion in patients with depression and panic disorder. *Biol Psychiatry.* 1989;25:873-878.
37. Lopez AL, Kathol RG, Noyes R. Reduction in urinary free cortisol during benzodiazepine treatment of panic disorder. *Psychoneuroendocrinology.* 1990;15:23-28.
38. Gurguis GNM, Mefford IN, Uhde TW. Hypothalamic-pituitary-adrenocortical activity in panic disorder: relationship to plasma catecholamine metabolites. *Biol Psychiatry.* 1991;30:502-506.
39. Axelrod J, Reisine TD. Stress hormones: their interaction and regulation. *Science.* 1984;224:452-459.

Conversions From Système International (SI) Units to Traditional Units (Modified From *The SI Manual in Health Care*)

System	Component	SI Reference Interval*	SI Unit	Conversion Factor (Divide by)	Traditional Reference Interval*	Traditional Unit
Plasma	Corticotropin (ACTH)	4-22	pmol/L	0.2202	20-100	pg/mL
Serum	Cortisol					
	8 AM	110-520	nmol/L	27.59	4-19	μg/dL
	4 PM	50-410	nmol/L	27.59	2-15	μg/dL
	Midnight	<140	nmol/L	27.59	<5	μg/dL

These reference values are not intended to be definitive since each laboratory determines its own values. They are provided for illustration only.

Mental Health Problems Among Homeless Mothers

Relationship to Service Use and Child Mental Health Problems

Bonnie T. Zima, MD, MPH; Kenneth B. Wells, MD, MPH; Bernadette Benjamin, MSc; Naihua Duan, PhD

Background: The purpose of this study was to describe the prevalence of psychological distress and probable lifetime mental disorders among homeless mothers, their use of services, and the relationship between maternal and child mental health problems.

Method: The study involved a cross-sectional assessment of 110 mothers and 157 children living in homeless shelters in Los Angeles County.

Results: The majority (72%) of sheltered homeless mothers reported high current psychological distress or symptoms of a probable lifetime major mental illness or substance abuse. However, few mothers (15%) in need of services received mental health care, and the main point of contact for those with a mental health problem was the general medical sector. Mothers with a probable mental disorder were also significantly more likely to have children with either depression or behavior problems.

Conclusions: Homeless mothers have a high level of unmet need for mental health services. The relationship between maternal and child problems underscores the need for homeless family interventions that promote access to psychiatric care for both generations.

(Arch Gen Psychiatry. 1996;53:332-338)

From the Departments of Psychiatry and Biobehavioral Sciences, the University of California at Los Angeles (Drs Zima and Wells); and RAND, Santa Monica, Calif (Ms Benjamin and Dr Duan).

HOMELESS families embody two generations at risk for mental health problems and limited access to care. In an earlier study, we reported that more than three fourths of homeless children in Los Angeles County suffered from at least one serious emotional or behavioral problem or severe academic delay, yet few received any mental health or special educational services.[1] In the present report, we focus on the mental health needs and service use among homeless mothers and explore the potential relationship between maternal and child mental health problems. If both generations have mental health problems, the policy implications include designing programs that integrate mental health services for mother and child.

Homeless mothers have a higher rate of mental disorders (50% to 80%) than housed impoverished mothers,[2-5] especially if they do not have custody of their children.[6-12] Rates of mental health service use, however, are much lower.[12-14] High rates of unmet need for mental health care are of clinical and policy concern because psychiatric disorders may increase the mother's vulnerability to homelessness,[6,15-19] victimization of violence,[20] and impaired parenting,[15,21,22] and may be associated with a greater risk for mental disorders among her children.[23-30]

The impact of mental disorders and psychological distress among homeless mothers may be exacerbated by multiple psychosocial stressors.[31-38] Homeless mothers living with children are younger,[11,39] less educated,[8] and more commonly dependent on public assistance[5,11,39] than other homeless women. Relative to domiciled low-income mothers, homeless mothers are more likely to be single parents with multiple children and to be separated from at least one child,[5,33,34,40,41] to have their first child during adolescence,[42] to have fewer social supports,[4,34,37,43] and to have traumatic histories of domestic violence,[3,4,16,44-46] child abuse,[3,4,16,44-46] and foster care placement.[3,16,47] Among these factors, we were particularly interested in how a history of separation from a child, number of social supports, and history of

See Methods on next page

METHODS

The design and methods of this study are described elsewhere.[1] All homeless family programs in Los Angeles County were screened by telephone for eligibility, and 22 emergency homeless family shelters were identified. An emergency shelter was defined as any program that allowed homeless families to sleep overnight, but for short-term stays only. Eligible shelters were selected in random order and surveyed twice between February and May 1991. Families were eligible if they had stayed at the shelter overnight and had at least one child between the ages of 6 and 12 years living with them. The parent who felt she or he knew the child better was interviewed. If there were more than two eligible children, two were randomly selected for interviews. The survey was translated and backtranslated into Spanish.

Parent and child interviews were conducted simultaneously at the shelter. Testing conditions varied, but the large majority of interviews were conducted in a quiet area of the shelter, such as an empty dining room, chapel, or meeting room. Parent interviews were conducted by trained lay interviewers, and all English-language child interviews were conducted by a child psychiatrist (B.T.Z.). Spanish-language child interviews were conducted by bilingual, bicultural lay interviewers with additional training in child measures. All lay interviewers received 3 weeks of training on the general administration of the survey, Diagnostic Interview Schedule (DIS) screener, and parent report assessments of child mental health problems. Bilingual children were tested in academic skills in both languages, and the best score was included in the analysis.

MEASURES

Adult

Questions on the history of homelessness and social support were adapted from the RAND Course of Homelessness Survey (M. A. Burnam, PhD, and P. Koegel, PhD, oral communication, March 12, 1992). Maternal homelessness was assessed by the amount of time homeless and by changes in residence of the oldest child. Maternal current health status was assessed using the five-item current health perception scale from the RAND Medical Outcomes Study (MOS) Short-Form General Health Survey, an instrument widely used in large medical outpatient samples.[53-55] Scores were transformed linearly to a scale of 0 to 100, with a cutpoint of 70 or below corresponding to poor current health. Psychological distress was assessed using the five-item Mental Health Inventory (MHI-5),[53,55] which performs well in screening primary care patients for psychiatric disorders.[56] The score was transformed linearly into a scale of 0 to 100, with a cutpoint of 67 or below corresponding to high psychological distress. Both scales have good reliability and construct validity.[53]

Parents were screened for major mental disorders using 24 items from the full DIS that were highly predictive of major psychiatric diagnoses in homeless adults.[57] The DIS screener has established cutpoints for high probability of having lifetime major depression, schizophrenia, and alcohol or drug abuse. Given the limitations of the DIS to detect true schizophrenia cases,[58] mothers who screened positive for schizophrenia were identified as having a probable psychotic disorder. For example, a mother screened positive for a probable psychotic disorder if she reported at least one psychotic symptom lasting more than 6 months that either had been diagnosed as a psychiatric illness or was not attributable to an organic cause. A mother screened positive for probable major depression if she endorsed feeling sad, blue, or depressed or had anhedonia for more than 2 weeks and during this period also experienced at least three neurovegetative symptoms, including suicidal ideation. If the mother endorsed being an excessive drinker, drinking more than a fifth of liquor per day, or drinking more than seven beers, drinks, or glasses of wine every day for at least 2 weeks, she was identified as having a high probability of a lifetime history of alcohol abuse. Use of health services for either a physical or mental problem in the prior 12 months was assessed using a four-item measure from the National Health Interview Survey.[59] Outpatient care was defined as a visit to a physician, health professional, or clinic, and inpatient care was defined as a hospital stay of at least 1 night.

Child

Major depressive symptoms over the past 2 weeks were assessed using the Children's Depression Inventory (CDI), a 27-item child self-report measure. A score above 9 is indicative of the need for psychiatric evaluation.[60] Serious behavior problems over the past 6 months were evaluated using the Child Behavior Checklist (CBCL), a 118-item parent report measure. The Child Behavior Checklist is norm-referenced for large populations, and socioeconomic status and race have little effect on scale scores.[61] A T-score of 60 or higher on the internalizing and externalizing behavior subscales corresponds to the 82nd percentile or borderline clinical range.

Receptive vocabulary skills were assessed using the Peabody Picture Vocabulary Test (PPVT), normed in English

Continued on next page

homelessness relate to maternal mental disorders. We focused on these variables because they reflect problem areas that are commonly experienced by homeless mothers with children and represent target areas for potential intervention.

Furthermore, psychosocial stressors of homelessness could increase the established association between maternal and child mental disorders,[23-30] especially if homeless mothers have low service use and thus high unmet need for mental health care. Homeless children living with their parents have been found to have a high prevalence of emotional and behavior problems and delays in development, visual motor skills, and receptive vocabulary,[1,9,48-52] but the link between these problems and maternal problems has seldom been studied. In a sheltered homeless sample, for example, parental distress was associated with child behavior problems.[48]

In this report, we describe the level of mental health need among homeless mothers with children, examine levels of service use, and explore whether maternal mental health problems are related to serious emotional problems and academic delays in their children, controlling and Spanish.[62] The child was asked to point to one of four pictures that best described a spoken word. Scores were normed by age using a large random sample representative of the national distribution of child age, sex, ethnicity, geographic region, and socioeconomic status. The Peabody Picture Vocabulary Test has high immediate retest reliability but only moderate (0.58) stability among disadvantaged child populations, indicating sensitivity to detect improvement of scores over time. Correlation between results on the Peabody Picture Vocabulary Test and other standardized vocabulary tests is strong. Scores at or below the 10th percentile for age were considered indicative of severe delay in receptive vocabulary.

Three reading skills were assessed using the reading subtest of the Woodcock-Johnson Language Proficiency Battery: (1) letter-word identification, (2) word attack (ability to pronounce nonsense words phonetically), and (3) passage comprehension.[63] Scores for each component were combined into a single reading score, a method that results in higher validity. The total reading score was normed for age and grade, using normative data from a large random sample representative of the national distribution of sex, race, occupation, geographic location, and type of community. Scores at or below the 10th percentile for age were considered indicative of a severe delay in reading skills. The Spanish version was scored using equated US norms, so that scores indicate the level of English proficiency that corresponds to the subject's demonstrated proficiency in Spanish.

DATA ANALYSIS

To estimate the prevalence of maternal health problems, we calculated the percentage of homeless mothers who exceeded the cutpoints on the current health status and psychological distress scales and their mean scores. To interpret the scores in terms of need for care, we compared them using a weighted *t* test with those of mothers below the poverty level who presented for outpatient care and with the subset of mothers who had depression, using the RAND MOS database adjusted for age.[64-66]

We estimated the prevalence of probable lifetime psychiatric disorders using the sensitivity, specificity, and positive predictive values of the screener cutpoint scores, as established in the Los Angeles skid row homeless population. The total number of cases that screened positive was multiplied by the positive predictive value and then divided by the sensitivity to estimate the number of true-positive cases. The positive predictive value is very high for substance abuse (0.96) and acceptable for severe mental disorder (0.52) and dual diagnosis (0.45).[57]

To identify predictors of maternal disorders, estimate service use, and relate maternal problems to child problems, we conducted bivariate analysis (χ^2 test of proportions for discrete variables and analysis of variance for continuous variables) and multiple regression analyses to control for confounding factors. We chose potential confounder variables that, based on prior studies,[67-76] were common characteristics of homeless families or were associated with established relationships to mental health problems in homeless or community samples. Specifically, for each dependent variable (poor current health, high psychological distress, and high probability of lifetime depression, psychosis, severe mental illness, alcohol abuse, drug abuse, substance abuse, and dual diagnosis), the predictor variables were sociodemographic characteristics (parent age, ethnicity, high school graduate, and income), history of homelessness (amount of time homeless and time since stable housing), number of adult social supports, and family structure variables (being without a partner, large family size, teenage motherhood, and being separated from at least one child).

Given the small sample size and large number of potential confounders, we reduced the set of confounders using the following exploratory analysis approach. Independent variables were entered into an interim model using the backward elimination process without correction for intracluster correlation. All significant variables at $P \leq .05$ were then entered using the stepwise method, followed by all other independent variables. The final model for each dependent variable included all significant predictors from the preliminary models and was corrected for intracluster correlation using the Huber method.[77] To guard against overinterpretation of significant but trivial findings, we required an adjusted odds ratio of 2 or greater and statistical significance at $P \leq .05$ for a variable to be classified as a predictor.

To examine the relationship between each maternal and child mental disorder, we controlled for parent sociodemographic characteristics and child age and sex as well as homeless history, social support, and family structure variables, because many of these factors could predict child problems.[78-82] The child data were weighted by the number of eligible children per family and adjusted for the intracluster correlation for children from the same family.[77]

To find the best specification of maternal psychiatric disorders as predictors, we conducted preliminary analyses using each separate disorder and selected the strongest predictors, reporting more specific variables, such as psychosis rather than severe mental illness, when both were significant. Inference statistics may overestimate the significance of these variables because of variable selection.

for sociodemographic characteristics, history of homelessness, social support, and family structure variables.

RESULTS

SAMPLE CHARACTERISTICS

Eighteen (82%) of the 22 eligible shelters participated, and interviews were completed for 98% (118/121) of the eligible families and all (N=169) eligible children. Parent and child characteristics are described in an earlier report.[1] The vast majority (93% [110/118]) of parents interviewed were women; 84% (n=92) of these women were from minority backgrounds, and 67% (n=74) had annual incomes below $10 000. More than one third (35% [n=39]) of the women had their first baby before age 18 years, and the mean number children per family was four (SD, two). Many families were fragmented; 38% (n=42) of the children had only one primary caregiver, and 31% (n=34) of the mothers were separated from at least one child. About half (53% [n=58]) of the women had two or fewer persons to whom they could turn for support,

Table 1. General Health and Level of Psychological Distress Among Homeless Mothers Compared With Poor Women Who Are Medical Outpatients

	Homeless Mothers		Poor Female Medical Outpatients*			
			Total		With Depression†	
	No. (%)	Mean (SE) Score	No. (%)	Mean (SE) Score	No. (%)	Mean (SE) Score
Poor current health‡	61/110 (55)	65 (2.4)	2455/3751 (65)	60 (1.1)	1215/1551 (78)	50 (1.9)§
High psychological distress‖	61/110 (55)	59 (2.2)	947/1813 (52)	63 (1.4)	670/765 (88)	46 (2.1)§

*From the RAND Medical Outcomes Study database,[64,65] restricted to women below the poverty level and adjusted for age.
†Determined using a brief screener for depression.[66]
‡Score of 70 or lower on a general health measure (scale, 0 to 100).
§*P*<.05.
‖Score of 67 or lower on a mental health inventory (scale, 0 to 100).

and 14% (n=15) reported children as their only social supports. While 25% (n=28) of mothers had no contact with any family member in the prior 60 days, 86% (84/98) had contact with at least one friend in the past 60 days. On average, mothers had been homeless 3 months (SD, 3 months) during the past year and had not lived in stable housing (≥30 continuous days) for 4 (SD, 7 months) of the prior 12 months.

MATERNAL GENERAL AND MENTAL HEALTH PROBLEMS

More than half of the homeless mothers reported poor current health and high levels of psychological distress (**Table 1**). Homeless mothers had levels of psychological distress and current health similar to those of poor, housed women who sought general medical outpatient services, but they had less distress and better general health than depressed outpatients.

Based on screener scales, we estimate that 21% of the homeless mothers had a probable lifetime severe mental illness (major depression or psychotic disorder), 16% had probable lifetime major depression, and 10% had probable lifetime psychotic disorder (**Table 2**). One quarter of the mothers had a probable lifetime substance abuse problem; specifically, 16% had an alcohol abuse problem, 18% had a drug abuse problem, and 6% had both a severe mental illness and a substance abuse problem. One third to one half of the mothers who screened positive had symptoms within the prior 6 months. In multiple regression analyses, being separated from at least one child was the only parental characteristic associated with a mental health problem, so that it was a significant predictor of high current psychological distress (odds ratio [OR], 2.8; 95% confidence interval [CI], 1.2 to 6.6; *P*=.02) and probable psychotic disorder (OR, 3.5; 95% CI, 1.2 to 10.7; *P*=.03).

Table 2. Homeless Mothers Screening Positive for High Probability of Psychiatric Disorders and Estimated True Prevalence of Disorders

	Exceeded Screener Cutpoints, No. (%)	Estimated True Prevalence, No. (%)*
Severe mental illness	40/110 (36)	23/110 (21)
Major depression	37/110 (34)	18/110 (16)
Episode within the past 6 mo	22/37 (59)	11/18 (61)
Psychotic disorder	16/110 (15)	11/110 (10)
Episode within the past 6 mo	6/16 (38)	4/11 (36)
Substance abuse	27/110 (25)	27/110 (25)
Alcohol abuse	18/110 (16)	17/106 (16)
Symptomatic within the past 6 mo	8/18 (44)	8/17 (47)
Drug abuse	18/110 (16)	20/110 (18)
Symptomatic within the past 6 mo	6/18 (33)	7/20 (35)
Dual diagnosis	12/110 (11)	6/100 (6)

*Prevalence estimates are corrected for the same likelihood to misclassify as found in the Los Angeles skid row homeless population.

UNMET NEED

Eleven percent (12/107) of the mothers had used any specialty mental health services in the past year, and such use was significantly higher among mothers with probable lifetime major depression (OR, 7.0; 95% CI, 1.3 to 39.0; *P*=.03) and psychotic disorder (OR, 6.3; 95% CI, 1.4 to 27.5; *P*=.02). Among mothers with symptoms during the past 12 months, only 43% (3/7) with probable psychotic disorder, 29% (8/28) with probable depression, and 29% (4/14) with a probable substance abuse problem had received any mental health services within the past year.

However, about half of the mothers had visited a physician, health professional, or clinic, and 21% (n=23) had stayed overnight in a hospital for treatment of a physical problem in the prior 12 months; use of outpatient medical services was independently associated with screening positive for psychosis (OR, 4.7; 95% CI, 1.2 to 17.9; *P*=.02), and inpatient medical hospitalization was independently associated with probable lifetime dual diagnosis (OR, 4.8; 95% CI, 1.4 to 16.8; *P*=.02). Among mothers with a high probability of psychiatric disorder in the past 12 months, 68% (19/28) with severe mental illness and 50% (7/14) with a substance abuse problem had used outpatient medical services, and 29% (8/28) with severe mental illness and 43% (6/14) with a substance abuse problem had been hospitalized for a physical problem.

Table 3. Prevalences and Odds Ratios of Child Problems by Highly Probable Lifetime Maternal Mental Disorders (N=157)*

Child Problem	Children (N=157), No. (%)	Maternal Problem	Odds Ratio (95% CI)	*t*	*P*
Depression	59 (38)	Schizophrenia	4.42 (2.10-9.28)	3.95	<.001
Internalizing behavior problem	34 (22)	Depression	3.27 (1.30-8.27)	2.54	.01
		Alcohol abuse	2.71 (1.05-7.01)	2.07	.04
Externalizing behavior problem	46 (29)	Depression	3.76 (1.62-8.74)	3.11	.002

**CI indicates confidence interval.*

RELATIONSHIP BETWEEN MATERNAL AND CHILD MENTAL DISORDERS

More than one third (38% [59/157]) of the homeless children required psychiatric evaluation for clinical depression, and child depression was associated with maternal probable lifetime psychosis (**Table 3**). Among children with depression, 25% (n=15) had mothers who screened positive for probable lifetime psychotic disorder. School-aged homeless children, for example, were four times more likely to require a psychiatric evaluation for depression if their mothers reported chronic psychotic symptoms than if their mothers did not report psychotic symptoms.

Twenty-two percent (34/157) of the homeless children required a clinical evaluation for an internalizing behavior problem that was associated with maternal probable lifetime depression and alcohol abuse. Among the children with an internalizing behavior problem, 56% (n=19) had mothers who screened positive for depression, and 26% (n=9) had mothers with a history of alcohol abuse. Homeless children were three times more likely to have an internalizing behavior problem if their mothers had a history of depressive symptoms, and almost three times more likely to have an internalizing behavior problem if their mothers had abused alcohol.

More than one quarter (46/157) of the homeless children scored in the borderline clinical range for an externalizing behavior problem (ie, hyperactivity, aggression, or delinquency) that was associated with maternal probable lifetime depression. Among the children who screened positive for an externalizing behavior problem, 54% (n=25) had mothers with a history of depressive symptoms, compared with 46% (n=21) whose mothers did not have depression. Homeless children were almost four times more likely to have an externalizing behavior problem if their mothers screened positive for lifetime major depression.

On academic measures, 45% (71/157) of the homeless children scored at or below the 10th percentile for receptive vocabulary, and 39% (61/157) performed at or below the 10th percentile for age in reading. Academic skill delays were not associated with maternal mental disorders.

COMMENT

The majority (72%) of sheltered homeless mothers in our study reported either high current psychological distress or symptoms of a probable lifetime major mental illness or substance abuse disorder. Homeless mothers had higher levels of psychological distress than the general population,[83] similar to those of poor women seeking outpatient general medical care. High psychological distress accounted for more than half of the total mental health problems and was moderately correlated with probable severe mental disorder (r=.43). Further research is needed to determine what high psychological distress represents in the absence of symptoms of a severe mental disorder, such as an acute response to homelessness, subthreshold disorders, or other unmeasured mental disorders.

Our results suggest, however, that mental disorders are overrepresented among homeless mothers, similar to findings from an earlier study.[2] Compared with women in the general population, homeless mothers were more than twice as likely to have had symptoms of major depression and four times as likely to have had a probable psychotic disorder during the past year.[84] Relative to poor housed women,[84] homeless mothers were almost five times as likely to have a problem with alcohol abuse and three times as likely to have a problem with drug abuse during the prior 12 months.

Despite this high need, we found that a minority (15%) of homeless mothers received mental health care. This rate of service use was similar to the rate among those in the general population with major depression and schizophrenia, and homeless mothers with a substance abuse problem were 2.5 times more likely to receive mental health services.[85] However, because homeless mothers had a prevalence of probable disorders two to six times greater than in the general population, our findings suggest greater absolute unmet need, particularly for homeless mothers with psychotic symptoms or a history of substance abuse. Further research should determine whether mental health services differ in their clinical appropriateness (untreated disorder) for homeless women and housed, poor women with psychiatric disorders.

The main point of contact with the health care system for homeless mothers was the general medical sector, suggesting that psychiatric evaluation and referral for mental health treatment should be coordinated with the provision of general medical services. Homeless mothers with a probable severe mental or substance abuse disorder during the past year were three to seven times as likely to use general medical services.[85] This is less surprising when one considers that the general health status of homeless mothers was poorer than that of the general population and similar to that of poor women using outpatient medical services.

Being separated from at least one child was the only characteristic we found to be associated with high psychological distress and high probability of lifetime psychotic disorder among homeless mothers. Psychiatric evaluations for these women should therefore include inquiry about separation from their children and its emotional impact. Whether separation from at least one child represents a response to maternal distress, exacerbates maternal symptoms, or reflects a temporary change in the family caused by being in a shelter merits exploration beyond the limits of our study's cross-sectional design.

The need to incorporate a psychiatric evaluation for both generations into intervention strategies for homeless families is underscored by our findings that maternal mental disorders are associated with child emotional or behavioral problems. Although the pattern of associations was consistent, we have less confidence in the relationships between specific maternal and child disorders and the strength of these associations, because of the use of screening instruments for disorders and the exploratory nature of the analysis. Furthermore, behavior problems may have been more likely to be reported by depressed mothers,[86-91] and because of greater disruption to the shelter milieu, externalizing behavior problems may have been more likely to be reported than internalizing behavior problems. The consistency of our general conclusion with the findings of prior research suggests, however, that greater effort should be made to identify mental disorders among homeless mothers and children.

Our study's main limitations are the lack of comprehensive structured psychiatric interviews and follow-up of homeless families. Prevalence estimates of maternal psychiatric disorder were adjusted for screener misclassification error standardized for a sample of predominantly homeless men and may overestimate, for example, the rate of substance abuse because of the screener's high positive predictive value. Compared with findings from an urban sample of homeless mothers using the full DIS,[11] however, the estimated prevalence of disorders in our study is similar except for a 9% greater estimate of psychosis. Because of the present study's cross-sectional design, the prevalence of chronic psychiatric symptoms and longer periods of homelessness may be overrepresented, and conclusions about the consequences of untreated mental disorders among homeless mothers cannot be made.

Findings of high levels of unmet need for mental health care should be used not to stigmatize homeless families but rather to support integration of mental health services for mothers and children with housing services[92] and primary care. Without timely intervention, homeless mothers with untreated mental disorders face the additional burden of caring for children and obtaining housing while suffering from psychiatric symptoms, and their children remain at greater risk for emotional problems.

Accepted for publication August 29, 1995.

This research was conducted under the Robert Wood Johnson Clinical Scholars Program at the University of California at Los Angeles, and data analysis was supported by grant 18945 from the Robert Wood Johnson Foundation, Princeton, NJ.

The views expressed are those of the authors and do not necessarily represent those of the Robert Wood Johnson Foundation.

The authors express their gratitude to the late Howard Freeman, PhD, for his outstanding mentorship; M. Audrey Burnam, PhD, and Paul Koegel, PhD, for their permission to use the abbreviated form of the Diagnostic Interview Schedule; Barbara Genovese, Enrique Godinez, Adam Oberweiser, and Monica Paez for their diligent data collection; and shelter staff and residents for their strong support that made this study possible.

Reprint requests to UCLA Neuropsychiatric Institute, 300 Medical Plaza, Room 1414, Los Angeles, CA 90095-6967 (Dr Zima).

REFERENCES

1. Zima BT, Wells KB, Freeman HE. Emotional and behavioral disorders and severe academic delays among homeless children in Los Angeles County. *Am J Public Health.* 1994;84:260-264.
2. Smith EM, North CS, Spitznagel EL. Alcohol, drugs, and psychiatric comorbidity among homeless women: an epidemiologic study. *J Clin Psychiatry.* 1993;54:82-87.
3. Wood D, Valdez RB, Hayashi T, Shen A. Homeless and housed families in Los Angeles: a study comparing demographic, economic, and family function characteristics. *Am J Public Health.* 1990;80:1049-1052.
4. Bassuk EL, Rosenberg L. Why does family homelessness occur? a case-control study. *Am J Public Health.* 1988;78:783-788.
5. Bassuk EL, Rubin L, Lauriat AS. Characteristics of sheltered homeless families. *Am J Public Health.* 1986;76:1097-1101.
6. Fischer PJ. Estimating the prevalence of alcohol, drug and mental health problems in the contemporary homeless population: a review of the literature. *Contemp Drug Probl.* 1989;16:415-452.
7. Johnson AK, Kreuger LW. Toward a better understanding of homeless women. *Soc Work.* 1989;34:537-540.
8. Burt MR, Cohen BE. Differences among homeless single women, women with children, and single men. *Soc Probl.* 1989;36:508-524.
9. Bassuk EL, Rosenberg L. Psychosocial characteristics of homeless children and children with homes. *Pediatrics.* 1990;85:257-261.
10. Bassuk EL. Who are the homeless families? characteristics of sheltered mothers and children. *Community Ment Health J.* 1990;26:425-434.
11. Smith EM, North CS. Not all homeless women are alike: effects of motherhood and the presence of children. *Community Ment Health J.* 1994;30:601-610.
12. Breakey WR, Fischer PJ, Kramer M, Nestadt G, Romanoski AJ, Ross A, Royall RM, Stine OC. Health and mental health problems of homeless men and women in Baltimore. *JAMA.* 1989;262:1352-1357.
13. North CS, Smith EM. A systematic study of mental health services utilization by homeless men and women. *Soc Psychiatry Psychiatr Epidemiol.* 1993;28:77-83.
14. Marshall EJ, Reed JL. Psychiatric morbidity in homeless women. *Br J Psychiatry.* 1992;160:761-768.
15. Shedlin MG. *The Health Care of Homeless Mothers and Children: Impact of a Welfare Hotel.* New York, NY: Medical and Health Research Association of New York City; 1989.
16. Knickman JR, Weitzman BC. *A Study of Homeless Families in New York City: Risk Assessment Models and Strategies for Prevention.* New York, NY: Human Resources Administration, Health Research Program, New York University; 1989;1.
17. Robertson MJ. Homeless women with children: the role of alcohol and other drug abuse. *Am Psychol.* 1991;46:1198-1204.
18. Weinreb LF, Bassuk EL. Substance abuse: a growing problem among homeless families. *Fam Community Health.* 1990;13:55-64.
19. Susser E, Moore R, Link B. Risk factors for homelessness. *Am J Epidemiol.* 1993;15:546-556.
20. Padgett DK, Struening EL. Victimization and traumatic injuries among the homeless: associations with alcohol, drug, and mental problems. *Am J Orthopsychiatry.* 1992;62:525-534.
21. Hausman B, Hammen C. Parenting in homeless families: the double crisis. *Am J Orthopsychiatry.* 1993;63:358-369.
22. Memmott RJ, Young LA. An encounter with homeless mothers and children: gaining an awareness. *Issues Ment Health Nurs.* 1993;14:357-365.
23. Beardslee WR, Keller MB, Lavori PW, Staley J, Sacks N. The impact of parental affective disorder on depression in offspring: a longitudinal follow-up in a nonreferred sample. *J Am Acad Child Adolesc Psychiatry.* 1993;32:723-730.
24. Weissman MM, Fendrich M, Warner V, Wickramaratne P. Incidence of psychiatric disorder in offspring at high and low risk for depression. *J Am Acad Child Adolesc Psychiatry.* 1992;31:640-648.

25. Radke-Yarrow M, Nottelmann E, Martinez P, Fox MB, Belmont B. Young children of affectively ill parents: a longitudinal study of psychosocial development. *J Am Acad Child Adolesc Psychiatry.* 1992;31:68-77.
26. Hammen C, Burge D, Burney E, Adrian C. Longitudinal study of diagnoses in children of women with unipolar and bipolar affective disorder. *Arch Gen Psychiatry.* 1990;47:1112-1117.
27. Canino GJ, Bird HR, Rubio-Stipec M, Bravo M, Alegria M. Children of parents with psychiatric disorder in the community. *J Am Acad Child Adolesc Psychiatry.* 1990;29:398-406.
28. Rutter M, Quinton D. Parental psychiatric disorder: effects on children. *Psychol Med.* 1984;14:853-880.
29. Rubio-Stipec M, Bird H, Canino F, Bravo M, Alegria M. Children of alcoholic parents in the community. *J Stud Alcohol.* 1991;52:78-88.
30. Greenfield SF, Swartz MS, Landerman LR, George LK. Long-term psychosocial effects of childhood exposure to parental problem drinking. *Am J Psychiatry.* 1993;150:608-613.
31. Goodman L, Saxe L, Harvey M. Homelessness as psychological trauma: broadening perspectives. *Am Psychol.* 1991;46:1219-1225.
32. Wagner J, Menke EM. Stressors and coping behaviors of homeless, poor, and low-income mothers. *J Community Health Nurs.* 1991;8:75-84.
33. Milburn N, D'Ercole A. Homeless women: moving toward a comprehensive model. *Am Psychol.* 1991;46:1161-1169.
34. Hagen JL, Ivanoff AM. Homeless women: a high-risk population. *Affilia.* Spring 1988;3:19-33.
35. Stoner MR. The plight of homeless women. *Soc Serv Rev.* 1983;57:565-581.
36. Hagen JL. Gender and homelessness. *Soc Work.* 1987;32:312-316.
37. Bassuk EL. The feminization of homelessness: families in Boston shelters. *Am J Soc Psychiatry.* 1987;7:19-23.
38. Bassuk EL. Social and economic hardships of homeless and other poor women. *Am J Orthopsychiatry.* 1993;63:340-347.
39. Winkleby MA, Boyce WT. Health-related risk factors for homeless families and single adults. *J Community Health.* 1994;19:7-23.
40. Roth L, Fox ER. Children of homeless families: health status and access to health care. *J Community Health.* 1990;15:275-284.
41. Institute of Medicine. *Homelessness, Health, and Human Needs.* Washington, DC: National Academy Press; 1988.
42. Mills C, Ota H. Homeless women with minor children in the Detroit metropolitan area. *Soc Work.* 1989;34:485-490.
43. McChesney KY. New findings on homeless families. *Fam Professional.* 1986; 1:165-174.
44. Browne A. Family violence and homelessness: the relevance of trauma histories in the lives of homeless women. *Am J Orthopsychiatry.* 1993;63:370-383.
45. D'Ercole A, Struening E. Victimization among homeless women: implications for service delivery. *J Community Psychol.* 1990;18:141-152.
46. Buckner JC, Bassuk EL, Zima BT. Mental health issues affecting homeless women: implications for intervention. *Am J Orthopsychiatry.* 1993;63:385-399.
47. Goodman LA. The prevalence of abuse in the lives of homeless and housed poor mothers: a comparison study. *Am J Orthopsychiatry.* 1991;61:489-500.
48. Masten AS, Miliotis D, Graham-Bermann SA, Ramirez ML, Neemann J. Children in homeless families: risks to mental health and development. *J Consult Clin Psychol.* 1993;61:335-343.
49. Parker RM, Rescorla LA, Finkelstein JA, Barnes N, Holmes JH, Stolley PD. A survey of the health of homeless children in Philadelphia shelters. *AJDC.* 1991; 145:520-526.
50. Rescorla L, Parker R, Stolley P. Ability, achievement, and adjustment in homeless children. *Am J Orthopsychiatry.* 1991;61:210-220.
51. Fox SJ, Barrnett RJ, Davies M, Bird HR. Psychopathology and developmental delay in homeless children: a pilot study. *J Am Acad Child Adolesc Psychiatry.* 1990;29:732-735.
52. Rafferty Y, Shinn M. The impact of homelessness on children. *Am Psychol.* 1991;46:1170-1179.
53. Stewart AL, Hays RD, Ware JE Jr. The MOS Short-Form General Health Survey: reliability and validity in a patient population. *Med Care.* 1988;26:724-735.
54. Wilken D, Hallam L, Doggett MA. Multidimensional measures. In: *Measures of Need and Outcome for Primary Health Care.* New York, NY: Oxford University Press; 1992:chap 7.
55. Jette AM, Davies AR, Cleary PD, Calkins DR, Rubenstein LV, Fink A, Kosecoff J, Young RT, Brook RH, Delbanco TL. The functional status questionnaire: reliability and validity when used in primary care. *J Gen Intern Med.* 1986;1: 143-149.
56. Berwick DM, Murphy JM, Goldman PA, Ware JE, Barsky AJ, Weinstein MC. Performance of a five-item mental health screening test. *Med Care.* 1991;29: 169-176.
57. Vernez G, Burnam MA, McGlynn EA, Trude S, Mittman BS. *Review of California's Program for the Homeless Mentally Disabled.* Santa Monica, Calif: RAND; 1988. Publication R-3631-CDMH.
58. Spengler PA, Wittchen HU. Procedural validity of standardized symptom questions for the assessment of psychotic symptoms: a comparison of the DIS with two clinical methods. *Compr Psychiatry.* 1988;29:309-322.
59. *National Health Interview Survey: Child Health Supplement, 1988* [computer data file and code book]. Washington, DC: National Center for Health Statistics; 1988.
60. Kovacs M. The Children's Depression Inventory (CDI). *Psychopharmacol Bull.* 1985;21:995-998.
61. Achenbach TM, Edelbrock CS. *Manual for the Child Behavior Checklist and Revised Behavior Profile.* Burlington: Dept of Psychiatry, University of Vermont; 1983.
62. Dunn LM, Dunn LM. *Peabody Picture Vocabulary Test—Revised.* Circle Pines, Minn: American Guidance Service; 1981.
63. Woodcock RW. *Woodcock-Johnson Language Proficiency Battery.* Allen, Tex: DLM Teaching Resources; 1984.
64. Tarlov AR, Ware JE, Greenfield S, Nelson EC, Perrin E, Zubkoff M. Medical Outcomes Study: an application of methods for evaluating the results of medical care. *JAMA.* 1989;262:925-930.
65. Wells KB, Stewart A, Hays RD, Burnam MA, Rogers W, Daniels M, Berry S, Greenfield S, Ware J. The functioning and well-being of depressed patients: results from the Medical Outcomes Study. *JAMA.* 1989;262:914-919.
66. Burnam MA, Wells KB, Leake B, Landsverk J. Development of a brief screening instrument for detecting depressive disorders. *Med Care.* 1988;26:775-789.
67. Holzer CE III, Shea BM, Swanson JW, Leaf PJ, Myers JK, George L, Bednarski P. The increased risk for specific psychiatric disorders among persons of low socioeconomic status: evidence from the Epidemiologic Catchment Area Surveys. *Am J Soc Psychiatry.* 1986;6:259-271.
68. Oakley A. Using medical care: the views and experiences of high-risk mothers. *Health Serv Res.* 1991;26:651-669.
69. Kessler RC, Neighbors HW. A new perspective on the relationships among race, social class, and psychologic distress. *J Health Soc Behav.* 1986;27:107-115.
70. Sue S. Community mental health services to minority groups: some optimism, some pessimism. *Am Psychol.* 1977;32:616-624.
71. Hauenstein EJ, Boyd MR. Depressive symptoms in young women of the Piedmont: prevalence in rural women. *Women Health.* 1994;21:105-123.
72. Triplett JL. Failure avoiders or success seekers? *Nurs Outlook.* September 1969; 17:68-71.
73. Children's Defense Fund. Births to teens. *Child Defense Fund Rep.* December 1994;16:7-11.
74. Gertler P, Rahman O, Feifer C, Ashley D. Determinants of pregnancy outcomes and targeting maternal health in Jamaica. *Soc Sci Med.* 1993;37:199-211.
75. Trad PV. Mental health of adolescent mothers. *J Am Acad Child Adolesc Psychiatry.* 1995;34:130-142.
76. Broadhead WE, Kaplan BH, James SA, Wagner EH, Schoenbach VJ, Grimson R, Heyden S, Tibblin G, Gehlbach SH. The epidemiologic evidence for a relationship between social support and health. *Am J Epidemiol.* 1983;117:521-537.
77. Huber PJ. *The Behavior of Maximum Likelihood Estimates Under Nonstandard Conditions.* Berkeley: University of California Press; 1967.
78. Najman JM, Bor W, Morrison J, Andersen M, Williams G. Child developmental delay and socio-economic disadvantage in Australia: a longitudinal study. *Soc Sci Med.* 1992;34:829-835.
79. Parker S, Greer S, Zuckerman B. Double jeopardy: the impact of poverty on early child development. *Pediatr Clin North Am.* 1988;35:1227-1240.
80. McLoyd VC, Wilson L. *The Strain of Living Poor: Parenting, Social Support, and Child Mental Health.* Cambridge, England: Cambridge University Press; 1991.
81. Kashani JH, Canfield LA, Borduin CM, Soltys SM, Reid JC. Perceived family and social support: impact on children. *J Am Acad Child Adolesc Psychiatry.* 1994;33:819-823.
82. Moilanen I, Rantakallio P. The single parent family and child's mental health. *Soc Sci Med.* 1988;27:181-186.
83. Stewart AL, Greenfield S, Hays RD, Wells KB, Rogers WH, Berry SD, McGlynn EA, Ware JE. Functional status and well-being of patients with chronic conditions: results from the Medical Outcomes Study. *JAMA.* 1989;262:907-913.
84. Robins LN, Regier DA, eds. *Psychiatric Disorders in America.* New York, NY: Free Press; 1991.
85. Regier DA, Narrow WE, Rae DS, Manderscheid RW, Locke BZ, Goodwin FK. The de facto US mental and addictive disorders service system: epidemiologic catchment area prospective 1-year prevalence rates of disorders and services. *Arch Gen Psychiatry.* 1993;50:85-94.
86. Estroff TW, Herrera C, Gaines R, Shaffer D, Gould M, Green AH. Maternal psychopathology and perception of child behavior in psychiatrically referred and child maltreatment families. *J Am Acad Child Adolesc Psychiatry.* 1984;23: 649-652.
87. Fergusson DM, Horwood LJ, Gretten ME, Shannon FT. Family life events, maternal depression, and maternal and teacher descriptions of child behavior. *Pediatrics.* 1985;75:30-35.
88. Friedlander S, Weiss DS, Traylor J. Assessing the influence of maternal depression on the validity of the Child Behavior Checklist. *J Abnorm Child Psychol.* 1986;14:123-133.
89. Griest DL, Wells KC, Forehand R. An examination of predictors of maternal perceptions of maladjustment in clinic-referred children. *J Abnorm Psychol.* 1979;88:277-281.
90. Jensen PS, Taylor J, Xenakis SN, Davis H. Child psychopathology rating scales and interrater agreement, I: parents' gender and psychiatric status. *J Am Acad Child Adolesc Psychiatry.* 1988;27:442-450.
91. Schaughency EA, Lahey BB. Mothers and fathers perceptions of child deviance: roles of child behavior, parental depression, and marital satisfaction. *J Consult Clin Psychol.* 1985;53:718-723.
92. Bassuk EL, Carman RW, Weinreb LF, ed. *Community Care for Homeless Families: A Program Design Manual.* Washington, DC: Interagency Council on the Homeless; 1990.

Psychiatric Diagnosis in Child and Adolescent Suicide

David Shaffer, MB, BS, FRCP, FRCPsych; Madelyn S. Gould, PhD, MPH; Prudence Fisher, MS; Paul Trautman, MD; Donna Moreau, MD; Marjorie Kleinman, MA; Michael Flory, PhD, MPH

Background: The age, sex, and ethnic distribution of adolescents who commit suicide is significantly different from that of the general population. The present study was designed to examine psychiatric risk factors and the relationship between them and demographic variables.

Methods: A case-control, psychologic autopsy study of 120 of 170 consecutive subjects (age, <20 years) who committed suicide and 147 community age-, sex-, and ethnic-matched control subjects who had lived in the Greater New York (NY) area.

Results: By using parent informants only, 59% of subjects who committed suicide and 23% of control subjects who met *DSM-III* criteria for a psychiatric diagnosis, 49% and 26%, respectively, had had symptoms for more than 3 years, and 46% and 29%, respectively, had had previous contact with a mental health professional. Best-estimate rates, based on multiple informants for these parameters, for suicides only, were 91%, 52%, and 46%, respectively. Previous attempts and mood disorder were major risk factors for both sexes; substance and/or alcohol abuse was a risk factor for males only. Mood disorder was more common in females, substance and/or alcohol abuse occurred exclusively in males (62% of 18- to 19-year-old suicides). The prevalence of a psychiatric diagnosis and, in particular, substance and/or alcohol abuse increased with age.

Conclusion: A limited range of diagnoses—most commonly a mood disorder alone or in combination with conduct disorder and/or substance abuse—characterizes most suicides among teenagers.

(Arch Gen Psychiatry. 1996;53:339-348)

THIS ARTICLE describes the psychopathologic characteristics, determined at "psychologic autopsy," of a substantial proportion of the 170 children and adolescents who committed suicide between June 1984 and May 1986, in New York, NY, and its surrounding area.

The seriousness of the problem of suicidal behaviors in adolescence has been well documented.[1] In 1992, 2150 children and adolescents younger than 20 years committed suicide in the United States.[2] The incidence of suicide among 15- to 19-year-old males has increased from just under 6/100 000 in 1965 to 17.8/100 000 in 1992.[2] The cumulative prevalence of suicide attempts in a representative population of adolescents[3] has been estimated at 3%. Large anonymous surveys have indicated that 2% of high school students have made a suicide attempt that required medical attention, with a substantially greater number making less medically serious attempts.[4]

In childhood and early adolescence, suicide is uncommon and occurs almost as often among females as males. The incidence among males increases through adolescence most rapidly after the age of 16 years.[2] In almost all countries, the male suicide rate has risen sharply during the last three decades.[5] In the United States, suicide is more common among white persons than among African-American individuals; however, since 1987, the incidence has increased most rapidly among young African-American males.[6] A principal goal of the present investigation was to understand these demographic patterns better by investigating their relationship to psychopathology, a well-established risk factor for suicide, in a representative group of teenage subjects who committed suicide and community

See Materials and Methods on next page

From the Division of Child Psychiatry, New York (NY) State Psychiatric Institute.

MATERIALS AND METHODS

The project was approved by the New York (NY) State Psychiatric Institute Ethical Review Board. Informed consent was obtained from all informants.

GEOGRAPHIC AREA

The area that was selected for study included the entire state of New Jersey, Litchfield, Fairfield, and New Haven Counties in Connecticut, and New York, Nassau, Suffolk, Putnam, Rockland, and Westchester Counties in New York State.

SUBJECTS

Adjudicated suicides that were committed by subjects (age, <20 years) in the above areas between June 1, 1984, and May 31, 1986, were identified by systematically reviewing all death certifications in the relevant medical examiner offices each week. One hundred seventy such suicides were recorded during this period. Deaths of an *undetermined* cause were not included. No attempt was made to second-guess suspicious accidents or to accept an informant's suggestions that an adjudicated suicide was really an accident or a murder.

Control subjects were identified from a stratified random sample that was drawn from the project study area. The stratification profile (sex, age, and race) was initially developed by using suicide mortality data from the same geographic area during the 3 years before the start of the study,[17] and it was then fine-tuned every 6 months to match the demographic characteristics of the current sample. Random-digit dialing was used to poll telephone subscribers to determine eligibility and willingness to receive information about the project. The research was described as a project concerning adolescent problems. The number of calls made within a county was proportional to the number of suicides in that county. One hundred ninety-six eligible control subjects were identified in this way, with 147 agreeing to participate.

The age, sex, and ethnic distribution of the subjects who committed suicide and control subjects are given in **Table 1**. The mean ages of males (16.9 years) and females (15.9 years) were not significantly different ($t_{27.6}$=.38 [based on separate variance estimates], P=.18). The modal age of the subjects who committed suicide was 18 years; only four subjects were 12 years or younger. Seventy-nine percent of the subjects who committed suicide were males. The male-to-female ratio increased from 0.75 for those subjects younger than 13 years, to 3.5 for those subjects in the 13- to 16-year-old age range, and to 4.9 for those subjects 17 years and older. Seventy percent of the subjects who committed suicide were white, 15% were Hispanic, and 11% were African American. Gender and age distributions did not differ significantly among ethnic groups. All demographic indexes were markedly different from those of the general population, and detailed comparisons will be provided in a future report (M.S.G., P.F., D.S., M. F., and M. Parides, PhD, and G. Todak, MSW, unpublished data, 1986). By design, control subjects did not differ significantly from the subjects who committed suicide in mean age, proportion older or younger than 17 years, sex, or ethnicity (Table 1).

The participation rate was 71%. Interview information was not obtained from informants for 50 suicides. Of these, nine relatives (5% of the total sample) could not be located, and the families of 41 (24%) were traced but refused to be interviewed. Forty-nine identified control subjects refused to be interviewed. Participants' and nonparticipants' suicides and controls did not differ significantly from each other in mean age, proportion older or younger than 17 years, sex, or ethnicity (Table 1). The socioeconomic status of nonparticipants was approximated by determining the proportion of the population within their residential zip code who received public assistance (1980 census data). Participants and nonparticipants did not differ on this measure.

ASSESSMENT METHODS

The interval between suicide and assessment ranged from 28 to 976 days (median, 159 days). Fifty-four percent of the interviews took place within 6 months and 92% within 1 year of the suicide. Most interviews took place in informants' homes. Information for both subjects who committed suicide and control subjects was obtained during the same time period.

Interviewers were masters- or doctoral-level psychologists and social workers who received systematic training on all instruments. Spanish-speaking interviewers were employed to interview Hispanic informants. All interviews were audiotaped and reviewed by a survey editor.

INFORMANTS

The information sources are described in **Table 2**.

Subjects Who Committed Suicide

Information about the victims was usually obtained from (1) a parent or another adult member of the victim's household at the time of death, (2) a sibling or friend no more than 5 years older than the victim who was nominated by the parent or caretaker, and (3) between one and three schoolteachers who were nominated by the parent or caretaker or by the school principal as being well informed about the subject's classroom behavior. Toxicology reports were obtained from the medical examiner's records in 97 (81%) of the interviewed subjects.

Control Subjects

Either a parent or caretaker was interviewed and, if the adolescent and parent consented, behavioral ratings were obtained from three schoolteachers. Information was obtained from the control adolescent, but it was not used in this report. To avoid biasing the parental report, parents of control subjects were assessed before the adolescent. When this was not possible, separate interviewers were assigned to adult and adolescent informants. Medical, psychiatric, and police reports were sought for suicides only and were used for best-estimate diagnoses (BEDs).

MEASURES

Symptom presence was assessed for the 3 months before death or in control subjects for the 3 months before contact by the research team. The interview determined the presence, onset, frequency, and interference with function of 205 symptom criteria for most of the disorders in the *DSM-III*[18] that affect children and adolescents and for a number of nondiagnostic symptoms. Developmental and autistic conditions were not assessed. The mood disorder questions were drawn from the Schedule for Affective Disorders and Schizophrenia[19] and the Schedule for Affective Disorders and Schizophrenia–Child Version.[20] Questions about psychotic symptoms were drawn from the Present State Examination.[21] The interview included 18 screening questions about substance and alcohol abuse (SAA) that were asked of all respondents. Conditional on their responses, an additional 20 questions were posed to inquire about complications and impairment attributable to alcohol and substance use. The interviewer was free to ask additional questions and was required to match responses to a symptom definition before assigning a rating. Interviewers were instructed not to make inferences about subjective states; they recorded the presence of a pathologic mood or thought only if the informant could recall a definite statement made by the subject that indicated its presence (eg, self-denigration required utterance of self-critical statements). Ratings of ambiguous responses were decided in conference.

Because of the low prevalence of individual diagnoses, five superordinate categories (mood, disruptive, SAA, anxiety, and miscellaneous) were created to facilitate data analysis. Obsessive-compulsive disorder was included among the anxiety disorders and attention-deficit disorder with hyperactivity among the disruptive disorders. Schizophrenia and eating disorders were ungrouped. A proportion of interviews were rerated from audiotapes and were then rescored by using the same computer algorithms. The κ coefficient of agreement between raters for any diagnosis was .85; for any mood disorder, it was .72; for any disruptive disorder, it was .58; for any SAA disorder, it was .76; and for anxiety disorders, it was .81.

A number of noncriterion symptoms (eg, hopelessness, perfectionism, self-damaging and explosive behaviors, running away, and being bullied) that have been linked to suicide in the literature[22,23] were also included in the symptom interview. Scales for perfectionism and aggressiveness (for 1 year) were constructed from candidate items in the symptom interview. These had satisfactory internal reliability (Cronbach's α was .71 for both). Hopelessness (for 3 months) was based on a report of repeated statements (eg, "no one can help me," "nothing will ever get better," "nothing is going to turn out right"); "morbid preoccupations" (for 3 months) were based on reports of brooding about a dead friend or relative or nonspecific concerns about "doom" or the "tragic" nature of life; the scale of self-damaging behaviors (for 3 months) was observed from reports of repetitive scratching, wrist cutting, head banging, hand biting, or hair pulling; and dangerous or reckless behaviors (for 1 year) were defined as activities "done for fun that most people regard as dangerous," including playing Russian roulette, playing chicken, and fast driving.

Parents and teachers completed appropriate versions of the Child Behavior Checklist.[24,25] The Children's Global Assessment Scale[26] impairment rating was made by the interviewer after reviewing all information. The entire assessment, including obtaining details of the circumstances leading to death, history, etc, took between 4 and 20 hours.

ASSIGNING A DIAGNOSIS

Nonblind BEDs[27] provided the most complete description of the suicides. They were assigned at a conference that was led by an experienced child psychiatrist (D.S., P.T., or D.M.) and were based on the narrative summary, original interview material, and unsummarized medical, educational, and police records. Case-control comparisons were based on blind parent informant data (common to both subjects who committed suicide and control subjects) that were assigned by computer to diagnostic algorithms. The BEDs were, as expected, significantly more prevalent (91%) than "parent informant–only" diagnoses (59%). Fifty-six percent of the best-estimate mood disorder cases, 54% of the best-estimate SAA cases, 46% of the best-estimate disruptive disorder cases, and 59% of the best-estimate anxiety disorder cases were identified by the parent-only algorithm.

DATING SYMPTOMS AND DISORDERS

Age at onset of any symptom that was present during the 3 months prior to death or interview was ascertained, and it was used to examine the order of appearance of symptoms. Parents were also asked the age when any emotional or behavioral problems were first noted, and this datum was taken to indicate the onset of a disorder. If symptom onset preceded the onset of a disorder, onset of disorder was adjusted to reflect the earliest date.

STATISTICAL METHODS

Logistic regression analyses were performed separately for each sex to assess the effect of a set of possible risk factors simultaneously and to account for shared associations that they might have with suicide. The specific variables included a previous suicide attempt, runaway behavior, recklessness, and the computer-generated, parent-informed diagnostic disorder groupings (mood, disruptive, substance abuse, and anxiety). All models were adjusted for possible confounding of socioeconomic status, age, and ethnicity (only African-American, white, and Hispanic subjects were analyzed). The socioeconomic status for each household was determined from the demographic information obtained at interview, by using Hollingshead's four-factor score.[28]

The models were fit in a stepwise fashion after inclusion of the demographic variables. The likelihood ratio tests were used to determine whether a variable added significantly to the fit or if its removal significantly worsened the fit of the model. Interactions that involved the significant main effects were also assessed.

Table 1. Demographic Characteristics of Participants and Nonparticipants*

Characteristic	Subjects Who Committed Suicide: Participants (n=120)	Subjects Who Committed Suicide: Nonparticipants (n=50)	Control Subjects: Participants (n=147)	Control Subjects: Nonparticipants (n=49)†
Age, y				
Mean	16.7	16.9	16.7	16.2
≤16	43 (36)	17 (34)	60 (41)	24 (49)
≥17	77 (64)	33 (66)	87 (59)	25 (51)
Sex				
M	95 (79)	37 (74)	116 (79)	39 (80)
F	25 (21)	13 (26)	31 (21)	10 (20)
Race or ethnicity				
White	84 (70)	29 (58)	111 (76)	35 (76)
African American	13 (11)	8 (16)	16 (11)	9 (20)
Hispanic	18 (15)	12 (24)	15 (10)	1 (2)
Other	5 (4)	1 (2)	5 (3)	1 (2)

*Data are given as the number (percentage) of subjects, except for mean age.
†Information on race not obtained for three nonparticipants.

Table 2. Information Sources*

Source	Subjects Who Committed Suicide (n=120)	Nonpsychiatric Control Subjects (n=147)
Interview with parent or other adult	118 (98)	145 (99)
Interview with peer, sibling, or proband	76 (63)	132 (90)
Educational record	88 (73)	81 (55)
Police or health records	75 (63)	16 (11)
All 4	47 (39)	8 (5)
3 only	35 (29)	75 (51)
2 only	26 (22)	53 (36)
1 only	10 (8)	11 (8)

*Data are given as the number (percentage) of subjects.

control subjects. The psychologic autopsy technique was used; this has been shown to be a robust method that is not unduly subject to bias attributable to the informant-affective state or death-evaluation interval.[7] Although there are several psychologic autopsy studies of child and adolescent suicides in the literature, most have been small,[8-13] with only two studying more than 50 cases; these are the uncontrolled Finnish National Study (n=53)[14,15] and the psychologic autopsy study of 67 subjects who committed suicide and community control subjects in an ethnically homogeneous area surrounding Pittsburgh, Pa, that was done by Brent et al.[16] Both studies reported high rates of psychopathology but, because of limited numbers, did not address age-, gender-, and ethnic-specific features.

In this study, multiple informants were assessed with a standardized assessment procedure. The suicides occurred in an ethnically diverse population that provided an opportunity to examine ethnic-specific differences. Although information was obtained from many sources, case-control comparisons were drawn by using information from parents only, to ensure a comparable information source for both groups.

RESULTS

PREVALENCE AND DURATION OF A PSYCHIATRIC DIAGNOSIS

The *prevalence* of the most common BEDs is presented in **Table 3**. More than 90% of subjects who committed suicide met criteria for at least one *DSM-III* psychiatric diagnosis. The most common diagnostic groups were mood, disruptive, and SAA disorders. Sixty-one percent of the subjects who committed suicide met criteria for a mood disorder (52% of these for major depressive disorder), 22% for dysthymia, 10% for adjustment disorder with depressed features, 4% for bipolar disorder, and 12% for depression not otherwise specified or another variant. All but five of the subjects who committed suicide with a disruptive disorder met criteria for conduct disorder. A substantial number of suicide victims (27% [32/119]) met criteria for an anxiety disorder, including nine with overanxious disorder of childhood, eight with one of the avoidant diagnoses (social phobia, avoidant disorder, or schizoid disorder), and seven with an adjustment disorder with "mixed emotional features." Five subjects who committed suicide had panic attacks: one met criteria for panic disorder, one for agoraphobia with panic disorder, one for panic disorder with separation anxiety, and two for panic attacks only. Four subjects who committed suicide had separation anxiety disorder, six had simple phobia, and one had obsessive-compulsive disorder. Schizophrenia was present in four patients (3%), and an eating disorder was present in five (4%).

Four percent of the subjects who committed suicide had an onset within 3 months prior to death, 13% between 3 and 12 months, 13% between 1 and 2 years, 18% from 3 to 5 years, and 32% more than 5 years. The proportion of subjects who committed suicide with an onset of 3 or more years before death was the same for those with a BED of disruptive (64%), substance abuse (65%), and mood disorders (56%).

Table 3. Prevalence of Psychiatric Diagnoses in Subjects Who Committed Suicide by Sex and Age and Comorbidity of Mood, Anxiety, Disruptive Disorder, and SAA Diagnostic Groups*

Diagnosis	Boys <17 y (n=30)	Boys ≥17 y (n=64)	Boys All (n=94)	Girls <17 y (n=12)	Girls ≥17 y (n=13)	Girls All (n=25)	All Subjects (N=119)
Prevalence of Psychiatric Diagnoses							
Mood disorders	17 (57)	39 (61)	**56** (60)	7 (58)	10 (77)	**17** (68)	**73** (61)
Major depression	5 (17)	19 (30)	**24** (26)	6 (50)	8 (62)	**14** (56)	**38** (32)
Dysthymia	5 (17)	11 (17)	**16** (17)	0	0	**0**	**16** (13)
Bipolar	0	3 (5)	**3** (3)	0	0	**0**	**3** (2)
Depression NOS	1 (3)	1 (2)	**2** (2)	0	1 (8)	**1** (4)	**3** (3)
Adjustment disorder with:							
Depressed mood	4 (13)	2 (3)	**6** (6)	1 (8)	0	**1** (4)	**7** (6)
Other	2 (7)	3 (5)	**5** (5)	0	1 (8)	**1** (4)	**6** (5)
Disruptive disorders	13 (43)	38 (59)	**51** (54)	6 (50)	3 (23)	**9** (36)	**60** (50)
Conduct	9 (30)	38 (59)	**47** (50)	6 (50)	2 (15)	**8** (32)	**55** (46)
Oppositional	0	1 (2)	**1** (1)	0	1 (8)	**1** (4)	**2** (2)
Attention-deficit	6 (20)	2 (3)	**8** (9)	1 (8)	0	**1** (4)	**9** (8)
Anxiety disorders	9 (30)	16 (25)	**25** (27)	4 (33)	3 (23)	**7** (28)	**32** (27)
Any substance abuse	3 (10)	36 (56)	**39** (42)	2 (17)	1 (8)	**3** (12)	**42** (35)
Alcohol	2 (7)	24 (38)	**26** (28)	0	0	**0**	**26** (22)
Drug	2 (7)	25 (39)	**27** (29)	2 (17)	1 (8)	**3** (12)	**30** (25)
Eating disorder	0	1 (2)	**1** (1)	1 (8)	3 (23)	**4** (16)	**5** (4)
Schizophrenia	1 (3)	2 (3)	**3** (3)	0	1 (8)	**1** (4)	**4** (3)
Miscellaneous	1 (3)	0	**1** (1)	0	0	**0**	**1** (1)
No diagnosis	5 (17)	4 (6)	**9** (10)	2 (17)	0	**2** (8)	**11** (9)
Comorbidity							
Single diagnosis							
Mood only	5 (17)	7 (11)	**12** (13)	1 (8)	5 (38)	**6** (24)	**18** (15)
Disruptive only	1 (3)	5 (8)	**6** (6)	1 (8)	0	**1** (4)	**7** (6)
Anxiety only	4 (13)	3 (5)	**7** (7)	1 (8)	1 (8)	**2** (8)	**9** (8)
Substance only	0	1 (2)	**1** (1)	0	0	**0**	**1** (1)
Mood comorbid							
Mood and disruptive	7 (23)	3 (5)	**10** (11)	2 (17)	3 (23)	**5** (20)	**15** (13)
Mood and anxiety	2 (7)	5 (8)	**7** (7)	2 (17)	1 (8)	**3** (12)	**10** (8)
Mood and substance	0	5 (8)	**5** (5)	0	1 (8)	**1** (4)	**6** (5)
Mood, disruptive, anxiety	0	1 (2)	**1** (1)	1 (8)	0	**1** (4)	**2** (2)
Mood, disruptive, substance	2 (7)	13 (20)	**15** (16)	1 (8)	0	**1** (4)	**16** (13)
Mood, anxiety, substance	0	1 (2)	**1** (1)	0	0	**0**	**1** (1)
Mood, disruptive, anxiety, substance	1 (3)	4 (6)	**5** (5)	0	0	**0**	**5** (4)
Other comorbid							
Disruptive and anxiety	2 (7)	0	**2** (2)	0	0	**0**	**2** (2)
Disruptive and substance	0	10 (16)	**10** (11)	1 (8)	0	**1** (4)	**11** (9)
Disruptive, anxiety, and substance	0	2 (3)	**2** (2)	0	0	**0**	**2** (2)
Other diagnoses not included above	1 (3)	0	**1** (1)	0	2 (15)	**2** (8)	**3** (3)
No diagnosis	5 (17)	4 (6)	**9** (10)	2 (17)	0	**2** (8)	**11** (9)

**Best-estimate method was used for both the prevalence of psychiatric diagnoses and comorbidity; for the former, the sum of disorders is greater than the total sample size because some individuals had more than one diagnosis. SAA indicates substance or alcohol abuse; NOS, not otherwise specified. Data are given as number (percentage) of the subjects.*

DEMOGRAPHIC FACTORS ASSOCIATED WITH A DIAGNOSIS

Age

Seventy-one percent of subjects who committed suicide were younger than 13 years; 86% of the 13- to 16-year-old and 95% of the 17- to 19-year-old subjects had a BED (χ^2_2 [*df*]=5.68, *P*=.06). The prevalence of most psychiatric diagnoses increased with age; exceptions were adjustment disorder with depressive features in males and disruptive disorder in females (these exceptions were more common in the younger subjects who committed suicide). The increase was especially striking for SAA in boys; this type of abuse was absent in those subjects 12 years and younger, and it was present in 12% of the 13- to 15-year-old subjects and in 62% of the 18- and 19-year-old subjects.

Sex

Substance abuse and dysthymia occurred almost exclusively in males. Major depression was twice as common in females.

Ethnicity

The rates of psychiatric disorder in white (93%) and Hispanic (89%) subjects were similar and higher than those among African-American (77%) subjects. A smaller pro-

Table 4. Noncriterion Symptoms in Subjects Who Committed Suicide and Control Subjects*

Symptom	Suicides, All Informants: Boys (n=91-94)	Suicides, All Informants: Girls (n=23 and 24)	Suicides, Parent Informant: Boys (n=78-81)	Suicides, Parent Informant: Girls (n=19)	Control Subjects, Parent Informant: Boys (n=112-115)	Control Subjects, Parent Informant: Girls (n=29)	Suicide Risk (Both Sexes), Parent Informant: χ^2‡	Suicide Risk (Both Sexes), Parent Informant: OR‡ (95% CI)	Suicide Risk, Parent Informant (Adjusted OR† [95% CI]): Boys	Suicide Risk, Parent Informant (Adjusted OR† [95% CI]): Girls
Recklessness	20/91 (22)	0/24	14/78 (18)	0/19	3/115 (3)	0/29	11.3§	7.93‖ (2.21-28.40)	5.33‖ (1.30-21.94)	...
Morbid preoccupation	14/91 (15)	4/24 (17)	5/78 (6)	1/19 (5)	0/115	0/29	6.6‖	...	...	...
Hopelessness	41/94 (44)	8/23 (35)	19/81 (24)	4/19 (21)	5/115 (4)	2/29 (7)	15.0§	8.85‖ (2.40-14.25)	...	...
Self-damage	7/94 (7)	1/23 (4)	5/81 (6)	0/19	0/115	0/29	5.1‖	...	...	...
Panic attack	4/94 (4)	1/23 (4)	3/81 (4)	1/19 (5)	0/115	0/29	3.6	...	...	...
Runaway	26/94 (28)	9/23 (39)	20/81 (25)	6/19 (32)	6/115 (5)	4/29 (14)	15.6§	4.71‖ (2.15-10.30)	3.99‖ (1.30-12.21)	4.26 (0.31-58.36)
Mean (SD)										
Aggressivity	1.28 (1.67)	1.08 (0.52)	0.89 (1.41)	0.32 (0.82)	0.28 (0.74)	0.28 (1.13)	t_{242}=3.61§¶		...	...
Perfectionism	0.78 (1.28)	1.78 (2.71)	0.53 (1.04)	0.95 (2.30)	0.43 (1.09)	0.52 (1.06)	*P*.31¶		...	...

*OR indicates odds ratio; CI, confidence interval. Data are given as the number (percentage) of the subjects.
†The ORs are adjusted for socioeconomic status, ethnicity, age, mood disorder, any disruptive disorder, and substance or alcohol abuse.
‡The χ^2 tests of associations and ORs are not adjusted for any other variables.
§P<.01.
‖P<.05
¶Tests are of differences between suicides and control subjects.

portion of African-American (23%) than white (42%) subjects who committed suicides were described as having SAA; this finding may be due to systematic underreporting. The number of subjects who committed suicide whose blood alcohol level was greater than 0.06 mg/dL was noted in the toxicology report without a corresponding report of SAA in the interview; it was greater among African-American subjects (38% [3/8]) than among white subjects (11% [4/38]). While this difference is not statistically significant, the power to detect significance was limited by small numbers. There were no significant differences in the rates of mood, anxiety, or disruptive disorder among the three ethnic groups.

SAA AND OTHER DIAGNOSES

The diagnosis of SAA was common in older males and almost invariably associated with either a mood or disruptive disorder, or both. Forty-one male suicides were comorbid for SAA and either mood or disruptive disorder, or both. Data that provided which disorder had appeared first were available for 37 of 41 subjects. Disruptive disorder appeared first in 18 of 19 triply comorbid cases. The diagnosis of SAA preceded mood disorder in five of six subjects who were comorbid for mood disorder and SAA, and disruptive disorder appeared first in seven of 12 subjects who were comorbid for disruptive disorder and SAA.

COMORBIDITY

Using the best-estimate method, 70% of the subjects who committed suicide had complex diagnostic profiles with comorbid diagnoses (Table 3). Mood disorder alone or in combination with disruptive and SAA disorders accounted for half of all subjects who committed suicide. The diagnosis of SAA was almost invariably present with another diagnosis—most commonly, a disruptive or mood disorder.

MISCELLANEOUS SYMPTOMS

Hopelessness, morbid concerns, and reckless and runaway behavior were only found in children with an Axis I diagnosis (**Table 4**). Thirty-four of 49 subjects who had committed suicide and expressed hopelessness met criteria for a mood disorder, seven of 18 subjects who had committed suicide and expressed morbid concerns had diagnoses of comorbid mood and disruptive disorder, seven had a diagnosis of mood disorder, and two had a diagnosis of a disruptive disorder only. Six of the eight subjects with self-damaging behavior had a diagnosis of comorbid mood and disruptive disorder. Ten of the 20 boys with a history of reckless behavior had a diagnosis of comorbid mood and disruptive disorder, six had a diagnosis of disruptive disorder alone, and three had a diagnosis of mood disorder alone. Among the 35 subjects who had committed suicide (30%) and had run away overnight at least once, two had a diagnosis of comorbid mood and disruptive disorder, 10 had a diagnosis of mood disorder, and seven had a diagnosis of disruptive disorder only. The only type of reckless behavior that was reported in more than one individual was driving excessively fast in an automobile. Despite the extensive overlap between the behaviors and these diagnostic groups, reckless and runaway behavior remain a significant predictor of suicide risk for boys after controlling for mood, disruptive, and substance abuse disorders. Our measure of perfectionism differed from these other symptoms in being equally common in subjects who committed suicide and control subjects and by having a weak relationship to diagnostic status.

SUBJECTS WHO COMMITTED SUICIDE AND CONTROL SUBJECTS WITH NO PSYCHIATRIC DIAGNOSIS

The 11 subjects who committed suicide (9%) who did not meet criteria for a BED were significantly younger (mean age, 14.61 years; SD, 3.56 years) than those with a diagnosis (mean age, 16.9 years; SD, 2.03 years) (t=3.36, df=117, P<.001). They did not differ in the scores for the Children's Global Assessment Scale and the total Child Behavior Checklist score or the rate of school suspensions from the control subjects without a diagnosis (n=110). More of the suicides without a BED (six [54.5%] of 11) had information from only one source, compared with subjects with BED.

PRIOR SUICIDE ATTEMPTS

Information on previous attempts was available for 112 subjects who committed suicide. Thirty-seven subjects (33%) had made a previous suicide attempt compared with only one control (P<.001). Subjects who made previous attempts were no more likely to have a psychiatric diagnosis than those subjects who had not made an attempt, but they were more likely to have a diagnosis of mood disorder (78%) than were those subjects who did not make attempts (53%) (corrected χ^2_1 [df]=5.55, P<.02). Previous attempts were nonsignificantly more common in females (50%) than in males (28%). This difference appeared to be related to the higher rate of mood disorder in females. Prior attempts in subjects who committed suicide without a mood disorder were as common in males (19%) as females (14%).

PREVIOUS PSYCHIATRIC TREATMENT

Lifetime Treatment

According to parental report, 46% of the subjects who committed suicide and 20% of the control subjects had had contact with a mental health professional before their death or evaluation. White subjects were significantly more likely to have received prior psychiatric treatment (57%) than either African-American (31%) or Hispanic (6%) subjects. The diagnostic profile of the subjects who committed suicide and who received treatment did not differ from the sample as a whole.

Recent Treatment

Significantly more (n=24 [21%]) of the subjects who committed suicide than control subjects (n=7 [5%]) had been evaluated or treated by a mental health professional during the 3 months before their death or evaluation (corrected χ^2_1 [df]=13.96, P<.001). Recent treatment rates did not vary with age or gender, but white subjects (26%) were significantly more likely to have received recent treatment than either African-American (15%) or Hispanic (0%) subjects (corrected χ^2_1 [df]=6.2, P=.045). Recent treatment was significantly more common in those subjects with a disruptive disorder (31%) and schizophrenia (75%) than in subjects with other diagnoses who committed suicide (Fisher's exact test, P=.027). Nine of the 24 subjects who committed suicide who had been recently treated (8% of all subjects) had been hospitalized, and eight (7% of all subjects) had been treated with psychotropic medications. Seven of the eight subjects who had committed suicide and had been treated with medication received this treatment during a hospital admission.

RISK FOR SUICIDE—COMPARISON WITH CONTROL SUBJECTS

Comparisons between subjects who committed suicide and control subjects were based on computer-generated diagnoses with symptoms reported by parents. Earlier reports of these data[29-31] variously employed nonblind best-estimate evaluations or broad diagnostic groupings only or symptom counts.

Univariate odds ratios (ORs) were calculated as unconditional maximum likelihood estimates to assess the association of individual diagnoses, previous suicide attempts, and ever running away on the risk of suicide (**Table 5**). All ORs, except bipolar disorder, were significantly different from 1 at the .05 level. For the group as a whole, the factors that best differentiated subjects who had committed suicide and control subjects were having made a previous attempt and diagnoses of mood disorder and SAA. A previous attempt and diagnoses of major depression and atypical depression were the strongest discriminators for males; previous attempt and mood disorder were the best discriminators for females.

A logistic regression analysis was undertaken on 177 males (70 subjects who committed suicide and 107 control subjects) and 45 females (18 subjects who committed suicide and 27 control subjects) for whom complete data were available.

Males

A previous attempt and diagnoses of mood disorder and SAA significantly increased the risk of suicide. There were no significant interactions. The adjusted (for the demographic variables and significant risk factors) ORs (and 95% confidence intervals [CIs]) were 19.4 (CI, 2.3 to 162.1) for having made a previous attempt, 7.8 (CI, 2.6 to 23.2) for a mood disorder, and 5.8 (CI, 1.6 to 20.6) for SAA. Runaway and reckless behavior were no longer significant risk factors in the final logistic regression model that included previous attempts.

Females

There was only one female (a control subject) who was positive for substance abuse so this diagnostic category was excluded from the analysis. Having made a previous attempt and having a mood disorder significantly increased the risk of suicide for females. The adjusted (for demographic variables and mood disorder) OR for having made a previous attempt was not precisely esti-

Table 5. Difference in Prevalence of Psychiatric Disorders and Selected Symptoms Between Subjects Who Committed Suicide and Control Subjects (Parent Information Only)*

	Boys				Girls				
Disorder or Symptom	Subjects Who Committed Suicide (n=81)	Control Subjects (n=115)	OR (95% CI)	Adjusted OR (95% CI)†	Subjects Who Committed Suicide (n=19)	Control Subjects (n=29)	OR (95% CI)	Adjusted OR (95% CI)†	All Subjects, OR (95% CI)
Mood disorders	31 (38.3)	6 (5.2)	11.26‡ (4.42-28.72)	7.81‡ (2.63-23.15)	9 (47.4)	1 (3.4)	25.2‡ (2.82-224.84)	20.80‡ (1.35-319.97)	12.10 (5.12-28.57)
Major depression	10 (12.3)	1 (0.9)	16.06‡ (2.01-128.13)	NE§	3 (15.8)	0	. . .	NE	19.87 (2.55-154.66)
Dysthymia	1 (1.2)	0	. . .	NE	0	0	. . .	NE	NE
Bipolar	0	1 (0.9)	. . .	NE	1 (5.3)	1 (3.4)	1.56 (0.09-26.48)	NE	0.67 (0.06-7.46)
Depression NOS	20 (24.7)	4 (3.5)	9.10‡ (2.97-27.83)	NE	5 (26.3)	0	. . .	NE	10.83 (3.63-32.32)
Disruptive disorders	25 (30.9)	14 (12.2)	3.22‡ (1.55-6.69)	¶	2 (10.5)	2 (6.9)	1.59 (0.20-12.36)	#	2.73 (1.38-5.40)
Conduct	22 (27.2)	11 (9.6)	3.53‡ (1.60-7.78)	NE	2 (10.5)	1 (3.4)	3.29 (0.28-39.14)	NE	3.21 (1.52-6.80)
Oppositional	11 (13.6)	4 (3.5)	4.36‡ (1.34-14.23)	NE	1 (5.3)	2 (6.9)	0.75 (0.06-8.90)	NE	2.91 (1.05-8.04)
Attention-deficit	0	1 (0.9)	. . .	NE	0	0	. . .	NE	. . .
Anxiety disorders	19 (23.5)	10 (8.7)	3.22‡ (1.41-7.36)	¶	3 (15.8)	6 (20.7)	0.72 (0.16-3.31)	#	2.08 (1.03-4.21)
Any substance abuse	20 (24.7)	5 (4.3)	7.21‡ (2.58-20.18)	5.76‡ (1.61-20.6)	0	1 (3.4)	. . .	NE	5.33 (2.05-13.85)
Alcohol	17 (21.0)	5 (4.3)	5.84‡ (2.06-16.59)	NE	0	0	. . .	NE	5.28 (1.88-14.87)
Drug	10 (12.3)	0	. . .	NE	0	1 (3.4)	. . .	NE	14.78 (1.86-117.46)
Eating disorder	0	0	. . .	NE	1 (5.3)	0	. . .	NE	NE
Schizophrenia	1 (1.2)	0	. . .	NE	0	0	. . .	NE	NE
Previous attempt‖	17 (23.9)	1 (0.9)	34.31‡ (4.45-264.70)	19.39‡ (2.32-162.13)	7 (38.9)	0	. . .	NE	NE
Ever run away	20 (24.7)	6 (5.2)	5.96‡ (2.27-15.63)	¶	6 (31.6)	4 (13.8)	2.88 (0.69-12.07)	#	3.04‡ (1.61-5.71)
Recklessness	14 (17.3)	3 (2.6)	7.95‡ (2.20-28.72)	¶	0	0	. . .	NE	NE
No diagnosis	33 (40.7)	89 (77.4)	4.98‡ (2.67-9.28)	NE	8 (42.1)	22 (75.9)	4.32‡ (1.24-15.03)	NE	0.14 (0.08-0.26)

**OR indicates odds ratio; CI, confidence interval; and NOS, not otherwise specified. Data for subjects are given as the number (percentage).*
†The ORs are adjusted for socioeconomic status, ethnicity, age, and other significant risk factors (see text).
‡P<.05.
§NE denotes not examined because diagnosis is redundant with supraordinate categories of mood and disruptive disorder.
‖Seventy-one suicides, 110 controls for boys; 18 suicides, 28 controls for girls.
¶Effect insignificant when adjusted for previous attempt, mood, and substance abuse.
#Effect insignificant when adjusted for mood disorder.

mable since none of the control subjects had made a previous attempt (Table 5), but it was clearly an important risk factor. The adjusted (for the demographic variables and previous attempts) OR for having a mood disorder was 20.80 although, because of the relative rarity of the outcome, the 95% CI extended from 1.4 to 320, indicating that precise estimation of the increased risk was not possible with this sample. No significant interactions were found.

COMMENT

Valuable features of this study include (1) a sample large enough to examine sex, ethnic, and age differences in psychopathology; (2) the use of both single and multi-informant strategies so that risk estimates would be derived from comparable information sources (parent only), while providing rich descriptive material from multiple sources; (3) the use of a standardized assessment battery; and (4) community control subjects. The principal limitations were the 71% interview completion rate, similar to that (74%) reported by Brent et al[16] but lower than that (94%) obtained in the Finnish study.[14] However, the moderate completion rate may not be a significant threat to validity because (1) suicides for whom informants were or were not available did not differ substantially on demographic or event variables and (2) a major reason for failing to locate survivors lay outside the individual characteristics of the suicides and was caused by a delay in identifying eligible suicides because of the backlog of work at one of the medical examiners' offices.

The 90% prevalence of psychiatric disorders is similar to that found in comparable studies in Pittsburgh[16] and Finland.[14,15] The small number of subjects without a psychiatric diagnosis who committed suicide were younger, and they were less likely to have been investigated comprehensively than subjects who committed suicide with a diagnosis. The prevalence (61%) of the most common psychiatric diagnosis, ie, mood disorder, is similar to the 64% that was found in the Finnish National Study,[14] and it is somewhat higher than the 49% prevalence reported in the Pittsburgh study[16] that did not include adjustment disorder with depressive features. There were three cases of bipolar disorder in the New York study and one in the Finnish studies compared with 18% in the Pittsburgh study. The discrepancy may be due a substantially different approach to handling diagnostic information or simply to chance in the relatively small samples.

The 50% of those who committed suicide who had a disruptive disorder was higher than the 20% rate that was found in the Finnish National Study[14] and the 36% reported in the Pittsburgh study.[16] Hopelessness and aggressivity were common in the suicides. Panic symptoms, in most instances, associated with a mood disorder, were reported in approximately 10% of the suicides but in no control subjects. One third of the suicides had a history of runaway behavior. Just under one third of the suicides were known to have made a prior suicide attempt, and a similar proportion had previously had contact with a mental health professional. The failure to show a relationship between suicide and perfectionism and the weak relationship between perfectionism and diagnosis may indicate that this is simply not a clinically significant construct. Comparable information is not available from other studies.

The older suicides were more likely to be male and to have a psychiatric disorder, especially SAA. It was our impression that young suicides were more likely to have committed suicide in the context of a misunderstanding about the likely consequences of a recent stress. However, the rarity of suicide in the very young is such that their distinctive risk factors can only be studied with an oversampling design.

DURATION AND COURSE OF DISORDER

Duration

More than one third of the New York suicides had an onset of symptoms more than 5 years before their death, and 4% had had a very recent onset. In the Pittsburgh study,[16] most mood disorders were of recent onset, whereas, in the present study, mood disorder duration was similar to that of other disorders.

Symptom Sequencing

The order in which symptoms appear has not been well described in the adolescent suicide literature, although Runeson[12] found that a high proportion of Swedish suicides had secondary SAA. In our examination of 37 subjects with comorbid mood and SAA and/or conduct disorder, the most common sequence was for conduct disorder to predate substance abuse, which predated mood disorder. Mood disorder predated SAA or the conduct disorder in only two subjects. These findings need to be interpreted cautiously. Information was obtained retrospectively through third-party informants who may have been ignorant of the onset of either the subjective symptoms of mood disorder or the covert symptoms of conduct disorder or SAA.

PSYCHOPATHOLOGY AND DEMOGRAPHICS

The epidemiology of suicide begs several questions: (1) Why is suicide less common in prepubertal children than in adolescents?[5,9,32] (2) Why is suicide so much more common in postpubertal males than in females? (3) Why have recent increases in the suicide rates been confined to males? Our findings suggest developmental changes in that the suicide rate reflects the developmental trajectories of its main risk factors (ie, mood and SAA disorders). In this study, SAA occurred significantly more often in males than females; SAA was present in about two thirds of 18- and 19-year-old male subjects who committed suicide. Given the ample evidence that the prevalence of SAA has increased in many countries during the past three decades[33,34] and the consistency of evidence that shows a relationship between suicide and alcohol abuse,[11,14,15] it would be reasonable to suggest that changes in youth suicide rates may be associated with changes in the prevalence of SAA. The recent stabilization of youth suicide rates is compatible with the reduction in rates of substance abuse in young persons.[33,34]

IMPLICATIONS

Approximately two thirds of the suicides bore one of three risk factors before their death: a prior suicide attempt, mood disorder, and SAA. Thirty-seven percent of the subjects had only one risk factor, 12% had two risk factors, and 7% had all three risk factors. Most suicides had had encounters with mental health professionals, but fewer than 10% had been treated with antidepressants and even fewer had been in a substance abuse program. These findings are, in some respects, encouraging. Along with observations in other studies of youth suicide,[9,11-14,16] these findings confirm that the potential for suicide is not present in all individuals and that young suicide victims are, in many respects, both remarkably similar to one another and very different to the general population. It should therefore be possible to fashion systematic screening surveys to identify adolescents at risk and, just as importantly, to devise professional education programs to improve the quality of treatment that they receive. Effective suicide prevention efforts that include both screening and professional education can be expected to reduce this lethal complication of two common conditions: mood disorder and SAA.

Accepted for publication July 27, 1995.

This work was supported by the Faculty Scholars Award 84-0954-84 from the William T. Grant Foundation, New York City, and by Research Training Grant T32 MH16434, Research Grants MH 38198-05A2, and Cen-

ter Grant MH 43878-A1 for The Center to Study Youth Depression, Anxiety, and Suicide from the National Institute of Mental Health, Washington, DC.

We acknowledge the assistance of the following medical examiners: Millard J. Hyland, MD, Leslie Lukash, MD, Sigmund M. Menchel, MD, Charles S. Hirsh, MD, Catherine Galvin, MD, Elliot Gross, MD, Robert Goode, MD, John M. Zarcone, DO, and Frederick Zugibe, MD.

Reprint requests to 722 W 168th St, New York, NY 10032 (Dr Shaffer).

REFERENCES

1. Rosenberg ML, Smith JC, Davidson LE, Conn JM. The emergence of youth suicide: an epidemiologic analysis and public health perspective. *Annu Rev Public Health.* 1987;8:417-440.
2. National Center for Health Statistics. *Vital Statistics of the United States.* Hyattsville, Md: Mortality Statistics Branch, US Dept of Health and Human Services; 1992:2(pts A & B).
3. Velez CN, Cohen P. Suicidal behavior and ideation in a community sample of children: maternal and youth reports. *J Am Acad Child Adolesc Psychiatry.* 1988;27:349-356.
4. Centers for Disease Control and Prevention. Behaviors related to unintentional and intentional injuries among high school students—United States, 1991. *MMWR Morb Mortal Wkly Rep.* 1992;41:760-772.
5. Shaffer D, Hicks R. The epidemiology of child and adolescent suicide. In: Pless B, ed. *The Epidemiology of Childhood Disorders.* New York, NY: Oxford University Press Inc; 1993:339-368.
6. Shaffer D, Gould M, Hicks R. Increasing rate of black suicide in the United States. *Am J Psychiatry.* 1994;151:1810-1812.
7. Brent DA, Perper JA, Kolko DJ, Zelenak JP. The psychological autopsy: methodological considerations for the study of adolescent suicide. *J Am Acad Child Adolesc Psychiatry.* 1988;27:362-366.
8. Sanborn DE, Sanborn CJ, Cimbolic P. Two years of suicide: a study of adolescent suicide in New Hampshire. *Child Psychiatry Hum Dev.* 1973;3:234-242.
9. Shaffer D. Suicide in childhood and early adolescence. *J Child Psychol Psychiatry.* 1974;15:275-291.
10. Dizmang M, Watson J, May P, Bopp J. Adolescent suicide at an Indian reserve. *Am J Orthopsychiatry.* 1974;44:43-49.
11. Shaffi M, Carrigan S, Whittinghill JR, Derrick A. Psychological autopsy of completed suicide in children and adolescents. *Am J Psychiatry.* 1985;142:1061-1064.
12. Runeson B. Mental disorder in youth suicide: *DSM-III-R* Axes I and II. *Acta Psychiatr Scand.* 1989;79:490-497.
13. Rich CL, Sherman M, Fowler RC. San Diego Suicide Study: the adolescents. *Adolescence.* 1990;25:855-865.
14. Marttunen MJ, Hillevi MA, Henriksson MM, Lonnqvist JK. Mental disorders in adolescent suicide: *DSM-III-R* Axes I and II diagnoses in suicides among 13- to 19-year-olds in Finland. *Arch Gen Psychiatry.* 1991;48:834-839.
15. Marttunen MJ, Hillevi MA, Lonnqvist JK. Adolescent suicide: endpoint of long-term difficulties. *J Am Acad Child Adolesc Psychiatry.* 1992;31:649-654.
16. Brent DA, Perper JA, Moritz G, Allman C, Friend A, Roth C, Schweers J, Balach L, Baugher M. Psychiatric risk factors for adolescent suicide: a case-control study. *J Am Acad Child Adolesc Psychiatry.* 1993;32:521-529.
17. National Center For Health Statistics. *Vital Statistics of the United States.* Hyattesville, Md: Mortality Statistics Branch, US Dept of Health and Human Services; 1966-1990:2(pts A & B).
18. American Psychiatric Association. *Diagnostic and Statistical Manual of Mental Disorders, Revised Third Edition.* Washington, DC: American Psychiatric Association; 1987.
19. Endicott J, Spitzer RL. A diagnostic interview: the Schedule for Affective Disorders and Schizophrenia. *Arch Gen Psychiatry.* 1978;35:837-844.
20. Chambers WJ, Puig-Antich J, Hirsch M, Paez P, Ambrosini PJ, Tabrizi MA, Davies M. The assessment of affective disorders in children and adolescents by semistructured interview: test-retest reliability of the Schedule for Affective Disorders and Schizophrenia for School-age Children–present episode version. *Arch Gen Psychiatry.* 1985;42:696-702.
21. Wing JK, Cooper JE, Sartorius M. *The Measurement and Classification of Psychiatric Symptoms: An Instruction Manual for the Present State Examination and CATEGO Programme.* New York, NY: Cambridge University Press; 1974.
22. Allebeck P, Allgulander C, Fisher LD. Predictors of completed suicide in a cohort of 50,465 young men: role of personality and deviant behavior. *BMJ.* 1988; 297:176-178.
23. Beck AT, Brown G, Berchick RJ, Stewart BL, Steer RA. Relationship between hopelessness and ultimate suicide: a replication with psychiatric outpatients. *Am J Psychiatry.* 1990;147:1577-1578.
24. Achenbach TM, Edelbrock CS. *Manual for the Child Behavior Checklist and Revised Profile.* Burlington, Vt: Dept of Psychiatry, University of Vermont; 1983.
25. Achenbach TM, Edelbrock CS. *Manual for the Teacher's Report Form and Teacher Version of the Child Behavior Profile.* Burlington, Vt: University of Vermont, Department of Psychiatry; 1986.
26. Shaffer D, Gould MS, Brasic J, Ambrosini P, Fisher P, Bird H, Alvwahlia S. A children's global assessment scale (CGAS). *Arch Gen Psychiatry.* 1983;40: 1228-1231.
27. Leckman JF, Sholomskas D, Thompson WD, Belanger A. Best estimate of lifetime diagnosis: a methodological study. *Arch Gen Psychiatry.* 1982;39:879-883.
28. Hollingshead AB. *Four-Factor Index of Social Status.* New Haven, Conn: Yale University; 1975.
29. Shaffer D. The epidemiology of teen suicide: an examination of risk factors. *J Clin Psychiatry.* 1988;49:36-41.
30. Gould MS, Shaffer D, Davies M. Truncated pathways from childhood: attrition in follow-up studies due to death. In: Robins L, Rutter M, eds. *Straight and Devious Pathways From Childhood to Adulthood.* New York, NY: Cambridge University Press; 1990:3-10.
31. Gould MS, Shaffer D, Fisher P, Kleinman M, Morishima A. The clinical prediction of suicide. In: Maris R, Berman L, eds. *Assessment and Prediction of Suicide.* New York, NY: Guilford Press; 1992:130-143.
32. Shaffer D, Fisher P. The epidemiology of suicide in children and young adolescents. *J Am Acad Child Adolesc Psychiatry.* 1981;20:545-565.
33. National Institute on Drug Abuse. *1985 National Household Survey on Drug Abuse: Main Findings.* Washington, DC: US Government Printing Office; 1988.
34. Kandel D. The social demographics of drug use. In: Bayer R, Oppenheimer GM, eds. *Confronting Drug Policy.* New York, NY: Cambridge University Press; 1993.

Personality Disorders Predict Onset of Axis I Disorders and Impaired Functioning Among Homosexual Men With and at Risk of HIV Infection

Jeffrey G. Johnson, PhD; Janet B. W. Williams, DSW; Raymond R. Goetz, PhD; Judith G. Rabkin, PhD; Robert H. Remien, PhD; Joshua D. Lipsitz, PhD; Jack M. Gorman, MD

Background: A longitudinal study was conducted to investigate whether personality disorders (PDs) increase risk for the development of future Axis I disorders and serious functional impairment among human immunodeficiency virus (HIV)–seropositive and HIV-seronegative homosexual men.

Method: Baseline assessments of PDs, Axis I disorders and symptoms, and Global Assessments of Functioning were conducted with a community sample of 107 (66 HIV-positive and 41 HIV-negative) homosexual men participating in a longitudinal study with semiannual interviews over 3 years.

Results: Logistic regression analysis indicated that PDs predicted onset of subsequent Axis I disorders after controlling for both HIV status and lifetime Axis I history (adjusted odds ratio, 4.31; *P*=.01; 95% confidence interval, 1.39 to 13.32). Of the 21 participants with PDs, 16 (76%) were subsequently diagnosed with Axis I disorders on at least one occasion. By contrast, only 36 (42%) of the 86 participants without PDs were subsequently diagnosed with Axis I disorders. Further, 33% of the participants with PDs, in comparison with only 8% of those without PDs, were assigned Global Assessments of Functioning scores of 50 or lower, indicating serious impairment during the postbaseline study period (adjusted odds ratio, 5.70; *P*<.005; 95% confidence interval, 1.66 to 19.53).

Conclusion: Personality disorders may contribute to increased risk for onset of Axis I disorders and serious impairment among homosexual men regardless of HIV serologic status.

(Arch Gen Psychiatry. 1996;53:350-357)

SINCE THE introduction of *DSM-III*,[1] a number of longitudinal studies have investigated the hypothesis that psychiatric patients with personality disorders (PDs) tend to have poorer outcomes than patients without PDs.[2,3] Research findings have confirmed that patients with PDs tend to have poorer treatment outcomes,[4-14] greater recurrence of Axis I disorders,[6,15] and higher risk for suicidal behavior[3,16,17] than patients without PDs. However, little research has examined the association between PDs and Axis I disorders among nonpatients,[18] in part because major epidemiological studies have assessed only one of the 10 *DSM-IV* PDs.[19,20] The findings that do exist indicate that nonpatients with PDs are more likely than nonpatients without PDs to have co-occurring Axis I disorders.[21,22] Results of the only prospective study to investigate the association between PD and change in Axis I symptoms among nonpatients indicated that PD symptoms predicted increases in Axis I symptoms.[23] As yet, no published studies have reported whether nonpatients with PDs are at risk of onset of either Axis I disorders or serious impairment. Insofar as PDs have been postulated, among both patients and nonpatients, to be stable and of long duration, to be inflexible and maladaptive, and to cause significant impairment or distress,[24] the extent to which PDs predict future Axis I symptoms among nonpatients is an issue that warrants investigation.

Within the nonpatient population, it is particularly important for research to determine whether PDs predict risk for onset of Axis I disorders and serious impairment among patients infected with human immunodeficiency virus (HIV) and persons at risk of HIV infection. Previous research has indicated that certain psychiatric disorders may be associated with both

From the Department of Psychiatry, Columbia University, and the New York State Psychiatric Institute (Drs Johnson, Williams, Goetz, Rabkin, Lipsitz, and Gorman) and the HIV Center for Clinical and Behavioral Studies, New York State Psychiatric Institute, New York City (Dr Remien).

See Subjects and Methods on next page

SUBJECTS AND METHODS

SUBJECTS

One hundred seven homosexual male subjects who volunteered to participate in a prospective study of factors associated with progression of HIV infection completed the measures described below during baseline assessment and follow-up assessments conducted every 6 months during the study period. This sample was a subset of a larger initial sample of 208 homosexual men who had participated in an assessment session 6 months earlier. Thirty-two HIV-negative subjects were recruited solely for participation in the earlier assessment session, while 69 subjects could not be followed up because of attrition or missed visits. All subjects had undergone HIV testing before study entry and knew their serologic status. Individuals with acquired immunodeficiency syndrome were excluded; thus, at baseline, all participants were either HIV-negative (n=41) or HIV-positive with absent to moderate physical symptoms (n=66). The mean (SD) age of the sample was 38 (8.02) years (range, 22 to 59 years); 87% were white; and 90% had 1 year or more of college education. Participants volunteered in response to announcements in newsletters and a newspaper with predominantly homosexual readership and by word of mouth.

MEASURES

The Brief Symptom Inventory (BSI)[32] is a 53-item self-report inventory of psychiatric symptoms that are each rated as follows: 0, not at all; 1, a little bit; 2, moderately; 3, quite a bit; or 4, extremely, to indicate how much that problem has bothered or distressed the subject during the past week. The inventory assesses generalized anxiety, phobic anxiety, depression, somatization, interpersonal sensitivity, obsessive-compulsive symptoms, hostility, paranoia, and psychoticism. The BSI also includes a composite measure, the Global Severity Index, which is the mean of the 53-item severity ratings. Research has indicated that the BSI has acceptable levels of reliability and validity.[32]

The GAF scale is a revision of the Global Assessment Scale[33,34] and comprises Axis V of *DSM-III-R*.[35] The GAF scale enables a clinician to evaluate a person's functioning during the past year on a scale from 1 to 100. While GAF scores of 70 and above signify positive mental health, GAF scores of 50 and below signify serious symptoms or impairment in social, occupational, or school functioning, and GAF scores below 40 are typically found among hospitalized psychiatric patients. Acceptable test-retest reliability has been reported for the GAF.[36]

The Beck Hopelessness Scale (BHS)[37] is a 20-item questionnaire that assesses negative expectations about the future and pessimism. The format is true/false, and half of the items are reverse scored. The range of possible scores is 0 to 20, with higher scores indicating greater hopelessness. The BHS has acceptable reliability, concurrent validity, and predictive validity.[37,38]

The Structured Interview Guide for the Hamilton Anxiety and Depression Rating Scales (SIGH-AD) was used because it has been demonstrated to increase the reliability of scale items.[39] A number of studies have demonstrated that the Hamilton Depression Scale (HAM-D)[40] has a high degree of reliability and validity.[41-43] The Hamilton Anxiety Scale (HAM-A)[44] was selected for this study because it assesses several types of anxiety and because it is widely used, enabling us to compare our findings with those of other studies.

The Structured Clinical Interview for *DSM-III-R* (SCID)[34,45] is a semistructured clinical interview that begins with an overview of the present illness and past episodes of psychopathology; it then inquires systematically about specific syndromes. One of the following ratings is assigned for each symptom assessed by the SCID, based on the subject's response: "inadequate information," "absent or false," "subthreshold," or "threshold." A subthreshold rating is assigned if the threshold for the criterion is almost, but not quite, met. The SCID was modified for this study to assess only mood, substance use, panic, generalized anxiety, and adjustment disorders. Adjustment disorder criteria were modified, so as to require both "impairment in occupational functioning or in usual social activities or relationships" and "significant mood disturbance and at least two symptoms associated with that mood disturbance." Acceptable levels of test-retest diagnostic reliability have been reported for the SCID.[36]

The SCID Personality Disorders (SCID-II)[46,47] is a 120-item, semistructured clinical interview that yields both PD diagnoses and the number of diagnostic criteria met for each of the *DSM-III-R* PDs. As with the SCID, one of the following ratings is assigned for each symptom assessed by the SCID-II, based on the subject's response: "inadequate information," "absent or false," "subthreshold," or "threshold." Acceptable levels of interrater diagnostic reliability, comparable with those obtained using other widely used structured clinical interviews, have been reported for the SCID-II.[48] When SCID-II diagnoses were compared with diagnoses obtained using other structured clinical interviews or the LEAD procedure, findings reported for the SCID-II were comparable with those obtained for other widely used structured clinical interviews.[49-51]

Continued on next page

HIV infection[25] and behavior facilitating HIV transmission.[26,27] It is of further significance that, while approximately 10% of adults in the community have PDs,[28] research indicates that the comparable prevalence rates for PDs are 19% to 36% among HIV-infected persons and 15% to 20% among persons at risk of HIV infection.[29-31] While it has been reported that HIV-infected persons with PDs are likely to have co-occurring Axis I disorders,[29-31] research has not yet examined whether PDs predict onset of future Axis I symptoms and serious impairment among persons with or at risk of HIV infection.

Therefore, as part of a prospective longitudinal study of the physical and psychological functioning of a sample of HIV-seropositive and HIV-seronegative homosexual men, we examined whether PDs increased risk for onset of Axis I disorders and/or serious impairment during a 3-year period, after HIV status and lifetime Axis I history were controlled statistically. Baseline assessments of PDs, Axis I symptoms, and Global Assessments of Functioning (GAF) were conducted, with follow-up assessments of Axis I symptoms and GAF every 6 months. Because overall PD symptom levels are thought by some researchers to be of greater

PROCEDURE

At baseline assessment, 6 months after subjects were recruited, informed consent obtained, and data collection initiated, participants were administered the above instruments. The SCID, SCID-II, and SIGH-AD were administered by master's level clinicians with extensive clinical experience. Training consisted of lectures, practice with videotapes, and supervised interviews monitored by an expert in diagnosis and structured interviewing. After every baseline interview was monitored, it was discussed with the interviewer so that final diagnostic decisions and severity ratings reflected consensus judgments between two clinicians. Each interviewer participated in 20 or more supervised interviews. Participants were readministered the BSI, GAF, BHS, SCID, and SIGH-AD every 6 months during the next 3.5 years. The BSI and BHS were mailed to participants 2 weeks before each appointment and were completed prior to each appointment. The GAF, SCID, SCID-II, and SIGH-AD were administered by trained clinicians who had access to each participant's previous diagnostic findings. The reader is referred to previous reports for a more detailed presentation of the study methodology.[52,53]

DATA ANALYTIC PROCEDURE

We began by conducting analyses of contingency tables to determine whether baseline PDs were associated with future Axis I disorders among (1) the total sample regardless of lifetime Axis I history, (2) participants with a lifetime history of corresponding Axis I disorders, and/or (3) participants without a lifetime history of corresponding Axis I disorders (**Table 1**). Odds ratios (ORs), ie, the frequency with which both disorders are present or absent, divided by the frequency with which either disorder appears alone, were computed for each contingency table. We then conducted an identical series of analyses to determine whether the presence of high PD symptom levels, regardless of diagnostic status, predicted onset of Axis I disorders (**Table 2**). Twenty-eight subjects with 11 or more threshold PD symptoms were identified as having high PD symptom levels; 18 (64%) of these subjects were diagnosed as having PD. This decision was taken because subjects with 11 or more threshold PD symptoms were in the top quartile. The median number of threshold symptoms was 5.0. In this and all subsequent analyses, lifetime Axis I history was defined as diagnosis, at baseline, with either a current or lifetime disorder. Similar analyses were conducted to determine whether cluster A (paranoid, schizoid, and schizotypal), cluster B (antisocial, borderline, histrionic, and narcissistic), and cluster C (avoidant, dependent, obsessive-compulsive, and passive-aggressive) PDs predicted onset of Axis I disorders.

Because so few individuals were diagnosed with a specific PD, subjects meeting subthreshold criteria were included, thus permitting these analyses to be conducted. Five, 18, and 14 participants were thus assigned threshold, or subthreshold, cluster A, B, and C diagnoses.

Similar analyses were conducted to determine whether the 21 participants with PD, and/or the 28 participants with high PD symptom levels, were at risk of subsequent clinically significant psychiatric symptoms (defined as a BHS score of ≥12, a GSI score of ≥1.35, an HAM-A score of ≥14, and/or an HAM-D score of ≥14 at least once, following baseline assessment) or serious impairment (defined as a GAF score of ≤50 at least once, following baseline assessment). To determine whether specific types of PD were associated with subsequent psychiatric symptoms and serious impairment, analyses were conducted to determine whether cluster A, B, and C PDs predicted onset of clinically significant psychiatric symptoms and serious impairment.

Logistic regression analyses were conducted to determine whether PD, and/or high PD symptom levels, predicted onset of Axis I disorders, clinically significant psychiatric symptoms, and/or serious impairment, after controlling for HIV status and lifetime Axis I history. In the first logistic regression analysis, baseline PD diagnostic status, HIV status, and lifetime Axis I history were the independent variables, and postbaseline diagnosis with Axis I disorders was the dependent variable. In the second logistic regression analysis, baseline PD symptom level, HIV status, and lifetime Axis I history were the independent variables, and postbaseline diagnosis with Axis I disorders was the dependent variable. In the third logistic regression analysis, PD diagnostic status, HIV status, and lifetime Axis I history were the independent variables, and significant postbaseline psychiatric symptoms were the dependent variable. In the fourth logistic regression analysis, baseline PD symptom level, HIV status, and lifetime Axis I history were the independent variables, and significant postbaseline psychiatric symptoms were the dependent variable. Because no subjects without prior Axis I disorders were assigned a postbaseline GAF score of 50 or less, logistic regression analyses controlling for lifetime Axis I history and involving GAF scores of 50 or less as the dependent variable could not be conducted. Therefore, logistic regression analyses were instead conducted with baseline PD symptoms and HIV status as the independent variables, and postbaseline GAF scores (≤50 vs >50) as the dependent variable.

prognostic value than categorical diagnoses, we also investigated whether the presence of substantial PD symptom levels, regardless of diagnostic status, predicted onset of Axis I disorders and serious impairment.

RESULTS

PREVALENCE OF PDs AND AXIS I DISORDERS

At baseline, 21 (20%) of the 107 participants were diagnosed as having PD, while 10 (9%) were diagnosed with current Axis I disorders. The numbers of subjects diagnosed as having a specific PD were, by category: avoidant (n=5), dependent (n=0), obsessive-compulsive (n=3), passive-aggressive (n=2), self-defeating (n=3), paranoid (n=2), schizotypal (n=2), schizoid (n=0), histrionic (n=2), narcissistic (n=2), borderline (n=0), antisocial (n=2), and not otherwise specified (n=4). During the study period, 55 participants (49%) were diagnosed as having current Axis I disorders on at least one occasion. The percentages of subjects diagnosed at least once with particular Axis I disorders were, by category, as follows: mood dis-

Table 1. Incidence of Axis I Disorders Subsequent to Baseline Assessment by Baseline Personality Disorder Status and Lifetime Axis I History*

Subjects	n	No Personality Disorders, No. (%) Total	No Personality Disorders, No. (%) With Subsequent Axis I Disorder	At Least One Personality Disorder, No. (%) Total	At Least One Personality Disorder, No. (%) With Subsequent Axis I Disorder	OR	95% CI
Any Subsequent Axis I Disorder							
All	**107**	**86**	36 (42)	**21**	16 (76)	4.44‡	1.49-13.24
With previous Axis I disorders	73	**57**	29 (51)	**16**	13 (81)	4.18§	1.08-16.28
With no previous Axis I disorders	34	**29**	7 (24)	**5**	3 (60)	4.71	0.65-34.20
Any Subsequent Anxiety Disorder							
All†	**107**	**86**	0 (0)	**21**	2 (10)	13.05‖	1.29-132.17
With previous anxiety disorders†	3	**1**	0 (0)	**2**	1 (50)	2.00	0.09-44.38
With no previous anxiety disorders†	104	**85**	0 (0)	**19**	1 (5)	9.05	0.78-105.10
Any Subsequent Mood Disorder							
All	**107**	**86**	11 (13)	**21**	7 (33)	3.41§	1.13-10.31
With previous mood disorders	39	**28**	8 (29)	**11**	5 (45)	2.08	0.49-8.82
With no previous mood disorders	68	**58**	3 (5)	**10**	1 (10)	2.04	0.19-21.81
Any Subsequent Substance Use Disorder							
All	**107**	**86**	16 (19)	**21**	8 (38)	2.69	0.96-7.58
With previous substance use disorders	59	**45**	14 (31)	**14**	7 (50)	2.21	0.65-7.53
With no previous substance use disorders	48	**41**	2 (5)	**7**	1 (14)	3.25	0.25-41.63

*OR indicates odds ratio; CI, confidence interval.
†To permit calculation of OR, one subject was added to each cell when cells included no cases; table prevalences do not reflect this adjustment.
‡$P<.005$ by χ^2 test.
§$P<.05$ χ^2 test.
‖$P\leq.01$ by χ^2 test.

orders (17%), anxiety disorders (2%), substance use disorders (22%), and adjustment disorders (19%). The percentages of subjects diagnosed with any Axis I disorder at follow-up assessments 1 through 7 were 20%, 18%, 14%, 13%, 17%, 10%, and 9%, respectively.

PDs AS PREDICTORS OF ONSET OF AXIS I DISORDERS

As Table 1 indicates, in the total sample, participants with PD were more likely than those without PDs to be diagnosed with subsequent anxiety, mood, and any Axis I disorders during the 3 years following baseline assessment. However, when subjects with and without previous Axis I disorders were considered separately, ORs did not reach statistical significance, perhaps owing to decreased statistical power that resulted from diminished sample size. Separate analyses revealed that cluster A PD did not predict onset of subsequent Axis I disorders. However, cluster B PD predicted onset of any Axis I disorder (OR=3.33; $P<.05$; 95% confidence interval [CI], 1.09 to 10.15), anxiety (OR=15.88; $P<005$; 95% CI, 1.54 to 42.18), and substance use disorders (OR=6.70; $P<.001$; 95% CI, 2.17 to 20.32). Additionally, cluster C PD predicted onset of any Axis I (OR=4.65; $P<.05$; 95% CI, 1.22 to 17.78) and mood disorders (OR=5.06; $P=.005$; 95% CI, 1.39 to 17.31).

As Table 2 indicates, in the total sample, subjects with 11 or more PD symptoms were more likely than those with 10 or less symptoms to be diagnosed with subsequent mood, substance use, and any Axis I disorders. Among participants with previous substance use disorders, those with 11 or more PD symptoms were more likely than those with 10 or less PD symptoms to be diagnosed with subsequent substance use disorders. However, in the remaining comparisons, when subjects with and without previous Axis I disorders were considered separately, ORs did not reach statistical significance.

Logistic regression analyses indicated that PD predicted onset of Axis I disorders, after controlling for HIV status and lifetime Axis I history (adjusted OR [aOR]=4.31; $P=.01$; 95% CI, 1.39 to 13.32). Lifetime Axis I history also predicted subsequent Axis I diagnoses (aOR=3.12; $P=.01$; 95% CI, 1.26 to 7.72), but HIV status and all interactions between the independent variables did not. The final logistic regression model was significant ($\chi^2=15.81$; $df=3$; $P=.001$). Baseline PD symptom level also predicted onset of Axis I disorders after controlling for HIV status and lifetime Axis I history (aOR=5.57; $P=.001$; 95% CI, 2.25 to 13.80). Human immunodeficiency virus status, lifetime Axis I history, and all interactions between the independent variables failed to predict subsequent Axis I diagnoses. The final logistic regression model was significant ($\chi^2=20.15$; $df=3$; $P<.001$).

PDs AS PREDICTORS OF FUTURE PSYCHIATRIC SYMPTOMS AND IMPAIRMENT

As **Table 3** indicates, PDs predicted onset of serious impairment (ie, postbaseline GAF scores of ≤50) but did not predict onset of significant psychiatric symptoms. Separate analyses indicated that cluster A and cluster C PDs did not predict onset of significant psychiatric symptoms or serious impairment. However, cluster B PD pre-

Table 2. Incidence of Axis I Disorders Subsequent to Baseline Personality Disorder Level and Lifetime Axis I History*

Subjects	n	≤10 Personality Disorder Symptoms, No. (%) Total	≤10 Personality Disorder Symptoms, No. (%) With Subsequent Axis I Disorder	≥11 Personality Disorder Symptoms, No. (%) Total	≥11 Personality Disorder Symptoms, No. (%) With Subsequent Axis I Disorder	OR	95% CI
Any Subsequent Axis I Disorder							
All	**107**	**79**	30 (38)	**28**	22 (79)	5.99‡	2.18-16.46
With previous Axis I disorders	73	**50**	23 (46)	**23**	19 (83)	5.58§	1.66-18.76
With no previous Axis I disorders	34	**29**	7 (24)	**5**	3 (60)	4.71	0.65-34.20
Any Subsequent Anxiety Disorder							
All†	**107**	**79**	0 (0)	**28**	2 (7)	8.89	0.87-89.13
With previous anxiety disorders†	3	**1**	0 (0)	**2**	1 (50)	2.00	0.09-44.38
With no previous anxiety disorders†	104	**78**	0 (0)	**26**	1 (4)	6.08	0.53-69.83
Any Subsequent Mood Disorder							
All	**107**	**79**	9 (11)	**28**	9 (32)	3.68‖	1.28-10.57
With previous mood disorders	39	**24**	6 (25)	**15**	8 (53)	3.43	0.87-13.52
With no previous mood disorders	68	**55**	3 (5)	**13**	1 (8)	1.44	0.14-15.13
Any Subsequent Substance Use Disorder							
All	**107**	**79**	11 (14)	**28**	13 (46)	5.36‡	2.01-14.26
With previous substance use disorders	59	**40**	9 (23)	**19**	12 (63)	5.90§	1.79-19.44
With no previous substance use disorders	48	**39**	2 (5)	**9**	1 (11)	2.31	0.19-28.73

*OR indicates odds ratio; CI, confidence interval.
†To permit calculation of OR, one subject was added to each cell when cells included no cases; table prevalences do not reflect this adjustment.
‡$P<.001$ by χ^2 test.
§$P<.005$ by χ^2 test.
‖$P\leq.01$ by χ^2 test.

Table 3. Clinically Significant Psychiatric Distress* and Global Assessments of Functioning Scores of ≤50† Subsequent to Baseline Assessment by Baseline Personality Disorder Status and Lifetime Axis I History‡

Subjects	n	No Personality Disorders, No. (%) Total	No Personality Disorders, No. (%) With Subsequent Distress/Impairment	At Least One Personality Disorder, No. (%) Total	At Least One Personality Disorder, No. (%) With Subsequent Distress/Impairment	OR	95% CI
Clinically Significant Postbaseline Psychiatric Symptoms*							
All	**107**	**86**	26 (33)	**21**	11 (52)	2.54	0.96-6.71
With previous Axis I disorders	73	**57**	22 (39)	**16**	10 (63)	2.65	0.84-8.33
With no previous Axis I disorders	34	**29**	4 (14)	**5**	1 (20)	1.56	0.14-17.80
Postbaseline Global Assessments of Functioning Score ≤50†							
All	**107**	**86**	7 (8)	**21**	7 (33)	5.64§	1.71-18.59
With previous Axis I disorders	73	**57**	7 (12)	**16**	7 (44)	5.56§	1.57-19.70
With no previous Axis I disorders	34	**29**	0 (0)	**5**	0 (0)	...	...

*Defined as any of the following: a Beck Hopelessness Scale score of ≥12, a Global Severity Index score of ≥1.35, a Hamilton Anxiety Scale score of ≥14, and/or a Hamilton Depression Scale score of ≥14 at least once, following baseline assessment.
†Indicates serious symptoms or seriously impaired functioning during the past year at least once, following baseline assessment.
‡OR indicates odds ratio; CI, confidence interval.
§$P<.005$ by χ^2 test.

dicted onset of significant psychiatric symptoms (OR=3.81; $P<.01$; 95% CI, 1.31 to 11.35). As **Table 4** indicates, the presence of 11 or more PD symptoms predicted onset of significant psychiatric symptoms but did not predict onset of serious impairment. Additional analyses revealed that (1) of the 14 individuals assigned GAF scores of 50 or less after baseline assessment, two (14%) had been assigned GAF scores of 50 or less at baseline and (2) of the 37 individuals with clinically significant psychiatric symptoms after baseline assessment, nine (24%) were so assessed at baseline.

Logistic regression analyses indicated that, while both HIV status (aOR=5.96; $P<.01$; 95% CI, 1.55 to 22.86) and lifetime Axis I history (aOR=4.53; $P<.01$; 95% CI, 1.49 to 13.75) predicted onset of significant psychiatric symptoms, PD did not do so after controlling for HIV status and lifetime Axis I history. The interactions between these variables did not predict subsequent Axis I symptoms. By contrast, PD symptom level predicted postbaseline psychiatric symptoms after controlling for HIV status and lifetime Axis I history (aOR=4.33; $P<.005$; 95% CI, 1.61 to 11.69). Human immunodeficiency virus status (aOR=3.52; $P=.01$;

Table 4. Clinically Significant Psychiatric Distress* and Global Assessments of Functioning Scores of ≤50† Subsequent to Baseline Assessment by Baseline Personality Disorder Symptom Level and Lifetime Axis I History‡

Subjects	n	≤10 Personality Disorder Symptoms, No. (%) Total	≤10 Personality Disorder Symptoms, No. (%) With Subsequent Distress/Impairment	≥11 Personality Disorder Symptoms, No. (%) Total	≥11 Personality Disorder Symptoms, No. (%) With Subsequent Distress/Impairment	OR	95% CI
Clinically Significant Postbaseline Psychiatric Symptoms*							
All	**107**	**79**	20 (25)	**28**	17 (61)	4.56§	1.83-11.36
With previous Axis I disorders	73	**50**	16 (32)	**23**	16 (70)	4.86‖	1.67-14.14
With no previous Axis I disorders	34	**29**	4 (14)	**5**	1 (20)	1.56	0.14-17.80
Postbaseline Global Assessments of Functioning Score of ≤50†							
All	**107**	**79**	8 (10)	**28**	6 (21)	2.42	0.76-7.74
With previous Axis I disorders	73	**50**	8 (16)	**23**	6 (26)	1.85	0.56-6.15
With no previous Axis I disorders	34	**29**	0 (0)	**5**	0 (0)	...	...

*Defined as any of the following: a Beck Hopelessness Scale score of ≥12, a Global Severity Index score of ≥1.35, a Hamilton Anxiety Scale score of ≥14, and/or a Hamilton Depression Scale score of ≥14 at least once, following baseline assessment.

†Indicates serious symptoms or seriously impaired functioning during the past year at least once, following baseline assessment.

‡OR indicates odds ratio; CI, confidence interval.

§$P<.005$ by χ^2 test.

‖$P<.005$ by χ^2 test.

95% CI, 1.29 to 9.61) and lifetime Axis I history (aOR=3.85; *P*<.05; 95% CI, 1.26 to 11.80) also predicted postbaseline psychiatric symptoms. Again, the interactions between these variables did not predict subsequent Axis I symptoms. Personality disorders predicted serious impairment during the postbaseline period after controlling for HIV status (aOR=5.70; *P*<.0025; 95% CI, 1.66 to 19.53). However, HIV status did not predict subsequent impairment. Neither PD symptom level, HIV status, nor their interaction predicted subsequent impairment.

COMMENT

The present findings that PDs predicted onset of future Axis I disorders and serious impairment are particularly striking because these findings were obtained after controlling for HIV status and lifetime history of Axis I disorders, as well as independent of the interaction of PDs with HIV status and Axis I history. These are the first published findings to demonstrate that persons in the community with PDs are at risk of onset of future Axis I disorders and serious impairment, whether or not they have had prior Axis I disorders. Insofar as approximately one in 10 adults suffers from PD,[28] our findings suggest that efforts directed toward increased recognition of PDs might have considerable benefit.

Also of substantial interest are our findings that the presence of high PD symptom levels was as effective as categorical PD diagnosis in predicting onset of Axis I disorders. Recently, there has been substantial debate regarding the validity of categorical PD, in comparison with dimensional assessments of the extent of PD symptoms.[54] Significantly, research has indicated that PD symptoms are associated with Axis I symptoms, regardless of whether PD diagnoses are assigned.[22,55] Nonetheless, because PD, but not elevated PD symptoms, predicted onset of serious impairment, our findings suggest that categorical and dimensional measures of PD symptoms may provide complementary sources of information.[54]

As in previous reports concerning the association between HIV status and Axis I symptoms,[30,50,56,57] HIV status failed to predict onset of Axis I disorders and serious impairment following baseline assessment. Interestingly, other researchers have reported that, among medical patients, impairment associated with mental disorders was comparable with or greater than that associated with chronic physical ailments.[58] Our findings suggest that PD and lifetime Axis I history may be more strongly associated with subsequent well-being than is HIV status and that improved recognition of PDs may assist in the prevention of future psychiatric disorders and serious impairment among HIV-infected persons.

Several issues that may affect the interpretation of the present findings merit consideration. First, our findings may not be generalizable to populations other than those investigated in this study, ie, HIV-seropositive or HIV-seronegative homosexual men. Second, the sample size did not permit us to examine relationships between specific PDs and specific Axis I disorders. A number of studies[59-61] have indicated that particular PDs may play a role in the course, origin, and/or treatment outcome of particular Axis I disorders. Third, few of the Axis I disorders diagnosed were severe, and many participants met diagnostic criteria on only one or two occasions. The unavailability of comparative data regarding the prevalence of Axis I disorders during a 3-year period in the nonpatient population limits somewhat the interpretation of our findings regarding rates of Axis I disorders in our sample. Fourth, because the interviewers had access to each subject's previous diagnostic evaluations, it is possible that their subsequent assessments were influenced by this access.

Finally, while our logistic regression findings indicated that PDs predicted onset of Axis I disorders after controlling for HIV status and lifetime Axis I history, it is of interest that our analyses of contingency tables indicated that participants with PDs were more likely to be diagnosed with specific Axis I disorders if they had previously suffered from a related Axis I disorder than if they had not. These findings suggest that the prediction of future Axis I disorders may be optimized by assessing both PD and lifetime Axis I history. However, even among participants without previous Axis I disorders, those with PDs tended to be more likely than those without PDs to develop subsequent Axis I disorders. Although the ORs, ranging from 2.0 to 11.86, were generally not statistically significant, this is likely due to the small sample size. Because the interaction between PD and lifetime Axis I history never predicted future psychiatric status in our logistic regression analyses, it appears most prudent to accept the logistic regression findings indicating that participants with PDs were more likely than those without PDs to develop psychiatric disorders, regardless of their lifetime Axis I history.

Accepted for publication September 29, 1995.

This study was supported in part by grant 1P50 MH 43520 from the National Institute of Mental Health/National Institute on Drug Abuse, Bethesda, Md (Principal Investigator: Anke A. Ehrhardt, PhD) and by Mental Hygiene Research Center grant MH30906-14 (Principal Investigator: Donald F. Klein, MD). Dr Johnson is an Aaron Diamond Foundation Fellow, and this study was supported by a grant from the Aaron Diamond Foundation, New York, NY.

The authors gratefully acknowledge the assistance of Jacob Cohen, PhD, in the data analysis reported in this article, as well as comments and suggestions provided by Anke Erhardt, PhD, and Robert Spitzer, MD, regarding the preparation of the manuscript.

Reprint requests to Biometrics Research Department, Unit 74, New York State Psychiatric Institute, 722 W 168th Street, New York, NY 10032 (Dr Johnson).

REFERENCES

1. American Psychiatric Association. *Diagnostic and Statistical Manual of Mental Disorders, Third Edition.* Washington, DC: American Psychiatric Association; 1980.
2. Drake RE, Vaillant GE. Introduction: longitudinal views of personality disorder. *J Pers Disord.* 1988;2:44-48.
3. Perry JC. Longitudinal studies of personality disorders. *J Pers Disord.* 1993; 7(suppl):63-85.
4. Andreoli A, Gressot G, Aapro N, Tricot L, Gognalons MY. Personality disorders as a predictor of outcome. *J Pers Disord.* 1989;3:307-320.
5. Black DW, Bell S, Hulbert J, Nasrallah A. The importance of Axis II in patients with major depression: a controlled study. *J Affect Disord.* 1988; 14:115-122.
6. Frank E, Kupfer DJ, Jacob M, Jarrett D. Personality features and response to acute treatment in recurrent depression. *J Pers Disord.* 1987;1:14-26.
7. Nurnberg HG, Raskin M, Levine PE, Pollack S, Prince R, Siegel O. Borderline personality disorder as a negative prognostic factor in anxiety disorders. *J Pers Disord.* 1989;3:205-216.
8. Perry JC. A prospective study of life stress, defenses, psychotic symptoms, and depression in borderline and antisocial personality disorders and bipolar type II affective disorder. *J Pers Disord.* 1988;2:49-59.
9. Pfohl B, Coryell W, Zimmerman M, Stangl D. Prognostic validity of self-report and interview measures of personality disorder in depressed inpatients. *J Clin Psychiatry.* 1987;48:468-472.
10. Pilkonis PA, Frank E. Personality pathology in recurrent depression: nature, prevalence, and relationship to treatment response. *Am J Psychiatry.* 1988; 145:435-441.
11. Reich JH. Effect of *DSM-III* personality disorders on outcome of tricyclic antidepressant–treated nonpsychotic outpatients with major or minor depressive disorder. *Psychiatry Res.* 1990;32:175-181.
12. Reich JH, Green AI. Effect of personality disorders on outcome of treatment. *J Nerv Ment Dis.* 1991;179:74-82.
13. Shea MT, Widiger TA, Klein MH. Comorbidity of personality disorders and depression: implications for treatment. *J Consult Clin Psychol.* 1992;60:857-868.
14. Ilardi SS, Craighead WE. Personality pathology and response to somatic treatments for major depression: a critical review. *Depression.* 1995;2:200-217.
15. Perry JC, Lavori PW, Pagano CJ, Hoke L, O'Connell ME. Life events and recurrent depression in borderline and antisocial personality disorders. *J Pers Disord.* 1992;6:394-407.
16. Raczek SW, True PK, Friend RC. Suicidal behavior and personality traits. *J Pers Disord.* 1989;3:345-351.
17. Stone MH, Hurt SW, Stone DK. The PI 500: long-term follow-up of borderline patients meeting *DSM-III* criteria, I: global outcome. *J Pers Disord.* 1987;1: 291-298.
18. Overholser JC. Aggregation of personality measures: implications for personality disorder research. *J Pers Disord.* 1992;6:267-277.
19. Kessler RC, McGonagle KA, Zhao S, Nelson CB, Hughes M, Eshleman S, Wittchen H, Kendler KS. Lifetime and 12-month prevalence of *DSM-III-R* psychiatric disorders in the United States: results from the National Comorbidity Survey. *Arch Gen Psychiatry.* 1994;51:8-19.
20. Robins LN, Regier DA. *Psychiatric Disorders in America.* New York, NY: Free Press; 1991.
21. Nestadt G, Romanoski AJ, Samuels JF, Folstein MF, McHugh PR. The relationship between personality and *DSM-III* Axis I disorders in the population: results from an epidemiological survey. *Am J Psychiatry.* 1992;149:1228-1233.
22. Zimmerman M, Coryell W. *DSM-III* personality disorder diagnoses in a nonpatient sample. *Arch Gen Psychiatry.* 1989;46:682-689.
23. Johnson JG, Bornstein RF. PDQ-R personality disorder scores and negative life events independently predict changes in SCL-90 psychopathology scores. *J Psychopathol Behav Assess.* 1991;13:61-72.
24. American Psychiatric Association: *Diagnostic and Statistical Manual of Mental Disorders, Fourth Edition.* Washington, DC: American Psychiatric Association; 1994.
25. Atkinson JH, Grant I, Kennedy CJ, Richman DD, Spector SA, McCutchan A. Prevalence of psychiatric disorders among men infected with human immunodeficiency virus. *Arch Gen Psychiatry.* 1988;58:859-864.
26. Lipsitz JD, Williams JBW, Rabkin JG, Remien RH, Bradbury M, Sadr W, Goetz R, Sorrell S, Gorman JM. Psychopathology in male and female intravenous drug users with and without HIV infection. *Am J Psychiatry.* 1994;151:1662-1668.
27. Lowry R, Holtzman D, Truman BI, Kann L, Collins JL, Kolbe LJ. Substance use and HIV-related sexual behaviors among US high school students: are they related? *Am J Public Health.* 1994;84:1116-1120.
28. Weissman MM. The epidemiology of personality disorders: a 1990 update. *J Pers Disord.* 1993;7(suppl):44-62.
29. Jacobsberg L, Frances A, Perry S. Axis II diagnoses among volunteers for HIV testing and counseling. *Am J Psychiatry.* 1995;152:1222-1224.
30. Johnson JG, Williams JBW, Rabkin JG, Goetz RR, Remien RH. Axis I psychiatric symptomatology associated with HIV infection and personality disorder. *Am J Psychiatry.* 1995;152:551-554.
31. Perkins DO, Davidson EJ, Leserman J, Liao D, Evans DL. Personality disorder in patients infected with HIV: a controlled study with implications for clinical care. *Am J Psychiatry.* 1993;150:309-315.
32. Derogatis LR, Melisaratos N. The Brief Symptom Inventory: an introductory report. *Psychol Med.* 1983;13:595-605.
33. Endicott J, Spitzer RL, Fleiss J, Cohen J. The Global Assessment Scale: a procedure for measuring overall severity of psychiatric disturbance. *Arch Gen Psychiatry.* 1976;33:766-771.
34. Spitzer RL, Williams JBW, Gibbon M. *Structured Clinical Interview for DSM-III-R (SCID).* New York, NY: New York State Psychiatric Institute, Biometrics Research Unit; 1987.
35. American Psychiatric Association. *Diagnostic and Statistical Manual of Mental Disorders, Revised Third Edition.* Washington, DC: American Psychiatric Association; 1987.
36. Williams JBW, Gibbon M, First MB, Spitzer RL, Davies M, Borus J, Howes MJ, Kane J, Pope HG, Rounsaville B, Wittchen H. The Structured Clinical Interview for *DSM-III-R* (SCID), II: multisite test-retest reliability. *Arch Gen Psychiatry.* 1992;49:630-636.
37. Beck AT, Weissman A, Lester D, Trexler L. The measurement of pessimism: the Hopelessness Scale. *J Consult Clin Psychol.* 1974;42:861-865.

38. Beck AT, Steer RA, Kovacs M, Garrison B. Hopelessness and eventual suicide: a 10-year prospective study of patients hospitalized with suicidal ideation. *Am J Psychiatry.* 1985;142:559-563.
39. Williams JBW. *The Structured Interview Guide for the Hamilton Anxiety and Depression Rating Scales (SIGH-AD).* New York, NY: Biometrics Research Dept, New York State Psychiatric Institute; 1988.
40. Hamilton M. A rating scale for depression. *J Neurol Neurosurg Psychiatry.* 1960;23:56-62.
41. Carroll BJ, Fielding JM, Blashki TG. Depression rating scales: a critical review. *Arch Gen Psychiatry.* 1988;45:742-747.
42. Hedlund JL, Vieweg BW. The Hamilton rating scale for depression: a comprehensive review. *J Oper Psychiatry.* 1979;10:149-165.
43. Rabkin JG, Klein DF. The clinical measurement of depressive disorders. In: A Marsella, R Hirschfeld, M Katz, eds. *The Measurement of Depression.* New York, NY: Guilford Press; 1987.
44. Hamilton M. The assessment of anxiety states by rating. *Br J Med Psychiatry.* 1959;32:50-55.
45. Spitzer RL, Williams JBW, Gibbon M, First, MB. The Structured Clinical Interview for *DSM-III-R* (SCID), I: history, rationale, and description. *Arch Gen Psychiatry.* 1992;49:624-629.
46. Spitzer RL, Williams JBW, Gibbon M. *Structured Clinical Interview for the* DSM-III-R *Personality Disorders (SCIDII).* Washington, DC: American Psychiatric Association; 1987.
47. First MB, Spitzer RL, Gibbon M, Williams JBW. The Structured Clinical Interview for *DSM-III-R* Personality Disorders (SCID-II), I: description. *J Pers Disord.* 1995;9:83-91.
48. First MB, Spitzer, RL, Gibbon M, Williams JBW, Davies M, Borus J, Howes MJ, Kane J, Pope HG Rounsaville B. The Structured Clinical Interview for *DSM-III-R* Personality Disorders (SCID-II), II: multi-site test-retest reliability study. *J Pers Disord.* 1995;9:92-104.
49. O'Boyle M, Self D. A comparison of two interviews for *DSM-III-R* personality disorders. *Psychiatry Res.* 1990;32:85-92.
50. Oldham JM, Skodol AE, Kellman HD, Hyler SE, Rosnick L, Davies M. Diagnoses of *DSM-III-R* personality disorders by two structured interviews: patterns of comorbidity. *Am J Psychiatry.* 1992;149:213-220.
51. Skodol AE, Oldham JM, Rosnick L, Kellman HD, Hyler SE. Diagnosis of *DSM-III-R* personality disorders: a comparison of two structured interviews. *Int J Meth Psychiatric Res.* 1991;1:13-26.
52. Williams JBW, Rabkin JG, Remien RH, Gorman JM, Ehrhardt AA. Multidisciplinary baseline assessment of homosexual men with and without human immunodeficiency virus infection, II: standardized clinical assessment of current and lifetime psychopathology. *Arch Gen Psychiatry.* 1991;48:124-130.
53. Gorman JM, Kertzner R, Todak G, Goetz RR, Williams JBW, Rabkin J, Meyer-Bahlburg HFL, Mayeux R, Stern Y, Lange M, Dobkin J, Spitzer R, Ehrhardt AA. Multidisciplinary baseline assessment of homosexual men with and without human immunodeficiency virus infection, I: overview of study design. *Arch Gen Psychiatry.* 1991;48:120-123.
54. Gunderson JG, Links PS, Reich JH. Competing models of personality disorders. *J Pers Disord.* 1991;5:60-68.
55. Overholser JC: Categorical assessment of the dependent personality disorder in depressed inpatients. *J Pers Disord.* 1991;5:243-255.
56. Chuang HT, Devins GM, Hunsley J, Gill MJ. Psychosocial distress and well-being among gay and bisexual men with human immunodeficiency virus infection. *Am J Psychiatry.* 1989;146:876-880.
57. Rosenberger PH, Bornstein RA, Nasrallah HA, Para MF, Whitaker CC, Fass RJ, Rice RR. Psychopathology in human immunodeficiency virus infection: lifetime and current assessment. *Compr Psychiatry.* 1993;34:150-158.
58. Wells KB, Stewart A, Hays RD, Burnam A, Rogers W, Daniels M, Berry S, Greenfield S, Ware J. The functioning and well-being of depressed patients: results from the Medical Outcomes Study. *JAMA.* 1989;262:914-919.
59. Brooner RK, Schmidt CW, Felch LJ, Bigelow GE. Antisocial personality disorder and HIV infection among intravenous drug abusers. *Am J Psychiatry.* 1993; 150:53-58.
60. O'Boyle M. Personality disorder and multiple substance dependence. *J Pers Disord.* 1993;7:342-347.
61. Johnson JG, Hyler SE, Skodol AE, Bornstein RF, Sherman M. Personality disorder symptomatology associated with adolescent depression and substance abuse. *J Pers Disord.* 1995;9:318-329.

Communication Disturbances in Schizophrenia and Mania

Nancy M. Docherty, PhD; Maddalena DeRosa; Nancy C. Andreasen, MD, PhD

Background: A "natural language" measure was developed for classifying type and severity of communication disturbance in the speech of psychotic patients by assessing their linguistic reference performance.

Methods: This measure was applied to speech samples of schizophrenic, manic, and nonpsychiatric subjects, and the groups were compared on levels and types of communication failures.

Results: The speech of the schizophrenic and manic subjects contained much higher frequencies of each of six types of communication failures than did the speech of the control subjects. Proportions of the different types of unclarity differed among the diagnostic groups.

Conclusions: This method provides a measure of overall severity of communication disturbance, discriminates the speech of schizophrenic and manic subjects from that of nonpsychiatric subjects, and reflects some differences in distribution of types of communication failure in schizophrenic vs manic patients. The measure may be helpful in elucidating cognitive weaknesses underlying psychotic communication failures.

(Arch Gen Psychiatry. 1996;53:358-364)

COMMUNICATION disturbances are fundamental symptoms of both schizophrenia and mania.[1,2] To study these phenomena, investigators have attempted to define them qualitatively and to develop methods for measuring their severity. For the most part, researchers have viewed psychotic disordered speech as reflective of disordered thinking and, therefore, have pursued ways of characterizing and measuring the underlying thought disorder. There is a large and very interesting literature on thought disorder, which can be only briefly mentioned here. Bleuler[1] described loosening of associations and autistic thinking as central to schizophrenic thought pathology. Vigotsky,[3] Sullivan,[4] and others noted an egocentric quality to psychotic speech, in that concepts are used in highly personalized and idiosyncratic, rather than conventional, ways, so that their meanings and associations are personally relevant but not socially shared (see also Harrow and Quinlan[5]). More recently, Spitzer[6] has used semantic priming paradigms to provide empirical evidence suggesting an overactivity or disinhibition of associative processes in schizophrenia. Other investigators[7,8] have focused on difficulties in abstraction and concept definition as the central deficit in psychotic thought disorder. As Goldstein and Scheerer[7] pointed out, concept formation difficulties may be associated with the schizophrenic patient's inability to separate figure from ground, ie, to distinguish between relevant or "essential" and irrelevant or "nonessential" characteristics of objects and situations. In line with these ideas, numerous laboratory studies have demonstrated conceptual overinclusion[5,9] and conceptual boundary disturbances[10,11] in people with schizophrenia. Harrow and Quinlan[5] created a measure of "bizarre-idiosyncratic thinking" that assesses several different facets of thought disorder. Johnston and Holzman[11] developed the Thought Disorder Index, a Rorschach test–based combination measure of thought disorder. These methods provide relatively comprehensive measures of thought disorder, as reflected in the speech generated in response to specific stimuli.

From the Departments of Psychiatry, Yale University School of Medicine, New Haven, Conn (Dr Docherty and Ms DeRosa), and University of Iowa School of Medicine, Iowa City (Dr Andreasen).

See Subjects and Methods on next page

SUBJECTS AND METHODS

SUBJECTS

The sample consisted of 38 schizophrenic and 24 manic inpatients, and 40 nonpsychiatric control subjects, randomly selected from a large group of participants in a study of thought, language, and communication at the University of Iowa.[2] The Schedule for Affective Disorders and Schizophrenia diagnostic interview was administered to all patient subjects, and diagnoses were determined by an independent psychiatrist using the Research Diagnostic Criteria (descriptive data are provided in **Table 1**). The diagnostic groups did not differ in gender distribution, level of education, or number of hospitalizations, but the manic patients were significantly older than the schizophrenic and nonpsychiatric subjects and their age at onset was later than that of the schizophrenic patients.

PROCEDURES

Speech Samples

All subjects were interviewed using a semistructured format. They were asked a series of open-ended questions about topics such as school, interests, family, religion, and political beliefs. The interviews were audiotaped, and the tapes transcribed. Ratings were done using the typewritten transcripts of the speech. These were the same speech samples that Hoffman et al[17] used for their analysis of differences in language structure, or "discourse trees," in schizophrenic vs manic speech.

Types of Communication Failures

The CDI is based on the concept of the unclear reference developed by Halliday and Hasan[23] and Rochester and Martin,[15] but we expanded on it in several ways. First, the threshold was lowered for designating a reference as unclear, including instances of subtly unclear meaning. Second, the concept of referent was extended to include the definitional meaning of a word or phrase, based on the premise that words themselves are references to objects or concepts (ie, "common knowledge"); thus, a word or phrase that is used in such a way that its definition in context is ambiguous or unknown is counted as unclear. Third, we included words and phrases other than nominals and pronominals, counting instances of unclear meaning of any word or phrase, whenever the unclear meaning impairs the comprehensibility of the speech. Fourth, we included instances of faulty word usage or grammatical structure, whenever the incorrect usage impairs the clarity of meaning of the utterance.

The speech samples were scored for instances of unclear meaning. Each instance was classified according to the apparent nature of the impediment to the communication of meaning. We counted instances of each of six types of communication failure. These types are described below, and examples are given. Unclear references are boldfaced.

1. *Vague references* are words or phrases that are unclear because they are overinclusive. They are scored only if their lack of specificity is important and significantly diminishes the meaning communicated by the utterance. They are not usually blatantly deviant, but they leave the listener with an amorphous and questionable impression, rather than a clearly communicated meaning.

1.1. *I'm hoping they don't get caught up in* ***some of the ills of our life, of our society.***

1.2. *It seems so, you know,* ***this, that, or the other.***

2. *Confused references* are unclear because they could refer to one of at least two clear-cut alternative referents, and the correct choice is not obvious. Confused references are often, but not always, pronouns.

2.1. *He stabbed the dude and I kicked* ***him.*** *I thought* ***he*** *punched* ***him.*** *I thought* ***he*** *was on the ground just acting like he was hurt.*

2.2. *My son has two children and my daughter has three.* ***The kids*** *have counted on me for a lot.*

3. *Missing information references* seem to assume that the listener has prior information that he or she does not have and should not be expected to have. Unqualified references to persons, places, or things unknown to the listener are classified here, as well as comparative references for which the basis of comparison is unknown.

3.1. *I like to work all right. Some of* ***those shops*** *were filthy. I liked* ***the bakeries,*** *some of* ***the shops*** *are clean.* (No prior mention of any shops or bakeries.)

3.2. *They let* ***George*** *go home, so why not me?* (No prior mention of George, and listener does not know him.)

3.3. *I love the place best in the winter. It's just a total* ***opposite*** *then.* (Missing information comparison; "oppo-

Continued on next page

Other investigators[12-18] have hypothesized that disordered speech is primarily reflective of deficits in linguistic functioning and have concentrated on studying deviances in the structure of the language that might be responsible for the loss of communicative power. Studies employing the "cloze" technique have demonstrated insufficient levels of redundancy and predictability in the speech of psychotic patients,[14] perhaps again related to egocentricity, or a diminished awareness on the part of the speaker of the information needed by the listener to understand the communication. Deficiencies in other structural elements of language such as mechanisms of cohesion and reference[15], depth of clausal embedding,[16] and organization and hierarchical ordering of clauses and speech segments[17] have been demonstrated in the speech of psychotic patients.

There is some debate between these two approaches to disordered speech, yet they clearly have areas of overlap. Comprehensive measures intended to assess formal thought disorder generally include anomalies of language structure and word usage, as well as elements of thought disorder such as concept formation, abstraction, and logical thinking deficits.[5,11] Johnston and Holzman,[11] for example, include "peculiar language" in their Thought Disorder Index, and, in fact, this is one of the most frequently scored categories in their system. Harrow and Quinlan,[5] in their measure of bizarre-idiosyncratic thinking, include "peculiar word form or use." Furthermore, those taking a structural approach to disordered speech do not deny that psychotic patients often show signs of disordered thinking in addition to language deviance.

site" in what way? Listener does not know the basis of comparison.)

4. *Ambiguous word meanings* are instances in which a word or phrase is used in such a way that its intended definitional meaning is uncertain. This does not include instances in which it seems that the wrong word has been chosen, but rather the word used could have a number of different meanings in its current context, and the correct meaning is not obvious.

4.1. *He was a man that was* **pow** *in a minute.* ("Pow" is unclear because the intended definitional meaning is uncertain. Does it mean he became violent easily, or he was a man of action, or...?)

4.2. *Those people don't belong on the earth. God will* ***get them.***

4.3. *I had a chance to* **grow** *with him but I got a divorce because I couldn't.*

5. *Wrong word references* are unclear because of a seemingly incorrect choice of word or phrase. The meaning of the utterance seems clear, but doubt is cast because of the use of an odd or apparently inappropriate word or expression.

5.1. *We've had our* **qualms** *about me bowling, but I've always won out.* (Does she mean "quarrels"?)

5.2. *I used to sit in the cafe, have something to eat, and just* **glare** *out into the night.* (Does he mean "stare"?)

6. *Structural unclarities* are instances in which meaning is unclear due to a breakdown or inadequacy of grammatical structure. Incorrect grammar is not scored unless it results in a loss of clarity of meaning.

6.1. *I got a sister in Buffalo, New York. I've been there . . . must have been about* ***twice since I was up there.***

6.2. *We went to Arizona. We stopped off lots of towns* ***between Chicago.*** (Spoken by a person living in Connecticut.)

Ratings of Communication Disturbance

Speech samples were rated by counting each instance of each type of communication failure as defined above. The entire interview was rated. The basic unit of analysis was the individual word or phrase, except in the case of structural unclarities, which generally involved nongrammatical or otherwise incomprehensible constructions of several words. These structural unclarities were delimited by clause boundaries as much as possible, using a best estimate when clause boundaries were unclear. Each instance of unclarity was classified as of only one type; multiple ratings were not applied to a single instance. In studies of natural language, amounts of speech produced vary widely among subjects. We controlled for differences among subjects in the amounts of speech generated by counting the number of words in each speech sample and calculating the number of each type of communication failure per 100 words of speech. Total CDI scores were computed by summing the counts of all six types of communication failure per 100 words of speech. Thus, the CDI ratings reported are frequency scores rather than absolute scores. Ratings were done by the first author (N.D.), blind to identity, diagnosis, symptom, and all other subject variables. A second rater, trained by the first author using speech samples from another study, blindly scored a randomly selected 20% of the speech samples for the present study. Interrater reliabilities for ratings of communication disturbance were as follows:

Communication Disturbance	**Intraclass *r***
Vague references	.73
Confused references	.88
Missing information references	.89
Ambiguous word meanings	.88
Wrong word references	.80
Structural unclarities	.93
Total Communication Disturbances	**.94**

Analysis

We calculated means and SDs for the ratings of communication failure in each diagnostic group. Assumptions regarding distributions and variances for analysis of variance (ANOVA) were not met by the data; therefore, we performed log transformations, which normalized the distributions and made the variances nearly equal. We then computed correlations between the different types of communication failures for the whole sample and one-way ANOVAs comparing the frequencies of each type of communication failure between diagnostic groups. We also computed proportions of each type of communication failure to the total communication disturbance score in each group and compared these proportions between groups. All results reported are two tailed.

It is difficult to separate out language processes from other thought processes in this group. Whereas aphasic individuals have specific language-related impairments that are not necessarily associated with more general cognitive deficits, those with psychotic language disturbances tend also to show cognitive failures in other domains. There may or may not be dysfunction in "language areas" of the brain in psychotic disorders, but there clearly is impairment in cognitive processes that are not considered to be specifically language related but that, nevertheless, are likely to have an impact on language performance. For example, some of the multiple cognitive impairments in areas such as memory, attention, and concept formation that have been noted in individuals with schizophrenia could be expected to impair their language functioning to some degree. In fact, scores on tests of attention[19-22] and working memory[22] have been found to correlate with severity of formal thought and communication disorder in schizophrenic patients. In a recent study of 48 schizophrenic outpatients,[22] poor performance on cognitive tests tapping working memory and poor performance on an auditory continuous performance task assessing sustained attention were associated with higher levels of communication disturbance, even when overall severity of illness was residualized out of the analysis. This supports the idea that deficits in working memory and attentional processes may underlie language symptoms to some extent.

The distinction between thought and language deviance in psychosis is not altogether on firm theoretical ground. We have approached the definition and measurement of psychotic communication disturbances from an angle that does not attempt to separate thought from language functioning. We have developed a method designed specifically to assess level and type of *communication* disturbance as such, ie, of clarity or unclarity of *meanings* in speech. Our method is based on the simple observation that communication failures result in large part from a speaker's use of words or phrases with meanings not shared by the listener. An instance of communication failure may be caused by a lack of knowledge on the part of the listener, or by unclarity on the part of the speaker. The latter is believed to be the problem in psychotic speech, ie, the speaker uses words and phrases in such a way that their meanings are not socially shared. The listener cannot determine their referents because of the idiosyncratic usage.

Rochester and Martin[15] have applied a number of measures of linguistic cohesion to the speech of schizophrenic subjects. Most of their measures essentially assess structural characteristics of language, as outlined by the linguists Halliday and Hasan[23]; however, their measure of unclear references directly reflects unclarity or ambiguity of meaning in speech, as well as lack of cohesiveness of structure. In their system, references are nominal or pronominal words or phrases that depend on previously presented information or on common knowledge in order to be understood. References are distinguished from other nominal groups that introduce new material into the discourse. Unclear references are those for which the referents are ambiguous or unknown. In contrast to other methods of assessing communication disturbance, this measure does not rely on assumptions that either thought disorder or structural language dysfunction necessarily underlie the communicative impairments. Unclear references directly represent communication failures, or failures in the conveyance of meaning by the speaker to the listener, in that a reference is designated as unclear if the listener is uncertain as to its referent or meaning. The frequency of unclear references in speech has been found to discriminate the speech of schizophrenic and manic subjects from that of nonpsychiatric control subjects.[15,24,25] It also has been found to correspond moderately highly with ratings of positive formal thought disorder on Andreasen's Thought, Language, and Communication scales[26] and with ratings on the disorganization scale of the Positive and Negative Syndrome Scale.[27,21]

Our experience with this measure suggests that it provides a relatively accurate assessment of overall clarity or unclarity of meaning in discourse. Speech segments that are perceived as difficult to follow generally contain frequent unclear references. However, we have observed that there are several different types of unclear reference within the definition by Rochester and Martin[15] that may have different origins or different cognitive substrata and also that there are a number of instances of communicative unclarity that are not captured by their measure. In the present study, we developed criteria for identifying and classifying a wider range of communication failures to create a more inclusive index of communication disturbances.

Table 1. Subjects' Descriptive Data*

Characteristics	Subjects: Schizophrenic	Manic	Control
n	38	24	40
Age, y	26±6	35±14	26±9
Female, %	39	54	38
Education, y	14±2	13±2	13±2
Previous hospitalizations, No. (range)	4±3 (1-12)	4±3 (0-10)	...
Age at onset, y	19±3	26±11	...

*Data are mean±SD.

Based on data from our earlier studies of language,[21,22,25,28] and using an expanded definition of referential unclarity, we catalogued and developed criteria for rating six different types of communication failures. We then applied the methods to "natural language" speech samples of psychotic and nonpsychiatric subjects, assessed the reliability of the ratings, and compared levels and types of communication disturbance between groups. As mentioned above, our measure, the Communication Disturbances Index (CDI), was designed to be inclusive to capture as many of the unclarities of meaning in speech as possible, including even subtle instances of communication failure. Therefore, we expected it to register low levels of communicative unclarity in the speech of the nonpsychiatric subjects as a group, higher levels in the psychotic subjects as a group, and a wide range in levels and types of disturbance between subjects within groups.

RESULTS

DESCRIPTIVE FINDINGS

Amounts of speech generated during the interview varied among subjects and between diagnostic groups: the schizophrenic group produced a mean of 1449 (±971) words; the manic subjects, 2468 (±1066) words; and the nonpsychiatric control subjects, 2117 (±805) words. Total CDI scores varied widely among subjects, ranging from 0.11 to 14.18 (instances of failure per 100 words). Means, SDs, and ranges for frequencies of communication failures in each of the diagnostic groups are presented in **Table 2**. Ambiguous word meanings were the type of communication failure most frequently rated in all groups, and scores on this variable were highest in the manic group. The schizophrenic subjects scored slightly higher than the manic subjects on all other categories of the CDI, and both patient groups scored higher than the nonpsychiatric subjects.

CORRELATIONS BETWEEN TYPES OF COMMUNICATION FAILURE

Using log-transformed data, we computed correlations between scores on the different types of communication failures. Most of the measures were moderately highly correlated with each other. These results are presented in **Table 3**. Vague references were the least closely

Table 2. Frequency of Communication Failures in the Speech of Schizophrenic, Manic, and Nonpsychiatric Subjects

Communication Failure	Subjects/Communication Failure Scores,* Mean±SD (Range): Schizophrenic (n=38)	Manic (n=24)	Control (n=40)	F†	P	Fisher PLSD‡
Vague references	0.18±0.17 (0-0.68)	0.15±0.15 (0-0.58)	0.11±0.10 (0-0.40)	4.87	.01	Schizophrenic>manic, control
Confused references	0.39±0.37 (0-1.36)	0.35±0.26 (0.06-1.07)	0.10±0.12 (0-0.53)	11.19	.0001	Schizophrenic, manic>control
Missing information references	0.60±0.49 (0-1.92)	0.57±0.89 (0-4.45)	0.12±0.12 (0-0.47)	34.49	.0002	Schizophrenic, manic>control
Ambiguous word meanings	1.01±0.96 (0.21-5.22)	1.14±0.96 (0.19-3.99)	0.30±0.24 (0-1.18)	30.95	.0001	Manic, schizophrenic>control
Wrong word references	0.41±0.83 (0-5.22)	0.27±0.18 (0-0.67)	0.13±0.13 (0-0.51)	14.09	.0001	Schizophrenic, manic>control
Structural unclarities	0.38±0.39 (0-1.87)	0.27±0.28 (0-1.22)	0.10±0.12 (0-0.57)	10.22	.0001	Schizophrenic, manic>control
Total Communication Disturbance	**3.0±2.5 (0.78-14.18)**	**2.8±2.1 (0.30-9.78)**	**0.86±0.59 (0.11-2.85)**	36.18	.0001	Schizophrenic, manic>control

*Communication failure scores are presented as instances per 100 words of speech.
†F values were computed using log-transformed scores.
‡PLSD indicates protected least significant difference test.

related to the other types of failure, but still were significantly correlated with most of the other ratings and with the total communication disturbance scores, $r=.45$, $P<.01$. These findings indicate that, for the most part, the various types of failures are associated with each other and with the larger construct of communication disturbance as we have defined it. Total CDI scores also were correlated with global ratings of thought, language, and communication disorder made by Andreasen's group in the original Iowa study,[26] $r=.60$, $P<.001$.

BETWEEN-GROUP DIFFERENCES

Communication Disturbances

Analyses of variance revealed significant between-group differences for every category of communication failure. On the measure of vague references, the schizophrenic patients scored higher (ie, showed more disorder) than the manic patients or the nonpsychiatric control subjects, who did not differ from each other. On the five remaining measures, and also on the total scores, the nonpsychiatric subjects scored lower (better) than either of the patient groups. The two patient groups did not differ significantly from each other. These findings are presented in Table 2.

Patterns of Communication Failures

We wanted to determine whether levels of overall communication disturbance in the different diagnostic groups reflected differences in *proportions* of the six types of communication failure in the speech. We formed ratios of ratings of each type of failure over ratings of total disturbance and performed ANOVAs comparing these ratios between groups. Control subjects showed a higher proportion of vague references in their communication failures than did either of the patient groups; manic subjects showed a higher proportion of ambiguous word meanings than did the schizophrenic or control subjects ($P<.06$, trend); and schizophrenic subjects showed a higher proportion of missing information references than did the control group. These results are presented in **Table 4**.

COMMENT

The CDI clearly discriminated speech of schizophrenic and manic patients from that of nonpsychiatric control subjects. The schizophrenic and manic groups scored about equally on the measure. Scores ranged widely within groups. The different types of communication failures were associated with each other, indicating that those subjects who made frequent unclear references of one kind were likely also to make frequent unclear references of other kinds.

The communication disturbances for the whole sample correlated with both positive and negative symptoms; however, these correlations were not significant within the diagnostic groups. This lack of significant correlations within groups is consistent with the schizophrenia literature indicating three relatively independent symptom dimensions: positive symptoms, negative symptoms, and disorganization symptoms.[29,30] It is also consistent with findings that cognitive symptoms tend to remain relatively stable even when psychotic symptoms remit[31] and with our own earlier findings that reference performance in schizophrenic patients (using the method of Rochester and Martin) tends to remain stable over time, even though more blatant forms of formal thought disorder vary with overall clinical state.[25]

Every speech sample contained some unclear references as defined by the CDI, and the errors were of the same six types in all three diagnostic groups. Ratings of these types of failures for the most part discriminated schizophrenic and manic subjects from control subjects, but did not discriminate between schizophrenic vs manic speakers. However, there were differences between diagnostic groups in the *proportions* of each type of communication failure. Communication failures in the speech of schizophrenic patients, compared with those in normal speech, were more likely to consist of references to information completely unknown to the listener (3.1. Some of *those shops* were filthy [no prior mention of any shops]). The manic subjects showed the highest proportion of unclarities owing to the use of words

Table 3. Correlations Between Frequencies of Six Types of Communication Failure in Schizophrenic, Manic, and Nonpsychiatric Subjects

	Type of Communication Failure					
Six Types of Communication Failures	**1**	**2**	**3**	**4**	**5**	**6**
1. Vague references	1					
2. Confused references	0.10	1				
3. Missing information references	0.22*	0.66†	1			
4. Ambiguous word meanings	0.37†	0.65†	0.77†	1		
5. Wrong word references	0.43†	0.43†	0.49†	0.58†	1	
6. Structural unclarities	0.34‡	0.43†	0.58†	0.61†	0.46†	1
Total Communication Disturbance	**0.45†**	**0.74†**	**0.83†**	**0.93†**	**0.63†**	**0.71†**

P<.05*.
†P<*.01*.
‡P<*.001*.

Table 4. Proportion of Each Type of Communication Failure to Total Communication Disturbance Scores in Schizophrenic, Manic, and Nonpsychiatric Subjects

	Subjects					
	Schizophrenic	**Manic**	**Control**	**F**	***P***	**Fisher PLSD***
Vague references	0.07 (±0.07)	0.06 (±0.05)	0.15 (±0.12)	9.3	.001	Control>schizophrenic, manic
Confused references	0.13 (±0.11)	0.14 (±0.08)	0.10 (±0.10)	1.6	.21	NS
Missing information references	0.21 (±0.12)	0.17 (±0.11)	0.14 (±0.10)	3.8	.02	Schizophrenic>control
Ambiguous word meanings	0.34 (±0.11)	0.41 (±0.14)	0.35 (±0.14)	3.0	.06	Manic>control, schizophrenic
Wrong word references	0.12 (±0.11)	0.11 (±0.07)	0.17 (±0.14)	2.2	.12	NS
Structural unclarities	0.12 (±0.08)	0.10 (±0.09)	0.10 (±0.09)	1.2	.30	NS
Total Communication Disturbance	**1.00**	**1.00**	**1.00**	. . .	. . .	. . .

**PLSD indicates protected least significant difference test; NS, not significant.*

that could be interpreted reasonably in more than one way (4.1. He was a man that was *pow* in a minute). The control subjects had the highest proportion of communication failures owing to vague, overinclusive references that were not sufficiently explicit to convey meaning adequately (1.2. It seems so, you know, *this, that, or the other*). The differences in relative contributions of the various types of failures rated here probably account in part for the oft-noted subjectively perceived between-group differences in unclear schizophrenic, manic, and normal speech. Other investigators have elucidated language-related diagnostic discriminators of schizophrenia and mania;[2,16,17] however, findings in this area have been limited and, as in the present study, between-group differences have essentially been quantitative in nature, with one group demonstrating more or less of a particular variable than the other group. To our knowledge, no quality or characteristic of speech has yet been defined that is unique to one or the other of these diagnoses.

The manic subjects produced the most speech during the interview, and the schizophrenic subjects the least. While we controlled for these differences in productivity by computing frequency scores, this method did not take into account the effect of possible differences in complexity on the number of communication failures in the sparser vs denser speech samples. In addition, our method counted the frequency of communication failures but did not rate the severity of each instance. Subtle and severe unclarities were rated equally. Those speech samples containing instances of severe failure generally contained very frequent failures as well; however, it is possible that adding the dimension of severity to each rated instance of failure would increase the power of the index to discriminate between groups. These are both questions for further inquiry.

Our current psychiatric diagnostic system perforce classifies disorders by combinations of symptoms, rather than by underlying processes.[32,33] Individuals assigned a diagnosis of schizophrenia or mania are heterogeneous in presentation, symptoms, language functioning, and cognitive profile. We believe that communication disturbances are caused, at least in part, by underlying cognitive weaknesses, which are associated, to some degree, with both schizophrenia and mania but which may vary more markedly among subjects than between diagnostic groups. We developed the CDI because we believed there was a need for a "natural language" measure of communication disturbance, which could effectively capture and quantify the level of clarity or unclarity of meaning in speech. Besides providing a global, inclusive measure of communication disturbance that can serve as an index of overall severity, the CDI also consists of separate categories of deviance, potentially related to specific areas of deficit in cognitive functioning. By virtue of this classification system, the measure may also prove useful in efforts to elucidate the cognitive underpinnings of specific types of communication disturbances. For example, missing information references may be associated with deficits in working memory, in that the speaker may be unable to maintain a discourse plan in memory long enough to complete it[22] or unable to remember clearly what he or she has presented vs what he or she has only thought.[34] Wrong word references and structural unclarities may reflect, in part, a general weakness in concept formation. Such hypotheses could be tested by assessing associations between the various types of communication disturbances and scores on tests of working memory, concept formation, and other potentially relevant areas of cognitive functioning.

Accepted for publication July 10, 1995.

Reprint requests to Department of Psychology, Kent State University, Kent, OH 44242 (Dr Docherty).

REFERENCES

1. Bleuler E. *Dementia Praecox, or the Group of Schizophrenias.* New York, NY: International Universities Press; 1911.
2. Andreasen NC, Grove WM. Thought, language and communication in schizophrenia: diagnosis and prognosis. *Schizophr Bull.* 1986;12;348-358.
3. Vigotsky L. Thought in schizophrenia. *Arch Neurol Psychiatry.* 1934;31:1063.
4. Sullivan HS. The language of schizophrenia. In: Kasanin JS, ed. *Language and Thought in Schizophrenia.* New York, NY: WW Norton Co Inc; 1944.
5. Harrow M, Quinlan DM. *Disordered Thinking and Schizophrenic Psychopathology.* New York, NY: Gardner Press; 1985.
6. Spitzer M. *The Psychopathology, Neuropsychology, and Neurobiology of Associative and Working Memory in Schizophrenia.* Heidelberg, Germany: Ruprecht-Karls-Universität, Psychiatrische Klinik; 1993.
7. Goldstein K, Scheerer M. Abstract and concrete behavior. *Psychol Monogr.* 1941;53:239.
8. Cameron N. Experimental analysis of schizophrenic thinking. In: Kasanin JS, ed. *Language and Thought in Schizophrenia.* New York, NY: WW Norton Co Inc; 1944.
9. Lovibond SH. The Object Sorting Test and conceptual thinking in schizophrenia. *Austral J Psychol.* 1954;6:52-70.
10. Blatt SJ, Ritzler BA. Thought disorder and boundary disturbances in psychosis. *J Consult Clin Psychol.* 1974;42:370-381.
11. Johnston MH, Holzman PS. *Assessing Schizophrenic Thinking.* San Francisco, Calif: Jossey-Bass; 1979.
12. Chaika E. A linguist looks at 'schizophrenic' language. *Brain Language.* 1974; 1:257-276.
13. Chaika EO. *Understanding Psychotic Speech: Beyond Freud and Chomsky.* Springfield, Ill: Charles C Thomas Publisher; 1990.
14. Salzinger K. *Schizophrenia: Behavioral Aspects.* New York, NY: John Wiley & Sons Inc; 1973.
15. Rochester SR, Martin JR. *Crazy Talk: A Study of the Discourse of Schizophrenic Speakers.* New York, NY: Plenum Press; 1979.
16. Morice R, McNichol D. Language changes in schizophrenia: a limited replication. *Schizophr Bull.* 1986;12:239-250.
17. Hoffman RE, Stopek S, Andreasen NC. A comparative study of manic vs schizophrenic speech disorganization. *Arch Gen Psychiatry.* 1986;43:831-838.
18. Sledge WH, Hoffman RE, Hawkins KA, Docherty NM, Quinlan DM, Rakfeldt J. Linguistic deviance in schizophrenia, preliminary report. In: Spitzer M, Maher B, eds. *Experimental Psychopathology.* New York, NY: Cambridge University Press. In press.
19. Nuechterlein KH, Edell WS, Norris M, Dawson ME. Attentional vulnerability indicators, thought disorder, and negative symptoms. *Schizophr Bull.* 1986;12: 408-426.
20. Harvey PD, Serper MR. Linguistic and cognitive failures in schizophrenia. *J Nerv Ment Dis.* 1990;178:487-493.
21. Docherty NM. Linguistic reference performance in the parents of schizophrenic patients. *Psychiatry.* 1995;58:20-27.
22. Docherty NM, Hawkins KA, Hoffman RE, Quinlan DM, Rakfeldt J, Sledge WH. Working, memory, attention, and communication disturbances in schizophrenia. *J Abnorm Psychol.* In press.
23. Halliday MAK, Hasan R. *Cohesion in English.* London, England: Longman; 1976.
24. Harvey PD. Speech competence in manic and schizophrenic psychoses: the association between clinically rated thought disorder and cohesion and reference performance. *J Abnorm Psychol.* 1983;92:368-377.
25. Docherty N, Schnur M, Harvey PD. Reference performance and positive and negative thought disorder: a follow-up study of manic and schizophrenic patients. *J Abnorm Psychol.* 1988;97:437-442.
26. Andreasen NC. Thought, language, and communication disorders. *Arch Gen Psychiatry.* 1979;36:1315-1330.
27. Kay SR, Opler LA, Fiszbein A. Positive and Negative Syndrome Scale (PANSS) for schizophrenia. *Schizophr Bull.* 1987;13:261-275.
28. Docherty NM, Evans IM, Sledge WH, Seibyl JP, Krystal JH. Affective reactivity of language in schizophrenia. *J Nerv Ment Dis.* 1994;182:98-102.
29. Liddle PF. The symptoms of chronic schizophrenia: a reexamination of the positive-negative dichotomy. *Br J Psychiatry.* 1987;151:45-151.
30. Bilder RM, Mukherjee S, Rieder RO, Pandurangi AK. Symptomatic and neuropsychological components of defect states. *Schizophr Bull.* 1985;11:409-417.
31. Sweeney JA, Haas GL, Keilp JG, Long M. Evaluation of the stability of neuropsychological functioning after acute episodes of schizophrenia: one-year follow-up study. *Psychiatry Res.* 1991;38:63-76.
32. Jeste DV, Kleinman JE, Potkin SG, Luchins DJ, Weinberger DR. Ex uno multi: subtyping the schizophrenic syndrome. *Biol Psychiatry.* 1982;17:199-222.
33. Weiss KM. Advantages of abandoning symptom-based diagnostic systems of research in schizophrenia. *Am J Orthopsychiatry.* 1989;39:324-330.
34. Rochester SR. Are language disorders in acute schizophrenia actually information-processing problems? In: Wynne LC, Cromwell RL, Matthysse S, eds. *The Nature of Schizophrenia.* New York, NY: John Wiley & Sons Inc; 1978.

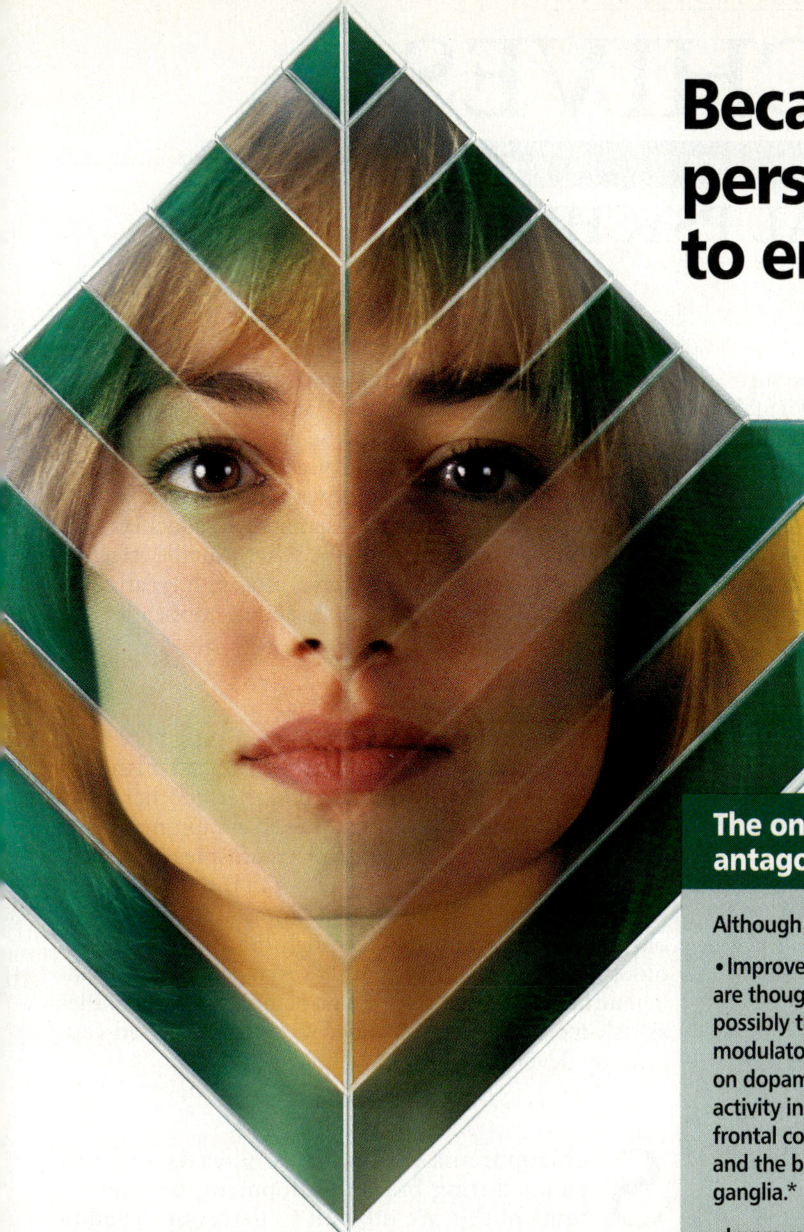

Because a whole person is waiting to emerge.

The only first-choice serotonin/dopamine antagonist (SDA).

Although the exact mechanism of action is unknown:

- Improvement of negative symptoms and lessened risk of EPS are thought to result from blockade of serotonin 5-HT_2 receptors, possibly through a modulatory effect on dopamine D_2 activity in the frontal cortex and the basal ganglia.*
- Improvement of positive symptoms is thought to result from blockade of dopamine D_2 receptors in the limbic system.*

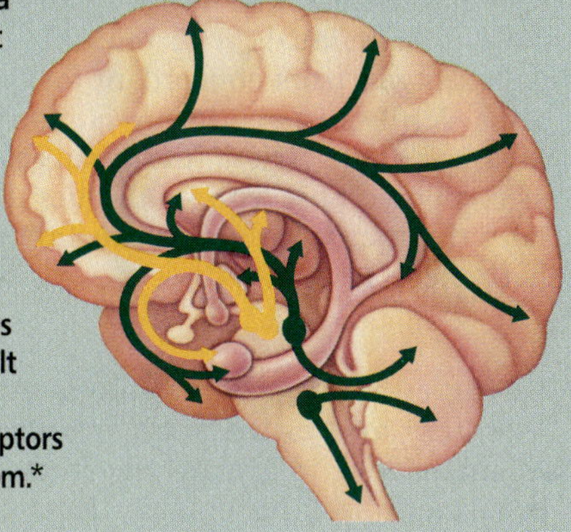

Dopaminergic system   Serotoninergic system

A first choice

1-, 2-, 3-, 4-mg tablets

Risperdal®

RISPERIDONE

Raising the standard of care.

*Ereshefsky L, Lacombe S. Pharmacological profile of risperidone. *Can J Psychiatry.* 1993;38(Suppl 3):S80-S88.

Please see the brief summary of Prescribing Information adjacent to this ad.

JANSSEN · PHARMACEUTICA · · RESEARCH FOUNDATION ·

SmithKline Beecham Pharmaceuticals

The brain mechanisms that underlie the symptoms of posttraumatic stress disorder (PTSD) remain unknown. In the first functional imaging study of PTSD to use a symptom provocation approach, **Rauch et al** (page 380) show the brain activity profile associated with a PTSD symptomatic state. Specifically, during the PTSD-provoked condition, the right-sided paralimbic and limbic regions, as well as the visual cortex, were activated, whereas Broca's area was deactivated. These results provide an initial glimpse at the brain systems that mediate PTSD symptoms. Future studies, with appropriate control groups, will be needed to determine the specificity of these findings to PTSD.

Can the clinical heterogeneity of depression be related to etiologic heterogeneity? In a population-based sample of female twins, **Kendler et al** (page 391) identified, by latent class analysis, 3 clinically significant depressive syndromes: mild typical depression, atypical depression, and severe typical depression. These syndromes tended to be stable in individuals with multiple episodes, and members of twin pairs concordant for depression had the same depressive syndrome far more often than expected by chance. These results suggest that depression is composed of several syndromes that are at least partially distinct from a clinical, longitudinal, and familial/genetic perspective.

Ling et al (page 401) compared the relative safety and efficacy of buprenorphine and methadone in a year-long study that involved 225 treatment-seeking opiate addicts. They found 8-mg/d buprenorphine to be comparable to 30-mg/d methadone, as measured by drug use and retention, but neither group performed as well as the 80-mg/d methadone group. The study validated buprenorphine as a safe and effective pharmacotherapy, but buprenorphine's optimal dose still needs to be established with further studies.

Cocaine abuse remains a serious and costly public health problem that has not yielded to conventional treatment approaches. In a randomized controlled trial in cocaine-abusing methadone patients, **Silverman et al** (page 409) found that patients receiving monetary vouchers (exchangeable for goods and services) for providing cocaine-free urine specimens achieved significantly longer durations of cocaine abstinence than patients who received vouchers on a noncontingent basis (controls). Presentation of vouchers contingent on cocaine-free urine specimens can be effective in the treatment of cocaine abuse, although creative efforts will be needed to develop practical applications of these procedures.

Laor et al (page 416) examined preschool children and their mothers following Scud missile attacks in Israel. Children and their mothers who were displaced by the attacks showed symptomatic levels that were higher than those of undisplaced participants whose homes remained intact in the area that was hit or in a more distant city. Symptoms of 3- and 4-year-old children correlated more strongly than those of 5-year-old children with their mothers' symptoms and inadequate family cohesion. The role of mothers and families as risk-modifying factors may decrease as the child's autonomy develops with increasing age.

Schizophrenia may have as its basis a disturbance during brain development, but indications of this are difficult to detect in the adult brain. Interstitial neurons of the white matter are remnants of a developmentally regulated population of cells that guides growing axons into the cerebral cortex and facilitates formation of connections. They usually die in large numbers. The study by **Akbarian et al** (page 425) shows that the surviving neurons, as detected by 3 different neuronal markers, are displaced deeper in the prefrontal white matter of a subpopulation of patients with schizophrenia. This may imply defective migration or a disturbed pattern of developmentally regulated cell death, leading to defective cortical circuitry. The cause of the pathologic abnormality remains to be determined.

Childhood-onset attention-deficit hyperactivity disorder (ADHD) predicts significant impairment in later life. In a 4-year follow-up study, **Biederman et al** (page 437) show that children with ADHD are at risk of developing behavioral, mood, and anxiety disorders along with impaired cognitive, familial, school, and psychosocial functioning.

Memory and attention abilities are impaired in many psychiatric disorders, including ADHD, yet pharmacological treatments for cognitive impairment remain limited. **Arnsten et al** (page 448) review studies of nonhuman primates that demonstrate that norepinephrine can enhance cognitive functioning through actions at α-2A-adrenergic receptors postjunctional to noradrenergic terminals in the prefrontal cortex. Selective α-2A-receptor agonists such as guanfacine improve working memory, lessen distractability, and calm behavior, with relatively few side effects.

The Fifth International Congress on Schizophrenia Research, held at Warm Springs, Va, April 8-12, 1995, convened 700 investigators from around the world to report their latest findings. Major topics that were covered included genetics (with particular emphasis on genetic-environmental interactions), epidemiology, phenomenology, brain imaging, neuropathy, neurochemistry, psychopharmacology, and psychosocial treatments for schizophrenia. Implications and directions for schizophrenia research that emanate from the conference are discussed in the article by **Buckley et al** (page 456).

A Symptom Provocation Study of Posttraumatic Stress Disorder Using Positron Emission Tomography and Script-Driven Imagery

Scott L. Rauch, MD; Bessel A. van der Kolk, MD; Rita E. Fisler, EdM; Nathaniel M. Alpert, PhD; Scott P. Orr, PhD; Cary R. Savage, PhD; Alan J. Fischman, MD, PhD; Michael A. Jenike, MD; Roger K. Pitman, MD

Background: Previous studies have used symptom provocation and positron emission tomography to delineate the brain systems that mediate various anxiety states. Using an analogous approach, the goal of this study was to measure regional cerebral blood flow changes associated with posttraumatic stress disorder (PTSD) symptoms.

Methods: Eight patients with PTSD, screened as physiologically responsive to a script-driven imagery symptom provocation paradigm, were exposed sequentially to audiotaped traumatic and neutral scripts in conjunction with positron emission tomography. Heart rate and subjective measures of emotional state were obtained for each condition. Statistical mapping techniques were used to determine locations of significant brain activation.

Results: Increases in normalized blood flow were found for the traumatic as compared with control conditions in right-sided limbic, paralimbic, and visual areas; decreases were found in left inferior frontal and middle temporal cortex.

Conclusions: The results suggest that emotions associated with the PTSD symptomatic state are mediated by the limbic and paralimbic systems within the right hemisphere. Activation of visual cortex may correspond to the visual component of PTSD reexperiencing phenomena.

(Arch Gen Psychiatry. 1996;53:380-387)

THE PURPOSE of this study was to explore the mediating neuroanatomy of posttraumatic stress disorder (PTSD) symptoms by measuring changes in relative regional cerebral blood flow (rCBF) associated with the PTSD symptomatic state. Recently, Rauch and colleagues reported the results of 2 positron emission tomographic (PET) studies using within-subject symptom provocation designs to explore the functional neuroanatomy of obsessive-compulsive disorder[1] and simple (small animal) phobia.[2] In the present study, similar methods were used to investigate the mediating neuroanatomy of PTSD symptoms.

Posttraumatic stress disorder is an anxiety disorder manifested by symptoms that can be reliably provoked. Script-driven imagery was first used by Lang[3] to study psychophysiologic responses associated with anxiety, and subsequently by Pitman et al[4] to study PTSD. For PTSD, the technique involves the preparation of "scripts" describing the subjects' past personal experiences (ie, "idiographic" scripts), including the traumatic experience(s) that caused their PTSD. The scripts are read one at a time to the subjects in the psychophysiology laboratory setting, where they are instructed to imagine the events that the scripts portray, while measures of heart rate, skin conductance, and facial electromyograms are recorded. In a series of 4 studies,[4-8] the physiologic responses in subjects with PTSD were found to be higher than the responses of control subjects during personal traumatic imagery.

Within the framework of Lang's network theory of emotion, Pitman[9] and Pitman and Orr[10] hypothesized that PTSD may be conceptualized as consisting of pathologic emotional networks that produce characteristic reexperiencing phenomena. Thus, PTSD network activation may occur "upon exposure to internal or external cues that symbolize or resemble aspects of the traumatic event."[11(p428)] To date, activation of such networks in PTSD

From Harvard Medical School (Drs Rauch, van der Kolk, Alpert, Orr, Savage, Fischman, Jenike, and Pitman), and the Department of Psychiatry, Massachusetts General Hospital (Drs Rauch, van der Kolk, Alpert, Savage, Fischman, and Jenike and Ms Fisler), Boston, Mass; and Veterans Affairs Medical Center, Manchester, NH (Drs Orr and Pitman).

See Patients and Methods on next page

PATIENTS AND METHODS

PATIENTS

Entry criteria included the *DSM-III-R* criteria for PTSD,[26] as determined by clinical interview and Structured Clinical Interview for *DSM-III-R*.[27] Inclusion criteria also required that patients be 18 to 65 years of age and right-handed (as established via the Edinburgh Inventory[28]). Furthermore, patients must have undergone psychophysiologic testing for PTSD and been classified as "physiologic responders," in accordance with a discriminant function derived from previous studies.[4-7] Exclusion criteria were presence of major medical illness or particular comorbid major psychiatric disorders (eg, organic mental disorder, psychoactive substance use disorder, any psychotic disorder, bipolar disorder, or multiple personality disorder). Patients were free of psychoactive drugs for 4 weeks or more before entry into the study. Patients were recruited via the Massachusetts General Hospital Trauma Clinic, Boston (n=6), and the Harvard Medical School Psychophysiology Laboratory at the Veterans Affairs Medical Center, Manchester, NH (n=2). This study was approved by the Subcommittees on Human Studies of the Massachusetts General Hospital and the Veterans Affairs Medical Center. Written informed consent was obtained from each patient.

The study population was composed of 8 patients (6 women and 2 men), with mean (±SE) age at study of 41.1±3.4 years (range, 25-55 years) (**Table 1**). Clinical evaluation determined the presence of comorbid psychiatric diagnoses in 6 of 8 patients. Patients were further clinically characterized using the Clinician-Administered PTSD Scale (CAPS),[29-31] Dissociative Experiences Scale,[32] Civilian Version of the Mississippi PTSD Scale,[33] and Impact of Events Scale–Revised.[34,35]

SCRIPTS

Scripts of patients' past personal events were prepared according to a published procedure.[4-6] Two traumatic scripts were developed, incorporating either 2 separate traumatic experiences (for multiple-blow trauma) or 2 aspects of the same traumatic experience (for single-blow trauma); 2 neutral scripts (eg, brushing one's teeth, emptying the dishwasher) were likewise developed. Each script was then audiotaped in a neutral voice for playback in the laboratory settings. All scripts were 30 to 40 seconds in duration.

EMOTIONAL STATE ANALOG SCALES

Each patient rated the severity of various emotional dimensions (eg, anxiety, fear, sadness, anger, guilt, and disgust) for each condition on separate subjective 0- to 10-point analog scales.[1,2,4-7] Anchor points were provided, where 0 indicated complete absence and 10, maximum possible for the specified emotion. With regard to reexperiencing phenomena during the study, each patient was asked which sensory modalities were involved (ie, visual, auditory, tactile, olfactory, and gustatory), and which were most prominent.

PSYCHOPHYSIOLOGIC SCREENING

Psychophysiologic assessments had previously been performed in accordance with published methods.[4-7] Classification as a "physiologic responder" was one entry criterion. In the psychophysiology laboratory setting, when tested with the identical scripts used in the PET study, the mean (±SE) responses were as follows: for heart rate, 19.7±3.5/min during traumatic scripts vs −2.6±1.5/min during neutral scripts (*df*=7, *t*=5.40, *P*=.002); for skin conductance, 3.08±0.69 microsiemens during traumatic scripts vs −0.47±0.44 microsiemens during neutral scripts (*df*=7, *t*=3.38, *P*=.02); and for frontalis muscle electromyograms, 7.63±2.78 μV during traumatic scripts vs −0.15±0.30 μV during neutral scripts (*df*=7, *t*=2.87, *P*=.03).

PET SYMPTOM PROVOCATION PARADIGM

After habituation to the PET suite environment, patients with PTSD were scanned 6 times. Two scans corresponded to the Traumatic condition (patients imagined the contents of a personal traumatic script), 2 scans corresponded to the Neutral condition (patients imagined the contents of a personal neutral script), and 2 scans corresponded to the Teeth-Clenching condition (patients imagined the contents of a neutral script while performing a teeth-clenching maneuver).

Each scan proceeded as follows: (1) each patient was reminded of instructions to lie still, breath through his or her nose, and allow himself or herself to focus on the contents of the script until after the scan was completed (each patient was also reminded to clench his or her teeth, only during the teeth-clenching scans); (2) an audiotape of the script was played to the patient from a stereocassette player placed on a stand straddling the patient's torso on the scanner bed (centered 1 m from the patient's head); (3) immediately following the end of the script, the PET camera was started, and it continued acquiring data for 90 seconds; (4) the final 60 seconds of PET camera data acquisition coincided with a 60-second period of tracer inhalation, and heart rate monitoring via finger plethysmography (n=4) or electrocardiography (n=4); (5) at the end of this period, PET data acquisition and radiolabeled gas flow were terminated; (6) at the end of each scan, the patient was immediately debriefed regarding his or her subjective experiences during the scan, as outlined above; (7) following a 10-minute tracer washout period, the next scan was performed, until the series of 6 scans was completed.

In all cases, the first 4 scans included 2 in the Traumatic condition and 2 in the Neutral condition. The order of scans was counterbalanced for the 6 female patients and randomized for the 2 male patients, in an effort to control for order effects. The Teeth-Clenching control scans were always the final 2 scans. We anticipated that some patients might not be able to tolerate the full series of 6 scans. Therefore, this design reflected our priority that all patients complete a full complement of Traumatic and Neutral scans; completion of the Teeth-Clenching condition was of secondary importance.

PET FACILITIES AND PROCEDURES

The PET facilities and procedures were similar to those previously described.[1,2]

PET Camera

A 15-slice whole-body tomograph (model PC4096, Scanditronix, General Electric, Milwaukee, Wis) was used in

Continued on next page

its stationary mode to acquire the PET data.[36] The slice geometry consists of contiguous slices with center-to-center distance of 6.5 mm (axial field equal to 97.5 mm) and axial resolution of 6.0-mm full-width half maximum. Image reconstruction was performed using a computed attenuation correction and a Hanning-weighted reconstruction filter set to yield 8.0-mm in-plane spatial resolution full-width half maximum. Additional corrections were made in the reconstruction process to account for scattered radiation, random coincidences, and counting losses due to dead time in the camera electronics.

Subject Positioning

Head alignment was made, relative to the canthomeatal line, using projected laser lines whose positions are known with respect to the slice positions of the scanner. An individually molded thermoplastic mask was used to minimize head motion. Once the head was in place, the patient was fitted with a pair of nasal cannulae and an overlying face mask, which were attached to radiolabeled gas inflow and vacuum, respectively.

Image Acquisition

First, transmission measurements were made using an orbiting pin source. Next, each PET data acquisition run consisted of 15 frames, the first 3 of 10 seconds' duration each and the remaining 12 of 5 seconds' duration each. Subjects began inhaling oxygen 15–labeled carbon dioxide 30 seconds after initiation of the scan and finished 60 seconds later. Frames 4 through 15 (corresponding to the 60 seconds of tracer inhalation) were summed after reconstruction to form images of relative blood flow.

The subjects were studied while continuously inhaling tracer quantities of oxygen 15–labeled carbon dioxide mixed with room air. The concentration of the delivered gas was 2960 MBq/L with a flow rate of 2 L/min, further diluted by free mixture with room air within the face mask, resulting in a rapidly rising count rate in the brain, reaching terminal count rates of 100 000 to 200 000 events per second. The radiation exposure for each subject participating in this study was less than 500 mrem effective dose equivalent. Previous work in the Massachusetts General Hospital Trauma Clinic and the Harvard Medical School Psychophysiology Laboratory at the Veterans Affairs Medical Center, using radial artery cannulation, has demonstrated that the integrated counts over inhalation periods up to 90 seconds is a linear function over the flow range of 0 to 130 mL/min per 100 g (N.M.A., unpublished data, 1991). Therefore, for data to be produced with units of flow relative to whole brain, no arterial access was necessary.

Image Processing

All brain images were corrected for interscan movement using an automated motion correction algorithm (similar to that of Woods et al[37]). The images were then transformed to the standard Talairach coordinate system.[1,2,38,39]

The mean concentration in each run was obtained as an area-weighted sum of the concentration of each slice and adjusted to a nominal value of 50 mL/min per 100 g, yielding normalized blood flow images. The data were then rescaled and smoothed with a 2-dimensional gaussian filter of 20 mm in width (full-width half maximum). These images were pooled over all subjects for each scanning condition, and pairwise subtractions were performed (within subject and between conditions), to yield images of the difference and SD. Then, paired t values were computed and converted into z scores, producing statistical parametric maps (SPMs).

Statistical Parametric Maps

Each SPM was inspected for regions of activation with z scores of 3.00 or greater, corresponding to a threshold of $P \leq .001$, uncorrected for multiple comparisons (ie, many pixels).[2,40] Interpretations of the results from PET activation studies can be substantially influenced by the selected threshold for statistical significance.[2] More stringent criteria have reflected a Bonferroni-type correction for multiple comparisons resulting in a threshold of z scores of 3.50 or greater to 3.75 or greater (depending on the number of pixels in the total search volume).[2,40] Conversely, less stringent criteria have included z scores of 1.96 or greater, reflecting uncorrected $P \leq .05$,[41] or variable thresholds (eg, $z \geq 2.00$)[1] corresponding to a Bonferroni-type correction based on the number of pixels contained within a priori regions of interest.[40] The approach adopted in the present study has the advantage of being moderately stringent while remaining unbiased with respect to a priori hypotheses.[2]

Statistical parametric maps of the Traumatic minus Neutral and Traumatic minus Teeth-Clenching conditions were inspected to identify foci of increased rCBF associated with the Traumatic condition. In cases in which either of these SPMs revealed a focus of activation above threshold, the maximum z scores for both SPMs were recorded. The SPM of the Teeth-Clenching minus Neutral condition was inspected to determine foci of increased rCBF attributable to extracranial blood flow sources or brain activations corresponding to facial muscle contraction. Finally, the SPM of the Neutral minus Traumatic condition was inspected to determine foci of *decreased* rCBF associated with the Traumatic condition.

has been inferred from self-report, as well as behavioral and peripheral physiologic responses.[8] In the present study, we sought to measure changes in rCBF corresponding to activation of these emotional memory networks.

We hypothesized that the PTSD symptomatic state would be associated with increased rCBF in the limbic and paralimbic systems because they are purported to mediate anxiety and other intense emotions.[2,12-16] Relevant brain structures include anterior cingulate, posterior medial orbitofrontal, and insular and anterior temporal cortex; the amygdala[10,16,17]; and the thalamus. Activation within territories involved in visual mental imagery were also predicted[1,2] (ie, dorsolateral prefrontal and visual cortex[18]). Finally, change in rCBF within the hippocampus was anticipated because of its purported role in explicit memory[16,19-21] and in PTSD.[22-24]

In the present study, we used script-driven imagery to achieve a PTSD symptomatic state and asymptomatic control states. By comparing PET rCBF profiles from the dif-

Table 1. Demographic and Clinical Data for Each Subject*

Subject No./ Sex/Age, y	Trauma	Other Diagnosis	CAPS Score	DES Score	M-PTSD Score	IOE Score
1/F/55	Childhood sexual abuse	None	69	13.9	122	87
2/F/25	Victim of domestic violence	MDD	63	40.6	160	79
3/F/40	Childhood sexual and physical abuse	MDD	93	27.0	133	65
4/F/44	Car accident, children died	MDD	74	6.5	127	80
5/M/44	Firefighter, witnessed burn victims	Panic disorder	56	15.5	119	38
6/F/46	Witnessed partner's death	None	87	11.6	111	86
7/F/30	Victim of sexual assault	Dissoc Dis NOS	56	12.3	119	71
8/M/45	Vietnam combat exposure	MDD	59	9.0	107	86

**CAPS indicates Clinician-Administered PTSD (Posttraumatic Stress Disorder) Scale[29-31]; DES, Dissociative Experiences Scale[32]; M-PTSD, Civilian Version of the Mississippi PTSD Scale[33]; IOE, Impact of Event Scale–Revised[34,35]; MDD, major depression; and Dissoc Dis NOS, dissociative disorder not otherwise specified. The mean±SE responses for CAPS score, DES score, M-PTSD score, and IOE score were 69.6±5.0, 17.1±4.0, 124.8±5.8, and 74.0±5.9, respectively.*

Table 2. Heart Rate and Subjective Emotion Analog Scale Scores During Neutral and Traumatic Imaging Conditions*

Variable	Neutral	Traumatic	*t*	*P*
Heart rate (beats/min)	65.8±4.6	76.0±4.5	7.15	<.001
Anxiety analog scale	0.2±0.1	9.6±0.2	38.19	<.001
Fear analog scale	0.0±0.0	9.0±0.3	27.50	<.001
Sadness analog scale	0.2±0.1	7.5±1.0	6.78	<.001
Disgust analog scale	0.0±0.0	6.8±1.5	4.60	.003
Anger analog scale	0.1±0.1	6.9±1.5	4.54	.003
Guilt analog scale	0.1±0.1	3.9±1.3	2.85	.03

**Data are given as mean±SE.*

ferent conditions, PTSD symptomatic state-dependent characteristics could be identified, and each patient could serve as his or her own control (ie, a within-subject design). A teeth-clenching control condition was included to control for extracranial muscle contraction artifacts.[2,25]

RESULTS

CLINICAL INDEXES

For the cohort, compared with the Neutral condition, the Traumatic condition was associated with significant increases in heart rate, and all subjective emotional state analog scale scores (**Table 2**). All patients confirmed that the emotional state achieved was reflective of their PTSD symptomatic state and that visual mental imagery represented the most prominent sensory component of the symptomatic state during the Traumatic condition. Some patients also reported the presence of imagery via other sensory modalities, though to a lesser degree than via the visual modality (tactile [n=3], olfactory [n=3]). Finally, all patients reported intense reexperiencing phenomena.

PET RESULTS

The study yielded a complete set of PET data: 16 scans for each of the 3 conditions (ie, Traumatic, Neutral, and Teeth-Clenching) from the 8 patients studied. Although the results reported reflect the findings from the entire cohort, analogous analyses were performed on the subgroup of 6 female patients and yielded an identical pattern of activation, but with generally lower *z* scores.

Initial inspection of the SPMs corresponding to the Traumatic minus Neutral condition and the Traumatic minus Teeth-Clenching condition were performed for all brain territories scanned (**Table 3** and **Figure**[42]). Activations with maximum pixel values reflecting *z* scores of 3.00 or greater for *both* subtractions were located within right posterior medial orbitofrontal cortex, right insular cortex, right anterior temporal pole, and right medial temporal cortex. Activations with maximum pixel values reflecting *z* scores of 3.00 or greater for the Traumatic minus Teeth-Clenching SPM, but not for the Traumatic minus Neutral SPM, were located within the right amygdala and anterior cingulate cortex. Suprathreshold activation within the amygdala was part of a large territory of contiguous activation extending through insular and anterior temporal cortex. Also, whereas activation was confined to right anterior cingulate cortex in the Traumatic minus Neutral SPM, the territory of activation extended bilaterally for the Traumatic minus Teeth-Clenching SPM. Activations with maximum pixel values reflecting *z* scores of 3.00 or greater for the Traumatic minus Neutral SPM, but not for the Traumatic minus Teeth-Clenching SPM, were located within right secondary visual cortex (Brodmann area 18), and bilateral precentral and postcentral gyri (multiple foci >3.30 for Traumatic minus Neutral; none ≥3.00 for Traumatic minus Teeth-Clenching). Inspection of the Teeth-Clenching minus Neutral SPM revealed multiple activations with maximum pixel values of 3.00 or greater only within precentral and postcentral gyri bilaterally, as well as at foci identified as outside brain.

Inspection of the SPM for Neutral minus Traumatic (**Table 4**), indicating *decreased* rCBF with symptom provocation, revealed activations with maximum pixel values reflecting *z* scores of 3.00 or greater within the left middle temporal cortex and the left inferior frontal cortex (Broca's area).

Inspection of mean difference images revealed that territories of significant activation reflected changes in rCBF of 2.5% to 5.5%; SEs for these foci ranged from 0.32 to 0.68 normalized blood flow units.

With regard to other a priori hypotheses, review of the SPMs revealed that no activations within hippocam-

Table 3. Brain Regions Exhibiting Significantly Increased Activation Associated With Provocation of PTSD Symptoms

Brain Region	Maximum Pixel Value, z Score*: Traumatic Minus Neutral	Maximum Pixel Value, z Score*: Traumatic Minus Teeth-Clenching	Maximum Pixel Coordinates†
Medial orbitofrontal cortex (right/posterior)	3.39‡	3.04‡	21, 10, −16
Insular cortex (right)	3.29‡	3.57‡	36, 0, −12
Anterior temporal pole (right)	3.25‡	3.54‡	43, −2, −12
Medial temporal cortex (right)	3.43‡	3.12‡	47, −26, −8
Secondary visual cortex (right, Brodmann area 18)	3.27‡	2.72	2, −68, 0
Amygdala (right)	2.82	3.58‡	21, −3, −12
Anterior cingulate cortex	2.62	3.11‡	6, 37, 4
Sensorimotor cortex (bilateral)	>3.30‡§	<3.00	(multiple foci)

*Values represent the actual maximum pixel value (in z score units) within the brain region from the statistical parametric map.

†Coordinates defining the location of the maximum pixel values within each brain region from the Traumatic minus Neutral statistical parametric map in Talairach space[38] are expressed as "x, y, z"; x>0 is right of the midsagittal plane, y>0 is anterior to the anterior commissure, and z>0 is superior to the intercommissural plane.

‡Regional activations with z scores ≥3.00, corresponding to P=.001 uncorrected for multiple comparisons.

§Activation in sensorimotor cortex was >3.30 in both precentral and postcentral gyri bilaterally for Traumatic minus Neutral, but also for Teeth-Clenching minus Neutral, and <3.00 for Traumatic minus Teeth-Clenching.

pus ($z \leq 2.88$), dorsolateral prefrontal cortex ($z \leq 2.68$ [decrease]), primary visual cortex ($z \leq 2.01$), or thalamus ($z \leq 2.28$) achieved the threshold for significance. The range of SEs at these foci (0.31-0.59) were comparable to those for the positive findings reported. Therefore, generally, these pertinent negative results failed to achieve significance due to lesser mean increases in rCBF (all <3%).

COMMENT

We found normalized rCBF increases during the PTSD symptomatic vs control conditions in right-sided limbic and paralimbic structures, including posterior medial orbitofrontal, insular, anterior temporal, medial temporal, and anterior cingulate cortex, as well as amygdala. We also found increases in right secondary visual cortex. Decreases in normalized rCBF during the PTSD symptomatic condition were found in left inferior frontal (Broca's area) and left middle temporal cortex. Teeth-clenching control data suggested that increased rCBF within precentral and postcentral gyri were attributable to brain activation associated with muscle contraction, and that artifacts due to blood flow from pericranial muscles were accurately localized outside brain. No statistically significant increases in rCBF were found in dorsolateral prefrontal cortex, primary visual cortex, or thalamus, and no significant change in rCBF was found within the hippocampus.

When exposed to trauma-related cues in the context of script-driven imagery, patients with PTSD who were studied via PET showed activation of the brain structures hypothesized to mediate intense emotion.[13] These PET rCBF findings represent a new class of information distinct from previously obtained psychophysiologic data.[8] The present data more directly reflect changes in brain activity that presumably mediate PTSD symptoms.

This study entailed a within-subject design and did not include any control group. Therefore, it is not possible to conclude that the observed pattern of activation is unique to PTSD symptoms. The activation paradigm involved cognitive procedures that are not necessarily specific to PTSD. For instance, it is possible that the results partially reflect the normal mediating anatomy of intense emotions or emotional memory. A qualitative review of the findings from this and prior studies[1,2] suggests that the limbic and paralimbic systems play a mediating role in the symptomatic state across various anxiety disorders. In this study, the PTSD symptomatic state was characterized by a constellation of negative emotions. One study of transient sadness in healthy women found rCBF increases in cingulate cortex, orbitofrontal cortex, striatum, and thalamus, and rCBF decreases in right temporal and bilateral occipital cortex.[43] One study of self-induced dysphoria found activation of inferior frontal and lateral orbitofrontal cortex; women exhibited bilateral activation, whereas the activations were predominantly left-sided for men.[44] A series of studies exploring brain glucose metabolic correlates of anxiety and hostility in normal subjects have implicated several regions, including anterior cingulate cortex.[45,46] Future research should include a quantitative analysis of symptom provocation data from various emotional states and subject populations. Future studies of PTSD should include a matched trauma-exposed non-PTSD group to evaluate the specificity of the current findings.

Limitations of the present study include the small number of subjects, their heterogeneity with respect to gender, and the presence of comorbid diagnoses. With only 2 male subjects, cross-gender generalizability of these results is tenuous, however their inclusion statistically strengthened the observed findings. Similarly, the heterogeneity with respect to traumatic stimuli confers greater generalizability to the results across PTSD. Subsequent studies could benefit from larger numbers of subjects and more homogeneous groups to test questions pertaining to differences between various PTSD subpopulations.

There are additional limitations intrinsic to the PET methods used.[1,2] The technique of signal normalization to whole brain, although reducing variance and obviating the issue of whole-brain P_{CO_2} correction, does not allow for detection of changes in whole-brain cerebral

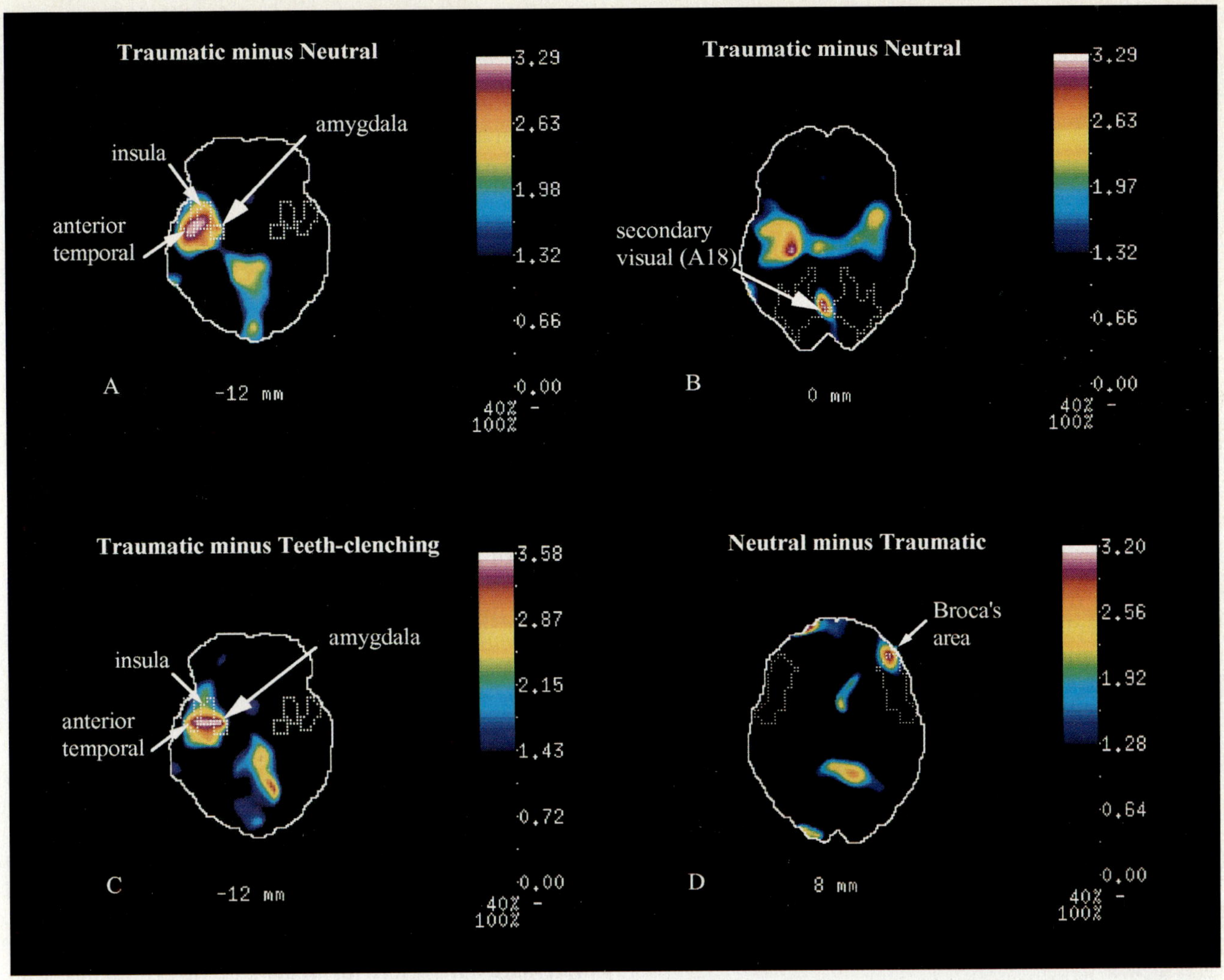

Positron emission tomography statistical parametric maps of Traumatic minus Control conditions for all subjects (N=8; 16 scans per condition) are displayed with a Sokoloff color scale in units of z score. White dashed outlines reflecting the boundaries of specified brain regions, as defined via a digitized version of the Talairach atlas,[42] are superimposed for anatomical reference. Whole-brain slice outlines are demarcated with solid lines. All images are transverse sections parallel to the intercommissural plane, shown in conventional neuroimaging orientation (top=anterior, bottom=posterior, right=left, left=right). Each transverse section is labeled with its z coordinate, denoting its position with respect to the intercommissural plane (superior >0). For the Traumatic minus Neutral condition, activation is located within right anterior temporal and insular cortex, the amygdala (panel A), and secondary visual cortex (panel B). Panel C, For the Traumatic minus Teeth-Clenching condition, the pattern of activation shown parallels that seen in panel B. Panel D, For the Neutral minus Traumatic condition, activation is located within left Broca's area (representing a decrease in relative blood flow associated with the Traumatic condition).

blood flow. It remains unclear whether changes in respiratory rate, P_{CO_2}, and whole-brain cerebral blood flow might confound findings in studies that rely on normalized cerebral blood flow values. Localization of activation is constrained by the spatial resolution of PET. Although head movement cannot be absolutely prevented, automated motion correction represents a major technical improvement.[1,2,37] Still, the potential for imperfectly corrected head motion combined with stereotaxic transformation represent potential sources of error in anatomic localization. In this study, the localization of activations within amygdala, anterior temporal pole, and insula cannot be made with certainty owing to these limitations. Nevertheless, the advantages of this technique remain: the capability to sum data across subjects and the superior statistical power of the SPM data analytic approach.

The teeth-clenching control results indicate that identified activations are not attributable to extracranial artifacts. They also suggest that our transformation and localization methods are effective at distinguishing between brain and extracranial sources. The Teeth-Clenching condition produced bilateral activation in primary sensorimotor cortex, similar to activations seen in the Traumatic condition but not the Neutral condition, which is consistent with psychophysiologic data documenting increased facial muscle contraction during traumatic vs neutral scripts. Moreover, this raises the possibility that the Teeth-Clenching condition represents a superior control for contrast with the Traumatic condition, since it, unlike the Neutral condition, controls for the cortical activation associated with facial muscle contraction.

The preponderance of right-sided brain findings for the Traumatic minus control conditions suggests a functional asymmetry in the mediating neuroanatomy of the PTSD symptomatic state. This is consistent with literature supporting the preferential role of the right hemisphere in anxiety and other adverse emotions.[47-49] In par-

Table 4. Brain Regions Exhibiting Significantly Decreased Activation Associated With Provocation of PTSD Symptoms

Brain Region	Maximum Pixel Value, z Score* Neutral Minus Traumatic	Maximum Pixel Coordinates†
Middle temporal cortex (left)	3.03‡	−61, −27, −8
Inferior frontal cortex (left Broca's area)	3.12‡	−43, 42, 8

*Values represent the actual maximum pixel value (in z score units) within the brain region from the statistical parametric map.

†Coordinates defining the location of the maximum pixel values within each brain region from the statistical parametric maps in Talairach space[38] are expressed as "x, y, z"; $x>0$ is right of the midsagittal plane, $y>0$ is anterior to the anterior commissure, and $z>0$ is superior to the intercommissural plane.

‡Regional activations with z scores ≥3.00, corresponding to $P=.001$ uncorrected for multiple comparisons.

ticular, the finding of right-sided anterior temporal activation replicates previous results in simple phobia,[2] as well as in patients with panic disorder.[25,50,51] Our findings also converge with a recent report of right dominant asymmetry in evoked potentials during recall of traumatic memories in a cohort of subjects with childhood trauma histories[52]; no such pattern was observed during recall of neutral memories or in a control cohort without history of childhood trauma.

It has been suggested that traumatic memories tend to be organized on a perceptual and affective level with limited semantic representation,[53-55] and tend to intrude as emotional or sensory fragments[11,56] related to the original event, with stability over time.[56-59] These observations have given rise to the notion that traumatic memories may be encoded differently than memories for ordinary events, possibly because of the high degree of emotional arousal at the time of consolidation.[53,60-65] Schacter[66] hypothesized that emotional memories are supported by a separate brain system. In this study, the activation of the amygdala supports its purported role in the pathogenesis of PTSD symptoms[16,17,67] and the proposed scheme of an amygdala-based emotional memory system.[20,62-64,66]

The finding of increased rCBF in secondary visual cortex during traumatic imagery suggests that activation of sensory brain structures might underlie reexperiencing phenomena in PTSD. Kosslyn et al[18] have shown that visual imagery is mediated by topographically organized visual cortex. Reexperiencing phenomena are to be distinguished from ordinary visual mental images; to the patient experiencing a flashback, it is "as if the traumatic event were recurring."[11(p428)] Such phenomena may require activation of visual cortex along with activation or deactivation of other brain regions.

The meaning of decreased rCBF in left-sided cortical territories during the Traumatic condition is unclear. The observed deactivation in Broca's area is consistent with the notion that patients with PTSD have difficulty cognitively structuring their traumatic experiences.[68,69]

The results of this study should be interpreted cautiously, pending replication. One recent PET study of PTSD, using a cognitive activation paradigm, an all-male combat veteran patient population with PTSD, and trauma-exposed non-PTSD controls, also found activations in anterior cingulate cortex and right amygdala, as well as deactivation in left Broca's area for selected contrasts in the PTSD group, and not in the control subjects.[70]

In summary, the present study demonstrated a pattern of changes in normalized rCBF associated with the PTSD symptomatic state, which includes increases in right-sided components of the limbic and paralimbic systems, as well as visual cortex, and decreases in left inferior frontal cortex. Future studies should seek to replicate these findings, to explore their specificity by including a trauma-exposed non-PTSD comparison cohort, and to integrate the relative merits of alternative experimental paradigms.

Accepted for publication October 26, 1995.

This study was supported in part by a Young Investigator Award from the National Alliance for Research on Schizophrenia and Depression, Chicago, Ill, grant MH01215 from the National Institute of Mental Health, Rockville, Md, and the Pfizer-sponsored Harvard-MIT Clinical Investigator Training Program, Cambridge, Mass (all to Dr Rauch); by grant 5T32CA09362 from the National Cancer Institute, Bethesda, Md (Drs Rauch and Savage); by the David Judah Research Fund, Boston, Mass (Drs Rauch, Savage, and Jenike); and by grants from the Veterans Affairs Medical Center, Manchester, NH, and grant MH48559 from the National Institute of Mental Health (Drs Orr and Pitman).

Presented in part at the 10th Annual Meeting of The International Society for Traumatic Stress Studies, Chicago, Ill, November 8, 1994.

The authors thank Dmitry Berdichevsky, MS, Linda Leahy, Avis Loring, and Steve Weise for technical contributions.

Reprints: Scott L. Rauch, MD, Department of Psychiatry, Massachusetts General Hospital—East, CNY-9130, 149 13th St, Charlestown, MA 02129.

REFERENCES

1. Rauch SL, Jenike MA, Alpert NM, Baer L, Breiter HCR, Savage CR, Fischman AJ. Regional cerebral blood flow measured during symptom provocation in obsessive-compulsive disorder using oxygen15–labeled carbon dioxide and positron emission tomography. *Arch Gen Psychiatry.* 1994;51:62-70.
2. Rauch SL, Savage CR, Alpert NM, Miguel EC, Baer L, Breiter HC, Fischman AJ, Manzo PA, Moretti C, Jenike MA. A positron emission tomographic study of simple phobic symptom provocation. *Arch Gen Psychiatry.* 1995;52:20-28.
3. Lang PJ. The cognitive psychophysiology of emotion: fear and anxiety. In: Tuma AH, Maser J, eds. *Anxiety and the Anxiety Disorders.* Hillsdale, NJ: Lawrence Erlbaum Associates; 1985:131-170.
4. Pitman RK, Orr SP, Forgue DF, de Jong JB, Claiborn JM. Psychophysiology of PTSD imagery in Vietnam combat veterans. *Arch Gen Psychiatry.* 1987;44:970-975.
5. Orr SP, Pitman RK, Lasko NB, Herz LR. Post-traumatic stress disorder imagery in World War II and Korean combat veterans. *J Abnorm Psychol.* 1993;102:152-159.
6. Pitman RK, Orr SP, Forgue DF, Altman B, de Jong JB, Herz LR. Psychophysiologic responses to combat imagery of Vietnam veterans with post-traumatic stress disorder vs. other anxiety disorders. *J Abnorm Psychol.* 1990;99:49-54.
7. Shalev AY, Orr SP, Pitman RK. Psychophysiologic assessment of traumatic imagery in Israeli civilian post-traumatic stress disorder patients. *Am J Psy-*

chiatry. 1993;150:620-624.
8. Orr SP. An overview of psychophysiological studies of PTSD. *PTSD Q.* 1994; 5:1-7.
9. Pitman RK. Post-traumatic stress disorder, conditioning, and network theory. *Psychiatr Ann.* 1988;18:182-189.
10. Pitman RK, Orr SP. Psychophysiology of emotional memory networks in posttraumatic stress disorder. In: McGaugh JL, Weinberger NM, Lynch G, eds. *Brain and Memory: Modulation and Mediation of Neuroplasticity.* New York, NY: Oxford University Press; 1995:75-83.
11. American Psychiatric Association. *Diagnostic and Statistical Manual of Mental Disorders, Fourth Edition.* Washington, DC: American Psychiatric Association; 1994.
12. Papez JW. Proposed mechanism of emotion. *Arch Neurol Psychiatry.* 1937; 38:725-743.
13. Mesulam M-M. Patterns in behavioral neuroanatomy: association areas, the limbic system, and hemispheric specialization. In: Mesulam M-M, ed. *Principles of Behavioral Neurology.* Philadelphia, Pa: FA Davis Co Publishers; 1985: 1-70.
14. Gorman JM, Liebowitz MR, Fyer AJ, Stein J. A neuroanatomical hypothesis for panic disorder. *Am J Psychiatry.* 1989;146:148-161.
15. Charney DS, Deutch AY, Krystal JH, Southwick SM, Davis M. Psychobiologic mechanisms of posttraumatic stress disorder. *Arch Gen Psychiatry.* 1993;50: 294-305.
16. van der Kolk BA. The body keeps the score: memory and the evolving psychobiology of posttraumatic stress. *Harvard Rev Psychiatry.* 1994;1:253-265.
17. Shalev AY, Rogel-Fuchs Y, Pitman RK. Conditioned fear and psychological trauma. *Biol Psychiatry.* 1992;31:863-865.
18. Kosslyn SM, Alpert NM, Thompson WL, Maljkovic V, Weise SB, Chabris CF, Hamilton SE, Rauch SL, Buonano FS. Visual imagery activates topographically organized visual cortex: PET investigations. *J Cogn Neurosci.* 1993;5:263-287.
19. Squire LR, Zola-Morgan S. The medial temporal lobe memory system. *Science.* 1991;253:2380-2386.
20. Squire LR. Mechanisms of memory. *Science.* 1986;232:1612-1619.
21. Zola-Morgan SM, Squire LR. The primate hippocampal formation: evidence for a time-limited role in memory storage. *Science.* 1990;250:288-290.
22. Bremner JD, Scott TM, Delaney RC, Southwick SM, Mason JW, Johnson DR, Innis RB, McCarthy G, Charney DS. Deficits in short-term memory in posttraumatic stress disorder. *Am J Psychiatry.* 1993;150:1015-1019.
23. Bremner JD, Seibyl JP, Scott TM, Southwick SM, Delaney RC, Mason JW, Scanley E, McCarthy G, Charney DS, Innis RB. Decreased hippocampal volume in posttraumatic stress disorder. In: Program and abstracts of the 145th annual meeting of the American Psychiatric Association; May 2-7, 1992; Washington, DC.
24. Semple WE, Goyer P, McCormick R, Morris E, Compton B, Muswick G, Nelson D, Donovan B, Leisure G, Berridge M, Miraldi F, Schulz SC. Preliminary report: brain blood flow using PET in patients with posttraumatic stress disorder and substance-abuse histories. *Biol Psychiatry.* 1993;34:115-118.
25. Drevets WC, Videen TO, MacLeod AK, Haller JW, Raichle ME. PET images of blood flow changes during anxiety: correction. *Science.* 1992;256:1696.
26. American Psychiatric Association. *Diagnostic and Statistical Manual of Mental Disorders, Third Edition, Revised.* Washington, DC: American Psychiatric Association; 1987.
27. Spitzer RL, Williams JBW, Gibbon M, First M. *Structured Clinical Interview for DSM-III-R (SCID).* Washington, DC: American Psychiatric Press; 1990.
28. Oldfield RC. The assessment and analysis of handedness: the Edinburgh Inventory. *Neuropsychologia.* 1971;9:97-113.
29. Blake DD, Weathers FW, Nagy LN, Kaloupek DG, Gusman F, Charney DS, Keane TM. The development of a Clinician-Administered PTSD Scale. *J Trauma Stress.* 1995;8:75-90.
30. Blake DD, Weathers FW, Nagy LN, Kaloupek DG, Klauminzer G, Charney DS, Keane TM. A clinician rating scale for assessing current and lifetime PTSD: the CAPS-1. *Behav Therapist.* 1990;13:187-188.
31. Weathers FW, Litz BT. Psychometric properties of the Clinician-Administered PTSD Scale, CAPS-1. *PTSD Res Q.* 1994;5:2-6.
32. Bernstein EM, Putnam FW. Development, reliability, and validity of a dissociation scale. *J Nerv Ment Dis.* 1986;174:727-735.
33. Keane TM, Caddell JM, Taylor KL. Mississippi Scale for Combat-Related Posttraumatic Stress Disorder: three studies in reliability and validity. *J Consult Clin Psychol.* 1988;56:85-90.
34. Weiss DF, Marmar CR, Metzler T, Ronfeldt H. Predicting symptomatic distress in emergency services personnel. *J Consult Clin Psychol.* 1995;63:361-368.
35. Weiss DF, Marmar CR. The Impact of Events Scale–Revised. In: Wilson JP, Keane TM, eds. *Assessing Psychological Trauma and PTSD: A Practitioner's Handbook.* New York, NY: Guilford Press. In press.
36. Kops ER, Herzog H, Schmid A, Holte S, Feinendegen LE. Performance characteristics of an eight-ring whole body PET scanner. *J Comput Assist Tomogr.* 1990;14:437-445.
37. Woods RP, Cherry SR, Mazziotta JC. Rapid automated algorithm for aligning and reslicing PET images. *J Comput Assist Tomogr.* 1992;16:620-633.
38. Talairach J, Tournoux P. *Co-Planar Stereotaxic Atlas of the Human Brain.* New York, NY: Thieme Medical Publishers Inc; 1988.
39. Alpert NM, Berdichevsky D, Weise S, Tang J, Rauch SL. Stereotactic transformation of PET scans by nonlinear least squares. In: Uemura K, Jones J, Lassen NA, Kanno I, eds. *Quantification of Brain Function: Tracer Kinetics and Image Analysis in Brain PET.* Amsterdam, the Netherlands: Elsevier Science Publishers; 1993:459-463.
40. Friston K, Frith C, Liddle P, Frackowiak R. Comparing functional (PET) images: the assessment of significant change. *J Cereb Blood Flow Metab.* 1991;11: 690-699.
41. Corbetta M, Miezin FM, Dobmeyer S, Shulman GL, Petersen SE. Selective and divided attention during visual discriminations of shape, color, and speed: functional anatomy by positron emission tomography. *J Neurosci.* 1991;11:2383-2402.
42. Talairach J, Szikla Z. *Atlas of Stereotactic Anatomy of the Telencephalon.* Paris, France: Masson et Cie; 1967.
43. George MS, Ketter TA, Parekh PI, Horowitz B, Herscovitch P, Post RM. Brain activity during transient sadness and happiness in healthy women. *Am J Psychiatry.* 1995;152:341-351.
44. Pardo JV, Pardo PJ, Raichle ME. Neural correlates of self-induced dysphoria. *Am J Psychiatry.* 1993;150:713-719.
45. Gottschalk LA, Buchsbaum MS, Gillin JC, Wu J, Reynolds CA, Herrera DB. Positron emission tomographic studies of the relationship of cerebral glucose metabolism and the magnitude of anxiety and hostility experienced during dreaming and waking. *J Neuropsychiatry.* 1991;3:131-142.
46. Gottschalk LA, Buchsbaum MS, Gillin JC, Wu J, Reynolds CA, Herrera DB. The effect of anxiety and hostility in silent mentation on localized cerebral glucose metabolism. *Compr Psychiatry.* 1992;33:52-59.
47. Ross ED. Modulation of affect and nonverbal communication by the right hemisphere. In: Mesulam M-M, ed. *Principles of Behavioral Neurology.* Philadelphia, Pa: FA Davis Co Publishers; 1985:239-258.
48. Silberman EK, Weingartner H. Hemispheric lateralization of functions related to emotion. *Brain Cogn.* 1986;5:322-353.
49. Tomarken AJ, Davidson RJ, Wheeler RE, Ross RC. Individual difference in anterior brain asymmetry and fundamental dimensions of emotion. *J Pers Soc Psychol.* 1992;64:676-687.
50. Reiman EM, Rachle ME, Butler FK, Herscovitch P, Robins E. A focal brain abnormality in panic disorder: a severe form of anxiety. *Nature.* 1984;310:683-685.
51. Reiman EM, Raichle ME, Robins E, Mintun MA, Fusselman MJ, Fox PT, Price JL, Hackman KA. Neuroanatomical correlates of a lactate-induced anxiety attack. *Arch Gen Psychiatry.* 1989;46:493-500.
52. Schiffer F, Teicher MH, Papanicolaou AC. Evoked potential evidence for right brain activity during recall of traumatic memories. *J Neuropsychiatry.* 1995; 7:169-175.
53. Janet P. *L'automatisme Psychologique.* Paris, France: Alcan; 1889.
54. Kardiner A. *The Traumatic Neuroses of War.* New York, NY: Hoeber; 1941.
55. van der Kolk BA, van der Hart O. The intrusive past: the flexibility of memory and the engraving of trauma. *Am Imago.* 1991;48:425-454.
56. van der Kolk BA, Fisler RE. Dissociation and the fragmentary nature of traumatic memories: overview and exploratory study. *J Trauma Stress.* 1995;8: 505-525.
57. Rainey RM, Aleem A, Ortiz A, Yaragani V, Pohl R, Berchow R. Laboratory procedure for the inducement of flashbacks. *Am J Psychiatry.* 1987;144:1317-1319.
58. Southwick SM, Krystal JH, Morgan CA, Johnson D, Nagy LM, Nicolaou A, Heninger GR, Charney DS. Abnormal noradrenergic function in posttraumatic stress disorder. *Arch Gen Psychiatry.* 1993;50:266-274.
59. van der Kolk BA, Blitz R, Burr WA, Hartmenn E. Nightmares and trauma: lifelong and traumatic nightmares in veterans. *Am J Psychiatry.* 1984;141:187-190.
60. Christianson SA. Emotional stress and eyewitness memory: a critical review. *Psychol Bull.* 1992;112:284-309.
61. Heuer F, Reisberg D. Vivid memories of emotional events: the accuracy of remembered minutiae. *Memory Cogn.* 1990;18:496-506.
62. LeDoux JE. Emotion as memory: anatomical systems underlying indelible neural traces. In: Christianson A, ed. *Handbook of Emotion and Memory.* Hillsdale, NJ: Lawrence Erlbaum Associates; 1992:269-288.
63. LeDoux JE, Romanski L, Xagoraris A. Indelibility of subcortical emotional memories. *J Cogn Neurosci.* 1991;1:238-243.
64. LeDoux JE. Information flow from sensation to emotion: plasticity of the neural computation of stimulus value. In: Gabriel M, Moore J, eds. *Learning Computational Neuroscience: Foundations of Adaptive Networks.* Cambridge, Mass: MIT Press; 1990:3-51.
65. Nilsson LG, Archer T. Perspective on animal learning and human memory. In: Nilsson LG, Archer T, eds. *Perspectives on Learning and Memory.* Hillsdale, NJ: Lawrence Erlbaum Associates; 1992:3-14.
66. Schacter DL. *Searching for Memory: The Brain, the Mind, and the Past.* New York, NY: Basic Books. In press.
67. Pitman RK, Orr SP, Shalev A. Once bitten, twice shy: beyond the conditioning model of PTSD. *Biol Psychiatry.* 1993;33:145-146.
68. van der Kolk BA. *Psychological Trauma.* Washington, DC: American Psychiatric Press; 1987.
69. van der Kolk BA, Ducey C. The psychological processing of traumatic experience: Rorschach patterns in PTSD. *J Trauma Stress.* 1989;2:259-274.
70. Shin LM, Kosslyn SM, McNally RJ, Pitman RK, Alpert NM, Rauch SL. A positron emission tomography study of combat-related post-traumatic stress disorder. Presented at the 10th Annual Meeting of The International Society for Traumatic Stress Studies; November 8, 1994; Chicago, Ill. Abstract.

A selective serotonin
reuptake inhibitor for OCD

LUVOX™

fluvoxamine maleate 50 mg & 100 mg SCORED TABLETS

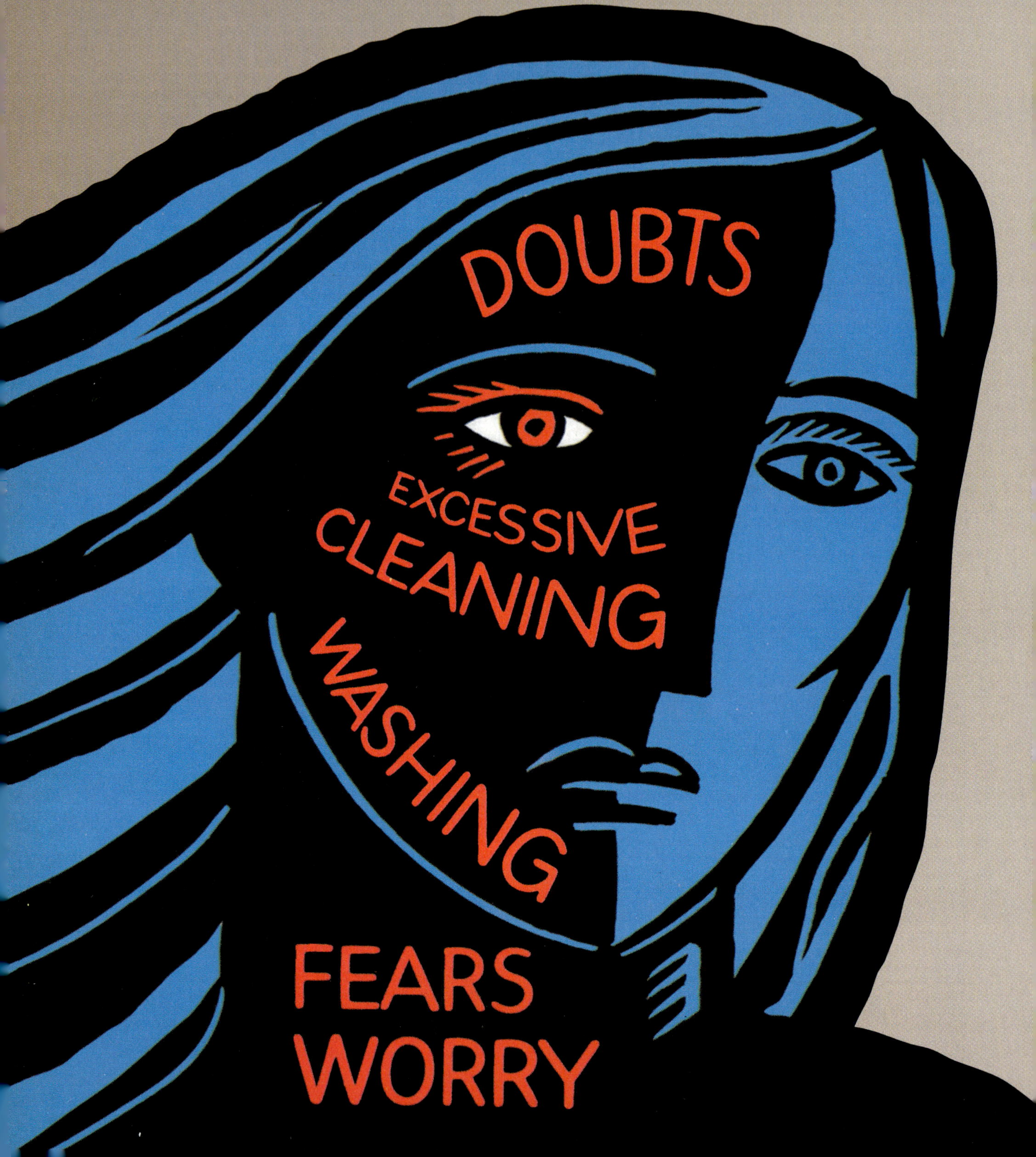

The Identification and Validation of Distinct Depressive Syndromes in a Population-Based Sample of Female Twins

Kenneth S. Kendler, MD; Lindon J. Eaves, PhD, DSc; Ellen E. Walters, MS; Michael C. Neale, PhD; Andrew C. Heath, DPhil; Ronald C. Kessler, PhD

Background: Depression, a clinically heterogeneous syndrome, may also be etiologically heterogeneous. Using a prospective, epidemiologic, and genetically informative sample of adult female twins, we identify and validate a typology of depressive syndromes.

Methods: Latent class analysis was applied to 14 disaggregated *DSM-III-R* symptoms for major depression reported over the last year by members of 1029 female-female twin pairs.

Results: Seven classes were identified, of which 3 represented clinically significant depressive syndromes: (1) *mild typical depression*, (2) *atypical depression*, and (3) *severe typical depression*. Severe typical depression was characterized by comorbid anxiety and panic, long episodes, impairment, and help seeking. Atypical depression was similar in severity to mild typical depression, but was characterized by increased eating, hypersomnia, frequent, relatively short episodes, and a proclivity to obesity. Individuals with recurrent episodes tended to have the same syndrome on each occasion. The members of twin pairs concordant for depression had the same depressive syndrome more often than expected by chance and this resemblance was greater in monozygotic than in dizygotic pairs.

Conclusion: In an epidemiologic sample of female twins, depression is not etiologically homogeneous, but is instead made up of several syndromes that are at least partially distinct from a clinical, longitudinal, and familial/genetic perspective.

(Arch Gen Psychiatry. 1996;53:391-399)

From the Departments of Psychiatry (Drs Kendler, Neale, and Eaves and Ms Walters) and Human Genetics (Drs Kendler and Eaves), Medical College of Virginia/Virginia Commonwealth University, Richmond; the Institute for Social Research, University of Michigan, Ann Arbor (Dr Kessler); and the Department of Psychiatry, Washington University School of Medicine, St Louis, Mo (Dr Heath).

DESPITE DECADES of research,[1-4] it is still uncertain whether depression is a homogeneous clinical syndrome and, if not, whether it is possible to identify meaningful and valid subtypes. From a methodologic perspective, typological studies of depression can be characterized in 4 ways. First, a wide array of the statistical methods have been used including factor analysis,[5-7] discriminant function analysis,[8,9] cluster analysis,[3,5,10] grade of membership analysis,[11-13] latent trait analysis,[14] and latent class analysis (LCA).[10,15-18] Second, samples have been ascertained in varying settings, including psychiatric hospitals,[5,10,15,19] outpatient clinics,[13] primary care practices,[9,14] and the general population.[7,11,12,16,17] Third, different assessment tools have been used including self-report checklists,[9] clinician completed rating scales,[8,13,19] and structured psychiatric interviews.[7,10-12,15-17] Fourth, efforts to validate the proposed typology have varied widely, from the examination of treatment response,[13] relapse rate,[10] pattern of psychiatric illness in relatives[10,13,19] to replication in a second sample.[16]

A small proportion of individuals affected with major depression (MD) are in specialist care,[20,21] and of these, few are hospitalized. Those seen in psychiatric treatment settings are not a random sample of those affected in the population, as they are more severely affected and more likely to demonstrate certain symptoms such as suicidal ideation.[22] Therefore, a "natural" typology of depressive syndromes may more likely emerge from epidemiologic samples.[16]

In this study, we examine a typology of depression based on an LCA of all depressive symptoms from the *DSM-III-R* criteria for MD as they occurred over the last year in a large sample of female twins from a population-based registry. We then attempt to empirically validate this typology.[23,24]

See Methods on next page

METHODS

SAMPLE AND ASSESSMENT METHODS

Data for the LCA analysis were collected from 2163 white female same-sex twins ascertained through a population-based twin registry in the state of Virginia.[25] Zygosity diagnoses were based on a series of standard questions, photographs, and in cases of uncertainty, DNA polymorphisms. In this report, we examine twins from the 1029 pairs of known zygosity (589 monozygotic [MZ] and 440 dizygotic [DZ]) where both twins had been personally interviewed and had responded to all symptom questions. The mean (±SD) age of this sample at initial interview was 30.1±7.5 years.

Information was collected from respondents on the occurrence during the year prior to interview of 20 individual symptoms. Fourteen of these symptoms were the disaggregated 9 "A Criteria" for MD in *DSM-III-R*[26] (**Table 1**) and were used in the latent class analysis. Six of the 9 criteria were represented by a single item. Two criteria were disaggregated into 2 items: criterion A4, insomnia and hypersomnia and criterion A5, psychomotor retardation and agitation. One criterion, A2, was disaggregated into 4 items: decreased appetite, increased appetite, decreased weight, and increased weight. The 6 remaining items reflected hopelessness, irritability, and the cognitive and somatic aspects of generalized anxiety and panic.

Symptoms were required to have a duration of at least 5 days. For each symptom that was reported as present, interviewers probed to determine if it was due to physical illness or medication. If this was the case, which occurred an average of 17.4% of the time across all symptoms, then the symptom was considered not present.

If only 1 symptom was reported, that single symptom was analyzed. If 2 or more symptoms were reported, the respondent was asked whether any of the symptoms co-occurred. If no, then the single more severe symptom determined by the twin was analyzed. If 2 or more symptoms co-occurred, this defined a syndrome. If only 1 syndrome was present in the last year, then this was analyzed. If 2 or more syndromes were present in the last year (which occurred in 14.6% of the sample), then we examined the syndrome with more symptoms, giving greater weight to depressive symptoms.

For the most prominent symptom or syndrome, respondents were asked a series of further questions including number of occurrences during the last year, longest duration, degree of impairment, and help seeking.

If twins responded to either of the 2 questions for generalized anxiety disorder (GAD) or panic, they were then asked, for the last year, questions assessing *DSM-III-R* criteria for GAD and panic disorder.

POTENTIAL VALIDATORS

In a separate section of the interview, respondents were asked about any history of MD, GAD, or panic disorder *prior* to the last year, as well as any lifetime history of phobia, bulimia, and alcoholism. The interview booklet was blindly reviewed by one of us (K.S.K.) and diagnoses were assigned using *DSM-III-R* criteria for the last year and prior to the last year. The GAD criteria were modified in 2 ways. First, the *DSM-III*[27] 1-month rather than 6-month minimum duration was used. Second, the diagnostic hierarchy, in which GAD could not be diagnosed if only present during a depressive episode, was dropped. Four phobia subtypes were examined.[28]

Body mass index (BMI represents a measure of weight in kilograms divided by the square of the height in meters) was calculated using self-report data. Significantly overweight and obese in this female population were defined, respectively, as a BMI of more than 23.8 and 28.6 or more.[29] Personality was assessed using an adapted version of the short form of Eysenck's Personality Questionnaire[30,31] obtained by a mailed questionnaire at least 1 year *prior* to the interview at which depressive symptoms were reported.

RESULTS

THE CLASSES: ENDORSED SYMPTOMS

Table 1 depicts the observed class membership and endorsement frequencies for all 14 depressive symptoms in the best fitting LCA model. Class 1 was the largest class, constituting 52.2% of the sample. Of the individuals in this class, two thirds denied any depressive symptoms in the last year and the remaining one third endorsed 1 symptom—most commonly depressed mood, feeling tired, or gaining weight.

Members of class 2—4.6% of the sample—endorsed on average (mean±SD) 2.3±1.0 individual symptoms. All reported increased appetite, the only other symptoms commonly endorsed being weight gain and depressed mood. None of these twins met *DSM-III-R* criteria for MD.[26]

The individuals in class 3, who made up 21.6% of the sample, endorsed 2.8±1.0 co-occurring symptoms, most commonly the "core" depressive symptoms of depressed mood or loss of interest and/or pleasure. Vegetative symptoms, except for tiredness, were rare. Only 3.8% of the individuals in this class met criteria for MD.

Members of class 4, who consisted of 7.2% of the sample, endorsed a mean (±SD) of 3.1±1.3 individual depressive symptoms. More than half of these twins endorsed decreased appetite and depressed mood, other commonly reported symptoms being weight loss, trouble sleeping, and feeling of tiredness. A diagnosis of MD was made for 2% of these twins.

Twins in class 5 made up 8.9% of the sample and reported a mean (±SD) of 6.3±1.3 co-occurring depressive symptoms. Nearly all twins in this class reported depressed mood and more than half described loss of interest and/or pleasure, decreased appetite, trouble sleeping, feelings of tiredness, and psychomotor agitation. More than 30% endorsed weight loss, guilt, and trouble concentrating. However, almost none of the twins in this class reported increased appetite or weight gain, and hypersomnia was also rare. Of the twins in this class, 66.1% met *DSM-III-R* criteria for MD.

Individuals in class 6, who constituted 3.9% of the sample, reported a mean (±SD) of 6.2±1.5 co-occurring depressive symptoms. Ninety-seven percent of these twins endorsed depressed mood and 80% loss of interest and/or pleasure. In contrast to class 5, these twins commonly re-

We also asked about the occurrence and dating of 9 "personal" and 22 "network" stressful life events (SLEs) over the month of the interview and the 12 preceding months.[32] To assess the relationships between SLEs and the depressive syndromes, we examined the frequency of "severe" SLEs in the month preceding or the month of onset of the depressive syndrome, severe events being defined as those 4 events that increased the risk of onset of *DSM-III-R* MD by at least 10-fold: assault, serious marital problems, divorce or break-up, and death of a close relative.[32]

In addition, an average (mean±SD) of 17±3.7 months after their initial interview, twins were reinterviewed by telephone with a 92.5% cooperation rate. This telephone interview contained the same assessment of last year symptoms used in their initial face-to-face interview.

STATISTICAL ANALYSIS

Typically, multivariate analyses in psychiatric genetics have been confined to linear structural modeling, as implemented by programs such as LISREL 7[33] and Mx.[34] Although these approaches have been fruitful, they emphasize a "dimensional" approach to psychiatric disorders. By contrast, LCA assumes that psychiatric disorders are, by their nature, "categorical."[35] Latent class analysis, which can probably be best characterized as a "categorical analog" of factor analysis, is based on the following major assumptions:

- There exist m (>1, to be determined) mutually exclusive and exhaustive classes of subjects within the population.
- The distribution of responses to each item is entirely determined by class membership.
- Within each class, responses to individual items are independent.

Using a FORTRAN program written by 1 of us (L.J.E.),[36] we applied LCA to a 2058×14-data matrix (individual twins × symptoms of the disaggregated 9 "A Criteria" for MD in *DSM-III-R*) and identified 7 classes (details available on request). Individual twins were then assigned class membership based on the likelihood of their particular response profiles. The median likelihood ratio between the most and next most likely class was 12.4; 75.1% of the sample was assigned to a class with a likelihood ratio of more than 3.0. This computer program, including the algorithm for class assignment, is available to interested researchers. The purpose of our study is to present these results for clinical and research considerations, and to test the validity of the classes so identified.

Data concerning the occurrence of symptoms in the 12 months after the initial interview were also available on a slightly smaller sample (n=1874) obtained from a follow-up interview conducted by telephone 1 year later. The solution for the first year of interview was imposed on the data from the second year to examine changes in class membership over time.

Exploratory analyses were then performed to examine characteristics of the classes of depressive episodes (eg, level of impairment, average duration, frequency), as well as comorbidity of the classes with other disorders. Comparisons of mean values of these descriptive variables among classes were performed using generalized linear models in SAS.[37] Multiple comparison tests using the GT2 method of Hochberg[38] were performed to more closely examine the differences among the means when the overall F test of the means was significant. Complete tables of these pairwise comparisons can be obtained from the senior author. Discussion of comparisons among classes is limited to 3 classes which, on examination, appeared to describe MD-like syndromes. In addition, classes were examined across twin pairs to examine possible familiality of class membership. To maximize our sample size of twin pairs concordant for a depressive syndrome, we examined class membership either at the first or second personal interview. If an individual had a depressive syndrome at each assessment, she was classified on the basis of her first episode.

ported *increased* appetite and weight gain, only rarely endorsing decreased appetite or weight loss. While insomnia was endorsed by over twice as many twins in class 5 as in class 6, hypersomnia was reported by over 3 times as many twins in class 6 as in class 5. While psychomotor agitation was considerably more common in members of class 5 compared with class 6, retardation was endorsed more frequently by twins in class 6 than in class 5. Forty-six percent of the twins in class 6 met *DSM-III-R* criteria for MD.

Individuals in class 7, who constituted only 1.6% of the sample, were far and away the most symptomatic, endorsing on average (mean±SD) 9.9±1.2 co-occurring depressive symptoms. *All* individuals in this class endorsed depressed mood, loss of interest and/or pleasure, psychomotor agitation, tiredness, and insomnia. Seventy percent or more also reported psychomotor retardation, trouble concentrating, and feelings of guilt. Decreased appetite, weight loss, and insomnia were reported considerably more frequently than increased appetite, weight gain, and hypersomnia. Nearly all individuals in this class (96.9%) met *DSM-III-R* criteria for MD.

Pairwise comparisons of all classes indicate that classes 5 through 7 are significantly different from all other classes for the percentage diagnosed with MD, while classes 2 through 4 did not differ. In addition, on average individuals in class 7 endorsed significantly more symptoms than subjects in any other class. Classes 5 and 6 did not significantly differ from each other in the average number of symptoms endorsed, but both had greater symptom frequencies than classes 1 through 4. Thus, classes 5 through 7 represent potential "clinical" depressive syndromes and we will refer to them as follows: class 5 "mild typical depression," class 6 "atypical depression," and class 7 "severe typical depression." While some of the subsequent analyses will examine all classes, others will be restricted to these 3 clinical classes.

THE CLASSES: OTHER CLINICAL CHARACTERISTICS

Table 2 examines clinical characteristics of the 7 classes as delineated by LCA. Age at interview differed significantly across all classes, largely due to a younger age of those in class 4. However, age did not differ in the 3 clinical classes. All classes, as well as the 3 clinical classes,

Table 1. Observed Class Membership and Endorsement Frequencies of 14 Depressive Symptoms in the Best Fitting Latent Class Model

	*DSM-III-R**	Prevalence by Class 1	2	3	4	5	6	7
Symptom								
Felt depressed	A1	0.15	0.28	0.61	0.53	0.99	0.97	1.00
Loss of interest and/or pleasure	A2	0.00	0.06	0.42	0.16	0.82	0.80	1.00
Decreased appetite	A3	0.00	0.00	0.00	0.91	0.58	0.05	0.69
Increased appetite	A3	0.00	1.00	0.00	0.02	0.01	0.64	0.19
Weight loss	A3	0.01	0.00	0.00	0.47	0.42	0.00	0.43
Weight gain	A3	0.06	0.44	0.04	0.01	0.00	0.60	0.14
Insomnia	A4	0.04	0.14	0.24	0.27	0.60	0.27	1.00
Hypersomnia	A4	0.00	0.00	0.08	0.02	0.12	0.41	0.24
Psychomotor agitation	A5	0.03	0.08	0.23	0.16	0.57	0.36	1.00
Psychomotor retardation	A5	0.00	0.05	0.11	0.04	0.28	0.30	0.73
Tired	A6	0.06	0.15	0.33	0.24	0.59	0.69	1.00
Guilt	A7	0.00	0.03	0.19	0.08	0.46	0.36	0.83
Trouble concentrating	A8	0.00	0.04	0.16	0.12	0.48	0.23	0.86
Suicide	A9	0.00	0.01	0.04	0.05	0.18	0.14	0.38
Observed class membership, %		52.2	4.6	21.6	7.2	8.9	3.9	1.6
N		1075	95	445	148	183	86	32
% Diagnosed MD by *DSM-III-R*		0.0	0.0	3.8	2.0	66.1	46.3	96.9
No. of symptoms, mean		0.4	2.3	2.8	3.1	6.3	6.2	9.9
No. of symptoms, ±SD		0.5	1.0	1.0	1.3	1.3	1.5	1.2

**The* DSM-III-R *"A Criteria" for major depression (MD) reflected by the individual symptoms.*

significantly differed for the other 4 characteristics. The typical clinical classes had a syndrome of longer duration than the nonclinical classes, while the class representing atypical depression did not differ in duration from the nonclinical classes. Among the clinical classes, severe typical depression had significantly longer episodes than either mild typical or atypical depression.

For number of episodes in the last year, the most deviant class was that with atypical depression, which had significantly more frequent episodes than mild typical depression but not severe typical depression. Both severe impairment and treatment seeking were reported significantly more frequently by the clinical than by the nonclinical classes and were significantly more common in those with severe typical depression than in those with mild typical or atypical depression, which did not, in turn, differ significantly from each other.

Endorsement rates for the 6 co-occurring additional symptoms, inquired of in all twins, are seen for all 7 classes in **Table 3**. The endorsement rates for all of these 6 symptoms differed significantly both across all 7 classes and within the 3 clinical classes. Those with severe typical depression endorsed all 6 of these symptoms significantly more frequently than those with mild typical or atypical depression. Cases with mild typical depression reported all of these symptoms more frequently than those with atypical depression, and this difference was significant for 3 of the 6 symptoms: hopeless, anxious, and tense. Of the 4 remaining classes, class 1 reported significantly lower rates of irritability, hopelessness, and anxiousness than all other classes. Among classes 2 through 4, no consistent pattern of differences in the 6 symptoms was detected.

Table 3 also depicts the frequency with which members of the 7 clinical classes had GAD or a panic disorder, diagnosed by *DSM-III-R* criteria, in the last year that *co-occurred* with their depressive syndrome. These rates differed significantly both across all 7 classes and within the 3 clinical classes. The results were particularly striking for GAD. While 78.1% of those with severe typical depression also met criteria for GAD during the depressive episode, the comparable figures for mild typical and atypical depression were 32% and 15%, respectively—all significantly different from one another.

THE CLASSES: LIFETIME PREVALENCE OF OTHER DISORDERS

Lifetime prevalence rates for alcoholism in the 3 clinical classes were similar: mild typical depression, 28.1%; atypical depression, 26.3%; and severe typical depression, 24.6%. For phobias, severe typical depression had substantially higher rates (59.4%) than either mild typical depression (42.6%) or atypical depression (48.8%). The difference between mild and severe typical depression approached significance (odds ratio [OR]=1.97, $P<.08$). We then examined specific phobic subtypes and found that the rates of neither animal nor social phobia distinguished the 3 clinical classes. However, compared with those with mild typical or atypical depression, individuals with severe typical depression had significantly higher lifetime prevalences of both agoraphobia and situational phobia. Twins with atypical depression had the highest lifetime prevalence of bulimia (19.0%), followed by those with severe typical (15.6%) and mild typical depression (6.6%). Compared with those with mild typical depression, twins with atypical depression were at a significantly increased risk for bulimia (OR=3.34, $P<.01$).

Table 2. Clinical Characteristics of the 7 Classes Delineated by Latent Class Analysis

Class	Longest Duration, d*	No. of Episodes, Last Year*	Age at Interview, y*	% Severe Impairment	% Seeking Treatment
1	...	...	30.2 (7.7)	4.4†	7.2‡
2	29.4 (55.6)	2.7 (2.8)	31.7 (7.5)	5.1†	13.7
3	23.4 (45.0)	2.7 (3.3)	29.8 (7.4)	11.1†	17.3
4	27.7 (57.1)	1.7 (1.4)	27.2 (6.9)	5.8†	12.2
5	59.7 (79.8)	2.7 (2.7)	30.8 (7.2)	22.4	31.7
6	42.6 (72.6)	3.6 (3.2)	31.1 (7.4)	16.3	25.6
7	111.5 (113.4)	2.3 (2.4)	30.8 (6.8)	43.8	56.3
F (*df*)§	20.6‖ (5, 977)	4.7‖ (5, 974)	5.1‖ (6, 2051)	...	...
F (*df*)¶	8.1‖ (2, 292)	3.6# (2, 292)	0.1 (2, 292)	...	...
χ^2_6§	...	...	...	71.1	113.2
χ^2_2¶	...	...	...	10.3#	9.9#

*Mean±SD.
†N smaller than class total, only those with 2 or more concurrent symptoms queried.
‡N smaller than class total, only those with 1 or more symptoms queried.
§Test over all 7 categories.
‖P<.001
¶Test only over the 3 categories representing "clinical" depression: classes 5, 6, and 7.
#P<.05.

BMI AND PERSONALITY

Because the typical and atypical depressive syndromes were most clearly distinguished by a different pattern of appetite and weight change, we investigated BMI. Body mass index differed significantly both across all 7 classes (F=15.65, *df*=6/2043, *P*=.000) and across the 3 clinical classes (F =17.79, *df*=2/289, *P*=.000). Body mass index was highly significantly greater in women with atypical depression (mean±SE, 26.0±0.6) than in either those with mild or severe typical depression (22.3±0.3 and 21.9±0.6, respectively). Of those with atypical depression, 60.0% were significantly overweight compared with 22.4% of those with mild and 18.8% of those with severe typical depression (χ^2=39.01, *df*=2, *P*=.000). Criteria for obesity were met by 28.9% of women with atypical depression and only 6.0% and 3.1% of those with mild and severe typical depression, respectively (χ^2=30.15, *df*=2, *P*=.000).

Although increased above those without major depressive symptoms, the levels of neuroticism did *not* differentiate between the 3 depressive classes (F=0.44, *df*=2/230, *P*=not significant). By contrast, of all 7 classes, those with atypical depression had the lowest level of extraversion, with scores on this dimension significantly differentiating the 3 clinical classes (F=3.85, *df*=2/230, *P*=.02).

THE CLASSES: PRIOR STRESSFUL LIFE EVENTS

The occurrence of severe SLEs was examined in the month prior to and the month of the onset of the depressive episode. In a random 2-month period in twins without clinical depressive syndromes, severe SLEs occurred 5.5% of the time. Severe SLEs were associated with the onset of mild typical, atypical, and severe typical depression at 20.4%, 20.0%, and 28.3% of the time, respectively. While the frequency of severe SLEs was increased above chance expectation in all of these 3 groups (χ^2=65.6, 40.0, and 40.7, respectively, all with *df*=1 and *P*=.000), they did not differ significantly from one another (χ^2=1.59, *df*=2, *P*=not significant).

THE CLASSES: LONGITUDINAL ANALYSES

We first examined whether the kind of depressive syndrome experienced in the year preceding the first interview predicted having any of the 3 clinical depressive syndromes in the year prior to the second interview. Compared with those in the "nonclinical classes" (1 through 4) at the first interview, the ORs for the clinical classes were mild typical depression, 3.89 (*P*=.000); atypical depression, 8.29 (*P*=.000); and severe typical depression, 6.06 (*P*=.000).

We next examined the 106 individuals who reported a syndrome in 1 of the 3 depressive classes in *both* the year prior to the first interview *and* the year prior to the second interview. As seen in **Table 4** (which shows the observed, expected, and χ^2 value for each of the 9 cells), the proportion of twins who had the same depressive syndrome during both periods of assessment substantially exceeded chance expectation (χ^2=17.69, *df*=4, *P*=.001). Examining only those twins with depressive syndromes during both years, the OR for having the *same* depressive class on both occasions was similar for mild typical depression (3.39) and atypical depression (5.78), but lower for severe typical depression (1.56).

THE CLASSES: LIFETIME HISTORY OF PSYCHIATRIC DISORDERS AND BMI IN CO-TWINS

Table 5 presents the ORs for the lifetime risk for psychiatric disorders in the co-twin of a twin in 1 depressive class compared with the co-twin of a twin in another depressive class. Compared with co-twins of twins with mild typical depression, co-twins of twins with severe typical depression were at increased lifetime risk for all the psychiatric disorders examined. The increase, however, did not reach significance for any disorder. Compared with co-twins of twins with atypical depression, co-twins of twins with severe typical depression were at increased risk for MD, alcoholism, panic disorder, pho-

Table 3. Endorsement Frequencies of Other Symptoms and Anxiety Disorders by Class

	Class 1	2	3	4	5	6	7	Overall, χ^2_6	Within Depressive Classes 5-7, χ^2_2
Other symptoms									
Irritable	7.4	28.4	29.7	16.2	58.5	46.3	78.1	393.1	9.8
Hopeless	5.0	14.7	23.4	16.9	69.4	55.6	96.9	629.1	18.8
Anxiety symptoms									
Anxious	16.6	27.4	42.9	39.2	71.6	50.0	90.6	342.4	20.4
Tense	2.8	4.2	12.1	7.4	36.6	22.5	90.6	443.9	45.6
Frightened	3.2	2.1	3.6	2.7	15.3	13.8	40.6	145.0	13.2
Heart racing	3.7	1.1	5.2	4.1	14.2	10.0	31.3	80.9	8.3
Anxiety disorders									
Generalized anxiety disorder (GAD) co-occur	5.3*	5.3	8.5	4.7	32.2	15.0	78.1	207.9	41.5
Panic co-occur	1.1*	1.1	2.5	1.4	7.7	5.0	18.8	41.4	5.9 (not significant)
GAD and/or panic	6.3*	6.3	9.9	5.4	36.1	17.5	78.1	201.7	36.7

Odds Ratios for Risk of Symptom or Disorder for Twin in Depressive Class (A) Compared With Risk of Disease for Twin in Depressive Class (B)

Class A/B	Irritable	Hopeless	Anxious	Tense	Frightened	Heart Race	GAD	Panic
5/6	1.24	1.51	2.64†	1.85‡	0.74	1.19	2.48†	1.02
7/5	1.83	11.65‡	6.32	8.82§	2.78†	1.98	6.80§	2.16
7/6	2.26	17.63†	16.69†	16.33§	2.06	2.36	16.84§	2.21

*Applies only to those who endorsed at least 1 depression symptom.
†$P<.01$.
‡$P<.05$.
§$P<.001$.

Table 4. Observed and Expected Values and χ^2 Statistics for Twins Who Were Classified in a Depressive Class From Symptoms Reported in the Year Before Both the First and Second Interview*

	Second Interview		
First Interview	Mild Typical	Atypical	Severe Typical
Mild typical	40 (32.3) 1.8	13 (19.5) 2.2	6 (7.2) 0.2
Atypical	7 (15.9) 5.0	18 (9.6) 7.4	4 (3.6) 0.1
Severe typical	11 (9.8) 0.1	4 (5.9) 0.6	3 (2.2) 0.3

*For each cell, the observed number is given, followed within parentheses by the expected value; beneath these, is the χ^2 value for that cell. Total number equals 106.

bias, and GAD but at decreased risk for bulimia. Again, there was no significant difference for any disorder. Compared with co-twins of twins with mild typical depression, co-twins of twins with atypical depression had a relatively similar risk for the psychiatric disorders examined, except for bulimia, where their risk was nearly tripled. This difference was statistically significant.

Compared with co-twins of twins in the nonclinical classes, BMI was significantly elevated in co-twins of twins with atypical depression (b=2.17, *t*=4.98, *P*=.000). The BMI was also significantly elevated in the co-twins of twins with mild typical depression, but the associated increase was about half as large as that seen in co-twins of twins with atypical depression (b=1.17, *t*=2.60, *P*=.01). By contrast, BMI was not elevated in co-twins of twins with severe typical depression (b=0.16, *t*=0.24, *P*=not significant).

CONCORDANCE OF SPECIFIC DEPRESSIVE SYNDROMES IN TWIN PAIRS

Including both years of assessment, the sample contained 94 twin pairs where both twins had had a mild typical, atypical, or severe typical depressive episode, 54 of whom were MZ and 38 DZ (**Table 6**). The MZ pairs demonstrated a much more significant concordance for class membership (χ^2=16.08, *df*=4, *P*=.001; κ=+0.55, reference 39) than did the DZ twins (χ^2=5.10, *df*=4, *P*=.28, κ=+0.37). Substantial concordances were found for all 3 clinical syndromes in the MZ twin pairs: mild typical OR, 5.9; atypical OR, 5.4; and severe typical OR, 15.7. The degree of twin similarity was less striking in the DZ pairs: mild typical OR, 1.3; atypical OR, 1.0; and severe typical OR, 5.4.

Table 7 presents a summary of the findings associated with the 3 clinical classes of mild typical, atypical, and severe typical depression.

COMMENT

SUBTYPES OF DEPRESSION AS IDENTIFIED BY LATENT CLASS ANALYSIS

Examining the pattern of symptom endorsement in the last year for the 14 disaggregated *DSM-III-R* criteria for MD in our epidemiologic sample of female twins, LCA identified 7 classes. The first 2 classes, which demonstrated few if any depressive symptoms, bore no apparent relationship to clinical depression.

Table 5. Odds Ratio for Lifetime Risk of Disease in Co-twin of Twin in Depressive Class (A) Compared With Risk to Co-twin of Twin in Depressive Class (B)*

Class A/B	MD	ALC	Panic	Phobia	Bulimia	GAD
Atypical/mild typical	1.01	1.05	1.23	0.89	2.80†	0.66
Severe typical/mild typical	1.25	1.05	1.62	1.62	1.65	2.20
Severe typical/atypical	1.23	1.03	1.36	2.03	0.59	3.21

**MD indicates major depression; ALC, alcoholism; and GAD, generalized anxiety disorder.*
†Significant at $P<.01$.

Table 6. Similarity for Specific Depressive Syndromes in Twin Pairs Where Both Members Reported a 'Clinical' Depression*

	Monozygotic Twin Pairs, Twin 2		
Twin 1	Mild Typical	Atypical	Severe Typical
Mild typical	25 (20.0)	4 (7.8)	1 (2.2)
	1.3	1.8	0.7
Atypical	9 (12.7)	9 (4.9)	1 (1.4)
	1.1	3.4	0.1
Severe typical	2 (3.3)	1 (1.3)	2 (0.4)
	0.5	0.1	7.2

	Dizygotic Twin Pairs, Twin 2		
Twin 1	Mild Typical	Atypical	Severe Typical
Mild typical	12 (12.5)	4 (3.5)	3 (3.0)
	0.0	0.1	0.0
Atypical	9 (7.2)	2 (2.0)	0 (1.7)
	0.4	0.0	1.7
Severe typical	4 (5.3)	1 (1.5)	3 (1.3)
	0.3	0.2	2.4

**For each cell, the observed number is given, followed within parentheses by the expected value; beneath these, is the χ^2 value for that cell.*

Table 7. Summary of Overall Results*

	Mild Typical	Atypical	Severe Typical
Severity of depression	Moderate	Moderate	Severe
Vegetative symptoms	Typical	Atypical	Typical
Length of episodes	Intermediate	Short	Long
Comorbid: GAD + panic	Sometimes	Infrequent	Often
Other lifetime disorders	...	↑ Bulimia	↑ Phobia
BMI	Normal	Increased	Normal
Extraversion	...	Decreased	...
Risk of illness in co-twin	...	↑ Bulimia?	↑ GAD
Predict future risk of depression	Increased	Increased	Markedly increased
Stability over time	Moderate	Moderate	Moderate
Concordance in affected MZ twin pairs	Moderate	High	High

**GAD indicates generalized anxiety disorder; BMI, body mass index; upward arrow, increased; question mark, nonsignificant trends; and MZ, monozygotic.*

The third and fourth classes, which together constituted 30% of the sample, reported depressive syndromes with 2 to 4 individual symptoms. Although almost none of these twins met criteria for MD, 10% reported incapacitation, 45% moderate impairment, and 15% sought professional help. These conditions were recurrent, typically lasting 3 to 4 weeks. We know relatively little about these syndromes of "minor depression disorder."

All the 3 remaining classes, 5 through 7, bore some resemblance to clinical depression. With respect to *severity*, classes 5 and 6 were similar and reflected a depressive syndrome of mild to moderate intensity. By contrast, class 7 was substantially more severe. However, the *pattern* of symptoms revealed a different grouping. While classes 5 and 7 were characterized by decreases in the vegetative functions of eating and sleeping, class 6 was characterized by increases.

VALIDATION OF THESE PUTATIVE SUBTYPES

We attempted to validate our putative typology of depression in several ways, the results of 5 of which are particularly noteworthy. First, we examined their co-occurrence with anxiety symptoms, which strongly discriminated all 7 classes and the 3 clinical classes. Uniformly, individuals with severe typical depression endorsed anxiety and panic symptoms at rates 2 to 4 times higher than the other 2 clinical classes. A similar pattern was seen with anxiety disorders. More than 75% of twins with severe typical depression had, at the same time, an anxiety syndrome diagnosable as either GAD or panic disorder. In this epidemiologic sample of women, severe depression rarely occurred *without* major symptoms of anxiety.

Second, we examined lifetime prevalence of other psychiatric disorders. Some differences were found. Severe typical depression had the highest prevalence rates of phobia, while the risk of bulimia was highest in atypical depression.

Third, the association between BMI and depressive class was particularly striking. On average, twins with atypical depression weighed 9 kg more than those with mild typical depression and 7.2 kg more than those with severe typical depression. Along with the association with bulimia, these findings suggest that individuals with atypical depression may have a vulnerability to excess eating under stress. Our results replicate the previous findings of Stunkard et al[40] that weight change during a depressive episode is strongly related to basal BMI. Body mass index was also substantially elevated in the co-twins of twins with atypical depression. These results suggest the intriguing hypothesis that familial/genetic factors that influence the vulnerability to atypical depression also influence the vulnerability to obesity. Alternatively, the liability to obesity may not be itself directly related to the risk for broadly defined depression. However, given that depression is manifest, then the clinical form of the disorder (ie, typical vs atypical vegetative features) may be influenced by the familial/genetic vulnerability to obesity.

Fourth, in a reinterview with the same twin sample, among twins with depressive syndromes at both assessments, a moderate and highly statistically significant concordance for depressive class was revealed. These results are consistent with previous findings that the direction of weight change is stable across depressive episodes.[40]

Fifth, among all twin pairs where both members had had a clinical depressive syndrome, there was a highly significant concordance for class membership. Furthermore, resemblance for depressive class was substantially greater in concordant MZ twin pairs than in concordant DZ twin pairs. These results suggest that the familial factors that influence the kind of depressive syndrome displayed by an affected individual are at least in part genetic. Given that these twins were assessed blindly by different interviewers, this result provides strong validation for our typology. Our findings suggest that, from a familial/genetic perspective, the syndrome of major depression is *not* etiologically homogeneous.

We are aware of only 1 previous study[41] that has addressed the familial/genetic relationship between typical and atypical depression. In a family history study of 330 patients with unipolar depression, Stewart et al[41] found that compared with relatives of probands with melancholia, relatives of probands with atypical depression had a significantly *lower* rate of typical MD and a significantly *higher* rate of atypical depression. These same authors also present results from a pilot family study showing a similar pattern of results. Also, since atypical depression has been previously characterized by selective antidepressant response to monoamine oxidase inhibitors,[41] it is of interest to note that Pare and Mack[42] suggest that response to monoamine oxidase inhibitors vs tricyclic antidepressants is correlated in pairs of relatives with MD.

'NEUROTIC' DEPRESSION

Previous work[43] suggests that, in this large epidemiologic sample of women, we should have found a syndrome of neurotic depression characterized by nonendogenous clinical features, personality abnormalities, life events prior to onset, and a personal and family history of alcoholism. Neuroticism was not increased in our twins with atypical depression, although they were more introverted. Stressful life events were slightly more common in those with severe typical depression—the syndrome with the most *endogenous* features. Neither alcoholism in the twin nor in her co-twin discriminated among the 3 clinical depressive syndromes. These results suggest that our typology of depression bears little resemblance to that proposed by Winokur.[43,44]

ATYPICAL DEPRESSION

The most striking result of these analyses was the identification, in an epidemiologic sample, of a class of patients characterized by atypical (ie, reverse) vegetative symptoms. More important, this class was both relatively stable over time and familial. The term "atypical depression" was first applied by West and Dally[45] to patients with nonendogenous clinical features and emotional reactivity whose depression responded to the monoamine oxidase inhibitor iproniazid. Since then, the term has been used to describe a variety of related syndromes. In addition to responsiveness to monoamine oxidase inhibitors, such patients are often characterized by reverse vegetative features, prominent anxiety, mood reactivity, rejection sensitivity, and intense lethargy.[41] We are aware of only 1 epidemiologic study of this syndrome based on the Epidemiologic Catchment Area study.[46] Defining atypical depression solely by overeating and oversleeping, Horwath and colleagues[46] found that it constituted 16% of all lifetime cases of MD and was associated with psychomotor slowing and comorbid panic disorder, drug abuse, and somatization disorder. Like us, Horwath et al found no significant association between atypical depression and alcoholism.

The syndrome labeled here as "atypical depression" shares some but not all features with those described previously. Most important, it is characterized by the reverse vegetative features of overeating and oversleeping. There is also modest evidence that, at least compared with cases with mild typical depression that are of similar overall severity, those with atypical depression more frequently report tiredness and psychomotor retardation.

Two features of atypical depression as found in this sample, however, were *not* consistent with previous formulations of this diagnostic category or with the results of the 1 previous epidemiologic study.[46] First, atypical depression in this sample was *not* characterized by prominent anxiety symptoms or disorders. In fact, anxiety symptoms were less common in atypical depressive cases than in those with either mild or severe typical depression. Second, several previous descriptions of atypical depression emphasized the stress-related nature of the syndrome. However, those with atypical depression in our sample were the *least* likely depressive class to have their episode preceded by an SLE.

LIMITATIONS

These results should be interpreted in the context of 4 potential methodologic limitations. First, the sample is solely women, mostly in early to middle adult life. Whether depressive symptoms in an epidemiologic sample of men, or an older sample of women, would yield similar classes is unknown.

Second, observations in twin pairs were not statistically independent as assumed by our LCA model. Previous simulations have suggested that this situation produces little bias in parameter estimation, but underestimates sampling error.[47]

Third, latent class membership is not an "all or none" phenomenon. The LCA program calculates, for all individuals, the likelihood of membership in each class. For some twins, 1 class was far and away the most likely, while for others, the difference in likelihood across 2 or more classes was small. We have conducted preliminary analyses including only those twins whose class could be assigned with confidence. While the stability of class assignment over time changed little, concordance for the clinical classes in MZ twin pairs increased. It may be useful to incorporate the confidence of class assignment in future LCA analyses.

Finally, while LCA can indicate whether a pattern of observed symptoms in a population is *consistent with* the existence of discrete latent classes, it cannot *prove* that such discrete classes exist.[35] For example, although we consider it unlikely, especially for mild typical and atypical depression, it is possible that the classes of depression observed in this sample reflect only differing points on a single underlying continuum of severity.

Accepted for publication January 5, 1996.

This work was supported by grants MH-40828, AA-09095, MH-49492, and MH-01277 from the National Institutes of Health, Bethesda, Md. The Virginia Twin Registry, established and maintained by W. Nance MD, PhD, and L. Corey, PhD, is supported by the National Institutes of Health grants HD-26746 and NS-31564.

Laura Karkowski-Shuman, PhD, assisted in the data analysis.

Reprints: Kenneth S. Kendler, MD, Psychiatric Genetics Research Program, Department of Psychiatry, Box 980710, Richmond, VA 23298-0710.

REFERENCES

1. Lewis AJ. Melancholia: a clinical survey of depressive states. *J Ment Sci.* 1934; 80:277-378.
2. Kendell RE. The classification of depressions: a review of contemporary confusion. *Br J Psychiatry.* 1976;129:15-28.
3. Paykel ES. Classification of depressed patients: a cluster analysis derived grouping. *Br J Psychiatry.* 1971;118:275-288.
4. Farmer A, McGuffin P. The classification of the depressions: contemporary confusion revisited. *Br J Psychiatry.* 1989;155:437-443.
5. Kiloh LG, Garside RF. Depression: a multivariate study of Sir Aubrey Lewis's data on melancholia. *Aust N Z J Psychiatry.* 1977;11:149-156.
6. Ryan ND, Puig-Antich J, Ambrosini P, Rabinovich H, Robinson D, Nelson B, Iyengar S, Twomey J. The clinical picture of major depression in children and adolescents. *Arch Gen Psychiatry.* 1987;44:854-861.
7. Muthen BO. Dichotomous factor analysis of symptom data. *Sociol Meth Res.* 1989;18:19-65.
8. Feinberg M, Carroll BJ. Separation of subtypes of depression using discriminant analysis, I: separation of unipolar endogenous depression from non-endogenous depression. *Br J Psychiatry.* 1982;140:384-391.
9. Sen B. An analysis of the nature of depressive phenomena in primary health care utilising multivariate statistical techniques. *Acta Psychiatr Scand.* 1987; 76:28-32.
10. Grove WM, Andreasen NC, Young M, Endicott J, Keller MB, Hirschfeld RMA, Reich T. Isolation and characterization of a nuclear depressive syndrome. *Psychol Med.* 1987;17:471-484.
11. Blazer D, Swartz M, Woodbury M, Manton KG, Hughes D, George LK. Depressive symptoms and depressive diagnoses in a community population: use of a new procedure for analysis of psychiatric classification. *Arch Gen Psychiatry.* 1988;45:1078-1084.
12. Woodbury MA, Manton KG. Grade of membership analysis of depression-related psychiatric disorders. *Sociol Meth Res.* 1989;18:126-163.
13. Davidson JRT, Woodbury MA, Zisook S, Giller EL Jr. Classification of depression by grade of membership: a confirmation study. *Psychol Med.* 1989;19: 987-998.
14. Goldberg DP, Bridges K, Duncan-Jones P, Grayson D. Dimensions of neuroses seen in primary-care settings. *Psychol Med.* 1987;17:461-470.
15. Young MA, Scheftner WA, Klerman GL, Andreasen NC, Hirschfeld RMA. The endogenous sub-type of depression: a study of its internal construct validity. *Br J Psychiatry.* 1986;148:257-267.
16. Eaton WW, Dryman A, Sorenson A, McCutcheon A. DSM-III major depressive disorder in the community: a latent class analysis of data from the NIMH Epidemiologic Catchment Area Programme. *Br J Psychiatry.* 1989;155:48-54.
17. Eaton WW, McCutcheon A, Dryman A, Sorenson A. Latent class analysis of anxiety and depression. *Sociol Meth Res.* 1989;18:104-125.
18. Eaton WW, Chilcoat H. The latent structure of anxiety and depression in treated and untreated samples of two US populations. In: Cooper B, Eastwood R, eds. *Primary Health Care and Psychiatric Epidemiology.* London, England: Routledge; 1992:307-318.
19. Zimmerman M, Coryell W, Pfohl B, Stangl D. An American validation study of the Newcastle Diagnostic Scale, II: relationship with clinical, demographic, familial and psychosocial features. *Br J Psychiatry.* 1987;150:526-532.
20. Shapiro S, Skinner EA, Kessler LG, Von Korff M, German PS, Tischler GL, Leaf PJ, Benham L, Cottler L, Regier DA. Utilization of health and mental health services: three epidemiologic catchment area sites. *Arch Gen Psychiatry.* 1984; 41:971-978.
21. Kessler RC, McGonagle KA, Zhao S, Nelson CB, Hughes M, Eshleman S, Wittchen H-U, Kendler KS. Lifetime and 12-month prevalence of *DSM-III-R* psychiatric disorders in the United States: results from the National Comorbidity Survey. *Arch Gen Psychiatry.* 1994;51:8-10.
22. Costello CG. The similarities and dissimilarities between community and clinic cases of depression. *Br J Psychiatry.* 1990;157:812-821.
23. Robins E, Guze SB. Establishment of diagnostic validity in psychiatric illness: its application to schizophrenia. *Am J Psychiatry.* 1970;126:983-987.
24. Kendler KS. The nosologic validity of paranoia (simple delusional disorder): a review. *Arch Gen Psychiatry.* 1980;37:699-706.
25. Kendler KS, Neale MC, Kessler RC, Heath AC, Eaves LJ. A population based twin study of major depression in women: the impact of varying definitions of illness. *Arch Gen Psychiatry.* 1992;49:257-266.
26. American Psychiatric Association: *Diagnostic and Statistical Manual of Mental Disorders, Third Edition, Revised.* Washington, DC: American Psychiatric Association; 1987.
27. American Psychiatric Association: *Diagnostic and Statistical Manual of Mental Disorders, Third Edition.* Washington, DC: American Psychiatric Association; 1980.
28. Kendler KS, Neale MC, Kessler RC, Heath AC, Eaves LJ. The genetic epidemiology of phobias in women: the inter-relationship of agoraphobia, social phobia, situational phobia and simple phobia. *Arch Gen Psychiatry.* 1992;49:273-281.
29. FAO/WHO/UNV Expert Consultations. *Energy and Protein Requirements.* Geneva, Switzerland: World Health Organization; 1985. Series No. 724.
30. Eysenck HJ, Eysenck SBG. *Manual of the Eysenck Personality Questionnaire.* London, England: Hodder & Stoughton; 1975.
31. Heath AC, Neale MC, Kessler RC, Eaves LJ, Kendler KS. Evidence for genetic influences on personality from self-reports and from informant ratings. *J Person Soc Psychol.* 1992;63:85-96.
32. Kendler KS, Kessler RC, Walters EE, MacLean CJ, Sham PC, Neale MC, Heath AC, Eaves LJ. Stressful life events, genetic liability and onset of an episode of major depression in women. *Am J Psychiatry.* 1995;152:833-842.
33. Joreskog KG, Sorbom D. *LISREL 7: A Guide to the Program and Applications.* 2nd ed. Chicago, Ill: SPSS Inc; 1989.
34. Neale MC. *Statistical Modelling With Mx.* Richmond: Department of Psychiatry, Medical College of Virginia/Virginia Commonwealth University; 1991.
35. Klein DN, Riso LP. Psychiatric disorders: problems of boundaries and comorbidity. In: Costello CG, ed. *Basic Issues in Psychopathology.* New York, NY: Guilford Press; 1993.
36. World Health Organization. *Composite International Diagnostic Interview Computer Programs (Version 1.1).* Geneva, Switzerland: World Health Organization; 1990.
37. SAS Institute. *SAS/STAT User's Guide, Version 6, Fourth Edition.* Cary, NC: SAS Institute Inc; 1990: vol 1 and 2.
38. Hochberg Y. Some conservative generalizations of the T-method in simultaneous inference. *J Multivar Anal.* 1974;4:224-234.
39. Fleiss JL, Cohen J. The equivalence of weighted kappa and the intraclass correlation coefficient as measures of reliability. *Educ Psychol Meas.* 1973;33: 613-619.
40. Stunkard AJ, Fernstrom MH, Price A, Frank E. Direction of weight change in recurrent depression: consistency across episodes. *Arch Gen Psychiatry.* 1990; 47:857-860.
41. Stewart JW, McGrath PJ, Rabkin JG, Quitkin FM. Atypical depression: a valid clinical entity? *Psychiatr Clin North Am.* 1993;16:479-495.
42. Pare CMB, Mack JW. Differentiation of two genetically specific types of depression by the response to antidepressant drugs. *J Med Genet.* 1971;8:306-309.
43. Winokur G. The validity of neurotic-reactive depression: new data and reappraisal. *Arch Gen Psychiatry.* 1985;42:1116-1122.
44. Winokur G. Unipolar depression: is it divisible into autonomous subtypes? *Arch Gen Psychiatry.* 1979;36:47-52.
45. West ED, Dally PJ. Effect of iproniazid in depressive syndromes. *BMJ.* 1959; 1:1491-1494.
46. Horwath E, Johnson J, Weissman MM, Hornig CD. The validity of major depression with atypical features based on a community study. *J Affect Disord.* 1992;26:117-126.
47. McGue R, Wette R, Rao DC. Evaluation of path analysis through computer simulation: effects of incorrectly assuming independent distribution of familial correlations. *Genet Epidemiol.* 1984;1:255-269.

ORIGINAL ARTICLE

A Controlled Trial Comparing Buprenorphine and Methadone Maintenance in Opioid Dependence

Walter Ling, MD; Donald R. Wesson, MD; Charles Charuvastra, MD; C. James Klett, PhD

Background: Buprenorphine is a partial agonist at the μ-opioid receptor that has been proposed as an alternative to traditional full agonist maintenance therapy for the treatment of opioid addiction. We report on a clinical trial in which the relative safety and efficacy of long-term fixed-dose buprenorphine maintenance was examined in comparison to low- and high-dose methadone maintenance.

Methods: Two hundred twenty-five treatment-seeking opioid addicts (46 women, 179 men) were randomly assigned to receive, in a double-blind manner, either 8 mg/d of buprenorphine, 30 mg/d of methadone, or 80 mg/d of methadone maintenance over a 1-year period. Objective and subjective measures of efficacy (urine toxicology, retention, craving, and withdrawal symptoms) were examined at the study midpoint and at termination, and safety data were tabulated over the entire 52-week study period.

Results: Patients assigned to high-dose methadone maintenance performed significantly better on measures of retention, opioid use, and opioid craving than either the low-dose methadone or the buprenorphine group at both 26-week and 52-week time points. Performance on these measures was virtually identical between the latter two groups. No serious adverse health effects attributable to buprenorphine were noted.

Conclusions: Buprenorphine maintenance at 8 mg/d appears to be less than optimally efficacious under the conditions of the present study. Continued research is needed to reconcile these findings with the more positive results reported by other investigative groups. There are no apparent health risks associated with long-term buprenorphine maintenance at this dosage.

(Arch Gen Psychiatry. 1996;53:401-407)

From the Los Angeles Addiction Treatment Research Center; Department of Psychiatry and Biobehavioral Sciences Substance Abuse Program, University of California, Los Angeles, and Substance Abuse Treatment Program, West Los Angeles VA Medical Center (Drs Ling and Charuvastra); MPI Treatment Services, Summit Medical Center, Oakland, Calif, and Department of Psychiatry, University of California, San Francisco (Dr Wesson).

OPIOID maintenance therapy remains the primary pharmacological approach for the treatment of opioid dependence. The benefits of maintenance therapy, including significant reductions in illicit opioid use, increases in treatment retention, and improved psychosocial functioning, have been clearly demonstrated within the methadone maintenance model.[1-7] Further, methadone maintenance therapy for opioid addiction has been shown to decrease the mortality and morbidity associated with illicit drug use,[1,8,9] dramatically diminish the transfer of the human immunodeficiency virus,[10-12] profoundly reduce criminal activity,[13-15] and normalize disruptions in immune and neuroendocrine function caused by heroin use.[16]

In spite of these benefits, methadone treatment is considered undesirable pharmacotherapy by a significant number of addicts and communities. Provision of an alternative opioid maintenance agent may help attract some of the over 500 000 untreated opioid addicts in the United States to maintenance pharmacotherapy. Levo-alpha-acetyl-methadol,[17] recently approved by the Food and Drug Administration (FDA), is one such alternative. The extensive evaluation of buprenorphine further illustrates the desire of the research and treatment community to find effective alternatives to methadone.

Buprenorphine, a partial opioid agonist at the μ receptor, is a potent analgesic that is available for clinical use as a sublingual tablet in many parts of the world and as an injectable form in the United States. The potential utility of buprenorphine for the treatment of opioid addiction was apparent in the definitive work of Jasinski et al,[18] who demonstrated that

See Patients and Methods on next page

PATIENTS AND METHODS

PATIENTS

The sample consisted of 225 patients who met *DSM-III-R* criteria for opioid dependence and who were seeking treatment at the Pizarro Treatment Clinic, an outpatient treatment facility located about 1 mile from downtown Los Angeles in California. The Pizarro Treatment Clinic serves an approximately 60% male patient population with an ethnic mix that is predominantly Hispanic (about 55%) but with moderate representation of African Americans (30%) and whites (15%).

Screening procedures were conducted at baseline by intake counselors. Volunteers aged 18 to 65, who were mentally competent to give informed consent, were accepted if they were in good general health and met the *DSM-III-R* diagnosis of opioid dependence and the FDA criteria for methadone maintenance treatment,[27] but were not currently enrolled in a methadone maintenance program. Patients were excluded if they had acute hepatitis or other acute medical conditions that seemed to contraindicate participation; if they met the *DSM-III-R* diagnosis of dependence on alcohol, sedative-hypnotics (including benzodiazepines), cocaine, or amphetamines; if they were currently using anticonvulsants, disulfiram, or neuroleptics daily; or if for some reason they could not reasonably be expected to remain available to attend clinic for the duration of the trial. Women of childbearing age were required to be practicing birth control, and those already pregnant or still nursing a child were excluded.

Patients were not paid for their participation, but medication and counseling services were provided free of charge. The informed consent documents and the study protocol were approved by the Institutional Review Board of Friends Medical Science Research, Inc. Patient enrollment began October 16, 1990, and was completed on schedule in September 1992.

METHODS

Drug Assignment

After screening for eligibility and baseline observations, including laboratory studies, patients were assigned to one of three fixed-dose treatment schedules in blocks of 15, using a computer-generated random numbers list. The treatments were methadone, 30 mg/d (M30); methadone, 80 mg/d (M80); and buprenorphine, 8 mg/d. In order to conduct the study in a double-blind fashion, each patient received both an oral and a sublingual form of medication, only one of which was active. Unit doses were prepared weekly by a contract research pharmacist who was the only individual locally who had knowledge of drug assignment.

Each dose of methadone was made to a volume of 40 mL and administered in a vehicle consisting of 0.2 mg denatonium benzoate per 1000 mL in a cherry syrup concentrate. Buprenorphine was initially obtained in powder form from the National Institute on Drug Abuse (NIDA) and put into solution by dissolving in 30% alcohol to form a buprenorphine concentration of 8 mg/mL. The 1-mL doses of buprenorphine were dispensed in 1.5-mL pediatric oral syringes. Placebo buprenorphine consisted of the 30% alcohol without added buprenorphine, and the methadone placebo consisted of the denatonium benzoate vehicle without methadone. During the last year of the study, unit doses of buprenorphine (also in 30% alcohol) and buprenorphine placebo were supplied by NIDA.

A preliminary evaluation of the effectiveness of the double-blind selection conducted early in the study revealed a general tendency (82%) for patients to assume that they were receiving buprenorphine (41 of 50). All 13 patients assigned to buprenorphine guessed correctly. Only one of the 17 high-dose methadone patients guessed correctly and two of this group guessed incorrectly that they were receiving low-dose methadone. Among the 20 patients on low-dose methadone, four guessed correctly, one guessed placebo, and another guessed 40 mg of methadone plus buprenorphine.

All doses of study medication were administered by the dispensing nurse. The oral dose was administered first, followed by the sublingual dose. Patients were instructed to delay swallowing the sublingual dose for up to 5 minutes to assure absorption and were observed by clinic staff for compliance.

To avoid possible withdrawal symptoms precipitated by the antagonistic action of buprenorphine during induction, the study drugs were not administered while the patient was under the acute influence of opioids. Before the first dose of medication, each patient completed a subjective checklist of opioid withdrawal symptoms and was examined by a staff physician for eligibility to begin treatment. The first dose of precoded medication consisted of either 2 mg of buprenorphine (and a methadone placebo) or 30 mg of methadone (and a buprenorphine placebo). Patients were observed for 2 hours after the initial dose. Buprenorphine was increased to 4 mg on day 2 and 8 mg on day 3. For patients assigned to the M80 group, the methadone dose was increased by 5 mg daily until the 80-mg dose was reached.

Since off-site administration of medication was not allowed, patients had to attend the clinic daily. If patients missed more than four consecutive clinic visits, they received half of their full dose on their first day back, three fourths on their second day back, and a full dose on their third day back. In general, patients who missed seven consecutive clinic visits were dropped from the study, but there were a few patients who were openly treated with 40 mg of methadone daily during a brief inpatient stay for concurrent illness. It was not necessary to break the double-blind code for any patient before the conclusion of the trial.

In terms of what was known of the safety of buprenorphine, it was not expected that there would be a problem in administering the drug for a full year. However, to ensure the safety of the participants, there was close medical monitoring throughout. Baseline observations included a complete physical examination and laboratory workup (complete blood cell count, urinalysis, serum chemistry, and electrocardiogram). The electrocardiogram was repeated every 3 months and the other laboratory tests were conducted monthly. The pregnancy status of the female patients was determined at baseline and monthly. One patient became pregnant during the trial and, according to the protocol, was dropped from the study without breaking the blind and was treated openly with methadone. It was later determined that she had been assigned to the M30 group.

OUTCOME MEASURES

Determining the relative efficacy of the three maintenance schedules in a study lasting a full year required some a priori decisions about the criteria that would be used to evaluate efficacy, as well as the time points at which efficacy would be assessed. On the basis of past experience, it was thought to be quite possible that a treatment advantage apparent in the short term would be completely obscured at the end of a year. Accordingly, it was decided to base our efficacy evaluation on the first 26 weeks and to consider safety issues over the entire year. It was also our intention to analyze the experience over the first 17 weeks for direct comparison with the results of the study by Johnson et al,[25] which had recently been completed. Hereafter, their study will be referred to as the ARC study.

The protocol identified four efficacy measures: days of retention in treatment, urinalysis for drugs of abuse, a patient measure of craving, and a checklist of opioid withdrawal symptoms. In calculating days of retention in treatment, patients were considered to be active participants until the day of their last study dose.

Urine specimens were collected in the morning three times weekly (Monday, Wednesday, and Friday) under direct observation or with the use of an FDA-approved, tamper-proof collecting system (Franklin Diagnostics, Cedar Knolls, NJ). For a few weeks at the beginning of the study, if a patient missed a scheduled collection, a specimen was collected the following day, but this procedure was soon abandoned in favor of the Monday/Wednesday/Friday collection only. Samples were analyzed for opioids in the form of morphine by fluorescence polarization immunoassay (FPI), using the Abbott Diagnostics TDX system (Irving, Tex). This method, which employs an antibody specific to morphine, is linked with mechanized fluorescence polarization. Controls and a fixed percentage of FPI-positive results were cross-confirmed by gas-liquid chromatography (GLC) or high-pressure liquid chromatography (HPLC). Assay morphine sensitivity for FPI was 30 ng/mL, and 0.1 to 1 ng/mL for GLC and HPLC. The first specimen obtained each week (usually on Monday) was also tested for the presence of other drugs of abuse (cocaine, amphetamines, benzodiazepines). The results of these urinalyses were not made known to anyone locally, but were transmitted electronically to a remote location (Maryland) for monitoring purposes. As a supplement to the urinalyses, patients provided a self-report of drug use weekly to a research technician.

To assess craving, patients were asked each week to estimate the maximum amount of opioid craving at any time during the past 7 days by making a mark on a 100-mm line designated as no craving at one end and maximum craving ever experienced at the other. Patients' summary scores were computed by counting the frequency of ratings below a cut point of 50 on the craving scale and were used for comparison.

Each week, patients were also asked to what extent they experienced opioid withdrawal symptoms or possible medication side effects during the previous week. This information was recorded on a symptom-sign checklist that had been used in several earlier multicenter clinical trials of levo-alpha-acetyl-methadol.[17] Specific symptom-signs were not enumerated, but when their presence was elicited by general questioning, there were additional probes to enable a judgment as to their severity, such as mild, moderate, or severe.

In addition to these measures directly relevant to safety and/or efficacy, data collection at baseline included the Addiction Severity Index[28] and a drug-use history. If patients were terminated from the study early, attempts were always made to repeat the laboratory studies and to determine the reason for termination.

All study patients received the same psychosocial and other treatment services. Each patient was assigned a primary counselor who coordinated psychosocial counseling services. All counselors had a college education and had received specialized training in drug and alcohol abuse counseling. In addition to regular contact with research staff, patients were encouraged to attend weekly individual counseling sessions that focused on crisis intervention and case management; few patients took advantage of the offer. However, since the study focused on pharmacological efficacy, no patients were discharged for nonattendance of counseling sessions. There was no difference between groups in the proportion of the number of sessions attended (P=.95). On average, patients attended 48% of possible sessions, each averaging 13.8 minutes.

There was concern during the planning of this study about randomizing patients to a fixed-dose maintenance schedule for a full year when past experience had shown that there would be patients in all three groups who would remain in the study without significant diminution of heroin use. Considering the dangers of human immunodeficiency virus infection associated with intravenous drug use, some of these patients clearly would need more aggressive treatment than would be provided by the fixed-dose design. The compromise adopted was to monitor urine results remotely to avoid breaking the blind but to inform the treatment physician whenever a patient obtained 12 consecutive urine samples positive for heroin (a missing urine sample was considered positive). The patient was then considered to be an early terminator. For purposes of computing retention, the last study day was the day the 12th positive urine sample was obtained. The study code was not broken for these patients. They, in effect, entered a new protocol that permitted escalating the dose of their assigned drug while still maintaining the double-blind selection.

DATA ANALYSIS

Retention rates were estimated by the Kaplan-Meier product limit method, and survival curves of the three groups were compared using the Wilcoxon rank sum test. Differences among groups in number of completers at various time points were evaluated by χ^2 analysis. Urine samples were considered to be opioid-free if the test reading was less than 300 mg/mL. Percent opioid-free urine samples were calculated for each patient by dividing the number of opioid-free urine samples by the number of urine samples scheduled for collection while that patient was still an active study participant (missing urine samples were also counted for inclusion in the denominator). A second dependent variable to evaluate opioid use, the treatment effectiveness score (TES),[29] consisted of the number of opioid-free urine samples obtained during the time frame being evaluated. The Kruskal-Wallis test was used to compare groups using these two urine-based outcome variables and the craving scale data. Statistical tests were considered to be significant at $P<.05$.

Demographic and Drug Use Variables*

	8-mg Buprenorphine Group (n=75)	30-mg Methadone Group (n=75)	80-mg Methadone Group (n=75)	Total (N=225)
Sex, No. (%)				
Male	54 (72)	63 (84)	62 (83)	**179** (80)
Female	21 (28)	12 (16)	13 (17)	**46** (20)
Race, No. (%)†				
White	14 (19)	8 (11)	10 (13)	**32** (14)
Black	20 (27)	18 (24)	6 (8)	**44** (20)
Hispanic	41 (55)	49 (65)	57 (76)	**147** (18)
Other	...	...	2 (2)	**2** (.8)
Age, y (±SD)	41.5 (9.9)	40.8 (9.4)	40.1 (9.2)	40.8 (9.5)
Education, y (±SD)	11.7 (2.0)	11.2 (1.9)	11.7 (2.0)	11.4 (2.0)
Heroin addiction, y (±SD)	15.9 (8.3)	18.2 (10.3)	19.0 (10.0)	17.7 (9.7)
No. of patients using intravenous cocaine in 30 days prior to study entry	57	59	50	**166**
Days of use (±SD)	8.21 (12.1)	7.85 (10.5)	7.44 (9.6)	7.85 (10.7)
No. of patients using crack cocaine in 30 days prior to study entry	21	13	17	**51**
Days of use (±SD)	7.19 (9.7)	6.0 (8.0)	3.59 (7.4)	5.69 (8.5)

**Ellipses indicate not applicable.*
†χ^2=15.1, df=6, P=.01.

daily dosages of 8 mg sublingually blocked the effects of subsequently administered morphine and did not appear to induce significant physical dependence. Mello and Mendelson's[19-21] extensive work in the animal and the clinical laboratory demonstrated that buprenorphine suppresses heroin self-administration by opioid-dependent primates and humans.

Buprenorphine appears to have many clinical advantages. It is acceptable to some heroin users who do not want or qualify for methadone maintenance.[22] Buprenorphine has a more favorable safety profile than methadone. Although buprenorphine is used intravenously by heroin addicts in countries where the sublingual tablet is available as an analgesic,[23] its abuse potential appears substantially lower than that for full agonists such as methadone or heroin. Buprenorphine may be less likely than other partial opioid agonists to precipitate opioid withdrawal, if given to patients already maintained on an opioid agonist such as methadone.[24]

See also page 409

Buprenorphine produces physical dependence of the opioid type. Because of buprenorphine's tight binding to the μ receptor, the onset of withdrawal symptoms after maintenance treatment is generally delayed for 24 hours or more and symptom intensity may not peak for 5 or more days. The overall intensity of withdrawal symptoms appears less intense than with methadone.

Several controlled clinical trials comparing the effectiveness of buprenorphine and methadone in maintenance treatment have been published[25,26] or are currently in some stage of completion. Since a variety of doses of each drug is represented in these studies, the aggregate results should provide a better understanding of the relative effectiveness of the two drugs. The purpose of the present study was to compare a dose of buprenorphine that was considered to be clinically optimal with two doses of methadone, one of which most would agree represents a relatively low dose (30 mg/d) and the other a relatively high dose (80 mg/d). Such a design also permitted another comparison of low- vs high-dose methadone, an issue that continues to be of some interest to clinicians.

RESULTS

SAMPLE CHARACTERISTICS

Three hundred ten patients were screened in order to achieve the target sample of 75 patients per group. There were three main reasons for exclusion. Twenty-two patients simply did not return to the clinic after the preliminary screening contact, another 21 had a medical condition that made them ineligible, and 21 had evidence of significant polydrug dependence (crack cocaine, four patients; benzodiazepines, one patient; and alcohol, 16 patients). The **Table** shows the demographics of the study patients. There were no baseline differences between groups except for race. Cox regression of all randomized patients using demographic and drug-use characteristics as covariates showed higher retention to be associated with increasing age (χ^2=6.08, *df*=1, *P*=.01). Nonsignificant associations were observed with gender (χ^2=0.01, *df*=1, *P*=.93), race (χ^2=4.58, *df*=2, *P*=.10), and duration of addiction (χ^2=3.83, *df*=1, *P*=.05).

EFFICACY RESULTS

The percentage of patients still active in the study over time is shown in the **Figure** for the full year. Applying the Wilcoxon rank sum test to the survival curves showed that over the first 26 weeks the M80 group had significantly better retention than both the M30 group (*P*=.04) and the buprenorphine group (*P*=.009). Over the entire

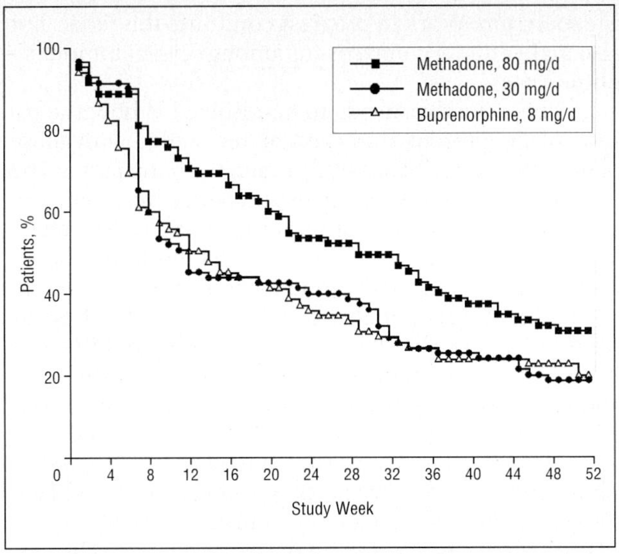

Patients in each group still in treatment at the end of each study week.

year, the M80 group had better retention than the M30 (*P*=.02) and buprenorphine groups (*P*=.009). The differences between the M30 and buprenorphine groups failed to achieve significance at either 26 weeks (*P*=.33) or 1 year (*P*=.44).

To evaluate retention in a different manner, the percentage of patients who completed 26 weeks of treatment was 52%, 40%, and 35% for the M80, M30, and buprenorphine groups, respectively. The overall comparison was not significant (χ^2=4.846, *df*=2, *P*=.09). Similarly, 31%, 19%, and 20% in each of the three groups, respectively, completed 52 weeks of treatment. These outcomes were not significantly different (χ^2=3.652, *df*=2, *P*=.16).

At one time or another during the projected 52-week period of maintenance treatment, 60 patients were terminated because they failed to give a single sample negative for opioids in any series of 12 consecutive scheduled urine samples: 29 in the M30 group, 16 in the M80 group, and 15 in the buprenorphine group. The three groups are significantly different in this respect (χ^2=8.319, *df*=2, *P*=.02), with the M30 group worse than both the M80 (χ^2=4.571, *df*=1, *P*=.03) and buprenorphine groups (χ^2=5.435, *df*=1, *P*=.02). Nearly all of these patients continued to receive their assigned study drug in a double-blind fashion for a longer period with varying amounts of dose escalation before their tenure in the study was terminated for a variety of other reasons. If these patients are considered to be members of the study until they finally terminated for other reasons, the retention figures at week 26 increase to 58%, 58%, and 44% for the M80, M30, and buprenorphine groups, respectively, and to 35%, 22%, and 23% at week 52. However, the overall comparison of the three groups at these two time points is still not significant.

The extent of opioid use by the three groups was analyzed using two outcome measures. Each patient had 1% more opioid-free scores reflecting opioid use after varying lengths of time during his or her tenure in the study. Over the first 26 weeks the means±SDs of these scores were 61.9±31.6 for the M80 group, 44.6±33.5 for the buprenorphine group, and 44.5±36.0 for the M30 group. The median scores were 72, 47, and 46, respectively. The comparison of the three groups by the Kruskal-Wallis test was significant (H=12.635, *df*=2, *P*=.002), with the M80 group better than both the M30 (H=8.882, *df*=1, *P*=.003) and buprenorphine (H=9.999, *df*=1, *P*=.002) groups. Over the entire 52 weeks, the means, standard deviations, and medians were virtually the same as after the first 26 weeks. Over 52 weeks, the groups were significantly different (H=11.131, *df*=2, *P*=.004), with the M80 group better than both the M30 (H=7.930, *df*=1, *P*=.005) and buprenorphine (H=8.698, *df*=1, *P*=.003) groups.

The use of the TES yielded essentially the same results. During the first 26 weeks of the study, the TES could take values between zero and 78 for any patient (three samples per week for 26 weeks). A score of 78 could only be achieved by a patient who stayed in the study for 26 weeks and gave the full complement of 78 urine samples, all of which were negative. There were three such patients in this study, one in each of the study groups. The means±SDs of the TES were 41.3±27.3 for the M80 group, 26.5±26.3 for the buprenorphine group, and 26.5±26.7 for the M30 group. The median scores for the three groups were 49, 16, and 24, respectively. The overall Kruskal-Wallis test was significant (H=14.366, *df*=2, *P*=.001) with the M80 groups superior to both the M30 (H=10.772, *df*=1, *P*=.001) and buprenorphine (H=10.654, *df*=1, *P*=.001) groups. Again, the results after 52 weeks were very similar to the 26-week results. The maximum score could be achieved by a patient who completed the study and gave 156 opioid-free urine samples. A single patient from the M80 group achieved this goal. The mean±SDs were 64.9±52.5 for the M80 group, 41.9±49.8 for the buprenorphine group, and 40.1±46.6 for the M30 group. The median scores were 59, 16, and 24, respectively. The groups differed significantly (H=12.159, *df*=2, *P*=.002), with the M80 group better than both the M30 (H=9.709, *df*=1, *P*=.002) and buprenorphine (H=8.358, *df*=1, *P*=.004) groups.

The same pattern of results was observed in the craving symptom data over 26 weeks (H=8.446, *df*=2, *P*=.02), with the M80 group showing less craving than either the M30 (H=4.794, *df*=1, *P*=.03) or buprenorphine (H=7.492, *df*=1, *P*=.006) groups and over 52 weeks (H=10.213, *df*=2, *P*=.006).

The expectation was that the extent to which patients experienced symptoms of opioid withdrawal would correspond roughly to the other efficacy data. As one way of testing this, we tallied the number of patients who were rated as experiencing moderate or severe discomfort at least once during their tenure in the study for each of 11 withdrawal symptoms, and evaluated these frequencies by a 2×3 χ^2 test. The three groups differed only on the symptom of nausea (χ^2=8.382, *df*=2, *P*=.02), with patients in the M30 group reporting this more frequently (29 of 75) than those in either the M80 (17 of 75) or buprenorphine (14 of 74) groups.

ADVERSE EVENTS

Numerous and diverse adverse events were recorded for each of the three groups. Many of these represented chronic conditions such as anemia, asthma, and controlled diabetes mellitus, or preexisting aches and pains, dental problems, and the like, which may or may not have prompted a visit to a health care provider. Another large set of events were the results of accidents (broken bones, burns, lacerations) that seemed to reflect a chaotic lifestyle (stab wounds, swollen and infected jaw due to assault, alcohol withdrawal) or, in other instances, the ordinary diseases of everyday life (ear infection). These minor problems were perhaps more frequent or intense because of the compromised health status of these patients.

Fourteen patients were hospitalized at one time or another, usually for brief periods. Two of these patients died. One male patient in the M30 group died of multiple stab wounds to the abdomen during an altercation that occurred after 43 days in the study, and the other died of cancer at his brother's home after a brief hospitalization. Overall, adverse events were about equally represented in all three groups, and no clustering of type of event was apparent.

COMMENT

This study has extended the safety evaluation of the 8-mg dose of buprenorphine to a full year, provided additional methadone benchmarks with which to evaluate the efficacy of buprenorphine, and increased the size and diversity of the experience base with buprenorphine.

There was confidence in the safety profile of buprenorphine before the study was undertaken. There was no expectation of serious adverse effects and none were found. At the clinical level, we believe buprenorphine to be a safe drug.

The evidence in this study supporting the efficacy of the 8-mg daily dosage of buprenorphine as a maintenance drug is, at best, indirect. The observed fact is that the outcomes of the buprenorphine group are almost identical to those of the M30 group. In the past we have argued that while 30 mg of methadone is a reasonable starting dose for most street addicts entering either detoxification or maintenance, it is a marginally effective maintenance dose for most. Schuster[30] has cautioned, for instance, that for many patients doses below 60 mg may not be adequate to prevent withdrawal symptoms or to provide blockade of intravenous heroin during the 24 hours between methadone doses.

What the study demonstrates with some certainty is that, as a group, patients can be expected to do better on 80 mg of methadone daily than they will on 30 mg of methadone or 8 mg of buprenorphine. They can be expected to stay in treatment longer, use less opioids, and have less craving. However, many individuals remained in treatment and reduced their heroin use to a clinically significant extent in all three groups.

At this stage in the development of buprenorphine as a maintenance treatment, the research interest is shifting from whether or not buprenorphine is effective to a search for the daily dosage that will be considered optimal for most patients. The tactic of this search to date has been to compare one or more doses of buprenorphine with one or more doses of methadone in an attempt to position buprenorphine on the methadone dosage spectrum. Work in progress continues this tactic, but also makes direct comparisons among several buprenorphine doses.

One issue that needs to be resolved is how the results of the present study can be reconciled with those of the ARC study.[25] That study evaluated outcomes in 162 patients during 17 weeks of maintenance treatment and concluded that 8 mg/d of buprenorphine was as effective as 60 mg/d of methadone, and that both were superior to 20 mg/d of methadone in reducing illicit opioid use and retaining patients in treatment. In the first 17 weeks of our study, there was essentially no difference in outcome between the M30 and buprenorphine groups, and the M80 group was unequivocally superior to both groups in retention and in measures of opioid use.

The difference in observed outcome of the buprenorphine groups in the two studies is not the issue. In fact, these outcomes are remarkably similar; retention was 42% in the ARC study and 44% in the current study. The percent of opioid-free urine samples was 58% in the ARC study and 58% in the current study.

There were four methadone doses represented in the two studies. The expectation was that the ARC 20-mg methadone dose group would have the worst outcomes and that our M80 group would have the best; those expectations are borne out. The ARC 20-mg methadone dose group had 20% retention and 29% opioid-free urine samples after 17 weeks, while our M80 group had 64% retention and 72% opioid-free urine samples. Where expectation failed was that the ARC 60-mg methadone dose group did so poorly (32% retention and 44% opioid-free urine samples) compared with our M30 group, which had 44% retention and 57% opioid-free urine samples.

The ARC study was meticulously designed, scrupulously conducted, and thoughtfully analyzed. The puzzling observation of the essential equivalence of the buprenorphine groups in the two studies and the apparent reversal in effectiveness of the 30- and 60-mg methadone groups very likely reflects chance variation. There are, of course, some implications for the conclusions of the ARC study concerning the adequacy of the 8-mg dose of buprenorphine. First, the observed differences between their 20-mg and 60-mg groups are not robust. In all of their comparisons of these two groups, only the difference in the percentage of opioid-free urine samples was significant ($P<.04$). Second, the fact that their 60-mg methadone and buprenorphine groups do not differ significantly does not support the inference that these two doses are equipotent. They may be roughly comparable. Discussion in terms of statistical power and confidence intervals might have helped put these results in better perspective.

It is our confident belief on the basis of this and other studies, as well as our clinical experience, that buprenorphine will, in due course, be declared a safe and effective drug for maintenance treatment of heroin addicts. However, it is our impression that 8 mg/d of buprenorphine is not an optimal dosage. Because of the excellent safety profile, there is no reason to believe a higher dose will not be well tolerated, and this might move the effectiveness of this promising drug into a more advantageous position in relation to standard methadone practice.

Accepted for publication November 1, 1995.

This research was supported by grant number R18 DA6082 from the NIDA to Friends Medical Science Research Center Inc, Baltimore, Md, and by an interagency agreement for medication development from the Medication Development Division of NIDA to the West Los Angeles VA Medical Center.

We thank Jeffrey Wilkins, MD, for overseeing the toxicologic laboratory. This article is dedicated to the memory of Daniel X. Freedman, chairman of our Scientific Advisory Group.

Reprint requests to Los Angeles Addiction Treatment Research Center, 10350 Santa Monica Blvd, Ste 340, Los Angeles, CA 90025 (Dr Ling).

REFERENCES

1. Ball JC, Ross A. *The Effectiveness of Methadone Maintenance Treatment: Patients, Programs, Services and Outcome.* New York, NY: Springer-Verlag; 1993.
2. Cooper JR, Altman F, Brown BS, Czechowicz D. *Research on the Treatment of Narcotic Addiction: State of the Art.* Rockville, Md: National Institute on Drug Abuse; 1983. Dept of Health and Human Services publication (ADM) 83-1281.
3. Hubbard RL, Marsden ME. Relapse to heroin, cocaine and other drugs in the first year after treatment. In: Tims FM, Leukfeld CG, eds. *Relapse and Recovery in Drug Abuse.* Washington, DC: US Government Printing Office; 1986: 157-166.
4. Sells SB, Dernaree RG, Hornick CW. *Comparative Effectiveness of Drug Abuse Treatment Modalities.* NIDA Services Research Administrative Report. Rockville, Md: National Institute on Drug Abuse; 1979.
5. Senay EC, Uchtenhagen A. Methadone in threatment of opioid depdence: a review of the world literature. In: Westermeyer J, Arif A, eds. *Methadone Maintenance in the Management of Opioid Dependence: An International Review.* New York, NY: Praeger Publishers; 1990:19-54.
6. Simpson DD. Treatment for drug abuse: follow-up outcomes and length of time spent. *Arch Gen Psychiatry.* 1981;38:875-880.
7. Uchtenhagen A. Policy and practice in methadone maintenance: an analysis of the worldwide experience. In: Westermeyer J, Arif A, eds. *Methadone Maintenance in the Management of Opioid Dependence: An International Review.* New York, NY: Praeger Publishers; 1990:55-74.
8. Capelhorn JRM, Bell J. Methadone dosage and retention of patients in methadone treatment. *Med J Aust.* 1991;154:195-199.
9. Segest E, Mygind O, Bay H. The influence of prolonged stable methadone maintenance treatment on mortality and employment: an 8-year follow-up. *International J Addict.* 1990;25:53-63.
10. Des Jarlais DC, Friedman SR, Hopkins W. Risk reduction for acquired immunodeficiency syndrome among intravenous drug users. *Ann Intern Med.* 1985; 103:755-759.
11. Dole VP. Methadone treatment and the acquired immunodeficiency syndrome epidemic. *JAMA.* 1989;262:1681-1682.
12. Drucker E. AIDS and addiction in New York City. *Am J Drug Alcohol Abuse.* 1986;12:165-181.
13. Dole VP, Robinson JW, Orraga J, Towns E, Searcy P, Caine E. Methadone treatment of randomly selected criminal addicts. *N Engl J Med.* 1969;280: 1372-1375.
14. Hubbard RL, Marsden ME, Rachal JV, Harwood HJ, Cavanaugh ER, Ginsburg HM. *Drug Abuse Treatment: A National Study of Effectiveness.* Chapel Hill, NC: University of North Carolina Press; 1989.
15. Hubbard RL, French MT. New perspectives on the benefit-cost and cost-effectiveness of drug abuse treatment. In: Cartwright WS, Kaple JM, eds. *Economic Costs, Cost-effectiveness, Financing and Community-Based Drug Treatment.* Washington, DC: US Government Printing Office; 1991:94-113. National Institute on Drug Abuse Research Monograph 113.
16. Kreek MJ. Using methadone effectively: achieving goals by application of laboratory, clinical and evaluation research and by development of innovative programs. In: Pickens RW, Leukefeld CG, Schuster CR, eds. *Improving Drug Abuse Treatment.* Washington, DC: US Government Printing Office; 1991:245-266. National Institute on Drug Abuse Research Monograph 106.
17. Ling W, Charuvastra VC, Kaim SC, Klett CJ. Methadyl acetate and methadone as maintenance treatments for heroin addicts: a Veterans Administration cooperative study. *Arch Gen Psychiatry.* 1976;33:709-720.
18. Jasinski DR, Pevnick JS, Griffith JD. Human pharmacology and abuse potential of the analgesic buprenorphine: a potential agent for treating narcotic addiction. *Arch Gen Psychiatry.* 1978;35:501-516.
19. Mello NK, Bree MP, Mendelson JH. Comparison of buprenorphine and methadone effects on opiate self-administration in primates. *J Pharmacol Exp Ther.* 1983;225:378-386.
20. Mello MK, Mendelson JH. Buprenorphine suppresses heroin use by heroin addicts. *Science.* 1980;27:657-659.
21. Mello MK, Mendelson JH, Kuehnle JC. Buprenorphine effects on human heroin self-administration: an operant analysis. *J Pharmacol Exp Ther.* 1982;223:30-39.
22. Resnick RB, Resnick E, Galanter M. Buprenorphine responders: a diagnostic subgroup of heroin addicts? *Prog Neuropyschopharmacol Biol Psychiatry.* 1991; 15:531-538.
23. San L, Torrens M, Castillo C, Porta M, de la Torre R. Consumption of buprenorphine and other drugs among heroin addicts under ambulatory treatment: results from cross-sectional studies in 1988 and 1990. *Addiction.* 1993; 88:1341-1349.
24. Strain EC, Preston KL, Liebson IA, Bigelow GE. Acute efffects of buprenorphine, hydromorphone and naloxone in methadone-maintained volunteers. *J Pharmacol Exp Ther.* 1992;261:985-993.
25. Johnson RE, Jaffe JH, Fudala PJ. A controlled trial of buprenorphine treatment for opioid dependence. *JAMA.* 1992;267:2750-2755.
26. Kosten TR, Schottenfeld R, Ziedonis D, Falcioni J. Buprenorphine versus methadone maintenance for opioid dependence. *J Nerv Ment Dis.* 1993;181:358-364.
27. Food and Drug Administration. *FDA Regulations in the Federal Register.* Washington, DC: Food and Drug Administration, March 2, 1989. 21 CFR Part 21.
28. McLellan AT, Luborsky L, O'Brien CP. Improved diagnostic instrument for substance abuse patients: the addiction severity index. *J Nerv Ment Dis.* 1985; 168:26-33.
29. Ling W. *Treatment Effectiveness Score as an Outcome Measure in Clinical Trials.* Washington, DC: National Institute on Drug Abuse. NIDA Research Monograph. In press.
30. Schuster C. An adequate dose is vital in checking the spread of AIDS. *NIDA Notes.* 1989;4:33.

Take The Next Logical Step.

Easy Access To The Information You Need

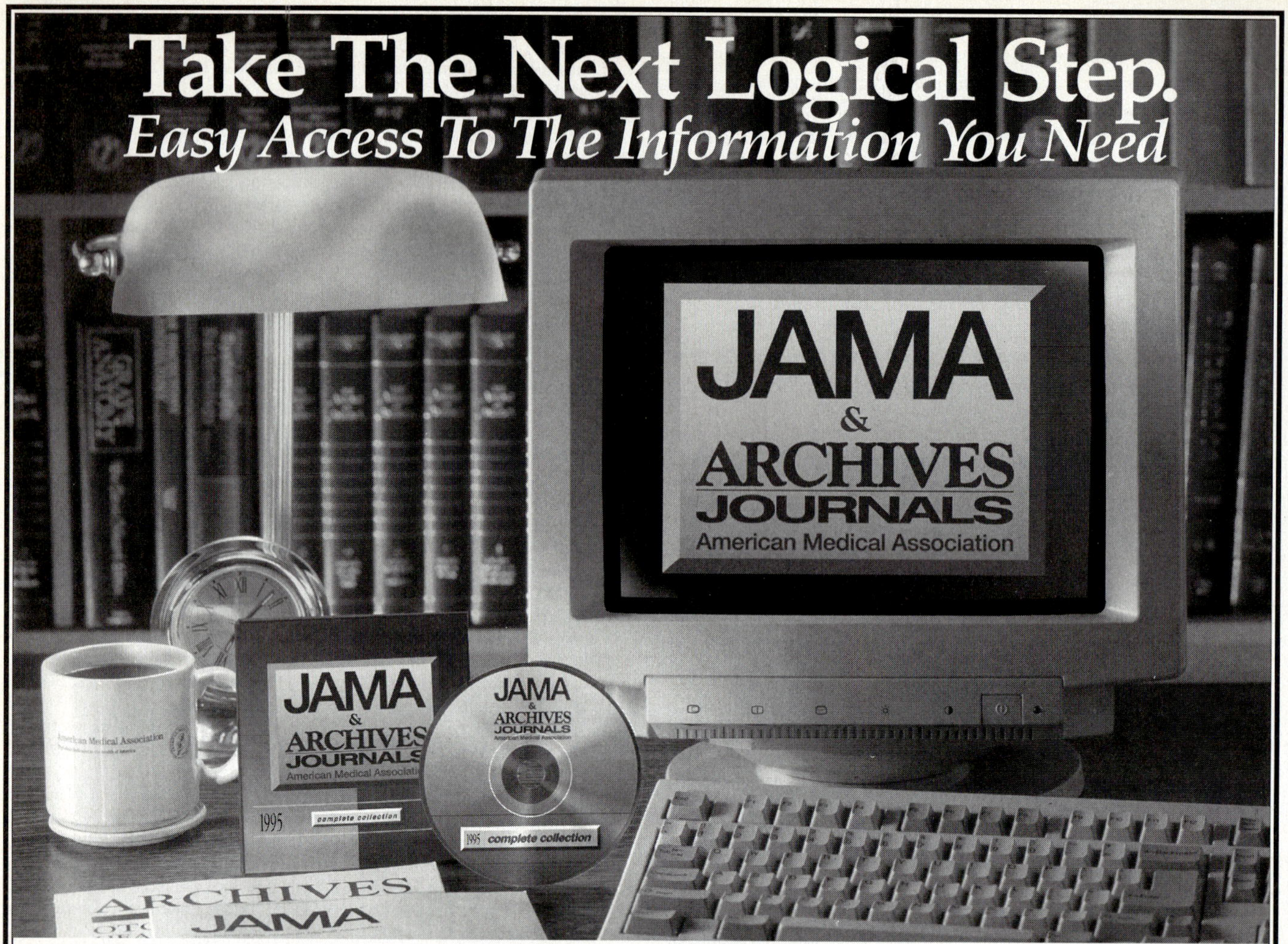

Introducing the complete JAMA & Archives Journals on CD-ROM. Superb reference materials have traditionally played a critical role in the practice of medicine. However, with the body of knowledge expanding so rapidly, along with increased pressures to maintain a broader base of expertise, conventional formats alone are no longer enough.

Now, with JAMA & Archives Journals on CD-ROM, you can easily search, cross-reference, print and save medical information from 10 of the world's most respected journals – right on your own computer. Plus, you have instant links to complete MEDLINE® references associated with the journal articles, along with a five-year JAMA & Archives Journals index.

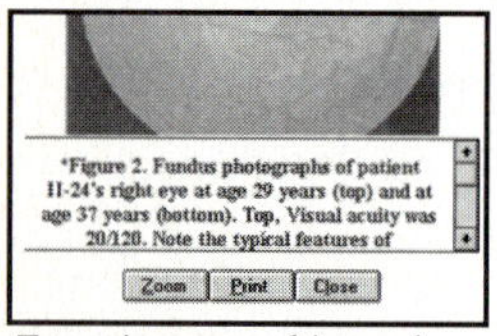

Zoom in on graphics and print complete articles.

An easy-to-use format, based on the journals themselves, makes the act of browsing the material very familiar. The powerful access capabilities quickly retrieve exactly the information you need.

Whether you're just beginning, or already well along in recognizing the ease of computer-based medical reference materials, JAMA & Archives Journals on CD-ROM is your next logical addition.

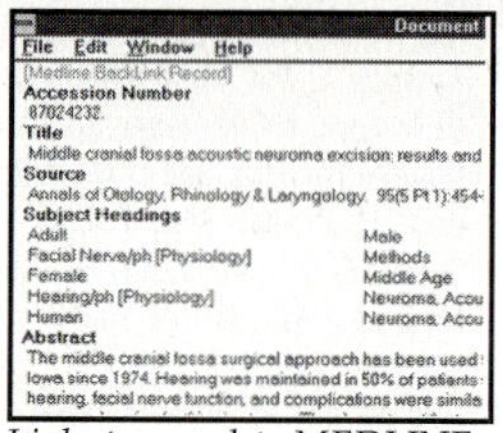

Links to complete MEDLINE references and 5-year abstracts.

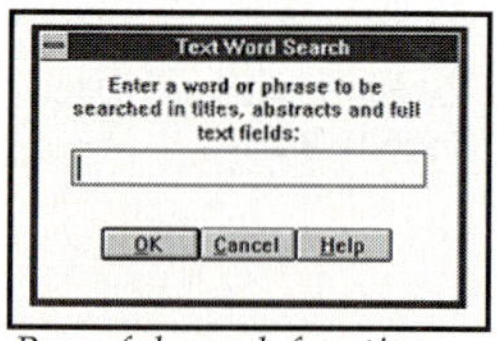

Powerful search functions can be performed by anyone.

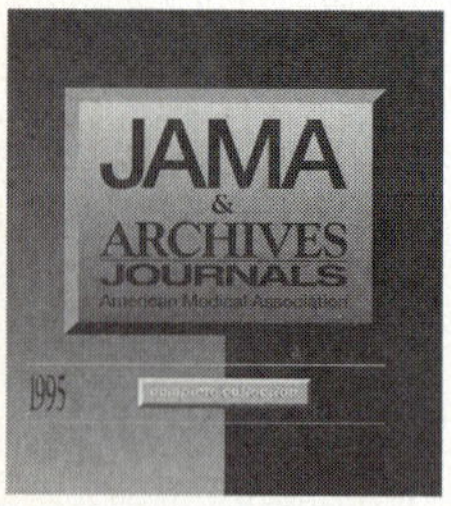

❏ **Yes, please send me**

JAMA & Archives Journals on CD-ROM

❏ 1995 Archival Disk **$150***
One disk includes editorial content from January-December 1995 for JAMA and all nine Archives Journals. 1995 Archival Disk will be shipped in February 1996.

❏ 1996 Quarterly Subscription **$250***
The first disk, containing editorial content for January through March 1996, will be shipped in April 1996. Each subsequent quarterly disk will be cumulative with the final disk in the subscription term containing the entire editorial content for 1996.

Minimum Windows System Requirements: 386-SX, 540 KB hard disk space, 4 MB RAM, VGA monitor. **Macintosh format not yet available.** OVID Software from OVID Technologies, Inc.

To order by phone, call

1-800-AMA-2350

Or, fax to **312-464-5831**

Mail coupon to: AMA Subscription Dept. CD, P.O. 10946, Chicago, IL 60610-0946

Please complete and return with your order:

Name

❏ MD/DO ❏ Other (please specify)__________

Address

City State

Country

Zip/Postal Code

Phone __________ Fax __________

❏ Check made payable to AMA ❏ VISA ❏ MC ❏ AmEx ❏ Optima

Card # __________

Exp. Date________ Signature__________

*Residents in AZ, CA, CT, DC, IL, IA, MN, NJ, NY, NC, WI, add required sales tax. In Canada, add GST. Contact AMA Subscription Dept for institution and foreign rates. Rates subject to change. Payment must accompany order. Nonrefundable.

P6FAB

Sustained Cocaine Abstinence in Methadone Maintenance Patients Through Voucher-Based Reinforcement Therapy

Kenneth Silverman, PhD; Stephen T. Higgins, PhD; Robert K. Brooner, PhD; Ivan D. Montoya, MD; Edward J. Cone, PhD; Charles R. Schuster, PhD; Kenzie L. Preston, PhD

Background: Chronic cocaine abuse remains a serious and costly public health problem. This study assessed the effectiveness of a voucher-based reinforcement contingency in producing sustained cocaine abstinence.

Methods: A randomized controlled trial compared voucher-based reinforcement of cocaine abstinence to noncontingent voucher presentation. Patients were selected from 52 consecutively admitted injecting heroin abusers in a methadone maintenance treatment program. Patients with heavy cocaine use during baseline period (N=37) participated. Except where otherwise indicated, the term *cocaine abuse* is used in this article in a generic sense and not according to the *DSM-III-R* definition. Patients exposed to abstinence reinforcement received a voucher for each cocaine-free urine sample (ie, negative for benzoylecgonine) provided three times per week throughout a 12-week period; the vouchers had monetary values that increased as the number of *consecutive* cocaine-free urine samples increased. Control patients received noncontingent vouchers that were matched in pattern and amount to the vouchers received by patients in the abstinence reinforcement group.

Results: Patients receiving vouchers for cocaine-free urine samples achieved significantly more weeks of cocaine abstinence (P=.007) and significantly longer durations of sustained cocaine abstinence (P=.001) than controls. Nine patients (47%) receiving vouchers for cocaine-free urine samples achieved between 7 and 12 weeks of sustained cocaine abstinence; only one control patient (6%) achieved more than 2 weeks of sustained abstinence. Among patients receiving vouchers for cocaine-free urine samples, those who achieved sustained abstinence (≥5 weeks) had significantly lower concentrations of benzoylecgonine in baseline urine samples than those who did not achieve sustained abstinence ($P \leq .01$). Patients receiving voucher reinforcement rated the overall treatment quality significantly higher than controls (P=.002).

Conclusion: Voucher-based reinforcement contingencies can produce sustained cocaine abstinence in injecting polydrug abusers.

(Arch Gen Psychiatry. 1996;53:409-415)

From the Addiction Research Center, Intramural Research Program of the National Institute on Drug Abuse, Baltimore, Md (Drs Silverman, Montoya, Cone, Schuster, and Preston); The Johns Hopkins University School of Medicine, Baltimore (Drs Silverman, Brooner, and Preston); and University of Vermont College of Medicine, Burlington (Dr Higgins). Dr Montoya is now affiliated with University of Antioquia, Medellín, Colombia. Dr Schuster is now affiliated with Wayne State University, Detroit, Mich.

DESPITE considerable efforts to control both supply and demand, cocaine abuse remains a serious public health problem. Intravenous cocaine abuse is a leading cause of the spread of acquired immunodeficiency syndrome (AIDS),[1,2] and cocaine abuse has been associated with increased rates of both crime[3] and death.[4] Unfortunately, there is no generally accepted treatment for cocaine abuse.[5-8] One promising intervention is reinforcement of drug abstinence in which patients receive tangible incentives that are contingent on providing objective evidence of drug abstinence.[9,10] An abstinence reinforcement system was recently developed for cocaine dependence in which patients receive vouchers exchangeable for goods and services for providing cocaine-free urine samples.[11-13] This system, used in combination with an intensive behavioral treatment program, has produced impressive outcomes in cocaine-dependent patients residing in a small metropolitan area.

The present study evaluated this reinforcement system in injecting cocaine–abusing patients receiving methadone maintenace treatment in an inner-city program. Cocaine abuse is a widespread clinical problem in inner-city methadone programs,[14-16] and so it is critical to determine the efficacy of the reinforcement intervention in this treatment context. Evaluation in patients receiving methadone treatment is also important because these

See Patients and Methods on next page

PATIENTS AND METHODS

PATIENTS

Participants were selected from 52 persons consecutively admitted over a 4-month period to methadone maintenance treatment at the Archway Clinic, Intramural Research Program, National Institute on Drug Abuse, Baltimore, Md. Patients participated if they used cocaine regularly during a baseline period. Except where otherwise indicated, the term *cocaine abuse* is used in this article in a generic sense and not according to the *DSM-III-R*[17] definition. Of the 52 patients, 47 completed the baseline period, and of these, 37 used cocaine regularly and therefore qualified for the study. Patients were screened for eligibility for methadone maintenance treatment by telephone followed by a 2-day screening process. Persons were eligible for methadone maintenance treatment if they were 18 to 65 years old, met Food and Drug Administration guidelines, and reported histories of injecting opiate use. Persons with major psychiatric or serious unstable medical illness were excluded. The study was approved by the institutional review board for human research, and patients gave informed written consent before participation.

PROCEDURES

Screening and Standard Treatment

Screening prior to entering treatment included the following: (1) Addiction Severity Index[18]; (2) National Institute of Mental Health Diagnostic Interview Schedule [19]; (3) Beck Depression Inventory[20]; (4) Symptom Check List-90–Revised[21]; and (5) Shipley Institute of Living Scale.[22] Throughout the study, patients received daily methadone, weekly individual counseling (45 minutes per week), and medical monitoring. The methadone dose of 50 mg was established by the fifth day of treatment. This dose was selected because it is a typical dose used in the United States.[23] Patients were strongly encouraged to attend counseling, wherein counselors emphasized abstinence from all drugs and promoted important lifestyle changes (eg, drug-free social support).

Urine and Breath Toxicology

Urine samples were collected Monday, Wednesday, and Friday of each week. The specimen collection process was observed through a one-way mirror and specimens were passed through an opening to a technician who measured specimen temperature. Samples were tested for cocaine (benzoylecgonine), opiates (morphine), benzodiazepines (oxazepam), phencyclidine (PCP), and marijuana, using the enzyme multiplication immunoassay technique (EMIT) (Syva Corp, Palo Alto, Calif). Samples were considered positive for cocaine, opiates, and benzodiazepines if concentrations were at or above 300 ng/mL, and for PCP and marijuana if concentrations were at or above 25 ng/mL and 50 ng/mL, respectively. Breath alcohol levels were assessed (Alco-Sensor III, Intoximeter Inc, St Louis, Mo) at the same times as urine sample testing. Urine aliquots were frozen at −30°C and later quantitatively analyzed for cocaine (TDx, Abbott Diagnostics, Abbott Park, Ill).[24] The lower limit for sensitivity of the assay for benzoylecgonine was 30 ng/mL.

Baseline Period

Patients participated in a baseline period that began on enrollment in treatment and continued until the patient provided 15 urine samples; this typically took 5 weeks. Patients who used cocaine regularly during the baseline (ie, at least three of the last 12 and two of the last six urine samples tested positive for cocaine) were then randomly assigned to the abstinence reinforcement or control group using minimum likelihood allocation.[25] This procedure stratified patients according to whether or not they were (1) heavy cocaine users (cocaine positive on all baseline urine samples); (2) light cocaine users (cocaine positive on only 50% or fewer of baseline urine samples); (3) male; (4) involved with a significant other who used drugs; (5) employed full-time; (6) on parole or probation. (See the "Voucher Period" section below for additional restriction on random assignment.) Patients in both groups then participated in a 12-week voucher period.

Voucher Period

On Monday, Wednesday, and Friday of each week of the voucher period, abstinence reinforcement patients received vouchers for providing cocaine-free urine samples according to two independent schedules.[11] Under the main schedule, patients received a voucher for each cocaine-free urine sample. The first cocaine-free urine sample earned a voucher worth $2.50; thereafter, vouchers increased in value by $1.50 for each consecutive cocaine-free urine sample. If the patient provided a cocaine-positive urine sample or failed to provide a scheduled urine sample, the patient did not receive a voucher and the value of the next earned voucher was reset to $2.50. Vouchers then increased in value in increments of $1.50 for each consecutive cocaine-free urine sample; if the patient provided six consecutive cocaine-free urine samples, the value of the voucher for the sixth urine sample increased to the highest value that the patient had achieved previously. This schedule provided escalating pay for sustained abstinence and was designed to promote long periods of sustained abstinence. Under a supplemental schedule, patients received a $10 bonus for every three consecutive cocaine-free urine samples. A patient who remained continuously abstinent for 12 consecutive weeks would earn a total of $1155 in vouchers. The vouchers were exchangeable for goods and services considered (by the first author) consistent with the patient's treatment goals; this was broadly defined and could include living necessities or educational or recreational items and activities. To exchange vouchers, patients made written requests to the treatment and research staff, and staff went into the community to make requested purchases.

Control patients received vouchers of comparable value and frequency as those of reinforcement patients, but independent of urinalysis results. Each control patient was yoked to a reinforcement patient who had already begun the voucher period. On every urine collection day numbered from 1 to 36 (three per week for 12 weeks) that the reinforcement patient earned a voucher for a cocaine-free urine sample, the control patient received a voucher of equal value for attending the clinic. To ensure that reinforcement patients would be available for the yoking procedure, the first six patients were assigned to the abstinence reinforcement group; after that, patients were randomly assigned as described above. Pairs of reinforcement and control patients were matched according to the stratification variables listed above. Control patients were told that (1) they would receive vouchers according to an unpredictable schedule, (2) they could not control when they would receive vouchers or how much they would be worth, and (3) the vouchers could be used to support their efforts to achieve cocaine abstinence by allowing them to purchase goods or services that might improve the quality of their lives. The rules for purchasing items were the same as those described above.

Exit Interview and Postintervention Period

At the completion of the voucher period, patients rated on a four-point scale (0, not at all, to 3, very much) whether the counseling, vouchers, and methadone were helpful in stopping their cocaine use, whether they would like to continue in the voucher condition if they could, and whether they had reduced or stopped their cocaine use during the voucher condition. They also compared on a five-point scale (from −2, much worse, to 2, much better) the drug abuse treatment they received during the study to other drug abuse treatments they had received in the past. Patients also indicated which of eight behaviors they had engaged in to reduce or stop their cocaine use (ie, attended Narcotics Anonymous meetings, avoided drug-using friends or relatives, avoided places where drugs were available, found new things to do, prayed for help from God, used willpower, spent more time with people who did not use drugs, threw away their "works," or none of these). Patients also completed the Beck Depression Inventory.[20] Standard methadone maintenance treatment along with urine and breath monitoring continued for 4 weeks after the voucher program was discontinued.

DATA ANALYSIS

Each patient was categorized as cocaine abstinent or cocaine positive for each week. A patient was abstinent only if all three samples for a week were cocaine negative based on EMIT results. Using the same definition, for each study week, each patient was categorized as abstinent from or positive for opiates, benzodiazepines, PCP, marijuana, and alcohol (breath testing). Missing urine samples were considered positive for all drugs. Secondary analyses were also conducted in which missing samples were considered positive only if a sample provided before or after the missing sample was positive. The results of the secondary analyses were essentially the same as the results of the primary analyses and will not be presented unless substantially discrepant from the primary analyses.

An analysis of variance (ANOVA) with group (reinforcement and control) as a factor was used to analyze the longest duration of sustained cocaine abstinence (ie, the largest number of consecutive weeks in which each patient was cocaine abstinent during the 12-week voucher period). Similar analyses were calculated for each of the other drugs.

A repeated-measures ANOVA (with Huynh-Feldt correction[26]) was calculated for cocaine abstinence by week with two factors: group (reinforcement and control) and time (weeks 1 through 17). Similar analyses were conducted for other drugs. Fisher's least significant difference planned comparisons[27,28] were used to compare the percentage of reinforcement and control patients who were cocaine abstinent for each of the study weeks. The percentages for all weeks were calculated based on the total number of patients initially entered into each group.

Fisher's least significant difference planned contrasts were used to compare mean percentage of reinforcement and control patients abstinent per week from each of the drugs tested during the 5-week baseline condition. Tukey's honestly significant difference post hoc contrasts were conducted to compare the mean percentage of subjects abstinent per week from each of the drugs tested averaged over the 12-week voucher period. The more conservative Tukey's test was used because we had no a priori assumptions that the voucher intervention would affect the use of substances other than cocaine.

For patients who remained in treatment for at least 1 month after the voucher period (n=15 [control patients]; n=15 [reinforcement patients]), analyses of urine data were conducted for that month similar to the ones described above.

Reinforcement and control groups were compared on all intake measures, exit interview responses, and voucher earnings. Categorical variables were analyzed using χ^2 tests (with continuity correction); continuous variables were analyzed using *t* tests.

Mean benzoylecgonine concentrations were calculated for baseline and voucher periods for individual patients; missing urine samples were omitted from calculations. Data were analyzed with a two-factor repeated-measures ANOVA, with group (reinforcement and control) and phase (baseline and voucher periods) as factors. Data from reinforcement group patients were further analyzed to compare patients who achieved substantial periods of sustained abstinence (≥5 weeks) and those who did not (<5 weeks). These groups were determined post hoc based on EMIT results. These data were analyzed with two-factor repeated-measures ANOVA with group (patients who achieved ≥5 weeks of sustained abstinence and patients who did not) and phase (baseline and voucher periods) as factors. Between-group comparisons were made using the Tukey test.

Pearson correlation coefficients (with Bonferroni's correction) were calculated between each intake characteristic and each of the two measures of cocaine use during the voucher period. No significant correlations were found.

Statistical tests were considered significant at $P \leq .05$ and were two-tailed. To correct for the number of intake characteristics compared (n=186) and the number of exploratory correlational analyses conducted (n=186), a Bonferroni corrected *P* value was used ($P \leq .001$).

patients tend to stay in treatment, presumably because of the methadone, which allows for evaluation of the effects of the voucher system on cocaine use with comparable retention rates across groups. While a previous study showed that voucher reinforcement improved treatment retention,[13] an important outcome in itself, it did not fully assess the effects of reinforcement contingencies on cocaine use independent of treatment retention.

RESULTS

PATIENT CHARACTERISTICS

Nineteen patients were assigned to the reinforcement group and 18 to the control group. At intake or during counseling all patients reported injecting cocaine and heroin. The **Table** shows characteristics of patients in the two groups based on data collected prior to the voucher period. These data show that the two groups appeared similar. The two groups differed ($P \leq .05$) on only two characteristics, race and SCL-90-R psychoticism scores, and those differences were not significant after a Bonferroni correction was made for the number of tests conducted. Correlational analyses between baseline characteristics and treatment outcome show that neither race (correlation between white patients and percent cocaine-free weeks, $r=.014$, $P=.94$; and between white patients and longest duration of cocaine abstinence, $r=-.028$, $P=.87$) nor scores on the psychoticism scale of the SCL-90-R (percent cocaine-free weeks, $r=.105$, $P=.55$; longest duration of cocaine abstinence, $r=.110$, $P=.53$) was associated with treatment outcome.

See also page 401

According to the Diagnostic Interview Schedule, 43% of patients met *DSM-III-R* lifetime criteria for cocaine dependence, 11% for cocaine abuse, and 25% for antisocial personality. Intake interviews appeared to grossly underestimate the frequency of cocaine abuse and dependence given the extremely high rates of cocaine use observed throughout the study. Underreporting of cocaine use is common in methadone programs,[29] and may result from the belief that programs exclude cocaine abusers from treatment.

RETENTION AND VOUCHER EARNINGS

Eighty-nine percent and 83% of patients in the abstinence reinforcement and control groups, respectively, were retained in treatment for all 12 weeks of the voucher period. Mean voucher earnings for the reinforcement ($426) and control ($357) groups were not significantly different. Control subjects had slightly lower earnings because they only received scheduled vouchers if they attended the clinic and therefore did not receive all available vouchers.

COCAINE USE

Reinforcement patients achieved significantly longer durations of sustained cocaine abstinence than controls (**Figure 1**; $F=13.5$; $df=1, 35$; $P<.001$). Very few pa-

Characteristics of Study Participants*

	Abstinence Reinforcement Group	Control Group
Mean age, y (±SE)	36.4 (1.6)	35.7 (1.3)
Married, %	16	11
≥12 y education, %	74	61
Race†		
% Black	26	67
% White	74	33
Past 30 days' income, $ (±SE)		
Illegal	563 (230)	556 (266)
Total	1238 (242)	1156 (290)
Usual employment pattern, %		
Employed full-time	47	39
Unemployed	37	44
Legal history		
Mean lifetime arrests (±SE)	9.79 (3.14)	7.56 (1.53)
Mean lifetime convictions (±SE)	5.6 (2.4)	3.5 (1.0)
Mean ASI composite scores (±SE)		
Medical	0.10 (0.06)	0.32 (0.10)
Employment	0.70 (0.08)	0.77 (0.05)
Alcohol	0.04 (0.01)	0.06 (0.03)
Drug	0.35 (0.02)	0.35 (0.02)
Legal	0.12 (0.04)	0.14 (0.05)
Family	0.23 (0.06)	0.24 (0.05)
Psychiatric	0.09 (0.04)	0.07 (0.03)
Baseline urine toxicology, % of samples positive per week (mean±SE)		
Benzodiazepines	27 (3)	20 (3)
Cocaine	99 (1)	97 (2)
Opiates	55 (4)	60 (5)
Phencyclidine	11 (0)	8 (2)
Marijuana	28 (3)	19 (3)
Mean total BDI score (±SE)	15 (2)	20 (3)
Mean SCL-90-R scores (±SE)		
Somatization	61 (2)	67 (2)
Obsessive-compulsive	60 (3)	63 (2)
Interpersonal sensitivity	58 (3)	60 (3)
Depression	64 (2)	68 (2)
Anxiety	60 (3)	65 (2)
Hostility	56 (3)	55 (2)
Phobic anxiety	53 (2)	57 (2)
Paranoid ideation	58 (3)	59 (3)
Psychoticism‡	54 (3)	64 (3)
Global Severity Index	63 (3)	67 (3)
Positive Symptom Distress Index	61 (2)	59 (2)
Positive Symptom Total	60 (3)	65 (2)
DIS score (% of patients with current diagnosis)		
Nicotine	53	61
Phobia	5	11
Posttraumatic stress disorder	11	0
Major depression	0	6
Dysthymia	0	6
Antisocial personality disorder	21	22
Bulimia	5	0
Alcohol	16	11
Cannabis	0	6
Amphetamine	0	6
Sedative	16	0
Cocaine	47	33
Heroin	100	100
Opioid	26	28
Gambling	5	0

*ASI indicates Addiction Severity Index[18]; BDI, Beck Depression Inventory[20]; SCL-90-R, Symptom Check List-90–Revised[21]; and DIS, Diagnostic Interview Schedule.[19]

†*P=.033.*

‡*P=.017;* P *values for other characteristics were not significant (*P*>.05).*

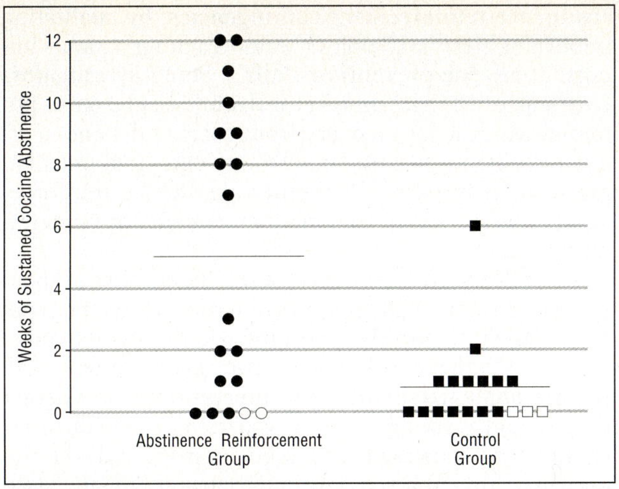

Figure 1. *Longest duration of sustained cocaine abstinence achieved during the 12-week voucher condition. Each point represents data for an individual patient; the lines represent group means. The 19 abstinence reinforcement patients are displayed in the left column (circles) and the 18 control patients in the right (squares). Open symbols represent patients who dropped out of the study early.*

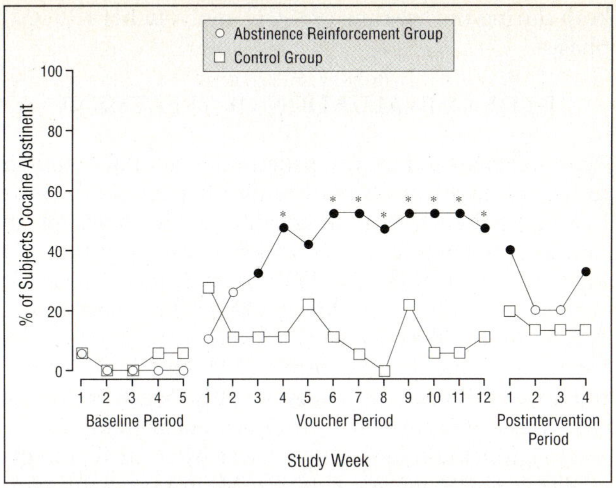

Figure 2. *Percentage of patients abstinent during 25 successive study weeks. A patient was considered cocaine abstinent for a given week if all of the three urine samples for that week were negative for cocaine. Solid circles and asterisks indicate the weeks on which the abstinence reinforcement group value differed significantly from the control group value according to planned comparisons based on a repeated-measures analysis of variance (P≤.05 and P≤.01, respectively). Data for the 4-week postintervention period are based on the urinalysis results from subjects who completed the entire 4-week postintervention period (15 control and 15 abstinence reinforcement subjects).*

tients in either group were abstinent during any baseline weeks, but the percentage of reinforcement patients who were cocaine abstinent increased progressively during the voucher period to a level significantly above that observed in the control group (**Figure 2**). A repeated-measures ANOVA revealed significant group (F=8.16; *df*=1, 35; *P*=.007) and group × time (F=5.45; *df*=16, 560; *P*<.001) effects. Repeated-measures ANOVA did not show an effect of the reinforcement intervention during the postintervention period; however, planned comparisons showed that significantly more reinforcement than control patients were cocaine abstinent on the first and last week of the postintervention period (Figure 2).

OTHER DRUG AND ALCOHOL USE

Tukey's post hoc contrasts indicated that the mean percent (± SE) of reinforcement patients abstinent per week from opiates during the voucher period (52%±2%) was significantly greater than controls (33%±4%) (*P*≤.01). Tukey's post hoc contrasts also showed that the mean percent of reinforcement patients abstinent per week from alcohol during the voucher period (78%±3%) was significantly greater than the percent of controls (60%±4%) (*P*≤.01).

The effects of the voucher intervention on benzodiazepine, marijuana, and PCP use is less clear since the primary and secondary analyses produced conflicting results: Tukey's post hoc contrasts based on primary analyses (missing samples considered positive) showed that the mean percent of reinforcement patients abstinent per week from benzodiazepines (57%), marijuana (57%), and PCP (72%) during the voucher period did not differ significantly from the mean percent of control patients abstinent from those substances (52%, 64%, and 57%, respectively). In contrast, based on the secondary analyses (missing samples considered positive only if a sample provided before or after the missing sample was positive), significantly (*P*≤.05) fewer reinforcement patients were abstinent from those substances (70%, 71%, and 88%, respectively) relative to controls (81%, 86%, and 98%, respectively). Finally, the repeated-measures ANOVA of urinalysis data from the 4-week postintervention period did not reveal any significant differences between the reinforcement and control patients for any of the drugs tested or for alcohol.

QUANTITATIVE URINALYSES

Urine benzoylecgonine concentrations (mean total ± SE) for the 5-week baseline were similar for the control (35 566±7076 ng/mL) and reinforcement (42 929±8092 ng/mL) groups. Compared to baseline, benzoylecgonine concentrations in the evaluation period were unchanged for the control group (to 40 357±9780 ng/mL) but were decreased by approximately one half for the reinforcement group (to 18 584±4527 ng/mL). Furthermore, there was a significant group by phase interaction (F=7.92; *df*=1, 35; *P*=.008), reflecting a lack of change in concentration from baseline to voucher phases in the control group but a substantial decrease in the experimental group.

Reinforcement group patients who achieved sustained cocaine abstinence (≥5 weeks; n=9) had mean (±SE) benzoylecgonine concentrations of 21 709±5669 ng/mL during baseline and 3142±1883 ng/mL during voucher phases. Reinforcement patients who failed to achieve sustained cocaine abstinence (<5 weeks; n=10) had mean (± SE) concentrations of 62 028±11 729 ng/mL during baseline and 32 483±5453 ng/mL during voucher phases. There were significant main effects of group (F=20.61; *df*=1, 17; *P*<.001) and phase (F=11.44; *df*=1, 17; *P*=.004). Tukey's post hoc test showed a significant difference between those patients who achieved 5 weeks or more of sustained abstinence and those who did not, both during the baseline ($P \leq .01$) and voucher ($P \leq .05$) phases.

PATIENT EVALUATION OF TREATMENT

Reinforcement and control patients did not differ on their ratings of the helpfulness of counseling and methadone in helping them stop their cocaine use; however, mean ratings of the helpfulness of vouchers were significantly higher (t=2.23; df=31; P=.033) for reinforcement (2.20) than for controls (1.33). Mean ratings of patients' desire "to continue in the voucher condition" were high for both the reinforcement and controls (2.89 and 2.73, respectively) and did not differ significantly. Mean ratings of the overall treatment by reinforcement patients (1.72) were significantly higher than those by control patients (0.93) (t=3.29; df= 31; P=.002). Mean ratings by reinforcement patients as to whether they had stopped or reduced their cocaine use during the voucher condition (2.33) were significantly higher than controls (1.60) (t=2.15; df= 31; P=.04). Finally, significantly more reinforcement patients (61%) than control patients (27%) indicated that they used "willpower" (t=2.04; df= 31; P=.05) to stop or reduce their cocaine use; no other differences on the exit interview measures were significant.

COMMENT

This study showed that voucher-based reinforcement[11-13] can produce sustained cocaine abstinence in inner-city injecting polydrug abusers in the context of standard methadone maintenance treatment. About half (47%) of the patients exposed to the reinforcement intervention achieved between 7 and 12 weeks of sustained cocaine abstinence, and overall concentrations of the cocaine metabolite benzoylecgonine decreased by 56%. In contrast, only one control patient (6%) achieved more than 2 weeks of sustained cocaine abstinence, and mean benzoylecgonine concentrations did not decrease. High retention rates for both groups allowed for a thorough evaluation of the effects of the intervention on cocaine use as determined by urinalyses. The reinforcement intervention was also associated with decreases in the use of opiates and alcohol, even though use of those substances was not explicitly targeted by the intervention. Patients gave favorable evaluations of the reinforcement intervention. The study also identified the aspect of the reinforcement system responsible for the observed effects: the contingent as opposed to noncontingent presentation of vouchers.

This study represents only an initial step in the development and application of an abstinence reinforcement technology, and a systematic program of research is needed. The current study employed a small sample size and was conducted in the context of a single treatment clinic, so it will be important to conduct studies on a larger scale, eg, in multisite clinical trials.

As with virtually all drug-abuse treatments, relapse to drug use was common in this study after the intervention was discontinued. Future investigations will have to explore methods of sustaining abstinence for longer periods of time, perhaps by extending the duration of the abstinence reinforcement contingencies, by facilitating important lifestyle changes,[30] or by teaching patients important relapse-prevention skills.[31] Some investigators have suggested that "short-term abstinence presents a potential window for recovery from cocaine dependency" during which other treatments may take hold and "begin to have impact."[32] Whether abstinence reinforcement can be used in this manner remains to be determined.

While the voucher intervention was effective in about half the patients, a large proportion of reinforcement patients failed to stop their cocaine use for any extended period. Whether those treatment-resistant patients will require qualitatively different interventions or whether they would respond to improved reinforcement interventions (eg, increased reinforcement magnitudes) is unknown at this point. Quantitative urinalysis suggested that the patients with the heaviest cocaine use were least likely to achieve long periods of sustained abstinence when exposed to the voucher intervention. While these quantitative urinalysis results are interesting, they must be interpreted cautiously, since changes in benzoylecgonine concentrations can result either from changes in the amount of cocaine use or from changes in temporal patterns of use. Nevertheless, future studies will have to explore alternative interventions for treatment-resistant patients, and the quantitative urinalyses may provide a means of identifying patients in need of those special interventions.

Systematic research is needed to develop practical applications of this technology, especially those that can use existing sources of funding. Viable applications could take a number of forms, some of which have not yet even been considered, and creative efforts will be needed to design and evaluate them. For example, abstinence reinforcement systems could be integrated into existing programs (eg, welfare) that provide financial support to drug abusers. Although government benefits have historically been provided to recipients on a noncontingent basis, many states are recognizing that public assistance benefits may be of greater value to recipients if they are used to promote important lifestyle changes. Thus, a growing number of states are adopting welfare-to-work programs in which benefits are given to recipients only if they engage in employment and employment-related behaviors.[33] Similarly, providing public assistance benefits contingent on verified drug abstinence could provide a cost-effective means of funding abstinence reinforcement on a large scale. One such application is currently being developed for the treatment of drug-abusing schizophrenic patients in which a portion of their monthly disability payment is being provided to patients on a daily basis, contingent on their abstinence from cocaine use.[34]

CONCLUSIONS

Cocaine abuse has not yielded to conventional treatments and may require novel approaches such as voucher-based abstinence reinforcement. While the potential benefits of reinforcement interventions are considerable, as described above, many issues remain unresolved. Of special concern is the issue of addressing the needs of patients who fail to achieve abstinence when exposed to contingent interventions. For this reason, the development and application of the technology should proceed cautiously, with careful and thorough scientific evaluation. Abstinence reinforcement interventions are amenable to empirically based development. Because abstinence reinforcement procedures are concrete, specific, and largely quantitative, they can be systematically and parametrically manipulated in the search for optimal parameters of efficiency and effectiveness. Those investigations can be guided by an extensive body of laboratory and clinical research on operant conditioning and reinforcement, from which the voucher-based abstinence intervention was derived. Finally, the abstinence reinforcement procedures are precisely reproducible, a feature that should facilitate their systematic and controlled dissemination.

Accepted for publication October 26, 1995.

This research was supported by the National Institute on Drug Abuse through its intramural research budget.

Presented in part at the 27th Annual Association for Advancement of Behavior Therapy Convention, Atlanta, Ga, November 19, 1993, and at the 56th Annual Scientific Meeting of the College on Problems in Drug Dependence, Palm Beach, Fla, June 20, 1994.

We thank research assistants Chris Johnson and Anna DeJesus, Addiction Research Center, National Institute on Drug Abuse, for their expert technical assistance; Linda Felch for statistical consultation and support; and the staff of the Archway Clinic for providing excellent patient care and assistance in implementing this protocol. We also thank Christopher Sheppard and Rosalind Jones for performing the quantitative urine assays.

Reprint requests to the National Institute on Drug Abuse, Division of Intramural Research, Clinical Trials Section, PO Box 5180, Baltimore, MD 21224 (Dr Preston).

REFERENCES

1. Friedman SR, Lipton DS, Stimel B. *Cocaine, AIDS, and Intravenous Drug Use.* New York, NY: Harrington Park Press; 1991:1-11.
2. Chaisson RE, Bacchetti P, Osmond D, Brodie B, Sande MA, Moss AR. Cocaine use and HIV infection in intravenous drug users in San Francisco. *JAMA.* 1989; 261:561-565.
3. De La Rosa M, Lambert EY, Gropper B, eds. *Drugs and Violence: Causes, Correlates, and Consequences.* Washington, DC: US Government Printing Office; 1990. NIDA Research Monograph 103.
4. *Drug Abuse: The Crack Cocaine Epidemic: Health Consequences and Treatment.* Washington, DC; General Accounting Office: 1991. GAO/HRD-91-55FS.
5. Johanson CE, Schuster CR. Cocaine. In: DJ Kupfer, FE Bloom, eds. *Psychopharmacology: The Fourth Generation of Progress.* New York, NY: Raven Press; 1995:1685-1697.
6. Gorelick DA. Pharmacologic therapies for cocaine addiction. In: Miller NS, Gold M, eds. *Pharmacological Therapies for Alcohol and Drug Addictions.* New York, NY: Marcel Dekker Inc; 1994:143-157.
7. Rawson RA, Obert JL, McCann MJ, Castro FG, Ling W. Cocaine abuse treatment: a review of current strategies. *J Subst Abuse.* 1991;3:457-491.
8. Rawson RA, McCann MJ, Hasson AJ, Ling W. Cocaine abuse among methadone patients: are there effective treatment strategies? *J Psychoactive Drugs.* 1994;26:129-136.
9. Stitzer ML, Higgins ST. Behavioral treatment of drug and alcohol abuse. In: Bloom FE, Kupfer DJ, eds. *Psychopharmacology: The Fourth Generation of Progress.* New York, NY: Raven Press; 1995:1807-1819.
10. Stitzer ML, Bigelow GE, Gross J. Behavioral treatments of drug abuse. In: *Treatments of Psychiatric Disorders: A Task Force Report of the American Psychiatric Association.* Washington, DC: American Psychiatric Association; 1989;2: 1430-1448.
11. Higgins ST, Delaney DD, Budney AJ, Bickel WK, Hughes JR, Feorg F, Fenwick JW. A behavioral approach to achieving initial cocaine abstinence. *Am J Psychiatry.* 1991;148:1218-1224.
12. Higgins ST, Budney AJ, Bickel WK, Hughes JR, Foerg F, Badger GJ. Achieving cocaine abstinence with a behavioral approach. *Am J Psychiatry.* 1993;150: 763-769.
13. Higgins ST, Budney AJ, Bickel WK, Foerg FE, Donham R, Badger GJ. Incentives improve outcome in outpatient behavioral treatment of cocaine dependence. *Arch Gen Psychiatry.* 1994;51:568-576.
14. Kosten TR, Gawin FH, Rounsaville BJ, Kleber HD. Cocaine abuse among opioid addicts: demographic and diagnostic factors in treatment. *Am J Drug Alcohol Abuse.* 1986;12:1-16.
15. Hanbury R, Sturiano V, Cohen M, Stimmel B, Aguillaume C. Cocaine use in persons on methadone maintenance. *Adv Alcohol Subst Abuse.* 1986;6:91-106.
16. Condelli WS, Fairbank JA, Dennis ML, Rachal JV. Cocaine use by clients in methadone programs: significance, scope, and behavioral interventions. *J Subst Abuse Treat.* 1991;8:203-212.
17. American Psychiatric Association. *Diagnostic and Statistical Manual of Mental Disorders, Revised Third Edition.* Washington, DC: American Psychiatric Association; 1987.
18. McLellan AT, Luborsky L, Cacciola J, Griffith J, Evans F, Barr HL, O'Brien CP. New data from the Addiction Severity Index: reliability and validity in three centers. *J Nerv Ment Dis.* 1985;173:412-423.
19. Robins LN, Helzer JE, Croughan J, Ratcliff KS. National Institute of Mental Health Diagnostic Interview Schedule: its history, characteristics, and validity. *Arch Gen Psychiatry.* 1981;38:381-389.
20. Beck AT, Steer RA. *Beck Depression Inventory Manual.* New York, NY: Psychological Corp; 1987.
21. Derogatis LR. *SCL-90-R Administration, Scoring & Procedures Manual–II for the Revised Version.* Towson, Md: Clinical Psychometric Research; 1977.
22. Zachary RA. *Shipley Institute of Living Scale, Revised Manual.* Los Angeles, Calif: Western Psychological Services; 1986.
23. D'Aunno T, Vaughn TE. Variations in methadone treatment practices: results from a national study. *JAMA.* 1992;267:253-258.
24. Cone EJ, Menchen SL, Mitchell J. Validity testing of the TDX cocaine metabolite assay with human specimens obtained after intravenous cocaine administration. *Forensic Sci Int.* 1988;37:265-275.
25. Aickin M. A program for balancing the allocation of subjects in a clinical trial. *Comput Biomed Res.* 1982;15:519-524.
26. Huynh H, Feldt LS. Estimation of the Box correction for degrees of freedom from sample data in randomized-block and split-plot designs. *J Educ Stat.* 1976; 1:69-82.
27. Keppel G. *Design and Analysis: A Researcher's Handbook.* 2nd ed. Englewood Cliffs, NJ: Prentice-Hall Inc; 1982:146-150.
28. Bruning JL, Kintz BL. *Computational Handbook of Statistics.* 2nd ed. Glenview, Ill: Scott Foresman & Co; 1977:113-116.
29. Sherman MF, Bigelow GE. Validity of patients' self-reported drug use as a function of treatment status. *Drug Alcohol Depend.* 1992;30:1-11.
30. Higgins ST, Budney AJ, Bickel WK, Badger GJ, Foerg FE, Ogden D. Outpatient behavioral treatment for cocaine dependence: one-year outcome. *Exp Clin Psychopharmacol.* 1995;3:205-212.
31. Carroll KM, Rounsaville BJ, Nich C, Gordon LT, Wirtz PW, Gawin F. One-year follow-up of psychotherapy and pharmacotherapy for cocaine dependence: delayed emergence of psychotherapy effects. *Arch Gen Psychiatry.* 1994;51:989-997.
32. Gawin FH, Kleber HD, Byck R, Rounsaville BJ, Kosten TR, Jatlow PI, Morgan C. Desipramine facilitation of initial cocaine abstinence. *Arch Gen Psychiatry.* 1989;46:117-121.
33. Friedlander D, Ricco J, Freedman S. *GAIN: Two-Year Impacts in Six Counties: California's Greater Avenues for Independence Program.* New York, NY: Manpower Demonstration Research Corp; 1993.
34. Shaner AE, Eckman TT, Roberts LJ, Wilkens JN, Tucker DE, Tsuang JW, Mintz J. Disability income, cocaine use, and repeated hospitalization among schizophrenic cocaine abusers. *N Engl J Med.* 1995;333:777-783.

ORIGINAL ARTICLE

Israeli Preschoolers Under Scud Missile Attacks

A Developmental Perspective on Risk-Modifying Factors

Nathaniel Laor, MD, PhD; Leo Wolmer, MA; Linda C. Mayes, MD; Abigail Golomb, MD; Donald S. Silverberg, MD; Ronit Weizman, MD; Donald J. Cohen, MD

Background: The devastating effects of traumatic events on children are modulated by risk and protective factors. This study examines the differential effects of traumatic displacement of preschool children and their families following Scud missile attacks on Israel during the Persian Gulf War.

Methods: Three groups participated in the study: families displaced after their houses were damaged, undisplaced families from the same neighborhood (without home damage), and families from a distant city that was threatened but not directly attacked. Data concerning the traumatic event, the child (personality, internalizing, externalizing, and stress symptoms), the mother (Symptom Checklist-90–Revised), and the family (Family Adaptability and Cohesion Evaluation Scales) were gathered 6 months after the end of the war.

Results: Displaced children and mothers showed higher externalizing and stress symptom levels compared with undisplaced and threatened subjects. Destruction of the house and displacement, but not mere distance from the missile impact, explained symptomatic behavior. Inadequate family cohesion predicted symptomatic reaction for 3- and 4-year-old children but not for older ones.

Conclusions: Both human and nonhuman factors contribute to the preschool child's adaptive mechanisms that regulate environmental stressful stimuli. These risk-modifying factors become more autonomous of caretakers with increasing age.

(Arch Gen Psychiatry. 1996;53:416-423)

From the Tel Aviv–Brull Community Mental Health Center (Drs Laor, Golomb, and Weizman and Mr Wolmer), Sourasky Medical Center (Dr Silverberg), and Department of Psychiatry, Sackler Faculty of Medicine, Tel Aviv University (Drs Laor and Weizman), Tel Aviv, Israel; and the Yale Child Study Center, New Haven, Conn (Drs Laor, Mayes, and Cohen).

CLINICIANS TREATING children during World War II[1] and researchers studying reactions to natural disasters[2] have described in detail the impact of stressful events on children. In the last two decades, more rigorous studies have also reported the effects of acute stressors on early development. A wide variety of stressors have been examined: sibling death[3]; natural disasters such as hurricanes,[4] floods,[5] and bushfires[6-8]; and provoked aggressive incidents such as the Holocaust,[9] parental murder,[10] sexual assault,[11] kidnapping,[12] sniper attacks,[13] and war.[14] While most of the children facing these stressful situations do not develop psychiatric illnesses, more careful study typically reveals the appearance of symptomatic stress reactions.[5,13,15] The symptoms include clinging and demanding behavior, sleep problems, fears and anxiety, irritability, regression, intrusive thoughts, restricted social and affective life, and concentration difficulties. Several investigators[5,6,16] have proposed grouping these symptoms in children according to the *DSM-III-R*[17] criteria for posttraumatic stress disorder (PTSD): reexperiencing, avoidance or numbing, and increased arousal. Terr's[15] description of children's reactions to traumatic events shows a similarity to PTSD as defined by *DSM-III-R* criteria for adults. According to Terr,[12] however, children usually do not exhibit a period of amnesia about the experience, alternations between denial and repetitive intrusive phenomena, or true flashbacks and dream reenactments. Furthermore, instead of showing common PTSD symptoms,[5] preschool children with a posttraumatic disorder more often exhibit loss of recently gained developmental skills, increased irritability or problems with wake-sleep cycles, and nonspecific distractability and lability. Moreover, this nonspecific behavioral disorganization is strongly influenced by parental reaction.[4,5]

The majority of studies on children's reactions to natural disasters and

See Subjects and Methods on next page

SUBJECTS AND METHODS

THE TRAUMATIC EVENT

The events leading to the missile attacks on Tel Aviv during the Persian Gulf War were initiated months before the actual missile attacks and ended months after. It started with the Iraqi invasion of Kuwait followed by the international warning (August 1990) and the final ultimatum of the US-led coalition (January 1991). In that period, gas masks were distributed to every person in Israel, including newborns in the delivery rooms of hospitals, and citizens prepared the necessary materials for sealing rooms against chemical attacks. Five missile attacks hit heavily populated neighborhoods in the greater Tel Aviv area, damaging over 7000 houses during the first 2 weeks of the war. Two of the missiles affected the populations studied in this article. The threat of the missiles (January through February 1991) brought about a radical change in the daily routine of the Israeli population, particularly in what were considered the target areas, ie, the major, heavily populated cities. The attacks were expected throughout the night. Thus, people were anxious to return home earlier and avoided evening outdoor activities. Each missile alert represented a genuine threat transmitted throughout the whole country. With each alert, families were required to gather fully masked in sealed rooms. The families under investigation (n=72) had homes destroyed by the missiles. These families were displaced and were offered refuge in "third-rate" hotels within the bounds of the hit zone. Hence, they were not spared the continuous stress of the war. Twenty-five percent of the houses were still uninhabitable 6 months after the attack. The mean period of displacement was 14 weeks (range, 2 to 30 weeks). At the time when the families returned home (August 1991), they were approached for participation in the follow-up study.

SUBJECTS

The subjects of the study were 230 preschool children and their mothers, divided into three groups. The experimental group (n=72) consisted of families whose houses were destroyed and who moved into hotels (displaced group). Two control groups were matched for socioeconomic status, the sex of the child, distance from the missile impact, and age. The first control group (n=81) came from families living in the same neighborhood as the experimental group (and at a similar distance from the missile strikes: range, 10 to 500 m), but whose houses remained intact (undisplaced group). The second control group (n=77) was selected from lists of families provided by the public health agency in the southern city of Beer Sheva, 120 km (70 miles) from the impact area; these families were under the threat of missile attack throughout the war (threatened group). No siblings were included in the sample. The subjects came from intact families from the bottom socioeconomic quartile of the Israeli population, which was defined by a scale operationalizing four criteria: professional status, educational level, income level, and housing density.[30] All families agreed to volunteer and take part in the study and they all signed an informed consent form.

PROCEDURES

Six months after the end of the Persian Gulf War, 90 families with preschool children (3 to 5 years old) included in the Tel Aviv municipality list of displaced families were asked to participate in the study. Seventy-two of these families agreed. The rest refused further contact. The two control groups were defined as described previously. Trained psychologists interviewed the mothers during a 2-hour session in which self-report measures provided information on the family, the event itself, symptoms related to the child and to the parent, personality of the child, and family cohesion and adaptability. Demographic data regarding the family (eg, age of parents, number of children), and information related to the event (length of the displacement, damage to the house, personal injuries, distance from the missile impact) were gathered by the Exposure to Event Questionnaire (available from the authors).

INSTRUMENTS

Mother's Symptoms

The mother's symptoms were measured by the Symptom Checklist-90–Revised (SCL-90-R) scales[31] and the Global Severity Index.

Continued on next page

traumatic situations have involved school-age children[7,8,12,13,18] or adolescents.[12,18,19] The higher verbal and conceptual capacities of older children permit the researcher to use interviews and self-report techniques that eliminate certain biases inherent in the parents' reports used in research with preschoolers.

The present study focuses on the relation between parental response to the traumatic event and the severity and persistence of the preschool child's acute symptoms. The assumption of the study is that parents play an important role in the development of a "protective matrix" in preschool-age children. The protective matrix consists of cultural, social, physical, familial, and personal adaptive mechanisms regulating environmental stressful stimuli. The younger the child, the more dependent he or she is on the immediate supportive environment, and thus the more vulnerable he or she is to stressful stimuli.

The notion that the developing mental apparatus is in need of buffering against the disorganizing effects of traumatic events goes back to Freud. He postulated[20,21] the existence of a superficial "protective shield," functioning as an external stimulus barrier, an envelope that passively filters stimuli and scales down the traumatic event to manageable intensity. Trauma was thus perceived as a massive break of this protective shield. To this day, this concept is central to the major theoretical formulations in the field.[22] A view of development as occurring within the parent-child dyad[23-26] calls for the replacement of the concept of the passive protective filter on the child's side with a more dynamic matrix that is constructed between parent and child. This matrix helps

Child's Symptoms and Personality

The following scales relating to the child's symptoms were used: (1) The Child Behavior Checklist (CBCL).[32] Based on research with Israeli preschool children,[33] items were grouped according to 10 behavioral clusters of symptoms: aggression, withdrawal, depression, delinquency, anxiety, odd behavior, immaturity, hyperactivity, somatic complaints, and unpopular behavior. A scale score was computed, averaging the items within each cluster. (2) The Preschool Children's Assessment of Stress Scale (PCASS) (available from the authors), which assesses the child's reaction as a result of a stressor (ie, the missile attack) based on parental reports (Cronbach's α=.89). Assessed in a semistructured interview are symptoms such as anxiety, fears, sleep problems, mood changes, loss of recently acquired developmental skills (eg, toilet training), and mood lability. (3) The Change of Functioning Scale (CFS) (also available from the authors), a 3-point scale (range, 9 to 27) assessing nine symptoms (separation; mood changes; fears; tension; problems with eating, sleeping, and toileting; general health; and level of maturity) (Cronbach's α=.90) was completed for three time points: the interview and, retrospectively, the war and prewar periods. The child's personality was studied by the Childhood Personality Scales.[34] This instrument assesses five personality factors: good attention, sociability, zestfulness, verbal expressiveness, and behavior modulation. (For psychometric information about the different factors, see Cohen et al.[34])

Family Functioning

The Hebrew version[35] of the Family Adaptability and Cohesion Evaluation Scales (FACES)[36] measured two central aspects of the family system's functioning: the capacity of the family to change its power structure, roles, and norms as a result of external and developmental pressures (adaptability) and the affective bonds between family members (cohesion). The model implies curvilinear relations between each dimension of the scale and adequate family functioning (for example, both too much and too little cohesion reflect inadequate functioning).

DATA ANALYSIS

Individual symptom scales from the CBCL and PCASS were submitted to 3 (displaced vs undisplaced vs threatened) × 3 (3- vs 4- vs 5-year-olds) × 2 (boys vs girls) analyses of variance (ANOVAs), and to Scheffé post hoc tests. Data concerning the CFS at three time points (within-subject) were analyzed by repeated-measures multivariate ANOVA. Because of the curvilinear characteristic of the FACES dimensions (extreme scores reflecting inadequate functioning), cohesion and adaptability scores were transformed into distance from the research sample's mean scores for these dimensions. Distance was the square power of the difference between the raw score and our sample's mean. It was then correlated with the mother's and child's symptom scales. In order to cluster statistically the data regarding children's symptoms, the symptom clusters of the two scales used (CBCL and PCASS) were entered into a principal components factor analysis with varimax rotation. Finally, regression analyses were performed to examine the relation between the severity and duration of the child's symptoms, the mother's symptoms, and family cohesion and adaptability. Because of multiple comparisons, significance level was set at .01 after Bonferroni adjustment.

the child regulate both external and internal stimuli. This study examines, among other things, the preschool-age child's growing capacity for such regulation.

The complementary pair of concepts "vulnerability" and "protection" is central to discussions concerning exposure to risk situations.[27] Three major factors are defined as protective for the child: the child's personal (internal) strength, the warmth and cohesion of the family, and the support provided from sources external to the nuclear family. Thus, it may be assumed that prewar psychopathology in the child and/or a parent reacting pathologically to the missile attack could lead to a more severe and prolonged reaction in the child. Conversely, the child's healthy adaptive mechanisms and adequately cohesive family may help regulate the protective matrix and prevent its collapse. In the same vein, speaking about a child living in a stress-resistant family, Baldwin et al[28] stated that " . . . such a child is shielded from many of the risks of the environment by a protective family that creates a low-risk proximal environment despite living in a high-risk distal environment."

The Scud missile attack on the city of Tel Aviv, Israel, during the Persian Gulf War served as an opportunity to study the effects of acute and continuous stress of war on a civilian population (see also Solomon et al[29]). We report on the impact of the destruction of the houses and resulting displacement of hundreds of preschool children and their families from their homes following the missile attacks. Three groups of children and their families living at different distances from the affected area were studied with an accent on three protective dimensions: the child's personality, the mother's profile and response to the event, and the family cohesion and adaptability. Further variables relating to the missile attack and the evacuation period were hypothesized to constitute risk factors affecting both the caretaker and the child. Our hypotheses were that (1) proximity predicts the children's symptomatic reactions; thus, children living in the area of Tel Aviv hit by missiles show more severe and prolonged responses compared with those living in a distant city that was under the threat of but not actually hit by them; (2) within the city of Tel Aviv, home destruction and displacement explain the children's pathological responses to the attack; (3) premorbid personality, parents' response, and family functioning are very relevant to the child's reactions following the traumatic event; and (4) younger children exhibit more symptoms in response to the event for longer periods of time, and the severity of their responses is related to the degree of parental anxiety and family cohesion.

Table 1. Distribution of Subjects According to Group, Age, and Sex*

Age, y	Displaced Boys	Displaced Girls	Undisplaced Boys	Undisplaced Girls	Threatened Boys	Threatened Girls	Total
3	5	18	7	21	9	18	**78**
4	13	10	16	11	14	10	**74**
5	12	14	12	14	11	15	**78**
Total	**30**	**42**	**35**	**46**	**34**	**43**	**230**

*For definition of groups, see the "Subjects and Methods" section of the text.

RESULTS

The distribution of children according to age, sex, and group is shown in **Table 1**.

MOTHER'S SYMPTOMS

The one-way ANOVA on the total SCL-90-R score revealed significant differences between the three groups of mothers (F[2,195]=8.73, $P<.0005$). The group of displaced mothers reported a more severe symptomatic reaction (mean±SD, 165.8±64.7) compared with both control groups of undisplaced and threatened mothers (133.0±41.3 and 132.2±47.8, respectively).

CHILD'S SYMPTOMS

There were no significant differences between boys and girls, and thus sex was not considered in further data analysis. Looking at the three groups of children, the displaced group was more symptomatic than the undisplaced and the threatened groups on the uncommunicative scale of the CBCL (F[2,229]=6.2, $P<.005$), and on all the PCASS scales: separation problems (F[2,229]=15.1, $P<.0001$), mood changes (F[2,228]=12.6, $P<.0001$), fears (F[2,227]=12.2, $P<.0001$), sleep difficulties (F[2,229]=24.2, $P<.0001$), regressive symptoms (F[2,220]=19.5, $P<.0001$), and tension (F[2,226]=16.4, $P<.0001$). Further, the displaced group scored higher than the threatened group on the CBCL aggression (F[2,229]=3.4, $P<.05$) and anxiety (F[2,229]=7.5, $P<.001$) domains.

When the three groups of children were pooled together, no significant age differences appeared in the symptomatic responses. However, significant group × age interactions were found for five CBCL symptom scales: aggression (F[4,221]=2.93, $P<.05$), uncommunicative (F[4,221]=2.97, $P<.05$), hyperactivity (F[4,220]=4.75, $P<.001$), unpopular behavior (F[4,220]=3.59, $P<.01$), and regression (F[4,209]=3.11, $P<.05$). These interactions show that within the 3-year-old group, displaced children showed more hyperactivity and uncommunicative behavior than the undisplaced group and more regressive symptoms than the threatened children. Among the 4-year-old children, the displaced group scored higher than the threatened children for the five symptom scales and higher than the undisplaced children for the hyperactivity and regression scales. In the 5-year-old group, no significant differences emerged between the three groups of children.

To identify more definable domains of maladaptation, a factor analysis was conducted using CBCL and PCASS symptom clusters. Items with a communality greater than .55 were considered. Three factors met the criteria of eigenvalue greater than or equal to 1, explaining 65.7% of the total variance: (1) Acting-out behavior. This factor, resembling the "externalizing" described by Achenbach and Edelbrock[32] was defined by the following symptom clusters of the CBCL: aggression, delinquency, hyperactivity, and odd, immature, and unpopular behavior (eigenvalue=8.92) and explained 49.5% of the total variance. (2) Anxiety and stress symptoms. This factor explained 10.7% of the variance (eigenvalue=1.93) and included the anxiety factor of the CBCL and problems with separation, mood changes, fears, tension, sleep, and regression from the PCASS. (3) Internalizing. The uncommunicative depression and somatic complaints scales of the CBCL defined the third factor, which explained 5.5% of the variance (eigenvalue=1.00) and resembled the CBCL "internalizing" factor. **Table 2** summarizes the means of these factors according to group and age.

A multivariate ANOVA found displaced children to suffer from more externalizing and stress symptoms compared with the two control groups. Compared with the control groups, displaced children's symptoms were also more strongly correlated to their mothers' symptoms. However, this was particularly observed in the 3- and 4-year-old groups and less in the older group of children (**Table 3**).

Using the mother's report on the CFS, severity of children's symptoms at three time points (before, during, and 6 months after the end of the war) was examined. Significant group differences appeared only during (F[2,227]=8.50, $P<.001$) and after the war (F[2,227]=30.64, $P<.001$). Scheffé post hoc tests revealed that symptom scores of displaced children were higher than those of the undisplaced and threatened children. Since the age × group interaction was not significant, the age groups were collapsed. The within-subject effect was statistically significant, reflecting overall changes in the scale score at the three time points (F[2,214]=114.75, $P<.001$). However, these changes were significantly different for the three groups (F[4,428]=11.19, $P<.001$). Mean scores of the different groups at the three time points are presented in the **Figure**.

No difference existed in the prewar retrospective assessment of the children for the three groups ($P>.05$). A significant increase in symptoms was experienced by the three groups during the war, especially for the displaced children. Six months after the end of the war, a decrease occurred in the three groups ($P<.001$). However, while both control groups returned to the prewar level, the displaced children remained significantly symptomatic.

FAMILY FUNCTIONING

To assess family structure and symptoms, Pearson correlations were computed between parameters of family functioning (cohesion and adaptability) and mother's symptoms

Table 2. Internalizing, Externalizing, and Stress Factors by Group and Age*

	Age, y								
	Displaced			Undisplaced			Threatened		
	3	4	5	3	4	5	3	4	5
Internalizing† (CBCL score), mean±SD	1.13±1.15	0.98±0.97	0.60±0.68	0.55±0.58	0.73±0.78	0.76±0.56	0.74±0.49	0.69±0.64	0.91±0.72
Externalizing‡ (CBCL score), mean±SD	3.39±2.05	3.50±2.36	2.63±1.57	2.42±1.46	2.29±1.36	2.70±2.07	2.87±1.56	2.07±1.17	2.44±1.37
Stress§ (PCASS and CBCL scores), mean±SD	43.4±19.6	44.3±18.7	39.2±16.9	31.4±13.4	25.5±10.1	30.4±14.5	27.3±13.5	24.1±11.5	26.8±9.0

*CBCL indicates Child Behavior Checklist[32]; PCASS, Preschool Children's Assessment of Stress Scale. For definition of groups, see the "Subjects and Methods" section of the text.

†$P>.05$.

‡$F(2,206)=3.04$, $P<.05$.

§$F(2,206)=25.2$, $P<.001$.

Table 3. Pearson Correlations Between Mothers' Symptoms (SCL-90-R) and Children's Symptom Domains According to Group and Age*

	Age, y								
	Displaced			Undisplaced			Threatened		
	3	4	5	3	4	5	3	4	5
Internalizing (CBCL)	.73†	.71†	.37‡	.25	.54‡	.50‡	.40‡	.11	.54‡
Externalizing (CBCL)	.80†	.79†	.43‡	.57‡	.32	.40‡	.39‡	.24	.43‡
Stress (PCASS and CBCL)	.52‡	.80†	.61‡	.22	.07	.39‡	.55‡	.52‡	.68†

*SCL-90-R indicates Symptom Checklist-90–Revised[31]; CBCL, Child Behavior Checklist[32]; and PCASS, Preschool Children's Assessment of Stress Scale. For definition of groups, see the "Subjects and Methods" section of the text.

†$P<.001$.

‡$P<.05$.

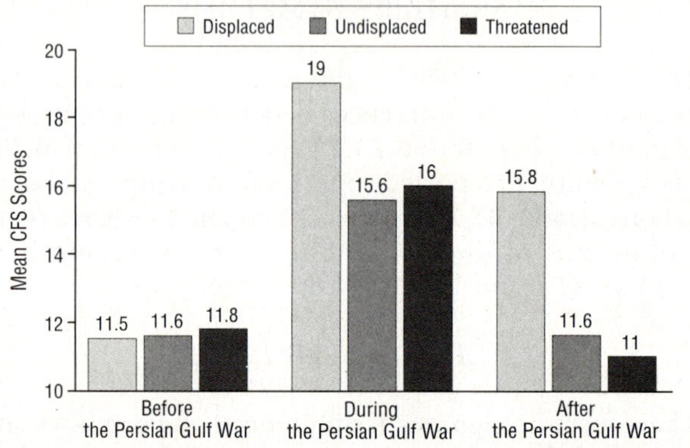

Change of functioning (CFS) scores at three time points. Data for before the war and during the war were obtained retrospectively.

(SCL-90-R domains) as well as between family functioning and child's symptom domains (PCASS and CBCL).

Within the displaced mothers' group, the more inadequate the family cohesion, the more they reported the following symptoms: somatization (r=.42), paranoia (r=.54), depression (r=.49), aggression (r=.45), interpersonal sensitivity (r=.43), and psychoticism (r=.56) (for all correlations, $P<.001$). Likewise, they reported more symptoms of compulsivity (r=.35), anxiety (r=.39), and phobia (r=.32) (for all correlations, $P<.005$). For the same group of mothers, there also were moderate positive correlations between inadequate adaptability and symptoms of somatization (r=.34), compulsivity (r=.31), and aggression (r=.30) (for all correlations, $P<.01$).

Within the undisplaced group of mothers, there were moderate positive correlations between inadequate family cohesion and a single subscale of the SCL-90-R (psychoticism, r=.35, $P<.005$). For the threatened group of mothers, the more inadequate the family cohesion, the more they reported symptoms of anxiety (r=.38), aggression (r=.38), somatization (r=.42), paranoia (r=.47), depression (r=.46), and psychoticism (r=.57) (for all correlations, $P<.001$). In both control groups, the adaptability dimension did not correlate significantly with any of the SCL-90-R symptom scales.

Whereas children's symptoms correlated with the cohesion dimension of the FACES, the picture was different for the older (5-year-old) as compared with the younger (3- and 4-year-old) subjects. In the former, only two marginally significant correlations ($P<.05$) were found, separation (r=.37) and sleep problems (r=.40) in the undisplaced group. The significant correlations for the 3- and 4-year-old groups (**Table 4**) show that the more inadequate the cohesion of the family, the more severe the child's symptomatic reaction.

Furthermore, the more inadequate the adaptability of the family, the more uncommunicative (r=.40) and hyperactive (r=.54) was the behavior of the displaced 3-year-old group; the more severe were symptoms of depression (r=.32), somatic complaints (r=.49), mood changes (r=.36), and fears (r=.36) in the undisplaced 3-year-old group; and the more regressive (r=.70) were 4-year-old children in the threatened group (for all correlations, $P<.05$).

INTEGRATIVE ASSESSMENTS

Using the three symptom domains previously defined (internalizing, externalizing, and stress) as dependent measures, we were able to look at the contribution of the fol-

Table 4. Pearson Correlations Between Inadequate Family Cohesion and Child's Symptoms*

	Age, y					
	Displaced		Undisplaced		Threatened	
	3	4	3	4	3	4
Internalizing						
Uncommunicativity	.44†	.38†	...	...	...	.41†
Depression	.61†	.50†	...	.66‡	...	...
Externalizing						
Immaturity	.40†	.40†	...	...	...	...
Aggression	.40†	.54†	...	...	...	...
Delinquency	.60‡	.56‡	...	...	...	...
Hyperactivity	.38†	.53†	...	...	...	...
Odd behavior	...	.60†	.35†	...	...	...
Unpopular behavior	...	.51†	...	...	...	.92‡
Mood changes	.38†	.36†	...	...	.49‡	...
Stress						
Anxiety	.50†	.50†	...	.36†	...	...
Fears	...	.38†	...	...	...	...
Regression	.41†	...	...	...	...	...
Sleep problems	...	...	.36†	.60‡	...	...
Separation problems	...	...	...	...	.37†	...

**High cohesion reflects inadequate family functioning. For definition of groups, see the "Subjects and Methods" section of the text. Ellipses indicate not significant.*

†$P<.05$.

‡$P<.005$.

Table 5. Multiple Regression Analyses of Children's Symptoms Against Five Sets of Variables

	Multiple r	Adjusted r^2	r^2 Change	F	P
Externalizing					
Child before the war	.75	.50	.50	8.73	<.001
Family	.78	.54	.04	8.10	<.001
The event	.82	.56	.02	6.00	<.001
Child during the war	.83	.57	.01	5.84	<.001
Mother's symptoms	.86	.62	.05	4.43	<.001
Internalizing					
Child before the war	.61	.28	.28	4.02	<.001
Family	.66	.33	.05	4.03	<.001
The event	.73	.38	.05	3.41	<.005
Child during the war	.76	.42	.04	3.66	<.001
Mother's symptoms	.83	.55	.13	5.20	<.001
Stress/Anxiety					
Child before the war	.41	.04	.04	1.36	>.05
Family	.48	.08	.04	1.50	>.05
The event	.70	.31	.23	2.76	<.01
Child during the war	.82	.56	.25	5.63	<.001
Mother's symptoms	.87	.66	.10	7.67	<.001

lowing sets of data to the prediction of symptoms 6 months after the end of the war: (1) the child before the war: age, personality, and symptoms as measured by the Childhood Personality Scales and the CFS; (2) family structure (FACES); (3) variables related to the stressful event: danger, exposure, injuries, damage to the house, and length of the evacuation period (Exposure to Event Questionnaire); (4) the child's symptoms during the war (CFS); and (5) the mother's symptoms after the war (total SCL-90-R score). The five sets of variables were entered in that order both to mirror the chronological order of events and to avoid masking the contribution of less correlated parameters (eg, prewar variables) by strongly correlated ones (eg, mother's symptoms) (**Table 5**).

Information related to child and family status before the war (age, personality, and family adequacy) did not predict the children's anxiety and stress symptoms 6 months after the war but did predict the presence of externalizing behavior and of internalizing symptoms. However, the other three sets of variables (pertaining to the war and its impact: nature of the event, child's symptoms during the war, and mother's symptoms after the event) when taken together, accounted for a significant amount of variance of the anxiety and stress factor (58%), similar to that explained by the five sets for the externalizing (62%) and internalizing (55%) symptoms.

COMMENT

Preschool children developed varied symptoms during the Persian Gulf War. Children whose houses were destroyed by missiles and were evacuated to hotels had the most symptomatic difficulties. Children under continuous threat but at a considerable distance from missile impact and children near the impact of the missiles reacted with similar severity. Six months after the end of the war, the displaced children remained highly symptomatic, primarily with clusters of externalizing and stress symptoms; the other children returned to their prewar level. These findings are consistent with other studies of preschool children's global and disorganized reactions to stressful events.[4,5] What factors determine a child's continuing reaction to a stressful event? Can these factors be explicitly identified and operationalized?

Our first two hypotheses related to the distance of the family's home from the missile impact and the effect of the destruction of the house and the displacement of the family. The present study shows significant differences between the stressful reactions of the two groups of children coming from the same neighborhood that was hit by missiles, those who were displaced and those who remained at home. Furthermore, our results indicate that both undisplaced groups (in the Tel Aviv neighborhood hit by missiles and in Beer Sheva, a city under threat of attack) returned to the same level of symptoms 6 months after the war. Thus, it seems that although it is an immediate risk factor,[11] distance from the physical impact does not explain pathological reaction 6 months after the war. As Anthony[37] concludes: "Exposure is clearly not the whole story; vulnerability and mastery also play integral roles in determining the response to stress."

Our first two hypotheses have been previously tested (see Pynoos et al[11,38] and Lonigan et al[39]). Comparisons between our current study and earlier reports must be made with caution owing to differences in the populations studied (preschool vs school-age children, respectively) and the instruments used (CBCL and stress measures vs PTSD–Reaction Index, respectively).

Pynoos and Nader[11] found a negative correlation between traumatic symptoms and personal distance from the event. Recently, Pynoos et al[38] showed that the destruction of the house as a result of an earthquake had no effect on the pathological reaction of the children. The difference between our results and those of Pynoos may relate to the fact that in the study by Pynoos, families were still displaced and separated and therefore had higher symptom levels. This may have reflected a ceiling effect, masking the impact of the physical destruction of the home on the well-being of the displaced children. A complementary explanation may involve the fact that Pynoos et al studied 8- to 16-year-old children, who are more autonomous than preschool children from both physical and mental perspectives. Older children are better able to confront adverse situations cognitively, affectively, and socially and therefore may be less dependent on their closest human and nonhuman environments for the regulation of their well-being[40] (see also Lonigan et al[39]). When the house is destroyed, younger children in particular may lean more heavily on support from parent and family. The parent's failure to contain the child's anxiety[41] and/or the pathological structure of the family[42] may contribute to the child's vulnerability. In reaction to stressful events, vulnerable children may exhibit more acute symptoms and recover from them more slowly. It is of importance to note that displaced mothers reported higher symptom levels as compared with those of the other groups. The mother's persistent symptoms may also contribute to the child's vulnerability.

Our third hypothesis predicted that children from families with inadequate functioning will exhibit more severe symptoms than those from families with normal functioning. This hypothesis was confirmed for the groups of 3- and 4-year-old displaced children. It is primarily the family's cohesion (which stands for the flexibility of the affective bonds that exist between its members) that determines its ability to withstand stressful events and not its adaptability (which stands for its capacity to change its power structure roles and norms). Since the cohesion function is not linear but curvilinear, it follows that both too cohesive and too loose ties within the family are risky for the well-being of the child. (These two poles of family structure may reflect those defined by Minuchin[43] as "enmeshed" and "disengaged," respectively.) The overly cohesive family, with loss of distance between the members and reduction in their sense of autonomy, may present a too compact and rigid system within which stress cannot be regulated and modified but merely transmitted from one member to the other. The undercohesive family as well, with its too loose matrix, cannot serve as a regulative network within which safety can be maintained for the family, as well as for the child.

Correlations between family cohesion and individual symptoms were only sporadically found in the control groups. This could be explained by the lower symptom scores and variance in children and mothers of these groups. For the displaced families, the significant (positive) correlations between a family's inadequate cohesion and child symptoms appeared within the 3- and 4-year-old groups and not within the 5-year-old group. Furthermore, we did not find overall age differences but did observe interaction effects between age and group. These were reflected in significant group differences for younger children and both lower and similar group symptom scores for older children. These results are in line with the review of Jensen and Shaw[44] concerning children as victims of war. Their review stressed the importance of affective, cognitive, and behavioral characteristics of older age as protective factors. Here, too, we see that at the age of 5 years, family cohesion ceases to serve as a risk factor. This may reflect a development of internal cohesion at this age. To complement this finding, when compared with the younger age groups, 5-year-old children showed significantly lower correlations between their symptom levels and their mothers' (Table 4). Both dynamic[45] as well as cognitive[46] psychological theories underscore the maturational leap that takes place around the age of 5 years. Physical development, cognitive abilities to process information (including stressful and traumatic stimuli), and affective individuation that makes the child less dependent on caretakers contribute to a more autonomous protective matrix.

Finally, some limitations of the present study should be mentioned. First, data regarding the children were not gathered directly from them and did not include measures of specific posttraumatic symptoms. This could result in biased information owing to mothers' reports. Second, some measures concerning the prewar personality and symptoms of the child were obtained retrospectively after the war. Third, although family functioning is generally considered a stable attribute, it too was assessed only after the war. Given the conditions of the "natural laboratory" within which we operated, some of these limitations are understandable but still constitute an inherent weakness in the design. However cautious the interpretation of our data should be, this study of young children's response to the Scud missile attacks provides a developmental perspective on the emergence and fate of trauma-related symptoms that calls for further elucidation.

Accepted for publication September 29, 1995.

This research was supported by a grant from the Spunk Foundation, New York, NY (Dr Laor).

Preliminary results included in this article were presented at the Annual Meeting of the American Academy of Child and Adolescent Psychiatry, San Antonio, Tex, October 26, 1993.

The authors appreciate the persistent commitment and support of Marianne Gerschel and are grateful to Samuel Ron, PhD, for his assistance and comments.

Reprint requests to Tel Aviv–Brull Community Mental Health Center, 9 Hatzvi St, Tel Aviv, Israel 67197 (Dr Laor).

REFERENCES

1. Freud A, Burlingham D. *War and Children.* New York, NY: International University Press; 1944.
2. Bloch DA, Silber E, Perry S. Some factors in the emotional reaction of children to disaster. *Am J Psychiatry.* 1956;113:416-422.
3. Applebaum DR, Burns GL. Unexpected childhood death: posttraumatic stress disorder in surviving siblings and parents. *J Clin Child Psychol.* 1991;20:114-120.

4. Sullivan MA, Saylor CF, Foster KY. Post-hurricane adjustment of preschoolers and their families. *Adv Behav Res Ther.* 1991;13:163-171.
5. Green BL, Korol M, Grace MC, Vary MG, Leonard AC, Gleser GC, Smitson-Cohen S. Children and disaster: age, gender, and parental effects on PTSD symptoms. *J Am Acad Child Adolesc Psychiatry.* 1991;30:945-951.
6. McFarlane AC. Posttraumatic morbidity of a disaster: a study of cases presenting for psychiatric treatment. *J Nerv Ment Dis.* 1986;174:4-14.
7. McFarlane AC. Posttraumatic phenomena in a longitudinal study of children following a natural disaster. *J Am Acad Child Psychiatry.* 1987;26:764-769.
8. McFarlane AC. Family functioning and overprotection following a natural disaster: the longitudinal effects of posttraumatic morbidity. *Aust N Z J Psychiatry.* 1987;21:210-218.
9. Kestenberg JS, Brenner I. Children who survived the Holocaust: the role of rules and routines in the development of the superego. *Int J Psychoanal.* 1986; 67:309-316.
10. Malmquist CP. Children who witness parental murder: posttraumatic aspects. *J Am Acad Child Adolesc Psychiatry.* 1986;25:320-325.
11. Pynoos RS, Nader K. Children's memory and proximity to violence. *J Am Acad Child Adolesc Psychiatry.* 1989;28:236-241.
12. Terr LC. Psychic trauma in children: observations following the Chowchilla schoolbus kidnapping. *Am J Psychiatry.* 1981;138:14-19.
13. Pynoos RS, Frederick C, Nader K, Arroyo W, Steinberg A, Eth S, Nunez F, Fairbanks L. Life threat and posttraumatic stress in school-age children. *Arch Gen Psychiatry.* 1987;44:1057-1063.
14. Chimienti G, Nasr JA, Khalifeh I. Children's reactions to war-related stress: affective symptoms and behavior problems. *Soc Psychiatry and Psychiatr Epidemiol.* 1989;24:282-287.
15. Terr LC. Childhood traumas: an outline and overview. *Am J Psychiatry.* 1991; 148:10-20.
16. Stuber ML, Nader K, Yasuda P, Pynoos RS, Cohen S. Stress responses after pediatric bone marrow transplantation: preliminary results of a prospective longitudinal study. *J Am Acad Child Adolesc Psychiatry.* 1991;30:952-957.
17. American Psychiatric Association. *Diagnostic and Statistical Manual of Mental Disorders, Revised Third Edition.* Washington, DC: American Psychiatric Association; 1987.
18. Handford H, Mayes S, Mattison R. Child and parent reactions to the Three Mile Island nuclear accident. *J Am Acad Child Adolesc Psychiatry.* 1986;25: 346-356.
19. Gleser GC, Green BL, Winget C. *Prolonged Psychosocial Effects of Disaster: A Study of Buffalo Creek.* New York, NY: Academic Press; 1981.
20. Freud S. *Beyond the Pleasure Principle.* London, England: The Hogarth Press; 1955.
21. Freud S. *Project for a Scientific Psychology.* London, England: The Hogarth Press; 1955.
22. Pynoos RS, Steinberg A, Wraith R. A developmental model of childhood traumatic stress. In: Cicchetti D, Cohen DJ, eds. *Developmental Psychopathology.* New York, NY: John Wiley & Sons Inc; 1995.
23. Loewald H. Instinct theory, object relations, and psychic structure formation. In: *Papers of Psychoanalysis.* New Haven, Conn: Yale University Press; 1980.
24. Stern D. *The Interpersonal World of the Infant.* New York, NY: Basic Books; 1985.
25. Winnicott DW. The theory of the parent-infant relationship. In: *The Maturational Process and the Facilitating Environment.* New York, NY: International University Press; 1965.
26. Solan R. 'Jointness' as integration of merging and separateness in object relations and narcissism. *Psychoanal Study Child.* 1991;46:337-352.
27. Anthony EJ. Risk, vulnerability, and resilience: an overview. In: Anthony EJ, Cohler BJ, eds. *The Invulnerable Child.* New York, NY: The Guilford Press; 1987.
28. Baldwin AL, Baldwin C, Cole RE. Stress-resistant families and stress-resistant children. In: Rolf J, Masten AS, Cicchetti D, Neuchterlein KN, Weintraub S, eds. *Risk and Protective Factors in the Development of Psychopathology.* Cambridge, Mass: Cambridge University Press; 1990.
29. Solomon Z, Laor N, Weiler D, Muller UF, Hadar O, Waysman M, Koslowsky M, Ben Yakar M, Bleich A. The psychological impact of the Gulf War: a study of acute stress in Israeli evacuees. *Arch Gen Psychiatry.* 1993;50:320-321.
30. Har-Paz H, Alterson Z, Ganani S, Hadad M, Fedida M. *City Neighborhoods: Physical, Demographic, and Socioeconomic Characteristics (1983-1984).* Tel Aviv, Israel: Tel Aviv Municipality Center for Economic and Social Research; 1986.
31. Derogatis LR. *SCL-90-R Manual.* Baltimore, Md: The Johns Hopkins University; 1977.
32. Achenbach TM, Edelbrock CS. *Manual for the Child Behavior Checklist and Revised Child Behavior Profile.* Burlington, Vt: University of Vermont; 1983.
33. Auerbach JG, Lerner Y. Syndromes derived from the Child Behavior Checklist for clinically referred Israeli boys aged 6-11: a research note. *J Child Psychol Psychiatry.* 1991;32:1017-1024.
34. Cohen DJ, Dibble E, Grawe JM. Fathers' and mothers' perceptions of children's personality. *Arch Gen Psychiatry.* 1977;34:480-487.
35. Teichman Y, Navon S. The evaluation of families: the Circumplex model. *Psychology* (Hebrew). 1990;2:36-46.
36. Olson DH. Circumplex Model VII: validation studies and FACES III. *Fam Process.* 1986;25:337-351.
37. Anthony EJ. The syndrome of the psychologically invulnerable child. In: Anthony EJ, Koupernik C, eds. *The Child in His Family: Children at Psychiatric Risk.* New York, NY: Wiley & Sons Inc; 1974.
38. Pynoos RS, Goenjian A, Tashjian M, Karakashian M, Manjikian R, Manoukian G, Steinberg A, Fairbanks LF. Posttraumatic stress reactions in children after the 1988 Armenian earthquake. *Br J Psychiatry.* 1993;163:239-247.
39. Lonigan CJ, Shannon MP, Taylor CM, Finch AJ, Salee FR. Children exposed to disaster, II: risk factors for the development of post-traumatic symptomatology. *J Am Acad Child Adolesc Psychiatry.* 1994;33:94-105.
40. Searls HF. *The Nonhuman Environment.* New York, NY: International University Press; 1960.
41. Pianta RC, Egeland B, Sroufe LA. Maternal stress and children's development: prediction of school outcomes and identification of protective factors. In: Rolf J, Masten AS, Cicchetti D, Neuchterlein KN, Weintraub S, eds. *Risk and Protective Factors in the Development of Psychopathology.* Cambridge, Mass: Cambridge University Press; 1990.
42. Rutter M. Psychosocial resilience and protective mechanisms. In: Rolf J, Masten AS, Cicchetti D, Neuchterlein KN, Weintraub S, eds. *Risk and Protective Factors in the Development of Psychopathology.* Cambridge, Mass: Cambridge University Press; 1990.
43. Minuchin S. *Families and Family Therapy.* Cambridge, Mass: Harvard University Press; 1974.
44. Jensen PS, Shaw J. Children as victims of war: current knowledge and future research needs. *J Am Acad Child Adolesc Psychiatry.* 1993;32:697-708.
45. Freud S. *The Ego and the Id.* London, England: The Hogarth Press; 1955.
46. Piaget J. *The Origins of Intelligence in Children.* New York, NY: International University Press; 1952.

Maldistribution of Interstitial Neurons in Prefrontal White Matter of the Brains of Schizophrenic Patients

Schahram Akbarian, MD, PhD; James J. Kim; Steven G. Potkin, MD; William P. Hetrick, PhD; William E. Bunney, Jr, MD; Edward G. Jones, MD, PhD

Background: The cortical subplate is a transitory structure involved in the formation of connections in developing cerebral cortex. Interstitial neurons, normally present in subcortical white matter (WM) of the adult brain, have escaped the programmed cell death that eliminates most subplate neurons. Previous investigations indicated a maldistribution of one population of interstitial neurons in the WM of brains of schizophrenic patients, suggesting a defect of the subplate during brain development.

Methods: Three histochemically or immunocytochemically defined neuronal populations were studied in WM beneath the middle frontal gyrus of 20 schizophrenic patients and 20 matched control subjects.

Results: Brains of schizophrenic patients showed significant changes in the distribution of the three neuronal populations: microtubule-associated protein 2 and nonphosphorylated neurofilament-immunoreactive neurons showed a decreased density in superficial WM and an increased density in deeper WM. Nicotinamide adenine dinucleotide phosphate–diaphorase neurons were reduced in superficial WM and showed variable densities in deeper WM. Thirty-five percent of the brains of schizophrenic patients but no brains of the control subjects showed a maldistribution of neurons toward deeper WM with at least two of the three markers. Changes in neuronal distribution were not linked to age, gender, autolysis time, or subtype of schizophrenia.

Conclusions: Selective displacement of interstitial WM neurons in the frontal lobe of brains of schizophrenic patients may indicate alteration in the migration of subplate neurons or in the pattern of programmed cell death. Both could lead to defective cortical circuitry in the brains of schizophrenic patients.

(Arch Gen Psychiatry. 1996;53:425-436)

From the Departments of Anatomy and Neurobiology (Drs Akbarian and Jones and Mr Kim) and Psychiatry and Human Behavior (Drs Potkin, Hetrick, and Bunney), University of California, Irvine.

DISRUPTION OF connections between neocortical association fields and other cortical and subcortical centers may play a key role in the symptoms of schizophrenia.[1] This hypothesis has been supported by results of in vivo brain imaging studies, especially when allied with findings from neuropsychological testing.[2,3]

Disturbances of cortical connectivity in schizophrenic patients may stem from perturbations of cortical development.[4,5] Epidemiological data have identified additional risk factors that increase the incidence of schizophrenia in offspring who are genetically at risk.[6-15]

During cortical ontogenesis, the subplate, which is a zone of early generated neurons and synaptic neuropil located immediately beneath the developing cerebral cortex, is thought to play a key role in the formation of cortical connections by providing guidance to developing afferent and efferent fibers.[16] The subplate is transitory, and its neurons undergo a programmed cell death that leads to the disappearance of many of them during the later stages of brain development.[17-19] In humans, this takes place during late fetal and early postnatal life.[20] However, many subplate neurons are spared from cell death and remain in the adult brain as the interstitial neurons of the white matter (WM).[21] Therefore, examination of the interstitial neurons of the adult WM might provide clues to potential defects of the subplate during brain development.

In previous investigations with a small sample of schizophrenic patients and control subjects, a selected subpopulation of WM neurons, recognized by histochemical

See Materials and Methods on next page

MATERIALS AND METHODS

ACQUISITION, STORAGE, AND FIXATION OF BRAIN TISSUE

Brains of 20 schizophrenic patients and 20 control subjects, matched for age, gender, and autolysis time, as described in detail in the **Table**, were used. The matching process was finished before all experimental procedures. Brain tissue was obtained from a brain bank in the Department of Anatomy and Neurobiology, University of California, Irvine. The diagnosis of schizophrenia and the determination of the particular symptom type, identified in the Table, was made before and after the deaths of the schizophrenic patients and control subjects by two board-certified psychiatrists. Diagnoses were made according to *DSM-III-R* criteria by using the best estimate diagnostic procedure from all available interview and medical record sources. These sources included prospective interviews with the subjects and/or postmortem interviews with a family member, significant other, and/or treating professional. Exclusion criteria for the schizophrenic patients and control subjects included a history of neurological illnesses with the exception of neuroleptic-induced seizures; positive blood tests for human immunodeficiency virus; neuropathological evidence of stroke, Alzheimer's disease, brain tumor, or vascular anomalies; and a history of, or evidence at autopsy of, severe drug abuse (eg, needle tracks, positive toxicology for substances of abuse). Moderate marijuana use and alcoholism or occasional recreational drug abuse were not exclusionary criteria, unless they confounded the Axis I diagnosis (eg, cocaine or amphetamine abuse resulting in psychosis).

The brains of control subjects were obtained from the coroner's office or the eye bank. The coroner's office or eye bank investigators determined that there had been no psychiatric illness in the subjects based on the findings from their investigative interview that included a discussion with family members or significant others. Medical, psychiatric, and neurological illnesses and medications were specifically inquired about. The absence of a psychiatric illness was further confirmed by results of a telephone interview with a family member, a review of available medical records, and/or consultation with the control subject's family physician.

Patients were matched by using the following order and criteria: (1) gender; (2) age±5 years (mean [±SD] age, 3.9±2.8 years); (3) autolysis time ±3.5 hours (mean [±SD] time, 3.9±2.8 hours); and, if possible, (4) cause of death. A computer program was used to identify potential control subjects as possible matches for the patients in the schizophrenic cohort. The brains of the control subjects were taken from a control brain repository that consisted of more than 100 cases. Of those cases identified by the computer, the composite records of the possible matches were carefully rereviewed to satisfy criteria for schizophrenia and normality, following which the best matches were selected.

Lack of a chronic degenerative process was confirmed in all brains by the absence of plaques and tangles in thioflavine S–stained sections. Procedures for removal and storage of the brains have been described previously.[22,32] In all sampling, fixation, and staining procedures, tissue from the brains of schizophrenic patients was processed together with tissue from the brains of the matched control subjects. For each brain, two blocks were cut from the middle third of the middle frontal gyrus (Brodmann's area 46) (**Figure 1**). Care was taken that the WM of all blocks was separated by a distance greater than 6 mm from the striatal gray matter and from the gray matter of adjacent cortical regions. The unfixed, frozen blocks were brought from −75°C up to 4°C during a period of 20 minutes. They were then fixed by immersion in 4% paraformaldehyde in 0.1-mol/L phosphate buffer (pH 7.4) for 20 hours, infiltrated with 30% sucrose, and refrozen in dry ice. Subsequent cytoarchitectonic analysis of thionin-stained sections confirmed the cytoarchitectonic features of area 46[33-35] in the cortex of the selected blocks. None of the brains showed freezing artifacts at the level of light microscopy; this finding is in accord with that of previous studies on frozen specimens derived from the same brain bank.[36] Brains of the schizophrenic patients and of the control subjects were stored at −75°C for a similar period (brains of schizophrenic patients, 2.2±0.3 years; brains of control subjects, 2.4±0.3 years; *P*=.63).

HISTOCHEMICAL PROCEDURES

Serial sections (thickness, 20 μm) were cut from each block on a freezing microtome. The plane of section was always perpendicular to the cortical surface, thus avoiding any hidden cortex in the walls of sulci that would confound subsequent gray matter or WM depth measurements. Sections were collected in chilled, 0.1-mol/L phosphate buffer and series at 140-μm intervals, mounted on slides, air-dried, and stained with thionin or with thioflavine S. Additional series of free-floating sections were stained by using the following protocols.

Immunohistochemical Studies

After repeated washing at room temperature in 0.1-mol/L phosphate buffer, endogeneous peroxidase activity was blocked by incubation in a mixture of 25% ethanol in 0.1-mol/L phosphate buffer (pH 7.4) that contained 0.3% hydrogen peroxide for 30 minutes at room temperature. Sections were then washed in phosphate buffer, preincubated at room temperature for 60 minutes in 0.1-mol/L phosphate buffer that contained 5% horse serum and 0.25% Triton X-100, and then incubated in a solution that contained 5% horse serum and 0.25% Triton X-100 and in a 1:500 concentration of the mouse monoclonal antibody SMI-32 (Sternberger Monoclonals Inc, Bethesda, Md), or in 1:500 concentration of the mouse monoclonal antibody SMI-52, which recognizes MAP-2 (Sternberger Monoclonals Inc). After 24-hour incubation at 8°C, sections were washed three times in 0.1-mol/L phosphate buffer (20 minutes each), incubated for 1 hour at room temperature in 0.1-mol/L phosphate buffer that contained 5% horse serum, 0.25% Triton X-100, and 1:200 biotinylated horse anti–mouse IgG (Vector Laboratories, Burlingame, Calif). Sections were washed three times in 0.1-mol/L phosphate buffer and stained by the avidin-biotin-peroxidase method (by using Vectastain ABC kits). Immunoreactivity was finally developed by incubation in 0.1-mol/L phosphate buffer that contained 0.02% 3,3′-diaminobenzidine tetrahydrochloride and 0.035% hydrogen peroxide. After repeated washings, sections were mounted and air-dried, counterstained with cresyl violet, dehydrated through ascending alcohols, cleared in xylene, and coverslipped with DPX (BDH Laboratory Supplies, Poole, England). From each brain, at least 10 sections were processed for SMI-32 immunostaining, and at least 10 sections were processed for MAP-2 immunoreactivity. In pilot experiments, the incubation time and the concentration of Triton X-100 and of the primary antibody were systematically varied. For tissue from each schizophrenic patient and control subject, optimal staining quality was achieved with the protocol described above. Control experiments were done by omitting either the primary or secondary antibody from the staining procedure. Staining was absent in both cases.

NADPH-d Histochemical Studies

Sections were repeatedly washed in 0.1-mol/L phosphate buffer, then preincubated in 0.1-mol/L TRIS buffer (pH 8.0) for 30 minutes, and transferred to a reaction solution that contained 1.2-mmol/L NADPH-d (N-1630, Sigma Chemical Co, St Louis, Mo), 30-mmol/L L-malic acid (tetrasodium salt), 0.3-mmol/L nitroblue tetrazolium (Sigma Chemical Co), 0.25% Triton X-100, and 1.2% dimethyl sulfoxide. Sections were incubated at 37°C in total darkness for 120 minutes; then these sections were repeatedly washed in 0.1-mol/L phosphate buffer, mounted on gelatin-coated slides, air-dried, dehydrated in alcohol, cleared in xylene, and coverslipped. At least 10 sections were processed from each brain. In addition, for each brain, systematic variations in the incubation time from 20 to 120 minutes in 10-minute steps were carried out. Reductions in the incubation time caused a uniform decrease in the staining intensity of neurons, with no apparent difference between schizophrenic and control tissue; this finding is in accord with previous findings.[22,23]

Double-Labeling Studies

Sections were first processed for NADPH-d histochemistry, as described above. Incubation time was systematically varied between 10 and 90 minutes in 10-minute steps. This produced numerous NADPH-d–positive neurons, with the typical somatodendritic morphology achieved at longer incubation times, but with a light blue color, which was required for the purposes of double labeling. After the histochemical reaction, sections were repeatedly washed in 0.1-mol/L phosphate buffer; then these sections were further processed for SMI-32 or MAP-2 immunostaining as described above.

NEURONAL COUNTING IN WM

All cell-counting procedures were performed without knowledge of the diagnosis. Camera lucida drawings were made at 15× magnification, showing the gray matter–WM border and profiles of blood vessels as internal landmarks. Red ink dots were placed in a grid on the coverslip as external landmarks. The layer VI–WM border was defined as the line of sudden, steep change in neuronal density. The subcortical WM was subdivided into six compartments: compartment WM-1 was the most superficial compartment from 0 to 1000 μm deep to layer VI; compartment WM-2 was 1000 to 2000 μm deep to the cortex; and the deeper WM was subdivided into successively deeper 1000-μm-wide compartments (WM-3 through WM-6), ending at WM-6 that consisted of WM more than 6000 μm deep to the overlying cortex. Sections were screened at ×200 magnification for labeled neurons. The position of each neuron was plotted on the drawings, by reference to the internal and external landmarks. The area of each compartment of a particular section was measured with a digitizing pad and commercially available software (SigmaScan [Jandel, San Rafael, Calif]), and the density of neurons for each compartment was calculated. Five measurements were made on each brain, each histochemical stain, and each compartment.

In sections that were processed for SMI-32 or MAP-2 immunohistochemistry, labeled neurons that were cut through the level of the nucleus were counted, and their diameters were measured with an eyepiece reticle. Because of the dark reaction product in NADPH-d–stained neurons, the nucleus could not be regularly identified; instead, whole-cell body counts were made. The somal size of NADPH-d–stained neurons did not differ between the brains of schizophrenic patients and control subjects.[22,23] None of the brains that were included in the present study showed immunostaining of glial cells with SMI-32 or for MAP-2. In the NADPH-d–processed sections, faint staining was present in the vascular endothelium, but only neurons showed the characteristic dark blue or black, Golgi-like staining pattern (**Figure 2**).

STATISTICAL ANALYSIS

Statistical analysis was performed with commercially available software (GBSTAT, Biodynamics Microsystems Inc, Silver Spring, Md, and BMDP, BMDP Statistical Software Inc, Los Angeles, Calif). For each case and neuronal subpopulation, the distribution was determined in the prefrontal WM. The term *distribution* refers to the topographical distribution of neurons across WM compartments and was analyzed by three different methods.

Regression Analysis

For each case, the mean cell density (neurons per square millimeter) was determined for each neuronal subpopulation and WM compartment. Because of the steady decline of neuronal densities from the superficial toward the deeper WM compartments, for each case and neuronal population, the distribution of neurons across the WM compartments was described by a simple regression function. For each of the three neuronal populations, the optimal regression was given by the power function $y=a*xb$ (equals the function: $\log y = \log a + b*\log x$), in which y is the cell density and x is the corresponding WM compartment. In this function, the constant b determines the slope of the curve and reflects the distribution of SMI-32, MAP-2, and NADPH-d neurons across WM compartments. For each case, the actual values of the constants b and a were computed, together with the corresponding correlation coefficient R of the power function and the corresponding level of significance. For the schizophrenic and control cohorts, the mean value, SD, and SE of the slope (constant b) and of the correlation coefficients were calculated. Based

Continued on next page

on previous observations,[22,23] it was hypothesized that the brains of schizophrenic patients would show a redistribution of neurons toward the deeper WM compartments (recognized by a less negative slope of the distribution curve, ie, a less negative value of the constant *b*). This hypothesis was tested by using a one-tailed pooled Student's *t* test.

Subgroup Criteria

In both cohorts, the individual values for the slopes of the distribution curves were normally (gaussian) distributed, according to the criteria of Sachs[37] ($P<.01$ to $P<.05$). In a gaussian distribution, the mean value marks the 50th percentile of the population, the sum of the mean value +1 SD marks the 84th percentile of the total population, and the subtraction of the mean value −1 SD marks the 16th percentile of the total population. To define a subgroup of schizophrenic patients and/or control subjects with evidence of abnormal subplate markers, the following operational criteria were selected: (1) a "substantial redistribution" of WM neurons toward the deeper WM compartments in an individual case was present if the values for two of the three neuronal subpopulations exceeded the 84th percentile of control subjects and if the value of the third population exceeded the 50th percentile of control subjects, and (2) a "substantial opposite redistribution" of WM neurons toward the superficial compartments in an individual case was present if the values for two of the three neuronal populations were below the 16th percentile of control subjects and if the value of the third population was below the 50th percentile of control subjects. The significance of differences in the frequency of cases with substantial redistribution between the schizophrenic and control cohort was tested by a two-tailed χ^2 test.

staining for nicotinamide adenine dinucleotide phosphate–diaphorase (NADPH-d) was shown to be displaced more deeply in the prefrontal and lateral temporal WM of the brains of the schizophrenic patients.[22,23] This finding raised the possibilities that the orderly migration of young neurons from the ventricular zone toward the territory of the future subplate could have been compromised, or that there could have been an alteration in the program of cell death in the subplate. Both of these mechanisms could potentially cause alterations in the development of normal cortical connectivity.

The previously studied NADPH-d cells are a subpopulation of a much larger group and, to demonstrate a major involvement of the embryonic subplate, it is essential to study the larger population of interstitial neurons. Several populations of interstitial neurons can be recognized by specific staining patterns or patterns of gene expression for various neurochemical markers.[19,24-26] Among these, neurons defined by immunoreactivity for microtubule-associated protein 2 (MAP-2) represent the largest fraction of subplate neurons[18] and, in the adult human brain, MAP-2 neurons are more numerous than NADPH-d neurons.[25] Another large population can be identified by immunostaining with the monoclonal antibody SMI-32,[27] which recognizes a nonphosphorylated epitope of the 160- and 200-kd neurofilament proteins.[28,29] It is also essential to study the potential defects of interstitial neurons in a much larger sample of brains of schizophrenic patients than previously available. The present study focused on the WM of the prefrontal cortex, which is thought to be primarily involved in the pathophysiology of schizophrenia.[30,31]

RESULTS

The neuronal distribution in the prefrontal WM of schizophrenic patients and control subjects was first compared by means of cohort analysis, to determine if there was an overall group difference in the distribution of the three subplate markers. Subsequently, the operational criteria were applied on each case and control, as described in the "Materials and Methods" section, to determine if a subgroup of schizophrenic patients and/or control subjects showed pronounced changes in interstitial cells.

MORPHOLOGY AND DISTRIBUTION OF MAP-2 NEURONS IN WM

In the subcortical WM of the middle frontal gyrus of all control subjects and schizophrenic patients, MAP-2–immunoreactive neurons were bipolar, with immunoreactivity in both somata and dendritic stems (Figure 2). In the brains of the control subjects, the mean (±SD) density of MAP-2 neurons was 48.5±10.4 neurons per square millimeter in compartment WM-1, 1.7±0.4 neurons per square millimeter in compartment WM-2; and 0.86±0.16, 0.66±0.12, 0.38±0.08, and 0.13±0.03 neurons per square millimeter in compartments WM-3, WM-4, WM-5, and WM-6, respectively (**Figure 3**). In the brains of the schizophrenic patients, there was a 31% decrease in the density of MAP-2 neurons in compartments WM-1 and WM-2 (Figure 3). There was a 9% and 12% decrease in the MAP-2 neuronal density in compartments WM-3 and WM-4, respectively. The decrease in the superficial compartments WM-1 through WM-4 in the middle frontal gyri of the schizophrenic patients was accompanied by an increased density of MAP-2 neurons in the deep compartments WM-5 and WM-6: in compartment WM-5, there was a 21% increase in comparison with that of the middle frontal gyri of the control subjects, and, in compartment WM-6, there was a 148% increase in comparison with that of the middle frontal gyri of the control subjects.

The distribution of MAP-2 neurons across WM compartments in each cohort was best described by the function $y=a*xb$ (equals the function: $\log y=\log a+b*\log x$), with *y* equal to the MAP-2 neuronal density and *x* equal to the WM compartment. The average correlation coefficient *R* for the distribution function in the control cohort was −0.92±0.01 ($P=.015\pm.002$), and, in the schizophrenic cohort, it was −0.86±0.01 ($P=.031\pm.005$). In both cohorts, the value of the slope of the distribution curve (constant *b*) was negative, owing to the steady decrease in MAP-2 neuronal density in successively deeper WM compartments (Figure 3). The mean value of *b* in

Clinical Data of Schizophrenic Patients and Control Subjects*

	Schizophrenic Patients							Control Subjects			
Pair	Sex	Age at Death, y	Autolysis, h	Age at Onset, y	Duration of Illness, y	Diagnosis	Cause of Death	Sex	Age at Death, y	Autolysis, h	Cause of Death
1	M	70	24.25	19	51	Schizophrenia, chronic paranoid	Cardiac	M	61	25.5	Cardiac
2	F	47	30.25	32	15	Schizophrenia, chronic paranoid	Suicide: gunshot wound to chest	F	51	26.5	Cardiac
3	M	32	26.5	16	16	Schizophrenia, chronic undifferentiated with childhood onset	Peritonitis	M	39	27.75	Cardiac arrest (traumatic)
4	F	69	7.3	35	34	Schizophrenia, chronic undifferentiated	Cardiac	F	69	7.25	Cardiac
5	M	55	21.15	20	35	Schizophrenia, chronic undifferentiated	Cancer	M	51	21.5	Cardiac
6	M	79	5	35	44	Schizophrenia, chronic paranoid	Cardiac	M	84	6	Cardiac
7	F	70	11.2	25	45	Schizophrenia, chronic undifferentiated	Cardiac	F	68	7	Respiratory failure
8	M	72	9	24	48	Schizophrenia, chronic undifferentiated	Cardiac	M	75	7.5	Cardiac
9	M	79	5.5	30	49	Schizophrenia, chronic paranoid	Cardiac	M	81	8	Cardiac
10	M	60	26	22	38	Schizophrenia, chronic undifferentiated	Cardiac	M	63	23.5	Cardiac
11	M	24	9	18	6	Schizophrenia, chronic undifferentiated	Suicide: gunshot wound to chest	M	30	7	Automobile accident
12	M	23	11	17	6	Schizophrenia, chronic paranoid	Suicide: overdose	M	21	17	Automobile accident
13	M	87	8.5	38	49	Schizophrenia, chronic undifferentiated	Cardiac	M	90	8.5	Cardiac
14	M	30	23	27	3	Schizophrenia, chronic paranoid	Suicide: jump from height	M	38	16	Cardiac
15	F	67	38.5	34	33	Schizophrenia, chronic paranoid	Cardiac	F	69	40.15	Cardiac
16	F	61	15	32	29	Schizophrenia, chronic paranoid	Undetermined	F	57	16.45	Cardiac
17	F	75	27.25	25	50	Schizophrenia, chronic paranoid	Pneumonia	F	85	21.5	Cardiac
18	F	58	7.5	25	33	Schizophrenia, chronic undifferentiated	Cardiac	F	56	8	Cardiac
19†	M	79	15	<64	>15	Schizophrenia, chronic undifferentiated	Pneumonia	M	78	11	Cardiac
20	M	40	13.5	33	7	Schizophrenia, chronic undifferentiated	Cardiac	M	41	18	Cardiac

*Brains were obtained from these patients and subjects for the matching process in this study.
†Records definitely document a 15-year duration of illness, but suggest a much longer duration.

the schizophrenic cohort was 30% larger in comparison with the mean of the control cohort (brains of schizophrenic patients, −2.17±0.29; brains of control subjects, −3.10±0.20). This difference was significant (*P*=.01). The increased (ie, less negative) value of the slope in the schizophrenic cohort was caused by the decreased density of MAP-2 neurons in the superficial WM compartments of the brains of the schizophrenic patients; this was accompanied by higher densities of MAP-2 neurons in the deeper WM (Figure 3).

MORPHOLOGY AND DISTRIBUTION OF SMI-32 NEURONS IN WM

In the subcortical WM of the brains of all control subjects and schizophrenic patients, SMI-32–stained neurons were bipolar or multipolar, with immunoreactivity in the dendritic stems and the cell somata (Figure 2). In the middle frontal gyri of the control subjects, the mean (±SD) density was 46.3±5.7 and 0.91±0.21 neurons per square millimeter in compartments WM-1 and WM-2, respectively. It was 0.38±0.12, 0.28±0.10, 0.21±0.08, and 0.06±0.02 neurons per square millimeter in compartments WM-3, WM-4, WM-5, and WM-6, respectively (Figure 3). In the middle frontal gyri of the schizophrenic patients, there was a 30% and 45% decrease in the density of SMI-32 neurons in compartments WM-1 and WM-2, respectively (Figure 3), and a 25%, 39%, and 38% decrease in compartments WM-3, WM-4, and WM-5, respectively, in comparison with that in the middle frontal gyri of the control subjects (Figure 3). There was a 66% increase in the numbers of SMI-32 neurons in compartment WM-6 of the middle frontal gyri of the schizophrenic patients (Figure 3).

The distribution of SMI-32 neurons across WM compartments in both cohorts is described by the distribution function $y=a*x^b$ (equals the function: $\log y=\log a+b*\log x$), with y equal to the SMI-32 neuronal density and x equal to the WM compartment. The average correlation coefficient R for this function in the brains of the schizophrenic patients was $-.89\pm.01$ ($P=.024\pm.004$), and, in the brains of the control subjects, it was $-.90\pm.01$ ($P=.021\pm.001$). In both cohorts, the value of the slope of the distribution curve (constant b) was negative, reflecting the continuous decrease in the density of SMI-32 neurons toward the deeper WM compartments. The brains of the schizophrenic patients had a 16% larger constant b than those of the control subjects, which was a significant difference (brains of schizophrenic patients, -3.39 ± 0.17; brains of control subjects, -3.92 ± 0.15; $P=.02$). The increased (ie, less negative) value of b in the schizophrenic patients in comparison with that of control subjects was caused by decreased densities of SMI-32 neurons in WM compartments WM-1 through WM-5 and an increased density in the deepest WM compartment, namely, WM-6.

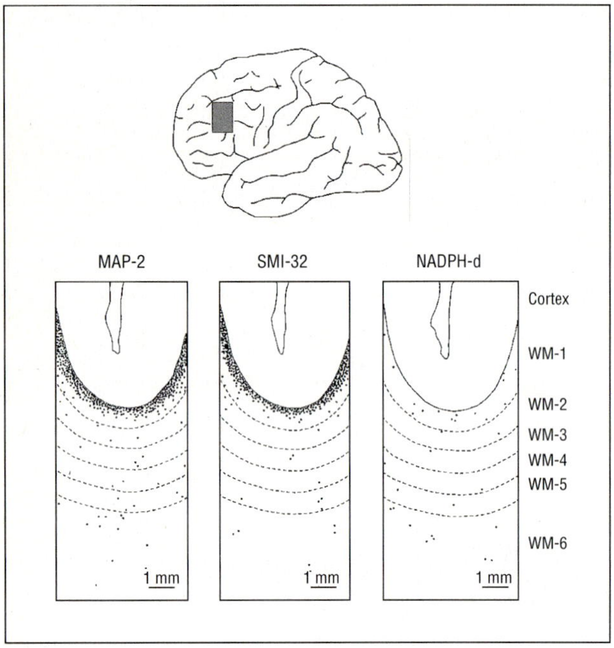

Figure 1. *Top, Location of the blocks taken from the superior frontal gyrus for quantitative analysis and the plane of section. Bottom, Camera lucida drawings of typical sections, stained as indicated, show the distributions of the interstitial cells of the white matter (WM) and the anatomical compartments of the WM used for counting neurons. Stained neurons in the cerebral cortex were not plotted. MAP-2 indicates microtubule-associated protein 2; NADPH-d, nicotinamide adenine dinucleotide phosphate–diaphorase.*

MORPHOLOGY AND DISTRIBUTION OF NADPH-d NEURONS IN WM

In the subcortical WM of the middle frontal gyri of the control subjects and schizophrenic patients, NADPH-d–positive neurons were multipolar and stained intensely dark blue or black (Figure 2). In the control cohort, the density of NADPH-d neurons was 1.83 ± 0.14, 0.67 ± 0.08, and 0.44 ± 0.05 neurons per square millimeter in compartments WM-1, WM-2, and WM-3, respectively. It was 0.26 ± 0.03, 0.25 ± 0.03, and 0.23 ± 0.03 neurons per square millimeter in compartments WM-4, WM-5, and WM-6, respectively (Figure 3). In the schizophrenic cohort, there was a 16%, 2%, and 20% decrease in compartments WM-1, WM-2, and WM-3, respectively, in comparison with that of the control cohort. In the middle frontal gyri of the schizophrenic patients, there was a 22%

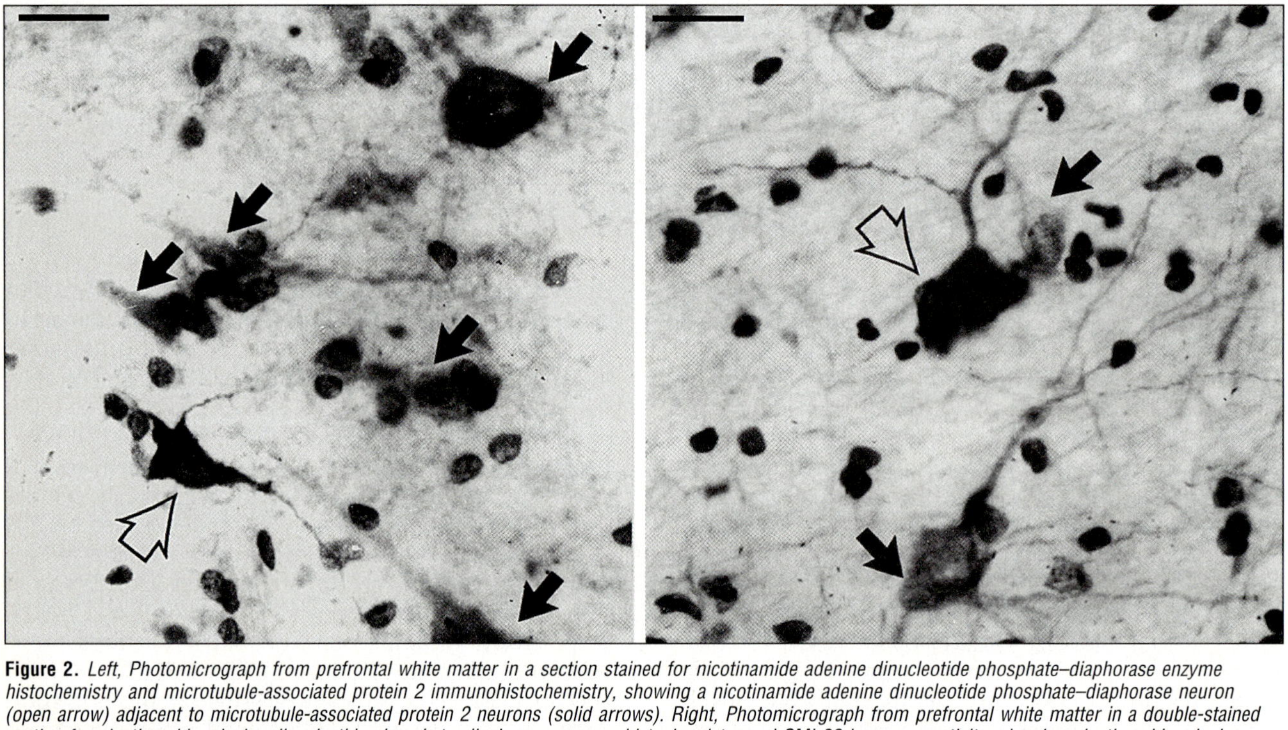

Figure 2. *Left, Photomicrograph from prefrontal white matter in a section stained for nicotinamide adenine dinucleotide phosphate–diaphorase enzyme histochemistry and microtubule-associated protein 2 immunohistochemistry, showing a nicotinamide adenine dinucleotide phosphate–diaphorase neuron (open arrow) adjacent to microtubule-associated protein 2 neurons (solid arrows). Right, Photomicrograph from prefrontal white matter in a double-stained section for nicotinamide adenine dinucleotide phosphate–diaphorase enzyme histochemistry and SMI-32 immunoreactivity, showing nicotinamide adenine dinucleotide phosphate–diaphorase neuron (open arrow) adjacent to SMI-32 neurons (solid arrows). Bars indicate 10 μm.*

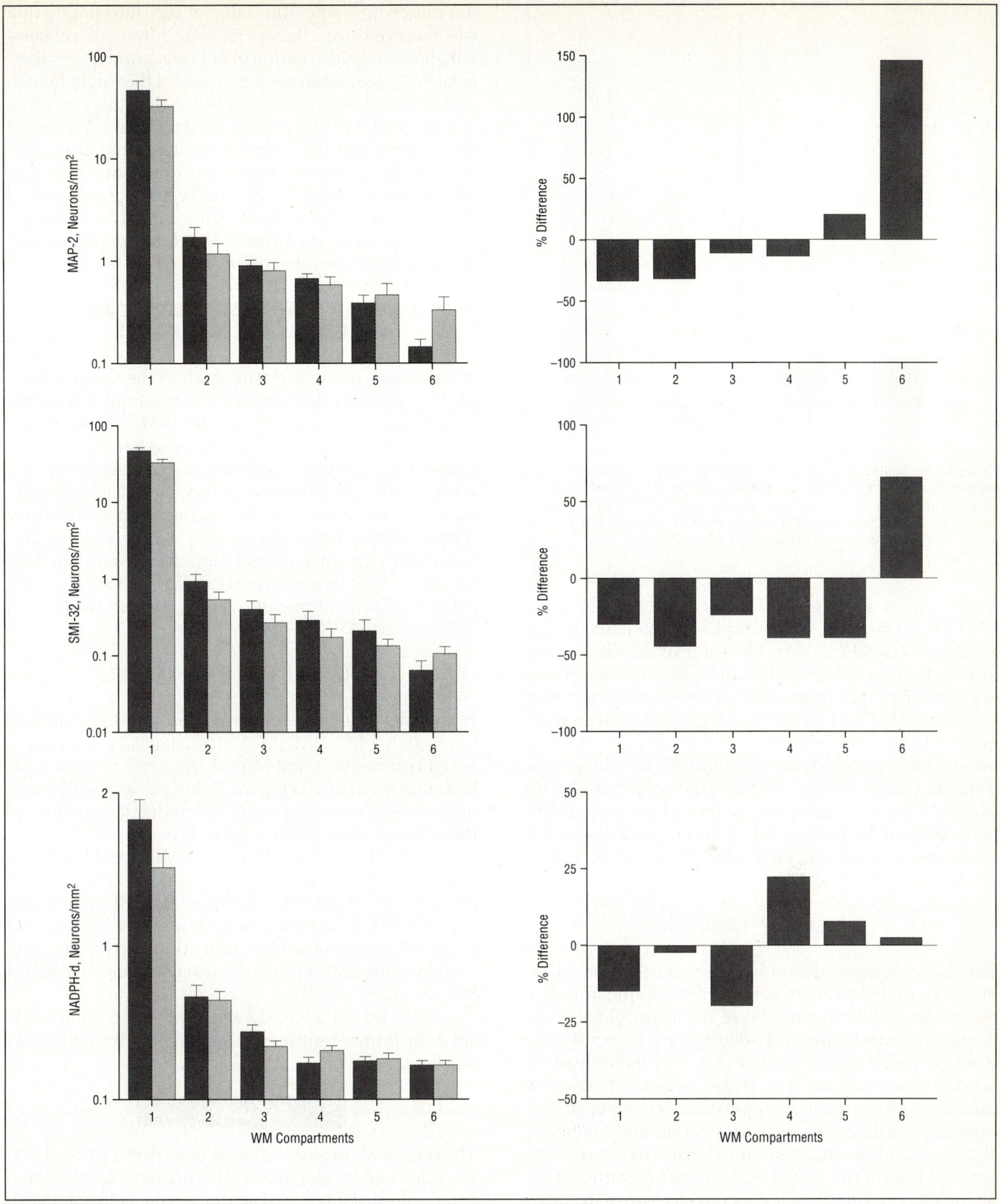

Figure 3. *Left, Density (neurons per square millimeter) of microtubule-associated protein 2 (MAP-2), SMI-32, and nicotinamide adenine dinucleotide phosphate–diaphorase (NADPH-d) neurons in white matter (WM) compartments 1 through 6. Data are shown as mean±SEM. Solid bars indicate brains of control subjects; shaded bars, brains of schizophrenic patients. The MAP-2 and SMI-32 neuron densities are shown as log scales. Right, Same data as those shown at left, now expressed in terms of percentage difference between brains of schizophrenic patients and control subjects.*

and 7% increase in compartments WM-4 and WM-5, respectively, in NADPH-d neuronal density, in comparison with that of the control subjects. In compartment WM-6, the difference between the two cohorts was less than 1%.

The distribution of NADPH-d neurons across WM compartments in each cohort is described by the function $y=a^*xb$ (equals the function: $\log y=\log a+b^*\log x$), with y equal to the NADPH-d neuronal density and x equal to the WM compartment. The average correlation coef-

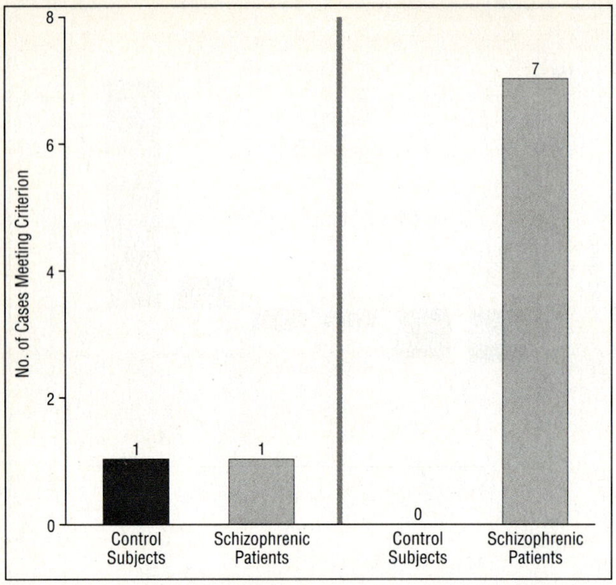

Figure 4. *The number of brains of schizophrenic patients and control subjects in which the distributions of at least two of the three neuronal subpopulations that were counted deviated by more than 1 SD from the mean. Left, Distribution toward the superficial white matter (>1 SD). Right, Distribution toward the deeper white matter (>1 SD).*

ficient *R* in the control cohort was −.90±.02 (*P*=.021±.006), and, in schizophrenic patients, it was −.90±.01 (*P*=.017±.004). The value of the slope of the distribution curve (constant *b*) in the control cohort was −1.28±0.08, and, in the schizophrenic cohort, it was −1.10±0.07. This 14% increase (ie, less negative value) in the schizophrenic cohort was significant (*P*=.05). The overall differences remained significant when the groups were treated as a between factor, ignoring matched pairs (MANOVA: F [15, 24]=2.08, *P*=.05). The overall differences remained significant when the groups were treated as a between factor, ignoring matched pairs (MANOVA: F [15, 24]=2.08, *P*=.05).

SUBGROUP ANALYSIS

The cohort analysis demonstrated that the distribution of interstitial WM neurons differed significantly between the middle frontal gyri of the schizophrenic patients and control subjects. To determine if there was variability among the middle frontal gyri of the individual schizophrenic patients and control subjects, the data for each case and neuronal subpopulation were grouped into categories as described in the "Materials and Methods" section. By definition, a substantial redistribution of WM neurons toward the deeper WM compartments in an individual case was present if the values for two of the three neuronal subpopulations exceeded the 84th percentile (mean+1 SD) of the brains of the control subjects and if the value for the third population exceeded the 50th percentile of the control subjects; this was found in seven of the brains of the schizophrenic patients (cases 1, 3, 7, 9, 10, 11, and 18) or 35% of the total schizophrenic cohort but was found in none of the brains of the control cohort (**Figure 4**). This difference between the two cohorts was significant (χ^2=8.49, *df*=1, *P*<.02). This result did not change when the value of the third population was removed from the operational criteria. A substantial opposite redistribution of neurons toward the superficial WM compartments was present if the values for two of the three populations were below the 16th percentile (mean−1 SD) of the control cohort and if the value of the third population was below the 50th percentile of the control cohort; this was found in the brain of one schizophrenic patient (case 15) and in the brain of one control subject (case 3), or in 5% of each cohort. This result did not change when the value of the third population was removed from the operational criteria.

DSM-III-R DIAGNOSIS AND GENDER, AGE, AND AUTOLYSIS TIME

In the brains of the subpopulation of the seven schizophrenic patients that showed a substantial redistribution of neurons toward the deeper WM compartments, three patients or 43% were diagnosed as having had paranoid-hallucinatory schizophrenia, and five patients or 71% were male. Of the remaining 13 schizophrenic patients, seven or 54% had paranoid-hallucinatory schizophrenia, and eight or 61% were male. The differences in age or autolysis time were less than 10% between the two populations of schizophrenic patients. None of these differences reached the level of significance (*P*>.4 to *P*>.8).

DOUBLE-LABELING STUDIES

In sections that were double-stained for MAP-2 immunoreactivity and NADPH-d histochemistry, numerous NADPH-d neurons and MAP-2 neurons lay closely adjacent to one another (Figure 2), but costaining of single neurons was not observed in the middle frontal gyri of the schizophrenic patients or control subjects.

In the double-labeled sections, SMI-32 and NADPH-d neurons were localized in close spatial proximity to each other in each brain (Figure 2). Occasionally, a dendrite of an NADPH-d neuron came in close contact with a soma or dendritic stem of an SMI-32 neuron. No neurons were costained for SMI-32 immunoreactivity and NADPH-d histochemical activity.

Costaining for SMI-32 and MAP-2 was not feasible since the primary antiserum samples were from the same species.

COMMENT

The results of the present study have demonstrated that the brains of schizophrenic patients have an abnormal composition of interstitial neurons in the prefrontal WM. The brains of a subgroup of schizophrenic patients that showed pronounced alterations in the distribution of WM neurons were identified. The large populations of MAP-2 and SMI-32 neurons showed an abnormal topographical distribution across WM compartments, recognized by a decreased cell density in WM up to 4000 and 5000 μm beneath the cortex and an increased cell density in the deeper WM. The NADPH-d neuronal population, which is separate from and a much smaller population than those defined by SMI-32 or MAP-2 immunoreactivity, was decreased in the superficial WM up to 3000 μm beneath the cortex and showed a slight increase in the deeper WM. This increase in the deeper WM was less than reported in an earlier study[22] with a smaller group of schizophrenic patients. These alterations in the topographical distribution of WM neurons were not accompanied by recognizable morphological changes in the individual neurons or in neurochemical-staining properties. The somal size of WM neurons also did not differ between the brains of schizophrenic patients and control subjects, as previously described.[22,23]

THE PRESENT study was initiated to determine if all major populations of interstitial WM neurons show an abnormal distribution in the prefrontal WM of brains of schizophrenic patients. The implication is that any alterations in the distribution of subcortical WM neurons would reflect an abnormality in their precursor structure, namely, the embryonic subplate, a transitory structure that consists of early maturing neurons and synaptic neuropil.[16,38-42] It is located immediately beneath the overlying cortex, and, in primates, it extends for several millimeters into the WM.[20] Most of the interstitial WM neurons of the adult brain are generated concurrently with the subplate neurons, before the generation of neurons of the cerebral cortex proper.[18,19,21,43-46] The interstitial WM neurons of the adult brain appear to be representatives of the subplate that escape the preprogrammed cell death that eliminates most subplate neurons.[16,18,19] In the present study, the three neuronal populations showed an abnormal distribution or density in the WM of the middle frontal gyri of schizophrenic patients, but changes in the MAP-2 population were most profound; MAP-2 immunoreactivity is expressed by the majority of subplate neurons[18] and by their derivatives in the adult brain,[19,25] so the finding implies that most former subplate neurons are affected.

The magnitude of the changes in the distribution of the NADPH-d neurons in the schizophrenic cohort of the present study was less severe in comparison with those reported in our earlier study.[22] In that study, a small sample that consisted of the brains of five schizophrenic patients and five control subjects was analyzed; three (60%) of the five schizophrenic patients showed a pronounced redistribution of NADPH-d neurons toward the deeper WM compartments, while, in the present study, seven (35%) of the brains of 20 schizophrenic patients showed a similar change in NADPH-d neuronal distribution. However, the size of the cohort of the present study was much larger than that of the earlier study, and it might be more representative of the general population of schizophrenic patients and control subjects and different subgroups of schizophrenic patients.

The reduction in the superficial WM neurons and the increase in the deeper WM neurons beneath the prefrontal cortex of schizophrenic patients might reflect an impairment of neuronal migration of future subplate neurons[43,47,48] early in the second trimester. A substantial defect in neuronal migration, however, would be likely to cause significant changes in cytoarchitecture and cell packing density in the overlying cortex proper, as well as in the WM, and might be accompanied by decreased gray matter volumes.[49,50] This was not observed in studies that were conducted on the same brains.[51] Analysis of the packing density and laminar distribution of cortical MAP-2 and SMI-32 neurons in the cohorts of the present study (S.A. and E.G.J., unpublished data, January 1995) did not show significant changes in the middle frontal gyri of schizophrenic patients, and other studies have reported modest, variable, or insignificant changes in cell density or volume of prefrontal cortex in the brains of schizophrenic patients.[52-66] In the absence of severe cytoarchitectural defects or volumetric changes of the prefrontal cortex, theories that explain the distorted distribution of prefrontal WM or former subplate neurons in the brains of schizophrenic patients by a defect in neuronal migration must assume that this disturbance affects rather selectively the neuronal population of the subplate and, to a lesser degree, or not at all, the cortical neuronal population.

An alternative explanation of the distorted distribution of interstitial WM neurons in schizophrenia could be an alteration in the pattern of cell death that normally occurs in the subplate. In the rodent brain, more than 80% of all subplate neurons die during ontogenesis[67]; however, the death of neurons in the cerebral cortex is less extensive and affects only 12% to 40% of the cortical neurons, depending on the cytoarchitectonic area.[68,69] Any alterations in the mechanisms of developmentally regulated cell death in schizophrenia could, therefore, primarily affect former subplate neurons, and these could have few or no major effects on the structure of the overlying cortex.

At present, the mechanisms that regulate programmed cell death of subplate neurons are not fully understood. A decrease in immunoreactivity for the low-affinity nerve growth factor receptor in the subplate coincides with the onset of massive cell death in this compartment[41,70,71]; this decrease suggests an inhibitory role for the low-affinity nerve growth factor receptor in the regulation of subplate cell death. A temporal or spatial alteration in the expression of the low-affinity nerve growth factor receptor or a related[72-74] molecule in the embryonic subplate of schizophrenic patients could potentially cause imbalances in the amount of subplate cell death, with an overshoot in the superficial compartments of the subplate and a compensatory decrease in the deeper regions of the subplate. In the outer, superficial subplate zones beneath the visual cortex of the monkey, cell death during the first postnatal months affects 20% of the MAP-2 neuronal population; however, during the same period, the death rate of MAP-2 neurons in the inner regions of the subplate is 70%.[75] An alteration in a similar pattern of subplate cell death could therefore readily explain the present results.

The human subplate is laid down from the beginning of the second trimester of pregnancy, reaches its maximum at the late second and early third trimester, and gradually diminishes in size during late pregnancy and early postnatal life.[20] Thus, the timing of several putative risk factors for schizophrenia, such as exposure to influenza virus during the second trimester,[9-12] coincides with the time during which the subplate is important for cortical development. Any disruption of the subplate potentially has severe consequences for the formation and maintenance of cortical connectivity because subplate neurons provide guidance for developing afferents that originate from the basal forebrain[76,77] and thalamus[78,79] and for efferent axons that grow along processes of the subplate neurons.[80-82] Selective destruction of the embryonic subplate causes a disorganized ingrowth of thalamocortical afferents[83-85] and a defect in the orderly formation of corticothalamic connections,[86] without changes in the overall structure and cytoarchitecture of the cortex.

Neurological disorders that are accompanied by diffuse defects of the WM are able to cause psychotic illness.[4,87-92] Therefore, could schizophrenia be caused by a primary lesion of the WM? The differential and opposite changes between the superficial and deep WM, reported in the present study, are not easily explained by theories based on degenerative lesions. Moreover, gliosis is not present in the cerebral cortex and in the subcortical WM of schizophrenic patients,[53,54,91,92] and imaging studies do not report gross abnormalities in the WM of the prefrontal cortex.[93-95] The reported reduction in the overall volume of the cerebral cortex[64] and the reported neuronal loss and volume reduction in the thalamus[96,97] may ultimately be based on an affection of the embryonic subplate during brain development, causing a defect in the orderly formation of the interconnections between the prefrontal cortex and the temporal association cortex[98,99] and their reciprocal connections with the thalamus.[100,101]

In the present study, the degree of alteration in the distribution of WM neurons among individual schizophrenic patients varied. One third of the schizophrenic patients showed more profound abnormalities than others. In this particular subpopulation of schizophrenic patients, a substantial defect of the embryonic subplate may be involved in the origin of schizophrenia. In the remaining schizophrenic patients, the evidence for dysfunction of the subplate is less compelling, and other causal factors (eg, a primary defect in glutamatergic or dopaminergic neurotransmission or a hitherto unknown developmental defect that is unrelated to the subplate) that could lead to prefrontal dysfunction in individual schizophrenic patients[2,3,102,103] have to be considered.

Accepted for publication September 13, 1995.

This study was supported by grants MH53674, MH54844, and NS21377 from the National Institutes of Health, US Public Health Service, Bethesda, Md, and by grants from the National Alliance for Research on Schizophrenia and Depression, Chicago, Ill (Dr Akbarian), and from the Stanley Foundation (Research Award from the National Alliance for the Mentally Ill, Arlington, Va) (Dr Jones).

We thank Phong Nguyen for technical assistance, the patients and families who participated in these studies, and the California Alliance for the Mentally Ill, Tustin. Resources for processing brains were provided by Wallace W. Tourtellotte, MD, PhD, and Iris Rosario at the National Neurological Research Specimen Bank, West Los Angeles (Calif) Veterans Affairs Hospital.

Reprint requests to Department of Anatomy and Neurobiology, University of California, Irvine, CA 92717 (Dr Jones).

REFERENCES

1. Mesulam MM, Geschwind N. On the possible role of neocortex and its limbic connections in the process of attention and schizophrenia: clinical cases of inattention in man and experimental anatomy in monkey. *J Psychiatr Res.* 1978;14:249-259.
2. Buchsbaum MS, Haier RJ, Potkin SG, Nuechterlein K, Bracha HS, Katz M, Lohr J, Wu J, Lottenberg S, Jerabek PA, Trenary M, Tafalla R, Reynolds C, Bunney WE Jr. Frontostriatal disorder of cerebral metabolism in never-medicated schizophrenics. *Arch Gen Psychiatry.* 1992;49:935-942.
3. Weinberger DR, Berman KF, Suddath R, Torrey EF. Evidence of dysfunction of a prefrontal-limbic network in schizophrenia: a magnetic resonance imaging and regional cerebral blood flow study of discordant monozygotic twins. *Am J Psychiatry.* 1992;149:890-897.
4. Hyde TM, Ziegler JC, Weinberger DR. Psychiatric disturbances in metachromatic leukodystrophy: insights into the neurobiology of psychosis. *Arch Neurol.* 1992;49:401-406.
5. Scheibel AB, Conrad AS. Hippocampal dysgenesis in mutant mouse and schizophrenic man: is there a relationship? *Schizophr Bull.* 1993;19:21-33.
6. Fish B, Marcus J, Hans SL, Auerbach JG, Perdue S. Infants at risk for schizophrenia: sequelae of a genetic neurointegrative defect: a review and replication analysis of pandysmaturation in the Jerusalem infant development study. *Arch Gen Psychiatry.* 1992;49:221-235.
7. Cannon TD, Mednick SA, Parnas J, Schulsinger F, Praestholm J, Vestergaard A. Developmental brain abnormalities in the offspring of schizophrenic mothers, I: contributions of genetic and perinatal factors. *Arch Gen Psychiatry.* 1993;50:551-564.
8. Susser ES, Lin SP. Schizophrenia after prenatal exposure to the Dutch hunger winter of 1944-1945. *Arch Gen Psychiatry.* 1992;49:983-988.
9. Mednick SA, Machon RA, Huttunen M, Bone D. Adult schizophrenia following prenatal exposure to an influenza epidemic. *Arch Gen Psychiatry.* 1988;45:189-192.
10. Kendell RE, Kemp IW. Maternal influence in the etiology of schizophrenia. *Arch Gen Psychiatry.* 1989;46:878-882.
11. Barr CE, Mednick SA, Munk-Jorgensen P. Exposure to influenza during gestation and adult schizophrenia. *Arch Gen Psychiatry.* 1990;47:869-874.
12. O'Callaghan E, Sham P, Takei N, Glover G, Murray RM. Schizophrenia after prenatal exposure to 1957 A2 influenza epidemic. *Lancet.* 1991;337:1248-1250.
13. DeLisi LE, Dauphinais ID, Gershon ES. Perinatal complications and reduced size of limbic brain structures in familial schizophrenia. *Schizophr Bull.* 1988;14:185-191.
14. McNeil TF. Obstetric factors and perinatal injuries. In: Tsuang MT, Simpson JC, eds. *Handbook of Schizophrenia: Nosology, Epidemiology, and Genetics.* New York, NY: Elsevier Science Publishing Co Inc; 1988;3:319-344.
15. Mednick SA, Cannon TD. Fetal development, birth and the syndromes of adult schizophrenia. In: Mednick SA, Cannon TD, eds. *Fetal Neural Development and Adult Schizophrenia.* New York, NY: Cambridge University Press; 1991:3-13.
16. Shatz CJ, Ghosh A, McConnell SK, Allendoerfer KL, Friauf E, Antonini A. Pioneer neurons and target selection in cerebral cortical development. *Cold Spring Harb Symp Quant Biol.* 1990;55:469-480.
17. Valverde F, Facal-Valverde MV. Postnatal development of interstitial (subplate) cells in the white matter of the temporal cortex of kittens: a correlated Golgi and electron microscopic study. *J Comp Neurol.* 1988;269:168-192.
18. Chun JJM, Shatz CJ. The earliest-generated neurons of cat cerebral cortex: characterization by MAP-2 and neurotransmitter immunohistochemistry during fetal life. *J Neurosci.* 1989;9:1648-1667.
19. Chun JJM, Shatz CJ. Interstitial cells of the adult neocortical white matter are the remnant of the early generated subplate neuron population. *J Comp Neurol.* 1989;282:555-569.
20. Kostovic I, Rakic P. Developmental history of the transient subplate zone in the visual and somatosensory cortex of the macaque monkey and human brain. *J Comp Neurol.* 1990;297:441-470.
21. Kostovic I, Rakic P. Cytology and time of origin of interstitial neurons in the white matter in infant and adult human and monkey telencephalon. *J Neurocytol.* 1980;9:219-242.

22. Akbarian S, Bunney WE Jr, Potkin SG, Wigal SB, Hagman JO, Sandman CA, Jones EG. Altered distribution of nicotinamide adenine dinucleotide phosphate–diaphorase cells in frontal lobe of schizophrenics implies disturbances of cortical development. *Arch Gen Psychiatry.* 1993;50:169-177.
23. Akbarian S, Viñuela A, Kim JJ, Potkin SG, Bunney WE Jr, Jones EG. Distorted distribution of nicotinamide adenine dinucleotide phosphate–diaphorase neurons in temporal lobe of schizophrenics implies anomalous cortical development. *Arch Gen Psychiatry.* 1993;50:178-187.
24. Hendry SHC, Jones EG, Emson PC. Morphology, distribution and synaptic relations of somatostatin- and neuropeptide Y-immunoreactive neurons in rat and monkey neocortex. *J Neurosci.* 1984;4:2497-2517.
25. Meyer G, Wahle P, Castaneyra-Perdomo A, Ferres-Torres R. Morphology of neurons in the white matter of the adult human neocortex. *Exp Brain Res.* 1992;88:204-212.
26. Jones EG, Huntley GW, Benson DL. Alpha calcium/calmodulin-dependent protein kinase II selectively expressed in a subpopulation of excitatory neurons in monkey sensory-motor cortex: comparison with GAD-67 expression. *J Neurosci.* 1994;14:611-629.
27. Campbell MJ, Morrison JH. Monoclonal antibody to neurofilament protein (SMI-32) labels a subpopulation of pyramidal neurons in the human and monkey neocortex. *J Comp Neurol.* 1989;282:191-205.
28. Sternberger LA, Sternberger NH. Monoclonal antibodies distinguish phosphorylated and nonphosphorylated forms of neurofilaments in situ. *Proc Natl Acad Sci U S A.* 1983;80:6126-6130.
29. Lee VM-Y, Otvos L Jr, Carden MJ, Hollosi M, Dietzschold B, Lazzarini RA. Identification of the major multiphosphorylation site in mammalian neurofilaments. *Proc Natl Acad Sci U S A. 1988;85:1998-2002.*
30. Zec RF, Weinberger DR. Brain areas implicated in schizophrenia: a selective overview. In: Nasrallah HA, Weinberger DR, eds. *The Handbook of Schizophrenia: the Neurology of Schizophrenia.* Amsterdam, the Netherlands: Elsevier Science Publishers; 1986;1:175-206.
31. Winn P. Schizophrenia research moves to the prefrontal cortex: meeting report. *Trends Neurosci.* 1994;17:265-268.
32. Tourtellotte WW, Berman K. Brain banking. In: Adelman G, ed. *Encyclopedia of Neuroscience.* Cambridge, Mass: Birkhauser Boston Inc; 1987;1:156-158.
33. Brodmann K. *Vergleichende Lokalisationslehre der Grosshirnrinde in Prinzipien dargestellt auf Grund des Zellenbaues.* Leipzig, Germany; J. A. Barth; 1909.
34. Walker AE. A cytoarchitectural study of the prefrontal area of the macaque monkey. *J Comp Neurol.* 1940;73:59-86.
35. Rajkowska G, Goldman-Rakic PS. Cytoarchitectonic definition of prefrontal areas in the human cortex, I: remapping of areas 9 and 46 using quantitative criteria. *Cereb Cortex.* In press.
36. Jones EG, Hendry SHC, Liu XB, Potkin SG, Tourtellotte WW. A method for fixation of previously fresh-frozen human adult and fetal brains that preserves histological quality and immunoreactivity. *J Neurosci Methods.* 1992; 44:133-144.
37. Sachs L. *Angewandte Statistik.* 7th ed. Berlin, Germany: Springer-Verlag; 1992: 422-424.
38. Marin-Padilla M. Early ontogenesis of the human cerebral cortex. In: Peters A, Jones EG, eds. *Cerebral Cortex: Development and Maturation of Cerebral Cortex.* New York, NY: Plenum Press; 1988;7:1-34.
39. Huntley GW, deBlas AL, Jones EG. $GABA_A$ receptor immunoreactivity in adult and developing monkey sensory-motor cortex. *Exp Brain Res.* 1990;82:519-535.
40. Schwartz ML, Goldman-Rakic PS. Prenatal specification of callosal connections in rhesus monkey. *J Comp Neurol.* 1991;307:144-162.
41. Meinecke DL, Rakic P. Low-affinity p75 nerve growth factor receptor expression in the embryonic monkey telencephalon: timing and localization in diverse cellular elements. *Neuroscience.* 1993;54:105-116.
42. Naeff B, Schlumpf M, Lichtensteiger W. Pre- and postnatal development of high-affinity [^{3}H]nicotine binding sites in rat brain regions: an autoradiographic study. *Dev Brain Res.* 1992;68:163-174.
43. Luskin MB, Shatz CJ. Cogeneration of subplate and marginal zone cells in the cat's primary visual cortex. *J Neurosci.* 1985;5:1062-1075.
44. Ferriero DM, Arcavi LJ, Sagar SM, McInthosh TK, Simon RP. Selective sparing of NADPH-diaphorase neurons in neonatal hypoxia-ischemia. *Ann Neurol.* 1988;24:670-676.
45. Ferrante RJ, Kowall NW, Beal MF, Richardson EP Jr, Bird ED, Martin JB. Selective sparing of a class of striatal neurons in Huntington's disease. *Science.* 1985;230:561-563.
46. Kowall NW, Beal MF. Cortical somatostatin, neuropeptide Y, and NADPH-diaphorase neurons: normal anatomy and alterations in Alzheimer's disease. *Ann Neurol.* 1988;23:105-114.
47. Rakic P. Mode of cell migration to the superficial layers of the fetal monkey neocortex. *J Comp Neurol.* 1972;145:61-84.
48. Rakic P. Neurons in rhesus monkey visual cortex: systematic relationship between time of origin and eventual disposition. *Science.* 1974;183:425-427.
49. Caviness VS Jr, Williams RS. Cellular pathology of the developing human nervous system. In: Katzman R, ed. *Congenital and Acquired Cognitive Disorders.* New York, NY: Raven Press; 1979:69-90.
50. Rakic P. Defects of neuronal migration and the pathogenesis of cortical malformations. *Prog Brain Res.* 1988;73:15-37.
51. Akbarian S, Kim JJ, Potkin SG, Hagman JO, Tafazzoli A, Bunney WE Jr, Jones EG. Gene expression for glutamic acid decarboxylase is reduced without loss of neurons in prefrontal cortex of schizophrenics. *Arch Gen Psychiatry.* 1995; 52:258-266.
52. Colon EJ. Quantitative cytoarchitectonics of the human cerebral cortex in schizophrenic dementia. *Acta Neuropathol (Berl).* 1972;20:1-10.
53. Benes FM, Davidson J, Bird ED. Quantitative cytoarchitectural analyses of the cerebral cortex of schizophrenics. *Arch Gen Psychiatry.* 1986;43:31-35.
54. Benes FM, McSparren J, Bird ED, SanGiovanni JP, Vincent SL. Deficits in small interneurons in prefrontal and cingulate cortices of schizophrenic and schizoaffective patients. *Arch Gen Psychiatry.* 1991;48:996-1001.
55. Daviss SR, Lewis DA. Calbindin- and calretinin-immunoreactive local circuit neurons are increased in density in the prefrontal cortex of schizophrenic subjects. *Neurosci Abstr.* 1993;19:201.
56. Selemon LD, Rajkowska G, Goldman-Rakic PS. Cytologic abnormalities in area 9 of the schizophrenic cortex. *Neurosci Abstr.* 1993;19:200.
57. Coggeshall RE. A consideration of neural counting methods. *Trends Neurosci.* 1992;15:9-13.
58. Pakkenberg B. Total nerve cell number in neocortex of chronic schizophrenics and controls estimated using optical dissectors. *Biol Psychiatry.* 1993; 34:768-772.
59. Heckers S, Heinsen H, Geiger B, Beckmann H. Hippocampal neuron number in schizophrenia. *Arch Gen Psychiatry.* 1991;48:1002-1008.
60. Scheibel AB, Kovelman JA. Disorientation of the hippocampal pyramidal cell and its processes in the schizophrenic patient. *Biol Psychiatry.* 1981;16:101-102.
61. Jakob H, Beckmann H. Prenatal development disturbances in the limbic allocortex of schizophrenics. *J Neural Transm.* 1986;65:303-326.
62. Arnold SE, Hyman BT, Van Hoesen GW, Damasio AR. Some cytoarchitectural abnormalities of the entorhinal cortex in schizophrenia. *Arch Gen Psychiatry.* 1991;48:625-632.
63. Andreasen N, Nasrallah HA, Dunn V, Olson SC, Grove WM, Ehrhardt JC, Coffman JA, Crossett JHW. Structural abnormalities in the frontal system in schizophrenia. *Arch Gen Psychiatry.* 1986;43:136-144.
64. Zipursky RB, Lim KO, Sullivan EV, Brown BW, Pfefferbaum A. Widespread cerebral gray matter volume deficits in schizophrenia. *Arch Gen Psychiatry.* 1992;49:195-205.
65. Breier A, Buchanan RW, Elkashef A, Munson RC, Kirkpatrick B, Gellad F. Brain morphology and schizophrenia: a magnetic resonance imaging study of limbic, prefrontal cortex, and caudate structures. *Arch Gen Psychiatry.* 1992;49: 921-926.
66. Wible CG, Shenton ME, Hokama H, Kikinis R, Jolesz FA, McCarley RW. A magnetic resonance imaging study of the prefrontal cortex in schizophrenia. *Biol Psychiatry.* 1993;33:316.
67. Woo TU, Beale JM, Finlay BL. Dual fate of subplate neurons in a rodent. *Cereb Cortex.* 1991;1:433-443.
68. Heumann D, Leuba G. Neuronal death in the development and aging of the cerebral cortex of the mouse. *Neuropathol Appl Neurobiol.* 1983;9:297-311.
69. Finlay BL, Slattery M. Local differences in the amount of early cell death in neocortex predict adult local specializations. *Science.* 1983;219:1349-1351.
70. Allendoerfer KL, Shelton DL, Shooter EM, Shatz CJ. Nerve growth factor immunoreactivity is transiently associated with the subplate neurons of the mammalian cerebral cortex. *Proc Natl Acad Sci U S A.* 1990;87:187-190.
71. Kordower JH, Mufson EJ. Nerve growth factor receptor-immunoreactive neurons within the developing human cortex. *J Comp Neurol.* 1992;323:25-41.
72. Itoh N, Yonehara S, Ishii A, Yonehara M, Mizushima S-I, Sameshima M, Hase A, Seto Y, Nagata S. The polypeptide encoded by the cDNA for human cell surface antigen Fas can mediate apoptosis. *Cell.* 1991;66:233-243.
73. Oehm A, Behrmann I, Falk W, Pawlita M, Maier G, Klas C, Li-Weber M, Richards S, Dhein J, Trauth BC, Ponsting H, Krammer PH. Purification and molecular cloning of the APO-1 cell surface antigen, a member of the tumor necrosis factor/nerve growth factor superfamily. *J Biol Chem.* 1992;267: 10709-10715.
74. Golstein P, Ojcius DM, Young JD. Cell death mechanisms and the immune system. *Immunol Rev.* 1991;121:29-65.
75. Mehra RD, Hendrickson AE. A comparison of the development of neuropeptide and MAP-2 immunocytochemical labeling in the macaque monkey visual

cortex during pre- and postnatal development. *J Neurobiol.* 1993;24:101-124.
76. Koh S, Loy R. Localization and development of nerve growth factor-sensitive rat basal forebrain neurons and their afferent projections to hippocampus and neocortex. *J Neurosci.* 1989;9:2999-3018.
77. Kostovic I, Goldman-Rakic P. Transient cholinesterase staining in the mediodorsal nucleus of the thalamus and its connections in the developing human and monkey brain. *J Comp Neurol.* 1983;219:431-447.
78. Friauf E, McConnell SK, Shatz CJ. Functional synaptic circuits in the subplate during fetal and early postnatal development of cat visual cortex. *J Neurosci.* 1990;10:2601-2613.
79. Callaway EM, Katz LC. Development of axonal arbors of layer IV spiny neurons in cat striate cortex. *J Neurosci.* 1992;12:570-582.
80. McConnell SK, Ghosh A, Shatz CJ. Subplate neurons pioneer the first axon pathway from the cerebral cortex. *Science.* 1989;245:978-982.
81. Kim GJ, Shatz CJ, McConnell SK. Morphology of pioneer and follower growth cones in the developing cerebral cortex. *J Neurobiol.* 1991;22:629-642.
82. De Carlos JA, O'Leary DDM. Growth and targeting of subplate axons and establishment of major cortical pathways. *J Neurosci.* 1992;12:1194-1211.
83. Gosh A, Antonini A, McConnell SK, Shatz CJ. Requirement for subplate neurons in the formation of thalamocortical connections. *Nature.* 1990;347:179-181.
84. Ghosh A, Shatz CJ. Involvement of subplate neurons in the formation of ocular dominance columns. *Science.* 1992;255:1441-1443.
85. Ghosh A, Shatz CJ. Segregation of geniculocortical afferents during the critical period: a role for subplate neurons. *J Neurosci.* 1994;14:3862-3880.
86. McConnell SK, Ghosh A, Shatz CJ. Subplate pioneers and the formation of descending connections from cerebral cortex. *J Neurosci.* 1994;14:1892-1907.
87. Shapiro EG, Lockman LA, Knopman D, Krivit W. Characteristics of the dementia in late-onset metachromatic leukodystrophy. *Neurology.* 1994;44:662-665.
88. Alzheimer A. Beitrag zur Kenntniss der pathologischen Neuroglia und ihrer Beziehungen zu AbbauvorgZngen im Nervengewebe. In: Nissl F, Alzheimer A, eds. *Histologische und histopathologische Arbeiten über die Grosshirnrinde.* Jena, Germany: Gustav Fischer; 1910:401-404.
89. Bruton CJ, Stevens JR, Frith CD. Epilepsy, psychosis, and schizophrenia: clinical and neuropathologic correlations. *Neurology.* 1994;44:34-42.
90. Mizukami K, Sasaki M, Suzuki T, Shiraishi H, Koizumi J, Ohkoshi N, Ogata T, Mori N, Ban S, Kosaka K. Central nervous system changes in mitochondrial encephalomyopathy: light and electron microscopic study. *Acta Neuropathol (Berl).* 1992;83:449-452.
91. Roberts GW, Colter N, Lofthouse R, Bogerts B, Zech M, Crow TJ. Gliosis in schizophrenia: a survey. *Biol Psychiatry.* 1986;21:1043-1050.
92. Roberts GW, Colter N, Lofthouse R, Johnstone EC, Crow TJ. Is there gliosis in schizophrenia? investigation of the temporal lobe. *Biol Psychiatry.* 1987;22:1459-1468.
93. Brown FW, Lewine RJ, Hudgins PA, Risch SC. White matter hyperintensity signals in psychiatric and nonpsychiatric subjects. *Am J Psychiatry.* 1992;149:620-625.
94. Williamson P, Pelz D, Merskey H, Morrison S, Karlik S, Drost D, Carr T, Conlon P. Frontal, temporal and striatal proton relaxation times in schizophrenic patients and normal comparison subjects. *Am J Psychiatry.* 1992;149:549-551.
95. Harvey I, Ron MA, Murray R, Lewis S, Barker G, McManus D. MRI in schizophrenia: basal ganglia and white matter T1 times. *Psychol Med.* 1991;21:587-598.
96. Andreasen NC, Arndt S, Swayze V II, Cizadlo T, Flaum M, O'Leary D, Ehrhardt JC, Yuh WTC. Thalamic abnormalities in schizophrenia visualized through magnetic resonance image averaging. *Science.* 1994;266:294-298.
97. Pakkenberg B. Pronounced reduction of total neuron number in mediodorsal thalamic nucleus and nucleus accumbens in schizophrenics. *Arch Gen Psychiatry.* 1990;47:1023-1028.
98. Jones EG, Powell TPS. An anatomical study of converging sensory pathways within the cerebral cortex of the monkey. *Brain.* 1970;93:793-820.
99. Pandya DN, Yeterian EH. Architecture and connections of cortical association areas. In: Peters A, Jones EG, eds. *Cerebral Cortex: Association and Auditory Cortices.* New York, NY: Plenum Press; 1985;4:1-61.
100. Jones EG. *The Thalamus.* New York, NY: Plenum Press; 1985.
101. Goldman-Rakic PS, Porrino LJ. The primate mediodorsal (MD) nucleus and its projection to the frontal lobe. *J Comp Neurol.* 1985;242:535-560.
102. Fuster JM. The prefrontal cortex and temporal integration. In: Peters A, Jones EG, eds. *Cerebral Cortex: Association and Auditory Cortices.* New York, NY: Plenum Press; 1985;4:151-172.
103. Tamminga CA, Thaker GK, Buchanan R, Kirkpatrick B, Alphs LD, Chase TN, Carpenter WT. Limbic system abnormalities identified in schizophrenia using positron emission tomography with fluorodeoxyglucose and neocortical alterations with deficit syndrome. *Arch Gen Psychiatry.* 1992;49:522-530.

Correction

Word Missing in Article Title. In the article by McGuffin et al, published in the February issue of the ARCHIVES (1996;53:129-136), the article title should have agreed with that listed on the cover and in the Table of Contents. The title should have read "A Hospital-Based Twin Registry Study of the Heritability of *DSM-IV* Unipolar Depression." The journal apologizes for its error.

A Prospective 4-Year Follow-up Study of Attention-Deficit Hyperactivity and Related Disorders

Joseph Biederman, MD; Stephen Faraone, PhD; Sharon Milberger, DSc; Jessica Guite; Eric Mick; Lisa Chen; Douglas Mennin; Abbe Marrs; Cheryl Ouellette; Phoebe Moore; Thomas Spencer, MD; Dennis Norman, EdD; Timothy Wilens, MD; Ilana Kraus, MD; James Perrin, MD

Background: Previous cross-sectional data showed that children and adolescents with attention-deficit hyperactivity disorder (ADHD) are at increased risk of comorbid conduct, mood, and anxiety disorders as well as impairments in cognitive, social, family, and school functioning. However, longitudinal data were needed to confirm these initial impressions.

Methods: Using *DSM-III-R* structured diagnostic interviews and raters blinded as to diagnosis, we reexamined psychiatric diagnoses at 1- and 4-year follow-ups in children with ADHD and controls. In addition, subjects were evaluated for cognitive, achievement, social, school, and family functioning.

Results: Analyses of follow-up findings revealed significant differences between children with ADHD and controls in rates of behavioral, mood, and anxiety disorders, with these disorders increasing markedly from baseline to follow-up assessments. In addition, children with ADHD had significantly more impaired cognitive, family, school, and psychosocial functioning than did controls. Baseline diagnosis of conduct disorder predicted conduct disorder and substance use disorders at follow-up, major depression at baseline predicted major depression and bipolar disorder at follow-up, and anxiety disorders at baseline predicted anxiety disorders at follow-up.

Conclusions: These results confirm and extend previous retrospective results indicating that children with ADHD are at high risk of developing a wide range of impairments affecting multiple domains of psychopathology such as cognition, interpersonal, school, and family functioning. These findings provide further support for the value of considering psychiatric comorbidity in both clinical assessment and research protocols involving children with ADHD.

(Arch Gen Psychiatry. 1996;53:437-446)

From the Pediatric Psychopharmacology Unit, Psychiatry Service (Drs Biederman, Faraone, Milberger, Spencer, and Wilens; Mss Guite, Chen, Marrs, Ouellette, and Moore; and Messers Mick and Mennin), Departments of Child Psychology (Dr Norman) and Pediatrics (Dr Perrin), Massachusetts General Hospital, Department of Psychiatry, Harvard Medical School (Drs Biederman, Faraone, Spencer, and Wilens), Harvard Institute of Psychiatry, Epidemiology, and Genetics, Department of Psychiatry, Harvard Medical School at Brockton–West Roxbury Veterans Affairs Medical Center and Massachusetts Health Center (Dr Faraone), Department of Epidemiology, Harvard School of Public Health (Dr Milberger), and Department of Pediatrics, Harvard Community Health Plan (Dr Kraus), Boston.

FOLLOW-UP STUDIES of children with attention-deficit hyperactivity disorder (ADHD) into adolescence and early adulthood indicate that ADHD frequently persists and is associated with significant psychopathological symptoms and dysfunction in later life.[1-13] The adolescent and young adult with ADHD is at risk of school failure, emotional difficulties, poor peer relationships, and trouble with the law.[9,14] However, relatively little is known about the risk factors that determine these poor outcomes. Notably, most prior longitudinal studies of children with ADHD have focused on the assessment of comorbid conduct disorder, delinquency, and substance abuse but have provided less information about other conditions that might predict poor outcome.

In addition to conduct disorder, children with ADHD frequently have mood and anxiety disorders.[15,16] Comorbidity complicates follow-up studies of ADHD. When 2 disorders co-occur (comorbidity), the outcomes of 1 disorder might be erroneously attributed to the other.[16] Since the presence of comorbidity can influence diagnosis, prognosis, treatment, and health care delivery,[17,18] it remains to be determined whether research findings previously reported in samples of children with ADHD are related to the ADHD itself, the presence of comorbid disorders, or the combination of both.[16,19]

For example, antisocial personality, delinquency, and substance use disorder outcomes consistently reported in samples of children with ADHD followed up to adolescence and young adulthood have also been reported in children with conduct disorder.[20] Since conduct disorder is a well-established comorbidity of ADHD,[15] these outcomes could be due to the presence of comorbid conduct disorder, not ADHD. For example, August et al[8] followed up boys with ADHD, with and without con-

Subjects and Methods on next page

duct disorder, into early adolescence. All of these children continued to have prototypical ADHD problems at a 4-year follow-up, but those with conduct disorder had additional problems with aggressive behavior, delinquency, and substance abuse.

We have previously reported cross-sectional data regarding psychiatric comorbidity, intellectual functioning, interpersonal deficits, and familial transmission in 140 children with ADHD and 120 control children.[21-25] In this article, we describe the clinical features of these children based on additional longitudinal data collected at 1- and 4-year follow-up assessments. Our goal was to reexamine prospectively the adolescent outcome of children with ADHD, attending to issues of antisocial and other comorbid psychiatric disorders. Based on our prior work,[21-29] we hypothesized that among children with ADHD, the presence of a comorbid disorder at baseline would predict the development of comorbidity-specific complications. We also hypothesized that the presence of a comorbid disorder at baseline would predict more impaired adaptive, school, and cognitive functioning and more aggressive psychiatric treatment in children with ADHD.

SUBJECTS AND METHODS

The original sample included a total of 260 children (a group of 140 children with ADHD and a group of 120 normal controls) chosen from psychiatric and pediatric settings.[21] These groups had 454 and 368 first-degree biological relatives, respectively. All probands were white, non-Hispanic boys between the ages of 6 and 17 years. Potential probands were excluded if they had been adopted or if their nuclear family was not available for study. We excluded children if they had major sensorimotor handicaps, psychosis, autism, or an estimated full-scale IQ of less than 80. To minimize the potential confounds of social adversity, we excluded subjects from the lowest socioeconomic class, as determined by Hollingshead-Redlich Socioeconomic Status. Each of the ADHD probands met diagnostic criteria for current ADHD at the time of the clinical referral; at the time of recruitment, each had active symptoms of the disorder. However, we did not require that ADHD be the referral problem that initially brought the child to the ascertainment source.

We selected psychiatrically referred ADHD probands from consecutive referrals to the Pediatric Psychopharmacology Unit at the Massachusetts General Hospital (MGH). We recruited normal controls from the Pediatric Ambulatory Service at MGH. The 3000 children who use this clinic make approximately 9000 visits each year. They come from the entire metropolitan Boston area. The Harvard Community Health Plan (HCHP) provided the pediatrically referred ADHD probands and pediatric controls. We recruited subjects from HCHP centers that serve approximately 32 000 pediatric patients from both inner-city and suburban areas.

ASCERTAINMENT PROCEDURE

A 3-stage ascertainment procedure selected the probands. For ADHD probands, the first stage was the patient's referral to a psychiatric or pediatric clinic resulting in a clinical diagnosis of ADHD by a child psychiatrist (n=154) or pediatrician (n=238), as recorded in the clinic record. Because these diagnoses had been made by many different clinicians using different clinical standards of diagnosis, we included a second, systematic screening using *DSM-III-R* criteria. This second stage confirmed the diagnosis of ADHD by screening all children positive at the first stage using a telephone questionnaire answered by their mothers. The questionnaire asked about the 14 *DSM-III-R* symptoms of ADHD. Eligible subjects meeting study entry criteria who consented to participate in additional assessments were recruited for the study. They received the comprehensive assessment battery described below. This assessment battery collected data for the final *DSM-III-R* diagnoses used in this article. Only patients who received a positive diagnosis of ADHD at all 3 stages were included in the final analysis.

We also screened potential normal controls in 3 stages. First, we selected patients referred to medical clinics for routine physical examinations. Second, we administered the *DSM-III-R* ADHD telephone questionnaire to the mothers of referred controls. Potential controls were deemed ineligible based on our exclusion criteria or because they met the telephone interview diagnosis of ADHD. Eligible subjects who consented to participate in additional assessments were recruited for the study; they received the same assessment battery as that used for the ADHD sample. We screened controls only for the presence of ADHD. Screening for other conditions is inappropriate; it could spuriously produce evidence for familial coaggregation between the screened conditions and ADHD.[30]

ASSESSMENT PROCEDURES

Probands and their relatives were assessed at baseline and then again 1 and 4 years later. We examined their parents at baseline only. All diagnostic assessments were based on *DSM-III-R* structured interviews. Psychiatric assessments of children relied on the Schedule for Affective Disorders and Schizophrenia for School-Age Children, Epidemiologic 4th Version (Kiddie-SADS-E).[31] Diagnoses were based on independent interviews with the mothers and direct interviews of probands and siblings, except that children younger than 12 years of age were not directly interviewed. Diagnostic assessments of parents were based on direct interviews with each parent using the Structured Clinical Interview for *DSM-III-R* (SCID).[32] To assess childhood diagnoses in the parents, we administered unmodified modules from the Kiddie-SADS-E. At baseline and year 1, the structured interviews assessed lifetime history of psychopathological symptoms; at year 4, these assessments reflected the interval since the prior assessment.

The assessment personnel were blinded as to proband diagnosis (ADHD or control) and ascertainment site (MGH or HCHP). All efforts were made to sequence the mothers' interviews about their children after the direct interviews with the mothers about themselves had been completed and to have different interviewers conduct the direct interviews of siblings and those with mothers about their children. All follow-up assessments were made with interviewers blinded as to prior assessments of the same subjects and their family members. We collected interview data about all siblings in both the control families and families with children with ADHD. At MGH, 89% of the parents were directly interviewed; at HCHP, 93% were directly interviewed. Ninety-five percent of all uninterviewed cases were fathers. When a parent was unavailable for interviewing, information was obtained by administering the SCID about the absent spouse to the available spouse. Information from 1 HCHP control father could not be obtained.

The interviewers had undergraduate degrees in psychology and were trained to high levels of interrater reliability. Before working independently, interviewers observed interviews by experienced interviewers and clinicians. They subsequently conducted at least 6 practice (nonstudy) interviews and at least 2 study interviews while being observed by senior interviewers. The principal investigator (J.B.) supervised the interviewers throughout the study.

We computed κ coefficients of agreement by having 3 experienced, board-certified child and adult psychiatrists diagnose subjects from audiotaped interviews made by the assessment staff. Based on 173 interviews, the median κ was 0.86. For the disorders of most relevance to this article, the κ's were 0.99 for ADHD, 0.93 for conduct disorder, 0.83 for major depression, and 0.94 for bipolar disorder. As Faraone et al[33] reported in detail, the 1-year test-retest κ's were 0.95 for ADHD, 0.67 for conduct disorder, 0.66 for major depression, 0.64 for multiple anxiety disorders, and 0.71 for bipolar disorder.

A committee of 4 board-certified child and adult psychiatrists resolved all diagnostic uncertainties. The committee members were blinded as to the subjects' ascertainment group, ascertainment site, all data collected from other family members, and all nondiagnostic data (eg, neuropsychological, psychosocial, and family functioning). As suggested by others,[34,35] we diagnosed major depression only if the depressive episode was associated with marked impairment. Since the anxiety disorders comprise many syndromes with a wide range of severity, we used 2 or more anxiety disorders to indicate the presence of a clinically meaningful anxiety syndrome.[36] For children older than 12 years, the diagnosticians combined data from direct and indirect interviews by considering a diagnostic criterion positive if it was endorsed in either interview.

Persistent ADHD was defined as having a lifetime diagnosis of ADHD at baseline and continuing to meet criteria for ADHD at either the year 1 or year 4 follow-up assessments. Meeting criteria for ADHD at follow-up was considered positive if the subject met criteria for a full diagnosis of ADHD or for a subthreshold diagnosis with significant impairment, as evidenced by a *DSM-III-R* Global Assessment of Functioning Scale score below 60.

In addition to psychiatric data, we assessed: (1) cognitive functioning, using subtests from the Wechsler Intelligence Scale for Children–Revised (WISC-R), the Wide Range Achievement Test–Revised, and the Gilmore Oral Reading test. (Interviewers were trained to administer these tests by a child clinical psychologist with extensive experience in the psychological assessment of children. A psychologist [D.N.] supervised the interviewers throughout the study.); (2) social functioning with the Global Assessment of Functioning Scale of the *DSM-III-R* and the Social Adjustment Inventory for Children and Adolescents (SAICA); and (3) Hollingshead-Redlich Socioeconomic Status and family intactness (no divorce or separation of parents in family of origin). School dysfunction was assessed by documenting repeated grades, placement in special classes, or the need for tutoring. These assessments were identical for baseline and follow-up assessments with 1 exception. At baseline, the Gilmore Oral Reading test assessed reading ability, but at the follow-up examinations we used the reading subtest of the Wide Range Achievement Test–Revised. All cognitive, school, and psychosocial assessments at follow-up were blinded as to baseline data collected on the same subjects.

Using the methods of Sattler,[37] we estimated full-scale IQ from the vocabulary and block design subtests and computed the freedom from distractibility IQ from the other subtests. All of our analyses of the Wechsler subtests use age-corrected scaled scores. As we did elsewhere,[24] we used the regression procedure recommended by Reynolds[38] to define learning disability.

STATISTICAL PROCEDURES

We first compared children with ADHD and control children on outcome in 3 domains: psychopathological abnormalities, intellectual and school functioning, and psychosocial functioning. We then stratified the ADHD sample based on the presence or absence of baseline diagnosis of conduct disorder, major depression, and multiple anxiety disorders and compared these subgroups with ADHD subjects without these disorders and also with controls. Bivariate analyses used the Pearson χ^2 test (for nominal variables), the Wilcoxon rank sum and signed rank tests (for continuous variables that were not normally distributed), and linear regression analysis for other variables. To statistically control analyses for potentially confounding variables (eg, social class, other comorbid disorders, baseline functioning) we used logistic or linear regression, depending on the scale of the variable. To reduce the probability of type 1 errors, we used .01 as our threshold of statistical significance.

RESULTS

At the 1-year follow-up, 130 of the 140 children with ADHD and 113 of the 120 normal controls seen at baseline were successfully recruited. The rates of successful 1-year follow-up did not differ between groups. At the 4-year follow-up, 128 (91%) of the 140 children with ADHD and 109 (91%) of the 120 normal controls seen at baseline were successfully recruited. The rates of successful follow-up at 4 years did not differ between groups. Of the 23 families lost to follow-up in year 4, 11 were from the psychiatric ascertainment sample (6 children with ADHD and 5 controls) and 12 from the HCHP ascertainment sample (6 children with ADHD and 6 controls). Twenty-one of the 23 families refused participation (11 children with ADHD and 10 controls) and 2 could not be traced at follow-up (1 from the ADHD group and 1 control). There were no significant differences between subjects successfully followed up and those lost to follow-up on each of the measures used in this study (all $P>.01$; detailed information available on request) (**Table 1**). Subjects lost to follow-up were not included in the analyses for this article. Therefore, the base-

Table 1. Demographic Information*

	Baseline		Year 1		Year 4	
	ADHD Group (N=128)	Control Group (N=109)	ADHD Group (N=126)	Control Group (N=106)	ADHD Group (N=128)	Control Group (N=109)
Mean (SD) age, y	10.6 (3.0)	11.6 (3.7)	11.7 (3.1)	12.7 (3.7)	14.4 (3.1)	15.2 (3.7)
Socioeconomic status, mean (SD)	1.9† (0.97)	1.5 (0.73)	...	...	...	...
Intactness, No. (%)‡	96 (75)	90 (82)	89 (70)	87 (80)	84 (66)	84 (77)
Diagnosis of ADHD, No. (%)	128 (100)	0 (0)	121 (96)	1 (1)	83 (65)	3 (3)

**ADHD indicates attention-deficit hyperactivity disorder; ellipses, not reassessed.*
†P<.01, t test.
‡Intactness indicates no divorce or separation of the child's parents.

Table 2. Cumulative Rates of Lifetime Diagnoses at Each Assessment*

	Baseline		Year 1		Year 4		
	ADHD Group, No. (%) (N=128)	Control Group, No. (%) (N=109)	ADHD Group, No. (%) (N=126)	Control Group, No. (%) (N=106)	ADHD Group, No. (%) (N=128)	Control Group, No. (%) (N=109)	Remission, ADHD Group, No. (%) (N=128)
Conduct disorder	28 (22)†	3 (3)	30 (24)†	4 (4)	36 (28)†‡	6 (6)	7 (25)
Oppositional disorder	83 (65)†	10 (9)	89 (71)†	12 (11)	93 (73)†‡	17 (16)‡	12 (15)
Any alcohol/drug abuse or dependence	3 (2)	7 (6)	6 (5)	9 (8)	19 (16)‡§	18 (17)‡§	1 (33)
Major depression (severe)	37 (29)†	2 (2)	53 (42)†‡	4 (4)	58 (45)†‡	6 (6)	9 (24)
Bipolar disorder	14 (11)†	0 (0)	22 (18)†‡	0 (0)	29 (23)†‡§	2 (2)	10 (71)
Multiple (≥2) anxieties	35 (27)†	5 (5)	42 (34)†‡	8 (7)	45 (35)†‡	10 (9)	5 (14)
Panic disorder	1 (1)	0 (0)	3 (2)	1 (1)	6 (5)	2 (2)	1 (100)
Agoraphobia	11 (9)†	1 (1)	18 (15)†‡	3 (3)	26 (20)†‡§	3 (3)	5 (45)
Overanxious disorder	39 (30)†	7 (6)	48 (38)†‡	8 (7)	56 (44)†‡§	10 (9)	17 (44)
Simple phobia	24 (19)†	5 (5)	31 (25)†‡	10 (9)	33 (26)†‡	10 (9)	11 (46)
Social phobia	16 (13)	4 (4)	23 (19)‡	7 (6)	31 (24)†‡§	9 (8)	6 (38)
Separation anxiety	37 (29)†	6 (6)	38 (30)†	7 (7)	39 (30)†	8 (7)	16 (43)
Obsessive-compulsive disorder	4 (3)	1 (1)	5 (4)	1 (1)	14 (11)†‡§	1 (1)	2 (50)
Tic disorder	22 (17)†	4 (4)	38 (30)†‡	5 (5)	42 (33)†‡	7 (6)	5 (23)
Enuresis	38 (30)†	15 (14)	42 (34)†	18 (17)	42 (33)†	18 (17)	8 (21)

**ADHD indicates attention-deficit hyperactivity disorder. At each follow-up the lifetime diagnosis was considered positive if it had been endorsed at the follow-up or any prior assessment.*
†P≤.01 vs controls by Pearson's χ^2 test.
‡P≤.01 vs baseline by McNemar's χ^2 test.
§P≤.01 vs year 1 by McNemar's χ^2 test.

line sample size in Table 1 reflects only those subjects who returned at 4-year follow-up.

There were no statistically significant differences between the ADHD and control samples in the age of the proband or percentage of intact families at each of the 3 assessments conducted. However, there were small but statistically significant differences in socioeconomic status between children with ADHD and controls (Table 1). Thus, all comparisons between the groups were statistically corrected for socioeconomic status.

PSYCHIATRIC OUTCOME

The lifetime psychiatric diagnoses of children with ADHD and comparison children at each assessment are given in **Table 2**. At each follow-up, we defined a lifetime diagnosis as positive if it had been endorsed at the follow-up assessment or at any prior assessment. Thus, increases in lifetime rates over the 4-year follow-up period reflect new onsets of disorders. At each assessment, children with ADHD were significantly more likely to have antisocial disorders (conduct disorder and oppositional defiant disorder), mood disorders (major depression and bipolar disorder), anxiety disorders (multiple anxiety disorder, overanxious disorder, separation anxiety disorder, agoraphobia, simple phobia), tic disorders (chronic tic disorder and Tourette's syndrome), and enuresis. Among subjects with ADHD, the rates of disruptive behavior disorders, mood and anxiety disorders, substance use disorders, and language disorder significantly increased from baseline to follow-up assessment. In contrast, among controls, the increase from baseline assessment was limited to oppositional defiant disorder and substance use disorder.

Fifteen percent of the ADHD probands had remission of ADHD during the follow-up period. The last column of Table 2 shows that remission rates were higher for subjects with conduct disorder (25%), major depression (24%), and multiple anxiety disorders (14%) than for subjects with other comorbid disorders. There were no significant differences in baseline rates of comorbid

Table 3. Cognitive Outcome*

	Baseline		Year 4	
	ADHD Group (N=128)	Control Group (N=109)	ADHD Group (N=128)	Control Group (N=109)
WISC-R subscale scores, mean (SD)				
Vocabulary	11.2† (3.2)	13.1 (2.6)	11.3† (2.9)	13.4 (2.6)
Block design	13.1† (3.8)	15.2 (3.3)	11.6†‡ (3.6)	13.6‡ (3.0)
Digit symbol	9.9† (3.6)	11.8 (2.6)	9.7† (3.4)	11.5 (2.9)
Digit span	9.0† (2.8)	10.7 (2.9)	9.6† (3.1)	11.8‡ (3.0)
Oral arithmetic	10.6† (3.2)	12.4 (2.9)	10.3† (3.0)	12.6 (3.0)
Estimated full-scale IQ	109.5† (13.5)	118.5 (10.1)	107.0†‡ (13.7)	116.6 (10.5)
Freedom from distractibility	98.9† (16.1)	111.2 (13.6)	97.9† (18.8)	112.6 (15.4)
Achievement scores				
WRAT arithmetic	96.8† (17.4)	111.3 (16.1)	93.4†‡ (18.3)	109.5 (15.7)
Gilmore/WRAT reading	93.1† (16.8)	100.6 (100.1)	102.0†‡ (16.3)	111.8‡ (10.0)
Learning disability, No. (%)				
Arithmetic	26 (21)	8 (8)	36 (30)†‡	11 (10)
Reading	22 (18)†	4 (4)	25 (21)†	4 (4)
School functioning, No. (%)				
Repeat grade	40 (31)†	12 (11)	47 (37)‡	17 (16)
Extra help	72 (56)†	27 (25)	109 (85)†‡§	39 (36)‡§
Special class	41 (32)†	1 (1)	59 (46)†‡§	2 (1)

*ADHD indicates attention-deficit hyperactivity disorder; WISC-R, Wechsler Intelligence Scale for Children–Revised; and WRAT, Wide Range Achievement Test.
†$P \leq .01$ vs controls by Pearson's χ^2 or *t* test.
‡$P \leq .01$ vs baseline by McNemar's χ^2 or paired *t* test.
§$P \leq .01$ vs year 1 by McNemar's χ^2 or paired *t* test.

disorders between ADHD probands who did and did not experience a remission of their ADHD (all $P>.05$).

COGNITIVE AND PSYCHOSOCIAL OUTCOMES

Table 3 shows that children with ADHD had significantly more impaired scores than controls at follow-up on all assessed subscales of the WISC-R. Both ADHD and control subjects showed small but significant decreases in block design scores from baseline to year 4. In addition, children with ADHD showed small but significant decreases in estimated full-scale IQ, and controls had a significant increase in digit span scores (Table 3).

Compared with controls, children with ADHD had significantly more impaired reading and arithmetic achievement scores and significantly higher lifetime rates of learning disabilities and school dysfunction (Table 3). For children with ADHD, arithmetic achievement scores decreased and lifetime rates of arithmetic disability, repeated grades, need for extra help, and placement in special classes significantly increased during the follow-up period (Table 3).

Table 4 shows that children with ADHD continued to manifest impaired psychosocial functioning both globally (as measured by the Global Assessment of Functioning Scale) as well as in individual domains (as measured by the SAICA). Moreover, the families of children with ADHD continued to manifest more impaired levels of cohesion and conflict on the Family Environment Subscales (FES) than controls. Children with ADHD not only continued to receive intense interventions ranging from counseling, pharmacotherapy, and combined counseling plus pharmacotherapy to psychiatric hospitalization at follow-up, but there was a marked increase for each of these interventions over time.

Most of the differences in outcome remained significant after controlling for the baseline score. However, in the cognitive domain, differences in block design, digit symbol, and full-scale IQ in year 4 became marginally significant ($.01<P<.05$). In the psychosocial domain, SAICA measures of peer activities and sibling problems (in year 1) and sibling problems in year 4 became marginally significant. Also, the FES expression differences in year 4 lost significance.

IMPACT OF COMORBIDITY AT BASELINE ON OUTCOME AT FOLLOW-UP

The comorbid disorders used to stratify the ADHD sample in **Table 5** through **Table 7** were not mutually exclusive. Ten children with ADHD had conduct disorder only, 15 had depression only, 14 had multiple anxiety disorders only, 7 had both conduct disorder and major depression, 6 had conduct and multiple anxiety disorders, 10 had depression and multiple anxiety disorders, and 5 had all 3 disorders. Because of this overlap in comorbid disorders, each table of results indicates which effects remained significant after correcting for other comorbidities.

Baseline conduct disorder significantly increased the risk for conduct and oppositional defiant disorders, bipolar disorder, and alcohol and drug dependence at follow-up (Table 5). Major depression at baseline predicted oppositional defiant disorder, major depression, bipolar disorder, and agoraphobia at follow-up. Multiple anxiety disorders at baseline increased the risk for

Table 4. Functional Outcome*

	Baseline		Year 1		Year 4	
	ADHD Group (N=128)	Control Group (N=109)	ADHD Group (N=126)	Control Group (N=106)	ADHD Group (N=128)	Control Group (N=109)
SAICA scores, mean (SD)						
School behavior	2.8† (0.78)	1.7 (0.67)	2.6† (0.71)	1.6 (0.70)	2.8† (0.69)	1.7 (0.68)
Spare-time activities	1.9† (0.56)	1.7 (0.53)	1.9† (0.67)	1.6 (0.59)	2.3†‡§ (0.61)	2.0‡§ (0.44)
Spare-time problems	2.2† (0.85)	1.4 (0.61)	2.1† (0.83)	1.3‡ (0.44)	2.1† (0.78)	1.4 (0.62)
Problems with peers	2.1† (0.85)	1.4 (0.53)	2.0† (0.79)	1.3 (0.54)	2.2† (0.76)	1.5 (0.56)
Problems with siblings	1.9† (1.1)	1.5 (0.81)	1.8†‡ (0.94)	1.4‡ (0.70)	2.2† (1.3)	1.6 (1.0)
Problems with parents	2.1† (0.82)	1.3 (0.50)	2.0† (0.87)	1.2 (0.47)	1.9† (0.79)	1.3 (0.48)
Global Assessment Scale score, mean (SD)	48.2† (7.5)	69.8 (10.0)	49.4† (7.1)	69.0 (8.7)	53.1†‡§ (7.9)	66.9‡ (7.6)
Family functioning score, mean (SD)						
Cohesion	44.0† (21.5)	53.6 (17.8)	...	...	48.8† (18.9)	58.3 (13.9)
Expression	47.6 (15.0)	51.9 (14.7)	...	...	52.0‡ (14.5)	54.5 (12.9)
Conflict	57.6† (13.0)	50.8 (13.3)	...	...	55.3† (11.2)	48.1 (11.8)
Treatment, No. (%)						
Counseling	90 (70)†	30 (28)	102 (80)†‡	41 (38)	106 (83)†‡§	46 (42)
Medication	42 (33)†	0 (0)	57 (45)†‡	0 (0)	73 (57)†‡§	0 (0)
Combination	72 (56)†	1 (1)	72 (56)†	1 (1)	83 (65)†‡§	1 (1)
Hospitalization	2 (2)	0 (0)	4 (3)	0 (0)	9 (7)†‡§	0 (0)

*ADHD indicates attention-deficit hyperactivity disorder; SAICA, Social Adjustment Inventory for Children and Adolescents; ellipses, not assessed.
†P≤.01 vs controls by Pearson's χ^2, t, or Wilcoxon rank sum test.
‡P≤.01 vs year 1 by McNemar's χ^2, paired t, or Wilcoxon signed rank test.
§P≤.01 vs baseline by McNemar's χ^2, paired t, or Wilcoxon signed rank test.

anxiety disorders. These differences remained significant after statistically correcting for other comorbidities and socioeconomic status. The children with noncomorbid ADHD had significantly higher rates of oppositional defiant, tic, and language disorders compared with controls.

As shown in Table 6, children with ADHD with and without psychiatric comorbidities at baseline differed significantly from controls at follow-up on measures of intellectual functioning, achievement, and school dysfunction. However, the presence of psychiatric comorbidity did not increase the level of impairment beyond that conferred by ADHD: the patients with noncomorbid ADHD performed as poorly on these measures as the patients with ADHD and comorbid disorders.

Baseline comorbid diagnoses predicted more impaired psychosocial functioning in the global measure of dysfunction indexed by the Global Assessment Scale (Table 7). However, despite more impaired functional scores on individual subscales of the SAICA in each comorbid ADHD group than in noncomorbid cases, most of these differences failed to attain statistical significance. The children with ADHD and no comorbidities still had substantial deficits in most areas of functioning compared with controls.

On the FES, the comorbid ADHD cases had poorer scores for family cohesion, expressiveness, and conflict compared with the children with noncomorbid ADHD. However, the differences failed to attain our threshold of statistical significance. The FES indexes of family dysfunction differed significantly between controls and comorbid ADHD cases, but the children with noncomorbid ADHD were indistinguishable from controls. We found similar effects for treatment (Table 7). Children with comorbid ADHD received more intensive treatment than noncomorbid ones, as shown by their higher rates of combined psychosocial and pharmacological approaches and psychiatric hospitalization. Notably, psychiatric hospitalization was observed exclusively among comorbid ADHD cases.

COMMENT

Our 4-year follow-up found that by midadolescence, children with ADHD were at very high risk of a wide range of adverse outcomes. As found in the baseline assessment, children with ADHD had markedly elevated rates of antisocial, mood, and anxiety disorders; more impaired intellectual and achievement scores; and more impaired school, interpersonal, and family functioning at follow-up. These longitudinal results confirm and extend our previous cross-sectional findings, indicating a wide range of psychopathological abnormalities and dysfunction among children with ADHD that includes not only antisocial disorders but extends to mood and anxiety disorders as well. The prospective demonstration of comorbidity as an important predictor of impaired outcome in ADHD stresses the importance of early recognition of comorbid disorders for prevention and early intervention strategies in children with ADHD.

The antisocial and substance use disorder outcomes of our subjects with ADHD are consistent with those reported by prior follow-up studies.[1-13,39] However, our findings also indicate that the risk for antisocial disorders and substance use disorders observed among children with ADHD was predicted by the comorbidity with conduct disorder at baseline and not by ADHD itself. In this regard, our results are consistent with other work showing a continuity of antisocial behavior through childhood and adolescence.[6,8,10,40] Taken together, these

Table 5. Diagnostic Outcome at 4-year Follow-up Based on Baseline Comorbid Diagnosis*

	Baseline Comorbid Diagnosis			
	Conduct Disorder, No. (%) (n=28)	Major Depression, No. (%) (n=37)	Multiple (≥2) Anxieties, No. (%) (n=35)	Noncomorbid ADHD, No. (%) (n=61)
Conduct disorder	**10 (36)†‡**	6 (16)	6 (17)	6 (10)
Oppositional disorder	**20 (71)†‡**	**25 (68)†‡**	19 (54)†	21 (34)†
Major depression (severe)	7 (27)†	**11 (32)†‡**	5 (16)†	4 (7)
Bipolar disorder	**8 (27)†‡**	**9 (23)†‡**	4 (10)	1 (1)
Multiple (≥2) anxieties	21 (9)†	**11 (30)†‡**	**12 (34)†‡**	1 (2)
Panic disorder	3 (11)†	2 (5)	4 (11)†‡	0 (0)
Agoraphobia	4 (14)†	**9 (24)†‡**	**10 (29)†‡**	1 (2)
Overanxious disorder	5 (18)†	10 (27)†	11 (31)†‡	5 (8)
Social phobia	4 (14)	9 (24)†	**11 (31)†‡**	3 (5)
Separation anxiety	3 (11)	6 (16)†‡	**8 (23)†‡**	0 (0)
Obsessive-compulsive disorder	2 (7)†	3 (8)†	5 (14)†	2 (3)
Alcohol dependence	**5 (18)‡**	3 (8)	1 (3)	2 (3)
Drug dependence	**4 (15)‡**	2 (5)	1 (3)	2 (3)
Tic disorder	6 (21)†	7 (19)†	8 (23)†	9 (15)†

ADHD indicates attention-deficit hyperactivity disorder. Boldface entries represent significant findings after correcting for socioeconomic status and other comorbidities using logistic regression. N=128 for all ADHD subjects; N=109 for all controls.

†$P \leq .01$ *vs controls by Pearson's* χ^2 *test.*

‡$P \leq .01$ *vs ADHD without the respective comorbid diagnosis (conduct disorder, major depression, or anxiety) by Pearson's* χ^2 *test.*

Table 6. Baseline Comorbidity and Cognitive and School Functioning at 4-year Follow-up*

	Baseline Comorbid Diagnosis			
	Conduct Disorder (n=28)	Major Depression (n=37)	Multiple (≥2) Anxieties (n=35)	Noncomorbid ADHD (n=61)
WISC-R subscales, mean (SD)				
Vocabulary	10.6† (3.7)	11.1† (3.0)	10.5† (3.4)	11.5† (2.8)
Block design	10.4† (3.1)	12.0 (3.9)	10.7† (4.2)	11.6† (3.5)
Digit symbol	9.9 (3.3)	8.9† (2.9)	8.7† (3.5)	10.4 (3.4)
Digit span	10.4 (3.7)	9.6† (3.7)	9.1† (2.7)	9.2† (2.8)
Oral arithmetic	9.6† (2.8)	10.4† (3.5)	9.9† (3.6)	10.4† (3.0)
Estimated full-scale IQ	102.6† (14.9)	107.3† (14.5)	103.0† (16.0)	108.0† (13.2)
Freedom from distractibility	99.8† (16.1)	98.0 (18.9)	92.7† (24.1)	99.1† (15.5)
Achievement scores, mean (SD)				
WRAT arithmetic	87.9† (16.9)	92.6† (20.3)	88.1† (18.7)	95.9† (17.4)
WRAT reading	99.6† (19.7)	99.9† (18.8)	99.2† (17.5)	103.7† (15.4)
Learning disability, No. (%)				
Arithmetic	5 (23)†	5 (18)	7 (24)†	9 (16)
Reading	2 (9)†	5 (18)†	2 (7)†	4 (7)†
School functioning, No. (%)				
Repeat grade	4 (14)	3 (8)	3 (9)	3 (5)
Extra help	13 (46)†	18 (49)†	22 (63)†	31 (51)†
Special class	10 (36)†	14 (38)†	14 (40)†	9 (15)†

ADHD indicates attention-deficit hyperactivity disorder; WISC-R, Wechsler Intelligence Scale for Children–Revised; and WRAT, Wide Range Achievement Test.

†$P \leq .01$ *vs controls by Pearson's* χ^2 *test or one-way analysis of variance.*

findings indicate that the antisocial and delinquent behaviors and substance abuse often reported in follow-up studies of boys with ADHD may be linked to childhood antisocial disorders rather than to the syndrome of ADHD per se.[8,25]

Our longitudinal findings challenge the notion that comorbidity with ADHD is limited to antisocial disorders. The children with ADHD had significantly higher rates of comorbid anxiety and mood disorders than controls, but the prevalence of these disorders rose significantly over the follow-up period. The results for depression and anxiety are consistent with epidemiological data showing their comorbidity with ADHD was not caused by referral artifacts. Although epidemiological studies have not addressed the comorbidity of ADHD with bipolar disorder, prior clinical and family studies suggest it may be a valid comorbidity.[41-44]

If the comorbid disorders at baseline had been due to misdiagnoses, overlapping symptoms, or epiphenomena of ADHD (eg, demoralization secondary to failure),

Table 7. Baseline Comorbidity and Functional and Treatment History Outcome at 4-year Follow-up*

	Baseline Comorbid Diagnosis				
	Conduct Disorder (n=28)	**Major Depression (n=37)**	**Multiple (≥2) Anxieties (n=35)**	**Noncomorbid ADHD (n=61)**	**Control Group (n=109)**
SAICA scores, mean (SD)					
School behavior	3.2† (0.7)	2.9† (0.8)	2.9† (0.8)	2.6† (0.7)	1.7 (0.7)
Spare-time activities	2.3 (0.6)	2.2 (0.6)	2.4† (0.7)	2.2 (0.5)	2.0 (0.4)
Spare-time problems	2.4† (0.8)	2.3† (0.8)	2.1† (0.7)	2.0† (0.8)	1.4 (0.6)
Problems with peers	2.5† (0.8)	2.4† (0.8)	2.3† (0.7)	2.1† (0.8)	1.5 (0.6)
Problems with siblings	2.3 (1.1)	2.1 (1.1)	2.0 (1.1)	2.3† (1.5)	1.7 (1.0)
Problems with parents	2.4†‡ (0.9)	2.2† (0.9)	1.8† (0.8)	1.8† (0.7)	1.3 (0.5)
Global Assessment Scale score, mean (SD)	**49.0**†‡ (7.9)	**49.1**†‡ (7.6)	49.7†‡ (7.7)	56.5† (7.0)	66.9 (7.6)
Family functioning score, mean (SD)					
Cohesion	43.8† (21.5)	44.2† (19.2)	43.7† (21.2)	54.1 (15.6)	58.2 (13.9)
Expression	52.7 (16.2)	48.5 (16.2)	50.0 (18.0)	54.6 (11.2)	54.5 (12.9)
Conflict	59.5† (10.3)	**60.4**† (10.0)	56.7† (11.7)	52.1 (10.6)	48.0 (11.9)
Treatment history, No. (%)					
Counseling	12 (43)†	17 (46)†	15 (43)†	28 (46)†	11 (9)
Medication	7 (25)†	10 (27)†	9 (26)†	22 (36)†	0 (0)
Combination	11 (39)†	17 (46)†	17 (49)†	21 (34)†	0 (0)
Hospitalization	3 (11)†	5 (14)†‡	2 (6)†	0 (0)	0 (0)

ADHD indicates attention-deficit hyperactivity disorder; SAICA, Social Adjustment Inventory for Children and Adolescents. Boldface entries represent significant findings after correcting for socioeconomic status and other comorbidities using logistic regression.

†P≤.01 vs controls by Pearson's χ^2, analysis of variance (ANOVA), or Kruskal-Wallis test.

‡P≤.01 vs ADHD without the respective comorbid diagnosis (conduct disorder, major depression, or anxiety) by Pearson's χ^2, ANOVA using the Scheffé multiple comparison, or Kruskal-Wallis test.

then we would expect all ADHD probands to be at risk of comorbidity, not only those who had the disorders at baseline. Although we did observe some incident cases, we also found that each comorbid disorder was a strong predictor of the same disorder at follow-up. The continuity of comorbid disorders over the 4-year follow-up supports the hypothesis that the comorbid conditions have the syndromatic status of disorders and are not mere epiphenomena of ADHD.

With one exception, comorbidities between ADHD with anxiety and mood disorders have not been systematically investigated by most research examining adolescent outcome in ADHD. However, Gittelman et al[9] reported negligible rates of depression and anxiety in children with ADHD followed up into adolescence. The different results between our study and that of Gittelman et al may reflect differences in sample composition: they studied *DSM-II*–defined hyperactive children, whereas our study used *DSM-III-R* criteria for ADHD. Moreover, in our initial ascertainment, we did not require ADHD to be the reason for referral or to be the predominant diagnosis, and we did not select subjects from an ADHD specialty clinic. In contrast, the subjects from the study of Gittelman et al had been referred by teachers because of behavior problems to a free research psychiatric clinic.

Our cognitive findings also confirmed the cross-sectional results[24,29] showing that, compared with normal controls, the children with ADHD were more likely to have learning disabilities, repeated grades, placement in special classes, and academic tutoring. They also had significantly lower scores on subtests of the WISC-R. These findings confirm the clinical observation that despite average or above-average WISC-R scores, many children with ADHD frequently do poorly in school. However, children with ADHD and psychiatric comorbidity did not differ markedly from other children with ADHD on other school dysfunction, achievement, and WISC-R measures. This suggests that the cognitive deficits in children with ADHD are the result of ADHD and not the associated comorbid disorders. This conclusion supports the work of Frick et al[45] and Frost et al.[46] Both studies found evidence for neuropsychological impairments that were specifically associated with ADHD and not with comorbid psychiatric disorders. This also conforms to Hinshaw's[47] idea that early intellectual problems are a core component of ADHD that are subsequently exacerbated by disruptive behavior.

Our results regarding psychosocial dysfunction confirm and extend the cross-sectional findings showing that children with ADHD are at significant risk of interpersonal deficits. As in the baseline assessment,[48] children with ADHD at follow-up had more impaired scores than controls on scales reflecting school behavior; use of spare time; and problems with peers, parents, and siblings. Subscales of the SAICA showed more impairment owing to psychiatric comorbidity. This finding highlights the potential for these associated disorders to further compromise the child's adaptive capabilities.

Our treatment history findings revealed an association between comorbidity and intensity of treatment. While rates of counseling and use of psychoactive drugs were highly prevalent in all subtypes of ADHD with and without comorbidity, combined psychosocial plus pharmacological approaches were much more prevalent among the comorbid subtypes. The most intensive treatment histories were observed among those with comorbid major depression and anxiety disorders. Psychiatric hospitalization was observed exclusively among the comorbid subtypes; major depression conferred the highest risk for subsequent psychiatric hospitalization. These findings stress the very high risk among children with comorbid ADHD for serious and, at times, life-threatening complications.

Our results showing that ADHD families have more conflict and are less cohesive are consistent with a body of literature documenting the critical role played by family environmental factors in children's mental health.[49-52] Although the directionality of risk remains unknown, these findings add to the literature on familial risk in ADHD documenting that children with ADHD often come from families that are disorganized and have a parent who exhibits psychopathological symptoms. These families may create pathogenic environments that cause or aggravate the disorder in the child.

Our results also provide evidence for the validity of the ADHD syndrome per se. Although our subjects with noncomorbid ADHD were not afflicted with the emotional and behavioral disruptions that accompany conduct, mood, and anxiety disorders, 51% required tutoring, 34% had repeated a grade, 15% had been placed in special classes, and 16% had a learning disability at the 4-year follow-up. Moreover, compared with controls, at the 4-year follow-up the children with noncomorbid ADHD had significantly poorer functioning on measures of intellectual ability, academic achievement, and psychosocial functioning. Thus, uncomplicated ADHD conferred a serious risk for persistent dysfunction in multiple domains; it may be less disruptive than its comorbid counterparts, but its potential for adverse consequences cannot be ignored.

Our results must be interpreted in the context of methodological limitations. Although our interviewers were blinded as to the diagnosis of the probands, parents were not. Another potential source of bias stems from the lack of direct psychiatric interviews with children younger than 12 years; this may have decreased the sensitivity of some diagnoses. This may especially be the case for internalizing disorders such as anxiety and depression. However, we found high rates of both these disorders in our study. Also, children younger than 12 years have limited expressive and receptive language abilities; they cannot easily sequence events in time and have difficulties with abstraction. Thus, there is a real question about whether their self-perceptions, memories, feelings, and reported behavior can be reliably assessed through self-report, especially as regards lifetime history of psychopathological symptoms.[53] Although limited, studies of interview techniques for children under the age of 12 years suggest that their responses are unreliable.[54] Another concern is that interviews with mothers about their children may have been subject to a halo effect (ie, a bias toward reporting a second illness in the presence of another). This could have led to an overestimation of the comorbidity between ADHD and other disorders.

Although diagnoses were made by a committee of board-certified child and adolescent psychiatrists, some caution in their interpretation is warranted. First, the baseline diagnoses were based on the child's lifetime history of psychopathological symptoms. The formulation of such diagnoses is a difficult process, especially in the context of comorbidity. However, in our own work, lifetime diagnoses have shown excellent interrater reliability (see "Subjects and Methods" section) and good to excellent test-retest reliability over a 1-year period.[33]

Although our results are likely to generalize to many of the children with ADHD seen in pediatric and psychiatric settings, we do not know if our results will generalize to children with ADHD in the general population. For example, our finding of a 23% lifetime rate of bipolar disorder should not be interpreted to mean that 23% of children with ADHD in the community will develop that disorder. The population risk will likely be lower, because clinical referrals tend to be more severe. Also, because we did not manipulate treatment as an independent variable, we cannot use our study to determine treatment effectiveness[55] or to describe the untreated course of ADHD.

Despite these limitations, in a large sample of adolescents with ADHD as determined by the *DSM-III-R* ascertained from pediatric and psychiatric facilities, we have prospectively confirmed and extended results from a baseline assessment. We have shown that at both a 1- and 4-year follow-up, high levels of comorbidity exist between ADHD and antisocial, mood, and anxiety disorders. Moreover, comorbidity at baseline significantly predicted an increased intensity of treatment and additional school, cognitive, and psychosocial impairments. Thus, our data provide further evidence for the validity of subgrouping by comorbidity and highlight the need for clinicians to consider comorbidity as a viable diagnostic option in their assessment of children.

Accepted for publication November 7, 1995.

This work was supported in part by grant RO1 MH41314-07 from the National Institute of Mental Health, Bethesda, Md (Dr Biederman).

Reprints: Joseph Biederman, MD, Pediatric Psychopharmacology Unit (ACC 725), Massachusetts General Hospital, Fruit Street, Boston, MA 02114.

REFERENCES

1. Weiss G, Minde K, Werry JS, Douglas V, Nemeth E. Studies on the hyperactive child, VIII: five-year follow-up. *Arch Gen Psychiatry.* 1971;24:409-414.
2. Cohen NJ, Weiss G, Minde K. Cognitive styles in adolescents previously diagnosed as hyperactive. *J Child Psychol.* 1972;13:203-209.
3. Minde K, Weiss G, Mendelson N. A five year follow-up study of 91 hyperactive school children. *J Am Acad Child Psychiatry.* 1972;11:595-610.
4. Hoy E, Weiss G, Minde K, Cohen N. The hyperactive child at adolescence: cognitive, emotional and social functioning. *J Abnorm Child Psychol.* 1978;6:311-324.
5. Hechtman L, Weiss G, Perlman T, Amsel R. Hyperactives as young adults: initial predictors of adult outcome. *J Am Acad Child Psychiatry.* 1984;23:250-260.
6. Loney J, Kramer J, Milich RS. The hyperactive child grows up: predictors of symptoms, delinquency and achievement at follow-up. In: Gadow KD, Loney J, eds. *Psychosocial Aspects of Drug Treatment for Hyperactivity.* Boulder, Colo: Westview Press; 1981:381-416.
7. Satterfield JH, Hoppe CM, Schell AM. A prospective study of delinquency in 110 adolescent boys with attention deficit disorder and 88 normal adolescent boys. *Am J Psychiatry.* 1982;139:795-798.
8. August GJ, Stewart MA, Holmes CS. A four-year follow-up of hyperactive boys with and without conduct disorder. *Br J Psychiatry.* 1983;143:192-198.

9. Gittelman R, Mannuzza S, Shenker R, Bonagura N. Hyperactive boys almost grown up, I: psychiatric status. *Arch Gen Psychiatry.* 1985;42:937-947.
10. Mannuzza S, Gittelman-Klein R, Horowitz-Konig P, Giampino TL. Hyperactive boys almost grown up, IV: criminality and its relationship to psychiatric status. *Arch Gen Psychiatry.* 1989;46:1073-1079.
11. Mannuzza S, Gittelman-Klein R, Addalli KA. Young adult mental status of hyperactive boys and their brothers: a prospective follow-up study. *J Am Acad Child Adolesc Psychiatry.* 1991;30:743-751.
12. Barkley RA, Fischer M, Edelbrock CS, Smallish L. The adolescent outcome of hyperactive children diagnosed by research criteria, I: an 8-year prospective follow-up study. *J Am Acad Child Adolesc Psychiatry.* 1990;29:546-557.
13. Hart E, Lahey B, Loeber R, Applegate B, Frick P. Developmental change in attention-deficit hyperactivity disorder in boys: a four-year longitudinal study. *J Abnorm Child Psychol.* 1995;23:729-749.
14. Weiss G, Hechtman L, Milroy T, Perlman T. Psychiatric status of hyperactives as adults: a controlled prospective 15-year follow-up of 63 hyperactive children. *J Am Acad Child Psychiatry.* 1985;24:211-220.
15. Biederman J, Newcorn J, Sprich S. Comorbidity of attention deficit hyperactivity disorder with conduct, depressive, anxiety, and other disorders. *Am J Psychiatry.* 1991;148:564-577.
16. Caron C, Rutter M. Comorbidity in child psychopathology: concepts, issues and research strategies. *J Child Psychol Psychiatry.* 1991;32:1063-1080.
17. Maser JD, Cloninger CR. Comorbidity of anxiety and mood disorders: introduction and overview. In: Maser JD, Cloninger CR, eds. *Comorbidity of Mood and Anxiety Disorders.* Washington, DC: American Psychiatric Press; 1990: 869.
18. Angold A, Costello EJ. Depressive comorbidity in children and adolescents: empirical, theoretical and methodological issues. *Am J Psychiatry.* 1993;150: 1779-1791.
19. Rutter M. Isle of Wight revisited: twenty-five years of child psychiatric epidemiology. *J Am Acad Child Adolesc Psychiatry.* 1989;28:633-653.
20. Robins LN, Helzer JE, Croughan J. *The National Institute of Mental Health (NIMH) Diagnostic Interview Schedule, Version III.* Rockville, Md: National Institute of Mental Health; 1981.
21. Biederman J, Faraone SV, Keenan K, Benjamin J, Krifcher B, Moore C, Sprich-Buckminster S, Ugaglia K, Jellinek MS, Steingard R, Spencer T, Norman D, Kolodny R, Kraus I, Perrin J, Keller MB, Tsuang MT. Further evidence for family-genetic risk factors in attention deficit hyperactivity disorder: patterns of comorbidity in probands and relatives in psychiatrically and pediatrically referred samples. *Arch Gen Psychiatry.* 1992;49:728-738.
22. Faraone S, Biederman J, Chen WJ, Krifcher B, Keenan K, Moore C, Sprich S, Tsuang M. Segregation analysis of attention deficit hyperactivity disorder: evidence for single gene transmission. *Psychiatry Genet.* 1992;2:257-275.
23. Biederman J, Faraone SV, Doyle A, Krifcher Lehman B, Kraus I, Perrin J, Tsuang MT. Convergence of the Child Behavior Checklist with structured interview-based psychiatric diagnoses of ADHD children with and without hyperactivity. *J Child Psychol Psychiatry.* 1993;34:1241-1251.
24. Faraone SV, Biederman J, Krifcher Lehman B, Spencer T, Norman D, Seidman L, Kraus I, Perrin J, Chen W, Tsuang MT. Intellectual performance and school failure in children with attention deficit hyperactivity disorder and in their siblings. *J Abnorm Psychol.* 1993;102:616-623.
25. Faraone SV, Biederman J, Chen WJ, Milberger S, Warburton RM, Tsuang MT. Genetic heterogeneity in attention deficit hyperactivity disorder: gender, psychiatric comorbidity and maternal ADHD. *J Abnorm Psychol.* 1995;104:334-345.
26. Biederman J, Faraone SV, Keenan K, Tsuang MT. Evidence of familial association between attention deficit disorder and major affective disorders. *Arch Gen Psychiatry.* 1991;48:633-642.
27. Biederman J, Faraone SV, Keenan K, Steingard R, Tsuang MT. Familial association between attention deficit disorder (ADD) and anxiety disorder. *Am J Psychiatry.* 1991;148:251-256.
28. Faraone SV, Biederman J, Keenan K, Tsuang MT. Separation of DSM-III attention deficit disorder and conduct disorder: evidence from a family-genetic study of American child psychiatric patients. *Psychol Med.* 1991;21:109-121.
29. Faraone S, Biederman J, Krifcher Lehman B, Keenan K, Norman D, Seidman L, Kolodny R, Kraus I, Perrin J, Chen W. Evidence for the independent familial transmission of attention deficit hyperactivity disorder and learning disabilities: results from a family genetic study. *Am J Psychiatry.* 1993;150:891-895.
30. Kendler KS. The super-normal control group in psychiatric genetics: possible artifactual evidence for coaggregation. *Psychiatry Genet.* 1990;1:45-53.
31. Orvaschel H, Puig-Antich J. *Schedule for Affective Disorder and Schizophrenia for School-Age Children: Epidemiologic 4th Version.* Fort Lauderdale, Fla: Nova University Center for Psychological Study; 1987.
32. Spitzer RL, Williams JB, Gibbon M, First MB. *Structured Clinical Interview for DSM-III-R: Non-Patient Edition (SCID-NP, Version 1.0).* Washington, DC: American Psychiatric Press; 1990.
33. Faraone S, Biederman J, Milberger S. How reliable are maternal reports of their children's psychopathology? one year recall of psychiatric diagnoses of ADHD children. *J Am Acad Child Adolesc Psychiatry.* 1995;34:1001-1008.
34. Gershon ES, Hamovit J, Guroff JJ, Dibble E, Leckman JF, Sceery W, Targum SD, Nurnberg JI Jr, Goldin LR, Bunney WE Jr. A family study of schizoaffective, bipolar I, bipolar II, unipolar, and normal control probands. *Arch Gen Psychiatry.* 1982;39:1157-1167.
35. Weissman MM, Gershon ES, Kidd KK, Prusoff BA, Leckman JF, Dibble E, Hamovit J, Thompson WD, Pauls DL, Guroff JJ. Psychiatric disorders in the relatives of probands with affective disorders. *Arch Gen Psychiatry.* 1984;41:13-21.
36. Biederman J, Rosenbaum JF, Hirshfeld DR, Faraone SV, Bolduc EA, Gersten M, Meminger SR, Kagan J, Snidman N, Reznick JS. Psychiatric correlates of behavioral inhibition in young children of parents with and without psychiatric disorders. *Arch Gen Psychiatry.* 1990;47:21-26.
37. Sattler JM. *Assessment of Children's Intelligence.* San Diego, Calif: Jerome M Sattler; 1988.
38. Reynolds CR. Critical measurement issues in learning disabilities. *J Special Ed.* 1984;18:451-476.
39. Klinteberg B, Andersson T, Magnusson D, Stattin H. Hyperactive behavior in childhood as related to subsequent alcohol problems and violent offending: a longitudinal study of male subjects. *Person Indiv Diff.* 1993;15:381-388.
40. Stewart MA, Cummings C, Singer S, deBlois CS. The overlap between hyperactive and unsocialized aggressive children. *J Child Psychol Psychiat.* 1981; 22:35-45.
41. Grigoroiu-Serbanescu M, Christodorescu D, Jipescu I, Totoescu A, Marinescu E, Ardeleau V. Psychopathology in children aged 10-17 of bipolar parents: psychopathology rate and correlates of the severity of the psychopathology. *J Affect Disord.* 1989;16:167-179.
42. Geller B, Fox L, Clark K. Rate and predictors of prepubertal bipolarity during follow-up of 6- to 12-year-old depressed children. *J Am Acad Child Adolesc Psychiatry.* 1994;33:461-468.
43. Biederman J, Wozniak J, Kiely K, Ablon S, Faraone S, Mick E, Mundy E, Kraus I. CBCL clinical scales discriminate prepubertal children with structured-interview derived diagnosis of mania from those with ADHD. *J Am Acad Child Adolesc Psychiatry.* 1995;34:464-471.
44. Wozniak J, Biederman J, Kiely K, Ablon S, Faraone S, Mundy E, Mennin D. Mania-like symptoms suggestive of childhood-onset bipolar disorder in clinically referred children. *J Am Acad Child Adolesc Psychiatry.* 1995;34:867-876.
45. Frick PJ, Lahey BB, Kamphaus RW, Loeber R, Christ MAG, Hart EL, Tannenbaum LE. Academic underachievement and the disruptive behavior disorders. *J Consult Clin Psychol.* 1991;59:289-294.
46. Frost LA, Moffitt TE, McGee R. Neuropsychological correlates of psychopathology in an unselected cohort of young adolescents. *J Abnorm Psychol.* 1989; 98:307-313.
47. Hinshaw SP. Externalizing behavior problems and academic underachievement in childhood and adolescence: causal relationships and underlying mechanisms. *Psychol Bull.* 1992;111:127-155.
48. Biederman J, Faraone S, Chen W. Social adjustment inventory for children and adolescents: concurrent validity in ADHD children. *J Am Acad Child Adolesc Psychiatry.* 1993;32:1059-1064.
49. Barkley RA. *Attention Deficit Hyperactivity Disorder: A Handbook for Diagnosis and Treatment.* New York, NY: The Guilford Press; 1990.
50. Palfrey JS, Levine MD, Walker DK, Sullivan M. The emergence of attention deficits in early childhood: a prospective study. *Developmental and Behavioral Pediatrics.* 1985;6:339-348.
51. Nichols PL, Chen TC. *Minimal Brain Dysfunction: A Prospective Study.* Hillsdale, NJ: Lawrence Erlbaum Associates Inc; 1981.
52. Mrazek P, Haggerty R, eds. *Reducing Risks for Mental Disorders.* Washington, DC: National Academy Press; 1994.
53. Loeber R, Green SM, Lahey BB, Stouthamer-Loeber M. Differences and similarities between children, mothers, and teachers as informants on disruptive child behavior. *J Abnorm Child Psychol.* 1991;19:75-95.
54. Achenbach TM, McConaughy SH, Howell CT. Child/adolescent behavioral and emotional problems: implications of cross-informant correlations for situational specificity. *Psychol Bull.* 1987;101:213-232.
55. Faraone SV, Simpson JC, Brown WA. Mathematical models of complex dose-response relationships: implications for experimental design in psychopharmacologic research. *Stat Med.* 1992;11:685-702.

The Contribution of α_2-Noradrenergic Mechanisms to Prefrontal Cortical Cognitive Function

Potential Significance for Attention-Deficit Hyperactivity Disorder

Amy F. T. Arnsten, PhD; Jenna C. Steere, MPH; Robert D. Hunt, MD

This article aims to review research in nonhuman primates demonstrating that norepinephrine can enhance the cognitive functioning of the prefrontal cortex through actions at α_2A-adrenergic receptors postjunctional to noradrenergic terminals. As prefrontal cortex cognitive deficits are prominent in several psychiatric disorders, including attention-deficit hyperactivity disorder, these basic findings may have relevance for the development of novel pharmacotherapies. *(Arch Gen Psychiatry. 1996;53:448-455)*

Symptoms of prefrontal cortex (PFC) dysfunction accompany many mental disorders, including schizophrenia, Korsakoff's amnesia, and attention-deficit hyperactivity disorder (ADHD). Numerous investigators have noted the similarity between patients with ADHD and patients with PFC lesions, and data suggest that alterations in the PFC and its related subcortical circuits may contribute to this disorder. In particular, researchers have focused on PFC interactions with the caudate[1-3] and the brain stem's dopamine (DA) and norepinephrine (NE) systems.[4] Attention-deficit hyperactivity disorder is generally treated with stimulant medication such as methylphenidate hydrochloride, which promotes catecholamine transmission, and researchers have posited that ADHD symptoms arise from impaired DA[5-8] and NE[7,9] transmission. Norepinephrine depletion in rodents results in increased distractibility,[10,11] suggesting that poor attention regulation in patients with ADHD may involve NE mechanisms. Motor hyperactivity has also been associated with NE depletion in rodent cortex.[7,12] This article reviews recent data from animal studies indicating a mechanism whereby NE can enhance the attentional, mnemonic, and inhibitory abilities of the PFC.

These findings may have relevance to our understanding of ADHD. Evidence from several laboratories indicates that NE can improve PFC function through actions at α_2-adrenergic receptors in the PFC. Although α_2-agonists such as clonidine have traditionally been thought to act at presynaptic (prejunctional) receptors, decreasing NE tone and lowering arousal, recent research has demonstrated the importance of NE actions *postsynaptic* (postjunctional) to NE terminals as well. Furthermore, the discovery of 3 subtypes of α_2-receptors (α_2A, α_2B, and α_2C) has indicated a mechanism whereby the various actions of α_2-agonists may be dissociated. Indeed, NE's beneficial actions in the PFC appear to result from stimulation of α_2A-receptors postjunctional to NE terminals. These findings from basic research suggest strategies for pharmacological treatment of disorders such as ADHD where PFC dysfunction is evident.

MANY ADHD SYMPTOMS RESEMBLE PFC DYSFUNCTION

Although ADHD is a complex and varied disorder, many investigators have noted the resemblance between patients with ADHD and subjects with lesions to the PFC.[13-19] The poor attention regulation, disorganized behavior, hyperactivity, and impulsivity found in ADHD can also be seen in humans[20-25] and animals[26-28] with PFC lesions, especially those involving the right hemisphere.[12,29] Lesions involving the

From the Section of Neurobiology, Yale Medical School, New Haven, Conn (Dr Arnsten and Ms Steere), and the Center for Attention and Hyperactivity Disorders, Nashville, Tenn (Dr Hunt).

right dorsal PFC produce deficits in sustaining attention regulation[22] and inhibiting responses to distracting stimuli.[30,31] In contrast, lesions to the right orbital PFC often produce deficits in the affective realm, such as immature behavior, lack of restraint, and increased motor activity.[32-34] Consistent with this profile, the right PFC has been shown to be smaller in patients with ADHD than it is in age-matched controls.[35] Neuropsychological testing of patients with ADHD also suggests that PFC dysfunction is involved in this disorder. Patients with ADHD are consistently impaired on tests of frontal lobe function (eg, Continuous Performance, Go/No-Go, and Stroop Interference tasks[18]) but not on the Posner task, a test of parietal attentional abilities.[36] Event-related potential studies have shown that patients with ADHD, like patients with PFC lesions, show reduced attention-related negativity during a selective attention task.[21,30,37] Imaging studies in patients with ADHD have shown a pattern of decreased activity in the PFC and striatum and increased activity in the posterior sensory/motor cortices,[2,38-40] which can be normalized by methylphenidate treatment.[2,38,41] Magnetic resonance imaging studies in patients with ADHD have shown decreased frontal lobe volume,[35] reversal of normal symmetry in the caudate nucleus,[3] and a smaller cross-sectional area of the rostral corpus callosum.[42,43] Thus, the PFC and its subcortical targets may contribute significantly to this disorder.

RESEARCH IN MONKEYS ELUCIDATES THE FUNCTIONAL CIRCUITRY OF THE PFC

Research in nonhuman primates indicates that the primary function of the PFC is to guide behavior by working memory.[44] In this context, the impulsive, disorganized, and distracted behavior of patients with ADHD can be viewed as an inability to regulate responses by internal representations. Understanding the neural circuits underlying these cognitive abilities may help to elucidate the etiology of ADHD.

Behavioral,[45] electrophysiological,[46,47] and anatomical[48-50] studies of the monkey cortex indicate the presence of parallel circuits through the PFC that subserve working memory functions for distinct modalities.[44] Most of this research has focused on the circuits subserving visuospatial working memory, as tested by the delayed-response task. Even small lesions to the PFC surrounding the principal sulcus (area 46) produce profound impairments on this task.[45,51] Electrophysiological studies have revealed neurons with topographically organized receptive fields for memories of spatial locations.[46] Anatomical studies demonstrated that area 46 shares reciprocal projections with the parietal association cortex (area 7), specialized for visuospatial processing[50]; the medial temporal lobe, important to memory abilities[52-54]; and the anterior cingulate cortex,[55] involved in organizing complex cognitive activity.[56,57] In addition, the PFC is thought to regulate motor behavior through its projections to the caudate nucleus[57,58] and premotor cortices.[59,60] Thus, it is ideally connected to regulate behavior according to memories of visuospatial information.[61,62]

Anatomical and electrophysiological findings suggest the existence of comparable circuits specialized for guiding behavior via different modalities of information.[44,47] For example, connections between the inferior temporal lobe and ventrolateral PFC mediate working memory for visual feature information.[54] Connections between the superior temporal cortex and anterior PFC may subserve a similar role in the auditory domain.[63,64] Goldman-Rakic[44] has speculated that these parallel circuits may extend to the orbital and medial PFC, which interconnect with the amygdala[65,66] and hypothalamus, and may serve the same function for affective behavior.[44] Thus, there appear to be circuits for guiding behavior by working memory in both the cognitive and emotional realms. Furthermore, studies of humans with PFC lesions suggest that these principles hold for both "overt" behaviors (motor responses) and "covert behaviors" such as perceptions, thoughts, and feelings.[44]

α_2-NORADRENERGIC MECHANISMS IMPROVE PFC FUNCTION IN MONKEYS

Reciprocal Connections Between the PFC and Locus Coeruleus (LC)

The PFC receives monoaminergic inputs from the brain stem,[67-70] and pharmacological studies suggest that PFC function is very sensitive to the neurochemical environment provided by these projections.[71] Although previous studies have often focused on the significance of DA input to the PFC,[71-74] the NE projection from the LC has an important influence on the PFC as well.[75,76] This projection appears to be reciprocal; the dorsolateral and dorsomedial PFC may supply the sole cortical afferents to the LC,[77] thus providing one of the few "intelligent" inputs to the LC. These anatomical findings suggest a special relationship between the PFC and LC, whereby PFC dysfunction may impair regulation of the LC and vice versa. Indeed, recent evidence in rodents indicates that lesions of the PFC disinhibit the LC,[78] a condition associated with poor stimulus responsivity in LC cells in monkeys.[79] Thus, enhancing PFC function may result in more appropriate regulation of the LC.

α_2-Agonists Improve PFC Function in Norepinephrine-Depleted Monkeys

Research in monkeys indicates that the NE projection to the PFC provides a vital influence on the cognitive functioning of this region. Depletion of NE and DA from the PFC results in marked spatial working memory deficits that are ameliorated by DA- or NE-agonist treatment.[71] Beneficial effects of α_2 NE agonists have been observed in young monkeys with experimentally induced NE depletion[80,81] or in aged monkeys with naturally occurring NE degeneration.[80,82,83] Performance of the delayed-response task can be improved by α_2-agonists such as clonidine, guanfacine, and UK-14304, and these improvements are blocked by α_2-antagonists but not by the α_1-

antagonist prazosin hydrochloride.[80,82,84] Furthermore, the α_2-antagonist yohimbine by itself impairs delayed-response performance in aged monkeys, while prazosin is without effect.[84] Taken together, this pharmacological profile is consistent with an α_2 mechanism but not an α_1, or imidazoline, site of drug action.[83]

Evidence for Drug Actions at the α_2A-Receptor Subtype

Three α_2 subtypes have now been cloned in humans: the α_2A, α_2B, and α_2C, the genes for which reside on chromosomes 10, 2, and 4, respectively.[85-87] This discovery suggests that the adverse effects of α_2-agonists may be dissociated from beneficial drug effects. The regional localization of messenger RNA (mRNA) for each subtype in rat brain encourages this possibility. For example, mRNA for the α_2B-receptor is found exclusively in the thalamus,[88,89] a major site for clonidine's sedative actions.[90] The nucleus tractus solitarius, thought to underlie the hypotensive actions of α_2-agonists,[91] contains both α_2A and α_2C mRNA.[88,89] Recent immunocytochemical studies of α_2A, α_2B, and α_2C receptor subtypes in the monkey brain have revealed that the α_2A subtype is densest in the PFC, including area 46, as well as in the LC.[92]

The effects of α_2-agonists in monkeys further indicate that their cognitive-enhancing, sedative, and hypotensive actions can be dissociated according to their relative affinities for each receptor subtype. Thus, the ability of an α_2-agonist to improve PFC function without adverse effects was found to correspond to its selectivity for the α_2A site: guanfacine>UK-14304 >clonidine>BHT920.[82,83] Thus, guanfacine was able to improve the delayed-response performance of aged monkeys without the sedative or hypotensive side effects accompanying clonidine administration. An α_2A mechanism is also supported by the finding that, unlike the α_2A, B, or C antagonist idazoxan, prazosin was ineffective in reversing beneficial effects. Prazosin has quite high affinity for the α_2B and α_2C subtypes (in addition to its α_1–receptor blocking properties) but has low affinity for the α_2A-receptor.[93,94]

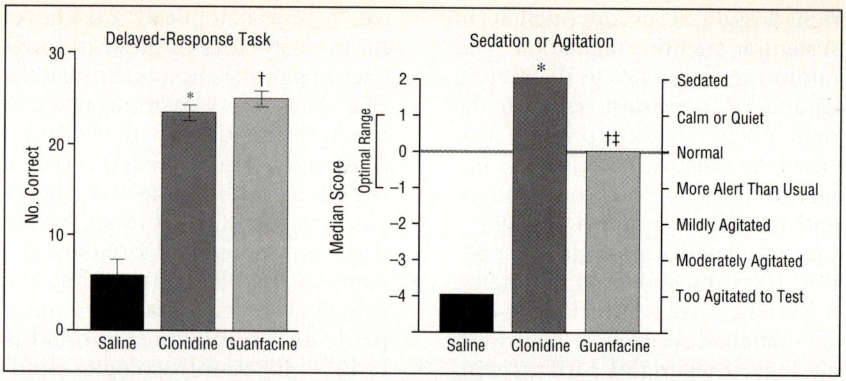

Figure 1. *Single doses of clonidine hydrochloride (0.05 mg/kg intramuscularly) and guanfacine (0.5 mg/kg intramuscularly) have calming effects in hyperactive, inattentive young monkeys during training on the delayed-response task. Left, Pretreatment with either clonidine or guanfacine significantly improved performance on the delayed-response task. Results represent mean±SEM number of trials correct out of a possible 30 trials. Asterisk indicates significantly different from saline,* $P=.03$*; dagger, significantly different from saline,* $P=.004$*. Right, Median sedation/agitation score determined during the delayed-response test session by an experimenter blind to drug treatment conditions. Following saline pretreatment, most young monkeys were too agitated to complete a test session (score of −4). Following clonidine pretreatment, animals completed the test session, but were rated as "sedated," ie, exhibiting drooping eyelids and slowed movements (score of 2). In contrast, the guanfacine-treated animals were able to complete a test session without evidence of sedation (median score of 0). Asterisk indicates significantly different from saline,* $P=.03$*; dagger, significantly different from saline,* $P=.005$*; double dagger, significantly different from clonidine,* $P=.004$.

A dissociation of cognitive vs sedative actions has recently been observed in young monkeys administered clonidine or guanfacine during delayed-response training.[95] These newly acquired animals were hyperactive and inattentive and rarely completed a test session following saline treatment. However, following single-dose administration of clonidine or guanfacine, performance of the task markedly improved (**Figure 1**, left). As with the aged animals, guanfacine improved performance without inducing the sedative effects found with clonidine (Figure 1, right). Guanfacine (0.1 to 0.7 mg/kg intramuscularly) has also been found to improve delayed-response testing accuracy in highly trained young monkeys with few adverse effects.[95]

The receptor subtype mechanisms underlying the sedative and hypotensive effects of α_2-agonists are currently being examined. Results from aged monkeys are suggestive of an α_2B or α_2C mechanism (order of potency for inducing hypotension or sedation was clonidine >BHT920>UK-14304>guanfacine).[82,83] These findings are consistent with the presence of α_2C mRNA in the nucleus tractus solitarius and α_2B mRNA in the thalamus, the brain regions thought to underlie the hypotensive and sedative effects of α_2-agonist treatment, respectively.[90,91]

Evidence for Actions at Postjunctional α_2-Receptors

Although most researchers have focused on the autoreceptor actions of α_2-agonists, such as inhibiting NE release and decreasing LC firing,[96] a very large portion of α_2-receptors are localized on non-NE cells that receive NE input.[88,92,97] Messenger RNA for α_2-receptors can be observed throughout most of the brain, indicating that diverse populations of cells are capable of making α_2-receptors.[88] Indeed, the induction of hypotension and sedation appears to involve drug actions at postjunctional receptors,[90,98] although global reduction in NE release may also contribute to sedative effects.[99]

The cognitive-enhancing properties of α_2-agonists also appear to involve actions at postjunctional receptors. Clonidine becomes more rather than less effective in young monkeys in whom the presynaptic element is destroyed or depleted with 6-OHDA (6-hydroxydopamine),[80] MPTP (1-methyl-4-phenyl-1,2,3,6-tetrahydropyridine),[100] or long-term reserpine administration.[81] Performance can also be improved by increasing endogenous NE stimulation of postsynaptic receptors with very-low-dose α_2-antagonist treatment.[101] Thus, the cognitive-enhancing actions of α_2-agonists result from actions at

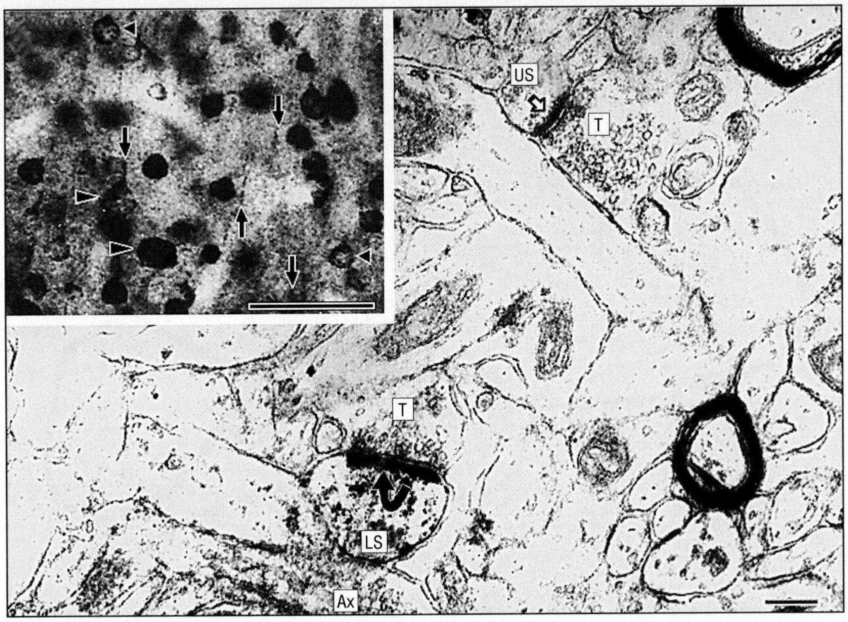

Figure 2. *An antibody directed against the human α_2A-adrenergic receptor recognizes neuronal elements in the monkey prefrontal cortex (area 46). Inset, Light micrograph shows sites immunoreactive for α_2A-adrenergic receptor in layer III of monkey prefrontal cortical tissue. Tissue was processed for immunocytochemistry using peroxidase reaction product as labels. Small puncta appear clustered over larger and smaller cell bodies (large and small arrowheads, respectively). In addition, apical dendrites appear faintly immunoreactive (arrows). Bar=50 μm. Electron micrograph shows the subcellular distribution of α_2A-adrenergic receptor in layer III. In this example, immunoreactivity is concentrated within a dendritic spine (labeled spine [LS]). Immunolabeling occurs over the perforated postsynaptic density as well as the extrasynaptic plasma membrane. The LS forms an asymmetric synaptic junction with an unlabeled terminal (T) and is contacted by another axon (Ax). US indicates unlabeled spine; bar=200 nm. Figure courtesy of Chiye Aoki, PhD, Center for Neural Science, New York University, NY.*

postjunctional receptors with an α_2A pharmacological profile.

Electron microscopic analysis of the monkey PFC has localized α_2A-immunoreactivity at postjunctional sites. α_2A-immunoreactivity was observed on nonadrenergic as well as noradrenergic neuronal terminals and dendrites and on glia[92] (**Figure 2**, inset). Closer examination revealed postjunctional α_2A-immunoreactivity over the postsynaptic membrane in traditional synaptic junctions (Figure 2), as well as over nonsynaptic membranes. These receptors may be the site of action for the beneficial effects of α_2-agonists on spatial working memory.

Evidence for PFC Mechanisms

Several lines of evidence support drug actions directly in the PFC. In young monkeys with 6-OHDA lesions restricted to the PFC, clonidine's potency directly relates to the degree of NE depletion in this region, a result consistent with drug actions at supersensitive, postjunctional receptors in the PFC.[80] Furthermore, α_2-agonists lose their efficacy when the PFC itself is ablated,[80] suggesting that this cortical machinery is necessary for α_2-agonists to have their beneficial effects. Intracortical infusion studies also support a PFC mechanism. Direct infusion of clonidine or guanfacine into the PFC, but not the nearby premotor cortex, improves delayed response performance in aged monkeys (A.F.T.A., unpublished data, 1988). Conversely, infusion of the α_2-antagonist yohimbine directly into the PFC impairs delayed-response performance under delay, but not no-delay (0 seconds) control conditions.[102] Preliminary evidence indicates that yohimbine infusions into the PFC impair oculomotor delayed response performance as well (T. Sawaguchi, oral communication, November 1995). Comparable infusions of the α_1-antagonist prazosin or the β-antagonist propranolol hydrochloride do not impair performance.[102] Furthermore, yohimbine infusions into the PFC significantly increase errors of commission[102] and impair Go/No-Go performance,[103] suggesting that endogenous α_2 stimulation is important for regulating the inhibitory abilities of the PFC. Finally, electrophysiological evidence indicates that yohimbine interferes with PFC neuronal firing, while clonidine enhances delay-related activity in PFC cells,[104] suggesting a cellular mechanism whereby these agents can affect PFC function.

The cognitive abilities of the PFC are particularly sensitive to α_2-receptor manipulation, while the functions subserved by posterior cortical regions appear less responsive to treatment. For example, clonidine or guanfacine have little effect on reference memory[80] or recognition memory,[105] tasks that depend on the inferior or medial temporal cortex, respectively. Similar negative effects have been seen when guanfacine is administered to rats performing a reference memory task.[106] In contrast, the α_2-agonists clonidine, guanfacine, or medetomidine hydrochloride administered to rats or monkeys have been shown to improve a variety of working memory tasks that use PFC abilities, such as delayed response,[82] delayed alternation,[80,107] and delayed match-to-sample with repeated stimuli.[108] α_2-Agonists are most effective under conditions of high interference or distraction when the PFC is challenged.[84,108,109] Indeed, even very low doses of guanfacine can protect the performance of aged monkeys from the deleterious effects of irrelevant stimulation (**Figure 3**).[84] These findings are consistent with NE depletion increasing distractibility,[10,11] emphasizing the importance of NE mechanisms in attention regulation. In summary, animal research has shown that α_2-agonists are especially effective in enhancing working memory performance under distracting conditions, and they have these effects through actions at postjunctional, α_2A-receptors in the PFC.

A HYPOTHETICAL MODEL OF α_2-AGONIST ACTION ON PFC CIRCUITS

Findings from various fields have suggested a speculative model whereby α_2-agonists may diminish distractibility[84] (**Figure 4**). Pyramidal cells of the dorsolateral PFC

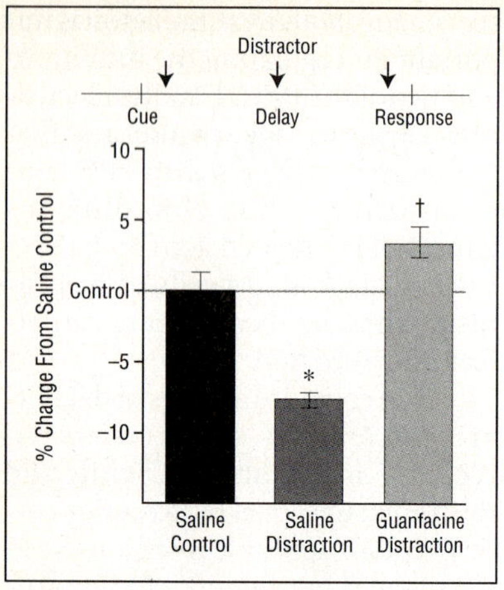

Figure 3. *Single doses of guanfacine (0.000011 to 0.0011 mg/kg intramuscularly) decreased distractibility in aged monkeys performing a delayed-response task. Results represent mean±SEM percent change from saline control performance. The distraction paradigm is schematically represented in the top graph; a distractor was presented during the beginning, middle, or end of the delay period on 9 of 30 trials in an unpredictable manner. When distractors were presented to saline-treated animals, performance decreased relative to control (nondistracting) conditions. If monkeys received guanfacine pretreatment, performance was no longer impaired under distracting conditions. Asterisk indicates significantly different from saline control,* P=.003; *dagger, significantly different from saline distraction condition,* P=.02. *(Figure adapted from Arnsten and Contant.[84])*

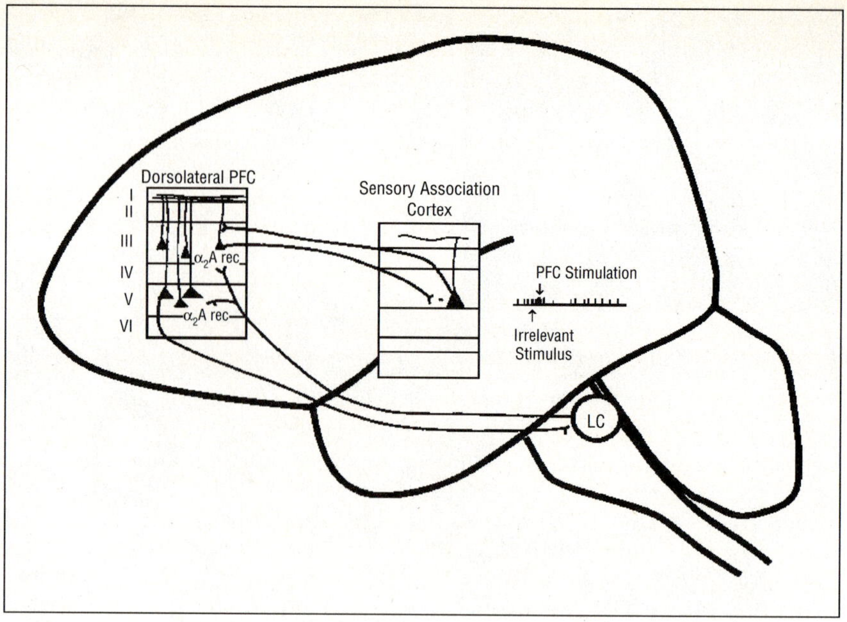

Figure 4. *A hypothetical model describing a possible mechanism whereby α_2A-adrenergic agonists such as guanfacine could improve dorsolateral prefrontal cortex (PFC) function and decrease distractibility. The model is based on findings from neuroanatomical, electrophysiological, and functional studies of the monkey prefrontal cortex, as described in the text. LC indicates locus coeruleus; rec, receptor.*

project back to sensory association cortices,[55,110] (Anne Morel, oral communication) and electrophysiological evidence indicates that these projections may inhibit the processing of irrelevant stimuli in the sensory cortices. For example, stimulation of the PFC in monkeys inhibits the response of auditory cortex neurons to tones that have no relevance to the animal.[111] (These data from nonhuman primates are schematically represented in Figure 4.) Electrophysiological studies of patients with PFC lesions suggest a similar mechanism in humans. Evoked potentials generated by the auditory cortices to irrelevant tones are disinhibited in patients with PFC lesions,[112] and comparable findings have been seen in other modalities.[23] These PFC circuits may provide the architecture to sculpt and protect the contents of working memory, thus lessening distractibility and improving concentration.

Inhibitory projections may be a general feature of frontal lobe circuitry, including the anterior cingulate cortex. For example, in addition to its connections with the PFC,[55] the anterior cingulate projects back to sensory association cortices, and stimulation of this region inhibits auditory cortical responses to acoustic stimulation.[113] Experiments using single-photon emission computed tomography, positron emission tomography, and functional magnetic resonance imaging have observed enhanced activity in the anterior cingulate during the Stroop interference paradigm[56,114,115] or during selective attention tasks.[116,117] Many of these studies have also shown PFC activation during these tasks, and, interestingly, they have concurrently observed decreased activity in posterior cortical areas. Indeed, increased activity in the frontal pole and anterior cingulate cortex was found to significantly correlate with decreased activity in the posterior sensory cortices.[114] Thus, the imaging data support the hypothesis that the anterior cortices regulate attention through inhibitory actions on the posterior cortices.

Norepinephrine may enhance these inhibitory circuits through its actions at α_2A-receptors on pyramidal cells (Figure 4). Electrophysiological studies in monkeys performing the delayed response task have shown that iontophoretic application of NE onto area 46 pyramidal cells enhances cue and delay-related firing relative to spontaneous firing.[72] More recently, either systemic or iontophoretic application of clonidine has been shown to enhance cue- and delay-related firing in PFC neurons, while yohimbine had the opposite effect.[104] If these PFC neurons project to sensory association cortices, α_2 stimulation would aid the inhibition of irrelevant sensory stimulation, thus providing a protective framework during the cueing and delay periods. Conversely, DA may improve PFC function through an inverse mechanism: intensifying the appropriate signal by exciting delay-related firing in cells with specific mnemonic fields.[72] These complementary catecholamine mechanisms would provide essential components for proper PFC function[71,80] and may underlie the beneficial effects of psychostimulant (eg, methylphenidate) medication as well.

Parallel mechanisms may extend to the ventromedial and orbital PFC, which have an even richer catecholamine innervation.[68-70] Lesions of the ventromedial PFC in rodents retard extinction of fear conditioning mediated by the amygdala,[118] suggesting that the ventromedial and/or orbital PFC can inhibit inappropriate emotional responses through its projections to subcortical limbic nuclei. Stimulation of these circuits may contribute to the behavioral calming induced by α_2-agonist treatment. This hypothesis is supported by preliminary evidence that guanfacine can improve object reversal performance in monkeys,[119] a task that is highly sensitive to orbital PFC lesions.

Finally, the model depicted in Figure 4 suggests that α_2 stimulation may benefit cognitive function by actions on reciprocal circuits between the PFC and LC. Preliminary evidence indicates that clonidine can decrease spontaneous LC firing and restore stimulus-evoked LC activity in a hyperactive monkey with a very high rate of baseline LC firing.[120] α_2-Agonists could enhance LC responding to relevant stimuli in two ways: direct effects on LC neurons, decreasing spontaneous firing relative to stimulus-evoked activity, and indirect beneficial effects on PFC function, thus improving PFC regulation of the LC. Both would result in more appropriate NE release throughout the forebrain.

THE EFFECTS OF α_2-AGONISTS IN PATIENTS WITH COGNITIVE DISORDERS

Studies of α_2-agonist effects on cognitive function in clinical populations indicate that these agents improve PFC cognitive functions in humans as well as in animals. Much of this research has been done with clonidine, as it is widely available and safe for human treatment. Clonidine has been shown to improve PFC cognitive tasks such as the Trails B, Word Fluency, and Stroop tasks in patients with schizophrenia[121] or Korsakoff's syndrome.[122,123] Single-photon emission computed tomography imaging studies of patients with Korsakoff's syndrome further support a PFC mechanism, as clonidine's beneficial effects on Word Fluency test performance correlated with increased regional cerebral blood flow in the left PFC, the cortical region most affiliated with performance of this task.[123] Clonidine also increased regional cerebral blood flow in the anterior cingulate cortex in these patients. Clonidine's beneficial effects in patients with Korsakoff's syndrome appear to result from actions at postjunctional receptors, as the drug has been most efficacious in those patients with the greatest NE loss.[124] Similar, but smaller, improvements have been observed in normal young adult volunteers given clonidine prior to performing a spatial working memory task.[125] Thus, α_2-agonists can mimic NE at postjunctional α_2-receptors and improve PFC function in both monkeys and humans.

These results in animals and humans suggest that α_2-agonists may be a useful treatment for PFC cognitive deficits. Clonidine has been explored in the treatment of ADHD, although its hypotensive and sedative adverse effects have seriously limited its clinical usefulness.[126,127] Research in animals suggests that more selective α_2A-agonists may provide a superior adverse effect profile. Based on guanfacine's beneficial effects in young and aged monkeys, open trials were initiated in patients with ADHD symptoms with encouraging results.[128,129] These positive findings have recently been replicated in an open trial,[130] but double-blind, placebo-controlled studies are clearly needed to establish efficacy.

In summary, animal research indicates that α_2A-adrenergic stimulation exerts an important, beneficial influence on PFC function. Thus, α_2A-agonists may provide one of the few pharmacological tools for improving working memory, behavioral inhibition, and attention regulation in patients with PFC dysfunction.

Accepted for publication December 10, 1995.

This work was supported by National Institute of Aging PHS grant AG06036 (Dr Arnsten).

We thank Chiye Aoki, PhD, and Patricia Goldman-Rakic, PhD, for their many helpful comments and Lisa Ciavarella and Tracy White for their technical support.

Reprints: Amy F. T. Arnsten, PhD, Section of Neurobiology, Yale Medical School, 333 Cedar St, New Haven, CT 06510-8001 (e-mail: Amy_Arnsten@qm.yale.edu).

REFERENCES

1. Roeltgen DP, Schneider JS. Task persistence and learning ability in normal and chronic low dose MPTP-treated monkeys. *Behav Brain Res.* 1994;60:115-124.
2. Lou HC, Henriksen L, Bruhn P, Borner H, Bieber Nielson J. Striatal dysfunction in attention deficit and hyperkinetic disorder. *Arch Neurol.* 1989; 46:48-52.
3. Hynd GW, Hern KL, Novey ES, Eliopulos D, Marshall R, Gonzalez JJ, Voeller KK. Attention deficit-hyperactivity disorder and asymmetry of the caudate nucleus. *J Child Neurol.* 1993;8:339-347.
4. Shaywitz BA, Klopper JH, Gordon JW. Methylphenidate in 6-hydroxydopamine-treated developing rat pups. *Arch Neurol.* 1978;35:463-469.
5. Shaywitz BA, Cohen DJ, Bowers MB. CSF monoamine metabolites in children with minimal brain dysfunction: evidence for alteration of brain dopamine. *J Pediatr.* 1977;90:67-71.
6. Shaywitz BA, Teicher MH, Cohen DJ, Anderson GM, Young JG, Levitt P. Dopaminergic but not noradrenergic modulation of hyperactivity and performance deficits in the developing rat pup. *Psychopharmacology.* 1984;82:73-77.
7. Raskin LA, Shaywitz BA, Anderson GM, Cohen DJ, Teicher MH, Liakis J. Differential effects of selective dopamine, norepinephrine or catecholamine depletion on activity and learning in the developing rat. *Pharmacol Biochem Behav.* 1983; 19:743-749.
8. Cook EH, Stein MA, Krasowski MD, Cox NJ, Olkon DM, Kieffer JE, Leventhal BL. Association of attention-deficit disorder and the dopamine transporter gene. *Am J Hum Genet.* 1995; 56:993-998.
9. Shekim WO, Dekirmenjian H, Chapel JL. Urinary MHPG excretion in minimal brain dysfunction and its modification by d-amphetamine. *Am J Psychiatry.* 1979;136:667-671.
10. Carli M, Robbins TW, Evenden JL, Everitt BJ. Effect of lesions to ascending noradrenergic neurons on performance of a 5-choice serial reaction task in rats: implications for theories of dorsal noradrenergic bundle function based on selective attention and arousal. *Behav Brain Res.* 1983;9:361-380.
11. Roberts DCS, Price MTC, Fibiger HC. The dorsal tegmental noradrenergic projection: an analysis of its role in maze learning. *J Comp Physiol Psychol.* 1976;90:363-372.
12. Pearlson GD, Robinson RG. Suction lesions of the frontal cerebral cortex in the rat induce asymmetrical behavioral and catecholaminergic responses. *Brain Res.* 1981;218:233-242.
13. Mattes JA. The role of frontal lobe dysfunction in childhood hyperkinesis. *Compr Psychiatry.* 1980;21:358-369.
14. Chelune GJ, Ferguson W, Koon R, Dickey TO. Frontal lobe disinhibition in attention deficit disorder. *Child Psychiatry Hum Dev.* 1986;16:221-234.
15. Gorenstein EE, Mammato CA. Performance of inattentive-overactive children on selected measures of prefrontal-type function. *J Clin Psychol.* 1989;45:619-632.
16. Loge DV, Staton RD, Beatty WW. Performance of children with ADHD on tests sensitive to frontal lobe dysfunction. *J Am Acad Child Adolesc Psychiatry.* 1989;29:540-545.
17. Benson DF. The role of frontal dysfunction in attention deficit hyperactivity disorder. *J Child Neurol.* 1991;6:S9-S12.
18. Barkley RA, Grodzinsky G, DuPaul GJ. Frontal lobe functions in attention deficit disorder with and without hyperactivity: a review and research report. *J Abnorm Child Psychol.* 1992;

20:163-188.
19. Shue KL, Douglas VI. Attention deficit hyperactivity disorder and the frontal lobe syndrome. *Brain Cogn.* 1992;20:104-124.
20. Drewe EA. Go/no-go learning after frontal lobe lesions in humans. *Cortex.* 1975;11:8-16.
21. Knight RT, Hillyard SA, Woods DL, Neville HJ. The effects of frontal cortex lesions on event-related potentials during auditory selective attention. *Electroencephalogr Clin Neurophysiol.* 1981;52:571-582.
22. Wilkins AJ, Shallice T, McCarthy R. Frontal lesions and sustained attention. *Neuropsychologia.* 1987;25:359-365.
23. Yamaguchi S, Knight RT. Gating of somatosensory input by human prefrontal cortex. *Brain Res.* 1990;521:281-288.
24. Brazelli M, Columbo N, Della Sala S, Spinnler H. Spared and impaired cognitive abilities after bilateral frontal damage. *Cortex.* 1994;30:27-51.
25. Della Sala S, Marchetti C, Spinnler H. The anarchic hand: a frontal-mesial hyperkinetic sign. In: Boller F, Grafman J, eds. *Handbook of Neuropsychology.* Amsterdam, Holland: Elsevier Science; 1994:233-255.
26. Butter CM, Snyder DR, McDonald JA. Effects of orbital frontal lesions on aversive and aggressive behaviors in rhesus monkeys. *J Comp Physiol Psychol.* 1970;72:132-144.
27. Bartus RT, Levere TE. Frontal decortication in rhesus monkeys: a test of the interference hypothesis. *Brain Res.* 1977;119:233-248.
28. Malmo RB. Interference factors in delayed response in monkeys after removal of frontal lobes. *J Neurophysiol.* 1942;5:295-308.
29. Mesulam M-M. A cortical network for directed attention and unilateral neglect. *Ann Neurol.* 1981;10:309-325.
30. Woods DL, Knight RT. Electrophysiological evidence of increased distractibility after dorsolateral prefrontal lesions. *Neurology.* 1986;36:212-216.
31. Chao LL, Knight RT. Human prefrontal lesions increase distractibility to irrelevant sensory inputs. *Neuroreport.* 1995;6:1605-1610.
32. Blumer D, Benson DF. Personality changes with frontal and temporal lobe lesions. In: Benson DF, Blumer D, eds. *Psychiatric Aspects of Neurologic Disease.* New York, NY: Grune & Stratton; 1975.
33. Stuss DT, Gow CA, Hetherington CR. 'No longer Gage': frontal lobe dysfunction and emotional changes. *J Consult Clin Psychol.* 1992;60:349-359.
34. Starkstein SE, Fedoroff P, Berthier ML, Robinson RG. Manic-depressive and pure manic states after brain lesions. *Biol Psychiatry.* 1991;29:149-158.
35. Hynd GW, Semrud-Clikeman M, Lorys AR, Novey ES, Eliopulos D. Brain morphology in developmental dyslexia and attention deficit disorder/hyperactivity. *Arch Neurol.* 1990;47:919-926.
36. Swanson JM, Posner M, Potkin S, Bonforte S, Youpa D, Fiore C, Cantwell D, Crinella F. Activating tasks for the study of visual-spatial attention in ADHD children: a cognitive anatomic approach. *J Child Neurol.* 1991;6:S119-S127.
37. Satterfield JH, Schell AM, Nicholas T, Backs RW. Topographic study of auditory event-related potentials in normal boys and boys with attention deficit disorder with hyperactivity. *Psychophysiology.* 1988;25:591-606.
38. Lou HC, Henriksen L, Bruhn P. Focal cerebral hypoperfusion in children with dysphasia and/or attention deficit disorder. *Arch Neurol.* 1984;41:825-829.
39. Lou HC, Henriksen L, Bruhn P. Focal cerebral dysfunction in developmental learning disabilities. *Lancet.* 1990;335:8-11.
40. Zametkin AJ, Liebenauer LL, Fitzgerald GA, King AC, Minkunas DV, Herscovitch P, Yamada EM, Cohen RM. Brain metabolism in teenagers with attention-deficit hyperactivity disorder. *Arch Gen Psychiatry.* 1993;50:333-340.
41. Matochik JA, Liebenauer LL, King CA, Szymanski HV, Cohen RM, Zametkin AJ. Cerebral glucose metabolism in adults with attention deficit hyperactivity disorder after chronic stimulant treatment. *Am J Psychiatry.* 1994;151:658-664.
42. Hynd GW, Semrud-Clikeman M, Lorys AR, Novey ES, Eliopulos D, Lyytinen H. Corpus callosum morphology in attention deficit-hyperactivity disorder: morphometric analysis of MRI. *J Learning Disabil.* 1991;24:141-146.
43. Giedd JN, Castellanos FX, Casey BJ, Kozuch P, King AC, Hamburger SD, Rapoport JL. Quantitative morphology of the corpus callosum in attention deficit hyperactivity disorder. *Am J Psychiatry.* 1994;151:665-669.
44. Goldman-Rakic PS. Circuitry of the primate prefrontal cortex and the regulation of behavior by representational memory. In: Plum F, ed. *Handbook of Physiology, The Nervous System, Higher Functions of the Brain.* Bethesda, Md: American Physiological Society; 1987;5:373-417.
45. Goldman PS, Rosvold HE. Localization of function within the dorsolateral prefrontal cortex of the rhesus monkey. *Exp Neurol.* 1970;27:291-304.
46. Funahashi S, Bruce CJ, Goldman-Rakic PS. Visuospatial coding in primate prefrontal neurons revealed by oculomotor paradigms. *J Neurophysiol.* 1990;63:814-831.
47. Wilson FAW, Ò Scalaidhe SP, Goldman-Rakic PS. Dissociation of object and spatial processing domains in primate prefrontal cortex. *Science.* 1993;260:1955-1958.
48. Selemon LD, Goldman-Rakic PS. Common cortical and subcortical target areas of the dorsolateral prefrontal and posterior parietal cortices in the rhesus monkey: evidence for a distributed network subserving spatially guided behavior. *J Neurosci.* 1988;8:4049-4068.
49. Cavada C, Goldman-Rakic PS. Posterior parietal cortex in rhesus monkey, I: parcelation of areas based on distinctive limbic and sensory corticocortical connections. *J Comp Neurol.* 1989;287:393-421.
50. Cavada C, Goldman-Rakic PS. Posterior parietal cortex in rhesus monkey, II: evidence for segregated corticocortical networks linking sensory and limbic areas with the frontal lobe. *J Comp Neurol.* 1989;287:422-445.
51. Funahashi S, Bruce CJ, Goldman-Rakic PS. Mnemonic coding of visual space in the monkey's dorsolateral prefrontal cortex. *J Neurophysiol.* 1989;61:331-349.
52. Goldman-Rakic PS, Selemon LD, Schwartz ML. Dual pathways connecting the dorsolateral prefrontal cortex with the hippocampal formation and parahippocampal cortex in the rhesus monkey. *Neuroscience.* 1984;12:719-743.
53. Martin-Elkins CL, Horel JA. Cortical afferents to behaviorally defined regions of the inferior temporal and parahippocampal gyri as demonstrated by WGA-HRP. *J Comp Neurol.* 1992;321:177-192.
54. Bates JF, Wilson FAW, Ò Scalaidhe SPO, Goldman-Rakic PS. Area TE connections with inferior prefrontal regions responsive to complex objects and faces. *Soc Neurosci Abstracts.* 1994;20:1054.
55. Schwartz ML, Goldman-Rakic PS. Single cortical neurones have axon collaterals to ipsilateral and contralateral cortex in fetal and adult primates. *Nature.* 1982;299:154-156.
56. Pardo JV, Pardo PJ, Janer KW, Raichle ME. The anterior cingulate cortex mediates processing selection in the Stroop attentional conflict paradigm. *Proc Natl Acad Sci U S A.* 1990;87:256-259.
57. Goldman PS, Nauta WJH. An intricately patterned prefronto-caudate projection in the rhesus monkey. *J Comp Neurol.* 1977;171:369-386.
58. Selemon LD, Goldman-Rakic PS. Longitudinal topography and interdigitation of corticostriatal projections in the rhesus monkey. *J Neurosci.* 1985;5:776-794.
59. McGuire PK, Bates JF, Goldman-Rakic PS. Interhemispheric integration, I: symmetry and convergence of the corticocortical connections of the left and right principal sulcus and the left and right supplementary motor area in the rhesus monkey. *Cereb Cortex.* 1991;1:390-407.
60. Bates JF, Goldman-Rakic PS. Prefrontal connections of medial motor areas in the rhesus monkey. *J Comp Neurol.* 1993;335:1-18.
61. Goldman-Rakic PS. Motor control function of the prefrontal cortex. In: Porter R, ed. *Motor Areas of the Cerebral Cortex.* Ciba Foundation Symposium No. 132. Chichester, England: Wiley & Sons; 1987:187-200.
62. Goldman-Rakic PS, Bates JF, Chafee MV. The prefrontal cortex and internally generated motor acts. *Curr Opin Neurobiol.* 1992;2:830-835.
63. Jones EG, Powell TPS. An anatomical study of converging sensory pathways within the cerebral cortex of the monkey. *Brain.* 1970;93:793-820.
64. Petrides M, Pandya DN. Association fiber pathways to the frontal cortex from the superior temporal region in the rhesus monkey. *J Comp Neurol.* 1988;273:52-66.
65. Aggleton JP, Burton MJ, Passingham RE. Cortical and subcortical afferents to the amygdala of the rhesus monkey (macaca mulatta). *Brain Res.* 1980;190:347-368.
66. Amaral DG, Price JL, Pitkznen A, Carmichael ST. Anatomical organization of the primate amygdaloid complex. In: Aggleton JP, ed. *The Amygdala: Neurobiological Aspects of Emotion, Memory and Mental Dysfunction.* New York, NY: Wiley-Liss Inc; 1992:1-66.
67. Porrino LJ, Goldman-Rakic PS. Brainstem innervation of prefrontal and anterior cingulate cortex in the rhesus monkey revealed by retrograde transport of HRP. *J Comp Neurol.* 1982;205:63-76.
68. Levitt P, Rakic P, Goldman-Rakic P. Region-specific distribution of catecholamine afferents in primate cerebral cortex: a fluorescence histochemical analysis. *J Comp Neurol.* 1984;227:23-36.
69. Lewis DA, Campbell MJ, Foote SL, Goldstein M, Morrison JH. The distribution of tyrosine hydroxylase-immunoreactive fibers in primate neocortex is widespread but regionally specific. *J Neurosci.* 1987;7:279-290.
70. Lewis DA, Morrison JH. The noradrenergic innervation of monkey prefrontal cortex: a dopamine beta hydroxylase immunohistochemical study. *J Comp Neurol.* 1989;282:317-330.
71. Brozoski TJ, Brown RM, Rosvold HE, Goldman PS. Cognitive deficit caused by regional depletion of dopamine in prefrontal cortex of rhesus monkey. *Science.* 1979;215:929-932.
72. Sawaguchi T, Matsumura M, Kubota K. Catecholaminergic effects on neuronal activity related to a delayed response task in monkey prefrontal cortex. *J Neurophysiol.* 1990;63:1385-1400.
73. Arnsten AFT, Cai JX, Murphy BL, Goldman-Rakic PS. Dopamine D1 receptor mechanisms in the cognitive performance of young adult and aged monkeys. *Psychopharmacology.* 1994;116:143-151.
74. Arnsten AFT, Cai JX, Steere JC, Goldman-Rakic PS. Dopamine D-2 receptor mechanisms contribute to age-related cognitive decline: the effects of quinpirole on memory and motor performance in monkeys. *J Neurosci.* 1995;15:3429-3439.
75. Berridge CW, Arnsten AFT, Foote SL. Noradrenergic modulation of cognitive function: clinical implications of anatomical, electrophysiological and behavioural studies in animal models. *Psychol Med.* 1993;23:557-564.
76. Coull JT. Pharmacological manipulations of the α-2 noradrenergic system: effects on cognition. *Drugs Aging.* 1994;5:116-126.

77. Arnsten AFT, Goldman-Rakic PGR. Selective prefrontal cortical projections to the region of the locus coeruleus and raphe nuclei in the rhesus monkey. *Brain Res.* 1984;306:9-18.
78. Sara SJ, Herve-Minvielle A. Inhibitory influence of frontal cortex on locus coeruleus. *Proc Natl Acad Sci U S A.* 1995;92:6032-6036.
79. Kubiak P, Ivanova S, Rajkowski J, Aston-Jones G. Contrasting responses of monkey locus coeruleus neurons to conditioned vs unconditioned stimuli: relationship to arousal, performance and vigilance. *Soc Neurosci Abstracts.* 1995;21:2092.
80. Arnsten AFT, Goldman-Rakic PS. α-2 Adrenergic mechanisms in prefrontal cortex associated with cognitive decline in aged nonhuman primates. *Science.* 1985;230:1273-1276.
81. Cai JX, Ma Y, Xu L, Hu X. Reserpine impairs spatial working memory performance in monkeys: reversal by the α-2-adrenergic agonist clonidine. *Brain Res.* 1993;614:191-196.
82. Arnsten AFT, Cai JX, Goldman-Rakic PS. The α-2 adrenergic agonist guanfacine improves memory in aged monkeys without sedative or hypotensive side effects: evidence for α-2 receptor subtypes. *J Neurosci.* 1988;8:4287-4298.
83. Arnsten AFT, Leslie FM. Behavioral and receptor binding analysis of the α-2 adrenergic agonist, UK-14304 (5 bromo-6 [2-imidazoline-2-yl amino] quinoxaline): evidence for cognitive enhancement at an α-2 adrenoceptor subtype. *Neuropharmacology.* 1991;30:1279-1289.
84. Arnsten AFT, Contant TA. α-2 adrenergic agonists decrease distractibility in aged monkeys performing the delayed response task. *Psychopharmacol.* 1992;108:159-169.
85. Kobilka BK, Matsui H, Kobilka TS, Yang-Feng TL, Francke U, Caron MG, Lefkowitz RJ, Regan JW. Cloning, sequencing, and expression of the gene encoding for the human platelet α-2-adrenergic receptor. *Science.* 1987:238:650-656.
86. Regan JW, Kobilka TS, Yang-Feng TL, Caron MG, Lefkowitz RJ, Kobilka BK. Cloning and expression of a human kidney cDNA for an α-2 adrenergic receptor subtype. *Proc Natl Acad Sci U S A.* 1988;85:6301-6305.
87. Lomasney JW, Lorenz W, Allen LF, King K, Regan JW, Yang-Feng TL, Caron M, Lefkowitz RJ. Expansion of the α-2 adrenergic family: cloning and characterization of a human α-2-adrenergic receptor subtype, the gene for which is located on chromosome 2. *Proc Natl Acad Sci U S A.* 1990;87:5094-5098.
88. Scheinin M, Lomasney JW, Hayden-Hixson DM, Schambra UB, Caron MG, Lefkowitz RJ, Fremeau RT. Distribution of α-2-adrenergic receptor subtype gene expression in rat brain. *Mol Brain Res.* 1994;21:133-149.
89. Nicholas AP, Pieribone V, Hökfelt T. Distributions of mRNAs for α-2-adrenergic receptor subtypes in rat brain: an in situ hybridization study. *J Comp Neurol.* 1993;328:575-594.
90. Buzsaki G, Kennedy B, Solt VB, Ziegler M. Noradrenergic control of thalamic oscillation: the role of alpha-2 receptors. *Eur J Pharmacol.* 1991; 3:222-229.
91. Reis DJ, Granata AR, Joh TH, Ross CA, Ruggiero DA, Park DH. Brain stem catecholamine mechanisms in tonic and reflex control of blood pressure. *Hypertension.* 1984;6(SII):7-15.
92. Aoki C, Go C-G, Venkatesan C, Kurose H. Perikaryal and synaptic localization of α-2A-adrenergic receptor-like immunoreactivity. *Brain Res.* 1994;650:181-204.
93. Uhlen S, Wikberg JES. Delineation of rat kidney α-2A and α-2B-adrenoceptors with [3H]RX821002 radioligand binding: computer modeling reveals that guanfacine is an α-2A-selective compound. *Eur J Pharmacol.* 1991; 202:235-243.
94. Marjamäki A, Luomala K, Ala-Uotila S, Scheinin M. Use of recombinant human α-2-adrenoceptors to characterize subtype selectivity of antagonist binding. *Eur J Pharmacol.* 1993;246:219-226.
95. Steere JC, Arnsten A. The alpha-2 noradrenergic agonist, guanfacine, improves delayed response performance and calms behavior in young monkeys: relevance to attention deficit disorder. *Soc Neurosci Abstracts.* 1994;20: 831.
96. Svensson TH, Bunney BS, Aghajanian GK. Inhibition of both noradrenergic and serotonergic neurons in brain by the alpha-adrenergic agonist clonidine. *Brain Res.* 1975;92:291-306.
97. U'Prichard DC, Bechtel WD, Rouot BM, Snyder SH. Multiple apparent α-noradrenergic receptor binding sites in rat brain: effect of 6-hydroxydopamine. *Mol Pharmacol.* 1979;16:47-60.
98. Van Zwieten PA, Timmermans PBMWM, Van Brummelen P. Role of alpha-adrenoceptors in hypertension and in antihypertensive drug treatment. *Am J Med.* 1984:17-25.
99. Berridge CW, Foote SL. Effects of locus coeruleus activation on electroencephalographic activity in neocortex and hippocampus. *J Neurosci.* 1991;11:3135-3145.
100. Schneider JS, Kovelowski CJ. Chronic exposure to low doses of MPTP, I: cognitive deficits in motor asymptomatic monkeys. *Brain Res.* 1990;519:122-128.
101. Arnsten AFT, Cai JX. Postsynaptic alpha-2 receptor stimulation improves memory in aged monkeys: indirect effects of yohimbine versus direct effects of clonidine. *Neurobiol Aging.* 1993; 14:597-603.
102. Li B-M, Mei Z-T. Delayed response deficit induced by local injection of the α-2 adrenergic antagonist yohimbine into the dorsolateral prefrontal cortex in young adult monkeys. *Behav Neural Biol.* 1994;62:134-139.
103. Li B-M, Hu X-T, Mei ZT. Prefrontal injection of the alpha-2-adrenergic antagonist yohimbine impairs performance of a delayed go/no-go task in monkeys. *Acta Physiol Sinica.* 1994;46:249-257.
104. Li B-M, Mei Z-T. Alpha-2 adrenergic modulation of prefrontal neuronal activity related to working memory in monkeys. Presented at the 3rd Congress of the Federal Asian and Oceanian Physiological Societies; 1995. Abstract S9-3(0).
105. Arnsten AFT, Goldman-Rakic PS. Analysis of α-2 adrenergic agonist effects on the delayed nonmatch-to-sample performance of aged rhesus monkeys. *Neurobiol Aging.* 1990;11:58 3-590.
106. Sirviö J, Riekkinen P, Vajanto I, Koivisto E, Riekkinen PJ. The effects of guanfacine, α-2 agonist, on the performance of young and aged rats in spatial navigation task. *Behav Neural Biol.* 1991;56:101-107.
107. Carlson S, Tanila H, Rama P, Mecke E, Pertovaara A. Effects of medetomidine, an α-2 adrenoceptor agonist, and atipamezole, and α-2 antagonist, on spatial memory performance in adult and aged rats. *Behav Neural Biol.* 1992; 58:113-119.
108. Jackson WJ, Buccafusco JJ. Clonidine enhances delayed matching-to-sample performance by young and aged monkeys. *Pharmacol Biochem Behav.* 1991;39:79-84.
109. Rama P, Hietanen JK. Alpha-2 adrenergic function and visual selective attention in monkeys. *Soc Neurosci Abstracts.* 1995;21:2092.
110. Morel A, Bullier J. Cortical connections of intraparietal and inferotemporal visual areas in the macaque monkey: a double-labeling study. *Abstracts Soc Neurosci.* 1989;15:111.
111. Alexander GE, Newman JD, Symmes D. Convergence of prefrontal and acoustic inputs upon neurons in the superior temporal gyrus of the awake squirrel monkey. *Brain Res.* 1976;116: 334-338.
112. Knight RT, Scabini D, Woods DL. Prefrontal cortex gating of auditory transmission in humans. *Brain Res.* 1989;504:338-342.
113. Müller-Preuss P, Newman JD, Jürgens U. Anatomical and physiological evidence for a relationship between the 'cingular' vocalization area and the auditory cortex in the squirrel monkey. *Brain Res.* 1980;202:307-315.
114. Bench CJ, Frith CD, Grasby PM, Friston KJ, Paulesu E, Frackowiak RSJ, Dolan RJ. Investigations of the functional anatomy of attention using the Stroop test. *Neuropsychologia.* 1993;31:907-922.
115. Casey BJ, Cohen JD, Noll DC, Forman S, Rapoport JL. Activation of the anterior cingulate during the Stroop conflict paradigm using functional MRI. *Soc Neurosci Abstracts.* 1993; 19:1285.
116. Roland PE. Metabolic measurements of the working frontal cortex in man. *Trends Neurosci.* 1984; 7:430-435.
117. Mangun GR, Heinze HJ, Burchert W, Hinrichs H, Scholz M, Münte TF, Gos A, Hundeshagen H, Gozzaniga MS, Hillyard SA. Combined PET and ERP studies of visual spatial selective attention in humans. *Soc Neurosci Abstracts.* 1993; 19:1285.
118. Morgan MA, Romanski LM, LeDoux JE. Extinction of emotional learning: contribution of medial prefrontal cortex. *Neurosci Lett.* 1993;163: 109-113.
119. Steere JC, Arnsten AFT. The alpha-2 noradrenergic agonist, guanfacine, improves visual object discrimination reversal in rhesus monkeys. *Soc Neurosci Abstracts.* 1995;21:195.
120. Rajkowski J, Ivanova S, Kubiak P, Aston-Jones G. Improved vigilance performance in monkey associated with altered locus coeruleus activity after clonidine. *Soc Neurosci Abstracts.* 1995;21:2092.
121. Fields RB, Van Kammen DP, Peters JL, Rosen J, Van Kammen WB, Nugent A, Stipetic S, Linnoila M. Clonidine improves memory function in schizophrenia independently from change in psychosis. *Schizophr Res.* 1988;1:417-423.
122. Mair RG, McEntee WJ. Cognitive enhancement in Korsakoff's psychosis by clonidine: a comparison with l-dopa and ephedrine. *Psychopharmacology.* 1986;88:374-380.
123. Moffoot A, O'Carroll RE, Murray C, Dougall N, Ebmeier K, Goodwin GM. Clonidine infusion increases uptake of Tc-exametazamine in anterior cingulate cortex in Korsakoff's psychosis. *Psychol Med.* 1994;24:53-61.
124. McEntee WJ, Mair RG. The Korsakoff syndrome: a neurochemical perspective. *Trends Neurosci.* 1990;13:340-344.
125. Coull JT, Middleton HC, Robbins TW, Sahakian BJ. Contrasting effects of clonidine and diazepam on tests of working memory and planning. *Psychopharmacology.* 1995;120:311-321.
126. Hunt RD, Minderaa RB, Cohen DJ. Clonidine benefits children with attention deficit disorder and hyperactivity: report of a double-blind placebo-crossover therapeutic trial. *J Am Acad Child Psychiatry.* 1985;24:617-629.
127. Hunt RD, Capper L, O'Connell P. Clonidine in child and adolescent psychiatry. *J Child Adolesc Psychiatry.* 1990;1:87-102.
128. Hunt RD, Arnsten AFT, Asbell MD. An open trial of guanfacine in the treatment of attention deficit hyperactivity disorder. *J Am Acad Child Adolesc Psychiatry.* 1995;34:50-54.
129. Chappell PB, Riddle MA, Scahill L, Lynch K, Schultz R, Arnsten AFT, Leckman JF, Cohen DL. Guanfacine treatment of comorbid attention deficit hyperactivity disorder and Tourette's syndrome: preliminary clinical experience. *J Am Acad Child Adolesc Psychiatry.* 1995;34:1140-1146.
130. Horrigan JP, Barnhill LJ. Guanfacine for treatment of attention-deficit hyperactivity disorder in boys. *J Child Adolesc Psychopharm.* 1995; 5:215-223.

Catching up on Schizophrenia

The Fifth International Congress on Schizophrenia Research, Warm Springs, Va, April 8-12, 1995

Peter F. Buckley, MD; Robert W. Buchanan, MD (Rapporteurs)
S. Charles Schulz, MD; Carol A. Tamminga, MD (Organizers)

It is axiomatic that the diversity and ingenuity of strategies in the study of schizophrenia bear testimony to the complexity of this disorder. Accordingly, the opportunity for investigators of diverse interests to share their latest findings and be informed of developments in key areas of science is critical to advance our understanding of schizophrenia. Nearly 700 investigators from around the world gathered at Warm Springs, Va, to present their data at the Fifth International Congress on Schizophrenia Research (April 8-12, 1995). This 5-day conference, held every other year alternating with the European Winter Workshop on Schizophrenia, is co-organized by S. Charles Schulz, MD, Case Western Reserve University, Cleveland, Ohio, and Carol Tamminga, MD, Maryland Psychiatric Research Center, University of Maryland at Baltimore. Drs Schulz and Tamminga first held the Congress in 1987 in Clearwater, Fla, with 170 investigators presenting. The Congress has flourished since then and is now the largest research meeting devoted solely to schizophrenia. The Congress organizers, the program coordinator (Jeffrey Lieberman, MD, Hillside Hospital, Glen Oaks, NY), and the Congress coordinator (Susan Nusbaum, Maryland Psychiatric Research Center) are congratulated on the success of this event and its contribution to fostering initiatives and collaborations within schizophrenia research.

The Congress acknowledges the talent and endeavors of researchers by two special awards. The William K. Warren Schizophrenia Research Award is given to senior investigators who have made outstanding contributions in the field. Past awardees are Seymour S. Kety, MD, Arvid Carlsson, MD, and William T. Carpenter, Jr, MD. The fourth William K. Warren Schizophrenia Research Award was presented at the meeting to Nikki Erlenmyer-Kimling, PhD, in recognition of the contribution of her studies of high-risk subjects to our understanding of the premorbid characteristics and development of schizophrenia. In a complementary fashion, the potential of junior investigators whose efforts and scientific development are critical to sustaining research on schizophrenia is acknowledged by the Congress' Young Investigator Award. With support from the National Institute of Mental Health, Rockville, Md, the Congress enabled 36 young scientists to attend and present their findings.

In addition to the broad range of research presented on schizophrenia, the Congress has a tradition of inviting experts from other areas of neuroscience and medicine to present the latest developments in their fields. This broader perspective helps ensure that psychiatric researchers remain fluent with and can integrate pertinent findings from other disciplines. Paul Greengard, PhD, delivered a plenary lecture on the complexity of interactions between the signal transduction pathways that subserve information processing at the cellular level. Carlton Gajdusek, MD, Nobel laureate in 1976, gave a provocative plenary lecture on the evolution of his studies on infectious amyloid protein molecules and the importance of these molecules in neuropsychiatric disorders; he was circumspect about the possible role of these agents in the eti-

From the Department of Psychiatry, Case Western Reserve University, Cleveland, Ohio (Dr Buckley); and the Department of Psychiatry, Maryland Psychiatric Research Center, University of Maryland, Baltimore (Dr Buchanan).

ology of schizophrenia. In another presentation that complemented an interesting session on genetic and environmental influences in schizophrenia, Timothy Rebbeck, MD, indicated that many of the molecular genetic approaches that are currently being applied to schizophrenia research have yielded important discoveries concerning the etiology and treatment of cancers, most notably breast carcinoma.

The purpose of this report is to provide a brief account of the proceedings of the meeting, highlighting some of its most salient findings, and to convey the themes and directions for schizophrenia research that emerged. Similar reports on the European counterpart meeting, the Winter Workshop on Schizophrenia, have previously proved useful in widely disseminating research information well before formal publication. It should be emphasized, however, that no attempt has been made to be exhaustive or inclusive; we based this review on our observations and notes of presentations at this Congress. In addition, details were confirmed, as necessary, through correspondence with the presenting authors.

GENETICS

In a report on the ongoing analysis of data from the Roscommon Family Study, Kenneth Kendler, MD, presented evidence for genetic linkage in schizophrenia (lod score of 3.4) at the p22-25 region of chromosome 6. The region is located near the HLA complex. The specificity of the markers used does not preclude the possibility that the linkage may be with a gene within the complex. Such a possibility would be of particular interest given the recent revival of immunovirological hypotheses of schizophrenia etiology. Charles Kaufmann, MD, emphasized the importance of this finding and reported that preliminary analyses from two other laboratories (using different statistical approaches) have also found a susceptibility locus on chromosome 6.

Several groups reported on the extent and variability in expression of coding sequences at dopamine (D_3, D_4) and serotonin (5-hydroxytryptamine 1C) receptor gene loci and attempted to relate these to clinical variables. Vishwajit Nimgaonkar, PhD, reported that allele expression at the D_3 receptor gene locus was associated with an increased risk for schizophrenia when one particular allele predominates, while another allele was associated with an earlier age at onset of illness. Other reports were less conclusive and, contrary to a previous report, did not detect any association between allele variation of dopamine or serotonin receptor loci and clinical response to clozapine. There was also much interest in the phenomenon of anticipation, wherein successive generations among multiplex schizophrenic families show a progressively more severe form of illness and an earlier age of onset. Anticipation has been demonstrated in a number of neuropsychiatric disorders (most notably in Huntington's disease) and is thought to occur because of genetic mutations in the expansion of unstable trinucleotide repeat sequences. Although this remains an attractive hypothesis to explain the variable genetic penetrance and perpetuation of schizophrenia in the face of low fecundity, no direct evidence for anticipation emerged either from clinical observation of large pedigrees or from the search for unstable DNA sequences. Also, the candidate gene approach (using the neural cell adhesion molecule [NCAM], Snap 25, and N-cadherin gene loci) as a genetic test of the neurodevelopmental hypothesis of schizophrenia failed to reveal any compelling associations.

The exploration of genetic phenocopies is a heuristic approach that was described by several groups. Jeremy Silverman, MD, reported that high ventricular brain ratio was predicted by the presence of a marker allele among nonaffected members of a well-documented family pedigree. In contrast, William Honer, MD, did not observe any relationship between familial factors and the expression of temporal lobe abnormality among their pedigrees. In an elegant study that sought to extend previous positron emission tomography (PET) research on the neuroanatomical substrates of phenomenological syndromes, Peter Liddle, MD, compared cerebral blood flow during a word fluency test between 10 obligate carriers for schizophrenia and four normal subjects. Obligate carriers demonstrated a pattern of temporal and parietal activation that was distinct from that of normal controls. More importantly, this activation was remarkably similar to the pattern previously observed in patients with chronic schizophrenia.

The importance of genetic factors was also highlighted in a study of childhood schizophrenia (Robert Asarnow, MD) that found a rate of schizophrenia four times higher among the first-degree relatives of childhood schizophrenia probands than among the relatives of adult-onset schizophrenia probands. The suggestion that childhood (early-onset) schizophrenia represents a more genetic form of illness is congruent with the notion of anticipation. Complementary findings were described in the New York High-Risk Project (Nikki Erlenmeyer-Kimling, PhD), in which 13% of the offspring of schizophrenic parents evaluated prospectively since 1971 manifested schizophrenia, in contrast to the absence of schizophrenia among the offspring of either affectively ill or normal parents. Thomas McNeil, MD, produced evidence suggesting that this diathesis may be apparent by the first week of life. He demonstrated that a subgroup of offspring of schizophrenic parents had reduced arousal and concomitant neurological deficits during a pediatric examination on the third to fourth day after birth. It is perhaps surprising, then, that genetic phenocopies are not more readily distinguishable either by clinical characteristics or by experimental paradigms, as Fuller Torrey, MD, commented in reporting on a detailed comparison of 27 monozygotic twin pairs discordant for schizophrenia with 13 concordant twin pairs. The limited discriminatory power of the familial-sporadic distinction, evidenced again by contrasting findings reported at the meeting, supports this observation. In summarizing the findings of the extensive National Institute of Mental Health twin study, Dr Torrey concluded that the results were most consistent with the hypothesis that genetic factors determine predisposition to schizophrenia, but environmental factors are required for expression of the illness. In this area, as in many areas of schizophrenia research, the jury is still out.

EPIDEMIOLOGICAL CHARACTERISTICS

The claim for maternal influenza infection as a risk factor for schizophrenia was advanced (beyond earlier debate) into the arena of etiopathological inquiry, suggesting a role for immunological mechanisms (particularly autoimmunity) in schizophrenia. Studies from the Institute of Psychiatry, London, England (Catherine Gilvarry, MD, and Padraig Wright, MD), provided evidence for increased rates of thyrotoxicosis and insulin-dependent diabetes mellitus among relatives of psychotic patients, excess of HLA-A2 among mothers of female patients, and excess of HLA-A9 in patients with schizophrenia. Consistent with the hypothesis that schizophrenia may be an autoimmune disorder, Meggin Hollister, PhD, presented data from the Danish Perinatal Cohort that showed a possible association between rhesus hemolytic disease and schizophrenia. Robert Yolken, MD, stressed the relevance of gene-viral interactions and demonstrated a strong homology for endogenous retrovirus sequences (representing both human and animal retroviruses) in the DNA from the ill cotwin among monozygous twins discordant for schizophrenia. The gene-viral hypotheses are of particular interest given the report of linkage to chromosome 6 (see above).

Presentations at this meeting and an enduring literature attest to the merit of exploring gender differences in schizophrenia. Lynn Marcinko, MD, reported more positive symptoms and poorer psychosocial functioning among men than among women in the *DSM-IV* field trials. Martin Harrow, PhD, concluded that the more favorable outcome for women in the Chicago Follow-up Study was strongly influenced by stringent diagnostic criteria and by the premorbid and life role characteristics of female patients. In contrast to the lack of gender differences in neuropsychological test performance, several magnetic resonance imaging (MRI) studies emphasized the predominance of gender differences in the occurrence of structural abnormalities, particularly within the temporal lobe of male patients. Declan G. M. Murphy, MD, proposed that the observed gender differences are the result of sexual dimorphism in brain aging. Additional longitudinal MRI studies are needed to address this important issue.

Sexual dimorphism was also invoked to explain the curious perpetuation of schizophrenia in the face of low fecundity among patients. John Waddington, DSc, reported increased fertility confined to the parents of male patients who had a prominent familial excess of schizophrenia. Anne Bassett, MD, in a study of fertility among patients and their siblings, found no evidence for increased fertility among siblings but rather a relative preservation of fertility in female (but not male) patients. Important clues to the nature of schizophrenia will doubtless emanate from the eventual resolution of this fertility conundrum.

PHENOMENOLOGICAL CHARACTERISTICS

The binary distinction of positive-negative symptoms and the three-syndrome (psychosis/reality distortion, deficit/psychomotor poverty, and thought disorder/disorganization) conceptualization were examined by several investigators. Three groups (Nadia Davies, MD, Sonia Dollfus, MD, and Patrick McGorry, MD) favored a four-factor solution. Dr Davies identified distinct factors of psychomotor poverty, disorganization, delusions, and hallucinations. Dr Dollfus described greater overlap of symptom clusters, with positive, negative, disorganized, and mixed groups. In an Australian study of first episode of functional psychoses, Dr McGorry identified separate factors of mania, depression, psychosis (a composite of negative, motor, and disorganization symptoms—Bleulerian features), and a combination of first-rank Schneiderian symptoms (delusions and hallucinations). When the analysis was confined to those with first-episode schizophrenia, the results were more consistent with the Bleulerian-Schneiderian two-factor solution; this solution was also advocated in a confirmatory factorial analysis by Helio Elkis, MD. Differences in patient sampling and particularly in the acuity of illness (but not in medication status, according to Loro White, MD) may account for these inconsistencies.

There were multiple posters and presentations addressing the structural and functional correlates of symptom complexes. The majority of studies suggest that abnormalities of frontal executive/attention measures are associated with psychomotor poverty (negative) symptoms, whereas disorganization is associated with measures of abnormalities in distractibility. In contrast, reality distortion (hallucinations and delusions) tend to be associated with temporal lobe dysfunction. Several presentations addressed the nature of insight and the subjective experience of psychotic phenomena in schizophrenia. Poor insight appears to be attributable to underlying cognitive impairments, particularly those of the frontal lobe region.

NEUROPATHOLOGICAL AND NEUROCHEMICAL FINDINGS

Presentations of postmortem morphometric and immunohistochemical data represented the renewed interest in schizophrenia pathological studies, no longer the graveyard of neuropathologists. In a carefully conducted study, Steven Arnold, MD, could not detect an increase in gliosis among elderly patients with schizophrenia compared with patients who had Alzheimer's disease or normal brain tissue. However, for the small subgroup of patients with schizophrenia who exhibited gliosis, the pattern was atypical of that observed in patients with Alzheimer's disease and was strongly associated with antemortem evidence of severe cognitive impairment. Joel Kleinman, MD, replicated some earlier findings of neuronal decrements in layers 2, 5, and 7 of the entorhinal cortex but did not observe the cellular disorganization described by Jacob and Beckmann. In an extension of earlier work on the cortical displacement of neurons containing reduced nicotinamide adenine dinucleotide phosphate diaphorase (NADPH-d), William E. Bunney, Jr, MD, reported that the expression of messenger RNA for glutamatic acid decarboxylase (the key enzyme in the synthesis of γ-aminobutyric acid [GABA]) was reduced in the prefrontal cortex in the absence of any quantitative evidence of cellular loss. It was suggested that this functional defect, perhaps manifest by perturbations in GABAergic transmissions, may explain in part the consistent observation of frontal lobe dysfunction in schizophrenia.

Focusing on a different neurotransmitter system and pathogenic model, Joseph T. Coyle, MD, gave an authoritative plenary lecture on excitotoxic cell death and the glutamate hypothesis of schizophrenia. He cited evidence for kainate neurotoxicity and for elevated N-acetyl-L-aspartate-L-glutamic acid (NAAG) in the parahippocampus of patients with schizophrenia and suggested that the clinical picture of illness progression might be related to indolent, apoptotic cell death consequent to oxidative damage. Although other investigators also presented data on N-methyl-D-aspartate (NMDA) and kainate glutamate receptor subunits, they generally posited a neurodevelopmental explanation for their findings. Christine Humphries, MD, reported reduced gene expression of messenger RNA for specific NMDA subunits, while Robert Kerwin, MD, found widespread reductions in messenger RNA for non-NMDA receptor subunits in medial temporal lobe structures. In addition, Dr Kerwin also reported, in postmortem autoradiographic studies, a selective decrement in the developmental isoform of the glutamate receptor subunit within the hippocampus of patients with schizophrenia. Future studies are required to resolve whether NMDA, non-NMDA, both, or neither class of glutamate receptor is primarily involved in the pathophysiological characteristics of schizophrenia. The studies are also of interest in light of recent ketamine infusion studies (see below) and the use of pharmacological agents that act at the glutamate receptor for the treatment of schizophrenia.

David Lewis, MD, presented findings from studies of the frontal cortex of monkeys that indicate that critical changes occur at puberty in the architecture of both pyramidal and dopaminergic neurons. This is congruent with notions of a time-dependent susceptibility to neurodevelopmental insults and to the later emergence of symptoms of schizophrenia. Barbara Lipska, PhD, reported further work on an animal model of schizophrenia, based on neonatal excitotoxic damage to the hippocampus. In response to environmental stress and particularly dopaminergic challenge (of haloperidol infusion), these rats exhibited a dysregulation (rather than purely up-regulation or down-regulation) of dopamine activity in the cortex and striatal regions. These findings are attractive since they speak to the complexity of dopaminergic interactions rather than solely reemphasizing the initial view of hyperdopaminergia as the biochemical hallmark of schizophrenia.

The distribution and selectivity of dopamine D_2-type receptors was investigated by several groups. Robert Lahti, PhD, confirmed the discrete location of D_4 receptors in cortical and limbic regions, with sparing of striatal regions. Ian Creese, PhD, described further developments in a novel in vivo approach to the elucidation of the behavioral effects of dopamine receptor stimulation. Antisense oligonucleotides are infused to selectively block a specific receptor; then the animal is exposed to a specific pharmacological or environmental challenge. Dr Creese noted that following amphetamine infusion, catalepsy was inhibited during antisense knockout of D_2 and D_3 but not D_4 receptors. This observation may hold relevance for the mechanism of action of antipsychotic agents or, alternatively, may explain the low propensity for extrapyramidal side effects with these agents.

ELECTROPHYSIOLOGICAL CHARACTERISTICS AND EYE MOVEMENTS

The strategy of using pharmacological probes to explore the neurobiological characteristics of schizophrenia was also evident in electrophysiological studies. Clozapine was found to be more effective than conventional neuroleptic agents in facilitating P50 auditory sensory gating, with risperidone having an effect intermediate between the two (Laurence Adler, MD). Clozapine (Yi Jin, MD) was also found to selectively increase theta and alpha activity in the frontoparietal cortex, an effect that was not found with haloperidol; the effect was hypothesized to be related to clozapine's serotonergic affinity in the cortex.

The validity of eye movement dysfunction as a trait marker for schizophrenia was emphasized from studies of normal college students with features of schizotypy (Gillian O'Driscoll, PhD), offspring of schizophrenic parents (David Rosenberg, PhD), adolescents with schizophrenia (Lee Friedman, PhD), and patients at variable stages of the illness (Michael Obuchowski, MA, and Gunvant Thaker, MD). In addition, presentations on the relationship of eye fixation, anhedonia, and the ability to recognize facial emotions suggested that affective blunting in schizophrenia reflects both an affective deficit and neuromotor dysregulation. Somewhat counterintuitively then, David Laporte, PhD, did not find that affect recognition was more impaired in patients with the deficit syndrome. This suggests that impairments in the perception of social cues do not underlie the decreased social drive observed in these patients.

NEUROIMAGING AND NEUROPSYCHOLOGICAL CHARACTERISTICS

First-episode schizophrenia figured prominently among MRI studies. In broad terms, those structural brain abnormalities common to chronic schizophrenia were also observed in this group, including a generalized deficit (loss vs hypoplasia?) of cortical gray matter in patients with first-episode schizophrenia (Kelvin Lim, MD). Using magnetic resonance spectroscopy, Perry Renshaw, MD, provided new evidence for a bilateral reduction in *N*-acetylaspartate (a neuronal cell body marker) in first-episode psychosis. Addressing the controversy of caudate nucleus enlargement in chronic schizophrenia, Matcheri Keshavan, MD, reported an increase in caudate volume between diagnosis and a 6- to 24-month follow-up MRI of patients with first-episode schizophrenia. These findings may reflect an antipsychotic drug action rather than illness progression. This is consistent with findings from Hillside Hospital of an 8% increase in caudate volume after first psychotic treatment among patients receiving conventional antipsychotic agents, while clozapine-treated patients exhibited a 10% reduction in caudate volume.

Refinements in neuroimaging have created functional imaging techniques characterized by a high level of complexity, as evidenced by presentations on MRI, MRI-PET coregistration, brain averaging, and analysis of cortical gyral patterns. John Gore, MD, gave a concise overview of the physics and clinical applications of functional MRI, a new modality whose coming-of-age within psychiatry was heralded by a number of presentations at this meeting. Functional MRI studies were largely concerned with validating this new and promising modality as a noninvasive technique for assessing cerebral blood flow and microcirculation of schizophrenia. In contrast, several sophisticated PET studies exemplified the potential of this neuroimaging technique for neurochemical/pharmacological studies (Jonathan Brodie, MD, Nora Volkow, PhD, and Carol Tamminga, MD). These approaches can yield valuable information on the in vivo pharmacokinetics and pharmacodynamics of antipsychotic medications and can provide the biochemical framework for dose-reduction strategies aimed at minimizing side effects while optimizing antipsychotic efficacy. Neuroimaging can also provide a window to directly visualize dopaminergic and other neurotransmitter systems. Both Marc Laruelle, MD, using 3-iodo-6-methoxybenzamide iodine 123–labeled single photon emission computed tomography, and Alan Breier, MD, using carbon 11–labeled raclopride PET, have proposed models for estimating synaptic dopamine concentrations. Both groups presented data consistent with the association of change in subjective mood state with synaptic dopamine following amphetamine challenge.

In concert with the increased focus on the possible causal role of glutamate in schizophrenia were the PET studies examining the effects of ketamine, an NMDA antagonist, on cerebral blood flow patterns in normal controls and patients with schizophrenia. Specific activation was noted in the limbic cortex of patients with schizophrenia (Adrienne Lahti, MD), whereas a diffuse pattern of cortical activation was observed in normal controls (Alan Breier, MD). These metabolic changes are of particular interest given the effects of ketamine infusion on symptoms and cognition in patients with schizophrenia (Adrienne Lahti, MD, John Krystal, MD, and Anil Malhotra, MD).

Attempts to link neurocognition with neuroanatomy often yielded conflicting results. Nancy Andreasen, MD, reported activation of frontal, parietal, and cerebellar (but not temporal) regions in normal persons during the performance of memory tasks. Rohan Ganguli, MD, showed selective deficits in temporal lobe activation, yet Deborah Yurgelun-Todd, PhD, found anomalous hyperactivation in the temporal lobe of patients relative to control subjects in response to a word-generation test during functional MRI.

Studies addressing neurocognition alone provided more homogeneous findings. It may be concluded from several presentations (Robert Bilder, PhD, Laura Flashman, PhD, John Kenny, PhD, Norbert Sobizack, MD, and John Sweeney, PhD) that memory deficits are prominent in schizophrenia, occur early in the illness, and are most often superimposed on a generalized pattern of cognitive dysfunction. Findings from a 1969-1970 Swedish conscription survey were presented by Anthony David, MD. One hundred ninety-five patients with an *ICD-8 (International Classification of Diseases, Eighth Revision)* diagnosis of schizophrenia identified out of a sample of 50 000 conscriptees showed deficits in verbal and visuospatial IQ score and in arithmetic. These impairments antedated the emergence of typical schizophrenic symptoms and represented an overall group shift to the left compared with the IQ distribution of normal conscriptees. Other studies (Barbara Cornblatt, PhD, Sanjay Gupta, MD, and Darren Mockler, MD) suggested that cognitive impairment, once established, does not appear to show progressive deterioration (in excess of the age-related decline for the normal population) over the course of the illness.

Several studies explored the significance of semantic priming in schizophrenia, wherein patients (particularly those who are thought disordered) perform better on information-processing tasks that test lexical associations. Deanna Barch, PhD, reported that priming effects in unmedicated patients were similar to (or less than) those in depressed patients or normal controls. Her group concluded that the enhanced priming effect was confined to medicated patients. In normal subjects, levodopa was shown to cause a decrement in the indirect priming effect from 4.7% to 1.2% (Manfred Spitzer, MD), suggesting that dopamine (and/or norepinephrine) may improve the signal-to-noise ratio in semantic priming. Increased facilitation of Stroop Color-Word Interference Test performance was associated with thought disorder but not other symptoms (Cameron Carter, MD). These (anomalous) cognitive "advantages" in patients provide a useful framework for examining the pathophysiological characteristics of cognitive deficits and for planning cognitive remediation strategies.

PSYCHOSOCIAL THERAPIES, PSYCHOPHARMACOLOGICAL CHARACTERISTICS, AND DRUG SIDE EFFECTS

In the face of the growing specter of managed care, several presentations advocated the use and effectiveness of Assertive Community Training (ACT) programs in the rehabilitation and relapse prevention of patients with severe forms of schizophrenia. Strategies to improve cognitive performance were also highlighted. However, it was unclear whether the effect of such cognitive remediation interventions can endure past the induction and treatment phases. It was disappointing to learn that in a preliminary report from a multicenter comparative study of haloperidol and clozapine (Alan Bellack, PhD), no advantage or synergy was found between clozapine and the psychosocial therapies. Stephen Marder, MD, also reported that the relapse rates in this study were indistinguishable between patients receiving social skills training and those receiving supportive group therapy.

Several reports suggested that a delay in treatment with antipsychotic medications may result in biologically deleterious effects, manifest by poor initial and subsequent poorer response to pharmacological treatment. Sally Szymanski, MD, reported that a longer duration of illness prior to initiation of treatment was related to poorer treatment response both in patients with first-episode schizophrenia and in patients with chronic illness. Richard Wyatt, MD, presented further evidence of the benefit of early intervention with antipsychotic treatment. In an analysis of first-admission patients from the original study of antipsychotic efficacy by May and colleagues, patients initially treated with antipsychotic agents during hospitalization did better at follow-up than those initially treated without antipsychotic agents, even though the latter group subsequently received adequate antipsychotic treatment. Similarly, Anthony Loebel, MD, highlighted the progressively protracted time to treatment response during subsequent relapses in patients with first-episode psychosis. Twelve patients had relapsed at least twice, with their mean±SD duration to remittance being 48.8±36.1, 58.2±34.9, and 85.4±65.5 days for the first, second, and third relapses, respectively. Jeffrey Lieberman, MD, advocated prompt pharmacological intervention with the hope that adequate treatment early in the illness might prevent the emergence of nonresponsivity and poor outcome that is seen in some patients. Although the efficacy of clozapine in treatment-refractory schizophrenia is compelling, he stressed that results from ongoing studies of clozapine in the treatment of early-stage schizophrenia are necessary before informed debate can occur on the wider use of clozapine. Of relevance here is an Austrian open-labeled study (Martina Hummer, MD) on the use of clozapine in patients with first-episode and chronic schizophrenia. This group noted a high percentage of treatment responders in both groups (63% for first-episode schizophrenia, 43% for chronic schizophrenia), with the best response seen at relatively low plasma clozapine levels (100 to 200 ng/mL). This report provides some initial evidence for the efficacy of clozapine in the early course of schizophrenia.

Other reports highlighted the effectiveness of clozapine in specific subgroups of treatment-refractory schizophrenic patients. Clozapine was shown to be of notable benefit for patients with water intoxication, for those with comorbid substance abuse, and for those with persistent aggressive behavior.

William T. Carpenter, Jr, MD, and Herbert Y. Meltzer, MD, debated several issues concerning the use of clozapine, including what was an appropriate duration for a clinical trial of clozapine. Dr Carpenter provided evidence to suggest that if a patient had not shown an adequate response by the end of 4 months of therapy, clozapine treatment should be discontinued. Dr Meltzer argued that the cost of savings and improvement along multiple dimensions of outcome during clozapine therapy should not be dismissed lightly and that a longer trial would be warranted in most cases. Despite a lively and interesting exchange, the debate was unresolved and was subsequently published in the *American Journal of Psychiatry*.

There was a dearth of comparative studies of the efficacy of clozapine and risperidone in chronic schizophrenia. Simon Altman, MD, reported that, in an open-labeled study, severely ill patients receiving clozapine (n=85) did best, with risperidone-treated patients (n=44) achieving an intermediate outcome between those receiving clozapine and those receiving conventional antipsychotic agents (n=42). Interestingly, when clozapine-treated patients relapsed and crossed over to risperidone therapy, 15% subsequently responded; in contrast, just under 40% of previously risperidone-treated patients subsequently responded to clozapine therapy. Jack Grebb, MD, commented on an 8-week double-blind Swiss study of clozapine and risperidone. Sixty-seven percent of risperidone-treated patients and 65% of clozapine-treated patients achieved a 20% or greater reduction in Positive and Negative Syndrome Scale score compared with their pretreatment evaluation. The conflicting results suggest that additional formal studies are needed comparing the relative efficacy of these two agents.

The results of augmentation strategies presented at this meeting were not encouraging. S. Charles Schulz, MD, reported that the addition of lithium to antipsychotic medication was ineffective for nonresponders in the collaborative Treatment Strategies in Schizophrenia Study. Robert W. Buchanan, MD, found no benefit for negative (or any) symptoms during a double-blind, placebo-controlled study of mazindol (a dopamine/noradrenaline reuptake inhibitor) augmentation of antipsychotic medication. During a brief open-labeled study, high-dose famotidine (a selective histaminergic antagonist) produced only a modest improvement in symptoms (Richard Rosse, MD). Jayashri Kulkarni, MD, demonstrated that adjunctive estrogen treatment in female schizophrenic patients resulted in a quicker initial response to antipsychotic medication, but this effect was lost after 1 month of treatment.

It has become a practice of the Congress to have pharmaceutical companies present data on novel and putative antipsychotic medications at various advanced stages of clinical investigation. These presentations serve to inform Congress participants of the latest advances in drug development, and in turn, they provide representatives of pharmaceutical companies with an opportunity to discuss issues of drug development with their academic colleagues. Progress reports were provided on risperidone, olanzapine, sertindole, seroquel, ziprasidone, SDZ-MAR 327, MDL 100 907, and NGD 94-1. Results to date are encouraging. Although many of these agents have favorable side-effect profiles, particularly with respect to extrapyramidal symptoms, information on their efficacy for treatment-resistant patients was limited.

Regarding the treatment of side effects, several studies confirmed the importance of illness-related factors in the genesis of tardive dyskinesia (TD). William Hoffman, MD, detected choreoathetoid movements (indistinguishable from TD) in 22% of neuroleptic-naive patients, an observation in agreement with the presentation of Wayne Fenton, MD, on dyskinesia in the preneuroleptic era. Dyskinetic patients in the Chestnut Lodge Study showed clinical evidence of cognitive impairment and prominent negative symptoms. Similarly, Miranda Chakos, MD, reported that the emergence of TD during the follow-up of patients with first-episode psychosis was predicted by ventriculomegaly and neuropsychological impairments. However, John Waddington, DSc, did not find MRI correlates of TD in a sample of patients with more chronic disease. Waddington did report similar associations with frontal lobe neuropsychological deficits and, interestingly, also with craniofacial dysmorphogenesis. Thus, TD may represent a discrete phenotypic expression of the illness and, more speculatively, of its neurodevelopmental origin in these patients. However, the morphological correlates of TD, if any, have not been consistently delineated.

John Kane, MD, delivered a plenary lecture on the incidence and risk factors of TD. He described the prospective, naturalistic study of TD at Hillside Hospital and reported that the incidence of TD in this large sample was just over 5.3% per year of neuroleptic therapy, with this rate remaining linear for the first 6 years. Sixty percent of patients who developed signs of TD had a later remittance of TD. Good prognostic indicators for remission included low neuroleptic dosage and few interruptions in neuroleptic treatment during the follow-up period.

CONCLUDING REMARKS

The neurodevelopmental etiopathological model of schizophrenia was probed from multiple standpoints ranging from neurochemistry to epidemiology, and it endured as a theme during the conference. However, the inconsistency across studies concerning many abnormal findings in schizophrenia and the absence of pathognomonic postmortem changes (the smoking gun, as Daniel R. Weinberger, MD, remarked) indicate the need for a complex conceptualization of neurodevelopmental arrest and encourage keeping an open mind toward other heuristic models. Robin Murray, MD, DSc, offered a reconciliation of disparate findings by suggesting that the schizophrenias may be divided into those exhibiting a severe, early-onset neurodevelopmental form, predominately in males; a relapsing form, occurring predominately in females, that overlaps with affective psychosis; and a late-onset, degenerative-type illness. Further comparisons between schizophrenia and affective disorder and between other, pathobiologically distinct conditions (eg, Alzheimer's disease, autism, and neurological disorders) should help to clarify the extent and expression of aberrant neurodevelopment in schizophrenia.

Refinements in psychopharmacological approaches and the potential of novel pharmacological approaches for probing the neurobiological characteristics of schizophrenia were much in evidence at the Congress. Pharmacological approaches to the investigation of the pathophysiological characteristics of schizophrenia are likely to become ever more important as newer, more specific agents become available.

Finally, the sophistication of the neuroscience armamentarium that is applicable to the study of schizophrenia is impressive. Neuroscience is advancing at a prodigious rate, particularly in the fields of genetics, neurochemistry, and neuroimaging. The benefits of such developments for schizophrenia research were evident at this Congress and suggest that our chances of overtaking schizophrenia will be maximized by integrating concepts and methods from multiple areas of biomedical research. However, the advances in psychosocial therapies and in service research, which were also prominent at this conference, should not be overshadowed by biomedical perspectives, particularly since the former often result in a more immediate impact for patients.

Accepted for publication September 21, 1995.

Correspondence to Department of Psychiatry, Case Western Reserve University, University Hospitals of Cleveland, 2040 Abington Rd, Cleveland, OH 44106 (Dr Buckley).

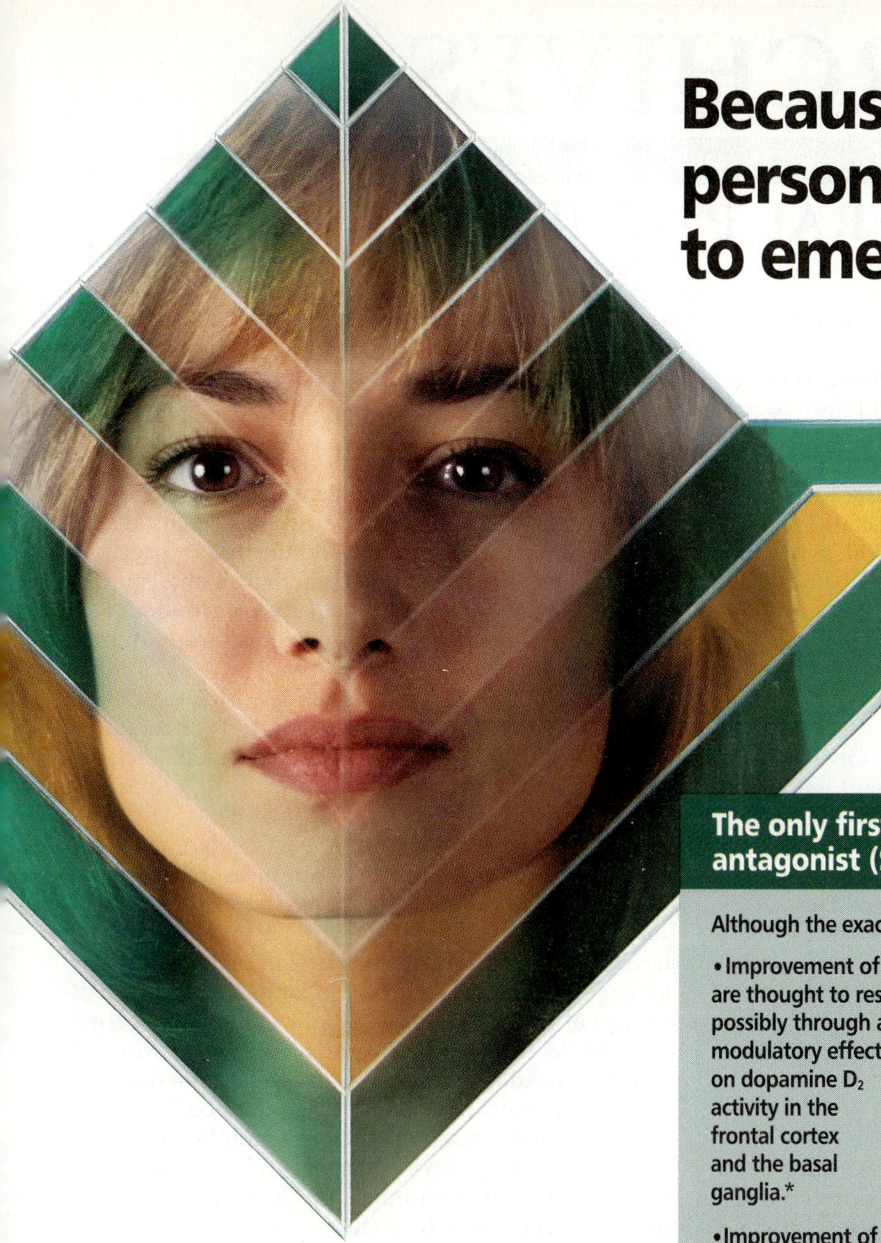

Because a whole person is waiting to emerge.

The only first-choice serotonin/dopamine antagonist (SDA).

Although the exact mechanism of action is unknown:

- Improvement of negative symptoms and lessened risk of EPS are thought to result from blockade of serotonin 5-HT_2 receptors, possibly through a modulatory effect on dopamine D_2 activity in the frontal cortex and the basal ganglia.*
- Improvement of positive symptoms is thought to result from blockade of dopamine D_2 receptors in the limbic system.*

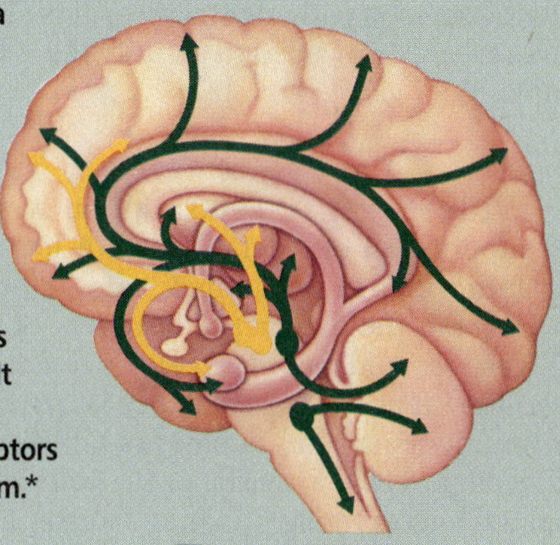

Dopaminergic system   Serotoninergic system

A first choice

1-,2-,3-,4-mg tablets

Risperdal®

RISPERIDONE

Raising the standard of care.

*Ereshefsky L, Lacombe S. Pharmacological profile of risperidone. *Can J Psychiatry.* 1993;38(Suppl 3):S80-S88.

Please see the brief summary of Prescribing Information adjacent to this ad.

JANSSEN · PHARMACEUTICA · RESEARCH FOUNDATION ·

SmithKline Beecham Pharmaceuticals

THIS MONTH IN

ARCHIVES OF GENERAL PSYCHIATRY

Since the 1970s, evidence has been accumulating that there may be an association between serious mental disorders and criminality. **Hodgins et al** (page 489) examined a Danish birth cohort followed to age 43. Proportionately more of the men and women with mental disorders who had been admitted to a hospital were convicted of criminal offenses than the men and women who were never admitted to a hospital. The offenders with mental disorders committed all types of offenses and, on average, as many as the nondisordered offenders. These findings emphasize again the need for further research on the relationship between mental disorders and crime.

The association between mental disorders and violence is one of the most important issues in forensic psychiatry. **Eronen et al** (page 497) studied a comprehensive group of homicide offenders in Finland to calculate odds ratios for the statistical risk increase associated with specific mental disorders. The study indicates that schizophrenia, personality disorders, and alcoholism significantly increase the odds ratio of homicide. However, the authors emphasize that only a minority of persons with mental disorders are violent, and future research is needed to identify these high-risk subgroups.

In 1994, over 800 000 women were under the supervision of federal, state, or local correctional authorities in the United States. However, little is known about the psychiatric disorders of these women. In the largest epidemiologic studies to date, **Teplin et al** (page 505) report the prevalence of psychiatric disorders among female jail inmates in Chicago, and **Jordan et al** (page 513) provide prevalance estimates for women felons entering prison in North Carolina. Teplin et al found that more than 80% of the women had had 1 or more psychiatric disorders, and substance abuse was the most common one. Most disordered women were in jail for minor offenses and could be treated in the community. Jordan et al had similar findings: compared with rates for women in the community in North Carolina, convicted women felons had higher rates of substance abuse and dependence, antisocial and borderline personality disorder, mood disorders, and exposure to extreme events. Because correctional facilities are mandated by law to provide needed treatment, psychiatry and the criminal justice system should work together to design jail and prison programs as well as community-based services. Increased mental health and substance abuse services may have the potential to reduce recidivism.

Alcoholic, impulsive violent offenders and fire setters are characterized by reduced central serotonin turnover rate. **Virkkunen et al** (page 523) report that a family history of paternal alcoholism with violence is associated with particularly low serotonin turnover rate among violent offenders. Low serotonin turnover rate, low sympathetic nervous system activity, and absence of the father from home during early childhood are variables that are predictive of recidivist violent criminality among alcoholic violent offenders and fire setters.

Inverse relationships between measures of central serotonin function and impulsive aggression, particularly in individuals with personality disorder, have been reported over the past 2 decades. **Coccaro et al** (page 531) report an inverse relationship between life history of impulse aggressive behavior and the peripheral platelet serotonin transporter in subjects with personality disorder. Numbers of central serotonergic 5-hydroxytryptamine transporters may be reduced in subjects with personality disorder who have prominent histories of impulsive aggressive behavior, and selected peripheral measures of serotonin may be useful in studying impulsive aggressive behavior.

Higley et al (page 537) used a nonhuman primate model to study low serotonin functioning in the central nervous system and aggressive behavior early in life as risk factors for adult violent behavior and subsequent survival to maturity. The rate of mortality was ascertained among free-ranging, male rhesus monkeys over a 4-year period after obtaining blood and cisternal cerebrospinal fluid (CSF) samples from subjects when they were 2 years old. Low CSF 5-hydroxyindoleacetic acid (5-HIAA) concentrations, frequent episodes of violent behavior, and high rates of risk taking were highly predictive of which subjects died or were presumed dead. These findings suggest that low CSF 5-HIAA quantified early in life is a powerful predictor of future excessive aggression, risk taking, and premature death among nonhuman primate males.

Violent crime is thought to develop when individuals possess both biological and social deficits. **Raine et al** (page 544) found that individuals with both neuromotor deficits at age 1 year and unstable families during adolescence (biosocial group) had double the rates of violent crime at age 21 relative to those with only biological risk factors (obstetric) or only social risk factors (poverty). These individuals also had significantly higher rates of behavioral and academic problems during adolescence.

In a community population, **Davidson et al** (page 550) found a history of attempted suicide in 15% of victims of sexual trauma after accounting for other known risk factors. Sexual trauma before age 16 was a particularly strong associative risk factor. Nearly all subjects in this study were women. Greater clinical awareness of these relationships is urged, and studies of causality are needed.

An Editorial by Peter Marzuk, MD, on the link between violence, crime, and mental illness is also included in this issue.

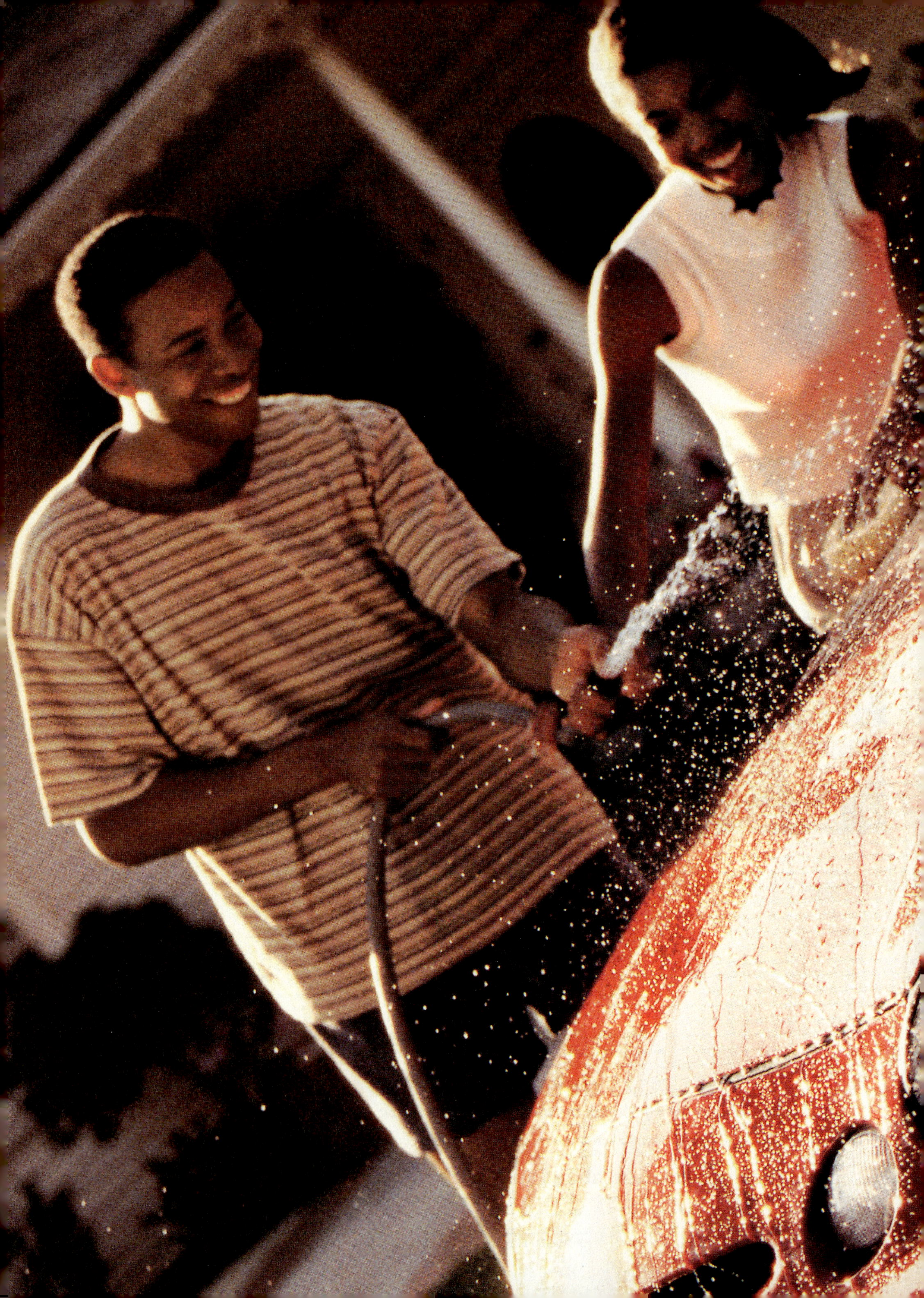

Violence, Crime, and Mental Illness

How Strong a Link?

A MAN DIAGNOSED with schizophrenia slashes 2 people to death with a sword and wounds 9 others aboard the Staten Island ferry. A woman who has schizophrenia kills a child and wounds 5 others in a schoolroom in Chicago. A man with bipolar disorder kills 7 coworkers and wounds 13 others in Kentucky. A man with schizophrenia shoots President Reagan and 3 others. A pilot, reportedly responding to auditory hallucinations, crashes a commercial airliner into Tokyo Bay. Perhaps more than any other type, violence by the mentally ill is feared by the public. It seems so senseless, so random, so unpredictable, so deadly. Somehow it is more reassuring to know that someone was shot to death in a grocery store robbery than stabbed to death by a deranged man.

Violence and mental illness have been topics of discourse for thousands of years. Socrates argued that the rate of mental disorders in Athens had to be low because there was so little violence in the city.[1,2] Benjamin Franklin argued before the Pennsylvania assembly in 1751 that ". . . the number of persons distempered in mind and deprived of their rational faculties has increased greatly in this province. Some of them going at large are a terror to their neighbors, who are daily apprehensive of the violence they may commit."[2,3]

Ironically, it is only in recent years that we mental health professionals and advocates for the mentally ill have begun to appreciate the association between violence and mental illness,[2,4] a link that has been recognized by the general public for centuries. What took us so long? Why were we so blind? There are several good reasons.

First, the studies purportedly showing a link between mental illness and violence have been unconvincing. They have been limited by unstandardized or vague definitions of violence, mental illness, or both; case finding that has largely relied on official records, which results in reporting biases; comparisons with populations who are not mentally ill that either have failed to account for demographic or situational variables or are altogether lacking them; and a design that almost by necessity has been retrospective.[4]

Second, the ways in which society handles the violent and the mentally ill vary over time within cultures and differ between cultures. In some countries, the mentally ill are largely confined to their homes by their families. In the United States, those with mental illnesses who are violent have been variously ignored, medicated, hospitalized, jailed, or even executed. Before the 1960s, many studies found that the arrest rate for those with mental illness was lower than that of the general population, which led to the typical mantra of mental health professionals that the mentally ill are no more likely to be violent than others.[5] Most of these studies were conducted when individuals with serious mental illness were routinely institutionalized for much of their lives. The deinstitutionalization policy of the 1960s shifted persons with serious disorders into the community and resulted in a marked increase in their rates of arrest.[6]

Third, it has only been in the last decade or two that the pervasive use of illicit psychoactive drugs, particularly cocaine, heroin, sedatives, and hallucinogens, along with alcohol, has increased the risk for violence among mentally ill persons, as it has once again for all persons.[7]

Fourth, we in the psychiatric field have been appropriately cautious about further stigmatizing the mentally ill with what was an apparently tenuous association with violence.[5] After all, perceived dangerousness and unpredictability are probably the most important sources of stigma for persons with mental illness,[8] affecting their choice of friends, academic advancement, job prospects, and living arrangements in the community.

In the last decade, however, the evidence showing a link between violence, crime, and mental illness has mounted. It cannot be dismissed; it should not be ignored. As Monahan[2] points out, most studies had examined rates of violence among the disordered, or rates of disorder among the violent. Typically, this has meant that persons were studied who already had been admitted to mental hospitals or already had been arrested, convicted, or incarcerated. More recently, studies have examined community samples, reducing selection bias, and convincing many of us that the link between violence and mental illness is indeed a real one.

In a 1990 study, Swanson and colleagues[9,10] used data from the Epidemiologic Catchment Area study. Compared with people who had no diagnoses of a mental disorder, the incidence of violence was 5 times higher among people with serious mental illnesses such as schizophrenia, major depression, and mania or bipolar disorder, and 12 to 16 times higher among persons with alcohol or substance use disorders, even after controlling for demographic factors.

In a well-designed study, Link and colleagues[11] in 1992 compared rates of arrest and self-reported violence in a sample of adults living in upper Manhattan who had never been in a mental hospital or sought help for a mental disorder with the rates of violence in samples of both inpatients and outpatients with mental disorders.

Many factors were controlled, including demographics, socioeconomic status, educational level, and family composition; the ethnic homogeneity, residential mobility, and homicide rates of the community; and differences in social desirability of the respondents, which might affect their willingness to disclose a history of violence. Although certain demographic features such as male sex, lower education, and residence in a district with a high homicide rate were related to the risk for being violent, patient groups were still much more likely than the nonpatient groups to be violent. When the presence of psychotic symptoms was controlled, the differences in recent violent behavior between the patients and the nonill community residents disappeared. Thus, the difference in rates of violence between those with mental illness and never-treated community residents is largely explained by the level of psychotic symptoms, not by the label of "mental patient." The differences remained significant even after the investigators controlled for use of alcohol and other drugs. It might be tempting to say that psychotic symptoms, themselves, cause persons to be violent. However, Link et al[11] also suggest that it may be the general public's typically fearful or angry reaction to psychotic symptoms that causes them to try to coerce or control the disturbed person, which often triggers the violence.

OUR THEME ISSUE ON VIOLENCE

In this issue of the ARCHIVES, 4 studies provide more evidence for a link between violence and crime and mental illness. All 4 have certain methodological limitations that should be borne in mind. Because they involve hospitalization and officially recorded violence (ie, arrests, convictions, incarcerations), they can incur selection bias. As Link et al[11] have pointed out, the deviant person may be "medicalized," that is, people who are violent may be more likely to be selected into a patient group by being hospitalized. Alternatively, the mentally ill may be "criminalized," that is, people who are mentally ill may be treated differently by police, be more likely to surrender or get caught, and in effect have higher rates of "official" crime but not of actual violence or illegal conduct. As a result, studies of this design are likely to have the greatest accuracy for those disorders or those crimes that are most likely to come to the attention of the authorities. This would include severe mental illnesses such as schizophrenia and the most serious crimes such as homicides. Persons with schizophrenia are probably more likely to be hospitalized in their lifetimes than persons with less severe mental disorders; thus we can be more assured that a study involving hospitalization will "capture" many persons with schizophrenia. On the other side of the coin, compared with other crimes, homicides are more likely to be discovered and reported.[12] In some countries, most homicides are solved and there is less police discretion involved in arresting a person for homicide than for disorderly conduct or nonviolent offenses. Thus, we can be more assured that a study involving official crime records will capture most incidents of homicide.

Three of these 4 studies in this issue use the Epidemiological Catchment Area study as a basis for comparison with rates of mental disorders in a community sample. While it is important to have comparisons with the general population, the communities represented in the Epidemiological Catchment Area data are not the exact communities from which the cases were drawn. Despite these limitations, the findings are quite noteworthy.

In the largest unselected birth cohort studied to date, Hodgins and colleagues[13] found that persons who had psychiatric hospitalizations in Denmark were 3 to 11 times more likely to have criminal convictions than persons who had never been hospitalized. Almost all diagnostic groups carried this increased risk for all types of crime, both violent and nonviolent. In the Finnish study by Eronen and colleagues,[14] the odds ratios of homicidal violence were substantially increased for both men and women with the diagnoses of schizophrenia, antisocial personality disorder, and alcoholism compared with the general population.

There are several strengths to these 2 studies. They are large. The Danish study involved 324 401 persons in the birth cohort who were followed up through age 43 years, beyond the period of highest risk for both violence and serious mental illnesses. The Finnish study examined almost 700 homicide offenders, who account for almost 70% of all known homicides in Finland in a 7-year period. Also, the official records in these countries are thought to be unequalled in the world in their quality.[15] Nonetheless, these studies must be interpreted in light of the distinctive societies in which they were conducted. Denmark and Finland have relatively homogeneous populations, low overall crime rates, and relatively uniform prosperity—characteristics that are very different from those of the United States or some other nations. They may also have different criminal justice, mental health, and social service systems and different attitudes about what to do with those who are violent, mentally ill, or both.

Two studies in this issue examined the rate of mental disorders among pretrial detainees in jail (Teplin and colleagues[16]) and convicted felons in prison (Jordan and colleagues[17]). The studies are all the more remarkable because all of those studied were women. Most studies of incarcerated persons have been of men,[18-20] and with good reason, since men commit the vast majority of crimes in every culture.[21] However, the rate at which women are entering the jail and prison system is increasing.[22] Moreover, studies in this issue[13,14] and elsewhere[23-25] suggest the sex ratio among the violent mentally ill is more nearly equal.

These studies had several strengths: they involved large numbers of randomly selected subjects, standardized diagnostic interview instruments, and comparisons with community samples. They were conducted in very different settings: an urban jail in Cook County, Illinois (Chicago) and a correctional institution in North Carolina, and yet they yielded rather similar findings. Among the jail detainees and convicted felons, 80% and 64%, respectively, met criteria for 1 or more lifetime disorders; 70% and 46%, respectively, were symptomatic within 6 months of interview. The most common disorders included alcohol or other drug abuse, antisocial or borderline personality disorder, posttraumatic stress symptoms, and major depression, the rates of which were significantly higher than the rates in the general population. Most of the subjects with psychiatric illness had been arrested for nonviolent crimes. Although the findings can say less about the statistical association between crime and psychiatric disorders, they clearly underscore the importance of ensuring adequate substance abuse and mental health services to incarcerated women (and to men as well).

RESEARCH INTO the neurobiology of violence has been fueled by the hope that a marker (anatomic, biochemical, or genetic) might provide us with a better understanding not only of the intrinsic causes of violence but of better ways to predict it. There is also the hope that medications could target the specific neural pathways that may go awry in mentally disordered individuals who are repeatedly violent.

The neuroanatomic and neurochemical pathways underlying violence are gradually being elucidated. Although by no means worked out, animal studies suggest that a propensity for aggression is governed by excitatory and inhibitory centers that include the orbitofrontal cortex, septal area, hippocampus, amygdala, caudate, thalamus, hypothalamus, midbrain, tegmentum, pons, and, somewhat surprisingly, the cerebellum.[26-28] Likewise, a series of excitatory and inhibitory neurotransmitters such as dopamine, γ-aminobutyric acid, and norepinephrine, as well as hormones, particularly of hypothalamic or gonadal origin, are involved in mediating aggression.[26-28] Research on the genetic underpinnings of violence is still in its infancy, if not still in utero, but a link between a particular type of impulsive violence and a point mutation in the monoamine oxidase A gene was recently discovered in one family.[29] Of course, the line of investigation that has received the most attention among psychiatrists has involved the association of hyposerotonergic functioning with impulsive violence. Three studies reported in this issue further cement this link.

Virkkunen and colleagues[30] extend their previous findings[31] that among male alcoholic violent offenders and fire setters, a low cerebrospinal fluid (CSF) concentration of 5-hydroxyindoleacetic acid (5-HIAA), the principal metabolite of serotonin, was associated with a family history that was positive for paternal violence and alcoholism. Moreover, in a follow-up period that averaged more than 4 years, recidivist violence in this population was associated with low CSF 5-HIAA and 3-methoxy-4-hydroxyphenylglycol concentrations, earlier parental absence, and the presence of brothers in the home. The study illustrates the larger principle that the best prediction models of recurrent violence will probably incorporate both biological and environmental variables, rather than either type alone. It also provides added support for the "low serotonin syndrome" proposed by this group.[32] In this conceptual model, a heritable defect in serotonergic functioning is temporarily relieved by alcohol intake, which only exacerbates the serotonin defect further and leads to violence.

The study of aggressive persons with personality disorders by Coccaro and colleagues[33] involves measurement of the platelet binding of tritiated paroxetine, a radioligand for the serotonin transporter. Because CSF is hard to obtain (among other reasons), many investigators have turned to platelet models because platelet serotonin transporter sites are reportedly identical in structure to the corresponding sites on serotonergic neurons.[34] In the past, most studies used tritiated imipramine as a radioligand, which may not reflect the full serotonin transporter population. In the study by Coccaro et al, a history of aggressive acts and physical assaults in response to provocation in these individuals with personality disorders was found to be inversely correlated with the Bmax values of tritiated paroxetine binding, which suggests another abnormality of serotonergic functioning in these patients.

In a study by Higley and colleagues,[35] free-ranging monkeys confined to an island off the coast of South Carolina were captured in food traps and had their CSF levels of various neurotransmitters measured. The animals were released and then tracked by direct visual observation or radio collars that emitted specific sound frequencies. At a 4-year follow-up of naturalistic observations, 91% of the subjects known or presumed dead came from the group with the 2 lowest quartiles of CSF 5-HIAA concentration. Subjects known to die because of aggressive encounters with other monkeys all came from the group in the lowest quartile. Interestingly, subjects that were captured more than once in food traps, that is, that took more risks than others, were also more aggressive and likely to suffer early mortality. The study will require confirmation, but it suggests that low CSF 5-HIAA may be a biological marker associated with future excess aggression and risk-taking, which leads to premature mortality. It is particularly striking how many of us humans die in aggressive encounters that we ourselves have provoked—a "victim-precipitated" homicide phenomenon noted by Wolfgang[36] decades ago. Such types of encounters are largely thought to be determined by environmental context and situational circumstances; it is intriguing to think there may be an underlying biological propensity. The study's "etho-ecological" design is also noteworthy. Brain and Haug[37] have argued wisely that the traditional approaches to studying animal behavior involve manipulating the animals' brains with surgery, implants, electrical stimulation, or injections and then observing their behaviors in tightly controlled situations in which the animals have few options other than to attack or fail to attack. Although the study by Higley et al[35] sacrificed tight experimental control, it allowed the animals to have a wider array of behaviors than they would otherwise have when confined to observational cages.

Low serotonin level has been linked with impulsive violence and suicidality as tightly as love and marriage or horses and carriages. Yet the link is not found in every study.[27] New ideas will be needed to push it further. One of the more intriguing ones involves the role of prior social experience in modifying serotonergic responses associated with "fight or flight" behaviors. In crayfish, the effect of serotonin on the neural circuit for tail-flip escape varied on the basis of the crayfish's social experience.[38] In socially dominant crayfish, serotonin reversibly enhanced the response to sensory stimuli of the lateral giant tail-flip command neuron, reversibly inhibited it in subordinate animals, and persistently enhanced it in socially isolated crayfish. Clearly, the serotonin story is far from complete.

TWO STUDIES in this issue[39,40] examine how the early environment may predispose some individuals to commit criminal and violent acts as adults. Raine and colleagues[39] found that a group of individuals studied from birth who had both early neuromotor deficits and unstable family environments had more than twice the rate of total crime than 2 other groups who suffered from either childhood poverty or birth complications alone.

In a large community sample, Davidson and colleagues[40] found that a self-reported history of sexual assault, particularly before the age of 16 years, was associated with a significantly increased lifetime rate of attempted suicide, after controlling for sex, age, education, posttraumatic stress symptoms, and psychiatric disorders. The study has a number of limitations, which are well outlined by the authors, including uncertainty about the temporal sequence between the assault and the attempted suicide. Although the finding requires replication, the study did assess a community sample, which eliminates some of the biases inherent in studying treatment-seeking clinical samples.

These 2 studies, along with the study by Virkkunen et al,[31] add to the growing body of evidence that certain events or situations that occur during critical developmental periods in childhood may predispose some individuals to be violent when they become adolescents or adults. Early misconduct characterized by aggression, stealing, lying, and dishonesty has been perhaps most strongly associated with later antisocial behaviors.[41] Familial criminal behavior appears to be another strong risk factor.[41] Other risk factors have included deficiencies in childhood health and neurologic status (prenatal or perinatal complications, minor physical anomalies, head injury, and exposure to toxins such as lead); early academic skills (IQ, learning disabilities, motor skills development); and family functioning and parenting style (child abuse, family discord, poor marital relations, large family size, and excessively punitive, restrictive, rejecting, or neglectful parents).[41] Superimposed on these are issues of culture, social class, and poverty.

After reading these studies in this issue, it is tempting to propose a wide range of early interventions that might include extensive prenatal care, nutritional programs, lead screening, home-visiting outreach programs, parenting classes, or preschool educational activities. It is unclear if any such expensive programs applied individually on a massive scale would result in any decrease in violence years hence. First, it is hard to prove that any of the early childhood risk factors cause violence, since most children with any one or several of them do not grow up to be violent adults.[41] The time delay between these factors and later violence, along with the potential for many intervening variables, makes proving causation more problematic.[41] Second, many of these factors are highly intercorrelated. While this does nothing to help us sort out which of these variables are truly independent, it does mean that there are probably a large number of children with many of them who presumably constitute a group with high risk for violence. It may be more likely that early interventions will be most successful if they are targeted to the highest risk group and then applied broadly in all spheres.[41] From the standpoint of preventing adult violence, it does little good to screen children for lead poisoning alone if they then have to return to families who abuse them.

WHAT MIGHT WE CONCLUDE?

It is critical that we place the link between violence and crime and mental illness in the proper perspective. The way in which we view this link will profoundly color our perception of how the criminal justice, mental health, and social service systems should interact. More important, our understanding of the nuances of the link is crucial if we are to ensure that stigmatization of persons with mental illness is not increased further.

First, I, like others in this field,[2,4] believe we must recognize that the link is a real one and that it persists even after controlling for demographic and probably socioeconomic variables. The link appears strongest for the severe mental illnesses, particularly those involving psychosis, and, as for those persons without diagnosed mental illness, it is increased by the use of alcohol and other psychoactive substances. It is likely that active symptoms, particularly distorted perceptions, faulty reasoning, and disordered modulation of affect are more important than the label of a specific diagnosis. This has important implications for the assessment of dangerousness in patients who are noncompliant with treatment.[5] Thus, it is likely that the violence associated with mental illness is not a fixed odds ratio, but rather varies with time, depending on symptoms and situations.[4] There are undoubtedly genetic, neurochemical, and neuroanatomical substrates that interact with early environmental influences in childhood that contribute additively, if not synergistically, to increase the risk for violence in persons with mental illness, particularly in those who repeat their violence. However, not all violence or crime perpetrated by mentally ill persons is the inevitable result of faulty brain wiring or bad upbringing. Clearly, violence and crime occur in a social, cultural, and situational context for the mentally ill as much as for the "normal" population. For example, mental patients drawn from the larger US society are more likely to be violent in psychiatric hospitals in the United States than patients drawn from Swedish or British society who are hospitalized in their respective institutions.[42] Social and moral rules about behavior, the likelihood of apprehension, the severity of punishment, the accessibility of firearms, the immediate availability of alcohol and other drugs, the characteristics of the physical setting, the personality of the people involved, the presence of racial and religious discrimination, economic inequality, poverty, and crowding all influence the likelihood of violence.[7]

It must be emphasized that the magnitude of the association between violence and mental illness, however statistically significant, is still modest when it is compared with other factors such as age, sex, educational level, or socioeconomic status. In short, violence would be reduced more effectively by a policy that locks up all men in the United States than by one that locks up all persons with mental illness. This theme issue focuses specifically on violence and mental illness. However, we must not forget that violent and criminal acts directly attributable to mental illness account for a very small proportion of all such acts in the United States, most of which involve drug deals, disputes, ongoing criminality, and domestic arguments. Most persons with mental illness are not criminals, and of those who are, most are not violent. They are probably more likely to be victims of violence themselves than to be perpetrators of it. Moreover, when they are violent, their families are more likely to be victims than are the unsuspecting persons on the street, in the workplace, in the school, or at the shopping mall.[43,44]

WHERE MIGHT WE GO?

Research on violence, crime, and mental illness must proceed. As all of us in the field know, it is not easy. First, there are the logistical hassles. The behavior is rare. The researcher studying it has to wait a long time to observe it, and when it does occur, it is at best unpleasant and at worst frightening or dangerous. Violent behavior is hard to manipulate experimentally on either an ethical level or a practical basis. There are many correlative and confounding factors that are virtually impossible to control. Then there are the political perils that confront the researcher at every turn, eg, that one will be accused of conservatism or liberalism, biological or environmental determinism, social control, genetic engineering, Darwinism, sexism, racism, stigmatization, perhaps even religious heresy.

Much of the criticism of violence research arises from the naive belief that there will be a sudden breakthrough, which, through misinterpretation for a narrow political agenda, will overturn social policy. This is unlikely, as the causes of violence, if they are ever to be found, will undoubtedly be complex and multifactorial. It is unlikely, for example, that a gene or biochemical defect will entirely explain most or even some violence. It is unlikely that violence will be found to be due to a single biochemical or environmental defect such that society must reduce the level of culpability or legal responsibility for those who are unlawful. It is also improbable, given all the neural pathways involved in violence, that a single drug will provide a treatment or a cure.

Although it may take decades to develop a unifying, coherent theory that explains the relation of violence to mental illness, most of us in the field believe certain strategies, if followed, may help put the puzzle pieces together.

First, more prospective studies of violence among mentally ill persons and demographically matched controls from the same community who are not mentally ill are needed to avoid the biases inherent in studying people already identified as mentally ill or criminal by virtue of their hospitalization, treatment, arrest, or incarceration.

Second, it may prove more fruitful to study temperaments, dimensional psychological traits such as impulsivity, and active symptoms such as hallucinations, delusions, or uncontrollable anger than specific categorical disorders such as schizophrenia, major depression, or alcoholism.[11]

Third, a typology of violent behavior is needed.[27] The violence perpetrated by a young man who holds up a convenience store for the eighth time is different from that of an elderly women who strikes out with her cane at perceived demons. Paradoxically, only by studying violence further can we type it, but only by typing it can we advance our study of it. The ideal nosology would be comprehensive but not unwieldy. Many proposed classifications measure different aspects such as the form of violence (physical vs verbal); the frequency (transient vs persistent)[45]; the perceived motive (instrumental vs hostile or defensive)[46,47]; the internal physiological changes of the perpetrator (targeted predatory behavior characterized by the absence of sympathetic arousal vs more diffuse, affective responses characterized by sympathetic arousal, vocalization, and affective display)[48]; or social purpose (economic vs systemic).[49]

Fourth, the genetic, neuroanatomical, and neurochemical underpinnings of violence require further exploration. While study of the serotonin system has yielded fruitful results, its interactions with other pathways, including the dopaminergic reward system, require examination. The recent discovery of a genetic strain of male mice that lacks neuronal nitric oxide synthase, and therefore lacks nitric oxidase and behaves in an unusually aggressive manner, suggests new neurotransmitter systems that warrant investigation.[50]

Fifth, we must study how violence, itself, begets further violence.[27] One of the strongest predictors of future violence, after all, is past violence. Most violent acts are committed by a small number of individuals who are recurrently violent—either the criminal recidivist or the mentally ill repeat offender. These studies would not only mitigate the problem with the low base rate of violence, but would be likely to have the greatest impact in reducing overall levels of violence in society. Does exposure to repeated violence in the community, news media, or entertainment media affect those who are repeatedly violent differently from those who are not? The link between violence and suicide, perhaps most vividly seen in cases of murder-suicide, also merits further exploration.[51]

Finally, it is increasingly apparent that violence cannot be explained exclusively by nature or nurture. Nor necessarily, does nature always precede nurture (remember the crayfish). New ideas about how the environment may restructure the brain must be entertained. For example, could either the perpetration of or exposure to repeated violence rewire neural circuits? Is there a kindling phenomenon in which cumulative effects of low-level stimulation over time lower the threshold for aggression and induce more violent responses later?[28] This will be particularly important in understanding how early developmental factors influence the risk of later violence.

HOW FAR CAN WE GO?

Perhaps we may recognize some day that not every act of violence and crime perpetrated by persons with mental illness has anything to do with biology, environment, or even mental illness. Some mentally ill persons, like everyone else, can be just plain mean sometimes. This statement is not meant to denigrate those with mental disorders. Rather, it is meant to recognize their fundamental humanness. Perhaps it is in our nature, whether we are mentally ill or not, to have a tremendous potential for goodness and a profound capacity for evil.

Peter M. Marzuk, MD
Associate Editor

I am particularly grateful to Kenneth Tardiff, MD, MPH, who has taught me much about the study of violence. I am also indebted to the thoughtful insights in the writings of A. Blumstein, P. Brain, P. Cook, F. Earls, B. Eichelman, J. Fagan, P. Goldstein, A. Kellerman, B. Link, C. Loftin, J. Mercy, J. Monahan, E. Mulvey, A. Reiss, H. Steadman, K. Tardiff, J. Q. Wilson, W. J. Wilson, M. Wolfgang, F. Zimring, and St Augustine.

REFERENCES

1. Rosen G. *Madness in Society: Chapters in the Historical Sociology of Mental Illness.* Chicago, Ill: The University of Chicago Press; 1968:100.
2. Monahan J. Mental disorder and violent behavior: perceptions and evidence. *Am Psychol.* 1992;47:511-521.
3. Deutsch A. *The Mentally Ill in America: A History of Their Care and Treatment From Colonial Times.* 2nd ed. New York, NY: Columbia University Press; 1949: 59.
4. Mulvey EP. Assessing the evidence of a link between mental illness and violence. *Hosp Community Psychiatry.* 1994;45:663-668.
5. Torrey EF. Violent behavior by individuals with serious mental illness. *Hosp Community Psychiatry.* 1994;45:652-662.
6. Rabkin J. Criminal behavior of discharged mental patients. *Psychol Bull.* 1979; 86:1-27.
7. Fagan J. Interactions among drugs, alcohol, and violence. *Health Aff (Millwood).* 1993;12:65-79.
8. Link BG, Cullen FT, Frank J, Wozniak JF. The social rejection of former mental patients: understanding why labels matter. *Am J Sociol.* 1987;92:1461-1500.
9. Swanson JW, Holzer CE, Ganju VK, Jono RT. Violence and psychiatric disorders in the community: evidence from the Epidemiologic Catchment Area survey. *Hosp Community Psychiatry.* 1990;41:761-770.
10. Swanson J. Mental disorder, substance abuse, and community violence. In: Monahan J, Steadman HJ, eds. *Violence and Mental Disorders: Developments in Risk Assessment.* Chicago, Ill: The University of Chicago Press; 1994.
11. Link BG, Andrews H, Cullen FT. The violent and illegal behavior of mental patients reconsidered. *Am Sociol Rev.* 1992;57:275-292.
12. Reiss AJ, Roth JA. Measuring and counting violent crimes and their consequences. In: Reiss AJ, Roth JA, eds. *Understanding and Preventing Violence.* Washington, DC: National Academy Press; 1993:404-429.
13. Hodgins S, Mednick SA, Brennan PA, Schulsinger F, Engberg M. Mental disorder and crime: evidence from a Danish birth cohort. *Arch Gen Psychiatry.* 1996;53:489-496.
14. Eronen M, Hakola P, Tiihonen J. Mental disorders and homicidal behavior in Finland. *Arch Gen Psychiatry.* 1996;53:497-501.
15. Wolfgang ME. Foreword. In: Mednick SA, Christiansen KO, eds. *Biosocial Bases of Criminal Behavior.* New York, NY: Gardener Press; 1977.
16. Teplin LA, Abram KM, McClelland GM. The prevalence of psychiatric disorder among incarcerated women: pretrial jail detainees. *Arch Gen Psychiatry.* 1996; 53:505-512.
17. Jordan BK, Schlenger WE, Fairbank JA, Caddell JM. Prevalence of psychiatric disorders among incarcerated women: convicted women felons entering prison. *Arch Gen Psychiatry.* 1996;53:513-519.
18. Teplin LA. The prevalence of severe mental disorder among male urban jail detainees: comparison with the Epidemiologic Catchment Area program. *Am J Public Health.* 1990;80:663-669.
19. Teplin LA. Psychiatric and substance abuse disorders among male urban jail detainees. *Am J Public Health.* 1994;8:290-293.
20. Lamb HR, Grant RW. The mentally ill in an urban county jail. *Arch Gen Psychiatry.* 1982;39:17-22.
21. Reiss AJ, Roth JA. Patterns of violence in American society. In: Reiss AJ, Roth JA, eds. *Understanding and Preventing Violence.* Washington, DC: National Academy Press; 1993:42-97.
22. Gilliard DK, Beck AJ. *Prisoners in 1993.* Washington, DC: Bureau of Justice Statistics; 1994. Bulletin NCJ-147036.
23. Tardiff K, Sweillam A. Assaultive behavior among chronic inpatients. *Am J Psychiatry.* 1982;139:212-215.
24. Binder RL, McNeil DE. The relationship of gender to violent behavior in acutely disturbed psychiatric patients. *J Clin Psychiatry.* 1990;51:110-114.
25. Tardiff K. The current state of psychiatry in the treament of violent patients. *Arch Gen Psychiatry.* 1992;49:493-499.
26. Elliot FA. Violence, the neurologic contribution: an overview. *Arch Neurol.* 1992; 49:595-603.
27. Eichelman B. Aggressive behavior, from laboratory to clinic: quo vadit? *Arch Gen Psychiatry.* 1992;49:488-492.
28. Garza-Trevino ES. Neurobiological factors in aggressive behavior. *Hosp Community Psychiatry.* 1994;45:690-699.
29. Brunner HG, Nelen M, Breakfield XO, Ropers HH, van Oost BA. Abnormal behavior associated with a point mutation in the structural gene for monoamine oxidase A. *Science.* 1993;262:578-580.
30. Virkkunen M, Eggert M, Rawlings R, Linnoila M. A prospective follow-up study of alcoholic violent offenders and fire setters. *Arch Gen Psychiatry.* 1996;53: 523-529.
31. Virkkunen M, De Jong J, Bartko J, Goodwin FK, Linnoila M. Relationship of psychobiological variables to recidivism in violent offenders and impulsive fire setters: a follow-up study. *Arch Gen Psychiatry.* 1989;46:600-603.
32. Linnoila M, Virkkunen M. Aggression, suicidality, and serotonin. *J Clin Psychiatry.* 1992;53(suppl 1):46-51.
33. Coccaro EF, Kavoussi RJ, Sheline YI, Lish JD, Csernansky JB. Impulsive aggression in personality disorder correlates with tritiated paroxetine binding in the platelet. *Arch Gen Psychiatry.* 1996;53:531-536.
34. Lesch KP, Wolozin BL, Murphy DL, Riederer P. Primary structure of the human platelet serotonin uptake site: identity with the brain serotonin transporter. *J Neurochemistry.* 1993;60:2319-2322.
35. Higley JD, Mehlman PT, Taub DM, Higley SB, Fernald B, Vickers J, Lindell SG, Suomi SJ, Linnoila M. Excessive mortality in young free-ranging male nonhuman primates with low cerebrospinal fluid 5-hydroxyindolacetic acid concentrations. *Arch Gen Psychiatry.* 1996;53:537-543.
36. Wolfgang ME. Victim-precipitated criminal homicide. *J Criminal Law Criminal Police Sci.* 1957;48:1-11.
37. Brain PF, Haug M. Hormonal and neurochemical correlates of various forms of animal 'aggression.' *Psychoneuroendocrinology.* 1992;17:537-551.
38. Yeh SR, Fricke RA, Edwards DH. The effect of social experience on serotonergic modulation of the escape circuit of crayfish. *Science.* 1996;217:366-369.
39. Raine A, Brennan P, Mednick B, Mednick SA. High rates of violence, crime, academic problems, and behavioral problems in males with both early neuromotor deficits and unstable family environments. *Arch Gen Psychiatry.* 1996; 53:544-549.
40. Davidson JRT, Hughes DC, George LK, Blazer DG. The association of sexual assault and attempted suicide within the community. *Arch Gen Psychiatry.* 1996; 53:550-555.
41. Buka S, Earls F. Early determinants of delinquency and violence. *Health Aff (Millwood).* 1993;12:46-63.
42. Lion JR, Reid WH, eds. *Assaults Within Psychiatric Facilities.* New York, NY: Grune & Stratton; 1983.
43. Straznickas KA, McNeil DE, Binder RL. Violence toward family caregivers by mentally ill relatives. *Hosp Community Psychiatry.* 1993;44:385-387.
44. Tardiff K. Characteristics of assaultive patients in private hospitals. *Am J Psychiatry.* 1984;141:1232-1235.
45. Krakowski MI, Czobor P. Clinical symptoms, neurological impairment, and prediction of violence in psychiatric inpatients. *Hosp Community Psychiatry.* 1994; 45:700-705.
46. Moyer KE. Kinds of aggression and their physiological basis. *Community Behav Biol A.* 1968;2:65-87.
47. Valzelli L. *Psychobiology of Aggression and Violence.* New York, NY: Raven Press; 1981.
48. Reis D. Central neurotransmitters in aggression. *Res Publ Assoc Res Nerv Ment Dis.* 1974;52:119-148.
49. Goldstein PJ, Brownstein HH, Ryan PJ, Bellucci PA. Crack and homicide in New York City, 1988: a conceptually based event analysis. *Contemp Drug Prob.* 1989;16:651-687.
50. Nelson RJ, Demas GE, Huang PL, Fishman MC, Dawson VL, Dawson TM, Snyder SH. Behavioral abnormalities in male mice lacking neuronal nitric oxide synthase. *Nature.* 1995;378:383-386.
51. Marzuk PM, Tardiff K, Hirsch CS. The epidemiology of murder-suicide. *JAMA.* 1992;267:3179-3183.

Mental Disorder and Crime

Evidence From a Danish Birth Cohort

Sheilagh Hodgins, PhD; Sarnoff A. Mednick, DrMed, PhD; Patricia A. Brennan, PhD; Fini Schulsinger, MD; Marianne Engberg, MD, PhD

Background: Evidence has accumulated since the mid 1960s from a number of different countries indicating an association between mental disorder and crime and particularly between the major mental disorders and violence. Registries in Denmark were used to identify a birth cohort and to document all psychiatric admissions and all criminal proceedings of the 324 401 members of this cohort up to the age of 43 years.

Methods: Persons who had been admitted to a psychiatric ward were assigned to a diagnostic category according to a hierarchy of principal discharge diagnoses. They were compared with persons never admitted to a psychiatric ward as to the prevalence, type, and frequency of criminal convictions.

Results: Women and men who had been hospitalized in psychiatric wards were more likely to have been convicted of a criminal offense than persons with no history of psychiatric hospitalization. The offenders who were hospitalized committed all types and, on average, as many offenses as did the never-hospitalized group of the same sex.

Conclusions: These findings confirm those from 2 other post–World War II Scandinavian birth cohorts that have found an association between psychiatric hospitalization and criminal convictions. They also concur with findings that patients discharged from psychiatric wards are more likely than other persons living in the same community to commit crimes and with results from North America showing elevated rates of major mental disorders among incarcerated offenders. Generalization of these findings is limited to nations with similar criminal justice, mental health, and social welfare systems.

(Arch Gen Psychiatry. 1996;53:489-496)

From the Department of Psychology, Université de Montréal, Quebec (Dr Hodgins); Department of Psychology (Dr Mednick) and Social Science Research Institute (Dr Brennan), University of Southern California, Los Angeles; Institute for Preventive Medicine, Kommunehospitalet, Copenhagen, Denmark (Drs Mednick and Schulsinger); and the Institute of Psychiatric Demography, Aarhus, Denmark (Dr Engberg).

EVIDENCE HAS been accumulating in recent years to indicate that persons who suffer from mental disorders are at increased risk of criminality generally, and at even greater risk of violent criminality. Since the 1960s, several follow-up studies of patients discharged from psychiatric wards have been conducted in the United States and Scandinavia. All have consistently found that proportionately more of the former patients than the nondisordered persons living in the same neighborhood had been convicted of offenses.[1-12] Further, follow-up studies of discharged patients document high rates of aggressive behavior.[12,13] Recent investigations of representative samples of US prison inmates[14-17] and Canadian penitentiary inmates[18] have revealed higher prevalence rates of mental disorders, particularly of the major mental disorders such as schizophrenia and major affective disorders, within these facilities than in the general population. Most of the major mental disorders were present before the current period of incarceration.[18,19] Four investigations conducted in Scandinavia and Canada documented even higher prevalence rates of major mental disorders among homicide offenders.[20-23] In addition, 2 investigations of Scandinavian birth cohorts followed up to ages 23[24] and 30[25] years compared the prevalence of convictions for criminal offenses among persons with and without admissions to psychiatric wards. All found higher rates of convictions among both men and women who had been admitted with a diagnosis of major mental disorder than among those with no admissions. In the largest of these studies,[25] it was found that the men and women with major mental disorders were at even greater risk to be convicted of violent than nonviolent offenses; that they had committed, on

See Methods on next page

METHODS

The person-register of Denmark, which includes data on everyone born in the country or who immigrates to Denmark, was screened to identify all persons born between January 1, 1944, and December 31, 1947. This procedure identified 358 180 individuals. When the subjects were 43 years old, the psychiatric register was screened to identify all the subjects' admissions to psychiatric wards, dates of admission and discharge, and discharge diagnoses (*International Classification of Diseases, Eighth Revision*). This register includes all admissions to all psychiatric wards within Denmark.[33] At the same time, the national police register was screened to identify all arrests and convictions. This register includes information on all criminal proceedings in Denmark. An eminent US criminologist, Marvin Wolfgang, has noted that "the criminal registry office in Denmark is probably the most thorough, comprehensive, and accurate in the Western world."[34] Findings reported here are based on court convictions for infractions of penal law. It was decided to use convictions rather than arrests because they require proof of guilt, are a more conservative measure of criminality, and may be less subject to bias that has been found to characterize at least one US police force.[35] Once the information from the psychiatric and criminal registers had been computerized, a third party named by the Minister of Justice merged the 2 tapes and de-identified the information. Excluded from the analyses presented here are 12 019 persons who had emigrated from Denmark before the end of the follow-up period and 11 761 persons for whom data were incomplete. Excluded as well were the 9999 persons who had died. Death rates varied by sex and by type of mental disorder.

The first step in the data analysis was to divide the subjects into 8 groups, 7 groups who had been admitted to a psychiatric ward at least once and 1 group who had never been admitted. The group with major mental disorders (MMD) included all subjects having at least 1 discharge diagnosis of schizophrenia, manic-depressive psychosis, psychogenic psychosis, or other psychosis. The group with mental retardation (MR) was defined to include all subjects with no diagnosis of an MMD who had a diagnosis of "oligophrenia." The group with organic disorders (ORG) included all subjects with no diagnosis of MMD or MR and who had a diagnosis of presenile or senile psychosis or psychosis due to vascular disease, syphilis, or epilepsy. The group with antisocial personality disorder (APD) included all subjects with no diagnosis of MMD, MR, or ORG with a diagnosis of antisocial personality disorder. The group with drug use disorders (DRG) included all subjects with no diagnosis of MMD, MR, ORG, or APD who had a diagnosis of drug addiction. The group with alcohol use disorders (ALC) included all subjects with no diagnosis of MMD, MR, ORG, APD, or DRG who had a diagnosis of alcoholism. The group with other mental disorders (OMD) included subjects who had been admitted to a psychiatric ward but who had no diagnosis of MMD, MR, ORG, APD, DRG, or ALC. Thus, the diagnostic groups were constructed using a hierarchy of diagnoses (MMD, MR, ORG, APD, DRG, ALC, OMD) and taking account of only 1 diagnosis per subject, the diagnosis that was highest in the hierarchy. The nondisordered group (NMD) included all subjects who had never been admitted to a psychiatric ward.

The cohort was composed of 158 799 women and 165 602 men who were alive and had been living in Denmark at least until their 43rd birthdays. Among the women, 2.5% (3900) of the subjects were assigned to the MMD group, 0.2% (318) to the MR group, 0.0004% (73) to the ORG group, 2.2% (3553) to the APD group, 0.2% (249) to the DRG group, 0.4% (568) to the ALC group, 1.7% (2771) to the OMD group, and 92.8% (147 367) to the NMD group. Among the men, 1.9% (3130) were assigned to the MMD group, 0.2% (297) to the MR group, 0.1% (101) to the ORG group, 1.9% (3069) to the APD group, 0.1% (208) to the DRG group, 1.0% (1731) to the ALC group, 0.9% (1486) to the OMD group, and 93.9% (155 580) to the NMD group.

A very strict definition of crime was used. All offenses in the penal code were included, except those referring to suicide and consensual sexual relations between persons of the same sex. All offenses against other laws, such as special laws, traffic laws, tax laws, and administrative laws were excluded. All crimes in the penal code were classified into 7 categories: violent offenses (all offenses involving interpersonal aggression or a threat thereof), theft of all kinds, fraud, vandalism, traffic offenses included in the criminal code (stealing a vehicle and driving it), all drug-related offenses, and all "other" criminal offenses.

Relative risk (RR) estimates for conviction of a criminal offense and for conviction of a violent offense were calculated, comparing each diagnostic group with the NMD group, who had never been admitted to a psychiatric ward. When examining types of crimes, mean numbers of offenses, and age at first conviction, each group was compared with the NMD group. The α levels of significance were adjusted using the Bonferroni formula to avoid errors due to multiple comparisons. These adjustments are noted on the tables or in the text.

average, more or as many offenses as nondisordered offenders of the same sex; and that they committed all types of offenses.

The purpose of the present investigation was to replicate and extend the previous findings in an effort to further understand the relations among the various mental disorders and criminality. To address this issue, the most powerful research design is to examine the prevalence and distribution of criminality and mental disorders in an unselected birth cohort. Consequently, this design was adopted. All criminal convictions and all admissions to psychiatric wards were examined for an unselected Danish birth cohort followed up to age 43 years.

This investigation corrected many of the weaknesses of the earlier birth cohort studies. The cohort was 24 times larger than the largest cohort studied to date, thereby increasing the validity of the findings and allowing for examination of more specific categories of mental disorders. The subjects in the present investigation had passed through the risk periods for criminality and for all mental disorders other than those associated with aging.[26] The age of the subjects would allow verifi-

Table 1. Percentages of Female and Male Subjects Registered for at Least 1 Crime

Group*	1959-1977 Percent	1959-1977 Relative Risk Estimate (95% Confidence Interval)	1978-1990 Percent	1978-1990 Relative Risk Estimate (95% Confidence Interval)
Female Subjects (N=158 799)				
NMD (n=147 367)	1.3	...	2.1	...
MMD (n=3900)	4.4	3.37 (2.89-3.93)	9.5	4.50 (4.06-4.99)
MR (n=318)	13.5	10.40 (7.85-13.78)	11.6	5.53 (4.08-7.51)
ORG (n=73)	4.1	3.16 (1.04-9.58)	9.6	4.56 (2.25-9.23)
APD (n=3553)	7.0	5.41 (4.76-6.15)	13.6	6.45 (5.90-7.06)
DRG (n=249)	8.8	6.80 (4.55-10.15)	23.7	11.27 (8.99-14.12)
ALC (n=568)	6.7	5.15 (3.77-7.02)	18.7	8.88 (7.45-10.58)
OMD (n=2771)	4.0	3.08 (2.55-3.72)	7.8	3.69 (3.23-4.22)
Male Subjects (N=165 602)				
NMD (n=155 580)	8.3	...	6.1	...
MMD (n=3130)	19.1	2.29 (2.13-2.47)	23.0	3.74 (3.49-3.99)
MR (n=297)	46.8	5.61 (4.97-6.34)	42.4	6.90 (6.03-7.89)
ORG (n=101)	27.7	3.32 (2.42-4.56)	31.7	5.15 (3.87-6.86)
APD (n=3069)	34.7	4.16 (3.95-4.38)	32.4	5.27 (4.99-5.57)
DRG (n=208)	45.2	5.42 (4.66-6.30)	46.2	7.50 (6.47-8.70)
ALC (n=1731)	29.1	3.48 (3.23-3.76)	35.8	5.82 (5.45-6.22)
OMD (n=1486)	20.6	2.47 (2.23-2.73)	16.7	2.71 (2.42-3.05)

**NMD indicates nondisordered group; MMD, major mental disorders; MR, mental retardation; ORG, organic disorders (see "Methods" section for more detailed explanation); APD, antisocial personality disorder; DRG, drug use disorders; ALC, alcohol use disorders; and OMD, other mental disorders. Ellipses indicate not applicable.*

cation of the often cited finding that persons with major disorders commit crimes later in life than do nondisordered individuals.[18,27-32] The present study also included all hospitalizations, even those ordered by a criminal court.

RESULTS

The national police data recording procedure changed in 1978, when a computerized system was instituted. We interviewed relevant police officials regarding any effects of this change and were informed that some arrests and convictions in 1978 may not be in the register owing to start-up errors. These errors were due to operator inexperience with the equipment and were not biased with respect to characteristics of offenders. It should also be noted that because of the ease of recording with the computerized system, more minor offenses were registered after 1978. To ensure that the results of the present investigation are valid, all analyses were conducted separately for the manual criminal register and for the computerized register.

PREVALENCE OF CRIMINALITY BY DIAGNOSTIC GROUP

The percentages of female and male subjects in each group who were convicted of at least 1 offense are presented in **Table 1**. For the early period, 1959 through 1977 (when files were recorded by hand), and for the later period, 1978 through 1990 (when the files were computerized), the RR ratios indicate that the differences between diagnostic groups and the nondisordered group are larger among the female subjects than among the male subjects. Among the women, all diagnostic groups were found to be at significantly increased risk of criminality compared with the NMD group, with RR estimates varying from 3.08 to 10.4 up to 1977 and from 3.69 to 11.27 from 1978 through 1990. Among the men, all diagnostic groups were found to be at significantly increased risk of a criminal conviction compared with the NMD group, with RR estimates varying from 2.29 to 5.61 for the period ending in 1977 and from 2.71 to 7.50 for the period from 1978 through 1990.

These same analyses (the percentages of men and women within each diagnostic group who were convicted of at least 1 crime and the corresponding RR estimates) were recalculated, dividing subjects into 4 groups according to their year of birth. The percentages of men and women within each diagnostic group who were convicted of at least 1 offense were found to be relatively stable across the 4 birth years and very similar to those presented for the entire cohort. The percentages of subjects within the 7 diagnostic groups who were convicted of an offense varied more across the 4 birth years among the female than among the male subjects. This is probably owing to the smaller number of female subjects who were convicted.

TYPES OF CRIMES

Table 2 and **Table 3** present the percentages of subjects in each group who were convicted of different types of offenses. As can be observed in these tables, among both the female and the male subjects and during both time periods, the offenders in the various diagnostic groups were convicted of all kinds of offenses. There is no evidence of specialization of crime by diagnostic groups.

Only the group differences that are statistically sig-

Table 2. Percentages of Female Subjects* Convicted for Different Types of Offenses, 1959-1977† and 1978-1990‡§

Group	Violent 1959-1977	Violent 1978-1990	Theft 1959-1977	Theft 1978-1990	Fraud 1959-1977	Fraud 1978-1990	Vandalism 1959-1977	Vandalism 1978-1990	Traffic 1959-1977	Traffic 1978-1990
NMD (n=147 367)	0.1	0.1	0.9	1.4	0.3	0.5	0	0	0.1	0
MMD (n=3900)	0.5	0.9	2.6	5.7	1.1	1.9	0.1	0.9	0.4	0.2
MR (n=318)	0.6	1.3	9.7	8.5	3.1	2.5	0.3	0.6	0.3	0
ORG (n=73)	0	0	4.1	5.5	1.4	5.5	0	0	0	0
APD (n=3553)	0.6	1.3	4.7	9.3	2.0	3.9	0.1	0.7	0.4	0.1
DRG (n=249)	0.8	1.6	6.4	17.3	3.2	8.8	0	1.2	0	0
ALC (n=568)	0.5	1.6	4.4	13.0	1.8	5.5	0	0.9	0.5	0.4
OMD (n=2771)	0.5	0.4	2.5	4.7	1.0	2.4	0	0.4	0.1	0

**See footnotes to Table 1 for explanation of abbreviations for subject groups.*

†χ^2 Comparisons for 1959-1977: NMD vs MMD: all comparisons P>.000 except drug P>.01; NMD vs MR: all comparisons P>.000 except violent P>.001, drug P>.005, and traffic P>.05; NMD vs ORG: all comparisons not significant (NS) except theft P>.005; NMD vs APD: all comparisons P>.000; NMD vs DRG: all comparisons P>.000 except vandalism and traffic, which are NS; NMD vs ALC: all comparisons P>.000 except others P>.005 and vandalism and drug which are NS; and NMD vs OMD: all comparisons P>.000 except others P>.01, vandalism P>.05, and traffic which is NS.

‡χ^2 Comparisons for 1978-1990: NMD vs MMD: all comparisons P>.000 except drug P>.001; NMD vs MR: all comparisons P>.000 except traffic, which is NS; NMD vs ORG: all comparisons NS except fraud P>.000 and theft P>.005; NMD vs APD: all comparisons P>.000; NMD vs DRG: all comparisons P>.000 except traffic, which is NS; NMD vs ALC: all comparisons P>.000 except drug P>.01; and NMD vs OMD: all comparisons P>.000 except traffic, which is NS.

§Note: Using the Bonferroni formula to correct for errors due to multiple comparisons in the 2 preceding footnotes, P=.05 becomes P=.007; P=.01 becomes P=.001; and P=.001 becomes P=.0001.

Table 3. Percentages of Male Subjects* Convicted for Different Types of Offenses, 1959-1977† and 1978-1990‡§

Group	Violent 1959-1977	Violent 1978-1990	Theft 1959-1977	Theft 1978-1990	Fraud 1959-1977	Fraud 1978-1990	Vandalism 1959-1977	Vandalism 1978-1990	Traffic 1959-1977	Traffic 1978-1990
NMD (n=155 580)	1.9	1.5	4.7	2.7	1.3	1.7	0.4	0.4	2.1	0.2
MMD (n=3130)	4.7	6.7	10.9	10.6	4.6	5.4	1.8	4.8	5.5	1.2
MR (n=297)	11.4	11.4	32.3	26.9	10.4	13.1	1.0	7.1	16.2	2.4
ORG (n=101)	5.0	4.0	20.8	20.8	5.9	7.9	1.0	5.9	8.9	1.0
APD (n=3069)	10.4	10.8	22.9	17.8	11.4	12.5	2.3	4.5	11.5	2.5
DRG (n=208)	11.5	13.0	35.1	31.3	13.0	15.9	4.3	7.2	18.8	4.8
ALC (n=1731)	8.1	10.0	18.8	18.3	7.5	11.8	1.7	4.6	9.4	2.2
OMD (n=1486)	4.6	4.7	11.7	7.2	4.9	5.2	1.1	1.4	5.5	0.8

**See footnotes to Table 1 for explanation of abbreviations for subject groups.*

†χ^2 Comparisons for 1959-1977: NMD vs MMD: all comparisons P>.000; NMD vs MR: all comparisons P>.000 except vandalism, which is not significant (NS); NMD vs ORG: all comparisons P>.000 except others P>.005, violent P>.05, and vandalism and drug, which are NS; NMD vs APD: all comparisons P>.000; NMD vs DRG: all comparisons P>.000; NMD vs ALC: all comparisons P>.000; and NMD vs OMD: all comparisons P>.000.

‡χ^2 Comparisons for 1978-1990: NMD vs MMD: all comparisons P>.000; NMD vs MR: all comparisons P>.000; NMD vs ORG: all comparisons P>.000 except violent P>.05, traffic P>.05, and drug, which is NS; NMD vs APD: all comparisons P>.000; NMD vs DRG: all comparisons P>.000; NMD vs ALC: all comparisons P>.000; and NMD vs OMD: all comparisons P>.000.

§Note: Using the Bonferroni formula to correct for errors due to multiple comparisons, P=.05 becomes P=.007; P=.01 becomes P=.001; and P=.001 becomes P=.0001.

nificant at levels corrected to account for multiple comparisons (7 per group) were accepted as indicating differences.

For the female subjects, for both time periods, proportionately more of the MMD group than the NMD group had been convicted of all types of offenses except those related to drugs. Proportionately more of the MR women than the NMD women were convicted for theft, fraud, van-

Drug		Others	
1959-1977	1978-1990	1959-1977	1978-1990
0	0	0.1	0.2
0.1	0.1	0.4	1.3
0.3	0.3	1.6	1.6
0	0	0	0
0.3	0.2	0.8	1.5
0.4	0.8	1.2	2.8
0	0.2	0.5	1.6
0.1	0.1	0.3	1.0

Drug		Others	
1959-1977	1978-1990	1959-1977	1978-1990
0.4	0.1	0.6	1.1
1.1	0.6	1.7	7.0
8.1	1.3	6.7	12.5
1.0	0	3.0	5.0
3.5	1.0	4.2	9.3
6.3	3.8	4.3	11.1
2.4	0.5	2.5	9.5
1.8	0.8	2.8	3.8

dalism, and offenses classified as "other" during the early period and for all types of offenses except those related to traffic during the later period. Proportionately more of the women in the ORG group than those in the NMD group were convicted of theft during the early period and of fraud and theft during the later period. Proportionately more of the APD women than the NMD women were convicted of all types of offenses during both the early and late periods. Proportionately more of the DRG women than the NMD women were convicted of all offenses except vandalism and traffic in the early period, and of all types of offenses except traffic during the later period. Proportionately more of the ALC women than the NMD women were convicted of all types of offenses except those classified as other, drug-related, and vandalism in the early period and of all types of offenses except those related to drugs during the later period. Proportionately more of the OMD women as compared with the NMD women were convicted of violence, theft, fraud, and drug-related offenses during the early period, and of all types of offenses except traffic during the later period.

Among the men, during both time periods, more of the MMD, APD, DRG, ALC, and OMD subjects compared with the NMD group had been convicted of all 7 types of offenses. This was also true of the MR group during the later period. During the early period, more of the MR subjects than the NMD subjects had been convicted of all types of offenses other than vandalism. More of the men in the ORG group than those in the NMD group had been convicted of theft, fraud, and traffic offenses during the early period and for theft, fraud, vandalism, and offenses classified as other during the later period.

Table 4 presents the percentages of subjects in each group who were convicted of at least 1 violent offense. The RR estimates indicate that for both women and men, all the diagnostic groups except the ORG group are at increased risk of violence compared with the NMD group. Among the ORG subjects, no woman had been convicted of a violent offense, and among the men the risk ratios and their confidence intervals indicate that there is no increased risk for violent offenses.

NUMBER OF OFFENSES

The average number of convictions of the offenders within each diagnostic group were compared with the average number of convictions of the same-sex NMD offenders. Only differences that were statistically significant at the P=.01 level after Bonferroni correction (P=.001) to protect against errors due to multiple comparisons are reported.

Among the female subjects, during the early period, only the APD subjects had accumulated, on average, more convictions for criminal offenses than the NMD subjects. During the later period, the MMD, APD, DRG, ALC, and OMD offenders accumulated, on average, more convictions than the NMD offenders. Among the men, during both time periods, the MMD, MR, APD, DRG, ALC, and OMD offenders accumulated, on average, more convictions than the NMD offenders.

AGE AT FIRST CONVICTION

The percentages of subjects in each group who were first convicted within 4 age periods (15-20, 21-30, 31-40, and ≥41 years) were examined. Once the level of significance was corrected to protect against chance findings

Table 4. Percentages of Female and Male Subjects Registered for at Least 1 Violent Crime

Group*	1959-1977 Percent	1959-1977 Relative Risk Estimate (95% Confidence Interval)	1978-1990 Percent	1978-1990 Relative Risk Estimate (95% Confidence Interval)
		Female Subjects (N=158 799)		
NMD (n=147 367)	0.1	...	0.1	...
MMD (n=3900)	0.5	5.86 (3.57-9.62)	0.9	8.66 (6.04-12.43)
MR (n=318)	0.6	7.99 (1.98-32.19)	1.3	11.81 (4.40-31.66)
ORG (n=73)	...	...	...	...
APD (n=3553)	0.6	7.86 (4.99-12.39)	1.3	12.15 (8.76-16.85)
DRG (n=249)	0.8	10.20 (2.54-41.06)	1.6	15.08 (5.63-40.36)
ALC (n=568)	0.5	6.71 (2.14-21.05)	1.6	14.87 (7.64-28.97)
OMD (n=2771)	0.5	5.96 (3.36-10.56)	0.4	3.39 (1.79-6.41)
		Male Subjects (N=165 602)		
NMD (n=155 580)	1.9	...	1.5	...
MMD (n=3130)	4.7	2.42 (2.06-2.84)	6.7	4.48 (3.91-5.14)
MR (n=297)	11.4	5.89 (4.29-8.10)	11.4	7.65 (5.56-10.52)
ORG (n=101)	5.0	2.55 (1.08-5.99)	4.0	2.65 (1.01-6.92)
APD (n=3069)	10.4	5.35 (4.80-5.97)	10.8	7.20 (6.46-8.04)
DRG (n=208)	11.5	5.94 (4.07-8.67)	13.0	8.67 (6.09-12.36)
ALC (n=1731)	8.1	4.19 (3.57-4.93)	10.0	6.68 (5.76-7.73)
OMD (n=1486)	4.6	2.36 (1.86-2.98)	4.7	3.15 (2.49-3.97)

**See footnotes to Table 1 for explanation of abbreviations for subject groups. Ellipses indicate not applicable.*

due to multiple comparisons, no group differences were evident.

COMMENT

In a large birth cohort followed up to age 43 years, it has been shown that individuals with a history of psychiatric hospitalization were more likely to have been convicted of a criminal offense than persons with no history of psychiatric hospitalization. This finding was true for both men and women. The results are very similar to those reported for a smaller Swedish birth cohort followed up to age 30 years. The present findings indicate that women in the MMD or MR groups are at even greater risk of violence than of criminality generally. On average, the offenders with a history of psychiatric hospitalization committed as many or more crimes than the never-hospitalized offenders. The results of the present investigation are also consistent with findings from follow-up studies of patients discharged from psychiatric wards to the community, of diagnostic studies of representative samples of convicted offenders in North America, and with diagnostic studies of unbiased cohorts of homicide offenders.

Consistent with our conservative approach, the present investigation was limited to an examination of criminal convictions, comparing subjects with mental disorders who were hospitalized with subjects never hospitalized. In the Danish system, decisions to convict an individual of a crime and to hospitalize someone for a mental disorder are independent, and consequently the interactions between the criminal justice and mental health systems do not explain the findings. In the present study and in the Swedish birth cohort study, a small number of offenses of psychotic subjects were not counted because the court considered these subjects to be too ill to prosecute. Because they were hospitalized, they would be categorized in the MMD group, but the offense would not have been counted. Considering that the present findings are limited to persons with mental disorders who were hospitalized, it is important to note that only the most severely disturbed patients receive inpatient care. Consequently, the proportions of subjects with different mental disorders who were hospitalized are thought to vary by the nature and severity of their disorder. Unfortunately, no data are available to test this proposition. Not only are hospitalized patients more severely disturbed than nonhospitalized patients with the same disorders, but patients who behave aggressively would be more likely to be hospitalized than would a quiet, nondisruptive individual with similar symptoms.[36] To date, only the diagnostic studies of convicted offenders have overcome this limitation (of using hospitalization as an indicator of mental disorder), yet the results of these studies concur with those from the present investigation and other studies that have examined the association between hospitalization and convictions.

The results of the present investigation are limited to a cohort raised after World War II. The present birth cohort study, the 2 others published to date,[24,25] the follow-up studies of patients discharged to the community, and the investigations of convicted offenders have all been conducted since 1970 and for the most part have included subjects born after World War II. There are almost no data that examine the association between mental disorder and criminality before the 1960s.[37] Prior to this time, individuals suffering from severe mental disorders were institutionalized for life. Since the 1960s, however, even persons with the most serious disorders are hospitalized for only short periods of time.[38] This change in policy in the mental health field coincided with an observed increase in crime among individuals with mental disorders.[39,40]

The subjects included in the present study, in the 2

other birth cohort studies, in the follow-up studies of discharged patients, and in the diagnostic studies of convicted offenders can be presumed to be the first generation of persons in modern times with major mental disorders to have been treated, for the most part, in the community. Further, they are the first generation to have received antipsychotic, antidepressant, and mood-stabilizing medications. Living in the community has often led to abuse of alcohol and drugs by persons with mental disorders. Among those with major mental disorders, rates of alcohol and drug use disorders exceed the rates among nondisordered individuals.[41] Alcohol and drug use increases the risk for criminality[42] and aggressive behavior[43] among both mentally disordered and nondisordered subjects. In discussing and examining this issue, it is important to distinguish between intoxication at the time of the offense and past and current secondary diagnoses of abuse or dependence. Most investigations fail to do so. Even when this information is available, its reliability and validity remain questionable. In the Swedish cohort study[10,42] and in the 4 published studies of unbiased cohorts or samples of homicide offenders,[20-23] both a history of substance abuse and intoxication were found to increase the risk for violent and nonviolent criminal behavior but failed to explain all of this behavior. In other words, recent findings suggest that the major disorders increase the risk for violent behavior, and this risk is further elevated by alcohol and drug use. For example, a recent Finnish study examined a cohort composed of 1423 homicide offenders. Schizophrenia with no secondary diagnosis of an alcohol use disorder increased the risk for homicide 7.3 times in men and 5.1 times in women. Schizophrenia with a secondary diagnosis of an alcohol use disorder increased the risk for homicide 17.2 times among men and 80.9 times among women.[22] Similar findings emerged from analyses of the Epidemiologic Catchment Area data on self-reported aggressive behavior, showing an increase in risk owing to major mental disorders in a pure form and an even greater increase in risk when the major mental disorder is combined with a substance use disorder.[43] It may also be that alcohol and other drugs in combination with certain medications lead to aggressive behavior in the presence of a major mental disorder.[44] It is important to note that the association that has been identified between substance use or abuse and criminality is not specific to subjects with major mental disorders.[45] As can be seen in Tables 2 and 3 of the present report, significant proportions of subjects with primary diagnoses of alcoholism and drug dependence committed violent offenses.

As noted, the associations between major mental disorders and criminality and violence have been documented among subjects who developed their disorders after the policy of deinstitutionalization was implemented in the mental health field. In addition to being the first generation of mentally disordered persons to be treated primarily in the community with neuroleptic medications, they may well be the first generation who during the fetal period were affected by alcohol, drugs, and medications taken by their mothers. These and other obstetrical factors have been linked to violence.[46,47]

The specific rates of crime reported in the present investigation cannot be generalized to other jurisdictions. The extent to which these results can be generalized to other jurisdictions depends in large part on the similarities of the respective criminal justice, mental health, and social service systems. Generalization of the findings will also be affected by variations in rates of premature death within different countries. It is known that the various mental disorders differentially increase rates of premature death,[48] and that antisocial subjects[49] and those with major disorders who commit crimes are at especially high risk of an early death.[50]

It has been shown in 1 jurisdiction of 1 country (United States) that the police discriminated against mentally ill subjects.[35] However, all the other evidence accumulated from several different countries suggests that it is possible, although highly unlikely, that both the police and the courts discriminate against the mentally disordered, so that for the same behavior a disordered person would be convicted and a nondisordered person not convicted. Both clinical lore and some data suggest that many instances of aggression on the part of patients are not reported to police.[51] Two US studies[12,52] show that mentally disordered subjects were less often arrested than others for certain violent offenses. Evidence suggests that the mentally disordered are not arrested for trivial offenses, but that they are arrested more often than the nondisordered because more of them behave aggressively more often.[12,13,53,54]

The relations between the various disorders and criminal behavior require further elucidation. For example, antisocial behavior at a young age, before the onset of a major mental disorder, has been reported in some proportion of subjects who develop major mental disorders and offend.[55-57] These results are consistent with findings from the present investigation and from prospective[58,59] and retrospective[56] studies indicating that aggressive and/or antisocial behavior characterizes a subgroup of children who develop schizophrenia later in life, with data from epidemiological investigations showing high rates of comorbid conduct disorder among children with affective disorders,[60] and with both retrospectively[61] and prospectively[62] collected data indicating that some proportion of men who develop bipolar disorder had evidence of a conduct disorder in childhood. The role played by alcohol and drug use and paranoid-type symptoms[63] in determining illegal behaviors may differ depending on the subject's history of antisocial behavior.[57]

It would be destructive for societies to allow the findings on the criminality of the mentally disordered and mentally retarded to be used to further stigmatize these individuals. Rather, these data can be used constructively to provide more adequate, appropriate, and humane care to individuals who, through no fault of their own, suffer from devastating disorders, and at the same time to protect society. We hope that the results of the present investigation will incite us to evaluate our understanding of the various mental disorders and to question current mental health policies. Describing the problem is the first step to solving it.

Accepted for publication February 21, 1996.

Reprints: Sheilagh Hodgins, PhD, Department of Psychology, Université de Montréal, CP 6128, Succursale Centre-ville, Montreal, Quebec H3C 3J7.

REFERENCES

1. Durbin JR, Pasewark RA, Albers D. Criminality and mental illness: a study of current arrest rates in a rural state. *Am J Psychiatry.* 1977;134:80-83.
2. Giovannoni JM, Gurel L. Socially disruptive behavior of ex-mental patients. *Arch Gen Psychiatry.* 1967;17:146-153.
3. Rappeport JR, Lassen G. Dangerousness arrest rate comparisons of discharged patients and the general population. *Am J Psychiatry.* 1965;121:776-783.
4. Rappeport JR, Lassen G. The dangerousness of female patients: a comparison of the arrest rate of discharged psychiatric patients and the general population. *Am J Psychiatry.* 1966;123:413-419.
5. Sosowsky L. *Violence and the Mentally Ill: Putting State Mental Hospitals Out of Business: The Community Approach to Treating Mental Illness in San Mateo County.* Berkeley: University of California Graduate School of Public Policy; 1974:13-33.
6. Sosowsky L. Crime and violence among mental patients reconsidered in view of the new legal relationship between the state and the mentally ill. *Am J Psychiatry.* 1978;135:33-42.
7. Sosowsky L. Explaining the increased arrest rate among mental patients: a cautionary note. *Am J Psychiatry.* 1980;137:1602-1605.
8. Steadman HJ, Cocozza JJ, Melick ME. Explaining the increased arrest rate among mental patients: the changing clientele of state hospitals. *Am J Psychiatry.* 1978;135:816-820.
9. Zitrin A, Hardesty AS, Burdock ET, Drossman AK. Crime and violence among mental patients. *Am J Psychiatry.* 1976;133:142-149.
10. Hodgins S. The criminality of mentally disordered persons. In: Hodgins S, ed. *Mental Disorder and Crime.* Newbury Park, Calif: Sage Publications Inc; 1993: 3-21.
11. Lindqvist P, Allebeck P. Schizophrenia and crime: a longitudinal follow-up of 644 schizophrenics in Stockholm. *Br J Psychiatry.* 1990;157:345-350.
12. Link BG, Andrews H, Cullen FT. The violent and illegal behaviour of mental patients reconsidererd. *Am Sociol Rev.* 1992;57:275-292.
13. Steadman HJ, Monahan J, Robbins PA, Applebaum P, Grisso T, Klassen D, Mulvey E, Roth L. From dangerousness to risk assessment: implications for appropriate research strategies. In: Hodgins S, ed. *Mental Disorder and Crime.* Newbury Park, Calif: Sage Publications Inc; 1993:22-39.
14. Collins JJ, Schlenger WE. The prevalence of psychiatric disorder among admissions to prison. Presented at the 35th Annual Meeting of the American Society of Criminology; November 1983; Denver, Colo.
15. Daniel AE, Robins AJ, Reid JC, Wilfley DE. Lifetime and six-month prevalence of psychiatric disorders among sentenced female offenders. *Bull Am Acad Psychiatry Law.* 1988;16:333-342.
16. Hyde PS, Seiter RP. *The Prevalence of Mental Illness Among Inmates in the Ohio Prison System.* Dept of Mental Health and the Ohio Dept of Rehabilitation and Correction Interdepartmental Planning and Oversight Committee for Psychiatric Services to Corrections; 1987.
17. Neighbors HW, Williams DH, Gunnings TS, Lipscomb WD, Broman C, Lepkowski J. *The Prevalence of Mental Disorder in Michigan Prisons.* Final report submitted to the Michigan Department of Corrections; 1987.
18. Hodgins S, Côté G. The prevalence of mental disorders among penitentiary inmates. *Canada's Mental Health.* 1990;38:1-5.
19. Teplin LA. The prevalence of severe mental disorder among male urban jail detainees: comparison with the epidemiologic catchment area program. *Am J Public Health.* 1990;80:663-669.
20. Gottlieb P, Gabrielsen G, Kramp P. Psychotic homicides in Copenhagen from 1959 to 1983. *Acta Psychiatr Scand.* 1987;76:285-292.
21. Lindqvist P. Criminal homicide in Northern Sweden 1970-1981: alcohol intoxication, alcohol abuse and mental disease. *Int J Law Psychiatry.* 1986;8:19-37.
22. Eronen M, Tiihonen J, Hakola P. Schizophrenia and homicidal behavior. *Schizophr Bull.* In press.
23. Côté G, Hodgins S. The prevalence of major mental disorders among homicide offenders. *Int J Law Psychiatry.* 1992;15:89-99.
24. Ortmann J. Psykisk afvigelse og kriminel adfaerd En undersogelse af 11533 maend fodt i 1953 i det metropolitane omrade Kobenhavn. *Forskningsrapport nr.17.* Copenhagen, Denmark: Justitsministeriet; 1981.
25. Hodgins S. Mental disorder, intellectual deficiency, and crime: evidence from a birth cohort. *Arch Gen Psychiatry.* 1992;49:476-483.
26. Robins LN, Helzer JE, Weissman MM, Orvaschel H, Gruenberg E, Burke JD Jr, Regier DA. Lifetime prevalence of specific psychiatric disorders in three sites. *Arch Gen Psychiatry.* 1984;41:949-958.
27. Häfner H, Böker W. *Crimes of Violence by Mentally Abnormal Offenders.* Cambridge, England: Cambridge University Press; 1982.
28. Pasewark RA, Bieber S, Bosten KJ, Kiser M, Steadman HJ. Criminal recidivism among insanity acquittees. *Int J Law Psychiatry.* 1982;5:365-374.
29. Hodgins S. Men found unfit to stand and/or not guilty by reason of insanity: criminal recidivism. *Can J Criminol.* 1987;29:51-70.
30. Hodgins S, Webster CD. *The Canadian Data Base: Patients Held on Lieutenant-Governors' Warrants.* Ottawa, Ontario: Department of Justice of Canada; 1992.
31. Walker N, McCabe S. *Crime and Insanity in England, II.* Edinburgh, Scotland: Edinburgh University Press; 1973.
32. Hodgins S, Côté G. The criminality of mentally disordered offenders. *Criminal Justice Behav.* 1993;28:115-129.
33. Munk-Jorgensen P, Kastrup M, Mortensen PB. The Danish psychiatric case register as a tool in epidemiology. *Acta Psychiatr Scand.* 1993;370(suppl):27-32.
34. Wolfgang ME. Foreword. In: Mednick SA, Christiansen KO, eds. *Biosocial Bases of Criminal Behavior.* New York, NY: Gardner Press; 1977.
35. Teplin L. Criminalizing mental disorder: the comparative arrest rate of the mentally ill. *Am Psychol.* 1984;39:794-803.
36. Monahan J, Steadman HJ. Crime and mental disorder: an epidemiological approach. In: Tonry M, Morris N, eds. *Crime and Justice: An Annual Review of Research.* Chicago, Ill: The University of Chicago Press; 1983:145-189.
37. Hodgins S, Lalonde N. Major mental disorders and crime: changes over time? In: Cohen P, Robins L, Slomkowski S, eds. *Where and When: Geographical and Historical Aspects of Psychopathology.* Mahwah, NJ: Lawrence Erlbaum Associates. In press.
38. Morrisey J, Goldman HH. Care and treatment of the mentally ill in the United States: historical developments and reforms. *Ann Am Acad Pol Soc Sci.* 1986; 484:12-27.
39. Rabkin JG. Criminal behaviour of discharged mental patients: a critical appraisal of the research. *Psychol Bull.* 1979;86:1-29.
40. Coid B, Lewis SW, Reveley AM. A twin study of psychosis and criminality. *Br J Psychiatry.* 1993;162:87-92.
41. Regier DA, Farmer ME, Rae DS, Locke BZ, Keith SJ, Judd LL, Goodwin FK. Comorbidity of mental disorders with alcohol and other drug abuse. *JAMA.* 1990;264:2511-2518.
42. Hodgins S. Violence in the severely mentally ill. *Arch Gen Psychiatry.* 1994; 51:71-72.
43. Swanson JW. Alcohol abuse, mental disorder, and violent behavior. *Alcohol Health Res World.* 1993;17:123-132.
44. Herrera JN, Sramek JJ, Costa JF, Roy S, Heh CW, Nguyen BN. High potency neuroleptics and violence in schizophrenics. *J Nerv Ment Disord.* 1988;176: 558-561.
45. Beaudoin MN, Hodgins S, Lavoie F. Homicide, schizophrenia and substance abuse or dependency. *Can J Psychiatry.* 1993;38:1-7.
46. Reiss AJ, Roth JA, eds. *Understanding and Preventing Violence.* Washington, DC: National Academy Press; 1993.
47. Raine A, Brennan P, Mednick SA. Birth complications combined with early maternal rejection at age 1 year predispose to violent crime at age 18 years. *Arch Gen Psychiatry.* 1994;51:984-988.
48. Tsuang MT, Woolson RF, Fleming JA. Premature deaths in schizophrenia and affective disorders: an analysis of survival curves and variables affecting the shortened survival. *Arch Gen Psychiatry.* 1980;37:979-983.
49. Hodgins S. Status at age 30 of children with conduct problems. *Stud Crime Crime Prev.* 1994;3:41-62.
50. Lidberg L, Wiklund N, Jakobsson SW. Mortality among criminals with suspected mental disturbance. *Scand J Soc Med.* 1989;17:59-65.
51. Ritchie JH, Dick D, Lingham R. *Report of the Inquiry Into the Care and Treatment of Christopher Clunis.* London, England: North East Thames and South East Thames Regional Health Authorities; 1994.
52. Steadman HJ, Felson RB. Self-reports of violence: ex-mental patients, ex-offenders, and the general population. *Criminol.* 1984;22:321-342.
53. Swanson JW, Holzer CE, Ganju VK, Jono RT. Violence and psychiatric disorder in the community: evidence from the epidemiologic catchment area surveys. *Hosp Community Psychiatry.* 1990;42:761-770.
54. Steadman HJ, Monahan J, Appelbaum PS, Grisso T, Mulvey EP, Roth LH, Robbins PC, Classen D. Designing a new generation of risk assessment research. In: Monahan J, Steadman HJ, eds. *Violence and Mental Disorder: Developments in Risk Assessment.* Chicago, Ill: The University of Chicago Press; 1994: 297-318.
55. Hodgins S. Major mental disorder and crime: an overview. *Psychol Crime Law.* 1995;2:5-17.
56. Hodgins S, Toupin J, Côté G. Schizophrenia and antisocial personality disorder: a criminal combination. In: Schlesinger LB, ed. *Explorations in Criminal Psychopathology: Clinical Syndromes with Forensic Implication.* Springfield, Ill: Charles C Thomas Publisher. In press.
57. Hodgins S, Côté G, Toupin J. Major mental disorder and crime: an etiological hypothesis. In: Cooke D, Forth A, Hare RD, eds. *Psychopathy, Theory, Research and Implications for Society.* Dortrecht, the Netherlands: Kluwer. In press.
58. Cannon TD, Mednick SA, Parnas J. Antecedents of predominantly negative- and predominantly positive-symptom schizophrenia in a high-risk population. *Arch Gen Psychiatry.* 1990;47:622-632.
59. Asarnow JR. Children at risk for schizophrenia: converging lines of evidence. *Schizophr Bull.* 1988;14:613-631.
60. Angold A, Costello EJ. Depressive comorbidity in children and adolescents: empirical, theoretical, and methodological issues. *Am J Psychiatry.* 1993;150: 1779-1791.
61. Manzano J, Salvador A. Antecedents of severe affective (mood) disorders: patients examined as children or adolescents and as adults. *Acta Paedopsychiatr.* 1993;56:11-18.
62. Carlson GA, Weintraub S. Childhood behavior problems and bipolar disorder: relationship or coincidence? *J Affect Disord.* 1993;28:143-153.
63. Link BG, Stueve A. Psychotic symptoms and the violent/illegal behavior of mental patients compared to community control. In: Monahan J, Steadman H, eds. *Violence and Mental Disorder: Developments in Risk Assessment.* Chicago, Ill: The University of Chicago Press; 1994:137-159.

Mental Disorders and Homicidal Behavior in Finland

Markku Eronen, MD; Panu Hakola, MD, PhD; Jari Tiihonen, MD, PhD

Background: Owing to the fact that Finnish police have been able to solve about 95% of all homicides during recent decades and because most homicide offenders are subjected to an intensive psychiatric evaluation, it was possible to examine data on 693 of 994 homicide offenders during an 8-year period.

Methods: The prevalences of mental disorders of the homicide offenders were used to calculate odds ratios (ORs) for the statistical increase in risk associated with specific mental disorders.

Results: The results indicate that schizophrenia increases the OR of homicidal violence by about 8-fold in men and 6.5-fold in women. Antisocial personality disorder increases the OR over 10-fold in men and over 50-fold in women. Affective disorders, anxiety disorders, dysthymia, and mental retardation did not elevate the OR to any significant extent (OR <5.0).

Conclusion: Homicidal behavior in a country with a relatively low crime rate appears to have a statistical association with some specific mental disorders classified according to *DSM-III-R* classifications.

(Arch Gen Psychiatry. 1996;53:497-501)

MENTALLY disturbed violent offenders are an ever-popular subject preoccupying the mass media, and the association between mental disorders and violent behavior has been taken into account in the legislation of all countries for centuries. The effect of violence on public health is also remarkable. In the United States about 24 000 homicides are committed every year, and homicide has been the second leading cause of death among 15- to 24-year-old Americans between 1979 and 1988.[1,2] The annual range of homicides in the United States has varied from 7.9 to 9.8 per 100 000 population, and in the United Kingdom from 1.5 to 2.5 per 100 000 population.[1] The mean annual rate of homicides in Finland between the years 1984 and 1991 was 130 homicides per year (range, 107 to 152 [2.14 to 3.04 per 100 000 population]).[3] When one considers the damage wrought by violence, one must remember that violence does not only affect the victim and his or her relatives, but also the offender and his or her family.

Until recently, many researchers have been skeptical that there is any relationship between mental disorders and violence, and they have claimed that when appropriate statistical control groups of sociodemographic factors are applied, any apparent association between violence and mental disorder disappears.[4] However, since epidemiological methods have improved, more reliable and scientifically valid data on the possible association between violence and mental illness have been obtained, indicating that such a relationship exists.[4-6]

Although calculation of odds ratios (ORs) for different risk factors has been widely used in several fields of medicine, this approach has not been applied thus far to study the quantitative risk for homicidal behavior associated with different mental disorders. With regard to risk factors for homicidal behavior, the increased risk for homicide related to gun ownership has been evaluated with an epidemiological approach.[7] A longitudinal study[8] of incident cases of schizophrenia in London, England, indicated that the rate ratio for violent offenses in men with

See Subjects and Methods on next page

From the Department of Forensic Psychiatry, University of Kuopio, Niuvanniemi Hospital, Kuopio, Finland.

SUBJECTS AND METHODS

During the period between January 1, 1984, and December 31, 1991, 1037 murders and manslaughters were committed in Finland (population 5 029 000, of which 1 947 000 are men and 2 113 000 are women older than 15 years).[11] The Finnish police force was able to solve 1005 (96.9%) of these homicides.[3] Of the total homicides, 922 were committed by male offenders and 83 by female offenders. One woman committed 3 homicides in a single violent episode, 1 man committed 5 homicides, 1 man committed 4 homicides, 2 men committed 3 homicides each, and 30 men committed 2 homicides each. This means that 994 individual homicide offenders were known to exist, if one assumes that the 32 unsolved homicides were committed by 32 separate offenders. Of the 32 unsolved cases, we estimated the male/female offender ratio to be the same as in cases of solved homicides. With this assumption, and by excluding the few offenses committed by the same person, we arrived at a final total of 910 male and 84 female homicide offenders. The Finnish courts of law ordered that a forensic psychiatric examination be conducted on 693 of these 994 offenders (69.7%). All homicide offenders are evaluated by a psychiatrist to provide information for the courts, which independently decide whether a detailed forensic psychiatric examination should be made. If the courts decide that there is any possibility the offender is not fully criminally responsible owing to a mental disorder, a full-scale forensic psychiatric examination will be ordered. This examination is made by a forensic psychiatrist, who is always a civil servant of the state (thus, he or she gets paid by the state and is expected to be as objective as possible). This examination is very thorough and includes exhaustive psychiatric evaluation, standardized psychological tests such as the Wechsler Adult Intelligence Scale, Rorschach test, Minnesota Multiphasic Personality Inventory, evaluation of physical condition with laboratory testing (basic blood tests, electroencephalography, and computed tomography of the head), and observation of the offender by the staff in the hospital, normally lasting from 4 to 8 weeks. After this examination, a very detailed report with the *DSM-III-R* diagnosis (before 1987, *DSM-III*) is presented by the forensic psychiatrist. He or she is advised to estimate what were the most severe mental disorders (psychoses > personality disorders > anxiety disorders or dysthymia), if any, from which the offender suffered during the commission of his or her offense. After the examination, the reports are scrutinized by the Finnish National Board of Medico-Legal Affairs by at least 2 independent psychiatrists and by at least 1 lawyer. If they disagree with the report, they send it back to the forensic psychiatrist for modification. These investigative reports are then filed with the Finnish Board of Medico-Legal Affairs. We studied all of these forensic psychiatric reports from January 1985 to December 1992 (because of bureaucratic delays, offenders were normally evaluated by a forensic psychiatrist 6 to 12 months after they had committed the crime). In our calculations we have considered all offenders from whom there were no forensic psychiatric reports available as not being mentally disordered or handicapped. The 32 offenders (3% of the total) who had not been identified by the police were also considered not to be mentally disordered.

In OR calculations we have used 1-month point prevalence rate estimates for *DSM-III* disorders, obtained from a large US epidemiological catchment area (ECA) study.[12] A recent Finnish study indicates that the prevalence rates of mental disorders in Finland do not differ greatly from the US prevalence rates.[13] For example, in Finland the prevalence rate for manic disorders was 0.4% (ECA study, 0.4%), and the prevalence of alcoholism was 4.9% for men and 0.9% for women (ECA study, 5.0% for men and 0.9% for women). The total number of schizophrenic patients in Finland, estimated on the basis of disability pensions and sickness allowances, was 26 098[14] (the estimated number based on the prevalence obtained from the ECA study was 28 400). The prevalence of mental retardation in Finland has been estimated to be 0.7%[15] (the estimate based on US data was 1.0%[16]). The prevalence estimates used for the anxiety disorders and dysthymia are based on the prevalence estimates in the ECA study. The approximations of the prevalences of personality disorders and other psychoses have been made on the bases of Finnish data.[13,17]

Odds ratio is defined as the odds of disease in exposed persons divided by the odds of disease in unexposed persons; OR = *ad/bc*. The 95% confidence interval (CI) for the OR can be obtained from the formula:

$$\exp\left[\ln(\mathrm{OR}) \pm 1.96\sqrt{\frac{1}{a}+\frac{1}{b}+\frac{1}{c}+\frac{1}{d}}\right],$$

where exp denotes the exponential function of the natural logarithm, ln.[18] To adjust for the confounding factor of age, indirect standardization was used. This was done by analyzing the proportion (percentage) of subjects in age groups of 18 to 24, 25 to 44, 45 to 65, and 65 years and older in the ECA[12] and in our sample of homicide offenders.

schizophrenia is 3.8. Schizophrenia also made a small independent contribution to the risk for acquiring a criminal record (hazard ratio =1.4). In Denmark, the OR for the risk increase for psychotic homicide was 6 in men and 16 in women.[9] The association between criminality and different categories of mental disorders (major mental disorder, substance abuse, and mental retardation) has been studied recently, but these categories were heterogeneous and contained several different disorders; therefore, this study did not reveal the association between crime and specific mental disorders classified according to the *DSM-III-R* or *International Classification of Diseases, Ninth Revision*.[10] The aim of this study was to investigate if there is any association between specific *DSM-III-R* disorders and homicidal behavior.

RESULTS

The **Table** shows the ORs and 95% CIs of risk increase for each *DSM-III-R* mental disorder among men and women. Our results reveal that there is an association between homicidal behavior and certain mental disorders classified according to the *DSM-III-R*. The mean ±SD age of male offenders was 34.0±11.5 years (range, 17-77

Odds Ratios (ORs) and 95% Confidence Intervals (CIs) of Risk Increase for Each Main Diagnosis of *DSM-III-R*–Classified Mental Disorders Among Male and Female Homicide Offenders in Finland, 1984-1991*

Diagnosis (*DSM-III-R*)	Sex	% Prevalence Among the General Population	No. of Subjects Among the General Population Older Than 15 y	No. (%) of Subjects Among Offenders	OR (Age-Adjusted OR)	95% CI
Schizophrenia and schizophreniform psychoses	Men	0.7 (0.8)	13 600 (16 500)	58 (6.4)	9.7 (8.0)	7.4-12.6 (6.1-10.4)
	Women	0.7 (0.97)	14 800 (20 500)	5 (6.0)	9.0 (6.5)	3.6-22.2 (2.6-16.0)
Other psychoses	Men	1-2 (estimate)	38 900	23 (2.5)	1.3 (minimum)	0.8-1.9
	Women	1-2 (estimate)	42 300	1 (1.2)	0.6 (minimum)	0.08-4.2
Major depressive episode	Men	1.6 (1.84)	31 200 (35 800)	27 (3.0)	1.9 (1.6)	1.3-1.8 (1.1-2.4)
	Women	2.9 (3.43)	61 300 (72 500)	5 (6.0)	2.1 (1.8)	0.9-5.2 (0.7-4.4)
Manic disorders	Men	0.3 (0.42)	5800 (8200)	0	...	...
	Women	0.4 (0.58)	8500 (12 300)	0	...	...
Anxiety disorders	Men	4.7 (4.78)	91 500 (93 060)	14 (1.5)	0.3 (0.3)	0.2-0.5 (0.2-0.5)
	Women	9.7 (10.8)	205 000 (228 000)	0	...	...
Dysthymia	Men	2.2 (2.5)	42 800 (48 700)	13 (1.4)	0.6 (0.6)	0.4-1.1 (0.3-1.0)
	Women	4.2 (4.4)	88 700 (93 000)	1 (1.2)	0.3 (0.3)	0.04-2.0 (0.04-1.9)
Personality disorders (all)	Men	5.0 (estimate)	97 000	313 (34.4)	10.0	8.7-11.5
	Women	5.0 (estimate)	106 000	30 (35.7)	10.5	6.7-16.4
Antisocial personality disorder†	Men	0.8 (1.08)	15 600 (21 000)	103 (11.3)	15.8 (11.7)	12.9-19.4 (9.5-14.4)
	Women	0.2 (0.28)	4200 (5900)	11 (13.1)	75.7 (53.8)	40.1-142.7 (28.5-101.5)
Alcoholism†	Men	5.0 (5.70)	97 400 (111 000)	357 (39.2)	12.3 (10.7)	10.7-14.0 (9.4-12.2)
	Women	0.9 (1.24)	19 000 (26 000)	27 (32.1)	52.2 (37.7)	33.0-82.5 (23.9-59.6)
Mental retardation‡	Men	1.0	19 500	11 (1.2)	1.2	0.9-2.2
	Women	1.0	21 300	2 (2.4)	2.4	0.6-9.9

**The population in Finland is 1 947 000 men and 2 113 000 women older than 15 years, 910 male and 84 female homicide offenders.*[3,11] *Point prevalences used are based to the 1-month point prevalence estimates for* DSM-III *disorders obtained from a large US epidemiological catchment area (ECA) study.*[12] *The numbers in parentheses are age-adjusted estimates, which are based on indirect standardization of the confound of age according to the ECA study.*[20]

†*Secondary diagnoses are also included. Alcoholism was the main diagnosis in 82 male and 3 female offenders; antisocial personality disorder was the main diagnosis in 73 male and 10 female offenders. The rest of these diagnoses were secondary (comorbid) diagnoses, and the offenders were in these cases counted also in their main diagnostic group.*

‡*The prevalence estimate is based on a compilation from a large number of empirical studies.*[16] *Six men and 2 women had a secondary diagnosis of mental retardation. The remaining diagnoses were main diagnoses.*

years). Schizophrenia increased the OR of a man to commit a homicide by 8-fold, and antisocial personality disorder or alcoholism increased it by over 10-fold. In the offenders with schizophrenia, there were 31 (49.2%) who suffered from paranoid schizophrenia. A major depressive episode increased the risk only slightly in men, and mental retardation did not elevate the risk at all. Since the diagnoses in the years 1985 and 1986 were based on the *DSM-III*, we calculated the corresponding ORs for the men of this group separately. The ORs and 95% CIs among them are as follows: schizophrenia, 7.4 (3.9-14.0); other psychoses, 1.5 (0.7-3.4); major depressive episode, 0.6 (0.2-2.5); manic disorders, 0; anxiety disorders, 0.7 (0.4-1.4); dysthymia, 1.5 (0.8-3.1); personality disorders, 11.5 (8.6-15.3); antisocial personality disorder, 5.8 (3.0-11.3); alcoholism, 12.9 (9.8-17.1); and mental retardation, 1.0 (0.2-4.0).

The mean ($\pm$SD) age of female offenders was 34.0 ± 12.3 years (range, 15-79 years). Our figures on female offenders emphasize the high risk, up to 40- to 50-fold, in women with alcoholism or antisocial personality disorder. Schizophrenia and all personality disorders altogether increase women's ORs by up to 6.5- to 10-fold. Major depressive episodes and mental retardation may cause a slight elevation of the risk, but this cannot be confirmed statistically with these data. When evaluating these ORs, it must be taken into account that, in general, the risk of a woman's committing a homicide is clearly lower than the risk associated with men.

COMMENT

Thanks to the exceptionally good homicide-solving percentage of Finnish police (96.9%), and because of the fact that most of the homicide offenders in Finland have been examined with a thorough forensic psychiatric evaluation, we have been able to estimate the risk of violence associated with certain psychiatric disorders. For example, in the United States, about one third of homicides remain unsolved,[1] which makes estimating the epidemiological background of homicidal behavior much more complicated than it is in Finland.

The OR calculations were made on the basis of the assumption that offenders on whom sufficient data were unavailable were considered as not mentally disordered. We also know that, occasionally, Finnish courts of law consider that offenders who obviously suffer from alcohol problems, antisocial personality disorder, anxiety disorders, or dysthymia do not need to be examined by the thorough forensic psychiatric evaluation we described. The Finnish legal system normally considers that alcoholism, antisocial personality disorder, and most anxiety disorders or dysthymia are not necessarily reasons to consider an offender to be not guilty by reason of insanity. This means that in this study we have probably omitted a few alcoholics and some offenders suffering from personality disorders and anxiety disorders or dysthymia as well. Because of the retrospective research method used, we did not have access to the offenders who had committed suicide after committing their act of violence. We assume we may have missed some of the subjects suffering from major depression who committed suicide immediately after their homicidal act. Thus, the calculated ORs must be regarded as minimum numbers. Nonetheless, it should be emphasized that Finnish courts of law almost invariably require a forensic psychiatric evaluation for obviously disturbed offenders, since almost all homicide offenders are examined by a psychiatrist. Therefore, the ORs for homicidal behavior are probably more valid for those subjects with major disorders than for subjects with less severe anxiety disorders, dysthymia, personality disorders, or mild alcoholism.

WE HAVE USED point prevalence rate estimates from US residents because there are no detailed *DSM-III-R* classification-based prevalence rates for an equivalent large Finnish population. Using a foreign database, which may not be entirely relevant to Finland, limits the accuracy of the ORs. In addition, the Diagnostic Interview Schedule, which was used in the ECA study, may not be as reliable in diagnosing subjects with psychotic symptoms as it is for the other disorders.[19] Even though prevalences in Finland may be slightly different, our results nonetheless demonstrate the increased ORs associated with several mental disorders. Thus, our data would suggest that in view of the above assumptions, the role of anxiety disorders, dysthymia, alcoholism, and personality disorders is probably slightly greater. Therefore, it is probable that anxiety disorders and dysthymia do not decrease the risk for homicidal behavior, as would seem to be the case from inspection of our ORs.

Since Finland is a racially homogeneous country, race and ethnicity were not adjusted for in the present study. More than 95% of the inhabitants and homicide offenders in Finland are white.[11] One could have used the prevalence estimates of nonblack and non-Hispanic subgroups of the ECA study[20] for our comparison. In most cases, this would have caused a minor increase in the ORs, since in the ECA the prevalence estimates for nonblack and non-Hispanic subgroups are, for most disorders, slightly lower than the estimates for the general ECA population. In addition, race and ethnicity data from the ECA do not include gender, and omitting the effect of gender would notably decrease the value of the presented ORs.

One important question that should be considered is whether there is causality between committing a crime and obtaining a diagnosis of a mental disorder. This "halo effect" could be a cause for notable measurement error or bias. However, although the index offense can on some occasions be one of the diagnostic criteria (eg, antisocial personality disorder), even in these cases the offender must fulfill several other criteria before the diagnosis can be confirmed. Also, the effect of the timing of the forensic examination could cause bias or measurement error. The effect of the delay between the crime and the forensic psychiatric examination has been minimized by advising the forensic psychiatrist to estimate the mental state of the offenders at the time they committed their offenses. For example, if the offender had no depression or mania at the time of the homicide, the main diagnosis of mania was not recorded, although he or she suffered from depression or mania during the forensic examination.

Another important question concerning the reliability of the data is the interrater reliability of the diagnoses. The diagnoses were made on the basis of an exhaustive clinical examination, standardized psychological tests, and observation of the offender by the hospital staff. If it were possible to regulate the legal system of the entire nation for scientific purposes for many years, one could attempt to achieve controlled interrater reliability with structured clinical interviews and thus further improve the reliability of the diagnoses. However, obtaining standardized conditions nationwide for almost a decade is extremely difficult, if not impossible, to achieve. Forensic psychiatric reports do not include standardized data of the socioeconomic status of the offenders. However, socioeconomic status can be either a cause or a consequence of psychopathological abnormalities. Thus, controlling socioeconomic status could even, to some extent, attenuate the relationship between mental disorders and homicide.

The Finnish ORs cannot be directly applied to countries with higher crime rates. Organized crime and drug abuse are not important factors in Finnish homicides, but alcohol abuse figures highly in Finnish violence.[21] In most cases, not only the offenders but also the victims had been intoxicated from alcohol when the violence took place. Our results suggest that severe alcohol dependence associated with an antisocial personality disorder clearly increases the risk for homicidal behavior. The data obtained from our preliminary study with a 1-year sample showed that 20 (95%) of 21 offenders with a diagnosis of antisocial personality disorder also fulfilled the criteria for type 2 alcoholism,[22] and we could predict that a very large proportion of our 103 men and 11 women with an antisocial personality disorder diagnosis in this 8-year sample were also type 2 alcoholics. This type of alcoholism is associated with alcoholism in male relatives, early onset of heavy alcohol abuse (before the age of 25 years), repeated violent behavior when drunk, loss of appetite during drinking, and dysfunction in serotonin metabolism.[23-25] These results are in agreement with those findings indicating that impulsive aggressive behavior is associated with malfunction of serotonergic neural networks.[26] Therefore, it is possible that new serotonin reuptake inhibitors might prove useful in the treatment of impulsive aggressive alcoholics, although only placebo-controlled trials can verify the potential benefits of this theoretically logical treatment. Recent studies have implied that serotonergic drugs and opioid antagonists may offer new effective ways to treat alcoholism,[27,28] and this may possibly be one of the most important biomedical aids in the prevention of homicidal behavior.

The results indicate that schizophrenia seems to multiply the OR of homicidal behavior by about 8-fold in men and 6.5-fold in women. We have previously proposed this in an earlier study with a 1-year sample,[22] and the present data support these preliminary results. Although psychiatrists have traditionally not been inclined to admit that there is an increased risk for violence associated with schizophrenia, we consider that such a risk truly exists. Since we have been able to use only a retrospective method in the present study, no direct conclusions of the causality and mental disorders should be made on the basis of these data. We also wish to emphasize that all patients with schizophrenia should not be considered to be violent, although there are minor subgroups of schizophrenic patients among whom the risk for violence may be remarkably high. Future research is needed to identify these high-risk subgroups among schizophrenic patients. At present we would estimate that this increase in risk could be associated with the paranoid form of schizophrenia and coexisting substance abuse. In addition, a history of previously committed violent acts seems to greatly elevate the risk for acting violently in the future.[29]

Accepted for publication October 26, 1995.

Reprints: Markku Eronen, MD, Department of Forensic Psychiatry, University of Kuopio, Niuvanniemi Hospital, FIN-70240 Kuopio, Finland.

REFERENCES

1. *International Crimes Statistics 1984-1991.* Lyons, France: International Criminal Police Organisation; 1986-1993.
2. Hammett M, Powell KE, O'Carroll PW, Clanton ST. Homicide surveillance: United States, 1979-1988. *MMWR CDC Surveill Summ.* 1992;41:1-33.
3. Central Statistical Office of Finland. *Criminality Known to the Police 1984-1991.* Helsinki, Finland: Valtion Painatuskeskus; 1985-1992.
4. Mental disorder and violent behavior: perceptions and evidence. *Am Psychol.* 1992;47:511-521.
5. Link BG, Andrews H, Cullen FT. The violent and illegal behavior of mental patients reconsidered. *Am Sociol Rev.* 1992;57:275-292.
6. Hodgins S. *Mental Disorder and Crime.* London, England: Sage Publications; 1993.
7. Kellerman AL, Rivara FP, Bushforth NB, Banton JG, Reay DT, Fransisco JT, Locci AB, Prodzinski J, Hackman BB, Somes G. Gun ownership as a risk factor for homicide in the home. *N Engl J Med.* 1993;7:1084-1091.
8. Wessely SC, Castle D, Douglas AJ, Tayler PJ. The criminal careers of the incident cases of schizophrenia. *Psychol Med.* 1994;24:483-502.
9. Gottlieb P, Cabrielsen G, Kramp P. Psychotic homicide in Copenhagen from 1959 to 1983. *Acta Psychiatr Scand.* 1987;76:285-292.
10. Hodgins S. Mental disorder, intellectual deficiency and crime. *Arch Gen Psychiatry.* 1992;49:476-483.
11. *Statistical Yearbook of Finland 1992.* Helsinki, Finland: The Statistics Centre of Finland; 1992.
12. Regier DA, Boyd JH, Burke JD, Rae DS, Myers JK, Kramer M, Robins LN, George LK, Karno M, Locke BZ. One-month prevalence of mental disorders in the United States: based on five epidemiologic catchment area sites. *Arch Gen Psychiatry.* 1988;45:977-986.
13. Lehtinen V, Veijola J, Lindholm T, Väisänen E, Moring J, Puukka P. *Mielenterveyden pysyvyys ja muutokset suomalaisilla aikuisilla.* [Stability and changes of mental health in the Finnish adult population.] Turku, Finland: Kansaneläkelaitoksen Julkaisuja Al-sarja; 1993.
14. *Statistical Yearbook of the Social Insurance Institution 1991.* Helsinki, Finland: Kansaneläkelaitoksen Julkaisuja; 1992.
15. Palo J, Jokelainen M, Kaste M, Teräväinen H, Waltimo O. *Neurologia.* Porvoo, Finland; 1988:462.
16. Lakin KC, Krantz GC, Bruininks RH, Clumpner JL, Hill BK. One hundred years of data on population of public residential facilities for mentally retarded patients. *Am J Ment Defic.* 1982;87:1-8.
17. Lehtinen V, Joukamaa M, Lahtela K, Raitasalo R, Jyrkinen E, Maatela J, Aromaa A. Prevalence of mental disorders among adults in Finland: basic results from the Mini Finland Health Survey. *Acta Psychiatr Scand.* 1990;81:418-425.
18. Dawson-Saunders B, Trapp RG, eds. *Basic & Clinical Biostatistics.* East Norwalk, Conn: Appleton & Lange; 1994:170.
19. Spitzer RL, Williams JB, Gibbon M, First MB. The Structured Clinical Interview for *DSM-III-R*, I: history, rationale and description. *Arch Gen Psychiatry.* 1992; 49:624-629.
20. Regier DA, Farmer ME, Rae DS, Myers JK, Kramer M, Robins LN, George LK, Karno M, Locke BZ. One-month prevalence of mental disorders in the United States and sociodemographic characteristics: the Epidemiologic Catchment Area study. *Acta Psychiatr Scand.* 1993;88:35-47.
21. Research Institute of Criminality in Finland. *Criminality in Finland 1990.* Helsinki, Finland: Haakapaino Oy; 1991.
22. Tiihonen J, Eronen M, Hakola P. Criminality associated with mental disorders and intellectual deficiency. *Arch Gen Psychiatry.* 1993;50:917-918.
23. Cloninger CR. Neurogenetic adaptive mechanisms in alcoholism. *Science.* 1987; 236:410-416.
24. Virkkunen M, DeJong J, Bartko J, Goodwin FK, Linnoila M. Relationship of psychobiological variables to recidivism in violent offenders and impulsive fire setters: a follow-up study. *Arch Gen Psychiatry.* 1989;46:600-603.
25. Irwin M, Shuckit M, Smith TL. Clinical importance of age at onset in type 1 and type 2 primary alcoholics. *Arch Gen Psychiatry.* 1990;47:320-324.
26. Coccaro EF, Siever LJ, Klar HM, Maurer G, Cochrane K, Cooper TB, Mohs RC, Davis KL. Serotonergic studies in patients with affective and personality disorders: correlates with suicidal and impulsive aggressive behavior. *Arch Gen Psychiatry.* 1989;46:587-599.
27. Naranjo CA, Sellers EM. Serotonin uptake inhibitors attenuate ethanol intake in problem drinkers. *Recent Dev Alcohol.* 1989;7:255-266.
28. O'Malley SS, Jaffe AJ, Chang G, Schottenfeld RS, Meyer RE, Rounsaville B. Naltrexone and coping skills therapy for alcohol dependence. *Arch Gen Psychiatry.* 1992;49:881-887.
29. Tiihonen J, Hakola P. Psychiatric disorders and homicide recidivism. *Am J Psychiatry.* 1994;151:436-438.

A selective serotonin
reuptake inhibitor for OCD

LUVOX™
fluvoxamine maleate 50 mg & 100 mg SCORED TABLETS

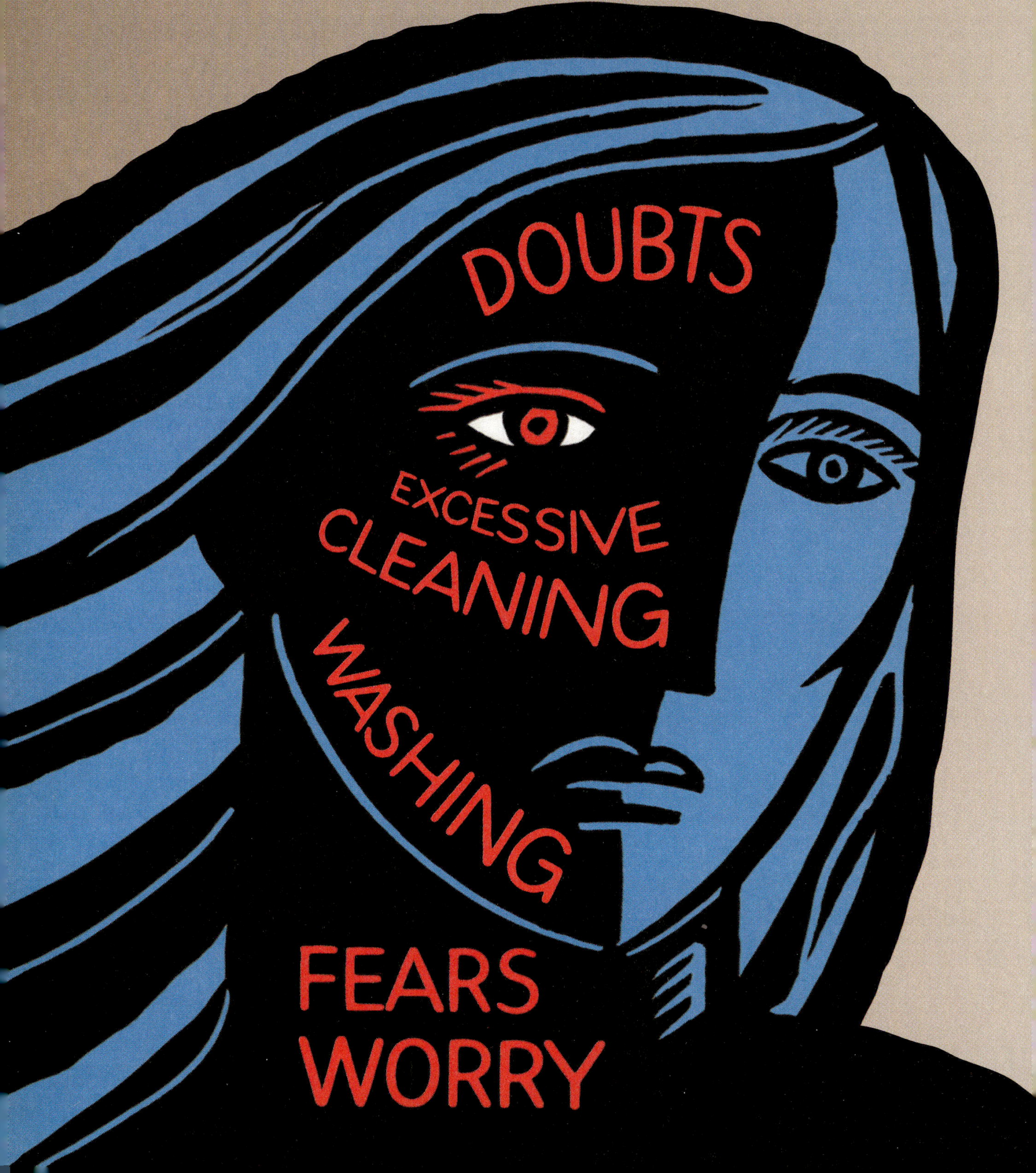

ORIGINAL ARTICLE

Prevalence of Psychiatric Disorders Among Incarcerated Women

I. Pretrial Jail Detainees

Linda A. Teplin, PhD; Karen M. Abram, PhD; Gary M. McClelland, PhD

Background: There are little epidemiologic data on psychiatric disorders of women in jails. Accurate data on female jail detainees are critical because of their increasing numbers and their unique treatment needs.

Methods: Using the Diagnostic Interview Schedule, independent interviewers assessed a randomly selected, stratified sample of 1272 female jail detainees awaiting trial in Chicago, Ill. We tabulated lifetime and 6-month prevalence rates of disorders by race or ethnicity (African American, non-Hispanic white, Hispanic), age, and education and compared the jail rates with general population rates for women in the Epidemiologic Catchment Area program. We also examined whether or not psychiatric disorder was associated with the severity of the detainee's current arrest charges.

Results: Over 80% of the sample met criteria for one or more lifetime psychiatric disorders; 70% were symptomatic within 6 months of the interview. The most common disorders were drug abuse or dependence, alcohol abuse or dependence, and post-traumatic stress disorder. Major depressive episode was the most prevalent major mental disorder. Rates were generally highest among non-Hispanic whites and among older detainees. Rates for all disorders were significantly higher than general population rates, except for schizophrenia. Most detainees with psychiatric disorders were arrested for nonviolent crimes.

Conclusion: These results suggest substantial psychiatric morbidity among female jail detainees.

(Arch Gen Psychiatry. 1996;53:505-512)

ACCURATE epidemiologic data on psychiatric disorders among correctional populations are required to determine service needs. The courts have mandated that inmates with mental disorders, whether in jail awaiting trial or sentenced to prison, be treated.[1-3] Ideally, they should receive care similar to that available in the community.[4] The jail is a critical place to gather psychiatric epidemiologic data, because it is the first point in the criminal justice process where serious offenders can be treated and less serious offenders (misdemeanants) can be diverted to the mental health system.

Psychiatric epidemiologic data are available for men in jail.[5-9] The most recent large-scale study found that 9% of male urban-jail detainees had a severe disorder (schizophrenia or major affective disorder) sometime during their lifetime; 6% had a "current" episode (within 2 weeks of their arrest).[5,6] These rates are two to three times higher than general population rates, even after controlling for demographic differences between the jail sample and the general population.[5] Substance use disorders were common.

However, data on men in jail cannot be generalized to women in jail because women in the general population have quite different diagnostic profiles.[10] Moreover, the related literature, studies of persons judged incompetent to stand trial or found not guilty by reason of insanity, suggests that psychiatric disorders may be even more prevalent among incarcerated women than among incarcerated men.[11-13]

See also page 513

There is little epidemiologic research on women in jail,[14,15] and prior studies have several methodological problems. First, most studies sampled jail inmates *referred* for treatment. Second, pre-

From the Psycho-Legal Studies Program, Department of Psychiatry, Northwestern University Medical School, Chicago, Illinois

See Subjects and Methods on next page

SUBJECTS AND METHODS

SUBJECTS AND SAMPLING PROCEDURES

Subjects were a randomly selected, stratified sample of 1272 female arrestees awaiting trial at the Cook County Department of Corrections (CCDOC) in Chicago, Ill, from 1991 through 1993. The sample was stratified by charge (misdemeanor or felony) and race or ethnicity (African American, non-Hispanic white, Hispanic, and other) to ensure adequate representation of key subgroups. Persons arrested for both misdemeanors and felonies were categorized as felons. Subjects were recruited and interviewed in the jail's intake area during routine intake processing. The Cook County Department of Corrections receives approximately 6400 female admissions per year.[23] Like other jails, the CCDOC is used solely for pretrial detention and for offenders sentenced to less than 1 year on misdemeanor charges. The CCDOC's population is similar to jails' nationwide, composed disproportionately of racial or ethnic minorities[24]: African American, 78.6%; non-Hispanic white, 14.8%; and Hispanic, 6.3%. We chose the CCDOC, because its population is demographically similar to other large urban jails[25] and because its size ensured adequate subject availability. Our sample (N=1272) allowed us to reliably detect disorders that have a base rate in the general population greater than or equal to 1.0%, with a power of .80.[26]

All post-arraignment detainees (excluding persons with gunshot wounds or other traumatic injuries) were eligible for the study, regardless of their psychiatric morbidity, state of drug or alcohol intoxication, or fitness to stand trial. Interviewers selected subjects using a list of random numbers as the detainees waited to be processed in the CCDOC intake area. The interviewers explained the project to potential subjects and assured them that all information gathered was strictly confidential. Detainees who agreed to participate signed a consent form and were paid $15 for the interview. Subjects were interviewed in private rooms in the CCDOC intake area.

Of the 1418 detainees randomly selected, only 59 (4.2%) refused to participate. Six of these individuals appeared to be mentally disorganized and possibly psychotic. Another 87 subjects (6.1%) agreed to participate but were unable to complete the interview, because they were ill (n=37), were diverted to other jail procedures (n=28), were not fluent in English and no bilingual interviewer was available (n=10), were too mentally disorganized (n=9), or presented a security risk (n=3). The total participation rate was 90%, and the final sample size was 1272.

PSYCHIATRIC DIAGNOSES

We used the National Institute of Mental Health Diagnostic Interview Schedule Version III-R (NIMH DIS-III-R) developed for the ECA program[27] for use by lay interviewers. We chose the DIS-III-R for four reasons. First, the DIS-III-R is a highly structured instrument, providing *DSM-III-R*[28] diagnoses (scored by computer), as well as rich descriptive data. Second, it has acceptable reliability (see Burke[29] and Helzer et al[30] vs Anthony et al[31]). Third, the DIS-III-R differentiates lifetime disorders (which may be remitted) from disorders in which symptoms are recent. Fourth, it allows us to compare our data with those from large community samples. Most interviews lasted between 1 and 3 hours, depending on the number of reported symptoms. Interviewers were female, had at least a master's degree, and were trained in the use of the DIS-III-R. Three interviewers were fluent in Spanish. Interviewer consistency was maintained via monitored mock interviews with scripted subjects.

The presence of one disorder did not preclude the diagnosis of another.[32] As in the ECA study, major affective and substance use disorders were scored *present* even if the disorders were mild (met minimal diagnostic criteria). The DIS-III-R assesses cognitive impairment with the Mini-Mental Status Examination. Because the Mini-Mental Status Examination can overestimate cognitive impairment among jail detainees[5] and may be culturally biased,[33] we counted subjects as cognitively impaired only if they met "severe" and "definite" criteria.

STATISTICAL ANALYSIS

Because we stratified our sample by charge and race or ethnicity, all prevalence parameter estimates were weighted to reflect the jail population's actual charge and racial or ethnic characteristics. All reported SEs and tests of significance have been corrected for design characteristics with the Taylor Series Expansion implemented in SUDAAN 6.4.[34] We used corrected χ^2 tests to assess differences in prevalence of specific psychiatric disorders by race or ethnicity, age, and education. Our level of significance for all tests was .05.

Our analysis for the ECA comparison had two steps. First, for each disorder, we estimated hierarchical log-linear models of jail-ECA differences holding age and race or ethnicity constant.[35] Second, we computed χ^2 tests for differences between jail and ECA rates within each subgroup of age and race or ethnicity. These tests have less statistical power than the log-linear analysis but allowed us to examine subgroup differences.

Our analysis of the relationship between current arrest charges and psychiatric status used χ^2 tests to compare each of the diagnostic groups (which can overlap) with the "no disorder" group.

vious studies used samples that were too small to generate reliable rates of less common psychiatric disorders (schizophrenia and major affective disorders). Third, many studies used nonstandardized instruments to assess psychiatric disorder.

Because no prior study has compared its findings with rates among women in the general population and controlled for demographic variables, we do not know if the observed rates of psychiatric disorder in jail are greater than would be expected by chance. Moreover, no study has examined the relationship between a detainee's psychiatric morbidity and the crime that precipitated her arrest. This information is pivotal to planning treatment strategies for jail detainees with mental disorders, because the severity of the alleged offense determines pretrial treatment options.[16-18]

Epidemiologic data on women in jail are essential because their numbers are increasing rapidly.[19] The female jail inmate population grew 138% between 1983 and 1989, compared with 72.7% for males.[20] The literature

Table 1. Demographic and Criminologic Characteristics of Female Jail Detainee Sample: Unweighted Data

Characteristics	n	%
Race/ethnicity		
African American	514	40.4
Non-Hispanic white	427	33.6
Hispanic	314	24.7
Other	17	1.3
Total	**1272**	**100**
Age, y		
17	26	2.0
18-20	143	11.2
21-25	309	24.3
26-29	259	20.4
30-34	270	21.2
35-50	247	19.4
51+	18	1.4
Education, y		
0-8	115	9.0
9-11	550	43.2
12	369	29.0
>12	238	18.7
Currently employed	271	21.3
Marital status		
Never married	791	62.2
Separated/divorced	322	25.3
Widowed	40	3.1
Married	118	9.3
No. of children		
0	282	22.2
1	258	20.3
2	266	20.9
3+	465	36.6
No. of prior arrests		
None	174	15.1
1	204	17.7
2+	777	67.3
Offense for which currently incarcerated		
Property offenses	441	34.8
Drug-related offenses	295	23.3
Violent crimes	201	15.9
Prostitution and soliciting	193	15.2
Traffic offenses	131	10.3
Other crimes	228	18.0

suggests that women in jail are even more disadvantaged than men in jail.[19-22]

This article presents prevalence estimates for 1272 female jail detainees awaiting trial by demographic subgroups (race or ethnicity, age, and education) for 10 psychiatric disorders: schizophrenia or schizophreniform disorder, manic episode, major depressive episode, dysthymic disorder, alcohol abuse or dependence, drug abuse or dependence, panic disorder, generalized anxiety disorder (GAD), posttraumatic stress disorder (PTSD), and antisocial personality disorder (ASPD). We compared these prevalence estimates with general population data collected in the Epidemiologic Catchment Area (ECA) program. We also examined current arrest charge by disorder.

RESULTS

DEMOGRAPHIC AND CRIMINOLOGIC CHARACTERISTICS

Table 1 describes the sociodemographic and criminologic characteristics of subjects. (These descriptive data are not weighted for the stratification criteria, race or ethnicity, and charge.) The sample comprised African Americans (40.4%), non-Hispanic whites (33.6%), Hispanics (24.7%), and others (1.3%). Subjects were between 17 and 67 years old (mean and median age, 28 years), with mean and median educational levels of 11 years. Most (78.7%) were not legally employed at the time of arrest. Nearly two thirds were never married. Nearly 80% had at least one child; 36.6% had three or more children. The most common arrest charges were for property crimes (34.8%) and drug crimes (23.3%). These demographic characteristics (other than the stratification variables) are similar to those in many large urban jails.[25]

PREVALENCE OF PSYCHIATRIC DISORDERS

Five subjects (0.4%) met criteria for severe cognitive impairment. Because cognitive impairment reflects the sub-

Table 2. Lifetime Prevalence of Specific Psychiatric Disorders Among Women Entering Jail by Race/Ethnicity

	Rate, % (SE)			
Disorder	Total (N=1272)	African American (n=514)	Non-Hispanic White (n=427)	Hispanic (n=314)
Severe disorders*	18.5 (1.4)	17.0 (1.7)	26.1 (2.1)	19.4 (2.2)
Schizophrenia/schizophreniform	2.4 (0.5)	2.3 (0.7)	2.6 (0.8)	3.5 (1.0)
Manic episode	2.6 (0.5)	2.3 (0.7)	4.1 (1.0)	2.5 (0.9)
Major depressive episode*	16.9 (1.3)	15.6 (1.6)	24.0 (2.1)	17.3 (2.1)
Dysthymia†	9.6 (1.0)	8.6 (1.2)	13.5 (1.7)	12.4 (1.9)
Substance abuse/dependence*	70.2 (1.6)	69.4 (2.0)	79.8 (1.9)	57.1 (2.8)
Alcohol abuse/dependence*	32.3 (1.6)	28.3 (2.0)	51.7 (2.4)	35.5 (2.7)
Drug abuse/dependence*	63.6 (1.7)	63.4 (2.1)	71.6 (2.2)	46.3 (2.8)
Panic disorder*	1.6 (0.4)	1.0 (0.4)	4.1 (1.0)	3.2 (1.0)
Generalized anxiety disorder	2.5 (0.5)	2.1 (0.6)	3.5 (0.9)	3.8 (1.1)
Post-traumatic stress disorder	33.5 (1.7)	32.7 (2.1)	35.1 (2.3)	38.6 (2.8)
Antisocial personality disorder*	13.8 (1.2)	12.1 (1.5)	20.8 (2.0)	17.4 (2.2)
Any of the above disorders*	80.6 (1.4)	80.2 (1.8)	86.1 (1.7)	73.0 (2.5)

*$P<.01$.
†$P<.05$.

ject's state only at the time of the interview, recency criteria do not apply, and, therefore, cognitive impairment is not reported in the tables.

Table 2 shows the lifetime prevalence of specific psychiatric disorders for the total sample and by race or ethnicity: 2.4% of the sample met *DSM-III-R* criteria for schizophrenia, 2.6% for manic episode, and 16.9% for lifetime major depressive episode. The most common disorders were drug abuse or drug dependence (63.6%), alcohol abuse or alcohol dependence (32.3%), and PTSD (33.5%). Nine cases are missing from the PTSD diagnosis because the subject found the event too upsetting to discuss; thus, the true rate of PTSD may be slightly higher. Over 80% of the sample had one of the lifetime disorders listed in Table 2. Table 2 also shows that rates differed by race or ethnicity for all disorders except schizophrenia, manic episode, generalized anxiety, and PTSD; non-Hispanic whites often had the highest rates.

Table 3 shows the 6-month prevalence of the disorders for the total sample and by race or ethnicity. These rates show the proportion of subjects who met the *DSM-III-R* diagnostic criteria for each disorder and who have experienced at least one symptom of the disorder within 6 months of the interview. Again, rates differed by race or ethnicity for most disorders, and non-Hispanic whites most often had the highest rates. The similarity be-

Table 3. Six-Month Prevalence of Specific Psychiatric Disorders Among Women Entering Jail by Race/Ethnicity

	Rate, % (SE)			
Disorder	Total (N=1272)	African American (n=514)	Non-Hispanic White (n=427)	Hispanic (n=314)
Severe disorders*	15.0 (1.2)	13.5 (1.5)	22.3 (2.0)	16.5 (2.1)
Schizophrenia/schizophreniform	1.8 (0.4)	1.5 (0.5)	2.6 (0.8)	2.9 (0.9)
Manic episode	2.2 (0.5)	2.1 (0.6)	2.9 (0.8)	1.5 (0.7)
Major depressive episode*	13.7 (1.2)	12.3 (1.5)	20.4 (2.0)	15.0 (2.0)
Dysthymia	6.5 (0.9)	5.9 (1.0)	8.8 (1.4)	7.9 (1.5)
Substance abuse/dependence*	60.1 (1.8)	59.2 (2.2)	69.7 (2.2)	48.1 (2.8)
Alcohol abuse/dependence*	23.9 (1.5)	21.3 (1.8)	35.5 (2.3)	28.2 (2.6)
Drug abuse/dependence*	52.4 (1.8)	53.0 (2.2)	56.5 (2.4)	35.3 (2.7)
Panic disorder†	1.4 (0.4)	1.0 (0.4)	3.0 (0.8)	2.6 (0.9)
Generalized anxiety disorder	2.2 (0.5)	1.9 (0.6)	3.3 (0.9)	3.5 (1.0)
Post-traumatic stress disorder	22.3 (1.5)	21.5 (1.8)	24.2 (2.1)	26.7 (2.5)
Antisocial personality disorder†	13.7 (1.2)	12.1 (1.5)	20.5 (2.0)	16.7 (2.1)
Any of the above disorders*	70.3 (1.6)	69.0 (2.0)	78.9 (2.0)	64.7 (2.7)

*$P<.01$.
†$P<.05$.

Table 4. Lifetime Prevalence of Specific Psychiatric Disorders Among Women Entering Jail and in the ECA: Age 18-25 y*

	African American			Non-Hispanic White		
	Rate, % (SE)†			Rate, % (SE)†		
Disorder	Jail (n=188)	ECA (n=354)	OR (95% CI)	Jail (n=123)	ECA (n=428)	OR (95% CI)
Severe disorders	17.2 (2.8)	8.8 (1.9)§	2.16 (1.18-3.96)	24.7 (3.9)	8.5 (1.5)¶	3.54 (2.01-6.24)
Schizophrenia/ schizophreniform	1.6 (0.9)	0.8 (0.4)	1.93 (0.46-8.13)	2.4 (1.4)	1.6 (0.6)	1.56 (0.39-6.18)
Manic episode‡	3.7 (1.4)	1.4 (0.7)	2.68 (0.80-8.93)	4.2 (1.8)	1.1 (0.5)	3.89 (1.03-14.67)
Major depressive episode	15.5 (2.7)	7.7 (1.9)‖	2.19 (1.14-4.20)	21.4 (3.7)	7.5 (1.4)¶	3.35 (1.84-6.10)
Dysthymia	7.6 (1.9)	3.6 (1.2)	2.17 (0.90-5.23)	13.5 (3.1)	3.6 (1.1)§	4.22 (1.89-9.41)
Substance abuse/dependence	59.9 (3.6)	14.4 (2.4)¶	8.90 (5.52-14.35)	71.3 (4.1)	13.7 (1.8)¶	15.65 (9.56-25.63)
Alcohol abuse/dependence	18.7 (2.9)	3.4 (1.1)¶	6.55 (3.07-13.98)	41.7 (4.5)	6.7 (1.3)¶	9.92 (5.73-17.20)
Drug abuse/dependence	52.5 (3.7)	13.6 (2.3)¶	6.99 (4.31-11.34)	64.0 (4.4)	10.0 (1.5)¶	15.96 (9.72-26.21)
Panic disorder	1.6 (0.9)	1.6 (0.8)	1.01 (0.22-4.61)	0.0 (. . .)	1.1 (0.4)	. . .
Antisocial personality disorder	12.5 (2.4)	2.0 (0.8)¶	6.87 (2.69-17.56)	27.6 (4.1)	1.2 (0.5)¶	30.33 (12.57-73.17)
Any of the above disorders	70.8 (3.3)	22.4 (2.8)¶	8.41 (5.37-13.16)	76.6 (3.8)	20.4 (2.2)¶	12.75 (7.78-20.90)

**N=1385. ECA indicates Epidemiologic Catchment Area; OR, odds ratios; and CI, confidence interval.*

†Log-linear models holding age and race constant for the combined sample of Tables 4 and 5 (N=4488, model df=24) show differences of all disorders to be significantly higher in the jail population at $P<.001$, except for schizophrenia/schizophreniform ($P<.10$) and panic disorder ($P<.02$).

‡The CI for manic episode among non-Hispanic whites does not overlap with 1.0 even though the difference of proportions test is not significant. The estimated asymptotic variance of the logged odds converges to its theoretical distribution more quickly than the χ^2 (Agresti,[35] 1990), so this test is slightly more efficient. The corrected Pearson χ^2 statistic is 2.52 ($P=.11$), and the corrected likelihood ratio χ^2 is 4.03 ($P=.04$).

§$P<.01$.
‖$P<.05$.
¶$P<.001$.

tween the data in Tables 2 and 3 shows that most subjects who had a lifetime disorder also had an episode within the past 6 months.

We also compared lifetime and 6-month diagnoses by age and education. Substance abuse or dependence and generalized anxiety disorders were least prevalent in the youngest age group (17 to 24 years old), and ASPD was most common among persons with less education (analyses are available from authors).

COMPARING FEMALE JAIL DETAINEES WITH WOMEN IN THE ECA PROJECT

Table 4 and **Table 5** compare the jail rates, controlling for race or ethnicity, and age with rates for women in the general household population from three combined ECA sites. Because our sample was urban, we used ECA data from the most urban sites: Baltimore, Md; Los Angeles, Calif; and St Louis, Mo. Because ECA's Wave I study did not include PTSD and generalized anxiety disorder, we did not include those disorders in this comparison.

Log-linear models holding age and race constant showed that the prevalence and the odds of all disorders were significantly higher at $P<.001$ in the jail than in the general population, except for schizophrenia or schizophreniform disorder ($P<.10$) and panic disorder ($P<.02$). Also, for most disorders, χ^2 tests found significant differences for each age and racial or ethnic subgroup. However, for schizophrenia or schizophreniform disorder and panic disorder, the rates were significantly higher in the jail than the ECA only in the older Hispanic subgroup. For manic disorder, the rates in jail were significantly higher than the ECA rates only in the older white subgroup.

The ECA used an earlier version of the DIS-III based on *DSM-III*[36] criteria. To check that the observed differences were not an artifact of diagnostic discrepancies, we rescored the jail data using criteria similar to the *DSM-III* and replicated the jail-ECA analyses. Results did not change using these adjusted criteria.

Hispanic		
Rate, % (SE)†		
Jail (n=134)	ECA (n=158)	OR (95% CI)
17.8 (3.3)	6.7 (2.4)§	3.03 (1.25-7.36)
2.9 (1.4)	1.4 (1.4)	2.11 (0.23-19.24)
2.2 (1.2)	0.9 (0.9)	2.46 (0.25-24.15)
15.7 (3.2)	4.4 (1.9)§	4.03 (1.49-10.88)
9.0 (2.5)	1.2 (0.6)§	8.07 (2.42-26.90)
58.2 (4.3)	7.9 (2.5)¶	16.30 (7.59-34.98)
30.4 (4.0)	5.7 (2.4)¶	7.19 (2.82-18.33)
48.7 (4.3)	4.1 (1.5)¶	22.41 (9.95-50.47)
3.9 (1.7)	0.0 (. . .)	. . .
23.2 (3.7)	1.2 (0.6)¶	25.91 (8.41-79.79)
68.7 (4.0)	12.9 (3.1)¶	14.75 (7.71-28.23)

THE RELATIONSHIP BETWEEN ARREST CHARGE AND PSYCHIATRIC DISORDER

We next examined the relationship between the subject's current major mental or substance use disorders and her most serious current charge. Because our goal was to determine the contemporaneous relationship between psychiatric disorder and arrest charge, we used the narrowest recency criteria the DIS-III-R provides: disorders were counted as present if the subject met criteria for the disorder and experienced at least one symptom within 2 weeks of the interview. Schizophrenia and manic episode were combined for analyses because there were too few cases to analyze each separately. Arrest charges were categorized into four mutually exclusive groups: violent felony, nonviolent felony, violent misdemeanor, or nonviolent misdemeanor. Because subjects may have more than one disorder, columns sum to more than 100%.

Table 6 describes how many subjects within each disorder group were arrested for each crime type (eg, 43.4% of subjects with drug use disorders were arrested for a nonviolent felony). There were no significant differences between any of the diagnostic groups and the no-disorder group. The difference between the schizophrenia or manic episode group and the no-disorder group was almost significant ($P<.11$). A post hoc power analysis showed that this difference would have been significant at the .05 level had the same difference been obtained with a larger sample of subjects with schizophrenia or manic episode (n=66). We also analyzed the data, collapsing disorder into mutually exclusive categories. Each subject was categorized by her most severe diagnosis, using the order shown in Table 6. The results (available from the authors) were the same.

COMMENT

Over 80% of the sample met criteria for one or more lifetime *DSM-III-R* psychiatric disorders; 70% were symptomatic within 6 months of the interview. Substance abuse or dependence was extremely prevalent overall, affecting over 70% of the sample, and 60% within 6 months of the interview. Drug abuse or dependence (predominantly heroin and cocaine) was the most prevalent disorder, irrespective of race or ethnicity, education, or age; over one half of all subjects had drug abuse or dependence within 6 months of the interview. The observed estimates may underestimate the true prevalence rates among these female jail detainees, particularly of severe mental disorders and substance abuse disorders, for three reasons. First, our sample excludes mentally ill persons who were not jailed because their charges were minor and were dismissed at pretrial arraignment. Second, the sample excludes 15 persons who appeared mentally disorganized and possibly psychotic but either refused to

Table 5. Lifetime Prevalence of Specific Psychiatric Disorders Among Women Entering Jail and in the ECA: Age 26-50 y*

Disorder	African American: Rate, % (SE)† Jail (n=312)	African American: Rate, % (SE)† ECA (n=815)	African American: OR (95% CI)	Non-Hispanic White: Rate, % (SE)† Jail (n=294)	Non-Hispanic White: Rate, % (SE)† ECA (n=1149)	Non-Hispanic White: OR (95% CI)
Severe disorders	16.6 (2.1)	9.7 (1.2)‡	1.85 (1.25-2.75)	26.5 (2.6)	14.2 (1.3)‖	2.18 (1.56-3.03)
Schizophrenia/ schizophreniform	2.8 (0.9)	2.7 (0.6)	1.05 (0.46-2.36)	2.8 (1.0)	2.3 (0.6)	1.21 (0.51-2.83)
Manic episode	1.6 (0.7)	1.3 (0.4)	1.19 (0.40-3.53)	3.8 (1.1)	1.1 (0.4)§	3.54 (1.46-8.60)
Major depressive episode	15.3 (2.0)	7.6 (1.1)‡	2.20 (1.44-3.38)	24.8 (2.5)	12.8 (1.2)‖	2.24 (1.60-3.15)
Dysthymia	8.9 (1.6)	4.7 (0.9)§	2.00 (1.14-3.52)	13.3 (2.0)	6.2 (0.8)‡	2.30 (1.48-3.57)
Substance abuse/dependence	77.2 (2.4)	10.8 (1.3)‖	28.12 (19.37-40.82)	84.8 (2.1)	10.4 (0.9)‖	48.21 (33.12-70.18)
Alcohol abuse/dependence	34.7 (2.7)	7.3 (1.1)‖	6.76 (4.56-10.03)	56.5 (2.9)	5.7 (0.7)‖	21.52 (15.31-30.25)
Drug abuse/dependence	72.1 (2.5)	4.6 (0.8)‖	54.07 (34.40-84.99)	76.8 (2.5)	6.6 (0.8)‖	47.03 (32.73-67.58)
Panic disorder	0.6 (0.5)	2.0 (0.6)	0.31 (0.07-1.43)	6.0 (1.4)	3.8 (0.7)	1.61 (0.87-2.99)
Antisocial personality disorder	12.1 (1.9)	1.7 (0.5)‖	8.14 (4.23-15.65)	18.7 (2.3)	1.5 (0.4)‖	14.66 (7.93-27.12)
Any of the above disorders	80.1 (2.3)	20.0 (1.7)‖	16.13 (11.41-22.80)	89.6 (1.8)	24.1 (1.5)‖	27.06 (18.02-40.64)

**N*=3103. ECA indicates Epidemiologic Catchment Area; OR, odds ratios; and CI, confidence interval.*

†*Log-linear models holding age and race constant for the combined sample of Tables 4 and 5 (N=4488, model df=24) show differences of all disorders to be significantly higher in the jail population at P<.001, except for schizophrenia/schizophreniform (P<.10) and panic disorder (P<.02).*

‡*P<.01.*

§*P<.05.*

‖*P<.001.*

Table 6. Distribution of Arrest Charges Among Women Entering Jail by Current Diagnosis*

Current Diagnosis	n	Felony, % Violent	Felony, % Nonviolent	Misdemeanor, % Violent	Misdemeanor, % Nonviolent
Schizophrenia/mania	38	34.5	35.9	6.5	23.1
Major depressive episode	134	16.9	42.6	2.6	37.9
Both drug and alcohol abuse/dependence	157	10.6	40.8	7.9	40.7
Drug abuse/dependence	554	8.7	43.4	4.5	43.3
Alcohol abuse/dependence	279	11.5	36.4	11.1	41.0
None of the above disorders	540	11.5	38.4	7.1	42.9
Total	1267	10.5	40.3	6.7	42.6

**Percents are row percents. Five subjects missing current charge information are excluded. One additional case is missing on "None of the above disorders." Tests compare each disorder to the "None of the above disorders" group (df=3). No test is significant at .05.*

participate or terminated the interview before it was finished. Third, underreporting of symptoms is endemic,[37] especially for disorders such as drug abuse. Thus, the true epidemiologic picture of arrestees and jail detainees is probably even more bleak than it appears.

The observed demographic patterns differ from those found in the ECA program, but they are similar to studies on men in jail and women in prison. The ECA study found that among women there were few significant differences between non-Hispanic whites and African Americans or between non-Hispanic whites and Mexican Americans.[38] In contrast, we found that non-Hispanic whites had the highest rates of most disorders. Our findings are remarkably similar to those of Jordan et al,[39] who conducted the largest epidemiologic study of convicted women in a US prison. Many rates in their study, eg, lifetime major depressive episode (18.0%), dysthymia (7.1%), and lifetime alcohol abuse or dependence (38.6%), were almost the same as the observed jail rates. Jordan et al also found racial differences substantially similar to those observed here: whites often had higher rates of specific psychiatric disorders than African Americans.

The relatively higher rates of disorder among white jail detainees may reflect biases against racial or ethnic minorities and the poor. African Americans and Hispanics have higher arrest rates than whites[40] and are poorer.[41] Thus, minorities, whether or not they have psychiatric disorders, may often be unable to afford bail or a lawyer who can obtain their immediate release. Whites with psychiatric disorders may be economically similar to minorities: too poor to afford bail or legal counsel.

The prevalence of major depressive episode and dysthymia is a significant problem in jails because suicide is the second most common cause of death.[24] Perhaps even more alarming is the prevalence of substance use disorders, particularly drug abuse or dependence. The high rates of drug use disorders may result, in part, from the "war on drugs," the National Drug Control Strategy, which mandates harsh penalties for drug crimes.[42] In the last decade, arrests for all offenses rose 27.7%, but arrests for

Hispanic		
Rate, % (SE)†		
Jail (n=165)	ECA (n=368)	OR (95% CI)
18.9 (3.1)	7.3 (1.5)‡	2.95 (1.63-5.34)
3.2 (1.4)	0.6 (0.4)§	5.45 (1.24-23.92)
2.4 (1.2)	0.4 (0.4)	6.91 (0.76-62.91)
17.1 (3.0)	6.8 (1.5)‡	2.81 (1.52-5.22)
14.5 (2.8)	7.0 (1.5)§	2.27 (1.20-4.28)
58.4 (3.8)	4.6 (1.2)‖	28.85 (15.69-53.03)
39.8 (3.8)	3.5 (1.1)‖	18.14 (9.16-35.92)
46.7 (3.9)	2.4 (0.8)‖	35.14 (16.95-72.88)
3.0 (1.3)	0.3 (0.2)§	12.47 (1.43-108.55)
13.5 (2.7)	1.3 (0.6)‖	11.77 (4.47-30.98)
65.1 (3.7)	15.1 (2.1)‖	10.49 (6.62-16.60)

drug violations rose 125.9%.[43] Once arrested, however, few detainees receive drug abuse services.[42] Although detainees do not have a constitutional right to substance abuse treatment,[44] drug abuse services are critical. Substance use disorders are serious illnesses, are often difficult to treat, and may complicate the treatment of other disorders. Although we will address the issue of comorbidity in future studies, our findings suggest that many detainees have more than one psychiatric disorder and that jails need treatment programs for persons with comorbidity.[45] Persons with both mental disorders and substance use disorders may be particularly vulnerable to arrest and recidivism.[46]

A striking percentage of women in jail had PTSD. These rates did not vary by race or ethnicity, age, or education. Most of these women were victims of rape or other violent assault. Untreated trauma can have severe psychological and behavioral repercussions.[47] The predominance of PTSD among female detainees is a relatively unexplored, but important, aspect of their mental health needs.

There was a nonsignificant trend for detainees with current schizophrenia or manic episode to be arrested more often for violent crimes than for detainees with no mental disorder. This trend appears to be consistent with work by Link and Steuve[48] which found an association between violence and psychotic symptoms involving threats or control-override. However, our data cannot be used to infer the overall relationship between violence and mental disorder for two reasons: detainee samples are biased samples of offenders (the underclass is more likely to be arrested and then jailed pretrial), and current charge is a poor indicator of criminal career.[49]

These data have critical implications for mental health services for women in jail. Sixty percent of detainees with schizophrenia or manic episode and 80% of those with major depressive episode were arrested for nonviolent crimes, often misdemeanors. Most often, subjects were jailed because they could not afford even the low bail usually required for misdemeanors. The American Bar Association recommends that persons with mental disorders who were arrested for misdemeanors be diverted to a mental health facility instead of arrested.[18] With appropriate community programs, nonviolent felons also could be treated outside the jail after pretrial hearings. Thus, many subjects could have been diverted at arrest. Unfortunately, community-based programs are rarely available for released jail detainees, who often have complicated diagnostic profiles and special treatment needs.[46,50]

The female jail census is at an all time high: nearly 50 000 nationwide.[24] Although the number of women in jail requiring treatment seems small, they are more impoverished[20] and even more underserved than are men in jail. Ironically, the relatively small number of women in jail makes the per capita cost too high to provide them with needed services.[51] Moreover, women have not benefited from many court decisions mandating improved treatment for men because court orders are often not binding beyond the specific prison or appellate region in which the case was decided.[52] Although the courts have mandated that female prisoners must have services equivalent to males[53-55] and must be provided adequate health care,[56-58] in practice they have been deprived.[14,59]

In summary, the jail is a potentially viable point of intervention or referral. In practice, however, the magnitude of inmate health problems far exceeds current budgetary outlays,[42] and few jails have resources to treat the mental disorders of their growing populations.[17,45,60] Psychiatry and the criminal justice system must allocate resources and design programs to reach women who are diverted at arrest, who need treatment while in jail, and who need liaison with community programs after they are released.

Accepted for publication September 21, 1995.

This work was supported by grants R01-MH45583 and R01-MH47994 from the National Institute of Mental Health, Rockville, Md.

We appreciate the cooperation of Cook County Sheriff Michael F. Sheahan and former Cook County Department of Corrections Executive Director J. W. Fairman, Jr, and we acknowledge the assistance and cooperation of Cermak Health Services of Cook County, especially Carl Alaimo, PsyD. We also acknowledge the outstanding efforts of our interviewers. We thank Laura Coats for her astute editing of the manuscript.

Reprint requests to the Psycho-Legal Studies Program, Department of Psychiatry, Northwestern University Medical School, 750 N Lakeshore Dr, Suite 900, Chicago, IL 60611 (Dr Teplin).

REFERENCES

1. *Bowring v Godwin*, 551 F2d 44 (4th Cir 1977).
2. *Estelle v Gamble*, 429 US 97 (1976).
3. *Jones v Wittenberg*, 323 F Supp 793 (ND Ohio 1971).

4. American Psychiatric Association. *Psychiatric Services in Jails and Prisons: Task Force Report 29.* Washington, DC: American Psychiatric Association; 1989.
5. Teplin LA. The prevalence of severe mental disorder among male urban jail detainees: comparison with the Epidemiologic Catchment Area program. *Am J Public Health.* 1990;80:663-669.
6. Teplin LA. Psychiatric and substance abuse disorders among male urban jail detainees. *Am J Public Health.* 1994;8:290-293.
7. Lamb HR, Grant RW. The mentally ill in an urban county jail. *Arch Gen Psychiatry.* 1982;39:17-22.
8. Glaser WF. Admissions to a prison psychiatric unit. *Aust N Z J Psychiatry.* 1985;19:45-52.
9. Valdiserri EV, Carroll KR, Hartl AJ. A study of offenses committed by psychotic inmates in a county jail. *Hosp Community Psychiatry.* 1986;37:163-166.
10. Robins LN, Helzer JE, Weissman MM, Orvaschel H, Gruenberg E, Burke JD Jr, Regier DA. Lifetime prevalence of specific psychiatric disorders in three sites. *Arch Gen Psychiatry.* 1984;41:949-958.
11. Steadman HJ. Insanity acquittals in New York: 1965-1978. *Am J Psychiatry.* 1980;137:321-326.
12. Steadman HJ, Monahan J, Hartstone E, Davis SK, Robbins PC. Mentally disordered offenders: a national survey of patients and facilities. *Law Hum Behav.* 1982;6:31-38.
13. Steadman, HJ, Rosenstein MJ, MacAskill RL, Manderscheid RW. A profile of mentally disordered offenders admitted to inpatient psychiatric services in the United States. *Law Hum Behav.* 1988;12:91-99.
14. Washington P, Diamond RJ. Prevalence of mental illness among women incarcerated in five California county jails. *Res Community Ment Health.* 1985; 5:33-41.
15. Lamb R, Grant RW. Mentally ill women in a county jail. *Arch Gen Psychiatry.* 1983;40:363-368.
16. Steadman HJ, Barbera SS, Dennis DL. A national survey of jail diversion programs for mentally ill detainees. *Hosp Community Psychiatry.* 1994;45:1109-1113.
17. Steadman HJ, McCarty DW, Morrissey JP. *The Mentally Ill in Jail: Planning for Essential Services.* New York, NY: The Guilford Press; 1989.
18. American Bar Association. *ABA Criminal Justice Mental Health Standards.* Washington, DC: American Bar Association; 1989.
19. Morris A. *Women, Crime and Criminal Justice.* New York, NY: Basil Blackwell; 1987.
20. US Department of Justice. *Women in Jail 1989.* Washington, DC: Bureau of Justice Statistics; 1992. Publication NCJ-134732.
21. Glick R, Neto V. *National Study of Women's Correctional Programs.* Washington, DC: US Government Printing Office; 1977.
22. Sanchez JE, Johnson BD. Women and the drugs-crime connection: crime rates among drug abusing women at Rikers Island. *J Psychoact Drugs.* 1987;19: 205-216.
23. Cook County Department of Corrections. *Long Range Master Plan Executive Summary.* Chicago, Ill: Cook County Department of Corrections; 1990.
24. US Department of Justice. *Jails & Jail Inmates 1993-94.* Washington, DC: Bureau of Justice Statistics; 1995. Publication NCJ-151651.
25. US Department of Justice. *Drug Use Forecasting Annual Report.* Washington, DC: National Institute of Justice; 1990.
26. Lazerwitz B. Sampling theory and procedures. In: Blalock HM Jr, Blalock AB, eds. *Methodology in Social Research.* New York, NY: McGraw Hill International Book Co; 1968:278-328.
27. Robins LN, Helzer JE, Croughan J, Ratcliff K. National Institute of Mental Health Diagnostic Interview Schedule: its history, characteristics and validity. *Arch Gen Psychiatry.* 1981;38:381-389.
28. American Psychiatric Association, Committee on Statistics. *Diagnostic and Statistical Manual of Mental Disorders, Revised Third Edition.* Washington, DC: American Psychiatric Association; 1987.
29. Burke JK. Diagnostic categorization by the Diagnostic Interview Schedule (DIS): a comparison with other methods of assessment. In: Barrett J, Rose R, eds. *Mental Disorders in the Community.* New York, NY: Guilford Press; 1986:255-285.
30. Helzer JE, Robins LN, McEvoy LT, Spitznagel EL, Stoltzman RK, Farmer A, Brockington IF. A comparison of clinical and Diagnostic Interview Schedule diagnoses. *Arch Gen Psychiatry.* 1985;42:657-666.
31. Anthony JC, Folstein M, Romanoski AJ, Von Korff MR, Nestadt GR, Chahal R, Merchant A, Brown H, Shapiro S, Kramer M, Gruenberg EM. Comparison of the lay Diagnostic Interview Schedule and a standardized psychiatric diagnosis. *Arch Gen Psychiatry.* 1985;42:667-675.
32. Boyd JH, Burke JD Jr, Gruenberg E, Holzer CE III, Rae DS, George LK, Karno M, Stoltzman R, McEvoy L, Nestadt G. Exclusion criteria of *DSM-III*: a co-occurrence of hierarchy-free syndromes. *Arch Gen Psychiatry.* 1984;41:983-989.
33. Burnam MA, Hough RL, Escobar JI, Karno M, Timbers DM, Telles CA, Locke BZ. Six-month prevalence of specific psychiatric disorders among Mexican Americans and non-Hispanic whites in Los Angeles. *Arch Gen Psychiatry* 1987;44: 687-694.
34. Shah BV, Barnwell BG, Hunt N, LaVange LM. *SUDAAN User's Manual.* Research Triangle Park, NC: Research Triangle Institute; 1992. Release 6.34.
35. Agresti A. *Categorical Data Analysis.* New York, NY: John Wiley & Sons Inc; 1990:228-232.
36. American Psychiatric Association, Committee on Statistics. *Diagnostic and Statistical Manual of Mental Disorders, Third Edition.* Washington, DC: American Psychiatric Association; 1980.
37. Hodgins S. Assessing mental disorder in the criminal justice system: feasibility versus clinical accuracy. *Int J Law Psychiatry.* 1995;18:15-28.
38. Robins LN, Regier DA, eds. *Psychiatric Disorders in America: The Epidemiologic Catchment Area Study.* New York, NY: The Free Press; 1991.
39. Jordan BK, Schlenger WE, Fairbank JA, Caddell JM. Prevalence of psychiatric disorders among incarcerated women, II: convicted women felons entering prison. *Arch Gen Psychiatry.* 1996;53:513-519.
40. US Department of Justice. *Crime in the United States.* Washington, DC: Federal Bureau of Investigation; 1990.
41. US Bureau of the Census. *Statistical Abstract of the United States (114th Edition).* Washington, DC: US Bureau of the Census; 1994:469.
42. American College of Physicians, National Commission on Correctional Health Care, American Correctional Health Services Association. The crisis in correctional health care: the impact of the National Drug Control Strategy on Correctional Health Services. *Ann Intern Med.* 1992;117:71-77.
43. Maguire K, Flanagan TJ. *Sourcebook of Criminal Justice Statistics 1990.* Washington, DC: US Government Printing Office; 1991.
44. Cohen F. *Legal Issues and the Mentally Disordered Prisoner.* Washington, DC: National Institute of Corrections; 1988.
45. Roesch R, Ogloff JRP, Eaves D. Mental health research in the criminal justice system: the need for common approaches and international perspectives. *Int J Law Psychiatry.* 1995;18:1-14.
46. Abram KM, Teplin LA. Co-occurring disorders among mentally ill jail detainees: implications for public policy. *Am Psychol.* 1991;46:1036-1045.
47. Herman J. *Trauma and Recovery.* New York, NY: Basic Books; 1992.
48. Link BG, Steuve A. Psychotic symptoms and the violent/illegal behavior of mental patients compared to community controls. In: Monahan J, Steadman HJ, eds. *Violence and Mental Disorder.* Chicago, Ill: University of Chicago Press; 1994:137-159.
49. Teplin LA, Abram KM, McClelland GM. Does psychiatric disorder predict violent crime among released jail detainees? a six-year longitudinal study. *Am Psychol.* 1994;49:335-342.
50. Teplin LA. Criminalizing mental disorder: the comparative arrest rate of the mentally ill. *Am Psychol.* 1984;39:794-803.
51. Feinman C. *Women in the Criminal Justice System.* 2nd ed. New York, NY: Praeger; 1986.
52. Leonard EB. Judicial decisions and prison reform: the impact of litigation on women prisoners. *Soc Probl.* 1983;31:45-58.
53. *Barefield v Leach,* No. 10282, Dist Ct New Mexico, Dec 18, 1974.
54. *Cooper v Morin,* 91 Misc 2d 302, 398 NYS2d 36 (Monroe County Sup Ct, 1977).
55. *Glover v Johnson,* 478 R Supp 1075 (ED Mich 1979).
56. *Newman v Alabama,* 349 F Supp 278 (MD Ala, 1972).
57. *Morales v Turman,* 383 R Supp 53 (ED Tex, 1974).
58. *Todaro v Ward,* 431 R. Supp 1129, SDNY, aff'd, 565 F2d 48 (2d Cir 1977).
59. Velimesis ML. Sex roles and mental health of women in prison. *Prof Psychol.* 1981;12:128-135.
60. Steadman HJ, ed. *Effectively Addressing the Mental Health Needs of Jail Detainees.* Seattle, Wash: National Coalition for the Mentally Ill in the Criminal Justice System; 1990.

ORIGINAL ARTICLE

Prevalence of Psychiatric Disorders Among Incarcerated Women

II. Convicted Felons Entering Prison

B. Kathleen Jordan, PhD; William E. Schlenger, PhD; John A. Fairbank, PhD; Juesta M. Caddell, PhD

Background: No unbiased estimates of the rates of psychiatric disorder among women prison inmates are available. Nonetheless, available data suggest that some psychiatric disorders are prevalent in this population. The objective of the study was to determine the rates, risk factors, and outcomes of specific psychiatric disorders among women prison inmates.

Methods: A virtual census of women felons (N=805) entering prison in North Carolina was assessed using in-person interviews. Assessments were conducted for 8 disorders, using the Composite International Diagnostic Interview as the primary assessment measure. For validation purposes, one quarter of the inmates were reassessed for 2 of these disorders, using structured clinical interviews.

Results: Inmates were found to have high rates of substance abuse and dependence and antisocial and borderline personality disorders compared with women in community epidemiologic studies. Rates among inmates were also somewhat elevated for mood disorders but not for anxiety disorders. The rate of reports of lifetime exposure to traumatic events was also high. Rates of disorder tended to be higher among white than among African American women.

Conclusion: High rates of substance abuse, psychiatric disorder, and psychological distress associated with exposure to traumatic events suggest that women in prison have a need for treatment for substance abuse and other mental health problems.

(Arch Gen Psychiatry. 1996;53:513-519)

From Research Triangle Institute, Research Triangle Park, NC, and Department of Psychiatry and Behavioral Sciences, Duke University Medical Center, Durham, NC.

On any given day in 1994, over 800 000 women were under supervision of correctional authorities in the United States.[1-3] This total includes women in jail, on probation, in prison, and on parole. Despite their now substantial numbers, women criminal offenders have received relatively little research attention. In this article, we present data from Research Triangle Institute's Women Inmates' Health Survey (WIHS), the first large-scale epidemiologic study of women prison inmates in the United States.

Several factors make this research particularly timely and important. For a number of years, the rate at which women enter prison has been increasing faster than the rate for men.[4] Furthermore, findings from prior studies[5-9] suggest that a variety of problems, including drug use and some psychiatric disorders, are more prevalent among women inmates than among men inmates. Also, because many women sentenced to prison have major child-rearing responsibilities, symptoms and sequelae of their psychiatric disorders, as well as their extended absence from the home, can contribute to the development of psychiatric disorders and behavior problems among their children.

Most of the existing data on psychiatric disorders among prison inmates are from studies whose samples included predominantly or completely male subjects. These studies[10-12] have found higher rates of at least some specific psychiatric disorders than are found in the general community population, with lifetime rates often reported to be 50% or more. The high rates, however, reflect in large part the high rates of antisocial personality disorder (ASPD) and substance abuse and dependence seen in male prisoners.

See also page 505

Previous studies of psychiatric disorder among women prisoners have had serious limitations that may have introduced bias into their estimates (eg, the use of small or nonprobability samples and nonstandardized assessments). Nevertheless, findings do suggest that, as with men inmates, substance abuse and dependence are much more prevalent among

See Methods on next page

METHODS

THE SAMPLE

Data for the WIHS were collected between July 1991 and November 1992 at the Correctional Institution for Women in Raleigh, NC. At the time of the study, all women felons newly sentenced to prison in North Carolina entered prison at this facility. (A felony is a serious criminal offense for which the minimum sentence is 1 year or longer.) During most of the months of data collection (and for 94% of the total WIHS sample), subjects composed a census of women entering prison for new felony charges. (Women were interviewed 5 to 10 days after entering prison.) For a few months during which incarcerations were unusually heavy, we selected a random sample of newly entering felons; for those months, we have used weights to adjust for the probability of selection.

We used a 2-stage study design.[22,23] In the first stage, 805 in-depth, face-to-face interviews, averaging 2½ hours in length, were conducted in private by professional survey interviewers. Written or witnessed consents were obtained for all interviews, and the response rate was 95%. In the second stage, one quarter of the survey interview respondents were reinterviewed by a mental health clinician to validate 2 of our survey assessment measures. This follow-up had a response rate of 99%.

We used data from the North Carolina site of the ECA for comparisons with community women because of the ECA sample's similarities to the WIHS sample with respect to geographic location and sociodemographic characteristics, both of which have been found to be related to rates of disorder.[24,25] Disorder in the ECA sample was assessed using the Diagnostic Interview Schedule (DIS)[26] and *DSM-III* criteria.[27]

MEASUREMENT OF PSYCHIATRIC DISORDER

The specific disorders that we assessed were major depressive episode, dysthymia, generalized anxiety disorder, posttraumatic stress disorder (PTSD), panic disorder, alcohol abuse and dependence, drug abuse and dependence, ASPD, and borderline personality disorder (BPD). We did not assess 2 other disorders often included in psychiatric epidemiologic studies: schizophrenia and manic episode (to allow diagnosis of bipolar disorder). We expected that the rates of these disorders would be quite low, while the interview time required to assess them would have been substantial.

As noted above, *DSM-III-R* criteria were used for all disorders.[21] Most of the disorders were assessed in the survey interview with the Composite International Diagnostic Interview (CIDI), a modification of the DIS developed by the World Health Organization (WHO).[28-30] The CIDI, however, does not have a module that assesses ASPD or PTSD, so we used the DIS ASPD module to assess ASPD in the survey interview. Although the DIS has been used to assess PTSD in a number of major epidemiologic studies, we have found unsatisfactory agreement with clinical assessments when used with subjects who are not seeking treatment. We did attempt to assess PTSD in the survey interview using another instrument (the Impact of Events Scale). However, the results did not correspond well to the clinical assessments of PTSD made in our follow-up study using the Structured Clinical Interview for *DSM-III-R*, Revised, Nonpatient Version (SCID-R, NP-V).[31] For this reason, we do not provide population prevalence rates of PTSD in this article.

Neither the CIDI nor the DIS assesses BPD. In the survey interview, we assessed this disorder with a modification of the BPD module of the Diagnostic Interview for Personality Disorder, Revised (DIPD-R).[32] This module uses *DSM-III-R* criteria for BPD and has been found to have satisfactory reliability.

In the follow-up interview, clinicians assessed BPD using the Diagnostic Interview for Borderlines, Revised (DIB-R).[33] We found good correspondence between the survey interview BPD diagnosis and the *DSM-III-R* scoring of the clinician-administered DIB-R. With respect to the DIB-R's *DSM-III-R* diagnosis, the survey measure of BPD had a sensitivity of 77% and a specificity of 81%.

For both the CIDI and DIS, current prevalence is the proportion of individuals who have met the diagnostic criteria for the disorder at some time in their lives and who have experienced at least 1 symptom of the disorder in the period defined as *current*. Therefore, those with current disorder are a subset of those with lifetime disorder. For the CIDI and DIS disorders, we defined "within the past 6 months" as current. The survey instrument that we used to assess BPD does not assess lifetime disorder and uses the past 2 years as current. Because of the chronic nature of personality disorders, the relatively young age of many of the participants, and the fact that BPD is assessed for its presence within the past 2 years, it is likely that the lifetime and current rates of BPD would be similar.

To test our hypothesis that exposure to extreme events would be prevalent in this population and that such exposure would be related to a number of disorders, such as PTSD, BPD, and substance abuse, we assessed exposure to trauma with a lengthy survey interview section that contained detailed questions about a full range of potentially traumatic events. The instrument was a modification of that used by Resnick and colleagues[34] in their national study of rape.

STATISTICAL ANALYSIS

We developed weights to adjust for the probability of selection in all analyses and conducted χ^2 tests to examine group differences in rates of disorder. We have noted the probabilities associated with the χ^2 for group differences that were statistically significant. When discussed in the text, significance refers to less than a .05 probability. The SAS software was used to develop the prevalence estimates, associated SEs, and the χ^2 values for **Table 1** through **Table 4**. The age or racial groupings for the ECA sample have not been presented elsewhere, so the study team developed the prevalence estimates shown in **Table 5**, using the North Carolina ECA data file. Because of the complex sampling design used for the ECA, the Survey Data Analysis (SUDAAN) software[35] was used to develop the estimates, SEs, χ^2 values, associated probabilities, odds ratios, and confidence intervals presented in Table 5. In these analyses, the standard ECA weights were used.

women inmates than among women in the general population.[13-17] Rates of ASPD also tend to be elevated among women inmates, although they are substantially lower than for male prisoners.[13-15] Rates of anxiety and mood disorders vary substantially across studies of women prison inmates.[13,14,16,18] In general, rates of anxiety disorders do not appear to be elevated among women inmates. The rates for mood disorders appear to be el-

Table 1. Proportion of Women Entering Prison in North Carolina With Selected Characteristics (Unweighted) (N=805)

Characteristics	No. (%)
Race	
White	280 (34.8)
African American	468 (58.1)
Hispanic (black or white)	27 (3.4)
Other	30 (3.7)
Age, y	
18-20	50 (6.2)
21-25	161 (20.0)
26-29	181 (22.5)
30-34	190 (23.6)
35-50	203 (25.2)
51+	20 (2.5)
Education, y	
<12	430 (53.5)
12	223 (27.7)
13+	151 (18.8)
Marital status	
Never married	327 (40.6)
Separated or divorced	184 (22.9)
Living as married	153 (19.0)
Married	106 (13.2)
Widowed	35 (4.3)
No. of children under 18 y	
0	243 (30.3)
1	204 (25.4)
2	167 (20.8)
3+	188 (23.4)
First time in prison	373 (46.3)
Incarcerated before age 18 y	117 (14.6)
Offense for which currently incarcerated*	
Drug-related offenses	311 (38.7)
Burglary, robbery, or theft	214 (26.7)
Forgery, fraud, or bad checks	210 (26.2)
Probation or parole violations	143 (17.9)
Violent assault and child abuse	98 (12.2)
Other	124 (15.4)

**Totals are more than 100% because inmates may be incarcerated for more than 1 offense.*

Table 2. Lifetime Prevalence of Specific Psychiatric Disorders Among Women Entering Prison in North Carolina (N=805)

	Rate, % (SE)		
Specific Psychiatric Disorder	Total	White	African American
Major depressive episode*	13.0 (1.2)	19.2 (2.4)	9.4 (1.4)
Dysthymia*	7.1 (0.9)	10.3 (1.9)	5.2 (1.0)
Generalized anxiety disorder†	2.7 (0.6)	4.6 (1.3)	1.8 (0.6)
Panic disorder*	5.8 (0.9)	8.7 (1.7)	4.2 (0.9)
Alcohol abuse and dependence*	38.6 (1.8)	47.8 (3.1)	33.3 (2.2)
Drug abuse and dependence	44.2 (1.8)	46.2 (3.1)	43.2 (2.3)
Antisocial personality disorder	11.9 (1.2)	13.5 (2.1)	10.2 (1.4)
Any lifetime disorder*	64.0 (1.8)	73.7 (2.7)	58.3 (2.3)

*$P<.01$.
†$P<.05$.

Table 3. Six-Month Prevalence of Specific Psychiatric Disorders Among Women Entering Prison in North Carolina (N=805)

	Rate, % (SE)		
Specific Psychiatric Disorder	Total	White	African American
Major depressive episode*	10.8 (1.1)	14.7 (2.2)	8.8 (1.3)
Generalized anxiety disorder	1.4 (0.4)	2.0 (0.9)	1.2 (0.5)
Panic disorder†	4.7 (0.8)	7.1 (1.6)	3.7 (0.9)
Alcohol abuse and dependence	17.1 (1.4)	19.9 (2.4)	15.4 (1.7)
Drug abuse and dependence	30.3 (1.7)	30.8 (2.8)	30.7 (2.2)
Antisocial personality disorder	11.9 (1.2)	13.5 (2.1)	10.2 (1.4)
Borderline personality disorder‡	28.0 (1.6)	27.2 (2.7)	29.0 (2.1)
Any current disorder	46.3 (1.8)	50.3 (3.1)	44.4 (2.4)

*$P<.01$.
†$P<.05$.
‡*Prevalence of borderline personality disorder is for 2 years, not 6 months.*

evated in some studies but not in others.

A further problem with previous studies of women inmates is that little attention was paid to sociodemographic characteristics and how such characteristics may be related to rates of disorder. Findings from the Epidemiologic Catchment Area (ECA) Study[19] suggest that rates of disorder may vary by age and/or racial groups, and other studies have found age and/or race differences for rates of disorder among male prison inmates: white men prison inmates are more likely to meet diagnostic criteria for a psychiatric disorder than are African American men inmates. This may result, at least in part, from the fact that African American men who engage in antisocial behavior have been found to be more likely to be arrested than white men who engage in similar behaviors.[20] Thus, white individuals may be less likely to be incarcerated than African American men unless they are very disturbed and/or antisocial.

The current study differs from most previous studies of women inmates in that it is a virtual census of women felons who entered prison from an entire state over a 17-month period. Unlike many previous studies, the WIHS used standardized instruments and the *DSM-III-R*[21] criteria to develop estimates of the rates of the specific psychiatric disorders.

RESULTS

Findings presented in Tables 1 through 4 are for WIHS sample members only. The variable "residence" in Table 4 represents the degree of urbanicity in the place where the woman grew up. Table 5 compares prevalence rates for the WIHS sample with rates for community women in North Carolina developed from ECA data.

DEMOGRAPHIC CHARACTERISTICS AND CRIMINAL JUSTICE VARIABLES

Table 1 presents the sociodemographic characteristics of the women in the inmate sample and information about their current and prior incarcerations. About 60% of the inmates were African American, while approximately 20% of North Carolina residents in 1991 and 1992 were African American. The major demographic differences among inmates between African Americans and whites were that African American women tended to have more children and were less likely to be married (data not shown.) Because only 3% of our sample was Hispanic, Tables 2 through 5 do not include a separate Hispanic category. Instead, Hispanics are included in the appropriate racial group (African American or white).

The women inmates were a little older than samples of men entering prison, with about half the sample 30 years old or older. In a similar study of men felons in North Carolina, about one quarter of the sample were 30 years of age or older.[36] Although the majority of respondents had fewer than 12 years of schooling, some had received a general equivalency diploma so that a slight majority of the sample had either a high school diploma or a general equivalency diploma. The most common offenses for which the women were in prison were drug offenses (eg, drug use, manufacture, or sale), and these were also the most common offenses for previous incarcerations. The category defined as "probation or parole violations" also includes other charges, such as weapons charges, gambling, liquor law violations, and resisting arrest, but most inmates in this category were incarcerated because of probation or parole violations. In contrast to the stereotype of prison inmates as violent and dangerous offenders, a rather small proportion (11%) of the women were incarcerated for a violent offense.

PREVALENCE OF THE SPECIFIC PSYCHIATRIC DISORDERS

Table 2 presents the lifetime prevalence of specific psychiatric disorders. About two thirds of the sample met *DSM-III-R* criteria for at least 1 of the disorders we assessed. The 2 substance-related disorders had the highest prevalence. Note that for all disorders, there is a trend for prevalence rates to be higher for whites; the racial differences are statistically significant for 5 of the 7 disorders.

Table 3 presents the estimates of the current prevalence rates of the specific disorders. Almost half of the women met current criteria for 1 or more of the *DSM-III-R* disorders we assessed. As with lifetime disorders, the substance use disorders and BPD were the most prevalent. (The *current* prevalence for BPD is higher than the *lifetime* rate for any other disorder except the substance use disorders; thus, BPD appears to be the third most prevalent lifetime disorder.) Again, there is a trend for rates of current disorder to be somewhat higher for whites than for African Ameri-

Table 4. Lifetime Prevalence of Specific Psychiatric Disorders for Women Entering Prison in North Carolina With Various Characteristics (N=805)

	Rate, % (SE)								
	Age, y			Residence			Education, y		
Specific Psychiatric Disorders	18-24 (n=168)	25-44 (n=595)	45-64 (n=41)	Rural (n=219)	Small Town (n=206)	City/ Urban (n=378)	<12 (n=430)	12 (n=223)	13+ (n=151)
Major depressive episode	14.3 (2.8)	12.4 (1.4)	17.4 (6.3)	14.0 (2.4)	15.8 (2.6)	10.8 (1.6)	12.5 (1.7)	9.9 (2.0)	19.1 (3.3)*
Dysthymia	3.8 (1.5)	7.4 (1.1)	15.3 (6.0)*	7.7 (1.9)	6.8 (1.8)	6.9 (1.4)	6.8 (1.3)	4.3 (1.4)	11.8 (2.7)*
Generalized anxiety disorder	2.3 (1.2)	2.9 (0.7)	2.3 (2.6)	3.1 (1.2)	4.2 (1.5)	1.7 (0.7)	2.8 (0.8)	2.2 (1.0)	3.2 (1.5)
Panic disorder	3.3 (1.4)	6.3 (1.0)	8.7 (4.7)	8.1 (1.9)	5.0 (1.6)	4.6 (1.1)	5.5 (1.2)	4.3 (1.4)	8.7 (2.4)
Alcohol abuse and dependence	39.0 (3.9)	38.3 (2.1)	41.3 (8.2)	32.1 (3.3)	45.3 (3.6)	38.9 (2.6)*	44.5 (2.5)	29.4 (3.1)	34.6 (4.0)†
Drug abuse and dependence	38.5 (3.9)	48.4 (2.1)	8.7 (4.7)†	34.5 (3.3)	40.7 (3.6)	51.8 (2.7)†	46.2 (2.5)	38.4 (3.3)	46.3 (4.2)
Antisocial personality disorder	16.6 (3.0)	11.3 (1.3)	2.2 (2.4)*	11.1 (2.2)	7.2 (1.9)	15.0 (1.9)*	15.7 (1.8)	6.5 (1.7)	8.7 (2.4)†

*P<.05.
†P<.01.

Table 5. Comparison of Lifetime Prevalence Rates for Women* Entering Prison in North Carolina and Women in the Household Population in 5 Counties in North Carolina†

	Rate, % (SE)							
	Age, 18-25 y							
	White				African American			
Specific Psychiatric Disorder	Prison (n=76)	ECA (n=134)	OR	95% CI	Prison (n=126)	ECA (n=113)	OR	95% CI
Mood disorder: major depression and dysthymia	18.8 (5.4)	7.1 (2.1)	3.0	1.1-8.5	11.1 (2.7)	6.4 (1.9)	1.8	0.6-5.5
Anxiety disorder: GAD and panic	5.2 (3.1)	8.2 (3.2)	0.6	0.1-2.8	5.3 (2.0)	22.1‡ (5.3)	0.2	0.1-0.5
Alcohol abuse and dependence	47.5 (6.0)	5.5‡ (2.3)	15.5	6.2-39.0	36.3 (4.5)	2.9‡ (1.7)	18.9	5.3-6.71
Drug abuse and dependence	46.2 (5.9)	9.6‡ (3.3)	8.1	3.2-20.5	37.0 (4.5)	1.4‡ (0.9)	40.8	10.1-165.5
Antisocial personality disorder	21.2 (4.7)	1.7‡ (1.2)	15.4	3.7-63.6	18.0 (3.8)	1.9‡ (1.9)	11.1	1.4-88.4

**Aged 18 to 50 years only.*
†*ECA indicates Epidemiological Catchment Area; OR, odds ratio; CI, confidence interval; and GAD, generalized anxiety disorder.*
‡*P<.01 for ECA or inmate comparison by age or racial group.*
§*Undefined because of zero prevalence in the ECA sample.*

cans (except for BPD), although the differences are statistically significant only for 2 disorders. For both African Americans and whites, the current prevalence rates for the Axis I disorders (other than substance abuse) did not differ substantially from the lifetime rates presented in Table 2. Because of the chronicity of the personality disorders, we would expect lifetime and current rates of ASPD to be similar. However, current and lifetime estimates of ASPD were identical in the WIHS because almost all of the women were convicted of a felony shortly before the interview, which is a sufficient condition for those meeting lifetime DIS criteria for ASPD to also meet criteria for current ASPD.

SOCIODEMOGRAPHIC CHARACTERISTICS AND PREVALENCE

Table 4 shows the association between selected sociodemographic characteristics and lifetime disorders. As is commonly found, ASPD was most prevalent among the youngest cohort. Alcohol use disorders and generalized anxiety disorder did not differ much between age groups, while drug abuse problems appeared to first increase with age then decline. There was a tendency for the prevalence of panic disorder to increase with age, although the differences were not statistically significant, perhaps because of the small cell size for the older group. The oldest age cohort also had the highest rates of mood disorders, although the large SE for the oldest group made the estimate unstable. Antisocial personality disorder and drug abuse and dependence were highest among those who grew up in an urban area, and the highest rate of alcohol use disorders was found among those growing up in small towns (the rate was also high for urban areas, however).

Antisocial personality disorder was highest among those with the least education. This is consistent with the *DSM-III-R* criteria for ASPD, which includes truancy, trouble with authorities, and engaging in such activities as fighting that are likely to get one expelled from school. Alcohol use disorders were most prevalent among those with low education. However, there was a tendency for all other Axis I disorders to be most prevalent among those with the highest education (although the rates for drug abuse and dependence were also high for those with low education). Despite the relatively small sample size of women with more than a high school education (and the associated large SEs), those with more than a high school education appeared to have significantly higher rates for the mood disorders.

COMPARISON OF PREVALENCE RATES FOR WOMEN INMATES AND COMMUNITY WOMEN IN NORTH CAROLINA

Table 5 compares rates of disorder, within race by age subgroups, for the women felons entering prison in North Carolina and women in the community in North Carolina. Rates of anxiety disorders tended to be lower among inmates than for community women, significantly so for African Americans. However, there was a trend for prevalence rates for all other disorders to be higher for women inmates than for community women. The odds ratios for 10 of the 20 inmate-community comparisons were greater than 5. The differences in rates for the mood disorders, although substantial, were significantly higher only for older whites. Probabilities associated with the χ^2 for both young whites and older African Americans were .07. It may well be that the differences between inmates and community women in these groups are real, but because of sample sizes, we did not have the power to detect the differences. The odds of inmates having a substance abuse disorder or ASPD were 5 to 25 times greater than for community women.

Because no assessment measure for BPD was included in the ECA instrumentation, no comparisons for this disorder are provided in Table 5. However, Swartz and colleagues[37] used items from the ECA instrumentation to develop a measure of this disorder. Their estimate for the prevalence of BPD in the community using the ECA sample was 1.8%. Even with a 1:3 male-female ratio that was found in the study by Swartz et al, the prevalence of BPD among women in the community would still be quite low in comparison with the prevalence among our women inmates (28%).

Rates of exposure to trauma were somewhat elevated among women inmates compared with a nationally representative sample of women, in which 69% reported lifetime exposure to trauma[38]: 78% of our sample reported

Age, 26-50 y							
White				African American			
Prison (n=200)	ECA (n=453)	OR	95% CI	Prison (n=354)	ECA (n=307)	OR	95% CI
21.6 (3.2)	11.5‡ (1.9)	2.1	1.3-3.6	12.2 (1.9)	7.6 (1.7)	1.7	1.0-3.0
14.1 (2.5)	12.3 (1.9)	1.2	0.7-2.0	5.9 (1.2)	20.6‡ (3.3)	0.2	0.1-0.4
48.2 (3.8)	1.9‡ (0.8)	47.3	19.0-117.4	32.5 (2.6)	2.8‡ (1.0)	16.8	7.7-36.8
48.6 (3.8)	4.1‡ (1.3)	22.1	10.8-45.2	46.2 (2.8)	1.8‡ (0.9)	46.8	16.0-137.1
11.5 (2.6)	0	§	§	7.7 (1.5)	0.8‡ (0.8)	10.6	1.4-82.2

experiencing at some time in their lives at least 1 event that met the *DSM-III-R* criteria for an extreme event (data not shown). Although we have not been able to develop an indicator of PTSD from the survey measure that matches well with the clinical diagnosis, reports of PTSD symptoms were high in this population: 30% of our sample reported both having experienced a traumatic event and having experienced 6 or more PTSD symptoms in the past 6 months.

COMMENT

It is not surprising that convicted women felons have high rates of those disorders that include acting out and engaging in illegal behaviors; ASPD, BPD, and substance abuse all appear to be elevated in comparison with community populations. We speculate that these disorders may be contributing factors in the criminal behavior that led to the incarceration of these women. Although comorbidity data are not presented here, many inmates had both a substance abuse and a personality disorder, which would tend to exacerbate the level of deviant behaviors.

With respect to other disorders, the women inmates had somewhat higher rates of mood disorders and somewhat lower rates of anxiety disorders than did the community women. Depression has been found to be elevated in people with ASPD when they are confined and the comorbidity of depression and BPD is substantial,[39] so the elevated rates of depression among women inmates are not inconsistent with a portrait of them as individuals who have "acted out" their distress while living in the community. The low rates of anxiety disorders also suggest that these women may act out their distress rather than internalizing it.

We should note that the rates for inmates were developed using *DSM-III-R* criteria,[21] while those for community women were developed using criteria from *DSM-III*.[27] Nevertheless, we think it unlikely that observed differences in estimates are due solely to differences between the 2 *DSM* versions. This position is supported by analyses conducted by Teplin and colleagues (and presented in this issue of the ARCHIVES[40]), in which mock *DSM-III* diagnoses for inmates were compared with diagnoses for ECA community women. The authors found that substantial rate differences remained between community and inmate women.

Because the ECA data were collected 10 years prior to the inmate data, the possibility exists that rate differences across studies reflect, in part, changes in rates of disorder over time. However, estimates of rates of disorder among community women based on data collected from 1990 to 1992 in the National Comorbidity Study[41] suggest that differences between community and inmate women would still obtain. In addition, national epidemiologic data suggest that, overall, the prevalence of drug use (including cocaine use) among the household population in the United States has decreased over the 10-year period between the ECA and WIHS,[42,43] while rates of drug use among women criminal offenders has stayed the same or increased.[44-46] Therefore, we would expect the differences in rates of the substance abuse disorders between community and inmate women would be at least as great if the ECA data had been collected in 1991-1992.

Moreover, our findings are remarkably similar to those of the study by Teplin et al[40] of women jail detainees conducted in 1991-1993. The similarities are surprising because the 2 studies deal with different populations. Most individuals housed in jails have been arrested for less serious offenses (eg, shoplifting), while individuals in prisons have been tried and convicted of felonies (ie, serious offenses). Because the type of offense for which an individual is arrested or convicted has been found to be related to the presence and type of psychiatric disorder with which he or she is diagnosed,[47] we would expect to find substantial rate differences between these 2 groups of inmates.

Not only were rates of disorders similar across the jail and prison studies, both studies also found that rates of disorder were higher for (non-Hispanic) whites than for African Americans for most disorders. The finding of higher rates of disorder for African American women than (non-Hispanic) white women in both studies suggests that among white women, only the most deviant or disturbed are likely to be incarcerated, whereas African American women may be incarcerated for less serious or frequent offenses, as was found for men in the ECA.

We suspect that an important reason for differences in rates between community women and women inmates is differences in exposure to psychological trauma. We think that the high rates of BPD, ASPD, and substance abuse, as well as PTSD symptoms, among women inmates may reflect, at least in part, these women's exposure to extreme events. We discuss elsewhere our finding that sexual abuse at or before age 10 years is a significant predictor of BPD in this sample.[48] Identifying the major psychosocial and biological risk factors for these disorders in this population, however, will require in-depth studies with prospective, longitudinal designs.

The high rates of exposure to psychological trauma experienced by women in this population, coupled with the association found in both our and previous studies between such trauma and the psychiatric disorders that were elevated among the women inmates, suggest that programs may be needed in women's prisons to address exposure to trauma and its sequelae. Many of the behaviors that appear to be related to being arrested and sent to prison, eg, impulsivity and use of illicit substances, are symptoms that are often associated with exposure to trauma and trauma-related disorders such as PTSD, BPD, and the substance abuse disorders. Additionally, because about half of the sample met the criteria for substance abuse and half of the sample were also incarcerated for drug-related charges, providing treatment for substance abuse problems should also be a high priority for prisons that serve women. Such treatment has the potential to reduce substance abuse and related problems including criminal activities.[49]

It is not clear how generalizable the findings from our North Carolina study are to women in other US prisons. Compared with female prison populations nationwide, our sample had a higher proportion of women incarcerated for drug-related crime and a smaller proportion of women incarcerated for violent crime.[7] Available data suggest that the rates of substance abuse and dependence and ASPD are at least as high in other women inmate populations as in ours, and in some studies[13] they have been found to be higher.

One important potential limitation of the study is that our findings rely mostly on retrospective self-reports. In general, it was our interviewers' impression that subjects were being frank and truthful (some even becoming distressed and tearful when discussing some experiences), and the inmates admitted to many socially undesirable behaviors. In addition, there was no gain to respondents for providing false information. However, potential problems related to recall and untruthfulness of retrospective self-reports are a limitation of this methodology.

To summarize, the WIHS is the first large-scale epidemiologic study on the prevalence of psychiatric disorders among women in prison. Using standardized assessment procedures, we found that convicted women felons had elevated rates of substance abuse disorders, BPD, ASPD, and depression. These findings suggest an important need for treatment among women in prison and identification of prisons as a potential site for secondary and tertiary preventive interventions.

Accepted for publication 21 September, 1995.

This study was supported in part by grant DA06387 from the National Institute on Drug Abuse, Washington, DC.

Reprints: B. Kathleen Jordan, PhD, Social and Behavioral Research Center, Research Triangle Institute, PO Box 12194, 3040 Cornwallis Rd, Research Triangle Park, NC 27709.

REFERENCES

1. Perkins CA, Stephan JJ, Beck, AJ. *Jails and Jail Inmates 1993-94.* Washington, DC: Bureau of Justice Statistics; 1995. BJS bulletin NCJ-151651.
2. Beck AJ, Gilliard DK. *Prisoners in 1994.* Washington, DC: Bureau of Justice Statistics; 1995. BJS bulletin NCJ-151654.
3. Beck AJ, Gilliard DK. *Results of 1994 Probation and Parole Data Surveys.* Washington, DC: Bureau of Justice Statistics; 1995. Advance press release for BJS bulletin NCJ-156432.
4. Gilliard DK, Beck AJ. *Prisoners in 1993.* Washington, DC: Bureau of Justice Statistics; 1994. BJS bulletin NCJ-147036.
5. Novick LF, Penna RD, Schwartz MS, Remmlinger E, Lowenstein R. Health status of the New York City prison population. *Med Care.* 1977;15:205-216.
6. Harlow CW. *HIV in US Prisons and Jails.* Rockville, Md: Bureau of Justice Statistics; 1993. BJS special report NCJ-143292.
7. Greenfeld LA, Minor-Harper S. *Women in Prison.* Rockville, Md: Bureau of Justice Statistics; 1991. BJS publication NCJ-127991.
8. Vlahov D, Brewer F, Castro KG, Narkunas JP, Salive ME, Ullrich J, Muñoz A. Prevalence of antibody to HIV-1 among entrants to US correctional facilities. *JAMA.* 1991;265:1129-1132.
9. Beck A, Gilliard D, Greenfeld L, Harlow C, Hester T, Jankowski L, Snell T, Stephan J, Morton D. *Survey of State Prison Inmates, 1991.* Rockville, Md: Bureau of Justice Statistics; 1993. BJS publication NCJ-136949.
10. Collins JJ, Schlenger WE. The prevalence of psychiatric disorder among admissions to prison. Presented at the American Society of Criminology 35th Annual Meeting; November 9-13, 1983; Denver, Colo.
11. Neighbors HW, Williams DH, Gunnings TS, Lipscomb WD, Broman C, Lepkowski J. *The Prevalence of Mental Disorder in Michigan Prisons: Final Report Submitted to the Michigan Department of Corrections.* Ann Arbor, Mich: University of Michigan, School of Public Health, Dept of Community Health Programs, Community Mental Health Program; 1987.
12. Hodgins S, Côté G. Prevalence of mental disorders among penitentiary inmates in Quebec. *Can Ment Health.* 1990;38:1-4.
13. Daniel AE, Robins AJ, Reid JC, Wilfey DE. Lifetime and six-month prevalence of psychiatric disorders among sentenced female offenders. *Bull Am Acad Psychiatry Law.* 1988;16:333-342.
14. Hurley W, Dunne MP. Psychological distress and psychiatric morbidity in women prisoners. *Aust N Z J Psychiatry.* 1991;25:461-470.
15. Robertson RG, Bankier RG, Schwartz L. The female offender: a Canadian study. *Can J Psychiatry.* 1987;32:749-755.
16. Denton B. Drug dependence and psychiatric morbidity among women prisoners: an Australian study. Presented at the 5th World Conference on Prison Health Care; June 1993; Brisbane, Australia.
17. Maden A, Swinton M, Gunn J. Women in prison and use of illicit drugs before arrest. *BMJ.* 1990;301:1133.
18. Scott NA, Hannum TE, Ghrist SL. Assessment of depression among incarcerated females. *J Pers Assess.* 1982;46:373-379.
19. Robins LN, Regier DA, eds. *Psychiatric Disorders in America: The Epidemiologic Catchment Area Study.* New York, NY: Free Press; 1991.
20. Robins LN, Tipp J, Przybeck T. Antisocial personality. In: Robins LN, Regier DA, eds. *Psychiatric Disorders in America: The Epidemiologic Catchment Area Study.* New York, NY: Free Press; 1991:258-290.
21. American Psychiatric Association. *Diagnostic and Statistical Manual of Mental Disorders, Third Edition, Revised.* Washington, DC: American Psychiatric Association; 1987.
22. Dohrenwend B, Shrout P. Toward the development of a two-stage procedure for case identification and classification in psychiatric epidemiology. *Res Commun Ment Health.* 1981;2:295-323.
23. Shrout PE, Skodol AE, Dohrenwend BP. A two stage approach for case identification and diagnosis: first stage instruments. In: Barrett JE, Rose RM, eds. *Mental Disorder in the Community.* New York, NY: Guilford; 1986;286-303.
24. Robins LN, Helzer JE, Weissman MM, Orvaschel H, Gruenberg E, Burke JD, Regier DA. Lifetime prevalence of specific psychiatric disorders in three sites. *Arch Gen Psychiatry.* 1984;41:949-958.
25. Blazer DK, George LK, Landerman R, Pennybacker M, Melville ML, Woodbury MA, Jordan BK, Locke B. Psychiatric disorders: a rural/urban comparison. *Arch Gen Psychiatry.* 1985;42:651-656.
26. Robins LN, Helzer JE, Croughan JL, Ratcliff KS. National Institute of Mental Health Diagnostic Interview Schedule: its history, characteristics and validity. *Arch Gen Psychiatry.* 1981;38:381-389.
27. American Psychiatric Association. *Diagnostic and Statistical Manual of Mental Disorders, Third Edition.* Washington, DC: American Psychiatric Association; 1980.
28. World Health Organization. *Composite International Diagnostic Interview (CIDI). Version 1.0.* Geneva, Switzerland: World Health Organization; 1990.
29. Robins LN, Wing J, Wittchen H-U, Helzer JE. The Composite International Diagnostic Interview: an epidemiologic instrument suitable for use in conjunction with different diagnostic systems and in different cultures. *Arch Gen Psychiatry.* 1988;45:1069-1077.
30. Wittchen H-U, Robins LN, Cottler LB, Sartorius N, Burke JD, Regier DA, Participants in the Multicentre WHO/ADAMHA Field Trials. Cross-cultural feasibility, reliability and sources of variance in the Composite International Diagnostic Interview (CIDI). *Br J Psychiatry.* 1991;159:645-653.
31. Spitzer RL, Williams JB, Gibbon M. *Structured Clinical Interview for DSM-III-R, Version NP-V.* New York, NY: New York State Psychiatric Institute, Biometrics Research Department; 1987.
32. Zanarini MC, Frankenburg FR, Chauncey DL, Gunderson JG. The Diagnostic Interview for Personality Disorders: interrator and test-retest reliability. *Compr Psychiatry.* 1987;28:467-480.
33. Gunderson JG, Kolb JE, Austin V. The Diagnostic Interview for Borderlines. *Am J Psychiatry* 1981;138:896-903.
34. Resnick MS, Kilpatrick DG, Freedy JR, Falsetti SA. Trauma assessment for adults. In: Miller TW, ed. *Stressful Life Events.* Madison, Conn: International Universities Press Inc. In press.
35. Research Triangle Institute. *SUDAAN Users' Manual: Release 6.4.* Research Triangle Park, NC: Research Triangle Institute; 1994.
36. Collins JJ, Schlenger WE, Jordan BK. Antisocial personality and substance abuse disorders. *Bull Am Acad Psychiatry Law.* 1988;16:187-198.
37. Swartz M, Blazer D, George L, Winfield I. Estimating the prevalence of borderline personality disorder in the community. *J Pers Disorder.* 1990;4:257-272.
38. Resnick HS, Kilpatrick DG, Dansky BS, Saunders BE, Best CL. Prevalence of civilian trauma and posttraumatic stress disorder in a representative national sample of women. *J Consult Clin Psychol.* 1993;61:984.
39. Widiger TA, Hyler SE. Axis I/Axis II interactions. In: Michels R, Cooper AM, Goze SB, Judd LL, Klerman GL, Solnit AJ, eds. *Psychiatry.* Philadelphia, Pa: JB Lippincott;1989.
40. Teplin LA, Abram KM, McClelland GM. The prevalence of psychiatric disorder among incarcerated women, I: pretrial jail detainees. *Arch Gen Psychiatry.* 1996; 53:505-512.
41. Kessler RC, McGonagle KA, Zhao S, Nelson CB, Hughes M, Eshleman S, Wittchen H-U, Kendler KS. Lifetime and 12-month prevalence of *DSM-III-R* psychiatric disorders in the United States: results from the National Comorbidity Survey. *Arch Gen Psychiatry.* 1994;51:8-19.
42. Miller JD, Cisin IH, Gardner-Keaton H, Harrell AV, Wirtz PW, Abelson HI, Fishburne PM. *National Survey on Drug Abuse: Main Findings 1982.* Rockville, Md: National Institute on Drug Abuse; 1982.
43. Substance Abuse and Mental Health Services Administration. *Preliminary Estimates From the 1992 National Household Survey on Drug Abuse (Advance Report No. 3).* Rockville, Md: Substance Abuse and Mental Health Services Administration; 1993.
44. Wellisch, J, Predergast, ML, Aglin, MD. *Drug-Abusing Women Offenders: Results of a National Survey.* Washington, DC: National Institute of Justice; 1994.
45. National Institute of Justice. *1988 Drug Use Forecasting Annual Report.* Washington, DC: National Institute of Justice; 1990. NCJ 122225.
46. National Institute of Justice. *1992 Drug Use Forecasting Annual Report: Drugs and Crime in America's Cities.* Washington, DC: National Institute of Justice; 1993. NCJ 142973.
47. Abram KM. The effect of concurring disorders on criminal careers: interaction of ASPD, alcoholism, and drug disorders. *Int J Law Psychiatry.* 1989;12:133-148.
48. Jordan BK, Schlenger WE, Caddell JM, Fairbank JA. Etiologic factors in the development of borderline personality disorder in a sample of convicted women felons. In: Zanarini M, ed. *The Role of Sexual Abuse Borderline Personality Disorder.* Washington, DC: American Psychiatric Association Press. In press.
49. Anglin MD, Hser Y. Treatment of drug abuse. In: Tonry M, Wilson JQ, eds. *Drugs and Crime.* Chicago, Ill: University of Chicago Press; 1990.

A Prospective Follow-up Study of Alcoholic Violent Offenders and Fire Setters

Matti Virkkunen, MD; Monika Eggert, MD; Robert Rawlings, MS; Markku Linnoila, MD, PhD

Background: This study investigated biochemical and family variables and predictors of recidivism among forensic psychiatric patients who had committed violent offenses or set fires.

Methods: One hundred fourteen male alcoholic violent offenders and fire setters were followed up for an average of 4.5 years after release from prison. At the beginning of their incarceration, the first half of the offenders were administered clinical diagnostic interviews, whereas the latter half received the Structured Clinical Interview for *DSM-III* (SCID) that was blind rated. A structured family history questionnaire was administered to all available first-degree relatives of offenders. The offenders also received lumbar punctures for monoamine metabolites, an oral glucose tolerance test, and a measurement of fasting plasma cholesterol level. At the end of the follow-up, the Finnish criminal registry was searched for recidivist crimes.

Results: Among all offenders, low cerebrospinal fluid (CSF) 5-hydroxyindoleacetic acid (5-HIAA) and homovanillic acid (HVA) concentrations were associated with a family history positive for paternal alcoholism with violence. Low plasma cholesterol concentration was associated with a family history positive for paternal alcoholism without violence. The recidivists, who committed violent offenses or set fires during the follow-up period, had low CSF 5-HIAA and 3-methoxy-4-hydroxyphenylglycol (MHPG) concentrations compared with those in nonrecidivists. Early family environments of the recidivists, compared with those of the nonrecidivists, were characterized by common paternal absence from and presence of brothers at home.

Conclusion: Among male alcoholic violent offenders and fire setters, low CSF 5-HIAA and HVA concentrations are strongly associated with a family history positive for paternal violence and alcoholism, while low fasting plasma cholesterol concentration is associated with a family history positive for paternal alcoholism. Recidivist violent offenders and fire setters are predicted by low CSF 5-HIAA and MHPG concentrations and a developmental history positive for early paternal absence from and presence of brothers in the family of origin.

(Arch Gen Psychiatry. 1996;53:523-529)

ACCURATELY predicting future violence is an extremely difficult task. Literature published during the last decade suggests that clinicians are becoming better predictors of future violence. This apparent improvement could, however, reflect a publication bias favoring positive findings,[1] and exercise of caution has been urged in using clinical judgment to predict violence.[2] Nevertheless, short-term, intensive observation of behavior, which can be carried out on an inpatient ward, may have relatively high predictive power for the following few days or weeks.[3-6] The paucity of studies with accurate long-term prediction of violence has been suggested to be partially caused by inappropriate selection of predictive variables.[7]

In a prior study,[8] we followed up 58 Finnish alcoholic violent offenders for an average of 3 years after release from prison. The biological variables, blood glucose nadir during an oral glucose tolerance test and cerebrospinal fluid (CSF) 5-hydroxyindoleacetic acid (5-HIAA) concentration showed relatively high sensitivity and specificity in predicting recidivist violent crimes. The present study combines the original sample of 58 with an additional sample of 56 violent offenders and fire setters and examines their outcomes after release from prison. All subjects had undergone an extensive forensic psychiatric evaluation at the time of their initial incarceration. This included a 4- to 6-week medication-free observation period on a locked forensic psychiatry ward; an oral glucose challenge test; quantitation of fasting plasma cholesterol concentration; and, on consenting offenders, a lumbar

From the Department of Psychiatry, University of Helsinki, Helsinki, Finland (Drs Virkkunen and Eggert), and Laboratory of Clinical Studies, Division of Intramural Clinical and Biological Research, National Institute on Alcohol Abuse and Alcoholism, Bethesda, Md (Mr Rawlings and Dr Linnoila).

See Subjects and Methods on next page

SUBJECTS AND METHODS

SUBJECTS

Subjects were 73 violent offenders and 41 fire setters, all were male, and their mean±SD age at the time of the initial forensic psychiatric examination was 31.9 ± 13.1 years. The mean±SD Wechsler Adult Intelligence full-scale IQ of the group was 97.3±16.4. Seven subjects, 3 fire setters and 4 violent offenders, had an IQ between 65 and 70. One of these subjects, an impulsive violent offender, had an XXY (Klinefelter) syndrome. An additional subject, an impulsive fire setter, had the XYY genotype. A nonimpulsive violent offender had sustained a closed head injury prior to the initial crime. The mean±SD height and weight of the subjects were 176.7±10.4 cm and 76.1±9.9 kg, respectively. The results of the studies performed during the initial forensic psychiatric examination of all but 5 schizophrenic subjects have been reported previously.[9,12-17] The schizophrenic subjects had remained incarcerated in a forensic psychiatry hospital at the time of the earlier follow-up study. In the present study, the duration of the follow-up for the 58 men who participated in our earlier follow-up study is more than twice as long as that in the earlier study.[8]

CHARACTERISTICS OF THE ORIGINAL CRIME

On the basis of the police report on the original crime, violent offenders were divided into impulsive (n=35) and nonimpulsive (n=38) groups. Impulsive offenders had killed or attempted to kill without premeditation. The victim was previously unknown to them, and there was no report of a provocation. The crime was not committed in the context of a robbery or burglary. The nonimpulsive violent offenses were premeditated and had a rationale to the offenders, according to their own admission. Furthermore, there was clear evidence of preparation for the crime such as procuring a weapon. The criteria used to categorize the violent offenses were identical to those used in our previous publications.[8,9,12-17]

Twenty-five fire setters were determined as impulsive and 16 as nonimpulsive. Impulsive fire setting was usually the result of a sudden fit of rage, which occurred typically while the fire setter was under the influence of alcohol. Fire setting was categorized as nonimpulsive when it was premeditated. The most common motivation for nonimpulsive fire setting was revenge. Fire setting for insurance fraud was used as an exclusion criterion. The offenses were categorized as impulsive or nonimpulsive by the senior forensic research psychiatrist (M.V.), who was blind to the results of any biochemical studies at the time. He knew, however, the criminal histories of the offenders.

METHODS

Psychiatric Diagnoses

Diagnoses were initially made based on the available information according to *DSM-III* criteria[18] by the same forensic research psychiatrist (M.V.). For this study, *DSM-III-R*[19] diagnoses were derived from medical records by the forensic research psychiatrist (M.V.) for the 51 subjects who were not interviewed, using a structured interview. At the time, he was aware of the criminal and medical histories of the offenders. Sixty-five offenders (34 violent offenders and 31 fire setters) were administered the structured diagnostic interview for *DSM-III-R*[10,19] by the junior research psychiatrist (M.E.) who was blind to the offenders medical and criminal records at the time of the interview. For all subjects, intermittent explosive disorder was diagnosed according to *DSM-III* criteria[18] to provide data comparable to our previous studies. To arrive at the diagnosis among the subjects, who were administered the structured interview, they were asked questions based on the items in *DSM-III*[12] used to make the diagnosis of intermittent explosive disorder. The interviews were blind rated by 2 research psychiatrists. When the diagnostic blind ratings by the 2 psychiatrists disagreed, the diagnosis was assigned by a senior research psychiatrist, who was blind to all other data except the diagnostic interview concerning the subject.

Family Variables

Family history was obtained using a structured questionnaire, which was sent to all living first-degree relatives of the offenders. It contains 12 groups of questions concerning (1) parents; (2) siblings; (3) spouse; (4) offspring; (5) second-degree relatives all of them eliciting information on each individual concerning physical and mental health, substance abuse and alcoholism, criminality, and time and cause of death (this information was checked against official death certificates) and concerning the offender with regard to (6) development and behavior up to the age of 14 years; (7) circumstances at home, including discipline, parenting, separations and divorces; (8) education, including interests, strengths and weaknesses, absenteeism and discipline (this information was checked against official school records); (9) employment history, including unemployment (this information was checked against official unemployment records); (10) mandatory military service (this information was checked against official military records); (11) character as an adult; and (12) unusual or disturbed behaviors after the age of 14 years. For each question, space was provided for a narrative answer by the relative. This questionnaire has been an integral part of the forensic psychiatric examination administered by the Department of Psychiatry, University of Helsinki, for the past 25 years. The same experienced social worker helped all the relatives of offenders and fire set-

puncture as an experimental procedure. The monoamine metabolites 5-HIAA, homovanillic acid (HVA) and 3-methoxy-4-hydroxyphenylglycol (MHPG) were quantitated in the samples of CSF. Family and developmental histories were obtained from first-degree adult relatives of the offenders, using a structured questionnaire.

The first objective of the present study was to explore associations between variables related to parental behavior, early family environment, and biochemical variables. The second objective was to corroborate or refute our earlier findings that biochemical and behavioral variables have predictive value for future violence and fire setting.[8,9] To improve diagnostic accuracy, everyone in the new sample and 7 subjects from the earlier sample were administered the Structured Clinical Interview for *DSM-III-R* (SCID).[10] The diagnoses were subsequently blind rated. To facilitate comparisons across predictive ters who participated in this study to fill out the questionnaire, when needed. (Copies of the questionnaire, in Finnish, are available from M.V.) A condition, circumstance, or behavior in a relative was accepted as positive only when reported independently by a minimum of 2 relatives. To increase reliability, this report contains only the data provided by first-degree adult relatives of the offenders and fire setters.

Using the family history questionnaire, we defined dichotomous behavioral variables (assigned values 0 when absent and 1 when present). These were used to construct 2 global measures called *parental behavior* and *family environment*. Parental behavior consisted of the sum of the values of the following 10 variables: paternal violence, paternal alcoholism, paternal depression, paternal major mental illness other than depression or alcoholism, paternal suicide, maternal alcoholism, maternal depression, maternal major mental illness other than depression, maternal suicide, and alcoholism among maternal grandfather and/or mother's brothers. The cell "maternal violence" had no entries and was omitted. Family environment was defined as the sum of the values of the following 5 variables: father dead, father away from home owing to divorce, mother away from home owing to divorce, brothers at home (all starting before 5 years of age), and alcoholic brother(s) at home. The cell "mother dead" had no entries (before 5 years of age) and was omitted. The 2 global measures were scaled in order from 0 for low risk to a larger number for higher risk (maximum score of 10 for parental behavior and score of 5 for family environment).

Follow-up

Outcome data were examined after a mean±SD follow-up period of 53.7±35.9 months after release from prison. The criminal registry of Finland was searched for repeated crimes at the end of the follow-up. This cumulative registry contains information concerning all criminal convictions since the age of 16 years. It is considered representative of the violent criminal population in Finland. This is primarily related to the fact that the conviction rate for violent offenses in Finland is very high. In 1994, it was more than 90% for murder and manslaughter and over 80% for aggravated assault.[20]

When new murders, manslaughters, attempted murders, attempted manslaughters, aggravated assaults, or fire settings were found, police reports and court documents were reviewed. For statistical analyses, the violent and fire-setting recidivists were combined into a single category of recidivists. Six subjects committed suicide during the follow-up: 4 were recidivists, and 2 were nonrecidivists. Suicides were verified from death certificates, which, in turn, were based on forensic autopsies in every case.

Biochemical Variables

CSF Samples. The CSF samples were obtained under medication-free conditions between 8 AM and 9 AM after the subjects had been maintained on a low-monoamine diet for at least a week.[13,16,17] Concentrations of the major metabolites of dopamine, norepinephrine and serotonin, HVA, MHPG, and 5-HIAA, respectively, were quantitated with high-performance liquid chromatography using electrochemical detection. The within-run and between-run coefficients of variation of the method were less than 10%.[21] All biochemical analyses were performed by personnel unaware of the clinical characteristics of the subjects.

Oral Glucose Tolerance Tests. Oral glucose tolerance tests were administered after a 12- to 16-hour overnight fast. At 8 AM, the subjects received 1 g/kg (in a volume of 4 mL/kg) of body weight of glucose solution, which they consumed as quickly as possible. Blood samples were collected before glucose administration and 30 minutes and 1, 2, 3, 4, and 5 hours afterward. Blood glucose concentrations were determined enzymatically.[17]

Plasma Cholesterol. Total plasma cholesterol obtained after an overnight fast was quantitated during the first week of hospitalization as a part of a routine clinical chemistry screening procedure.

Statistical Analyses

Relationships between biochemical and behavioral variables were examined with the Spearman rank order correlations. Group differences were tested by using the nonparametric Mann-Whitney U test and Kruskal-Wallis test for continuous variables and the χ^2 test for dichotomous variables. The recidivist and nonrecidivist classification accuracy was examined by using ROC analysis in a logistic regression. The logistic regression was used because the discriminating variables were both continuous and discrete (hence, not multivariate normal). The ROC curve is presented with the y-axis measuring sensitivity and the x-axis measuring 1–specificity. The area under the curve computed in the ROC analysis is a useful measure of classification accuracy that is not dependent on the cut point chosen in the logistic regression or the a priori probabilities (prevalences) in the 2 populations. The area under the curve can be interpreted as the probability of correctly classifying a randomly selected pair of subjects from the set of pairs in groups 1 and 2. Because of the large number of statistical tests that were computed, the level of significance, α, was set to equal .01. Bonferroni correction of the level of α was used in the post hoc analyses where appropriate. All statistical analyses were performed using the BMDP software.[22] Because of missing data, the cell sizes differ from one analysis to another.

studies, which often employ different prior probabilities, receiver operating characteristic (ROC) analyses were used. In this type of analysis, the area under the curve equals the likelihood at which a clinician would rate a randomly selected, recidivist violent individual more likely to be a recidivist than a randomly selected nonrecidivist violent individual.[1,11] The detailed family and developmental histories permitted preliminary analyses on the roles of nature vs nurture in repetitious interpersonal violence, as well as fire setting among alcoholic offenders.

RESULTS

PSYCHIATRIC DIAGNOSES

Diagnoses based on either the SCID-R (n=65) or the clinical interviews (n=49) are indicated in **Table 1**. Com-

Table 1. Lifetime Psychiatric Diagnoses of Violent Offenders and Fire Setters Who Participated in the Follow-up Study*

Disorder	Violent Offenders (n=73) Impulsive (n=35)	Violent Offenders (n=73) Nonimpulsive (n=38)	Fire Setters (n=41) Impulsive (n=25)	Fire Setters (n=41) Nonimpulsive (n=16)	Total (N=114)
DSM-III-R Axis I disorder					
Alcohol dependence	33	25	19	12	**89**
Alcohol abuse	4	7	3	6	**20**
Sedative-hypnotic-anxiolytic dependence	1	2	1	0	**4**
Opioid dependence	1	0	0	0	**1**
Cannabis dependence	0	0	1	0	**1**
Major depressive disorder	0	0	6	3	**9**
Bipolar disorder	0	0	1	0	**1**
Dysthymic disorder	3	8	1	3	**15**
Schizophrenia	0	5	0	0	**5**
Social phobia	0	1	2	2	**5**
Panic disorder	0	0	0	1	**1**
Obsessive-compulsive disorder	0	0	0	1	**1**
Intermittent explosive disorder	12	0	18	0	**30**
DSM-III-R Axis II personality disorders					
Antisocial	20	8	5	1	**34**
Borderline	20	4	11	2	**37**
Narcissistic	2	0	0	0	**2**
Paranoid	5	6	4	0	**15**
Schizotypal	0	0	1	0	**1**
Schizoid	0	0	2	2	**4**
Avoidant	0	1	4	3	**8**
Dependent	0	3	1	2	**6**
Passive-aggressive	0	2	0	1	**3**
NOS	2	2	1	0	**5**
No Axis II disorder	5	6	7	3	**21**

**Subjects can have more than one diagnosis. NOS indicates not otherwise specified.*

pared with the clinical diagnoses, the SCID-R increased the number of diagnoses per subject. The prevalence of the primary diagnoses was, however, very similar in the 2 halves of the sample.[8]

BIOLOGICAL AND FAMILY VARIABLES

The overall mean±SD concentrations of the biochemical variables were as follows: CSF 5-HIAA, 67.0±29.3 pmol/mL (n=113); CSF HVA, 194.5±82.8 pmol/mL (n=101); CSF MHPG, 31.5±10.8 pmol/mL (n=103); lowest blood glucose, 2.8±0.6 mmol/L (n=112); and fasting plasma cholesterol, 5.7±1.3 mmol/L (n=112). The overall mean±SD scores of the family history variables were as follows: parental behavior, 1.2±1.1 (n=112), and family environment, 1.2±0.8 (n=113).

INTERACTIONS BETWEEN BIOLOGICAL AND FAMILY VARIABLES

The significant correlations at the $P=.01$ level were between the parental behavior score and CSF 5-HIAA, $r=-0.37$; parental behavior score and CSF HVA, $r=-0.26$; and parental behavior score and plasma cholesterol concentrations, $r=-0.24$. To examine relations among the component variables included in the composite of the parental behavior score, we utilized Mann-Whitney tests. For CSF 5-HIAA, the 2 variables significant at the $P=.01$ level were paternal violence and paternal alcoholism. For CSF HVA concentration, the variables significant at the $P=.01$ level were paternal violence for CSF HVA concentration and paternal alcoholism for fasting plasma cholesterol concentration. Because there was only 1 father who was violent but nonalcoholic, we computed a 1-way analysis of variance, which consisted of the following cells: paternal violence and paternal alcoholism, paternal nonviolence and paternal alcoholism, and paternal nonviolence and nonalcoholism. The Kruskal-Wallis test results for CSF 5-HIAA, CSF HVA, and plasma cholesterol concentrations were significant at the $P=.01$ level. The significant Bonferroni corrected pairwise comparisons at the $P=.01$ level for CSF 5-HIAA and CSF HVA were between paternal violence and paternal alcoholism and both paternal nonviolence and paternal alcoholism and paternal nonviolence and paternal nonalcoholism. Hence, the most important family variable associated with low CSF 5-HIAA and CSF HVA concentrations was paternal violence combined with paternal alcoholism (**Table 2**). The significant Bonferroni corrected pairwise comparison at the $P=.01$ level for fasting plasma cholesterol concentration was between paternal nonviolence and paternal alcoholism and paternal nonviolence and paternal nonalcoholism (Table 2).

QUALITY OF CRIMES AND PATERNAL FAMILY HISTORY

Thirty of the crimes committed by sons of violent alcoholic fathers were coded as impulsive, and 3 were coded as nonimpulsive. The respective numbers for the sons of all nonviolent fathers were 29 and 47 ($\chi^2[df=1]=25.8$; $P<.01$).

Table 2. Biological Variables as a Function of Paternal Family History*

Biological Variables	Paternal Violence and Paternal Alcoholism	Paternal Nonviolence and Paternal Alcoholism	Paternal Nonviolence and Paternal Nonalcoholism
CSF 5-HIAA, pmol/mL	45.3±19.1† [34]	88.1±31.1 [17]	73.2±26.3 [60]
CSF HVA, pmol/mL	149.1±60.7† [30]	284.5±81.4 [17]	204.5±80.0 [52]
Plasma cholesterol, mmol/L (mg/dL)	5.4±1.2 (209.0±46.4) [34]	5.1±0.8‡ (197.4±31.0) [17]	6.0±1.4‡ (232.2±54.2) [60]

**CSF indicates cerebrospinal fluid; 5-HIAA, 5-hydroxyindoleacetic acid; and HVA, homovanillic acid. Data are mean±SD; number of subjects in each group is indicated in brackets.*

†P<.01 compared with each of the other 2 means.

‡P=.01 compared with each other.

Table 3. Biological and Family History Variables Among Recidivists and Nonrecidivists

Variables*	Recidivists Mean	Recidivists SD	Recidivists N	Nonrecidivists Mean	Nonrecidivists SD	Nonrecidivists N	Mann-Whitney *U* Test Score	*P*
Biological								
5-HIAA, pmol/L	50.8	21.7	28	72.5	29.9	83	667.5	.001
HVA, pmol/L	165.6	76.1	25	205.5	83.6	74	652.0	.03
MHPG, pmol/L	27.0	10.1	26	33.1	10.7	75	657.0	.01
LBG, mmol/L (mg/dL)	2.7 (48.6)	0.5 (9.0)	28	2.8 (50.4)	0.6 (10.8)	82	988.5	.27
Cholesterol, mmol/mL (mg/dL)	5.6 (216.8)	1.0 (38.7)	28	5.7 (220.6)	1.4 (54.2)	82	1063.5	.56
Family history								
Parental behavior	1.6	1.1	27	1.1	1.1	83	1409.0	.04
Family environment	1.6	0.8	28	1.1	0.8	83	1569.5	.003

**5-HIAA indicates 5-hydroxyindoleacetic acid; HVA, homovanillic acid; MHPG, 3-methoxy-4-hydroxyphenylglycol; and LBG, lowest blood glucose level.*

RECIDIVISM

Two subjects, who committed suicide without committing violent or fire setting crimes after release from prison, were excluded from the following analyses. The variables that differed between the recidivists and nonrecidivists at the $P=.01$ level according to the Mann-Whitney U test were CSF 5-HIAA, CSF MHPG, and the family environment score. The recidivists had significantly lower CSF 5-HIAA and CSF MHPG concentrations and higher family environment scores than did the nonrecidivists (**Table 3**).

To examine the contribution of the 5 components of the family environment score to predict recidivism, we computed Pearson χ^2 tests. The only significant components at the $P=.01$ level were father away due to divorce and brothers at home. Both of these conditions applied more often to the recidivists than the nonrecidivists (**Table 4**).

To derive an equation to predict recidivism, a logistic regression equation with the variables CSF 5-HIAA, CSF MHPG, and family environment was used. The predictive ability of the equation was examined by using an ROC curve and the measure of the area under the ROC curve. The 3 predictor variables were entered according to a forward stepwise method. The resultant order of entry was CSF 5-HIAA, family environment, and CSF MHPG. The tests for the regression coefficients were significant at the $P=.01$ level for CSF 5-HIAA and family environment and at the $P=.02$ level for CSF MHPG. The conclusion to be drawn from this analysis is that CSF 5-HIAA and family environment made significant independent contributions to the prediction of recidivism, while CSF MHPG's contribution was approaching this level. The area under the curve was 0.78 (**Figure**), which indicates that the predictor variables in combination were able to correctly classify a recidivist-nonrecidivist pair 78% of the time.

COMMENT

PREDICTION OF RECIDIVISM

The present findings derived from the enlarged sample generally agree with the results of our earlier study[8] on the prediction of violent recidivism and recidivist fire setting. In both studies, CSF 5-HIAA concentration made a major contribution to the prediction equation. The lower the CSF 5-HIAA concentration, the more likely the offender was to become a recidivist. The similarities of the findings between the earlier and the current expansion study attest to their general robustness among the population of Finnish alcoholic violent offenders. Even though the patients have been selected by the courts for forensic psychiatric examination, with inherent biases involved in the legal proceedings, the present sample is representative of the general Finnish population involved in recidivist homicidal violent criminality. In a study on a complete cohort of recidivist homicidal offenders in Finland, Tiihonen and Hakola[23] found 85% to fulfill criteria for early-onset alcoholism and antisocial personality disorder, and the remaining 15% for schizophrenia. The data may also have some relevance for the United States because, in a prospective follow-up study of American adolescents with disruptive behavioral disorders, similiar to the present findings, Kruesi et al[24] found low CSF 5-HIAA concentration to predict future violence. Furthermore, in a nonhuman primate model of violent be-

Table 4. Family Environment Variables Among Recidivists and Nonrecidivists

Family Environment	Recidivists	Nonrecidivists	χ^2	*df*	*P**
Father away due to divorce					
Yes	9	10	6.0	1	.01
No	19	73			
Brothers at home					
Yes	25	54	6.0	1	.01
No	3	29			

*Pearson test.

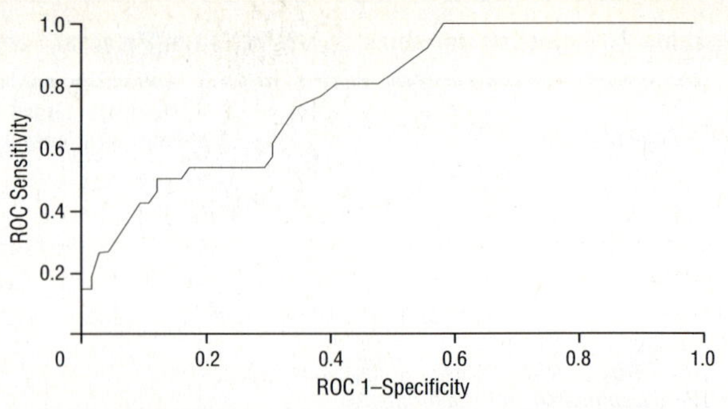

Receiver operating characteristic (ROC) curve to predict recidivist violent crimes and arson. The variables, that contributed independently to the prediction were cerebrospinal fluid 5-hydroxyindoleacetic acid and 3-methoxy-4-hydroxyphenylglycol concentrations and early family environment. AUC indicates area under the curve.

havior among *Rhesus* monkeys, a low CSF 5-HIAA concentration was predictive of early migration of young males from their groups of origin.[25] Moreover, among the migrating young males, it carried a very high risk for mortality because of repeated fighting.[26]

In the present study, CSF MHPG concentration made a modest independent contribution, at the $P=.02$ level, to the equation predicting violence. The lower the CSF MHPG concentration, the more likely the offender was to become a recidivist. Ninety percent of CSF MHPG is derived from peripheral norepinephrine metabolism[27]; thus, it represents an integrated biochemical indicator of sympathetic nervous system activity. Therefore, the present results are also compatible with the findings of Raine et al,[28] who found that low autonomic arousal was predictive of future violent criminality.

Although findings by Virkkunen et al[17,29] of low blood glucose nadir during an oral glucose tolerance test were replicated among the recidivist fire setters (data not shown), there was no difference in the mean blood glucose nadir between the overall recidivist and nonrecidivist groups. Thus, different from our earlier study,[8] a low blood glucose nadir did not contribute to predicting recidivist criminality in the present sample. Diets with reduced cholesterol content and low plasma cholesterol level have been associated with an increased incidence of suicidality,[30,31] homicidality,[32] and antisocial personality disorder[33,34] in humans and aggression in nonhuman primates.[35] In the present study, a low fasting plasma cholesterol concentration was not predictive of outcome during the follow-up. It was, however, associated with a family history positive for paternal alcoholism. Such a positive family history among the general population may be associated with increased incidence of violent and suicidal behaviors.[36]

INTERACTIONS BETWEEN BIOCHEMICAL AND FAMILY VARIABLES

A striking finding among the violent offenders and fire setters was that a family history positive for both paternal violence and alcoholism was associated with very low CSF 5-HIAA concentrations. This observation is in apparent agreement with the recent adoption study by Cadoret et al[37] and the family studies by Mattes and Fink[38] and Moss et al,[39] all of whom found that paternal aggression, violence, and impaired impulse control, behaviors that in other studies have been strongly associated with low CSF 5-HIAA levels,[16,40,41] were contributing to similar behaviors in the sons. According to these authors, the transmission seems to be at least partially genetic. In our sample, the last point is possibly supported by many of the fathers being absent from the home during the early childhood of the sons. Thus, they were unlikely to have served as role models to be imitated, or to be in a position to physically abuse their sons. Interestingly, low central serotonin turnover rate, as indicated by low CSF 5-HIAA levels, is highly heritable among nonhuman primates.[42]

FAMILY ENVIRONMENT

The more common presence of brothers in the home during the childhood of the recidivist offenders, which coincided with the lack of fathers, may have been conducive to learning destructive conflict resolution strategies. The importance of a chaotic family environment with patterns of child abuse and neglect for the development of habitually violent behaviors during childhood and adulthood has been previously emphasized by Widom[43] and Dodge et al,[44] respectively. In the study by Widom, however, fewer than a fifth of the boys raised in such chaotic environments grew up to be violent adolescents. Clearly, both genetic and environmental variables can contribute to untoward outcomes, such as violent criminality,[45] as attested to by the independent and significant contributions by the biological and early family environment variables to the results of the ROC analysis for the prediction of recidivism in the present data set.

CAVEATS

The present study has some severe limitations. Because the sample was collected in Finland between 1981 and 1990, structured diagnostic interviews in Finnish were available to be administered only to the latter half of the subjects. The early clinical interviews were performed by M. V., who knew the subjects histories at the time of the interviews. This may be an obvious source of bias, even though when the clinical diagnoses on antisocial personality disorder and alcohol dependence were made, the SCID-R diagnoses showed more than 90% agreement (M.V., M.E., and M.L., unpublished data, August 1995). As expected, the SCID-R was conducive to having more diagnoses per subject. To reduce bias, we were very careful to protect the blind of the biochemical data from the clinical investigators until the final merging of the databases. Finally, because the subjects represent a non-randomly selected group with homicidal violent behaviors, the data have to be generalized conservatively. This is particularly true concerning any generalizations to the American population because of the different patterns of violent crime in America and Finland.

CONCLUSION

The present study suggests that a positive family history for paternal violence and alcoholism is associated with reduced central serotonin and dopamine turnover rates. The reduced central serotonin turnover rate, in combination with low norepinephrine turnover rate and paternal absence from and the presence of brothers at home during early childhood, is predictive of impulsive, recidivist violent behavior among violent offenders and fire setters.

Accepted for publication March 11, 1996.

The authors are grateful to Michael Eckardt, PhD, and William Z. Potter, MD, PhD, for their constructive criticisms of the manuscript; Andrea S. Hobbs for preparation and editorial assistance; and Carmelita Duenas for typing. The SCID-R interview data were entered into the computer by Marie Watters, MSW, and blind rated by Susan Goodson, MD, and Wendol Williams MD. Differences in diagnostic ratings were settled by Gerald L. Brown, MD.

Reprints: Markku Linnoila, MD, PhD, Laboratory of Clinical Studies, DICBR National Institute on Alcohol Abuse and Alcoholism, NIH Bldg 10, Room 3C103, 10 Center Dr, MSC 1256, Bethesda, MD 20892-1256.

REFERENCES

1. Mossman D. Assessing predictions of violence: being accurate about accuracy. *J Consult Clin Psychol.* 1994;4:783-792.
2. Lidz CW, Mulvey EP, Gardner WP. The accuracy of the predictions of violence to others. *JAMA.* 1993;269:1007-1011.
3. Monahan J. The prediction of violent behavior: toward a second generation of theory and policy. *Am J Psychiatry.* 1984;141:10-15.
4. Monahan J. Risk assessment of violence among the mentally disordered: generating useful knowledge. *Int J Law Psychiatry.* 1988;11:249-257.
5. McNiel DE, Binder RL. Predictive validity of judgements of dangerousness in emergency civil commitment. *Am J Psychiatry.* 1987;144:197-200.
6. McNiel DE, Binder RL, Greenfield TK. Predictors of violence in civilly committed psychiatric patients. *Am J Psychiatry.* 1988;145:965-970.
7. Monahan J, Steadman HJ. Toward a rejuvenation of risk assessment research. In: Monahan J, Steadman HJ, eds. *Violence and Mental Disorder: Developments in Risk Assessment.* Chicago, Ill: University of Chicago Press; 1994:1-17.
8. Virkkunen M, DeJong J, Bartko J, Goodwin FK, Linnoila M. Relationship of psychobiological variables to recidivism in violent offenders and impulsive fire setters: a follow-up study. *Arch Gen Psychiatry.* 1989;46:600-603.
9. DeJong J, Virkkunen M, Linnoila M. Factors associated with recidivism in a criminal population. *J Nerv Ment Dis.* 1992;180:543-550.
10. Spitzer RL, Williams JB, Gibbon M. Structured Clinical Interview for *DSM-III-R.* New York, NY: Biometrics Research Department, New York State Psychiatric Institute; 1987.
11. Hanley JA, McNeil MJ. The meaning and use of the area under a receiver operating characteristic (ROC) curve. *Radiology.* 1982;13:29-36.
12. Virkkunen M,. DeJong J, Bartko J, Linnoila M. Psychobiological concomitants of history of suicide attempts among violent offenders and impulsive fire setters. *Arch Gen Psychiatry.* 1989;46:604-606.
13. Virkkunen M, Rawlings R, Tokola R, Poland RE, Guidotti A, Nemeroff C, Bissette G, Kalogeras K, Karonen S-L, Linnoila M. CSF biochemistries, glucose metabolism, and diurnal activity rhythms in alcoholic, violent offenders, fire setters, and healthy volunteers. *Arch Gen Psychiatry.* 1994;51:20-27.
14. Virkkunen M, Kallio E, Rawlings R, Tokola R, Poland RE, Guidotti A, Nemeroff C, Bissette G, Kalogeras K, Karonen S-L, Linnoila M. Personality profiles and state aggressiveness in Finnish alcoholic, violent offenders, fire setters, and healthy volunteers. *Arch Gen Psychiatry.* 1994;51:28-33.
15. Linnoila M, DeJong J, Virkkunen M. Family history of alcoholism in violent offenders and impulsive fire setters. *Arch Gen Psychiatry.* 1989;46:613-616.
16. Linnoila M, Virkkunen M, Scheinin M, Nuutila A, Rimon R, Goodwin FK. Low cerebrospinal fluid 5-hydroxyindoleacetic acid concentration differentiates impulsive from nonimpulsive violent behavior. *Life Sci.* 1983;33:2609-2614.
17. Virkkunen M, Nuutila A, Goodwin FK, Linnoila M. Cerebrospinal fluid monoamine metabolites in male arsonists. *Arch Gen Psychiatry.* 1987;44:241-247.
18. American Psychiatric Association, Committee on Nomenclature and Statistics. *Diagnostic and Statistical Manual of Mental Disorders, Third Edition.* Washington, DC: American Psychiatric Association; 1980.
19. American Psychiatric Association, Committee on Nomenclature and Statistics. *Diagnostic and Statistical Manual of Mental Disorders, Third Edition Revised.* Washington, DC: American Psychiatric Association; 1987.
20. Oikeuspoliittinen Tutkimuslaitos. *Rikollisuustilanne 1994.* Helsinki, Finland: Hakapaino Oy; 1996:142-143.
21. Scheinin M, Chang W-H, Kirk K, Linnoila M. Simultaneous determination of 3-methoxy-4-hydroxyphenylglycol, 5-hydroxyindoleacetic acid and homovanillic acid in cerebrospinal fluid with high performance liquid chromatography using electrochemical detection. *Anal Biochem.* 1983;131:246-253.
22. Statistical Software Inc. *BMDP.* Los Angeles: University of California Press; 1992.
23. Tiihonen J, Hakola P. Psychiatric disorders and homicide recidivism. *Am J Psychiatry.* 1994;151:436-438.
24. Kruesi MJP, Hibbs ED, Zahn TP, Keysor CS, Hamburger SD, Bartko JJ, Rapoport JL. A two-year prospective follow-up study of children and adolescents with disruptive behavior disorders: prediction by cerebrospinal fluid 5-hydroxyindoleacetic acid, homovanillic acid, and autonomic measures? *Arch Gen Psychiatry.* 1992;49:429-435.
25. Mehlman PT, Higley JD, Faucher I, Lilly AA, Taub DM, Vickers J, Suomi SJ, Linnoila M. Correlation of CSF 5-HIAA concentration with sociality and the timing of emigration in free-ranging primates. *Am J Psychiatry.* 1995;152:907-913.
26. Higley JD, Mehlman PT, Taub DM, Higley SB, Fernald B, Vickers J, Suomi SJ, Linnoila M. Excessive mortality in young male nonhuman primates with low CSF 5-HIAA concentrations. *Arch Gen Psychiatry.* 1996;53:537-543.
27. Kopin IJ, Gordon EK, Jimerson DC, Polinsky RJ. Relation between plasma and cerebrospinal fluid levels of 3-methoxy-4-hydroxyphenylglycol. *Science.* 1983; 219:73-75.
28. Raine A, Venables PH, Williams M. Relationship between central and autonomic measures of arousal at age 15 years and criminality at age 24 years. *Arch Gen Psychiatry.* 1990;47:1003-1007.
29. Virkkunen M. Reactive hypoglycemic tendency among arsonists. *Acta Psychiatr Scand.* 1984;69:445-452.
30. Engelberg H. Low serum cholesterol and suicide. *Lancet.* 1992;339:727-729.
31. Golier JA, Marzuk PM, Leon AC, Weiner MA, Tardiff K. Low serum cholesterol and attempted suicide. *Am J Psychiatry.* 1995;152:419-423.
32. Virkkunen M. Serum cholesterol levels in homicidal offenders: a low cholesterol level is connected with a habitually violent tendency under the influence of alcohol. *Neuropsychobiology.* 1983:10:65-69.
33. Virkkunen M. Serum cholesterol in antisocial personality. *Neuropsychobiology.* 1979;5:27-30.
34. Freedman DS, Byers T, Barrett DH, Stroup NE, Eaker E, Monroe-Blum H. Plasma lipid levels and psychologic characteristics of men. *Am J Epidemiol.* 1995; 141:507-517.
35. Kaplan JR, Shively CA, Fontemont B, Morgan TM, Howell SM, Manuck SB, Muldoon MF, Mann J. Demonstration of an association among dietary cholesterol, central serotonergic activity, and social behavior in monkeys. *Psychosom Med.* 1994;56:479-484.
36. Cloninger CR, Bohman M, Sigvardsson S. Inheritance of alcohol abuse: cross-fostering analysis of adopted men. *Arch Gen Psychiatry.* 1981;38:861-868.
37. Cadoret RJ, Yates WR, Troughton E, Woodsworth G, Stewart M. Adoption study demonstrating two genetic pathways to drug abuse. *Arch Gen Psychiatry.* 1995; 52:42-52.
38. Mattes JA, Fink M. A family study of patients with temper outbursts. *J Psychiatr Res.* 1987;21:249-255.
39. Moss HB, Merzich A, Yao JK, Gavaler J, Martin CS. Aggressivity among sons of substance-abusing fathers: association with psychiatric disorder in the father and son, paternal personality, pubertal development, and socioeconomic status. *Am J Drug Alcohol Abuse.* 1995;21:195-208.
40. Brown GL, Goodwin FK, Ballenger JC, Goyer PF, Major LF. Aggression in humans correlates with cerebrospinal fluid amine metabolites. *Psychiatry Res.* 1979;1:131-139.
41. Agren H, Mefford IN, Rudorfer M, Linnoila M, Potter WZ. Interactive neurotransmitter systems: a non-experimintal approach to the 5HIAA-HVA correlation in human CSF. *Psychiatry Res.* 1986;20:175-193.
42. Higley JD, Thompson WT, Champoux M, Goldman D, Hasert MF, Kraemer GW, Scan Ian JM, Suomi SJ, Linnoila M. Paternal and maternal genetic and environmental contributions to CSF monoamine metabolites in rhesus monkeys (*Macaca mulatta*). *Arch Gen Psychiatry.* 1993;50:615-623.
43. Widom C. The cycle of violence. *Science.* 1989;244:160-166.
44. Dodge KA, Bates JE, Pettit GS. Mechanisms in the cycle of violence. *Science.* 1990;250:1678-1683.
45. DiLalla LF, Gottesman II. Biological and genetic contributors to violence: Widom's untold tale. *Psychol Bull.* 1991;109:125-129.

ORIGINAL ARTICLE

Impulsive Aggression in Personality Disorder Correlates With Tritiated Paroxetine Binding in the Platelet

Emil F. Coccaro, MD; Richard J. Kavoussi, MD; Yvette I. Sheline, MD; Jennifer D. Lish, PhD; John G. Csernansky, MD

Background: To examine the relationship between binding parameters of the platelet central serotonergic (5-HT) transporter and measures of aggression and impulsivity in adult human subjects.

Methods: Maximal number of platelet tritiated paroxetine binding sites (Bmax) and dissociation constant (Kd) values were measured in patients with personality disorder (n=24) and healthy volunteers (n=12). Measures of aggression and impulsivity included the total score and aggression subscale of the Life History of Aggression, the Motor Aggression factor and the assault subscale of the Buss-Durkee Hostility Inventory, and the total score and motor impulsivity subscale of the Barratt Impulsiveness Scale.

Results: The Bmax, but not Kd, values of platelet tritiated paroxetine binding was inversely correlated with the Life History of Aggression total score and aggression score and with the Buss-Durkee Hostility Inventory assault score in patients with personality disorder but not in healthy volunteer subjects. This relationship was independent of influences of factors related to depression, global function, or history of alcoholism or drug abuse.

Conclusions: Reduced numbers of platelet 5-HT transporter sites may covary with life history of aggressive behavior in patients with personality disorder. This may represent another abnormality in 5-HT function in individuals with personality disorder and aggressive behavior.

(Arch Gen Psychiatry. 1996;53:531-536)

From the Clinical Neuroscience Research Unit, Department of Psychiatry, Medical College of Pennsylvania and Hahnemann University, Philadelphia (Drs Coccaro, Kavoussi, and Lish); and Department of Psychiatry, Washington University School of Medicine, St Louis, Mo (Drs Sheline and Csernansky).

EVIDENCE OF a significant relationship between indexes of central serotonergic (5-HT) system function and impulsive aggressive behavior in adult human subjects has been accumulating for more than a decade. First, inverse correlations between cerebrospinal fluid 5-hydroxyindolacetic acid (CSF 5-HIAA) concentrations and history of aggressive behavior were reported in men with personality disorder[1,2] and in men with alcohol abuse.[3] Second, reduced CSF 5-HIAA concentrations were reported in impulsive, compared with nonimpulsive, male violent offenders.[4,5] Third, inverse correlations between prolactin responses to 5-HT agents (eg, fenfluramine hydrochloride, *m*-chlorophenylpiperazine hydrochloride) and historical and self-rated measures of aggression and impulsivity or irritability were reported in men with personality disorder.[6,7] In addition to these findings in humans, similar inverse relationships between either CSF 5-HIAA[8,9] or prolactin responses to fenfluramine[10] and assessments reflective of overt aggression have been reported in nonhuman primates.

The 5-HT measures used in biological studies of aggression in adult human subjects to date have been only measures reflective of central physiological events.[11] This is in contrast to biological studies of suicidal behavior, where presynaptic and postsynaptic receptor elements have been examined in both postmortem brain tissue and peripheral antemortem platelet tissue.[12] While postmortem studies of aggression may be difficult to complete because of the methodological complexities of accurately ascertaining aggressive behavior through psychological autopsy, antemortem studies using platelet tissue may be easily performed prospectively in a group of well-defined subjects with aggressive and nonaggressive tendencies. Platelet measures of 5-HT–related receptor elements include binding studies of postsynaptic 5-HT-2a receptor and presynaptic serotonin uptake inhibitor (eg,

See Subjects and Methods on next page

SUBJECTS AND METHODS

SUBJECTS

The subjects in this study were 24 healthy outpatient subjects (16 men, 8 women) diagnosed with 1 or more *DSM-III-R*[16] personality disorders and 12 healthy volunteer subjects (6 men, 6 women) without *DSM-III-R* Axis I or II disorder. Subjects with personality disorder were recruited from newspaper advertisements that sought individuals who considered themselves to have difficulty controlling their aggressive tendencies and other individuals willing to participate in biological studies of personality. The mean±SD age of the personality disorder sample was 33.4±9.7 years (range, 21-50 years). Healthy volunteers were also recruited by newspaper advertisement. The mean age of the healthy volunteer sample was 25.5±4.8 years (range, 21-38 years). Written informed consent, using an Institutional Review Board–approved consent document, was obtained from all subjects after all procedures were fully explained.

DIAGNOSTIC AND MEDICAL EVALUATION

Axis I and II diagnoses in all 37 subjects were made using the *DSM-III-R* (diagnosis of alcoholism was made by modified Research Diagnostic Criteria as in previous reports[6]) and were assigned through a best-estimate process[17,18] performed by 2 psychiatrists (E.F.C., R.J.K.) and 3 psychologists (J.D.L., M. E. Berman, L. Y. Weinberg), based on information obtained through interviews by a trained clinician using the Schedule for Affective Disorders and Schizophrenia[19] and the Structured Interview for the Diagnosis of Personality Disorder,[20] clinical interviews by a research psychiatrist, and all other available clinical data. One best-estimator (J.D.L., M. E. Berman, L. Y. Weinberg) reviewed all available information and summarized this information in a written narrative report with suggested diagnoses. This written report was then reviewed, and final consensus best-estimate diagnoses (all Axis I and II diagnoses both current and past as an adult) were assigned by the best-estimate board. By inclusion criteria, all subjects with personality disorder met *DSM-III-R* criteria for at least 1 personality disorder. All but 6 met criteria for specific personality disorders; these 6 were diagnosed with "personality disorder not otherwise specified." Of those subjects meeting criteria for specific personality disorders, the average number of personality disorder diagnoses was 1.4±0.6 per subject (range, 1-3). The frequencies of the personality disorder diagnosis by cluster were as follows: (1) dramatic cluster, n=12 (borderline, n=5; histrionic, n=5; narcissistic, n=3; antisocial, n=3); (2) anxious cluster, n=6 (avoidant, n=3; obsessive-compulsive, n=3; passive-aggressive, n=1); (3) eccentric cluster, n=3 (paranoid, n=2; schizoid, n=1). Twelve subjects with personality disorder had 1 concurrent Axis I disorder at the time of the study. The frequency of these Axis I disorders was as follows: intermittent explosive disorder, n=4; depressive disorder not otherwise specified, n=3; social phobia, n=3; dysthymia, n=2; and simple phobia, n=1. Sixteen of the subjects with personality disorder also had a history (ie, currently in full remission) of an Axis I disorder as an adult. The number of these past Axis I disorders averaged 1.3±1.3 per subject (range, 1-5 disorders). The frequency of these disorders was as follows: alcoholism, n=6; drug abuse/dependence, n=7 (cocaine, n=4; marijuana, n=3; amphetamine, n=2; hallucinogens, n=1; polysubstance dependence, n=1); major depressive episode, n=5; depressive disorder not otherwise specified, n=5; dysthymia, n=1. Finally, 6 subjects with personality disorder had neither a current nor a past Axis I diagnosis as an adult. Healthy volunteer subjects were found to be free of current or lifetime psychopathological abnormalities through the best-estimate process. Medical health was documented by medical history, physical examination, electrocardiogram, blood analysis (including platelet count), serum chemistry analysis (including hepatic profile), thyroid function tests, and urinalysis (including a comprehensive drug screen). Subjects with evidence of any current medical (including hematologic) illness, whether or not medication was required, were not enrolled in this study.

GENERAL PREPARATION FOR STUDY

Only 3 of the 37 subjects, all in the personality disorder group, had any history of treatment with psychotropic agents. One patient reported a history of treatment with sertraline hydrochloride (50 mg once daily for 2 months) but had discontinued treatment 17 days prior to the study; 1 reported treatment with diazepam, chlorpromazine hydrochloride, and imipramine (intermittently over the previous 6 years) but had discontinued treatment 6 months prior to the study; and 1 reported treatment with fluoxetine hydrochloride (for 3 years) but had discontinued treatment 1 year prior to the study. These subjects did not differ from the remaining subjects on any demographic, behavioral, or biological variable. Subjects were instructed to remain drug free for 2 weeks prior to the study, to follow a low monoamine diet for at least 3 days prior to the study, and to fast, without smoking, after midnight the night before the study. Subjects were informed that initial and follow-up urine toxicologic screening would be performed randomly just prior to the study; illicit drug use was not detected in any subject reported herein. Female subjects were all studied within the first 10 days of the follicular phase of the menstrual cycle.

PLATELET STUDY

All blood samples for platelet study were obtained between 9 and 9:30 AM through a 20-gauge indwelling intravenous catheter that was in place for the purposes of other biological studies being performed in our unit. Twenty milliliters of venous blood was collected in a plastic syringe and transferred to vacutainer collection tubes containing ethylenediaminetetraacetic acid (EDTA). Samples were kept

tritiated imipramine hydrochloride and tritiated paroxetine) binding sites. Although the platelet constitutes a peripheral site and does not share the same microenvironment as central 5-HT neurons, platelet 5-HT transporter sites have been reported to be structurally identical to corresponding sites on serotonergic neurons in the brain.[13,14] Accordingly, assessment of these binding sites on the platelets of aggressive individuals may yield important information about corresponding sites on 5-HT neurons in the brain. In this study we chose tritiated par-at room temperature and processed to obtain platelet pellets within 3 hours. Platelet harvesting was performed by centrifuging samples for 10 minutes at 900 rpm at room temperature. The platelet-rich plasma samples were then removed by plastic pipette, divided into 3 aliquots in polypropylene sample tubes, and recentrifuged for 15 minutes at 3400 rpm at room temperature. The supernatants were discarded and the platelet pellets were washed twice with a buffer solution and centrifuged again at 3400 rpm for 15 minutes at room temperature. After discarding the final supernatant, the platelet pellets in their polypropylene tubes were immediately frozen at −70°C until assay at the Washington University School of Medicine in the laboratory of 2 of the coauthors (J.G.C. and Y.I.S.). In this laboratory, the frozen platelet pellets were resuspended in 5 mL of 5-mmol/L TRIS and 0.1% EDTA (pH 7.5) and homogenized (20 strokes), using a Teflon pestle and glass homogenization tube. The homogenates were centrifuged at 50 000g for 15 minutes at 4°C. The pellets were resuspended in 5 mL of ice-cold incubation buffer (50- mmol/L TRIS, 120-mmol/L sodium chloride, 5-mmol/L potassium chloride, 2-mmol/L magnesium chloride, and 0.05% ascorbic acid, pH 7.3) and homogenized again with pestle and glass tube; the resulting suspension was assayed. Protein concentration was determined using the BioRad Protein Assay (Bio-Rad, Richmond, Calif) with bovine gamma globulin as the protein standard. Specific binding of tritiated paroxetine (NEN DuPont, Wilmington, Del) was determined at 6 concentrations (range, 0.05 to 1.0-nmol/L) in the presence and absence of 1-μmol/L fluoxetine (Eli Lilly & Co, Indianapolis, Ind). Incubations were performed in microcentrifuge tubes at 37°C for 20 minutes and contained 20 μg platelet membrane protein, 10 μL incubation buffer or fluoxetine, and 10 μL tritiated paroxetine and incubation buffer, bringing the total volume to 1 mL. The samples were rapidly filtered through prewetted Whatman GF/B (Whatman, Hillsboro, Ore) filters. Filters were rinsed twice with 4 mL of ice-cold TRIS/bovine serum albumin buffer and placed in 12×75-mm polypropylene tubes for scintillation counting. These data were transformed by Scatchard analysis (EBDA-LIGAND software, Elsevier-Biosoft, Cambridge, England) to determine receptor density and dissociation constant (Kd) values in each sample. Only samples in which the correlation coefficient of the Scatchard analysis exceeded 0.75 were used in the data analysis. The mean±SD for these correlation coefficients in this study was 0.935±0.054 (range, 0.782-0.998).

BEHAVIORAL MEASURES

Interview (Life History of Aggression [LHA]) and self-report measures of aggression (Buss-Durkee Hostility Inventory [BDHI][21]) and impulsivity (Barratt Impulsiveness Scale-Version 11 [BIS-11][22]) were used in this study.

The LHA assessment was completed by a research psychiatrist after a semistructured interview with the subject and consideration of other available clinical data, as in previous studies.[6] The LHA represents a revision of the Brown-Goodwin Life History of Aggression.[1] It was revised by us so that aggressive behavior directed toward others through verbal outbursts, directed toward inanimate objects, and directed toward the self could be assessed, as well as aggression manifested by "temper tantrums" and "direct assault against others." The LHA differs from the original assessment[1] also in that the rater evaluates the items with a range of 0 to 5 rather than 0 to 4. The LHA has good internal consistency (α=.81) and good interrater reliability (intraclass correlation, 0.95) and stability from 2 to up to 12 months (intraclass correlation, 0.82). Principal-components analysis of the LHA (M. E. Berman, unpublished observations, 1996) supports the presence of 3 subscales: (1) aggression (5 items), including temper tantrums, general history of fighting, assault against others, assault against inanimate objects, and verbal argumentativeness; (2) self-injurious and suicidal behavior (2 items); and (3) antisocial behavior and consequences of aggressive behavior (4 items) including antisocial behavior not involving law enforcement, antisocial behavior involving law enforcement, disciplinary action during the school years, and disciplinary action in the workplace.

The BDHI[21] is a well-known, 75-item, true-false questionnaire composed of 2 main factors (Motor Aggression and Hostility) and 8 subscales. The Motor Aggression factor is composed of 4 subscales: assault (direct [against people]), indirect (assault against objects), verbal (assault through vocalization), and irritability (readiness to react with negative affect). The Hostility factor is composed of 2 subscales: resentment and suspiciousness. Remaining subscales include negativism and guilt.

The BIS-11[22] is another well-known, 34-item, Likert-type self-report questionnaire containing 3 subscales related to motoric, cognitive, and nonplanning impulsivity. Scores for the BIS-11 were available in all but 6 subjects.

The 21-item Hamilton Depression Rating Scale (HAM-D21)[23] was used to assess severity of current depressive symptoms; HAM-D21 data were available in all but 2 subjects. Global function of subjects was assessed by the Global Assessment of Function scale (GAF).[16]

STATISTICAL ANALYSIS

The primary behavioral variables tested were as follows: LHA total score and the aggression subscale; BDHI Motor Aggression factor and the assault subscale; and BIS-11 total score and the motor impulsivity subscale. All other behavioral variables were considered secondary variables. The primary biological variables tested were Bmax and Kd for platelet tritiated paroxetine binding. Comparisons between groups were performed by *t* test, with correction for unequal variances where necessary, or 1-way analysis of variance as appropriate. Correlations were performed by Pearson correlation. Correlations with secondary behavioral variables were adjusted for multiple comparisons with Bonferroni correction. All reported *P* values are 2-tailed.

oxetine, rather than tritiated imipramine, as the radioligand for the platelet 5-HT transporter. Based on preclinical data, tritiated paroxetine appears to be more sensitive and selective than tritiated imipramine as a radioligand for the 5-HT transporter.[15]

RESULTS

With regard to sex, there were no significant differences in either group in tritiated paroxetine binding parameters, age, GAF, HAM-D21, LHA, BDHI, or BIS-11 scores, or the presence of current (or past) Axis I disorders. Mean±SD values for demographic features and parameters of platelet tritiated paroxetine binding for subjects with personality disorder and healthy volunteer subjects are displayed in the **Table**. Healthy volunteers differed significantly from subjects with personality disorder with regard to age (younger), sex (more women), global functioning (higher GAF score), aggression (lower LHA and BDHI scores), and depression (lower HAM-D21 scores). With the exception of LHA total score, LHA aggression, BDHI assault, and HAM-D21 scores, however, no significant relationships were noted between platelet tritiated paroxetine binding parameters and age, sex, season of study, or GAF scores in the total subject group or in the personality-disordered group.

Despite the absence of categorical differences in parameters of platelet tritiated paroxetine binding parameters between the groups, there was a statistically significant inverse correlation between Bmax values and LHA total score ($r=-0.48$, $P=.02$) and LHA aggression ($r=-0.50$, $P=.01$; **Figure**) scores among subjects with personality disorder (n=24) but not among healthy volunteer subjects (LHA total score, $r=0.13$, $P>.60$; LHA aggression, $r=0.18$, $P>.55$). An inverse correlation with the LHA antisocial behavior and consequences of antisocial behavior subscale was noted, but this did not reach statistical significance ($r=-0.39$, $P=.06$). No correlation was found with the LHA self-injury and suicidal behavior factor ($r=-0.01$, $P=.96$); however, only 2 patients in the sample received any score on this subscale. While there was a nonsignificant inverse correlation between Bmax values and BDHI Motor Aggression factor scores ($r=-0.30$, $P=.15$) in the subjects with personality disorder, the correlation between Bmax values and BDHI assault scores was statistically significant ($r=-0.45$, $P=.03$); in normal healthy volunteers, these correlations were similarly inverse, but not statistically significant (BDHI motor aggression, $r=-0.34$, $P=.31$; BDHI assault, $r=-0.35$, $P=.28$). In subjects with personality disorder, the remaining BDHI subscales each demonstrated inverse, though nonsignificant, correlations with Bmax values (indirect assault, $r=-0.32$, $P=.12$; verbal assault, $r=-0.18$, $P=.40$; irritability, $r=-0.12$, $P=.55$). Despite a positive correlation between Bmax and Kd values ($r=0.42$, $P=.04$), no correlation was found between Kd values and LHA total score ($r=0.01$, $P=.96$); LHA aggression ($r=-0.02$, $P=.94$); BDHI Motor Aggression factor ($r=0.09$, $P=.69$); or BDHI assault scores ($r=-0.16$, $P=.45$).

An inverse correlation between HAM-D21 scores and platelet tritiated paroxetine Bmax values in the subjects with personality disorder was nearly statistically significant ($r=-0.42$, n=22, $P>.05$). However, this was owing to the presence of 4 subjects whose HAM-D21 scores were greater than 4 (8, 11, 11, and 14); HAM-D21 scores of the remaining 18 subjects ranged from 0 to 4. The correlation between platelet tritiated paroxetine Bmax values and LHA aggression scores among the 18 subjects with personality disorder and HAM-D21 scores lower than 4 (n=18) remained statistically significant ($r=-0.47$, $P=.05$); the corresponding correlation for BDHI assault score approached significance ($r=-0.43$, $P=.07$). Similarly, the relationship between these LHA aggression scores and Bmax values remained significant ($r=-0.57$, $P=.01$) among subjects without a current mood disorder diagnosis (ie, without major depression, dysthymia, or depressive disorder not otherwise specified); the corresponding correlation for BDHI assault scores approached significance ($r=-0.41$, $P=.09$). This indicates that an inverse correlation between, at least, LHA aggression scores and platelet tritiated paroxetine Bmax values was present even in the absence of clinically significant depressive symptoms or a diagnosable current mood disturbance. There was no significant relationship noted between Bmax values and the presence of a life history of major depression or of a less severe mood disorder (ie, dysthymia or depressive disorder not otherwise specified). Also, there was no relationship between platelet tritiated paroxetine Bmax values and life history of alcoholism or drug abuse/dependence.

Despite a strong positive correlation between the BIS-11 total score with LHA total score ($r=0.72$, $P=.001$),

Bmax and Kd Values for Tritiated Paroxetine Binding, Behavioral Scores, and Demographic Features for the Personality Disordered (PD) and Healthy Volunteer Subjects*

	Patients With PD (n=24)	Normal Controls (n=12)	*P*
Bmax, fmol/mg	1124.0±368.8	1024.9±510.1	.509
Kd, nmol/L	0.35±0.22	0.33±0.11	.728
LHA aggression	10.4±7.1	3.5±2.8	.001
BDHI assault	4.3±3.0	2.0±1.6	.026
BIS-11 impulsivity	43.1±20.0	34.0±14.9	.187
HAM-D21 score	2.5±4.4	0.3±0.5	.023
GAF score	58.9±9.5	86.0±6.0	.001
Age, y	33.6±9.9	25.5±4.8	.020
M/F, No.	16/8	6/6	.050

**Bmax indicates maximal number of platelet tritiated paroxetine binding sites; Kd, affinity constant for platelet tritiated paroxetine binding sites; LHA aggression, aggression subscale of the Life History of Aggression; BDHI assault, assault subscale of the Buss-Durkee Hostility Inventory; BIS-11, total score for Barratt Impulsiveness Scale; HAM-D21, 21-Item Hamilton Depression Rating Scale; and GAF, Global Assessment of Function. Unless otherwise indicated, values are expressed as mean±SD.*

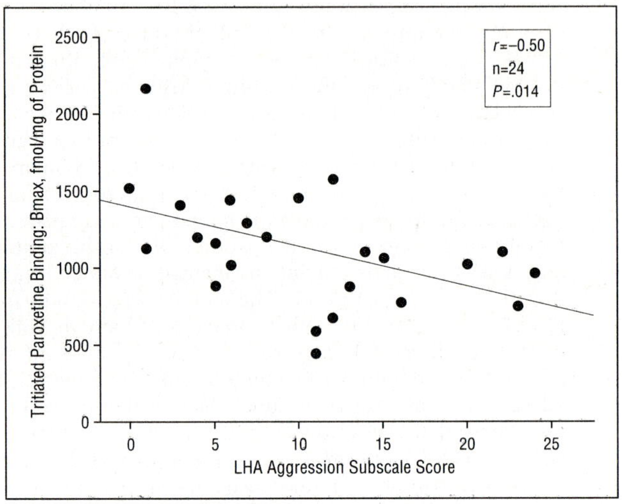

Correlation between maximal number of platelet tritiated paroxetine binding sites (Bmax) and Life History of Aggression (LHA) scores in 24 individuals with DSM-III-R *personality disorder.*

LHA aggression (r=0.65, P=.004), and the BDHI Motor Agression factor (r=0.70, P=.001) in subjects with personality disorder, there were no significant correlations between platelet tritiated paroxetine binding parameters and BIS-11 total score (r=−0.05, P=.83) or motor impulsivity subscale (r=−0.10, P=.70) score. There were no significant correlations between platelet tritiated paroxetine binding parameters and the remaining BIS-11 subscales of impulsiveness: cognitive impulsivity (r=0.05, P=.83) or non-planning impulsivity (r=−0.07, P=.79). Finally, there were no significant correlations between any platelet and BIS-11 variables in the healthy volunteer sample.

COMMENT

These data suggest that a history of aggressive acts and a tendency to respond to provocation with physical assaultiveness in individuals with personality disorder covaries with the number, and not the affinity, of platelet 5-HT uptake sites as assessed using tritiated paroxetine. Notably, the correlation between Bmax values for tritiated paroxetine binding and life history of aggression was independent of global functioning, state depression, or current or life history of mood disorder, alcoholism, or drug abuse. Thus, it is unlikely that this relationship simply represents an epiphenomenon of another psychopathological condition among the patients in this sample.

The absence of similar inverse correlations among the healthy normal volunteers may be accounted for by the limited range in scores for the life history of aggression measure (eg, LHA aggression) and/or the small size of this subject group (eg, BDHI assault). The absence of an overall difference in Bmax values between subjects with personality disorder and healthy volunteers suggests that there are no platelet 5-HT transporter abnormalities in subjects with personality disorder as a group. Rather, these data suggest that there is a relationship between a dimension of aggression and variables related to the platelet 5-HT transporter site. This is consistent with other data relevant to biological variables and personality in individuals with personality disorder.[6,24,25]

Nearly all binding studies of the platelet 5-HT uptake site in psychiatric subjects have been conducted with tritiated imipramine, mostly in depressed subjects. Overall, these studies have yielded mixed evidence of an abnormality of the 5-HT uptake site in depression[26] and suicidality.[27] This may be because tritiated imipramine binding does not reflect the full 5-HT transporter population. Ablation of 5-HT terminals only eliminates 50% of tritiated imipramine binding in the rat brain.[28] Furthermore, tritiated imipramine has a lower affinity than tritiated paroxetine for the platelet uptake site, and this can be more easily confounded by residual drug and other nuisance variables. Accordingly, tritiated imipramine binding does not appear as sensitive or as selective a marker for 5-HT uptake sites as first reported.[15] In contrast, tritiated paroxetine is 100 times more avid than tritiated imipramine for the 5-HT uptake site.[29,30] Its distribution in mouse brain closely follows that of 5-HT itself.[31] In addition, chemical ablation of 5-HT terminals reduces tritiated paroxetine binding between 60% and 90%, depending on the toxin used (60%-90% for *p*-chloroamphetamine, 70% for 3,4-methylenedioxyamphetamine, and 90% for 5,7-dihydroxytryptamine[29,32,33]). Accordingly, tritiated paroxetine appears to be a more sensitive and selective radiolabel for the 5-HT uptake site in brain and in platelets than tritiated imipramine.[15]

The physiological effects of reducing the numbers of presynaptic 5-HT transporter sites on central 5-HT neurons are unknown. However, reports of a positive correlation between the maximum velocity (Vmax) of platelet 5-HT uptake and Bmax of platelet tritiated paroxetine binding in healthy volunteers[34,35] suggest that reduced numbers of 5-HT transporter sites would be associated with a reduction in 5-HT uptake. There are several likely consequences for a reduction in 5-HT uptake. First, by reducing the amount of 5-HT returned to the cytosol, the catabolism of 5-HT to 5-HIAA by monoamine oxidase[36] could be reduced. This could partially account for the reduction in 5-HIAA of the brains of suicide victims and in the CSF of depressives, suicide attempters, and individuals with impulsive aggressive behaviors.[37] Second, reduced 5-HT uptake could be associated with a chronic and relative increase in synaptic concentration of 5-HT. This could lead to a reduction in the sensitivity of terminal 5-HT autoreceptors,[38] a greater release of 5-HT per neuronal impulse,[39] and, ultimately, a subsensitivity of various postsynaptic 5-HT receptors. Depending on the degree to which these alterations occur, a reduction in 5-HT transporter sites or uptake could be associated with a reduction in net central 5-HT neurotransmission, as has been reported in both depressed[6,40] and impulsive-aggressive[6,41] patients.

The present findings are consistent with findings of reduced platelet tritiated imipramine Bmax values in a mixed population of aggressive, "mentally handicapped," institutionalized residents compared with healthy volunteers without a personal or family history of psychiatric disorder[42]; reduced platelet tritiated imipramine Bmax values in adolescents with conduct disorder[43]; and an inverse correlation between platelet tritiated imipramine Bmax values and measures of aggression in impulsive-aggressive children.[44] It is possible that measures of aggression correlate inversely with platelet indexes of 5-HT transporter number across the life cycle as well as in subjects with mental disorders other than personality disorder.

These data are also consistent with the inverse correlation reported for Vmax values and impulsivity scores in a population of aggressive adults.[45] While we found a significant inverse correlation with aggression but not impulsivity, LHA aggression and BDHI aggression scores were correlated with BIS-11 impulsiveness scores in this sample. Accordingly, the more aggressive the subject, the more impulsive as well.

The limited potential of platelet receptor data to reflect the characteristics of analogous structures in the brain has always been problematic.[46] This is because platelets are not neurons and do not exist within neural networks. However, recent studies from 2 laboratories have confirmed that the amino acid sequence of the 5-HT transporter protein expressed in platelets and in 5-HT neurons is identical.[13,14] Thus, it is possible that some pathophysiological abnormalities linked to the 5-HT transporter protein and level of expression would occur in parallel in platelets and in the brain. While platelets and central

5-HT neurons are exposed to different local environments, observations of reduced Bmax values for tritiated imipramine binding on the platelets of suicide attempters[27] and on the 5-HT neurons of violent suicide victims[47,48] seem to support this hypothesis.

Accepted for publication September 7, 1995.

This project was supported in part by National Institutes of Mental Health grants RO1MH49678 and KO2MH00951 (Dr Coccaro). The authors acknowledge Mitchell E. Berman, PhD, and Lauren Y. Weinberg, MS, for their contributions to the best-estimate procedures involved in the final assignment of subject diagnosis. Also noted are the technical contributions of Michelle Stozek, Michael Oakes, Miranda Ellis, and Jaime Jackson.

Reprints: Emil F. Coccaro, MD, Clinical Neuroscience Research Unit, Department of Psychiatry, Medical College of Pennsylvania, 3200 Henry Ave, Philadelphia, PA 19129.

REFERENCES

1. Brown GL, Goodwin FK, Ballenger JC, Goyer PF, Major LF. Aggression in humans correlates with cerebrospinal fluid amine metabolites. *Psychiatry Res.* 1979;1:131-139.
2. Brown GL, Ebert MH, Goyer PF, Jimerson DC, Klein WJ, Bunney WE, Goodwin FK. Aggression, suicide, and serotonin: relationships to CSF amine metabolites. *Am J Psychiatry.* 1982;139:741-746.
3. Limson R, Goldman D, Roy A, Lamparski D, Ravitz B, Adinoff B, Linnoila M. Personality and cerebrospinal fluid monoamine metabolites in alcoholics and controls. *Arch Gen Psychiatry.* 1991;48:437-441.
4. Linnoila M, Virkkunen M, Scheinin M, Nuutila A, Rimon R, Goodwin FK. Low cerebrospinal fluid 5-hydroxyindolacetic acid concentration differentiates impulsive from nonimpulsive violent behavior. *Life Sci.* 1983;33:2609-2614.
5. Virkkunen M, Rawlins R, Tokola R, Poland RE, Guidotti A, Nemeroff C, Bisssette G, Kalogeras K, Karonen SL, Linnoila M. CSF biochemistries, glucose metabolism, and diurnal activity rhythms in alcoholics, violent offenders, fire setters, and healthy volunteers. *Arch Gen Psychiatry.* 1994;51:20-27.
6. Coccaro EF, Siever LJ, Klar HM, Maurer G, Cochrane K, Cooper TB, Mohs RC, Davis KL. Serotonergic studies in patients with affective and personality disorder: correlates with suicidal and impulsive aggressive behavior. *Arch Gen Psychiatry.* 1989;46:587-599.
7. Moss HB, Yao JK, Panzak GL. Serotonergic responsivity and behavioral dimensions in antisocial personality disorder with substance abuse. *Biol Psychiatry.* 1990;28:325-338.
8. Higley JD, Mehlman PT, Taub DM, Higley SB, Suomi SJ, Linnoila M, Vickers JH. Cerebrospinal fluid monoamine and adrenal correlates of aggression in free-ranging rhesus monkeys. *Arch Gen Psychiatry.* 1992;49:436-441.
9. Mehlman PT, Higley JD, Faucher I, Lilly AA, Taub DM, Vickers J, Suomi SJ, Linnoila M. Low CSF 5-HIAA concentrations and severe aggression and impaired impulse control in non-human primates. *Am J Psychiatry.* 1994;151:1485-1491.
10. Botchin MB, Kaplan JR, Manuck SB, Mann JJ. Low versus high prolactin responders to fenfluramine challenge: marker of behavioral differences in adult male cynomolgus macaques. *Neuropsychopharmacology.* 1993;9:93-99.
11. Coccaro EF. Impulsive aggression and central serotonergic system function in humans: an example of a dimensional brain-behavioral relationship. *Int J Clin Psychopharmacol.* 1992;7:3-12.
12. Coccaro EF, Astill J. Central serotonergic function in parasuicide. *Prog Neuropsychopharmacol Biol Psychiatry.* 1990;14:663-674.
13. Ramamoorthy S, Bauman AL, Moore KR, Han H, Yang-Feng T, Chang AS, Ganapathy V, Blakely RD. Antidepressant- and cocaine-sensitive human serotonin transporter: molecular cloning, expression, and chromosomal localization. *Proc Natl Acad Sci U S A.* 1993;90:2542-2546.
14. Lesch K-P, Wolozin BL, Murphy DL, Riederer P. Primary structure of the human platelet serotonin uptake site: identity with the brain serotonin transporter. *J Neurochemistry.* 1993;60:2319-2322.
15. Marcusson J, Ross SB. Binding of some antidepressants to the 5-hydroxytryptamine transporter in brain and platelets. *Psychopharmacology.* 1990;102:145-155.
16. American Psychiatric Association. *Diagnostic and Statistical Manual of Mental Disorders, Third Edition, Revised.* Washington, DC: American Psychiatric Association; 1987.
17. Leckman JF, Sholomskas D, Thompson WD, Belanger A, Weissman MM. Best estimate of lifetime psychiatric diagnosis: a methodological study. *Arch Gen Psychiatry.* 1982;39:879-883.
18. Klein DN, Ouimette PC, L Kelly HS, Ferro T, Riso LP. Test-retest reliability of a team consensus best-estimate diagnoses of Axis I and II disorders in a family study. *Am J Psychiatry.* 1994;151:1043-1047.
19. Spitzer RL, Endicott J. *Schedule for Affective Disorders and Schizophrenia.* NY State Psychiatric Institute; New York: 1978.
20. Pfohl B, Zimmerman M. *Structured Interview for the Diagnosis of DSM-III-R Personality Disorders.* Iowa City; University of Iowa College of Medicine: 1989.
21. Buss AH, Durkee A. An inventory for assessing different kinds of hostility. *J Consult Psychol.* 1957;21:343-348.
22. Barratt ES. Factor analysis of some psychometric measures of impulsiveness and anxiety. *Psychol Reports.* 1985;16:547-554.
23. Guy W. *ECDEU Manual for Psychopharmacology.* Washington, DC: Superintendent of Documents, US Government Printing Office; 1976. US Dept of Health, Education, and Welfare publication ADM 76-338.
24. Coccaro EF, Lawrence T, Trestman R, Gabriel S, Klar HM, Siever LJ. Growth hormone responses to intravenous clonidine challenge correlates with behavioral irritability in psychiatric patients and in healthy volunteers. *Psychiatry Res.* 1991;39:129-139.
25. Seiver LJ, Amin F, Coccaro EF, Bernstein DP, Kavoussi RJ, Kalus O, Horvath TB, Warne P, Davidson M, Davis KL. Plasma homovanillic acid in schizotypal personality disorder. *Am J Psychiatry.* 1991;148:1246-1248.
26. Langer SZ, Galzin AM, Poirier MF, Loo H, Sechter D, Zarifian E. Association of ^{3}H-imipramine and ^{3}H-paroxetine binding with the 5-HT transporter in brain and platelet: relevance to studies in depression. *J Receptor Res.* 1987;7:499-525.
27. Marazziti D, DeLeo D, Conti L. Further evidence supporting the role of the serotonin system in suicidal behavior: a preliminary study of suicide attempters. *Acta Psychiatr Scand.* 1989;80:322-324.
28. Dawson TM, Wamsley JK. Autoradiographic localization of ^{3}H-imipramine binding sites: association with serotonergic neurons. *Brain Res Bull.* 1983;11:325-334.
29. Habert E, Graham D, Tahraoui L, Claustre Y, Langer SZ. Characterization of ^{3}H-paroxetine binding to rat cortical membranes. *Eur J Pharmacol.* 1985;118:107-114.
30. Mellerup E, Plenge P. High affinity binding of ^{3}H-paroxetine and ^{3}H-imipramine to rat neuronal membranes. *Psychopharmacology.* 1986;89:436-439.
31. Scheffel U, Hartig PR. In vivo labeling of serotonin uptake sites with ^{3}H-paroxetine. *J Neurochemistry.* 1989;52:1605-1612.
32. DeSouza EB, Kuyatt BL. Autoradiographic localization of ^{3}H-paroxetine-labeled serotonin uptake sites in rat brain. *Synapse.* 1987;1:488-496.
33. Marcusson J, Bergstrom M, Eriksson K, Ross SB. Characterization of ^{3}H-paroxetine binding in rat brain. *J Neurochem.* 1988;50:1783-1790.
34. Maguire K, Tuckwell V, Pererira A, Dean B, Singh B. Significant correlation between ^{14}C-5-HT uptake by and ^{3}H-paroxetine binding to platelets from healthy volunteers. *Biol Psychiatry.* 1993;34:356-360.
35. Nankai M, Yamada S, Yoshimoto S, Watanabe A, Mori H, Asai K, Toru M. Platelet ^{3}H-paroxetine binding in control subjects and depressed patients: relationship to serotonin uptake and age. *Psychiatry Res.* 1994;51:147-155.
36. Kuhn DM, Wolf W, Youdim MBH. Serotonin neurochemistry revisited: a new look at some old axioms. *Neurochem Int.* 1986;2:141-154.
37. Asberg M, Schalling D, Traksman-Bendz L, Wagner A. Psychobiology of suicide, impulsivity, and related phenomena. In: Meltzer HY, ed. *Psychopharmacology: Third Generation of Progress.* New York, NY: Raven Press; 1987:655-688.
38. Blier P, de Montigny C, Chaput Y. Modifications of the serotonin system by antidepressant treatments: implication for the therapeutic response in major depression. *J Clin Psychopharmacol.* 1987;7(suppl):24S-35S.
39. Aghajanian GK. Feedback regulation of central monoaminergic neurons: evidence from single cell recording studies. In: Youdim MBH, Lovenberg W, Shaman DF, Langnado JR, eds. *Essays in Neurochemistry and Neuropharmacology.* New York, NY; Wiley & Sons: 1978;3:1-33.
40. O'Keane V, Dinan TG. Prolactin and cortisol responses to D-fenfluramine in major depression: evidence for diminished responsivity of central serotonergic function. *Am J Psychiatry.* 1991;148:1009-1015.
41. O'Keane V, Moloney E, O'Neill H, O'Connor A, Smith C, Dinan TG. Blunted prolactin responses to D-fenfluramine in sociopathy: evidence for subsensitivity of central serotonergic function. *Br J Psychiatry.* 1992;160:643-646.
42. Marazziti D, Rotondo A, Presta S, Panioli-Guadagnucci ML, Palego L, Conti L. Role of serotonin in human aggressive behavior. *Aggressive Behav.* 1993;9:347-353.
43. Stoff DM, Pollock L, Vitiello B, Behar D, Bridger WH. Reduction of ^{3}H-imipramine binding sites on platelets of conduct disordered children. *Neuropsychopharmacology.* 1987;1:55-62.
44. Birmaher B, Stanley M, Greenhill L, Twomey J, Gavrilescu A, Rabinovich H. Platelet imipramine binding in children and adolescents with impulsive behavior. *J Am Acad Child Adolesc Psychiatry.* 1990;29:914-918.
45. Brown CS, Kent TA, Bryant SG, Gevedon RM, Campbell JL, Felthous AR, Barratt ES, Rose RM. Blood platelet uptake of serotonin in episodic aggression. *Psychiatry Res.* 1989;27:5-12.
46. Murphy DL, Mellow AM, Sunderland T, Aulahk CS, Lawlor BL, Zohar J. Strategies for assessing serotonin in humans. In: Coccaro EF, Murphy DL, eds. *Serotonin in Major Psychiatric Disorders.* Washington, DC: American Psychiatric Press; 1990.
47. Stanley MS, Viggilio J, Gershon S. Tritiated imipramine binding sites are decreased in the frontal cortex of suicides. *Science.* 1982;216:1337-1339.
48. Gross-Isseroff R, Israeli M, Biegon A. Autoradiographic analysis of tritiated imipramine binding in the human brain post mortem: effects of suicide. *Arch Gen Psychiatry.* 1989;46:237-241.

Excessive Mortality in Young Free-Ranging Male Nonhuman Primates With Low Cerebrospinal Fluid 5-Hydroxyindoleacetic Acid Concentrations

J. Dee Higley, PhD; Patrick T. Mehlman, PhD; Sue B. Higley; Beth Fernald; James Vickers, DVM; Stephen G. Lindell; David M. Taub, PhD; Stephen J. Suomi, PhD; Markku Linnoila, MD, PhD

Background: The purpose of this study was to assess the impact of central serotonin turnover rate on survival to adulthood among nonhuman primates living in a large, free-ranging colony.

Methods: The rate of mortality was ascertained over a 4-year period after obtaining blood and cisternal cerebrospinal fluid (CSF) samples from 49 free-ranging, 2-year-old prepubertal male rhesus monkeys. Cerebrospinal fluid was assayed for 5-hydroxyindoleacetic acid (5-HIAA), norepinephrine, 3-methoxy-4-hydroxyphenylgycol, and homovanillic acid. Blood plasma was assayed for adrenocorticotropic hormone, cortisol, and testosterone. Following the sampling of body fluids, records of scars and wounds and aggressive encounters were used to rank the subjects from low to high in aggressiveness. Direct observations of aggressive behavior were collected from 27 of the subjects over a 3-month period.

Results: Four years later, 6 of the 49 subjects were known to be dead and an additional 5 had been missing for more than 2 years and were presumed dead. The CSF 5-HIAA concentrations were predictive of which subjects died, with 46% of the subjects with low CSF 5-HIAA concentrations dead or presumed dead. None of the subjects from the highest CSF 5-HIAA concentration quartile were dead or missing. Indeed, 91% of the dead subjects came from the 2 lowest quartiles of CSF 5-HIAA concentrations. Direct observations of aggressive behavior showed that dead or missing subjects had initiated escalated aggression, a measure of unrestrained aggression that has a high probability of trauma or injury, at a higher rate than subjects that were known to be alive. The cause of death could be ascertained for 6 of the 11 missing subjects. The 4 subjects that were known to die as a consequence of aggressive encounters came from the lowest quartile of CSF 5-HIAA concentrations and had been rated as more aggressive during their initial capture. Subjects captured more than once possessed lower CSF 5-HIAA concentrations, were rated as more aggressive, and were more likely to suffer early death than those captured only once.

Conclusion: These findings suggest that low CSF 5-HIAA concentrations quantified early in life is a powerful biological predictor of future excessive aggression, risk taking, and premature death among nonhuman primate males.

(Arch Gen Psychiatry. 1996;53:537-543)

From the Section on Neurochemistry and Neuroendocrinology, Laboratory of Clinical Studies, Division of Intramural and Clinical Biological Research, National Institute of Alcohol Abuse and Alcoholism (Drs J. D. Higley and Linnoila and Mr Lindell), and Laboratory of Comparative Ethology, National Institute of Child Health and Human Development (Ms S. B. Higley and Dr Suomi), Bethesda, Md; Laboratory Animal Breeders and Services Inc, Yemassee, SC (Drs Mehlman and Taub and Ms Fernald); and the Food and Drug Administration, Bethesda (Dr Vickers).

SUBSTANTIAL evidence has accumulated showing that many men with low cerebrospinal fluid (CSF) 5-hydroxyindoleacetic acid (5-HIAA) concentrations exhibit excessive aggression and high rates of violence.[1-3] Similarly, among nonhuman primates, high rates of wounding, violence, and inappropriate aggression are frequently observed in subjects with low CSF 5-HIAA concentrations.[4-8] Past research shows that interindividual differences in CSF 5-HIAA are among the most stable of biochemical traits,[6,7,9,10] stabilizing early in life before aggression is first expressed and remaining relatively stable into adulthood.[6,9,11] No studies, however, have quantified CSF 5-HIAA early in life and followed subjects longitudinally to assess outcomes such as the rate of mortality.

To address the possibility of premature deaths among subjects with low CSF 5-HIAA concentrations, over the past 4 years, we have longitudinally studied a group of male rhesus macaques with known CSF 5-HIAA concentrations. The animals were 2 years old (middle- to late-childhood-age in human terms) when the study began. The surviving subjects are now 6-year-old young adults. Most male rhesus macaques migrate from their social group of origin to new social groups during adolescence.[12] This is a dangerous period of life for young male macaques,

See Subjects and Methods on next page

SUBJECTS AND METHODS

SUBJECTS

During November or December of 1989 and 1990, single CSF and blood samples were obtained from each of 49 young male subjects (28 in 1989, 21 in 1990; average age 28.2±1.6 SD months), chosen from a population of 4500 rhesus macaques maintained as a free-ranging, food-provisioned breeding colony located on a 475-acre South Carolina sea island. There are no predators of rhesus macaques on the island. There are 12 feeding corrals (10-25 m wide and 4 m high), equally distributed across the island, that are used each day to feed the monkeys throughout the year. On the first day of each 5-day trapping period, the corrals were baited with the monkeys' food rations and the doors that are used each day to enter and exit were closed, transforming the corrals into traps. The monkeys voluntarily jump into the traps but are precluded from exiting by the high walls. While the trapping methodology is passive (ie, the subjects decide whether or not to enter), at the age that the subjects were sampled, our analyses of each monoamine and hormone have shown that this provides a population distribution that is normal, and the mean of this population is similar to those obtained in the laboratory. This population has been longitudinally studied since their initial sampling in either 1989 or 1990 and has been reported on in previous publications. (Methods of capture, aggressiveness rating methodology, and assay information are described in more detail in a previous publication.[4]) These observations, however, represent new data that were not reported before.

METHODS

Physiological Measures

Anesthesia was induced with ketamine hydrochloride (10 mg/kg). Immediately thereafter, subjects were weighed, and CSF and blood were drawn from each subject. Two milliliters of cisternal CSF was removed, and the sample was immediately placed and maintained on dry ice. Blood samples were obtained via venipuncture, and the plasma was frozen and stored with the CSF at a temperature of −70°C. Cerebrospinal fluid was assayed for 5-HIAA, norepinephrine (NE), 3-methoxy-4-hydroxyphenylgycol, and homovanillic acid. Blood plasma was assayed for adrenocorticotropin, cortisol, and testosterone by Hazelton Biotechnologies (Vienna, Va) using radioimmunoassays.[23]

Ratings for Aggressivity

During the capture, brief descriptive written notes were made to record any aggressive acts that the subjects perpetrated or received. These included both aggression to and from other conspecifics or aggression directed to the experimenters. Following the removal of CSF and blood, each subject was examined by the senior author (J.D.H.) or another technician, and a written record was made of the frequency, severity, and patterns of wounds (eg, contusions, tooth marks, nips, canine slashes, and scars with the numbers and locations of each on the body). A photo was taken of each subject to record wound severity, extensiveness of scars, and general condition.

In 1989, 2 different primatologists, each with more than year of intensive experience observing nonhuman primate behavior (>1 and >4 years, respectively), and in 1990, 3 different primatologists, each with more than 1 year of experience and blind to the monkeys' monoamine and hormone status, were asked to rank the monkeys within each year from the most to the least aggressive based on the following criteria: (1) written descriptive notes of aggression observed during capture, when available; (2) frequency, severity, and patterns of wounding; and (3) the photograph of the monkey. Ratings were made at the time of each animal's capture, prior to the field observation period. Within-rater reliability was statistically assessed by correlating the 2 ratings made by each primatologist (r=0.686, and r=0.836, P<.001, df=1,44). Between-rater reliability was statistically assessed by correlating each primatologists' mean aggressivity rating using Pearson correlation coefficient tests, and it was above chance level of similarity (r=0.868, P<.001, df=1,44). We, therefore, averaged the raters' rankings for aggressivity, and all analyses reported use this average rank score. Insufficient information existed to rate 3 of the 49 subjects for aggressiveness. Eleven subjects jumped into the traps in both 1989 and 1990. All monkeys on the island are repeatedly captured from birth. Thus, the additional capture in 1990 of these 11 subjects should not have affected any of the variables measured. For subjects captured in both 1989 and 1990, only the rating and biochemical values from the first capture were used. One subject received numerous wounds around the time of the first capture; thus, we used values from his second capture. For biochemical variables whose means differed between 1989 and 1990, a regression equation was used to statistically partial out the between-year differences.

Objective Observations of Aggressive Behavior

Following recovery from anesthesia, all subjects were released with other members of their group within their home range area. Prior to their release, 27 of the subjects were fitted with a radio transmitter collar that emitted a unique frequency. Thereafter, these 27 subjects could be located and identified in the field for quantitative behavioral observations by means of a radio telemetry receiver. Quantitative behavioral scores were obtained from these 27 subjects, using an objective aggressive behavior scoring system. The scores were obtained by means of direct visual observation, either aided or unaided by binoculars, depending on the distance from the observer. Observations of aggres-

with adolescent males involved in many aggressive encounters[13,14] and a high rate of mortality from aggression (between 30% and 50% are killed or disappear and are presumed to die between 24 and 72 months of age).[15-17] While some males migrate early in adolescence when their growth acceleration is just beginning,[18] other subjects are able to delay migration until they are fully mature and more socially sophisticated.[19] An additional benefit of delaying migration is that older brothers and other familiar conspecifics may have migrated to nearby troops, facilitating an immigrant's integration into a new social group.[20,21] In our study population, the mean age of emigration is 52.4 months,[18] consistent with that found in other studies.[20] While males with high CSF 5-HIAA consive behavior were conducted from June 1 to August 25, 1991, by 2 observers who had been trained together by the second author (P.T.M.). Direct observations of aggressive behavior were obtained from these 27 subjects. Because they could not be located and identified, quantitative observations of aggressive behavior could not be performed on the 22 subjects without collars. Thus, the biochemical data obtained in 1989 or 1990 from the other 22 subjects could only be correlated with the aggressive ratings obtained at the time of capture and mortality status. Interobserver reliability tests for the behaviors collected from the subjects with radio collars were conducted at the beginning, the midpoint, and the end of the study. In the 3 tests, both observers simultaneously scored the same subject for a 15-minute observation session. In terms of interrater reliability, Cohen κ tests indicated a consistent 0.95 or better interrater agreement. Both behavioral observers were blind to all biochemical data.

Observations of aggression were scored as frequency data, falling into 1 of 4 categories of increasing intensity: (1) displacements, (2) stationary threats, (3) chases, and (4) physical assaults. Displacements were scored when the subject physically moved toward another individual and the latter moved from its position (often occurring at food and water stations). Stationary threats included all threat gestures, such as stares, open-mouth threats, head bobs, ground slaps, etc, that were displayed while the subject remained in a stationary position. Chases were scored when the subject chased another individual and the other individual fled (often screaming and exhibiting submissive gestures). Physical assaults were scored for all contact aggression (ie, when the subject bit, hit, or slapped another individual). Whenever a sequence of aggressive behaviors was observed (eg, stationary threat, chase, and then bite), only the most intense aggressive act was scored (eg, physical assault). To control for the rate of activity and frequency of social encounters, a derived variable, escalated aggression, was calculated by dividing the total number of chases and physical assaults by the total number of aggressive acts (1-4 above). For any subject, the escalated aggression score therefore represents the proportion of aggressive acts that escalated into the 2 most intense forms of aggression.

Assessing Mortality Rate

Throughout the year, all monkey groups on the island are monitored by a team of 5 to 7 behavioral technicians and 1 to 3 graduate researchers. During each month, an island-wide census of all animals is obtained by these observers who record the location and group membership of all subjects. Subjects are identified by their unique individual identification numbers, which are tattooed on the face, chest, and leg for easy recognition. Where necessary, binoculars are used. Observers are generally familiar with their own census group, which facilitates identification. Subjects that are not located on 1 census are specifically identified as missing, and all observers then make locating these subjects their top priority during the following census. Island census records show subjects as dead if they have not been sighted for more than 1 year, and, without exception, subjects missing for more than 1 year have never been observed again. Extensive observations and regular weekly censuses of the study subjects were made by 2 observers during the summer months beginning in June 1991 and continuing through August 1994.

For the purposes of this study, we used a more conservative criterion for death by extending it to subjects' not having been sighted for more than 2 years. The period of assessment for death began with the 1989 sample and continued through the end of August 1994. At the end of August 1994, all missing subjects that were classified as dead or presumed dead had been missing for more than 2 years, and no other subjects had been missing for more than 1 year. Neither the rate of mortality nor concentrations of the neurotransmitter metabolites and hormones were significantly correlated with any of several potentially confounding variables (eg, age, size, time to capture, and time of day). Four of the 11 dead or presumed dead subjects had radio collars, and the radio collars were useful in locating 2 of these 4 dead subjects. Necropsies or direct observations determined the cause of death in 6 of the 11 dead subjects.

Data Analyses

Rate of mortality was assessed for all of the subjects that had been previously captured (ie, for subjects both with and without radio collars). To statistically assess the probability of early death as a function of low CSF 5-HIAA concentrations, subjects were divided into quartiles of low, mid-low, mid-high, and high CSF 5-HIAA concentrations. Divisions were made by first splitting the population into 2 groups, above and below the mean; median splits were then made of each group. The χ^2 test was used to statistically assess the differential probability of death for each of the quartiles. The ratings for aggression made during the initial capture were available for both the radio-collared and non–radio-collared animals. For the 27 subjects with radio collars, the behaviors, overall aggression (ie, the summed frequency for each subject of all 4 types of aggression), and the derived variable, escalated aggression, were used to assess differential rates of aggression among the dead and living subjects. To assess differences between subjects with multiple captures and single captures, subjects from 1989 were coded as captured or not captured in 1990, and these groupings were used to statistically compare differences between groups on each variable. For all analyses, *t* tests, Kruskal-Wallis tests, or Pearson correlation coefficients were computed. In all tests 2-tailed probabilities were used with a $P<.05$ criterion unless otherwise noted.

centrations remain in their troops until they are older than this normative age of migration,[19] males with low CSF 5-HIAA concentrations typically migrate from their social group of origin when they are younger and often not yet fully mature.[18]

A number of studies have shown that subjects with low CSF 5-HIAA concentrations receive disproportionately frequent wounds, are rated high in aggressivity, exhibit acts of violence, are isolated socially, and probably as a result migrate from their natal troops at an earlier age.[4-8,18,19,22] These studies have shown that subjects with low CSF 5-HIAA concentrations are not necessarily more aggressive in all ways than subjects with higher CSF 5-HIAA concentrations. However, they are more likely

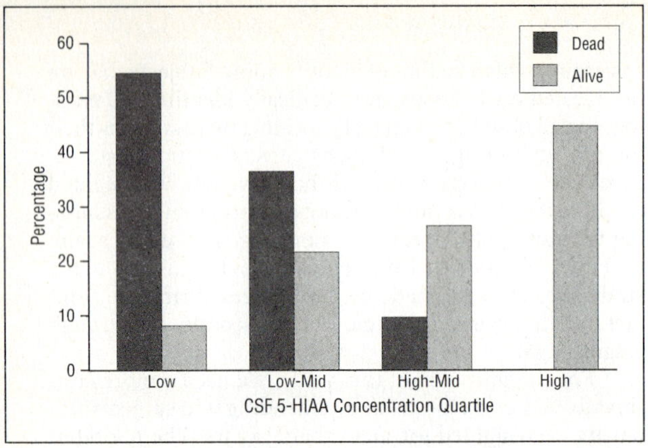

Figure 1. *The percentage of subjects dead (both known and presumed) or alive 4 years after a cerebrospinal fluid (CSF) sample was obtained to quantify 5-hydroxyindoleacetic acid (5-HIAA) concentrations. Subjects are grouped in quartiles according to CSF 5-HIAA concentrations. Units of 5-HIAA concentrations are in picomoles per milliliter. The figure shows a monotonic increase in death rates with lower quartiles. None of the subjects from the highest quartile died over the course of the study.*

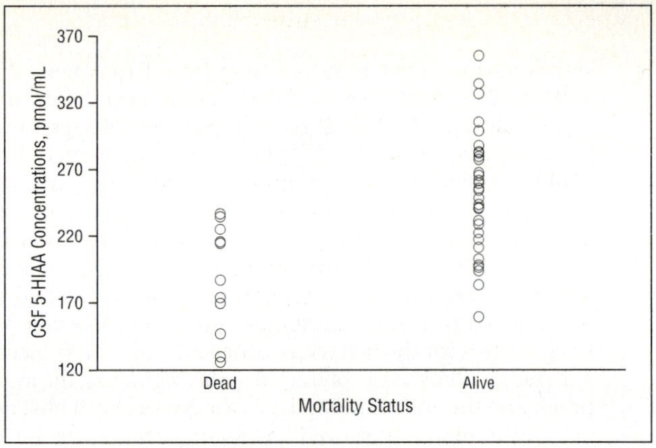

Figure 2. *A scatterplot showing cerebrospinal fluid 5-hydroxyindoleacetic acid (CSF 5-HIAA) concentrations from the first capture in 1989 or 1990. Subjects from 1989 and 1990 are grouped according to whether they are alive or dead (both known and presumed).*

to engage in aggression that escalates from a controlled low intensity to unrestrained aggression with a high probability of wounding and trauma. Once this escalated aggression begins, it is more likely to continue until wounding occurs. Moreover, within this free-ranging population of macaques, individual CSF 5-HIAA levels are relatively stable between years. For example, CSF 5-HIAA concentrations obtained from the same individuals 1 year apart correlate with each other at $r > 0.50$.[7] Based on these findings, we hypothesized that subjects with low CSF 5-HIAA concentrations would show disproportionally high rates of mortality during the period that most males migrate from their social groups of origin.

Subjects with low CSF 5-HIAA concentrations also exhibit evidence of impaired impulse control, such as unprovoked, spontaneous, long, dangerous leaps between the treetops.[8,18] This trait of impulsivity is thought to underlie in part the differences in aggression that are seen between subjects with low and high CSF 5-HIAA concentrations.[8,18] The population of monkeys from which we selected our subjects are trapped annually; however, not all subjects are captured during these trappings. As the subjects age, the number of males that are captured during the annual trappings decreases. While some subjects avoid the traps, others are trapped with regularity. About 50% of our subjects were trapped twice, once in 1989, and again in 1990. All the subjects captured in 1989 and again in 1990 had recently experienced the trapping procedure. In 1990, we were able to test differences between subjects with low and high CSF 5-HIAA levels in rates of reentering the traps. In 1990, we tested specifically whether subjects with low CSF 5-HIAA levels would exhibit evidence of impaired impulse control by disproportionately reentering the traps where they had been captured in 1989.

RESULTS

Of the 49 subjects sampled, 11 were considered dead (the bodies of 6 subjects were recovered; the remaining 5 were not observed for 2 years and were thus presumed dead), and CSF 5-HIAA concentrations were predictive of these early deaths. The χ^2 analyses showed that subjects in the 2 low CSF 5-HIAA concentration quartiles were more likely to die prematurely (χ^2=14.68, P<.002; **Figure 1**). Indeed, only 1 subject whose CSF 5-HIAA level was above the mean suffered early death. None of the subjects from the highest quartile died or were missing during this period. The 11 subjects that died or had not been sighted for over 2 years had significantly lower CSF 5-HIAA levels during their first capture than the subjects that remained alive (t=3.79, df=1,47, P<.0004; **Figure 2**). Direct observations of aggressive behavior showed that subjects that had died engaged in high rates of escalated aggression (t=2.02, df=1,25, P<.05); they also exhibited a trend to engage in more overall aggression (t= 1.74, df=1,25, P<.10).

When the 6 subjects, whose bodies had been recovered for necropsy, were compared with the subjects that were still alive, deaths were still predicted by low CSF-5-HIAA concentrations, with subjects that had died having lower CSF 5-HIAA concentrations during their first capture (t=2.87, df=1,42, P<.007; mean±SD CSF 5-HIAA concentrations: dead, 194.0±41.4; alive, 248.1±43.0). Of the 6 subjects with death records, 4 were killed in a fight or died from fight-related wounding. The other 2 died from illnesses. Subjects that died as a consequence of violence had significantly lower CSF 5-HIAA concentrations than the subjects that were alive (t=2.76, df=1,40, P<.01; mean±SD CSF 5-HIAA levels: death from aggression, 185.3±46.8; alive, 248.0±42.9). The CSF 5-HIAA concentrations of the 2 subjects that died from illness did not differ statistically from subjects that were still alive (t=1.97, df=1,38, P<.40; mean±SD CSF 5-HIAA levels: dead from illness, 211.5±33.2; alive, 248.0±42.9). When the ratings for aggressiveness from the first capture were compared, the 4 subjects killed in fights had been rated as being significantly more aggressive than the subjects that remained alive (Mann-Whitney U = 2.11, df=1,40, P<.03, mean±SD rating for aggressivity: dead by aggression; 24.7±6.7; alive, 15.3±8.1). Ratings for aggression were unrelated to death from illness (P>.90). Direct observations of aggressive behavior were obtained from too few of the subjects whose deaths were known to result from aggression to perform statistical comparisons.

MORTALITY RATE AND OTHER NEUROTRANSMITTER METABOLITES OR HORMONES

Of the other neurotransmitter metabolites and hormones that were measured, only CSF NE levels were correlated with mortality status (**Table 1**). The CSF NE concentrations were higher in the 511 subjects that were presumed dead (t=2.79, df=1,47, P<.01), in the 6 subjects that were known to be dead (t=2.12, df=1,47, P<.04), and in the 4 subjects that were known to have died from aggression (t=2.07, df=1,40, P=.05) than in the subjects that were still alive. This was, however, attributable to a significant negative correlation between NE and 5-HIAA levels (r=−0.34, df=1,48, P<.05; see **Table 2** for between-biochemical correlations). The relationship between CSF NE levels and death disappeared when the correlation between CSF 5-HIAA and NE levels was statistically controlled by simultaneously entering CSF NE and 5-HIAA levels as independent variables and death as the dependent variable in a multiple regression. When both were entered, only CSF 5-HIAA levels were statistically correlated with death (CSF 5-HIAA level partial r=−0.43, P<.003; CSF NE level partial r=−0.19, P>.20). Similarly, when a χ^2 test was used to test for differential death rates by CSF NE level quartiles, the results failed to approach statistical significance when the residuals from the 5-HIAA–NE levels' regression were used (χ^2<2.26, P>.50). None of the other neurotransmitter metabolites or hormones were correlated with the aggression ratings (P>.20). None of the comparisons involving other neurotransmitter metabolites or hormones approached statistical significance (P>.25).

REPEATED CAPTURES, NEUROTRANSMITTER MEBABOLITES, HORMONES, AND MORTALITY RATE

When the subjects captured in 1989 were classified as to whether they were captured again in 1990, the 11 subjects captured in both years had significantly lower CSF 5-HIAA concentrations than the 17 who avoided captured in 1990 (t=2.30, df=1,24, P<.03). Subjects captured in both years were also rated as more aggressive than those not captured in 1990 (t=2.08, df=1,24; P<.05). Similarly, subjects that were known to be dead (ie, whose bodies had been recovered for necropsy[n=4]) and those known to have died from aggression (n=2) were more likely to have undergone multiple captures (known to be dead: χ^2=5.06, df=1,27, P<.03; dead from aggression, χ^2=2.77, df=1,25, P<.09), although this last relationship was only of trend level significance. None of the other variables or neurotransmitter metabolites or hormones were related to repeated capture.

Table 1. Each of the Neurotransmitter Metabolites and Hormones by Mortality Status*

	Mortality Status of Subjects		
Neurotransmitter or Hormone	Alive (n=38)	Dead (n=11)	Dead From Aggression (n=4)
HVA	1759.1 (357.1)	1623.6 (308.7)	1664.3 (316.4)
NE	3.9 (1.2)	4.8 (0.8)	5.0 (1.1)
MHPG	157.1 (29.3)	162.1 (45.4)	152.3 (49.2)
ACTH	140.6 (99.9)	112.9 (52.4)	121.1 (55.6)
Cortisol	75.9 (58.0)	91.9 (62.4)	85.2 (41.5)
Testosterone	38.4 (29.3)	47.8 (32.7)	44.7 (19.4)

Values are expressed as mean (SD). HVA indicates homovanillic acid; NE, norepinephrine; MPHG, 3-methoxy-4-hydroxyphenylglycol; and ACTH, adenocorticotropin.
†*Both known and presumed.*

COMMENT

As predicted, 2-year-old subjects with low CSF 5-HIAA concentrations, that also exhibited high concurrent ratings for aggressivity and engaged in high rates of escalated aggression, were more likely to die at an early age as a result of violence. Our findings concerning overall mortality rates are consistent with other studies showing high rates of death during the period of life when nonhuman primate males migrate from their social groups of origin.[12] However, our findings also suggest that the rate of death is not randomly distributed across the overall male population. Instead, it appears that subjects with low CSF 5-HIAA concentrations are much more likely to die during this period of life than the rest of the male population. Subjects with low CSF 5-HIAA concentrations also exhibited other risky behaviors that may have contributed to their deaths. When compared with subjects with higher CSF 5-HIAA concentrations, they mi-

Table 2. The Between-Neurotransmitters and Hormones Correlations With Their Respective Probability and Sample Size*

	CSF 5-HIAA	CSF HVA	CSF NE	CSF MHPG	Plasma ACTH	Plasma Cortisol
HVA (n=49)	0.43, <.002					
NE (n=49)	−0.34, <.02	0.01, <.94				
MHPG (n=49)	0.02, <.90	0.33, <.02	0.04, <.77			
ACTH (n=48)	−0.07, <.62	−0.11, <.46	0.31, <.03	0.13, <.39		
Cortisol (n=48)	−0.06, <.69	0.02, <.88	0.10, <.50	0.39, <.006	0.14, <.35	
Testosterone (n=45)	0.01, <.93	−0.06, <.70	0.01, <.93	0.42, <.004	0.37, <.01	0.40, <.005

All values are expressed as correlation coefficient and probability (r, P). HVA indicates homovanillic acid; NE, norepinephrine; MPHG, 3-methoxy-4-hydroxyphenylglycol; ACTH, adrenocorticotropin; and 5-HIAA, 5-hydroxyindoleacetic acid.

grated at an earlier age[18] when they were less able to defend themselves and were presumably less socially sophisticated. They were also more likely to take life-threatening risks, such as spontaneous jumping at dangerous heights when moving from tree to tree.[7,18] This previously reported finding is consistent with results from the present study showing that subjects with low CSF 5-HIAA concentrations were more likely to enter the traps and thus were captured more often. Such risk-taking behavior might have contributed to the early deaths. For example, the male with the lowest CSF 5-HIAA concentration was the first subject to be killed. He was 3 years old and weighed less than half of a mature adult male. The night before his death, two of us (J.D.H. and P.T.M.) observed this young male repeatedly attack a pair of fully mature males. This vignette suggests how excessive risk-taking and aggressiveness might have contributed to the wounds and trauma that produced the high death rate among many of the males with low-CSF 5-HIAA concentrations.

While there are explanations other than risk taking and excessive aggression that could account for these premature deaths, we note that there is no evidence that the nonhuman primates with low CSF 5-HIAA concentrations are less coordinated or less skilled as fighters than their peers of an identical age. Indeed, in other studies we have observed that they climb through the trees, and are as active as the subjects with high CSF 5-HIAA concentrations,[8,18] and their high rates of escalated aggression are not the result of passive victimization.[8,18] They initiate the aggression, often at inappropriate targets such as high-ranking subjects or much larger adult males, and once aggression has started, it is more likely to escalate to injurious intensity. High CSF 5-HIAA concentrations, on the other hand, appear to be protective of early death. While this is at least in part because young males with high CSF 5-HIAA concentrations are unlikely to engage in life-threatening aggression, they also have other qualities that may protect them. When compared with subjects with low CSF 5-HIAA concentrations, they receive more social support[18] and are less likely to engage in impulsive behaviors such as long leaps between trees at great heights.[8] Low rates of social support and increased impulsivity may have also contributed to some of the deaths among the subjects with low CSF 5-HIAA concentrations whose bodies were not recovered for necropsy.

These findings on nonhuman primates parallel findings from a study of rates of early death among 73 mixed diagnosis, male inpatients who consented to provide a CSF sample between 1976 and 1990.[24] Of those 73, 12 have died since the original sampling, and 7 of the 12 died before the age of 40. The 7 who died before the age of 40 had significantly lower CSF 5-HIAA concentrations than the surviving patients. Six of the 7 subjects who died before the age of 40 died either from violent causes (homicide or suicide) or from accidents that had suspicious causes (ie, suicide could not be ruled out).[24] These findings suggest that low CSF 5-HIAA concentrations may be a marker for early death among humans as well.

These differential death rates associated with CSF 5-HIAA concentrations pose an interesting question. Since CSF 5-HIAA concentration among rhesus monkeys is highly heritable[25] and most of these subjects die at an early age when they are barely capable of producing offspring, how is the phenotype maintained in the environment? Studies are under way to assess whether these subjects reach reproductive status at a particularly early age and if they produce more offspring during their short period of reproductive activity.

The data presented show that young male nonhuman primates with low CSF 5-HIAA concentrations are at a high risk for early death. This study and others suggest that this high mortality rate in subjects with low CSF 5-HIAA concentrations may be a result of such factors as impaired impulse control, excessive risk taking, and early migration from the social group of origin. Research is under way to investigate factors that maintain this phenotype in the population.

Accepted for publication March 11, 1996.

The research subjects that composed this study are part of a breeding colony supported by the Food and Drug Administration (FDA) contract 223-89-1101 made to Laboratory Animal Breeders and Services Inc (LABS), Yemassee, SC, which supports the colony.

The authors would like to thank Alan Dodson; Maribeth Champoux, PhD; Isabelle Faucher; Martin Kriete, DVM; and Kristin Zajicek who assisted in the data collection. Staff and research were supported by intramural research funding from the National Institute of Alcohol Abuse and Alcoholism and the National Institute of Child Health and Human Development, Bethesda. We thank the FDA for its authorization to conduct the research. A research protocol was approved by the National Institutes of Health (NIH), Bethesda, Md, and LABS' Institutional Animal Care and Use committees in accordance with and as required by the Animal Welfare Act.

Reprints: J. Dee Higley, PhD, NIH Animal Center, Building 112, PO Box 529, Poolesville, MD 20837.

REFERENCES

1. Virkkunen M, Linnoila M. Psychobiology of violent behavior. *Clin Neuropharmacology.* 1992;15:233A-234A.
2. Virkkunen M, Kallio E, Rawlings R, Tokola R, Poland RE, Guidotti A, Nemeroff C, Bissette G, Kalogeras K, Karonen SL, Linnoila M. Personality profiles and state aggressiveness in Finnish alcoholic, violent offenders, fire setters, and healthy volunteers. *Arch Gen Psychiatry.* 1994;51:28-33.
3. Virkkunen M, Rawlings R, Tokola R, Poland RE, Guidotti A, Nemeroff C, Bissette G, Kalogeras K, Karonen SL, Linnoila M. CSF biochemistries, glucose metabolism, and diurnal activity rhythms in alcoholic, violent offenders, fire setters, and healthy volunteers. *Arch Gen Psychiatry.* 1994;51:20-27.
4. Higley JD, Mehlman PT, Taub DM, Higley SB, Vickers JH, Suomi SJ, Linnoila M. Cerebrospinal fluid monoamine and adrenal correlates of aggression in free-ranging rhesus monkeys. *Arch Gen Psychiatry.* 1992;49:436-441.
5. Higley JD, Linnoila M, Suomi SJ. Ethological contributions: experiential and genetic contributions to the expression and inhibition of aggression in primates. In: Hersen M, Ammerman RT, Sisson L, eds. *Handbook of Aggressive and Destructive Behavior in Psychiatric Patients.* New York, NY: Plenum Press; 1994:17-32.
6. Higley JD, King ST, Hasert MF, Champoux M, Suomi SJ, Linnoila M. Stability of interindividual differences in serotonin function and its relationship to aggressive wounding and competent social behavior in rhesus macaque females. *Neuropsychopharmacology.* 1996;14:67-76.

7. Higley JD, Mehlman PT, Poland RE, Faucher I, Taub DT, Vickers J, Suomi SJ, Linnoila M. A nonhuman primate model of violence and assertiveness: CSF 5-HIAA and CSF testosterone correlate with different types of aggressive behaviors. *Biol Psychiatry.* In press.
8. Mehlman PT, Higley JD, Faucher I, Lilly AA, Taub DM, Suomi S, Linnoila M. Low CSF 5-HIAA concentrations and severe aggression and impaired impulse control in nonhuman primates. *Am J Psychiatry.* 1994;151:1485-1491.
9. Higley JD, Suomi SJ, Linnoila M. A longitudinal assessment of CSF monoamine metabolite and plasma cortisol concentrations in young rhesus monkeys. *Biol Psychiatry.* 1992;32:127-145.
10. Kraemer GW, Ebert MH, Schmidt DE, McKinney WT. A longitudinal study of the effect of different social rearing conditions on cerebrospinal fluid norepinephrine and biogenic amine metabolites in rhesus monkeys. *Neuropsychopharmacology.* 1989;2:175-189.
11. Higley JD, Suomi SJ, Linnoila M. A nonhuman primate model of Type II excessive alcohol consumption? low CSF 5-HIAA concentrations and diminished social competence correlate with excessive alcohol consumption. *Alcohol Clin Exp Res.* In press.
12. Higley JD, Suomi SJ. Effect of reactivity and social competence on individual responses to severe stress in children: investigations using nonhuman primates. In: Pfeffer CR, ed. *Intense Stress and Mental Disturbance in Children.* Washington, DC: American Psychiatric Press Inc. 1996:1-69.
13. Bernstein IS, Ehardt CL. Age-sex differences in the expression of agonistic behavior in rhesus monkey (*Macaca mulatta*) groups. *J Comp Psychol.* 1985; 99:115-132.
14. Hausfater G. Intergroup behavior of free-ranging rhesus monkeys (*Macaca mulatta*). *Folia Primatol.* 1972;18:78-107.
15. Dittus WPJ. The evolution of behaviors regulating density and age-specific sex ratios in primate population. *Behaviour.* 1979;69:265-302.
16. Drickamer LC. A ten-year summary of reproductive data for free-ranging *Macaca mulatta. Folia Primatol.* 1974;21:61-80.
17. Meikle BB, Vessey SH. Maternal dominance rank and lifetime survivorship of male and female rhesus monkeys. *Behav Ecol Sociobiol.* 1988;23:379-383.
18. Mehlman P, Higley JD, Faucher I, Lilly AA, Taub DM, Vickers JH, Suomi S, Linnoila M. Correlation of CSF 5-HIAA concentrations with sociality and the timing of emigration in free-ranging primates. *Am J Psychiatry.* 1995;152:907-913.
19. Kaplan JR, Fontenot MB, Berard J, Manuck SB, Mann JJ. Delayed dispersal and elevated monoamine activity in free-ranging rhesus monkeys. *Am J Primatol.* 1995;35:229-234.
20. Drickamer LC, Vessey SH. Group changing in free-ranging male rhesus monkeys. *Primates.* 1973;14:249-254.
21. Vessey SH, Meikle DB, Drickamer LC. Demographic and descriptive studies at La Parguera, Puerto Rico. *P R Health Sci J.* 1989;8:121-127.
22. Raleigh MJ, McGuire MT. Serotonin, aggression, and violence in vervet monkeys. In: Masters RD, McGuire MT, eds. *The Neurotransmitter Revolution.* Carbondale, Ill: Southern Illinois University Press; 1994:129-145.
23. Abraham GE, Buster JE, Teller RC. Radioimmunoassay of plasma cortisol. *Anal Lett.* 1972;5:757-766.
24. Faustman WO, Ringo DL, Faull KF. An association between low levels of 5-HIAA and HVA in cerebrospinal fluid and early mortality in a diagnostically mixed psychiatric sample. *Br J Psychiatry.* 1993;163:519-521.
25. Higley JD, Thompson WW, Champoux M, Goldman D, Hasert MF, Kraemer GW, Scanlan JM, Suomi SJ, Linnoila M. Paternal and maternal genetic and environmental contributions to cerebrospinal fluid monoamine metabolites in rhesus monkeys (*Macaca mulatta*). *Arch Gen Psychiatry.* 1993;50:615-623.

High Rates of Violence, Crime, Academic Problems, and Behavioral Problems in Males With Both Early Neuromotor Deficits and Unstable Family Environments

Adrian Raine, PhD; Patricia Brennan, PhD; Birgitte Mednick, PhD; Sarnoff A. Mednick, PhD, DM

Background: It is commonly assumed that individuals with both biological and psychosocial deficits are more likely to become criminal, but there is surprisingly little empirical support for this assumption. We test the hypothesis that a group with biosocial risk factors are more likely to develop behavioral and academic problems in adolescence and violent criminal offending in adulthood compared with groups with only biological or only social risk factors.

Methods: Hypotheses were tested on a sample of 397 male subjects, using obstetric and early neuromotor measures collected in the first year of life; family, social, demographic, and behavioral measures at age 17 to 19 years; and criminal data at 20 to 22 years of age.

Results: Cluster analysis of the risk factors indicated a group with obstetric risk factors only, a group with poverty risk factors only, and a biosocial group with both early neuromotor deficits and unstable family environments. The biosocial group had more than double the adult violence, theft, and total crime rates of the other 2 groups and had significantly more behavioral and academic problems in adolescence.

Conclusions: When early neuromotor deficits and negative family factors cluster together, individuals are particularly likely to become criminal and violent compared with those with only poverty or only obstetric risk factors. Because this biosocial group accounted for 70.2% of all crimes committed in the entire sample, early interventions that tackle these deficits might significantly reduce violence.

(Arch Gen Psychiatry. 1996;53:544-549)

A LONG-STANDING view held by many criminologists is that while biological processes may play a minor role in predisposing to crime in a small, disturbed subgroup of offenders, social factors are the primary determinants of crime.[1-4] This traditional perspective is currently being challenged by a biosocial approach to crime,[5-13] an approach that has its roots in the earlier criminological literature.[14,15] In addition to arguing that one subgroup commits crimes largely because of social factors, while another subgroup commits crime largely because of biological factors, this biosocial approach theorizes that a substantial third subgroup of subjects can be identified who commit crime largely because of both social and biological predispositions to crime.[16] There are surprisingly few convincing empirical examples of the biosocial approach, primarily because strong studies require both social and biological measures to be prospectively collected on large samples.

One recent study on 4269 live male births[16] provides strong support for a biosocial approach, showing that maternal rejection of the child in the first year was found to statistically interact ($P<.001$) with birth complications in predicting to criminal violence at age 18 years. Subjects with both birth complications and maternal rejection made up only 4.4% of the sample but accounted for 18% of all violent crimes committed by the entire sample of 4269. There are some limitations to this study: (1) it dealt only with 1 biological and 1 social risk factor for violence; (2) official crime data were only available during adolescence; and (3) no other measures were available to validate the official crime data, such as ratings by parents of early behavior problems.

The present study attempts to address some of the above-mentioned limitations. Approximately 10% of the original sample of 4269 males used by Raine et al[16] were randomly selected for further follow-up at ages

See Subjects and Methods on next page

From the Departments of Psychology (Drs Raine, Brennan, and S. A. Mednick) and Education (Dr B. Mednick) and Social Science Research (Drs Brennan and S. A. Mednick), University of Southern California, Los Angeles; and Institute of Preventive Medicine, Copenhagen, the Netherlands (Dr S. A. Mednick).

17 to 19 years on a wider array of social, family, and biological variables than were available on the original sample. Additional variables included income and unemployment, marital conflict, family instability, and parental crime.[17] In addition, official crime data on the subjects were available for a longer follow-up period than in the original study, while new data on maternal ratings of behavioral and academic problems at ages 17 to 19 years were also available.

SUBJECTS AND METHODS

SUBJECTS

Subjects were drawn from a larger initial cohort of 4269 males born in the maternity department of the State University Hospital (Rigshospitalet) in Copenhagen, Denmark, between September 1959 and December 1961.[16,17] Ten percent (n=423) of this larger sample were randomly selected to participate in a long-term follow-up at ages 17 to 19 years, which took place between 1977 and 1979. In total, 397 males (93%) made up the follow-up sample employed in the current study, with 7% of subjects being unavailable because of refusal to participate, death, and emigration.[17] Informed consent for human investigation was obtained from the parents. Only data for male subjects were analyzed because the low rates of crime and violence in female subjects precluded meaningful statistical analyses.

Analyses indicated that the subjects who were included in the 17- to 19-year follow-up were virtually identical with the larger population in terms of mother's age at birth, birth order, family size, and marital stability (see Baker and Mednick[17]). Comparisons with the general Danish population indicated that although the follow-up sample was representative of the entire range of the national socioeconomic status (SES) distribution, mean SES was slightly lower because the original cohort included a disproportionate number of unwed, low-SES mothers from poorer inner-city areas of Copenhagen. The Rigshospitalet had also had referred mothers who were expected to experience difficult deliveries irrespective of mothers' social background.[17] Consequently, the follow-up sample was similar to the national population with the exception that it comprised (*1*) women of lower SES and (*2*) women with difficult pregnancies who were expected to have birth complications.

METHODS

Biological Measures

Data on all biological measures were collected prospectively. They were available for all 397 subjects and have previously been shown to be relevant to crime and delinquency.[22-26] Each weighted frequency scale was based on multiple items coded on a 1- to 5-point scale developed through the collaboration of American and Danish obstetricians and pediatric neurologists.[17,27] In all cases, higher scores on these scales indicate poorer biological status. Full details of these scales are provided by Baker and Mednick,[17] while brief details are given below.

Pregnancy complications were recorded and rated as early as possible in pregnancy during mothers' attendance at the hospital's antenatal clinic. The same physician conducted all prenatal examinations to help ensure uniform coding of obstetric histories. Examples of items include bacterial infection (scored 1), placenta previa (scored 5).

Birth complications and conditions were recorded at the time of delivery by an obstetrician assisted by a midwife.[16] Examples include ruptured perineum (scored 1), umbilical chord prolapse (scored 5).

Nonmaturity scale consisted of items concerning the neonate's physical maturity at birth (gestation, birth weight). Examples include birth stage 34 to 35 weeks and weight 2500 to 3000 g (scored 1); birth stage less than 28 weeks and weight less than 1000 g (scored 5).

Neurological status (days 1 and 5) was established by a full neonatal neurological examination conducted at days 1 and 5 by a pediatrician. Examples include shivering, restlessness, and frog position (scored 1); repeated cyanosis attacks (scored 5).

Motor development (1 year) was examined by a team of 3 pediatricians on the child's first birthday at the pediatric outpatient department of the State University Hospital. The protocol for the examinations was developed by a joint team of Danish and American pediatricians representing both clinical and research expertise. Examples include does not stand with support or crawl until 11 to 12 months (scored 1), does not hold head up until after 9 months (scored 5).

Psychosocial, Family, and Demographic Measures

Psychosocial variables were selected and constructed from this data set on the basis of their relevance to criminal behavior.[28-34] The psychosocial and family data were retrospectively obtained from a 2-hour interview with the mother at the 17- to 19-year follow-up. Interviews were conducted by a trained psychiatric social worker at the mother's home, while family size and birth order data were confirmed with reference to the Danish National Population Register. Data on early maternal rejection were collected from a psychosocial interview conducted with the mother when the child was 1 year old.

Early maternal rejection is described in full by Raine et al.[16] Briefly, its measure was based on factor scores derived from a factor of "Early Child Rejection" based on items with the following loadings: public institutional care of infant (0.68), attempt to abort fetus (0.65), and unwanted pregnancy (0.44). *Public care* was defined as placement of the infant for care into a full-time public institution for more than 4 months of the first year. High scores indicate relatively greater rejection.

Social, economic, educational, employment, and living status was measured on the basis of the following 7 items drawn from the psychosocial interview with the mother: mother's occupation, father's occupation, periods of unemployment, periods of economic hardship, mother's years of education, number of rooms per person, and conditions of home furnishings. Full details of the derivation of these variables were reported by Baker and Mednick.[17] Scores on each of the items were transformed to z scores and summed to form an overall scale, which, for ease of reference, was labeled "social deprivation," with high scores indicating greater deprivation; coefficient α for this scale was .77.

Marital conflict was measured using 9 items derived from the psychosocial interview of the mother and consisted of disagreements between parents concerning child raising, sharing of household chores, money, problems with

Continued on next page

in-laws, spare time activities, sexual problems, jealousy, other problems, and 1 partner always giving in during an argument. Mothers rated each item on a 1- to 4-point scale (1, no disagreements, and 4, major disagreements) for the longest spousal relationship they had been in since the subject was born. The item concerning 1 partner always giving in during an argument was rated on a 1- to 4-point scale (1, very untrue, and 4, very true). High scores indicate high levels of marital conflict; coefficient α for this scale was .84.

Family instability measured by the extent of disruption to the family was indexed by 3 items taken from the mother's psychosocial interview as follows: (1) number of marriages of mother in child's first 18 years, (2) number of changes in the family constellation of the household (defined as a movement in or out of the house by an adult member) up to age 18 years, and (3) number of years father lived in the household (fewer years indicated greater instability). High scores indicated relatively greater family instability; coefficient α for this scale was .66.

Parental crime was coded on the basis of how many parents (0, 1, or 2) had been arrested for an offense, as indicated by registration in the Danish National Criminal Register (see below).

Behavioral Outcome Measures

Criminal Offending. Criminal status for all 397 subjects was assessed in 1981, when offspring were aged 20 to 22 years, by a search of the Danish National Criminal Register in which all police contacts and court decisions involving Danish citizens are recorded. This is viewed as one of the most comprehensive and accurate registers in the Western world.[17,35]

Three indexes of criminal offending were constructed: (1) violence, (2) thievery, and (3) total offending. The definition of *violence* used by the National Academy of Sciences Panel on the Understanding and Control of Violence ("behaviors by individuals that intentionally threaten, attempt, or inflict physical harm on others"[6(p2)]) was used. Consequently, *violent crime* was defined by arrests for the following offenses: murder, attempted murder, assault (including domestic assault), rape, robbery and armed robbery, illegal possession of a weapon, and threats of violence. In contrast, *thievery* was defined as all types of property offending, including theft, breaking and entering, shoplifting, fraud, forgery, blackmail, and embezzlement. In addition, a third index of *total criminal offending* was compiled, in which all index offenses were included. Index offenses consisted of violence, thievery, sexual offenses (including prostitution and pimping), drug offenses, and narcotics offenses. In total, 23.9% of the sample were registered for a criminal index offense, 19.4% had a registration for thievery, and 8.6% had a registration for violence.

Ratings of Behavioral and Academic Problems. These measures consisted of maternal ratings of the subject's behavioral and academic functioning at ages 17 to 19 years, using a 1- to 3-point scale (1, never; 2, sometimes; and 3, often). Ratings were available on 394 of the 397 subjects. Specifically, 4 scales were constructed to estimate these behaviors as follows:

1. The *Externalizing behavioral problems* scale consisted of the following 5 items: aggressive, irritable, disobedient, lying, and restless/hyperactive. Higher scores indicated greater externalizing problems; coefficient α for this scale was .65.
2. The *Internalizing behavioral problems* scale consisted of the following 4 items: lonely, nervous, very passive, and often teased. Higher scores indicated greater internalizing problems; coefficient α for this scale was 0.60.
3. The *Total behavior problems* scale consisted of the 9 items making up the above 2 scales summated to create this overall measure of behavior problems that had an internal reliability of 0.71.
4. The *Academic problems* scale consisted of the following 6 items: repeated a grade, needed tutoring, attended special classes, poor math class achievement, poor language class achievement, and poor Danish class achievement. Items were coded so that high scores on the scale indicated relatively more academic problems; coefficient α for this scale was 0.74.

Statistical Analyses

Cluster Analysis of Risk Variables. To assess whether coherent subgroups of subjects could be identified based on the risk factors, the 5 biological and 5 psychosocial risk variables were subjected to cluster analysis using SPSS (Statistical Package for the Social Sciences [SPSS Inc, Chicago, Ill]). Cluster analysis has numerous advocates in the field of psychopathology and psychiatry,[18,19,20] and there have been over 1000 cluster analytic studies published in the past 10 years in psychiatry, psychology, and medicine. Cluster analysis is a classification technique that statistically seeks out naturally occurring homogeneous subgroups within a population on the basis of the characteristics used to identify the groups (in this case, social and biological risk factors for crime). Consequently, 1 main advantage of this technique over other multivariate techniques lies in its ability to define groups using statistical algorithms as opposed to predetermined cutoffs imposed by the experimenter.

Variables were first transformed to z scores to standardize measures before entry into an agglomerative hierarchical cluster analysis. Ward's method was used to optimize minimum variance between clusters in conjunction with a squared Euclidean distance measure to assess similarity between subjects. Inspection of fusion coefficients and the dendrogram were used to help identify the number of clusters.[18,21]

The 3-cluster solution produced groups that were approximately equal in size and were defined by social variables only, biological variables only, and both biological and social variables. To help clarify the identity of the 3 clusters, analyses of variances were conducted on the biological and social risk variables.

Treatment of Missing Data. Sample sizes for the analyses on behavioral and academic problems varied slightly as a function of missing data (n=393, n=396, and n=373). Consequently, all analyses were recalculated on the reduced sample of 373. Results were identical to analyses reported above, with exactly the same configuration of main effects and between-groups differences.

Cluster analysis was employed to more objectively assess what specific subgroups may exist based on the wide array of social and biological risk variables available.[18-21] According to the way in which pregnant women were referred to the hospital (see the "Methods" section), it was anticipated that cluster analysis would define a group having socioeconomic deficits only, and a group with obstetric deficits only. In addition, it was hypothesized that if a subgroup was also

Table 1. Mean (SD) and Least Significant Difference Comparisons* of Biological and Social *z*-Transformed Variables for the Biosocial, Obstetric, and Poverty Clusters

Measures	Cluster: 1: Biosocial (n=176)	2: Obstetric (n=106)	3: Poverty (n=115)	*F*	Least Significant Difference
Biological					
Pregnancy	−0.34 (0.70)	0.85 (1.11)	−0.33 (0.76)	76†	2>1,3
Delivery	−0.32 (0.83)	0.84 (1.13)	−0.28 (0.62)	67†	2>1,3
Prematurity	−0.17 (0.68)	0.65 (1.40)	−0.35 (0.64)	38†	2>1,3
Motor	0.18 (0.95)	0.25 (1.2)	−0.53 (0.66)	25†	1,2>3
Neurological	0.20 (1.29)	−0.06 (0.69)	−0.26 (0.67)	7.7‡	1>2,3
Social					
Poverty	−0.50 (0.73)	0.15 (0.92)	0.68 (0.97)	68†	3>2>1
Family instability	0.46 (1.10)	−0.29 (0.75)	−0.51 (0.58)	50†	1>2,3
Marital conflict	0.39 (1.01)	−0.10 (0.91)	−0.49 (0.80)	32†	1>2>3
Rejection	0.39 (1.25)	−0.30 (0.64)	−0.32 (0.50)	27†	1>2,3
Parent crime	0.28 (1.4)	−0.14 (0.49)	−0.30 (0.23)	13†	1>2,3

*All P<.05.
†P<.001.
‡P<.005.

Table 2. Summary Characteristics of the Biosocial, Obstetric, and Poverty Clusters*

Risk Factors	Cluster: 1: Biosocial (n=176)	2: Obstetric (n=106)	3: Poverty (n=115)
Social			
Poverty			+
Marital conflict	+		−
Maternal rejection	+		
Family instability	+		
Parental crime	+		
Biological			
Neurological problems	+		
Slow motor development	+	+	−
Pregnancy complications		+	
Birth complications		+	
Nonmaturity		+	

**Plus sign indicates risk factor present; minus sign, relatively* lower *marital conflict and* faster *motor development.*

delineated that possessed both social and biological risk factors for crime, this biosocial subgroup would commit more crime and have more behavioral and academic problems than subgroups that possessed social predispositions only or biological predispositions only.

RESULTS

DESCRIPTION OF CLUSTERS

Results of the cluster analysis are shown in **Table 1**, and the defining characteristics of each cluster are shown in **Table 2**.

Cluster 1 (n=176) was characterized by neurological problems in the first week of life (P>.005), slow motor development at age 1 year (P<.001), early maternal rejection (P<.001), family conflict (P<.001), family instability (P<.001), and criminal parent (P<.001). Because this cluster had both biological and social risk factors for crime development, this subgroup is labeled "biosocial."

Cluster 2 (n=106), in contrast, was defined solely in terms of biological deficits, including relatively greater pregnancy complications (*P*<.001), birth complications (*P*<.001), prematurity (*P*<.001), and slower motor development (*P*<.001). For referencing purposes, this subgroup was labeled "obstetric."

Cluster 3 (n=115) was characterized by having relatively more negative social, economic, educational, employment, and living status characteristics compared with those in the other 2 groups (*P*<.001). It was thus labeled "poverty," although it should be noted that subjects also possess 2 positive features by virtue of having relatively *lower* marital discord (*P*<.001) and *faster* motor development (*P*<.001). This group is characterized by the social deficit of poverty, in contrast to the social characteristics of the biosocial group that specifically pertain to the domain of unstable, conflictual, or criminal family environment.

SUBGROUP DIFFERENCES ON CRIMINAL OUTCOME MEASURES

Rates of criminality in the 3 subgroups were compared using χ^2 analyses. Results of these analyses for total criminal offending, thievery, and violence are illustrated in the **Figure**.

For total criminal offending, groups differed in rates of crime (χ^2=14.3, *df*=2, *P*<.001). A breakdown of this overall group difference using 2×2 χ^2 analyses indicated that the biosocial group had significantly higher rates of crime (33%) than both the obstetric (17.9%) (χ^2=7.5, *df*=1, *P*<.006) and poverty (15.7%) (χ^2=10.8, *df*=1, *P*<.001) groups that did not differ from each other (*P*>.65). Parental crime per se does not account for the high crime rates in the biosocial group, which still had higher crime rates than the other 2 groups after removing the influence of parental crime.

For thievery, groups differed in rates of crime (χ^2=18.6, *df*=2, *P*<.001). A breakdown of this overall effect indicated that the biosocial group had significantly higher thievery rates (29%) than both the obstetric group (12.5%) (χ^2=10.5, *df*=1, *P*<.002) and the poverty group (11.3%) (χ^2=12.7, *df*=1, *P*<.001) that did not differ from each other (*P*>.82).

For violent offending, the overall analysis was significant (χ^2=7.4, *df*=2, *P*<.03). A breakdown of the overall effect indicated that the biosocial group had significantly higher violence rates (12.5%) than the poverty group (3.5%) (χ^2=7.0, *df*=1, *P*<.009). Although the biosocial group had higher violence rates than the obstetric group (7.5%), this difference was not statistically significant (χ^2=1.7, *df*=1, *P*>.19). Obstetric and poverty groups did not differ significantly on violence (*P*>.82).

SUBGROUP DIFFERENCES ON BEHAVIORAL AND ACADEMIC PROBLEMS

Table 3 provides means and SDs for behavioral and academic problems in the biosocial, obstetric, and poverty clusters. Full details of 1-way analysis of variance and individual group comparisons for these variables are also given in Table 3. Briefly, the biosocial cluster had significantly more academic, externalizing, and internalizing behavior problems than did the poverty cluster (*P*<.05) and significantly more behavior problems than the obstetric group (*P*<.05).

COMPARISONS WITH SUBJECTS WITH NEITHER BIOLOGICAL NOR SOCIAL DEFICITS

The cluster analysis did not produce a group low on all risk factors. To compare the biosocial cluster with such a group of "normal controls," subjects who were scored below the mean on *all* variables that defined the biosocial group (see Table 2) were drawn from obstetric and poverty clusters to form this normal control group (n=44). Results of these analyses confirmed that the biosocial group had significantly higher rates of total criminal offending than normal controls (33.1% vs 2.3%; χ^2=17.0, *df*=1, *P*<.001), of thievery (29.1% vs 0.0%; χ^2=16.7, *df*=1, *P*<.001), and of violence (12.6% vs 2.3%; χ^2=4.0, *df*=1, *P*<.05).

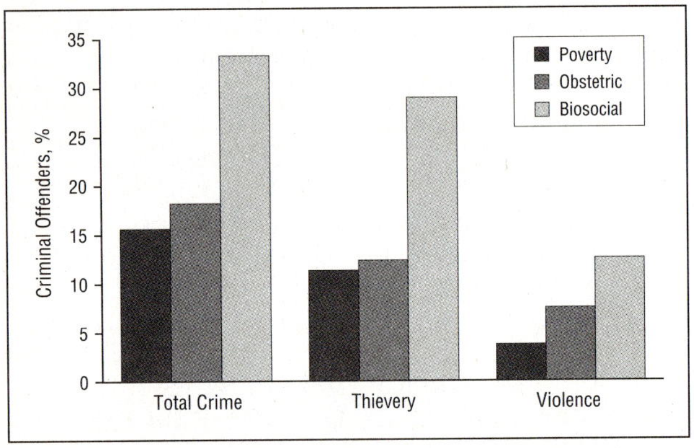

Percentages of poverty, obstetric, and biosocial cluster members who become thieves and violent criminal offenders by ages 20 to 22 years.

COMMENT

The key finding from this article is that rates of crime are particularly high in a subgroup of subjects who possess both biological (early neuromotor deficits) and psychosocial (unstable family environments) risk factors for crime. This biosocial group had 2.0 times the level of total crime of the other 2 groups, 2.5 times the level of thievery, and 2.3 times the level of violence. The fact that the biosocial group also showed significantly more mother-reported behavioral and academic problems than the other 2 groups provides additional support for the findings based on official crime records. An important next step in this line of research would be to generalize findings from a Danish population to a more heterogeneous US population.

Results confirm the presence of a subgroup with both biological and social predispositions to crime and provide some support for the conceptual importance of a biosocial approach to crime. Although the importance of this biosocial approach has been frequently acknowledged, there have been surprisingly few convincing empirical demonstrations of its validity.[36-38] Although purely biological and purely social research on crime may continue to be productive, this study suggests that one of the major future advances in understanding crime causation will be derived from a biosocial approach. As such, social researchers cannot continue to ignore the research findings of biological researchers and vice versa.

One interesting result of the study is that the poverty group, which was characterized by multiple social, economic, educational, employment, and living status problems, had the *lowest* rates of crime relative to the other 2 groups. This finding challenges the traditional stereotype of poverty and crime going hand in hand and instead suggests that such associated stigmatization of all

Table 3. Mean (SD),* Analyses of Variance (ANOVAs), and Group Comparisons for Behavioral and Academic Problems in Biosocial, Obstetric, and Poverty Clusters

	Cluster				
Problems	1: Biosocial (n=176)	2: Obstetric (n=106)	3: Poverty (n=115)	*F* by 1-Way ANOVAs	Group Comparisons by *t* Test
Academic	9.5 (2.6)	9.1 (2.7)	8.5 (1.8)	4.9†	1>3
Behavioral					
Total behavioral	15.5 (3.5)	14.5 (3.3)	13.3 (2.7)	16.6‡	1>2>3
Externalizing	8.8 (2.3)	8.2 (2.1)	7.6 (1.7)	12.0§	1>2>3
Internalizing	6.7 (1.9)	6.3 (1.9)	5.7 (1.6)	9.8§	1,2>3

*P<.05.
†P<.01.
‡P<.001.
§P<.0001.

poor, underserved populations, although not intentional, is unjustified. Crime was probably not elevated in this impoverished but resilient group compared with the other 2 groups because parents had a relatively more satisfactory and harmonious marital life and the children had relatively faster (not slower) motor development in infancy. As such, this socially impoverished group possessed 1 biological and 1 social protective factor against crime development. This is a potentially important finding in that good parenting and good early health development may compensate for the otherwise ill effects of low income and unemployment.

Findings have potentially important implications for treatment and intervention programs. The fact that biological and psychosocial factors converged in the group with high crime rates (biosocial cluster) indicates that tackling one or the other or both of these components could reduce crime and violence. At the biological level, better postnatal care could help early neurological and motor deficits to be identified and remediated before they translate into child behavior problems, cognitive deficits, school failure, and ultimately criminal behavior.[39,40] Alternatively, tackling the psychosocial half of the biosocial equation could be equally effective. School interventions aimed at educating young adolescents on parent-child management, conflict resolution in the family, and family planning may help reduce rates of later marital conflict, family instability, and child rejection, which are critical components of the biosocial cluster.[41,42] Because the biosocial group accounted for 70.2% of all crimes committed in the sample, successful intervention could, in theory, have a major effect in reducing rates of crime and violence. Because several of the variables making up the biosocial cluster (eg, neurological and motor development, maternal rejection) reflect very early (year 1) life processes, interventions may be most effectively employed in early childhood rather than in adolescence or early adulthood. Experimental intervention studies are first needed, however, to establish the causal significance of biosocial risk factors.

Accepted for publication February 27, 1996.

This research was conducted with the support of Research Scientist Development awards K02 MH01114-01 and 5 K05MH00619-08 from the National Institute of Mental Health, Washington, DC (Drs Raine and S. A. Mednick), and a grant from the Harry Frank Guggenheim Foundation, New York, NY (Dr Brennan).

Reprints: Adrian Raine, PhD, Department of Psychology, SGM Building, University of Southern California, Los Angeles, CA 90089-1061.

REFERENCES

1. Farrington DP. Early predictors of adolescent aggression and adult violence. *Violence Victims.* 1989;4:79-100.
2. McCord J. Long-term perspectives on parental absence. In: Robins LN, Rutter M, eds. *Straight and Devious Pathways From Childhood to Adulthood.* Cambridge, Mass: Cambridge University Press; 1990:116-134.
3. Loeber R, Stouthamer-Loeber M. Family factors as correlates and predictors of juvenile conduct problems and delinquency. In: Tonry M, Morris N, eds. *Crime and Justice.* Chicago, Ill: Chicago University Press; 1986;7:29-149.
4. Reiss AJ, Roth JA, eds. *Understanding and Preventing Violence.* Washington, DC: National Academy Press; 1993.
5. Denno DJ. *Biology, Crime and Violence: New Evidence.* Cambridge, Mass: Cambridge University Press; 1989.
6. Earls F. Not fear, not quarantine, but science: preparation for a decade of research to advance knowledge about causes and control of violence in youths. *J Adolesc Health.* 1991;12:619-629.
7. Eichelman B. Aggressive behavior: from laboratory to clinic. *Arch Gen Psychiatry.* 1992;49:488-492.
8. Elliott F. Violence: a product of biosocial interactions. *Bull Am Acad Psychiatry Law.* 1988;16:131-143.
9. Eysenck HJ, Gudjonsson GH. *The Causes and Cures of Criminality.* New York, NY: Plenum Press; 1989.
10. Jeffery CR. An interdisciplinary theory of criminal behavior. In: Laufer WS, Adler F, eds. *Advances in Criminological Theory.* New Brunswick, NJ: Transaction Press; 1989:69-87.
11. Lewis DO. From abuse to violence: psychophysiological consequences of maltreatment. *J Am Acad Child Adolesc Psychiatry.* 1992;31:383-391.
12. Mednick SA, Christiansen KO. *Biosocial Bases of Criminal Behavior.* New York, NY: Gardner; 1977.
13. Raine A. *The Psychopathology of Crime: Criminal Behavior as a Clinical Disorder.* San Diego, Calif: Academic Press; 1993.
14. McCord W, McCord J. *The Psychopath: An Essay on the Criminal Mind.* Princeton, NJ: Van Nostrand; 1964.
15. Glueck S, Glueck T. *Unraveling Juvenile Delinquency.* Cambridge, Mass: Harvard University Press; 1950.
16. Raine A, Brennan P, Mednick SA. Birth complications combined with early maternal rejection at one year predispose to violent crime at age 18 years. *Arch Gen Psychiatry.* 1994;51:984-988.
17. Baker RL, Mednick BR. *Influences on Human Development: A Longitudinal Analysis.* Boston, Mass: Kluwer; 1984.
18. Everitt BS. *Cluster Analysis.* 3rd ed. New York, NY: Halstead Press; 1993.
19. Hinshaw SP. On the distinction between attentional deficits/hyperactivity and conduct problems/aggression in child psychopathology. *Psychol Bull.* 1987; 101:443-463.
20. Kaufman L, Rousseuw PJ. *Finding Groups in Data: An Introduction to Cluster Analysis.* New York, NY: John Wiley & Sons Inc; 1990.
21. Aldenderfer MS, Blashfield RK. *Cluster Analysis.* Beverly Hills, Calif: Sage; 1984.
22. Elliott F. Violence: the neurologic contribution: an overview. *Ann Neurol.* 1992; 49:595-603.
23. Lewis DO, Shanock SA, Balla DA. Perinatal difficulties, head and face trauma, and child abuse in the medical histories of seriously delinquent children. *Am J Psychiatry.* 1979;136:419-423.
24. Lewis DO, Pincus JH, Bard B, Richardson E, Prichep LS, Feldman M, Yeager C. Neuropsychiatric, psycho-educational, and family characteristics of 14 juveniles condemned to death in the United States. *Am J Psychiatry.* 1988;145:584-589.
25. Pincus JH, Tucker GL. Violence in children and adults: a neurological view. *J Am Acad Child Psychiatry.* 1978;17:277-288.
26. Werner EE, Smith RS. *Overcoming the Odds: High Risk Children From Birth to Adulthood.* Ithaca, NY: Cornell University Press; 1992.
27. Mednick SA, Mura E, Schulsinger F, Mednick B. Perinatal conditions and infant development in the children of schizophrenic parents. *Soc Biol.* 1971;18:5103-5113.
28. Farrington DP. Childhood aggression and adult violence: early precursors and later life outcomes. In: Pepler DJ, Rubin KH, eds. *The Development and Treatment of Childhood Aggression.* Hillsdale, NJ: Erlbaum; 1991:5-29
29. Lahey BB, Hartdagen SE, Frick PJ, McBurnett K. Conduct disorder: parsing the confound relation to parental divorce and antisocial personality. *J Abnorm Psychol.* 1988;97:334-337.
30. McCord JM. A longitudinal view of the relationship between paternal absence and crime. In: Gunn J, Farrington DP, eds. *Abnormal Offenders, Delinquency, and the Criminal Justice System.* New York, NY: John Wiley & Sons Inc; 1982:113-127.
31. Offord DR. Family background of male and female delinquents. In: Gunn J, Farrington DP, eds. *Abnormal Offenders, Delinquency, and the Criminal Justice System.* New York, NY: John Wiley & Sons Inc; 1982:129-151
32. Robins LN. Sturdy childhood predictors of adult outcomes: replication from longitudinal studies. In: Barratt JE, Rose RM, Klerman GL, eds. *Stress and Mental Disorder.* New York, NY: Raven Press; 1979:219-235.
33. Rutter M, Giller H. *Juvenile Delinquency: Trends and Perspectives.* Harmondsworth, England: Penguin; 1983.
34. Wilson JQ, Herrnstein RJ. *Crime and Human Nature.* New York, NY: Simon and Schuster; 1985.
35. Wolfgang ME. Foreword. In: Mednick SA, Christiansen KO, eds. *Biosocial Bases of Criminal Behavior.* New York, NY: Gardner; 1977.
36. Cloninger CR, Gottesman II. Genetic and environmental factors in antisocial behavioral disorders. In: Mednick SA, Moffitt TE, Stack S, eds. *The Causes of Crime: New Biological Approaches.* Cambridge, Mass: Cambridge University Press; 1987.
37. Raine A, Venables PH. Classical conditioning and socialization: a biosocial interaction. *Personality Individual Differences.* 1981;2:273-283.
38. Brennan P, Mednick SA, Kandel E. Congenital determinants of violent and property offending. In: Pepler DJ, Rubin, eds. *The Development and Treatment of Childhood Aggression.* Hillsdale, NJ: Erlbaum; 1993:81-92.
39. Drillien CM. *The Growth and Development of the Prematurely Born Infant.* Baltimore, Md: Williams and Williams; 1964.
40. McMillan HL, MacMillan JH, Offord DR, Griffith L. Primary prevention of child physical abuse and neglect: a critical review. *J Child Psychol Psychiatry.* 1994;35:835-856.
41. Offord DR. Prevention of behavioral and emotional disorders in children. *J Child Psychol Psychiatry.* 1987;28:9-19.
42. Offord DR, Boyle MH, Racine YA, Fleming JE. Outcome, prognosis, and risk in a longitudinal follow-up study. *J Am Acad Child Adolesc Psychiatry.* 1992;31: 916-923.

The Association of Sexual Assault and Attempted Suicide Within the Community

Jonathan R. T. Davidson, MD; Dana C. Hughes, RN, PhD; Linda K. George, PhD; Dan G. Blazer, MD, PhD

Background: Lifetime community rates of attempted suicide were compared between those who reported a history of sexual assault and a control group without such a history.

Methods: The 2918 respondents in the Duke University Epidemiological Catchment Area Study were placed into groups with reported sexual assault (n=67) and those with no known history of such (n=2851). Multivariate and bivariate procedures were used to examine the relation between sexual assault and attempted suicide.

Results: Subjects reporting a history of sexual assault were more likely to be female, younger, and to report higher rates of lifetime suicide attempt and posttraumatic stress symptoms; no differences were found in the number of chronic medical disorders, major depression, substance abuse or substance dependence, or panic attacks. Nine (14.9%) of the 67 index group subjects reported a suicide attempt, 4 of whom reported their first sexual assault as occurring before age 16 years. A sexual assault history was associated with increased prevalence of lifetime suicide attempt after controlling for sex, age, education, posttraumatic stress symptoms, and psychiatric disorder. Findings were similar in the female-only subsample (n=1778). For women, the odds of attempting suicide was 3 to 4 times greater when the first reported sexual assault occurred prior to age 16 years compared with age 16 years or older.

Conclusions: Sexual assault is associated with an increased lifetime rate of attempted suicide. In women, a history of sexual trauma before age 16 years is a particularly strong correlate of attempted suicide.

(Arch Gen Psychiatry. 1996;53:550-555)

SEXUAL TRAUMA has been associated with impaired social, interpersonal, and sexual functioning; increased rates of attempted suicide; and psychiatric morbidity in adult life.[1-11] In a community-based sample, we have previously[12] found increased rates of attempted suicide in individuals meeting criteria for the full posttraumatic stress disorder diagnosis, as well as those with subthreshold symptoms of posttraumatic stress. This finding, which was not explained by the presence of lifetime major depression, stimulated further interest in the relations between psychological trauma and suicide attempts. Previous investigators[13-15] have shown that suicidality may be influenced by a variety of factors including sex, age, marital status, education, race, and physical and psychiatric illnesses, particularly major depression, substance abuse, and panic disorders. Thus, a study that finds a significant association between any single variable and suicide attempt must be interpreted in the context of whether other known correlates of suicidality explain the observed association.

In this article, we examine the association between a history of sexual assault and the lifetime occurrence of attempted suicide in an adult community-based population living in the Piedmont region of North Carolina. The primary question addresses whether a history of sexual assault retains its association with suicidality if the effects of other known correlates of suicidality and symptoms associated with a traumatic event are controlled. The secondary question concerns whether age at first reported sexual assault (eg, age <16 years vs 16+ years) is related to risk of suicidality after controlling for other correlates.

See Subjects and Methods on next page

From the Departments of Psychiatry and Behavioral Sciences (Drs Davidson, George, and Blazer) and Sociology (Dr George), and School of Nursing (Dr Hughes), Duke University Medical Center, Durham, NC.

SUBJECTS AND METHODS

SUBJECTS

The data were drawn from 2918 adult community respondents in North Carolina who participated in Wave I and Wave II of the National Institute of Mental Health Epidemiological Catchment Area survey conducted by Duke University.[16-18] Subjects who lived within a 5-county area were selected via a multistage sampling design.[16-18] Elderly residents (ages 60 years and older) were oversampled. Of all individuals selected for the community survey, 79% participated in the Wave I survey (3921 household residents; 502 institutionalized individuals). Seventy-nine percent of the Wave I household residents participated in the follow-up survey 1 year later (n=3115). In addition to the 806 household respondents who refused to be interviewed at Wave II, 197 subjects were dropped from this report for a variety of reasons (available on request). This yielded a sample of 2918 household respondents with complete data on the variables of interest.

Dropouts exhibited greater likelihood of being younger, less well educated, and unmarried and more frequently attempted suicide and experienced panic attacks.

METHODS

Data Collection

Data were obtained in a 2-hour structured face-to-face interview, which included the Diagnostic Interview Schedule–Version III.[19]

Respondents were asked about demographic characteristics, history of sexual assault, history of suicide attempt, posttraumatic stress symptoms, substance abuse or substance dependency, depression, anxiety, and chronic medical disorders.

Lifetime history of suicide attempt was the dependent variable of interest in this study. Although recency of suicide attempt was asked, age at first suicide attempt was not.

Reported sexual assault was the primary independent variable of interest. Subjects were asked as to the occurrence of sexual assault by means of the following question or statement: One event which people often report as a serious one in their lives is that of being sexually assaulted. Have you ever been in a situation in which you were pressured into doing more sexually than you wanted to do, that is, a situation in which someone pressured you, against your will, into forced contact with the sexual parts of your body or their body?

Subjects were asked their age at the first forced sexual contact as well as the number of forced sexual contacts before age 16 years and at age 16 years or older. The 2918 respondents selected for this study were separated into 2 groups: those who reported a history of sexual assault (n=67) and those without a known history of sexual assault (n=2851).

Because it is important to determine if sexual assault itself or only the symptoms associated with a traumatic event explain the relation between sexual trauma and suicidality, we controlled for the presence of posttraumatic stress symptoms in the multivariate models examined. Subjects were asked as to the occurrence of trauma-related symptoms, according to the following 9 questions, each of which was prefaced by the following statement:

Did you ever see something that frightened you so much or had something so frightening happen to you that you

1. . . . kept seeing it over again, just as you began to fall asleep, or would suddenly act as if you were in the middle of it all over again?
2. . . . were jumpy and easily startled even by a small noise?
3. . . . felt you had to stay on guard and wouldn't let yourself get involved in other things?
4. . . . wouldn't let yourself fall asleep or had trouble sleeping?
5. . . . had trouble concentrating?
6. . . . had much less feeling for the people you normally cared about?
7. . . . afterwards, lost interest in activities that meant a lot to you before?
8. . . . felt ashamed of still being alive after it was over?
9. . . . avoided doing anything that would remind you of it?

Subjects' Categorization

Respondents with posttraumatic stress symptoms were categorized into above or below threshold. Symptoms were

Continued on next page

RESULTS

Sixty-seven respondents (2.9%) reported lifetime sexual assault: 21 (1%) before age 16 years and 44 (1.8%) at or beyond 16 years of age. Age at first assault was unavailable in 2 instances. Of the male subjects in the study, only 5 (0.6%) reported having been sexually assaulted, whereas among women, 62 (4.8%) reported such an assault. The total number of times victims were pressured into sexual contact ranged from 1 time (60%) to 40 or more times (5%). Twelve victims reported 3 or more incidents. Data were missing on this question for 8 victims.

Bivariate associations between sexual assault history and demographic characteristics are shown in **Table 1**. Respondents with a history of sexual assault were more likely to be female and in the 25- to 44- and 45- to 64-year-old age groups. Differences between the 2 groups were not statistically significant with respect to ethnicity, marital status, or level of education.

Bivariate associations between history of sexual assault and comorbidity are shown in **Table 2**. Respondents with a history of sexual assault, compared with those without, reported higher rates of suicide attempt (14.9% vs 1.4%) and posttraumatic stress symptoms (45.2% vs 14.3%). Differences between the 2 groups were statistically significant for both the subthreshold and suprathreshold trauma symptoms. However, differences were not statistically significant on the prevalence rates of chronic medical disability, major depression, substance threshold if at least 1 of the symptoms had either been reported to a physician, resulted in taking medication, or interfered with activities. Cases were considered below threshold if none of these held true, but at least 1 posttraumatic stress symptom had been endorsed during the subject's lifetime. The subthreshold trauma and suprathreshold trauma symptom variables were derived, respectively, by summing the number of trauma-related symptoms that respondents in each of the 2 subgroups reported experiencing during their lifetime. The subthreshold and suprathreshold trauma symptom variables were used in the bivariate analysis. A single dummy variable was created for the presence of both subthreshold and suprathreshold posttraumatic stress symptoms for the regression models, as the number of respondents in the suicide attempt group (n=42) limited the total number of independent variables that should be entered into a single logistic regression model to ensure stability of the parameter coefficients in the model.

Other independent variables examined in this study were known correlates of suicidality.[13-15] The demographic variables examined were sex, chronological age (ages, 18-24, 25-44, 45-64, and 65+ years), years of completed education (0-11, 12, and 13-17+ years), race (white vs nonwhite), and marital status (married vs not married). Age and education were analyzed as categorical variables in the cross-tabulation analyses and as continuous variables in the multivariate logistic regression models.

Chronic physical illness was also examined, by assigning a value of 1 to each of 13 conditions if the respondent reported being bothered at least a little by the condition and a value of 0 if the respondent was not bothered by the condition or did not have it.

Lifetime psychiatric comorbidity was evaluated with respect to 4 disorders associated with suicidality: major depression, alcohol abuse or dependence, other drug abuse or dependence, and panic attacks. In the multivariate logistic models in which we controlled for alcohol and other drug abuse or dependence, the disorders were combined into a single variable, as we were restricted to a limited number of independent variables that we could enter into the model. In our preliminary analyses, panic disorder was not associated with attempted suicide, which, we thought, resulted from the low number of positive cases. We therefore substituted panic attacks for panic disorder to see if there was an association between panic attacks and sexual assault or suicide attempt.

Data Analysis

The χ^2 test was used to assess bivariate associations between group membership (sexual assault vs no sexual assault) and demographic characteristics, psychiatric comorbidity, medical comorbidity, and suicide attempt. Lifetime history of suicide attempt was then regressed on the selected independent variables in a series of logistic regression models, so we could determine if history of sexual assault entered as a dummy variable was associated with suicide attempt when known correlates of suicidality including sex, age, education, posttraumatic stress symptoms, and 1 of the following 4 comorbid conditions: major depression, substance abuse or dependence (alcohol and/or other drug), panic attacks, or chronic medical disability were examined. In each model, the interaction between sexual assault and the comorbid condition was also entered as an independent variable.

The general rule of thumb suggests there be a minimum of 5 to 6 respondents per parameter estimate in the model and that the total number of suggested respondents not exceed the number of respondents in the smaller of the 2 groups composing the dependent variable. Although we entered 7 independent variables into each of the regression models, we feel certain that the stability of the models was not compromised as the results were similar across the 2 samples, ie, all respondents and female-only group and across the models for the 4 comorbidity conditions.

Data were weighted to adjust for (1) the unequal probability of selection in the initial survey, (2) the oversample of elderly, (3) demographic characteristics of the geographical region sampled according to the 1980 US Census Report, and (4) attrition at Wave II Epidemiological Catchment Area.[17] Given the likelihood of underestimation of SEs for respondent items in complex multistage sampling designs, all statistically significant associations were reanalyzed with the design effect taken into consideration.[20,21] Only those factors that maintained their statistically significant association are reported as significant in this study. Weighting the data and correcting for the design effects allowed us to generalize to the adult population living in the sampling area. In this study, unless otherwise stated, raw numbers are taken from unweighted data, whereas percentages are derived from weighted data.

abuse or dependence (alcohol and/or other drug), and panic attacks.

Bivariate associations between the demographic and comorbidity variables with a lifetime history of suicide attempt were also examined (data not shown). Respondents in the suicide attempt group were more likely to be female (90.4% vs 53.9%; χ^2=12.4, df=1, P<.01) and younger (ages 18-24 years, 29.4% vs 14.8%; ages 25-44 years, 59.5% vs 42.3%; ages 45-64 years, 7.8% vs 27.5%; and ages 65+ years, 3.3% vs 15.4%; χ^2=12.2, df=3, P<.01).

Respondents with a history of suicide attempt differed from those with no history, were statistically different on 2 of the comorbidity variables: suprathreshold trauma symptoms (42.0% vs 7.5%; χ^2=7.3, df=1, P<.01) and major depression (36.1% vs 3.5%; χ^2=6.8, df=1, P<.01). Respondents in these 2 groups were not significantly different on race, marital status, education, subthreshold trauma symptoms, chronic medical disability, substance abuse or dependence, or panic attacks.

Almost one third (30.2%) of the index group, 2 of whom were male, indicated that their first assault occurred before age 16 years. The mean±SD age at first reported sexual assault was considerably younger in those who had attempted suicide than in those who had not (12.6±7.24 years [range, 6-32 years] vs 18.1±6.95 years [range, 5-57 years]; F=6.81, P=.01).

We assessed the association between history of sexual assault and suicidality controlling for posttraumatic stress symptoms and other known demographic and comorbidity correlates of suicidality. Given the limited num-

Table 1. Demographic Characteristics of Subjects With and Without Lifetime History of Sexual Assault (SA)

Characteristic	Subjects, Weighted %: With SA (n=67)*	Subjects, Weighted %: Without SA (n=2851)	χ^2	*df*
Female	90.4	53.5†	27.6	1
White	55.8	44.2	0.7	1
Married	59.8	62.2	0.1	1
Education, y				
<12	17.9	35.8		
12	29.8	29.4	5.8	2
>12	52.3	34.8		
Age, y				
18-24	19.6	15.0		
25-44	66.5	42.2†	19.3	3
45-64	12.6	27.4		
65+	1.3	15.4		

*First sexual assault at age less than 16 years (n=21) and at age 16 years or older (n=44); for 2 cases, age at first sexual assault missing.
†P<.001.

Table 2. Comorbidity for Subjects With and Without Lifetime History of Sexual Assault (SA)

Characteristic	Subjects, Weighted %: With SA (n=67)*	Subjects, Weighted %: Without SA (n=2851)	χ^2	*df*
Suicide attempt	14.9	1.4†	4.0	1
Trauma symptoms	45.2	14.3‡	9.9	1
Trauma symptoms subthreshold	19.3	6.7*†	4.7	1
Trauma symptoms suprathreshold	25.9	7.6‡	6.7	1
Chronic medical disability	32.8	28.7	0.3	1
Major depression	12.4	3.8	2.3	1
Substance abuse/dependency:				
alcohol and/or drug	15.5	9.9	0.9	1
Alcohol abuse/dependency	12.0	9.4	0.2	1
Drug abuse/dependency	3.56	1.0	1.1	1
Panic attacks	7.1	3.5	0.8	1

*First sexual assault at age less than 16 years (n=21) and at age 16 years or older (n=44); for 2 cases, age at first sexual assault missing.
†P<.05.
‡P<.01.

ber of suicide attempters, we were restricted on the number of variables that we could enter into the regression model. We believed that it was imperative to enter sex, age, and education into each of the models examined. Because we wanted to examine the differential contribution of the sexual assault event vs symptoms associated with trauma, we entered the latter as a dummy variable. Finally, we controlled for comorbid conditions as well as their interaction with reported sexual assault. However, only 1 comorbid disorder or condition and its interaction with history of sexual assault was entered into a single model. Thus, 4 logistic regression models were examined with the full sample of respondents and again for female-only subsample.

The regression of suicide attempt on reported sexual assault controlling for sex, age, education, post-traumatic stress symptoms, major depression is shown in **Table 3**. Respondents with a history of sexual assault were 6 times more likely to report a suicide attempt controlling for other variables in the model. Depression was associated with increased odds for reporting a suicide attempt. The interaction of major depression and sexual assault history was not statistically significant (odds ratio [OR] = 0.6, 95% confidence interval [CI] = 0.06-6.7). Findings were similar for the full sample and the female-only subsample.

Results were similar in both total sample and female-only subsample when panic attacks and substance abuse or dependence were the comorbidity variables entered into the model: for attempted suicide in association with panic attacks, OR=6.66 (95% CI=2.25-18.70, *P*<.02) and OR=6.86 (95% CI=2.37-19.66, *P*<.001), respectively; and for substance abuse or dependence, OR=7.40 (95% CI=2.32-23.49, *P*<.001) and OR=7.03 (95% CI=2.30-21.48, *P*<.001), respectively. The association between chronic medical disorder and suicide attempt was not significant.

Another set of models examined the female-only subsample to determine if a history of first sexual assault before age 16 years was related to an increased OR for attempting suicide. Findings for the demographics, post-traumatic stress symptoms, the comorbidity variable, and its interaction with sexual assault were similar to those reported for the female-only subsample in Table 3. With major depression in the model, the OR for a suicide attempt when a victim's first sexual assault occurred before age 16 years compared with age 16 years or older was 12.43 (95% CI=2.86-54.05, *P*<.001) vs 3.06 (95% CI=0.07-13.33, *P*=.13). With substance abuse or dependence in the model, the OR for attempted suicide when first sexual assault reportedly occurred before age 16 years compared with age 16 years or older was 13.2 (95% CI=3.48-50.04, *P*<.001) vs 3.78 (95% CI=1.06-13.52, *P*=.04). Finally, when panic attacks was the comorbid disorder entered into the model, the OR for a first sexual assault before age 16 years compared with age 16 years or older was 11.94 (95% CI=3.22-44.40, *P*<.001) vs 3.67 (95% CI=1.01-13.38, *P*=.05).

COMMENT

Our study has shown a clear association between reported sexual trauma and reported suicide attempt, an association that hitherto has not been well established by means of community-based studies, with 1 exception,[13] in which 1 in 5 victims of sexual assault was found to have made a suicide attempt. In our study, the association between sexual assault and attempted suicide remains statistically significant after controlling for the effects of other potential risk factors. A strikingly increased risk for suicide attempt was found in women whose first sexual assault occurred before age 16 years. While major depression, substance abuse or dependence, and panic attacks are all separately associated with an increased odds of suicide attempt, sexual assault remained significantly associated with suicidal behavior.

Table 3. Association of Attempted Suicide With History of Sexual Assault Controlling for Demographic Characteristics, Posttraumatic Stress Symptoms, and Major Depression*

Characteristic	OR (95% CI) All Respondents (n=2918)	OR (95% CI) Females Only (n=1778)
Female: 1, yes	6.84† (1.39-33.37)	. . .
Age: younger, higher score; OR per year	1.08‡ (1.03-1.12)	1.07‡ (1.03-1.12)
Education: fewer years, higher score; OR per year	1.35‡ (1.18-1.55)	1.32‡ (1.17-1.49)
Major depression: 1, yes	12.17† (4.23-35.11)	14.59‡ (4.85-43.71)
Trauma symptoms: 1, yes	2.81† (1.21-6.51)	2.89† (1.24-6.70)
Ever sexually assaulted: 1, yes	5.89† (1.71-20.18)	6.36‡ (1.81-22.30)

*The interaction between major depression and history of sexual assault was not statistically significant for either sample. OR indicates odds ratio; CI, confidence interval.
†$P<.02$.
‡$P<.001$.

Our findings are of importance to practitioners, given that suicide attempts are associated with increased health service utilization (eg, emergency department and hospitalization services) and, in 10% of cases,[13] eventually associated with a completed suicide. Victims of sexual assault also visit health care providers more often for physical and mental health symptoms.[22] In assessing suicide potential, it may be important to ask about earlier sexual assault.

With so few male individuals reporting sexual assault, we cannot speak to the importance of gender with respect to sexual assault and suicidality. Others[23,24] have reported that women who experience early sexual abuse exhibit low self-esteem, self-blame, difficulties with trust, and symptoms of depression. Further studies are needed to determine whether gender is related to the symptomatic sequelae of sexual abuse.

Although we believe that the association between sexual trauma and suicide attempt is not an artifact of the analysis, there are some limitations to the study, as follows.

1. Deletion of respondents with incomplete data could have biased our findings. We argue, however, that the impact of dropping out these respondents reduced, rather than increased, the strength of the association that we would have found between sexual assault and suicidality. We base this on the fact that differences between respondents included in, and excluded from, the study were found on only 1 of the comorbidity variables. If dropouts had been retained, panic attacks would possibly have been an even more significant risk factor for suicide attempt. This, however, seems unlikely given the strength of the OR for panic attacks observed for both the full sample and the female-only subsample.

2. A more serious limitation is our inability to elicit the age at suicide attempt; thus, we do not know whether sexual assault preceded a suicide attempt. It is more probable that the victims of sexual trauma whose first sexual assault occurred before age 16 years did not attempt suicide until after age 16 years. Kilpatrick and colleagues[3] noted that when suicide attempts occurred in rape victims, they generally followed the trauma.

3. Sexual trauma may have been underreported, which would mean that some subjects were classified as false negatives. We do not know the impact this may have on our findings. In Los Angeles, Calif, Sorenson et al[25] reported a 16.7% lifetime rate of any sexual assault in women and 9.4% in men. These are substantially higher than the rates of sexual assault in our sample. Whether there are regional differences in readiness to report trauma or whether other factors in the Los Angeles sample, such as race and location, account for the differences is difficult to establish.

4. The greater importance of the traumatic event compared with the presence of posttraumatic stress symptoms may be caused by differential recall between the event itself and symptoms thereof. Possibly, subjects had a stronger recall of the trauma than the ensuing symptoms. There is also the possibility that younger women are better able to recall and/or disclose incidents of sexual trauma than their older counterparts, thereby explaining the observed age difference between the groups. We found that victims of sexual assault were younger, as did Sorenson et al.[8] On the other hand, Mullen et al[5] found that age did not distinguish subjects with childhood sexual abuse histories vs those without. Others[26-28] have noted that younger women report more childhood sexual assault. Both different methods of inquiry and regional differences should be taken into account before concluding whether cohort effects exist.

5. Systematic assessment of personality disorders was not undertaken, and it remains possible that the association between sexual assault and suicide attempt is explained by Axis II comorbidity.

6. All data are based on self-report and therefore lack external corroboration as to authenticity.

7. Subject response is clearly shaped by the form in which the questions are presented. The Epidemiological Catchment Area Study was not designed specifically to assess the relation between suicide attempts and sexual trauma.

Notwithstanding the above limitations, we believe that our study demonstrates that sexual trauma is associated with lifetime suicide attempt, that this association is not explained by other risk factors, and that it is particularly strong in women who reported a sexual assault before age 16 years. The immensely damaging effect of such an event cannot be stressed too strongly, particularly in individuals with other vulnerability factors, such as family dysfunction, genetic or familial vulnerability to psychopathological states, and other developmental problems. We need to maintain awareness that a relation does exist between suicide attempt and sexual trauma and that this is not confined merely to treatment seeking clinical samples, but that it holds true in community samples as well. Our data do not inform as to which came first, and subsequent work could well be directed at tracing the path that links sexual trauma and attempted suicide.

Accepted for publication January 12, 1996.

This study was supported by grants U01MH35386 (Dr Blazer) and R01MH43756 (Dr George) from the Public Health Service, Washington, DC.

Reprints: Jonathan R. T. Davidson, MD, Department of Psychiatry, Anxiety and Traumatic Stress Program, Box 3812, Duke University Medical Center, Durham, NC 27710.

REFERENCES

1. Kolb LC. Chronic posttraumatic stress disorder implications of recent epidemiological and neuropsychological studies. *Psychol Med.* 1989;10:821-824.
2. Kolb LC. Posttraumatic stress disorder in Vietnam veterans. *N Engl J Med.* 1976;6:641-642.
3. Kilpatrick DG, Best CL, Veronen LJ, Amick AE, Villeponteux LA, Ruff GA. Mental health correlates of criminal victimization: a random community survey. *J Consult Clin Psychol.* 1985;53:866-873.
4. Wyatt GE. The sexual abuse of Afro-American and white American women in childhood. *Child Abuse Negl.* 1985;9:50-59.
5. Mullen PE, Martin JL, Anderson JC, Romans GE, Herbison GP. Childhood sexual abuse and mental health in later life. *Br J Psychiatry.* 1993;163:721-732.
6. Winfield I, George LK, Swartz M, Blazer DG. Sexual assault and psychiatric disorders among a community sample of women. *Am J Psychiatry.* 1990;147: 335-341.
7. Siegel JM, Sorenson SB, Golding JM, Burnam MA, Stein JA. The prevalence of childhood sexual assault: the Los Angeles Epidemiological Catchment Area Project. *Am J Epidemiol.* 1987;126:1141-1153.
8. Sorenson SB, Stein JA, Siegel JM, Golding JM, Burnam MA. The prevalence of adult sexual assault: the Los Angeles Epidemiological Catchment Area Project. *Am J Epidemiol.* 1987;126:1154-1164.
9. Sheldrick C. Adult sequelae of child sexual abuse. *Br J Psychiatry.* 1991;158 (suppl 10):55-62.
10. Burnam MA, Stein JA, Golding JM, Siegel JM, Sorensen SB, Forsythe AB, Telles CA. Sexual assault and mental disorders in a community population. *J Consult Clin Psychol.* 1988;56:843-850.
11. Mullen PE, Romans-Clarkson SE, Walton VA, Herbison GP. Impact of sexual and physical abuse on women's mental health. *Lancet.* 1988;941-845.
12. Davidson JRT, Hughes DC, Blazer DG, George LK. Posttraumatic stress disorder in the community: an epidemiological study. *Psychol Med.* 1991;21:713-721.
13. Stevenson JM. Suicide. In: Talbott JA, Hales RE, Yudofsky SC, eds. *Textbook of Psychiatry.* Washington, DC: American Psychiatric Press; 1988:1021-1035.
14. Weissman MM, Klerman GL, Markowitz JS, Ouellette R. Suicidal ideation and suicide attempts in panic disorder and attacks. *N Engl J Med.* 1989;321:1209-1214.
15. Johnson J, Weissman MM, Klerman GL. Panic disorder, comorbidity, and suicide attempts. *Arch Gen Psychiatry.* 1990;47:805-808.
16. Blazer DG, George LK, Landerman RG, Pennybacker M, Melville ML, Woodbury M. Manton KG, Jordan K, Locke B. Psychiatric disorders. *Arch Gen Psychiatry.* 1985;42:651-656.
17. Eaton WW, Kessler LG, eds. *Epidemiological Field Methods in Psychiatry: The NIMH Epidemiological Catchment Area Program.* Orlando, Fla: Academic Press Inc; 1985.
18. Blazer DG, Swartz M, Woodbury M, Manton KG, Hughes DC, George LK. Depressive symptoms and depression diagnoses in a community population. *Arch Gen Psychiatry.* 1988;45:1078-1084.
19. Robins LN, Helzer JE, Croughland JL, Williams JBW, Spitzer RL. *NIMH Diagnostic Interview Schedule–Version III.* Rockville, Md: National Institutes of Mental Health; 1981. Public Health Service (PHS) publication PHS ADM-T-42-3.
20. Kessler LG, Folsom R, Royall R, Forsythe A, McEvoy L, Holzer CE, Rae DS, Woodbury M. Parameter and variance estimation. In: Eaton WW, Kessler LG, eds. *Epidemiological Field Methods in Psychiatry: The NIMH Epidemiological Catchment Area Program.* Orlando, Fla: Academic Press Inc; 1985:327-348.
21. Shah BV, Folsom R, Harrell RE, Dillard CN. *RTI Logit: Procedure for Logistic Regression on Survey Data.* Research Triangle Park, NC: Research Triangle Institute; 1987.
22. Golding JM, Stein JA, Siegel JM, Burnam MA, Sorensen SB. Sexual assault history and use of health and mental health services. *Am J Commun Psychol.* 1988;16:625-644.
23. Mullen PE, Romans-Clarkson SE, Martin JL, Anderson JD. The long-term effects of sexual assault on women's mental health. *N Z Med J.* 1989;102:633-634.
24. Mullen PE, Martin JL, Anderson JC, Romans SE, Herbison GP. The effect of child sexual abuse on social interpersonal and sexual freedom in adult life. *Br J Psychiatry.* 1994;165:35-47.
25. Sorenson SB, Siegel JM, Golding JM, Stein JA. Repeated sexual victimization. *Violence Victims.* 1991;6:299-308.
26. Bagley C, Ramsay R. Sexual abuse in childhood: psychosocial outcomes and implications for social work practice. *J Soc Work Hum Sexual.* 1986;4:33-47.
27. Russell DEH. *Sexual Exploitation: Rape Child Sexual Abuse, and Work Place Harassment.* Beverly Hills, Calif: Sage Publications; 1984.
28. Siegel JM, Golding JM, Stein JA, Burnam MA, Sorensen SB. Reactions to sexual assault: a community study. *J Interpers Violence.* 1990;6:229-246.

Correction

Reprint Address Missing. In the article titled "Enhanced Sensitivity of Pituitary β-Endorphin to Ethanol in Subjects at High Risk of Alcoholism" (1996;53:250-257), the address for reprints was omitted. Correspondence and requests for reprints should be directed to Christina Gianoulakis, PhD, Douglas Hospital Research Centre, 6875 LaSalle Blvd, Verdun, Quebec, Canada H4H 1R3. The ARCHIVES regrets the error.

MANUSCRIPT CRITERIA AND INFORMATION

Submit manuscripts to Jack D. Barchas, MD, Editor, *Archives of General Psychiatry,* Cornell Medical Center, Dept of Psychiatry, Box 171, 525 E 68th St, Room F2315, New York, NY 10021. Manuscripts are received with the understanding that they are not under simultaneous consideration by another publication, have not been published previously, and have the approval of each author. Accepted manuscripts become the permanent property of the ARCHIVES. They may not be republished without permission from the publisher (AMA).

Editing. Copyediting follows AMA style and requires corresponding author approval. The authors are responsible for all statements made in their work, including changes made by the copy editor and authorized by the corresponding author.

Reprints. Forms for ordering are included with the edited typescript sent for approval. Reprints are shipped 6 to 8 weeks after publication.

Cover Letter

- In the cover letter, designate one author as correspondent and provide a complete address and telephone and fax numbers.

- For a manuscript to be reviewed, considered, or edited, the following statement must be signed by *all* authors:

"I have been sufficiently involved in this work to take public responsibility for its validity and final presentation as an original publication. I can and will provide documentation of my work upon reasonable request and I have fulfilled the obligations for full disclosure and authorship as described by *Archives of General Psychiatry*. . . ." This signed statement must conclude with *one* of the two following sentences: "Accordingly, I hereby transfer, assign, or otherwise convey all copyright ownership to the AMA in the event such work is published by the AMA." [OR] "No copyright ownership can be transferred since this work was produced in the course of my official duties as a US government officer or employee."

Manuscript Preparation[1,2]

- Submit an original double-spaced typescript and 7 copies.
- **Manuscripts will not be returned after the review process.** Unpublished manuscripts will be destroyed.
- Type—double-spaced throughout (including references)—on one side only of 8½ × 11-in white bond paper. Number all pages. Do not justify right-hand margins. Use a printer of at least letter quality.
- The length of the text of the manuscript (not including abstract, tables, figures, or references) should be under 5000 words. Include a word count of the text on the title page.
- Titles should be short, specific, and descriptive, emphasizing the main point of the article. Avoid a two-part title, if at all possible. Do not number the title, eg, I or Part I. Title length, including punctuation and spaces, ideally should be under 100 characters and must not exceed 200 characters.
- The title page should list full names, degrees, academic affiliations and their locations, and the name and address to whom reprint requests should be sent. If the paper was presented at a meeting, include the organization, place, and date of presentation. Acknowledgment of grant or drug company support should also be made on this page.
- Include a structured abstract of 250 words or less that states the Background, Methods, Results, and Conclusions in four sections labeled as such.
- Use Système International (SI) measurements throughout the manuscript.
- Use generic names of drugs, unless the specific trade name is directly relevant to the study design or discussion.
- Do not use abbreviations in the title or abstract. Limit their use in the text.
- *Do not use footnotes or appendixes.* Such materials should either be incorporated into the text or offered to interested readers on request.
- Include a statistical analysis section under *Methods* that fully describes the application of each statistical procedure used. If a test is used that is not commonly presented in the ARCHIVES, briefly describe its purpose and how it is to be interpreted. Results should report the test statistic (eg, χ^2, F or *t* value), degrees of freedom, and *P* value. Measures of central tendency (eg, means) should be accompanied by measures of variability (eg, standard deviations). In the cover letter, state the name of your statistical consultant, if appropriate.
- Acknowledge fully any material taken from other publications, and submit written permission from the owner to reprint in any language or form without limitation.
- Tables and figures should provide substantive data and not merely illustrate the text. While the main finding of a table or figure may be discussed in the narrative, the table or figure should not duplicate the text. Although no specific guideline can be applied to all articles, the number and length of tables and figures should be kept to a minimum.

Tables. Double-space on separate sheets of 8½ × 11-in white bond paper. Title each one and number them in the order of their citation in the text. If a table must be continued, repeat the title on a second sheet, followed by "(cont)." Any explanatory notes to be printed with the table must be typed single-spaced beneath the table.

Figures. Once manuscripts are accepted, two sets of professionally prepared, high-resolution color transparencies are required for all color figures. For black and white art, two sets of professionally prepared glossy prints are required. If color figures are necessary, the ARCHIVES may pay part of the expense with the balance to be borne by the author.

- Number figures according to their order in the text. Type the figure number, proper orientation (eg, top), name of the senior author, and an abbreviated title on a gummed label; affix it to the back of the print.
- Double-space legends (maximum length, 40 words) on a separate sheet of 8½ × 11-in paper.

References. References should be carefully selected to acknowledge previous work or to document a specific point. They should not be exhaustive. Number references in the order they are mentioned in the text; do *not* alphabetize. In text, tables, and legends, identify references with superscript arabic numbers. Double-space, follow AMA style and abbreviate names of journals according to *Index Medicus*. List all authors and/or editors. Citation accuracy is the responsibility of the author.

Examples:

1. DuBois RN, Lazenby AJ, Yardley JH, Hendrix TR, Bayless TM, Giardiello FM. Lymphocytic enterocolitis in patients with 'refractory sprue.' *JAMA*. 1989;262:935-937.

2. Ritchie JM, Greene NM. Local anesthetics. In: Gilman AG, Goodman LS, Rall TW, Murad F, eds. *The Pharmacological Basis of Therapeutics*. 7th ed. New York, NY: Macmillan Publishing Co Inc; 1985:309-310.

Informed Consent and Confidentiality. A statement of informed consent for human investigation should be made. Authors must ensure that patient confidentiality is in no way breached. Do not use real names, initials, or disclose information that might identify a particular subject.

Obligations for Full Disclosure and Authorship[3,4]

Previous Publications. Manuscripts that are submitted must not have been previously published in *whole* or *substantial part* and must not be simultaneously under consideration elsewhere. This policy applies to the essential contents, tables, or figures, but does not apply to abstracts. Authors must disclose in their cover letters if the submitted manuscript contains any data or material that have already been published or are in press, submitted, or nearly submitted. Copies of closely related manuscripts should be submitted to the Editor for examination.

Financial Disclosure. At the time of initial submission, each author should disclose any financial arrangement he or she has with companies who either have products featured in the manuscript or with companies that produce competing products. These arrangements include, but are not limited to, company support, consultantships, patent rights, stock ownership, or other equity interests. Such arrangements do not constitute grounds for automatic rejection of the manuscript. Financial information will be held in confidence. If the manuscript is accepted for publication, the Editor and the author(s) will confer about the way this information will be communicated to the readers. Reviewers are also expected to notify the Editor of their own financial arrangements involving companies whose products (or competing products) are featured in the manuscripts they agree to review.

Other Disclosures. Authors should disclose to the Editor at the time of submission any special circumstances, vested interests, or sources of bias that might affect the integrity of the reported information. These disclosures also apply to referees.

Authorship does not require expertise in every aspect of the work. It does mean that each author within his or her own limits has exerted sufficient reasonable effort to vouch for the validity of the entire work and to bear public accountability for maintaining the integrity of the scientific information communicated. Each author must have had enough substantial involvement in generating and formulating the published product to bear such accountability. More than six authors requires a statement of justification in the cover letter.

Letters to the Editor

Letters to the Editor will be considered for publication if they are accompanied by a cover letter stating they are "for publication." Their purpose should be to comment on articles published in the ARCHIVES or to provide significant news that can be conveyed in a short format. The Editor reserves the right to edit the material prior to publication.

Letters intended for publication *must* follow manuscript preparation guidelines (eg, double-spaced, copyright transfer). They generally should not exceed 750 words. Include 3 copies. Illustrative material is not usually accepted; brief tables may occasionally be considered. Authors will receive only a brief acknowledgment of acceptance or rejection.

Review Process

A submitted manuscript will be acknowledged by postcard and assigned a manuscript number, which is to be used in all further correspondence. Manuscripts are reviewed and given a priority based upon their originality, scientific merit, appropriateness of statistical analyses, importance of their findings, significance for the field, lucidity, interest to readers, suitability for publication, and the journal's current portfolio. All reviewers remain anonymous and are expected to maintain the curtain of strict confidentiality. After the review process has been completed, authors will be informed by mail of the Editor's decision.

References

1. Iverson CL, Dan BB, Glitman P, et al. *American Medical Association Manual of Style*. 8th ed. Baltimore, Md: Williams & Wilkins; 1988.

2. International Committee of Medical Journal Editors. Uniform requirements for manuscripts submitted to biomedical journals. *Ann Intern Med*. 1988;108:258-265.

3. Freedman DX. The meaning of full disclosure. *Arch Gen Psychiatry*. 1988;45:689-691.

4. Freedman DX. Megamultiple authorship. *Arch Gen Psychiatry*. 1982;39:351.

Checklist

____ (1) Cover letter including all information deemed necessary for the editor's review.

____ (2) Statement on copyright and authorial responsibility, signed by *all* authors.

____ (3) Corresponding author identified and address and telephone and fax numbers provided.

____ (4) Original manuscript (including structured abstract, references, legends, tables, and figures) plus 7 copies.

____ (5) Word count of text only (not including abstract, tables, references) on the title page.

____ (6) Right-hand margin unjustified.

____ (7) Copies of publications considered to be helpful for the review process or that bear on any possible overlap of published data.

Professional Opportunities

Physician Recruitment

Psychiatry
Multiple Specialties/Group Practice
Locum Tenens Wanted
Graduate Training/Residencies/Fellowships
Chiefs/Department Heads/Directors
Academic/Faculty
CME Corner
Courses/Symposia/Seminars
Practices For Sale
Notices

1996 Physician Recruitment Rates

Regular	1x	1.15/wd	*3x	1.05/wd
Bold	1x	1.30/wd	*3x	1.20/wd

*In order to receive the 3 time frequency price, the request must be made upon initial placement. The minimum charge is 20 words. A word consists of one or more letters surrounded by space on each side.

For information on display advertising and our network buys contact an account representative.

Policy

Orders for classified advertising must be submitted in writing. Although the American Medical Association believes the classified advertisements in these pages to be from reputable sources, the Association does not investigate the offers made and assumes no liability concerning them. Acceptance of advertising is restricted to professional opportunities, practices for sale, and medical office space available. The Association reserves the right to decline, withdraw, or edit advertisements at its discretion. Every care is taken to avoid mistakes but responsibility cannot be accepted by the Association for clerical or printer's errors.

Reply Box Service

Confidential box numbers are available for an additional $20 per issue, plus the words - Box ____, c/o AGNP.

When responding to a box number, please send to Archives of General Psychiatry, Box ____, c/o AGNP, 515 N State St, Chicago, IL 60610.

Cancellations/Changes

Cancellations/changes must be received in writing at least 25 days prior to the date of the issue. In order to expedite, please fax to 312-464-5909 to the attention of your account representative.

General Information

To contact a Physician Recruitment Advertising account representative, call 312-464-2475/2490/2491/4485 or **800-AMA-2260.** Or fax your insertion order to **312-464-5909**. Mail your materials to **AMA Physician Recruitment Advertising, 12th Floor, 515 N State St, Chicago, IL 60610.**

Psychiatry

TEXAS, the SOUTHEAST, and the SUNBELT STATES- There are Excellent Private Practice Opportunities Available in Psychiatry. Major Cities and Rural Communities Are Available.

Call 1-800-284-4560/Houston 713-493-2797

Or send CV to:
P.O. Box 42314
Houston, TX 77242-2314
FAX 713-493-2234

Reuben Bronstein & Associates

Locum Tenens Wanted

HKA LOCUM TENENS is looking for quality general psychiatry physicians to do Locum Tenens. We have opportunities coast-to-coast. We furnish Occurrence Malpractice Insurance (no tail necessary). Please call **HKA LOCUM TENENS at (800)226-6347, Extension AM7.1.**

© 1995 MAILSTAR

For more **Professional Opportunities** please refer to the **Physician Recruitment** sections in ***JAMA*** and ***AMNews***.

THIS MONTH IN
ARCHIVES
OF
GENERAL PSYCHIATRY

Aylward et al (page 577) used magnetic resonance imaging (MRI) to measure caudate volumes in patients with obsessive-compulsive disorder (OCD) who did not have neurological signs and in normal comparison subjects. They observed similar structural imaging measures between the groups. A meta-analysis of the functional imaging (blood flow and metabolism) literature of patient-control baseline studies further indicated that caudate abnormality was not strongly supported when global brain metabolic rates were accounted for. Contrasted with the current study, the reduced caudate volume with ventricular enlargement that has been observed in some reports may reflect OCD heterogeneity and may be related to severity of associated neurological symptoms.

Murphy et al (page 585) investigated whether there are sex differences in the effect of aging on human regional brain volumes using MRI and on regional cerebral metabolism for glucose by positron emission tomography. They found significant sex differences in the aging of language areas; hippocampus; and frontal, temporal, and parietal lobes. These brain regions are essential to intellectual functioning and are implicated in neuropsychiatric disorders. Thus, these findings may explain some of the age-sex differences in human cognition and response to brain injury and disease.

The mediating neuroanatomy of OCD is incompletely understood and has not been investigated using the new tomographic technique of functional MRI. **Breiter et al** (page 595) used MRI for patients with OCD and normal volunteers during control and provoked conditions. Patients showed activation in medial orbitofrontal, lateral frontal, anterior temporal, anterior cingulate, and insular cortex, as well as caudate, lenticulate, and amygdala. Normal subjects did not exhibit activation in any brain area. These results are consistent with past imaging studies of OCD; however, paralimbic and limbic activations were more prominent in the current study.

Attention-deficit hyperactivity disorder (ADHD) is the most common psychiatric diagnosis in children and has substantial public health impact. In the largest anatomic study to date, **Castellanos et al** (page 607) compared MRIs of boys with ADHD to those of healthy matched controls with respect to volumes and symmetries for a dozen brain regions. They found significant differences in subjects with ADHD, predominantly in the right prefrontal-striatal-pallidal structures. This first comprehensive morphometric analysis extends the relevance of this circuit to pediatric subjects and, if replicated, may provide a brain-based marker of ADHD.

Frazier et al (page 617) used MRI to quantify volumes of specific brain regions in children with early-onset schizophrenia (before age 12) and in matched controls. Children with schizophrenia had a smaller total cerebral volume and midsagittal thalamic area. In addition, a larger caudate, putamen, and globus pallidus were seen as well as a trend toward larger ventricles. The brain anatomic abnormalities found in childhood-onset schizophrenia are similar to those described for adults with schizophrenia, supporting continuity between very early-onset and later-onset disease.

It has long been suspected that there may be structural brain abnormalities in patients with OCD, but until recently no techniques allowed for precise volumetric measurements of brain regions. **Jenike et al** (page 625) compared whole-brain structures in 10 female patients with OCD and 10 female controls who were matched for handedness, age, weight, education, and verbal IQ. Compared with controls, patients with OCD had significantly less total white matter and significantly greater total cortex volumes. Such widespread volumetric white matter differences suggest a widely distributed structural brain abnormality in OCD.

Understanding cognitive abnormalities in schizophrenia may improve our understanding of its mechanisms. **O'Leary et al** (page 633) used positron emission tomography to test the integrity of the distributed brain systems that control selective attention. When the patients were given competing auditory stimulation to both ears (dichotic listening), they consistently had less blood flow in the superotemporal gyrus than healthy normal volunteers and were unable to shift blood flow to their right hemisphere in response to attentional demands. Dysfunction in the brain circuitry that controls arousal, attention, and information processing may explain the fundamental cognitive deficits in schizophrenia.

Ho et al (page 645) measured the rate of glucose use in different areas of the brain during the first period of non–rapid eye movement sleep. Whole-brain glucose metabolism was 47% higher in the depressed patients compared with normal controls, suggesting that the patients were "overaroused" compared with normal controls. The greatest increases in metabolic rate were in the areas of the brain that have been implicated in the control of emotions and memory; the limbic system, especially the cingulate gyrus, amygdala, and hippocampus. In addition, the metabolic rate in the posterior portion of the cerebral cortex in the occipital and temporal areas was elevated. In contrast, the metabolic rate in the middle frontal cortex was relatively less elevated in the patient group.

A Commentary on brain imaging by John Mazziotta, MD, is also included in this issue on page 574.

Notice to Authors

Electronic publication by authors or by their institutions of articles appearing or scheduled to appear in this journal—on the World Wide Web or via any other electronic means—constitutes a violation of the American Medical Association's exclusive and permanent ownership of copyright to all articles published in the *Archives of General Psychiatry*. **Effective immediately, articles that have already been electronically published are not eligible for publication in the ARCHIVES.**

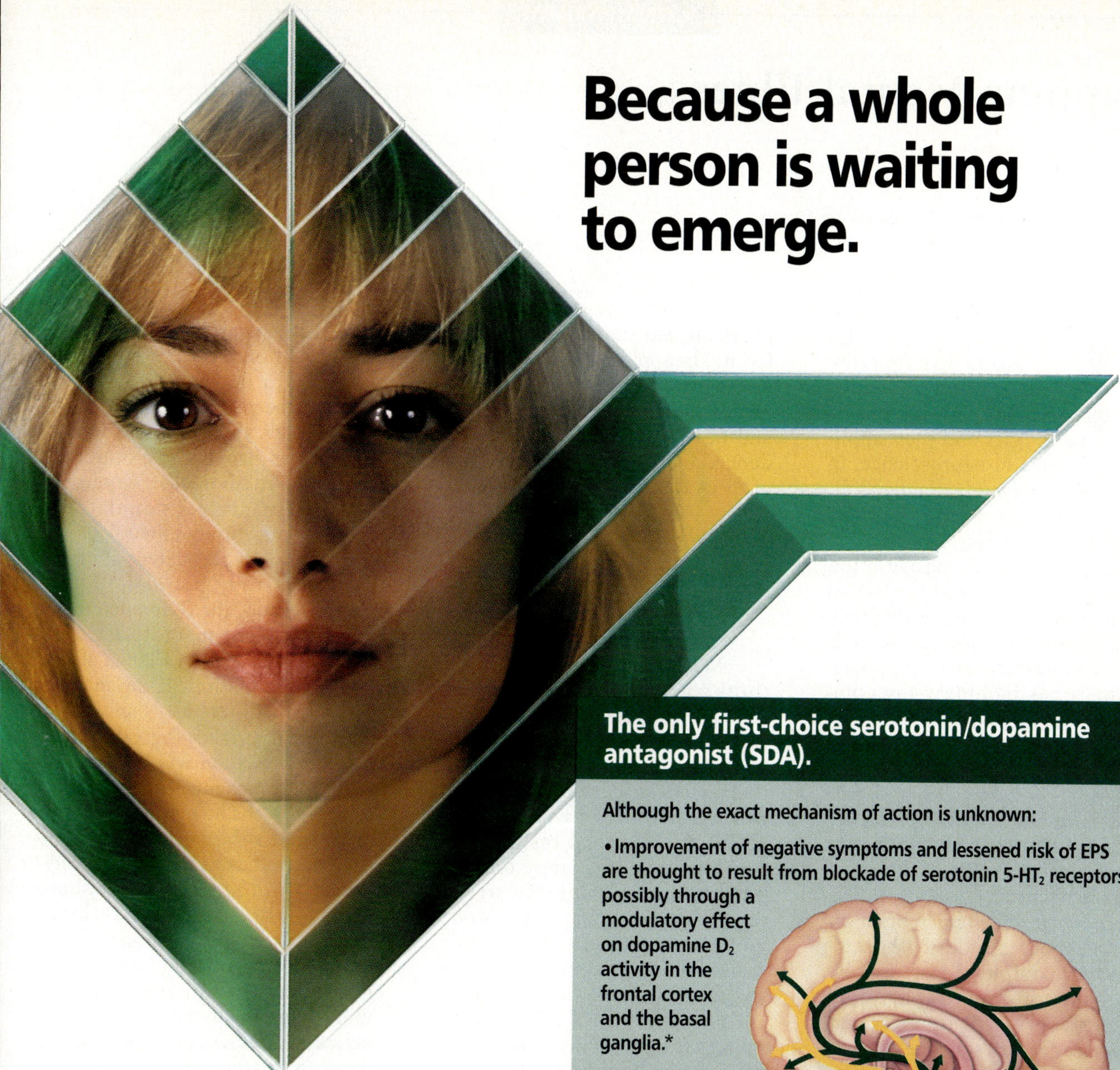

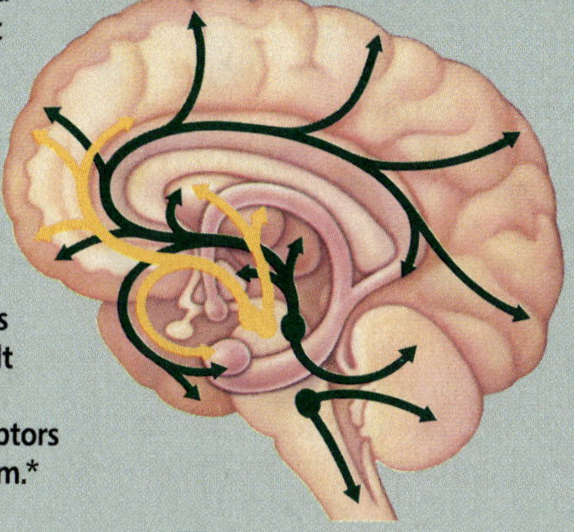

Dopaminergic system
Serotoninergic system

Mapping Mental Illness

A New Era

Where the telescope ends, the microscope begins.
Which of the two has the grander view?

Les Miserables, Victor Hugo, 1862

THIS ISSUE of the ARCHIVES reflects the explosion of neuroimaging technologies and their application to clinical neuroscience, in this case, to the study of mental illness. Since the invention of x-ray computed tomography 20 years ago,[1] a progressive array of constantly improving structural and functional imaging techniques has been developed to study the human brain in vivo. The modern structural imaging methods include x-ray computed tomography, magnetic resonance imaging, and magnetic resonance angiography. As discussed in several articles in this issue,[2-7] these techniques are of increasing value for investigating the morphometric structure of the human brain when it is healthy and diseased. Functional human brain imaging methods include single photon emission computed tomography, positron emission tomography, functional magnetic resonance imaging, magnetic resonance spectroscopy, optical intrinsic signal imaging, electroencephalography, and magnetoencephalography. These techniques provide insights into the physiology, neurochemistry, and neuropharmacology of the brain, as discussed in the articles by Aylward et al,[2] Murphy et al,[3] and Breiter et al.[4]

Techniques are constantly being developed to evaluate the structure and function of the human brain during life, and the spatial and temporal resolution of existing methods have progressively improved. Further, a transition has occurred in modern neuroimaging from the basic development of instrumentation to the application of these techniques to studies of normal brain function and the diseases that affect it. The application of these methods to persons who have mental illnesses and addictions is an exciting and rapidly maturing field, as evidenced by the articles in this issue of the ARCHIVES.

See also pages 577, 585, 595, 607, 617, and 625

When examining current thinking on brain structure and function in patients with psychiatric disorders, the following question should be asked: What will these modern neuroimaging techniques provide in the way of pathophysiological insights and new avenues of therapy for such patient populations? Current dogma suggests that there exist few consistent, macroscopic abnormalities of the brain that characterize psychiatric disorders or addictions. This belief leads to the conclusion that these disorders have a functional or pathophysiological origin. This concept is reinforced by the fact that drugs are effective in reducing or eliminating symptoms in patients with psychiatric disease and can also produce psychoses and alterations of mood or thought as side effects or when they are used inappropriately.

An argument against a functional or neurochemical basis for most psychiatric disorders would be difficult to substantiate. However, can macroscopic structural abnormalities be dismissed as nonexistent in such illnesses? Populations of limited size have been examined in most studies of brain anatomy in patients who have mental illnesses. In general, accurate estimates of the morphometric variance in normal populations have not been used. In vivo imaging methods vs earlier postmortem techniques provide the opportunity to learn about the structural variance of normal populations and the opportunity to study larger patient groups. To detect a difference in a study population vs a control group, the difference must have sufficient magnitude to be observed above the variance of the control population. If the magnitude of the difference is small and the control variance is great, a large patient population will be required to detect the change. Although the variance in the structural anatomy of normal subjects is unknown, evidence indicates that it is considerable. In imaging investigations, this variance comprises subject movement, improper subject alignment and registration, and instrumentation artifact, as well as the underlying anatomical differences between individuals.[8-12] Because of these problems, a simple, qualitative analysis of cross-sectional images would be unlikely to detect any but the most obvious differences between patients and control subjects. However, quantitative or probabilistic approaches seem likely to produce new insights.[13-15] Techniques using meta-analysis of multiple, previous investigations have the advantage of increasing the population size but must contend with differences in methodologies and patient populations employed in the original studies.[2] Thus, all neuroimaging techniques, both structural and functional, should be employed in protocols that optimize the detection sensitivity of patient populations from control subjects and do so in an environment where the range of variance in both populations is understood.

Modern functional imaging techniques provide in vivo data about neurochemistry and neurophysiology in patients who have mental illnesses and addictions. When properly employed, these techniques produce information about the spatial location and extent of abnormalities related to state and trait in patient populations. They can also supply clues about the functional neuroanatomy of specific psychiatric symptoms, such as hallucinations.[16,17] Positron emission tomography, single photon emission computed tomography, magnetic resonance spectroscopy, and functional magnetic resonance imaging have the capacity to evaluate the entire intracranial contents in a single study and the spatial resolution to provide excellent estimates about where abnormalities exist in patients with psychiatric disorders. Temporal information about synchrony and network interactions within pathological circuits can be provided by techniques such as electroencephalography and magnetoencephalography. The registration and alignment of data sets from structural, functional, and temporally sensitive methods will provide the best composite perspective on the sites and timing of such abnormalities.[18] After gaining knowledge about the location of such abnormalities, more invasive techniques and basic molecular and cellular neurobiology must be used to understand how abnormalities in these regions cause psychiatric disorders and to understand the mechanisms that underlie them.

To optimize the yield from human in vivo neuroimaging studies, investigators must obtain insights from and collaborate with basic neuroscientists. First, the use of carefully designed, neuropsychological paradigms, developed over extended periods and associated with a wealth of behavioral data, provide an important and readily available resource for use in the design and development of neurobehavioral imaging paradigms. The combination of cognitive tasks, neuropharmacological manipulations, and neuroimaging measurements can test hypotheses that have been developed to explain the signs and symptoms of mental illness and the drug therapies that minimize them.[19]

Second, the extension of macroscopic neuroimaging into the microscopic domain will link human neuroimaging techniques in patients and basic science explorations. This extension may occur directly by technological evolution[20] or may occur by the development of bridging technologies that have the capacity to image the entire brain at a macroscopic resolution (approximately 1 mm in all dimensions) and at the cellular level (approximately 10 μm in all dimensions).[21] By using a careful study design, molecular neurobiological insights about the genetics of psychiatric disease can be linked to the phenotypic expression of these disorders by the combined use of neuroimaging techniques and behavioral assessment. Neuroimaging methods that do not require invasive instrumentation can now be applied in genetically at-risk or presymptomatic populations.[22,23]

Third, the merger of basic science disciplines and modern neuroimaging, when applied to diseases, optimizes the value of both. By performing parallel experiments using neuroimaging techniques in patients and in animal models of diseases, such animal models can be validated or refuted. Valid animal models can then be used appropriately when experiments in human subjects would either be impractical or unethical.

The optimized use of structural and functional neuroimaging methods in the study of mental illness can provide new pathophysiological and pharmacological classifications of patients. These findings can be related to the genetic and cellular pathophysiology of disorders that affect the brain in precise ways. The pathophysiological classification of patients should help provide better and more efficient treatment selections for individual patients and refined, neurobiologically based classification schemes for psychiatric disorders and addictions, in general.

The ability to study the normal, living, human brain with high spatial and temporal resolution is a valuable prelude to the investigation of patient populations using the same tools. Mountcastle[24] stated succinctly, "Function is not the reciprocal of deficit." Modern, in vivo neuroimaging techniques have the ability to answer the "what," "where," "when," and "how" questions of normal brain function and mental illness.[25] We need to apply these methods in ways that are appropriate to their use and communicate the results amongst ourselves in a manner that leads to the most comprehensive and rapid insights into the cause and treatment of these human disorders.

John C. Mazziotta, MD, PhD
Director of Brain Mapping
Department of Neurology
UCLA School of Medicine
710 Westwood Plaza, Room 1-240
Los Angeles, CA 90095
(e-mail: mazziotta@loni.ucla.edu)

REFERENCES

1. Hounsfield GN. Computerized transverse axial scanning (tomography), I: description of system. *Br J Radiol.* 1973;46:1016-1022.
2. Aylward EH, Harris GJ, Hoehn-Saric R, Barta PE, Machlin SR, Pearlson GD. Normal caudate nucleus in obsessive-compulsive disorder assessed by quantitative neuroimaging. *Arch Gen Psychiatry.* 1996;53:577-584.
3. Murphy DGM, DeCarli C, McIntosh AR, Daly E, Mentis MJ, Pietrini P, Szczepanik J, Schapiro MB, Grady CL, Horwitz B, Rapoport SI. Sex differences in human brain morphometry and metabolism: an in vivo quantitative magnetic resonance imaging and positron emission tomography study on the effect of aging. *Arch Gen Psychiatry.* 1996;53:585-594.
4. Breiter HC, Rauch SL, Kwong KK, Baker JR, Weisskoff RM, Kennedy DN, Kendrick AD, Davis TL, Jiang A, Cohen MS, Stern CE, Belliveau JW, Baer L, O'Sullivan RL, Savage CR, Brady TJ, Jenike MA, Rosen BR. Functional magnetic resonance imaging of symptom provocation in obsessive-compulsive disorder. *Arch Gen Psychiatry.* 1996;53:595-606.
5. Castellanos FX, Giedd JN, Marsh WL, Hamburger SD, Vaituzis AC, Dickstein DP, Sarfatti SE, Vauss YC, Snell JW, Lange N, Kaysen D, Krain AL, Ritchie GF, Rajapakse JC, Rapoport JL. Quantitative brain magnetic resonance imaging in attention-deficit hyperactivity disorder. *Arch Gen Psychiatry.* 1996;53:607-616.
6. Frazier JA, Giedd JN, Hamburger SD, Albus KE, Kaysen D, Vaituzis C, Rajapakse JC, Lenane MC, McKenna K, Jacobsen LK, Gordon CT, Breier A, Rapoport JL. Brain anatomic magnetic resonance imaging in childhood-onset schizophrenia. *Arch Gen Psychiatry.* 1996;53:617-624.

7. Jenike MA, Breiter HC, Baer L, Kennedy DN, Savage CR, Olivares MJ, O'Sullivan RL, Shera DM, Rauch SL, Keuthen N, Rosen BR, Caviness VS, Filipek PA. Cerebral structural abnormalities in obsessive-compulsive disorder: a quantitative morphometric magnetic resonance imaging study. *Arch Gen Psychiatry.* 1996;53:625-632.
8. Tramo MJ, Loftus WC, Thomas CE, Green RL, Mott LA, Gazzaniga MS. Surface area of human cerebral cortex and its gross morphological subdivisions: in vivo measurements in monozygotic twins suggest differential hemisphere effects of genetic factors. *J Cogn Neurosci.* 1995;7:292-301.
9. Pfefferbaum A, Mathalon DH, Sullivan EV, Rawles JM, Zipursky RB, Lim KO. A quantitative magnetic resonance imaging study of changes in brain morphology from infancy to late adulthood. *Arch Neurol.* 1994;51:874-887.
10. Steinmetz H, Herzog A, Schlaug G, Huang Y, Jäncke L. Brain (a)symmetry in monozygotic twins. *Cereb Cortex.* 1995;5:296-300.
11. Loftus WC, Tramo MJ, Gazzaniga MS. Cortical surface modeling reveals gross morphometric correlates of individual differences. *Hum Brain Mapping.* 1995;3:257-270.
12. Kulynych JJ, Vladar K, Jones DW, Weinberger DR. Gender differences in the normal lateralization of the supratemporal cortex: MRI surface-rendering morphometry of Heschl's gyrus and the planum temporale. *Cereb Cortex.* 1994;4:107-118.
13. Andreasen NC, Arndt S, Swayze V, Cizaldo T, Flaum M, O'Leary D, Ehrhardt JC, Yuh WTC. Thalamic abnormalities in schizophrenia visualized through magnetic resonance image averaging. *Science.* 1994;266:294-298.
14. Hyde TM, Stacey ME, Coppola R, Handel SF, Rickler KC, Weinberger DR. Cerebral morphometric abnormalities in Tourette's syndrome: a quantitative MRI study of monozygotic twins. *Neurology.* 1995;45:1176-1182.
15. Mazziotta JC, Toga AW, Evans A, Fox P, Lancaster J. A probabilistic atlas of the human brain: theory and rationale for its development. *NeuroImage.* 1995;2:89-101.
16. Silbersweig DA, Stern E, Schnorr L, Frith CD, Ashburner J, Cahill C, Frackowiak RSJ, Jones T. Imaging transient, randomly occurring neuropsychological events in single subjects with positron emission tomography: an event-related count rate correlational analysis. *J Cereb Blood Flow Metab.* 1994;14:771-782.
17. Cohen MS, Green MF. Where the voices come from: imaging of schizophrenic auditory hallucinations. *Soc Neurol.* 1995;21:259.
18. Woods RP, Mazziotta JC, Cherry SR. MRI-PET registration with automated algorithm. *J Comput Assist Tomogr.* 1993;17:536-546.
19. Dolan RJ, Fletcher P, Frith CD, Friston KJ, Frackowiak RSJ, Grasby PM. Dopaminergic modulation of impaired cognitive activation in the anterior cingulate cortex in schizophrenia. *Nature.* 1995;378:180-182.
20. Jacobs RE, Frasier SE. Magnetic resonance microscopy of embryonic cell lineages and movements. *Science.* 1994;263:681-684.
21. Toga AW, Ambach KL, Quinn B, Shankar K, Schluender S. Post-mortem anatomy. In: Toga AW, Mazziotta JC, eds. *Brain Mapping: The Methods.* San Diego, Calif: Academic Press Inc; 1996: 169-190.
22. Small GW, Mazziotta JC, Collins MT, Baxter LR, Phelps ME, Mandelkern MA, Kaplan A, La Rue A, Adamson CF, Chang L, Guze BH, Corder EH, Saunders AM, Haines JL, Pericak-Vance MA, Roses AD. Apolipoprotein E type 4 allele and cerebral glucose metabolism in relatives at risk for familial Alzheimer disease. *JAMA.* 1995;273:942-947.
23. Mazziotta JC, Phelps ME, Pahl JJ, Huang SC, Baxter LR, Riege WH, Hoffman JM, Kuhl DE, Lanto AB, Wapenski JA, Markham CH. Reduced cerebral glucose metabolism in asymptomatic subjects at risk for Huntington's disease. *N Engl J Med.* 1987;316:357-362.
24. Mountcastle V. The evolution of ideas concerning the function of the neocortex. *Cereb Cortex.* 1995;5:289-295.
25. Wood CC. Human brain mapping in both time and space. *Hum Brain Mapping.* 1993/1994;1 (No. 4):iii-vi.

Correction

Error in Figure and Text. In the article titled "The Obsessive-Compulsive Drinking Scale: A New Method of Assessing Outcome in Alcoholism Treatment Studies," published in the March ARCHIVES (1996;53:225-231), the symbols used in Figure 3 were incorrect. Figure 3 is reprinted correctly here. In addition, on page 230, in Figure 5, the label on the x-axis should have read as follows: "OCDS Compulsive Subscale." We regret these errors.

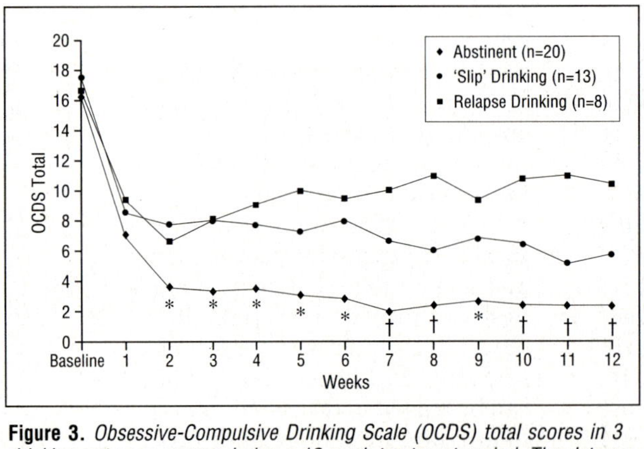

Figure 3. *Obsessive-Compulsive Drinking Scale (OCDS) total scores in 3 drinking outcome groups during a 12-week treatment period. The data are plotted with the use of the last point carry forward substitution for missing data. Asterisk indicates* P<.05 *for the abstinent group vs the slip and relapse groups (Student-Newman-Keuls multiple-group comparisons); dagger, all groups differ from each other at* P<.05.

ORIGINAL ARTICLE

Normal Caudate Nucleus in Obsessive-compulsive Disorder Assessed by Quantitative Neuroimaging

Elizabeth H. Aylward, PhD; Gordon J. Harris, PhD; Rudolf Hoehn-Saric, MD; Patrick E. Barta, MD, PhD; Steven R. Machlin, MD; Godfrey D. Pearlson, MB, BS

Background: Prior neuroimaging studies have not consistently demonstrated a structural or functional abnormality of the caudate nucleus in patients with obsessive-compulsive disorder (OCD). However, there is theoretical support for some associated dysfunction of the caudate nucleus.

Methods: We examined volumes of the caudate nucleus and putamen with magnetic resonance imaging in 24 patients with adult-onset OCD and 21 control subjects, group-matched on age, race, education, and sex. Patients were relatively free from tics. To evaluate function (metabolism or blood flow) of the caudate nucleus, we performed a quantitative review, including a meta-analysis, of normalized data from functional neuroimaging studies that compared patients who had OCD with normal control subjects.

Results: All structural basal ganglia measures failed to exhibit differences between patients with OCD and matched normal control subjects. Patients did not demonstrate evidence of ventricular enlargement. Quantitative meta-analysis of the functional neuroimaging literature did not demonstrate a consistent abnormality of the caudate nucleus.

Conclusions: We did not observe evidence of a structural abnormality of the caudate nucleus in patients with OCD. Prior reports of a structural aberration of the caudate nucleus were mixed. We also did not find strong support for relative caudate metabolic or perfusion dysfunction in the literature, although increased function in the frontal cerebral cortex was identified. The heterogeneous nature of this disorder may account for inconsistencies between studies. For example, ventricular enlargement or reduced caudate volume or blood flow might be evident in patients with soft neurological signs (eg, tics), while patients in the current study were relatively free from tics. Although theories of OCD suggest a dysfunction of the caudate nucleus, the structural and functional neuroimaging literature has not consistently verified this.

Arch Gen Psychiatry. 1996;53:577-584

THE HALLMARK characteristics of obsessive-compulsive disorder (OCD) are an inability to suppress repetitive, intrusive thoughts, and performance of repetitive actions.[1] These symptoms are distressful to the patient, and result in interference with home, school, and interpersonal functioning.

While theories of OCD include dysfunction of the basal ganglia,[2-5] neuroimaging studies of caudate structure and function have not demonstrated consistent differences between patients with OCD and control subjects, although hyperfrontal function has been commonly observed. Neuroimaging results with regard to the structure and function of the caudate nucleus in patients with OCD are briefly summarized here, with a thorough evaluation of prior studies to follow in the "Comment" section below.

Structural imaging studies of the caudate nucleus in patients with OCD have used either x-ray computed tomography or magnetic resonance imaging (MRI). In several studies, caudate nuclei in patients with OCD exhibited normal area, volume, or signal intensity compared with those in normal control subjects.[6-8] One study reported a relatively increased right-sided caudate volume in patients with OCD,[9] although another research team observed a reduced caudate volume (detected with MRI)[10] that was consistent with a prior report of a reduced caudate volume (detected with computed tomogra-

From the Departments of Psychiatry and Behavioral Sciences (Drs Aylward, Hoehn-Saric, Barta, Machlin, and Pearlson) and Mental Hygiene (Dr Pearlson) and Division of Psychiatric Neuro-Imaging (Drs Aylward, Barta, and Pearlson), The Johns Hopkins University, Baltimore, Md, and the Neuroimaging Research Laboratory, Department of Psychiatry, Tufts University School of Medicine/New England Medical Center, Boston, Mass (Dr Harris).

See Patients, Control Subjects, and Methods on next page

PATIENTS, CONTROL SUBJECTS, AND METHODS

Twenty-four patients who met *DSM-III-R* and Research Diagnostic Criteria for OCD participated in this imaging study. Patients who were enrolled in this imaging study were recruited for participation as part of a controlled drug study, and they were evaluated in the psychiatric outpatient department at The Johns Hopkins Hospital, Baltimore, Md. Demographic and clinical information are presented in **Table 1**. All patients had clinical onset of OCD after the age of 18 years (mininum age, 18 years; maximum age, 30 years), and they were symptomatic for at least 1 year. Before scanning, patients were free of medications for 4 weeks to 2 years (mean, 21 weeks) to allow washout for the controlled drug treatment study. Seven patients had never received any medication, while the remaining patients had been receiving tricyclic antidepressants (n=12), monoamine oxidase inhibitors (n=4), serotonergic reuptake inhibitors (n=5), benzodiazepines (n=5), or buspirone hydrochloride (n=1). Eight patients had been receiving several of these medications. Eligibility criteria included Yale-Brown Obsessive Compulsive Scale (YBOC)[21] scores of 16 or higher, and National Institute of Mental Health Global Severity[22] scores of 7 or higher. Comorbidity was assessed through a complete history and mental status examination, with particular attention to depression. Patients were excluded from the study if they had Hamilton Depression Rating Scale[23] scores greater than 16 or had met criteria for major depression before the onset of OCD. Eleven patients had a history of major depression, but none was depressed at the time of this study. Comorbidity consisted of generalized anxiety disorder (n=14), panic disorder (n=1), social phobias (n=2), and simple phobias (n=3).

The following additional exclusion criteria were used: histories of central neurological disorder (including head trauma that led to unconsciousness for more than 1 hour), histories of tics (1 patient reported intermittent mild blinking tics that were not present at examination), histories of substance abuse (obtained through a structured interview—patients were excluded if they acknowledged drug use during the past year or if they had a lifetime history that warranted a *DSM-III-R* diagnosis of substance abuse or dependence), or histories of schizoid personality disorder (excluded because patients were recruited for a controlled drug study and patients with schizoid personality disorder are poor responders to treatment).

Twenty-one control subjects were recruited for this study from the community, and some of these subjects were hospital employees (Table 1). The group of control subjects did not differ significantly from the group of patients on age, race, education, or sex. Potential comparison subjects were excluded from the study according to the same criteria that were used for the patients or if they had histories of any Axis I psychiatric disorders.[12,24,25] Informed consent was obtained from all subjects. Nineteen of the patients with OCD and all control subjects were included in a prior methodological report that examined a correlation between the bicaudate ratio (BCR) and caudate volume in several subject populations.[26]

MAGNETIC RESONANCE IMAGING

All patients with OCD and control subjects underwent scanning with a 1.5-T MRI scanner (Signa, General Electric, Milwaukee, Wis). An initial high-quality 3-mm sagittal series was used for slice orientation. The anterior commissure–posterior commissure line was identified. An interleaved dual-echo series (repetition and echo times, 2500 and 30/80 milliseconds, respectively; thickness, 5 mm; field of view, 24 cm; resolution, 256×256) was then obtained parallel to the anterior commissure–posterior commissure line.

The MRI images were displayed on a computer workstation, and these images were rated blind to diagnosis. Basal ganglia were interactively outlined, and areas that were so defined were summed across slices and multiplied by slice thickness to yield volumes. Brain volume and cerebrospinal fluid (CSF) volumes were computed with semiautomated software that was developed in-house.[27]

Axial proton-density scans were used for the head of the caudate nucleus and putamen volume measurements.

phy) in severely affected patients with childhood-onset OCD.[11]

See also pages 574, 585, 595, 607, 617, and 625

Functional neuroimaging studies that have used positron emission tomography (PET) or single photon emission computed tomography (SPECT) did not demonstrate abnormalities of the caudate nucleus in most studies when relative caudate measures, normalized to correct for global metabolic group differences, were used (see "Comment" section).[12-18] One study observed a decreased perfusion of the caudate nucleus with 1 SPECT radioactive tracer, but a normal caudate nucleus with another radioligand.[19] Another research group observed normal glucose metabolism of the caudate nucleus (detected with PET) in 1 study,[17] but increased metabolism of the caudate nucleus in a later report.[20]

In the current study, MRI morphometric measures of the basal ganglia and the whole brain were calculated to assess whether the caudate nucleus was structurally normal in patients with OCD. Combined with a comprehensive analysis of prior structural and functional imaging studies, these results may help to clarify the status of caudate neuroimaging findings in OCD observed to date.

RESULTS

The MRI measures of subcortical volumes, global brain and CSF volumes, and BCRs were similar between groups (**Table 3**) Furthermore, no laterality differences (all $P>.30$) were observed by using the following asymmetry index (equation 5) for caudate and putamen volumes:

$$\text{(5)} \quad \text{Asymmetry Index}=(L-R)/[0.5\times(L+R)]$$

Two-way ANOVA revealed no significant effects for diagnosis, gender, or a gender×diagnosis interaction with

The **Figure** displays caudate and putamen boundaries that were drawn on an MRI scan that was taken of a control subject. The head of the caudate nucleus was measured in all slices superior to the anterior commissure and inferior to the body of the caudate nucleus. The borders of the head of the caudate nucleus were defined laterally by the anterior limb of the internal capsule and medially by the frontal horn or body of the lateral ventricle.

The putamen was measured in the 3 slices in which it was largest. Boundaries were defined anteromedially by the anterior limb of the internal capsule, posteromedially by the globus pallidus or genu and posterior limb of the internal capsule, and laterally by the external capsule and claustrum.

The BCR, an indicator of enlargement of the lateral ventricles at the frontal horns, is a linear measure of the intercaudate distance at the most narrow part of the frontal horns, divided by the width of the brain along the same line and multiplied by 100.[26,28] Intracranial and CSF volumes were measured as estimates of brain size and global atrophy, respectively, by using highly reliable semiautomated methods that have been previously described in detail.[27]

Interrater reliability was established for each measure. Two raters measured 32 scans separately. Intraclass correlations were as follows: 0.91 for the right side of the caudate nucleus, 0.85 for the left side of the caudate nucleus, 0.83 for the right side of the putamen, 0.86 for the left side of the putamen, 0.92 for the BCR, 0.99 for the brain volume, and 0.99 for the CSF volume.

STATISTICAL ANALYSES

The MRI measures for patients with OCD were compared with those of control subjects by using 2-tailed *t* tests. Two-way analysis of variance (ANOVA) was used to assess gender effects and the interaction between gender and diagnosis. Regression analysis was used to compare imaging measures with clinical data.

In addition to questions of the structure of the caudate nucleus in patients with OCD addressed in the current MRI study, there is further relevant controversy over whether the caudate nucleus is functionally abnormal in patients with OCD. Therefore, we examined the literature and performed an objective quantitative evaluation of caudate function (metabolism or blood flow) that was measured by using PET or SPECT. We performed a meta-analysis that compared and combined prior studies. To make measurements comparable across studies, normalized values were used (ie, the ratio of the caudate nucleus to the reference region reported in each study). Values were taken directly from studies that reported an analysis of normalized data.[12,16,17,19,20] For other articles that reported only absolute values for regional and global measures,[13-15,18] normalized values were calculated for each subject group from the data presented (ie, the ratio of the caudate nucleus to the normalization region [equation 1]), and the SD estimates were calculated by converting the respective absolute SD value into a proportion of the mean values for the caudate nucleus (equation 2):

(1) Normalized Mean Value=Absolute Caudate Mean/Absolute Reference Mean

(2) Normalized SD=Absolute SD/Absolute Caudate Mean

For the meta-analysis, the normalized mean value for each measure was adjusted so that the control mean value was equal to 1.00. This was accomplished for each measure by dividing each mean value (and each SD proportionately) by the respective mean control value (equation 3).

(3) Meta-analysis Values=Each Measure (Mean and SD)/Relative Control Mean

Each study's values were then weighted to reflect the number of subjects in each study and combined (with N=105 for patients with OCD and N=143 for control subjects [equation 4]):

(4) Weighted Average=$[\Sigma(\text{Value}_i \times N_i)/\Sigma N_i]$, for i=1 to 9 (for each study)

For each comparison (individual studies and meta-analysis), statistical analysis was performed by using unpaired 2-tailed *t* tests.[29] These values are presented in **Table 2**.

basal ganglia measures. Age did not correlate significantly with the caudate volume for the whole sample or for either diagnostic group separately. The putamen volume declined significantly with age for the combined sample ($r=-0.33$, n=45, $P<.03$) and for the control subjects ($r=-0.49$, n=21, $P<.03$), but not for the patients with OCD ($r=-0.26$, n=24, $P>.20$).

Regression analysis demonstrated a direct correlation in patients with OCD between the putamen volume and National Institute of Mental Health Global Severity score ($r=0.54$, n=24, $P<.006$) and between the caudate volume and the Hamilton Depression Rating Scale score ($r=0.41$, $P<.05$), but no correlations were observed with the Yale-Brown Obsessive Compulsive Scale total score or with the obsessions or compulsions subscores (all $P>.10$). Duration of illness did not correlate with basal ganglia volumes (all $P>.40$), nor did age at onset, although there was a trend toward an inverse correlation with the caudate volume ($r=-0.39$, $P=.06$).

The division of the patients with OCD into subgroups based on a history of depression (11 of 24 patients had a history of depression, although none were depressed at the time of this study) did not demonstrate basal ganglia volume differences (all $P>.60$). Likewise, imaging measures were similar between subjects who had never received medications (7 of 24 patients) and those who had been receiving medications (all $P>.30$).

Findings from the meta-analysis of the functional neuroimaging literature of patient-control baseline studies in OCD did not support consistent caudate metabolic or perfusion abnormality (patients with OCD [N=105], control subjects [N=143], Table 2).

COMMENT

We observed normal caudate nucleus size in patients with OCD compared with that in matched normal control subjects. No volumetric group differences were observed on any measure in this study. Asymmetry measures of the caudate nucleus and putamen were also similar be-

Table 1. Demographic and Clinical Characteristics for OCD and Control Groups*

Characteristic	Group	
	OCD (n=24)	Control (n=21)
Age, y	34.4±9.8†	31.1±10.4
Level of education, y	14.3±3.9	16.4±4.9
Race	W (n=24)	W (n=20); B (n=1)
Gender	M (n=17); F (n=7)	M (n=14); F (n=7)
Age at clinical onset, y	21.9±4.5	...
Score		
YBOC scale, total	25.8±5.0	...
NIMH Global Severity	9.2±1.5	...
Hamilton Depression Rating Scale	10.2±4.3	...

*OCD indicates obsessive-compulsive disorder; YBOC, Yale-Brown Obsessive Compulsive; and NIMH, National Institute of Mental Health.
†Data are given as the mean±SD.

tween subject groups. There was no evidence of ventricular enlargement in patients with OCD, as measured by the BCR or CSF volume. A review of the literature indicates that structural neuroimaging reports of caudate nucleus size have been mixed, and the preponderance of functional neuroimaging studies have reported normal relative caudate nucleus activity in patients with OCD.

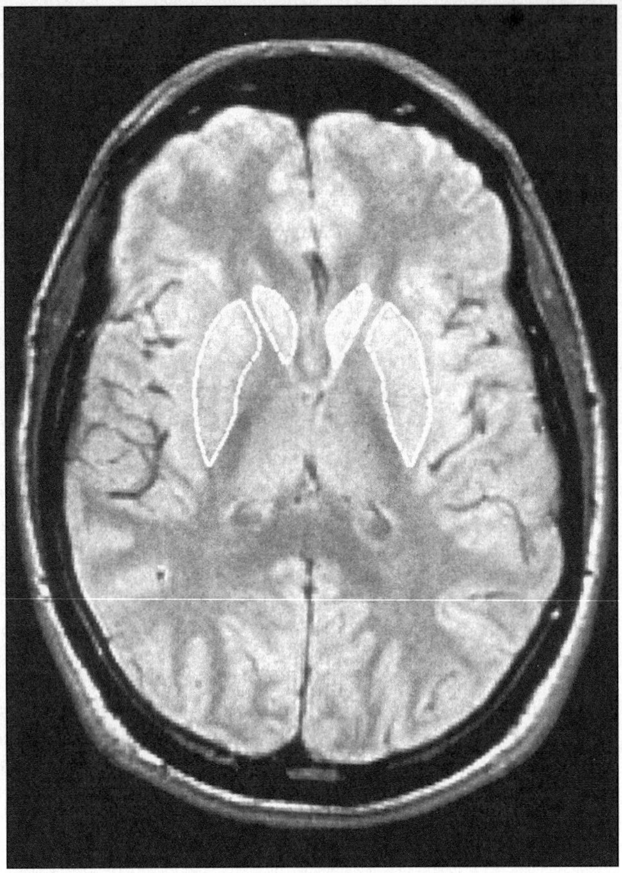

Magnetic resonance transaxial image at the level of the basal ganglia in a control subject depicts the outline of the caudate nucleus and putamen as measured for this study.

STRUCTURAL IMAGING OF THE CAUDATE NUCLEUS IN OCD

Results from quantitative MRI and x-ray computed tomography studies of the caudate nucleus in patients with OCD and normal control subjects are summarized in **Table 4**. Our findings agree with those of other studies that have reported normal caudate nucleus size in patients with OCD.[7,8] However, there were 2 studies that reported small caudate nuclei in patients with OCD, and these observations require further comment.[10,11]

In an MRI volumetric study, Robinson and associates[10] reported that patients with OCD had smaller caudate nuclei than did normal control subjects. However, their patient population also displayed considerably more ventricular enlargement, while those in the current study did not. In the current study, we observed only 3.6% group differences in measures of lateral ventricle width (BCR) and CSF volume. In contrast, Robinson et al[10] reported that lateral ventricles were, on average, 27.5% greater, and frontal horns were 24.3% greater in patients with OCD (although a high variance made these differences not statistically significant).

The imaging literature is inconsistent with regard to the presence of ventricular enlargement in patients with OCD (Table 4). Several studies, including the current one, did not find statistically significant evidence of ventricular enlargement in patients with OCD.[7,10,11,30] One research team reported an increased ventricular-brain ratio in 1 study,[31] but this finding was not replicated in a later report.[11] However, that later study[11] and others[10,30] reported some degree of increased ventricular size in patients with OCD that was not statistically significant because of a high variance of the ventricular measures. Such variability may be partly explained by the findings of another research team that reported significant lateral ventricular enlargement in patients with OCD who had high examination scores for soft neurological signs, but normal ventricles in patients with OCD who had low soft neurological sign scores (eg, those in the current study).[8] Thus, the heterogeneity of OCD, particularly pertaining to concomitant neurological abnormalities,[32] may explain why some reports observed ventricular enlargement while others found normal brain structure in patients with OCD.

One research team reported a reduced caudate volume (detected with computed tomography) in men who were suffering from childhood-onset OCD.[11] These patients consisted of a severely affected sample.[33] Furthermore, the childhood-onset version of OCD likely differs in origin and comorbidity from adult-onset OCD,[34] although differences could alternately be owing to developmental or severity effects. While the patients in the current, adult-onset OCD study were relatively free of tics, of 54 patients with childhood-onset OCD in another study, 59% experienced tics or Tourette disorder, with a higher incidence among males (67% had history of tics, 22% experienced Tourette disorder); most of these patients also had codiagnoses of anxiety disorder, attention-deficit hyperactivity disorder, or oppositional-conduct disorder.[35] These investigators concluded that Tourette dis-

Table 2. Normalized PET and SPECT Relative Caudate Measures From OCD Patient-Control Baseline Studies*

Study, y	Neuroimaging Method	Normalizing Region	Side	Patients With OCD	Control Subjects	t†	df, No.	P
Harris et al,[12] 1994	SPECT, HMPAO	Mean cortex	R	0.88±0.05	0.90±0.05	−0.94	16	>.2
			L	0.91±0.02	0.91±0.02	−0.3	10 OCD; 8 control	>.2
Rubin et al,[19] 1992‡	SPECT, HMPAO	Cerebellum	R	0.75±0.08	0.81±0.03	−2.13	18	.05
			L	0.76±0.07	0.81±0.05	−1.93	10 OCD; 10 control	>.05
	SPECT, xenon 133	Absolute	...	...	...	...	10 OCD;10 control	>.05
Benkelfat et al,[20] 1990	PET, FDG	Mean gray matter	R	1.05±0.12	0.97±0.11	1.71	36	>.05
			L	1.12±0.13	1.02±0.11	2.28	8 OCD; 30 control	.04
Nordahl et al,[17] 1989	PET, FDG	Mean gray matter	R	0.98±0.06	0.96±0.11	0.56	36	>.2
			L	1.03±0.10	1.01±0.11	0.58	8 OCD; 30 control	>.2
Swedo et al,[16] 1989	PET, FDG	Mean cortex	R	1.10±0.12	1.06±0.13	0.96	34	>.2
			L	1.13±0.13	1.18±0.13	−1.15	18 OCD; 18 control	>.2
Perani et al,[18] 1995§	PET, FDG	Mean cortex	Mean caudate	1.11±0.14	1.10±0.11	0.2	24; 11 OCD; 15 control	>.2
Baxter et al,[14] 1988§	PET, FDG	Ipsilateral hemispheric mean	R	1.28±0.15	1.27±0.24	0.11	18	>.2
			L	1.22±0.14	1.22±0.22	Small	10 OCD; 10 control	>.2
Baxter et al,[13] 1987§	PET, FDG	Ipsilateral hemispheric mean	R	1.29±0.20	1.25±0.15	0.6	26	>.2
			L	1.24±0.19	1.21±0.16	0.45	14 OCD; 14 control	>.2
Martinot et al,[15] 1990§	PET, FDG	Mean cortex	Mean basal ganglia	1.08±0.24	1.09±0.18	−0.1	22; 16 OCD; 8 control	>.2
Cumulative weighted meta-analysis	...	Control=1.00 for each study	L	1.01±0.13	1.00±0.11	0.65	246	>.2
			R	1.00±0.13	1.00±0.11	Small	105 OCD; 143 control	>.2

*PET indicates positron emission tomography; SPECT, single photon emission computed tomography; OCD, obsessive-compulsive disorder; HMPAO, technetium Tc99m hexamethyl-propylene amine oxime; NS, not significant; and FDG, fludeoxyglucose F 18.

†t values calculated according to the method of Matthews and Farewell.[29(p117)]

‡Reported paired t tests with lower P values. Ellipses indicate numbers were not provided.

§These studies did not report normalized values; normalized mean and SD were calculated from caudate divided by normalizing region absolute values.

order and childhood-onset OCD are not easily distinguished and, in some cases, may be alternative manifestations of the same underlying illness. Patients with Tourette disorder also had reduced caudate volumes (detected with MRI) compared with those in matched normal control subjects,[36] and other disorders that involve involuntary movement (eg, Huntington disease) are associated with a reduced caudate volume as well.[28,37] Thus, the high prevalence of neurological movement abnormalities (eg, tics and Tourette disorder), and the severity and comorbidities that arise from cases of childhood-onset OCD, may be related to the abnormality of the caudate nucleus that was observed by Luxenberg and associates.[11] An increased incidence of tics is often observed in patients with OCD, however, and the exclusion of patients with tics from the current study may have biased our results toward observation of normal caudate nucleus and normal ventricle size. To resolve this question, further studies that examine the relationship among OCD, tics, and basal ganglia anatomy are needed.

The results of the current study suggest that OCD symptom severity is not solely responsible for the reduced basal ganglia size that has been observed in other studies. In the current study, increased OCD symptom severity was associated with increased putamen volume, and the caudate volume was greater in subjects with higher depression scale scores, although no subject was clinically depressed.

Most studies, including the current one, reported similar caudate nucleus size asymmetry in both patients with OCD and normal control subjects.[7,8,10,11] One morphometric MRI report noted caudate asymmetry only in control subjects, with caudate volume symmetry in OCD, leading to an increased right-sided caudate volume in patients with OCD.[9] A potential confounding factor in that study was that the groups were not sex-matched, and differences observed in caudate symmetry may have been related in part to group gender composition. However, similar findings were observed in an MRI study of Tourette syndrome (a neurological disorder that often expresses obsessive-compulsive symptoms); this MRI

Table 3. MRI Measurements for OCD and Control Groups*

MRI Measurements†	Group: OCD (n=24)	Group: Control (n=21)	t (df=43)‡
Caudate nucleus			
L side	2.64±0.77§	2.51±0.60	0.63
R side	2.61±0.75	2.43±0.64	0.85
Putamen			
L side	4.46±0.55	4.41±0.50	0.31
R side	4.60±0.50	4.49±0.38	0.88
Total brain	1468±136	1464±161	0.09
Total CSF	98.1±39.4	101.8±42.5	0.31
BCR	8.6±2.1	8.3±1.8	0.49

*MRI indicates magnetic resonance imaging; OCD, obsessive-compulsive disorder; CSF, cerebrospinal fluid; and BCR, bicaudate ratio.

†Measurements are presented as volumes, in milliliters.

‡All P>.40 (not significant for all t values).

§Data are displayed as the mean±SD.

Table 4. Quantitative Structural Imaging Caudate and Lateral Ventricle Findings From OCD Patient-Control Studies*

Source, y	Structural Imaging	Mean±SD Age at Onset, y	Patient With OCD, No.	Control Subjects, No.	Lateral Ventricles†	Caudate Finding
Present study	MRI, volume	21.9±4.5	24 (17 men)	21 (14 men)	BCR, % CSF NS (+4%)	NS
Stein et al,[8] 1993	CT, volume	17.8±11.0	16 (10 men)	8 (3 men)	High SS (+60%)‡; low SS, NS (+12%)	NS
Kellner et al,[7] 1991	MRI, area	Not reported (mean age, 40 y; duration, 2+ y)	12 (7 men)	12 (7 men)	Intracaudate ratio, NS (−2%)	NS
Scarone et al,[9] 1992	MRI, volume	20.7±7.8	20 (8 men)	16 (10 men)	...	OCD (R)>control (R)‡ OCD (L)=control (L)= OCD (R)
Robinson et al,[10] 1995	MRI, volume	18.4±7.4	26 (14 men)	26 (16 men)	NS (+28%)	OCD<control‡
Luxenberg et al,[11] 1988	CT, volume	10±3.9§ (childhood onset)	10 (all men)	10 (all men)	NS (+19%)	OCD<control‡
Behar et al,[31] 1984	CT, area	10±3.9§ (childhood onset)	16 (13 men)	16 (13 men)	(+105%)‡	...
Insel et al,[30] 1983	CT, area	19.7±8.7	10 (6 men)	10 (6 men)	NS (+16%)	...
Garber et al,[6] 1989‖	MRI, T_1	18±9	32 (20 men)	14 (9 men)	...	T_1 symmetry for both OCD and control
Calabrese et al,[38] 1993‖	MRI, T_1	20.7±7.8	20 (8 men)	16 (10 men)	...	Control T_1 symmetry, OCD T_1 asymmetry‡

*OCD indicates obsessive-compulsive disorder; MRI, magnetic resonance imaging; BCR, bicaudate ratio; %CSF, cerebrospinal fluid percentage; NS, not significant (>.05); CT, computed tomography; and SS, soft neurological signs.

†For group of patients with OCD, the mean percent difference from control subjects is given in parentheses.

‡$P<.05$.

§Age at onset estimated from the study of Flament et al[33] (description of 19 patients from the same clinic).

‖These studies reported caudate T_1 signal intensity, not measures of caudate size.

study also reported that patients had basal ganglia symmetry, while control subjects had asymmetrical caudate volume.[36] Other MRI studies examined asymmetry in image T_1 signal intensity in patients with OCD and normal control subjects. In 1 study, caudate symmetry existed for both groups,[6] although another study observed T_1 asymmetry in the group with OCD.[38]

FUNCTIONAL IMAGING OF THE CAUDATE NUCLEUS IN OCD

While MRI and computed tomography enable the observation of caudate structure, PET and SPECT can be used to study caudate function (ie, metabolism and blood flow). Since there is a theoretical framework for an abnormality of the caudate nucleus in OCD,[2-5] we evaluated the functional imaging literature to determine whether there may be abnormal caudate function despite the observation of normal OCD caudate structure in the current study. However, findings from functional neuroimaging patient-control baseline studies do not well support an abnormality of the caudate nucleus in patients with OCD.[39]

The PET data can be presented as absolute metabolic values (in milligrams per 100 mL per minute) or as relative regional measures that are normalized to a reference value (eg, the cortical mean). While 4 studies found no significant global absolute metabolic differences between patients with OCD and control subjects,[16-18,20] 1 research group reported increased absolute global metabolism in patients with OCD,[13,14] and another team reported global absolute hypometabolism in patients with OCD.[15] In the presence of differences in the global absolute metabolic rate, a difference in regional absolute measures could also exist; however, this difference may not be regionally specific, and it may merely reflect the overall global group difference that is observed. Therefore, to assess objectively the literature and to use comparable measures among studies, normalized, relative measures (ratios) were compared and combined into a meta-analysis (see Table 2 for data and the "Statistical Analyses" subsection of the "Patients, Control Subjects, and Methods" section for details on calculations).

The meta-analysis results, combining data from available functional neuroimaging studies of OCD, indicated similar caudate function (~1% differences) between patients with OCD and control subjects (Table 2). Most researchers observed normal relative caudate function after normalizing for global metabolism.[12-18] In studies that reported whole-brain absolute metabolic differences, similar caudate absolute "differences," either increases[13,14] or decreases,[15] disappeared after accounting for global group metabolic values. One research group found normal caudate function in 1 study of 8 patients with OCD,[17] but increased left-sided caudate metabolism in a follow-up study of 8 patients with OCD—5 of whom were also in the first study.[20] One SPECT report by Rubin and associates[19] found normal absolute basal ganglia perfusion by using the tracer xenon 133; however, they found decreased bilateral caudate perfusion and a trend toward decreased left-sided putamen perfusion by using the blood flow tracer technetium Tc99m hexamethyl-propylene amine oxime. Since several groups have reported enlarged lateral ventricles[8,10,31] or reduced caudate nucleus size[10,11] in some patients with OCD, if the population studied by Rubin and colleagues[19] exhibited either, or a combination, of these abnormalities, such structural deficits could also be reflected as a reduced caudate radioactive tracer signal on the functional image. However, structural images on these subjects, to test this hypothesis, were unavailable.

Functional activation studies observed a right-sided caudate increase in response to obsessive-compulsive symptom provocation,[40,41] a right-sided caudate decrease with pharmacological or behavioral therapy,[2] or a left-sided caudate decrease with drug treatment,[42] although other studies did not observe a change in the caudate nucleus with pharmacotherapy.[18,43] Some caution is warranted in interpreting the results of these studies as they do not observe responses of matched normal control subjects to similar stimuli. Changes in the caudate nucleus do not demonstrate that the caudate nucleus is abnormal at baseline. Researchers who observed a caudate decrease with clinical treatment[2,42] also reported a normal relative caudate function at baseline.[13,14,17] Thus, changes in the caudate nucleus do not necessarily mean that the caudate nucleus is abnormal at baseline, or that caudate changes are a direct, or abnormal, result of provocation or therapy. For example, changes in the caudate nucleus may result from excitatory input from the frontal cortex.

Contrasted with negative findings in most studies of caudate function, an increased relative activity was reported in the medifrontal,[2,16,19,24] right frontal,[12,16,17,20] anterior cingulate,[16,18] and orbitofrontal[13,14,17,19,20] cortex in patients with OCD. These findings are consistent with theories of a prefrontal abnormality that is involved in OCD physiologic and psychiatric dysfunction.[44-46] Hyperfrontal function was inversely correlated with anxiety in patients with OCD,[12,24] suggesting that these observations do not merely reflect heightened anxiety in patients with OCD. Pharmacological agents that block serotonergic reuptake reduced obsessive-compulsive symptoms and reduced hyperfrontal function.[18,20,25,43,47]

CONCLUSIONS

Although the structural and functional neuroimaging literature does not consistently substantiate involvement of the caudate nucleus, there is a theoretical framework for caudate dysfunction as an integral feature of OCD, perhaps by way of a frontal cortex–basal ganglia–thalamus–frontal cortical circuit.[2-5] Other evidence for an association of OCD and basal ganglia abnormalities include the strong association of Tourette disorder[35] and Sydenham chorea[48] with OCD. The limited neuroimaging support does not refute the possibility of caudate dysfunction in patients with OCD, but merely indicates that whatever abnormality might exist in the caudate nucleus has not been consistently appreciable with neuroimaging to date. Moreover, findings from a recent family study of patients with OCD confirmed that OCD is a heterogeneous condition,[32] and the degree of basal ganglia abnormality may differ in subgroups, particularly in relation to severity of neurological signs. Subtle abnormalities of basal ganglia connectivity with other regions, or perhaps aberrant modulation between frontal regions and the basal ganglia, could be a component of OCD pathology; however, it need not be associated with an abnormal caudate nucleus size, metabolic rate, or blood flow, and therefore, it might not be consistently visible to MRI, PET, or SPECT.

Accepted for publication January 1, 1996.

This work was supported in part by grants MH40391 and MH437775 from the National Institutes of Health, Bethesda, Md, by grant DA05317 from the National Institute on Drug Abuse, Bethesda, by grant RR0722 from the National Institutes of Health Division of Research Resources/The Johns Hopkins Outpatient Clinical Research Center, Baltimore, Md, and by The Johns Hopkins Interdisciplinary Committee on Nuclear Magnetic Resonance Research (Dr Pearlson).

Presented in part as a poster at the 145th Annual Meeting of the American Psychiatric Association, Washington, DC, May 2-7, 1992.

Reprints: Gordon J. Harris, PhD, New England Medical Center, Box 1007, 750 Washington St, Boston, MA 02111.

REFERENCES

1. American Psychiatric Association. *Diagnostic and Statistical Manual of Mental Disorders, Third Edition, Revised.* Washington, DC: American Psychiatric Association; 1987.
2. Baxter L Jr, Schwartz JM, Bergman KS, Szuba MP, Guze BH, Mazziotta JC, Alazraki A, Selin CE, Ferng HK, Munford P, Phelps ME. Caudate glucose metabolic rate changes with both drug and behavior therapy for obsessive-compulsive disorder. *Arch Gen Psychiatry.* 1992;49:681-689.
3. Modell JG, Mountz JM, Curtis GC, Greden JF. Neurophysiologic dysfunction in basal ganglia/limbic striatal and thalamocortical circuits as a pathogenetic mechanism of obsessive-compulsive disorder. *J Neuropsychiatry Clin Neurosci.* 1989;1:27-36.
4. Rapoport JL. Obsessive compulsive disorder and basal ganglia dysfunction. *Psychol Med.* 1990;20:465-469.
5. Wise SP, Rapoport JL. Obsessive-compulsive disorder: is it basal ganglia dysfunction? In: Rapoport JL, ed. *Obsessive-compulsive Disorder in Children and Adolescents.* Washington, DC: American Psychiatric Press Inc; 1988:327-344.
6. Garber HJ, Ananth JV, Chiu LC, Griswold VJ, Oldendorf WH. Nuclear magnetic resonance study of obsessive-compulsive disorder. *Am J Psychiatry.* 1989;146:1001-1005.
7. Kellner CH, Jolley RR, Holgate RC, Austin L, Lydiard RB, Laraia M, Ballenger JC. Brain MRI in obsessive-compulsive disorder. *Psychiatry Res.* 1991;36:45-49.
8. Stein DJ, Hollander E, Chan S, DeCaria CM, Hilal S, Liebowitz MR, Klein DF. Computed tomography and neurological soft signs in obsessive-compulsive disorder. *Psychiatry Res.* 1993;50:143-150.
9. Scarone S, Colombo C, Livian S, Abbruzzese M, Ronchi P, Locatelli M, Scotti G, Smeraldi E. Increased right caudate nucleus size in obsessive-compulsive disorder: detection with magnetic resonance imaging. *Psychiatry Res Neuroimag.* 1992;45:115-121.
10. Robinson D, Wu H, Munne RA, Ashtari M, Alvir JM, Lerner G, Koreen A, Cole K, Bogerts B. Reduced caudate nucleus volume in obsessive-compulsive disorder. *Arch Gen Psychiatry.* 1995;52:393-398.
11. Luxenberg JS, Swedo SE, Flament MF, Friedland RP, Rapoport J, Rapoport SI. Neuroanatomical abnormalities in obsessive-compulsive disorder detected with quantitative x-ray computed tomography. *Am J Psychiatry.* 1988;145:1089-1093.
12. Harris GJ, Hoehn-Saric R, Lewis RW, Pearlson GD, Streeter C. Mapping of SPECT regional cerebral perfusion abnormalities in obsessive-compulsive disorder. *Hum Brain Map.* 1994;1:237-248.
13. Baxter LR, Phelps ME, Mazziotta JC, Guze BH, Schwartz JM, Selin CE. Local cerebral glucose metabolic rates in obsessive-compulsive disorder: a comparison with rates in unipolar depression and in normal controls. *Arch Gen Psychiatry.* 1987;44:211-218.
14. Baxter LR, Schwartz JM, Mazziotta JC, Phelps ME, Pahl JJ, Guze BH, Fairbanks L. Cerebral glucose metabolic rates in non-depressed patients with obsessive-compulsive disorder. *Am J Psychiatry.* 1988;145:1560-1563.
15. Martinot JL, Allilaire JF, Mazoyer BM, Hantouche E, Huret JD, Legaut-Demare

F, Deslauriers AG, Hardy P, Pappata S, Baron JC, Syrota A. Obsessive-compulsive disorder: a clinical, neuropsychological, and positron emission tomography study. *Acta Psychiatr Scand.* 1990;82:233-242.

16. Swedo SE, Schapiro MB, Grady CL, Cheslow DL, Leonard HL, Kumar A, Friedland R, Rapoport SI, Rapoport J. Cerebral glucose metabolism in childhood-onset obsessive-compulsive disorder. *Arch Gen Psychiatry.* 1989;46:518-523.
17. Nordahl TE, Benkelfat C, Semple WE, Gross M, King AC, Cohen RM. Cerebral glucose metabolic rates in obsessive compulsive disorder. *Neuropsychopharmacology.* 1989;2:23-28.
18. Perani D, Colombo C, Bressi S, Bonfanti A, Grassi F, Scarone S, Bellodi L, Smeraldi E, Fazio F. [18F]FDG PET study in obsessive-compulsive disorder: a clinical/metabolic correlation study after treatment. *Br J Psychiatry.* 1995;166: 244-250.
19. Rubin RT, Villanueva-Meyer J, Ananth J, Trajmar PG, Mena I. Regional xenon 133 cerebral blood flow and cerebral technetium 99m HMPAO uptake in unmedicated patients with obsessive-compulsive disorder and matched control subjects. *Arch Gen Psychiatry.* 1992;49:695-702.
20. Benkelfat C, Nordahl TE, Semple WE, King C, Murphy DL, Cohen RM. Local cerebral glucose metabolic rates in obsessive-compulsive disorder. *Arch Gen Psychiatry.* 1990;47:840-848.
21. Goodman WK, Price LH, Rasmussen SA, Mazure C, Fleischmann RL, Hill CL, Heninger GR, Charney DS. The Yale-Brown Obsessive Compulsive Scale. *Arch Gen Psychiatry.* 1989;46:1006-1016.
22. Insel TR, Murphy DL, Cohen RM, Alterman I, Kilts C, Linnoila M. Obsessive-compulsive disorder: a double-blind trial of clomipramine and clorgyline. *Arch Gen Psychiatry.* 1983;40:605-612.
23. Hamilton M. Development of a rating scale for primary depressive illness. *Br J Soc Psychol.* 1967;6:278-296.
24. Machlin SR, Harris GJ, Pearlson GD, Hoehn-Saric R, Jeffery P, Camargo EE. Elevated medial-frontal cerebral blood flow in obsessive-compulsive patients: a SPECT study. *Am J Psychiatry.* 1991;148:1240-1242.
25. Hoehn-Saric R, Pearlson GD, Harris GJ, Machlin SR, Camargo EE. Effects of fluoxetine on regional cerebral blood flow in obsessive-compulsive patients. *Am J Psychiatry.* 1991;148:1243-1245.
26. Aylward EH, Schwartz J, Machlin S, Pearlson GD. Bicaudate ratio as a measure of caudate volume on MR images. *AJNR Am J Neuroradiol.* 1991;12: 1217-1222.
27. Harris GJ, Rhew EH, Noga JT, Pearlson GD. A user-friendly method for rapid brain and CSF volume calculation using transaxial MRI images. *Psychiatry Res Neuroimag.* 1991;40:61-68.
28. Harris GJ, Pearlson GD, Peyser CE, Aylward EH, Roberts J, Barta PE, Chase GA, Folstein SE. Putamen volume reduction on magnetic resonance images exceeds caudate changes in mild Huntington's disease. *Ann Neurol.* 1992;31: 69-75.
29. Matthews DE, Farewell VT. *Using and Understanding Medical Statistics.* Basel, Switzerland: S Karger Publishers; 1988.
30. Insel TR, Donnelly EF, Lalakea ML, Alterman IS, Murphy DL. Neurological and neuropsychological studies of patients with obsessive-compulsive disorder. *Biol Psychiatry.* 1983;18:741-751.
31. Behar D, Rapoport JL, Berg CJ, Denckla MB, Mann L, Cox C, Fedio P, Zahn T, Wolfman MG. Computerized tomography and neuropsychological test measures in adolescents with obsessive-compulsive disorder. *Am J Psychiatry.* 1984;141:363-369.
32. Pauls DL, Alsobrook JP, Goodman W, Rasmussen S, Leckman JF. A family study of obsessive-compulsive disorder. *Am J Psychiatry.* 1995;152:76-84.
33. Flament MF, Rapoport JL, Berg CJ, Sceery W, Kilts C, Mellstrom B, Linnoila M. Clomipramine treatment of childhood obsessive-compulsive disorder: a double-blind controlled study. *Arch Gen Psychiatry.* 1985;42:977-983.
34. Flament MF. Recent findings in childhood onset obsessive compulsive disorder. In: Hollander E, Zohar J, Marazziti D, Oliver B, eds. *Current Insights in Obsessive Compulsive Disorder.* New York, NY: John Wiley & Sons Inc; 1994: 23-40.
35. Leonard HL, Lenane MC, Swedo SE, Rettew DC, Gershon ES, Rapoport JL. Tics and Tourette's disorder: a 2- to 7-year follow-up of 54 obsessive-compulsive children. *Am J Psychiatry.* 1992;149:1244-1251.
36. Peterson B, Riddle MA, Cohen DJ, Katz LD, Smith JC, Hardin MT, Leckman JF. Reduced basal ganglia volumes in Tourette's syndrome using three-dimensional reconstruction techniques from magnetic resonance images. *Neurology.* 1993;43:941-949.
37. Aylward EH, Brandt J, Codori AM, Mangus RS, Barta PE, Harris GJ. Reduced basal ganglia volume associated with the gene for Huntington's disease in asymptomatic at-risk persons. *Neurology.* 1994;44:823-828.
38. Calabrese G, Colombo C, Bonfanti A, Scotti G, Scarone S. Caudate nucleus abnormalities in obsessive-compulsive disorder: measurements of MRI signal intensity. *Psychiatry Res.* 1993;50:89-92.
39. Harris GJ, Pearlson GD, Hoehn-Saric R. Single photon emission computed tomography in obsessive-compulsive disorder. *Arch Gen Psychiatry.* 1993;50: 498-501.
40. Rauch SL, Jenike MA, Alpert NM, Baer L, Breiter HCR, Savage CR, Fischman AJ. Regional cerebral blood flow measured during symptom provocation in obsessive-compulsive disorder using oxygen 15–labeled carbon dioxide and positron emission tomography. *Arch Gen Psychiatry.* 1994;51:62-70.
41. McGuire PK, Bench CJ, Frith CD, Marks IM, Frackowiak RSJ, Dolan RJ. Functional anatomy of obsessive-compulsive phenomena. *Br J Psychiatry.* 1994; 164:459-468.
42. Benkelfat C, Murphy DL, Zohar J, Hill JL, Grover G, Insel TR. Clomipramine in obsessive-compulsive disorder: further evidence for a serotonergic mechanism of action. *Arch Gen Psychiatry.* 1989;46:23-28.
43. Swedo SE, Pietrini P, Leonard HL, Schapiro MB, Rettew DC, Goldberger EL, Rapoport SI, Rapoport JL, Grady CL. Cerebral glucose metabolism in childhood-onset obsessive-compulsive disorder: revisualization during pharmacotherapy. *Arch Gen Psychiatry.* 1992;49:690-694.
44. Baxter LR. PET studies of cerebral function in major depression and obsessive-compulsive disorder: the emerging prefrontal cortex consensus. *Ann Clin Psychiatry.* 1991;3:103-109.
45. Hoehn-Saric R, Benkelfat C. Structural and functional brain imaging in obsessive-compulsive disorder. In: Hollander E, Zohar J, Marazziti D, Olivier B, eds. *Current Insights in Obsessive-compulsive Disorder.* New York, NY: John Wiley & Sons Inc; 1994:183-211.
46. Insel TR. Toward a neuroanatomy of obsessive-compulsive disorder. *Arch Gen Psychiatry.* 1992;49:739-744.
47. Hoehn-Saric R, Harris GJ, Pearlson GD, Cox CS, Machlin SR, Camargo EE. A fluoxetine-induced frontal lobe syndrome in an obsessive-compulsive patient. *J Clin Psychiatry.* 1991;52:131-133.
48. Swedo SE. Sydenham's chorea: a model for childhood autoimmune neuropsychiatric disorders [clinical conference]. *JAMA.* 1994;272:1788-1791.

ORIGINAL ARTICLE

Sex Differences in Human Brain Morphometry and Metabolism: An In Vivo Quantitative Magnetic Resonance Imaging and Positron Emission Tomography Study on the Effect of Aging

Declan G. M. Murphy, MD; Charles DeCarli, MD; Andrew R. McIntosh, PhD; Eileen Daly; Marc J. Mentis, MD; Pietro Pietrini, MD; Joanna Szczepanik, MA; Mark B. Schapiro, MD; Cheryl L. Grady, PhD; Barry Horwitz, PhD; Stanley I. Rapoport, MD

Background: There are significant age and sex effects in cognitive ability and brain disease. However, sex differences in aging of human brain areas associated with nonreproductive behavior have not been extensively studied. We hypothesized that there would be significant sex differences in aging of brain areas that subserve speech, visuospatial, and memory function.

Methods: We investigated sex differences in the effect of aging on human brain morphometry by means of volumetric magnetic resonance imaging and on regional cerebral metabolism for glucose by positron emission tomography. In the magnetic resonance imaging study, we examined 69 healthy right-handed subjects (34 women and 35 men), divided into young (age range, 20 to 35 years) and old (60 to 85 years) groups. In the positron emission tomography study, we investigated 120 healthy right-handed subjects (65 women and 55 men) aged 21 to 91 years.

Results: In the magnetic resonance imaging study, age-related volume loss was significantly greater in men than women in whole brain and frontal and temporal lobes, whereas it was greater in women than men in hippocampus and parietal lobes. In the positron emission tomography study, significant sex differences existed in the effect of age on regional brain metabolism, and asymmetry of metabolism, in the temporal and parietal lobes, Broca's area, thalamus, and hippocampus.

Conclusions: We found significant sex differences in aging of brain areas that are essential to higher cognitive functioning. Thus, our findings may explain some of the age-sex differences in human cognition and response to brain injury and disease.

Arch Gen Psychiatry. 1996;53:585-594

THERE HAS been a substantial increase in the number of humans who reach old age, and by the year 2010 the proportion of the population aged more than 65 years will grow by 30%.[1] This has led to an increasing number of people who experience age-related cognitive decline, late-life diseases, such as Alzheimer's disease (AD), late-onset forms of anxiety and affective disorders, and psychotic disorders.[2,3] Furthermore, this same change in population demography has been accompanied by the realization that there may be significant sex differences in age-related cognitive decline[4-6] and in various age-related neuropsychiatric conditions, including AD[7] and late-onset schizophrenia.[8,9] However, research has focused mainly on mechanisms underlying sex differences in reproductive behavior, and not on sex differences in aging of human brain areas associated with higher cognition.

Postmortem studies reported sex differences in human regional brain weight, area, volume, and asymmetry.[10-15] In general, females have a smaller brain volume with less striking anatomic asymmetries in temporal lobe regions. Postmortem studies that examined sex differences in brain aging found that brain weight decreases in the fifth and sixth decades of life in women compared with the sixth and seventh decades of life in men[16]; in contrast, the area of corpus callosum decreases significantly with age in men but not women.[17] Computed tomographic studies have reported significant gender differences in age-associated ventricular enlargement.[18,19] A precipitous increase in ventricular volume begins in the fifth decade in men and the sixth decade in women.[18] However, once the atrophy process is started, its

See Subjects and Methods on next page

From the Laboratory of Neurosciences, National Institute on Aging, National Institutes of Health, Bethesda, Md.

SUBJECTS AND METHODS

SUBJECTS

All subjects were participants in a clinical program on brain aging conducted by the Laboratory of Neurosciences of the National Institute on Aging, Bethesda, Md. All were recruited from a relatively affluent area of Maryland; some volunteered because they were already aware of our program from friends and/or media news items, and others were recruited by advertisements in local newspapers. Every subject was rigorously screened[29] to exclude illnesses that could affect brain function, and all had normal results of a structured neurologic and cognitive examination,[31] urine and blood tests (including serology), chest radiography, and electrocardiography. All were medication free for at least 4 weeks before study. Informed consent was always obtained, and the research was approved by the National Institute on Aging institutional review board (National Institutes of Health protocol 80-AG-26).

We studied 69 subjects by MR imaging (34 women and 35 men) and 120 by PET (65 women and 55 men). All subjects were right handed, and men and women did not differ significantly in age or intelligence (**Table 1**). Recruitment difficulties and scanner availability in the MR imaging study led to relatively few middle-aged volunteers, and so subjects were divided into young (age range, 20 to 35 years) and old (60 to 85 years) groups. Of the young subjects, 15 were women (mean±SD age, 27±4 years) and 21 were men (25±2 years), and of the old subjects, 19 were women (68±6 years) and 14 were men (72±6 years). Our PET data set was larger than our MR imaging set, and, in the PET study, the mean (±SD) age of the 65 women was 52±23 years (range, 21 to 91 years) and that of the 55 men was 54±22 years (range, 21 to 90 years).

NEUROPSYCHOLOGICAL TESTING

The Wechsler Adult Intelligence Scale[32] was administered as an omnibus test of language and visuospatial functions and was scored to yield full-scale IQs.

MR IMAGING

The MR imaging of the brain was performed on a 0.5-T scanner (Picker Instruments, Cleveland, Ohio) and on a 1.5-T scanner (General Electric Medical System, Milwaukee, Wis).

The 0.5-T scanner was used to quantify volumes of cranium, lobar brain matter, ventricular and peripheral cerebrospinal fluid, and caudate, lenticular, and thalamic nuclei. Volumes of cranium, cerebral hemispheres, lobar brain, cerebellum, and ventricular and peripheral cerebrospinal fluid were acquired from 6-mm-thick contiguous coronal slices (repetition time, 2000 milliseconds; echo time, 20 milliseconds) obtained perpendicular to the inferior orbitomeatal line. The caudate, lenticular, and thalamic nuclei were measured from 7-mm-thick, contiguous axial slices (repetition time, 2000 milliseconds; echo time, 20 milliseconds) obtained from the foramen magnum to vertex, parallel to the inferior orbitomeatal line.[33]

The 1.5-T MR imaging was used to measure volumes of the amygdala, hippocampus, and parahippocampal gyrus, and data were obtained from 5-mm-thick contiguous coronal slices (repetition time, 400 milliseconds; echo time, 20 milliseconds) obliquely centered at and parallel to the sylvian fissure. Hippocampal sequences were available in 25 men (13 young and 12 old) and 23 women (11 young and 12 old). There were no significant differences in age or intelligence between those who did and those who did not undergo hippocampal MR imaging.

Data were analyzed with a computer system (VAX 11/750, Digital Equipment Corp, Landover, Md) and an image array processor (Gould 8400, Vicom Inc, Fairfax, Va) after being displayed on a television monitor. Scans were analyzed without knowledge of the subject's clinical status. Right and left caudate, lenticular, and thalamic nuclei, hippocampus, amygdala, parahippocampal gyrus, and lobar volumes were traced using a method that has been previously described.[29] Also, a segmentation analysis[33] was used to determine volumes of brain matter and ventricular and peripheral cerebrospinal fluid. The frontal lobe was defined as all supratemporal structures anterior to the aqueduct of Sylvius. Temporal lobe volume was traced from the anterior pole of the temporal lobe to the aqueduct of Sylvius. The superior temporal lobe boundary was defined as a straight line drawn from the angle of the medial temporal lobe, where it attaches to the temporal stem, to the midpoint of the operculum; dura of the middle cranial fossa was then traced around each temporal lobe to complete the region. Parietal lobe was defined as the brain matter posterior to the aqueduct of Sylvius, extending to the medial transverse fissure of striate cortex. The remaining caudal portions of the cerebral hemispheres were defined as parieto-occipital. Hippocampus and amygdala were traced by means of an adaptation of the criteria of Watson et al[34]—namely, we did not trace the hippocampus any further posterior than the aqueduct of Sylvius. Parahippocampal gyrus was also traced anterior to the aqueduct of Sylvius; its inferolateral boundary was defined by the collateral sulcus, its superior boundary by the subiculum, and its medial boundary by the entorhinal cortex.

The volume of each region was calculated by multiplying the summed pixel cross-sectional areas by slice thickness. Women were significantly shorter than men and had a smaller head size. Thus, to control for the relationship of cerebral volume to head size, brain volumes were normalized as a percentage of the traced intracranial volume. Brain asymmetries were calculated by dividing right-left volumes of a structure by total intracranial volume.

velocity increases with age more rapidly in women than in men.[19] Magnetic resonance (MR) imaging studies of sex differences in brain aging are in disagreement. Some found no sex difference,[20] whereas others[21,22] reported that men have a greater age-related loss of brain volume than women, and that age-related atrophy is asymmetric in men but symmetric in women. However, no study has examined sex differences in age-related effects on all brain lobar regions—including parietal and occipital lobes in addition to frontal and temporal lobes and subcortical nuclei (lenticular, caudate, and thalamic)—and examined hippocampus and amygdala as separate structures.

See also pages 574, 577, 595, 607, 617, and 625

Intrarater and interrater reliabilities were determined for all brain regions of interest (ROIs) traced by the operators as part of this analysis. Highly significant interrater and intrarater reliabilities were obtained in all cases. The interrater correlation coefficients were $F>4.0$ and $P<.01$.[35]

PET STUDY

The rCMRglc values were obtained by means of PET with (18F)-2-fluoro-2-deoxy-D-glucose. Studies were performed on a tomograph (Scanditronix PC-1024-7B, Uppsala, Sweden) that can simultaneously acquire data from seven slices and that has an in-plane resolution of 6 mm and an axial resolution of 10 mm. Before scanning, each subject underwent radial artery catheterization, and arterial blood samples obtained during the procedure were used to measure plasma glucose concentrations and radioactivity.

Scans were carried out with lights dimmed and the patient's eyes and ears covered to reduce sensory input, and a thermoplastic mask was fitted to maintain positioning in the scanner. A multislice transmission scan was performed at two interleaved levels for attenuation correction at the beginning of each scan. Two methods of acquiring transmission data were used. Postprocessing techniques, based on internal standards, were used to ensure comparability. Forty-five minutes after injection of 185 MBq of (18F)-2-fluoro-2-deoxy-D-glucose, two interleaved emission scans were obtained at the same level as transmission scans. Fourteen slices were acquired, parallel to the externally defined inferior orbitomeatal line.

Data from the scans were analyzed with the use of a template of 8-mm-diameter circular ROIs to sample metabolic rates from cortical and subcortical areas.[36] Each template slice was matched to a slice from the patient's scan. Brooks' modification[37] of the operational equation of Sokoloff et al was used to calculate rCMRglc in each ROI, with the use of a lumped constant of 0.418.[38] Scans were analyzed by members of the PET Unit of the Laboratory of Neurosciences; interrater reliability coefficients[35] for the regions analyzed ranged from 0.87 to 0.99.

We previously reported[29,30,39] significant effects of the X chromosome and sex steroids on verbal and visuospatial abilities and on structure and metabolism of parietal, superior parietal, temporal, midtemporal, and occipital cortex, hippocampus, and lenticular, caudate, and thalamic nuclei. Therefore, to decrease the number of statistical comparisons, and thus the chance of generating false-positive (type 1) errors, regional metabolic rates were averaged[36] into total values for these ROIs and Broca's and Wernicke's areas. We have previously defined[36] Broca's and Wernicke's areas on a slice 45 mm above the inferior orbitomeatal line as an inferior frontal region (premotor; ROI 12) and a superior temporal region (superior temporal; ROI 13), respectively. Hippocampus was defined on a slice 35 mm above the inferior orbitomeatal line as a posterior medial temporal region (ROI 10) and was a composite measure including parahippocampal gyrus. Only absolute metabolic rates (milligrams per 100 g per minute) were evaluated.

Right-left cerebral metabolic asymmetries were examined with the following equation, where R=rCMRglc in a right-sided region and L=rCMRglc in the homologous left-sided region: % metabolic asymmetry $=\{(R-L)/[(R+L)/2]\}\times 100$.

Anterior-posterior ratios were calculated for Broca's-Wernicke's area by the same equation but substituting the terms *Broca* and *Wernicke* for *right* and *left*, respectively.

STATISTICS

In the MR imaging study, statistical comparisons were carried out only on brain volumes normalized to intracranial volume to correct cerebral volume to head size because men had significantly bigger heads than women—and head size is directly proportional to brain size. Age (young vs old), sex (male vs female), and age×sex interactions were studied by an analysis of variance for unbalanced cells,[40] and a Student-Newman-Keuls multiple range post hoc correction for multiple comparisons.[40] The level of statistical significance was defined as $P<.05$.

Statistical comparisons in the PET study were carried out on absolute metabolic rates and not ratios because the denominator (whole-brain glucose metabolism) changes with age, but there is no uniform relationship between age-related changes in whole-brain glucose metabolism and ROIs. Thus, changes in ratios would not accurately reflect changes in the numerator (regional glucose metabolism). For example, if regional glucose metabolism of caudate does not change with age, but whole-brain metabolism decreases, then an artifactual increase in caudate metabolism would be reported with the use of ratios.

Metabolic activity was compared by means of a univariate multiple regression with age, sex, and age×sex interaction as the predictor variables.[41] This regression method is mathematically identical to a two-way analysis of variance with regard to age, sex, and their interaction as factors. The advantage of the regression equation is that we were able to keep age as a continuous variable because of the wide age distribution of our sample (20 to 91 years). The level of statistical significance was defined as $P<.05$. For brain ROIs that showed significant age-related sexual dimorphism, nonlinear trends were assessed by testing if a quadratic regression equation significantly improved the proportion of variance accounted for compared with a linear regression equation.[41] Also, for brain ROIs that showed a significant age×sex interaction, the Johnson-Neyman technique was used to define regions where the regression lines for the two groups significantly differed.[42]

Changes in bulk volume of brain tissue can be measured by MR imaging, and this may not reflect changes in neuronal metabolism and function. In contrast, single photon emission computed tomography and positron emission tomography (PET) allow measurement of cerebral blood flow and regional cerebral metabolic rates for glucose (rCMRglc). Sex differences have been reported in cerebral blood flow by means of single photon emission computed tomography,[23-25] and in cerebral blood flow and rCMRglc by means of PET.[23,26-28] However, there are no published reports on sex differences in age-related effects on metabolism of the healthy human brain.

Our aim was to determine whether the effect of aging differed between sexes on brain morphometry by means of in vivo MR imaging, and on rCMRglc by means

Table 1. Characteristics of Male and Female Subjects*

Variable	Subjects in MR Imaging Study: Men (n=35)	Subjects in MR Imaging Study: Women (n=34)	Subjects in PET Study: Men (n=55)	Subjects in PET Study: Women (n=65)
Age, y	44±23	50±21	54±22	52±23
Education, y	17±1	16±1	17±1	16±1
Wechsler full-scale IQ	122±12	123±11	128±12	123±14
Wechsler verbal IQ	122±12	123±13	129±13	124±15
Wechsler performance IQ	123±13	120±12	124±12	120±13
Blood pressure, mm Hg				
Systolic	125±14	118±18	125±14	118±18
Diastolic	75±9	73±11	75±9	73±11
Pulse, beats/min	68±8	72±8	68±8	72±8
Height, cm	174±8	159±9†	170±7	156±8†
Weight, kg	74±11	60±9†	74±11	60±9†
Head size (intracranial volume, cm^3, as measured by MR imaging)	1557±119	1403±114†	...	...

*MR indicates magnetic resonance; PET, positron emission tomography. Values are group means±SDs. Between-group comparisons were carried out with Student's *t* tests.
†*P*<.001.

of PET and (18F)-2-fluoro-2-deoxy-D-glucose. We previously reported significant and differential effects of the X chromosome and sex steroids on the brain.[29,30] The X chromosome is involved in development and aging of gray matter in association with the neocortex, but sex steroids modulate this effect and are crucial to the development and aging of the hippocampus. Thus, in this study, we hypothesized that sex would significantly influence age-related differences in brain morphometry and glucose metabolism, particularly in areas implicated in higher cognition and neuropsychiatric disorders.

RESULTS

Our analysis of variance and regression analysis simultaneously examined sex differences, age-related changes, and age×sex interactions. Interpretation of the main effects for age or sex are confounded if there is a significant age×sex interaction on the variable in question.[41] Therefore, the results are presented first for variables that showed only a main effect of sex or age without an interaction, and then for measures that showed an age×sex interaction.

MR IMAGING STUDY

Sex

Women had a significantly larger volume of thalamic and caudate nuclei than men (**Table 2**). In contrast, right-left asymmetry of lateral ventricles was significantly greater in men than women.

Age

There were significant age-related decrements in brain-matter volumes of cerebellum, cerebral hemispheres, parieto-occipital lobe, parahippocampal gyrus, and subcortical nuclei (amygdala, thalamic, and caudate) (Table 2). Furthermore, there were significant bilateral increases in volume of ventricular and peripheral cerebrospinal fluid. In contrast, there was no significant age-related decrease in volume of the temporal lobe.

Age by Sex

Men had a significantly greater age-related decrease than women in brain-matter volume of cerebral hemispheres and frontal and temporal lobes (Table 2). In contrast, women had a significantly greater decrease than men in volume of the parietal lobes and hippocampus, and a significantly greater increase in volume of the third ventricle. Furthermore, there were significant sex differences in the right-left asymmetry of age-related decreases in frontal lobe volume—the right decreased more than the left in men, but the left decreased more than the right in women.

PET STUDY

Sex

Right-left metabolic asymmetry of frontal lobe metabolism was significantly less in women than men. Interpretation of all the other significant sex differences noted in **Table 3** are confounded because of significant age×sex interactions (**Table 4**).

Age

There were significant age-related decrements in glucose metabolism of whole-brain, frontal, temporal, and parietal ROIs (Table 4). Also, these metabolic decrements were significantly asymmetric in parietal (left more affected than right) and frontal (right more affected than left) lobes, and language areas (Broca's more than Wernicke's area).

Age by Sex

Women had a significantly greater age-related metabolic decline than men in thalamus (Table 4) and hippocampus (**Figure**); thalamic metabolism of women was significantly higher than that of men until 24 years of age,

Table 2. Brain Matter and Cerebrospinal Fluid (CSF) Volumes in Young and Old Subjects*

	% of Intracranial Volume				*P*		
Structure	Young Men (n=21)	Old Men (n=14)	Young Women (n=15)	Old Women (n=19)	Sex Effect	Age Effect, Men + Women	Age × Sex Interaction
Brain Matter Volume							
Cerebellum							
Total	10.7±1.02	10.2±1.01	11.0±0.98	10.3±1.09	.55	.02	.67
Hemispheres							
Total	75.5±2.01	69.8±2.67	74.2±1.68	70.9±2.17	.84	<.001	.02
R	37.7±1.05	34.8±1.29	37.1±0.94	35.2±1.29	.68	<.001	.06
L	37.5±1.01	34.7±1.37	36.8±0.90	35.1±1.27	.51	<.001	.06
Frontal lobe							
Total	37.4±2.04	33.1±2.27	36.6±1.72	35.5±3.00	.18	<.001	<.01
R	18.8±1.03	16.5±1.11	18.3±0.91	17.9±1.51	.15	<.001	<.01
L	18.6±1.06	16.6±1.20	18.4±0.88	17.6±1.54	.25	<.001	.03
Parietal lobe							
Total	17.5±1.64	17.7±1.76	18.5±2.05	16.2±2.40	.63	.03	.01
R	8.78±0.87	8.88±0.83	9.29±1.16	8.02±1.31	.58	.02	<.01
L	8.73±0.79	8.84±1.03	9.17±0.94	8.17±1.15	.70	.05	.02
Temporal lobe							
Total	10.2±0.65	9.62±0.83	9.50±0.85	9.81±0.91	.15	.33	.02
R	5.21±0.39	4.87±0.54	4.84±0.49	5.05±0.53	.36	.48	.02
L	5.01±0.35	4.75±0.36	4.66±0.43	4.76±0.52	.09	.29	.08
Parieto-occipital lobe							
Total	10.0±1.21	9.07±1.56	9.23±1.05	8.82±1.75	.13	.03	.43
R	4.94±0.57	4.50±0.83	4.65±0.72	4.23±0.78	.12	<.01	.93
L	5.10±0.77	4.57±0.86	4.59±0.63	4.59±1.07	.22	.14	.21
Parahippocampal gyrus†							
Total	0.37±0.06	0.31±0.04	0.41±0.05	0.33±0.07	.07	<.001	.57
R	0.18±0.03	0.15±0.03	0.20±0.03	0.16±0.04	.18	<.001	.32
L	0.19±0.04	0.16±0.03	0.21±0.03	0.18±0.04	.07	<.01	.98
Caudate nucleus							
Total	0.76±0.12	0.74±0.18	0.88±0.11	0.77±0.12	.03	.04	.16
R	0.39±0.06	0.37±0.09	0.44±0.07	0.38±0.06	.03	.04	.18
L	0.38±0.07	0.38±0.10	0.43±0.05	0.39±0.07	.04	.28	.18
Lenticular nucleus							
Total	1.02±0.13	0.87±0.24	1.10±0.22	0.92±0.16	.15	<.001	.65
R	0.50±0.07	0.43±0.13	0.56±0.13	0.43±0.10	.27	<.001	.30
L	0.51±0.07	0.44±0.13	0.55±0.11	0.49±0.09	.11	.01	.82
Thalamic nucleus							
Total	0.94±0.15	0.87±0.15	1.02±0.11	0.94±0.11	.02	.04	.87
R	0.48±0.07	0.43±0.07	0.50±0.06	0.47±0.06	.04	.03	.40
L	0.46±0.09	0.44±0.09	0.52±0.06	0.47±0.06	.02	.04	.32
Amygdala†							
Total	0.24±0.05	0.20±0.03	0.27±0.06	0.20±0.04	.29	<.001	.29
R	0.12±0.03	0.09±0.03	0.14±0.03	0.09±0.03	.30	<.001	.22
L	0.13±0.02	0.10±0.02	0.14±0.03	0.10±0.02	.43	<.001	.56
Hippocampus†							
Total	0.33±0.05	0.29±0.05	0.43±0.06	0.28±0.06	<.01	<.001	<.01
R	0.17±0.03	0.14±0.03	0.22±0.04	0.14±0.03	.02	<.001	<.01
L	0.16±0.02	0.14±0.03	0.22±0.03	0.14±0.03	<.001	<.001	<.001
Ventricular and Peripheral CSF Volumes							
Lateral ventricle							
R	0.42±0.20	1.11±0.61	0.50±0.19	0.89±0.35	.43	<.001	.08
L	0.44±0.35	1.23±0.72	0.43±0.18	0.92±0.39	.14	<.001	.17
Third ventricle	0.09±0.02	0.18±0.04	0.10±0.02	0.14±0.06	.12	<.001	.04
Peripheral CSF							
Total hemispheres	10.8±1.88	14.7±2.76	11.6±1.25	14.3±2.56	.66	<.001	.28
R hemisphere	5.20±0.87	7.09±1.44	5.58±0.58	6.80±1.21	.80	<.001	.20
L hemisphere	5.25±1.03	7.17±1.41	5.50±0.65	7.00±1.33	.86	<.001	.44
R-L Brain Matter and CSF Asymmetries, $\times 10^{-2}$‡							
Cerebral hemisphere	0.24±0.47	0.01±0.42	0.30±0.62	0.09±0.43	.55	.08	.96
Frontal lobe	0.15±0.47	−0.08±0.41	−0.05±0.47	0.31±0.58	.51	.51	.02
Temporal lobe	0.20±0.35	0.12±0.39	0.18±0.36	0.28±0.53	.52	.80	.37
Parietal lobe	0.05±0.30	0.04±0.63	0.13±0.52	−0.15±0.53	.65	.21	.26
Parieto-occipital lobe	−0.16±0.60	−0.07±0.66	0.06±0.85	−0.35±0.64	.91	.32	.14
Ventricular CSF	−0.02±0.23	−0.12±0.23	0.07±0.09	−0.03±0.14	.04	.07	.96
Peripheral CSF	−0.05±0.32	−0.09±0.33	0.08±0.26	−0.19±0.46	.85	.09	.18

**Values are group means±SDs. All volumes are 100×(cubic centimeter structure/cubic centimeter total intracranial volume). Brain asymmetries were calculated by dividing R-L structure by total intracranial volume.*

†N=13 young and 12 old men, 11 young and 12 old women.

‡Brain asymmetries were calculated by dividing R-L structure by total intracranial volume.

Table 3. Mean Cerebral Metabolic Rates for Glucose in Men and Women*

Region of Interest	Rate, mg/100 g of Brain per Minute: Men (n=55)	Women (n=65)	P
Global gray matter	8.32±0.17	8.34±0.16	.17
Brain	6.37±0.14	6.46±0.13	.13
Frontal			
R total	8.51±0.19	8.51±0.17	.12
L total	8.66±0.19	8.61±0.18	.26
Parietal			
R total	8.49±0.20	8.70±0.17	.34
L total	8.54±0.21	8.76±0.18	.53
R superior	8.48±0.20	8.73±0.18	.37
L superior	8.47±0.22	8.77±0.19	.70
Temporal			
R total	7.56±0.15	7.65±0.14	.07
L total	7.67±0.17	7.74±0.15	.32
R middle	7.87±0.16	8.02±0.15	.11
L middle	8.06±0.17	8.21±0.15	.49
Hippocampus			
R	6.72±0.14	6.59±0.14	.03
L	6.62±0.14	6.50±0.14	.02
Broca's area			
R	9.05±0.21	8.99±0.20	.21
L	9.20±0.23	9.20±0.19	.51
Wernicke's area			
R	8.35±0.18	8.43±0.16	.11
L	8.57±0.18	8.50±0.17	.49
Occipital association			
R	7.97±0.16	7.90±0.14	.25
L	7.94±0.18	7.91±0.14	.33
Caudate			
R	9.00±0.22	9.21±0.21	.20
L	9.26±0.22	9.52±0.19	.16
Lenticular			
R	9.32±0.18	9.29±0.18	.14
L	9.39±0.20	9.36±0.18	.22
Thalamic			
R	8.66±0.23	8.75±0.21	<.01
L	8.79±0.23	8.88±0.21	<.01
R-L Asymmetry of Cerebral Glucose Metabolism, ×10⁻²†			
Frontal	−1.64±0.47	−1.21±0.37	.04
Parietal	−0.45±0.66	−0.50±0.50	.25
Superior parietal	−0.41±1.07	0.02±0.90	.06
Temporal	−1.36±0.74	−1.13±0.57	.03
Midtemporal	−2.25±1.01	−2.33±0.74	.03
Broca's area	−1.33±1.39	−2.43±0.96	.04
Wernicke's area	−2.63±0.81	−0.84±0.74	.03
Occipital	−1.67±1.01	−1.26±0.77	.89
Anteroposterior Asymmetry of Cerebral Glucose Metabolism, ×10⁻²†			
Broca/Wernicke			
L	6.50±0.01	7.69±0.92	.73

*All values are mean±SD. Regional cerebral metabolic rates for glucose (rCMRglc) were measured with (18F)-2-fluoro-2-deoxy-D-glucose and positron emission tomography.

†Right-left metabolic asymmetries were determined according to the following equation, where R=rCMRglc in a right-sided region and L=rCMRglc in the homologous left-sided region: % metabolic asymmetry=(R−L)/[(R+L)/2]×100. Anteroposterior metabolic asymmetries were calculated by the same equation as above but substituting the terms Broca and Wernicke for right and left, respectively.

whereas their hippocampal metabolism became significantly lower than that of men at 70 years of age. Also, there were significant age-related sex differences in right-left metabolic asymmetry of the temporal lobes until age 26 years (Table 4, Figure) and of the parietal lobes and Broca's area from age 60 and 75 years, respectively. Generally, compared with women, age-related declines in metabolism in men were greater in the left than the right (Table 4); whereas, in women, the aging effect was either equal in the two hemispheres or greater in the right than the left (Table 4). A quadratic fit was not significantly better than a linear fit in all brain regions that demonstrated significant age-related sex difference.

COMMENT

Our report of age-related brain atrophy and an age-related decrease in glucose metabolism, as well as regional differences in age-related brain atrophy and metabolism, replicate previous results from our laboratory.[33,43,44] Also, our MR imaging finding of significant sex differences in age-related brain atrophy supports, and adds to, the findings of Gur et al[21] and Cowell et al.[22] In the PET study, we found significant sex differences in age effects on metabolism in some of the same regions in which MR imaging demonstrated morphometric differences. Thus, some metabolic findings may have been influenced by sex differences in brain atrophy. Because not all subjects who underwent MR imaging had PET, we cannot directly address this issue. However, Grady and Rapoport[44] reported that age-related decreases in brain glucose metabolism are still significant after atrophy correction, and in the present study we found that regions that are anatomically close (eg, temporal lobe and Wernicke's and Broca's areas) had significant differences in age- and sex-related effects. Thus, our metabolic findings cannot be fully explained by sex differences in brain atrophy, although this probably accounts for some results.

We found a significant sex difference in age-related hippocampal volume loss, but the groups did not start from an identical baseline—hippocampal volume in young women was larger than that in men but was similar in old women and men. This result will need to be replicated in a larger sample. However, this MR imaging finding of significant sex differences in age-related loss of hippocampal volume is supported by our PET results, in a relatively large sample, which found significant sex differences in age-related decreases in hippocampal glucose metabolism. Thus, women have a significantly larger age-related decrease than men in hippocampal cellular glucose metabolism, and this may lead to greater atrophy and volume loss.

Our subjects were recruited locally, medication free, highly intelligent, and healthy. Thus, they do not represent the whole population, and our findings may not be generalizable. However, the selection of healthy subjects reduces the confounding effect of even mild physical disease on age-related changes in brain morphometry and metabolism.[45-47] Thus, our results may give a better measure of intrinsic age- and sex-related differences in the brain.

Cognitive abilities decline with advancing age,[48-50] but not all capabilities are equally affected. Most verbal capacities are preserved (including memory) until a very advanced age,[51,52] whereas visuospatial abilities and

Table 4. Age × Sex Differences in Brain Glucose Metabolism*

Region of Interest	Difference, mg/100 g of Brain per Minute per Decade: Men + Women (n=120)	Men (n=55)	Women (n=65)	P: Age Effect, Men + Women	Age Effect, Men	Age Effect, Women	Age × Sex Effect
Global gray matter	−0.24±0.06	−0.14±0.10	−0.33±0.08	<.001	.16	<.001	.13
Brain	−0.20±0.05	−0.12±0.08	−0.27±0.07	<.001	.15	<.001	.14
Frontal							
R total	−0.31±0.06	−0.19±0.10	−0.43±0.08	<.001	.07	<.001	.08
L total	−0.34±0.07	−0.25±0.10	−0.43±0.09	<.001	.02	<.001	.18
Parietal							
R total	−0.28±0.07	−0.22±0.10	−0.33±0.09	<.001	.04	<.001	.42
L total	−0.33±0.07	−0.30±0.11	−0.36±0.09	<.001	.01	<.001	.65
R superior	−0.31±0.07	−0.26±0.11	−0.36±0.09	<.001	.02	<.001	.48
L superior	−0.36±0.07	−0.35±0.12	−0.37±0.10	<.001	<.01	<.001	.91
Temporal							
R total	−0.18±0.06	−0.07±0.09	−0.28±0.07	<.01	.42	<.001	.07
L total	−0.22±0.06	−0.16±0.09	−0.28±0.08	<.001	.09	<.001	.31
R middle	−0.15±0.06	−0.06±0.09	−0.24±0.08	.02	.53	<.01	.13
L middle	−0.26±0.06	−0.23±0.09	−0.30±0.08	<.001	.01	<.001	.58
Hippocampus							
R	−0.10±0.05	0.04±0.08	−0.25±0.07	.06	.60	<.01	<.01
L	−0.10±0.05	0.05±0.08	−0.25±0.07	.06	.55	<.001	<.01
Broca's area							
R	−0.34±0.08	−0.21±0.12	−0.48±0.09	<.001	.07	<.001	.05
L	−0.40±0.08	−0.36±0.13	−0.44±0.09	<.001	.02	<.001	.08
Wernicke's area							
R	−0.22±0.06	−0.11±0.10	−0.32±0.08	<.001	.28	<.001	0.10
L	−0.23±0.07	−0.17±0.10	−0.29±0.09	<.001	.10	<.001	0.37
Occipital association							
R	−0.07±0.06	0.01±0.09	−0.16±0.08	.20	.97	.05	.18
L	−0.08±0.06	−0.01±0.01	−0.15±0.08	.19	.90	.06	.28
Caudate							
R	−0.15±0.09	−0.05±0.13	−0.25±0.12	.08	.68	.03	.25
L	−0.13±0.08	−0.03±0.12	−0.23±0.10	.11	.81	.03	.23
Lenticular							
R	−0.12±0.08	0.01±0.13	−0.25±0.10	.13	.94	.01	.10
L	−0.10±0.08	0.01±0.11	−0.20±0.10	.21	.95	.04	.17
Thalamic							
R	−0.04±0.09	0.19±0.13	−0.28±0.12	.61	.14	.02	<.01
L	−0.01±0.09	0.23±0.13	−0.25±0.12	.91	.08	.04	<.01
Difference in R-L Asymmetry of Cerebral Glucose Metabolism per Decade, ×10⁻²†							
Frontal	−0.33±0.16	0.65±0.26	0.01±0.21	.04	.01	.97	.05
Parietal							
Total	0.60±0.22	0.87±0.36	0.33±0.28	<.01	.02	.24	.23
Superior	0.24±0.31	1.02±0.46	−0.53±0.43	.44	.03	.22	.02
Temporal							
Total	0.57±0.24	1.13±0.40	0.02±0.32	.03	<.01	.94	.03
Middle	1.33±0.33	2.05±0.51	0.61±0.42	<.001	<.001	.23	.03
Broca's area	0.55±0.46	1.64±0.78	−0.54±0.54	.24	.04	.32	.02
Wernicke's area	0.16±0.31	0.70±0.46	−0.37±0.42	.60	.13	.38	.09
Occipital	0.49±0.36	0.49±0.58	0.49±0.43	.17	.40	.27	.99
Difference in Anteroposterior Ratio of Cerebral Glucose Metabolism per Decade, ×10⁻²†							
Broca/Wernicke							
R	−1.22±0.44	−0.86±0.71	−1.58±0.55	<.01	.23	<.01	.44
L	−1.60±0.41	−1.79±0.67	−1.41±0.50	<.001	.01	<.01	.59

**Difference per decade in mean absolute glucose metabolism, regional cerebral metabolic rate for glucose (rCMRglc), and R-L and anteroposterior asymmetry, as measured by positron emission tomography in male and female subjects. All values are mean±SD. Metabolic activity was compared by a univariate multiple regression with age, sex, and age × sex interaction as the predictor variables.*

†R-L metabolic asymmetries were determined according to the following equation, where R=rCMRglc in a right-sided region and L=rCMRglc in the homologous left-sided region: % metabolic asymmetry=(R−L)/[(R+L)/2]×100. Anteroposterior metabolic asymmetries were calculated by the same equation as above but substituting the terms Broca *and* Wernicke *for right and left, respectively.*

memory decline steadily throughout adulthood.[52-55] Women[4-6] have significantly less age-related decline than men in verbal memory, whereas men have significantly better preservation of visuospatial abilities, including visuoconceptual, constructional, and memory tasks. Performance on recognition tasks for visual stimuli is related to metabolic asymmetry in the parietal lobes,[56] and aging is associated with lateralized effects on cerebral blood

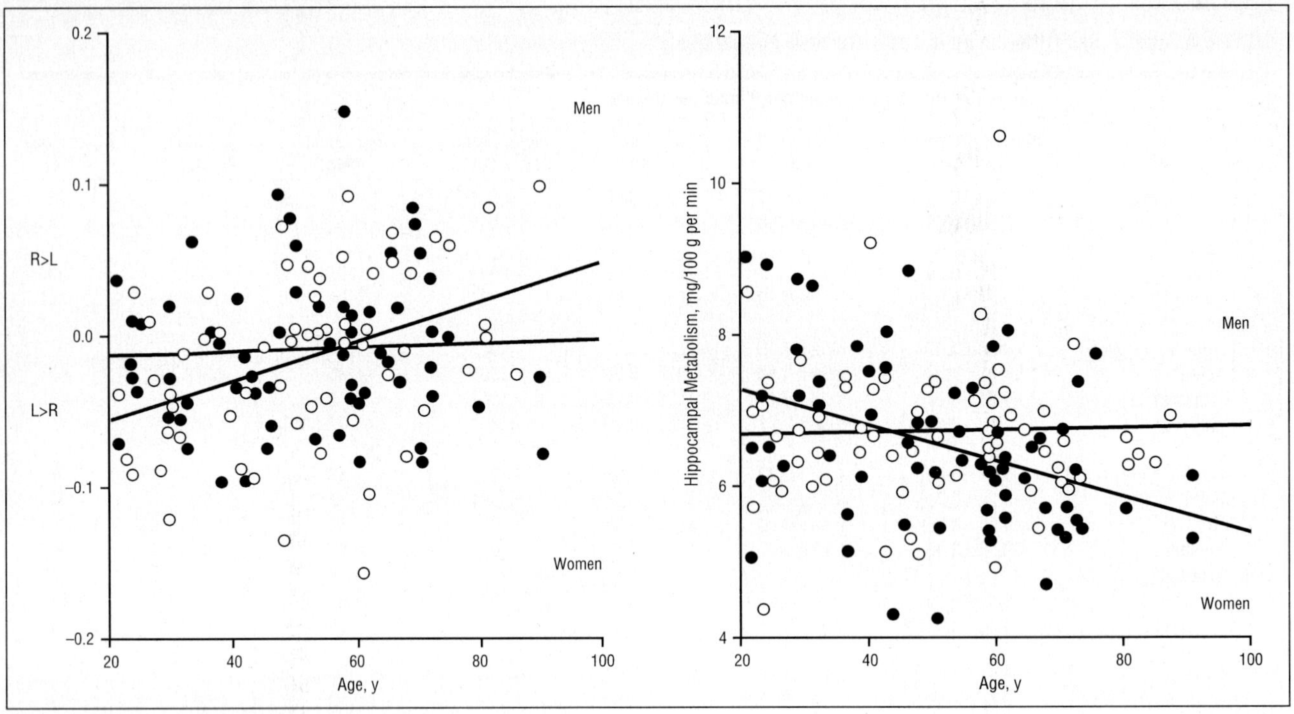

Effect of aging on right-left asymmetry of temporal lobe (left) and absolute glucose metabolism of the hippocampus (right) as measured by positron emission tomography in male (open circles) and female (solid circles) subjects.

flow.[57] Horwitz et al[58] suggested that decreased integration of metabolic function within parietal areas, and between frontal and parietal areas, may be associated with some age-related neuropsychological deficits. In this study, we found significant sex differences in age-related effects on morphometry and metabolism of brain regions involved in cognitive functions that also show significant age-related sex differences, and so these findings may be related. We are currently examining whether sex differences in age-related changes in cognitive ability and changes in brain morphometry and metabolism are related in a longitudinal study.

The timing, and biologic basis, for development of cerebral asymmetry is controversial. Human cerebral asymmetries are present at the 20th week of gestation[59] and well established by the 36th week.[60] However, it is unknown whether human brain asymmetry changes over the life span, and it has been proposed that specification of cerebral dominance is completed by birth,[61] age 5 years,[62] or puberty,[63-65] or continues to develop over the life span.[66] A Y chromosomal responsibility for development of cerebral asymmetry has been suggested,[67] but the X chromosome's importance is implied by studies of sex chromosome aneuploidies. For example, males with 49,XXXXY (Klinefelter syndrome) have better visuospatial than verbal skills,[68,69] girls with 47,XXX have delayed language and cognitive development,[70-73] and females with Turner's syndrome show X chromosome dosage effects on brain morphometry and cognitive ability.[29,30] Moreover, sex steroids are also implicated in the development of brain asymmetry. Some authors[74] proposed that in men testosterone modulates connectivity in an already asymmetric brain, and that low levels of testosterone lead to less functional asymmetry, whereas others[75,76] suggested that high levels of testosterone produce less functional asymmetry.

We found that right-left lateralization and anteroposterior ratios of brain metabolism undergo sex-dependent, age-related linear changes. Age-related changes in sex steroid concentrations are not linear, and we have reported sex chromosome dosage effects on structure and function of human association neocortex[29,30] and sex steroid effects on development of human hippocampus and memory function.[29,30] Thus, lateralized brain metabolism is not static but changes across the life span, and it may be genetically determined. Of course, other factors (such as hormone milieu) may modify aging of particular brain regions (eg, hippocampus and parietal cortex).[30] Also, this study was cross sectional rather than longitudinal and so could only address age-related differences and not changes during the life span of an individual.

Development of asymmetry in brain function is of relevance to human brain disease, eg, Crow[77] hypothesized that schizophrenia is secondary to an arrest of development of the primary asymmetry in Wernicke's area. Also, both aging and sex affect cerebral asymmetry because a lesion in left temporoparietal (Wernicke's) cortex produces different aphasia types by age[66] and aphasic symptoms in right-handed men but not in women.[78] Conversely, left anterior damage[78] causes aphasia more often in women than men.

The significant sex differences we found in age-related effects on the human brain may interact with a superimposed pathologic process and contribute to sex differences in brain disorders, because they occur in regions that are associated with higher cognitive function and that are implicated in age-related brain diseases (including AD and late-onset schizophrenia).

Women may have a higher age-adjusted prevalence and incidence of AD than men.[7,79-85] Furthermore, women with AD perform significantly worse than men in some visuospatial[86] and memory[87] tests. We found that women had significantly more age-related decline in hippocampal metabolism and parietal lobe volume than men, and both brain regions are involved in memory and visuospatial function and in neuropathologic abnormalities in AD.[88-93] Thus, sex differences in aging of brain regions implicated in AD may contribute to sex differences in its symptoms. Nevertheless, others[94] found that in AD rCMRglc does not differ significantly between sexes—although this may reflect the small number of women older than 65 years they studied (N=5).

In late-onset schizophrenia, the male-female ratio (3:20) in patients older than 75 years exceeds that in the elderly population,[95] and some have proposed that this is secondary to loss of the antidopaminergic effect of estrogens.[96,97] However, schizophrenia is associated with structural and metabolic abnormalities in a number of brain regions (including the hippocampus),[98] and we found that women had a significantly larger age-related decrease in hippocampal metabolism and volume than men. Thus, sex differences in late-onset schizophrenia may be secondary to differences in age-related decreases in volume and metabolism of brain regions implicated in the disease. Furthermore, previous reports of sex differences in the brain structure of schizophrenics (see Castle and Murray[99] for a review) may reflect normal sex differences in the brain rather than the effects of schizophrenia per se.

In conclusion, we found significant sex differences in age-related effects on human brain morphometry and metabolism in regions known to subserve higher cognitive function. Our findings may explain some sex differences in age-related cognitive decline and may interact with superimposed pathologic processes to contribute to sex differences in human brain diseases.

Accepted for publication September 6, 1995.

Reprint requests to Department of Psychological Medicine, Section on Mental Impairment, Institute of Psychiatry, DeCrespigny Park, Denmark Hill, London SE5 8AF, United Kingdom (Dr Murphy).

REFERENCES

1. Stanford PE, Du Bois BC. Gender and ethnicity patterns. In: Birren JE, Sloane RB, Cohen GD, eds. *Handbook of Mental Health and Aging.* 2nd ed. San Diego, Calif: Academic Press; 1992:99-119.
2. Myers GC. Demography of aging. In: Binstock RH, George LK, eds. *Handbook of Aging and Social Sciences.* San Diego, Calif: Academic Press; 1990:19-44.
3. Manton KG. Mortality and morbidity. In: Binstock RH, George LK, eds. *Handbook of Aging and Social Sciences.* San Diego, Calif: Academic Press; 1990: 59-90.
4. Zelinski EM, Gilewski MJ, Schaie KW. Individual differences in cross-sectional and 3-year longitudinal memory performance across the adult life span. *Psychol Aging.* 1993;8:176-186.
5. West RL, Crook TH, Barron KL. Everyday memory performance across the life span: effects of age and noncognitive individual differences. *Psychol Aging.* 1992;7:72-82.
6. Wiederholt WC, Cahn D, Butters N, Salmon DP, Kritz-Silverstein D, Barrett-Connor E. Effects of age, gender and education on selected neuropsychological tests in an elderly community cohort. *J Am Gerontol Soc.* 1993;41:639-647.
7. Zhang M, Katzman R, Salmon D, Jin H, Goujun C, Wang Z, Qu G, Grant I, Yu E, Levy P, Klauber MR, Liu WT. The prevalence of dementia and Alzheimer's disease in Shanghai, China: impact of age, gender and education. *Ann Neurol.* 1990;27:428-437.
8. Rector NA, Seeman MV. Auditory hallucinations in women and men. *Schizophr Res.* 1992;7:233-236.
9. Hambrecht M, Maurer K, Häfner H. Gender differences in schizophrenia in three cultures: results of the WHO collaborative study on psychiatric disability. *Soc Psychiatry Psychiatr Epidemiol.* 1992;27:117-121.
10. Pakkenberg H, Voigt J. Brain weight of the Danes: a forensic material. *Acta Anat.* 1964;56:297-307.
11. Clark S, Kraftsik R, Van der Loos H, Innocenti GM. Forms and measures of adult and developing human corpus callosum: is there sexual dimorphism? *J Comp Neurol.* 1989;280:213-230.
12. Witelson SF. Hand and sex differences in the isthmus and genu of the human corpus callosum: a post-mortem morphological study. *Brain.* 1989;112:799-835.
13. Allen LS, Hines M, Shryne JE, Gorski RA. Two sexually dimorphic cell groups in the human brain. *J Neurosci.* 1989;9:497-506.
14. Geschwind N, Levitsky W. Human brain: left-right asymmetries in temporal speech region. *Science.* 1968;161:186-187.
15. Witelson SF, Kigar DL. Sylvian fissure morphometry and asymmetry in men and women: bilateral differences in relation to handedness in men. *J Comp Neurol.* 1992;323:326-340.
16. Hubbard B, Anderson J. Sex differences in age-related brain atrophy. *Lancet.* 1983;1:1447-1448.
17. Witelson SF. Sex differences in neuroanatomical changes with aging. *N Engl J Med.* 1991;325:211-212.
18. Kaye JA, DeCarli CD, Luxenberg JS, Rapoport SI. The significance of age-related enlargement of the cerebral ventricles in healthy men and women measured by quantitative computed x-ray tomography. *J Am Geriatr Soc.* 1992; 40:225-231.
19. Takeda S, Matsuzawa T. Age-related brain atrophy: a study with computed tomography. *J Gerontol.* 1985;40:159-163.
20. Coffey CE, Wilkinson WE, Parashos IA, Soady SAR, Sullivan RJ, Patterson LJ, Figiel GS, Webb MC, Spritzer CE, Djang WT. Quantitative cerebral anatomy of the aging human brain: a cross-sectional study using magnetic resonance imaging. *Neurology.* 1992;42:527-536.
21. Gur RC, Mozley PD, Resnick S, Gottlieb GL, Kohn M, Herman G, Atlas S, Grossman R, Berretta D, Erwin R, Gur RE. Gender differences in age effect on brain atrophy measured by magnetic resonance imaging. *Proc Natl Acad Sci U S A.* 1991;88:2845-2849.
22. Cowell PE, Turetsky BI, Gur RC, Grossman RI, Shtasel DL, Gur RE. Sex differences in aging of the human frontal and temporal lobes. *J Neurosci.* 1994; 14:4748-4756.
23. Gur RC, Gur RE, Obrist WD, Hungerbuhler JP, Younkin D, Rosen AD, Skolnick BE, Reivich M. Sex and handedness differences in cerebral blood flow during rest and cognitive activity. *Science.* 1982;217:659-661.
24. Devous MES, Stokely EM, Chehabi HH, Bonte FJ. Normal distribution of regional cerebral blood flow measured by dynamic single-photon emission tomography. *J Cereb Blood Flow Metab.* 1986;3:95-104.
25. Rodrigues G, Warkentin S, Risberg J, Rosadini G. Sex differences in regional cerebral blood flow. *J Cereb Blood Flow Metab.* 1988;8:783-789.
26. Baxter LRJ, Mazziotta JC, Phelps ME, Seline CE, Guze BH, Fairbanks L. Cerebral glucose metabolic rates in normal human females versus normal males. *Psychiatr Res.* 1987;21:237-245.
27. Yoshii F, Barker WW, Chang JY, Loewenstein D, Apicella A, Smith D, Boothe T, Ginsberg MD, Pascal S, Duara R. Sensitivity of cerebral glucose metabolism to age, gender, brain volume, brain atrophy and cerebrovascular risk factors. *J Cereb Blood Flow Metab.* 1988;8:654-661.
28. Gur RC, Mozeley LH, Mozley DP, Resnick SM, Karp JS, Alavi A, Arnold SE, Gur RQ. Sex differences in regional cerebral glucose metabolism during a resting state. *Science.* 1995;267:528-531.
29. Murphy DGM, DeCarli CD, Daly E, Haxby JV, Allen G, White BJ, McIntosh AR, Powell CM, Horwitz B, Rapoport SI, Schapiro MB. X chromosome effects on female brain: a magnetic resonance imaging study of Turner's syndrome. *Lancet.* 1993;342:1197-1200.
30. Murphy DGM, Allen G, Haxby JV, Largay KA, Daly E, White BJ, Powell CM, Schapiro MB. The effects of sex steroids, and the X chromosome, on female brain function: a study of the neuropsychology of adult Turner syndrome. *Neuropsychologia.* 1994;132:1309-1323.
31. Kaye JA, May M, Atack JR, Daly E, Sweeney DL, Beal MF, Kaufman S, Milstein S, Friedland RP, Rapoport SI. Cerebrospinal fluid neurochemistry in the myoclonic subtype of Alzheimer's disease. *Ann Neurol.* 1988;24:647-650.
32. Wechsler DA. *Wechsler Adult Intelligence Scale.* New York, NY: Psychological Corp; 1955.
33. Murphy DGM, DeCarli CD, Schapiro MB, Rapoport SI, Horwitz B. Age related differences in volumes of subcortical nuclei, brain matter, and cerebrospinal fluid in healthy men as measured with MRI. *Arch Neurol.* 1992;49:839-849.
34. Watson C, Andermann F, Gloor P, Jones-Gotman M, Peters T, Evans A, Olivier A, Melanson D, Leroux G. Anatomic basis of amygdaloid and hippocampal volume measurement by magnetic resonance imaging. *Neurology.* 1992;42: 1743-1750.
35. Bartko JJ, Carpenter WT. On the methods and theory of reliability. *J Nerv Ment Dis.* 1986;163:307-317.
36. Kumar A, Schapiro MB, Grady CL, Haxby JV, Wagner E, Salerno JA, Friedland

RP, Rapoport SI. High-resolution PET studies in Alzheimer's disease. *Neuropsychopharmacology.* 1991;4:35-46.
37. Brooks RA. Alternative formula for glucose utilization using labeled deoxyglucose. *J Nucl Med.* 1982;23:538-539.
38. Huang SC, Phelps ME, Hoffman EJ, Sideris K, Selin CJ, Kuhl DE. Non-invasive determination of local cerebral metabolic rate of glucose in man. *Am J Physiol.* 1980;238:E69-E82.
39. Murphy DGM, Mentis MJ, Grady C, Haxby J, Horwitz B, Rapoport SI, Schapiro MB. The effect of the X chromosome and sex steroids on human brain development. *Biol Psychiatry.* 1993;33(suppl 6A):107. Abstract.
40. *SAS Users Guide: Basics Version 5.* 5th ed. Cary, NC: SAS Inc; 1985.
41. Pedhazur EJ, Schmelkin LP. *Measurement, Design, and Analysis: An Integrated Approach.* Hillsdale, NJ: Lawrence Erlbaum Assoc; 1991.
42. Karpman MB. Comparing non-parallel regression lines with the parametric alternative to analysis of covariance using SPSS-X or SAS: the Johnson-Neyman technique. *Educ Psychol Meas.* 1986;46:639-644.
43. DeCarli CD, Murphy DGM, Gillette JA, Haxby JV, Teichberg D, Schapiro MB, Horwitz B. Lack of age-related differences in temporal lobe volume of very healthy adults. *Am J Neuroradiol.* 1994;15:689-696.
44. Grady CL, Rapoport SI. Cerebral metabolism in aging and dementia. In: Birren JE, Sloane RB, Cohen GD, eds. *Handbook of Mental Health and Aging.* 2nd ed. San Diego, Calif: Academic Press; 1992:201-228.
45. Salerno JA, Murphy DGM, Horwitz B, DeCarli CD, Haxby JV, Rapoport SI, Schapiro MB. Brain atrophy in hypertension: a volumetric magnetic resonance imaging study. *Hypertension.* 1992;20:340-348.
46. Kozachuk WE, DeCarli C, Schapiro MB, et al. White matter hyperintensities in dementia of Alzheimer's type and in healthy subjects with and without cerebrovascular risk factors: a magnetic resonance imaging study. *Arch Neurol.* 1990;47:1306-1310.
47. Mentis MJ, Salerno JA, Horwitz B, Grady CL, Schapiro MB, Murphy DGM, Rapoport SI. Reduction of functional neuronal connectivity in long-term treated hypertension. *Stroke.* 1994;25:601-607.
48. Botwinick J. Intellectual abilities. In: Birren JE, Schaie KW, eds. *Handbook of the Psychology of Aging.* New York, NY: Van Nostrand Reinhold; 1977:580-605.
49. Horn JL, Donaldson G. On the myth of intellectual decline in adulthood. *Am Psychol.* 1976;31:701-709.
50. Salthouse TA. *Adult Cognition.* New York, NY: Springer-Verlag; 1982.
51. Birren JE, Butler RN, Greenhouse SW, Sokoloff L, Yarrow MR. Interdisciplinary relationships: inter-relations of physiological, psychological and psychiatric findings in healthy elderly men. In: Birren JE, Butler RN, Greenhouse SW, Sokoloff L, Yarrow MR, eds. *Human Aging: A Biological and Behavioral Approach.* Bethesda, Md: US Dept of Health, Education, and Welfare, Public Health Services; 1963:283-305. National Institutes of Health, National Institute of Mental Health.
52. Wechsler D. *The Measurement and Appraisal of Adult Intelligence.* 4th ed. Baltimore, Md: Williams & Wilkins; 1958.
53. Arenberg D. Differences and changes with age in the Benton Visual Retention Test. *J Gerontol.* 1978;33:435-540.
54. Eisdorfer C, Busse EW, Cohen LD. The WAIS performance of an aged sample: the relationship between verbal and performance IQ's. *J Gerontol.* 1959;14:197-201.
55. Koss E, Haxby JV, DeCarli C, Schapiro MB, Friedland RP, Rapoport SI. Patterns of performance preservation and loss in healthy aging. *Dev Neuropsychol.* 1991;7:99-113.
56. Berardi A, Haxby JV, Grady CL, Rapoport SI. Asymmetries of brain glucose metabolism and memory in the healthy elderly. *Dev Neuropsychol.* 1991;7:87-97.
57. Gur RC, Gur RE, Obrist WD, Skolnick BE, Reivich M. *Arch Gen Psychiatry.* 1987;44:617-621.
58. Horwitz B, Duara R, Rapoport SI. Age differences in intercorrelations between regional cerebral metabolic rates for glucose. *Ann Neurol.* 1986;19:60-67.
59. Weinberger DR, Luchins DJ, Morihisa MD, Wyatt RJ. Asymmetrical volumes of the right and left frontal and occipital regions of the human brain. *Ann Neurol.* 1982;11:97-100.
60. Chi JG, Dooling EC, Gilles FH. Gyral development of the human brain. *Ann Neurol.* 1977;1:86-93.
61. Kinsbourne M, Hiscock M. Does cerebral dominance develop? In: Segalowitz S, Gruber F, eds. *Language Development and Neurological Theory.* New York, NY: Academic Press; 1977:171-191.
62. Krashen SD. Lateralization, language learning, and the critical period: some new evidence. *Lang Learning.* 1973;23:63-74.
63. Basser LS. Hemiplegia of early onset and the faculty of speech with special reference to the effects of hemispherectomy. *Brain.* 1962;85:427-460.
64. Lenneberg E. *Biological Foundations of Language.* New York, NY: John Wiley & Sons; 1967.
65. Zangwill O. *Cerebral Dominance and Its Relation to Psychological Function.* Springfield, Ill: Charles C Thomas Publisher; 1960.
66. Brown J, Jaffe J. Hypothesis on cerebral dominance. *Neuropsychologia.* 1975;13:107-110.
67. Taylor DC. Mechanisms of sex differentiation: evidence from disease. In: Ghesquiere J, Martin RD, Newcombe F, eds. *Human Sexual Dimorphism.* London, England: Taylor and Francis; 1988:169-189.
68. Curfs LMG, Schreppers-Tijdink A, Wiegers A, Borghgraef M, Fryns JP. The 49,XXXXY syndrome: clinical and psychological findings in five patients. *J Ment Defic Res.* 1990;34:277-282.
69. Borghgraef M, Fryns JP, Smeets E, Marien J, Van Den Berghe H. The 49,XXXXY syndrome: clinical and psychological follow-up data. *Clin Genet.* 1988;33:429-434.
70. Pennington B, Puck M, Robinson A. Language and cognitive development of 47 XXX females followed since birth. *Behav Genet.* 1980;10:31-41.
71. Robinson A, Lubs HA, Nielsen J, Sorensen K. Summary of clinical findings: profiles of children with 47,XXY, 47,XXX, and 47,XYY karyotypes. In: Robinson A, Lubs H, Bergsma D, eds. *Sex Chromosome Aneuploidy: Prospective Studies in Children.* New York, NY: Alan R Liss Inc; 1979:124-125.
72. Nielsen J, Sorenson AM, Sorenson K. Mental development of unselected children with sex-chromosome abnormalities. *Hum Genet.* 1981;59:324-332.
73. Netley CT, Rovet J. Relations between a dermatoglyphic measure, hemispheric specialization, and intellectual abilities in 47,XXY males. *Brain Cogn.* 1987;6:153-160.
74. Witelson SF. Neural sexual mosaicism: sexual differentiation of the human temporoparietal region for functional asymmetry. *Psychoneuroendocrinology.* 1991;16:131-153.
75. Geschwind N, Galaburda AM. Cerebral lateralization: biological mechanisms, associations, and pathology, II: a hypothesis and a program for research. *Arch Neurol.* 1985;42:521-552.
76. Geschwind B, Galaburda AM. Cerebral lateralization: biological mechanisms, associations, and pathology, I: a hypothesis and a program for research. *Arch Neurol.* 1985;42:428-459.
77. Crow TJ. Temporal lobe asymmetries as the key to the etiology of schizophrenia. *Schizophr Bull.* 1990;16:433-443.
78. Kimura D. *Neuromotor Mechanisms in Human Communication.* Oxford Psychology Series; Broadbent DE, Makintosh NJ, McGaugh JL, Treisman A, Tulving E, Weiskrantz L, eds. New York, NY: Oxford University Press; 1993;20.
79. Jorm AF, Korten AE, Henderson AS. The prevalence of dementia: a quantitative integration of the literature. *Acta Psychiatr Scand.* 1987;76:465-479.
80. Akesson HO. A population study of senile and arteriosclerotic psychoses. *Hum Hered.* 1969;19:546-566.
81. Mölsä PK, Marttila RJ, Rinne UK. Epidemiology of dementia in a Finnish population. *Acta Neurol Scand.* 1982;65:541-552.
82. Schoenberg BS, Kokmen E, Okazaki H. Alzheimer's disease and other dementing illnesses in a defined United States population: incidence rates and clinical features. *Ann Neurol.* 1987;22:724-729.
83. Kokmen E, Chandra V, Schoenberg BS. Trends in incidence of dementing illness in Rochester, Minnesota, in three quinquennial periods, 1960-1974. *Neurology.* 1988;38:975-980.
84. Katzman R, Aronson M, Fuld P, Kawas C, Brown T, Morgenstern H, Frishman W, Gidez L, Eder H, Ooi WL. Development of dementing illness in an 80-year-old volunteer cohort. *Ann Neurol.* 1989;25:317-324.
85. Aronson MK, Ooi WL, Geva DL, Masur D, Blau A, Frishman W. Dementia: age-dependent incidence, prevalence, and mortality in the old old. *Arch Intern Med.* 1991;151:989-992.
86. Buckwalter JG, Sobel E, Dunn ME, Diz MM, Henderson VW. Gender differences on a brief measure of cognitive functioning in Alzheimer's disease. *Arch Neurol.* 1993;50:757-760.
87. Henderson VW, Buckwalter JG. Gender-associated cognitive deficits in Alzheimer's disease. *Neurology.* 1994;44:90-96.
88. Squire LR. Memory and the hippocampus: a synthesis from findings with rats, monkeys, and humans. *Psychol Rev.* 1992;99:195-231.
89. O'Keefe J, Nadel L. *The Hippocampus as a Cognitive Map.* Oxford, England: Clarendon Press; 1978.
90. Parkinson JK, Murray E, Mishkin M. A selective mnemonic role for the hippocampus in monkeys: memory for the location of objects. *J Neurosci.* 1988;8:4159-4167.
91. Haxby JV, Grady CL, Horwitz B, Ungerleider LG, Mishkin M, Carson RE, Herscovitch P, Schapiro MB, Rapoport SI. Dissociation of object and spatial visual processing pathways in human extrastriate cortex. *Proc Natl Acad Sci U S A.* 1991;88:1621-1625.
92. Hansen LA, DeTerasa R, Davies P, Terry RD. Neocortical morphometry, lesion counts, and choline acetyltransferase levels in the age spectrum of Alzheimer's disease. *Neurology.* 1988;38:48-54.
93. Khatchaturian ZS. Diagnosis of Alzheimer's disease. *Arch Neurol.* 1985;42:1097-1104.
94. Small GW, Kuhl DE, Riege WH, Fujikawa DG, Ashford JW, Metter EJ, Mazziotta JC. Cerebral glucose metabolic patterns in Alzheimer's disease: effect of gender and age at dementia onset. *Arch Gen Psychiatry.* 1989;46:527-532.
95. Castle DJ, Murray RM. The epidemiology of late-onset schizophrenia. *Schizophr Bull.* 1993;19:691-701.
96. Seeman MV, Lang M. The role of estrogens in schizophrenia gender differences. *Schizophr Bull.* 1990;16:185-194.
97. Salokangas RK. First-contact rate for schizophrenia in community psychiatric care: consideration of the oestrogen hypothesis. *Eur Arch Psychiatry Clin Neurosci.* 1993;242:337-346.
98. Suddath RI, Christison GW, Torrey EF, Casanova MF, Weinberger DR. Anatomical abnormalities in the brains of monozygotic twins discordant for schizophrenia. *N Engl J Med.* 1990;146:464-472.
99. Castle DJ, Murray RM. The neurodevelopmental basis of sex differences in schizophrenia. *Psychol Med.* 1991;21:565-575.

ORIGINAL ARTICLE

Functional Magnetic Resonance Imaging of Symptom Provocation in Obsessive-compulsive Disorder

Hans C. Breiter, MD; Scott L. Rauch, MD; Kenneth K. Kwong, PhD; John R. Baker, PhD; Robert M. Weisskoff, PhD; David N. Kennedy, PhD; Adair D. Kendrick; Timothy L. Davis, MS; Aiping Jiang, PhD; Mark S. Cohen, PhD; Chantal E. Stern, DPhil; John W. Belliveau, PhD; Lee Baer, PhD; Richard L. O'Sullivan, MD; Cary R. Savage, PhD; Michael A. Jenike, MD; Bruce R. Rosen, MD, PhD

Background: The new technique of functional magnetic resonance imaging was used to investigate the mediating neuroanatomy of obsessive-compulsive disorder symptoms.

Methods: Ten patients with obsessive-compulsive disorder and 5 normal subjects were studied via functional magnetic resonance imaging during control and provoked conditions. Data analysis entailed parametric and nonparametric statistical mapping.

Results: Statistical maps (nonparametric; $P<10^{-3}$) showed activation for 70% or more of patients with obsessive-compulsive disorder in medial orbitofrontal, lateral frontal, anterior temporal, anterior cingulate, and insular cortex, as well as caudate, lenticulate, and amygdala. No normal subjects exhibited activation in any brain region.

Conclusions: Results of functional magnetic resonance imaging were consistent with past studies of obsessive-compulsive disorder that used other functional neuroimaging modalities. However, paralimbic and limbic activations were more prominent in the present study.

Arch Gen Psychiatry. 1996;53:595-606

Obsessive-compulsive disorder (OCD) is a common psychiatric condition that remains incompletely understood. Positron emission tomography (PET)[1-11] and single photon emission computed tomography (SPECT)[12,13] studies have predominantly compared brain activation between patients with OCD and control subjects, as well as within patients with OCD before and after therapy. Building on xenon inhalation research,[14] 2 recent PET studies used within-subject symptom provocation paradigms.[10,11] Findings across studies have been heterogeneous; however, a convergent pattern suggests dysfunction within caudate, thalamus, anterior cingulate, and orbitofrontal cortex.[9,15,16]

With SPECT and PET, exposure to ionizing radiation limits the number of scans performed on a single subject during a calendar year. Consequently, PET and SPECT studies have, until recently,[11] pooled data across subjects. With the development of functional magnetic resonance imaging (fMRI), a new imaging modality not dependent on ionizing radiation, individual subjects can now be studied repeatedly without absolute limits to exposure duration or frequency.

Functional magnetic resonance imaging was first reported in 1991 with the use of the paramagnetic contrast agent gadolinium[17] and subsequently with non–contrast-based techniques.[18,19] One noncontrast method, BOLD (the blood oxygen level–dependent),[20,21] has been used to investigate normal cognitive,[22,23] motor,[18,19,24-27] and sensory[18,19,26,28] functions. Our pilot study reported its first use to evaluate psychopathology.[29] The BOLD technique is sensitive to T_2*-weighted signal alterations resulting from change of hemoglobin in an oxy- state, which is diamagnetic, to a deoxy- state, which is paramagnetic.[30,31] Cerebral blood flow and volume increase regionally during neuronal activation. At such times, local oxygen delivery exceeds oxygen utilization, and the net amount of deoxyhemoglobin decreases, leading to an

From the Nuclear Magnetic Resonance Center, Department of Radiology (Drs Breiter, Rauch, Kwong, Baker, Weisskoff, Kennedy, Jiang, Stern, Belliveau, O'Sullivan, and Rosen and Mr Davis), and Department of Psychiatry (Drs Breiter, Rauch, Baer, O'Sullivan, Savage, and Jenike and Ms Kendrick), Massachusetts General Hospital and Harvard Medical School, Boston; and Department of Neurology, UCLA Medical Center, Los Angeles, Calif (Dr Cohen).

See Subjects and Methods on next page

SUBJECTS AND METHODS

SUBJECTS

Forty-four fMRI studies were performed on 13 patients with OCD and 6 normal volunteers. Because of computer malfunctions and/or operator errors (8 studies) and unacceptable motion artifacts (17 studies), only 19 studies from 10 patients with OCD and 5 control subjects could be analyzed. Replicate studies were available for 4 patients with OCD.

Ten patients were recruited from the Massachusetts General Hospital OCD Unit, Boston. All met *DSM-III-R* criteria for OCD, without comorbid diagnoses on Axis I or II. Patients had been ill at least 1 year, with a mean±SD Yale-Brown Obsessive Compulsive Scale score of 13.5±7.8.[39,40] Five patients had contamination obsessions with washing compulsions, while 5 had doubting obsessions with checking compulsions, or sexual obsessions without compulsions. Normal volunteers had no psychiatric diagnosis or history of psychiatric treatment by clinical screen (H.C.B.). For the OCD and control groups, respectively, the mean±SD age was 41.2±12.3 years and 28.8±5.8 years (t=1.47, P=.22), and the mean education was 15.7±2.6 years and 16.4±2.7 years (t=0.32, P=.77). Normal subjects were medication free, while 9 of 10 patients with OCD were taking antiobsessional medications (**Table 1**). All subjects were strongly right-handed.[41] No subject had a history of head trauma, neurologic symptoms, or medical problems that had potential central nervous system sequelae. All were willing to be repeatedly provoked during experiments. Written informed consent, approved by the Massachusetts General Hospital Subcommittee on Human Studies, was obtained from each subject.

SYMPTOM PROVOCATION PARADIGM

Subjects were scanned in a baseline control condition followed by a provoked (ie, symptomatic) condition. This "off-on" paradigm entailed imaginal flooding and in vivo exposure.[14,42,43] Before scanning, the paradigm was discussed with each subject and individually tailored. Scanning began with subjects holding in their left hand an innocuous stimulus while imagining it and its innocuous implications. Subjects understood that halfway through scanning, the innocuous stimulus would be taken from their left hand and a provocative one substituted. Substitution would occur during the last 6 seconds of the baseline control interval, accompanied by a verbal reminder to visualize the provocative object and its threatening implications.

During previous studies,[10,29] patients remained symptomatic long after provocation, precluding use of an on-off design. Accordingly, studies were performed twice during each scan session, with timing between studies determined by the clinical intervention needed to return subjects to baseline (eg, washing subjects' hands with soap and water or alcohol). When subjects could not return to baseline despite multiple interventions, scanning was repeated from that higher baseline.

Ten-point, self-report, analog scales were administered before and after each functional scan to quantify the severity of anxiety and obsessionality.[10]

STIMULI

For each experiment, innocuous and provocative stimuli were matched for sensory, motor, and cognitive components so that they differed only in meaning to subjects and affective state evoked (Table 1 and **Table 2**). Provocative stimuli were developed for the 5 patients with contamination obsessions such that they also provoked normal subjects. In these experiments, after subjects observed stimulus preparation, sanitary versions were substituted for the actual experiment (unbeknownst to the subject). Universally aversive stimuli included (1) tissue soaked in toilet water, (2) plastic bags from contaminated waste barrels, and (3) tissue with nose effluvium. Innocuous stimuli were "clean" versions of the same objects (eg, tissue soaked in tap water, new plastic bags).

Stimuli for the 5 noncontamination patients with OCD were likewise individually tailored to provoke symptoms optimally and matched with innocuous stimuli to control for sensory, motor, and cognitive brain processes. One provocation example was a school picture of a patient's nephew (the object of the patient's sexual and violent obsessions), matched with a picture of that child's parent as the innocuous stimulus (Table 1).

IMAGING

Subjects were scanned on an instascan device (1.5-T Signa, General Electric Co, Milwaukee, Wis; modified by Advanced NMR Systems, Wilmington, Mass) with a quadrature head coil (General Electric Co). Initially, they were fitted with the head coil, then moved into the magnet cylinder via a mechanical table. The magnet aperture was 100 cm. Subjects could see out of the magnet by using a mirror. A pillow, foam padding, and Velcro straps were used to minimize subject movement in the head coil. Before scanning, all subjects were allowed to habituate to feelings of confinement.

A sagittal localizer scan was performed first to orient, for subsequent scans, 14 contiguous coronal slices extending from the frontal pole past the thalamus (**Figure 1**). Next, a spoiled gradient recall (SPGR) T_1-weighted flow-compensated scan (resolution, 1.6×1.6×7 mm) was obtained as an angiogram. The third scan was a T_2-weighted echo planar spin-echo sequence. Finally, functional scanning used a gradient-echo T_2*-weighted sequence (repetition time, 3000 milliseconds; echo time, 50 milliseconds; flip angle, 90°; field of view, 40×20 cm; in-plane resolution, 3.125×3.125 mm; through-plane resolution, 7 mm).[29] Images were acquired interleaved. Each functional study collected data over 4 minutes; complete sets of brain images were obtained every 3 seconds, yielding full data sets for 80 separate time points.

MOTION CORRECTION

Data were motion-corrected by means of an algorithm[44] after the work of Woods et al.[45] For each voxel, the algorithm minimized the variance of the ratio between a reference image and all subsequent images. Images were sequentially registered to the first image via 6 transformation variables for rotation about and translation along 3 coordinate axes. These variables were summarized as an average displacement function with time. Motion-corrected images were then created by reslicing the original image sets after the derived transformation function was applied. This process corrupted the first and last slices of the image stack. The transformation function generated a mean maximal movement scalar and mean movement correction value. With adoption of a conservative approach to the problem addressed by Hajnal et al,[46] data sets that evidenced any motion after attempted motion correction were excluded from further analysis.

STATISTICAL ANALYSES

Statistical analyses sought the presence and anatomical localization of significant differences in activation between control and provoked states for each subject.

Determination of Significant Change: Statistical Mapping

Determination of significant change in functional neuroimaging is an area of active research,[47-50] particularly for fMRI. In this study, we used voxel-by-voxel statistical mapping, which is widely used in PET.[49,51] With fMRI, it remains unclear whether parametric or nonparametric statistics are most appropriate.[52] Therefore, we analyzed both nonparametric and parametric statistical maps for each experiment without averaging between experiments or subjects.

Statistical maps for fMRI reflect statistical analysis across time points for each voxel. In the parametric case, an unpaired Student *t* statistic compares the mean of time points in the control condition vs the mean of time points in the provoked condition. In the nonparametric case, a Kolmogorov-Smirnov (KS) statistic[53] compares 2 samples of time points without assuming normal population distribution. It evaluates the maximum difference between cumulative distribution functions for each experimental condition.[53] Both parametric and nonparametric maps reflect change significance (ie, the likelihood that the null hypotheses is true), rather than change magnitude.

For this study, both KS and *t* statistics were implemented without adjusting degrees of freedom. At the repetition time used, little correlation existed between data points, making the degrees of freedom nearly equal to the number of samples (ie, $df=36$ for 40 time points). To first approximation, data point independence resulted since most signal fluctuations were not caused by hemodynamic response, but rather by "thermal" noise of the subject (which was white) or by other nonneuronal sources, such as blood and cerebrospinal fluid pulsations and involuntary patient motion.[54-57] Since the final 6 seconds of the neutral condition involved instructions regarding stimulus switching, both statistical approaches dropped the last 2 time points during the neutral condition.

Both parametric and nonparametric maps were smoothed, by means of a 2-dimensional center-weighted kernel analogous to a Hamming filter, so that each voxel was correlated with neighboring voxels. This altered effective spatial resolution to $6 \times 6 \times 7$ mm^3. Statistical maps were transformed to $-\log(p)$ maps and translated into color. Both types of statistical maps were assigned a threshold at selected *P* values; thus, voxels that corresponded to a *P* value greater than the threshold were excluded from further analysis.

For both statistical maps, *P* values are uncorrected. They do not account for multiple comparisons, nor do they fully address issues of temporal and spatial nonindependence. To deal with multiple comparisons, Bonferroni corrections were calculated for each voxel, despite such corrections being extremely stringent.[49] Given approximately 12 000 voxels in 12 usable motion-corrected slices, we derived a Bonferroni-corrected significance threshold of $P<10^{-7}$ ($P<[.01/12\,000]=10^{-7}$).

To protect further against type I error, we adopted a 2-dimensional cluster constraint. On the basis of anatomy, we selected a cluster of at least 5 side-connected voxels for brain cortex and 3 contiguous voxels for subcortical gray matter, requiring all voxels to exceed the threshold. These cluster constraints are affected by concomitant use of a smoothing kernel and by cross-correlation of pixel signal intensity introduced by the Fourier data acquisition. The decrease in type I error resulting from this analysis has recently been estimated by Foreman and colleagues.[58] For example, with our filtering, requiring all pixels to exceed $P<10^{-3}$ produces a per-pixel probability of detecting false-positive pixels of 3×10^{-5} in 5-pixel clusters. Our cluster sizes were small relative to brain regions sampled. Specifically, the cortical cluster was approximately 0.3 cm^3 compared with the volume of an average cortical parcellation unit of 6 cm^3 based on gyral topography.[59] Similarly, the subcortical cluster was approximately 0.2 cm^3 compared with an average volume of 3 cm^3 for such structures as the amygdala.[60]

With the use of these cluster constraints, both nonparametric and parametric maps (**Table 3**) were given thresholds at *P* values of 10^{-3}, 10^{-7}, and 10^{-10}. Signal intensity vs time curves were examined for each significant activation to estimate mean signal change between conditions and to confirm that activation did not precede stimulus presentation. Finally, statistical maps were compared with SPGR angiograms to determine overlapping territories of increased signal. Angiograms were scaled to the resolution of the functional images. Activations with any pixel overlapping an angiogram vascular structure were eliminated from further analysis. If activation was adjacent to but not overlapping the vascular structure, it was considered an activation of parenchymal origin.

A Priori Hypotheses: Regions of Interest

A priori we hypothesized that provoked patients with OCD would exhibit activation within the following regions of interest (ROIs): anterior medial and posterior medial[10] along with total medial[1-5,7] orbital gyri, lateral frontal cortex (inferior, middle, and/or superior frontal gyri),[4,6,7] anterior cingulate cortex,[4,7,8,10] caudate,[1,2,5,7,8,10] lenticulate,[5,10] and temporal cortex.[14] We further hypothesized that dominant (ie, left) motor strip and cerebellar vermis would not activate because subjects held all stimuli in the left hand, and previous PET and SPECT studies in OCD had not reported such findings.[1-14] These ROIs were a priori "control regions" to help distinguish widespread activation from global brain activation. Finally, we predicted a different activation pattern in normal subjects than in patients with OCD (ie, lacking activation in some or all a priori ROIs).

Continued on next page

Anatomic Localization

Statistical maps were first superimposed over high-resolution T_2-weighted images for anatomic localization. The high-resolution structural images were scaled to functional image resolution. A priori ROIs and a priori control ROIs were systematically inspected on parametric and nonparametric maps at 3 levels of significance thresholding. Both maps were inspected post hoc for unexpected activation according to cluster and Bonferroni criteria described above. T_2-weighted high-resolution scans involved an echo planar sequence similar to that of the functional scans and demonstrated the same regions of susceptibility artifact, primarily as signal dropout. Putative activations overlapping susceptibility artifact on T_2-weighted images could not be anatomically localized and might be artifactual; they were not tabulated as findings.

A second means of anatomic localization involved translation of activation foci from laboratory coordinates into Talairach coordinates[61] by computerized algorithm. Talairach translation entailed 3 steps. (1) The sagittal localizer scan was rotated and translated relative to Talairach orientation with the anterior commissure (AC), posterior commissure (PC), and midsagittal plane used as references. (2) Talairach scaling with the use of 6 pairwise linear scaling domains (lateral margins×2, frontal and occipital poles, superior and inferior margins) were imposed on the sagittal localizer scan for proportional scaling. (3) Machine measures of translation, rotation, and scaling from sagittal localizer to flow oblique, as well as functional scan, were then used for proportional scaling of the functional scan. One translation between flow oblique and functional scan was manually determined in the instascan blip (y) direction. Talairach dimensions were as follows: AC to superior extent (74 mm); AC to inferior extent (43 mm); AC to lateral margin (67 mm); AC to anterior pole (70 mm); AC to PC distance (24 mm); and PC to posterior pole (79 mm). By convention, for each region of activation across multiple slices, the locus translated into Talairach coordinates was the voxel with the most significant *P* value within the multiple clusters in that region.

increase in apparent T_2 relaxation time, or T_2^*, resulting in a local increase in magnetic resonance signal.[19,21,32]

Regional changes in brain hemodynamics are detectable by both conventional and echo-planar modified magnetic resonance imaging scanners, although the latter[33] has potential temporal resolution to 100 milliseconds. This superior temporal resolution is meaningfully limited by the hemodynamic response time of 1.5 to 2 seconds.[19,34,35] High temporal resolution, along with high spatial resolution and capacity for scanning subjects repeatedly, distinguish fMRI from other tomographic brain imaging modalities.[36,37]

In the present study, we used fMRI to image symptom provocation in individual patients with OCD and normal control subjects. As with our previous PET symptom provocation studies of OCD and simple phobia,[10,38] this fMRI study evaluated only positive signal changes. The present study is distinguished from our previous work in that normal control subjects as well as patients with OCD were studied; more aversive, "universally provocative" stimuli were used to provoke patients and control subjects; fMRI was used; both parametric and nonparametric statistical analyses were used in individual subjects; and a subgroup of subjects were scanned on multiple occasions to evaluate test-retest reliability.

See also pages 574, 577, 585, 607, 617, and 625

This study sought to address several questions. With fMRI, what is the pattern of positive activation in the OCD symptomatic vs control state? Is there similar activation in matched normal subjects? How do fMRI results compare with published PET and SPECT data on OCD? Do fMRI results differ depending on data analytic methods used? Are fMRI results reproducible within and between subjects? What are the implications for future research?

RESULTS

Individually tailored stimuli effectively provoked symptoms (Tables 1 and 2). Among patients, OCD analog scale scores reflected increased OCD symptoms during provoked (6.4±2.7) vs baseline (2.3±2.0) conditions (mean±SD difference, 4.2±2.5; paired t=5.3, P<.001, 2-tailed). For normal subjects, OCD analog scale scores also increased during provoked (3.0±2.8) vs baseline (1.0±1.4) conditions, although not as much (mean±SD difference, 2.0±1.4; paired t=3.2, P<.03, 2-tailed). Similarly, anxiety analog scale scores increased for both OCD (mean±SD difference, 3.0±2.8; paired t=3.0, P<.02) and normal (mean±SD difference, 1.4±1.1; paired t=2.8, P<.05) groups.

Seventeen of 36 otherwise acceptable studies were excluded because of uncorrectable movement (ie, movement >1.5 mm). For the 19 remaining studies, there was a *mean maximal* movement across patients with OCD of 0.59 mm, requiring *mean* movement correction of 0.25 mm. At least 1 scan was excluded from every patient and control subject, indicating that movement was not isolated to a particular subgroup of subjects. Furthermore, excluded scans were not associated with either higher or lower OCD analog scores.

The KS maps for normal controls showed no statistically significant activation in any brain region, even with liberal statistical thresholds ($P<10^{-3}$; Table 3). In contrast, at the same thresholding, 70% or more of patients with OCD exhibited significant activation within the following a priori ROIs (Table 3, **Figure 2**): bilateral anterior and posterior medial orbital gyri; bilateral superior, middle, and inferior frontal gyri; bilateral anterior cingulate cortex; bilateral temporal cortex; right caudate; and left lenticulate. No patient with OCD exhibited significant activation within a priori control ROIs. However, post hoc analyses found activation in 70% or more of patients with OCD in left insula and bilateral amygdaloid complex. Signal change amplitude varied by region across all 10 patients, being maximal on average in the left anterior orbital cortex (6.0%±3.3%) and least on average in the right caudate (1.4%±.9%). Typically, regional signal intensity changes occurred within 3 seconds of stimulus presentation.

For KS maps, with more stringent thresholds ($P<10^{-7}$) approximating Bonferroni correction, 70% or more of patients with OCD activated the right posterior and left anterior medial orbital gyri; left superior frontal, left middle frontal, and right inferior frontal cortex; and bilateral temporal cortex. Post hoc analysis showed no other activation at this stringent criterion.

With the most stringent threshold of KS maps ($P<10^{-10}$), no brain region activated for 70% or more of patients with OCD, although 50% or more did activate the left anterior and right posterior medial orbitofrontal cortex, along with the left superior frontal cortex. For *t* maps, spatial distribution of activation in patients with OCD resembled the KS maps. However, their *P* values were shifted 3 to 4 orders of magnitude compared with the KS maps (Table 3). Thus, *t* maps with a threshold at $P<10^{-7}$ resembled KS maps with a threshold at $P<10^{-3}$, and *t* maps with a threshold at $P<10^{-10}$ resembled KS maps with a threshold at $P<10^{-7}$.

Replicate data were available for 4 patients with OCD, allowing preliminary examination of test-retest reliability (**Table 4**). The time interval between test and retest ranged from 20 minutes (same scanning session) to 33 days. A binary criterion based on the presence or absence of activation within the ROI from KS maps with a threshold at $P<10^{-7}$ was used. All 4 patients exhibited good replication for the 23 regions inspected, ranging from 17 of 23 to 21 of 23 regions showing replication. Instances of nonreplication between scans predominantly reflected initial positive activation with subsequent failure to activate.

To characterize intersubject variability of activation location, the mean and SD for x, y, and z Talairach coordinates were determined for each regional activation (**Table 5**). This procedure was completed for 8 of 10 patients with OCD, since sagittal localizer data were not saved for 2. Standard deviations for each coordinate indicated intersubject variability per activation site. In most cases, SDs were less than ±1 cm, while in some, such as the x coordinate for the lenticulate, variability across subjects was large.

COMMENT

Functional magnetic resonance imaging of patients with OCD and normal control subjects showed a pattern of activation associated with the OCD symptomatic vs baseline state. For KS maps with a threshold at $P<10^{-3}$, a priori regions active in 70% or more of patients with OCD included bilateral anterior and posterior medial orbital gyri; bilateral superior, middle, and inferior frontal gyri; bilateral anterior cingulate cortex; bilateral temporal cortex; right caudate; and left lenticulate. Post hoc analyses demonstrated activation for 70% or more of patients with OCD in the left insula and bilateral amygdaloid complex.

Despite widespread activation, no patients with OCD activated a priori control ROIs. Therefore, observed patterns did not reflect global nonspecific activation. Global activation with fMRI can result from tachycardia, hyperventilation, venous filling, and cerebrospinal fluid motility. The long–repetition time echo-planar sequence we used minimizes the effect of velocity change for macroscopic flowing protons (ie, blood or cerebrospinal fluid) on signal intensity. Furthermore, motion correction reduces bulk motion from such sources as respiratory excursions.

In all cases, the activation pattern distinguished patients with OCD from control subjects, who did not show significant activation at $P<10^{-3}$. Additional studies are necessary, however, to determine whether such findings are specific to OCD.

Data were analyzed with parametric (*t* maps) and nonparametric (KS maps) statistics, and across a range of significance thresholds. Activation patterns were similar regardless of statistical method, and, as might be expected given fewer inherent assumptions, the nonparametric approach was more conservative than the parametric approach.

For KS maps with a threshold at $P<10^{-7}$ (the Bonferroni correction), 70% or more of patients with OCD showed activation in the right posterior and left anterior medial orbital gyri; left superior frontal, left middle frontal, and right inferior frontal cortex; and bilateral temporal cortex. Post hoc analysis showed no other activation. With a threshold of $P<10^{-10}$, no brain regions exhibited activation for 70% or more of patients with OCD. In contrast, for *t* maps, patients with OCD did show significant activation at $P<10^{-10}$, resembling the pattern of KS maps with a threshold at $P<10^{-7}$.

When patients with OCD were scanned multiple times, the activation patterns suggested good test-retest reliability. Of 4 pairs of test-retest studies, one replicated 21 of 23 regions, while 3 replicated 17 to 18 of 23 regions. These last 3 subjects had similar analog scale ratings across studies, suggesting that activation variability between scans was unlikely to be related to OCD state differences. As with any activation study, the observed variability may be attributable to imaging technology, paradigm implementation, or biological substrate under study.

In contrast to test-retest measures of intrasubject variability, no direct tests of intersubject variability were performed. Indirect indications of intersubject variability include the proportion of patients who demonstrated activation per region, and SDs of Talairach coordinates for each activation. Talairach coordinates

Table 1. Challenge Stimulus, Symptom Provoked, and Resulting Change in OCD and Anxiety Scale Scores After Provocation for Each Subject*

Patient No.	Challenge Stimulus		Symptom Type	OCD Score			
	Innocuous	Provocative		Rest	Provocation	Difference	Rest
1	Clean towel	Towel in toilet water	Contamination obsessions	5	7	2	5
2	New tissue	Nose effluvium in tissue	Contamination obsessions	4	7	3	4
	Same as above	Same as above	Same as above	3	7	4	3
3	Sterile gauze	Gauze wiped around toilet	Contamination obsessions	3	7	4	5
	Same as above	Same as above	Same as above	5	8	3	6
4	Sterile gauze	Nose effluvium in gauze	Contamination obsessions	5	10	5	5
5	Clean towel	Tower in toilet water	Contamination obsessions	2	4	2	2
6	Sheet from nursery without needles	Sheet from laundry with mixed-in used needles	Checking obsessions	0	3	3	0
7	Picture of nephew's parent	Picture of nephew and sexual imagery	Sexual/violent obsession	0	10	10	0
8	Picture of pet dog	Picture of man in underwear	Homosexual obsession	3	6	3	2
	Same as above	Same as above	Same as above	1	7	6	2
9	Clean envelope	Envelope associated with illicit drugs	Drug obsession	1	7	6	2
	Same as above	Same as above	Same as above	1	7	6	1
10	Pot in dishwasher	Pot with boiling water	Checking obsession	0	2	2	0
Mean±SD	...	...	...	2.4±1.9	6.7±2.2	4.3±2.2	2.7±2.1

*OCD indicates obsessive-compulsive disorder.

Table 2. Challenge Stimulus and Resulting Change in OCD and Anxiety Scale Scores After Provocation for Each Normal Subject*

Normal Subject No.	Challenge Stimulus		OCD Score			Anxiety Score		
	Innocuous	Provocative	Rest	Provocation	Difference	Rest	Provocation	Difference
1	Clean plastic bag	Contaminated waste bag	0	1	1	0	0	0
2	Clean towel	Towel with toilet water	0	1	1	0	1	1
3	Clean towel	Towel with toilet water	0	1	1	2	3	1
4	Clean tissue	Tissue with nose effluvium	2	5	3	2	5	3
5	Sterile gauze	Gauze with toilet water	3	7	4	3	5	2
Mean±SD	...	...	1.0±1.4	3.0±2.8	2.0±1.4	1.4±1.3	2.8±2.3	1.4±1.1

*OCD indicates obsessive-compulsive disorder.

(Table 5) characterized spatial variability by SDs of 1.0 cm or less for most regions. This is consistent with the spatial resolution after movement correction, image smoothing, and Talairach transformation (see below). Anatomic localization sometimes demonstrated substantial variability, as along y- and z-axes for frontal gyri and anterior cingulate cortex. Such examples likely reflect relatively large anterior to posterior and inferior to superior dimensions for some regions, and differential mapping of functionally homologous subterritories between subjects.

Alternatively, disparity in localization may reflect functional subterritories being activated differentially between subjects, as might occur with the lenticulate.

Despite promising preliminary findings, this study has several limitations. Although within-subject design provides some internal control, 9 of 10 patients with OCD were taking medication during scanning, in contrast to none of the control subjects. Therefore, differences in activation patterns could be attributable to medication rather than diagnosis. Four reports have addressed this issue with respect to OCD.[5,7,8,62] In 3 of these reports, serotonergic reuptake inhibitors significantly decreased or normalized regional glucose metabolic rates seen in untreated patients. In the fourth report,[62] fluoxetine treatment was associated with a decrease in the blood flow to frontal cortex in patients with OCD. Given these 4 reports, regional increases in patients' fMRI signal found by this study were unlikely to have been caused by medication effects, particularly since it was the symptom expression in each subject, despite ongoing medication treatment, that was being imaged.

Study limitations also include imperfect matching of patient and control groups on age, gender, and education, along with unequal magnitudes of symptom

Anxiety Score: Provocation	Anxiety Score: Difference	Medication	Total Daily Dose, mg
6	1	Fluoxetine	60
6	2	Fluoxetine	20
7	4	...	...
7	2	Fluoxetine	80
8	2	...	...
10	5	Sertraline hydrochloride	200
4	2	Fluoxetine	120
2	2	Clomipramine hydrochloride	75
10	10	Fluoxetine	120
5	3	Paroxetine	60
5	3	...	...
1	1	Paroxetine	60
0	1	...	...
1	1	None	...
5.1±3.3	2.7±2.4	...	...

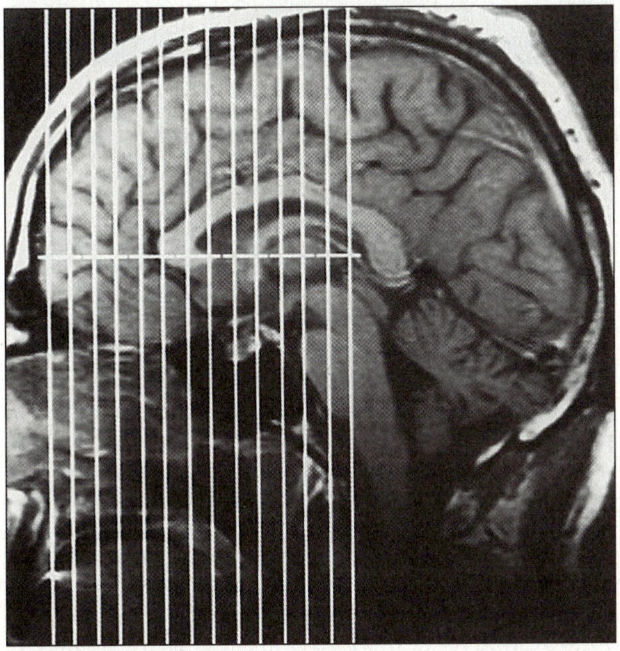

Figure 1. *Example of a midsagittal slice from an anatomic localizer scan with superimposed slice prescription for the 14 contiguous slices used in the functional magnetic resonance imaging experiment.*

Table 3. Proportions of Patients With OCD and Control Subjects Showing Regional Activation*

	Normal: KS Statistic (10^{-3})†	OCD: KS Statistic (10^{-3})†	OCD: KS Statistic (10^{-7})†	OCD: *t* Test (10^{-7})†
Regional Activation (A Priori)				
Orbital frontal cortex				
Right				
Anterior	0/5	10/10	5/10	9/10
Posterior	0/5	8/10	7/10	7/10
Left				
Anterior	0/5	10/10	9/10	10/10
Posterior	0/5	7/10	6/10	8/10
Gyrus superioris				
Right	0/5	10/10	5/10	7/10
Left	0/5	9/10	8/10	8/10
Gyrus medialis				
Right	0/5	10/10	6/10	7/10
Left	0/5	8/10	7/10	6/10
Gyrus inferioris				
Right	0/5	9/10	7/10	7/10
Left	0/5	7/10	2/10	5/10
Cingulate cortex				
Right	0/5	8/10	4/10	7/10
Left	0/5	10/10	6/10	8/10
Temporal cortex				
Right	0/5	10/10	7/10	10/10
Left	0/5	9/10	7/10	9/10
Caudate				
Right	0/5	8/10	5/10	6/10
Left	0/5	5/10	4/10	4/10
Lenticulate				
Right	0/5	6/10	4/10	5/10
Left	0/5	8/10	4/10	5/10
Additional Regions (Post Hoc)				
Insula				
Right	0/5	6/10	3/10	4/10
Left	0/5	8/10	2/10	5/10
Amygdaloid complex				
Right	0/5	9/10	5/10	6/10
Left	0/5	9/10	6/10	8/10
Control Regions (A Priori)				
Primary motor cortex				
Left	0/5	0/10	0/10	0/10
Cerebellar vermis				
Right	0/5	0/10	0/10	0/10
Left	0/5	0/10	0/10	0/10

**Based on Kolmogorov-Smirnov (KS) maps;* t *map included for comparison. OCD indicates obsessive-compulsive disorder.*
†*P value threshold.*

provocation between them. Indeed, differences in severity of symptomatic distress could partially account for altered brain activation between groups. Another consideration involves the heterogeneity of patient symptoms. The OCD group included subjects with diverse symptoms, which could reflect different neuronal substrates and produce disparate fMRI results.

Other study limitations may reflect the general state of fMRI research and its application to psychiatric illness. All subjects moved. With the use of a conservative criterion, 17 of 36 otherwise acceptable studies were excluded for excessive movement. Given 3.125×3.125-mm pixels with 7-mm slices, movement of 50% or more in-plane resolution or more than 20% through-plane resolution produced movement artifact despite attempted correction. Furthermore, motion correction of 19 studies with correctable movement

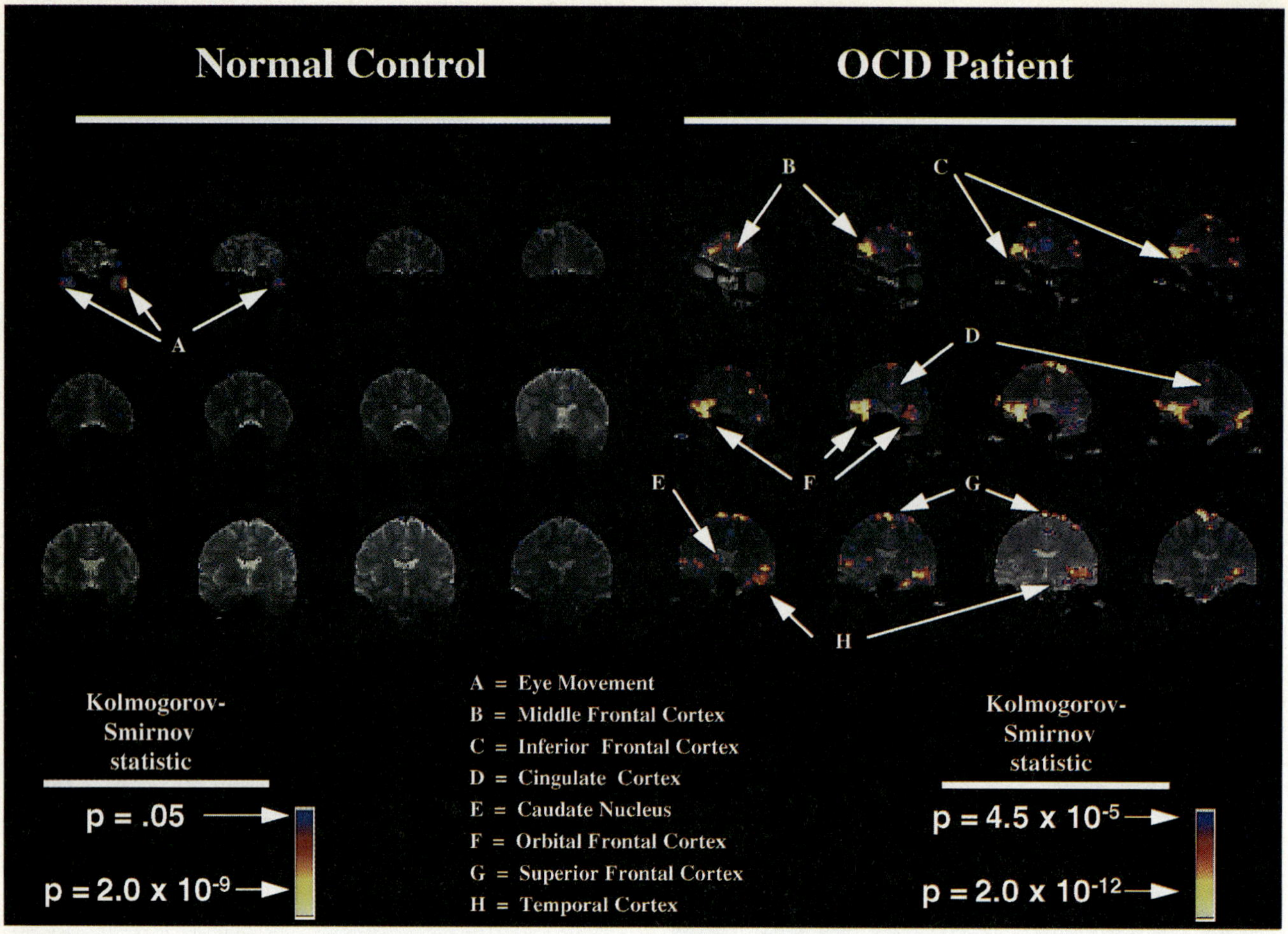

Figure 2. *Results for 1 normal subject and 1 patient with obsessive-compulsive disorder (OCD) (normal subject 2 and patient 9 [trial B]), juxtaposed for comparison. The gradient echo functional data are shown as a -log (p) map (Kolmogorov-Smirnov statistic) in color, superimposed over a T_2-weighted high-resolution instascan image in gray tone, for anatomical reference. Twelve contiguous slices are shown for each subject. The threshold for the control subject is at a lower level to emphasize the absence of activation, while the patient's threshold is at a more stringent level ($P<10^{-7}$, approximating Bonferroni-corrected $P<.01$).*

reduced spatial resolution an average of 0.14 mm in 3 dimensions. To smooth any residual effects for these 19 studies, statistical mapping used a 2-dimensional in-plane filter. Given motion correction and smoothing, overall spatial resolution became 6.39×6.39×7.14 mm, a resolution comparable with that of PET.

Movement is problematic for fMRI, particularly as fMRI can involve sampling of small voxels over short intervals, use of nonisotropic voxel dimensions, and acquisition of interleaved images. For fMRI there are at least 5 identifiable sources of motion. The first is motion between separate scanning sessions, the second is that of head relaxation or fatigue between experimental runs. The third involves motion between epochs in 1 run (ie, between neutral and obsessive state), while the fourth involves movement between time points. The fifth results from movement during acquisition of a stack of slices over 1 repetition time interval. This last form of motion is difficult to correct when fMR images are acquired interleaved, as in this study. Interleaving implies acquisition of slice 13 long before slices 12 and 14, leading to potentially nonlinear movement effects, since oversampled and undersampled regions of space cannot be compensated. At present, the relatively low yield of interpretable data can limit use of this fMRI technique, particularly for psychiatric populations with tics, dyskinesias, or agitation.

Finally, fMRI research awaits consensus about data analysis. In this study we attempted a conservative approach, with stringent motion correction criteria, parametric and nonparametric statistical mapping, cluster constraints, and statistical thresholding inclusive of a Bonferroni-type correction for multiple comparisons. Work is still needed to determine optimal statistical methods for fMRI, particularly to evaluate temporal differences in activation over distributed neural systems.

Despite its limitations and the relative infancy of fMRI, this study produced results remarkably consistent with previous neuroimaging of OCD, such as our previous PET symptom provocation study.[10] The present fMRI study found activation in 70% or more of patients with OCD (KS maps, $P<10^{-7}$) in the same quadrants of medial orbitofrontal cortex as that PET study. At the lower threshold (KS maps, $P<10^{-3}$), it replicated the PET observation of right caudate activation. Overall, it found less consistent activation of deep gray matter at high statistical thresholds than the

PET study; this may reflect differential effects on signal acquisition for cortical vs subcortical regions. At variance with our PET study, but in agreement with the findings of Zohar et al,[14] fMRI detected bilateral anterior temporal cortex activation in 70% or more of patients with OCD. Further at odds with the PET study, fMRI detected (KS maps, $P<10^{-3}$) different laterality of lenticulate activation and new amygdaloid and insular activations. Disparity in activation pattern between the 2 studies could reflect differences in the paradigms; more intensely provocative stimuli were used in this fMRI study than before.[10,14]

This fMRI study noted extensive paralimbic and limbic system activation. Two regions, medial orbitofrontal cortex and anterior temporal cortex, were observed at the Bonferroni threshold and have been reported in other neuroimaging studies of OCD. In contrast, insular cortex and amygdala activations were noted at the most liberal significance threshold and might represent type I error in the fMRI study or type II error in our PET study, which did not detect them. The fMRI data are presented as proportions of individuals who demonstrated activation. Data presented in this form reduce the risk of type II error from averaging across small numbers of subjects, while enhancing sensitivity to laterality findings. Data presented in this form also reduce potential for type II errors resulting from heterogeneity of activation location (see SDs for the Talairach coordinates, Table 5) caused by between-subject differences. In addition, compared with PET, the slightly superior spatial resolution of this fMRI application might help protect against type II errors for activation of small structures (eg, amygdala).

Paralimbic regions are associated with autonomic responses when electrically stimulated in humans and animals.[63-65] Together with the limbic system, the paralimbic belt is hypothesized to mediate strong emotions. As a link between the limbic system and the heteromodal association cortex, paralimbic structures are theorized to be important for assessing and responding to behavioral significance of external stimuli.[63] In another PET study, our group found widespread activation of paralimbic structures during simple phobic symptom provocation[38]; these subjects were also provoked to a state of severe anxiety. One might surmise paralimbic recruitment during anxiety symptom provocation to be a quantitative rather than a qualitative issue.

In contrast to recent PET studies of intense emotional states in normal subjects,[66-68] this fMRI study did not detect activation of paralimbic or other brain structures during provocation of normal controls. Perhaps greater statistical power by signal averaging techniques or collection of additional time points is necessary for detecting, by fMRI, activation associated with affect in normal controls. All three PET studies involving internally generated emotions in normal controls demonstrated activation of paralimbic and limbic structures observed in patients with OCD with this fMRI study. Such similarities raise the possibility that obsessional states use circuitry similar to that of sadness in normal subjects and might involve some dys-

Table 4. Test and Retest Results for 4 Patients With Obsessive-compulsive Disorder*

	Test/Retest Result			
	Patient 2	Patient 3	Patient 8	Patient 9
Regional Activation (A Priori)				
Orbital frontal cortex				
Right	−/−	+/+	+/+	+/+
Left	−/−	+/+	+/+	+/+
Lateral frontal cortex				
Gyrus superioris				
Right	−/−	+/+	+/+	+/+
Left	−/−	+/+	+/+	+/+
Gyrus medialis				
Right	+/−	+/+	+/+	+/+
Left	+/−	+/+	+/+	+/+
Gyrus inferioris				
Right	+/−	+/+	+/+	+/+
Left	−/+	−/−	−/−	+/+
Cingulate cortex				
Right	−/−	+/+	+/−	−/−
Left	+/−	−/+	+/−	+/−
Temporal cortex				
Right	−/−	+/+	+/+	−/+
Left	−/−	+/+	+/+	−/+
Caudate				
Right	−/−	+/+	+/+	+/+
Left	−/−	+/+	+/−	+/−
Lenticulate				
Right	−/−	−/−	+/+	+/+
Left	−/−	+/+	+/−	+/−
Control (A Priori)				
Primary motor cortex				
Left	−/−	−/−	−/−	−/−
Cerebellar vermis				
Right	−/−	−/−	−/−	−/−
Left	−/−	−/−	−/−	−/−
Additional Regions (Post Hoc)				
Insula				
Right	−/−	−/−	+/+	+/+
Left	−/−	−/−	+/−	+/+
Amygdaloid complex				
Right	+/−	−/−	+/−	−/−
Left	−/−	−/+	+/+	+/+
Time interval between test and retest	20 min	20 min	7 d	33 d

*From Table 1; Kolmogorov-Smirnov map, $P<10^{-7}$.

function of internal emotional regulation or emotional memory.[69] These considerations are tempered, though, by experimental differences in paradigms and the many regional activations that were not shared by these 3 studies and the present fMRI study.

In summary, this fMRI study found that patients with OCD exhibited isocortical (lateral frontal), paralimbic (medial orbital gyrus, anterior cingulate, temporal cortex, and insular cortex), limbic (amygdala), and striatal (caudate and lenticulate) activations in association with OCD symptoms. Consistent with the phenomenology of the disorder and convergent with previous OCD research, these results implicate brain systems involved with both cognition and emotion.[10,70] Despite unresolved issues regarding statistical

Table 5. Talairach Localization of Regional Activations in 8 Patients With Obsessive-compulsive Disorder*

	Talairach Coordinate (±SD)			No. of Patients
	X	Y	Z	
Orbital frontal cortex				
Right				
Anterior	30.1 (±3.8)	42.8 (±13.2)	−10.4 (±2.5)	8
Posterior	28.6 (±6.6)	24.2 (±4.4)	−12.7 (±4.9)	7
Left				
Anterior	−22.6 (±13.0)	39.1 (±9.3)	−13.0 (±3.2)	8
Posterior	−22.2 (±13.2)	19.2 (±5.5)	−14.2 (±3.6)	5
Gyrus superioris				
Right	17.4 (±8.6)	18.0 (±20.8)	57.2 (±11.8)	7
Left	−11.6 (±5.1)	1.7 (±17.6)	65.2 (±8.6)	7
Gyrus medialis				
Right				
Anterior	35.2 (±10.3)	41.6 (±16.2)	10.6 (±19.5)	5
Posterior	38.5 (±5.1)	12.5 (±12.9)	44.2 (±6.8)	6
Left				
Anterior	−25.0 (±4.6)	51.5 (±9.8)	13.8 (±19.2)	6
Posterior	−36.3 (±3.3)	12.7 (±9.4)	39.2 (±28.5)	6
Gyrus inferioris				
Right	42.6 (±12.1)	21.1 (±11.6)	3.3 (±9.7)	8
Left	−40.3 (±7.0)	20.2 (±9.1)	1.0 (±16.2)	7
Cingulate cortex				
Right	4.2 (±3.7)	22.0 (±22.3)	17.3 (±19.7)	7
Left	−5.3 (±4.0)	32.0 (±11.7)	12.3 (±14.6)	7
Temporal cortex				
Right				
Anterior (Brodmann area 38)	41.0 (±10.0)	11.7 (±5.5)	−25.6 (±8.5)	7
Medial	24.0 (±6.6)	−7.9 (±8.0)	−30.1 (±6.1)	8
Left				
Anterior (Brodmann area 38)	−30.3 (±6.9)	12.2 (±3.4)	−33.0 (±5.1)	6
Medial	−24.4 (±9.7)	−7.9 (±6.2)	−27.6 (±7.5)	7
Caudate				
Right	11.3 (±2.9)	−4.5 (±11.3)	19.5 (±1.7)	4
Left	−11.3 (±3.2)	11.7 (±10.1)	10.7 (±6.5)	3
Lenticulate				
Right	15.4 (±14.1)	−2.6 (±6.8)	−2.0 (±4.7)	5
Left	−14.5 (±17.8)	4.5 (±9.3)	−2.2 (±6.6)	6
Insula				
Right	44.3 (±8.3)	0.7 (±10.2)	5.0 (±9.4)	7
Left	−37.0 (±7.6)	6.4 (±8.6)	3.2 (±3.6)	7
Amygdaloid complex				
Right	22.0 (±7.6)	−8.8 (±9.9)	−15.3 (±4.6)	6
Left	−22.0 (±7.9)	−9.2 (±5.4)	−19.8 (±5.5)	5

**Based on Kolmogorov-Smirnov maps;* P *value threshold,* 10^{-3}.

analysis and movement, fMRI appears to be a promising tool for investigation of psychiatric disease given its ability to assess subjects repeatedly and to generate statistical power for analyses within individuals.

Accepted for publication January 3, 1996.

This study was supported in part by grant 5T32CA09362-11 from the National Cancer Institute, Bethesda, Md, and Young Investigator Awards from the National Alliance for Research on Schizophrenia and Depression, Chicago, Ill (Drs Breiter and Rauch), and the David Judah Research Fund, Charlestown, Mass. Dr Breiter received supplemental support from the Ethel Dupont Warren Fund and the Livingston Fund at Harvard Medical School, Boston, Mass.

We thank Terry Campbell and Linda Leahy for their technical assistance and Thomas Brady, MD, for his help with research design.

Reprints: Hans C. Breiter, MD, Massachusetts General Hospital–NMR Center, Second Floor, 149 13th St, Charlestown, MA 02129 (e-mail: hansb@nmr.mgh.harvard.edu).

REFERENCES

1. Baxter LR, Phelps ME, Maziotta JC, Guze BH, Schwartz JM, Selin SE. Local cerebral metabolic rates in obsessive-compulsive disorder. *Arch Gen Psychiatry.* 1987;44:211-218.
2. Baxter LR, Schwartz JM, Mazziotta JC, Phelps ME, Pahl JJ, Buze BE, Fairbanks L. Cerebral metabolic rates in non-depressed patients with obsessive-compulsive disorder. *Am J Psychiatry.* 1988;145:1560-1563.
3. Nordahl TE, Benkelfat C, Semple WE, Gross M, King AC, Cohen RM. Cerebral glucose metabolic rates in obsessive-compulsive disorder. *Neuropsychopharmacology.* 1989;2:23-28.
4. Swedo SE, Schapiro MB, Grady CL, Cheslow DL, Leonard HL, Kumar A, Friedland R, Rapoport SI, Rapoport JL. Cerebral glucose metabolism in childhood-

onset obsessive-compulsive disorder. *Arch Gen Psychiatry.* 1989;46:518-523.
5. Benkelfat C, Nordahl TE, Semple WE, King AC, Murphy DL, Cohen RM. Local cerebral glucose metabolic rates in obsessive-compulsive disorder: patients treated with clomipramine. *Arch Gen Psychiatry.* 1990;47:840-848.
6. Martinot JL, Allilaire JF, Mazoyer BM, Hantouche E, Huret JD, Legaut-Demare F, Deslauriers AG, Hardy P, Pappata S, Baron JC, Syrota A. Obsessive-compulsive disorder: a clinical, neuropsychological and positron emission tomography study. *Acta Psychiatr Scand.* 1990;82:233-242.
7. Swedo SE, Pietrini P, Leonard HL, Schapiro MB, Rettew DC, Goldberger EL, Rapoport SI, Rapoport JL, Grady CL. Cerebral glucose metabolism in childhood-onset obsessive-compulsive disorder: revisualization during pharmacotherapy. *Arch Gen Psychiatry.* 1992;49:690-694.
8. Baxter LR, Schwartz JM, Bergman KS, Szuba MP, Guze BH, Mazziotta JC, Alazraki A, Selin CE, Ferng H-K, Munford P, Phelps ME. Caudate glucose metabolic rate changes with both drug and behavior therapy for obsessive-compulsive disorder. *Arch Gen Psychiatry.* 1992;49:681-689.
9. Baxter LR. Neuroimaging studies of obsessive-compulsive disorder. *Psychiatr Clin North Am.* 1992;15:871-884.
10. Rauch SL, Jenike MA, Alpert NM, Baer L, Breiter HCR, Savage CR, Fischman AJ. Regional cerebral blood flow measured during symptom provocation in obsessive-compulsive disorder using ^{15}O-labeled CO_2 and positron emission tomography. *Arch Gen Psychiatry.* 1994;51:62-70.
11. McGuire PK, Bench CJ, Frith CD, Marks IM, Frackowiak RS, Dolan RJ. Functional anatomy of obsessive-compulsive phenomena. *Br J Psychiatry.* 1994; 164:459-468.
12. Machlin SR, Harris GJ, Pearlson GD, Hoehn-Saric R, Jeffery P, Camargo EE. Elevated medial-frontal cerebral blood flow in obsessive-compulsive patients: a SPECT study. *Am J Psychiatry.* 1991;148:1240-1242.
13. Rubin RT, Villanueva-Meyer J, Anath J, Trajmar PG, Mena I. Regional xenon 133 cerebral blood flow and cerebral technetium Tc 99m-HMPAO uptake in unmedicated patients with obsessive-compulsive disorder and matched normal control subjects: determination by high-resolution single-photon emission computed tomography. *Arch Gen Psychiatry.* 1992;49:695-702.
14. Zohar J, Insel TR, Berman KF, Foa EB, Hill JL, Weinberger DR. Anxiety and cerebral blood flow during behavioral challenge. *Arch Gen Psychiatry.* 1989; 46:505-510.
15. Insel TR. Toward a neuroanatomy of obsessive-compulsive disorder. *Arch Gen Psychiatry.* 1992;49:739-744.
16. Rauch SL, Jenike MA. Neurobiological models of obsessive-compulsive disorder. *Psychosomatics.* 1993;34:20-32.
17. Belliveau JW, Kennedy DN, McKinstry RC, Buchbinder BR, Weisskoff RM, Cohen MS, Vevea JM, Brady TJ, Rosen BR. Functional mapping of the human visual cortex by magnetic resonance imaging. *Science.* 1991;254:716-719.
18. Brady TJ. Future prospects for MR imaging. *Proc Soc Magn Reson Med.* 1991; 1:2.
19. Kwong KK, Belliveau JW, Chesler DA, Goldberg IE, Weisskoff RM, Poncelet BP, Kennedy DN, Hoppel BE, Cohen MS, Turner R, Cheng HM, Brady TJ, Rosen BR. Dynamic magnetic resonance imaging of human brain activity during primary sensory stimulation. *Proc Natl Acad Sci U S A.* 1992;89: 5675-5679.
20. Ogawa S, Lee T, Nayak A, Glynn P. Oxygenation-sensitive contrast in magnetic resonance image of rodent brain at high magnetic fields. *Magn Reson Med.* 1990;14:68-78.
21. Ogawa S, Tank DW, Menon R, Ellermann JM, Kim SG, Merkle H, Ugurbil K. Intrinsic signal changes accompanying sensory stimulation: functional brain mapping using MRI. *Proc Natl Acad Sci U S A.* 1992;89:5951-5955.
22. McCarthy G, Blamire AM, Rothman DL, Gruetter R, Shulman RG. Echo-planar magnetic resonance imaging studies of frontal cortex activation during word generation in humans. *Proc Natl Acad Sci U S A.* 1993;90:4952-4956.
23. Cohen JD, Forman SD, Braver TS, Casey BJ, Servan-Schreiber D, Noll DC. Activation of the prefrontal cortex in a nonspatial working memory task with functional MRI. *Hum Brain Mapping.* 1994;1:293-304.
24. Bandettini PA, Jesmanowicz A, Wong EC, Hyde JS. Processing strategies for time-course data sets in functional MRI of the human brain. *Magn Reson Med.* 1993;30:161-173.
25. Menon RS, Ogawa S, Tank DW, Ugurbil K. 4 tesla gradient recalled echo characteristics of photic stimulation-induced signal changes in the human primary visual cortex. *Magn Reson Med.* 1993;30:380-386.
26. Rao SM, Binder JR, Bandettini PA, Hammeke TA, Yetkin FZ, Jesmanowica A, Lisk L, Morris GL, Mueller WM, Estowski LD, Wong EC, Haughton VM, Hyde JS. Functional magnetic resonance imaging of complex human movements. *Neurology.* 1993;43:2311-2318.
27. Kim S-G, Ashe J, Georgopoulos AP, Merkle H, Ellemann JM, Menon RS, Ogawa S, Ugurbil K. Functional imaging of the human motor cortex at high magnetic field. *J Neurophysiol.* 1993;69:297-302.
28. Binder JR, Rao SM, Hammeke TA, Yetkin FZ, Jesmanowicz A, Bandettini PA, Wong EC, Estkowski LD, Goldstein MD, Haughton VM, Hyde JS. Functional magnetic resonance imaging of human auditory cortex. *Ann Neurol.* 1994;35: 662-672.
29. Breiter HC, Kwong KK, Baker JR, Belliveau JW, Davis TL, Baer L, O'Sullivan RM, Rauch SL, Savage CR, Cohen MS, Weisskoff RM, Brady TJ, Jenike MA, Rosen BR. Functional magnetic resonance imaging of symptom provocation in patients with obsessive compulsive disorder versus controls. *Proc Soc Magn Reson Med.* 1993;1:58. Abstract.
30. Pauling L, Coryell CD. The magnetic properties and structure of hemoglobin, oxyhemoglobin and carbonmonoxyhemoglobin. *Proc Natl Acad Sci U S A.* 1936; 22:210.
31. Thulborn KR, Waterton JC, Matthew PM, Radda GK. Oxygenation dependence of the transverse relaxation time of water protons in whole blood at high field. *Biochim Biophys Acta.* 1982;714:265.
32. Bandettini PA, Wong EC, Hinks RS, Tikofsky RS, Hyde JS. Time course EPI of human brain function during task activation. *Magn Reson Med.* 1992;25:390-397.
33. Cohen MS, Weisskoff RM. Ultra-fast imaging. *Magn Reson Imaging.* 1991;9: 1-37.
34. Blood AJ, Narayan SM, Toga AW. Stimulus parameters influence magnitude and time course of optical intrinsic responses in rodent barrel cortex. *Proc Soc Neurosci.* 1994;2:1422. Abstract.
35. Narayan SM, Blood AJ, Toga AW. Functional neural-vascular congruence over somatosensory cortex. *Proc Soc Neurosci.* 1994;2:1422. Abstract.
36. Cohen MS, Bookheimer S. Localization of brain function with magnetic resonance imaging. *Trends Neurosci.* 1994;17:268-277.
37. David A, Blamire A, Breiter H. Functional magnetic resonance imaging: a new technique with implications for psychology and psychiatry. *Br J Psychiatry.* 1994;164:2-7.
38. Rauch SL, Savage CR, Alpert NM, Miguel EC, Baer L, Breiter HC, Fischman AJ, Manzo PA, Moretti C, Jenike MA. A positron emission tomographic study of simple phobic symptom provocation. *Arch Gen Psychiatry.* 1995;52:20-28.
39. Goodman WK, Price LH, Rasmussen SA, Mazure C, Fleischmann RL, Hill CL, Heninger GR, Charney DS. The Yale-Brown Obsessive Compulsive Scale (YBOCS), I: development, use, and reliability. *Arch Gen Psychiatry.* 1989;46:1006-1011.
40. Goodman WK, Price LH, Rasmussen SA, Mazure C, Delgado P, Heninger GR, Charney DS. The Yale-Brown Obsessive Compulsive Scale (YBOCS), II: validity. *Arch Gen Psychiatry.* 1989;46:1012-1016.
41. Oldfield RC. The assessment and analysis of handedness: the Edinburgh inventory. *Neuropsychologia.* 1971;9:97-113.
42. Marks IM. Review of behavioral psychotherapy, I: obsessive-compulsive disorders. *Am J Psychiatry.* 1981;138:584-592.
43. Baer L. *Getting Control: Overcoming Your Obsessions and Compulsions.* Boston, Mass: Little Brown & Co; 1991:33-127.
44. Jiang A, Kennedy DN, Baker JR, Weisskoff RM, Tootell RBH, Woods RP, Benson RR, Kwong KK, Brady TJ, Rosen BR, Belliveau JW. Motion detection and correction in functional MR imaging. *Hum Brain Mapping.* 1995;3:1-12.
45. Woods RP, Cherry SR, Mazziotta JC. Rapid automated algorithm for aligning and reslicing PET images. *J Comput Assist Tomogr.* 1992;16:620-633.
46. Hajnal J, Myers R, Oatridge A, Schwieso J, Young I, Bydder G. Artifacts due to stimulus correlated motion in functional imaging of the brain. *Magn Reson Med.* 1994;31:283-291.
47. Fox PT, Mintun MA, Riemann EM, Raichle ME. Enhanced detection of focal brain responses using intersubject averaging and change-distribution analysis of subtracted PET images. *J Cereb Blood Flow Metab.* 1988;8:642-653.
48. Friston KJ, Frith CD, Liddle P, Dolan RJ, Lamertsma AA, Frackowiak RJ. The relationship between global and local changes in PET scans. *J Cereb Blood Flow Metab.* 1990;10:458-466.
49. Friston K, Frith C, Liddle P, Franckowiak R. Comparing functional PET images: the assessment of significant change. *J Cereb Blood Flow Metab.* 1991;11: 690-699.
50. Worsley KJ, Evans AC, Marrett S, Neelin P. A three-dimensional statistical analysis for CBF activation studies in human brain. *J Cereb Blood Flow Metab.* 1992; 12:900-918.
51. Fox PT, Mintun ME. Non-invasive functional brain mapping by change-distribution analysis of averaged PET images of $H_2{}^{15}O$ tissue activity. *J Nucl Med.* 1989;30:141-149.
52. Baker JR, Hoppel BE, Stern CE, Kwong KK, Weisskoff RM, Rosen BR. Dynamic functional imaging of the complete human cortex using gradient echo and asymmetric spin-echo echo-planar magnetic resonance imaging. *Proc Soc Magn Reson Med.* 1993;3:1400. Abstract.
53. Press WH, Flannery BP, Teulolsky SA, Vetterling WT. *Numerical Recipes: The Art of Scientific Computing.* New York, NY: Cambridge University Press; 1986: 472-475.

54. Davis TL, Weisskoff RM, Kwong KK, Boxerman JL, Rosen BR. Temporal aspects of fMRI task activation: dynamic modeling of oxygen delivery. *Proc Soc Magn Reson Med.* 1994;1:69.
55. Boxerman JL, Weisskoff RM, Kwong KK, Davis TL, Rosen BR. The intravascular contribution to fMRI signal change: modeling and diffusion-weighted in vivo studies. *Proc Soc Magn Reson Med.* 1994;2:619.
56. Baker JR, Weisskoff RM, Stern CE, Kennedy DN, Jiang A, Kwong KK, Kolodny LB, Davis TL, Boxerman JL, Buchbinder BR, Wedeen VJ, Belliveau JW, Rosen BR. Statistical assessment of functional MRI signal change. *Proc Soc Magn Reson Med.* 1994;2:626.
57. Boxerman JL, Weisskoff RM, Rosen BR. The effects of water permeability, red blood cell velocity and agent compartmentalization on susceptibility-contrast relaxivity. *Proc Soc Magn Reson Med.* 1994;2:1008. Abstract.
58. Foreman SD, Cohen JD, Fitzgerald M, Eddy WF, Mintun MA, Noll DC. Improved assessment of significant activation in functional magnetic resonance imaging (fMRI): use of a cluster-size threshold. *Magn Reson Med.* 1995;33:636-647.
59. Rademacher J, Galaburda AM, Kennedy DN, Filipek PA, Caviness VS. Human cerebral cortex: localization, parcellation, and morphometry with magnetic resonance imaging. *J Cogn Neurosci.* 1992;4:352-373.
60. Filipek PA, Richelme C, Kennedy DN, Caviness VS. The young adult human brain: an MRI-based morphometric analysis. *Cereb Cortex.* 1994;4:344-360.
61. Talairach J, Tournoux P. *Co-planar Stereotaxic Atlas of the Human Brain.* New York, NY: Thieme Medical Publishers Inc; 1988.
62. Hoehn-Saric R, Pearlson GD, Harris GJ, Machlin SR, Camargo EE. Effects of fluoxetine on regional cerebral blood flow in obsessive-compulsive patients. *Am J Psychiatry.* 1991;148:1243-1245.
63. Mesulam M-M. Patterns in behavioral neuroanatomy: association areas, the limbic system, and hemispheric specialization. In: Mesulam M-M, ed. *Principles of Behavioral Neurology.* Philadelphia, Pa: FA Davis Co; 1985:1-70.
64. Kaada BR. Cingulate, posterior orbital, anterior insular and temporal pole cortex. In: Magoun HW, ed. *Neurophysiology.* Baltimore, Md: Waverly Press; 1960:1345-1372.
65. Kaada BR, Pribram KH, Epstein JA. Respiratory and vascular responses in monkeys from temporal pole, insula, orbital surface and cingulate gyrus. *J Neurophysiol.* 1949;12:348-356.
66. Reiman EM, Lane RD, Ahern GL, Schwartz GE, Davidson RJ, Yun LS. Neuroanatomical correlates of normal human emotion. *Proc Soc Neurosci.* 1993;19:371. Abstract.
67. Pardo JV, Pardo PJ, Raichle ME. Neural correlates of self-dysphoria. *Am J Psychiatry.* 1993;150:713-719.
68. George MS, Ketter TA, Parekh PI, Horwitz B, Herscovitch P, Post RM. Brain activity during transient sadness and happiness in healthy women. *Am J Psychiatry.* 1995;152:341-351.
69. LeDoux JE. Emotion and the amygdala. In: Aggleton JP, ed. *The Amygdala: Neurobiological Aspects of Emotion, Memory, and Mental Dysfunction.* New York, NY: Wiley-Liss Inc; 1992:339-351.
70. Baer L, Jenike MA. Introduction. In: Jenike MA, Baer L, Minichiello WE, eds. *Obsessive-compulsive Disorders: Theory and Management.* 2nd ed. Chicago, Ill: Year Book Medical Publishers; 1990:3-9.

Quantitative Brain Magnetic Resonance Imaging in Attention-Deficit Hyperactivity Disorder

F. Xavier Castellanos, MD; Jay N. Giedd, MD; Wendy L. Marsh; Susan D. Hamburger, MA, MS; A. Catherine Vaituzis; Daniel P. Dickstein; Stacey E. Sarfatti; Yolanda C. Vauss; John W. Snell, PhD; Nicholas Lange, PhD; Debra Kaysen; Amy L. Krain; Gail F. Ritchie, MSW; Jagath C. Rajapakse, PhD; Judith L. Rapoport, MD

Background: Anatomic magnetic resonance imaging (MRI) studies of attention-deficit hyperactivity disorder (ADHD) have been limited by small samples or measurement of single brain regions. Since the neuropsychological deficits in ADHD implicate a network linking basal ganglia and frontal regions, 12 subcortical and cortical regions and their symmetries were measured to determine if these structures best distinguished ADHD.

Method: Anatomic brain MRIs for 57 boys with ADHD and 55 healthy matched controls, aged 5 to 18 years, were obtained using a 1.5-T scanner with contiguous 2-mm sections. Volumetric measures of the cerebrum, caudate nucleus, putamen, globus pallidus, amygdala, hippocampus, temporal lobe, cerebellum; a measure of prefrontal cortex; and related right-left asymmetries were examined along with midsagittal area measures of the cerebellum and corpus callosum. Interrater reliabilities were .82 or greater for all MRI measures.

Results: Subjects with ADHD had a 4.7% smaller total cerebral volume ($P=.02$). Analysis of covariance for total cerebral volume demonstrated a significant loss of normal right>left asymmetry in the caudate ($P=.006$), smaller right globus pallidus ($P=.005$), smaller right anterior frontal region ($P=.02$), smaller cerebellum ($P=.05$), and reversal of normal lateral ventricular asymmetry ($P=.03$) in the ADHD group. The normal age-related decrease in caudate volume was not seen, and increases in lateral ventricular volumes were significantly diminished in ADHD.

Conclusion: This first comprehensive morphometric analysis is consistent with hypothesized dysfunction of right-sided prefrontal-striatal systems in ADHD.

Arch Gen Psychiatry. 1996;53:607-616

From the Child Psychiatry Branch, National Institute of Mental Health, Bethesda, Md (Drs Castellanos, Giedd, Rajapakse, and Rapoport and Mss Marsh, Hamburger, Vaituzis, Vauss, Kaysen, Krain, and Ritchie); the Department of Neurosurgery, University of Virginia, Charlottesville (Dr Snell); and the National Institute of Neurological Disorders and Stroke, Bethesda (Dr Lange). Mr Dickstein is a medical student, Brown University, Providence, RI, and Ms Sarfatti is an undergraduate student, University of Pennsylvania, Philadelphia.

ATTENTION-DEFICIT hyperactivity disorder (ADHD) is the most common psychiatric disorder of children, affecting approximately 5% of the school-age population[1] and accounting for over 40% of clinic referrals.[2-4] Family, twin, and adoption studies implicate genetic factors as etiologic, but evidence for environmentally mediated fetal brain insult has also been reported.[5-7] Prospective longitudinal studies[8-10] indicate that up to 50% of subjects with ADHD continue to experience impairment from some symptoms of the disorder, if not the full syndrome, in adolescence and early adulthood and that ADHD is a risk factor for conduct disorder, antisocial personality disorder, and substance abuse.

Neuropsychological studies suggest that the core deficit in ADHD is a failure to inhibit or delay motor responses,[11] while sensory detection or early information processing is intact.[12,13] Phenomenological and neuropsychological studies[14-18] have implicated prefrontal dysfunction in ADHD. In light of findings of partial left visual field "neglect," deficits on delayed response tasks, and poor gating of irrelevant stimuli, Heilman and colleagues[19] proposed a right-sided dysfunction of frontal-striatal circuitry for ADHD. This relatively specific anatomic hypothesis received support from early imaging studies. Lou and colleagues,[20] using xenon blood flow in a heterogeneous group of patients with ADHD, found striatal hypoperfusion particularly on the right side, which was reversed by methylphenidate. Subsequent functional imaging studies have been less clear. Using positron emission tomography, Zametkin and colleagues reported decreased 2-deoxy-2[^{18}F]-glucose uptake in adults with ADHD,[21] particularly in frontal regions, but this was not replicated for adolescent subjects with ADHD.[22,23] Further, positron emission tomographic studies of short- and long-term stimulant drug

See Subjects and Methods on next page

SUBJECTS AND METHODS

SUBJECTS

Normal Controls

Fifty-five healthy male subjects (mean age, 12.0 years; range, 5.5 to 17.8 years) were recruited from the community. Screening included telephone interview; parent and teacher rating scales; and in-person assessment, which included physical and neurological examinations, the 12 handedness items from the Revised Physical and Neurological Examination for Subtle Signs,[35] structured psychiatric interview using the Child and Parent Diagnostic Interview for Children and Adolescents,[36] Child Behavior Checklist,[37] Conners Parent and Teacher Rating Scales,[38] the Vocabulary and Block Design subtests of the Wechsler Intelligence Scale for Children–Revised (WISC-R),[39] and Wide Range Achievement Test–Revised.[40] Group means were substituted for two subjects from each diagnostic group who did not undergo psychological assessment. Family psychiatric history for first- and second-degree relatives was ascertained from one or both parents. Individuals with physical, neurological, or lifetime history of psychiatric abnormalities, or who had any first-degree relatives or greater than 20% of second-degree relatives with major psychiatric disorders, were excluded. Approximately five candidates were screened for each one enrolled, with the most common exclusions being family psychiatric history, Conners Teacher Hyperactivity ratings greater than 1 SD above published age norms,[38] and probable psychiatric diagnosis based on structured interviews.[36]

Subjects With ADHD

Fifty-seven male subjects with ADHD (mean age, 11.7 years; range, 5.8 to 17.8 years) were recruited for a National Institute of Mental Health ADHD pharmacotherapy study within a specialized day treatment program. Fifty-three of them had been previously treated with psychostimulants, and 56 participated in a 12-week double-blind trial of methylphenidate, dextroamphetamine, and placebo, as described elsewhere.[41] A previous study[34] used 50 of these patients and 48 of the control subjects. Inclusion criteria were a history of hyperactive, inattentive, and impulsive behaviors that were impairing in at least two settings (home, school, or day program) and a Conners Teacher Hyperactivity rating greater than 2 SDs above age mean.[38] The *DSM-III-R*[42] diagnosis of ADHD was based on the Diagnostic Interview for Children and Adolescents with a parent and the patient, and Conners Parent and Teacher Rating Scales.[38] Exclusion criteria were a full-scale WISC-R IQ of less than 80, evidence of medical or neurological disorders on examination or by history, Tourette's disorder, or any other Axis 1 psychiatric disorder, with the exception of mild-moderate conduct disorder (n=9) or oppositional defiant disorder (n=20). Two subjects met criteria for mild anxiety disorders, and nine subjects had specific learning disorders meeting Axis II diagnostic criteria, confirmed for reading disorder by discrepancy ($z>1.65$) between Woodcock-Johnson Psychoeducational Battery and WISC-R standard scores.[43,44]

Assent from the child and written consent from the parents were obtained. The National Institute of Mental Health Institutional Review Board approved the protocol.

METHODS

Behavioral Measures

Behavioral measures for patients were obtained after at least 4 weeks off psychoactive medications. Conduct and hyperactivity factors were extracted from the Conners Parent and Teacher Rating Scales.[38,45] The Continuous Performance Test (CPT)[46] yielded omission (CPT-O) and commission (CPT-C) errors.

MRI Image Acquisition

All subjects were scanned on the same scanner (1.5-T GE Signa, Oxford Instruments Inc, Oxford, England). T_1-weighted images with contiguous 1.5-mm sections in the axial and sagittal planes and 2.0-mm sections in the coronal plane were obtained using three-dimensional spoiled gradient–recalled echo in the steady state. Imaging parameters were as follows: echo time, 5 milliseconds; repetition time, 24 milliseconds; flip angle, 45°; acquisition matrix, 256×192; number of excitations, 1; and field of view, 24 cm. Vitamin E capsules, wrapped in gauze and placed in each auditory meatus, were used to help standardize head placement. A third capsule was taped to the lateral aspect of the left inferior orbital ridge. The capsules are readily identifiable on MRI and were used to define a reference plane and to verify laterality. The patient's head was aligned in a padded head holder, so that a narrow guide light passed through each capsule. A sagittal-localizing plane was acquired and from this a multiecho axial series. If all three capsules were not contained within a single axial section, the patient was realigned until this criterion was met. Subjects were scanned in the evening to facilitate sleep. Younger children brought blankets and stuffed animals and were read to by their parents. Three normal children (ages, 5, 7, and 11 years) and two boys with ADHD (ages, 6 and 10 years) were unable to complete the scan because of claustrophobia or excessive anxiety. Scans for two normal boys had excessive motion artifact and were omitted. No sedation was used for normal subjects. Approximately 15 of the subjects with ADHD were sedated with oral lorazepam (2 mg) or chloral hydrate (2 g). Further details are provided elsewhere.[47]

Image Analysis

Clinical Interpretation. T_2-weighed images were also obtained for evaluation by a clinical neuroradiologist. Two control subjects had an increased T_2 signal in the left semiovale and right parietal lobe, respectively. One subject with ADHD who had a subarachnoid cyst in the right temporal fossa with decrease in volume of the right temporal cortex was excluded. No other gross abnormalities were reported. All raters were blind to subjects' characteristics.

Cerebrum and Cerebellar Quantification. After standardizing spatial orientation using midline anterior and posterior commissures (AC-PC line) and the interhemispheric fissure, a novel image analysis technique was used to remove the brain from the intracranial cavity and quantify the cerebral and cerebellar hemispheres.[48] This method models the brain surface as an elastically deformable structure and uses an energy minimization function to bring template surfaces into close correspondence with those of the individual brain. The resulting image was then edited section by section to remove artifacts (dura or eyeballs). This technique has been validated by comparison with postmortem specimens and with volumes obtained from conventional section-by-section hand-tracing through all axial sections on which brain matter is visible (intraclass correlation [ICC] =.95). Further details are provided elsewhere.[47,48]

Due to variability in gyral and sulcal patterns, prefrontal brain volume was estimated.[49] A coronal plane perpendicular to the AC-PC line was used to determine the volume of brain in front of the most anterior point of corpus callosum for both left and right hemispheres, excluding temporal lobe. This anterior frontal region overlaps primarily with prefrontal cortex, but it also includes subcortical white matter. Intrarater ICC for this semiautomated measure was .98.

Subcortical Gray Matter. The caudate (head and body) and putamen were manually outlined from coronal sections on a Macintosh II FX workstation using NIH Image (version 1.55).[50] Since the sum of areas from the odd- and even-numbered sections correlated highly for the first 20 subjects (ICC = .98), subsequent outlining was done on every other section. Intrarater reliability (ICC = .89 and .85 for caudate and putamen, respectively) was assessed initially and periodically during analyses to monitor potential operator drift. Interrater ICCs were .88 and .84 for caudate and putamen, respectively.

Globus pallidus, bounded medially by internal capsule and laterally by putamen, was also measured on coronal sections, but included every section, beginning 2 mm anterior to anterior commissure and proceeding posteriorly for a total of 14 mm. Limiting sampling to this domain, which encompassed almost the entire globus pallidus in the majority of subjects, was necessary to achieve adequate intrarater (ICC = .85) and interrater (ICC = .82) reliabilities. This measure does not distinguish internal and external segments.

Temporal Lobe Structures. Measures of temporal lobe, amygdala, and hippocampus were manually traced in the coronal plane. The temporal lobe is readily separated from frontal and parietal lobes by the sylvian fissure. The temporal stem was divided by a line connecting the most inferior point of the insular cisterns to the most lateral point of the hippocampal fissure. The coronal section including the posteriormost aspect of the corpus callosum was arbitrarily designated the temporal lobe posterior boundary (inclusive).[49] The section containing the most anterior portions of the mammillary bodies was used as the amygdala-hippocampus boundary.[51] Intrarater and interrater ICCs for amygdala were .89 and .86; for hippocampus, .89 and .87; and for temporal lobe, .99 and .98, respectively.

Lateral Ventricles. Lateral ventricular volumes were measured in the coronal plane using an operator-supervised thresholding technique that required little subjectivity, yielding high intrarater and interrater reliabilities (ICC=.99).

Midsagittal Area Measures. Corpus callosum area was obtained from a single midsagittal section reconstructed from the axial series. Resectioning allows more precise designation of the midsagittal plane than choosing a "best" midsagittal section.[47] Using the three-dimensional data set, a line was drawn to bisect the cerebral hemispheres in the axial plane. From this line, a midsagittal image was reconstructed in the same plane as the AC-PC line. Criteria to confirm a midsagittal orientation were patency of the cerebral aqueduct and presence of the septum pellucidum. An elliptical region of interest was drawn, and, within this region, a supervised thresholding technique was used to determine the corpus callosum perimeter x-y coordinates. These coordinates were saved and analyzed along radial lines to compute areas of seven subregions: rostrum, genu, rostral body, anterior midbody, posterior midbody, isthmus, and splenium, as defined by Witelson.[52] Intrarater ICC averaged .92 for the corpus callosum subdivisions.

For quantification of the cerebellar vermian lobules, we resectioned the axial series to determine the midsagittal plane with reference to vermian structures.[53] *Total midsagittal area* was defined as the sum of vermian lobules I-V, VI-VII, and VIII-X.[54] Intrarater ICC for midsagittal cerebellar area was .86.

Statistical Analysis

Volumetric measurements of the right and left brain regions (anterior frontal region, caudate, putamen, globus pallidus, lateral ventricles, amygdala, hippocampus, temporal lobe, and cerebellum) were analyzed by two-way repeated-measures analyses of covariance (ANCOVA) (BMDP P2V software program[55]) with diagnosis as the between-subjects factor, side (right and left) as the repeated factor, and total cerebral volume (TCV) as the covariate. *Percent asymmetry* was defined as $\{(R-L)/[(R+L)/2]\}\times 100$. Midsagittal cerebellar and corpus callosal areas and symmetries for bilateral structures were analyzed by one-way ANCOVA with TCV as the covariate. Since the diagnostic groups also differed significantly in IQ subscores, all analyses were retested by ANCOVA with both WISC-R Vocabulary score and TCV as covariates. Vocabulary subscore was chosen because it has the highest correlation to full-scale IQ[39] and because we measured it directly, although results were unchanged when short-form full-scale IQ (combining Vocabulary and Block Design)[56] was used. Bonferroni tests were used to determine post hoc significance of least-square adjusted means.[57]

The relations between volumetric and asymmetry measures and behavioral and demographic variables were examined with Pearson's correlations except for CPT errors (CPT-O and CPT-C), which were nonparametric and for which we used Spearman's correlations (SAS Version 6.07, SAS Institute Inc, Cary, NC). Partial correlations controlled for potentially confounding variables such as age or IQ. Because of the large number of comparisons, we set α=.01 for correlations. Age-related changes in regions that differed significantly between groups were examined with linear regression. After significance testing with linear regression, linearity and constant variance assumptions were relaxed by use of a "local regression" procedure that retained subtle nonlinearities in the data (a "supersmoother")[58] to yield curvilinear fits to the scatter plots of structure volumes by age, diagnosis, and side, as shown in **Figure 1** and **Figure 2**.

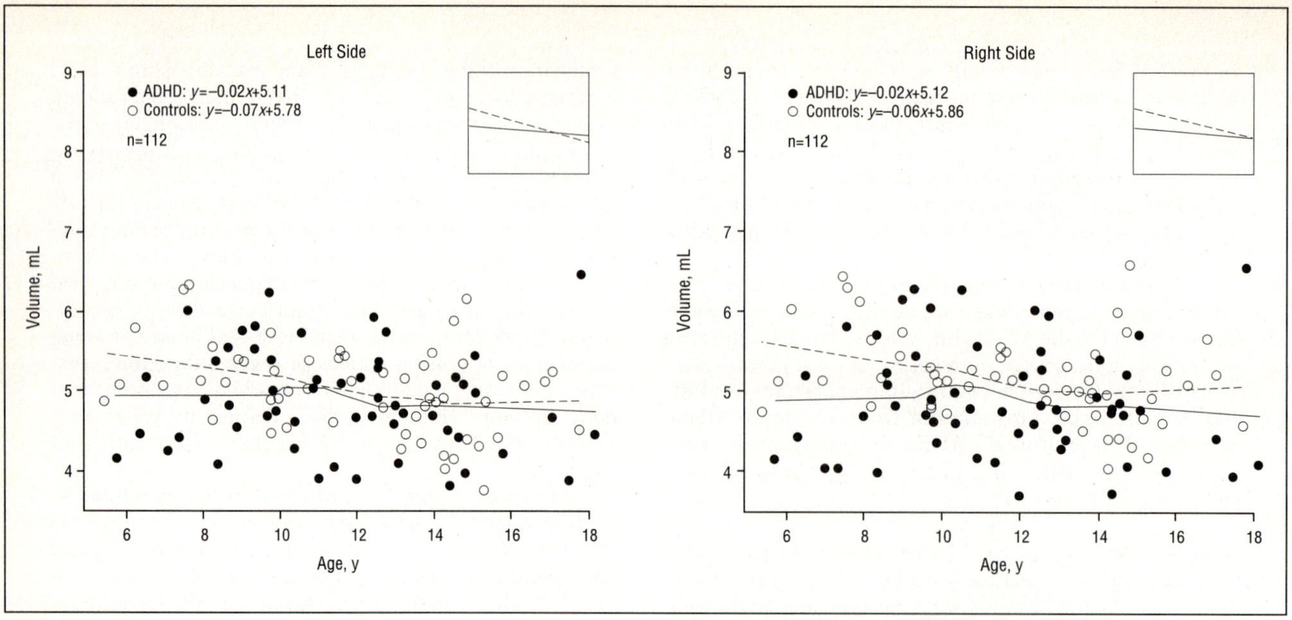

Figure 1. *Volumes of caudate nuclei in relation to age for 57 boys with attention-deficit hyperactivity disorder (ADHD) and 55 healthy control subjects. Local regression lines for each group are indicated in the main plot; linear regression coefficients and lines appear in the upper portion of the graph.*

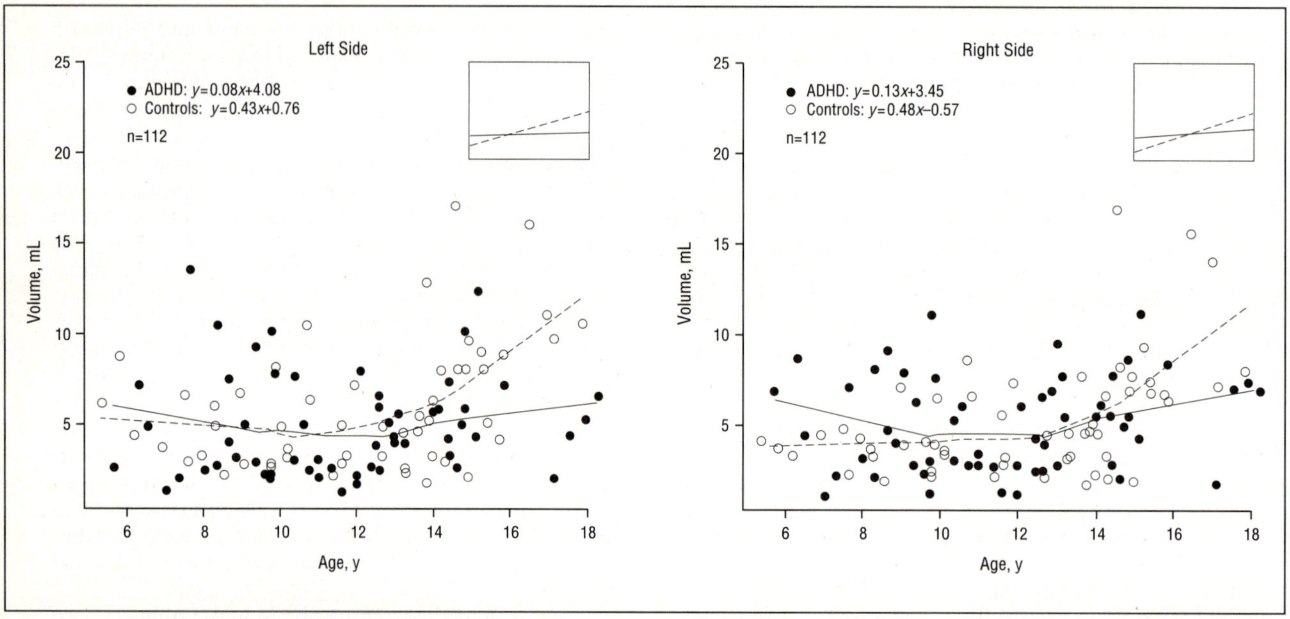

Figure 2. *Volumes of lateral ventricles in relation to age for 57 boys with attention-deficit hyperactivity disorder (ADHD) and 55 healthy control subjects. Local regression lines for each group are indicated in the main plot; linear regression coefficients and lines appear in the upper portion of the graph.*

treatment in adults with ADHD did not produce consistent changes.[24,25]

Early computed tomographic studies of children with ADHD reported nonspecific abnormalities[26,27] that were not confirmed when quantitative techniques and an appropriate contrast group were employed.[28] In a series of magnetic resonance imaging (MRI) studies with seven to 11 children with ADHD compared with control subjects, Hynd and colleagues reported a narrower right frontal cortex,[29] smaller total midsagittal corpus callosum area,[30] and a reversal of "normal" (reported to be left>right) caudate asymmetry based on a single 5-mm axial section.[31] Two other groups[32,33] also reported significantly smaller callosal areas in patients with ADHD. However, neither group found differences in total corpus callosum midsagittal area: one found differences in the rostrum and rostral body[32]; the other, only in the splenium.[33] Both studies used small samples (18 and 15 subjects per diagnostic group, respectively), and the latter found a significant difference only in the splenium when five stimulant nonresponders were combined with 10 stimulant responders.

In a subsequent report,[34] the present authors com-

See also pages 574, 577, 585, 595, 617, and 625

Table 1. Demographic Characteristics of Boys With ADHD and Controls*

Characteristics	ADHD (n=57)	Controls (n=55)
Age, y	11.65±2.97	12.03±3.06
Height, cm	147.62±17.45	153.75±19.33
Weight, kg	41.72±16.80	46.21±16.54
Tanner stage	2.19±1.65	2.38±1.63
Handedness, % right-handed	81	87
WISC-R subscales scores		
Vocabulary	11.89±3.22	13.84±2.87†
Block Design	11.86±3.48	13.44±2.69‡
WISC-R Full-Scale IQ	109.21±17.47	. . .
Estimated Full-Scale IQ§	110.84±17.19	121.09±13.34†
Conners Teacher Rating Scale hyperactivity ratings (0-3)		
Teacher	1.65±0.72	0.31±0.47†
Parent	2.03±0.75	0.33±0.34†
DSM-III-R diagnoses, No.		
ADHD	57	
Conduct disorder	9	
Oppositional defiant disorder	20	
Learning disorders	9	
Anxiety disorders	2	
Enuresis	11	

**ADHD indicates attention-deficit hyperactivity disorder; WISC-R, Wechsler Intelligence Scale for Children–Revised.*

†*P*<.001.

‡*P*<.01.

§*Short Form Full-Scale IQ using WISC-R Vocabulary and Block Design subscales.*[56]

pared MRI caudate volumes in 50 boys with ADHD and 48 normal boys. In contrast to findings by Hynd et al,[31] a normal right>left caudate asymmetry was found for controls, which was absent in subjects with ADHD (*P*=.001). The strengths of this study included a large sample size, well-characterized patients who were sufficiently impaired to participate in controlled stimulant trials, 2-mm coronal sections to minimize partial voluming effects, and a wide age range (6 to 18 years) that provided a developmental perspective.

Herein, we present a comprehensive morphometric MRI study for an expanded sample. We hypothesized right-sided frontal-striatal abnormalities, and we included contrast regions for which no abnormalities were hypothesized. Thus, the present study compared cerebral, prefrontal, and basal ganglia (caudate, putamen, and globus pallidus) volumes and corpus callosum area for which abnormalities were predicted, as well as exploratory analyses of cerebellar, temporal lobe, amygdala, and hippocampal volumes and midsagittal cerebellar areas.

RESULTS

SUBJECTS

Table 1 presents patient and control characteristics. There were no significant group differences in age, height, weight, Tanner pubertal stage, or handedness. Scores of WISC-R Vocabulary and Block Design subscale and full-scale scores were higher for control subjects (*P*<.01), although for both groups, subtests and estimated full-scale scores were above average (subscore population mean, 10±3).

MORPHOMETRY

Total cerebral volume was significantly smaller for ADHD on analysis of variance (F[1,110]=5.69, *P*=.02; not shown). Right hemispheric volume was larger than left for both groups (F[1,110]=24.33, *P* = .001), but the between-group disparity was larger for the right (5.2%) than for the left hemisphere (4.2%) (F[1,110]=4.62, *P*=.03). Total cerebral volume was used as a covariate for all subsequent analyses.

As shown in **Table 2**, there was a significant (*P*=.02) diagnosis-by-side interaction for the anterior frontal region. Post hoc testing revealed that the groups differed significantly in right anterior frontal volume (*P*<.05).

Total caudate volume also did not differ between groups. The loss of normal right>left caudate asymmetry in ADHD (reflected in the significant side-by-diagnosis interaction, *P*=.006) was due to reduced right caudate volume for the subjects with ADHD (*P*<.05, by Bonferroni test). This loss of asymmetry was seen across our entire age range (data not shown).

The left putamen was larger than the right for both groups, and there were no diagnostic differences with respect to volume or symmetry.

Although both the main effect of diagnosis and the interaction of diagnosis by side are significant for the globus pallidus, differences between groups were, again, most prominent for the right-sided structure (adjusted between-group difference of 10.3% on the right vs 4.3% on the left side). There were no age-related changes for globus pallidus volumes or symmetry. As **Table 3** shows, the absolute magnitude of the right globus pallidus between-group difference, while highly significant (interaction *P*=.005), is only 0.12 mL.

Since some prior studies[59-61] discuss the lenticular nucleus as a unit (globus pallidus plus putamen), our data include statistics for this measure (Tables 2 and 3 and **Table 4**). The lenticular nucleus retains the left>right asymmetry of the putamen; no diagnostically relevant differences were seen.

Midsagittal area was calculated for total corpus callosum and seven subregions.[32,52] Only total measurements appear in Table 4, but no significant group differences were found for total region or any subregion.

Cerebellar volume was significantly smaller in ADHD, although the groups did not differ in midsagittal cross-sectional area.[53]

Temporal lobe measures revealed a robust right>left asymmetry for both groups but no group effects. While ANCOVA suggested smaller amygdala volume for ADHD (*P*=.07), unlike our other findings, this was not significant when Vocabulary IQ subscale score and TCV were covaried (*P*=.19). Overall lateral ventricular volume did not differ between groups, but the left lateral ventricle was significantly smaller for ADHD than for control subjects.

SYMMETRY

Analysis of symmetry indexes is a common way of comparing bilateral structures, although it is comparable to a side-by-diagnosis interaction. Symmetry indexes and ANCOVA statistics are presented in Table 4 primarily for comparison to other data sets. A *positive* symmetry index in-

Table 2. Repeated Measures ANCOVA for Diagnosis, Side, and Diagnosis by Side Interactions for Brain Volumes of 57 Boys With ADHD and 55 Controls*

	Diagnosis		Side		Diagnosis×Side		
	F	P	F	P	F	P	Comment
Anterior frontal region	0.95	.33	3.42	.07	**5.64**	**.02**	Control>ADHD only on right
Caudate	0.32	.58	**11.56**	**.001**	**7.94**	**.006**	Control>ADHD only on right
Putamen	0.25	.62	**119.91**	**.0001**	0.27	.6	...
Globus pallidus	**6.79**	**.01**	0.17	.68	**8.04**	**.005**	Control>ADHD right and left; effect larger on right
Lenticular nucleus	1.80	.18	**78.86**	**.0001**	3.13	.08	...
Cerebellum	**3.97**	**.05**	3.60	.06	1.81	.18	Control>ADHD
Temporal lobe	2.57	.11	**25.54**	**.0001**	0.43	.51	...
Amygdala	3.43	.07	**8.60**	**.004**	3.01	.09	...
Hippocampus	2.10	.15	**10.1**	**.002**	1.11	.30	...
Lateral ventricles	1.09	.30	3.69	.06	**4.61**	**.03**	Control>ADHD only on left; control left>control right

**ANCOVA indicates analysis of covariance (covarying for total cerebral volume; df=1,104-110, due to missing data); ADHD, attention-deficit hyperactivity disorder. Statistically significant values are boldfaced.*

Table 3. Unadjusted and Adjusted Mean Volumes for 57 Boys With ADHD and 55 Controls*

	Volume, mL							
	Unadjusted Means±SDs				Adjusted Least Square Means†			
	Left		Right		Left		Right	
	ADHD	Controls	ADHD	Controls	ADHD	Controls	ADHD	Controls
Cerebral volume	557.38±58.2	581.64±65.3	561.52±58.8	592.19±63.2	...	...	...	...
Anterior frontal region	80.03±15.6	82.83±15.2	79.41±14.7	87.84±13.2	81.82	80.93	81.20	85.94
Caudate	4.87±0.6	4.99±0.6	4.88±0.7	5.14±0.5	4.93	4.92	4.95	5.07
Putamen	5.50±0.6	5.60±0.5	5.26±0.5	5.39±0.4	5.53	5.57	5.29	5.35
Globus pallidus	1.13±0.2	1.18±0.2	1.10±0.1	1.22±0.2	1.13	1.18	1.10	1.22
Lenticular nucleus	6.63±0.6	6.79±0.6	6.36±0.6	6.61±0.5	6.66	6.76	6.40	6.58
Cerebellum	77.28±11.4	86.31±16.6	80.30±11.9	86.83±17.3	78.65	84.86	81.67	85.38
Temporal lobe	84.13±9.3	88.68±11.9	87.46±9.5	93.01±10.3	85.32	87.46	88.66	91.79
Amygdala	2.23±0.5	2.34±0.5	2.29±0.5	2.56±0.5	2.25	2.33	2.30	2.55
Hippocampus	4.57±0.7	4.55±0.4	4.75±0.7	4.65±0.5	4.61	4.51	4.79	4.60
Lateral ventricles	4.96±2.8	5.90±3.5	5.00±2.6	5.22±3.2	4.96	5.90	5.00	5.22

**ADHD indicates attention-deficit hyperactivity disorder.*
†Adjusted for total cerebral volume.

dicates right>left and is seen for control subjects for all structures except for putamen, lenticular nuclei, and ventricles. Significant decreases in asymmetry are noted for the boys with ADHD in the cerebral hemispheres, anterior frontal region, caudate, and globus pallidus.

AGE-RELATED CHANGES

Caudate volume decreases with age for control subjects between 6 and 12 years old in this cross-sectional analysis. This is reflected in a significant negative slope (for right plus left caudate, $\beta=-0.12$ mL/y, $P=.01$), which is greater in magnitude than in subjects with ADHD ($\beta=-0.03$ mL/y, $P=.60$), although between-group differences were not significant ($z=1.16$, $P>.20$). Figure 1 presents these data along with local regression curves, with linear regressions shown in inset boxes.

Since ventricular volumes change significantly with age in normal male subjects in this age group,[47,59] age-related effects were examined. Ventricular volume increased significantly with age for normal male subjects ($\beta=0.48$ and 0.43 mL/y for right and left ventricles, $P<.001$ and $P=.002$, respectively), while for subjects with ADHD, there were no significant age-related changes (right $\beta=.13$ mL/y, $P=.21$; left $\beta=.08$ mL/y, $P=.51$). Slopes for right, left, and total ventricular volumes differed significantly between diagnostic groups ($z=1.96$, 2.07, and 2.12, respectively; $P<.05$).

A "super-smoother" analysis of lateral ventricular volume detected a significant slope change point at age 11 years for the normal boys. Prior to that age, the nonsignificant age slope was 0.08 mL/y, increasing to 2.19 mL/y after age 11 years ($P=.03$).[58] No significant age changes in slope were seen for the ADHD group (see Figure 2).

ABILITY TO DISTINGUISH BETWEEN GROUPS

A stepwise discriminant function using jackknife validation was performed, which included all measures (in-

Table 4. Unadjusted and Adjusted Means and ANCOVA for Subjects With ADHD and Controls*

Measures	Unadjusted Means±SDs: ADHD (n=57)	Unadjusted Means±SDs: Controls (n=55)	Adjusted Least Square Means†: ADHD (n=57)	Adjusted Least Square Means†: Controls (n=55)	ANCOVA: F	ANCOVA: *P*
Total cerebral volume, mL	1118.90±116.3	1173.83±127.2	...	...	...	...
Area measures, mm^2						
Cerebellum	1135.31±154.0	1171.18±116.0	1142.00	1164.12	0.72	.40
Corpus callosum	625.54±83.2	630.69±79.9	630.93	624.89	0.16	.69
Symmetry measures, %‡						
Cerebrum	0.7±2.4	1.9±3.3	...	...	...	...
Anterior frontal region	−0.6±16.0	6.3±14.3	−0.79	6.46	**5.81**	**.02**
Caudate	0.09±5.4	2.9±4.5	0.26	2.77	**6.89**	**.01**
Putamen	−4.4±4.3	−3.9±4.0	−4.41	−3.97	0.31	.58
Globus pallidus	−2.4±11.3	3.4±9.5	−2.55	3.56	**9.06**	**.003**
Lenticular nucleus	−4.1±4.4	−2.6±3.8	−4.13	−2.61	3.57	.06
Cerebellum	3.8±13.3	0.4±11.7	3.81	0.47	1.81	.18
Temporal lobe	3.9±8.3	5.3±9.5	3.76	5.19	0.63	.43
Amygdala	2.3±22.4	9.3±23.6	2.10	9.53	2.66	.11
Hippocampus	4.0±9.4	1.8±10.0	4.10	1.70	1.56	.21
Lateral ventricles	0.5±29.9	−11.5±30.2	−0.39	−10.51	3.05	.08

**ANCOVA indicates analysis of covariance; ADHD, attention-deficit hyperactivity disorder.*
†Adjusted for total cerebral volume; df=*1,104-110 due to missing data.*
‡Percentage of asymmetry defined as {(R−L)/[(R+L)/2)]}×100. Statistically significant values are boldfaced.

cluding asymmetry scores). Right globus pallidus volume, caudate symmetry, and left cerebellum volume emerged, in that order, as significant, independent predictors of group membership. These three measures correctly classified 72% of 106 subjects (the number of subjects was smaller owing to missing data; 78% of the subjects with ADHD, and 65% of the control subjects) and together accounted for 27% of total variance. When TCV was forced in as the first variable, the classification remained virtually unchanged, with 72% of subjects (75% of subjects with ADHD, 69% of control subjects) correctly classified and 29% of total variance accounted for.

ANATOMIC-BEHAVIOR CORRELATIONS

Within the ADHD group, Full-Scale WISC-R IQ score correlated with total cerebral volume (n=57, *r*=.32, *P*=.01) and with right and left prefrontal regions (*n*=55, *r*=.43, and r=.40, respectively, *P*<.003). Within the relatively restricted range of the healthy control subjects, similar, but attenuated, correlations were also found (right prefrontal regions correlated significantly with Vocabulary (n=52, *r*=.33, *P*=.016), while left prefrontal correlations were not significant (*r*=.20).

Correlations within the ADHD group between regions differing across groups and ratings of ADHD severity, demographics (Hollingshead socioeconomic status), perinatal risk taken from the Diagnostic Interview for Children and Adolescents,[62] as well as a measure of learning disability (reading discrepancy score)[43] showed a significant association (at α<.01) between caudate asymmetry index and prenatal, perinatal, and infancy complications (n=47, *r*=-.42, *P*=.003). Decreased (normal) caudate asymmetry was associated with increasing perinatal risk in the ADHD group and not in the healthy boys.

IQ-MATCHED ANALYSIS

Analysis of variance was also performed for a subgroup of ADHD and control subjects matched by WISC-R Vocabulary score. The groups thus defined, composed of 44 subjects with ADHD and 55 normal control boys, did not differ significantly on age, height, weight, Tanner pubertal stage, Block Design score, or full-scale IQ (short-form for control subjects).[56] The results were virtually identical to those shown in Tables 2 through 4 except that the group difference in total cerebral volume (diagnosis analysis of variance F[1,97]=1.87, *P*=.17) was no longer significant.

COMMENT

This is the first comprehensive regional morphometric analysis of ADHD and age-matched healthy boys. Using large samples, thin MRI sections, and highly reliable measurement algorithms, we found subtle yet statistically robust hypothesized between-group differences in the right anterior frontal region[14-16,18] (approximating prefrontal gray and white matter volumes), right caudate,[17,19,31,34] and globus pallidus,[63] most prominently on the right side. Unexpectedly, we did not replicate prior reports of differences in corpus callosum,[30,32,33] nor did we find expected differences in putaminal volume or symmetry. Exploratory analyses were generally negative except in lateral ventricles, where age-related changes appear to diverge, and in cerebellar volume.

Our groups differed significantly in IQ scores. Since IQ differences may be intrinsic to ADHD,[64] we did not covary IQ (or its surrogate, Vocabulary) in primary analyses.[65] However, results were essentially unchanged after covarying IQ alone, when combined with TCV (data not presented), or when IQ-matched subgroups were compared. It is also worth noting that while socioeconomic status correlated significantly with full-scale IQ in ADHD subjects (n=52, $r=-.43$, $P=.001$), it did not correlate significantly with any brain regions, including total cerebral volume.

In normal adults, three independent groups have now reported right>left caudate asymmetry.[66-68] In the largest of these studies, as with our pediatric normative study,[47] the magnitude of the asymmetry is also quite modest (3.9% in normal male subjects), but the level of statistical significance is very high ($F[1,179]=84$, $P<.001$).[68] Lateral ventricles were significantly larger on the left side for our normal subjects, as was also noted in adult samples.[68,69] Lack of normal asymmetry has been reported in neuropsychiatric disorders linked to early neurodevelopmental deviations,[70-72] including dyslexia,[73,74] Tourette's disorder,[60,61] and schizophrenia.[49,66,75] We found diagnostic differences in asymmetry in our measures of prefrontal cortex, caudate, globus pallidus, and lateral ventricles as well as in the cerebral hemispheres. We speculate that an early, presumably fetal, event affecting normal development of asymmetry is etiologically related to ADHD. In this respect, the significant correlation between decreased normal caudate asymmetry and a measure of pregnancy, delivery, or infancy complications is of great interest. If replicated, the "markers" for ADHD reported here may be useful for future high-risk, genetic, and treatment studies.

There are several limitations of this study. The absence of true boundaries for most brain regions necessitates manual tracing of individual sections. When clear boundaries are adopted, highly reliable morphometry is possible. However, arbitrary boundaries inherently limit validity. For example, some groups only quantify the head of the caudate,[76] whereas we included both head and body, but not the tail. Likewise, in globus pallidus, we limited our mensuration to a seven-slice "frame," which did not always include the entire structure. Thus, in spite of blind and reliable ratings, diagnostic differences may not be strictly comparable across studies.

Given the variability of sulcal and gyral patterns between even genetically identical individuals[77,78] and current methodological limits, valid subdivision of cortical regions was not feasible. Our estimate of anterior frontal region is susceptible to between-group shape differences in corpus callosum and includes both gray and white matter, which diverge with increasing age.[59,79] The findings of age-related changes in lateral ventricular and caudate volumes suggest that, in ADHD, a more general process possibly linked to synaptic pruning[80] may continue into adolescence. A prospective longitudinal study of patients and control subjects is under way to validate these maturational differences. Technical advances are needed for gray-white segmentation and quantification of other relevant regions, such as nucleus accumbens, anterior cingulate gyrus, and thalamus.

Because almost all (93%) subjects with ADHD had been exposed to stimulants, we cannot be certain that our results are not drug related. A replication study with stimulant-naive boys with ADHD is under way. Our findings for male individuals, if replicated, need to be extended to female individuals with ADHD.

The differences that we found in the caudate and not in the putamen are consistent with preclinical studies implicating caudate lesions in hyperactivity.[81,82] The lack of differences in putaminal volumes between subjects with ADHD and control subjects is consistent with the hypothesis that the ADHD-relevant corticostriatal-thalamocortical circuits are those that link the caudate and prefrontal regions such as orbital-frontal cortex,[11] rather than the parallel circuits linking the putamen and motor or supplementary motor cortex,[83] which have been linked to Tourette's disorder.[60,61]

Comorbidity between ADHD and oppositional defiant disorder, conduct disorder, and with specific learning disorders is well established.[1,2,84,85] It has been argued that most of the impairment associated with ADHD is actually owing to comorbid conditions and that ADHD is merely a variant of normal exuberant behavior.[86] We examined this question by comparing all measures in our 55 control subjects with those in the 48 subjects with ADHD without a specific learning disability and in the 28 boys with ADHD who did not have either oppositional defiant disorder or conduct disorder. In both cases, all of our hypothesized findings remained statistically significant. In fact, despite decreasing our ADHD sample by half, this subanalysis was even more robust for the 28 subjects with ADHD and without comorbid disruptive behavior disorders. Finally, although our groups did not differ in handedness, we reanalyzed our results for only strongly right-handed subjects and found no differences from our primary analyses for this subset of 46 boys with ADHD and 48 control subjects.

Reports on morphologic characteristics of the corpus callosum morphometry in ADHD have been inconsistent. Three independent groups, using small samples, found diagnostic differences in three different regions. In the present large sample, we fail to replicate our own[32] and our colleagues'[30,33] work. Our sample was relatively "clean," with only nine subjects (16%) having had specific learning disorders. The possibility that corpus callosal differences may be more pertinent to comorbidity with developmental disorders should be explored.[87,88]

There were no diagnostically relevant differences in the total temporal lobe, amygdala, or hippocampus. Since the amygdala and hippocampus partially overlap when measured in the coronal plane, the volumes that we obtained are not independent, and our negative findings should not be taken as definitive. However, we hypothesized that temporal lobe structures would not differentiate the groups based on reports of intact posterior parietal[89] and temporal lobe performance[90] in ADHD in the face of subtle deficits in tasks that require prefrontal involvement.[90-93]

Decreased cerebellar volume, if replicated, is intriguing in light of recent anatomic,[94] clinical,[95-97] and functional[98] results, suggesting that the cerebellum may have a prominent role in cognitive processes and executive functioning.[99,100]

In summary, we have found decreased volume of several candidate brain regions previously hypothesized to be involved in the pathophysiology of ADHD, ie, prefrontal cortex,[14-16,18] caudate nucleus,[17,19,31,34] and globus pallidus,[63] predominantly on the right side. These support other converging evidence that a lack of normal asymmetry mediates the expression of ADHD.[19,88,101-103] In humans, the functional significance of basal ganglia asymmetry is unknown. Interestingly, a study of rats not demonstrating the usual behavioral side preference reported them to be "the most active and the poorest overall learners on all tasks studied."[104] Lateralized rodent behavior has been associated with asymmetric basal ganglia neurochemistry.[104-108] These observations led to the suggestion that rats that exhibit low behavioral asymmetry may serve as an animal model of ADHD.[109] Other indirect evidence for the right-hemisphere abnormality in ADHD comes from positron emission tomographic studies in normal adults, in which the right hemisphere was preferentially activated in vigilance tasks.[110,111] In ADHD, subtle left-hemisphere "neglect" is normalized by administration of methylphenidate.[102,103,112,113] The significance of basal ganglia asymmetry is being examined in functional imaging studies.

Accepted for publication August 29, 1995.

This study was supported in part by a grant from the Gulton Foundation, Tenafly, NJ.

The authors would like to acknowledge Wayne Rasband for customizing image analysis software and Janet Hunter, MD, for technical assistance.

Reprints: F. Xavier Castellanos, MD, Child Psychiatry Branch, National Institute of Mental Health, Building 10, Room 6N240, 10 Center Dr, MSC 1600, Bethesda, MD 20892-1600.

REFERENCES

1. Szatmari P. The epidemiology of attention-deficit hyperactivity disorder. *Child Adolesc Psychiatr Clin North Am.* 1992;1:361-371.
2. Anderson JC, Williams S, McGee R, Silva PA. *DSM-III* disorders in preadolescent children: prevalence in a large sample from the general population. *Arch Gen Psychiatry.* 1987;44:69-76.
3. Bird HR, Canino G, Rubio-Stipec M, Gould MS, Ribera J, Sesman M, Woodbury M, Huertas-Goldman S, Pagan A, Sanchez-Lacay A. Estimates of the prevalence of childhood maladjustment in a community survey in Puerto Rico: the use of combined measures. *Arch Gen Psychiatry.* 1988;45:1120-1126.
4. Offord DR, Boyle MH, Szatmari P, Rae-Grant NI, Links PS, Cadman DT, Byles JA, Crawford JW, Blum HM, Byrne C. Ontario Child Health Study, II: six-month prevalence of disorder and rates of service utilization. *Arch Gen Psychiatry.* 1987;44:832-836.
5. Nichols PL, Chen TC. *Minimal Brain Dysfunction: A Prospective Study.* Hillsdale, NJ: Erlbaum; 1981.
6. Minde K, Webb G, Sykes D. Studies on the hyperactive child, VI: prenatal and perinatal factors associated with hyperactivity. *Dev Med Child Neurol.* 1968; 10:355-363.
7. Milberger S, Biederman J, Faraone SV. Pregnancy, delivery and infancy complications and attention deficit hyperactivity disorder: issues of gene-environment interaction. In: Alessi N, Porter S, eds. *Scientific Proceedings of the Annual Meetings.* Washington, DC: American Academy of Child & Adolescent Psychiatry; 1994;10:66. Abstract.
8. Weiss G, Hechtman L, Milroy T, Perlman T. Psychiatric status of hyperactives as adults: a controlled prospective 15-year follow-up of 63 hyperactive children. *J Am Acad Child Psychiatry.* 1985;24:211-220.
9. Gittelman R, Mannuzza S, Shenker R, Bonagura N. Hyperactive boys almost grown up, I: psychiatric status. *Arch Gen Psychiatry.* 1985;42:937-947.
10. Mannuzza S, Klein RG, Bessler A, Malloy P, LaPadula M. Adult outcome of hyperactive boys: educational achievement, occupational rank, and psychiatric status. *Arch Gen Psychiatry.* 1993;50:565-576.
11. Barkley RA. Impaired delayed responding: a unified theory of attention deficit hyperactivity disorder. In: Routh DK, ed. *Disruptive Behavior Disorders in Childhood.* New York, NY: Plenum Press; 1994:11-57.
12. Van der Meere J, Sergeant J. Acquisition of attention skill in pervasively hyperactive children. *J Child Psychol Psychiatry.* 1988;29:301-310.
13. Sergeant J, Van der Meere JJ. Ritalin effects and information processing in hyperactivity. In: Greenhill LL, Osman BB, eds. *Ritalin: Theory and Patient Management.* New York, NY: Mary Ann Liebert Inc; 1991:1-13.
14. Pontius AA. Dysfunction patterns analogous to frontal lobe system and caudate nucleus syndromes in some groups of minimal brain dysfunction. *J Am Med Wom Assoc.* 1973;28:285-292.
15. Mattes JA. The role of frontal lobe dysfunction in childhood hyperkinesis. *Compr Psychiatry.* 1980;21:358-369.
16. Benson DF. The role of frontal dysfunction in attention deficit hyperactivity disorder. *J Child Neurol.* 1991;6(suppl):S9-S12.
17. Levy F. The dopamine theory of attention deficit hyperactivity disorder (ADHD). *Aust N Z J Psychiatry.* 1991;25:277-283.
18. Gualtieri CT, Hicks RE. Neuropharmacology of methylphenidate and a neural substrate for childhood hyperactivity. *Psychiatr Clin North Am.* 1985;8:875-892.
19. Heilman KM, Voeller KKS, Nadeau SE. A possible pathophysiologic substrate of attention deficit hyperactivity disorder. *J Child Neurol.* 1991;6(suppl):S76-S81.
20. Lou HC, Henriksen L, Bruhn P, Borner H, Nielsen JB. Striatal dysfunction in attention deficit and hyperkinetic disorder. *Arch Neurol.* 1989;46:48-52.
21. Zametkin AJ, Nordahl TE, Gross M, King AC, Semple WE, Rumsey J, Hamburger SD, Cohen RM. Cerebral glucose metabolism in adults with hyperactivity of childhood onset. *N Engl J Med.* 1990;323:1361-1366.
22. Zametkin AJ, Liebenauer LL, Fitzgerald GA, King AC, Minkunas DV, Herscovitch P, Yamada EM, Cohen RM. Brain metabolism in teenagers with attention-deficit hyperactivity disorder. *Arch Gen Psychiatry.* 1993;50:333-340.
23. Ernst M, Liebenauer LL, King AC, Fitzgerald GA, Cohen RM, Zametkin AJ. Reduced brain metabolism in hyperactive girls. *J Am Acad Child Adolesc Psychiatry.* 1994;33:858-868.
24. Matochik JA, Nordahl TE, Gross M, Semple WE, King AC, Cohen RM, Zametkin AJ. Effects of acute stimulant medication on cerebral metabolism in adults with hyperactivity. *Neuropsychopharmacology.* 1993;8:377-386.
25. Matochik JA, Liebenauer LL, King AC, Szymanski HV, Cohen RM, Zametkin AJ. Cerebral glucose metabolism in adults with attention deficit hyperactivity disorder after chronic stimulant treatment. *Am J Psychiatry.* 1994;151:658-664.
26. Bergström K, Bille B. Computed tomography of the brain in children with minimal brain damage: a preliminary study of 46 children. *Neuropaediatrie.* 1978;9:378-384.
27. Caparulo BK, Cohen DJ, Rothman SL, Young JG, Katz JD, Shaywitz SE, Shaywitz BA. Computed tomographic brain scanning in children with developmental neuropsychiatric disorders. *J Abnorm Child Psychol.* 1981;20:338-357.
28. Shaywitz BA, Shaywitz SE, Byrne T, Cohen DJ, Rothman S. Attention deficit disorder: quantitative analysis of CT. *Neurology.* 1983;33:1500-1503.
29. Hynd GW, Semrud-Clikeman M, Lorys AR, Novey ES, Eliopulos D. Brain morphology in developmental dyslexia and attention deficit disorder/hyperactivity. *Arch Neurol.* 1990;47:919-926.
30. Hynd GW, Semrud-Clikeman M, Lorys AR, Novey ES, Eliopulos D, Lyytinen H. Corpus callosum morphology in attention-deficit hyperactivity disorder: morphometric analysis of MRI. *J Learn Disabil.* 1991;24:141-146.
31. Hynd GW, Hern KL, Novey ES, Eliopulos D, Marshall R, Gonzalez JJ, Voeller KKS. Attention deficit hyperactivity disorder and asymmetry of the caudate nucleus. *J Child Neurol.* 1993;8:339-347.
32. Giedd JN, Castellanos FX, Casey BJ, Kozuch P, King AC, Hamburger SD, Rapoport JL. Quantitative morphology of the corpus callosum in attention deficit hyperactivity disorder. *Am J Psychiatry.* 1994;151:665-669.
33. Semrud-Clikeman M, Filipek PA, Biederman J, Steingard R, Kennedy D, Renshaw P, Bekken K. Attention-deficit hyperactivity disorder: magnetic resonance imaging morphometric analysis of the corpus callosum. *J Am Acad Child Adolesc Psychiatry.* 1994;33:875-881.
34. Castellanos FX, Giedd JN, Eckburg P, Marsh WL, Vaituzis AC, Kaysen D, Hamburger SD, Rapoport JL. Quantitative morphology of the caudate nucleus in attention deficit hyperactivity disorder. *Am J Psychiatry.* 1994;151:1791-1796.
35. Denckla MB. Revised physical and neurological examination for subtle signs. *Psychopharmacol Bull.* 1985;21:773-800.
36. Welner Z, Reich W, Herjanic B, Jung KG, Amado H. Reliability, validity, and parent-child agreement studies of the Diagnostic Interview for Children and Adolescents (DICA). *J Am Acad Child Adolesc Psychiatry.* 1987;26:649-653.
37. Achenbach T, Edelbrock C. *Manual for the Child Behavior Checklist and Revised Child Behavior Profile.* Burlington, Vt: University of Vermont, Dept of Psychiatry; 1983.
38. Werry JS, Sprague RL, Cohen MN. Conners' Teacher Rating Scale for use in drug studies with children: an empirical study. *J Abnorm Child Psychol.* 1975; 3:217-229.
39. Wechsler D. *Manual for the Wechsler Intelligence Scale for Children–Revised.* New York, NY: The Psychological Corp; 1974.
40. Jastak S, Wilkinson GS. *Wide Range Achievement Test, Revised Edition.* Wilmington, Del: Jastak Assessment Systems; 1984.
41. Elia J, Borcherding BG, Rapoport JL, Keysor CS. Methylphenidate and dextroamphetamine treatments of hyperactivity: are there true nonresponders? *Psychiatry Res.* 1991;36:141-155.
42. American Psychiatric Association. *Diagnostic and Statistical Manual of Mental Disorders, Revised Third Edition.* Washington, DC: American Psychiatric Association; 1987.
43. Reynolds CR. Critical measurement issues in learning disabilities. *J Special Educ.* 1984;18:451-476.
44. Frick PJ, Kamphaus RW, Lahey BB, Loeber R, Christ MA, Hart EL, Tannenbaum LE. Academic underachievement and the disruptive behavior disorders. *J Consult Clin Psychol.* 1991;59:289-294.
45. Goyette CH, Conners CK, Ulrich RF. Normative data on revised Conners Parent and Teacher Rating Scales. *J Abnorm Child Psychol.* 1978;6:221-236.
46. Rosvold HE, Mirsky AF, Sarason I, Bransome ED, Beck LH. A continuous performance test of brain damage. *J Consult Psychol.* 1956;20:343-350.
47. Giedd JN, Snell JW, Lange N, Rajapakse JC, Kaysen D, Vaituzis AC, Vauss YC, Hamburger SD, Kozuch PL, Rapoport JL. Quantitative magnetic resonance imaging of human brain development: ages 4-18. *Cereb Cortex.* In press.
48. Snell JW, Merickel MB, Ortega JM, Goble JC, Brookeman JR, Kassell NF.

Boundary estimation of complex objects using hierarchical active surface templates. *J Pattern Recogn.* In press.
49. Bilder RM, Wu H, Bogerts B, Degreef G, Ashtari M, Alvir JM, Snyder PJ, Lieberman JA. Absence of regional hemispheric volume asymmetries in first-episode schizophrenia. *Am J Psychiatry.* 1994;151:1437-1447.
50. Rasband W. *NIH Image Manual.* Bethesda, Md: National Institutes of Health; 1993.
51. Shenton ME, Kikinis R, Jolesz FA, Pollak SD, Lemay M, Wible CG, Hokama H, Martin J, Metcalf D, Coleman M. Abnormalities of the left temporal lobe and thought disorder in schizophrenia: a quantitative magnetic resonance imaging study. *N Engl J Med.* 1992;327:604-612.
52. Witelson SF. Hand and sex differences in the isthmus and genu of the human corpus callosum. *Brain.* 1989;112:799-835.
53. Courchesne E, Yeung-Courchesne R, Egaas B. Methodology in neuroanatomic measurement. *Neurology.* 1994;44:203-208.
54. Courchesne E, Press GA, Murakami J, Berthoty D, Grafe M, Wiley CA, Hesselink JR. The cerebellum in sagittal plane: anatomic-MR correlation, I: the vermis. *AJNR Am J Neuroradiol.* 1989;10:659-665.
55. Dixon WJ, Brown MB, Engelman L, Jennrich, eds. *PMDP Statistical Software Manual.* Berkeley: University of California Press; 1990.
56. Silverstein AB. A short short form of the WISC and WAIS for screening purposes. *Psychol Rep.* 1967;20:682.
57. SAS Institute Inc. *SAS Language and Procedures: Usage, Version 6, First Edition.* Cary, NC: SAS Institute Inc; 1989.
58. Hastie T, Tibshirani R. *Generalized Additive Models.* London, England: Chapman and Hall; 1990.
59. Jernigan TL, Trauner DA, Hesselink JR, Tallal PA. Maturation of human cerebrum observed in vivo during adolescence. *Brain.* 1991;114:2037-2049.
60. Singer HS, Reiss AL, Brown JE, Aylward EH, Shih B, Chee E, Harris EL, Reader MJ, Chase GA, Bryan N, Denckla MB. Volumetric MRI changes in basal ganglia of children with Tourette's syndrome. *Neurology.* 1993;43:950-956.
61. Peterson B, Riddle MA, Cohen DJ, Katz LD, Smith JC, Hardin MT, Leckman JF. Reduced basal ganglia volumes in Tourette's syndrome using three-dimensional reconstruction techniques from magnetic resonance images. *Neurology.* 1993;43:941-949.
62. Sprich-Buckminster S, Biederman J, Milberger S, Faraone SV, Lehman BK. Are prenatal complications relevant to the manifestations of ADD? issues of comorbidity and familiality. *J Am Acad Child Adolesc Psychiatry.* 1993;32:1032-1037.
63. Voeller KKS. Toward a neurobiologic nosology of attention deficit hyperactivity disorder. *J Child Neurol.* 1991;6(suppl):S2-S8.
64. Halperin JM, Gittelman R. Do hyperactive children and their siblings differ in IQ and academic achievement? *Psychiatry Res.* 1982;6:253-258.
65. Meehl PE. Nuisance variables and the ex post facto design. In: Radner M, Winokur S, eds. *Analyses of Theories and Methods of Physics and Psychology.* Minneapolis, Minn: University of Minnesota Press; 1970:373-402.
66. Breier A, Buchanan RW, Elkashef A, Munson RC, Kirkpatrick B, Gellad F. Brain morphology and schizophrenia: a magnetic resonance imaging study of limbic, prefrontal cortex, and caudate structures. *Arch Gen Psychiatry.* 1992;49:921-926.
67. Peterson BS, Riddle MA, Cohen DJ, Katz LD, Smith JC, Leckman JF. Human basal ganglia volume asymmetries on magnetic resonance images. *Magn Reson Imaging.* 1993;11:493-498.
68. Flaum M, Swayze V, 2nd, O'Leary DS, Yuh WTC, Ehrhardt JC, Arndt SV, Andreasen NC. Brain morphology in schizophrenia: effects of diagnosis, laterality and gender. *Am J Psychiatry.* 1995;152:704-714.
69. Filipek PA, Richelme C, Kennedy DN, Caviness VS, Jr. The young adult human brain: an MRI-based morphometric analysis. *Cereb Cortex.* 1994;4:344-360.
70. Chi JG, Dooling EC, Gilles FH. Gyral development of human brain. *Ann Neurol.* 1977;1:86-93.
71. Weinberger DR, Luchins DJ, Morihisa J, Wyatt RJ. Asymmetrical volumes of the right and left frontal and occipital regions of the human brain. *Neurology.* 1982;11:97-100.
72. de Lacoste MC, Horvath DS, Woodward DJ. Possible sex differences in the developing human fetal brain. *J Clin Exp Neuropsychol.* 1991;13:831-846.
73. Galaburda AM, Geschwind N. Anatomical asymmetries in the adult and developing brain and their implications for function. *Adv Pediatr.* 1981;28:271-292.
74. Kushch A, Gross-Glenn K, Jallad B, Lubs H, Rabin M, Feldman E, Duara R. Temporal lobe surface area measurements on MRI in normal and dyslexic readers. *Neuropsychologia.* 1993;31:811-821.
75. Woodruff PWR, Murray RM. The aetiology of brain abnormalities in schizophrenia. In: Ancill R, ed. *Schizophrenia: Exploring the Spectrum of Psychosis.* New York, NY: John Wiley & Sons Inc; 1994:95-114.
76. Krishnan KR, McDonald WM, Escalona PR, Doraiswamy PM, Na C, Husain MM, Figiel GS, Boyko OB, Ellinwood EH, Nemeroff CB. Magnetic resonance imaging of the caudate nuclei in depression: preliminary observations. *Arch Gen Psychiatry.* 1992;49:553-557.
77. Rademacher J, Caviness VS, Steinmetz H, Galaburda AM. Topographical variation of the human primary cortices: implications for neuroimaging, brain mapping, and neurobiology. *Cereb Cortex.* 1993;3:313-329.
78. Weinberger DR, Berman KF, Torrey EF. Correlations between abnormal hippocampal morphology and prefrontal physiology in schizophrenia. *Clin Neuropharmacol.* 1992;15(suppl 1, pt A):393A-394A.
79. Jernigan TL, Archibald SL, Berhow MT, Sowell ER, Foster DS, Hesselink JR. Cerebral structure on MRI, I: localization of age-related changes. *Biol Psychiatry.* 1991;29:55-67.
80. Jernigan TL, Tallal P. Late childhood changes in brain morphology observable with MRI. *Dev Med Child Neurol.* 1990;32:379-385.
81. Fulton JF. *Frontal Lobotomy and Affective Behavior: A Neurophysiological Analysis.* New York, NY: WW Norton & Co; 1951.
82. Yoshida M, Nagatsuka Y, Muramatsu S, Niijima K. Differential roles of the caudate nucleus and putamen in motor behavior of the cat as investigated by local injection of GABA antagonists. *Neurosci Res.* 1991;10:34-51.
83. Alexander GE, Crutcher MD. Functional architecture of basal ganglia circuits: neural substrates of parallel processing. *Trends Neurosci.* 1990;13:266-271.
84. Bird HR, Gould MS, Staghezza BM. Patterns of diagnostic comorbidity in a community sample of children aged 9 through 16 years. *J Am Acad Child Adolesc Psychiatry.* 1993;32:361-368.
85. Kanbayashi Y, Nakata Y, Fujii K, Kita M, Wada K. ADHD-related behavior among non-referred children: parents' ratings of *DSM-III-R* symptoms. *Child Psychiatry Hum Dev.* 1994;25:13-29.
86. Schrag P, Divoky D. *The Myth of the Hyperactive Child and Other Means of Thought Control.* New York, NY: Pantheon Books; 1975.
87. Leonard CM, Voeller KK, Lombardino LJ, Morris MK, Hynd GW, Alexander AW, Andersen HG, Garofalakis M, Honeyman JC, Mao J, Agee OF, Staab EV. Anomalous cerebral structure in dyslexia revealed with magnetic resonance imaging. *Arch Neurol.* 1993;50:461-469.
88. Rumsey J. The biology of developmental dyslexia. *JAMA.* 1992;7:912-915.
89. Swanson JM, Posner M, Potkin S, Bonforte S, Youpa D, Fiore C, Cantwell D, Crinella F. Activating tasks for the study of visual-spatial attention in ADHD children: a cognitive anatomic approach. *J Child Neurol.* 1991;6(suppl):S119-S127.
90. Shue KL, Douglas VI. Attention deficit hyperactivity disorder and the frontal lobe syndrome. *Brain Cogn.* 1992;20:104-124.
91. Gorenstein EE, Mammato CA, Sandy JM. Performance of inattentive-overactive children on selected measures of prefrontal-type function. *J Clin Psychol.* 1989;45:619-632.
92. Chelune GJ, Ferguson W, Koon R, Dickey TO. Frontal lobe disinhibition in attention deficit disorder. *Child Psychiatry Hum Dev.* 1986;16:221-234.
93. Grodzinsky GM, Diamond R. Frontal lobe functioning in boys with attention-deficit hyperactivity disorder. *Dev Neuropsychol.* 1992;8:427-445.
94. Middleton FA, Strick PL. Anatomical evidence for cerebellar and basal ganglia involvement in higher cognitive function. *Science.* 1994;266:458-461.
95. Botez MI, Botez T, Elie R, Attig E. Role of the cerebellum in complex human behavior. *Ital J Neurol Sci.* 1989;10:291-300.
96. Levinson HN. The diagnostic value of cerebellar-vestibular tests in detecting learning disabilities, dyslexia, and attention deficit disorder. *Percept Mot Skills.* 1990;71:67-82.
97. Akshoomoff NA, Courchesne E, Press GA, Iragui V. Contribution of the cerebellum to neuropsychological functioning: evidence from a case of cerebellar degenerative disorder. *Neuropsychologia.* 1992;30:315-328.
98. Raichle ME, Fiez JA, Videen TO, MacLeod AK, Pardo JV, Fox PT, Petersen SE. Practice-related changes in human brain functional anatomy during nonmotor learning. *Cereb Cortex.* 1994;4:8-26.
99. Akshoomoff NA, Courchesne E. A new role for the cerebellum in cognitive operations. *Behav Neurosci.* 1992;106:731-738.
100. Houk JC, Wise SP. Distributed modular architectures linking basal ganglia, cerebellum, and cerebral cortex: their role in planning and controlling action. *Cereb Cortex.* 1995;5:95-110.
101. Malone MA, Kershner JR, Swanson JM. Hemispheric processing and methylphenidate effects in attention-deficit hyperactivity disorder. *J Child Neurol.* 1994;9:181-189.
102. Malone MA, Couitis J, Kershner JR, Logan WJ. Right hemisphere dysfunction and methylphenidate effects in children with attention-deficit/hyperactivity disorder. *J Child Adolesc Psychopharmacol.* 1994;4:245-253.
103. Malone MA, Kershner JR, Siegel L. The effects of methylphenidate on levels of processing and laterality in children with attention deficit disorder. *J Abnorm Child Psychol.* 1988;16:379-395.
104. Glick SD, Jerussi TP, Zimmerberg B. Behavioral and neuropharmacological correlates of nigrostriatal asymmetry in rats. In: Harnad S, Doty RW, Goldstein L, eds. *Lateralization in the Nervous System.* New York, NY: Academic Press; 1977:213-249.
105. Drew KL, Lyon RA, Titeler M, Glick SD. Asymmetry in D-2 binding in female rat striata. *Brain Res.* 1986;363:192-195.
106. Zimmerberg B, Mattson S, Riley EP. Impaired alternation test performance in adult rats following prenatal alcohol exposure. *Pharmacol Biochem Behav.* 1989;32:293-299.
107. Afonso D, Santana C, Rodriguez M. Neonatal lateralization of behavior and brain dopaminergic asymmetry. *Brain Res Bull.* 1993;32:11-16.
108. Rodriguez M, Santana C, Afonso D. Maternal ingestion of tyrosine during rat pregnancy modifies the offspring behavioral lateralization. *Physiol Behav.* 1994;55:607-613.
109. Shenker A. The mechanism of action of drugs used to treat attention-deficit hyperactivity disorder: focus on catecholamine receptor pharmacology. *Adv Pediatr.* 1992;39:337-382.
110. Cohen RM, Semple WE, Gross M, Holcomb HH, Dowling MS, Nordahl TE. Functional localization of sustained attention: comparison to sensory stimulation in the absence of instruction. *Neuropsych Neuropsychol Behav Neurol.* 1988;1:3-20.
111. Pardo JV, Fox PT, Raichle ME. Localization of a human system for sustained attention by positron emission tomography. *Nature.* 1991;349:61-64.
112. Voeller KKS, Heilman KM. Attention deficit disorder in children: a neglect syndrome? *Neurology.* 1988;38:806-808.
113. Voeller KKS. Right-hemisphere deficit syndrome in children. *Am J Psychiatry.* 1986;143:1004-1009.

ORIGINAL ARTICLE

Brain Anatomic Magnetic Resonance Imaging in Childhood-Onset Schizophrenia

Jean A. Frazier, MD; Jay N. Giedd, MD; Susan D. Hamburger, MA, MS; Kathleen E. Albus; Debra Kaysen; A. Catherine Vaituzis; Jagath C. Rajapakse, PhD; Marge C. Lenane, MSW; Kathleen McKenna, MD; Leslie K. Jacobsen, MD; Charles T. Gordon, MD; Alan Breier, MD; Judith L. Rapoport, MD

Background: Early-onset schizophrenia (first psychotic symptoms by age 12 years) has been the subject of a small number of studies, and its biological continuity with later-onset disorder has not been established. In this study, quantitative anatomic brain magnetic resonance images of children and adolescents with early-onset schizophrenia were compared with those of matched controls. Brain abnormalities in childhood-onset schizophrenia were examined in relation to those reported for later-onset schizophrenics.

Methods: Anatomic brain magnetic resonance imaging scans were obtained for 21 patients (mean±SD age, 14.6±2.1 years; range, 10 to 18 years) with childhood-onset schizophrenia (13 males, eight females) and 33 age-, sex-, height-, and weight-matched normal controls. Quantitative measurements were obtained for the cerebrum, anterior frontal region, lateral ventricles, thalamus, caudate, putamen, and globus pallidus.

Results: Total cerebral volume and midsagittal thalamic area were smaller in the patients (analysis of variance, $P=.002$, and analysis of covariance, $P=.03$, respectively); the caudate, putamen, and globus pallidus were larger in the patients (analysis of covariance, $P=.05$, $P=.007$, and $P<.001$, respectively); and the lateral ventricles tended to be larger in the patients (analysis of covariance, $P=.06$). Globus pallidus enlargement correlated with neuroleptic exposure and with age of onset of psychosis. The magnitude of abnormalities compared with controls was similar to that reported in adult studies, although there was a trend toward relatively smaller cerebral volumes for the childhood-onset group compared with controls.

Conclusion: Brain anatomic abnormalities in childhood-onset schizophrenia are similar to those reported for adult populations, indicating overall continuity between these rare childhood cases and the adult schizophrenia populations.

Arch Gen Psychiatry. 1996;53:617-624

CHILDHOOD-ONSET schizophrenia (defined as onset of psychotic symptoms by age 12 years, the age of pubertal onset)[1,2] is rare, having 1/50th the prevalence of later-onset disease.[3-6] An apparent increased prevalence prior to the 1970s was probably caused by psychotic disorders of childhood (including autism) being diagnosed as childhood schizophrenia. In 1971, Kolvin and colleagues' landmark studies[7] distinguished autism (psychosis before age 3 years) from schizophrenia (psychosis after age 5 years). Several subsequent studies have also documented very-early-onset schizophrenia as symptomatically similar to the adult-onset disorder.[2,8-11] However, it remains unknown whether childhood-onset schizophrenia reflects a pathophysiologic process separate from or continuous with adult schizophrenia.[7-8,11-14]

Clinical and neuropsychological studies of childhood-onset populations present compelling evidence for continuity, but there have been few neurobiological investigations of the disorder. In schizophrenic adults, there is considerable evidence for abnormal brain anatomy; most consistently, reduced medial temporal lobe, enlarged ventricles, dilation of the third ventricle, and smaller brain volume, with recent reports of enlarged basal ganglia and thalamic abnormalities.[15-28] Brain magnetic resonance imaging (MRI) measures therefore are particularly relevant to the question of continuity between early- and later-onset cases.

Only a few case reports and studies with small numbers of patients have addressed brain developmental patterns in childhood-onset cases.[29-31] Woody and colleagues[29] (1987) described a 10-year-old prepubertal boy with well-documented *DSM-III* schizophrenia whose MRI showed enlargement of the ventricles and cisterna magna with a hypoplastic (or atrophied) left cerebellum. Hendren and colleagues[31] (1991)

From the Child Psychiatry Branch (Drs Frazier, Giedd, Rajapakse, Jacobsen, and Rapoport and Mss Hamburger, Albus, Kaysen, Vaituzis, and Lenane) and Experimental Therapeutics (Dr Breier), National Institute of Mental Health, Bethesda, Md; Department of Psychiatry and Behavioral Sciences, Northwestern University Medical School, Chicago, Ill (Dr McKenna); and Child Psychiatry Division, University of Maryland at Baltimore (Dr Gordon). Dr Frazier is now with the Psychiatry Department, Massachusetts General Hospital, Harvard Medical School, Boston.

See Methods on next page

METHODS

SUBJECTS

Subjects were recruited nationally through professional and patient advocacy groups for an inpatient study involving a double-blind trial of haloperidol and clozapine.[32] Inclusion criteria were *DSM-III-R* diagnosis of schizophrenia,[33] psychotic symptoms documented by age 12 years, age 6 to 18 years, and full-scale IQ score of 70 or above. Medical or neurological diseases were exclusionary. Subjects had to have had at least two unsuccessful previous neuroleptic trials because of either intolerable side effects or nonresponse, as required for clozapine treatment.

From 450 charts, 105 patients and their families were screened in person. Admission to the study followed a 6-hour meeting, including review of old charts, clinical interviews with parents and child, and structured interviews using sections of the Schedule for Affective Disorders and Schizophrenia for School-Age Children–Epidemiologic Version[34] and the Diagnostic Interview for Children and Adolescents, Revised.[35] Those with a primary diagnosis of major affective disorder with psychotic features were excluded. Seventy-five children and adolescents who did not meet *DSM-III-R* criteria for schizophrenia were excluded after the screening process. Thirty children received the diagnosis of schizophrenia. Four children did not participate because of parental decision and two children were determined to have onset of psychosis after age 12 years during the screening and did not qualify for the study. Twenty-four of the 30 children have been studied to date.

Magnetic resonance imaging scans were obtained for 21 of the 24 enrolled patients; one patient was unable to comply with the scanning process and two others had not yet been scanned at the time this report was written. Thirteen patients were male and eight were female. Their mean±SD age at admission was 14.6±2.1 years (range, 10 to 18 years), and their mean age of onset of psychosis was 10.2±1.5 years (range, 7 to 12 years). All patients were pubertal at the time of admission (mean±SD Tanner score, 3.9±1.1; range, 2 to 5).[36] The group had considerable prior neuroleptic therapy (24.3±17.5 months) and hospitalization (8.0±10.6 months). Three (14%) of the 21 patients had a first-degree relative with definite or probable schizophrenia. Parents had considerable education. Eleven (52%) of the fathers and nine (43%) of the mothers had at least partial college training. The socioeconomic status was generally middle class. The mean full-scale IQ (FSIQ) score for the 14 patients who could be tested at the NIH was 82.1±16.8. Seven patients could not be adequately tested because of the severity of their illness and inability to comply, although all had demonstrated normal educational and developmental achievement before onset of psychosis, with a mean FSIQ of 87.3±16.6 for the seven subjects who had formal testing on the Wechsler Intelligence Scale for Children–Revised (WISC-R) prior to their arrival at the NIH. Rating scores on the Brief Psychiatric Rating Scale (BPRS), Scale for the Assessment of Negative Symptoms (SANS), Scale for the Assessment of Positive Symptoms (SAPS), and Bunney-Hamburg psychosis subscale during the fourth week of the drug-free period were obtained on all subjects and used in correlational analyses involving all measured brain structures that differed significantly between patients and controls.[37-40] Interrater reliabilities (intraclass correlation [ICC]) assessed by two separate sets of child psychiatrists at two separate points in the study (C.T.G. and K.M., and K.M. and J.A.F.; one physician was consistent across both reliability assessments) were .64 and .90 for the BPRS, .81 and .92 for the SANS, .91 and .87 for the SAPS, and .81 and .91 for the Bunney-Hamburg psychosis subscale.

Thirty-three healthy comparison subjects (mean age, 14.6±1.6 years; 22 male and 11 female) matched for age, sex, and handedness were recruited from the community through advertisements.[26,41] There were no significant height, weight, or Tanner stage differences between the groups. Screening procedures included a physical and neurological examination; Child and Parent Diagnostic Interview for Children and Adolescents[42]; Child Behavior Checklist[43]; the Vocabulary, Block Design, and Digit Span subtests of the WISC-R; Conners parent and teacher questionnaires[44,45]; and the 12 handedness items from the Physical and Neurological Examination for Subtle Signs.[46] Any physical or neurologic disorder, a lifetime history of any psychiatric disorder, or a history of major psychiatric disorder in first-degree relatives was exclusionary. Subject and control characteristics are summarized in **Table 1**.

The study was explained to the subjects and their parents. Written assent was obtained from the child and written informed consent from the parents. The protocol was approved by the Institutional Review Board at the National Institute of Mental Health, Bethesda, Md.

DRUG EXPOSURE

Antipsychotic doses at the time of admission and total lifetime antipsychotic exposure (summed doses×length of trials) were obtained via chart review and converted to chlorpromazine equivalents for correlational analyses.[47]

MRI PROTOCOL

Subjects were scanned on a 1.5-T Signa scanner (General Electric, Milwaukee, Wis) located at the NIH Clinical Center, Bethesda, Md. A three-dimensional spoiled gradient recalled echo in the steady-state imaging sequence (time to echo, 5 milliseconds; time to repeat, 24 milliseconds; flip angle, 45°; acquisition matrix, 192×256; number of excitations, 1; and field of view, 24 cm) was used to obtain T_1-weighted images with a slice thickness of 1.5 mm in the axial and sagittal planes and 2.0 mm in the coronal plane. Head position was controlled for using vitamin E capsules as external markers (one in the meatus of each ear and one taped to the left inferior orbital ridge, assuring that all three were visible in the same axial reference plane). Rotation in the other plane was controlled by aligning the nose to the 12-o'clock position. Head movement was minimized by placing foam padding on the sides of the subjects' heads. Scans were performed in the evening to promote subjects falling asleep in the scanner. Sedation with chloral hydrate (1.5 to 2.0 g by mouth) or lorazepam (1.0 to 2.0 mg by mouth) was used for seven childhood schizophrenia subjects.

IMAGE ANALYSIS

A neuroradiologist reviewed all scans. No abnormalities were noted for the control group. Clinical MRI readings of the childhood-onset schizophrenia group recorded enlargement of the left lateral ventricle for one subject and a focal area of increased signal in the left frontal white matter for one other subject. These subjects were retained in the data set. An image analysis program (Image 1.6) developed at the NIH was used.[48] All MRI scans of subjects and controls were rated blind.

Cerebral Volume

Brain spatial orientation was first standardized using the midline anterior and posterior commissures and the interhemispheric fissure. A novel image analysis technique, using an active surface template of the brain to incorporate prior knowledge of brain anatomy to supplement MRI signal intensity characteristics, was then employed to quantify the left and right cerebral hemispheres. This method models the brain surface as an elastically deformable structure while using successive iterations of an energy minimization function to enforce constraints on curvature and topology. After this procedure, the images were edited in the axial plane slice by slice by experienced raters to remove remaining artifacts, such as eyeballs or patches of dura. Intraclass correlations for the volumes of the edited brains were .99 for interrater reliability and .95 compared with volumes derived from more conventional slice-by-slice manual tracing technique through all axial slices on which brain matter is visible (**Table 2**). Further details are provided elsewhere.[49,50]

Anterior Frontal Volume

A region designated as "anterior frontal" was defined as all brain matter anterior to a coronal plane intersecting the anterior-most point of the corpus callosum. The orientation of the plane was further standardized to be perpendicular to a line connecting the midline anterior and posterior commissures. Interrater ICC for this semiautomated measure was .97.

Lateral Ventricle Volume

Lateral ventricular volumes were calculated by summing area measurements from all coronal planes on which ventricles were visible using an operator-supervised thresholding technique available in the Image 1.6 program.[48] Because of the semiautomated technique and clear distinction of cerebrospinal fluid from surrounding tissue, interrater reliability was extremely high (ICC, .99).

Subcortical Gray Matter Volumes

The caudate and putamen were manually outlined from all coronal slices on which they were visible. Both structures were traced along the gray matter–white matter border, and along the ventricle–gray matter border for the medial aspect of the caudate. The tail of the caudate, defined as the portion inferior to the head and body, was not included, nor was the nucleus accumbens. Since the sum of areas from the odd-numbered slices for the first 20 subjects correlated highly with the sum of the areas from the even-numbered slices (ICC, .98), subsequent outlining was done on every other slice and then multiplied by a slice thickness of 4 mm to derive volume. Interrater reliability (ICC, .88 and .84 for the caudate and putamen, respectively) was assessed initially and then periodically during the analyses to monitor potential "drift" in operator measurements.

The globus pallidus was also measured on coronal sections, but this measurement included every slice, beginning 2 mm anterior to the anterior commissure and proceeding posteriorly for a total of 14 mm. Our methods were not sufficient to differentiate internal from external components of the globus pallidus. Limiting sampling to the 14-mm domain described improved interrater reliability (ICC, .86) and encompassed the entire globus pallidus in the majority of subjects.

A symmetry index of basal ganglia structures was calculated by the following formula: (right−left)/[(right+left)/2].

Because volumetric quantification of the thalamus is beyond our current methods, the thalamus was manually outlined from a single midsagittal slice reconstructed from the axial series. Reslicing from the axial series allows more precise designation of the midsagittal plane than choosing a "best" midsagittal slice from the sagittal series. The ICC of interrater reliability for the thalamic area was .85.

DATA ANALYSIS

To examine group differences between patients and controls, *t* tests, analyses of covariance (ANCOVA), and χ^2 analyses were used, depending on data distribution and type. Comparisons were made on all demographic variables (gender, age, height, weight, Tanner stage, handedness, and cognitive measures) as well as the absolute values of the brain regions of interest. Because the childhood-onset schizophrenia cohort had significantly smaller total cerebral volume, ANCOVA controlling for cerebral volume was used in one-way or two-way (group-by-side) repeated-measures analyses, with Duncan post hoc comparisons. The Statistical Analysis System[51] was used for the above procedures. Pearson correlations were computed between (1) patient MRI measures with values significantly different from those of controls and (2) clinical measures, including age at study; age of onset; duration of illness; FSIQ score; week 4 off-drug baseline ratings on the SANS, SAPS, BPRS, and Bunney-Hamburg psychosis subscale; and neuroleptic exposure in chlorpromazine equivalents (admission and lifetime).

All tests were two-tailed, and the Greenhouse-Geiger correction factor was used where appropriate. P=.05 constituted significance, and P<.1 constituted a trend.

Standardized scores (z scores) were created for anatomic brain measures that were statistically different from those of controls; z scores were also created for the analagous structures reported for adults, to compare the degree of deviance for adult and child patients relative to their respective control groups.[18-21,24-26,28] For each structure, adult MRI studies done at different academic centers were chosen for comparison. Each study was done on a 1.5-T scanner and had a relatively large number of subjects (n≥25). A z score was created for each adult study, and then a mean z score was calculated for each structure. A z score difference between adults and children was calculated using the following formula: (mean adult z score−mean child z score)/$\sqrt{2}$.[52]

Table 1. Demographic Characteristics of Patients With Childhood-Onset Schizophrenia and Healthy Controls*

Measure	Schizophrenics (n=21)	Normal Controls (n=33)	P (t test)
Age, y	14.6 (2.1)	14.6 (1.6)	.65
Height, cm	164 (10)†	166 (14)	.52
Weight, kg	61.2 (17.6)	56.1 (11.8)	.17
Tanner stage	3.9 (1.1)	3.8 (1.4)	.78
Right-handed, No. (%)	15 (71)	28 (85)	.20‡
WISC-R subtests			
Vocabulary	7.3 (3.3)§	12.9 (2.8)	<.001
Block Design	9.4 (4.3)‖	13.3 (2.8)	<.001
Age at onset of psychosis, y	10.2 (1.5)	...	...
Neuroleptic exposure, mo	24.3 (17.5)	...	...
Hospitalization, mo	8.0 (10.6)	...	...
Age at first hospitalization, y	11.8 (2.2)	...	...

*Unless otherwise indicated, values are mean (SD). WISC-R indicates Wechsler Intelligence Scale for Children–Revised.
†n=20.
‡χ^2=1.7.
§n=15.
‖n=14.

completed quantitative MRIs for 37 psychiatric inpatients (age 5 to 14 years), but only six carried schizophrenia "spectrum" diagnoses (including schizophrenia, schizophreniform disorder, and other psychosis). Interestingly, three of six psychotic children had larger left ventricular frontal horns than did a comparison group of 31 children with other diagnoses. Similarly, Schultz and colleagues[30] (1983) reported ventricular enlargement in 15 schizophrenic/schizophreniform patients (mean±SD age, 16.5±1.7 years, with a mean duration of illness of 13 months), with no correlation with duration of illness or prior treatment.

The present report is on anatomic brain MRI morphologic characteristics of a group of children and adolescents with schizophrenia who had onset of psychotic symptoms by age 12 years.[12-14] Quantitative MRI measures of basal ganglia, thalamus, ventricular size, ventricular brain ratio, anterior frontal volume, and total cerebral volume are reported for the first 21 cases scanned at the National Institutes of Health (NIH). Based on the similar phenomenologic characteristics and family history pattern in this cohort and adult cohorts,[12] the authors hypothesized that there would be an anatomic brain pattern similar to that seen in adult populations. We further speculated that there might be more striking or severe brain abnormalities in this cohort as a possible explanation for the unusual age of presentation.

See also pages 574, 577, 585, 595, 607, and 625

RESULTS

Compared with controls, patients with childhood schizophrenia had a smaller cerebral volume, and even when the smaller cerebral volume was taken into account with ANCOVA, they had a smaller thalamic area, robust increases in basal ganglia volumes, and a larger lateral ventricular volume. These results are summarized in **Table 3** and **Table 4**.

Table 2. Childhood-Onset Schizophrenia Brain Magnetic Resonance Imaging Study Reliabilities for Operator-Assisted Measures

Structure	Intraclass Correlation Coefficient: Intrarater	Interrater
Cerebrum	.98	.99
Anterior frontal	.98	.97
Ventricles	.99	.99
Caudate	.89	.88
Putamen	.85	.84
Globus pallidus	.86	.82
Thalamus (area)	.86	.85

VOLUME MEASUREMENTS

Cerebrum

Schizophrenic children had a total cerebral volume 9.2% smaller than that of normal controls (*t*=3.01, *df*=52, *P*=.004). Both the right and left hemispheres were smaller than in normal controls (*t*=2.64, *df*=51, *P*=.004, and *t*=2.99, *df*=51, *P*=.01, respectively). Males had greater total cerebral volume than females in both the study and normal control groups (*t*=3.7, *df*=19, *P*=.002, and *t*=2.9, *df*=31, *P*=.006, respectively).

Anterior Frontal

Anterior frontal volume did not differ significantly between groups.

Ventricles

Schizophrenic subjects had a trend toward larger lateral ventricles bilaterally than controls (F[1, 50]=3.61, *P*=.06). The ventricular brain ratio was increased for schizophrenics (*t*=2.22, *df*=51, *P*=.03).

Subcortical Structures

All basal ganglia structures were enlarged in the patient group (Table 4). Subjects with schizophrenia had a larger total caudate than normal controls (ANCOVA: F[1, 50]=4.07, *P*=.05), predominantly on the left side. The normal caudate asymmetry (right greater than left) was decreased for patients (*t*=2.21, *df*=28, *P*=.04), the only significant asymmetry difference observed in this study.

Study subjects had a robust increase in globus pallidus total volume (F[1, 51]=16.07, *P*<.001). Finally, the putamen was larger for subjects with schizophrenia (F[1, 50]=5.44, *P*=.007).

Thalamus

The midsagittal area of the thalamus was 17.2% smaller for subjects with schizophrenia (*t*=2.82, *P*=.007; ANCOVA: F[1, 52]=5.44, *P*=.02).

Table 3. Mean Brain Volumes for Patients With Childhood-Onset Schizophrenia (n=21) and Normal Controls (n=33)

	Volume			
	Unadjusted Mean (SD)		Adjusted Least-Square Mean*	
Structure	Schizophrenics	Controls	Schizophrenics	Controls
Ventricles				
Right	7.06 (3.2)	5.87 (3.0)	7.40	5.66
Left	8.45 (4.5)	6.83 (3.4)	8.79	6.62
Anterior frontal				
Right	71.8 (26.2)	84.0 (14.7)	78.4	79.9
Left	71.4 (11.9)	82.9 (14.9)	74.7	80.8
Caudate				
Right	5.05 (0.7)	5.07 (0.6)	5.22	4.97
Left	5.03 (0.5)	4.89 (0.6)	5.20	4.79
Globus pallidus				
Right	1.49 (0.2)	1.31 (0.2)	1.52	1.29
Left	1.38 (0.2)	1.20 (0.2)	1.41	1.18
Putamen				
Right	5.67 (0.8)	5.49 (0.6)	5.86	5.38
Left	5.67 (0.8)	5.46 (0.8)	5.86	5.35
Thalamus (arca)	120.70 (29.5)	148.83 (39.1)	122.39	147.75
Cerebrum	1049.7 (116.8)	1155.9 (132)	...	...

Adjusted for total cerebral volume.

Table 4. ANOVA and Repeated-Measures ANCOVA for Brain Volumes in Childhood-Onset Schizophrenia*

		Diagnosis		Side Effects		Diagnosis × Side Effects	
Structure	Test†	F	*P* (2-Tailed)	F	*P*	F	*P*
Anterior frontal	ANOVA	10.14	.003 (N>S)	2.07	.16	0.02	.90
	ANCOVA	2.07	.16				
Ventricles	ANOVA	2.23	.14	12.16	.001 (L>R)	0.40	.53
	ANCOVA	3.61	.06 (S>N)				
Caudate	ANOVA	0.16	.69	8.27	.006 (R>L)	5.05	.03 (S: R=L, N: R>L)
	ANCOVA	4.07	.05 (S>N)				
Globus pallidus	ANOVA	11.12	.002 (S>N)	32.44	<.001 (R>L)	0.01	.94
	ANCOVA	16.07	<.001 (S>N)				
Putamen	ANOVA	1.07	.31	0.29	.59	0.20	.66
	ANCOVA	7.78	.007 (S>N)				

**ANOVA indicates analysis of variance; ANCOVA, analysis of covariance; S, schizophrenics; and N, normal controls.*
†The ANCOVA covaries for total cerebral volume.

COMPARISON WITH REPORTS ON LATER-ONSET DISORDER

The *z* score comparison of the effect size of differences from controls in brain volumes between this childhood-onset cohort and adult-onset schizophrenia studies showed no significant differences (P=.09 to .94) (**Table 5**). There was a trend, however, toward a difference from adults for the total cerebral volume in this cohort (P=.09). While the thalamic area was decreased in the childhood-onset schizophrenia patients, the difference from adult patients was not significant.

CLINICAL CORRELATES

Clinical correlates were evaluated for all MRI measures that differed significantly from control values. Seven correlations were significant (**Table 6**). There was a significant negative correlation between total cerebral volume and week 4 off-drug rating for negative symptoms with the SANS and with the Bunney-Hamburg psychosis subscale. The putamen showed a negative correlation with week 4 off-drug Bunney-Hamburg psychosis subscale score. The thalamic area also demonstrated a negative correlation with negative symptoms on the SANS. Most notable was the consistent relationship between globus pallidus volume and chlorpromazine equivalent medication dose at admission, age at time of study, and age of onset. There also was a trend toward a negative correlation between caudate volume and chlorpromazine equivalent medication dose at admission and total lifetime chlorpromazine equivalent dose.

COMMENT

Anatomic MRI brain measures of children with very-early-onset schizophrenia exhibit a pattern of abnormalities similar to that reported for adult populations. Children with early-onset schizophrenia have smaller cerebral volumes, smaller thalamic area, and enlarged basal ganglia structures, with a trend toward enlarged ventricles. Similar findings have been amply documented in adults.[17,19,20,23-28,53-65]

The effect size found in this cohort was generally similar to that observed for adult populations. Standardized differences were compared using *z* scores; this was the only way to directly compare measures of the child cohort with measures in adult cohorts. This type of comparison, however, is crude at best because of numerous methodological differences between studies.

The trend toward smaller total cerebral volume (using *z* score comparison) in this cohort suggests that children with schizophrenia may have a bigger lesion compared with their controls than is the case among adults with schizophrenia compared with their controls. The trend toward smaller total cerebral volume may indicate a greater central nervous system insult in the population with very-early-onset schizophrenia that might predispose these children to early development of psychotic symptoms. However, this trend toward smaller total cerebral volume is confounded by the lower IQ score and possible selection bias in this childhood-onset schizophrenia cohort.

A limitation of the study is that the schizophrenic children and normal controls could not be matched on IQ score, given the relatively poor performance of the cohort on the WISC-R vocabulary subtest. This is a potential confounding factor, as in normals there is an established relationship between IQ score and brain size.[41] However, the possible relationship between lower IQ score and smaller brain size is not necessarily a confounding factor, as lower IQ score may be an integral manifestation of the disorder, with its compromise in brain function and thought processes. In the childhood-onset schizophrenia cohort there was no correlation between scores on the WISC-R subtests and total cerebral volume, although there was a positive correlation between scores on both the Vocabulary and Block Design subtests and total cerebral volume in the control group. Also, the healthy subjects were likely to have higher-than-average WISC-R subtest scores because of our strict exclusion criteria for neurologic, medical, or psychiatric illness.

In addition, all of our subjects were nonresponders to typical neuroleptic therapy, which may mean we selected patients with inherently more severe illness. Crow,[66] for example (1985), has suggested that neuroleptic nonresponders may have greater brain abnormalities than neuroleptic responders. However, while the present cohort was severely ill, the phenomenologic characteristics, sex ratio, and premorbid histories of this population[67] resembled those described for more "typical" childhood cohorts.[2,7-10] Therefore, our findings may in fact be representative of children with schizophrenia.

The enlargement of the globus pallidus showed some relationship to current and previous medication therapy. Because of the number of correlations run on these data, a number of correlations would have been expected to be significant by chance. However, there is a consistent pattern of association between drug exposure and volume of the globus pallidus. Chakos and colleagues[23]

Table 5. Comparison of Effect Size of Differences From Normal Controls of Brain Volumes Between Adults and Children With Schizophrenia

	z Score			
Structure	Adult	Child	Difference*	*P* (2-Tailed)
Total cerebral[19, 21, 28]	−0.74	−3.09	1.67	.09
Ventricles[18, 21, 26]	2.62	1.47	1.15	.25
Thalamus[18, 26]	−0.92	−3.0	1.47	.14
Caudate[21, 24-26]	0.52	0.41	0.08	.94
Putamen[24, 25]	1.62	0.87	0.53	.60
Globus pallidus[24]	2.44	4.0	1.11	.27

*(Mean Adult *z* Score − Mean Child *z* Score)/$\sqrt{2}$.

Table 6. Clinical Correlates of Anatomic Brain Volume Measurements for Childhood-Onset Schizophrenia (n=21)*

	r/P						
Correlate	Total Cerebral	Ventricular Brain Ratio	Ventricles	Globus Pallidus	Caudate	Putamen	Thalamus
Age at study	.03/.91	−.29/.22†	−.27/.26†	**.48/.03**	−.20/.40†	.08/.75†	.19/.43
Age at onset	−.16/.50	−.30/.21†	−.24/.32†	**.53/.01**	−.04/.88†	.15/.54†	−.27/.24
Duration of illness	.08/.73	−.26/.28†	−.28/.24†	.22/.35	−.18/.44†	.05/.82†	.18/.43
Chlorpromazine equivalent at admission	−.12/.61†	.19/.43†	.15/.53†	**.49/.03†**	−.42/.07†	−.13/.60†	.11/.65†
Lifetime chlorpromazine equivalent	−.33/.17†	.11/.66†	.02/.94†	.30/.20†	−.41/.08†	−.07/.77†	.04/.88†
Full-scale IQ score	−.03/.92‡	−.21/.46§	−.16/.59§	.02/.95‡	.25/.38§	.14/.62§	−.11/.69‡
Brief Psychiatric Rating Scale total score	−.26/.17†	.10/.69‖	.01/.97‖	.36/.12†	−.26/.29‖	−.13/.60‖	−.06/.82†
Scale for the Assessment of Negative Symptoms total score	**−.63/.004‖**	−.05/.84¶	−.16/.52¶	.36/.13‖	−.14/.58¶	−.39/.11¶	**−.57/.01‖**
Scale for the Assessment of Positive Symptoms total score	−.41/.08†	.17/.48‖	.09/.71‖	.30/.20†	−.35/.14‖	−.07/.79‖	−.24/.31†
Bunney-Hamburg psychosis subscale score	**−.50/.02†**	−.15/.54‖	−.23/.35‖	.13/.60†	−.29/.24‖	**−.54/.02‖**	−.31/.18†

*Boldface indicates significant correlation.
†*n*=20.
‡*n*=15.
§*n*=14.
‖*n*=19.
¶*n*=18.

(1994) report a similar relationship between prior medication and caudate volume.

Animal studies have shown clear microscopic effects of typical neuroleptics in the striatum, with hypertrophy of mitochondria and small increases in neuronal cell size and striatal terminals.[68-70] Additionally, rat studies indicate that microscopic changes seen in the striatum are at least partially reversible with drug washout.[68] Typical neuroleptics and atypical neuroleptics, such as clozapine, affect different receptor populations[71] and have different effects on release of γ-aminobutyric acid in the basal ganglia.[72] In keeping with these preclinical data and the recent report by Chakos and colleagues[73] of differences in caudate volume in patients who underwent MRI scans while taking typical antipsychotics and then underwent rescanning while taking clozapine, there is also some evidence of basal ganglia normalization for a subset of patients in our cohort who underwent rescanning after 2 years of clozapine maintenance therapy.[74]

The association of enlarged globus pallidus with later age of onset is interesting. However, because there is no significant correlation between age of onset and neuroleptic dose, the association between neuroleptic dose at admission and globus pallidus size remains significant.

Alternatively, larger basal ganglia volumes in the present cohort might be seen as representing "abnormal pruning" in the patient population.[75-79] This appears unlikely, however, because the increase in volume occurs in structures that do not change at puberty in the normal child population (globus pallidus) as well as in those that do (putamen and caudate).[49]

The finding of smaller thalamic area is consistent with the recent findings of smaller thalamic area[28] and thalamic abnormalities[27] in adult patients. As discussed by Andreasen et al[27] (1994), lesions in the midline thalamus might explain complex symptoms involved in the psychotic process of schizophrenia, given the role of the thalamus in filtering sensory input.

Finally, we do not believe that these data reflect a nonspecific pattern for neurodevelopmentally impaired children. A large cohort of 60 males with attention deficit hyperactivity disorder (aged 4 to 18 years) and matched controls examined with identical procedures did not share the pattern of abnormalities seen in the present study.[80,81] This ADHD contrast group is particularly relevant, as six patients (29%) in this cohort had clear signs and symptoms of attention deficit hyperactivity disorder premorbidly.[67]

Further research on these rare cases will have important implications for later-onset schizophrenia. Given substantial data supporting a neurodevelopmental basis for schizophrenia,[82-89] the findings of this study raise important questions about whether there is evidence for late brain maturational shifts in those with childhood-onset schizophrenia. These questions can only be addressed, however, with a larger sample, including younger subjects who can be scanned closer to the time of onset. It is possible that scans at the time of onset would show more striking quantitative differences.

The larger purpose of the study of childhood-onset schizophrenia is to find clues as to the very early onset of the illness. Studies of other MRI parameters, including regional myelination, temporal lobe, and cerebellar lobular measures, are in progress, and these may be found to be unusual or deviant in the population with childhood-onset schizophrenia. The present report provides the most compelling neurobiological data to date concerning the continuity between childhood-onset schizophrenia and later-onset schizophrenia.

Accepted for publication September 13, 1995.

The authors thank David Pickar, MD, for his helpful comments and Yolanda C. Vauss, MA, Wendy L. Marsh, Roy Perlis, and Daniel P. Dickstein for their assistance.

Reprint requests to Child Psychiatry Branch, National Institute of Mental Health, Room 6N240, Bldg 10, MSC 1600, 10 Center Dr, Bethesda, MD 20902-1600 (Dr Rapoport).

REFERENCES

1. Werry JS. Child and adolescent (early onset) schizophrenia: a review in light of *DSM-III-R*. *J Autism Dev Disord.* 1992;22:601-624.
2. Green WH, Padron-Gayol M, Hardesty AS, Bassiri M. Schizophrenia with childhood-onset: a phenomenological study of 38 cases. *J Am Acad Child Adolesc Psychiatry.* 1992;31:976-986.
3. Beitchman JH. Childhood schizophrenia: a review and comparison with adult-onset schizophrenia. *Psychiatr Clin North Am.* 1985;8:793-814.
4. Kramer M. Population changes and schizophrenia. In: Wynne LC, Cromwell RL, Matthysse S, eds. *The Nature of Schizophrenia: New Approaches to Research and Treatment.* New York, NY: John Wiley & Sons Inc; 1978:1970-1985.
5. Karno M, Norquist GS. Schizophrenia: epidemiology. In: Kaplan HI, Sadock BJ, eds. *Comprehensive Textbook of Psychiatry IV.* 5th ed. Baltimore, Md: Williams & Wilkins; 1989;1:699-704.
6. Gottesman I. *Schizophrenia Genesis: The Origins of Madness.* New York, NY: WH Freeman & Co; 1991.
7. Kolvin I, Ounsted C, Humphrey M, Mcnay A. The phenomenology of childhood psychoses. *Br J Psychiatry.* 1971;118:385-395.
8. Watkins JM, Asarnow RF, Tanguay PE. Symptom development in childhood onset schizophrenia. *J Am Acad Child Adolesc Psychiatry.* 1988;6:865-878.
9. Russell AT, Bott L, Sammons C. The phenomenology of schizophrenia occurring in childhood. *J Am Acad Child Adolesc Psychiatry.* 1989;28:399-407.
10. Volkmar F, Cohen D, Hoshino V, Rende R, Paul R. Phenomenology and classification of the childhood psychoses. *Psychol Med.* 1988;18:191-201.
11. Murray RM, O'Callaghan E, Castle DJ, Lewis SH. Neurodevelopmental approach to the classification of schizophrenia. *Schizophr Bull.* 1992;18:319-332.
12. Gordon CT, Frazier JA, McKenna K, Giedd JN, Zametkin A, Zahn T, Hommer D, Hong W, Kaysen D, Albus K, Rapoport JL. Childhood-onset schizophrenia: an NIMH study in progress. *Schizophr Bull.* 1994;20:697-713.
13. McKenna K, Gordon CT, Rapoport JL. Childhood-onset schizophrenia: timely neurobiological research. *J Am Acad Child Adolesc Psychiatry.* 1994;33:771-781.
14. McKenna K, Gordon CT, Lenane M, Kaysen D, Fahey K, Rapoport JL. Looking for childhood-onset schizophrenia: the first 71 cases screened. *J Am Acad Child Adolesc Psychiatry.* 1994;33:636-644.
15. Marsh L, Suddath RL, Higgins N, Weinberger DR. Medial temporal lobe structures in schizophrenia: relationship of size to duration of illness. *Schizophr Res.* 1994;11:225-238.
16. Shenton ME, Kikinis R, Jolesz FA, Pollak SD, LeMay M, Wible CG, Hokama H, Martin J, Metcalf D, Coleman M, McCarley RW. Abnormalities of the left temporal lobe and thought disorder in schizophrenia: a quantitative magnetic resonance imaging study. *N Engl J Med.* 1992;327:604-612.
17. Andreasen NC, Nasrallah HA, Dunn V, Olson SC, Grove WM, Ehrhardt JC, Coffman JA, Crossett JHW. Structural abnormalities in the frontal system in schizophrenia: a magnetic resonance imaging study. *Arch Gen Psychiatry.* 1986;43:136-144.
18. Andreasen NC, Ehrhardt JC, Swayze VW, Alliger RJ, Yuh WTC, Cohen G, Ziebell S. Magnetic resonance imaging of the brain in schizophrenia. *Arch Gen Psychiatry.* 1990;47:35-44.
19. Breier A, Buchanan RW, Elkashef A, Munson RC, Kirkpatrick B, Gellad F. Brain morphology and schizophrenia: a magnetic resonance imaging study of limbic, prefrontal cortex, and caudate structures. *Arch Gen Psychiatry.* 1992;49:921-926.
20. Weinberger DR, Wyatt RJ. Cerebral ventricular size: a biological marker for subtyping chronic schizophrenia. In: Usdin E, Handen J, eds. *Biological Markers in Psychiatry and Neurology.* Elmsford, NY: Pergamon Press Inc; 1982:505-512.
21. DeLisi LE, Hoff AL, Schwartz JE, Shields GW, Halthore SN, Gupta SM, Henn FA, Anand AK. Brain morphology in first-episode schizophrenic-like psychotic patients: a quantitative magnetic resonance imaging study. *Biol Psychiatry.* 1991;29:159-175.
22. Bilder RM, Wu H, Bogerts B, Degreef G, Ashtari M, Alvir JMJ, Snyder PJ, Lieberman JA. Absence of regional hemispheric volume asymmetries in first-episode schizophrenia. *Am J Psychiatry.* 1994;151:1437-1447.
23. Chakos MH, Lieberman JA, Bilder RM, Borenstein M, Lerner G, Bogerts B, Wu H, Kinon B, Ashtari M. Increase in caudate nuclei volumes of first-episode schizo-

phrenic patients taking antipsychotic drugs. *Am J Psychiatry.* 1994;151:1430-1436.
24. Elkashef AM, Buchanan RW, Gellad F, Munson RC, Breier A. Basal ganglia pathology in schizophrenia and tardive dyskinesia: an MRI quantitative study. *Am J Psychiatry.* 1994;151:752-755.
25. Swayze VW, Andreasen NC, Alliger RJ, Yuh WTC, Ehrhardt JC. Subcortical and temporal structures in affective disorder and schizophrenia: a magnetic resonance imaging study. *Biol Psychiatry.* 1992;31:221-240.
26. Jernigan TL, Zisook S, Heaton RK, Moranville JT, Hesselink JR, Braff DL. Magnetic resonance imaging abnormalities in lenticular nuclei and cerebral cortex in schizophrenia. *Arch Gen Psychiatry.* 1991;48:881-890.
27. Andreasen NC, Arndt S, Swayze V, Cizadlo T, Flaum M, O'Leary D, Ehrhardt JC, Yuh WTC. Thalamic abnormalities in schizophrenia visualized through magnetic resonance image averaging. *Science.* 1994;266:294-297.
28. Flaum M, Swayze VW, O'Leary DS, Yuh WTC, Ehrhardt JC, Arndt SV, Andreasen NC. Brain morphology in schizophrenia: effects of diagnosis, laterality and gender. *Am J Psychiatry.* 1995;152:705-714.
29. Woody RC, Boylard K, Eisenhauer G, Altschuler L. CT scan and MRI findings in a child with schizophrenia. *J Child Neurol.* 1987;2:105-110.
30. Schultz SC, Koller MM, Kishore PR, Hamer RM, Gehl JJ, Friedel RO. Ventricular enlargement in teenage patients with schizophrenia spectrum disorder. *Am J Psychiatry.* 1983;140:1592-1595.
31. Hendren RL, Hodde-Vargas JE, Vargas LA, Orrison WW, Dell L. Magnetic resonance imaging of severely disturbed children: a preliminary study. *J Am Acad Child Adolesc Psychiatry.* 1991;30:466-470.
32. Frazier JA, Gordon CT, McKenna K, Lenane M, Jih D, Rapoport JL. An open trial of clozapine in 11 adolescents with childhood-onset schizophrenia. *J Am Acad Child Adolesc Psychiatry.* 1994;33:658-663.
33. American Psychiatric Association. *Diagnostic and Statistical Manual of Mental Disorders, Revised Third Edition.* Washington, DC: American Psychiatric Association; 1987.
34. Orvaschell H, Tabrizi MA, Chambers W. *Schedule for Affective Disorders and Schizophrenia for School-Age Children–Epidemiologic Version (Kiddie-SADS-E).* 3rd ed. New York, NY: New York State Psychiatric Institute and Yale University School of Medicine; 1980.
35. Reich W, Welner Z. *Diagnostic Interview for Children and Adolescents–RC (DSM-III-R Version), Revised Version V-R.* St Louis, Mo: Washington University; 1988.
36. Nelson WE. Developmental pediatrics. In: Behrman RE, Vaughan VC, eds. *Nelson Textbook of Pediatrics.* 12th ed. Philadelphia, Pa: WB Saunders Co; 1983:40-42.
37. Bunney WE, Hamburg DA. Methods for reliable longitudinal observation of behavior. *Arch Gen Psychiatry.* 1963;9:114-128.
38. Overall JE, Gorham DR. The Brief Psychiatric Rating Scale. *Psychiatry Res.* 1962;10:799-812.
39. Andreasen NC. *The Scale for the Assessment of Negative Symptoms (SANS).* Iowa City: University of Iowa; 1983.
40. Andreasen NC. *The Scale for the Assessment of Positive Symptoms (SAPS).* Iowa City: University of Iowa; 1984.
41. Andreasen NC, Flaum M, Swayze VS, O'Leary DS, Alliger R, Cohen G, Ehrhardt J, Yuh TC. Intelligence and brain structure in normal individuals. *Am J Psychiatry.* 1993;150:130-134.
42. Welner Z, Reich W, Herjanic B, Jung KG, Amado H. Reliability, validity, and parent-child agreement studies of the Diagnostic Interview for Children and Adolescents (DICA). *J Am Acad Child Adolesc Psychiatry.* 1987;26:649-653.
43. Achenbach TM, Edelbrock CS. *Manual for Child Behavior Checklist and Revised Behavior Profile.* Burlington: Dept of Psychiatry, University of Vermont; 1983.
44. Connors CK. Rating scales in drug studies with children. *Psychopharmacol Bull.* 1973:24-29. Special issue.
45. Goyett CH, Connors CK, Ulrich RF. Normative data on the revised Connor's parent and teacher rating scales. *J Abnorm Child Psychol.* 1978;6:221-236.
46. Denkla MB. Revised Physical and Neurological Examination for Subtle Signs. *Psychopharmacol Bull.* 1985;21:773-800.
47. Hyman SE, Arana GW. Anti-psychotic drugs. In: *Handbook of Psychiatric Drug Therapy.* Boston, Mass: Little Brown & Co Inc; 1991:4-36.
48. Rasband W. *Image (1.6).* Bethesda, Md: National Institutes of Health; 1993.
49. Giedd JN, Snell JW, Lange N, Rajapaks JC, Kaysen D, Vaituzis C, Vauss YC, Hamburger SD, Kozuch PL, Rapoport JL. Quantitative magnetic resonance imaging of human brain development: ages 4-18. *Cortex.* In press.
50. Snell JM, Merickel MB, Ortega JM, Goble JC, Brookeman JR, Kassell NF. Boundary estimation of complex objects using hierarchical active surface templates. *J Pattern Recognition.* In press.
51. *SAS Language and Procedures: Usage, Version 6, First Edition.* Cary, NC: SAS Institute Inc; 1989.
52. Altman DG. *Practical Statistics for Medical Research.* London, England: Chapman & Hall; 1991.
53. Weinberger DR, Bigelow LB, Kleinman JE. Cerebral ventricular enlargement in chronic schizophrenia: an association with poor response to treatment. *Arch Gen Psychiatry.* 1980;37:11-13.
54. Bogerts B, Meertz E, Schonfeldt-Bausch R. Basal ganglia and limbic system pathology in schizophrenia: a morphometric study of brain volume and shrinkage. *Arch Gen Psychiatry.* 1985;42:784-791.
55. Bogerts B. Recent advances in the neuropathology of schizophrenia. *Schizophr Bull.* 1993;19:431-445.
56. Heckers S, Heinsen H, Heinsen Y, Beckmann H. Cortex, white matter, and basal ganglia in schizophrenia: a volumetric postmortem study. *Biol Psychiatry.* 1991; 29:556-566.
57. Lieberman JA, Alvir JMJ, Woerner M, Degreef G, Bilder RM, Ashtari M, Bogerts B, Mayerhoff DI, Geisler SH, Loebel A, Levy DL, Hinrichsen G, Szymanski S, Chakos M, Koreen A, Borenstein M, Kane JM. Prospective study of psychobiology in first-episode schizophrenia at Hillside Hospital. *Schizophr Bull.* 1992;18:351-371.
58. Lieberman JA, Bogerts B, Degreef G, Ashtari M, Lantos G, Alvir J. Qualitative assessment of brain morphology in acute and chronic schizophrenia. *Am J Psychiatry.* 1992;149:784-794.
59. Lieberman JA, Jody D, Alver JMJ, Levy DL, Bogerts B, Degreef G, Mayerhoff DI, Cooper T. Brain morphology, dopamine, and eye-tracking abnormalities in first-episode schizophrenia. *Arch Gen Psychiatry.* 1993;50:357-368.
60. Meltzer HY. Biological studies in schizophrenia. *Schizophr Bull.* 1987;13:77-111.
61. Pakkenberg B. Stereological quantitation of human brains from normal and schizophrenic individuals. *Acta Neurol Scand.* 1992;suppl 137:20-33.
62. Stevens JR. An anatomy of schizophrenia? *Arch Gen Psychiatry.* 1973;29:177-189.
63. Stevens JR. Clinicopathologic correlations in schizophrenia. *Arch Gen Psychiatry.* 1986;43:715-716.
64. Buchanan RW, Breier A, Kirkpatrick B, Elkashef A, Munson RC, Gellad F, Carpenter WT. Structural abnormalities in deficit and nondeficit schizophrenia. *Am J Psychiatry.* 1993;150:59-65.
65. Degreef G, Ashtari M, Bogerts B, Bilder RM, Jody DN, Alvir JMJ, Lieberman JA. Volumes of ventricular system subdivisions measured from magnetic resonance images in first-episode schizophrenic patients. *Arch Gen Psychiatry.* 1992;49: 531-537.
66. Crow TJ. The two-syndrome concept: origins and current status. *Schizophr Bull.* 1985;1:471-486.
67. Alaghband-Rad J, McKenna K, Gordon CT, Albus KE, Hamburger SD, Rumsey JM, Frazier JA, Lenane MC, Rapoport JL. Childhood-onset schizophrenia: the severity of premorbid course. *J Am Acad Child Adolesc Psychiatry.* 1995;34:1273-1283.
68. Roberts RC, Gaither LA, Gao X, Kashap SM, Tamminga CA. Ultrastructural correlates of haloperidol-induced oral dyskinesias in rat striatum. *Synapse.* 1995; 20:234-243.
69. Benes FM, Paskevich PA, Domesick VB. Haloperidol-induced plasticity of axon terminals in rat substantia nigra. *Science.* 1983;221:969-971.
70. Benes FM, Paskevich PA, Davidson J, Domesick VB. The effects of haloperidol on synaptic patterns in the rat striatum. *Brain Res.* 1985;329:265-274.
71. Van Tol HHM, Bunzow JR, Guan H-C, Sunahara RK, Seeman P, Niznik HB, Civelli O. Cloning of the gene for a human dopamine D_4 receptor with high affinity for the antipsychotic clozapine. *Nature.* 1991;350:610-614.
72. Drew KL, O'Connor WT, Kehr J, Ungerstedt U. Regional specific effects of clozapine and haloperidol on GABA and dopamine release in rat basal ganglia. *Eur J Psychiatry.* 1990;187:385-397.
73. Chakos MH, Lieberman JA, Alvir J, Bilder R, Ashtari M. Caudate nuclei volumes in schizophrenic patients treated with typical antipsychotics and clozapine. *Lancet.* 1995;343:456-457.
74. Frazier JA, Giedd JN, Albus KE, Alaghband-Rad J, Lenane MC, McKenna K, Breier A, Rapoport JL. Childhood-onset schizophrenia: brain MRI rescan after 2 years of clozapine maintenance treatment. *Am J Psychiatry.* 1996;153:564-566.
75. Huttenlocher PR. Synaptic density in human frontal cortex: developmental changes and effects of aging. *Brain Res.* 1979;163:195-205.
76. Huttenlocher PR, deCourten C, Gare LJ, Van Der Loos H. Synaptogenesis in human visual cortex: evidence for synapse elimination during normal development. *Neurosci Lett.* 1982;33:247-252.
77. Feinberg I. Cortical pruning and the development of schizophrenia. *Schizophr Bull.* 1990;16:567-568.
78. Feinberg I. Schizophrenia and late maturational brain changes in man. *Psychopharmacol Bull.* 1982;18:29-31.
79. Feinberg I. Schizophrenia: caused by a fault in programmed synaptic elimination during adolescence? *Psychiatry Res.* 1982-1983;17:319-334.
80. Castellanos FX, Giedd JN, Marsh WL, Hamburger SD, Vaituzis AC, Dickstein DP, Sarfatti SE, Vauss YC, Snell JW, Lange N, Kaysen D, Krain AL, Ritchie GF, Rajapakse JC, Rapoport JL. Quantitative brain magnetic resonance imaging of the brain in attention-deficit hyperactivity disorder. *Arch Gen Psychiatry.* 607-616.
81. Castellanos FX, Giedd JN, Eckburg P, Marsh WL, Vaituzis C, Kaysen D, Hamburger SD, Rapoport JL. Quantitative morphology of the caudate nucleus in attention deficit hyperactivity disorder. *Am J Psychiatry.* 1994;151:1791-1796.
82. Weinberger DR. Implications of normal brain development for the pathogenesis of schizophrenia. *Arch Gen Psychiatry.* 1987;44:660-669.
83. Weinberger DR. Schizophrenia as a neurodevelopmental disorder: a review of the concept. In: Hirsch SE, Weinberger DR, eds. *Schizophrenia.* London, England: Blackwood Press; 1995:294-323.
84. Fish B. Neurobiologic antecedents of schizophrenia in children. *Arch Gen Psychiatry.* 1977;34:1297-1313.
85. Murray RM, Lewis SW. Is schizophrenia a neurodevelopmental disorder? *Br J Psychiatry.* 1987;295:681-682.
86. Mednick SA, Cannon TD, Barr CE, Lyon M, eds. *Fetal Neural Development and Adult Schizophrenia.* Cambridge, England: Cambridge University Press; 1991.
87. Bloom FE. Advancing a neurodevelopmental origin for schizophrenia. *Arch Gen Psychiatry.* 1993;50:224-227.
88. Keshavan MS, Anderson S, Pettegrew JW. Is schizophrenia due to excessive synaptic pruning in the prefrontal cortex? the Feinberg hypothesis revisited. *J Psychiatr Res.* 1994;28:239-265.
89. Andreasen NC. The mechanisms of schizophrenia. *Curr Opin Neurobiol.* 1994; 4:245-251.

Cerebral Structural Abnormalities in Obsessive-compulsive Disorder

A Quantitative Morphometric Magnetic Resonance Imaging Study

Michael A. Jenike, MD; Hans C. Breiter, MD; Lee Baer, PhD; David N. Kennedy, PhD; Cary R. Savage, PhD; Michael J. Olivares; Richard L. O'Sullivan, MD; David M. Shera, MS; Scott L. Rauch, MD; Nancy Keuthen, PhD; Bruce R. Rosen, MD, PhD; Verne S. Caviness, MD, PhD; Pauline A. Filipek, MD

Background: A previous pilot study of only posterior brain regions found lower white-matter volume in patients with obsessive-compulsive disorder than in normal control subjects. We used new cohorts of patients and matched normal control subjects to study whole-brain volume differences between these groups with magnetic resonance imaging–based morphometry.

Methods: Ten female patients with obsessive-compulsive disorder and 10 female control subjects, matched for handedness, age, weight, education, and verbal IQ, underwent magnetic resonance imaging with a 3-dimensional volumetric protocol. Scans were blindly normalized and segmented by means of well-characterized semiautomated intensity contour mapping and differential intensity contour algorithms. Brain structures investigated included the cerebral hemispheres, cerebral cortex, diencephalon, caudate, putamen, globus pallidus, hippocampus, amygdala, third and fourth ventricles, corpus callosum, operculum, cerebellum, and brain stem. Anterior to posterior neocortical regions, including precallosum, anterior pericallosum, posterior pericallosum, and retrocallosum, with adjacent white matter were also measured. Volumes found different between groups were correlated with Yale-Brown Obsessive Compulsive Scale score and Rey-Osterieth Complex Figure Test measures.

Results: Confirming results of our earlier pilot study and expanding the findings to the whole brain, patients with obsessive-compulsive disorder had significantly less total white matter but, in addition, significantly greater total cortex and opercular volumes. Severity of obsessive-compulsive disorder and nonverbal immediate memory correlated with opercular volume.

Conclusions: Replication of volumetric white-matter differences suggests a widely distributed structural brain abnormality in obsessive-compulsive disorder. Whereas determining the etiogenesis may require research at a microscopic level, understanding its functional significance can be further explored via functional neuroimaging and neuropsychological studies.

Arch Gen Psychiatry. 1996;53:625-632

Obsessive-compulsive disorder (OCD) is a common and often disabling syndrome. Prevalent in 2% to 3% of the world population,[1,2] it involves episodic obsessions that may lead to anxiety-dispelling compulsions (ie, such repetitive behaviors as washing and checking). Symptoms, described as senseless and unpleasant by patients, typically emerge around the second to third decade of life, have a familial incidence of 20% to 35%, and frequently overlap with motor tic symptoms.[3] Cognitively, patients show impaired visuospatial and nonverbal memory functions.[4-6] Obsessions and compulsions are remarkably resistant to treatment with psychodynamic therapeutic approaches but are often quite responsive to pharmacologic intervention.[3]

Several neuroimaging case reports have noted lesions in the caudate nucleus in occasional patients,[7-10] but studies of large cohorts of patients with OCD have not shown such findings to be common.[11-15] One computed tomographic study of men with OCD found decreased caudate volumes,[12] and computed tomographic studies of adolescents of both sexes have reported increased ventricle-to-brain ratios.[13] Higher-resolution magnetic resonance (MR) imaging studies, however, have not replicated these findings.[14,15]

The above findings have led investigators to postulate that OCD results directly from brain abnormalities that might

From the Departments of Psychiatry (Drs Jenike, Breiter, Baer, Savage, O'Sullivan, Rauch, and Keuthen and Messrs Olivares and Shera) and Radiology (Drs Breiter, Kennedy, Rauch, and Rosen), Nuclear Magnetic Resonance Center (Drs Breiter, Kennedy, O'Sullivan, and Rosen), and Department of Neurology (Drs Kennedy, Caviness, and Filipek), Massachusetts General Hospital and Harvard Medical School, Boston.

See Subjects and Methods on next page

SUBJECTS AND METHODS

SUBJECTS

Ten right-handed[20] female patients from the OCD Clinic and Research Unit at Massachusetts General Hospital, Boston, were assessed with the Structured Clinical Interview for *DSM-III-R*,[21] met *DSM-III-R* criteria for OCD,[22] and had no other psychiatric, medical, or neurologic illnesses. All patients had scores greater than 10 on the Yale-Brown Obsessive Compulsive Scale[23,24] at the time of imaging (mean±SD, 17.6±5.6).

The patients were matched for age, weight, years of education, and estimated verbal IQ to 10 right-handed female control subjects. The estimated verbal IQ score was calculated according to performance on the Information, Vocabulary, and Similarities subtests of the Wechsler Adult Intelligence Scale–Revised.[25] No control subject had current or past medical, neurologic, or *DSM-III-R* psychiatric illnesses as assessed by the Structured Clinical Interview for *DSM-III-R*. All patients and control subjects completed nonverbal memory testing with the Rey-Osterrieth Complex Figure Test.[26,27] Performance on this test was evaluated on 3 measures: figure copy (a measure of construction ability), immediate recall (a measure of immediate nonverbal memory), and 30-minute delayed recall (a measure of long-term nonverbal memory). All figures were scored without knowledge of group membership, according to the system described by Lezak.[27]

MORPHOMETRIC ANALYSES

MR Image Acquisition

After routine sagittal scout scanning, coronal 3-dimensional T_1-weighted spoiled gradient echo MR imaging was performed on all patients with OCD and control subjects at McLean Hospital, Belmont, Mass (1.5-T Signa MR System, General Electric Co, Milwaukee, Wis). Imaging variables were as follows: repetition time, 50 milliseconds; echo time, 9 milliseconds; flip angle, 50°; field of view, 24 cm; slice thickness, contiguous 3.0 mm; matrix, 256×256; and averages, 1.[28] Coronal T_2-weighted sequences were also performed, with the following variables: repetition time, 2000 milliseconds; echo time, 30/80 milliseconds; field of view, 24 cm; slice thickness, 5 mm/2.5 mm skip; matrix, 256×192; and averages, 1. Imaging was performed by 1 investigator (H.C.B.), and quality assurance signal-to-noise tests were completed by means of a phantom after each scanning session.

Positional Normalization and Image Segmentation

After transfer by magnetic tape to the Center for Morphometric Analysis at Massachusetts General Hospital, each native T_1-weighted 3-dimensional MR image was randomized and then positionally normalized. A standard 3-dimensional brain coordinate system was imposed on each scan,[29,30] with points of reference including the midpoints of the decussations of the anterior and posterior commissures and the midsagittal plane.[31] Each native scan was then resliced into normalized 3.0-mm coronal and 1.0-mm sagittal scans for subsequent segmentation.

On each normalized coronal plane, anatomic segmentation was performed by 1 researcher (M.J.O.) and independently verified by a second (P.A.F.), both of whom were unaware of the identity and diagnosis of the subject whose scan was being analyzed. Segmentation methods used well-characterized semiautomated intensity contour mapping and differential intensity contour algorithms.[32-38] Methods for positional normalization and image segmentation have been described in detail elsewhere.[39-42]

Anatomic Definitions

The brain structures measured for this study included the following: cerebral hemispheres; cortex; white matter; caudate; putamen; globus pallidus; central gray nuclei (including diencephalon and mesencephalon); hippocampus (including subiculum); amygdala; operculum; lateral third and fourth ventricles; corpus callosum; cerebellum; and brain stem. These structures were defined on each scan according to routine Center for Morphometric Analysis anatomic definitions, which have previously been described in detail.[42]

On the midline 1.0-mm normalized sagittal slice, the corpus callosum was segmented in continuum, which was then subdivided into 7 regions according to Witelson.[43] The measures obtained included total corpus callosum area, anterior-to-posterior length, mean corpus callosum thickness, and areas of the 7 individual subregions.

According to Center for Morphometric Analysis definitions, neocortical "pericallosal" regions with adjacent structures were subsequently delineated based on visualization of the corpus callosum in the normalized coronal plane: precallosal, defined as all slices anterior to the corpus callosum; anterior pericallosal, defined as all slices that showed the corpus callosum anterior to and not including the anterior commissure; posterior pericallosal, defined as all slices that showed the corpus callosum posterior to and including the anterior commissure; and retrocallosal, defined as all slices posterior to the corpus callosum (**Figure 1**). The anterior and posterior pericallosal regions were further divided into superior, inferior, and temporal regions, as follows: by a line connecting the sylvian fissure with the tip of the superior circular insular sulcus and the tip of the lateral ventricle and by a second line connecting the sylvian fissure with the tip of the inferior circular insular sulcus and the hippocampus or amygdala (**Figure 2**).[41]

Volumetric Analysis

The absolute volume of each structure was summed from all outlines in all planes where that structure appeared by multiplying the number of voxels by each voxel volume, as determined by the imaging variables.[33,35,39,40,42]

Statistical Analysis

Analyses were conducted in several steps. First, we looked for differential laterality in volumes between the 2 groups. Finding no evidence of this, we pooled the left plus right structural volumes for all regions. We then looked for either global or regional cerebral volume differences. Next, we looked for volumetric differences between the groups in any structures by a conservative criterion.

Because of the large number of measures resulting from volumetric MR image segmentation, we used either the conservative Bonferroni correction or an overall significant multivariate analysis of variance for each set of analyses to control for type I error. In exploratory analyses, we correlated OCD symptom severity and memory scores with only those volumes that significantly differed between groups. All analyses were conducted with SAS and SYSTAT statistical packages.

be detectable with modern neuroimaging techniques.[16-18] With the advent of precise structural morphometric MR imaging analytic techniques, it is now possible to investigate brain structures accurately in an effort to gain information about possible neurologic substrates of psychiatric disorders. In an earlier pilot study, we applied MR imaging–based morphometry to the posterior parieto-occipital ("retrocallosal") region (Figure 1) and found decreased white-matter volume in 6 patients with OCD when compared with 8 control subjects, despite both groups having similar total cerebral volumes.[19]

To study entire-brain anatomic differences further in patients with OCD compared with well-characterized control subjects, in the present study we applied whole-brain volumetric MR imaging in entirely new matched cohorts of 10 patients with OCD and 10 control subjects. Our primary a priori hypothesis was that white-matter volume would be significantly lower in patients with OCD than in control subjects. For exploratory analyses, we also collected measures of OCD symptom severity and nonverbal memory to assess their relationships to volumetric measures. Previous neuropsychological studies have consistently demonstrated impairment of nonverbal memory in OCD.[4-6] However, these deficits have never been correlated with underlying brain volumetric measures.

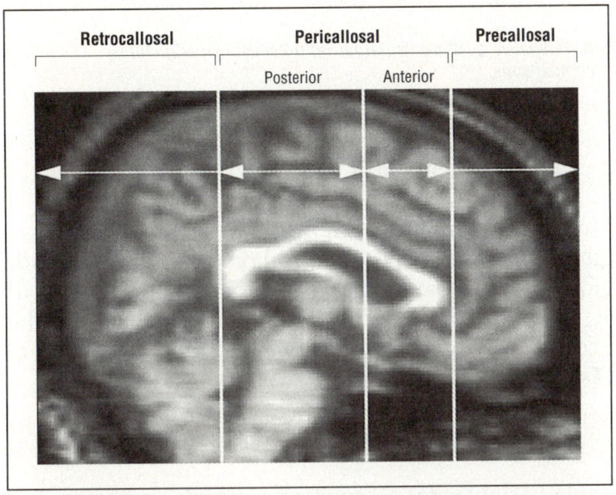

Figure 1. *Neocortical pericallosal regions: precallosal, slices anterior to corpus callosum; anterior pericallosal, slices visualizing corpus callosum anterior to and not including anterior commissure; posterior pericallosal, slices posterior to and including anterior commissure; and retrocallosal, all slices posterior to corpus callosum.*

RESULTS

DEMOGRAPHIC AND NEUROPSYCHOLOGICAL MEASURES

Patients with OCD and control subjects did not significantly differ in mean (±SD) age (patients with OCD, 31.6±8.7 years; control subjects, 28.5±11.4 years; $t[18]=0.7, P=.50$), weight (patients with OCD, 66.3±22.1 kg; control subjects, 65.6±9.9 kg; $t[18]=0.2, P=.81$), years of education (patients with OCD, 13.7±2.2 years; control subjects, 14.9±1.7 years; $t[18]=1.0, P=.33$), or estimated verbal IQ (patients with OCD, 116.9±14.8; control subjects, 118.5±17.5; $t[18]=0.2, P=.83$). Therefore, all analyses presented below were conducted without the use of these variables as covariates. (Analyses of covariance that used age and years of education as covariates produced identical results.)

See also pages 574, 577, 585, 595, 607, and 617

On the Rey-Osterrieth Complex Figure Test, performance of patients with OCD was slightly impaired relative to that of control subjects for the copy condition ($t[18]=2.0, P=.06$) and significantly impaired for the immediate ($t[18]=2.4, P=.02$) and delayed ($t[18]=2.5, P=.02$) recall conditions. None of the measures in this test correlated with the Yale-Brown Obsessive Compulsive Scale severity measure (all $P>.35$).

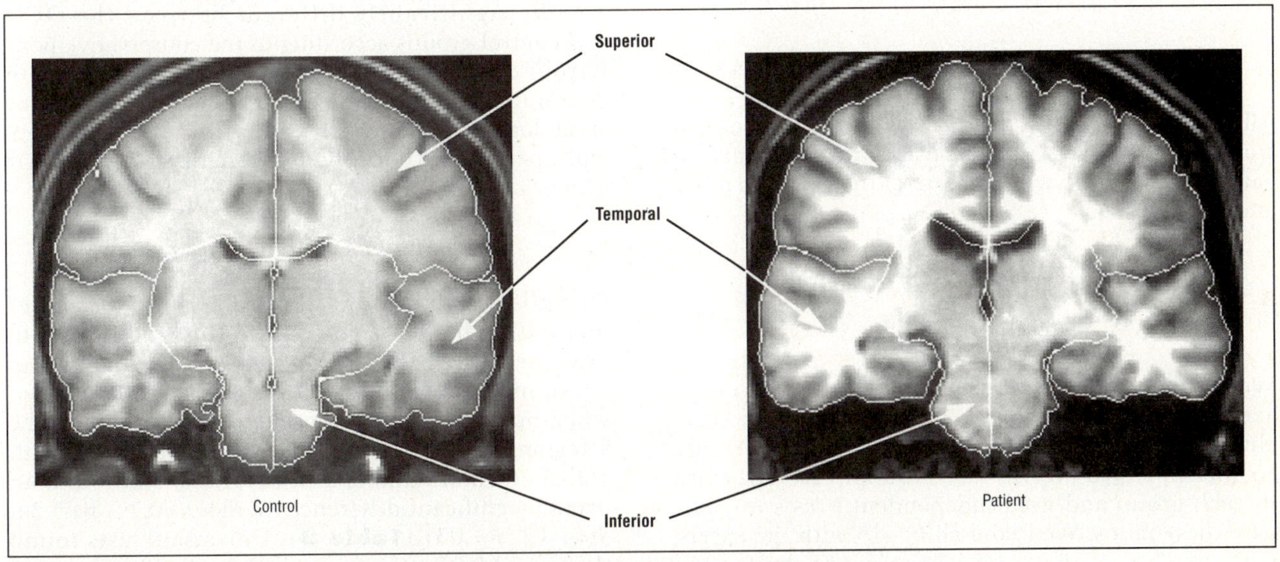

Figure 2. *Anterior and posterior pericallosal regions divided into superior, inferior, and temporal regions.*

Table 1. Comparison of Structures in OCD and Control Groups by Laterality Coefficient and Percentage of Total Cerebral Volume*

Structure	Laterality Coefficient† OCD (n=10)	Control (n=10)	t(18)	P	% of Total Cerebral Volume OCD (n=10)	Control (n=10)	t(18)	P
Cerebrum	0.006±0.010	0.001±0.012	1.13	.27	100.0	100.0	. . .	. . .
Cerebral cortex	−0.002±0.017	−0.007±0.015	0.76	.45	60.87±1.86	56.91±2.82	3.69	.001‡
Cerebral white matter	0.044±0.029	0.033±0.020	0.93	.36	27.82±2.09	32.56±3.43	3.71	.001‡
Cerebellum	−0.002±0.005	−0.011±0.007	0.95	.35	12.53±1.07	13.04±0.78	1.21	.24
Cerebellar cortex	0.016±0.024	0.011±0.036	0.033	.73	10.72±0.94	10.84±0.78	0.31	.75
Cerebellar white matter	−0.113±0.083	−0.128±0.102	0.036	.72	1.81±0.18	2.20±0.19	4.64	<.001‡
Lateral ventricle	−0.084±0.142	−0.100±0.140	0.25	.80	1.96±0.68	1.48±0.47	1.81	.08
Thalamus	−0.008±0.021	−0.028±0.044	1.25	.22	1.89±0.12	1.90±0.19	0.03	.96
Caudate	0.026±0.041	0.065±0.045	1.97	.06	0.73±0.11	0.81±0.11	1.72	.10
Lenticulate	0.008±0.049	−0.011±0.043	0.99	.33	1.19±0.08	1.20±0.15	0.16	.87
Putamen	0.018±0.052	−0.006±0.048	1.10	.28	0.88±0.06	0.87±0.11	0.18	.85
Pallidum	−0.015±0.132	−0.029±0.104	0.25	.80	0.31±0.02	0.33±0.05	0.89	.38
Hippocampus	0.021±0.106	−0.029±0.074	1.23	.23	0.82±0.10	0.75±0.08	1.59	.12
Amygdala	−0.026±0.200	0.051±0.162	0.96	.34	0.48±0.13	0.53±0.10	0.95	.35
Insula	−0.034±0.056	−0.092±0.071	1.97	.06	1.58±0.10	1.51±0.19	0.98	.33
Operculum	−0.092±0.125	−0.116±0.089	0.49	.62	2.60±0.15	2.30±0.22	3.55	.002‡

*Values are given as mean±SD. OCD indicates obsessive-compulsive disorder.
†[(L−R)/(L+R)]×100. Positive coefficients represent larger left-hemisphere structures; negative coefficients, larger right-hemisphere structures.
‡Significant by Bonferroni correction (P<.003) for 15 comparisons in each set of comparisons.

Table 2. Global and Regional Cerebral Volumes*

Region	Control	OCD	t(18)	P
Global	1181.3±83.1	1207.1±92.9	0.7	.52
Prefrontal	163.5±12.9	162.1±16.8	0.2	.83
Anterosuperior pericallosal	122.2±24.0	131.7±15.9	1.0	.30
Anteroinferior pericallosal	62.8±9.8	67.9±8.7	1.2	.23
Anterotemporal pericallosal	28.8±5.2	29.6±6.9	0.3	.76
Posterosuperior pericallosal	253.3±24.9	259.9±45.3	0.4	.68
Posteroinferior pericallosal	84.3±5.8	83.4±7.2	0.2	.77
Posterotemporal pericallosal	140.5±13.2	144.7±15.2	0.6	.51
Retrocallosal	325.7±28.3	327.3±28.6	0.1	.90
Cerebellar	153.8±10.8	150.5±7.4	0.7	.44

*Values are given as mean±SD. OCD indicates obsessive-compulsive disorder. Multivariate analysis of variance was not significant (Wilks λ=0.98, F[1,18]<1, P=.59).

CLINICAL MR IMAGE INTERPRETATIONS

All 20 MR images in both patients with OCD and control subjects were clinically read as normal by 1 investigator (B.R.R.), who was unaware of the subject's name and diagnosis.

MORPHOMETRIC ANALYSES

Laterality Measures

We compared left-right asymmetry in the 2 groups and found no significant ($P<.05$) differences in laterality between the groups. We calculated the laterality coefficient as $[(L-R)/(L+R)]\times 100$ for each structure in each group and used independent t tests to compare these ratios. We found all $P>.15$ with the exception of the caudate and insula (both $P=.06$) (**Table 1**).

Regional Cerebral Volumes

Multivariate analysis of covariance of the 9 major regions demarcated by the morphometric analyses, with global cerebral volume as a covariate, found no overall significant difference in cerebral volumes between the groups (Wilks $\lambda=0.98$, $F=0.30$, $df=1,18$, $P=.59$) (**Table 2**).

Structural Volume Comparisons

Table 1 (right side) compares the groups on pooled (left plus right) volumes for all major structures that were analyzed, with the volume of each structure expressed as a percentage of the total cerebrum.

For the volumes of these 15 structures, we found 4 to be significantly different between the OCD and control groups according to the conservative Bonferroni criterion for 15 tests of $P<.003$; these were cerebral white matter and cerebellar white matter (both lower in patients with OCD) and cerebral cortex and operculum (both higher in patients with OCD) (Table 1).

White-Matter Differences by Region

Our pilot study[19] found retrocallosal white-matter diminution in OCD. To confirm this finding and to examine further the possibilities of abnormalities in white matter in other brain regions, we compared white-matter volumes between groups for each of the 9 regions by multivariate analysis of covariance, with global cerebral volume as a covariate, and found an overall significant difference (Wilks $\lambda=0.77$, $F=5.34$, $df=1,18$, $P=.03$) (**Table 3**). Univariate tests found that in addition to retrocallosal white matter and cerebellar white matter, there was also a signifi-

Table 3. White-Matter Volumes by Region*

Region	Control	OCD	t(18)	P
Cerebellar	26.0±3.3	21.7±1.4	3.6	.001
Retrocallosal	108.2±21.6	86.9±16.9	2.4	.02
Posteroinferior pericallosal	30.6±4.0	27.3±2.2	2.2	.03
Posterosuperior pericallosal	100.5±18.6	88.9±16.4	1.4	.15
Anterotemporal pericallosal	2.8±1.0	2.2±0.9	1.4	.16
Prefrontal	46.7±8.1	42.1±6.2	1.4	.17
Posterotemporal pericallosal	34.7±7.2	30.6±5.5	1.4	.17
Anteroinferior pericallosal	16.9±4.0	15.5±3.0	0.9	.36
Anterosuperior pericallosal	45.3±10.2	42.1±5.9	0.8	.39

Values are given as mean±SD. OCD indicates obsessive-compulsive disorder. Multivariate analysis of variance was significant (Wilks λ=0.77, F[1,18]=5.3, P=.03).

cant decrease in posterior inferior pericallosal white matter.

Although the 6 other regions also showed smaller white-matter volumes in the OCD group, none of these reached statistical significance with this sample size.

EXPLORATORY ANALYSES

To generate hypotheses for future studies with larger samples, we conducted a number of analyses without a priori hypotheses.

Corpus Callosum Area and Length

We found no significant difference in area of the corpus callosum (P=.57), but there was a significant difference in length between the groups, with patients with OCD having, on average, longer corpus callosa (patients with OCD, 78.3±7.1 mm; control subjects, 72.0±3.8 mm; t[18]=2.5, P=.02). Despite the significant difference in length of the corpus callosa, which are used to mark off the retrocallosal area in morphometric analysis, there were no significant differences in volumes of the retrocallosal or anterior and posterior pericallosal regions (Table 2). We found no relationship between corpus callosum length and volume of global cortex or white matter in either patients with OCD (r=0.05, P=.89) or control subjects (r=0.43, P=.22).

Correlation of Clinical Measures and Volumes

In the 10 patients with OCD, we correlated the score on the Yale-Brown Obsessive Compulsive Scale, a measure of clinical severity of OCD, with volumes of the 4 structures found significantly different between the 2 groups (ie, cerebral cortex, cerebral white matter, operculum, and cerebellar white matter). Of these 4 structures, only opercular volume was significantly related to OCD severity (r=−0.66, P=.03), suggesting that patients with greater opercular volume had less severe symptoms at the time of testing. Similarly, in the patients, opercular volume was significantly positively related to Rey-Osterrieth Complex Figure Test immediate recall (r=0.64, P=.04), suggesting that patients with greater opercular volume had better memory performance. These correlations must be interpreted cautiously, since P values were not corrected for multiple tests, and when the more conservative nonparametric measure of association, Kendall τ, was used, neither reached the P<.05 level of statistical significance (τ=−0.40 and τ=0.33, respectively).

COMMENT

When individual brain regions were compared, patients with OCD had significantly less white matter in posteroinferior pericallosal, retrocallosal, and cerebellar regions (and trends toward decreased white matter in all other areas) than carefully matched control subjects. Among gray-matter structures, only the operculum was found to be larger in patients with OCD.

The primary limitation of this study is the modest number of subjects, which, although common in neuroimaging research, limits statistical power. Also, findings cannot be generalized to other populations, such as males with OCD. The strengths of the study include well-characterized patients with OCD, a carefully matched control group, blinded data analyses, and a design that provided clinical and neuropsychological measures that could be correlated with structural findings. Restriction of our sample to right-handed female patients with OCD and normal control subjects who were closely matched limits generalizability of our findings; however, by using such homogeneous groups, we are able to draw statistically reliable conclusions from significant differences with our sample size. In many previous MR imaging studies, mixed cohorts of patients were studied; in some, both men and women were combined even though there is now considerable evidence that there are sex differences in brain morphometry.[42] As in all neuroimaging studies with relatively small samples, nonsignificant differences must be interpreted cautiously, since they may reflect the high risk of type II error.

Findings that replicate or converge with results from previous research are most convincing. The finding of reduced posterior white matter replicates our previous pilot report in patients with OCD.[19] However, larger retrocallosal cortex volume was not found in the pilot study. This discrepancy might be attributed to the smaller number of subjects and/or less stringent matching on education in the earlier pilot cohort. The white-matter reductions in the present study do not appear to be localized to the retrocallosal region, since we found significant white-matter reductions in 2 other regions as well. The most conservative interpretation is that white matter is globally decreased in this cohort, with lack of statistical significance in many regions because of type II error.

The cortex–to–white matter ratio was larger in patients with OCD than in control subjects. During brain development, neurons, dendrites, axons, and synapses are first produced in excess, and then some are maintained while others are eliminated[44,45]; thus, normal brain development yields a decreasing ratio of gray to white matter.[45-49] Cell death during normal development of the central nervous system has been reported in many locations, including the cerebellum[50] and cerebral cortex.[51-53] Some failure in normal programmed cell death in the developing brain may contribute to greater amounts of cerebral cortex in patients with OCD, although this is clearly speculative.[44,54-57]

In the developing brain, the presence of transient juvenile projections that are eventually eliminated or pruned suggests an enormous potential for developmental plasticity. Perhaps a cerebral insult could produce localized brain damage in 1 region and another compensates by maintaining some of its juvenile projections that, under normal circumstances, would have been eliminated. These retained circuits might help compensate for deficits produced by an insult, but they may also result in other difficulties, such as obsessional symptoms. It has been hypothesized that psychosurgical operations for treatment of severe OCD improve symptoms by interfering with "overactive" or inappropriately modulated circuits in the brain.[58-66] Such circuits could theoretically result from impaired neuronal pruning during development.

The major contributing factor to the changing ratio of cortex to white matter is increasing myelination as the human brain develops.[67-71] Myelination, hypothesized to reflect functional maturity of the brain,[68,72-75] is the principal determinant of both volume increase [44] and increases in brain weight[76] during the postnatal years, and it continues throughout the fourth decade of life.[68-70,77-81] This may be particularly relevant since the mean age at onset of OCD symptoms is in late adolescence or early adult years.[82] All the basic elements required for cognition are acquired by the developing brain by the early teenage years; nevertheless, in later years, young adults improve the speed, capacity, and ability of their mental functions beyond the age at which somatic growth has already stopped.[77] In the central nervous system, myelination is accomplished by oligodendrocytes, and anything that interferes with or modifies their function could result in reduced amounts of myelin in the brain.[76,83-90]

Opercular volume was increased and negatively correlated with OCD symptoms, while positively correlated with immediate nonverbal memory. This pattern suggests that increased opercular volume might serve a compensatory function in OCD. However, given that these findings are novel and solely correlational, further speculation about these complex relationships must await additional data.[91-93]

The significance of the finding that half of the patients with OCD had a corpus callosum longer than that of any control subject is not known. A similar finding has been reported from MR imaging studies of schizophrenic patients compared with control subjects (see David[94] for a review), and there is indirect evidence of specific functional abnormality of excessive callosal transfer in schizophrenia, although its role in the pathogenesis of psychiatric symptoms remains unspecified.[94,95] It remains to be determined whether the longer corpus callosa are related in some fundamental way to the finding of generalized white-matter diminution in patients with OCD. It is of interest that Peterson et al,[96] using MR imaging morphology, recently reported that "worst-ever motor tic symptoms" in patients with Tourette syndrome correlated highly (r=0.88) with the length of the corpus callosum.

The caudate nucleus has been implicated in the pathophysiology of OCD, with the strongest support coming from the functional neuroimaging literature.[97-100] In the current study, we did not find a statistically significant decrease in caudate size for patients with OCD vs controls (P=.10), although the sample sizes in the present study provided adequate statistical power for detecting only large effect sizes.

In summary, this study found evidence of globally reduced white matter and increased gray matter in women with OCD vs matched normal controls. Increased opercular volume in patients with OCD was found to be negatively correlated with OCD symptom severity and positively correlated with immediate nonverbal memory. Trends toward reduced volume and decreased normal asymmetry were also noted in the caudate nuclei of patients with OCD. Further blurring the distinction between neurologic and psychiatric illnesses, replication of volumetric white-matter differences suggests a widely distributed structural brain abnormality in OCD. Additional morphometric studies will be necessary to evaluate this phenomenon in males, as well as to assess subcortical structures fairly. Whereas determination of the etiogenesis of the white-matter abnormality may require research at a microscopic level, eg, by postmortem histology or molecular biological techniques, understanding its functional significance can be further explored via functional neuroimaging and neuropsychological studies.

Accepted for publication September 29, 1995.

This study was supported in part by the David Judah Research Fund, Boston, Mass (Drs Jenike, Baer, Breiter, and Rauch and Mr Olivares); grants NS 20489 and NS 24279 from the National Institute of Neurological Disorders and Stroke, and grant HD 27802 from the National Institute of Child Health and Human Development (Drs Filipek and Kennedy), Bethesda, Md; and grant T32CA09502 from the National Institutes of Health, Bethesda (Dr Breiter). Dr Kennedy also holds a Fairway Trust Fellowship. Dr Breiter was supported in part by a National Association for Research on Schizophrenia and Depression Young Investigator Award.

We thank Jack M. Fletcher, PhD, for his commentary and technical assistance, and Perry Renshaw, MD, PhD, for use of the McLean Hospital MR imager.

Corresponding author: Michael A. Jenike, MD, Massachusetts General Hospital Psychiatric Neuroscience Program, Massachusetts General Hospital—East, Ninth Floor, 149 13th St, Charlestown, MA 02129 (e-mail: jenike@psych.mgh.harvard.edu).

REFERENCES

1. Myers JK, Weissman MM, Tischler GL, Holzer CE, Leaf PJ, Orvaschel H, Anthony JC, Boyd JH, Burke JD Jr, Kramer M. Six-month prevalence of psychiatric disorders in three commitments. *Arch Gen Psychiatry.* 1984;41:959-967.
2. Robins LN, Helzer JE, Weissman MM, Orvaschel H, Gruenberg E, Burke JD Jr, Regier DA. Lifetime prevalence of specific psychiatric disorders in three sites. *Arch Gen Psychiatry.* 1984;41:949-958.
3. Jenike MA, Baer L, Minichiello WE. *Obsessive Compulsive Disorders: Theory and Management.* 2nd ed. Chicago, Ill: Year Book Medical Publishers; 1990.
4. Boone KB, Ananth J, Philpott L, Kaur A, Djenderedjian A. Neuropsychological

characteristics of nondepressed adults with obsessive-compulsive disorder. *Neuropsychiatry Neuropsychol Behav Neurol.* 1991;4:96-109.
5. Christensen KJ, Kim SW, Dysken MW, Hoover KM. Neuropsychological performance in OCD. *Biol Psychiatry.* 1992;31:4-18.
6. Zielinski CM, Taylor MA, Juzwin KR. Neuropsychological deficits in obsessive-compulsive disorder. *Neuropsychiatry Neuropsychol Behav Neurol.* 1991;4:110-126.
7. Laplane D, Widlocher D, Pillon B, Baulac M, Binoux F. Comportement compulsif d'allure obsessionnelle par necrose circonscrite bilaterale apllidopstriatale. *Rev Neurol.* 1981;137:269-276.
8. Weilburg J, Mesulam MM, Weintraub S, Buonnano F, Jenike MA, Stakes JW. Focal striatal abnormalities in a patient with obsessive-compulsive disorder. *Arch Neurol.* 1989;46:233-235.
9. Laplane D, Baulac M, Widlocher D, Dubois B. Pure psychic akinesia with bilateral lesions of basal ganglia. *J Neurol Neurosurg Psychiatry.* 1984;47:377-385.
10. Williams AC, Owen C, Heath DA. A compulsive movement disorder with cavitation of caudate nucleus. *J Neurol Neurosurg Psychiatry.* 1988;51:447-448.
11. Garber HJ, Ananth JV, Chiu LC, Griswold VJ, Oldendorg WH. Nuclear magnetic resonance study of obsessive-compulsive disorder. *Am J Psychiatry.* 1988;146:1001-1005.
12. Luxenberg JS, Swedo SE, Flament AF, Friedland RP, Rapaport JL, Rapaport SI. Neuroanatomical abnormalities in obsessive-compulsive disorder detected with quantitative x-ray computed tomography. *Am J Psychiatry.* 1988; 145:1089-1093.
13. Behar D, Rapoport JL, Berg CJ, Denckla MB, Mann L, Cox C, Fedio P, Zahn T, Wolfman MG. Computerized tomography and neuropsychological test measures in adolescents with obsessive-compulsive disorder. *Am J Psychiatry.* 1984;141:363-368.
14. Kellner CH, Jolley RR, Holgate RC, Austin L, Lydiard RB, Laraia M, Ballenger JC. Brain MRI in obsessive-compulsive disorder. *Psychiatry Res.* 1991;36: 45-49.
15. Scarone S, Colombo C, Livian S, Abbruzzese M, Ronchi P, Locatelli M, Scotti G, Smeraldi E. Increased right caudate nucleus size in obsessive-compulsive disorder: detection with magnetic resonance imaging. *Psychiatry Res.* 1992; 45:115-121.
16. Jenike MA. Obsessive-compulsive disorder: a question of a neurologic lesion. *Compr Psychiatry.* 1984;25:298-304.
17. Insel TR, Winslow JT. Neurobiology of obsessive compulsive disorder. *Psychiatr Clin North Am.* 1992;15:813-824.
18. Baxter LR. Neuroimaging studies of obsessive compulsive disorder. *Psychiatr Clin North Am.* 1992;15:871-884.
19. Breiter HCR, Filipek PA, Kennedy DN, Baer L, Pitcher D, Olivares M, Renshaw P, Caviness VS, Jenike MA. Retrocallosal white matter abnormalities in patients with obsessive-compulsive disorder. *Arch Gen Psychiatry.* 1994;51: 663-664.
20. Oldfield RC. The assessment and analysis of handedness: the Edinburgh Inventory. *Neuropsychologia.* 1971;9:97-114.
21. Spitzer RL, Williams JBW, Gibbon M, First MD. *Structured Clinical Interview for* DSM-III-R *(SCID).* New York, NY: New York State Psychiatric Institute, Biometrics Research; 1987.
22. *Diagnostic and Statistical Manual of Mental Disorders, Third Edition, Revised.* Washington, DC: American Psychiatric Association; 1987:245-247.
23. Goodman WK, Price LH, Rasmussen SA, Mazure C, Fleischmann R, Hill C, Henninger GR, Charney DS. The Yale-Brown Obsessive Compulsive Scale, I: development, use, and reliability. *Arch Gen Psychiatry.* 1989;46:1006-1011.
24. Goodman WK, Price LH, Rasmussen SA, Mazure C, Delgado P, Heninger GR, Charney DS. The Yale-Brown Obsessive Compulsive Scale, II: validity. *Arch Gen Psychiatry.* 1989;46:1012-1016.
25. Wechsler D. *Wechsler Adult Intelligence Scale–Revised.* Cleveland, Ohio: Psychological Corp; 1981.
26. Osterrieth P, Rey A. Le test de copie d'une figure complex. *Arch Psychol.* 1944;30:205-221.
27. Lezak MD. *Neuropsychological Assessment.* 2nd ed. New York, NY: Oxford University Press; 1983.
28. Filipek PA, Kennedy DN, Caviness VS. Morphometric analysis of central nervous system neoplasms. *Ann Neurol.* 1989;26:461.
29. Filipek PA, Kennedy DN, Caviness VS. A method of morphometric analysis of the human brain based upon magnetic resonance imaging. *Ann Neurol.* 1988; 24:356.
30. Alpert NM, Bradshaw JF, Kennedy D, Correia JA. The principal axes transformation: a method for image registration. *J Nucl Med.* 1990;31:1717-1722.
31. Talairach J, Tournoux P. *Co-planar Stereotaxic Atlas of the Human Brain.* New York, NY: Thieme Medical Publishers Inc; 1988.
32. Kennedy DN. *A System for Three-Dimensional Analysis of Magnetic Resonance Images.* Cambridge, Mass: Dept of Nuclear Engineering, Massachusetts Institute of Technology; 1986. Thesis.
33. Kennedy DN, Nelson AC. Three-dimensional display from cross-sectional tomographic images: an application to MRI. *IEEE Trans Med Imag.* 1987;6: 134-140.
34. Kennedy DN, Filipek PA, Caviness VS. Semi-automated image segmentation in multi-slice magnetic resonance images. *Proc Soc Magn Reson Med.* 1987; 6:378.
35. Kennedy DN, Filipek PA, Caviness VS. Anatomic segmentation and volumetric calculation in nuclear magnetic resonance imaging. *IEEE Trans Med Imag.* 1989;8:1-7.
36. Kennedy DN, Kennedy SK, Filipek PA, Caviness VS. Morphometric characterization of brain shape by Fourier analysis. *Proc Soc Magn Reson Med.* 1988;7:993.
37. Kennedy DN, Filipek PA, Caviness VS. Fourier shape analysis of anatomic structures. In: Byrnes JS, Byrnes JL, eds. *Recent Advances in Fourier Analysis and Its Applications.* Dordrecht, the Netherlands: Kluwer Academic Publishers; 1990:17-28.
38. Kennedy DN, Rowell D, Filipek PA, Caviness VS. Neural system segmentation of three-dimensional magnetic resonance brain images. *Proc Soc Magn Reson Med.* 1989;8:983.
39. Filipek PA, Kennedy DN, Caviness VS, Rossnick SL, Spraggins TA, Starewicz PM. Magnetic resonance imaging-based brain morphometry: development and application to normal subjects. *Ann Neurol.* 1989;25:61-67.
40. Filipek PA, Kennedy DN, Caviness VS, Rossnick SL, Spraggins TA, Starewicz PM. MRI-based morphometry: development and application to normal controls. *Ann Neurol.* 1989;25:61-67.
41. Filipek PA, Kennedy DN, Caviness VS. Neuroimaging. In: Boller F, Grafman J, eds; Rapin I, Segalowitz S, topic eds. *Handbook of Neuropsychology, Vol 6: Child Neuropsychology.* Amsterdam, the Netherlands: Elsevier Science Publishers; 1992:301-329.
42. Filipek PA, Richelme C, Kennedy DN, Caviness VS. The young adult human brain: an MRI-based morphometric analysis. *Cereb Cortex.* 1994;4:344-360.
43. Witelson SE. Age and sex differences in the isthmus and genu of the human corpus callosum: a postmortem morphological study. *Brain.* 1989;112:799-835.
44. Innocenti GM. *The Development of Projections From Cerebral Cortex: Progress in Sensory Physiology.* Heidelberg, Germany: Springer-Verlag; 1991:12.
45. Jacobson M. Neuronal death and neurotrophic factors. In: *Developmental Neurobiology.* 3rd ed. New York, NY: Plenum Press; 1991:311-358.
46. Ernst M. Über Untergang von Zellen während der normalen Entwicklung bei Wirbeltieren. *Z Anat Entwicklungsgesch.* 1926;79:228-262.
47. Glücksmann A. Development and differentiation of the tadpole eye. *Br J Ophthalmol.* 1940;24:153-178.
48. Glücksmann A. Cell deaths in normal vertebrate ontogeny. *Biol Rev.* 1951; 26:59-86.
49. Glücksmann A. Cell death in normal development. *Arch Biol.* 1965;76:419-437.
50. Janowska JS, Finlay BL. Cell degeneration in early development of the forebrain and cerebellum. *Anat Embryol.* 1983;167:439-447.
51. Finlay BL, Slattery M. Local differences in the amount of early cell death in neocortex predict adult local specializations. *Science.* 1983;219:1349-1351.
52. Heumann D, Leuba G. Neuronal death in the development and aging of the cerebral cortex of the mouse. *Neuropathol Appl Neurobiol.* 1983;9:297-311.
53. Price DJ, Blakemore C. Regressive events in the postnatal development of association projections in the visual cortex. *Nature.* 1985;316:721-724.
54. Innocenti GM, Clarke S, Koppel H. Transitory macrophages in the white matter of the developing visual cortex, II: development and relations with axonal pathways. *Dev Brain Res.* 1983b;11:55-66.
55. Innocenti GM, Koppel H, Clarke S. Transitory macrophages in the white matter of the developing visual cortex, I: light and electron microscopic characteristics and distribution. *Dev Brain Res.* 1983a;11:39-55.
56. Clarke PGH. Identical populations of phagocytes and dying neurons revealed by intravascularly injected horseradish peroxidase, and by endogenous glutaraldehyde-resistant acid phosphatase, in the brains of chick embryos. *Histochem J.* 1984;16:955-969.
57. Beard J. The history of a transient nervous apparatus in certain Ichthyopsida: an account of the development and degeneration of ganglion-cells and nerve fibres. *Zool Jahrb Abt Morphol.* 1896;9:1-106.
58. Modell JG, Mountz JM, Curtis GC, Greden JF. Neurophysiologic dysfunction in basal ganglia/limbic striatal and thalamocortical circuits as a pathogenetic mechanism of obsessive-compulsive disorder. *J Neuropsychiatry Clin Neurosci.* 1989;1:27-36.
59. Rees WL. The value and limitations of psychosurgery in the treatment of psychiatric illness. *Psychiatr Neurol Neurochir.* 1973;76:323-334.

60. Greenblatt M, Solomon HC. Survey of nine years of lobotomy investigations. *Am J Psychiatry.* 1952;109:262-265.
61. Lewin W. Selective leukotomy: a review. In: Laitinen LV, Livingston KI, eds. *Surgical Approaches in Psychiatry.* England: Medical and Technical Publishing Co; 1973.
62. Tippin J, Henn FA. Modified leukotomy in the treatment of intractable obsessional neurosis. *Am J Psychiatry.* 1982;139:1601-1603.
63. Mitchell-Heggs N, Kelly D, Richardson A. Stereotactic limbic leucotomy: a follow-up at 16 months. *Br J Psychiatry.* 1976;128:226-240.
64. Martuza RL, Chiocca EA, Jenike MA, Giriunas IE, Ballantine HT. Stereotactic radiofrequency thermal cingulotomy for obsessive compulsive disorder. *J Neuropsychiatry Clin Neurosci.* 1990;2:331-336.
65. Jenike MA, Baer L, Ballantine HT, Martuza RL, Tynes S, Giriunas I, Buttolph L, Cassem N. Cingulotomy for refractory obsessive-compulsive disorder: a long-term follow-up of 33 patients. *Arch Gen Psychiatry.* 1991;48:548-555.
66. Chiocca EA, Martuza RL. Neurosurgical therapy of the obsessive-compulsive disorder. In: Jenike MA, Baer L, Minichiello WE, eds. *Obsessive Compulsive Disorders: Theory and Management.* 2nd ed. Chicago, Ill: Year Book Medical Publishing; 1990.
67. Looney GA, Elberger AJ. Myelination of the corpus callosum in the cat: time course, topography, and functional implications. *J Comp Neurol.* 1986;248: 336-347.
68. Yakovlev PI, Lecours AR. The myelogenetic cycles of regional maturation of the brain. In: Minkowski A, ed. *Regional Development of the Brain in Early Life.* Oxford, England: Blackwell Scientific Publications; 1967:3-70.
69. Jernigan TL, Tallal P. Late childhood changes in brain morphology observable with MRI. *Dev Med Child Neurol.* 1990;32:379-385.
70. Valk J, Knaap MS, eds. *Magnetic Resonance of Myelin, Myelination and Myelin Disorders.* Berlin, Germany: Springer Verlag; 1989:9-21.
71. Martin E, Kikinis R, Zuerrer M, Boesch C, Briner J, Kewitz G, Kaelin P. Developmental stages of human brain: an MR study. *J Comput Assist Tomogr.* 1988;12:917-922.
72. Van der Knaap MS, Valk J, Bakker CJ, Schooneveld M, Faber JAJ, Willemse J, Gooskens RHJM. Myelination as an expression of the functional maturity of the brain. *Dev Med Child Neurol.* 1991;33:849-857.
73. Flechsig P. Developmental (myelogenetic) localisation of the cerebral cortex in the human subject. *Lancet.* 1901;2:1027-1029.
74. Tilney F, Casamajor L. Myelinogeny as applied to the study of behavior. *Arch Neurol Psychiatry.* 1924;12:1-16.
75. Langworthy OR. Development of behavior patterns and myelinization of the nervous system of the human fetus and infant. *Contrib Embryol.* 1933;24:3-57.
76. Jacobson M. *Neuroglial Ontogeny.* 3rd ed. New York, NY: Plenum Press; 1991: 95-142.
77. Pujol J, Vendrell P, Junque C, Marti-Vilalta JL, Capdevila A. When does human brain development end? evidence of corpus callosum growth up to adulthood. *Ann Neurol.* 1993;34:71-75.
78. Barkovich AAJ, Kjos BO. Normal postnatal development of the corpus callosum as demonstrated by MR imaging. *Am J Neuroradiol.* 1988;9:487-491.
79. Barkovich AJ, Kjos BO, Jackson DE, Norman K. Normal maturation of the neonatal and infant brain: MR imaging at 1.5 T. *Radiology.* 1988;166:173-180.
80. Curnes JT, Burger PC, Djang WT, Boyko OB. MR imaging of compact white matter pathways. *AJNR Am J Neuroradiol.* 1988;9:1061-1068.
81. Benes FM, Turtle M, Khan Y, Farol P. Myelination of a key relay zone in the hippocampal formation occurs in the human brain during childhood, adolescence, and adulthood. *Arch Gen Psychiatry.* 1994;51:477-484.
82. Minichiello WE, Baer L, Jenike MA, Holland A. Age of onset of major subtypes of obsessive-compulsive disorder. *J Anxiety Disord.* 1990;4:147-150.
83. Phillips RJP. Jimpy, a totally new sex-linked gene in the house mouse. *Z Vererbungsl.* 1954;86:322-326.
84. Sidman RL, Dickie MN, Appel SH. Mutant mice (quaking and jimpy) with deficient myelination in the central nervous system. *Science.* 1964;144:309-311.
85. Bartlett WP, Skoff RP. Expression of the jimpy gene in the spinal cords of heterozygous female mice, II: oligodendroglial and endothelial cell hyperplasia. *Dev Brain Res.* 1989;47:1-11.
86. Dobbing J. The influence of early nutrition on the development and myelination of the brain. *Proc R Soc Lond Ser B.* 1963;159:503-509.
87. Wiggins RC. Myelin development and nutritional insufficiency. *Brain Res Rev.* 1982;4:151-175.
88. Lai M, Lewis PD, Patel AJ. Effects of undernutrition on gliogenesis and glial maturation in rat corpus callosum. *J Comp Neurol.* 1980;193:965-972.
89. Clos J, Legrand J, Limozin N, Dalmasso C, Laurent G. Effects of abnormal thyroid state and undernutrition on carbonic anhydrase and oligodendroglia development in the rat cerebellum. *Dev Neurosci.* 1982;5:243-251.
90. Clos J, Legrand C, Legrand J, Ghandour MS, Labourdette G, Vincendon G, Gombos G. Effects of thyroid state and undernutrition on S100 protein and astroglia development in rat cerebellum. *Dev Neurosci.* 1982;5:285-292.
91. Prats JM, Garaizar C, Uterga JM, Urroz MJ. Operculum syndrome in childhood: a rare cause of persistent speech disturbance. *Dev Med Child Neurol.* 1992;34:359-364.
92. Mao CC, Coull BM, Golper LAC, Rau MT. Anterior operculum syndrome. *Neurology.* 1989;39:1169-1172.
93. Heilman KM, Bowers D, Speedie L, Coslett HB. Comprehension of affective and nonaffective prosody. *Neurology.* 1984;34:917-921.
94. David AS. Callosal transfer in schizophrenia: too much or too little? *J Abnorm Psychol.* 1993;102:573-579.
95. Schaefer GB, Thompson JN, Bodensteiner JB, Hamza M, Tucker RR, Marks W, Gay C, Wilson D. Quantitative morphometric analysis of brain growth using magnetic resonance imaging. *J Child Neurol.* 1990;5:127-130.
96. Peterson BS, Leckman JF, Duncan JS, Wetzles R, Riddle MA, Hardin MT, Cohen DJ. Corpus callosum morphology from magnetic resonance images in Tourette's syndrome. *Psychiatry Res Neuroimag.* 1994;55:85-99.
97. Baxter LR, Phelps ME, Mazziotta JC, Guze BH, Schwartz JM, Selin CE. Local cerebral glucose metabolic rates in obsessive-compulsive disorder. *Arch Gen Psychiatry.* 1987;44:211-218.
98. Baxter LR Jr, Schwartz JM, Bergman KS, Szuba MP, Guze BH, Mazziotta JC, Alazraki A, Selin CE, Ferng HK, Munford P. Caudate glucose metabolic rate changes with both drug and behavior therapy for obsessive-compulsive disorder. *Arch Gen Psychiatry.* 1992;49:681-689.
99. Rauch SL, Jenike MA, Alpert NM, Baer L, Breiter HCR, Savage CR, Fischman AJ. Regional cerebral blood flow measured during symptom provocation in obsessive-compulsive disorder using oxygen 15–labeled CO_2 and positron emission tomography. *Arch Gen Psychiatry.* 1994;1:62-70.
100. Insel TR. Toward a neuroanatomy of OCD. *Arch Gen Psychiatry.* 1992;49: 739-744.

ORIGINAL ARTICLE

Auditory Attentional Deficits in Patients With Schizophrenia

A Positron Emission Tomography Study

Daniel S. O'Leary, PhD; Nancy C. Andreasen, MD, PhD; Richard R. Hurtig, PhD; Marilyn L. Kesler; Margaret Rogers, PhD; Stephen Arndt, PhD; Ted Cizadlo; G. Leonard Watkins, PhD; Laura L. Boles Ponto, PhD; Peter T. Kirchner, MD; Richard D. Hichwa, PhD

Background: Patients with schizophrenia have frequently been found to perform poorly on tasks requiring selective attention, defined as the ability to focus attention on relevant information while simultaneously ignoring irrelevant stimuli. This study explores the brain mechanisms mediating attentional processing in patients with schizophrenia by measuring their regional cerebral blood flow (rCBF) with positron emission tomography using [^{15}O]water as they performed tasks that differed systematically in attentional demand.

Methods: Ten schizophrenic patients (either neuroleptic-naive or withdrawn from medication) (patient group) and 10 normal volunteers (control group) performed auditory target detection tasks. Different types of auditory stimuli (environmental sounds, meaningless speech sounds, and words) were presented either binaurally (ie, same sounds in both ears) or dichotically (simultaneous and different sounds in the 2 ears). In dichotic conditions, subjects were instructed to focus on either their left or right ear.

Results: Initial subtraction-based image analyses sought significant rCBF changes anywhere in the brain. Patients consistently had less significant activation than controls in right superotemporal gyrus (STG). Follow-up analyses used regions of interest traced on individual magnetic resonance images to precisely measure rCBF in STG. Unlike controls, patients had higher rCBF in the left STG during all activation conditions.

Conclusions: The abnormal task-related rCBF asymmetry in STG of schizophrenic patients may indicate an isolated temporal lobe deficit, but it may also indicate abnormality in the thalamocortical circuitry mediating selective attention and/or in the brain systems that integrate auditory processing in the 2 hemispheres.

Arch Gen Psychiatry. 1996;53:633-641

From the Mental Health Clinical Research Center (Drs O'Leary, Andreasen and Arndt, Ms Kesler, and Mr Cizadlo), Departments of Psychiatry (Dr Andreasen), Speech Pathology and Audiology (Dr Hurtig), and Radiology (Dr Kirchner), and Positron Emission Tomography Imaging Center (Drs Watkins, Boles Ponto, and Hichwa), University of Iowa Hospitals and Clinics, Iowa City; and Department of Speech and Hearing Sciences, University of Washington, Seattle (Dr Rogers).

PATIENTS WITH schizophrenia perform abnormally on cognitive tasks ranging from early attentional gating to full-scale IQ.[1-3] Despite nearly a century of research,[4,5] however, there is no consensus concerning the neural basis of the multiple cognitive deficits of schizophrenia. Magnetic resonance imaging (MRI) studies have reported abnormalities in a variety of brain regions,[6,7] suggesting that the cognitive abnormalities of schizophrenia may have multiple causes. An alternative possibility is based on the fact that brain function is mediated by circuits that connect spatially distributed anatomical regions.[8] It has been suggested in a number of models[9,10] that schizophrenia involves dysfunction in various components of this circuitry. Using a novel technique of MRI averaging,[11] our group has recently proposed that the multiple symptoms and cognitive abnormalities of schizophrenia may be explained by dysfunction in the thalamus and in other circuitry mediating attention.

The proposal that schizophrenia results from abnormalities in attention-related circuitry fits well with neuropathological findings of abnormalities in the thalamus[12-14] and in structures such as the cingulate gyrus,[15] which may be part of a distributed attentional network.[16,17] The proposal is also in line with theories that schizophrenia is characterized by dysfunction in an "attentional filter."[1,18,19] Broadbent[20-22] proposed that such a filter normally protects limited-capacity brain systems from overload by selecting relevant information for processing and by inhibiting irrelevant stimuli. Dysfunction in the filter could lead to abnormali-

See Subjects and Methods on next page

SUBJECTS AND METHODS

SUBJECTS

Ten *DSM III-R*–diagnosed,[40] right-handed schizophrenic patients, 9 men and 1 woman (patient group) and 10 normal volunteers matched as a control group for gender, age, handedness, and parental socioeconomic status (**Table 1**) participated in the study. Controls were recruited from the community by newspaper advertisement and were paid for their participation. They were screened by telephone for history of psychiatric illness, neurological disorder, head injury, and alcohol or drug abuse and further screened using an abbreviated version of the Comprehensive Assessment of Symptoms and History,[41] a structured interview and recording instrument.

METHODS

Diagnosis

Diagnoses were established by consensus of at least 2 research psychiatrists and were based on cross-sectional and longitudinal information contained in the Comprehensive Assessment of Symptoms and History. Three of the patients were assessed during their first hospitalization and had never received neuroleptic medication. The remaining patients had been receiving neuroleptic medication an average of 55 months (SD=68) and underwent a 3-week drug wash prior to PET imaging while they were inpatients at the University of Iowa Mental Health Clinical Research Center (MHCRC). Patients were selected from among patients consecutively admitted to the MHCRC who were right-handed and had normal hearing. All subjects gave informed consent to participate in the study, which was approved by the University of Iowa Internal Review Board.

Patients and controls had normal hearing thresholds in both ears assessed with an audiometer. All patients and controls also had a right ear advantage on a dichotic task involving free report of consonant-vowel pairs, suggesting that they had left hemispheric dominance for language.

Activation Tasks

During the PET study, subjects were supine, with eyes closed. Ambient noise was attenuated approximately 80% by foam earphones (E-A-R TONE, Cabot Safety Corp, Indianapolis, Ind), inserted into the subjects' auditory canals, which were used to present the tape-recorded stimuli. All activation conditions required detection of a specified target within a sequence of stimuli. The subject pressed a thumb switch, mounted in a small device held in the right hand, either away from ("a target was detected"), or toward the palm ("no target"). Responses were recorded on a lap-top computer.

Detailed information concerning stimulus characteristics may be found in a previous report.[34] Briefly, each activation task used 1 of 3 types of auditory stimuli presented either binaurally or dichotically: environmental sounds (eg, a car horn), meaningless consonant-vowel-consonant (CVC) speech sounds (eg, bot), and CVCs that are English words (eg, dog). Seven stimuli (in binaural conditions) or pairs of stimuli (in dichotic conditions) were presented with an interstimulus interval of 300 milliseconds, followed by a tone burst, cueing the subject to respond if a target was detected in the preceding sequence. The target was a specific stimulus in the environmental sounds and CVC conditions but was any animal name in the words condition (there were 6 possibilities) to require that subjects process the words semantically. All stimuli were digitally edited to have equal RMS intensity and presented at 70-dB SPL. Dichotic stimulus pairs were digitally aligned for onset. All tasks started 90 seconds before image acquisition and continued for a total of 400 seconds (40 trials). There were 22 targets in each condition. A baseline task consisting of tone bursts (once every 10 seconds) was used during the first and last injections. The subjects responded with a thumb press on hearing the tone.

Image Acquisition and Reconstruction

On arrival at the PET Center, subjects had a 20-gauge arterial catheter placed in the radial artery of the left arm and a 20-gauge venous catheter in the antecubital vein of the right arm. Subjects were positioned in the PET scanner with laser light guides aligned at the orbital-meatal line (indicating the center of the lowest slice). The subject's head was loosely taped to a foam-lined head holder made of rigid plastic. Subjects were repositioned using the laser light guides before each injection, which were repeated at approximately 15-minute intervals. During the activation conditions, subjects were asked to close their eyes and to remain as motionless as possible. Between tasks, subjects remained in the scanner but were permitted to move to minimize discomfort. We found that the patients tolerated this procedure better than a more restrictive head holder. Head movement between scans was corrected by registration of the PET image from each injection to the subject's MRI (see below).

Once the subject was positioned, a transmission scan was performed for attenuation correction of the emission images, using a rotating rod source of germanium 68. This was followed by a sham injection using the baseline reaction time task. During the sham, all procedures were identical to an image acquisition condition from the subject's perspective, but no tracer was injected and no arterial blood was drawn. The sham helped to reduce the subject's anxiety and consequent higher overall CBF that had been found during the first injection.

Subjects performed 9 auditory tasks in the following order: sham, baseline task; 1, first baseline task; 2, dichotic environmental sounds, attend left; 3, dichotic CVCs, attend left; 4, dichotic CVCs, attend right; 5, dichotic words, attend right; 6, binaural words; 7, binaural environmental sounds; and 8, second baseline task. Radiation exposure considerations limited the study to 8 injections, which precluded use of all possible combinations of stimuli in a single experiment. The baseline task was presented first and last to assess possible changes in rCBF across the PET session

ties in perception and thought owing to an inability to exclude irrelevant stimuli.

Studies of attentional filtering often used dichotic presentation in which different stimuli are presented through earphones to the 2 ears (eg, "dog" to the right ear and "ball" simultaneously to the left ear), with the subject instructed to monitor 1 ear.[23] Theories concerning attentional filters have evolved a great deal since Broadbent's because of fatigue or anxiety. The effects of binaural vs dichotic presentation were assessed using environmental sounds and words. Subjects attended in a manner consistent with presumed hemispheric dominance in these dichotic conditions (to the right for words and to the left for environmental sounds). Changes in rCBF attributable to attend-left vs attend-right condition were assessed using dichotically presented CVCs. A fixed task order was used to reduce error variance that would be introduced by randomization and to make the task transitions as easy as possible for the schizophrenic patients to understand. Only 1 task dimension (ie, stimulus type, binaural vs dichotic mode of presentation, or direction of attention) changed from one activation condition to the next, so that the task requirements could be easily explained. One of the patients in the present study completed only 6 of the tasks. A later study used a different fixed order of presentation to assess order effects.

Each activation condition involved the injection of 75 mBq of [^{15}O]water through the venous catheter. Regional CBF was measured using the autoradiographic [^{15}O]water method[42-44] with a scanner (GE4096PLUS, General Electric, Milwaukee, Wis). Arterial blood was sampled from the arterial catheter to allow calculation of tissue perfusion (in milliliters per minute per 100 g). Fifteen sections (6.5 mm center to center) were acquired with an intrinsic in-plane resolution of 8-mm full-width half-maximum and a 10-cm axial field of view. More detailed information concerning image acquisition and reconstruction may be found in a previous report.[45]

Image Analysis

The quantitative PET rCBF images were transferred to the Image Processing Laboratory of the University of Iowa MHCRC for analysis, using locally developed software.[46,47] Image registration used software that performed a least-squares minimization to fit the surface of the PET and MRI.[47,48] Images from each of the 8 PET conditions were independently fit, without operator intervention, to the MRIs. Each coregistration met a quantitative criterion, and 2 independent raters then rated the fit for each PET condition. The registration procedure was rerun if required until an adequate fit was achieved. The MRIs were contiguous, 1.5-mm thick coronal MR sections acquired on a 1.5-T scanner (Signa, General Electric). Parameters of the MRI acquisition were a spoiled grass sequence with flip angle of 40°, echo time (TE) of 5 milliseconds, repetition time (TR) of 24 milliseconds, and 2 excitations.

Data Analysis

Two independent but conceptually related analysis strategies were pursued. An initial function of interest (FOI) analysis that did not involve a priori regional hypotheses was performed on the entire PET image. This analysis used a statistical mapping approach based on within-subject image subtraction and across-subject averaging. Brain landmarks on the MRIs were used to place each brain into a standardized coordinate space.[49] An 18-mm Hanning filter was applied to the registered PET images for each condition to reduce residual anatomical variability. The images were normalized for whole-brain blood flow on a voxel-by-voxel basis. Within-subject subtraction of the final baseline condition from each activation condition was then performed, followed by across-subject averaging of the subtraction images and computation of pixel-by-pixel *t* tests of the rCBF changes (**Figure 1**).

Significant regions of activation were calculated on the *t* map images, using a technique that corrects for the large number of *t* tests performed, the lack of independence between voxels, and the resolution of the processed PET images.[50] In keeping with the usage of the Montreal group who developed the technique,[50] a *t* value of 3.61 was considered to be statistically significant ($P<.001$, 1-tailed, uncorrected). Data are reported in tables by showing the location of the voxel with the highest *t* value in each significant area, using coordinates from the atlas of Talairach and Tournoux[49] and region names. Discussion will be limited to regions in which a cluster of contiguous pixels with *t* values above 3.61 resulted in a volume greater than 1 mL. The only exception is for homologous regions of the left and right superotemporal gyri (STG), which are reported to illustrate the changes in activation in these regions.

The significant rCBF changes found in the FOI analyses were almost exclusively localized in the left and right STG. Because the FOI approach results in a considerable loss of anatomical resolution, a second analysis used a region of interest (ROI) approach to explore significant rCBF changes found in the FOI analysis. For this analysis, manual tracings were made of the left and right STG on each subject's MRIs, using a locally developed software package,[46] which permits tracing on any one of 3 orthogonal views of the resampled MRI (Figure 1). Traces on any one view are telegraphed to the others, allowing accurate identification of brain landmarks, using 3-dimensional shape information. Mean rCBF within the traced region was calculated for each injection on the coregistered PET images.

Tracings were made on every other coronal slice (1 mm thick) on MRIs aligned and resampled into a standard orientation. The traces included gray and white matter of the STG, with a straight line connecting the deepest point of the superotemporal sulcus to the deepest point of the circular sulcus. The anterior boundary was the most anterior point on the transverse gyrus of Heschl (**Figure 2**). The posterior boundary was defined by a horizontal line drawn on the sagittal view passing through the most posterior point of the posterior ramus of the sylvian fissure. The traced region extended to the most posterior coronal slice containing the telegraphed projection of this line. The values reported below are from regions traced by 1 operator. However, interrater reliability of rCBF within ROIs traced by a second operator was good (r=0.96).

The traced ROI included Heschl gyrus and the planum temporale, but excluded the ascending ramus of the sylvian fissure. Heschl gyrus includes primary auditory cortex.[51] The planum, which is immediately posterior to Heschl gyrus, has been found to be larger on the left in the majority of right-handers[52-54] and may be the structural substrate for language lateralization. The ROI included Brodmann areas 22, 41, and 42.

initial model,[24,25] but dichotic monitoring remains useful for assessing selective attention. Recent dichotic studies generally support the concept of a filtering deficit in schizophrenia. Patients typically have deficits on tasks requiring focused attention but additionally show disproportionately large deficits attributable to distraction from stimuli presented to the nonattended ear.[26,27]

Dichotic tasks are frequently used to assess "cere-

Table 1. Demographic Characteristics of Patient and Control Groups and Clinical Characteristics of Patients*

Characteristics	Patients (n=10)	Controls (n=10)
Demographic		
Mean age, y	33.4 (4)	30.2 (8.2)
M:F ratio	9:1	9:1
Mean education, y		
Subject	13.2 (1.1)	14.7 (1.8)
Father	13.6 (3.9)	14.3 (3.3)
Clinical		
Mean age at onset, y	22.8 (5.4)	...
Mean duration of illness, mo	137.1 (68.5)	...
Mean age at first hospitalization, y	23.3 (4.4)	...
Mean No. of hospitalizations	7.3 (8.5)	...

Values in parentheses are SDs.

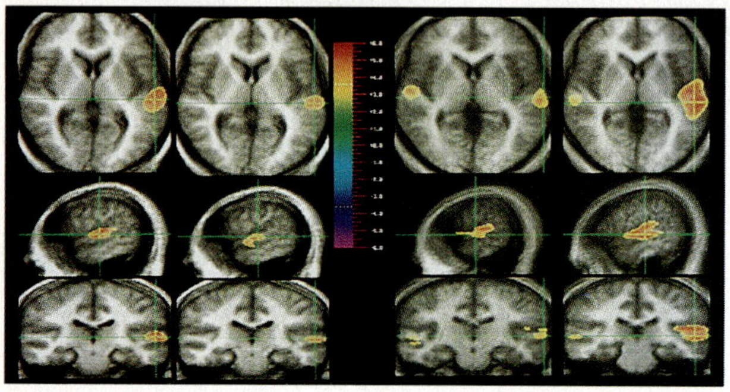

Figure 1. *Axial, sagittal, and coronal views showing significant* t *values (in color) for binaural and dichotic words conditions overlaid on the average magnetic resonance image for schizophrenic patients (2 columns on left) and controls (2 columns on right). Note the similarity of the pattern of activation in binaural and dichotic conditions in the patients, in contrast to the change in asymmetric activation in the controls.*

bral laterality," as well as selective attention. Right-handed subjects typically have a right ear advantage for dichotically presented speech sounds. This is thought to result from the high density of fibers from the right ear to the language-dominant left hemisphere and from inhibition of ipsilateral input from the left ear to the left hemisphere. Language stimuli presented to the left ear are presumed to be transmitted initially to the right hemisphere, but then they must be transferred to the left hemisphere via the corpus callosum, resulting in degradation of left ear stimuli and a subsequent right ear advantage.[28,29] Dichotic studies of cerebral laterality in schizophrenia have had mixed results.[30-32]

The present study assessed the hypothesis that patients with schizophrenia would exhibit deficits on tasks requiring selective attention, defined as the ability to focus attention on stimuli presented on a relevant auditory channel while ignoring stimuli presented simultaneously on another channel.[33] A previous study by our group[34] used auditory monitoring tasks in conjunction with positron emission tomography (PET) to assess the effects of attention on regional brain blood flow (rCBF) in normal controls. We anticipated that rCBF in patients would show the same bilateral pattern of activation found by our own and other studies of normal volunteers[35-39] during binaural conditions, which required

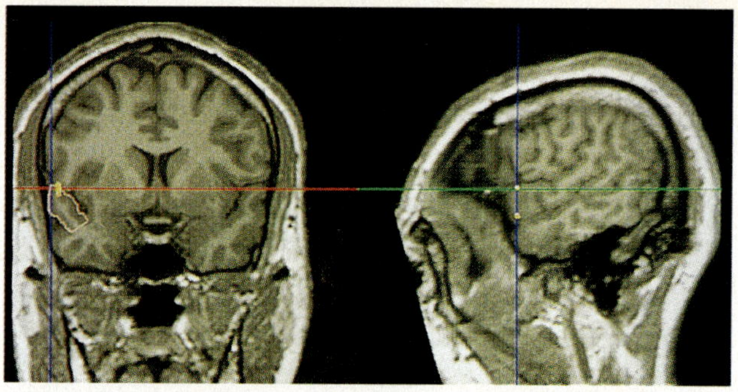

Figure 2. *Most anterior section of the right superotemporal gyrus region of interest of 1 individual that were traced on every other coronal section (1 mm thick) on alternating sections in the left and right hemisphere. Regional cerebral blood flow in the regions of interest was then obtained from the coregistered positron emission tomographic images.*

the ability to focus attention on auditory stimuli but did not require inhibition of competing auditory stimuli. We hypothesized that schizophrenic patients would show abnormal patterns of rCBF, coincident with poorer behavioral performance, in dichotic-monitoring conditions.

RESULTS

FOI ANALYSIS

Table 2 and Figure 1 present the results of the FOI analysis. Patients were similar to controls in showing significant regions of activation exclusively in STG. Patients differ from controls, however, in that task-related activations are primarily in the left hemisphere, whereas controls show activations in both left and right hemispheres, which change according to task demands.

The pattern of rCBF change exhibited by patients during binaural conditions indicates that they process both types of stimuli (environmental sounds and words) predominantly in their left hemispheres. The maximal *t* values were greater on the left, and the region of significant activation was many times bigger in the left than in the right STG in the patient group. The control group, in contrast, exhibited roughly symmetric increases in rCBF in the left and right STG when attending to binaurally presented environmental sounds and words.

The patients also showed a different pattern of task-related rCBF change from that in the controls in the dichotic conditions. Inspection of Table 2 indicates that for patients, dichotic presentation of environmental sounds and words resulted in very similar patterns of activation to that seen when the stimuli were binaurally presented (Figure 1). Compared with the binaural presentation of these stimuli, the patient group did not exhibit the large increase of activated volume in the left STG shown by the controls in the dichotic attend-right words condition, nor did it exhibit the decrease in the volume of the left STG activation during the dichotic attend-left environmental sounds condition. The patient group exhibited the same lack of right STG activation during the dichotic presentation of these stimuli as during the binaural conditions.

In the 2 dichotic CVC conditions, the patient group showed a nearly identical pattern to that of controls when attending right but a different pattern in the attend-left con-

Table 2. Function of Interest Analysis for Schizophrenic Patients and Controls*

Location	Patients (n=10)					Controls (n=10)				
			Coordinates‡					Coordinates‡		
	t	Size,† mL	*x*	*y*	*z*	*t*	Size,† mL	*x*	*y*	*z*
Binaural Conditions										
Environmental sounds										
Left STG	6.2	2.3	−50	−25	4	5.3	3.5	−44	−23	3
Right STG	4.9	0.7	57	−24	−2	5.1	4.2	47	−8	−6
Words										
Left STG	5.5	2.2	−55	−24	4	5.2	3.7	−57	−31	7
Right STG	3.8	0.1	57	−17	−3	5.0	3.9	54	−13	0
Dichotic Conditions										
Environmental sounds: attend left										
Left STG	7.0	4.3	−50	−29	4	4.1	0.2	−48	−28	8
Right STG	4.4	0.4	56	−20	2	4.7	1.8	43	−36	9
Right anterior STG	. . .	. . .	. . .	. . .	. . .	5.2	3.0	43	−1	−6
Words: attend right										
Left STG	6.6	3.5	−54	−24	5	7.0	10.0	−52	−28	2
Right STG	4.4	0.4	54	−16	−3	4.6	0.7	56	−24	0
Left STG	. . .	. . .	. . .	. . .	. . .	4.9	1.1	−44	−2	−9
CVC: attend left										
Left STG	7.0	7.4	−55	−26	4	5.2	1.5	−52	−25	6
Right STG	5.2	1.4	52	−19	−2	5.1	5.5	45	−32	12
CVC: attend right										
Left STG	8.5	8.0	−55	−24	3	6.6	11.1	−55	−21	5
Right STG	. . .	. . .	. . .	. . .	. . .	4.7	1.8	54	−17	0

Values presented are from a subtraction of the second baseline condition from each of the activation conditions. STG indicates superotemporal gyrus; CVC, consonant-vowel-consonant.

†*Volume of region in which contiguous pixels have a t value of 3.61 or greater.*

‡*In coordinates from Talairach and Tournoux,[47] x = No. of millimeters left (−) or right (+) of the interhemispheric fissure; y = No. of millimeters posterior (−) or anterior (+) to a coronal plane through the anterior commissure, and z = No. of millimeters superior (+) or inferior (−) to a horizontal plane through the anterior commissure.*

dition. In the patient group, attend-right condition resulted in a large (8-mL) region of increased rCBF in the left STG with the largest *t* value near that in controls (*x*, *y*, *z* locations: −55, −24, and 3 for patients and −55, −21, and 5 for controls, respectively). In coordinates from Talairach and Tournoux,[47] *x* = No. of millimeters left (−) or right (+) of the interhemispheric fissure, *y* = No. of millimeters posterior (−) or anterior (+) to the anterior commissure, and *z* = No. of millimeters inferior (−) or superior (+) to the anterior commissure. During the attend-left condition, the patients again exhibited a large (7.4-mL) region of activation in the left STG. In contrast, controls had a reversal of rCBF asymmetry in the activated volume in STG during the attend-left compared with the attend-right condition.

In summary, across all conditions, the pattern of activation in STG in the patient group was strongly asymmetric, with a consistent region of activation in the left STG but relatively little change from baseline in rCBF in right STG for any task. Left STG activation was normal in the patients during binaural conditions and during the dichotic attend-right CVC condition, but rCBF in the left STG of the patients did not show the attention-related changes exhibited by the control group in the other dichotic conditions.

ROI ANALYSIS

The ROI analysis used the excellent anatomical resolution of the MRIs to assess with greater specificity the rCBF changes found using the FOI approach. The ROI analysis also allowed direct statistical comparison of rCBF changes in the patient and control groups. **Table 3** summarizes these results.

The ROI data are largely consistent with the results of the FOI analysis, except for the relative symmetry of the left and right rCBF in the patient's ROI data in the binaural conditions. The FOI analysis showed greater left than right activation in STG for the patients in both binaural conditions. The discrepancy may be attributable to the fact that the rCBF values in Table 3 are averaged across the entire volume of tissue in STG, whereas the FOI analysis identifies regions showing the greatest change.

To directly compare rCBF in STG in patient and control groups, a mixed design 2 (patients vs controls)-by-2 (hemisphere) analysis of variance (ANOVA) was computed for each injection. The analyses used absolute rCBF, but the pattern of results was similar when rCBF was normalized by average rCBF in the whole brain. The main effect of group did not reach significance for any injection. There was a significant hemisphere by group interaction in the attend-right CVC condition ($F[1,18]=5.24$, $P<.03$). As shown in Table 3, controls had nearly equal rCBF in the left and right STG in this condition, whereas patients had higher rCBF in the left than in the right STG. There was a significant hemisphere by group interaction for the dichotic environmental sounds condition ($F[1,18]=4.35$, $P<.05$), resulting from controls hav-

Table 3. Mean Blood Flow in Left and Right STG in Schizophrenic Patients and Controls*

Condition	Patients (n=10) Left STG	Patients (n=10) Right STG	Controls (n=10) Left STG	Controls (n=10) Right STG
First baseline	52.6 (11.8)	50.2 (6.7)	52.8 (6.8)	53.1 (8.0)
Binaural				
Environmental sounds	51.5 (9.2)	51.7 (8.2)	52.8 (8.4)	55.2 (8.0)
Words	53.4 (15.0)	52.8 (10.9)	55.2 (10.8)	57.8 (11.2)
Dichotic				
Environmental sounds: attend left	56.2 (11.9)	54.9 (11.3)	51.3 (9.7)	55.3 (8.1)
CVC: attend left	56.0 (13.3)	54.8 (9.3)	57.6 (11.3)	60.9 (10.7)
CVC: attend right	55.7 (11.3)	51.5 (7.7)	56.4 (10.6)	56.3 (9.6)
Words: attend right	53.2 (12.6)	52.3 (10.8)	57.3 (12.5)	55.9 (9.8)
Second baseline	49.8 (10.4)	49.3 (9.2)	47.2 (7.5)	48.6 (8.1)

Mean Blood Flow, mL/min per 100 g

STG indicates superotemporal gyrus; CVC, consonant-vowel-consonant. Values in parentheses are SDs.

Table 4. Percentage of Correct Behavioral Responses for Patients and Controls*

Condition	Correct Behavioral Responses, % Patients (n=10)	Correct Behavioral Responses, % Controls (n=10)	*t* Value and Significance Level
Binaural			
Environmental sounds	82.2 (23.9)	96.6 (4.0)	*t*=1.8, *P*=.11†
Words	80.4 (21.8)	91.1 (20.0)	*t*=1.1, *P*=.28
Dichotic			
Words: attend right	54.6 (23.8)	74.0 (36.8)	*t*=1.3, *P*=.22
CVC: attend right	53.7 (39.7)	80.0 (37.3)	*t*=1.6, *P*=.13
CVC: attend left	53.5 (33.1)	90.0 (26.5)	*t*=2.7, *P*=.02
Environmental sounds: attend left	52.2 (37.6)	84.5 (29.6)	*t*=2.0, *P*=.07

**CVC indicates consonant-vowel-consonant. Values in parentheses are SDs.*
†Test for inhomogeneity of variance was significant for binaural environmental sounds condition, and the unequal variances t *test was used for this condition.*

ing higher rCBF in the right than in the left STG, whereas patients had higher left than right rCBF. There was also a marginally significant hemisphere by group interaction in the attend-left CVCs condition ($F[1,18]=3.71$, $P<.07$), which again resulted from controls having higher rCBF in right STG during the attend-left condition, whereas patients had higher rCBF in the left STG.

The ROI analysis is consistent with the FOI analysis in suggesting that patients have an inability to shift blood flow rCBF in the left and right hemispheres in response to changing task demands. Patients with schizophrenia had consistently higher rCBF in the left than in the right STG during all activation conditions, whereas controls had higher rCBF in the right STG for every condition, except for the 2 dichotic conditions in which attention was directed to the right ear.

POSSIBLE CONFOUNDING VARIABLES

To assess whether the FOI and ROI findings may have been influenced by confounding factors, several subsidiary analyses were performed. A 2 (group)-by-8 (injection) ANOVA of mean whole-brain blood flow for the patients and controls showed a marginally significant effect of injection ($F[1,7]=2.79$, $P<.07$), a nonsignificant group effect, and a nonsignificant group by injection interaction. There is, therefore, no evidence of a difference between the patient and control groups in whole-brain blood flow.

The regions traced on the MRIs in the left and right STG had a mean volume of 15.1 mL (SD=0.36) for the left and 14.7 mL (SD=0.27) for the right STG in the patients. The corresponding values for the controls were 15.8 mL (SD=0.26) and 16.9 mL (SD=0.32), respectively, for left and right STG. A 2 (group)-by-2 (hemisphere) ANOVA found no significant main effects or interactions, indicating that the left and right STG had similar volumes in the 2 groups, and that there was no significant asymmetry in the volume of the left and right STG in either group.

The percentage of correct responses (hits plus correct rejections) for patients and controls in each condition are given in **Table 4**. A completely random performance would yield 50% correct. The performance data indicated that the patients did well with binaural stimuli but had greater difficulty with the dichotic tasks. Analysis of the percent correct data for patient vs control groups revealed that they differed significantly on the dichotic CVC attend-left condition ($t=2.7$, $P<.02$) and had marginally significant differences on the dichotic environmental sounds attend-left condition ($t=-2.0$, $P<.07$). Inspection of individual performance scores for each condition revealed that 9 of the 10 patients performed above chance on the binaural tasks, but only 5 patients

Table 5. Blood Flow in Left and Right STG in Schizophrenic Patients With Good (n=5) and Poor (n=5) Performance on Dichotic and Binaural Tasks*

	Performers			
	Good (n=5)		Poor (n=5)	
Condition	Left STG	Right STG	Left STG	Right STG
First baseline	56.6 (15.1)	52.7 (8.0)	48.6 (6.5)	47.5 (4.5)
Binaural				
Words	59.1 (20.5)	57.7 (14.5)	47.7 (4.5)	47.9 (2.3)
Environmental sounds	54.0 (12.3)	53.4 (11.6)	49.0 (5.5)	50.1 (3.5)
Second baseline	53.1 (13.0)	53.0 (13.0)	47.2 (3.8)	46.4 (4.3)
Dichotic				
Environmental sounds: attend left	60.4 (13.7)	59.5 (14.9)	52.0 (9.3)	50.4 (3.6)
CVC: attend left	60.1 (17.8)	57.8 (11.7)	51.9 (6.1)	51.9 (6.1)
CVC: attend right	61.4 (12.3)	54.8 (8.3)	49.9 (7.4)	48.1 (6.1)
Words: attend right	58.2 (16.2)	58.0 (12.3)	48.2 (6.5)	46.7 (5.9)

**STG indicates superotemporal gyrus; CVC, consonant-vowel-consonant. Values in parentheses are SDs.*

performed better than chance on any dichotic task. **Table 5** lists rCBF in the left and right STG in a subgroup of patients whose mean performance was well above chance, along with data for the remaining patients. The group of patients with good performance had higher rCBF than the group with poor performance in every condition, but both groups had higher rCBF in the left than in the right STG for the majority of the activation conditions.

The 5 patients who performed above chance had a mean of 80.5% correct on the 4 dichotic conditions in comparison with a mean of 82.1% for the 10 controls. A 2 (group)-by-2 (left vs right STG) ANOVA was computed for each of the dichotic conditions to assess differences between the 10 controls and these 5 patients. The attend-right CVC condition had a significant group-by hemisphere interaction ($F[1,13]=14.1$, $P<.002$), resulting from higher left than right rCBF in the patient group in comparison with nearly equal left-right rCBF in controls. There was also a trend for a group-by hemisphere interaction in the attend-left CVC condition ($F[1,13]=3.5$, $P<.08$), resulting from the patient group having higher rCBF in the left than the right STG, whereas the control group had the opposite pattern. These analyses, although preliminary because of the small number of patients, suggest that even schizophrenic patients who are able to perform the dichotic tasks at normal levels have abnormal rCBF asymmetries in STG.

COMMENT

Both FOI and ROI analyses provided convergent evidence of abnormalities in rCBF in the STG of 10 schizophrenic patients receiving no medication in comparison with 10 controls. The FOI analyses showed less activation of auditory cortices in the right STG in the patient than in the normal group during binaurally presented auditory tasks requiring focused attention, whereas left STG activation was similar in the 2 groups. During dichotically presented tasks requiring inhibition of competing input as well as focused attention, there was evidence from FOI and ROI analyses of abnormal rCBF in both left and right STG in the patients. The rCBF and behavioral findings are consistent with a large number of studies showing that patients with schizophrenia have deficits on any task requiring attention, as well as a more specific deficit in the sort of attentional filtering required by dichotic tasks.[1,2,18,19,26,27,55]

BINAURAL TASKS

The finding of less-than-normal activation of right STG in the patients during binaural tasks was unanticipated. Patients performed normally on the tasks, which required focused attention to detect auditory targets. The FOI analysis showed significant changes in the left STG in these conditions in the patient group at nearly identical locations to changes observed in the controls (Table 2). The ROI analysis indicated that flow rCBF within the left STG was similar in the patient and control groups (Table 3), providing no evidence that the left STG was overactivated.[56] However, there were only small changes in right STG from baseline rCBF in the binaural conditions for the patients, whereas in the control group the right STG activation was equivalent to that in their left STG.

The bilateral activation of STG in the normal controls during the processing of language and nonlanguage stimuli is consistent with functional imaging studies from other centers.[35-38] The imaging findings are in line with evidence from studies of unilateral brain damage and from cognitive studies of cerebral lateralization,[57] which indicate that normal language processing takes place simultaneously in the left and right hemispheres. Chiarello[57] has recently suggested that the 2 hemispheres normally use different semantic systems. While the left hemisphere makes a rapid selection of a single meaning, the right hemisphere maintains a wider set of meanings over a longer period, permitting verbal input to be interpreted within the overall context of discourse. Since context was irrelevant in the present study in the word task, efficient performance could be mediated by the left hemisphere. The possibility that patients with schizophrenia routinely rely exclusively on left hemisphere strategies could explain the many unusual features of schizophrenic language,[58] although this possibility is clearly speculative at present.

DICHOTIC TASKS

The control group showed large changes in STG during the dichotic tasks, which were consistent with the direction of attention to their right and left ears. Similar modulation of rCBF was exhibited by the patient group only on the task requiring that attention be directed to the right ear for a CVC target. For patients, the dichotic words condition showed no difference in the pattern of rCBF from the binaural words condition. During the dichotic conditions requiring attention to their left ear, the patients failed to show the increase in the activated region of right STG and the decrease in left STG activation exhibited by the control group. The possibility that the abnormal patterns of rCBF resulted from the patients not performing the dichotic tasks was examined by an ROI analysis using only patients who performed well on the dichotic tasks. Despite the lack of power resulting from the small sample size (n=5), the ROI analysis found significant differences from the normal pattern of rCBF asymmetry in this subgroup of patients during dichotic tasks.

A number of PET studies have demonstrated that attention modulates rCBF in normal controls and that rCBF changes are similar in the left and right hemispheres.[59,60] Laberge[59] discusses the PET evidence and argues that thalamocortical and corticothalamic connections are involved in attentional filtering. He suggests that reciprocal connections between the pulvinar nucleus of the thalamus and cortical sensory regions mediate enhancement of cortical activity through a positive feedback loop. The lack of activation of right STG during tasks requiring attention to left ear input in the schizophrenic patients in the present study could, therefore, have resulted from an abnormality in the feedback loop between the right thalamus and the right STG. However, structural and functional abnormalities in STG have been reported in patients with schizophrenia[7,61-69] in addition to the thalamic abnormalities noted above.[11-14] Whether the lower task-related activation of right STG in schizophrenic patients resulted from abnormalities in thalamus, in STG, or in their interconnections cannot be determined with the in vivo imaging data available in the present study.

Our group, as well as others (reviewed in Andreasen et al[70]), has previously found less than normal activation of the frontal lobes in patients with schizophrenia. Abnormal rCBF or metabolism has also been found in a variety of other cortical locations in patients with schizophrenia,[71] as have abnormal correlational patterns between brain regions.[66,72] These widespread abnormalities may indicate that schizophrenia involves multiple mechanisms and variable regional abnormalities. An alternative, and more parsimonious, possibility is that the multiple functional abnormalities reported in patients with schizophrenia reflect a primary abnormality in the circuitry that mediates arousal, attention, and information processing. The abnormalities in cortical function found in the present study and in other imaging studies of patients with schizophrenia may be the localized, downstream effects of a more generalized abnormality of the thalamocortical circuitry controlling the integrated function of multiple regions of the left and right hemispheres.

Accepted for publication January 3, 1996.

Reprints: Nancy C. Andreasen, MD, PhD, Department of Psychiatry, Mental Health Clinical Research Center, 200 Hawkins Dr 2911 JPP, Iowa City, IA 52242-1057.

REFERENCES

1. Braff DL. Information processing and attention dysfunctions in schizophrenia. *Schizophr Bull.* 1993;19:233-259.
2. Nuechterlein KH, Dawson ME. Information processing and attentional function in the developmental course of schizophrenic disorders. *Schizophr Bull.* 1988; 10:160-203.
3. Kolb B, Whishaw IQ. Performance of schizophrenic patients on tests sensitive to left or right frontal, temporal, or parietal function in neurological patients. *J Nerv Ment Dis.* 1983;17:435-443.
4. Bleuler E; Zinkin J, trans. *Dementia Praecox of the Group of Schizophrenias.* New York, NY: International Universities Press; 1950.
5. Kraeplin E; Barclay RM, trans. *Dementia Praecox and Paraphrenia.* New York, NY: Robert E. Krieger; 1919.
6. Pearlson GD, Marsh L. Magnetic resonance imaging in psychiatry. In: Andreasen NC, ed. *Review of Psychiatry.* Washington, DC: American Psychiatric Press; 1993.
7. Flaum M, Swayze VW, O'Leary DS, Yuh WTC, Ehrhardt JC, Arndt SA, Andreasen NC. Brain morphology in schizoprenia: effects of diagnosis, laterality and gender. *Am J Psychiatry.* 1995;152:704-714.
8. Goldman-Rakic PS. Circuitry of primate prefrontal cortex and regulation of behavior by representational memory. In: Plum F, Mountcastle V, eds. *Handbook of Physiology.* Bethesda, Md: American Physiological Society; 1987;5:373-417.
9. Swerdlow NR, Koop GF. Dopamine, schizophrenia, mania, and depression: toward a unified hypothesis of cortico-striato-pallido-thalamic function. *Behav Brain Sci.* 1987;10:197-245.
10. Carlsson M, Carlsson A. Schizophrenia: a subcortical neurotransmitter imbalance syndrome. *Schizophr Bull.* 1990;16:425-443.
11. Andreasen NC, Arndt S, Swayze V, Cizadlo T, Flaum M, O'Leary D, Ehrhardt J, Yuh WTC. Thalamic abnormalities in schizophrenia visualized through magnetic resonance image averaging. *Science.* 1994;266:294-298.
12. Bogerts B. Recent advances in the neuropathology of schizophrenia: *Schizophr Bull.* 1993;19:431-445.
13. Pakkenberg B. Pronounced reduction of total neuron number in mediodorsal thalamic nucleus and nucleus accumbens in schizophrenics. *Arch Gen Psychiatry.* 1990;47:1023-1028.
14. Shapiro RM. Regional neuropathology in schizophrenia: where are we? where are we going? *Schizophr Res.* 1993;10:187-239.
15. Benes FM, McSparren J, Bird ED, SanGiovanni JP, Vincent SL. Deficits in small interneurons in prefrontal and cingulate cortices of schizophrenic and schizoaffective patients. *Arch Gen Psychiatry.* 1991;48:996-1001.
16. Posner MI, Peterson SE. The attention system of the human brain. *Ann Rev Neurosci.* 1990;13:25-42.
17. Mesulam MM. Large-scale neurocognitive networks and distributed processing for attention, language and memory. *Ann Neurol.* 1990;28:597-612.
18. McGhie A, Chapman J. Disorders of attention and perception in early schizophrenia. *Br J Med Psychol.* 1961;34:103-116.
19. Silverman J. The problem of attention in research and theory on schizophrenia. *Psychol Rev.* 1964;71:352-379.
20. Broadbent DE. *Perception and Communication.* London, England: Pergamon Press; 1958.
21. Broadbent DE. *Decision and Stress.* London, England: Academic Press; 1971.
22. Broadbent DE. Task combination and selective intake of information. *Acta Psychol.* 1982;50:253-290.
23. Cherry EC. Some experiments on the recognition of speech, with one and with two ears. *J Acoust Soc Am.* 1953;25:975-979.
24. Allport A. Attention and control: have we been asking the wrong questions? a critical review of 25 years. In: *Attention and Performance.* Hillsdale, NJ: L. Erlbaum; 1993:183-218.

25. Johnston WA, Dark VJ. Selective attention. *Ann Rev Psychol.* 1986;37:43-75.
26. Spring B, Weinstein L, Freeman R, Thompson S. Selective attention in schizophrenia. In: Steinhaurer SR, Gruzelier JH, Zubin J, eds. *Handbook of Schizophrenia.* Amsterdam, the Netherlands: Elsevier Science Publishing Co Inc; 1991; 5:371-396.
27. Bruder GE. Dichotic listening in psychiatric patients. In: Hugdahl K, ed. *Handbook of Dichotic Listening: Theory, Methods and Research.* New York, NY: John Wiley & Sons Inc; 1988.
28. Bryden MP. An overview of the dichotic listening procedure and its relation to cerebral organization. In: Hugdahl K, ed. *Handbook of Dichotic Listening: Theory, Methods and Research.* New York, NY: John Wiley & Sons Inc; 1988:1-43.
29. Kimura D. Functional asymmetry of the brain in dichotic listening. *Can J Psychol.* 1961;15:156-165.
30. Wexler BE, Giller Jr EL, Southwick S. Cerebral laterality, symptoms, and diagnosis in psychotic patients. *Biol Psychiatry.* 1991;29:103-116.
31. Lerner J, Nachson, Carmon A. Responses of paranoid and non-paranoid schizophrenics in a dichotic listening task. *J Nerv Ment Dis.* 1977;164:247-253.
32. Goode DJ, Manning AA, Middeleton JF. Cortical laterality and asymmetry of the Hoffmann reflex in psychiatric patients. *Biol Psychiatry.* 1981;16:1137-1151.
33. Parasuraman R, Davies DR. *Varieties of Attention.* Orlando, Fla: Academic Press; 1984.
34. O'Leary DS, Andreasen NC, Hurtig RR, Hichwa RD, Watkins GL, Boles Ponto LL, Rogers M, Kirchner PT. A positron emission tomography study of binaurally and dichotically presented stimuli: effects of level of language and directed attention. *Brain Lang.* 1996;53:20-39.
35. Howard D, Patterson K, Wise R, Brown D, Friston K, Weiller C, Frackowiak R. The cortical location of the lexicons. *Brain.* 1992;115:1769-1782.
36. Price C, Wise R, Ramsay S, Friston K, Howard D, Patterson K, Frackowiak R. Regional response differences within the human auditory cortex when listening to words. *Neurosci Lett.* 1992;146:179-182.
37. Wise R, Chollet F, Hadar U, Friston K, Hoffner E, Frackowiak R. Distribution of cortical neural networks involved in word comprehension and word retrieval. *Brain.* 1991;114:1803-1817.
38. Zatorre RJ, Evans AC, Meyer E, Gjedde A. Lateralization of phonetic and pitch discrimination in speech processing. *Science.* 1992;256:846-849.
39. Binder JR, Rao SM, Hammeke TA, Yetkin FZ, Jesmanowicz A, Bandettini RA, Wong EC, Estkowski LD, Goldstein MD, Haughton VM, Hyde JS. Functional magnetic resonance imaging of human auditory cortex. *Ann Neurol.* 1994;35: 662-672.
40. American Psychiatric Association. *Diagnostic and Statistical Manual of Mental Disorders, Third Edition, Revised.* Washington, DC: American Psychiatric Association; 1987.
41. Andreasen NC, Flaum M, Arndt S. The Comprehensive Assessment of Symptoms and History (CASH): an instrument for assessing psychopathology and diagnosis. *Arch Gen Psychiatry.* 1992;49:615-623.
42. Ginsberg MD, Lockwood AH, Busto R, Finn R. A simplified in vivo autoradiographic strategy for the determination of regional cerebral blood flow by positron emission tomography: theoretical considerations and validation studies in the rat. *J Cereb Blood Flow Metab.* 1982;2:89-98.
43. Raichle ME, Martin WRW, Herscovitch P. Brain bloodflow measured with H215O, II: implementation and validation. *J Nucl Med.* 1983;24:790-798.
44. Herscovitch P, Markham J, Raichle ME. Brain blood flow measured with intravenous H215O, I: theory and error analysis. *J Nucl Med.* 1983;24:782-789.
45. Hurtig RR, Hichwa RD, O'Leary DS, Boles Ponto LL, Narayana S, Watkins GL, Andreasen NC. Effects of timing and duration of cognitive activation in [^{15}O]water PET studies. *J Cereb Blood Flow Metab.* 1994;14:423-430.
46. Andreasen NC, Cohen G, Harris G, Cizadlo T, Parkikinen J, Rezai K, Swayze VW. Image processsing for the study of brain structure and function: problems and programs. *J Neuropsychiatry Clin Neurosci.* 1992;4:125-133.
47. Cizadlo T, Andreasen NC, Zeien G, Rajarethinam R, Harris G, O'Leary DS, Swayze V, Arndt S, Hichwa R, Ehrhardt J, Yuh WTC. Image registration issues in the analysis of multiple-injection 150H20 PET studies: BRAINFIT. *Proc SPIE Intl Soc Opt Eng.* 1994;2168:423-430.
48. Pelizzari CA, Chen GTY, Spelbring DR, Weichselbaum RR, Chen CT. Accurate three-dimensional registration of CT, PET, and/or MR images of the brain. *J Comput Assist Tomogr.* 1989;13:20-26.
49. Talairach J, Tournoux P. *Co-Planar Stereotaxic Atlas of the Human Brain: 3-D Proportional System: An Approach to Cerebral Imaging.* New York, NY: Georg Thieme Verlag; 1988.
50. Worsley KJ, Evans AC, Marrett S, Neelin P. A three-dimensional statistical analysis for CBF activation studies in human brain. *J Cereb Blood Flow Metab.* 1992; 12:900-918.
51. Liegeois-Chauvel C, Musolino A, Chauvel P. Localization of the primary auditory area in man. *Brain.* 1991;114:139-153.
52. Geschwind N, Levitsky W. Human brain: left-right asymmetries in temporal speech region. *Science.* 1968;161:186-187.
53. Galaburda AM, Le May M, Kemper TL, Geschwind N. Right-left asymmetries in the brain: structural differences between the hemispheres may underlie cerebral dominance. *Science.* 1978;199:852-856.
54. Steinmetz H, Rademacher J, Yanxiong H, Hefter H, Zilles KM, Thron A, Freund HJ. *J Comput Assist Tomogr.* 1989;13:996-1005.
55. Posner MI, Early TS, Reiman EM, Pardo PJ, Dhawan M. Asymmetries in hemispheric control of attention in schizophrenia. *Arch Gen Psychiatry.* 1988;45: 814-821.
56. Gur RE. Left hemisphere dysfunction and left hemisphere overactivation in schizophrenia. *J Abnorm Psychol.* 1978;7:63-66.
57. Chiarello C. Interpretation of word meanings by the cerebral hemispheres: one is not enough. In: Schwanenflugel PJ, ed. *The Psychology of Word Meanings.* Hillsdale, NJ: Lawrence Erlbaum Associates Inc; 1991:251-278.
58. Andreasen NC, Hoffman RE, Grove WM. Mapping abnormalities in language and cognition. In: Alpert M, ed. *Controversies in Schizophrenia.* New York, NY; Guilford; 199-226.
59. Laberge D. Thalamic and cortical mechanisms of attention suggested by recent positron emission tomographic experiments. *J Cognit Neurosci.* 1990;2: 358-372.
60. Roland P. *Brain Activation.* New York, NY: Wiley-Liss; 1993.
61. Barta PE, Pearlson GD, Tune LE, Powers RE, Richards SS. Auditory hallucinations and smaller superior temporal gyrus volume in schizophrenia. *Am J Psychiatry.* 1990;147:1457-1462.
62. Barta PE, Pearlson GD, Tune LE, Powers RE, Richards SS. Superior temporal gyrus volume in schizophrenia. *Schizoph Res.* 1990;3:22.
63. Shenton ME, Kikines R, Jolesz FA, Pollak SD, Lemay M, Wible CG, Hokama H, Martin J, Metcalf D, Coleman M. Abnormalities of the left temporal lobe and thought disorder in schizophrenia: a quantitative magnetic resonance imaging study. *N Engl J Med.* 1992;327:604-612.
64. McCarley RW, Shenton ME, O'Donnell BF. Auditory P300 abnormalities and left posterior superior temporal gyrus volume reduction in schizophrenia. *Arch Gen Psychiatry.* 1993;50:190-197.
65. Friston KJ, Liddle PF, Frith CD, Hirsch SR, Frackowiak RSJ. The left medial temporal region and schizophrenia: a PET study. *Brain.* 1992;115:367-382.
66. Liddle PF, Friston KJ, Frith CD, Hirsch SR, Jones T, Frackowiak RSJ. Patterns of cerebral blood flow in schizophrenia. *Br J Psychiatry.* 1992;60:179-186.
67. Liddle PF, Friston KJ, Frith CD, Frackowiak RSJ. Cerebral blood flow and mental processes in schizophrenia. *J R Soc Med.* 1992;85:224-226.
68. Rossi A, Strata P, Mattei P, Cupillari M, Bozzao A, Galluci M, Casacchia M. Planum temporale asymmetry in schizophrenia: a magnetic resonance imaging study. *Schizophr Res.* 1992;7:19-22.
69. Falkai P, Bogerts B, Schneider T, Greve B, Pfeiffer U, Pilz K, Gonsiorzcyk C, Majtenyi C, Ovary I. Disturbed planum temporale asymmetry in schizophrenia: a quantitative post-mortem study. *Schizophr Res.* 1995;14:161-176.
70. Andreasen NC, Rezai K, Alliger R, Swayze VW, Flaum M, Kirchner P, Cohen G, O'Leary DS. Hypofrontality in neuroleptic-naive patients and in patients with chronic schizophrenia: assessment with xenon 133 single-photon emission computed tomography and the Tower of London. *Arch Gen Psychiatry.* 1992;49: 943-958.
71. Gur RE, Pearlson GD. Neuroimaging in schizophrenia research. *Schizophr Bull.* 1993;19:337-353.
72. Volkow ND, Wolf AP, Brodie JD, Cancro R, Overall JE, Rhoades H, Van Gelder P. Brain interactions in chronic schizophrenics under resting and activation conditions. *Schizophr Res.* 1988;1:47-53.

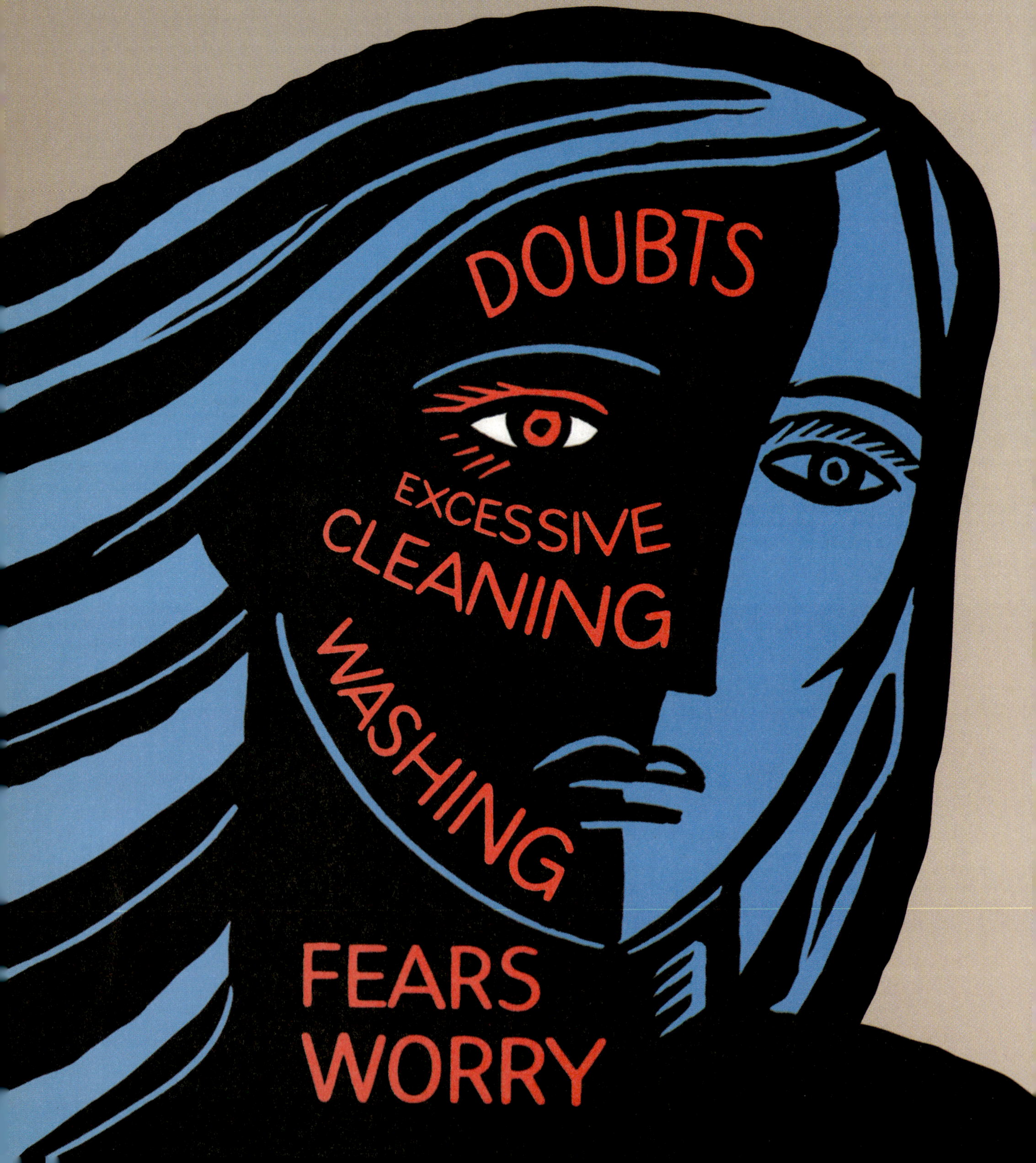
DOUBTS
EXCESSIVE
CLEANING
WASHING
FEARS
WORRY

ORIGINAL ARTICLE

Brain Glucose Metabolism During Non–Rapid Eye Movement Sleep in Major Depression

A Positron Emission Tomography Study

Andrew P. Ho, MD; J. Christian Gillin, MD; Monte S. Buchsbaum, MD; Joseph C. Wu, MD; Lennert Abel, MD; William E. Bunney, Jr, MD

Background: Depression is characterized by several sleep-related abnormalities shortly before and after sleep onset, such as prolonged sleep latency, loss of stage 3-4 sleep, reduced rapid eye movement (REM) latency, increased nocturnal core body temperature, and abnormal hormone secretion patterns. Sleep deprivation is associated with a temporary improvement in depression. We hypothesized that depressed patients may be "overaroused" and that absolute cerebral glucose metabolism would be elevated during the first nocturnal non-REM sleep period in depressed patients compared with normal controls. In addition, since hypofrontality (greater metabolic activity in occipital compared with frontal cortical activity) has been reported in waking positron emission tomographic studies of depressed patients compared with controls, we predicted significant hypofrontality in depressed patients during the first non-REM period.

Methods: Positron emission tomography with fludeoxyglucose F 18 was used to compare 10 unmedicated men with unipolar depression with 12 normal men during the first non-REM sleep period at normal bedtime.

Results: Whole-brain absolute metabolic rate during non-REM sleep was significantly elevated (+47%) in patients compared with controls. Mean absolute cerebral glucose metabolic rate was also higher in every area of the brain in patients compared with normal controls. The greatest significant mean increases were in the posterior cingulate and amygdala (+44%), hippocampus (+37% to +43%), occipital and temporal cortex (+33% to +34%), and pons (+33%). Relative metabolic rates in specific neroanatomical areas, however, varied considerably both within the patient group and between patients and controls. Patients showed significant hypofrontality, particularly in the medio-orbital frontal cortex, compared with controls. Patients also showed significant reductions of relative metabolic rate in the anterior cingulate, caudate, and medial thalamus compared with controls.

Conclusions: These findings provide further support for the hyperarousal hypothesis of some types of major depressive disorder. Abnormal patterns of cerebral metabolism during non-REM sleep in depressed patients confirmed earlier waking findings of decreased relative frontal and abnormal limbic metabolic activity and striatal metabolism in association with posterior cortical increases.

Arch Gen Psychiatry. 1996;53:645-652

Depressed patients often show prolonged sleep latency, reduced stage 3-4 (delta) sleep during the first non–rapid eye movement (non-REM) period, short REM latency, and increased duration and ocular activity during the first REM period.[1-4] In addition, they have elevated core body temperature and abnormalities in the nocturnal secretion of cortisol, growth hormone, and prolactin.[5-13] Moreover, many depressed patients experience brief antidepressant benefits following total or partial sleep deprivation.[14-18]

Nevertheless, the brain mechanisms responsible for disturbed sleep in depression remain elusive.[3,19,20] We report herein the first study, to our knowledge, of functional brain imaging during sleep in depression. We measured the localized cerebral glucose metabolism rate (CGMR) with positron emission tomography (PET) during the first non-REM period and addressed 3 important issues.

We tested the hyperarousal theory[21] of depression, which is supported by the following findings: (1) physiological measures of sleep in depression (eg, short, shallow, and fragmented sleep or enhanced REM sleep) and elevated core body temperature are consistent with overactivity of arousal systems, underactive sedation systems, or sleep satiety[14,19,21]; (2) the an-

See Subjects and Methods on next page

From the Department of Psychiatry, University of California, and Department of Veterans Affairs Medical Center, San Diego (Drs Ho and Gillin); Neuroscience PET Center, Department of Psychiatry, Mount Sinai School of Medicine, New York, NY (Drs Buchsbaum and Abel); and Department of Psychiatry and Human Behavior, University of California, Irvine (Drs Wu and Bunney).

SUBJECTS AND METHODS

SUBJECTS

Ten outpatients with unipolar depression were compared during the first non-REM period with the 12 normal controls previously described in our earlier study of CGMR[45] (**Table 1**). The diagnoses of major depressive disorder (without significant comorbid diagnoses) in the patients or no psychiatric disorder in the normal controls were made with the Structured Clinical Interview for *DSM-III-R*.[51] All subjects were in good physical health and had not used psychoactive substances for at least a month as determined by medical history, physical examination, and blood and urine drug tests. Patients and controls were paid a $100 honorarium and all provided written consent.

Since the study required subjects to remain in non-REM sleep for 32 minutes after the infusion of fludeoxyglucose F 18 (FDG), patients were excluded if they had severe depression, marked sleep disturbance, or very short REM latencies. Thus, the final sample of patients had relatively mild depression as assessed by both the Hamilton Rating Scale for Depression[52,53] and polygraphic sleep recordings (Table 1).

METHODS

Subjects first spent an adaptation night in individual sleep rooms to become accommodated to polygraphic sleep recordings (the "first-night" effect) and PET scan laboratory conditions, including a sham intravenous line. They then had a night of baseline sleep recording to characterize their sleep, according to the visual scoring criteria.[54]

On the night of the PET scan, 1 intravenous line was placed in each arm, with a 3-m extension outside the sleep rooms to allow for injection and sampling of venous (arterialized) blood without disturbance of sleep. Subjects retired between 9 and 11 PM and were injected with 5 mCi of FDG (1-5 mL, depending on time, over 30-60 seconds) into 1 arm 3 to 5 minutes after the onset of non-REM sleep (stage 2). From the other arm, heat-arterialized venous samples were obtained for FDG pharmacokinetics and glucose measurement. Subjects were awakened 32 to 45 minutes after the injection of FDG. Starting about 10 minutes later, scans were performed with both shadow and septa shields in a configuration with a measured in-plane resolution of 7.6 and resolution of 10.9 mm in the axial dimension. Images were acquired at 1-cm intervals. Three additional subjects were excluded from data analysis because they failed to maintain non-REM sleep for more than 75% of the 32-minute FDG uptake period.

Regional absolute (micromoles of glucose uptake per 100 g of brain per minute) and relative CGMR were calculated as described previously.[45] Whole-brain average CGMR was calculated as an average of all pixels within slice edges. The relative CGMR was calculated as regional absolute rate divided by slice-average metabolic rate except in the pons, where whole-brain instead of slice-average rate was used. Brain regions were defined with a circumferential 8-mm-thick cortical peel[45] and 7.1-mm^2 stereotaxic box methods.[45]

STATISTICAL ANALYSIS

Data were assessed by analyses of variance (ANOVA) and covariance, 2-tailed *t* tests, and linear regression (Biomedical Data Processing, Statistical Software Inc, Los Angeles, Calif).[55] Since CGMR data were obtained in 2 groups (normal and depressed), 2 hemispheres (left and right), and structures grouped on anatomical dimensions (eg, lateral/medial and anterior/posterior), multivariate ANOVA with independent groups and repeated dimensions was used for main group comparisons. This strategy limited the number of statistical procedures, helping to reduce type I error. All significant ($P<.05$) group interactions are reported. Follow-up ANOVA and 2-tailed *t* tests were performed to characterize significant group differences and interactions.

tidepressant benefits of sleep deprivation may result from sedation produced by prolonged wakefulness[20,21]; and (3) a study of daytime naps in depressed patients suggested that later benefits of antidepressant medications were directly correlated with prolonged sleep latency during the naps (usually interpreted as a measure of arousal).[22] Consistent with the overarousal hypothesis, the antidepressant response to overnight sleep deprivation is associated with daytime elevated baseline CGMR or cerebral blood flow in limbic structures compared with both depressed nonresponders and normal subjects.[23-26]

The CGMR may be abnormal in some of the same anatomical areas during both non-REM sleep and wakefulness in depressed patients; for example, hypofrontality or a reduced ratio of frontal to occipital activity.[27-34]

Positron emission tomography studies in normal and depressed subjects may clarify the neurobiological features of the first non-REM period in depression. Recent studies have implicated the thalamus, basal forebrain, hypothalamus, and mesencephalic tegmentum in the regulation of non-REM sleep and cortical electroencephalogram (EEG) synchronization, as well as in wakefulness, REM sleep, and cortical EEG desynchronization.[35-40] Cerebral metabolism is reduced during non-REM sleep compared with wakefulness and REM sleep,[39,40] as shown by decreased CGMRs in the monkey,[41,42] cat,[43] rat,[44] and normal human subjects[45-47]; decreased cerebral blood flow in humans[48-50]; and decreased cerebral oxygen consumption in humans.[49,50]

RESULTS

SLEEP MEASURES

In keeping with their relatively mild depression, patients showed minimal sleep disturbance on the baseline night relative to controls (Table 1). (The REM latency was not assessed on the PET study night since subjects were awakened before the first REM period.) The percentage of delta sleep during the PET study was slightly higher in depressed than in control subjects. Both sleep latency on the PET study night and percentage of waking during the FDG uptake period were significantly greater in patients than in controls. Since age and percentage of waking may contribute to differences in brain metabolism, they were en-

Table 1. Subject and Sleep Measurements*

	Normal Controls (n=12)	Depressed Patients (n=10)	*P*
Sex	All male	All male	. . .
Handedness	All right-handed	All right-handed	. . .
HRSD-24[53] score	. . .	25±9	. . .
HRSD-17[52] score	. . .	17±9	. . .
Age, y	26±8	33±10	.06
Sleep latency, min	10±12	47±40	.01
REM latency, min†	98±33	87±41	.74
Delta sleep, %	38±31	46±39	.70
Waking, %	5±7	12±9	.04

*HRSD-24 indicates 24-item Hamilton Rating Scale for Depression; HRSD-17, 17-item Hamilton Rating Scale for Depression. All data are presented as mean±SD unless otherwise indicated. Ellipses indicate not applicable.

†Baseline night; all other sleep measures are taken from the fludeoxyglucose F 18 night.

tered as covariates in additional analyses; however, the results were unchanged. Additional analyses with an age-matched subgroup of depressed and normal subjects (n=7 for each) also produced essentially the same results. Since these statistical controls did not affect the results, data are presented for the entire sample.

WHOLE-BRAIN METABOLISM

The whole-brain CGMR was significantly higher (47%) in the depressed patients than in the control group (22.7±8.2 vs 14.7±4.0 μmol of glucose uptake per 100 g/min; *P*=.01, 2-tailed *t* test; **Figure**). Mean absolute CGMR was higher in every anatomical area examined in depressed patients compared with controls. No significant correlation was found between depression severity (Hamilton Rating Scale for Depression score), REM latency, or age and whole-brain CGMR within the depressed group. Percentage of delta sleep during FDG uptake was negatively correlated with whole-brain CGMR in the depressed group (*r*=−0.73, *P*=.01) and at trend levels in the normal group (*r*=−0.50, *P*=.10).

CORTEX

Mean overall cortical CGMR was significantly higher (+30%) during non-REM sleep in depressed patients than in normal controls (24.3±6.6 vs 18.6±5.5 μmol of glucose uptake per 100 g/minute; **Table 2**), especially in the occipital (+34%) and temporal (+33%) lobes, and least in the parietal (+28%) and frontal (+25%) lobes.

Compared with the normal controls, the depressed patients showed hypofrontality whether assessed by absolute (0.99±0.16 vs 1.11±0.17; F=26.19, *df*=1,20, *P*<.001) or relative data (F=20.8, *df*=1,20, *P*<.001). Hypofrontality was significantly more marked in the medio-orbital than in the dorsolateral frontal lobe (group by area interaction in absolute CGMR, F=21.0, *df*=1,20, *P*<.001). Even though the absolute CGMR in the medio-orbital frontal cortex was nonsignificantly higher in depressed than in control subjects, the relative rates (region of interest compared with slice) were significantly lower:

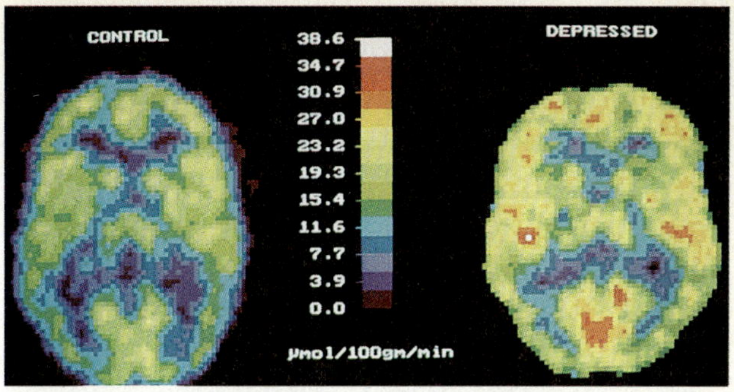

Representative examples of positron emission tomographic scans for local cerebral glucose metabolic rate (micromoles of glucose uptake per 100 g of brain per minute) in a normal control subject and a depressed patient during the first nocturnal non-REM period.

Table 2. Cortical Areas: Absolute Glucose Metabolic Rates in Depressed Patients and Normal Control Subjects*

Lobe	Normal Controls	Depressed Patients	Difference, %
Frontal	20.1±5.6	25.2±6.9	+25
Parietal	19.3±6.1	24.8±6.9	+28
Temporal	16.3±4.1	21.7±5.9	+33
Occipital	19.1±5.3	25.5±6.7	+34

*Data are presented as mean±SD μmoles of glucose uptake per 100 g of brain per minute. Group: F=5.2; df>+1,20; P<.03. Group × lobe: F=3.74; df=3,18; P<.03.

1.13±0.2 in patients vs 1.30±0.15 in controls (F=28.8, *df*=1,20, *P*<.001).

LIMBIC SYSTEM

Depressed patients had a significantly higher (+37%) mean absolute CGMR in limbic structures (anterior, superior, and retrosplenal [posterior] cingulate gyrus, amygdala, and superior and inferior hippocampus) than normal controls (20.5±7.9 vs 15.0±5.7 μmol of glucose uptake per 100 g/min; F=7.57, *df*=1,20, *P*<.02; **Table 3**). Glucose metabolism in depressed patients was greatest in the posterior cingulate (+44%), inferior hippocampus (+43%), and amygdala (+44%) and least in the anterior cingulate (+6%) (Table 3).

Relative activity in the anterior cingulate was lower in the depressed patients than in controls (−21%), whereas other limbic areas were relatively more active in the depressed patients (from +2% to +8%). In a follow-up analysis of the 3 regions of the cingulate gyrus, significant group by area interactions were found for both absolute (F=3.88, *df*=1.99,39.79, *P*<.03) and relative measures (F=6.46, *df*=1.56,31.21, *P*<.001).

THALAMUS AND BASAL GANGLIA

We divided the thalamus into 4 regions (anterior, lateral, posterior, and medial). Since the areas are small, only 1 box from each region on each hemisphere was measured. No statistically significant group effect was found for absolute values (Table 3), but a significant group by area interaction emerged for relative CGMR (F=3.64,

Table 3. Absolute and Relative Glucose Metabolic Rates in Depressed Patients and Normal Control Subjects in Limbic System and Absolute Rates in the Thalamus*

	Normal Controls	Depressed Patients	Difference, %
Absolute Metabolic Rates†			
Anterior cingulate	21.2±4.4	22.4±8.7	+6
Superior cingulate	16.0±6.5	20.7±7.3	+29
Posterior cingulate	18.3±3.7	26.4±8.0	+44
Amygdala	11.6±2.9	16.7±4.4	+44
Superior hippocampus	17.2±4.1	23.6±6.4	+37
Inferior hippocampus	9.2±2.3	13.2±3.1	+43
Relative Metabolic Rates‡			
Anterior cingulate	1.24±0.11	0.98±0.22	−21
Superior cingulate	0.91±0.20	0.93±0.18	+2
Posterior cingulate	1.11±0.22	1.19±0.22	+7
Amygdala	0.86±0.15	0.89±0.08	+3
Superior hippocampus	0.98±0.17	1.05±0.24	+7
Inferior hippocampus	0.62±0.08	0.67±0.06	+8
Absolute Metabolic Rates§			
Anterior thalamus	21.0±6.9	24.9±8.0	+19
Lateral thalamus	18.0±4.6	22.6±7.3	+26
Posterior thalamus	15.5±5.1	19.1±5.3	+23
Medial thalamus	23.5±7.1	24.9±7.2	+2

*Metabolic rate is presented as mean±SD micromoles of glucose uptake per 100 g of brain per minute.
†Group: $P<.02$, $F=7.57$, df=1,20. Group × area: $P<.05$, $F=2.36$, df=5,100.
‡Group × area: $P<.002$, $F=4.29$, df=5,100.
§Analysis of variance (group × area): $P=.24$, $F=1.46$, df=2.54, 50.88.

Table 4. Absolute and Relative Glucose Metabolic Rates in Depressed Patients and Normal Control Groups in the Caudate, Putamen, and Globus Pallidus*

	Normal Controls	Depressed Patients	Difference, %
Absolute Metabolic Rates†			
Caudate			
Left	23.6±5.5	25.7±6.4	+9
Right	24.7±5.5	27.2±9.1	+10
Putamen			
Left	22.9±5.6	26.1±5.9	+14
Right	22.4±6.1	26.4±7.6	+18
Globus pallidus			
Left	15.7±2.7	20.5±6.1	+31
Right	18.3±4.0	19.6±5.6	+7
Relative Metabolic Rates‡			
Caudate			
Left	1.33±0.08	1.12±0.13	−16
Right	1.39±0.06	1.16±0.19	−17
Putamen			
Left	1.13±0.09	1.15±0.09	−12
Right	1.27±0.14	1.16±0.16	−9
Globus pallidus			
Left	0.90±0.10	0.89±0.14	−1
Right	1.05±0.19	0.85±0.09	−19

*Metabolic rate is presented as mean±SD micromoles of glucose uptake per 100 g of brain per minute.
†Analysis of variance (group × area × hemisphere): $P<.04$, $F=4.01$, df=1.54,30.9.
‡Analysis of variance (group × area × hemisphere): $P<.009$, $F=5.33$, df=1.93,38.6.

$df=2.63,52.62$, $P<.02$), suggesting that the medial thalamus is relatively more hypometabolic than the other 3 thalamic areas in depressed patients than in controls.

Examination of the head of caudate, putamen, and globus pallidus revealed significantly higher absolute CGMR and lower relative CGMR in the depressed vs the normal group (**Table 4**). Relative hypometabolism was most severe in the right globus pallidus (−19%) and bilateral caudate nucleus (−16% left, −17% right) in depressed patients than in controls. A statistically significant hemispheric asymmetry was found in the globus pallidus, where the mean absolute and relative CGMR was greater on the right than on the left for the controls but showed an opposite effect in the patients (Table 4).

PONTINE BRAIN STEM

The depressed group had a significantly higher absolute localized CGMR than the normal group in the entire pons (12.0±4.1 vs 9.0±3.7 μmol of glucose uptake per 100 g/minute; $F=6.19$, $df=1,20$, $P<.02$). Neither group by structure interactions nor relative (to whole brain) metabolic rate differences proved to be significant.

COMMENT

HYPERAROUSAL

The results confirm our a priori hypotheses of elevated whole-brain CGMR and hypofrontality in major depression during the first non-REM period. Furthermore, a significantly higher absolute CGMRs were found in the cerebral cortex, limbic structures, and pons. In previous studies of unipolar depression during daytime waking states, the global CGMR either did not differ significantly from that in normal subjects[28,49] or was decreased.[30]

Interestingly, the elevated CGMR occurred in the absence of the characteristic sleep abnormalities (eg, shortened REM sleep latency or decreased delta sleep) that have been linked to major depression. Neither age nor wakefulness accounted for the increased metabolic rate. Our data suggest that the CGMR, like core body temperature,[6-8] is elevated in depressed patients compared with controls during nocturnal sleep but not during daytime wakefulness. On the basis of brain size compared with whole-body size, cerebral metabolism contributes a disproportionate share of whole-body glucose and oxygen metabolism.[50] Since systemic glucose utilization is highly correlated with cerebral glucose metabolism during non-REM sleep, elevated core body temperature during sleep in depressed patients may reflect increased rates of cerebral glucose metabolism.

Localized CGMR was not uniformly elevated throughout the brain in depressed patients compared with normal controls. Cortical metabolism was more elevated in occipital and parietal regions than in frontal regions, resulting in significant hypofrontality. In addition, limbic structures (especially posterior cingulate, amygdala, and hippocampus) and pons were significantly more metabolically active in depressed patients than in controls. Several midline structures as well as neostriatum were less activated in depressed patients than in controls, including reduced relative metabolic rates within the medio-orbital frontal cortex, medial thalamus, anterior cingulate, putamen, and head of the caudate.

Further studies are needed to confirm our finding of elevated CGMR during the first non-REM period in depressed patients. Potential problems with our study design include the following: (1) patients were studied after data had been acquired from the normal controls; (2) patients were not well matched for age with the controls; (3) increased wakefulness during the uptake period could account for increased CGMR in depression; and (4) all subjects were men. Nevertheless, the findings were not altered by the application of statistical controls for age and wakefulness; furthermore, they do not appear to represent drift over time in measurement techniques.

HYPOFRONTALITY

Consistent with most studies in awake depressed subjects,[27-34,56] the sleeping depressed patients showed hypofrontality, especially in the medio-orbital frontal cortex. Although several previous studies suggested that hypometabolism during daytime wakefulness might be predominantly left-sided, no statistically significant hemispheric asymmetry emerged for any cortical, limbic, or thalamic area in this study. Support for a possible mood-related role of the frontal cortex is provided by Pardo et al,[57] who found increased blood flow to inferior and orbital frontal areas in normal subjects instructed to experience sadness; Drevets et al,[58] who showed increased blood flow to left prefrontal cortex in depressed subjects; and reports of depression after frontal lobe strokes[59] or in association with Parkinson disease.[60,61]

Hypofrontality has been reported in functional imaging studies of schizophrenia,[62-65] but no PET sleep studies have yet been carried out in schizophrenia. While the dorsolateral frontal lobe has been more widely studied in schizophrenia, some recent studies have demonstrated more severe medial than lateral hypometabolism.[63,65] A relatively decreased rate of metabolism in medial frontal areas may be associated with emotional states, such as withdrawal and apathy,[66-69] that are common in both schizophrenia and depression.

The inferior frontal lobe or basal forebrain modulates non-REM sleep.[35,37,70] Thus, diminished metabolic activity in this area may be associated with poor maintenance of non-REM sleep and may play a role in the loss of delta sleep often observed in depression, schizophrenia, and other medical and psychiatric disorders.

ANTERIOR CINGULATE AND LIMBIC STRUCTURES

The anterior cingulate was the only limbic area with a significantly lower relative metabolic rate during sleep in depressed patients than in controls. In other limbic areas, such as the superior and posterior cingulate, both absolute and relative CGMR were elevated in depressed patients compared with control subjects. In a study performed during subject wakefulness, Bench et al[34] similarly reported decreased cerebral blood flow to the left anterior cingulate and increased cerebral blood flow in the left posterior cingulate in depressed patients. It is notable that the anterior cingulate most directly connects with the medio-orbital frontal cortex, an area that we found to be significantly hypometabolic. Further, increased activity during wakefulness in all 3 portions of the cingulate, as measured by glucose[23] and D,L-hexamethylpropyleneamide oxime,[24,26] predicted the antidepressant response to sleep deprivation.

CAUDATE, PUTAMEN, AND THALAMUS

Bilateral relative hypometabolism in caudate and putamen characterized depressed patients during non-REM sleep. Previous PET studies of waking depressed patients also observed relative hypometabolism in bilateral caudate.[27,32,58,60] It may be relevant that cortical inputs to the caudate originate predominantly from the orbital frontal cortex, anterior cingulate, and prefrontal cortex, suggesting the role of relative hypometabolism in this neuronal circuitry in the pathophysiological mechanisms of depression.

The relative hypometabolism found in the putamen parallels that in the caudate. Both structures are part of the ventral striatum and receive similar cortical inputs. The globus pallidus showed an elevated absolute metabolic rate (+30%) in depressed patients in the left hemisphere and a reduced relative metabolic rate (−19%) in the right hemisphere. Consequently, there was a reversal of the right greater than left pattern found in the controls. Interestingly, increased blood flow in the left globus pallidus during a sad mood induction task has been reported in normal subjects.[71] The globus pallidus receives inhibitory input from the caudate and putamen and projects inhibitory output to both dorsomedial thalamus and the anterior part of the ventrolateral nucleus.

PHYSIOLOGICAL AND PATHOPHYSIOLOGICAL FEATURES OF NON-REM SLEEP

Although we found a significant negative correlation between CGMR and delta sleep in the depressed patients but not in the controls, previous studies in normal subjects reported that CGMR,[46,47] cerebral blood flow,[48,49] and cerebral metabolic rate for oxygen[49] were lower during deep sleep (stages 3-4) than during light sleep (stage 2). We recently found that the rates of protein synthesis in rhesus monkeys assessed by the ^{14}C-leucine method are positively correlated with the amount of delta sleep in specific areas of the brain, including the basal forebrain, globus pallidus, optic chiasm, preoptic area, and supraoptic nucleus. These observations could suggest that, during non-REM sleep, CGMR would be even greater and protein synthesis even less in patients with more severe depression and lower levels of delta sleep than were found in the present sample. Because our data confirmed the correlation between EEG arousal and cerebral metabolic hyperactivity, a more sensitive computer analysis of sleep EEG might identify subtle abnormalities such as stage transitions, delta and spindle frequency, and delta sleep distribution in the depressed group.

While the depressed patients may have had higher waking levels of anxiety than the normal controls, both groups were in non-REM sleep while studied. It is not clear whether anxiety in normal subjects actually increases CGMR,[63] but a diagnosis of generalized anxiety disorder might contribute to increased occipital metabolic rate. While sex effects on metabolism may also be present, both our patient and comparison groups were all men.[72,73] However, sex-related metabolic differences in affective disorders have not been reported.

The physiological mechanisms underlying normal non-REM sleep and its EEG characteristics are incompletely understood. Many neuroanatomical areas are implicated in non-REM sleep, including the cerebral cortex, basal forebrain, anterior hypothalamus, area postrema, and thalamus, whereas projections from the posterior hypothalamus, dorsal tegmentum, and reticular activating system maintain cortical desychronization during wakefulness and REM sleep and reduce delta EEG activity during non-REM sleep. Nevertheless, no single center has been shown to be uniquely necessary for non-REM sleep, REM sleep, or wakefulness. Some central neurons are as active during non-REM sleep as during wakefulness, but their discharge patterns differ dramatically between states. According to Steriade et al,[37,38] 3 different EEG rhythms characterize non-REM sleep. Slow oscillations (<1 Hz) are generated within neocortical areas, sleep spindles (7-14 Hz) within the reticular thalamic nucleus, and at least one component of delta waves (1-4 Hz) by thalamocortical cells. The other component of delta waves is cortical in origin since it survives thalamectomy. The slow cortical oscillations apparently gate the thalamic-generated spindles and delta waves. Within the thalamus, the reticular nucleus plays a pivotal role in orchestrating and coordinating the rhythmic electrical activity of the thalamus and cortex during non-REM sleep. As non-REM sleep progresses, depolarizing input to the thalamus diminishes from basal forebrain, brain stem, posterior hypothalamus, and other areas. As thalamocortical neurons progressively hyperpolarize, their firing rates first approximate the spindle frequency and later the delta frequencies. The thalamocortical cells presumably synchronize the activity of large ensembles of neocortical cells at frequency rates that are detected with scalp electrodes.

To our knowledge, functional brain imaging techniques have not been applied to non-REM sleep in the context of newer neurophysiological models of sleep regulation. In our 2-deoxyglucose study of non-REM sleep in the monkey, however, the thalamic reticular nucleus showed one of the greatest reductions in glucose utilization during non-REM sleep compared with drowsy wakefulness (−40%),[42] consistent with its important role in the regulation of thalamocortical activity during non-REM sleep. Because of the limitations of temporal and anatomical resolution of PET studies in humans, our current data cannot fully address the specific implications of neurophysiological models for the regulation of non-REM sleep.

In a xenon inhalation study comparing stages 1 and 2 sleep at sleep onset with wakefulness, Meyer et al[48] reported increased cerebral blood flow in narcoleptic patients and decreased flow in normal controls. They speculated that an active metabolic process is involved in sleep induction in patients with narcolepsy compared with normal controls.

These findings are relevant to the present study since both narcoleptic and depressed patients typically have short REM latency. Although narcoleptic and depressed patients share short REM latency, the former fall asleep quickly and the latter fall asleep slowly. Comparisons of metabolic rates just before sleep onset in these 2 groups would be of interest.

The pathophysiological mechanisms responsible for the sleep abnormalities of depression are obscure. One hypothesis is that cholinergic circuits from basal forebrain and dorsal tegmentum are overactive, thereby depolarizing neurons within the thalamic reticular nucleus. This process theoretically increases cortical EEG arousal, decreases low-frequency and high-amplitude EEG, induces short REM latency, and possibly enhances cerebral metabolism during non-REM sleep.[74,75] Overactivity of tegmental cholinergic projections to thalamus could be secondary to disinhibition of serotonergic or noradrenergic input from dorsal raphe and locus ceruleus, respectively.[36,76,77]

In summary, our findings demonstrated increased absolute CGMR during the first nocturnal non-REM period in whole brain, cortex, specific limbic structures, anterior lateral and posterior thalamus, and pons in depressed patients compared with normal controls. Although all areas surveyed showed higher mean absolute metabolic rates in depressed patients than in controls, several midline areas were relatively less increased, including the medial thalamus, anterior cingulate, neostriatum, and medio-orbital frontal lobe. Indeed, the anterior cingulate and the medio-orbital portion of the frontal lobe showed a significantly decreased relative metabolic rate in depressed patients compared with normal controls. As predicted, hypofrontality, which has been commonly found during wakefulness in depressed patients, was present during non-REM sleep in depressed patients in contrast to normal controls. Further research is needed to confirm our findings, determine their diagnostic specificity and sensitivity, assess their clinical significance, and search for their underlying pathophysiological mechanisms.

Accepted for publication January 30, 1996.

This research was supported by National Institute of Mental Health grant MH 23910 to Dr Buchsbaum; the Brain Imaging Committee of the University of California, Irvine; the Veterans Affairs Research Service; the University of California, San Diego, Mental Health Clinical Research Center (grant MH 30914); and National Institute of Mental Health grant MH 387838 to Dr Gillin.

The authors thank M. Steriade, MD, DSc, for very helpful comments on an earlier version of this article. Chuck Tang provided computer system and programming support. Madeline Rose and Laura Sutton, RN, provided research nursing support and Caroline Ruiz assisted with sleep recording methods. Paul Jerabek, PhD, provided nighttime FDG. Dee Harvey provided administrative support.

Reprints: J. Christian Gillin, MD, Psychiatry Service (116A), San Diego Department of Veterans Affairs Medical Center, 3350 La Jolla Village Dr, San Diego, CA 92161.

REFERENCES

1. Benca RM, Obermeyer WH, Thisted RA, Gillin JC. Sleep and psychiatric disorders: a meta-analysis. *Arch Gen Psychiatry.* 1992;49:651-668.

2. Gillin JC, Dow BM, Thompson P, Parry B, Tandon R, Benca R. Sleep in depression and other psychiatric disorders. *Clin Neurosci.* 1993;1:90-96.
3. Gillin JC. The neurobiology of sleep: potential relevance to psychiatric disorders. *Biol Psychiatry.* In press.
4. Nofzinger EA, Buysse DJ, Reynolds CF III, Kupfer DJ. Sleep disorders related to another mental disorder (nonsubstance/primary): a DSM-IV literature review. *J Clin Psychiatry.* 1993;54:244-255.
5. Souêtre E, Wehr TA, Sack DA, Kreb B, Darcourt G. 24-hour profiles of body temperature and plasma TSH in bipolar patients during depression and during remission and in normal controls subjects. *Am J Psychiatry.* 1988;145:1133-1137.
6. Avery DH, Wildschiodtz G, Smallwood RG, Rafaelsen OJ. REM latency and core temperature relationships in primary depression. *Acta Psychiatr Scand.* 1986;74:269-280.
7. Avery D, Wildschiodtz G, Rafaelsen OJ. REM latency and temperature in affective disorder before and after treatment. *Biol Psychiatry.* 1982;17:463-470.
8. Elsenga S, van den Hoofdakker R. Body core temperature and depression during total sleep deprivation in depressives. *Biol Psychiatry.* 1988;24:531-540.
9. Poland RE, McCracken JT, Luchmansingh P, Tondo L. Relationship between REM sleep latency and nocturnal cortisol concentrations in depressed patients. *J Sleep Res.* 1992;1:54-57.
10. Steiger A, von Bardeleben U, Guldner J, Lauer C, Rothe B, Holsboer F. The sleep EEG and nocturnal hormonal secretion studies on changes during the course of depression and on effects of CNS-active drugs. *Prog Neuropsychopharmacol Biol Psychiatry.* 1993;17:125-137.
11. Steiger A, Guldner J, Colla-Muller M, Friess E, Sonntag A, Schier T. Growth hormone-releasing hormone (GHRH)-induced effects on sleep EEG and nocturnal secretion of growth hormone, cortisol and ACTH in patients with major depression. *J Psychiatr Res.* 1994;28:225-238.
12. Jarrett DB, Kupfer DJ, Miewald JM, Grochocinski VJ, Franz B. Sleep-related growth hormone secretion is persistently suppressed in women with recurrent depression: a preliminary longitudinal analysis. *J Psychiatr Res.* 1994;28:211-223.
13. Voderholzer U, Laakmann G, Wittmann R, Daffner-Bujia C, Hinz A, Haag C, Baghai T. Profiles of spontaneous 24-hour and stimulated growth hormone secretion in male patients with endogenous depression. *Psychiatry Res.* 1993; 47:215-227.
14. Vogel GW, Vogel F, McAbee RS, Thurmond AJ. Improvement of depression by REM sleep deprivation: new findings and a theory. *Arch Gen Psychiatry.* 1980;37:247-253.
15. Gillin JC. The sleep therapies of depression. *Prog Neuropsychopharmacol Biol Psychiatry.* 1983;7:351-364.
16. Wu JC, Bunney WE Jr. The biological basis of an antidepressant response to sleep deprivation and relapse: review and hypothesis. *Am J Psychiatry.* 1990; 147:14-21.
17. Hillman E, Kripke DF, Gillin JC. Sleep restriction, exercise and bright lights: alternate therapies for depression. In: Tasman A, Kaufmann C, Goldfinger S, eds. *American Psychiatric Press Review of Psychiatry: Treatment of Refractory Affective Disorder.* 9th ed. Washington, DC: American Psychiatric Press; 1990:132-144.
18. Leibenluft E, Wehr TA. Is sleep deprivation useful in the treatment of depression? *Am J Psychiatry.* 1992;149:159-168.
19. Gillin JC, Sitaram N, Wehr T, Duncan W, Post RM, Murphy DL, Mendelson WB, Wyatt RJ, Bunney WE Jr. Sleep and affective illness. In: Post RM, Ballenger J, eds. *Neurobiology of Mood Disorders.* Baltimore, Md: Williams & Wilkins; 1984:157-189.
20. Borbély M. The S-deficiency hypothesis of depression and the two process model of sleep regulation. *Pharmacopsychiatry.* 1987;20:23-39.
21. van den Burg W, van den Hoofdakker RH. Total sleep deprivation on endogenous depression. *Arch Gen Psychiatry.* 1975;32:1121-1125.
22. Kupfer DJ, Gillin JC, Coble PA, Spiker DG, Shaw D, Holtzer B. REM sleep, naps and depression. *Psychiatry Res.* 1981;5:195-203.
23. Wu JC, Gillin JC, Buchsbaum MS, Hershey T, Johnson JC, Bunney WE Jr. Effect of sleep deprivation on brain metabolism of depressed patients. *Am J Psychiatry.* 1992;149:538-543.
24. Ebert D, Feistel H, Barocka A. Effects of sleep deprivation on the limbic system and the frontal lobes in affective disorders: a study with Tc-99m-HMPAO SPECT. *Psychiatry Res Neuroimaging.* 1991;40:247-251.
25. Volk S, Kaendler SH, Weber R, Georgi K, Maul F, Hertel A, Pflug B, Hoer G. Evaluation of the effects of total sleep deprivation on cerebral blood flow using single photon emission computerized tomography. *Acta Psychiatr Scand.* 1992; 86:478-83.
26. Ebert D, Feistel H, Barocka A, Kaschka W. Increased limbic flood flow and total sleep deprivation in major depression. *Psychiatry Res Neuroimaging.* 1994; 55:101-109.
27. Baxter LR, Phelps ME, Mazziotta JC, Schwartz JM, Gerner RH, Selin CE, Suminda RM. Cerebral metabolic rates for glucose in mood disorders. *Arch Gen Psychiatry.* 1985;42:441-447.
28. Baxter LR, Jeffrey MS, Phelps ME, Mazziotta JC, Guze BH, Selin CE, Gerner RH, Sumida RM. Reduction of prefrontal cortex glucose metabolism common to three types of depression. *Arch Gen Psychiatry.* 1989;46:243-250.
29. Hurwitz TA, Clark C, Murphy E, Klonoff H, Martin WRW, Pate BD. Regional cerebral glucose metabolism in major depressive disorder. *Can J Psychiatry.* 1990;35:684-688.
30. Martinot JL, Hardy P, Feline A, Hurel JD, Mazoyer B, Attar-Levy D, Pappata S, Syrota A. Left prefrontal glucose hypometabolism in the depressed state: a confirmation. *Am J Psychiatry.* 1990;147:1313-1317.
31. Rubin E, Sackeim HA, Prohovnik I, Moeller JR, Schnur DB, Mukherjee S. Regional cerebral blood flow in mood disorders, IV: comparison of mania and depression. *Psychiatry Res Neuroimaging.* 1995;61:1-10.
32. Buchsbaum MS, Wu J, DeLisi LE, Holcomb H, Kessler R, Johnson J, King AC, Hazlett E, Langston K, Post RM. Frontal cortex and basal ganglia metabolic rates assessed by positron emission tomography with [^{18}F]2-deoxyglucose in affective illness. *J Affect Disord.* 1986;10:137-152.
33. Buchsbaum MS, DeLisi LE, Holcomb HH, Cappelletti J, King AC, Johnson J, Hazlett E, Dowling-Zimmerman S, Post RM, Morihisa J, Carpenter W, Cohen R, Pickar D, Weinberger DR, Margolin R, Kessler RM. Anteroposterior gradients in cerebral glucose use in schizophrenia and affective disorders. *Arch Gen Psychiatry.* 1984;41:1159-1166.
34. Bench CJ, Friston KJ, Brown RG, Scott LC, Frackowiak RSJ, Dolan RJ. The anatomy of melancholia: focal abnormalities of cerebral blood flow in major depression. *Psychol Med.* 1992;22:607-615.
35. Buzsaki G, Bickford R, Ponomareff G, Thal LJ, Mandel R, Gage FH. Nucleus basalis and thalamic control of neocortical activity in the freely moving rat. *J Neurosci.* 1988;8:4007-4026.
36. Jones BE. Paradoxical sleep and its chemical/structural substrates in the brain. *Neuroscience.* 1991;40:637-656.
37. Steriade M, Dossi RC, Nunez A. Network modulation of a slow intrinsic oscillation of cat thalamocortical neurons implicated in sleep delta waves: cortically induced synchronization and brainstem cholinergic suppression. *J Neurosci.* 1991;11:3200-3217.
38. Steriade M, Contreras D, Amzica F. Synchronized sleep oscillations and their paroxysmal developments. *Trends Neurosci.* 1994;17:199-208.
39. Franzini C. Brain metabolism and blood flow during sleep. *J Sleep Res.* 1992; 1:3-16.
40. Madsen PL. Blood flow and oxygen uptake in the human brain during various states of sleep and wakefulness. *Acta Neurol Scand.* 1993;88(suppl 148):5-25.
41. Kennedy C, Gillin JC, Mendelson WB, Suda S, Miyaoka M, Ito M, Nakamura RK, Storch FI, Pettigrew K, Mishkin M, Sokoloff L. Local cerebral glucose utilization in nonREM sleep. *Nature.* 1982;297:325-327.
42. Nakamura R, Kennedy C, Gillin JC, Suda S, Ito M, Storch FI, Mendelson W, Sokolof L, Mishkin M. Hypnogenic center theory of sleep: no support from metabolic mapping in monkeys. *Brain Res.* 1983;268:372-376.
43. Ramm P, Frost BJ. Cerebral and local glucose cerebral metabolism in the cat during slow wave and REM sleep. *Brain Res.* 1986;365:112-124.
44. Ramm P, Frost BJ. Regional activity in rat brain during sleep wake activity. *Sleep.* 1983;6:196-216.
45. Buchsbaum MS, Gillin JC, Wu J, Haslett E, Sicotte N, Dupont R, Bunney WE Jr. Regional cerebral glucose metabolic rate in human sleep assessed by positron emission tomography. *Life Sci.* 1989;45:1349-1356.
46. Maquet P, Dive D, Salmon E, Sadzot B, Franco G, Poirier R, Franck G. Cerebral glucose utilization during stage 2 sleep in man. *Brain Res.* 1992;571:149-153.
47. Maquet P, Dive D, Salmon E, Sadzot B, Franco G, Poirrier R, Von Frenckell R, Frank G. Cerebral glucose utilization during sleep wake cycle in man determined by positron tomography and ^{18}F-2-fluoro-2-deoxy-D-glucose method. *Brain Res.* 1990;513:136-143.
48. Meyer JS, Ishikawa Y, Hata T, Karacan I. Cerebral blood flow in normal and abnormal sleep and dreaming. *Brain Cogn.* 1987;6:266-294.
49. Madsen PL, Schmidt JF, Wildschiodtz G, Friberg L, Holm S, Vorstrup S, Lassen NA. Cerebral oxygen metabolism and cerebral blood flow in humans during deep sleep and rapid-eye-movement sleep. *J Appl Physiol.* 1991;70:2597-2601.
50. Boyle PJ, Scott JC, Krentz AJ, Nagy RJ, Comstock E, Hoffman C. Diminished brain glucose metabolism is a significant determinant for falling rates of systemic glucose utilization during sleep in normal humans. *J Clin Invest.* 1994; 93:529-535.
51. American Psychiatric Association. *Diagnostic and Statistical Manual of Mental Disorders, Third Edition, Revised.* Washington, DC: American Psychiatric Association; 1987.
52. Hamilton M. Development of a rating scale for primary depressive illness. *Br J Soc Clin Psychol.* 1967;6:278-296.
53. Guy W, ed. *ECDEU Assessment Manual for Psychopharmacology, Revised.* Washington, DC; Dept of Health, Education and Welfare; 1976. DHEW publication ADM 76-338.
54. Rechtschaffen A, Kales M. *A Manual of Standardized Terminology, Techniques, and Scoring System for Sleep Stages of Human Subjects.* Washington, DC: Public Health Service; 1968.
55. Dixon WJ. *BMD Biomedical Computer Programs.* Los Angeles: University of California Press; 1982.
56. Buchsbaum MS, Cappelletti J, Ball R, Hazlett E, King AC, Johnson J, Wu J, DeLisi LE. Positron emission tomographic image measurement in schizophrenia and affective disorders. *Ann Neurol.* 1984;15(suppl):S157-S165.
57. Pardo JV, Pardo PJ, Raichle ME. Neural correlates of self-induced dysphoria. *Am J Psychiatry.* 1993;150:713-719.
58. Drevets WC, Videen TO, Price JL, Preskorn SH, Carmichael ST, Raichle ME. A functional anatomical study of unipolar depression. *J Neurosci.* 1992;12:3628-3641.
59. Robinson RG, Boston JD, Starkstein SE, Price TR. Comparison of mania and depression after brain injury: causal factors. *Am J Psychiatry.* 1988;145:172-178.
60. Mayberg HS, Starkstein SE, Sadzot B, Preziosi T, Andrezejewski PL, Dannals RF, Wagner HN, Robinson RG. Selective hypometabolism in the inferior frontal lobe in depressed patients with Parkinson's disease. *Ann Neurol.* 1990;28:57-64.
61. Ring HA, Bench CJ, Trimble MR, Brooks DJ, Frackowiak RSJ, Dolan RJ. Depression in Parkinson's disease: a positron emission study. *Br J Psychiatry.*

1994;165:333-339.
62. Buchsbaum MS. The frontal lobes, basal ganglia, and temporal lobes as sites for schizophrenia. *Schizophr Bull.* 1993;16:379-389.
63. Buchsbaum M. Positron emission tomography and brain activity in psychiatry. In: Oldham JM, Riba MB, Tasman, A, eds. *Review of Psychiatry.* Washington, DC; American Psychiatric Press: 1993;12:461-485.
64. Andreasen NC, Rezai K, Alliger R, Swayze VW, Flaum M, Kirchner P, Cohen G, O'Leary DS. Hypofrontality in neuroleptic-naive patients and in patients with chronic schizophrenia. *Arch Gen Psychiatry.* 1992;49:943-958.
65. Weinberger DR, Berman KF, Illowsky BP. Physiological dysfunction of the dorsolateral prefrontal cortex in schizophrenia, III: a new cohort and evidence for a monoaminergic mechanism. *Arch Gen Psychiatry.* 1988;45:609-615.
66. Siegel BV Jr, Buchsbaum MS, Bunney WE Jr, Gottschalk LA, Haier RJ, Lohr JB, Lottenberg S, Najafi A, Nuechterlein KH, Potkin SG, Wu JC. Cortical-striatal-thalamic circuits and brain glucose metabolic activity in 70 unmedicated male schizophrenic patients. *Am J Psychiatry.* 1993;150:1325-1336.
67. Barbas H, Pandya DN. Patterns of connections of the prefrontal cortex in the rhesus monkey associated with cortical architecture. In: Levin HS, Eisenberg HM, Benton AL, eds. *Frontal Lobe Functions and Dysfunctions.* Oxford, England: Oxford University Press; 1991:35-58.
68. Mayberg HS, Solomon DH. Depression in Parkinson's disease: a biochemical and organic viewpoint. *Adv Neurol.* 1995;65:49-60.
69. Cummings JL. Frontal-subcortical circuits and human behavior. *Arch Neurol.* 1993;50:873-880.
70. Szymusiak R, Iriye T, McGinty D. Sleep-waking discharge of neurons in the posterior lateral hypothalamic area of cats. *Brain Res Bull.* 1989;23:111-120.
71. Schneider F, Gur RE, Mozley LH, Smith RJ, Mozley PD, Censits DM, Alavi A, Gur RC. Mood effects on limbic blood flow correlate with emotional self-rating: a PET study with oxygen-15 labeled water. *Psychiatry Res Neuroimaging.* In press.
72. Baxter LR, Mazziotta JC, Phelps ME, Selin CE, Guge BH, Fairbanks L. Cerebral glucose metabolic rates in normal females versus normal males. *Psychiatry Res.* 1987;21:237-245.
73. Andreason PJ, Zametkin AJ, Guo AC, Baldwin P, Cohen RM. Gender-related differences in regional cerebral glucose metabolism in normal volunteers. *Psychiatry Res.* 1994;51:175-183.
74. Gillin JC, Sutton L, Ruiz C, Kelsoe J, Dupont RM, Darko D, Risch C, Golshan S, Janowsky D. The cholinergic rapid eye movement induction test with arecoline in depression. *Arch Gen Psychiatry.* 1991;48:264-270.
75. Sitaram N, Nurnberger J, Gershon E, Gillin JC. Faster cholinergic REM sleep induction in euthymic patients with primary affective illness. *Science.* 1980; 208:200-202.
76. Luebke JI, Greene RW, Semba K, Kamondi A, McCarley RW, Reiner PB. Serotonin hyperpolarizes cholinergic low-threshold burst neurons in the rat laterodorsal tegmental nucleus in vitro. *Proc Natl Acad Sci U S A.* 1992;89: 743-747.
77. Bhatti T, Gillin JC, Golshan S, Clark C, Demodena A, Schlosser A, Stahl S, Kelsoe J, Rapaport H. The effect of a tryptophan-free amino acid drink on sleep and mood in normal controls. *Sleep Res.* 1995;24:153.

Retinoid Dysregulation May Result in Abnormal Expression of Glutamic Acid Decarboxylase in Schizophrenia

Akbarian et al[1] argue convincingly for abnormal expression of the enzyme glutamic acid decarboxylase (GAD) in the prefrontal cortex of a small sample of schizophrenic brains compared with controls. The authors suggest 4 mechanisms to account for this intriguing finding: (1) a genetic defect in the GAD protein, (2) a pathogenic agent, (3) a developmental defect in cell circuitry resulting in hypoactivity of the prefrontal cortex, and (4) a second-trimester environmental insult affecting the development of the cortical subplate. Except for mutation in the *GAD* gene, each of these mechanisms could be the result of abnormal function of the vitamin A (retinoid) cascade.

Review of the action and metabolism of genes of the retinoid cascade in relation to schizophrenia indicates that, in addition to controlling for neuronal migration and anterior and posterior positional development of the central nervous system, retinoids are present in all areas of the brain, particularly those areas innervated by dopaminergic neurons. Retinoic acid (RA), the final morphogenetic derivative of vitamin A, has been shown to regulate the expression of many of the neurotransmitters. Other retinoid genes are crucial to the developmental integrity of brain segmentation and structure. Retinoic acid is highly teratogenic in excess, producing severe congenital abnormalities of the forebrain, hindbrain, and ventricles, abnormalities that have been found, but to a much lesser degree, in schizophrenic brains.[2] Since mammals are unable to synthesize retinoid de novo and must acquire it from the maternal circulation through the placenta, maternal retinoid excess or deficit may profoundly alter the developing fetus, with particular effects in the second trimester, the time of highest fetal sensitivity to retinoids[3] and the time of neuronal migration and development of the cortical subplate.

Retinoic acid regulates the expression of a great variety of genes through characteristic base-pair (bp) sequences of DNA in the genes that bind to the nuclear RA receptors.[4] In a sequence of 2.79 kb of murine *GAD65* genomic DNA, which represents 151 bp of exon and intron sequence, and 2.64 kb of 5′ flanking DNA, a sequence motif of a putative RA response element is found in the 5′ flanking region (Catherine S. Pinal, PhD, personal communication, July 7, 1995). Although the manner and extent to which RA controls the expression of GAD remains to be determined, the presence of a DNA sequence resembling a major retinoid regulatory element in the *GAD* gene suggests that retinoids may be important in the expression of GAD.

Although mutations of the genes that are specific to the retinoid cascade are probably lethal, and none, to my knowledge, have been identified in humans to date, there are several ubiquitous proteins involved in retinoid metabolism that exhibit multiple allelic variants, of which some are pathogenic and others normal. These include transthyretin, which carries retinol bound to retinol-binding protein across the blood–cerebrospinal fluid barrier; the alcohol dehydrogenases, which convert retinol to retinal; the aldehyde dehydrogenases, which convert retinal to RA; and albumin, which binds RA. Apolipoprotein E is also involved in retinoid transport. Analogous to the vulnerability hypothesis regarding apolipoprotein E in Alzheimer's disease,[5] common normal allelic variants of these ubiquitous genes, working singly or in epistasis, may subtly alter the exquisite regulation that is required for proper homeostasis of retinoids in ways that may increase vulnerability to schizophrenia.

Taken together, I have argued that retinoid dysregulation is worthy of consideration as a possible etiologic factor in schizophrenia in this case, as it may relate to control of the expression of GAD.

Ann B. Goodman
Nathan S. Kline Institute for Psychiatric Research
Orangeburg, NY 10962

1. Akbarian S, Kim JJ, Potkin SG, Hagman JO, Tafazzoli A, Bunney WE Jr, Jones ED. Gene expression for glutamic acid decarboxylase is reduced without loss of neurons in prefrontal cortex of schzophrenics. *Arch Gen Psychiatry.* 1995;52:258-266.
2. Goodman AB. Chromosomal locations and modes of action of genes of the retinoid (vitamin A) system support their involvement in the etiology of schizophrenia. *Am J Med Genet (Neuropsychiatr Genet).* 1995;60:335-348.
3. Satre MA, Ugen KD, Kochhar DM. Developmental changes in endogenous retinoids during pregnancy and embryogenesis in the mouse. *Biol Reprod.* 1992;46:802-810.
4. Langston AW, Gudas LJ. Identification of a retinoic acid responsive enhancer 3′ of the murine homeobox gene *Hox-1.6. Mech Dev.* 1992;38:217-228.
5. Strittmatter WJ, Weisgraber KH, Goedert M, Saunders AM, Huang D, Corder EH, Dong LM, Jakes R, Alberts MJ, Gilbert JR, Han S-H, Hulatte C, Einstein G, Schmechel DE, Pericak-Vance MA, Roses AD. Hypothesis: microtubule instability and paired helical filament formation in the Alzheimer disease brain are related to apolipoprotein E genotype. *Exp Neurol.* 1994;125:163-171.

Venlafaxine in Obsessive-compulsive Disorder

In a contribution to the January 1995 issue of the ARCHIVES comparing the efficacy and tolerability of clomipramine, fluoxetine, fluvoxamine, and sertraline, Greist et al,[1] using a method of meta-analysis, found all 4 agents to be effective in the treatment of patients who have obsessive-compulsive disorder (OCD). Whereas all 4 are serotonin-transport inhibitors, clomipramine, with its noradrenergic transport–inhibition component, most notably showed an efficacy advantage. With regard to this finding, Greist et al stated, "It seems that something may be missing in fluoxetine, fluvoxamine, and sertraline that clomipramine contains." They posed the question, "Will agents such as . . . venlafaxine hydrochloride, which have selective and potent serotonin and noradrenergic transport inhibition and a better side-effect profile than clomipramine, work well in treating OCD?" I wish to respond by reporting our limited experience with venlafaxine therapy in such patients.

Research that we have conducted suggests that the preliminary answer to this question is yes. Venlafaxine is a novel phenylethylamine compound with a dual mechanism of action similar to that of clomipramine, which suggests an anti–obsessive-compulsive application, but venlafaxine produces fewer and less serious side effects as a result of its lack of affinity for muscarinic, histaminergic, and α_1-adrenergic receptors.

We recently performed a small, double-blind, placebo-controlled trial of venlafaxine in 30 outpatients who had OCD, the results of which have not been published yet (data on file, Institute for Bio-Behavioral Therapy and Research and Wyeth-Ayerst Research, 1995). Patients who had a positive score on the Hamilton Rating Scale for Depression were eliminated from the trial, and the active drug was titrated rapidly up to 225 mg/d and given during an 8-week period. Although critical ratings of avoidance and scores on the Clinical Global Impressions scale showed no significant differences between the 2 groups (P=.29 and P=.52, respectively), there were significant improvement trends in the patients treated with venlafaxine across 7 periods for both parameters (P<.001).

Of the 30 patients in our study (16 taking venlafaxine and 14 taking placebo), 8 patients (2 taking venlafaxine and 6 taking placebo) discontinued therapy. Venlafaxine proved beneficial in 6 patients who had OCD, while in 3 patients the condition remained unchanged and in 5 others the condition became worse. In contrast, none of the patients treated with placebo showed improvement. In addition, in these studies we noted an effect-size trend in favor of venlafaxine. The dropout rate was higher in the placebo group, suggesting that the active compound was exerting a beneficial effect.

We believe that the number of patients who might have benefited from treatment with venlafaxine would have been higher if the study had been carried out for a longer duration than was called for in the protocol (8 weeks) and if higher dosages of venlafaxine than that used (225 mg/d) had been employed. The duration of treatment in the studies reported by Greist et al ranged from 10 to 13 weeks and included mean daily dosages of fluoxetine, sertraline, and fluvoxamine at or near the manufacturers' recommended maximums for treating patients who have depression. The positive trends that we observed might have yielded statistically significant results had our study been longer and included higher venlafaxine dosages.

Furthermore, Zajecka et al[2] showed that venlafaxine titrated to a dosage of 375 mg/d over 5 weeks improved symptoms of OCD in 1 patient who had both OCD and major depression (refractory to other agents), although symptoms of depression in this patient did not improve.

The rationale for the use of venlafaxine therapy in patients who have OCD is related to the observation that OCD is mediated by serotonergic activity.[3] As a potent inhibitor of serotonin reuptake, venlafaxine may affect this pathway. In addition, as Greist et al point out in their comments, management of OCD in many patients may require a "salubrious combination" of serotonin and noradrenergic transport inhibition. Venlafaxine also inhibits the reuptake of norepinephrine.

A potential benefit of using venlafaxine in the management of OCD is its favorable safety profile. In our study, only 1 patient in the venlafaxine group discontinued treatment because of an adverse reaction, a burning sensation following urination (which may or may not have been related to treatment). Although some early studies reported increases in systolic and diastolic blood pressure levels after use of venlafaxine,[4,5] we observed no such increases in any of our 16 patients taking venlafaxine.

Obviously, because of the limited scope of our study, further research is needed before it can be determined if venlafaxine is safe and effective in the treatment of OCD. Based on the theory that the addition of norepinephrine-reuptake inhibition enhances the management of OCD and on our preliminary findings, we believe that venlafaxine is effective in the treatment of OCD.

Jose A. Yaryura-Tobias, MD
Fugen A. Neziroglu, PhD
Institute for Bio-Behavioral Therapy and Research
935 Northern Blvd, Suite 102
Great Neck, NY 11021

1. Greist JH, Jefferson JW, Kobak KA, Katzelnick DJ, Serlin RC. Efficacy and tolerability of serotonin transport inhibitors in obsessive-compulsive disorder: a meta-analysis. *Arch Gen Psychiatry.* 1995;52:53-60.
2. Zajecka JM, Fawcett J, Guy C. Coexisting major depression and obsessive-compulsive disorder treated with venlafaxine. *J Clin Psychopharmacol.* 1990; 10:152-153.
3. Yaryura-Tobias JA, Bebirian RJ, Neziroglu FA, Bhagavan HN. Obsessive-compulsive disorders as a serotonergic defect. *Res Commun Psychol Psychiatry Behav.* 1977;2:279-286.
4. Fabre LF, Punam III HP. An ascending single-dose tolerance study of WY-45,030, a bicyclic antidepressant, in healthy men. *Curr Ther Res.* 1987;42: 901-909.
5. Schweizer E, Weise C, Clary C, Fox I, Rickels K. Placebo-controlled trial of venlafaxine for the treatment of major depression. *J Clin Psychopharmacol.* 1991;11:233-236.

In reply

Yaryura-Tobias and Neziroglu have thoughtfully presented their experience with a small, double-blind, placebo-controlled trial of venlafaxine as a treatment for OCD. They note trends toward efficacy and suggest that the failure to find statistically significant differences is related to the short duration of their trial (8 weeks) and low doses of venlafaxine hydrochloride (225 mg/d, maximum dose).

They are correct that a longer duration of treatment would be needed to conclude that venlafaxine was ineffective as a treatment for OCD, as most potent serotonin-reuptake inhibitors studied to date have showed continued improvement beyond 8 weeks. Whether higher doses of venlafaxine are needed is less clear, and their assertion that mean daily doses of fluoxetine and sertraline were "at or near the manufacturers' recommended maximum for treating patients who have depression" is inaccurate. Both fluoxetine and sertraline were effective at low doses (20 and 50 mg/d, respectively) and exhibited a flat dose-response curve across fixed doses studied and only statistically insignificant trends for greater improvement at higher doses. Treating patients with greater than 225 mg of venlafaxine per day will increase the risk of blood pressure elevations found at higher doses.

Earlier studies in populations of comparable size have found treatment with clomipramine[1] and fluvoxamine[2] significantly more effective than placebo, but these studies were of longer duration.

In addition to the positive case report by Zajecka et al,[3] which the authors cite, Ananth and colleagues[4] recently reported 2 other positive responses to venlafaxine in patients who had not responded to or failed to tolerate other potent serotonin reuptake inhibitors.

While it is appealing to speculate about mechanisms by which venlafaxine and other medications may produce beneficial effects in OCD, the clinical touchstone for any treatment for any disorder remains the randomized controlled trial. It is gratifying that Yaryura-Tobias and Neziroglu qualify their enthusiasm about venlafaxine as an effective treatment for OCD by describing their "belief," rather than knowledge, at this stage in our study of this compound. As they indicate, more definitive trials are needed to define the strengths and limitations of venlafaxine as a treatment for OCD.

John H. Greist, MD
Dean Foundation for Health Research and Education
University of Wisconsin
8000 Excelsior Dr, Suite 302
Madison, WI 53717-1914

1. Greist JH, Jefferson JW, Rosenfeld R, Gutzmann LD, March JS, Barklage NE. Clomipramine and obsessive compulsive disorder: a placebo-controlled double-blind study of 32 patients. *J Clin Psychiatry.* 1990;51:292-297.
2. Jenike MA, Hyman S, Baer L, Holland A, Minichiello WE, Buttolph L, Summergrad P, Seymour R, Ricciardi J. A controlled trial of fluvoxamine in obsessive-compulsive disorder: implications for a serotonergic theory. *Am J Psychiatry.* 1990;147:1209-1215.
3. Zajecka JM, Fawcett J, Guy C. Coexisting major depression and obsessive-compulsive disorder treated with venlafaxine. *J Clin Psychopharmacol.* 1995; 10:152-153.
4. Ananth J, Burgoyne K, Smith M, Swartz R. Venlafaxine for treatment of obsessive-compulsive disorder. *Am J Psychiatry.* 1995;152:1832.

Professional Opportunities

Physician Recruitment

Academic/Faculty

FACULTY POSITION IN PSYCHIATRIC NEUROIMAGING RESEARCH: The University of North Carolina School of Medicine at Chapel Hill is seeking candidates for a tenured (or tenure track) faculty position to provide leadership in neuroimaging research for the Department of Psychiatry and the Mental Health and Neuroscience Clinical Research Center. Candidates should have an MD or PHD, postdoctoral training in psychiatry or psychology together with expertise in morphologic/morphometric and/or functional magnetic resonance imaging and spectroscopy and a documented record of accomplishment in the area of psychosis and/or affective disorders research. The successful candidate will work in collaboration with a team of MHCRC investigators from both the University of North Carolina and Duke University, and will be expected to obtain support to develop his or her independent research as well. Faculty appointment and salary will be commensurate with the candidate's level of experience and accomplishment. Interested applicants should send a curriculum vitae, statement of research interests and three letters of reference to Jeffrey A. Lieberman, MD, Vice Chairman, Department of Psychiatry, Chair of Search Committee, Campus Box #7160, University of North Carolina School of Medicine, Chapel Hill, NC 27599-7160. The search will be continued until the successful candidate is found.

CALL 800 AMA-2260
for rate and deadline information.

Psychiatry

TEXAS, the SOUTHEAST, and the SUNBELT STATES- There are Excellent Private Practice Opportunities Available in Psychiatry. Major Cities and Rural Communities Are Available.

Call 1-800-284-4560/Houston 713-493-2797

Or send CV to:
P.O. Box 42314
Houston, TX 77242-2314
FAX 713-493-2234

Reuben Bronstein
& Associates

Locum Tenens Wanted

HKA LOCUM TENENS is looking for quality general psychiatry physicians to do Locum Tenens. We have opportunities coast-to-coast. We furnish Occurrence Malpractice Insurance (no tail necessary). Please call **HKA LOCUM TENENS at (800)226-6347, Extension AM7.1.**

© 1995 MAILSTAR

R E A C H

29,400 physicians monthly
with
Archives of General Psychiatry.

National Institute on Alcohol Abuse and Alcoholism (NIAAA)
and the
Office of Alternative Medicine (OAM)
National Institutes of Health (NIH)
Bethesda, Maryland

The NIAAA and OAM invites motivated and highly qualified physicians to apply for a unique three year research fellowship. Research protocols will examine the efficacy of acupuncture and alternative medicine techniques on alcohol relapse utilizing state-of-the-art neurochemical and neuroimaging techniques. Training in acupuncture and neuroimaging techniques and core courses curriculum provided by both the Clinical Center at the NIH and the OAM will complement the rich intellectual environment of the NIH. The BC/BE applicant must have completed an accredited residency program and must be licensed to practice medicine.

Applicants should send a letter of interest, CV and three letters of recommendation to Markku V. Linnoila, MD, PhD, Scientific Director, National Institute on Alcohol Abuse and Alcoholism, Bldg 10, Rm 3C103, 10 Center Drive MSC 1256, Bethesda, MD 20892-1256. For more information call Joseph R. Hibbeln, MD, Chief, Outpatient Clinic, NIAAA, 301-443-2716 or JHIBBELN@DICBR.NIAAA.NIH.GOV.

Deadline for receipt of applications: August 1, 1996.

NIH is an Equal Opportunity Employer.

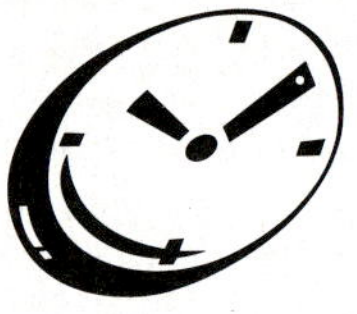

browse.
anytime you want - it's free

1·800·233·9330

The most comprehensive source of practice opportunities in the known world is available to you toll free, 24 hours a day.

Browse through recorded profiles of opportunities from 5 continents *(most in the U.S.)*. Then transmit a confidential response to the opportunities you choose. No salesman. No strings.

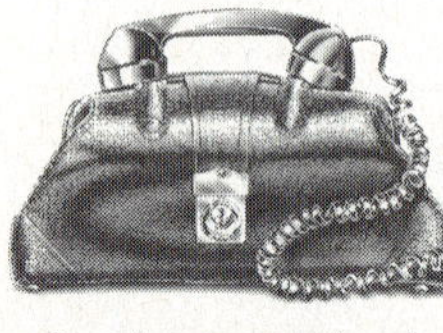

The Practice Opportunity Line
We're on call for you.

from Physician's Market Information Center **1·800·423·1229**

The Osler Institute
Board Review Courses

Presented by The Osler Institute and Finch University of Health Sciences/ The Chicago Medical School

Psychiatry Written Boards
October 14-19, 1996 – Chicago

Psychiatry Oral Boards
October 14-19, 1996 – Chicago
November 12-14, 1996 – Dallas

Child and Adolescent
May 11-16, 1996 – Austin, Texas
Aug. 31-Sept. 5, 1996 – Columbus, Ohio

Geriatric Psychiatry
September 5-8, 1996 – Atlanta
November 1-4, 1996 – Chicago

Call Today: 1-800-356-7537

ARCHIVES OF GENERAL PSYCHIATRY

In a 2-year, placebo-controlled study, **Sass et al** (page 673) studied the effects of acamprosate (calcium bisacetylhomotaurinate) on long-term abstinence in alcohol-dependent patients. Significantly more patients started on treatment with acamprosate remained abstinent and their duration of abstinence was longer during treatment. Only minor adverse effects were reported. Drug treatment was withdrawn after 1 year without rebound phenomena and the treatment advantage was maintained after another year of follow-up.

Two heritable forms of alcoholism were identified in the Stockholm Adoption Study in 1981 by Cloninger et al in Sweden. Type 1 alcoholism had adult onset and rapid progression of dependence without criminality, whereas type 2 had teenage onset of repeated social and legal problems from alcohol abuse. Now, an independent study by **Sigvardsson et al** (page 681) with different adoptees has confirmed that type 1 and type 2 alcoholism are clinically distinct forms of the disease, with causes that are independent but not mutually exclusive. This study encourages distinguishing these 2 types of alcoholics, both in research and in treatment.

The relapse rate of panic disorder after drug treatment is distressingly high. To a standard regimen with clomipramine, **Wiborg and Dahl** (page 689) added brief dynamic psychotherapy aimed at the patients' psychosocial vulnerability. The relapse rate in the group with added psychotherapy was significantly lower during 9 months of observation after the end of treatment. The result indicates that a combined treatment of drug and brief dynamic psychotherapy can give a better outcome over time in panic disorder.

The remaining articles are part of a joint publication venture with the Journal of Consulting and Clinical Psychology (JCCP) *to report the implicatons of advances in psychotherapy and psychopharmacologic treatments on the health care policy debate. The current issue of the* ARCHIVES *contains the series on psychosocial treatments; the complementary series on psychopharmacologic advances appears in the current issue of* JCCP. *An editorial by Beutler, Barchas, and Marzuk (page 670) describes this special series of articles.*

How many and which individuals, with which psychiatric disorders, receive (or do not receive) mental health services from which professionals in what settings? What is known about those individuals in need of mental health services and how they access these services? What are the professional affiliations and service sites of mental health professionals? **Howard et al** (page 696) summarize current knowledge about actual utilization of psychotherapy services relative to the needs of patients and the professional background of therapists.

Russell and Orlinsky (page 708) sketch the history of research on behavioral and nonbehavioral psychosocial treatments. They describe 4 major phases of investigative focus: an establishment of research (1927-1954); a search for scientific rigor (1955-1969); an expansion and organization (1970-1984); and a consolidation and reformulation (1984-present). Illustrative findings from process and outcome studies, innovative techniques for meta-analyses, the study of therapist-client interactions, and critical discourses about clinical significance are shown to have relevance for crafting well-informed mental health care policies.

The role of psychotherapy in the treatment of depression is a subject of debate as the health care system changes. **Clarkin et al** (page 717) review the evidence of the efficacy of psychotherapy in the treatment of depression in controlled designs with relatively homogeneous groups of therapists and patients. Whereas, the efficacy of psychotherapy argues for its place in an evolving health care system, the specific ways in which psychotherapy is used will probably be determined by effectiveness studies that examine the impact of psychotherapy on heterogeneous groups of depressed patients as delivered by clinicians in a multitude of treatment settings.

Barlow and Lehman (page 727) review the recent "explosive" growth in effective psychosocial treatments for anxiety disorders. Although these approaches are promising, the authors conclude that much still remains to be learned about how well these approaches will work in the variety of health care settings and how best they can be integrated with effective drug treatments.

McCrady and Langenbucher (page 737) discuss specific, effective case identification and empirically based treatments that have been developed for alcoholism. They conclude that 4 elements of a reformed health care system—universal insurance coverage for alcoholism treatment; early detection and triage in medical, legal, and employment settings; a flexible service mix emphasizing early, brief, outpatient, and intermittent long-term care; and provider incentives to offer sound treatment—will produce substantial economic benefits for alcoholics, their families, and society at large.

Crits-Cristoph and Siqueland (page 749) summarize the findings from studies of psychosocial treatments for drug dependence. The existing data suggest that substance abuse treatment should be intensive, involve multiple treatment approaches to address the variety of problems encountered (eg, employment, financial) by substance abusers, and target coexisting psychiatric problems when they are present. Although the field is new, relapse prevention techniques and community reinforcement approaches for adults, as well as family focused treatments for adolescents with substance dependence, appear promising.

Correction

Incorrect Street Address. In the article, titled "Prevalence of Psychiatric Disorders Among Incarcerated Women: I. Pretrial Jail Detainees," published in the June issue of the ARCHIVES (1996;53:505-512), the address for reprints (p 511) was slightly incorrect. The street number and name should have read "710 N Lake Shore Dr, Suite 900" **not** "750 N Lakeshore Dr, Suite 900."

EDITORIAL

The Contribution of Psychotherapy and Pharmacotherapy Research to National Mental Health Care

Introduction to the Special Series

This Editorial appears in virtually identical form in the current issues of the Journal of Consulting and Clinical Psychology *and the* Archives of General Psychiatry.

THE COLLECTION of psychotherapy and pharmacotherapy articles in this issue represents 1 part of a 2-part series, conjointly published by the *Archives of General Psychiatry* and the *Journal of Consulting and Clinical Psychology*. The idea for this series was conceived when the editors of these 2 journals met at a retreat sponsored by the National Institute of Mental Health for journal editors. One topic of discussion was the then-impending specter of nationalized health care. As editors of behavioral science journals, we found that we shared a common interest in ensuring that any national mental health care program would embody the treatments that have been shown in sound research studies to be effective and efficient. In the intervening time, the press of impending nationalized health care has waned, but our enthusiasm for the issues involved and for this joint project has not. Moreover, these issues assume greater urgency in the current climate of managed care. Thus we offer now, in joint issues of the 2 journals, what we think represents a summary of the current state of empirical knowledge regarding the treatment of 4 major conditions: major depression, anxiety disorders, alcoholism, and other drug abuse.

See also pages 696, 708, 717, 727, 737, and 749

Both journals have published a wide range of articles about treatments for mental illness. The current series presents, for the readership of *Archives of General Psychiatry*, articles that review the role and development of psychotherapeutic research. It is being published under the guest editorship of Larry E. Beutler, PhD, the editor of the *Journal of Consulting and Clinical Psychology*. Concomitantly, the series in the *Journal of Consulting and Clinical Psychology* summarizes the status of biomedical and psychopharmacological research on treatment. It is being published under the guest editorship of Jack D. Barchas, MD, and Peter M. Marzuk, MD, the editor and associate editor, respectively, of the *Archives of General Psychiatry*. We recognize that dividing research on this plane is arbitrary in some ways, and we were reminded of that fact repeatedly when reviewers critiqued articles within each series. We urge the readers of each journal to seek out the other for the complete set.

This publication of a coordinated set of articles in major journals of clinical psychology and psychiatry is to our knowledge unprecedented. We are hopeful that a less obvious agenda underlying this project than that of simply transmitting knowledge across disciplines becomes apparent to the respective audiences. The 3 of us share a common concern about the combative atmosphere that often has characterized the relationships between the disciplines of psychiatry and clinical psychology. While there are many reasons for the struggles that occur between our respective groups, we think that we all share a common interest in developing and advancing the best treatment possible for those who suffer from emotional and behavioral disorders. We also think that the disciplines share a common commitment to ensure that these treatments are founded in good science. With these common values, we believe that many if not most of the differences that separate our disciplines can be overcome by communication among the scientists and practitioners within and between each field. We hope that this coordinated joint publication facilitates this process.

The current series in the *Archives of General Psychiatry* presents a summary of empirical research on psychosocial interventions for each of the 4 areas. The initial 2 articles in this series are designed to acquaint the reader, who may be unfamiliar with research in this area, with a history of the field and the nature of psychosocial service delivery. Accordingly, the article by Howard et al[1] establishes the nature of mental health service delivery problems. Reviewing epistemological data, these authors emphasize both the importance of mental health problems and the necessity of utilizing the widest array of effective resources that may be available. Emphasizing the broad spectrum of care, they describe the role of both inpatient and outpatient services, routes to treatment, and implications for the distribution of mental health practitioners.

The article by Russell and Orlinsky[2] introduces the converging history of behavioral and psychotherapeutic research on the problems of national health care. These authors summarize the history of research on psychosocial treatments, setting the stage for the subsequent discussions of specific types of disorders. Accordingly, Clarkin et al[3] review the status of empirical research on the psychotherapy of depression. They present a range of treatment models, evidence of the efficacy and differential effectiveness of these treatments, and implications for a comprehensive model of psychotherapy-induced change in depressive disorders.

The presentation on depression is followed by a critical review of research on anxiety disorders. Barlow and Lehman[4] describe the nature of effective treatments for each anxiety disorder as distinguished by the *DSM-IV*. This area of research has provided valuable information that can guide both future research and the application of intervention guidelines to the treatment of anxiety disorders. They emphasize that the contemporary direction of research must both address the need for effectiveness data and seek the means to apply the information we have garnered in health care programs.

McCrady and Langenbucher[5] address the status of psychosocial research in alcoholism. Alcohol abuse, if not the most important of the mental health problems, is certainly the one that affects the most lives. Thus, McCrady and Langenbucher's disclosure that there are effective interventions and assessment procedures available sounds an optimistic note on a condition that is often thought to be beyond the range of effective treatment. This article emphasizes important developments in the initiation of treatments that include marital and family members and address the specific needs of the individuals involved. Indeed, their comments resonate with earlier ones in pointing out the need for services that range in level of intensity and the type of procedures employed to improve the "fit" between treatment and patient.

The article by Crits-Christoph and Siqueland,[6] while being the last in this series, is by no means least in importance. These authors echo, perhaps at a reduced tempo, the optimistic notes set by the preceding papers, that psychosocial interventions offer hope for making real change in the serious problems of substance abuse. They note both the difficulties of retaining and treating individuals with cocaine and opiate abuse problems, but also note several promising directions in which psychotherapies have been helpful. Sounding an important caution to those who might wish to develop managed or nationalized health care policies, they emphasize that substance abuse problems are chronic and require intensive interventions. They also stress the importance of addressing the complexity of individual patterns, comorbid conditions, and personal characteristics. Obviously, effective interventions must focus on the specific needs and behavior patterns of those affected by drug abuse, and make the treatments a better fit to each patient than they have been traditionally.

THE CURRENT SERIES in the *Journal of Consulting and Clinical Psychology* presents a summary of empirical research on pharmacological interventions for each of the 4 areas. In the first article, Wells and Sturm[7] make the important point that drugs that have been deemed efficacious have often been studied in ideal treatment settings. Typically, the patients studied have no major coexisting medical or psychiatric problems, the providers are highly trained specialists, treatment follows specific protocols, and the patients incur no treatment costs. They argue compellingly that to inform the health policy debate more data are needed about how effective pharmacotherapy is when it is provided in the "real" world of usual care. Using data from the Medical Outcomes Study as an example of this problem, they examine differences in the rate of use of antidepressant medications by type of payment and provider specialty, whether antidepressant treatment is effective in improving the functional outcomes of patients treated under prevailing usual care, and whether improving the quality of medication management improves cost-effectiveness. Research in this area is critical as the United States' health care delivery system increasingly relies on prepaid managed care and primary care providers.

In another article, Kupfer and Thase[8] focus on mood disorders, which, if left untreated, have a profound impact on quality of life and economic productivity. They describe the goals of pharmacological interventions during different stages of treatment: acute, continuation, and maintenance phases. They review a wide range of pharmacological treatments including tricyclic antidepressants, monoamine oxidase inhibitors, selective serotonin reuptake inhibitors, and newer drugs such as nefazadone hydrochloride and venlafaxine hydrochloride. In addition, they discuss the role of augmentation strategies for patients refractory to standard treatments and the increasing use of pharmacotherapy in treating persons with chronic forms of depression. They conclude by highlighting some of the limitations of lithium therapy in bipolar disorder and the indications for use of anticonvulsants.

Lydiard et al[9] review the efficacy of pharmacological agents used to treat anxiety disorders. Pharmacological treatments are most established for panic disorder and obsessive-compulsive disorder, but may be useful in social phobia and generalized anxiety disorder. In contrast, only certain symptoms of posttraumatic stress disorder may be responsive to drugs. The authors stress the need to obtain long-term outcome data, to understand the complex role of other disorders that are comorbid with anxiety disorders, to develop new regimens for the treatment of refractory patients, and to conduct further research on therapies that combine pharmacological treatment with behavioral and cognitive approaches.

In separate articles, Schuckit[10] and O'Brien[11] review the postdetoxification pharmacotherapy of alcohol dependence and substance abuse, respectively. Both authors stress that pharmacological interventions are effective in these disorders only if they are part of a comprehensive long-term treatment package that includes behavioral, cognitive, counseling, and rehabilitative procedures.

Schuckit[10] introduces the reader to important issues and caveats involved in evaluating drug trials in alcoholism (and presumably substance abuse). These include the episodic nature of these disorders, marked variability among patients' prognoses, dosages of medications used, the atmosphere in which treatment is provided, and difficulties inherent in assessing outcome. He examines the biological rationale for the development of drugs to treat alcoholism, specifically the effect of these drugs on systems believed to mediate drinking behaviors, such as the opiate, serotonergic, dopaminergic, and γ-aminobutyric acid (GABA) pathways. He concludes that certain drugs such as naltrexone, buspirone hydrochloride, and acamprosate hold promise, but believes that there is currently no justification for their routine use in all patients with alcoholism.

O'Brien[11] stresses the important shift in drug treatment rationale from prior emphasis on tolerance and dependence to loss of control over drug-taking. Pharmacotherapy is particularly helpful in treating patients who have comorbid psychiatric disorders. Treatments are better established to aid in rehabilitating persons with nicotine and opiate dependence than in treating persons with other addictions. He stresses that no treatment has been clearly demonstrated to benefit persons dependent on cocaine, cannabinoids, nonalcoholic sedatives, or hallucinogens.

In conclusion, it should be emphasized that neither set of articles provides the full picture of either research on that disorder or the nature of effective treatments. We think, however, that a more complete picture can be obtained if the 2 series are taken as complementary views of what is known and what can be done to increase the effectiveness of treating these disorders. We hope that the suggestions provided in these series will be taken seriously as representing an opportunity for collaboration among behavioral scientists and clinicians, facilitating knowledge transfer among the professions and the health care industry, and offering some promising directions in which contemporary and evolving health care systems might develop to maximize both cost savings and quality.

Larry E. Beutler, PhD
Editor, Journal of Consulting and Clinical Psychology
Jack D. Barchas, MD
Editor, Archives of General Psychiatry
Peter M. Marzuk, MD
Associate Editor

REFERENCES

1. Howard KI, Cornille TA, Lyons JS, Vessey JT, Lueger RJ, Saunders, SM. Patterns of service utilization. *Arch Gen Psychiatry.* 1996;53:696-703.
2. Russell RL, Orlinsky DE. Psychotherapy research in historical perspective: implications for mental health care policy. *Arch Gen Psychiatry.* 1996;53:708-715.
3. Clarkin JF, Pilkonis PA, Magruder KM. Psychotherapy of depression: implications for reform of the health care system. *Arch Gen Psychiatry.* 1996;53:717-723.
4. Barlow DH, Lehman C. Advances in the psychosocial treatment of anxiety disorders: implications for national health care. *Arch Gen Psychiatry.* 1996;53:727-735.
5. McCrady BS, Langenbucher JW. Alcohol treatment and health care reform. *Arch Gen Psychiatry.* 1996;53:737-746.
6. Crits-Cristoph P, Siqueland L. Psychosocial treatment for drug abuse: selected review and recommendations for national health care. *Arch Gen Psychiatry.* 1996;53:749-756.
7. Wells KB, Sturm R. Informing the policy process: from efficacy to effectiveness data on pharmacotherapy. *J Consult Clin Psychol.* 1996;64:638-645.
8. Kupfer DJ, Thase ME. Recent developments in the pharmacology of mood disorders. *J Consult Clin Psychol.* 1996;64:646-659.
9. Lydiard RB, Brawman-Mintzer O, Ballenger JC. Recent developments in the psychopharmacology of anxiety disorders. *J Consult Clin Psychol.* 1996;64:660-668.
10. Schuckit MA. Recent developments in the pharmacotherapy of alcohol dependence. *J Consult Clin Psychol.* 1996;64:669-676.
11. O'Brien CP. Psychopharmacology of substance abuse. *J Consult Clin Psychol.* 1996;64:677-686.

Announcement

Free Patient Record Forms Available

Patient record forms are available free of charge to ARCHIVES readers by calling or writing FORMEDIC, 12D Worlds Fair Dr, Somerset, NJ 08873-9863, telephone (908) 469-7031.

Relapse Prevention by Acamprosate

Results From a Placebo-Controlled Study on Alcohol Dependence

Henning Sass, MD; Michael Soyka, MD; Karl Mann, MD; Walter Zieglgänsberger, MD

Background: The effectiveness of acamprosate (calcium bisacetylhomotaurinate) as a treatment to maintain abstinence in alcohol-dependent patients was assessed for 1 year.

Methods: After short-term detoxification, 272 patients participated in a randomized, double-blind, placebo-controlled study. Patients received routine counseling and either the study medication or placebo for 48 weeks; they were followed up for another 48 weeks without medication. Statistical analysis was performed according to the intention-to-treat principle.

Results: Patients who were receiving acamprosate showed a significantly higher continuous abstinence rate within the first 60 days of treatment compared with patients who were assigned to placebo treatment (67% vs 50%) until completion of the treatment period (43% vs 21%, log rank $P=.005$), and they had a significantly longer mean abstinence duration of 224 vs 163 days, or 62% vs 45% days abstinent ($P<.001$); however, there was no difference in psychiatric symptoms. Of the patients who were receiving acamprosate, 41% had dropped out, whereas 60% of the placebo-treated patients dropped out of the study. Few side effects (mainly diarrhea and headache) were recorded. At the end of a further 48 weeks without receiving study medication, 39% and 17% of the acamprosate- and placebo-treated patients, respectively, had remained abstinent ($P=.003$).

Conclusion: Acamprosate proved to be a safe and effective aid in treating alcohol-dependent patients and in maintaining the abstinence of patients during 2 years.

Arch Gen Psychiatry. 1996;53:673-680

From the Psychiatric Clinic, Rheinisch Westfälische Technische Hochschule, Aachen, Germany (Dr Sass); the Psychiatric Hospital, University of Munich (Germany) (Dr Soyka); the Department of Psychiatry, University of Tübingen (Germany) (Dr Mann); and the Max Planck–Institute of Psychiatry, Munich (Dr Zieglgänsberger). Members of the Prevention of Relapse With Acamprosate in the Management of Alcoholism Study Group appears on page 679.

VARIOUS STUDIES have focused on those neurotransmitter and receptor systems that may be implicated in the development of alcohol tolerance and dependence. Research into the interaction of ethanol with dopaminergic,[1] serotonergic,[2] and γ-aminobutyric acid–ergic (GABAergic) systems and glutamate–*N*-methyl-D-aspartate[3] and opiate receptors has opened up new approaches into the pharmacotherapy for alcoholism. Efforts to increase the abstinence rate in alcoholic patients by using benzodiazepines[4] or lithium carbonate[5] have had limited success, but serotonin (5-hydroxytryptamine) reuptake inhibitors[6-8] and naltrexone[9,10] have yielded more promising results. More recent studies show that acetyl-3-aminopropanesulfonic acid as calcium bisacetylhomotaurinate (acamprosate) was found to suppress alcohol intake[11] in animal studies without an alteration in alcohol toxicity.[12]

Acamprosate is an analogue of homocysteic acid, which is the structural analogue of L-glutamic acid in which the carboxyl group is substituted by a sulfonyl group. Homocysteic acid meets most criteria for an endogenous ligand that is active at the *N*-methyl-D-aspartate receptor.[13] The finding that acamprosate showed affinity for both $GABA_A$ and $GABA_B$ receptors[14] in some in vitro preparations was previously interpreted as evidence for an involvement of GABAergic mechanisms in the action of acamprosate.[14-17] Furthermore, some previous findings pointed at a possible opiate antagonistic action.[18] However, more recent studies suggest that acamprosate lowers neuronal excitability by reducing the postsynaptic efficacy of excitatory amino acid (EAA) neurotransmitters and not by enhancement of GABAergic inhibition; it has been shown to

See Patients and Methods on next page

PATIENTS AND METHODS

Two hundred seventy-two newly detoxified alcohol-dependent patients (136 in each group) who were recruited from 12 centers in Germany gave their informed consent to take part in a randomized, double-blind, placebo-controlled study (total duration: 96 weeks, with a 48-week treatment [acamprosate or placebo] phase and a subsequent 48-week posttreatment follow-up). All centers were psychiatric outpatient clinics; most of these clinics had specialized alcohol treatment facilities. Two centers included less than 10 patients, 8 centers included between 10 and 30 patients, and 2 centers included more than 30 patients. Sealed envelope randomization with balance by blocks of 8 (4 per study medication) was used to obtain equal numbers per treatment group at each center. Assessors from the different centers had a common training before the study commenced. A patient may have been assessed by different assessors at different occasions. The study protocol was reviewed and approved by the local ethics committees.

Screening included medical, alcohol, and drug histories and various other instruments, including neuropsychological testing. All patients met at least 5 *DSM-III-R* criteria for alcohol dependence and were alcohol-dependent according to the Munich Alcoholism Test.[26] A family history (first-degree biological relative) was obtained from the patient, not from structured interviews or family members. Patients with mental or psychiatric impairment or disease that required psychotropic medication or a stay in a psychiatric clinic, multiple-drug misuse, or severe neurological or physical disorders (eg, liver cirrhosis, hyperparathyroidism) were excluded.

Patients had to be completely abstinent from any alcohol consumption for a minimum of 14 days and a maximum of 28 days and free of withdrawal symptoms before they could be admitted into the study. This period corresponded with the inpatient detoxification therapy period that included pharmacotherapy (mainly clomethiazole or benzodiazepines).

Treatment consisted of counseling or psychotherapy according to the routine practices of the participating centers, to which blinded study medication or placebo was added as adjuvant therapy. Hence, the counseling and psychotherapy were not standardized between centers, maintaining the naturalistic approach of the study design; however, for each center, all patients received similar therapy. Supportive group or individual therapy of a behavioral rather than a dynamic approach, with a mean frequency of once per week and a mean duration of 1 hour per session, was given during a mean duration of 18 weeks. Thereafter, patients joined contact groups that met once every 2 weeks for the remaining period of treatment.

At inception of this study, 2 completed acamprosate trials had used between 1332 and 2500 mg/d according to body weight.[17,23] In this study, medication comprised tablets that either contained 333 mg of acamprosate or placebo of an identical appearance; these tablets were dispensed throughout 48 weeks as follows: body weight (≥60 kg), 1998 mg/d as 2 tablets 3 times daily; body weight (<60 kg), 1332 mg/d as 4 tablets (2 tablets in the morning, 1 at midday, and 1 in the evening). Because of previously reported gastric side effects (mainly diarrhea, gastric colic, or nausea), physicians could reduce the dosage from 6 to 4 tablets per day if adverse events occurred. In the absence of described withdrawal symptoms, study medication was abruptly stopped after the treatment phase without any tapering of dosage. The use of concomitant

attenuate postsynaptic activity of EAA agonists in neocortical neurons, indicating a potential for modifying the behavioral manifestation that may be associated with alcohol intoxication.[19-21]

In pharmacological studies in animals, acamprosate has been shown to be devoid of hypnotic, anxiolytic, or muscle relaxant properties that distinguish it from barbiturates and benzodiazepines. There is no evidence of any antidepressant or other psychotropic effect (W. M. Herrmann, MD, unpublished data, January 1990). In trials that involved detoxified alcoholic patients,[17,22-24] acamprosate treatment was associated with a decrease in alcohol consumption. These and other published studies[8-10] have been of 3 to 6 months' duration when relapse from abstinence is most frequent.[25] Alcohol-drinking behavior in such trials typically defines a relapse in terms of the time to resumption of clinically significant drinking.[9,10,17,24] This trial combined naturalistic principles to classical experimental design in a large, long-term, comparative study during 2 years.[25]

RESULTS

The mean age in the placebo-treated group (109 males and 27 females) was 40.5 years (range, 21-65 years); in the active medication–treated group (102 males and 34 females), 41.9 years (range, 21-58 years). Statistical analysis of the demographical characteristics did not reveal any departure from homogeneity between the treatment groups (Table 1). The baseline mean scores for variables that were related to alcoholism were similar between treatment groups (**Table 3**), except for 2 variables: the mean GGT level, which was lower in the active medication–treated group ($P=.008$), and the level of education, which was higher in the placebo-treated group ($P=.03$). A family history of alcoholism—less in the acamprosate-treated group—approached statistical significance ($P=.06$).

TREATMENT PERIOD

Of 272 patients, 134 (49.3%) remained in the study after 1 year. Fifty-seven patients who were being treated with acamprosate (41.9%) and 81 patients who were receiving placebo (59.6%) were withdrawn (χ^2, $P=.01$, **Table 4**). For 8 of the 9 recorded reasons for dropout, the difference between the 2 treatment groups was not more than 1.6%. The only significant difference was owing to 45 placebo-treated patients (33.1%) and 20 acamprosate-treated patients (14.7%) who were "unwilling to continue" treatment. Of them, 30 (67%) of the 45 patients who were receving placebo and 8 (40%) of the 20 patients who were taking acamprosate had recorded relapse events at some time point before withdrawal from psychotropic medication (antidepressants, neuroleptics, benzodiazepines, barbiturates) or other medications (eg, disulfiram or clomethiazole) was not permitted. If the necessity for short-term administration (<3 days) arose, it was recorded, and if for longer, patients were withdrawn.

The investigators assessed the patients 10 times during the trial: every 4 weeks for the first 12 weeks and thereafter every 12 weeks. One week of extra study medication was provided for late appointments. A patient's declaration of drinking behavior was verified by the results of a Breathalyzer test and γ-glutamyltransferase (GGT) levels in every case, and by interviewing a family member if possible (**Table 1**). A GGT level of twice the upper limit of normal was considered as suggestive of a relapse. To be considered abstinent, these criteria and the physicians' own impression had to be concordant. If not, patients were deemed to be nonabstinent.

The primary outcome criteria was based on absolute abstinence, which was defined as no alcohol consumption and assessed by the time to the first drink, continuous abstinence, abstinent-relapse rates at individual visits, and cumulative abstinence duration (CAD). Duration of the relapse was a secondary criterion; it was recorded as a drinking period that lasted less than 24 hours or 24 to 72 hours or as a "continuous" drinking period that lasted more than 72 hours. Patients who missed a visit but returned for the subsequent visit were allowed to continue in the protocol; however, they were deemed to be nonabstinent for the missed visit (the worst-case scenario presumed for missing data). When patients skipped a visit or dropped out, they, their family, or their general practitioner were contacted by telephone or in writing to obtain reasons for absence, information on drinking behavior, and attempted returns to the treatment program.

Other assessments included aspartate and alanine aminotransferase levels, the mean erythrocyte volume, and the carbohydrate-deficient transferrin level by using a radioimmunoassay technique. Craving was measured by a 200-mm visual analogue scale that ranged from no desire (0) to an uncontrollable desire (200); this scale was completed by the patient in the presence of the physician. Compliance with medication was measured by urinalysis of acamprosate levels and by counting the tablets that were returned.

Statistical analysis (significance level, 5%) primarily followed the intention-to-treat (ITT) principle,[27] which considers any randomized patient who took at least 1 dose of the trial medication as eligible for the analysis[28]; however, per protocol (receiving treatment) analysis was also done. Patients who missed a visit or were withdrawn from the study were deemed to be nonabstinent for the time that data were not available; however, for comparison, an additional analysis that considered missing data as missing was also performed on the drinking data at each visit (**Table 2**). The main criterion (the time from commencement of study therapy until the first drink) was analyzed by life-table and Kaplan-Meier survival analysis, censoring missing data (log rank test). Cross-tabulations of drinking behavior was tested by the χ^2 test. The total number of days that a patient was free of alcohol was calculated as the CAD[28] and the percent abstinent days. For this, the denominator was the actual duration of treatment that, owing to public holidays and late appointments, was approximately 22 days longer than the prescribed protocol time of 48 weeks for the treatment period and 96 weeks for the total period. For early withdrawals, the period after withdrawal was considered as one of nonabstinence. The Wilcoxon-Mann-Whitney *U* test was used because of the pronounced top-and-bottom effects of the data that rendered *t* tests inadequate.

the study. Therefore, it appears that the 17.7% differential attrition across the treatment cells was mainly owing to 16.2% more patients being treated with placebo than with acamprosate who relapsed and withdrew. Seven acamprosate-treated patients and 5 placebo-treated patients were rehospitalized for a second detoxification period and were withdrawn for this reason. More than 50% of patients who were not attending visits could be reached by telephone to obtain information on their drinking behavior.

Determination of the GGT levels was done on equal percentages (91%-100%, depending on the visit) of patients in the 2 treatment groups. Despite the difference in the mean values for the GGT levels between treatment groups, the number of individual patients who had GGT values above the normal reference range corresponded closely with the number of patients who had relapses, except for the first visit at 4 weeks after detoxification, when many GGT values did not normalize yet. After that, 81% to 100% of patients who self-reported relapses had GGT values above normal, without a statistical difference between treatment groups. However, the percentage of patients who had GGT values above the protocol-stipulated threshold of twice the upper limit of normal was much smaller; however, this was also equally distributed between treatment groups: 51% of acamprosate-treated patients and 47% of placebo-treated patients who had relapses had values above twice the upper limit of normal. Family declarations on drinking behavior were obtained in only 30% to 41% of recorded patient assessments. The Breathalyzer test never identified an undeclared relapse. The biggest difference between the number of self-reports of relapse and the number based on self-reports plus the additional criteria (GGT values, family interviews, and Breathalyzer test results combined) was 4 patients in the acamprosate-treated group at the 24-week visit, when 23 patients self-reported drinking but 27 were considered to have had a relapse. During the entire treatment period, 22 additional relapse recordings were made that were not self-reports: 10 for patients who were being treated with acamprosate and 12 for patients who were receiving placebo, without a statistical difference between groups.

ABSOLUTE ABSTINENCE

Time to First Relapse

During the first 60 days, a difference developed between the 2 groups; this difference led to an earlier relapse rate in the placebo-treated group (**Figure**). Throughout the 48-week treatment period, the mean±SD number of days to the first relapse was 165.2±143.8 days (median, 131 days) in the acamprosate-treated group and

Table 1. Baseline Demographical Data*

Variable	Treatment: Placebo (n=136)	Treatment: Acamprosate (n=136)
Mean±		
Age, y	40.5±8.6	41.9±8.4
Weight, kg	73.9±13	72.3±12
No. (%) of patients		
Sex		
M	109 (80)	102 (75)
F	27 (20)	34 (25)
Civil status		
Single	34 (25)	36 (26)
Married	67 (50)	58 (43)
Divorced	32 (24)	39 (29)
Widowed	3 (2)	3 (2)
Living status		
Alone	46 (34)	57 (42)
With companion	90 (66)	79 (58)
Employment status		
Unemployed	37 (27)	35 (26)
Laborer	44 (32)	42 (31)
Employee	37 (27)	38 (28)
Self-employed	11 (8)	9 (7)
Other	7 (6)	12 (8)

*None of the variables were statistically significantly different between treatment groups.

112.3±126.5 days (median, 45 days) in the placebo-treated group. At the end of the treatment period, 44.8% of the patients who completed treatment in the acamprosate-treated group and 25.3% in the placebo-treated group had never had a relapse; this yielded a statistically significant difference in both the ITT sample (log rank P=.005) and the per protocol sample (log rank P=.009).

Relapse Rate per Visit

Since the above method does not detect abstinent periods after a first relapse, relapse rates for periods between subsequent visits were recorded at each visit. For example, the ITT and per protocol results for the first and last assessments on study medication are shown in Table 2 (top, at week 4; bottom, at week 48). Two different ITT approaches were used: one considered missing values as missing (χ^2 value "i"), and the other considered missing values as treatment "failures" together with relapses (χ^2 "ii"). At the last visit with the patients receiving medication, 43% of the acamprosate-treated patients and 21% of the placebo-treated patients (ITT sample, P=.001) and 78% and 55%, respectively, of the per protocol sample (P=.01) were abstinent.

Total Duration of All Abstinent Periods

The CAD is the total number of abstinent days and could equally be expressed as the percentage of days that a patient received treatment. During the 48 weeks of treatment, in the ITT analysis, the mean±SD CAD in the acamprosate-treated group was 224.62±136.61 days (median, 270 days) or 62.4% days abstinent; this was significantly more than the 162.03±132.19 days (median, 135 days) or 45.3% days abstinent in the placebo-treatd group (P=.001). The per protocol sample yielded values of 209.71 and 150.93 days, respectively (P=.001), for the acamprosate- and placebo-treated groups.

Table 2. Patients Who Had Relapses or Who Were Abstinent or Missing During the First 4 Weeks and Last 12 Weeks While They Were Receiving Study Medication*

Category	ITT Sample†: Acamprosate	ITT Sample†: Placebo	Per Protocol Sample‡: Acamprosate	Per Protocol Sample‡: Placebo
First 4 Weeks				
Abstinence	98 (72)	83 (61)	98 (82)	82 (71)
Relapse	22 (16)	33 (24)	21 (18)	33 (29)
Missing	16 (12)	20 (15)	0	0
Last 12 Weeks				
Abstinence	58 (43)	28 (21)	50 (78)	26 (55)
Relapse	21 (15)	27 (20)	14 (22)	21 (45)
Missing	57 (42)	80 (59)	0	0

*ITT indicates intention to treat. Data are given as the number (percentage) of patients. For the ITT sample, findings from χ^2 analysis were as follows: first 4 weeks, P=.14 (statistical testing performed on 3 categories of abstinence, relapse, and missing) and P=.05 (statistical testing performed on 2 categories of success or failure [success=abstinence, failure=relapse+missing]); last 12 weeks, P=.001 (statistical testing performed on 3 categories of abstinence, relapse, and missing) and P<.001 (statistical testing performed on 2 categories of success or failure [success=abstinence, failure=relapse+missing]). For the per protocol sample, findings from χ^2 analysis were as follows: first 4 weeks, P=.05; last 12 weeks, P=.01.

†For the ITT sample, the numbers of patients were as follows: first 4 and last 12 weeks, N=272 (acamprosate treatment [n=136] and placebo treatment [n=136]).

‡For the per protocol sample, the numbers of patients were as follows: first 4 weeks, N=234 (acamprosate treatment [n=119] and placebo treatment [n=115]); last 12 weeks, N=111 (acamprosate treatment [64] and placebo treatment [n=47]).

Duration of Individual Relapses

More patients with short-term relapses (<24 hours) were recorded at the early visits, and more patients with long-term relapses (>72 hours) were found at the later visits (**Table 5**). A higher frequency of continuous relapse was observed in the placebo-treated group at the 4-, 8-, and 36-week visits; it was statistically significant at week 8 and near significance at week 24.

Linear Regression Analysis

Findings from a linear regression analysis confirmed no significant effect of age, sex, level of education, marital status, living alone or not, a family history of alcoholism, the duration of alcoholism, and a baseline GGT value on the main criteria. The influence of the 3 baseline inhomogeneities on the main outcome criterion was also analyzed individually, but no statistically significant effect on outcome was seen.

Other Outcome Measures

Because of the high dropout rate, the sample sizes were small at the end of the treatment period. The mean±SD

Table 3. Baseline Data Relating to Diagnosis and History of Alcoholism*

Variable	Treatment: Placebo (n=136)	Treatment: Acamprosate (n=136)
Score (maximum, 9), *DSM-III-R*†	7.92±1.17	1.78±1.28
VAS score (0-200 mm), craving†	87.63±47.64	85.88±50.05
No. of previous detoxifying treatments‡		
None	42 (31)	40 (29)
1-2	58 (43)	61 (44)
3-4	20 (15)	17 (12)
≥5	16 (11)	18 (15)
Duration of alcoholism, y†	10.36±6.60	10.44±5.77
Last daily intake before detoxification†		
Intake, mL/d	284.38±146.64	271.55±147.48
Intake, g/d	227.50±117.31	217.24±117.98
Family history of alcoholism‡§		
No	98 (72)	111 (82)
Yes	38 (28)	25 (18)
Education‡§		
No school certificate	2 (2)	1 (1)
Special school	4 (3)	2 (2)
Grammar school	21 (15)	13 (9)
Junior secondary	58 (43)	85 (62)
Senior secondary	51 (37)	35 (26)
Level		
GGT, IU/L†; patients with values above normal‡§	89.48±118.28; 90 (66)	62.58±92.69; 69 (51)
MCV, fL†; patients with values above normal‡	96.71±5.44; 47 (35)	96.38±5.31; 43 (32)
CDT, IU/L†	20.54±10.53	20.83±13.58

**VAS indicates visual analogue scale; GGT, γ-glutamyltransferase; MCV, mean corpuscular volume; and CDT, carbohydrate-deficient transferrin.*

†Data are given as the mean±SD.

‡Data are given as the number (percentage) of patients.

§No statistically significant differences were identified for any of these variables, except for near significance for family history (P=.06), and significance for the level of education (P=.03), and the GGT level (P=.008).

Table 4. Reasons for Dropout

Termination Status	Treatment, No. (%) of Patients: Placebo (n=136)	Treatment, No. (%) of Patients: Acamprosate (n=136)
Reason for early termination		
Severe adverse event	1 (0.7)	2 (1.5)
Concurrent illness	1 (0.7)	0
Death	1 (0.7)	2 (1.5)
Rehospitalization for relapse	5 (3.7)	7 (5.1)
Unavailable for follow-up	28 (20.6)	26 (19.1)
Unwilling to continue	45 (33.1)	20 (14.7)
Noncompliance	0	0
Concomitant medication	0	0
Other protocol violation	0	0
Subtotal of dropouts	**81** (59.6)	**57** (41.9)
Patients with normal termination	55 (40.4)	79 (58.1)
Total	**136 (100)**	**136 (100)**

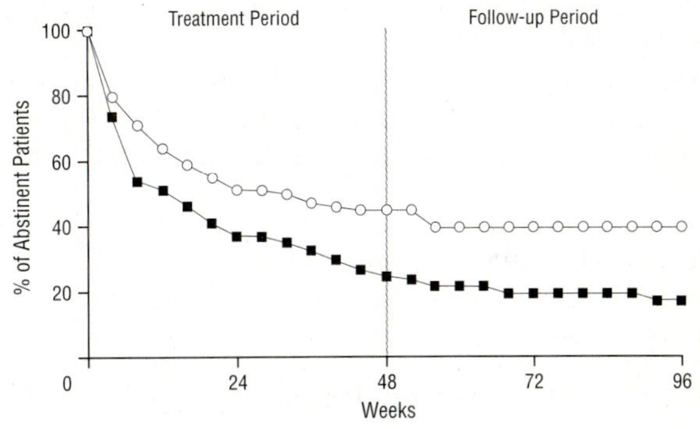

Kaplan-Meier survival analysis (survival function estimate). Continuous abstinence for the treatment and follow-up periods. Curve with open circles indicates acamprosate treatment; curve with shaded squares, placebo treatment.

GGT values at week 48 were 26±32 U/L (median, 16 U/L [n=75]) in the acamprosate-treated group and 49±75 U/L (median, 27 U/L [n=49]) in the placebo-treated group; however, a difference was already present at baseline. The mean±SD carbohydrate-deficient transferrin at week 48 in the acamprosate-treated group was 16.14±11.56 U/L (median, 13.05 U/L [n=59]), and in the placebo-treated group, 21.28±18.79 U/L (median, 15.15 U/L [n=46]), without a significant difference between groups (*P*=.10). The mean±SD corpuscular volume was 90.59±4.8 fL (n=76) in the acamprosate-treated group, and 91.67±5.7 fL (n=51) in the placebo-treated group (*P*=.25). The visual analogue scale for craving showed a wide variability and did not correlate with drinking behavior. After 48 weeks, the mean±SD score for the acamprosate-treated group was 65.3±41.6 mm (n=78), and for the placebo-treated group, 70.6±38.5 mm (n=54), without a significant difference. During the first month of treatment, 20% of the patients who were receiving acamprosate and 29% of the patients who were receiving placebo attended Alcoholics Anonymous meetings and, at the last visit, 14% and 13%, respectively, attended Alcoholics Anonymous meetings, without a significant difference between the groups. Urinalysis for acamprosate indicated the presence of acamprosate in 82% of the patients who abstained and in 67% of the patients who had relapses. The pill count of returned boxes showed only 3% to 6% of boxes with more tablets returned than were expected by the prescribed dosage, without a statistical difference between groups.

FOLLOW-UP PERIOD

After termination of study medication, 134 patients entered the 48-week follow-up period: 79 acamprosate-treated patients and 55 placebo-treated patients. Of them, a further 13 patients who were taking acamprosate and 17 who were receiving placebo dropped out during the second year; this left 104 patients to complete the entire 96-week period (66 acamprosate-treated patients and 38 placebo-treated patients).

On the life table, the progression in the 2 groups appeared to be similar: 5% to 6% of the patients in each group had relapses during the second year (Figure). No rebound phenomenon was noted after cessation of therapy

Table 5. Duration of Individual Relapse Episodes*

Weeks	Drug Treatment	Duration of Relapse Episode <24 h	24-72 h	Continuous
4	Acamprosate	50	30	20
	Placebo	47	17	37
8	Acamprosate	55	40	5
	Placebo	35	21	45
12	Acamprosate	25	40	35
	Placebo	29	33	38
24	Acamprosate	26	39	35
	Placebo	31	31	39
36	Acamprosate	27	35	39
	Placebo	23	9	68
48	Acamprosate	5	48	48
	Placebo	20	36	44

**No statistically significant differences between treatment groups were demonstrated. Data are given as the percentages of patients who had relapses at each visit.*

with acamprosate. At the end of the follow-up period, 39.9% of the remaining patients who were taking acamprosate and 17.3% of the patients who were receiving placebo had never had a relapse (log rank $P=.003$). The mean±SD CAD for the 2-year period was 387.14±280.52 days (median, 405 days), or 54% abstinent days, in the acamprosate-treated group; in the placebo-treated group, the mean±SD CAD was 250.95±244.63 days (median, 136 days), or 35% abstinent days (ITT, $P<.001$).

ADVERSE EVENTS

Adverse symptoms were reported most frequently during the first 4 weeks of medication and were evenly distributed between the 2 treatment groups: 41 in each group, of which 15 adverse events were rated as severe (acamprosate-treated group, 8; placebo-treated group, 7). The severe adverse events in the acamprosate-treated group were 2 cases of depression, 2 cases of tiredness, 1 case each of gastric hemorrhage, abdominal discomfort, myocardial infarction, and dislocated shoulder. Diarrhea and headache were the most frequently reported adverse effects: 10 patients of the acamprosate-treated group and 11 of the placebo-treated group reported mild or moderate diarrhea, and 7 of the acamprosate-treated patients compared with 9 placebo-treated patients reported mild or moderate headaches. Five percent of patients had a dose reduction of study medication because of adverse events, without a significant difference between treatment groups. Two patients (1 in each treatment group) committed suicide by hanging. No psychotropic adverse events of any significance and no withdrawal symptoms after cessation of the study medication were recorded.

COMMENT

Previous studies throughout periods of up to 3 months have reported lower relapse rates in alcoholic patients who were treated with acamprosate.[22-24] The present data during 2 years are consistent with these results and show better relapse control and retention in the study in detoxified alcohol-dependent patients who received acamprosate from the early postweaning phase. The difference between the 2 treatments developed during the treatment interval from 30 to 90 days; however, it was sustained for the remainder of the dosing phase and the following 1-year follow-up period without study medication. Acamprosate appeared to be well tolerated and without signs of psychotropic side effects or potential for abuse or dependence.

Differential attrition occurred between treatment groups. This complicated the interpretation of the data; however, it also suggested better retention as a potential treatment effect of the study medication, and seemed to be supportive of findings from previous studies that showed that compliance might be considered a valid predictor of treatment outcome.[29] The difference in the patient retention rate is predominantly owing to 16.2% of the patients in the placebo-treated group who were unwilling to continue further treatment, after they had had earlier relapse episodes (Table 4). There were 24 more acamprosate-treated patients (17 in the per protocol sample) who reached the end of the treatment medication phase. Hence, it was decided to determine whether the better outcome in the acamprosate-treated group was related to a specific relapse prevention effect of the drug or to a nonspecific benefit due to longer participation in a supportive treatment program.

If the latter positive retention effect was the only or primary effect, the number of patients who completed the study and who abstained would be bigger in the acamprosate-treated group than in the placebo-treated group; however, the abstinent rate would be the same for both. However, the abstinent rates in the acamprosate- and placebo-treated groups were 78% and 55%, respectively; these rates suggested a relapse prevention effect, not as a result of but probably contributing to the retention effect. Furthermore, retention rate is not expected to influence the time to the first relapse and CAD. The median time to the first relapse was 131 days with acamprosate treatment and 45 days with placebo treatment, and after the 1-year treatment, 45% of retained patients who were receiving acamprosate had never had a relapse compared with 25% of the placebo-treated patients. The mean CAD was 62 days longer in the acamprosate-treated group, and data on the duration of individual relapses showed that a higher percentage of the placebo-treated patients had a continuous relapse during the first 8 weeks.

The difference in abstinence rates remained significant during the 48-week follow-up period, with a drop of 5% to 6% in both groups, and no rebound phenomenon was noted. This could suggest that at or before termination of study medication, the conditions of the patients were sufficiently stabilized to control possible rebound relapse. Another hypothesis is that the pharmacodynamic effect or the need for acamprosate could have diminished over time, as neurotrans-

Members of the Prevention of Relapse With Acamprosate in the Management of Alcoholism Study Group*

Participating Centers and Investigators

Psychiatric University Clinic, Munich, Germany: H. Hippius, MD; D. Dieterle, MD. **Medical University, Lübeck, Germany:** H. Dilling, MD; T. Wetterling, MD; U. John, MD; R. D. Kanitz, MD; C. Veltrup, MD. **Psychiatric University Clinic, Tübingen, Germany:** M. Büscher, MD; E. Richartz, MD; B. Overberg, MD. **Catholic University, Essen-Borbeck, Germany:** K. D. Segerath, MD; J. Haseke, MD; H. Landefeld, MD. **Psychiatric University Clinic, Hamburg, Germany:** J. Gross, MD; N. Krauss, MD; U. Niedermeyer, MD. **Psychiatric Clinic, Schwerin, Germany:** H. Graf von Keyserlingk, MD; C. Kretschmar, MD; E. Gienke, MD. **Psychiatric Clinic, Eltville, Germany:** S. Haas, MD; H. G. Bialonski, MD. **Psychiatric University Clinic, Münster, Germany:** R. Toelle, MD; G. Buchkremer, MD; T. Poehlke, MD; A. Öskent, MD. **University Clinic, Homburg/Saar, Germany:** B. Ziegler, MD; W. Trabert, MD. **Psychiatric University Clinic, Leipzig, Germany:** R. Weise, MD; T. Kroh, MD. **Psychiatric Clinic, Magdeburg, Germany:** V. Kielstein, MD. **Psychiatric University Clinic, Würzburg, Germany:** J. Böning, MD.

mitters were physiologically adapted to the conditions of prolonged abstinence. Additional clinical studies that assessed particular coping mechanisms or more detailed behavioral aspects might address this question more adequately.

To enhance external validity, Moos and colleagues[30] defended naturalistic trials in alcoholism in which real-life processes were allowed to interfere with treatment. The design of this trial attempted to introduce this concept in a controlled, double-blind, multicenter study. Centers maintained their usual treatment programs and simply added double-blind study medication. Follow-up of dropouts, patient motivation to remain in the trial, and general treatment conditions were not significantly different from the daily routine of the participating alcohol treatment centers.

CERTAIN LIMITATIONS OF THE DESIGN

Certain limitations of this design were encountered: the number of patients included per center was not equal, and there was no standardization of counseling and psychotherapy between centers. Although a biasing influence cannot be completely excluded, the number of patients included by each center was balanced between treatment groups, and in all centers, a treatment effect that favored acamprosate was observed.

OTHER METHODOLOGICAL ISSUES THAT AROSE IN THIS STUDY

The design seemed to be adequate to measure an outcome measure of abstinence defined as no alcohol consumption, but detailed data on the severity of relapses, including the number of drinks per day and the percentage of heavy-drinking days, probably require more close and frequent observations in a more experimental trial design. Furthermore, the relatively low incidence of a positive family history, recorded at baseline assessment, could have been owing to the fact that more rigorous, structured interviews were not used. The markers of alcohol intake (the GGT and mean corpuscular volume values) did not clearly corroborate the acamprosate advantage in the data on consumption. This may be attributed to the growing number of missing values as the year continued, the variability of the individual laboratory tests, and the lack of specificity of absolute GGT and mean corpuscular volume values. All patients were between 2 to 4 weeks abstinent for initial detoxification periods; however, the exact number of days was not recorded, and, accordingly, the influence of individual variation of this period on outcome could not be established. It might be argued that the lower mean GGT value at baseline could have slightly favored the acamprosate-treated group, but statistical analysis could not identify any significant biasing influence. The lack of clinical correlation with GGT values might be partially explained by the high interpatient variability of GGTs and that the other markers, including baseline carbohydrate-deficient transferrin, showed no difference between treatment groups. The higher mean GGT value in the placebo-treated group did not result in more patients who were considered to have a relapse, probably because of the too low sensitivity of the chosen threshold value of twice the upper limit of normal—only approximately 50% of all patients who had relapses had GGT levels above this value. The higher education level in the placebo-treated group might also have influenced the outcome, but statistical analysis could not detect biasing influences due to any of the baseline inhomogeneities.

Animal and human data indicate that EAAs, especially glutamate, play a major role in the development of alcohol dependence and craving.[31-33] Long-term alcohol treatment increases the density of *N*-methyl-D-aspartate receptors and voltage-sensitive Ca^{2+} channels in neurons, whereas $GABA_A$ receptor–mediated actions are reduced.[34-36] These changes provide a plausible explanation for the hyperactivity that is observed during alcohol withdrawal and resembles, in some respects, grand mal seizures.[35] There is evidence that the repeated occurrence of withdrawal seizures leads to a more rapid development of withdrawal and more severe withdrawal syndromes.[36-38]

Acamprosate appears to reduce hyperexcitation from EAAs (eg, glutamate).[19] Neuronal hyperactivity during withdrawal may induce the activation of transcriptional modulators that are encoded by immediate early genes through kindlinglike mechanisms. Acamprosate reduces the expression of transcriptional modulators and alters EAA receptor gene expression in withdrawal and postwithdrawal periods.[38,39] Through such actions, it could counteract the long-lasting changes in latent neuronal hyperexcitability following long-term alcohol abuse.[40] The clinical lack of dependence is in accordance with findings from recent animal experiments that showed that acamprosate, in contrast to the N-methyl-D-aspartate receptor antagonist dizocilpine maleate (MK-801), does not substitute for ethanol or act as a discriminative stimulus.[41]

The features of the ideal pharmacological adjunct to alcoholism treatment are still undefined; Volpicelli et al[10] suggested decreased craving or motivation to drink, prevention or blocking of positive or negative reinforcement when drinking occurs, and freedom from adverse physical and emotional consequences. Future research should investigate whether acamprosate could fulfill these criteria. In our study, it has proved its efficacy in relapse prevention in a comprehensive treatment setting. Other open questions are the ideal starting time and duration of treatment and possible combination with other psychotropic medication.

Accepted for publication January 12, 1996.

The study was sponsored by the Lipha Company, Essen, Germany.

The authors thank Marc Schuckit, MD, Veterans Affairs Medical Center, San Diego, Calif, and Jonathan Chick, MD, Royal Edinburgh (Scotland) Hospital, for their helpful comments in reviewing the text. The statistical analysis was performed by Albrecht Müller, PhD, Medidata GmbH Company, Constance, Germany, and the clinical reporting was done by Adriaan Potgieter, MD. The study was monitored by A. Leibstein, PhD, and K. Wiedey, MD.

Reprints: Henning Sass, MD, Psychiatric Clinic, RWTH, Pauwelsstrasse 30, D-52057 Aachen, Germany.

REFERENCES

1. DiChiara G, Imperato A. Drugs abused by humans preferentially increase synaptic dopamine concentrations in the mesolimbic system of freely moving rats. *Proc Natl Acad Sci U S A.* 1988;85:5274-5278.
2. Engel JA, Enerback C, Fahlke C, Hulthe H, Hard E, Johannssen K, Svensson L, Soderpalm B. Serotonergic and dopaminergic involvement in ethanol intake. In: Naranjo CA, Sellers EM, eds. *Novel Pharmacological Interventions for Alcoholism.* New York, NY: Springer-Verlag NY Inc; 1990:68-82.
3. Lovinger DM, White G, Weight FF. Ethanol inhibits NMDA-activated ion current in hippocampal neurons. *Science.* 1989;243:1721-1724.
4. Nutt D, Adinoff B, Linnoila M. Benzodiazepines in the treatment of alcoholism. In: Galanter M, ed. *Recent Developments in Alcoholism: Treatment Research.* New York, NY: Plenum Press; 1989;7:283-313.
5. Fawcett J, Clark DC, Gibbons RD, Aageson CA, Pisani VD, Tilkin JM, Sellers D, Stutzman D. Evaluation of lithium therapy for alcoholism. *J Clin Psychiatry.* 1984;45:494-499.
6. Jaffe JH, Kranzler HR, Ciraulo DA. Drugs used in the treatment of alcoholism. In: Mendelson JH, Mello NK, eds. *Medical Diagnosis and Treatment of Alcoholism.* New York, NY: McGraw-Hill International Book Co; 1992:421-461.
7. Sellers EM, Higgins GA, Sobell MB. 5-HT and alcohol abuse. *Trends Pharmacol Sci.* 1992;13:69-75.
8. Naranjo CA, Kadlec KE, Sanhueza P, Woodley-Remus D, Sellers EM. Fluoxetine differentially alters alcohol intake and other consummatory behaviors in problem drinkers. *Clin Pharmacol Ther.* 1990;47:490-498.
9. O'Malley SS, Jaffe AJ, Chang G, Schottenfeld RS, Meyer RE, Rounsaville B. Naltrexone and coping skills therapy for alcohol dependence: a controlled study. *Arch Gen Psychiatry.* 1992;49:881-887.
10. Volpicelli JR, Alterman AI, Hayashida M, O'Brien CP. Naltrexone in the treatment of alcohol dependence. *Arch Gen Psychiatry.* 1992;49:876-880.
11. Boismare F, Daoust M, Moore ND, Saligaut C, Lhuintre JP, Chretien P, Durlach J. A homotaurine derivative reduces the voluntary intake of ethanol by rats: are cerebral GABA receptors involved? *Pharmacol Biochem Behav.* 1984;21:787-789.
12. Le Magnen J, Tran G, Durlach J, Martin C. Lack of effects of Ca-acetyl homotaurinate on chronic and acute toxicities of ethanol in rats. *Alcohol.* 1987;4:103-108.
13. Knöpfel TH, Zeise ML, Cuenod M, Zieglgänsberger W. L-Homocysteic acid but not L-glutamate is an endogenous *N*-methyl-D-aspartic acid receptor preferring agonist in rat neocortical neurons in vitro. *Neurosci Lett.* 1987;81:188-192.
14. Chabenat C, Chretien P, Daoust M, Moore ND, Andre D, Lhuintre JP, Saligaut C, Boucly P, Boismare F. Physicochemical, pharmacological and pharmacokinetic study of a new GABAergic compound, calcium acetylhomotaurinate. *Methods Find Exp Clin Pharmacol.* 1988;10:311-317.
15. Daoust M, Lhuintre JP, Saligaut C, Moore ND, Flipo JL, Boismare F. Noradrenaline and GABA brain receptors are co-involved in the voluntary intake of ethanol by rats. *Alcohol Alcohol.* 1987;(suppl 1):319-322.
16. Daoust M, Legrand E, Gewiss M, Heidbreder C, De Witte P, Tran G, Durbin P. Acamprosate modulates synaptosomal GABA transmission in chronically alcoholized rats. *Pharmacol Biochem Behav.* 1992;41:669-674.
17. Lhuintre JP, Daoust M, Moore ND, Chretien P, Saligaut C, Tran G, Boismare F, Hillemand B. Ability of calcium di-acetylhomotaurine, a GABA agonist, to prevent relapse in weaned alcoholics. *Lancet.* 1985;1:1014-1016.
18. Le Magnen J, Tran G, Durlach J, Martin C. Lack of effects of Ca-acetylhomotaurinate on chronic and acute toxicities of ethanol in rats, *Alcohol.* 1987;4:103-108.
19. Zieglgänsberger W, Zeise M. Calcium di-acetylhomotaurinate which prevents relapse in weaned alcoholics decreases the action of excitatory amino acids in neocortical neurons of the rat in vitro. In: Sellers EM, Naranjo CA, eds. *Novel Pharmacological Interventions for Alcoholism.* New York, NY: Springer-Verlag NY Inc; 1992:337-341.
20. Zeise M, Kasparow S, Capogna M, Zieglgänsberger W. Acamprosate (calcium homotaurinate) decreases postsynaptic potentials in the rat neocortex: possible involvement of excitatory amino acid receptors. *Eur J Pharmacol.* 1993;231:47-52.
21. Zeise HL, Madamba SG, Siggins GR, Putske J, Zieglgänsberger W. The anticraving substance acamprosate reduces glutamatergic synaptic transmission and a high-threshold calcium current in neocortical and hippocampal neurons. *Alcohol Clin Exp Res.* 1994;8:2. Abstract.
22. Hillemand B, Lhuintre JP, Steru L, Daoust M, Moore ND. Essai thérapeutique multicentrique du N-bis-acétylhomotaurinate de calcium (Ca Aota) dans le traitement de l'alcoolo-dépendent. *Rev Alcohol.* 1989;34:9-28.
23. Lhuintre JP, Moore ND, Tran G, Steru L, Langrenon S, Daoust M, Parot P, Ladure P, Libert C, Boismare F, Hillemand B. Acamprosate appears to decrease alcohol intake in weaned alcoholics. *Alcohol Alcohol.* 1990;25:613-622.
24. Pelc I, Le Bon O, Verbanck P, Lehert P, Opsomer L. Calcium-acetylhomotaurinate for maintaining abstinence in weaned alcoholic patients: a placebo-controlled double-blind multicenter study. In: Naranjo CA, Sellers EM, eds. *Novel Pharmacological Interventions for Alcoholism.* New York, NY: Springer-Verlag NY Inc; 1992:348-352.
25. Meyer RE. Prospects for a rational pharmacotherapy of alcoholism. *J Clin Psychiatry.* 1989;50:403-412.
26. Feuerlein W, Ringer C, Küfner H, Antons K. Diagnosis of alcoholism: the Munich Alcoholisms Test (MALT). In: Galanter M, ed. *Currents of Alcoholism.* New York, NY: Grune & Stratton; 1980;7:137-147
27. Gillings D, Koch G. The application of the principle of intention to treat to the analysis of clinical trials. *Drug Inform J.* 1991;25:411-424.
28. Lehert P. Review and discussion of statistical analysis of controlled clinical trials in alcoholism. *Alcohol Alcohol.* 1993;(suppl 2):157-163.
29. Fuller RK. Assessment of treatment outcome. *Alcohol Alcohol.* 1991;(suppl 1):519-522.
30. Moos RH, Finney JW, Cronkite RC. *Alcoholism Treatment, Context, Process and Outcome.* New York, NY: Oxford University Press Inc; 1990.
31. Charness ME. Molecular mechanisms of ethanol intoxification, tolerance, and physical dependence. In: Mendelson JH, Mello NK, eds. *Medical Diagnosis and Treatment of Alcoholism.* New York, NY: McGraw-Hill International Book Co; 1992:155-199.
32. Samson HH, Harris RA. Neurobiology of alcohol abuse. *Trends Pharmacol Sci.* 1992;13:206-211.
33. Ollat H, Parvez H, Parvez S. Alcohol and central neurotransmission. *Neurochem Int.* 1988;3:275-300.
34. Littleton JM, Brennan C, Bouchenafa O. The role of calcium flux in the central nervous system actions of ethanol. *Ann N Y Acad Sci.* 1991;625:388-394.
35. Hofman PL, Tabakoff B. The role of the NMDA receptor in ethanol withdrawal. In: Jansson B, Jörnvall J, Rydberg U, Terenius L, Vallee BL, eds. *Towards a Molecular Basis of Alcohol Use and Abuse.* Basel, Switzerland: Birkhäuser Verlag; 1994:61-70.
36. Ballenger JC, Post RM. Kindling as a model for alcohol withdrawal syndromes. *Br J Psychiatry.* 1978;133:1-4.
37. Becker HC, Hale RL. Repeated episodes of ethanol withdrawal potentiate the severity of subsequent withdrawal seizures: an animal model of alcohol withdrawal 'kindling.' *Alcohol Clin Exp Res.* 1993;17:94-98.
38. Grant KA, Valverius P, Hudspith M, Tabakoff B. Ethanol withdrawal seizures and the NMDA-receptor complex. *Eur J Pharmacol.* 1990;176:289-296.
39. Zieglgänsberger W, Hauser C, Putzke J, Spanagel R, Wetzel C. The enhanced excitability of central neurons following chronic alcohol intake is reduced by acamprosate. *Alcohol Alcohol.* 1995;30:C10.22.
40. Littleton J. Acamprosate in alcohol dependence: how does it work? *Addiction.* 1995;90:1179-1188.
41. Spanagel R, Zieglgänsberger W, Hundt W. Acamprosate and alcohol, III: effects on alcohol discrimination. *Eur J Pharmacol.* 1996;305:51-56.

Replication of the Stockholm Adoption Study of Alcoholism

Confirmatory Cross-Fostering Analysis

Sören Sigvardsson, PhD; Michael Bohman, MD; C. Robert Cloninger, MD

Background: Two forms of alcoholism with distinct clinical features and mode of inheritance were first distinguished in the Stockholm Adoption Study. This involved a large sample of children born in Stockholm, Sweden, who were adopted at an early age and reared by nonrelatives. Type 1 alcoholism had adult onset and rapid progression of dependence without criminality, whereas type 2 had teenage onset of recurrent social and legal problems from alcohol abuse.

Methods: A replication study was carried out with 577 men and 660 women born in Gothenburg, Sweden, and adopted at an early age by nonrelatives. The genetic and environmental backgrounds of the adoptees were classified by the exact procedures calibrated by discriminant analysis in the original study.

Results: Both type 2 and severe type 1 alcoholism were confirmed as independently heritable forms of alcoholism in male adoptees. The lifetime risk of severe alcoholism was increased 4-fold in adopted men with both genetic and environmental risk factors characteristic of type 1 alcoholism compared with the others (11.4% vs 3.0%). Neither genetic nor environmental risk factors for type 1 alcoholism by themselves were sufficient to cause alcoholism. In contrast, the risk of type 2 alcoholism was increased 6-fold in adopted sons with a type 2 genetic background compared with others, regardless of their postnatal environment (10.7% vs 2.0%). The sons with a type 2 genetic background in the replication sample had no excess of type 1 alcoholism, and vice versa. There was no increased risk of mild abuse in adopted men regardless of their genetic or environmental background.

Conclusion: Type 1 and type 2 alcoholism are clinically distinct forms of alcoholism with causes that are independent but not mutually exclusive.

Arch Gen Psychiatry. 1996;53:681-687

TWO FORMS of alcoholism with distinct clinical features and modes of inheritance were first distinguished in the Stockholm Adoption Study.[1,2] This subdivision was identified in a large population of consecutive births by means of multivariate methods of classification. The inheritance of alcoholism was studied in 913 Swedish women and 862 Swedish men adopted by nonrelatives at an early age. Lifetime records of alcohol abuse and related behaviors were available for the adoptees and all their biological and adoptive parents. Information about the biological parents and the postnatal environments of the adoptees disclosed clinical and etiological heterogeneity among the alcoholics. Type 1 alcoholism was clinically characterized by adult onset (age of 20 years or older) and rapid progression from mild abuse to severe alcohol dependence with little or no criminality. Type 2 alcoholism was associated with teenage onset of recurrent social and legal problems from alcohol abuse. These 2 forms of alcoholism were initially distinguished in terms of their pattern of inheritance.[1-3] The risk of type 1 alcoholism was increased only when there was a combination of a characteristic genetic background and a characteristic environmental background. Consequently, the average effect of genetic factors on type 1 alcoholism was weak, accounting for 38% of the variability of liability in mild cases and 25% in severe cases. In contrast, the liability to type 2 alcoholism was 90% heritable in men but was seldom expressed in women. The type of alcoholism in the biological parents increased the risk of the same type

From the Department of Social Medicine, University of Umeå, Umeå, Sweden (Drs Sigvardsson and Bohman), and the Departments of Psychiatry and Genetics, Washington University School of Medicine, St Louis, Mo (Dr Cloninger).

See Subjects and Methods on next page

SUBJECTS AND METHODS

SAMPLE AND DESCRIPTIVE DATA

The same sampling and assessment methods used in the original Stockholm Adoption Study[1,2] were applied in this replication study except that the children selected were born elsewhere in Sweden. The replication population includes all children born to single women in Gothenburg, Sweden, from 1930 through 1949 who were adopted at an early age by nonrelatives. No subjects in this study were part of the original Stockholm study. Subjects were excluded because of placement after 3 years of age, placement with relatives, or uncertain paternity, as in the previous work. This yielded a replication sample of 577 adopted men and 660 adopted women. The adoptees ranged in age from 28 to 47 years at the time of last information, which was 1977, as in the original study.

Data about the adoptees and their biological and adoptive background were obtained from multiple sources, as detailed in previous work.[1,3] Briefly, these included (1) data about the ages, occupations, and places of residence of both biological and adoptive parents from a register of child welfare officer appointments; (2) registrations of alcohol abuse, supervision, and treatment of alcoholics as kept by the Temperance Board; (3) registrations for criminal convictions in the criminal register; and (4) registrations about diagnoses and hospitalization as kept by local agencies of the National Health Insurance, as in the Stockholm Adoption Study. Temperance Board registrations for illegal manufacture or sale of alcohol were not considered evidence of alcohol abuse in either the original or the replication study. This multisource method has been estimated to have a sensitivity of 70% and high specificity for alcoholism diagnosed by all sources, including personal psychiatric interviews.[9]

CLASSIFICATION OF THE ADOPTEE'S ALCOHOL ABUSE

Adoptees were classified according to their lifetime record of alcohol abuse in exactly the same manner as defined in the Stockholm Adoption Study based on the clinical studies by Kaij.[7] Adoptees with 4 or more Temperance Board registrations, compulsory treatment, or psychiatric hospitalization with a diagnosis of alcoholism were classified as severe type 1 alcoholics. Adoptees with only a single Temperance Board registration and no treatment were classified as mild type 1 alcoholics. Adoptees with 2 or 3 Temperance Board registrations without treatment for alcoholism were classified as type 2 alcoholics.

CLASSIFICATION OF THE GENETIC AND ENVIRONMENTAL BACKGROUNDS

The genetic background of each adoptee in the replication sample was classified by means of information about the biological parents only and according to the discriminant function derived in original Stockholm population (the calibration sample). The genetic background was classified as type 1 (mild or severe), type 2 (moderate), or neither based on information about the biological parents' alcohol abuse, criminality, and occupational status, as specified in the original report.[1] Briefly, type 1 genetic background was characterized by adult onset of recurrent alcohol abuse with little or no criminality in biological mothers and fathers, whereas type 2 genetic background was characterized by teenage onset of both recurrent criminality and recurrent alcohol abuse in the biological father.

The postnatal environmental background was classified as mild type 1, severe type 1, and type 2 based on information about the adoptive parents and the adoptee's preplacement experiences, as specified in the original report.[1] Briefly, the rearing environment predicted to increase the risk of severe type 1 alcoholism was characterized by the adoptive father having an unskilled occupation. The environment predicted to be associated with mild type 1 alcoholism was characterized by early adoptive placement into a middle-class home. The environment predicted to increase risk of type 2 alcoholism was characterized by little preplacement medical care and late placement in the adoptive home.

STATISTICAL ANALYSES

Discriminant analysis was used to classify both the genetic and environmental backgrounds in accord with the functions derived in previous research.[1] All individuals in the population were assigned to their most probable background group by the Fisher linear classification method. The classification functions were derived (ie, calibrated) in the Stockholm Adoption Study and applied without modification to the replication sample.[24] Version 4.0 of the SPSS program for personal computers was used for discriminant analysis.[24]

Odds ratios (ORs) and their 95% confidence intervals (CIs) were computed by means of PROC FREQ in the SAS computer program, version 6.07.[25] The logit estimate of the 95% CI was computed. The tests of predicted hypotheses were considered confirmed as significant only if their probability of occurring by chance was less than 5%. We report significance levels based on 2-tailed tests, which is conservative in a replication study, but no other observed differences would have been judged significant by 1-tailed tests. Hence, ORs are significantly greater than unity when the lowest point of the 95% CI is greater than 1.0.

of alcoholism and no other forms of psychopathology in their adopted-away children, with 1 exception; type 2 alcoholic fathers increased the risk of somatization disorder, but not alcoholism or other psychopathology, in the daughters.[1-4]

The hypothesis of 2 alcoholic subtypes stimulated widespread interest and was extensively cited for its strengths. One important strength of the study was that the sample was large and based on an entire population of consecutive birth cohorts. In contrast, earlier adoption studies of alcoholism[5,6] involved comparisons of fewer than 100 cases and highly selected controls, and had produced contradictory results that could be attributed to selection artifacts.[3] A second important strength was that the adoptees and all their parents were assessed for their entire lifetime for alcohol abuse by means of systematic records. Third, the classification of alcohol abuse in the adoptees used multiple sources of data that were highly accurate in classifying alcohol abuse. This multisource method was validated by detailed clinical studies, including personal psychiatric interviews.[7-9] Fourth, the genetic and environmental backgrounds were classified by multivariate methods that are statistically efficient and similar to the polythetic criteria approach adopted in modern diagnostic systems beginning with *DSM-III*.[10]

Despite these strengths, the evidence for the hypothesis was criticized in 2 major ways.[11] First, the diagnosis of alcoholism was based on multivariate analysis of registry data, rather than conventional diagnostic criteria for alcoholism based on direct interviews.[12,13] Nevertheless, later clinical studies that used interviews confirmed the validity of the distinction by means of standard diagnostic criteria[14-17] and showed its utility for prediction of individual differences in clinical course,[18] response to treatment,[19] personality,[15,20,21] and neurobiological markers.[21,22]

The second major criticism was that it was implausible, or at least surprising, that qualitatively different types of alcoholics could be distinguished by separating a group of adoptees who were intermediate in severity of alcohol abuse (ie, the type 2 alcoholics with a moderate number of problems) from others who were more extreme in severity (mild type 1 or severe type 1).[11,13] After clinical observations about the relations between registration for problems and clinical diagnosis, the adoptees' alcohol abuse had been divided into subgroups with mild, moderate, and severe problems.[7] An unexpected empirical finding of the Stockholm Adoption Study was that the genetic background of the mild abusers was the same as that of the severe abusers, whereas the moderate abusers had a different genetic background.[1] To explain this unexpected finding, we hypothesized that individuals with a type 1 genetic background, which was characteristic of both mild and severe abusers, were predisposed to progress rapidly from mild to severe alcohol dependence if they continued drinking frequently to relieve anxiety.[21,23] In contrast, we hypothesized, individuals with a type 2 genetic background, which was characteristic of moderate abusers, were predisposed to seek euphoriant stimulation from alcohol, leading to recurrent social problems and only gradual development of severe dependence. Skeptics questioned this hypothesis, but independent clinical studies showed that type 1 alcoholism often progressed rapidly to dependence accompanied by medical complications, such as liver disease. Such progression is characteristic of female alcoholics and male relatives of female alcoholics.[15] The differences between subtypes in course of illness and response to treatment were confirmed in Sweden and the United States.[16-19] Despite this corroborating evidence, the differences in genetic and environmental backgrounds of these groups were questioned as possible artifacts of complex multivariate classification procedures, which always require independent replication before they should be accepted.[11,13]

In this study, we tested the replicability of the original findings and interpretations of the Stockholm Adoption Study by carrying out a strict replication trial. Subjects were selected and classified according to exactly the same procedures as in the original experiment. The findings and conclusions of the original and the replication experiments are presented side by side to facilitate comparison.

Table 1. Inheritance of Susceptibility to Alcohol Abuse in Stockholm and Replication Adoption Studies

Alcohol Abuse in Biological Parents		Alcohol Abuse in Adoptees, No. (%)	
Father	Mother	Stockholm	Replication
		Adopted Men	
No	No	571 (14.7)	469 (12.8)
Yes	No	259 (22.4)*	78 (23.1)*
No	Yes	23 (26.0)*	22 (31.8)*
Yes	Yes	9 (33.3)*	8 (12.5)*
		Adopted Women	
No	No	577 (2.8)	546 (1.1)
Yes	No	285 (3.5)	106 (0.9)
No	Yes	29 (10.3)†	7 (0.0)
Yes	Yes	22 (9.1)†	1 (0.0)

Sons with alcoholic biological parents were more likely than others to abuse alcohol in the Stockholm study (odds ratio, 1.7; 95% confidence interval, 1.2-2.5) and in the replication study (odds ratio, 2.2; 95% confidence interval, 1.3-3.6).

†Daughters with alcoholic biological mothers were more likely than others to abuse alcohol in the Stockholm study (9.8% vs 2.8%; P<.01).

RESULTS

The relationship between any lifetime alcohol abuse in the biological parents and their adopted-away sons is shown in **Table 1** for the original Stockholm study and for the replication sample. According to the Stockholm study, the 291 sons with alcoholic biological parents were more likely than the 571 others to abuse alcohol (23.0% vs 14.7%; OR, 1.7; 95% CI, 1.2-2.5). This prediction was confirmed in the replication sample. The 108 adopted-away sons with at least 1 alcoholic parent had a higher risk of alcohol abuse (24.1%) than the 469 other sons (12.8%), giving an OR in men of 2.2 (95% CI, 1.3-3.6).

The inheritance of lifetime alcohol abuse was also examined in the 660 adopted-away daughters (Table 1). In the Stockholm study, alcohol abuse in only the biological father did not increase the risk of alcohol abuse in the 285 adopted-away daughters compared with the risk in daughters of parents with no abuse (3.5% vs 2.8%). This prediction was confirmed in the replication sample: the 106 adopted-away daughters of alcoholic fathers had no increased risk of alcohol abuse compared with the daughters of 2 nonabusing parents (0.9% vs 1.1%). Furthermore, in the Stockholm study, the daughters of alcoholic mothers were more likely than other daughters to abuse alcohol (9.8% vs 2.8%; $P<.01$). There were too few such daughters (n=8) to test this prediction in the replication sample.

In the Stockholm study, the 99 sons with a type 2 genetic background were more likely to have type 2 abuse than the 763 others (17.2% vs 2.5%; OR, 8.1; 95% CI, 4.1-16.2) but not type 1 abuse (12.1% vs 13.5%; OR, 0.9; 95% CI, 0.5-1.7). Both of these predictions were con-

Table 2. Confirmatory Cross-Fostering Analysis: Risk of Type 2 Alcohol Abuse in 577 Men From Replication Study Classified According to Stockholm Study Discriminant Functions

Type 2 Genetic Background	Type 2 Environmental Background	Stockholm Men			Replication Men		
		No.	% Type 1	% Type 2	No.	% Type 1	% Type 2
No	No	567	14.4	1.9	333	11.4	2.4
No	Yes	196	10.7	4.1	160	10.6	1.3
Yes	No	71	9.9	16.9*	59	16.9	6.8*
Yes	Yes	28	17.9	17.9*	25	8.0	20.0*

Sons with type 2 genetic background were more likely to be type 2 abusers than others in the Stockholm calibration sample (odds ratio, 8.1; 95% confidence interval, 4.1-16.2) and in the replication sample (odds ratio, 5.8; 95% confidence interval, 2.3-14.7).

Table 3. Confirmatory Cross-Fostering Analysis: Severe Type 1 Alcohol Abuse in 577 Men From Replication Study Classified According to Stockholm Study Discriminant Functions

Type 1 Genetic Background	Severe Environmental Background	Stockholm Men		Replication Men	
		No.	% Severe	No.	% Severe
No	No	376	4.3	363	3.0
No	Yes	72	4.2	44	2.3
Yes	No	328	6.7	135	3.0
Yes	Yes	86	11.6*	35	11.4*

Risk was significantly increased compared with all others in the Stockholm study (odds ratio, 2.4; 95% confidence interval, 1.1-4.9) and in the replication study (odds ratio, 4.2; 95% confidence interval, 1.3-13.5).

Table 4. Confirmatory Cross-Fostering Analysis: Mild Type 1 Alcohol Abuse in 577 Men From Replication Study Classified According to Stockholm Study Discriminant Functions

Type 1 Genetic Background	Mild Environmental Background	Stockholm Men		Replication Men	
		No.	% Mild	No.	% Mild
No	No	341	6.7	295	7.8
No	Yes	107	5.6	112	9.8
Yes	No	323	6.5	121	7.4
Yes	Yes	91	15.4*	49	8.2†

Risk was significantly increased compared with all others in the Stockholm study (15.4% vs 6.5%; P<.01), but not in the replication study (8.2% vs 8.1%).

†*Risk was not increased compared with all others in the replication study (8.2% vs 8.1%).*

firmed in the replication sample (**Table 2**). The 84 adopted sons with a type 2 genetic background were more often type 2 abusers than were the 493 others (10.7% vs 2.0%; OR, 5.8; 95% CI, 2.3-14.7). Likewise, the sons with a type 2 genetic background in the replication sample had no excess of type 1 alcoholism (14.3% vs 11.2%; OR, 1.3; 95% CI, 0.7-2.6).

In the Stockholm study, the adopted-away sons were at increased risk for severe type 1 alcoholism only if they had *both* a type 1 genetic background and a severe environmental background (**Table 3**). In the Stockholm study, the risk was significantly increased in those with both genetic and environmental risk compared with all others (11.6% vs 5.3%; OR, 2.4; 95% CI, 1.1-4.9). This prediction was confirmed in the replication study. The risk of severe type 1 alcoholism was increased in the 35 adopted-away men with both genetic and environmental risk factors compared with all others (11.4% vs 3.0%; OR, 4.2; 95% CI, 1.3-13.5).

Likewise, in the Stockholm study, the adopted sons were at increased risk for mild type 1 alcoholism only if they had both a type 1 genetic background and a mild environmental background (**Table 4**). The risk of mild abuse was significantly increased in those with both genetic and environmental risk compared with all others in the Stockholm study (15.4% vs 6.5%; *P*<.01). However, this prediction was *not* confirmed in the replication study. There was no increased risk of mild abuse in the 49 adopted-away men predicted to have both the type 1 genetic background and mild environmental risk based on the Stockholm classification functions (8.2% vs 8.1%).

To understand this discrepancy, the risk of mild type 1, severe type 1, and type 2 alcoholism was examined in detail in those predicted to have a type 1 genetic background according to the Stockholm classification functions. **Table 5** shows that there was the predicted increase in severe type 1 alcoholism and the predicted lack of differences in the risk of type 2 alcoholism. Nevertheless, there was no increase in mild abuse regardless of genetic or environmental background in the replication sample with the use of the original Stockholm classification functions.

This discrepancy might be explained by possible unreliable detection of mild type 1 abuse, which was defined by a single Temperance Board registration. Alternatively, men with type 1 genetic backgrounds in the replication sample may have been influenced by other genetic or environmental factors, leading to severe abuse. To test these possibilities, an exploratory cross-fostering analysis was carried out to identify the genetic and environmental factors that might predict mild type 1 alcoholism in the replication sample. In other words, the weights of the possible explanatory variables were optimized in the replication sample, rather than using the weights estimated in the original study in Stockholm. The classification based on only the replication sample is summarized in **Table 6**. This showed that the measured variables about the

Table 5. Confirmatory Cross-Fostering Analysis: Mild and Severe Type 1 Alcohol Abuse in 577 Men From Replication Study Classified According to Stockholm Study Discriminant Functions

Type 1 Genetic Background	Mild or Severe Environmental Background	Male Adoptees Observed			
		No.	% Mild	% Severe	% Type 2
No	No	251	6.8	2.8	3.6
No	Mild	112	9.8	3.6	4.5
No	Severe	44	13.6	2.3	2.3
Yes	No	86	9.3	1.2	2.3
Yes	Mild	49	8.2	6.1	2.0
Yes	Severe	35	2.9	11.4*	2.9

The 35 men with both genetic and environmental backgrounds were more often severe type 1 abusers than others were.

Table 6. Exploratory Cross-Fostering Analysis: Mild Type 1 Alcohol Abuse in 577 Men From Replication Study

Type 1 Genetic Background	Mild Environmental Background	Male Adoptees Observed	
		a/N*	% Mild Abuse
No	No	41/509	8.1
No	Yes	2/22	9.1
Yes	No	4/45	8.8
Yes	Yes	0/1	0.0

**a denotes number of abusers; N, total number at risk.*

biological and adoptive parents were not predictive of mild abuse in the adopted children, even when they were optimized in the replication sample itself. Essentially, those with a type 1 genetic background in the replication sample were mainly at risk for severe, but not mild, alcoholism.

Besides the type 1 genetic background, the only variable associated with severe abuse in the Stockholm Adoption Study was low occupational status in the adoptive father. In the Stockholm sample, the occupational status of the biological fathers of the type 1 alcoholics did not differ from that of the biological fathers of nonalcoholics. However, among the 46 men with a type 1 genetic background in the replication study, 36 also had at least 1 father (biological and/or adoptive) who was an unskilled laborer (**Table 7**). This difference is noteworthy because the occupational status of adult adoptees was equally correlated with that of their biological father and of their adoptive father ($r=0.12$, $P<.01$), both in the Stockholm study and in the replication study. The confounding of predisposition to both type 1 alcoholism and low occupational status in the replication sample may account for the adopted men with a type 1 genetic background in the replication sample having an increased risk for severe, but not mild, alcoholism.

COMMENT

This is the first time that the distinction between genetic subtypes of any psychiatric disorder has been validated by a strict confirmatory test of an explicit multivariate classification procedure. Specifically, this replication study confirms that type 1 and type 2 alcoholism are clinically distinct forms of alcoholism that are inherited as a consequence of independent processes. In our replication study of adoptees, the original conclusions of the Stockholm Adoption Study[1] about type 2 alcoholism and severe type 1 alcoholism were confirmed. Both type 2 alcoholism and severe type 1 alcoholism were shown to be heritable in male adoptees. Severe alcoholism was shown to result from the combination of a type 1 genetic background and factors predisposing to unskilled occupational status. Neither low social status nor a type 1 genetic background alone was sufficient to cause alcoholism. Other conclusions of the Stockholm Adoption Study about the inheritance of alcoholism in women and mild alcoholism in men could not be tested because of inadequate numbers of subjects with relevant predisposing factors.

There was no excess of type 2 alcoholism in adopted children with type 1 backgrounds, or vice versa, in either the original Stockholm study or this replication study. However, this independence does not mean that type 1 and type 2 alcoholism are discrete and separate diseases. Although there was no *increase* in the risk of type 1 alcoholism in those with backgrounds characteristic of type 2, neither was there a *decrease* in its risk. In fact, given the substantial risk of type 1 alcoholism in the general population, both alcoholic subtypes are expected to occur often in the same families, as shown in Tables 2 and 5.

In this replication study, mild alcohol abuse was not predictably increased in the adopted men regardless of their genetic or environmental backgrounds. The simplest explanation would be that mild alcohol abuse, which is defined by single registrations by the Temperance Board, is not reliably measured or consistently heritable. This is supported by exploratory cross-fostering analysis in the replication sample (Table 6) showing that mild abuse was not significantly predicted by measured information about the biological or adoptive parents, even when variable weights were optimized in the replication sample itself. However, mild abuse was significantly heritable in the adoptees born in Stockholm, who also had a higher prevalence of type 1 alcoholism in their biological parents than adoptees born in Gothenburg. Alternatively, the adopted men with type 1 genetic backgrounds in Gothenburg may have also inherited other characteristics that predisposed them to an increased severity of alcoholism. For example, there are suggestions (see Table 7) in the Gothenburg replication sample that men with a type 1 genetic background were more likely to be lacking in heritable capacity and/or socially mediated opportunities for skilled employment than was observed in those in the Stockholm sample.

In any case, recurrent type 1 or recurrent type 2 alcohol abuse in biological parents was predictive of

Table 7. Interaction of Type 1 Genetic Background With Unskilled Occupational Status of Biological and Adoptive Parents and Risk of Severe Type 1 Abuse in Replication Study

Type 1 Genetic Background	Unskilled Genetic Background	Unskilled Environmental Background	Male Adoptees Observed a/N*		% Severe
No	No	No	5/199		2.5
No	Yes	No	3/197	8/332	2.4
No	No	Yes	1/53		
No	Yes	Yes	4/82		
Yes	No	No	0/10		0.0
Yes	Yes	No	4/19	7/36	19.4†
Yes	No	Yes	1/3		
Yes	Yes	Yes	2/14		

**a denotes number of abusers; N, total number at risk.*

†The 36 sons with type 1 alcoholic background who also had biological and/or adoptive parents who were unskilled workers were more likely to be severe alcoholics than others were (odds ratio, 9.8; 95% confidence interval, 3.6-26.4).

recurrent alcohol abuse of the same type in their adopted-away sons in both the Stockholm and Gothenburg samples. The replication findings strongly demonstrate that type 1 and type 2 alcoholism are influenced by independent, but not mutually exclusive, processes. If type 1 and type 2 alcoholism are not separate diseases, what is meant by our conclusion that they are clinically distinct forms of alcoholism caused by independent neuroadaptive processes? Elsewhere we have shown that the initiation, maintenance, and cessation of drinking and smoking have different causal antecedents. The initiation of drinking at an early age is associated with the heritable temperament traits of high novelty seeking, low harm avoidance, and low reward dependence.[21,26,27] This configuration of temperaments is characteristic of the antisocial temperament type,[28] which is associated with increased risk of type 2 alcoholism,[26] early conduct disorder,[29,30] and adolescent multiple-substance abuse.[31] Such individuals begin and continue drinking alcohol for its euphoriant effects.[18] In contrast, high harm avoidance inhibits the initiation of drinking but increases the risk of becoming dependent after heavy drinking has become frequent.[27] Such individuals with high harm avoidance usually drink alcohol for relief of anxiety, as is characteristic of type 1 alcoholics.

These temperament dimensions have been shown to be independently inherited.[32-34] Accordingly, it was expected and confirmed that all possible combinations of temperament dimensions occur,[28,35,36] providing extensive heterogeneity in the emotional predisposition for drinking and other activities.[27] Harm avoidance and novelty seeking appear to have predominant roles in predisposing to type 1 and type 2 alcoholism, respectively, but interact with other aspects of temperament, character, and the environment in the development of alcoholism and related psychopathology.[37,38] The psychobiology of personality in relation to alcoholic subtypes has been reviewed elsewhere.[39,40]

Some limitations of this study should be considered. Gothenburg is second to Stockholm in population size and was the most comparable available site for a replication study. Nevertheless, less registered alcohol abuse in the biological parents was identified in Gothenburg than in Stockholm, as shown in Table 1. In particular, type 1 alcoholism was much less frequent in parents in Gothenburg (29%) than in those in Stockholm (48%) (Table 4). Also, the adopted women from Gothenburg were more often reared in areas with less alcohol abuse regardless of genetic background than were the women from Stockholm (Table 1). Fortunately, cross-fostering analysis stratifies both the genetic and environmental risk factors so that such differences are taken into account. Cross-fostering analysis minimizes the impact of such distributional differences or selective placement on the observed pattern of inheritance. The replicability of our findings in men encourages future use of multivariate cross-fostering analysis. However, there were too few alcoholic mothers and adopted women in the Gothenburg sample to allow tests of the replicability of findings from the Stockholm Adoption Study about maternal inheritance of alcoholism in women,[4] but the heritability of alcoholism in women has been confirmed in female twins in the United States.[41,42]

In summary, the distinction between type 1 and type 2 alcoholism in Swedish adoptees is replicable. Similar evidence of genetic heterogeneity has also been demonstrated in male and female twins in the United States.[42] Our adoption data indicate that the subtypes are clinical manifestations of independent but not mutually exclusive etiological processes. The relief of anxiety and activation of euphoria are complementary neuroadaptive mechanisms that can each promote the development of alcoholism. The differences in age at onset, symptoms, course, and mode of inheritance of type 1 and type 2 forms of alcoholism can be well explained in terms of the interactions of individual experiences with the heritable dimensions of personality.

Accepted for publication February 13, 1996.

This study was supported in part by the Swedish Medical Research Council and by grants AA-7982 and AA-8028 from the National Institute on Alcoholism and Alcohol Abuse and grants MH-31302 and MH-46276 from the National Institute of Mental Health, National Institutes of Health, Bethesda, Md.

We thank Tordh Ohlsson for assistance in data management and Thomas R. Przybeck, PhD, for assistance in statistical analysis.

Reprints: C. Robert Cloninger, MD, 4940 Children's Pl, St Louis, MO 63110.

REFERENCES

1. Cloninger CR, Bohman M, Sigvardsson S. Inheritance of alcohol abuse: cross-fostering analysis of adopted men. *Arch Gen Psychiatry.* 1981;38:861-868.
2. Bohman M, Sigvardsson S, Cloninger CR. Maternal inheritance of alcohol abuse: cross-fostering analysis of adopted women. *Arch Gen Psychiatry.* 1981;38: 965-969.
3. Cloninger CR, Bohman M, Sigvardsson S, von Knorring A-L. Psychopathology in adopted-out children of alcoholics: the Stockholm Adoption Study. *Recent*

Dev Alcohol. 1985;3:37-51.

4. Bohman M, Cloninger CR, von Knorring A-L, Sigvardsson S. An adoption study of somatoform disorders, III: cross-fostering analysis and genetic relationship to alcoholism and criminality. *Arch Gen Psychiatry.* 1984;41:872-878.
5. Roe A, Burks B. Adult adjustment of foster children of alcoholic and psychotic parentage and the influence of the foster home. In: *Memoirs of the Section on Alcohol Studies.* New Haven, Conn: Yale University; 1945.
6. Goodwin DW, Schulsinger F, Moeller N, Hermansen L, Winokur G, Guze SB. Drinking problems in adopted and non-adopted sons of alcoholics. *Arch Gen Psychiatry.* 1974;31:164-169.
7. Kaij L. *Alcoholism in Twins: Studies on the Etiology and Sequels of Abuse of Alcohol.* Stockholm, Sweden: Almqvist & Wiksell; 1960.
8. Kaij L. Biases in a Swedish social register of alcoholics. *Soc Psychiatry.* 1970; 5:216-218.
9. Ojesjo L. Prevalence of known and hidden alcoholism in the revisited Lundby population. *Soc Psychiatry.* 1980;15:81-90.
10. Committee on Nomenclature and Statistics, American Psychiatric Association. *Diagnostic and Statistical Manual of Mental Disorders, Third Edition.* Washington, DC: American Psychiatric Association; 1980.
11. Searles JS. The role of genetics in the pathogenesis of alcoholism. *J Abnorm Psychol.* 1988;97:153-167.
12. Murray RM, Clifford CA, Gurling HMD. Twin and adoption studies: how good is the evidence for a genetic role? *Recent Dev Alcohol.* 1983;1:25-48.
13. Littrell J. The Swedish studies of the adopted children of alcoholics. *J Stud Alcohol.* 1988;49:491-515.
14. Gilligan SB, Reich T, Cloninger CR. Etiologic heterogeneity in alcoholism. *Genet Epidemiol.* 1987;4:395-414.
15. Gilligan SB, Reich T, Cloninger CR. Alcohol-related symptoms in heterogeneous families of hospitalized alcoholics. *Alcohol Clin Exp Res.* 1988;12: 671-678.
16. Cloninger CR, Sigvardsson S, von Knorring A-L, Bohman M. The Swedish studies of the adopted children of alcoholics: reply to Littrell. *J Stud Alcohol.* 1988; 49:516-521.
17. Babor TF, Hofmann M, DelBoca FK, Hesselbrock V, Meyer RE, Dolinsky ZS, Rounsaville B. Types of alcoholics, I: evidence for an empirically derived typology based on indicators of vulnerability and severity. *Arch Gen Psychiatry.* 1992;49:599-608.
18. Nordstrom G, Berglund M. Different patterns of successful long-term adjustment in genetically defined subtypes of alcoholics. *Alcohol Alcohol.* 1987; suppl 1:401-405.
19. Litt MD, Babor TF, DelBoca FK, Kadden RM, Cooney NL. Types of alcoholics, II: application of an empirically derived typology to treatment matching. *Arch Gen Psychiatry.* 1992;49:609-614.
20. Von Knorring L, von Knorring A-L, Smigan L, Lindberg U, Edholm M. Personality traits in subtypes of alcoholics. *J Stud Alcohol.* 1987;48:523-527.
21. Cloninger CR. Neurogenetic adaptive mechanisms in alcoholism. *Science.* 1987; 236:410-416.
22. Von Knorring A-L, Bohman M, von Knorring L, Oreland L. Platelet MAO activity as a biological marker in subgroups of alcoholism. *Acta Psychiatr Scand.* 1987;72:51-58.
23. Sigvardsson S. *Alcohol Abuse and Criminality: A Cross-fostering Study of Gene-Environment Interaction.* Umeå, Sweden: Umeå University; 1982. Dissertation.
24. SPSS Inc. *Statistical Package for the Social Sciences for Personal Computers (SPSS/PC): Version 4.0.* Chicago, Ill: SPSS Inc; 1989.
25. SAS Institute Inc. *SAS Technical Report P-229, SAS/STAT Software: Changes and Enhancements, Release 6.07.* Cary, NC: SAS Institute Inc; 1992.
26. Cloninger CR, Sigvardsson S, Bohman M (1988). Childhood personality predicts alcohol abuse in young adults. *Alcohol Clin Exp Res.* 1988;12:494-505.
27. Cloninger CR, Sigvardsson S, Przybeck TR, Svrakic DM. Personality antecedents of alcoholism in a national area probability sample. *Eur Arch Psychiatry Clin Neurosci.* 1995;245:239-244.
28. Cloninger CR. A systematic method for clinical description and classification of personality variants. *Arch Gen Psychiatry.* 1987;44:573-588.
29. Sigvardsson S, Bohman M, Cloninger CR. Structure and stability of childhood personality: prediction of later social adjustment. *J Child Psychol Psychiatry.* 1987;38:929-946.
30. Tremblay RE, Pihl RO, Vitaro F, Dobkin PL. Predicting early onset of male antisocial behavior from preschool behavior. *Arch Gen Psychiatry.* 1994;54:732-739.
31. Wills TA, Vaccaro D, McNamara G. Novelty seeking, risk taking, and related constructs as predictors of adolescent substance use: an application of Cloninger's theory. *J Subst Abuse.* 1994;6:1-20.
32. Heath AC, Cloninger CR, Martin NG. Testing a model for the genetic structure of personality: a comparison of the personality systems of Cloninger and Eysenck. *J Pers Soc Psychol.* 1994;66:762-775.
33. Svrakic NM, Svrakic DM, Cloninger CR. A general quantitative theory of personality: fundamentals of a self-organizing psychobiological complex. *Dev Psychopathol.* 1996;8:247-272.
34. Stallings MC, Hewitt JK, Cloninger CR, Heath AC, Eaves LJ. Genetic and environmental structure of the Tridimensional Personality Questionnaire: three or four primary temperament dimensions? *J Pers Soc Psychol.* In press.
35. Cloninger CR, Przybeck TR, Svrakic DM. The Tridimensional Personality Questionnaire: U.S. normative data. *Psychol Rep.* 1991;69:1047-1057.
36. Svrakic DM, Whitehead C, Przybeck TR, Cloninger CR. Differential diagnosis of personality disorders by the seven-factor model of temperament and character. *Arch Gen Psychiatry.* 1993;50:991-999.
37. Cloninger CR. A unified biosocial theory of personality and its role in the development of anxiety states. *Psychiatr Dev.* 1986;3:167-226.
38. Cloninger CR, Svrakic DM, Przybeck TR. A psychobiological model of temperament and character. *Arch Gen Psychiatry.* 1993;50:975-989.
39. Cloninger CR. The psychobiology of social cooperation. *Nat Med.* 1995;1:623-625.
40. Cloninger CR, Adolfsson R, Svrakic NM. Mapping genes for human personality. *Nat Genet.* 1996;12:3-4.
41. Pickens RW, Svikis DS, McGue M, Lykken DT, Heston LL, Clayton PJ. Heterogeneity in the inheritance of alcoholism: a study of male and female twins. *Arch Gen Psychiatry.* 1991;48:19-28.
42. Kendler KS, Neale M, Heath AC, Kessler RC, Eaves LJ. A twin-family study of alcoholism in women. *Am J Psychiatry.* 1994;151:707-715.

Does Brief Dynamic Psychotherapy Reduce the Relapse Rate of Panic Disorder?

Ida M. Wiborg, PhD; Alv A. Dahl, MD, PhD

Background: Although panic disorder can be effectively alleviated by drug treatment, the relapse rate is high. By adding brief dynamic psychotherapy focused on the psychosocial vulnerability of patients with panic disorder to an established drug treatment regimen, we hypothesized that this would result in a lower relapse rate after pharmacotherapy.

Methods: Patients with panic disorder (defined by *DSM-III-R*) were randomized to treatment with either clomipramine for 9 months (n=20), or clomipramine for 9 months combined with 15 weekly sessions of brief dynamic psychotherapy (n=20). Measures of anxiety and depression were collected at intake and at regular intervals. The patients had blind follow-up interviews at 6, 12, and 18 months after beginning treatment.

Results: All patients in both groups became free of panic attacks within 26 weeks of the start of treatment. On termination of pharmacotherapy, the relapse rate was significantly higher in the clomipramine-only group during the follow-up period. There were significantly lower scores for most anxiety measures in the clomipramine plus psychotherapy group at the 9-month follow-up.

Conclusion: The addition of brief dynamic psychotherapy to treatment with clomipramine significantly reduces the relapse rate of panic disorder compared with clomipramine treatment alone.

Arch Gen Psychiatry. 1996;53:689-694

THE CENTRAL feature of panic disorder (PD) is unexpected attacks of intense anxiety associated with multiple physical phenomena. Anticipatory anxiety and agoraphobia are frequent secondary features of PD.[1] Antidepressants and some benzodiazepines are effective drugs for the treatment of PD with and without agoraphobia.[2-9] A drawback of such treatment is that a substantial number of patients suffer a full or partial relapse after the treatment is terminated. As Ballenger[4] observed, research evidence is limited and generally contradictory as to the proportion of patients who relapse, so that reported figures vary from 20% to 30%[10] to 70% to 90%.[11,12] Different definitions of relapse may account for these variations. No standard definitions of relapse and remission have yet been agreed on.[13]

The cumulative effects of a combination of drug therapy and psychotherapy could reduce the relapse rate of PD compared with drug treatment alone. So far, few systematic studies have examined the efficacy of combined pharmacological and psychotherapeutic treatments for PD. Most studies have examined combinations of tricyclic antidepressants or placebo with various psychological techniques, usually exposure therapy. Four such studies included a direct comparison with pharmacotherapy alone.[14-16] Three of them combined imipramine or placebo and 1 studied alprazolam or placebo with exposure-based therapy vs exposure alone. All studies used samples composed exclusively of agoraphobic patients. The rationale of combined treatment was that psychotherapy alone was ineffective in reducing panic attacks, but, when combined with a panic-blocking drug, both could be helpful in reducing avoidance behavior and anticipatory anxiety. Telch and Lucas[17] calculated the effect size of these studies on some major clinical outcome measures, among them panic attacks, anticipatory anxiety, avoidance behavior, and levels of disability. They found that combined treatment offered a significant, but modest, overall short-term advantage over drug treatment alone for antici-

See Subjects and Methods on next page

From the Research Unit, Aker Hospital, Division of Psychiatry, University of Oslo, Oslo, Norway.

SUBJECTS AND METHODS

SUBJECTS

Patients suffering from PD, with and without agoraphobia, and who were between 18 and 50 years of age were recruited from physicians, psychiatric outpatient clinics, and by self-referral. The study design had 2 treatment groups: a clomipramine group (CG) and a clomipramine plus BDP group (CPG).

Fifty-seven outpatients were screened by 2 independent investigators using the Structured Clinical Interview for *DSM-III-R* (SCID, Axis I).[27] A self-rating instrument, Personality Diagnostic Questionnaire-Revised,[28] was administered to check for the occurrence of personality disorders.

Patients were excluded if they had any of the following: personality disorders, psychosis, alcohol/substance abuse, eating disorders, primary major depression, agoraphobia with or without panic attacks, pregnancy, lactation, or significant medical illnesses at evaluation.

Forty patients (23 women and 17 men) entered the study. All patients included met *DSM-III-R*[29] criteria for PD with and without agoraphobia. Patients were required to have a PD intensity of at least 1 panic attack per week in the 3-week period before inclusion into the study.

Thirty patients suffered from severe PD, which meant that they had had at least 8 panic attacks during the past month and 10 patients suffered from moderate PD, indicating at least 3 panic attacks during the same period.[27]

Eight patients had PD without agoraphobia; 6 had mild agoraphobia resulting in some avoidance, but otherwise lived a relatively normal life; 20 had moderate agoraphobia that led to a constricted lifestyle; and 6 had severe agoraphobia that had made them nearly or completely housebound.[27]

Comorbid disorders were generalized anxiety disorder in 3 patients; social phobia in 3 patients; hypochondriasis in 3 patients; simple phobia in 14 patients; a secondary major depressive episode in 2 patients; and secondary obsessive-compulsive disorder in 2 patients.

The age range of the patients was 21 to 49 years. All patients were medically examined and found to be in good physical health.

TREATMENT

After obtaining informed consent, patients were randomized to the CG (n=20) or the CPG (n=20) using computerized random number generator and sealed envelopes. Therapy with psychotropic medications other than anxiolytics was discontinued 2 weeks prior to treatment start.

During the step-up phase for clomipramine, benzodiazepines were allowed. The reason for this was 2-fold: first, increase of panic attacks at the beginning of clomipramine treatment was reported as both frightening and demotivating by a high proportion of the patients. Second, by allowing benzodiazepines, patients acknowledged such usage more readily rather than taking them secretly.[26] Seven patients reported irregular use of benzodiazepines at intake. During the first month of clomipramine treatment, 6 patients in the CG and 5 in the CPG took benzodiazepines. Two patients in each group used these drugs irregularly for about 6 months. One patient in the CG reported use at the 18-month follow-up.

Prior to randomization, patients met individually with a clinician (I.M.W.). She informed them about PD, the treatment with clomipramine, and the panic diary, and gave them a popular booklet about PD.

Medication treatment followed a flexible step-up procedure, and the dose was increased until maximum benefit was achieved (maximum, 150 mg/d). If adverse effects became too bothersome, dose increases were slowed or the dose reduced. Medication administration lasted for 36 weeks with a slow stepwise reduction during the last 6 weeks before termination.

Patients assigned to the CG were treated by general practitioners (GPs) according to a manual written by us. All GPs limited their interaction with the patients to "contact as usual" and met the patients weekly for 12 weeks. Clomipramine treatment was started during the first week of treatment. Patients were not allowed to undergo additional psychotherapy or behavior therapy.

Patients assigned to the CPG received BDP given by one of us (I.M.W.), who is a clinical psychologist well trained in this treatment method. Brief dynamic psychotherapy consisted of 1 weekly visit for 15 weeks. Three sessions of BDP were given prior to the start of pharmacotherapy. This was done to emphasize that BDP was the most important part of the combined treatment. Clomipramine was prescribed to the CPG by a psychiatrist who had no further contact with the patients.

patory anxiety, avoidance behavior, and levels of disability, but not for panic attacks. Only 3 of the studies produced long-term data, and these data showed no advantage for combined treatment.[18,19] Whether a combination of 2 effective treatment methods reduces the relapse rate in PD is still an unsettled issue.

To our knowledge, there are no controlled studies of the efficacy of a combination of pharmacotherapy and psychodynamic psychotherapy vs pharmacotherapy alone in PD. It is well known that the onset of PD often occurs after a period of stressful life events.[20-25] We hypothesized that brief dynamic psychotherapy (BDP) could make patients with PD less vulnerable to the psychosocial factors that trigger recurrence of PD after termination of drug treatment. Modigh et al[26] have demonstrated the effectiveness of clomipramine in PD. Our study was designed to test the hypothesis that compared with clomipramine alone, the combination of clomipramine and BDP would be more effective in reducing the relapse rate of PD after treatment end.

RESULTS

No significant group differences were found with respect to demographics (**Table 1**), sex, or illness characteristics. The majority of patients were between 25 and 28 years of age, well educated, and more than half of them were employed. The mean±SD duration of PD in the CG was 3.1±3.3 years, and in the CPG, 3.2±3.6 years (range, 6-204 months and 6-264 months, respectively). The mean±SD age at first panic attack was 28.6±7.9 and 25.9±7.3 years, respectively.

The BDP manual, compiled by one of us (I.M.W.), was developed on concepts and techniques from Davanloo,[30] Malan,[31-33] and Strupp and Binder.[34]

Based on extensive experience with patients with PD before the study, the authors have the following formulation of the central psychodynamic issues: patients with PD readily submit to other people. They do not express self-assertive behavior or negative feelings out of fear of not being liked, loved, or accepted. These interpersonal patterns are repetitions of earlier behavioral patterns with significant others and had originally served a self-protective function. These patterns now interfere with autonomous adult functioning and cause stress in interpersonal relationships. The unconscious conflict between need for approval and fear of punishment for self-assertiveness is therefore the focus of BDP.

The goal of the psychotherapy was to help the patient to develop insight into the origins and determinants of the dysfunctional patterns. This insight was needed to acquire more adaptive patterns of interpersonal relatedness. The therapist focused on the identification and working through of the dysfunctional patterns as they emerged in the past, the present, and the transference. The work included all the technical elements of dynamic psychotherapy: clarification, confrontation, and interpretation of the patients' resistance, defensive styles, and associated isolated affects.

We hypothesized that the acquisition of more adaptive interpersonal relatedness would reduce the risk for a relapse when the patients became exposed to interpersonal stress. Patients with agoraphobia were not encouraged to expose themselves to provocative situations.

ASSESSMENTS

Assessment measures were obtained at intake (before randomization), at each weekly treatment visit, and at 6, 12, and 18 months after treatment start.

The Hopkins Symptom Checklist (SCL-90)[35] and The State-Trait Anxiety Inventory[36] were administered to assess the patients' overall symptoms and proneness to anxiety at intake. In addition, the evaluators assessed global severity of illness using the Global Assessment Scale[37] and Clinical Global Impressions (CGI).[38]

At each weekly visit the patients were given the same package of self-report instruments. Panic attacks were monitored by a diary beginning at 2 weeks before start of treatment. Based on the diary, patients registered the weekly number of panic attacks (situational and unexpected) using the Panic Attack and Anxiety Scale,[2] their duration and intensity, and limited-symptom attacks together with anticipatory anxiety and fear intensity.

Further assessments used were the Hamilton Rating Scale for Anxiety (HAM-A)[39]; the Sheehan Disability Scale (SDS)[2]; the Phobia Scale (Modified Marks-Sheehan),[40] measuring panic-related phobias; a subscale of the Patient's Status (PSS)[41] evaluating overall illness severity; the Hamilton Rating Scale for Depression (HAM-D)[42]; and the Medical Events Checklist,[43] registering adverse effects of clomipramine.

At the 6-, 12-, and 18-month follow-up, patients completed the same self-report evaluations together with the SCL-90.

FOLLOW-UP

At 6, 12, and 18 months patients were assessed by an evaluator (A.A.D.) who was blind to treatment group, using the CGI and a structured follow-up interview. The interview included information about remission and relapse of both PD and other diagnoses; frequency and severity of panic attacks; degree of anticipatory anxiety and panic-related phobia; social, work, family, and somatic impairment; global severity; and type and frequency of interval psychological and medical treatment, medication, and outcome. Only outcome data from the 18-month follow-up are included in this article.

STATISTICAL ANALYSIS

Categorical data were examined using cross-tabulations and χ^2 tests. When comparing the treatment groups with respect to a continuous efficacy variable, a 2-tailed Wilcoxon rank-sum test was applied. For some continuous efficacy variables a significant difference was observed between the groups at the start of the treatment visits. To adjust for this initial difference, analysis of covariance (ANCOVA) was conducted. To adjust for initial differences between the groups when comparing relapse rate, logistic regression analysis was used. In each significance test an α level of .05 was applied. All data analysis were conducted using SPSS software, version 6.1 (Chicago, Ill).

At intake, no significant differences between the groups were found in overall symptom intensity (SCL-90), SCL-90 depression and anxiety subscales, anxiety proneness (The State-Trait Anxiety Inventory), or global severity of illness (Global Assessment Scale and CGI) (**Table 2**).

There were no significant differences at the start of the treatment visits using the following tests: Panic Attack and Anxiety Scale, Phobia Scale, disability in work (SDS), and PSS. However, the CG had significantly higher mean scores on HAM-A (P=.01), HAM-D (P=.04) and disability in family and social life (SDS) (P=.04 and P=.02, respectively).

When the groups were compared at the end of the treatment visits and at the 18-month follow-up, we adjusted for these initial differences with ANCOVA. No significant difference in slope was found between the groups in the analysis of HAM-A, HAM-D, and SDS social/leisure and family/home subscales (P>.20). Even with this conservative approach, the differences between the groups were still significant on HAM-A and SDS social/leisure and family/home subscales (P<.05), but not on HAM-D.

DOSAGES

No significant differences in mean dosages were found between the groups during the treatment visits and at the 6-month follow-up. The highest mean±SD dose in the CG was 113.3±31.6 mg and in the CPG, 107.5±41.4 mg. Compliance with clomipramine treatment in both groups was controlled by patient report and not by measurement of serum clomipramine concentration.

Table 1. Demographic Characteristics of Samples*

	CG (n=20)	CPG (n=20)
Age, y		
Mean±SD	32.8±8.2	30.6±6.3†
Median	32	28.5
Range	22-49	21-49
Sex, No. (%)		
F	13 (65)	10 (50)
M	7 (35)	10 (50)
Marital status, No. (%)		
Never married	8 (40)	8 (40)
Cohabitating	7 (35)	2 (10)
Married	3 (15)	8 (40)
Divorced	2 (10)	2 (10)
Education, No. (%)		
Less than high school	2 (10)	1 (5)
High school only	2 (10)	2 (10)
Semiprofessional	8 (40)	9 (45)
College graduate or beyond	8 (40)	8 (40)
Employment status, No. (%)		
Employed	14 (70)	12 (60)
Unemployed	2 (10)	3 (15)
Student	4 (20)	5 (25)

**CG indicates clomipramine group; CPG, clomipramine plus brief dynamic psychotherapy group.*

†The 2 groups did not show a statistically significant difference on any of the variables.

To examine tolerance to clomipramine, we compared mean ratings on the Medical Events Checklist. Patients in the CG reported significantly more adverse effects from the start of drug treatment to end of the treatment visits than patients in the CPG (33.9±12.8 vs 23.4±12.8) (P=.007) and (16.5±14.2 vs 6.1±4.1) (P=.009).

DROPOUTS

All patients completed the weekly treatment visits and the follow-up examinations. Four patients were incompletely treated according to the protocol, since they received clomipramine for less than 36 weeks. Two patients in the CG stopped taking clomipramine at weeks 12 and 16, respectively, and 2 patients in the CPG at weeks 3 and 26 owing to adverse effects.

IMPROVEMENT RATINGS

No patients recorded no panic attacks in the 2 weeks before the start of treatment. At the end of the treatment visits, all patients (100%) in the CPG were free of panic attacks compared with 15 (75%) in the CG. However, all patients in the CG were panic-free at the 6-month follow-up. All patients, therefore, had a time period when the diagnostic critera for PD no longer were fulfilled.

On the follow-up examinations relapse was defined as fulfilling the *DSM-III-R* diagnostic criteria for PD after a period of at least 8 weeks when the patient did not have panic attacks. According to this definition, 15 patients (75%) in the CG and 4 patients (20%) in the CPG relapsed during the 9 months between the end of medication treatment and the 18-month follow-up. Most relapses (74%) occurred between 2 and 3 months after discontinuation of treatment with clomipramine. Ten (91%) of 11 patients in the CG suffering from severe PD with moderate to severe agoraphobia relapsed compared with 1 (9%) of 11 patients in the CPG. This corresponds to an odds ratio for relapse in the CG of 8.0 and in the CPG of 0.2. Medication was resumed if patients had panic attacks for at least 1 month.

To determine whether the low relapse rate in the CPG could be due to the initial differences in HAM-A, HAM-D, and SDS social/leisure and family/home subscales, we adjusted for these differences using logistic regression analysis. The difference in relapse rate between the groups was still highly significant (adjusted for HAM-A, P=.004; HAM-D, P=.004; SDS social/leisure subscale, P=.002; and SDS family/home subscale, P=.001).

Remission of PD was defined as having CGI and PSS scores of 1 or 2 ("very significant improvement" or "significant improvement"); no panic attacks in the 9 months between end of medication treatment and the 18-month follow-up; and no remedication. Sixteen patients (80%) in the CPG and 5 (25%) in the CG fulfilled these remission criteria.

At the 18-month follow-up, patients in the CPG showed significantly greater global improvement on CGI (P=.001) and PSS (P<.001) than patients in the CG. They also had a significantly greater reduction in symptom levels and disability on most measurements.

Although patients in the CG also showed improvement at the 18-month follow-up on the different measurements, their improvement was mainly owing to the fact that 14 patients (70%) were back taking effective medication compared with 4 patients (20%) in the CPG.

Four patients in the CG who relapsed had additional psychological treatment for PD in the 9-month interval between the end of medication therapy and the 18-month follow-up compared with no patients in the CPG.

Patients in the CG suffering from comorbid generalized anxiety disorder, obsessive-compulsive disorder, hypochondriasis, and simple phobia were still complaining of these disorders at the 18-month follow-up. In the CPG, patients with generalized anxiety disorder, hypochondriasis, simple phobia, and social phobia experienced a slight symptomatic improvement.

COMMENT

We found a significantly higher relapse rate for the CG than the CPG during 9 months of follow-up after the end of medication therapy. The 75% relapse rate of the CG is consistent with the rates found in previous drug studies. Since a study of a similar combined treatment group has not previously been reported, we cannot compare the 20% relapse rate in that group directly with other studies. Patients with PD treated with a combination of clomipramine plus BDP have a much better outcome on all measures, including panic attacks, anticipatory anxiety, avoidance behavior, and disability, compared with other combined studies.[14-16]

The significant difference in relapse rates between the groups can be explained in several ways. The result

Table 2. Treatment Group Comparisons*

	Intake			Start Visits			End Visits			18-mo Follow-up		
	CG	CPG	*P*	CG	CPG	*P*	CG	CPG	*P*	CG	CPG	*P*
SCL-90	1.3±0.4	1.1±0.4	.99	...	...	...	...	...	...	0.8±0.7	0.3±0.3	.04
STAI												
Trait	49.5±10.6	49.5±12.0	.94	...	...	...	...	...	...	...	...	...
State	34.4±10.1	30.9±8.8	.15	...	...	...	...	...	...	...	...	...
CGI	4.1±1.1	4.0±1.1	.92	...	...	...	...	...	...	2.4±1.7	0.6±1.1	.001
GAS	57.1±13.8	60.7±5.1	.18	...	...	...	...	...	...	...	...	...
PAAS (total)	...	...		6.4±3.2	6.1±2.7	.80	0.8±2.1	0.0±0.0	.02	2.1±2.4	0.6±1.6	.02
Situational attacks	...	...		1.9±1.7	2.4±2.6	.63	0.5±1.5	0.0±0.0	.08	2.2±3.6	0.3±1.1	.004
Duration	...	...		7.7±10.2	17.5±28.7	.57	2.3±5.7	0.0±0.0	.08	6.7±20.1	10.5±40.5	.18
Intensity	...	...		4.5±3.9	3.2±3.5	.29	0.9±2.2	0.0±0.0	.08	2.2±3.6	0.5±1.6	.10
Spontaneous attacks	...	...		4.6±3.0	3.6±2.1	.58	0.3±0.8	0.0±0.0	.08	0.9±1.1	0.4±1.3	.03
Duration	...	...		16.3±18.3	27.5±24.0	.10	5.5±15.0	0.0±0.0	.08	4.0±13.5	2.3±7.3	.67
Intensity	...	...		4.8±3.8	5.6±2.1	.58	1.0±2.6	0.0±0.0	.08	1.0±12.4	0.5±1.6	.60
LSA	...	...		2.9±5.4	2.4±5.7	.96	0.5±2.2	0.1±0.2	.92	3.8±15.6	0.3±1.1	.33
Anticipatory anxiety	...	...		73.2±29.1	61.3±28.4	.23	24.3±27.4	4.2±5.4	.01	22.8±22.3	7.6±17.3	.02
Fear intensity	...	...		7.3±2.6	6.4±2.2	.27	3.2±2.8	1.1±2.3	.003	2.9±2.6	1.1±1.7	.008
PS	...	...		7.3±2.6	6.4±2.2	.70	2.6±3.3	1.1±1.1	.002	2.8±2.5	1.0±2.4	.005
HAM-A	...	...		30.3±10.9	21.8±9.2	.01	16.0±10.0	5.5±4.7	.001	15.6±12.0	7.7±5.8	.03
HAM-D	...	...		18.9±7.2	14.2±7.8	.05	7.4±6.1	3.6±2.7	.70	7.3±8.8	2.9±3.2	.14
SDS work	...	...		6.8±2.7	5.4±3.3	.22	3.0±2.7	1.2±1.5	.02	2.7±3.0	1.0±1.8	.01
SDS social/leisure	...	...		7.0±2.6	4.8±3.2	.02	3.6±2.9	1.1±0.9	.001	2.8±2.9	1.2±2.0	.03
SDS family/home	...	...		4.7±2.8	3.1±2.9	.04	2.5±2.1	0.8±1.1	.009	1.9±1.9	0.9±1.2	.05
PSS	...	...		4.3±1.4	4.0±1.3	.40	2.0±1.1	1.4±0.5	.03	2.2±1.1	1.2±0.7	<.001

**CG indicates clomipramine group; CPG, clomipramine plus brief dynamic psychotherapy group; SCL-90, Symptom Checklist-90[35]; STAI, The State-Trait Anxiety Inventory[36]; CGI, Clinical Global Impressions[38]; GAS, Global Assessment Scale[37]; PAAS, Panic Attack and Anxiety Scale[2]; LSA, limited-symptom attack; PS, Phobia Scale[40]; HAM-A, Hamilton Rating Scale for Anxiety[39]; HAM-D, Hamilton Rating Scale for Depression[42]; SDS, Sheehan Disability Scale[2]; PSS, Patient's Status Scale[41]; and ellipses, not given. All scores given as mean±SD.*

could be owing to group differences. The randomization, however, produced highly comparable samples. No significant differences were found on any characteristics between the groups nor on any measurements, except for HAM-A, HAM-D, and SDS social/leisure and family/home subscales obtained at the start of treatment visits. These differences, which remained even when we adjusted for them statistically, indicated an initial group difference that favored the outcome of the CPG. A possible explanation of these findings could be expectation bias caused by a more positive expectation of the patients concerning combined treatment. A representative population study in Norway showed that people had significantly greater trust in a combination of drugs and supportive talks than in drugs alone.[44] It is also a common clinical observation in BDP that patients initially have great expectations concerning psychotherapy.[45] In contrast, patients in the CG knew after randomization that they would be treated by a GP rather than by the experienced psychologist who had evaluated them, and that they would receive only medication with limited opportunity to discuss interpersonal issues.

The significant difference between the 2 groups in reporting adverse effects during the treatment visits could be explained along the same lines. In the CG, clomipramine was the main treatment, and the GPs were told to give "contact as usual," which meant that physical symptoms were a common topic during consultations. Consequently, this could have led to a stronger focus on patients' reactions to clomipramine. On the other hand, in the CPG patients were told that the psychotherapy was the main treatment modality. To emphasize this, the clomipramine component was first introduced during the fourth week of treatment. By then, patients were already informed about all common adverse effects. Good rapport and a trusting relationship with the psychotherapist probably reduced the significance of the adverse effects, and, therefore, they reported fewer than the CG patients.

The outcome differences between the 2 groups could also be attributed to the covert use of benzodiazepines, since previous studies have suggested that such use can be responsible for pill-placebo response.[46] There is a possibility that some patients, although denying they were doing so, were taking such medication at the 18-month follow-up, since we did not do serum drug screenings. However, patients had to consult physicians outside the study to ask for such drugs. Physicians in Norway are very restrictive in prescribing benzodiazepines, and the follow-up examinations were thorough and done by the same experienced psychiatrist. We therefore hold this explanation to be unlikely. We have few reasons to believe that the remitting patients in the CPG used medication covertly and certainly not more than those in the CG.

It is possible that the low relapse rate in the CPG is because of the BDP and its facilitation through pharmacotherapy. In our experience, patients with PD have a too high level of psychological distress to be able to work on the issues addressed by BDP without concommitant medication that reduces the frequency and intensity of panic attacks. The combined treatment could have maximized the patients' confidence by the amelioration of panic attacks and by the opportunity to change their maladaptive interpersonal patterns. In our view, BDP had a favorable impact on the psychosocial vulnerability of patients with PD, but we did not use an instrument to measure this in our study design.

Our study had several limitations. First, the treatment groups were small. Second, 1 psychotherapist carried out all the BDP. This makes it unclear whether the influence of BDP is attributable to the therapist, the therapy, or a combination of the 2. Other researchers have also reported a positive effect of BDP in PD, indicating that this therapy modality may be the decisive factor.[47]

This study strongly suggests that clomipramine in combination with BPD is effective in reducing the relapse rate in PD compared with treatment with clomipramine alone. The CPG had generally significantly better outcome on most measures at follow-up 9 months after termination of the drug treatment.

From this study we cannot claim that BDP has any advantage compared with other modalities of psychotherapy in reducing the relapse rate of PD after drug treatment. However, we hypothesize that BDP reduces psychosocial vulnerability associated with PD. Since the relapse rate of PD after pharmacotherapy alone is disturbingly high, more studies are needed to find ways to bring this rate down. The alternative might be long-term drug treatment.

Accepted for publication February 5, 1996.

This study was supported by grants from The Norwegian Research Council for Science and the Humanities, Oslo, Josef & Haldis Andresen's Legacy, and Anders Jahre's Legacy.

The authors acknowledge Leiv Sandvik of Medstat Research for his statistical advice and the staff of the Sinsen Community Psychiatric Center for their support and assistance in carrying out this study.

Reprints: Ida M. Wiborg, PhD, Research Unit, Gaustad Hospital, PO Box 33, Gaustad, 0320 Oslo, Norway.

REFERENCES

1. Klein DF, Gorman JM. A model of panic and agoraphobia development. *Acta Psychiatr Scand Suppl.* 1987;335:87-95.
2. Sheehan DV. Tricyclic antidepressants in the treatment of panic and anxiety disorders. *Psychosomatics.* 1986;27(suppl 11):10-16.
3. Sheehan DV. *The Anxiety Disease.* New York, NY: Bantam Books Inc; 1986.
4. Ballenger JC. Overview of the pharmacotherapy of panic disorder. In: Wolfe BE, Maser JD, eds. *Treatment of Panic Disorder: A Consensus Development Conference.* Washington, DC: American Psychiatric Press; 1994:59-72.
5. Ballenger JC. Efficacy of benzodiazepines in panic disorder and agoraphobia. *J Psychiatr Res.* 1990;24(suppl 2):15-25.
6. Sheehan DV. Benzodiazepines in panic disorder and agoraphobia. *J Affect Disord.* 1987;13:169-181.
7. Noyes R, DuPont RL, Pecknold JC, Rifkin A, Rubin RT, Swinson RP, Ballenger JC, Burrows GD. Alprazolam in panic disorder and agoraphobia: results from a multicenter trial, II: patient acceptance, side effects, and safety. *Arch Gen Psychiatry.* 1988;45:423-428.
8. Liebowitz MR, Fyer AJ, Gorman JM, Campeas R, Levin A, Davies SR, Goetz D, Klein DF. Alprazolam in the treatment of panic disorder. *J Clin Psychopharmacol.* 1986;6:13-20.
9. Beauclair L, Fontaine R, Annable L, Holobow N, Chouinard G. Clonazepam in the treatment of panic disorder: a double-blind, placebo-controlled trial investigating the correlation between clonazepam concentrations in plasma and clinical response. *J Clin Psychopharmacol.* 1994;14:111-118.
10. Zitrin CM, Klein DF, Woerner MG, Ross DC. Treatment of phobias, I: comparison of imipramine hydrochloride and placebo. *Arch Gen Psychiatry.* 1983;40:125-138.
11. Noyes R, Garvey MJ, Cook BL. Follow-up study of patients with panic disorder and agoraphobia with panic attacks treated with tricyclic antidepressants. *J Affect Disord.* 1989;16:249-257.
12. Noyes R, Garvey MJ, Cook BL, Suelzer M. Controlled discontinuation of benzodiazepine treatment for patients with panic disorder. *Am J Psychiatry.* 1991;148:517-523.
13. Shear MK, Maser JD. Standard assessment for panic disorder research. *Arch Gen Psychiatry.* 1994;51:346-354.
14. Mavissakalian M, Michelson L, Dealy RS. Pharmacological treatment of agoraphobia: imipramine versus imipramine with programmed practice. *Br J Psychiatry.* 1983;143:348-355.
15. Telch MJ, Agras WS, Taylor CB, Roth WT, Gallen CC. Combined pharmacological and behavior treatment for agoraphobia. *Behav Res Ther.* 1985;23:325-335.
16. Marks IM, Swinson RP, Basoglu M, Kuch K, Noshirvani H, O'Sullivan G, Lelliot PT, Kirby M, McNamee G, Sengun S, Wickwire K. Alprazolam and exposure alone and combined in panic disorder with agoraphobia: a controlled study in London and Toronto. *Br J Psychiatry.* 1993;162:776-787.
17. Telch MJ, Lucas RA. Combined pharmacological and psychological treatment of panic disorder: current status and future directions. In: Wolfe BE, Maser JD, eds. *Treatment of Panic Disorder: A Consensus Development Conference.* Washington, DC: American Psychiatric Press; 1994:177-197.
18. Cohen SD, Monteiro W, Marks IM. Two-year follow-up of agoraphobics after exposure and imipramine. *Br J Psychiatry.* 1984;144:276-281.
19. Mavissakalian M, Michelson L. Two-year follow-up of exposure and imipramine treatment of agoraphobia. *Am J Psychiatry.* 1986;142:1032-1036.
20. Faravelli C. Life events preceding the onset of panic disorder. *J Affect Disord.* 1985;9:103-105.
21. Faravelli C, Pallanti S. Recent life events and panic disorder. *Am J Psychiatry.* 1989;146:622-626.
22. Roy-Byrne PP, Geraci M, Uhde TW. Life events and course of illness in patients with panic disorder. *Am J Psychiatry.* 1986;143:1033-1035.
23. Roy-Byrne PP, Geraci M, Uhde TW. Life events and the onset of panic disorder. *Am J Psychiatry.* 1986;143:1424-1427.
24. Roy-Byrne PP, Geraci M. Uhde TW. Life events obtained via interview: the effect of time of recall on data obtained in controls and patients with panic disorder. *J Affect Disord.* 1987;12:57-62.
25. Roy-Byrne PP, Uhde TW. Exogenous factors in panic disorder: clinical and research implications. *J Clin Psychiatry.* 1988;49:56-61.
26. Modigh K, Westberg P, Eriksson E. Superiority of clomipramine over imipramine in the treatment of panic disorder: a placebo-controlled trial. *J Clin Psychopharmacol.* 1992;12:251-261.
27. Spitzer RL, Williams JBW. Revised diagnostic criteria and a new structured interview for diagnosing anxiety disorder. *J Psychiatr Res.* 1988;22:55-86.
28. Hyler SE, Rieder RO. *PDQ-R: Personality Diagnostic Questionnaire-Revised.* New York, NY; New York State Psychiatric Institute: 1987.
29. American Psychiatric Association. *Diagnostic and Statistical Manual of Mental Disorders, Third Edition, Revised.* Washington, DC: American Psychiatric Association; 1987.
30. Davanloo H, ed. *Basic Principles and Techniques in Short-Term Dynamic Psychotherapy.* New York, NY: Spectrum; 1978.
31. Malan D. *The Frontier of Brief Psychotherapy.* New York, NY: Plenum Medical Books; 1976.
32. Malan D. *The Frontier of Brief Psychotherapy: An Example of the Convergence of Research and Clinical Practice.* New York, NY: Plenum Press; 1976.
33. Malan D. *Individual Psychotherapy and the Science of Psychodynamics.* London, England: Butterworth; 1979.
34. Strupp HH, Binder JL. *Psychotherapy in a New Key: A Guide to Time-Limited Dynamic Psychotherapy.* New York, NY: Basic Books Inc Publishers; 1984.
35. Derogatis LR. *SCL-90: Administration Scoring and Procedures Manual-1 For the (Revised) Version.* Baltimore, Md: Clinical Psychometrics Research Unit, John Hopkins University School of Medicine; 1977.
36. Spielberger C, Gorsuch A, Lushene R. *The State-Trait Anxiety Inventory.* Palo Alto, Calif: Consulting Psychologist Press; 1970.
37. Endicott J, Spitzer RL, Fleiss JL, Cohen J. The Global Assessment Scale: a procedure for measuring overall severity of psychiatric disturbance. *Arch Gen Psychiatry.* 1976;33:766-771.
38. Guy W. *ECDEU Assessment Manual for Psychopharmacology.* Rockville, Md: National Institute of Mental Health; 1976. Publication 76-338.
39. Hamilton M. The assessment of anxiety by rating. *Br J Med Psychol.* 1959;32:50-55.
40. Sheehan DV. *The Anxiety Disease.* New York, NY: Bantam Books; 1986.
41. *Panic Disorder: Patient's Status.* Kalamazoo, Mich; The Upjohn Co: 1990. Reference 94-1557-41 01/90. Self-report questionnaire.
42. Hamilton M. A rating scale for depression. *J Neurol Neurosurg Psychiatry.* 1960;23:56-62.
43. *Panic Disorder: Medical Events Checklist.* Kalamazoo, Mich; The Upjohn Co: 1990. Reference 94-1557-37 01/90. Interview-based questionnaire.
44. Hamre P, Dahl AA, Malt U. Public attitudes to the quality of psychiatric treatment, psychiatric patients, and the prevalence of mental disorder. *Nord Psychiatr J.* 1994;48:275-281.
45. Ursano RJ, Sonnenberg SM, Lazar SG. *Psychodynamic Psychotherapy.* Washington, DC: American Psychiatric Press; 1991;102.
46. Clark DB, Taylor CB, Roth WT, Hayward C, Ehlers A, Margraf J, Agras WS. Surreptitious drug use by patients in a panic disorder study. *Am J Psychiatry.* 1991;36:130-138.
47. Millrod B, Shear MK. Psychodynamic treatment of panic: three case histories. *Hosp Community Psychiatry.* 1991;42:311-312.

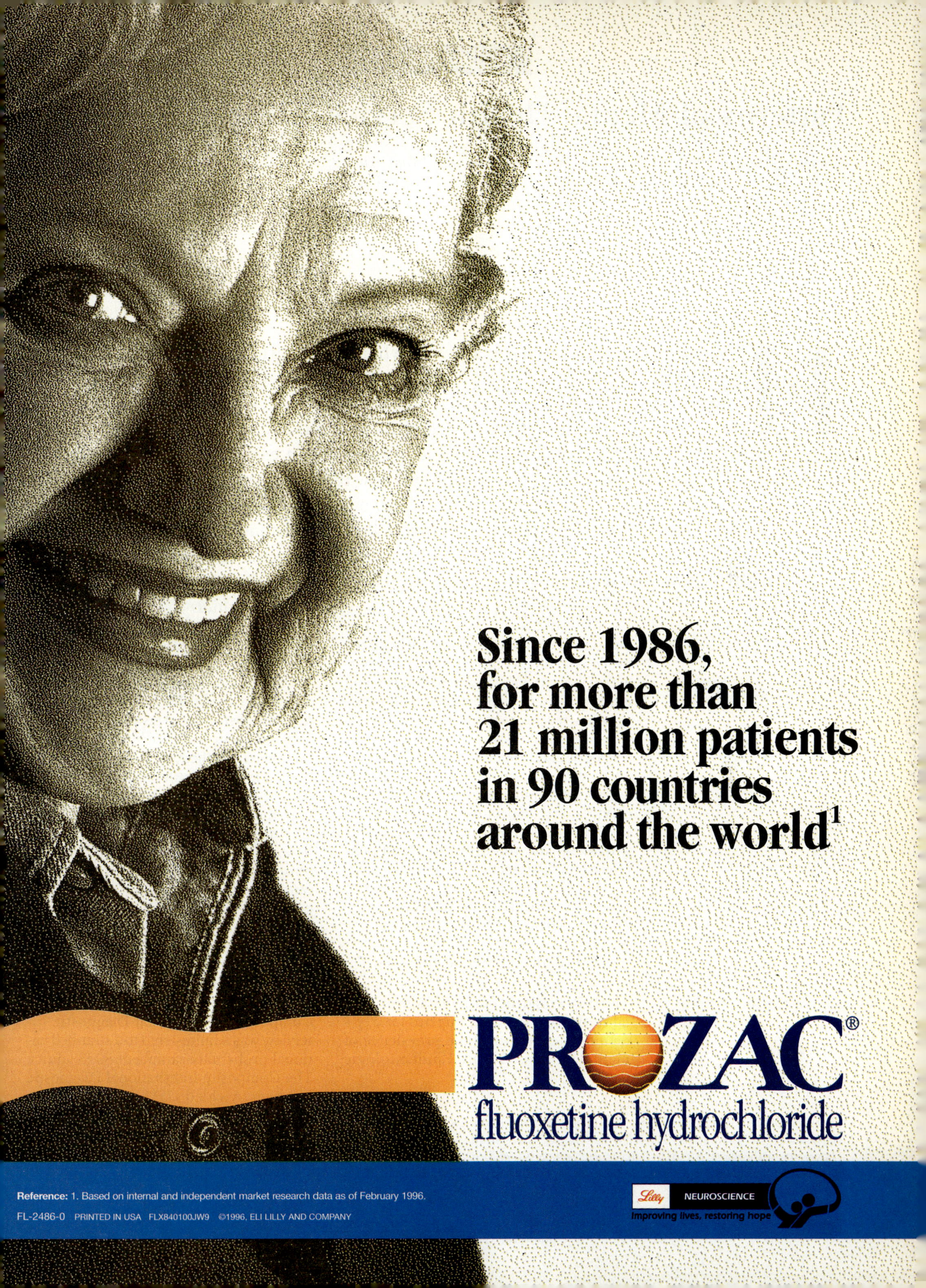
Since 1986,
for more than
21 million patients
in 90 countries
around the world[1]
PROZAC®
fluoxetine hydrochloride
Reference: 1. Based on internal and independent market research data as of February 1996.
FL-2486-0 PRINTED IN USA FLX840100JW9 ©1996, ELI LILLY AND COMPANY
Lilly NEUROSCIENCE
Improving lives, restoring hope

Patterns of Mental Health Service Utilization

Kenneth I. Howard, PhD; Thomas A. Cornille, PhD; John S. Lyons, PhD; John T. Vessey, PhD; Robert J. Lueger, PhD; Stephen M. Saunders, PhD

How many and which individuals, with which psychiatric disorders, receive (and do not receive) mental health services from which professionals in what settings? This question falls within the purview of mental health services research, which is a multidisciplinary field that brings together the methodologies of epidemiology, econometrics, and clinical research. First, in this article, we present an explication of what is known about those individuals in need of psychotherapy and how they access services. Next, we describe the numbers, professional affiliations, and service sites of professionals who are engaged in the practice of psychotherapy. We summarize our current knowledge about the actual utilization of psychotherapy services relative to the needs of patients and the professional background of therapists. Finally, we identify aspects of psychotherapy service utilization that are, as yet, unaddressed.

Arch Gen Psychiatry. 1996;53:696-703

National health policy is dependent on the availability of information about the characteristics and distribution of illnesses and effective services. In the mental health field, services research has combined the efforts of economists, sociologists, epidemiologists, anthropologists, and clinical investigators to provide information with regard to the public need for mental health services, the distribution and accessibility of these services, the types of service providers, and the utilization and benefits of these services.

THE NEED FOR MENTAL HEALTH SERVICES

Prevalence of Mental Illnesses

The 1978 President's Commission on Mental Health[1] provided the impetus for 2 epidemiologic studies of the prevalence of mental illness: (1) the Epidemiologic Catchment Area (ECA) Program and (2) the National Comorbidity Survey (NCS).

The ECA survey produced data from 5 sites between 1980 and 1985. Household and institutional residents older than 18 years were surveyed[2,3] with regard to their need for, their seeking, and their obtaining mental health services. In the first wave, 20 291 adults were interviewed with regard to outpatient mental health service utilization; 6 months later, household residents were interviewed via telephone; and 1 year later, 79.1% of the sample were reinterviewed.[4] The ECA Program used the Diagnostic Interview Schedule[5] to provide accurate identification and classification of mental health problems.

The second major epidemiologic study was the NCS, which was conducted between 1990 and 1992.[6] The Composite International Diagnostic Interview was administered to a stratified national probability sample of 8098 adults. The Composite International Diagnostic Interview yielded *DSM-III-R* diagnoses, and more diagnostic categories were included in this survey than in the ECA Program.

The findings of the ECA Program and the NCS are shown in **Table 1**. Both con-

From the Departments of Psychology, Northwestern University, Evanston, Ill (Dr Howard), Florida State University, Tallahassee (Dr Cornille), and Marquette University, Milwaukee, Wis (Drs Lueger and Saunders), and the Department of Psychiatry, Northwestern University Medical School, Chicago, Ill (Drs Lyons and Vessey).

Table 1. Prevalence of Mental Illness and Treatment per 100 Persons*

Use	Any Disorder	Major Depression	Anxiety Disorders	Drug Use Disorders	Alcohol Disorders
ECA Program					
1-y prevalence	28	5	13	3	7
% of diagnosed obtaining any service in past year	29	54	33	30	22
% of diagnosed obtaining MHP service in past year	13	29	15	14	11
Lifetime prevalence	30-40	4-7	11-25	6-7	12-17
NCS					
1-y prevalence	30	10	17	4	10
% of diagnosed obtaining any service in past year	21	...	...	...	...
% of diagnosed obtaining MHP service in past year	12	...	...	...	...
Lifetime prevalence	48	17	25	12	24
% of diagnosed obtaining any service during lifetime	42	...	...	...	...
% obtaining service from MHP, ever in lifetime	26	...	...	...	...

ECA indicates Epidemiologic Catchment Area; MHP, mental health professional; and NCS, National Comorbidity Survey. Proportion of subjects who obtained services for specific diagnoses were not described in the NCS. Data are given as percentages.

cluded that about 30% of adults will experience a diagnosable mental illness in any given year.[4,6] The ECA and NCS results differed (with the NCS reporting consistently higher rates) in their reports of the rates of anxiety disorders (13% vs 17%), alcohol use disorders (7% vs 10%), and major depression (5% vs 10%). With regard to lifetime prevalence, the ECA data suggested that 30% to 40% of all persons had experienced a mental illness at some time in their life. The NCS yielded a higher figure, finding that almost half of all respondents reported that they had had at least 1 disorder at some time in their lives. A possible explanation for the discrepancies in the prevalence rates is that the NCS and ECA diagnostic interviews were different in wording and degree of probing.

Regardless of differences in methods and prevalence rates, however, the results of the ECA Program and the NCS confirmed that the mental illnesses are highly comorbid: more than 60% of the ECA respondents with at least 1 lifetime disorder and 56% of the NCS respondents with at least 1 lifetime disorder had 2 or more disorders.[4,6] Taken together, the results indicate that mental illness is widespread and chronic.

Those Persons With Psychiatric Diagnoses Who Do Not Use Mental Health Services

These studies[4,6] also are consistent in identifying substantial unmet mental health needs. In the ECA Program, more than 70% of persons with a recent mental health or addiction disorder received no services to treat that problem, and only 13% reported that they obtained treatment from a mental health professional (MHP).[4] Similarly, the NCS found that about 79% of individuals with a recent disorder obtained no services, and only about 12% of persons with a recent disorder had obtained some service from an MHP in the past year.[6]

Persons with a major depression were the most likely to receive any services and MHP services in particular. However, only about one fourth of the respondents with a recent major depression had obtained MHP services in the past year. Although the treatment rate of the anxiety disorders was about 33%, there was a wide variability across the specific anxiety disorders. Treatment rates of phobia, by far the most common anxiety disorder, were less than 1 in 3, whereas almost 60% of the 1% of respondents who were diagnosed as having a panic disorder obtained services. Respondents with substance use disorders were the least likely to obtain services.[4]

Those Persons Who Sought Mental Health Services

A secondary analysis of the ECA data set[7,8] described the effect of having a diagnosable psychiatric disorder on the likelihood of making a visit to an MHP. From **Table 2**, it can be seen that having a disorder tripled the likelihood of making a visit to an MHP. However, less than 25% of those persons with a disorder ever made such a visit. A number of demographic variables were associated with psychotherapy utilization (**Table 3**). For example, those persons with the highest level of education were the least likely to have a psychiatric disorder, but they were the most likely to seek outpatient specialty mental health services given the presence of such a disorder. This same inverse relationship was true of race and income as well, but not so strongly.

Klerman and Weissman[9] suggested that there are 3 major classes of consumers of psychotherapy: (1) individuals with a diagnosed illness of fairly long standing, (2) individuals who have trouble coping with stressful life events, and (3) individuals who are interested in achieving a greater measure of success or life satisfaction. Only the first of these 3 groups is likely to have a diagnosable major psychiatric disorder (Axis I). The second group may have an adjustment disorder diagnosis or a phase of life (V code) problem. The third group of consumers would be unlikely to qualify for any *DSM* diagnosis.

Table 2. Lifetime Probability of Making at Least 1 Visit to a Mental Health Specialist*

Demographic Variable	No *DSM* Disorder In Lifetime	At Least 1 *DSM* Disorder in Lifetime
Gender		
M	.070	.201
F	.082	.254
Education		
Grammar school or less	.039	.110
Some high school	.054	.202
High school graduate	.058	.246
Some college	.105	.351
College graduate	.150	.432
Marital status		
Married	.065	.209
Widowed	.037	.101
Separated or divorced	.172	.347
Never married	.088	.273
Race		
W	.087	.274
Non-W	.054	.165
Income, $		
<10 000	.068	.205
10 000-14 999	.073	.230
15 000-19 999	.091	.250
20 000-24 999	.085	.309
25 000-34 999	.093	.297
≥35 000	.141	.371
Age, y		
18-20	.072	.246
21-30	.081	.263
31-40	.137	.367
41-50	.107	.335
51-60	.087	.238
61+	.041	.096

Data from the Epidemiologic Catchment Area survey from 1980 to 1984.

Table 3. Lifetime Probability of Having a *DSM-III* Diagnosis and Probability of Making a Mental Health Visit Given the Presence of a Diagnosis*

Demographic Variable	At Least 1 Diagnosis in Lifetime	At Least 1 Visit in Lifetime (Given a Diagnosis)
Gender		
M	.382	.201
F	.348	.254
Education		
Grammar school or less	.470	.110
Some high school	.389	.202
High school graduate	.314	.246
Some college	.311	.351
College graduate	.289	.432
Marital status		
Married	.314	.209
Widowed	.362	.101
Separated or divorced	.491	.347
Never married	.375	.273
Race		
W	.329	.274
Non-W	.426	.165
Income, $		
<10 000	.411	.205
10 000-14 999	.350	.230
15 000-19 999	.331	.250
20 000-24 999	.327	.309
25 000-34 999	.313	.297
≥35 000	.285	.371
Age, y		
18-20	.309	.246
21-30	.390	.263
31-40	.398	.367
41-50	.377	.335
51-60	.361	.238
61+	.330	.096

Data from the Epidemiologic Catchment Area survey from 1980 to 1984.

Howard and Orlinsky[10] described 3 characteristics that are relevant to utilization as follows: (1) the degree and type of psychopathology, (2) the degree of pathology-proneness (ie, the vulnerabilities or deficits that increase the probability of experiencing psychopathology), and (3) environmental stress. Consistent with these various classifications, Hough et al[11] used the ECA data to estimate that in any given year about 1% of the US population who did not have a current *DSM-III-R* diagnosis would make at least 1 visit to a mental health specialist. Of the 7 million people who made a visit to a mental health specialist in a 6-month period, 4 million had a current diagnosis, 1 million had a past diagnosis, and 2 million had never qualified for a *DSM-III-R* diagnosis.[11,12]

Routes to Mental Health Services

Utilization of mental health services has been linked to distress, education, marital status, and race.[8,13,14] Since these variables are likely to be indicators of different psychological phenomena, there is a need for a better understanding of the process that individuals go through in seeking professional help.[15]

The routes to mental health services can be understood through 2 overlapping "person-centered" processes (**Figure**): (1) intrapersonal decisions about the presence of the illness and what to do regarding it[16] and (2) interpersonal or external behaviors to surmount treatment barriers and to negotiate "pathways" into the service sector.[15]

The help-seeking process has multiple steps, including recognizing that there is a problem, deciding external help is necessary, and contacting the service sector.[17-19] The recognition that there is a problem is neither easy[17] nor automatic,[20,21] and it represents a formidable barrier to accessing care.[22] Many people resist recognizing that a problem exists or attributing the problem to psychological factors or mental illness. For example, 1 survey found that of the 19% of adults who had high depressive scores, two thirds denied that they felt depressed.[18]

Prochaska et al[23] proposed a multistage model of the change process: at the first of these, namely, the "precontemplation" stage, the individual lacks sufficient awareness of the problem and is thus unlikely to try to change. Persons in this stage are less likely to enter treatment programs and are less likely to experience successful change.[24]

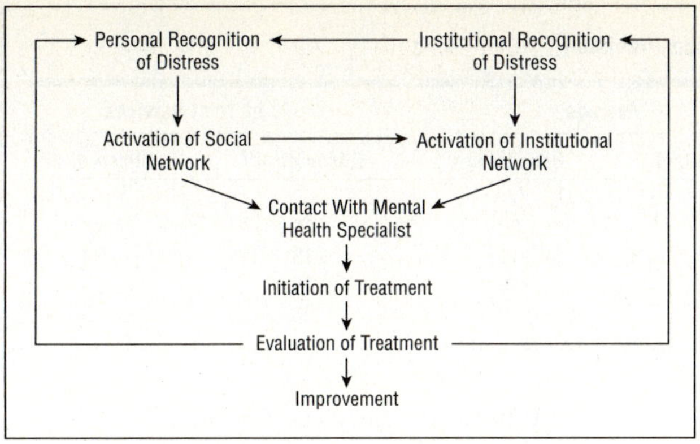

Modified generic clinical pathway for all mental health services.

The decision that professional intervention is necessary is largely influenced by consultation with informal help sources—the first and generally preferred resource.[17,18,25,26] The social network helps the individual to recognize and define the problem,[27] and to decide what, if any, action needs to be taken.[28] Some social networks are supportive of mental health services and encourage members to seek help; other networks are not so inclined and will, in effect, be a barrier to obtaining professional help.

A person's social network, in itself, may provide sufficient resources.[29] The ECA investigators explicitly acknowledged this "newly defined sector," composed of self-help groups, friends, and relatives, and they labeled it as the voluntary support network. They reported that the voluntary support network was the only source of service for 15% of all respondents with diagnosable conditions who sought any services.[4]

Many persons who obtain services from an MHP have been referred by medical providers.[17,30] Furthermore, a large proportion of mentally ill persons who seek professional services do so only within the general medical sector.[4,6] Some have perceived or labeled emotional distress as physical symptoms,[31] but most have explicitly chosen a general medical provider for mental health service.[12] However, it is unclear whether such treatment is generally adequate.[32]

Following problem recognition and definition, the next step in the process of seeking mental health services is deciding whether such help is acceptable, necessary, and potentially helpful. Receptivity to mental health services has been found to be low in both relatively old and relatively young subjects, less educated persons, and less affluent individuals.[33,34] Admitting a need for help has been found to be especially difficult for shy persons[35] and those persons with high self-esteem.[36] Stigma concerning mental health treatment continues to be a substantial barrier to seeking treatment. Veroff et al[25] examined the reasons people did not seek professional help even though, in retrospect, they realized that they could have benefited from such help. Fear of what others would think was a common barrier. In a substudy of the ECA Program, Leaf et al[37] found that 80% of respondents were highly receptive to mental health services, but that 83% reported at least 1 barrier (eg, upsetting a family member) to their own personal utilization of such services. Despite claims that the general public's attitude toward the mental health professions has become more positive,[38] it appears that one's attitude toward such services and one's willingness to utilize them are quite distinct.

Table 4. Estimated Number of Professionals Providing Services

Profession	Estimated Total No.	Estimated No. Active	Source, y
Mental health			
Specialty providers			
Psychiatrists	44 255	33 200	Olfson et al,[42] 1994
Psychologists	56 000	42 000	Dial et al,[43] 1990
Social workers	60 000	45 000	Robiner,[44] 1991
Other mental health providers			
Family therapists	. . .	28 000	VandenBos et al,[45] 1991
Psychiatric nurses	. . .	3000	Knesper et al,[46] 1985
Primary care physicians	. . .	116 642	Knesper et al,[46] 1985

The decision to consult a mental health provider does not guarantee that any services will be received. Numerous studies have shown that patients will drop out after scheduling an initial appointment or after only 1 visit.[39] Although resource-related barriers (eg, availability and affordability) undoubtedly interfere with the help-seeking process at this point, other factors, as yet not understood, are involved. For example, Ware et al[40(p1098)] found that "even with generous coverage of outpatient mental health services, the great majority of those who need care do not receive care." It seems that person-centered barriers play a major role in perpetuating the gap between service need and utilization.

The mental health service provision system continues to do a poor job in eliminating the barriers of stigma and ignorance about the benefits of mental health treatments.

SERVICE PROVIDERS

Several studies of mental health service providers yield information on the professional activities of providers, the setting in which services are provided, the types of problems that are addressed, and the characteristics of the services that are provided. Knesper et al[41] surveyed psychiatrists, psychologists, and social workers by using stratified sampling procedures on lists of professional organizations (eg, National Register of Health Care Providers, Washington, DC) for 1983. They obtained reports from 2038 psychiatrists, 2028 psychologists, 1106 social workers, and 768 primary care physicians about their practice patterns, patients, and services. Olfson et al[42] examined the practice patterns of psychiatrists by using data collected from 3 sources: (1) the Professional Activities Survey of members of the American Psychiatric Association, Washington, DC, that yielded usable data

Table 5. Distribution of Professionals' Efforts in Mental Health Service Provision

Profession	Weekly Direct Treatment, h	% of Hours	Average		% of Total Services	
			Patients/d	Patients/mo	Olfson et al[47]	Olfson et al[42]
Psychiatrists	33	70	10	39	19	48
Psychologists	24	57	6	16	13	34
Social workers	21	55	6	16	15	39
Primary care physicians	12	23	1	0	53	0

from 16 135 psychiatrists; (2) the Client/Patient Sample Survey,[43] which used a stratified sample of 1308 outpatient mental health service organizations; and (3) the National Ambulatory Medical Care Surveys that were conducted in 1980, 1985, and 1989, and included 424 psychiatrists and 2245 primary care physicians.

How Many Professionals in the Mental Health Specialty Sector Provide Mental Health Services?

The estimated numbers of professionals who provided mental health services in the late 1980s is presented in **Table 4**. There were about 120 000 mental health specialty providers (psychiatrists, psychologists, and social workers).[42-44] An equal number of primary care physicians were actively providing mental health services.[45] The numbers of other professionals (eg, family therapists and psychiatric nurses) were more difficult to estimate because they were either relatively new professions in independent mental health provision or were not uniformly defined by degrees or licensure.[46]

How Are the Efforts of Mental Health Service Providers Distributed?

Mental health professionals typically have multiple roles and practices in multiple settings. As can be seen in **Table 5**, psychiatrists spent the major proportion of their workweek in direct treatment. Psychologists and social workers spent a little more than half their time providing treatment. Primary care physicians reported that they spent 23% of their workweek providing mental health services. Psychiatrists saw more patients in a typical day than did psychologists or social workers. In a typical month, psychiatrists saw 39 different patients, and psychologists and social workers each saw 16 different patients.

Within organizations that have multiple mental health specialty professions represented among the providers, psychiatrists were involved in the treatment of 48% of outpatients, and social workers, psychologists, nurses, and other MHPs were involved with 39%, 24%, 15%, and 21% of outpatients, respectively.[47] Overall, primary care physicians, psychiatrists, social workers, and psychologists provided 53%, 19%, 15%, and 13% of all mental health services, respectively.[48] However, professional activities overlapped in services to an individual patient; for example, two thirds of the patients who were treated by psychiatrists also were treated by other MHPs.[47]

Where Are Services Provided?

Of the 1.3 million outpatients who were treated for at least 1 month in mental health specialty *organizations* in 1986, 56% were treated in interdisciplinary mental health service centers, 17% were treated in independent mental health clinics, 14% were treated in general hospital mental health clinics, 6% were treated in Veterans Affairs medical center clinics, 4% were treated in state and county mental hospital clinics, and 3% were treated in private psychiatric hospital clinics.[47] The sample of providers described by Knesper et al[46] indicated that 72% of patients were seen in a private office setting, 16% were seen in community mental health centers, 4% were in medical school clinics, and 4% were seen in public hospitals.

Approximately half of practicing psychiatrists primarily provided services in private office settings,[42,46] and another 14% practiced secondarily in private office settings. About 25% of psychiatrists were primarily employed in public service settings, and about 20% of psychiatrists were employed in private psychiatric or general hospital settings. Psychologists primarily were employed in private office settings and secondarily in public care settings. About half of social workers were employed in private office settings, and 40% were employed in public care settings. Most primary care physicians offered mental health services in private office settings.[46]

What Patient Problems Are Seen by Different Providers?

Of 12 272 patients described by mental health providers,[46] all disorders were seen more frequently in private office practice settings. Patients with less severe psychological and emotional problems were predominant in the caseloads of every provider group. Seventy-five percent of patients in the caseloads of psychologists and social workers had less severe conditions, and about a half of psychiatrists' caseloads included patients with less severe disorders. Patients with more serious disorders were more likely to be seen in public hospitals and community mental health settings.

With regard to diagnoses, 23% of the sample were diagnosed as having major depression or mania, 46% had a diagnosis of neurosis, anxiety, or personality disorders, and 5% were diagnosed as substance abusers.[49] By contrasting diagnoses and settings, depressive, anxiety, and substance use disorders respectively accounted for 17%, 8%, and 3% of all patients who were treated in spe-

Table 6. Duration of Psychotherapy by Provider Type*

Provider	Total No.	No. of Sessions 1-2	3-10	11-20	21+
Total nonpsychiatric physicians	39	72	50	35	22
Primary care	13	23	18	10	6
Other physicians	26	49	31	25	15
Total MHPs	50	15	39	57	66
Psychiatry	16	6	12	17	21
Clinical psychologists	19	6	15	23	24
Other MHPs	15	3	12	17	21
Unknown	11	13	11	8	12

Data adapted from Olfson and Pincus,[51] 1994. Percentages reflect within-duration category by overall provider type (eg, 72% of 1- to 2-session durations are provided by nonpsychiatric physicians, who make up 39% of mental health service providers). MHPs indicates mental health professionals.

cialty mental health service provision organizations.[49] For patients who were receiving treatment in mental health service organizations, patients with depression were most likely to be treated in a multiservice setting (eg, a community mental health center [33%] or a general hospital clinic [27%]); service recipients with anxiety disorders were most likely to be treated in a Veterans Affairs medical center (38%) or a general hospital program (21%); and patients with a substance use disorder were most likely to be treated in a Veterans Affairs medical center (33%) or a multiservice mental health organization (28%).[47]

Patients with depressive disorders, neurosis, anxiety, personality disorders, and substance use disorders were most likely to be seen by primary care physicians in any 60-day period. The figures for patients with depression were comparable with those based on a more focal study of 617 depressed patients[50]; this study indicated that 60% of patients with depression were seen in a general medical clinic, 21% were seen by a psychologist or other nonmedical therapist, and 20% were seen by a psychiatrist. Patients with depressive disorders were most likely to be seen by both a psychiatrist and another mental health specialty provider (44%), but 40% were only seen by a mental health specialty provider other than a psychiatrist. Nearly equal proportions of patients with anxiety disorders were likely to be seen by a nonpsychiatrist mental health specialty provider (41%) or an interdisciplinary combination of a psychiatrist and another mental health provider (39%). Patients with substance use disorders were most likely to be seen by mental health specialty providers other than psychiatrists (69%), or a combination of psychiatrists and another specialty provider (24%).

What Services Are Supplied by Providers?

By using data from the 1987 National Medical Expenditure Survey, Olfson and Pincus[51] analyzed the provision of psychotherapy by mental health specialty providers and primary care physicians. In this analysis, psychotherapy was defined as any talking therapy of any duration throughout any period. By this definition, mental health specialty providers supplied half of all psychotherapy visits (50%), general medical professionals provided 39% of all such visits, and the professional status of providers for 11% of visits was unknown. Of the patients who were treated exclusively by psychiatrists, 55% received individual psychotherapy, whereas 70% of the patients who were treated by nonpsychiatrist mental health professionals received individual psychotherapy.

UTILIZATION OF MENTAL HEALTH SERVICES

Patients who were treated by a provider who was in the specialty mental health sector tended to receive treatment of a longer duration (**Table 6**). Nearly two thirds of psychotherapies that lasted for more than 20 sessions were provided by mental health specialists, with roughly one fifth of such treatment episodes provided by nonpsychiatric physicians. These findings appear to apply to all specialty mental health providers.[51] For shorter-term patients (1 or 2 visits), only 15% received services from a specialty mental health provider. For longer-term patients (>20 visits), 66% were seen by a specialty provider.

Most of the psychotherapy provided by general medical professionals was of a brief duration—less than 3 sessions. The effective dose of psychotherapy for most patients has been shown to be 4 to 8 sessions.[52] Therefore, it is likely that few patients who receive psychotherapy from general medical professionals receive an effective treatment dose.

Olfson and Pincus[51] estimated the number of visits of psychotherapy for depression, anxiety, and substance use. Similar patterns of treatment length were observed for these disorders—the majority of patients received less than 10 sessions of treatment, regardless of diagnosis. However, about one fourth of the patients received more than 20 sessions of treatment. Patients with depression were likely to attend 10 or fewer sessions (54%), but 27% attended more than 20 sessions. For patients with anxiety disorders, 55% were seen for 10 or fewer sessions, and 21% attended more than 20 sessions. For patients with substance use disorders, 54% were seen for 10 or fewer sessions, and 23% were seen for more than 20 sessions.

Taube et al[13] reported that income, education, and insurance coverage were among the best predictors of the duration of outpatient treatment. Landerman et al[53] demonstrated that the presence of any insurance coverage increased the probability of seeking treatment. However, in the RAND study, insurance limits on the duration of care were inversely related to the duration of treatment—20-session limits were associated with longer average stays than unlimited co-pay coverage.[54] It is clear that efforts to study utilization should include a minimum standard data set that includes gender, age, education, income, and insurance coverage, since each of these variables appears to influence decisions with regard to the use of mental health services.

COMMENT

While this review provides an overview of mental health service utilization, several important areas are not addressed. For example, little is known about alternative routes to recovery from mental illnesses or the natural course of these illnesses. What happens to the symptoms of people who do not recognize that they have diagnosable mental health problems? It is likely that many persons who have a problem have developed coping strategies without professional intervention.

Litwak[55] suggested that people deal effectively with problems when they use a combination of informal and formal support systems. The formal systems (eg, mental health services) are best able to respond to needs that require higher levels of skill, and these systems typically operate within a well-organized scheduled routine. Informal systems (eg, families, neighbors, and friends) seem better equipped to deal with problems that require little professional training and demand frequent, flexible responses. Much more information is needed about the fit between the informal and formal networks that assist persons to recover from a mental illness. Informal systems can serve either as barriers to treatment or facilitators of recovery. What are the mechanisms that facilitate the transition from the exclusive use of informal networks for dealing with a mental illness to the use of some combination of formal and informal intervention?

Many persons with mental illnesses begin the process of receiving formal services through nonpsychiatric physicians. These physicians provide almost half of all mental health services. One growing movement has been the partnership between primary care physicians and MHPs (eg, the expansion of family systems medicine in the past decade). How large this movement is and what effect it has on utilization are not known.

We have provided an overview of "the facts" about service utilization, in particular which clinicians are providing what services to which persons with which mental illnesses in what settings. No attempt has been made here to address the "why" of the current status of mental health services or "how" services need to be tailored to meet the unmet needs of mentally ill persons best. The implications for the design and interpretation of treatment research are clear, however. The review that we have provided allows investigators to evaluate the generalizability of any findings from a clinical trial (at least in terms of the representativeness of the patients, therapists, and setting).

Services research provides important information about patterns of service needs and utilization. However, we need to expand our knowledge about which methods of intervention that have been efficacious in controlled settings are most transferable for use by specifically trained psychotherapists in clinical practice with clearly identified patients. Information is needed about the extent to which specific treatment modalities are perceived as more acceptable by potential patients for dealing with specific problems.

We must examine research reports for evidence about the specificity of the results that have been reported on particular groups of patients. For example, Scogin and McElreath[56] reviewed published research about the effectiveness of psychosocial treatment of depression among older adults. By using meta-analysis, they summarized 17 studies that examined the effect of psychotherapy on geriatric depression. They found that elderly persons responded as well to treatment as did younger persons, and no specific modality of treatment was found superior to other modalities. Their summary of the studies, however, did not report sociodemographic characteristics of the patients (eg, gender, ethnic origin, and economic status) or the settings in which the treatment was provided (eg, private practice, medical setting, community mental health center, or social service center). To translate these research findings into useful information for clinical service and policymaking, we need to explore the extent to which they apply to specific subgroups in specific settings.

The dictum of Paul[57] about the examination of the contributions of the clinician, the patient, the modality, and the setting to the outcome of treatments still needs to be addressed in a systematic manner. Such a systematic review might include the development of a multidimensional matrix that allows the placement of existing findings in the context of the 4 key elements of psychotherapy research: patient, clinician, modality, and setting. This process of organizing outcomes by key elements would accomplish 2 important tasks: (1) it would facilitate the consolidation of the existing information about the efficacy, effectiveness, and efficiency of specified treatments and (2) it would increase our awareness of gaps in our knowledge about mental health services research. This information could be used to inform the next generation of both researchers and clinicians about the direction to be taken in both clinical research and service provision.

Accepted for publication April 22, 1996.

This work was partially supported by grants RO1 MH42901 and KO5 MH00924 from the National Institute of Mental Health, Rockville, Md.

We are grateful for the statistical work of Bruce Briscoe, and the helpful comments of the Northwestern/Chicago (Ill) Psychotherapy Research Group.

Corresponding author: Kenneth I. Howard, PhD, Department of Psychology, Northwestern University, 2025 Sheridan Rd, Evanston, IL 60205-2710.

REFERENCES

1. The President's Commission on Mental Health and Illness, eds. *Report to the President From the President's Commission on Mental Health.* Washington, DC: US Government Printing Office; 1978;1.
2. Regier DA, Myers JK, Kramer M, Robins LN, Blazer DG, Hough RL, Eaton WW, Locke BZ. The NIMH Epidemiologic Catchment Area Program. *Arch Gen Psychiatry.* 1984;41:934-941.
3. Eaton WW, Holzer CE, Von Korff M, Anthony JC, Helzer JE, George L, Burnam MA, Boyd JH, Kessler LG, Locke BZ. The design of the Epidemiologic Catchment Area surveys: the control and measurement of error. *Arch Gen Psychiatry.* 1984;41:942-948.
4. Regier DA, Narrow WE, Rae DS, Manderscheid RW, Locke BZ, Goodwin FK. The de-facto US mental and addictive disorders service system: Epidemiologic Catchment Area prospective 1-year prevalence rate of disorders and services. *Arch Gen Psychiatry.* 1993;50:85-94.
5. Karno M, Hough RL, Burnam MA, Escobar JI, Timbers DM, Santana F, Boyd JH. Lifetime prevalence of specific psychiatric disorders among Mexican Americans and non-Hispanic whites in Los Angeles. *Arch Gen Psychiatry.* 1987;44: 695-701.
6. Kessler RC, McGonagle KA, Zhao S, Nelson CB, Hughes M, Eshleman S, Wittchen H, Kendler KS. Lifetime and 12-month prevalence of *DSM-III-R* psychiatric dis-

orders in the US: results from the National Comorbidity Survey. *Arch Gen Psychiatry.* 1994;51:8-19.
7. Vessey JT. *Determining Utilization of Mental Health Services.* Evanston, Ill: Northwestern University; 1991.
8. Vessey JT, Howard KI. Who seeks psychotherapy? *Psychotherapy.* 1993;30: 546-553.
9. Klerman GL, Weissman MM. An epidemiologic view of mental illness, mental health, and normality. In: Offer D, Sabshin M, eds. *Normality and the Life Cycle.* New York, NY: Basic Books Inc Publishers; 1984:315-344.
10. Howard KI, Orlinsky DE. Psychotherapeutic processes. *Annu Rev Psychol.* 1972; 23:615-668.
11. Hough RL, Landsverk JA, Karno M, Burnam MA. Utilization of health and mental health services by Los Angeles Mexican Americans and non-Hispanic whites. *Arch Gen Psychiatry.* 1987;44:702-709.
12. Shapiro S, Skinner EA, Kessler LG, von Korff M, German PS, Tischler GL, Leaf PJ, Benham L, Cottler L, Regier DA. Utilization of health and mental health services: three Epidemiologic Catchment Area sites. *Arch Gen Psychiatry.* 1984; 41:971-978.
13. Taube CA, Kessler LG, Burns BJ. Estimating the probability and level of ambulatory mental health services. *Health Serv Res.* 1986;21:321-340.
14. Olfson M, Pincus HA. Outpatient psychotherapy in the United States, I: volume, costs, and user characteristics. *Am J Psychiatry.* 1994;151:1281-1288.
15. Rogler LH, Cortes DE. Help-seeking pathways: a unifying concept in mental health care. *Am J Psychiatry.* 1993;150:554-561.
16. Mechanic D. The experience and expression of distress: the study of illness behavior and medical utilization. In: Mechanic D, ed. *Handbook of Health, Health Care, and the Health Professions.* New York, NY: Free Press; 1982:591-607.
17. Saunders SM. Applicants' experience of the process of seeking psychotherapy. *Psychotherapy.* 1993;30:554-564.
18. Yokopenic PA, Clark VA, Aneshensel CS. Depression, problem recognition and professional consultation. *J Nerv Ment Dis.* 1983;171:15-23.
19. Kadushin C. *Why People Go to Psychiatrists.* New York, NY: Atherton Publishing Co; 1969.
20. Mechanic D. *Mental Health and Social Policy.* 2nd ed. Englewood Cliffs, NJ: Prentice-Hall International Inc; 1980.
21. Horwitz AV. *The Social Control of Mental Illness.* Orlando, Fla: Academic Press Inc; 1981.
22. Regier DA, Hirschfeld RMA, Goodwin FK, Burke JD, Lazar JB, Judd LL. The NIMH Depression Awareness, Recognition, and Treatment Program: structure, aims, and scientific basis. *Am J Psychiatry.* 1988;145:1351-1357.
23. Prochaska JO, DiClemente CC, Norcross JC. In search of how people change. *Am Psychol.* 1992;47:1102-1114.
24. Prochaska JO, Norcross JC, Fowler JL, Follick MJ, Abrams DB. Attendance and outcome in a work-site weight control program: processes and stages of change as process and predictor variables. *Addict Behav.* 1992;17:35-45.
25. Veroff JB, Kulka RA, Douvan E. *Mental Health in America: Patterns of Help-Seeking From 1957 to 1976.* New York, NY: Basic Books Inc Publishers; 1981.
26. Tinsley HEA, de St Aubin TM, Brown MT. College students' help-seeking preferences. *J Counsel Psychol.* 1982;29:523-533.
27. Whitt HP, Meile RL. Alignment, magnification and snowballing processes in the definition of symptoms of mental illness. *Soc Forces.* 1985;63:682-697.
28. Horwitz AV. The pathways into psychiatric treatment: some differences between men and women. *J Health Soc Behav.* 1977;18:169-178.
29. Thoits PA. Social support as coping assistance. *J Consult Clin Psychol.* 1986; 54:416-423.
30. Gater R, Goldberg D. Pathways to psychiatric care in South Manchester. *Br J Psychiatry.* 1991;159:90-96.
31. Schurman RA, Kramer PD, Mitchell JB. The hidden mental health network: treatment of mental illness by nonpsychiatric physicians. *Arch Gen Psychiatry.* 1985;42:89-94.
32. Munoz RF, Hollon SD, McGrath E, Rehm LP, VandenBos GR. On the AHCPR Depression in Primary Care Guidelines: further considerations for practitioners. *Am Psychol.* 1994;49:42-61.
33. Waxman HM, Carner EA, Klein M. Underutilization of mental health services by community elderly. *Gerontologist.* 1984;24:23-30.
34. Leaf PJ, Livingston MM, Tischler GL, Weissman MM, Holzer CE, Myers JK. Contact with health professionals for the treatment of psychiatric and emotional problems. *Med Care.* 1985;23:1322-1337.
35. Zimbardo PG. *Shyness: What Is It, What to Do About It.* Reading, Mass: Addison-Wesley Publishing Co; 1977.
36. Miller WR. Motivation for treatment: a review with special emphasis on alcoholism. *Psychol Bull.* 1985;98:84-107.
37. Leaf PJ, Livingstone Bruce M, Tischler GL. The differential effect of attitudes on the use of mental health services. *Soc Psychiatry Psychiatr Epidemiol.* 1986; 21:187-192.
38. Murstein BI, Fontaine FA. The public's knowledge about psychologists and other mental health professionals. *Am Psychol.* 1993;48:829-845.
39. Sue S, McKinney HL, Allen DB. Predictors of the duration of therapy for clients in the community mental health system. *Community Ment Health J.* 1976; 12:365-375.
40. Ware JE, Manning WG, Duan N, Wells KB, Newhouse JP. Health status and the use of outpatient mental health services. *Am Psychol.* 1984;39:1090-1100.
41. Knesper DJ, Wheeler JRC, Pagnucco DJ. Mental health services providers' distribution across counties in the United States. *Am Psychol.* 1984;39:1424-1434.
42. Olfson M, Pincus HA, Dial TH. Professional practice patterns of U.S. psychiatrists. *Am J Psychiatry.* 1994;151:89-95.
43. Dial TH, Tebbutt R, Pion GM, Kohout J, VandenBos G, Johnson M, Schervish PH, Whiting L, Fox J, Merwin EI. Human resources in mental health. In: Manderschied RW, Sonnenschein MA, eds. *Mental Health, United States.* Rockville, Md: National Institute of Mental Health; 1990:196-215.
44. Robiner WN. How many psychologists are needed? a call for a national psychology human resource agenda. *Profes Psychol Res Pract.* 1991;22:427-440.
45. VandenBos GR, DeLeon PH, Belar CD. How many psychological practitioners are needed? it's too early to know! *Profes Psychol Res Pract.* 1991;22:441-448.
46. Knesper DJ, Pagnucco DJ, Wheeler JRC. Similarities and differences across mental health service providers and practice settings in the United States. *Am Psychol.* 1985;40:1352-1369.
47. Olfson M, Klerman GL, Pincus HA. The roles of psychiatrists in organized outpatient mental health settings. *Am J Psychiatry.* 1993;150:625-631.
48. Knesper DJ, Pagnucco DJ. Estimated distribution of effort by providers of mental health services to U.S. adults in 1982 and 1983. *Am J Psychiatry.* 1987; 144:883-888.
49. Knesper DJ, Belcher DT, Cross JC. Variations in the intensity of psychiatric treatment across markets for mental health services in the United States. *Health Serv Res.* 1988;22:797-819.
50. Rogers WH, Wells KB, Meredith LS, Sturm R, Burnam MA. Outcomes for adult outpatients with depression under prepaid or fee-for-service financing. *Arch Gen Psychiatry.* 1993;50:517-525.
51. Olfson M, Pincus HA. Outpatient psychotherapy in the United States, II: patterns of utilization. *Am J Psychiatry.* 1994;151:1289-1294.
52. Howard KI, Kopta SM, Krause MS, Orlinsky DE. The dose-response relationship in psychotherapy. *Am Psychol.* 1986;41:159-164.
53. Landerman LR, Burns BJ, Schwartz MS, Wagner HR, George LK. The relationship between insurance coverage and psychiatric disorders in predicting use of mental health services. *Am J Psychiatry.* 1994;151:1785-1790.
54. Manning WG, Leibowitz A, Goldberg G. A controlled study of the effect of a pre-paid group practice on use of services. *N Engl J Med.* 1984;310:1505-1510.
55. Litwak E. *Helping the Elderly: the Complementary Roles of Informal Networks and Formal Systems.* New York, NY: Guilford Press; 1988.
56. Scogin F, McElreath L. Efficacy of psychosocial treatments for geriatric depression: a quantitative review. *J Consult Clin Psychol.* 1994;62:69-74.
57. Paul GL. Strategy of outcome research in psychotherapy. *J Consult Clin Psychol.* 1967;31:109-118.

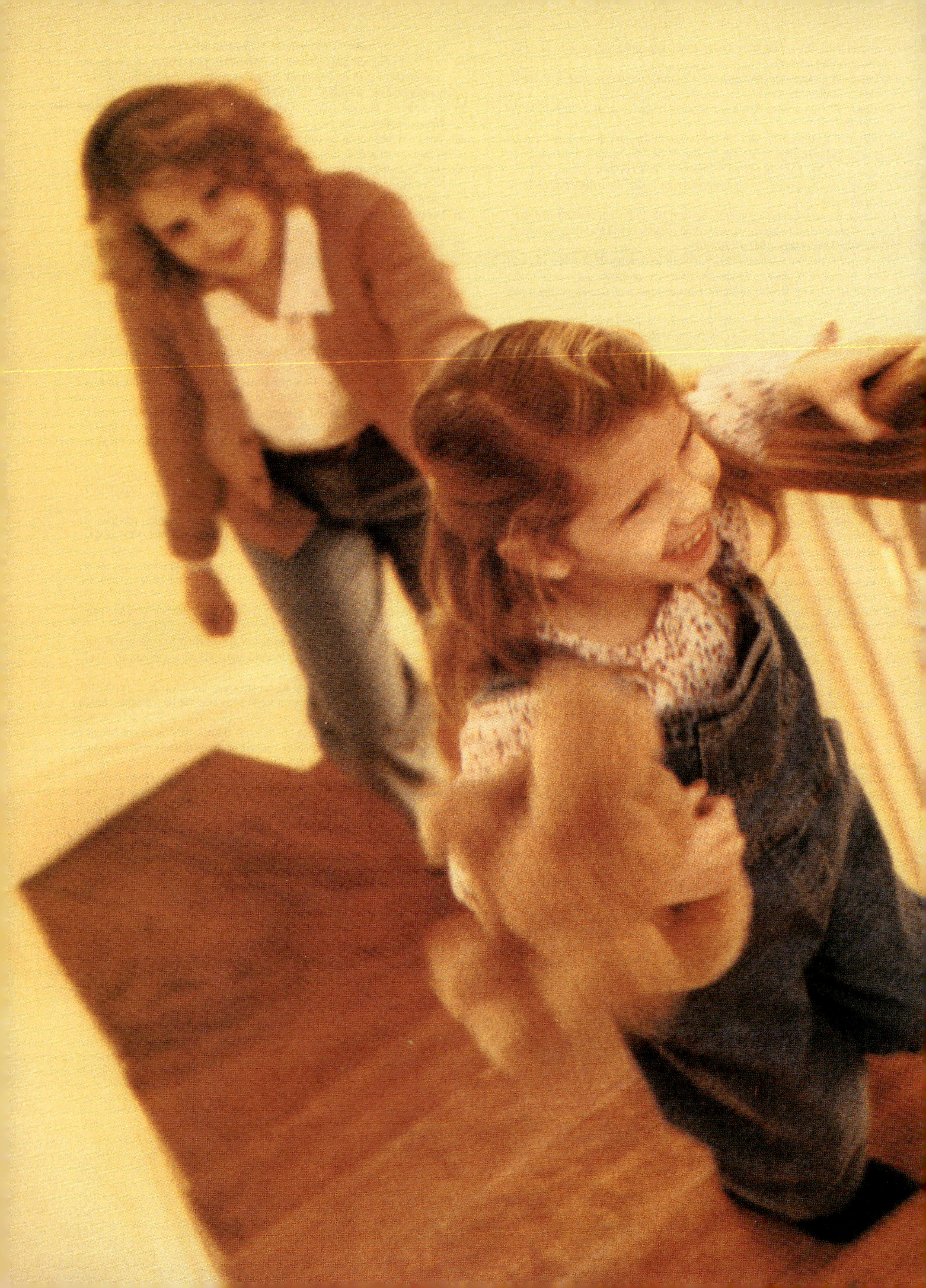

Psychotherapy Research in Historical Perspective

Implications for Mental Health Care Policy

Robert L. Russell, PhD; David E. Orlinsky, PhD

This article is a sketch of the historical development of the field of behavioral and nonbehavioral therapy research. Four phases are characterized: (1) establishing scientific research (1927-1954), (2) searching for scientific rigor (1955-1969), (3) expansion and organization (1970-1983), and (4) consolidation and reformulation (1984-present). Continuities between and key developments within successive phases are outlined, with emphasis given to methodological innovations. The corroboration of select findings about process and outcome and the development of several critical discourses within the third and fourth phases have implications for the provision of mental health care and for policy discussions.

Arch Gen Psychiatry. 1996;53:708-715

Psychotherapy research has been conducted for more than 50 years.[1,2] Its influence on clinical practices and mental health care policy has been inconsistent. Even in medicine, however, relations among research, health care, and health care policy are often encumbered.[3] This is instructive, for medical research and the sciences on which it is based have been established for much longer than psychotherapy research and its parent discipline, psychology. Nevertheless, psychotherapy research has advanced and can inform practitioners and those responsible for crafting policy.

The history of psychotherapy research divides into 4 phases. The first phase lasted from 1927 to 1954. Its main task was to demonstrate the feasibility of investigating psychotherapy scientifically. The second phase lasted from 1955 through 1969. A growing number of behaviorally, dynamically, and experientially oriented investigators developed new methods for studying psychotherapy. They were motivated by skeptics like Eysenck[4,5] and Levitt,[6,7] who challenged the effectiveness of dynamically oriented treatments, and by the growth of behavioral treatments, which seemed equally as or more effective than traditional therapies.[8,9]

The third phase, from 1970 to 1983, was one of expansion, differentiation, and organization. It was marked by the integration of cognitive principles within behavioral and nonbehavioral therapies and by new methods to assess the overall effectiveness of treatments. The fourth phase can be dated from about 1984 to the present. Researchers extended and consolidated past successes and explored more systematically the integrative and eclectic therapies.[10,11] In addition, researchers more actively attempted to demonstrate the relevance of their work to practitioners, third-party payers, and policymakers.[12] Concurrently, some mainstream researchers stimulated a countercurrent of interest in alternative research strategies that were focused on treatment processes.[13]

Characterizations of these research phases provide a context for summarizing research findings and critical discourses that should inform debates about mental health care policy.

HISTORY OF PSYCHOTHERAPY RESEARCH

Phase I (Circa 1927-1954): Establishing Scientific Research

Freud's oeuvre has provided the foundation for dynamically oriented therapies.

From the Department of Psychology, Loyola University Chicago, Ill (Dr Russell), and the Committee on Human Development, University of Chicago (Dr Orlinsky).

The works of Watson, Pavlov, Thorndike, and Skinner have provided the foundation for behavioral therapies. The earliest research publications, appearing in the 1920s, contained statistical tabulations of outcomes in a few clinics,[14] although single-case research reports did appear.[15] Elementary outcome research continued until 1940, nearly halted during the war, and resumed in full during the 1950s. At that time, the growth of psychologies of learning (eg, those of Guthrie, Hull, and Skinner) and the widening of psychologists' roles to include not only testing, but also the provision of treatment, allowed behavioral therapies to augment and compete with the dominant psychodynamically oriented therapies.

Competition between treatment types was sparked by Eysenck.[4] Empirical research, he argued, did not validate claims that psychodynamic treatments were more efficacious than control conditions. In addition, Skinner[16] and Wolpe[17] argued that other treatments, derived more directly from scientific experimentation than their analytic counterparts, might be more effective.

Simultaneous with debates about efficacy, process research began with the use of phonographic recordings to investigate client-centered counseling sessions in the 1940s.[18] The investigators accumulated enough research by the late 1940s to be featured in the *Journal of Consulting Psychology* (1949). In 1949, Rogers and his coworkers at the University of Chicago Counseling Center organized one of the first long-term programs of process and outcome research.

Other early research programs were the Psychotherapy Research Unit established by Jerome Frank[19] and his coworkers at The Johns Hopkins Medical School and the Menninger Project established by Karl Menninger.[20] By this time, other pioneers (eg, Edward Bordin, Lester Luborsky, and William Snyder) were engaged in investigations. Shortly thereafter, phase I reached a climax with the publication of 2 research anthologies,[21,22] and a book about therapy research edited by Rogers and Dymond.[23] Together with Eysenck's review and rejoinders to it,[24,25] these works signaled the end of the first phase. This period was marked by the advent of competitors to psychoanalytic orthodoxy and by applications of scientific method in the study of all types of psychotherapy.

Phase I was a success. Researchers demonstrated how psychotherapy could be brought from private offices into the purview of scientific study. Investigators had measured feelings, perceptions, behaviors, and thoughts, agreeing, as Rogers and his colleagues did, "that Thorndike's dictum is essentially correct—that 'anything that exists, exists in some quantity that can be measured.'"[26]

Phase I pioneers demonstrated that session recordings could "capture" psychotherapeutic phenomena for scientific investigation, and psychometric and statistical techniques could be used to quantify and test hypotheses. Eysenck's negative appraisal raised questions about the scientific legitimacy of dynamic psychotherapy—questions that were formulated in terms of evidence and that could only be answered in terms of evidence. The search for scientific legitimacy was, of course, under way before Eysenck's critique, but its appearance galvanized researchers to respond with more and better investigations.

Phase II (Circa 1955-1969): Searching for Scientific Rigor

Modern studies of psychotherapy were launched around 1950, and their numbers increased vigorously from 1955 to 1969. Phase II contained extensions of earlier efforts by younger workers among the pioneers (eg, Edward Bordin, Jack Butler, Fred Fiedler, Jerome Frank, Lester Luborsky, William Snyder, and Hans Strupp), and the work of a new generation (eg, Allen Bergin, Sol Garfield, Eugene Gendlin, Arnold Goldstein, Donald Kiesler, Maurice Lorr, Joseph Matarrazo, Morris Parloff, and Charles Truax).

In addition, rapid growth in behavior therapies occurred[27] and was indexed in *The Annual Review of Psychology*. Volumes in the early 1960s made little mention of behavior therapy. However, Matarrazo[28] recognized "that behavior therapy was established as an 'important new force' and 'was here to stay,'" [27(p15)] and Dittman[29] characterized it as a viable new school with its own journal.

The central task of phase II was to further build and solidify a rigorously scientific field of study. Therefore, study of *process* involved developing objective methods for measuring recorded therapy events, and study of *outcomes* involved devising controlled comparative outcome research and analogue studies, which afforded researchers optimum experimental control, use of graduate students rather than "professional therapists," and a large pool of subjects. Studies were conducted in accordance with logical positivism or empiricism, which asserted that only the physically measurable dimensions of observable events could be objects of scientific study. Thus, the preferred research data became measures of overtly observable (and mechanically recordable) behaviors of the patient and therapist during therapy sessions and scores on experimental tasks, tests, or behavioral recording forms that were administered before and after treatment. Although these practices dovetailed closely with behavior therapy, researchers of every type of therapy applied them in their studies.

Consequently, participants' reports of experiential states were avoided unless they could be directly linked to externally observed behaviors. Consensually validated perceptions by nonparticipant observers were considered scientifically trustworthy. This view of scientific work was reinforced by a general commitment to nomothetic group designs (especially controlled experimentation) and to the associated Fisherian statistical methodology (mainly the Student *t* test and analysis of variance, Pearson correlations, and their nonparametric parallels).

Outcome studies, then, consisted mainly of pretreatment-posttreatment experimental designs, in which the patient's problem behavior or descriptive psychopathologic characteristics were evaluated once at intake and at the end of treatment, with a follow-up assessment (if possible) occurring later. The basic logic of these designs required that treated groups be compared, in degree of change from pretreatment to posttreatment, with control groups that were presumably equivalent in all relevant respects. These assessments were usually elaborate, involving interviews and batteries of objective tests. Practicality encouraged 2 or, in the infrequent case, 3 such evaluations, implying that changes due to treatment were linear in form.

In process studies, researchers focused on speech behaviors that could be readily quantified from audio recordings (eg, ratios of adjectives to verbs, grammatical categories of speech, or amount of time spent speaking). Because recordings could be replayed, researchers studied these verbal behaviors in detail (eg, by using sentences, "thought units," or chronological periods as rating units). Recordings quickly accumulated, each containing hundreds of units, and researchers soon possessed more material than they knew how to analyze. Session transcriptions and ratings were extremely time-consuming. Consequently, time-sampling strategies were developed (eg, random selection of 5-minute time intervals). The measurements based on these samples were typically averaged (often for whole groups of patients or therapists) in the hope of forming a reliable estimate for the specified aspect of the therapeutic process.

Unfortunately, the process indexes that resulted from such investigations seemed removed from clinical experience, from theories of discourse, and from the theoretical constructs of treatment that had inspired them.[30] Active ingredients in behavior therapy, such as verbal reinforcement, were found in dynamic and experiential therapies as well.[31-33] Moreover, research was initiated on systematic desensitization, and dismantling research techniques were devised to assess the role of relaxation in it.[27,34-36] In fact, while the quantity of research on traditional therapies grew modestly in the 1960s, the quantity of research on behavioral therapies grew with "exponential drama" from 1964 to 1969.[14(p254)] Behavioral treatments also spread, as illustrated by the use of token economies in state and Veterans Administration hospitals.[37]

Although process studies proliferated during phase II, most of the studies were of client-centered treatments that tested the validity of Rogers' formulation of the necessary and sufficient conditions of therapeutic change.[38] Paradoxically, although Rogers' theory emphasized the client's experience of the "facilitative conditions" (eg, therapist empathy, unconditional positive regard, and congruence), positivist biases led researchers to use nonparticipant observational measures of therapist behavior. Nevertheless, research results showed the importance of the relationship in client-centered therapy.[39]

Overall, phase II was marked by expansion of the research community and growing respect for its scientific endeavors. Several research trends were established. For example, Paul's call for greater specificity[9] dovetailed with Kiesler's exposure of psychotherapy uniformity myths,[40] each suggesting multidimensional analysis of "what treatment, by whom, is most effective for this individual with that specific problem, and under which set of circumstances."[9(p111)] Furthermore, there were enough investigators to create a need for communication beyond what was possible in journals. Conferences were organized in 1958, 1961, and 1966 by the American Psychological Association, with support from the National Institute of Mental Health (NIMH), at which behavioral and nonbehavioral researchers were invited to explore basic research issues and to publish their research.[41-43] In addition, a new journal, *Psychotherapy: Theory, Research, and Practice,* was established in 1963. Phase I and II research had begun to coalesce and conferences in the late 1950s and 1960s signaled that the field had achieved scientific respectability.

Phase III (Circa 1970-1983): Expansion and Organization

The field continued to expand as younger researchers sought and won inclusion in the tradition. One strategy to quicken inclusion was the founding of the Association for the Advancement of Behavior Therapy in 1966 and the Society for Psychotherapy Research in 1969. These organizational developments were paralleled by the appearance of books surveying the first 2 phases[44,45] and by new journals focusing on behavior therapy, including modeling,[46] operant, and conditioning procedures (eg, the *Journal of Applied Behavioral Analysis* in 1968 and *Behavior Therapy* and the *Journal of Behavior Therapy and Experimental Psychiatry* in 1970).

The pursuit of methodological rigor was facilitated by the publication of key texts on experimental and quasi-experimental designs.[47,48] This pursuit probably contributed to viewing process and outcome research as separable. For example, Kiesler published a book entirely devoted to observational methods in process research.[49] In 1975, Waskow and Parloff[50] organized experts for the NIMH to provide a handbook on outcome measures. These works signaled the coalescence of a research mainstream committed to programs of objective, quantitative, and, when possible, experimental studies. Development during phase III involved expansion and refinement within the methodological mainstream, although a subcurrent of phenomenologically oriented research on therapeutic process began to gain recognition.[51,52]

In the mainstream, comparative outcome studies were state-of-the-art,[53] were systematically reviewed,[54] and included psychosocial and pharmacological interventions. By the end of the decade, plans developed at the NIMH for an ambitious controlled clinical trial to compare psychosocial and pharmacological treatments of depression.[55] The NIMH study involved strenuous effort to specify, control, and differentiate the treatments given to patients through the development of formal treatment manuals and evaluations of process to ensure treatment integrity. Concurrently, family therapy, health psychology and behavioral medicine, behavioral assessment, and psychotherapeutic integration and technical eclecticism were extending their influence throughout the treatment and research communities.[56-60] Major achievements of this period were summarized in the second and third editions of the *Handbook of Psychotherapy and Behavior Change.*[11,61]

A transformation in how the field's findings would be accumulated also occurred. Traditionally, reviewers would narratively report, and perhaps tally, their impressions of research successes and failures. This practice was transformed by the introduction of meta-analysis,[62] which enabled reviewers to assess overall treatment effectiveness by averaging and combining the magnitude of effect sizes in each study in the sample. The effectiveness of psychotherapy could be estimated by 1 quantitative index.

The first meta-analysis was encouraging, providing evidence that most forms of psychosocial treatments were effective. Replications of the first meta-analytic findings and refinements in the method itself appeared. In fact, meta-analytic techniques, based as they often are on effect sizes rather than probability levels, began to change reporting practices in outcome studies. Interest in the magnitude of differences between treated and control subjects at outcome was subtly relativizing the field's obsession with differences that were only assessed statistically.

After the mid-1970s, new impetus was provided for process research by 3 developments. First, single-case experimental designs were refined and applied principally in the study of behavioral therapies. Their application allowed researchers to better control extraneous factors that confounded comparison studies of large groups and to isolate the mechanisms of different therapies. These designs also allowed researchers to dismantle single treatment packages to identify their active and inactive components and to test different combinations.[63,64]

Second, reformulation of the therapeutic relationship as a "working alliance" with distinguishable components stimulated construction of new instruments and their application in process studies.[65] Third, reviewers of process studies imposed taxonomic order on the hundreds of studies using content analysis that had accumulated.[66,67] Such order enabled researchers to discern the association between types of patient and therapist speech behavior and therapeutic involvement and improvement. Together with sophisticated circumplex models and ratings of interactional behavior,[68] these developments helped researchers to study the therapeutic relationship and other facets of process that could be related to outcome.

Phase IV (Circa 1984-Present): Consolidation and Reformulation

Before phase IV, researchers had demonstrated methods that made scientific research on processes and outcomes possible, accumulated evidence that treatments produced improvements at outcome and follow-up over and above control conditions, and described change mechanisms that were embedded in treatment processes. Pursuit of these tasks persists in phase IV. However, current researchers have produced several new trends by reinterpreting some traditional tasks and by harnessing new methods to pursue them. In addition, phase IV has spawned critical dialogues that counterpoise different philosophies of science and their associated methods of inquiry.

Demonstrations of new or refinements in old quantitative and qualitative methods have been intense over the last decade. Innovation can be glimpsed at every level, from overarching meta-analytic reviews to microanalyses of body movements in treatment. We cannot review all of these developments, but will instead highlight a few that seem relevant to mental health care policy discussions.

Developments in meta-analytic techniques have reopened the question of treatment effectiveness, as methodological (eg, design quality) and content variables (eg, therapist effects) have been shown to mediate or moderate differences between treatment and control conditions.[69,70] Moreover, some evidence suggests that the advantages of treatment over control conditions in laboratory efficacy studies are not replicated when assessing treatment effectiveness in typical field settings.[71] Thus, outcome questions have been particularized during phase IV.

Phase IV researchers have also reframed the question of outcomes to relate to the clinical significance of treatments. Definitional issues took precedence—what is clinical significance, how should it be defined, and by whom? Statistical tradition provided the first proposals for defining and assessing clinical significance. The approach is based on social comparison (eg, posttreatment means are assessed for their distance from the mean of a "healthy" population on some measure of psychosocial functioning). Some criterion score is stipulated—1 or 2 SDs—and a treatment is considered clinically significant if the treated group mean crosses the criterion.[72] Researchers are no longer satisfied showing that treatments are statistically superior to control conditions, but are now compelled to assess the degree to which treated groups approximate the healthy population. The same logic applies, obviously, when comparing alternative treatments with each other. In the first meta-analyses assessing the clinical significance of treatments, however, it was demonstrated that use of different reference healthy populations resulted in different appraisals of the clinical significance of a treatment.[73] Because the assessment of clinical significance requires a healthy comparison group, a deeper link between outcome and epidemiological research must be established.

The emphasis on the study of clinical significance and effectiveness parallels other developments in methodology. Skepticism with randomized clinical trials as the preferred or exclusive model for clinical research has grown. It is widely recognized that random assignment of small samples to various treatment conditions does not guarantee equal distribution of relevant variables across conditions.[74] This is a serious problem, especially when multiple replication studies are uncommon. Consequently, researchers have turned to systematically conducted naturalistic studies to assess treatment effectiveness and clinical significance.

With naturalistic studies has come the need for new strategies for disaggregating client samples based on relevant pretreatment characteristics. Concern with pretreatment variables and with prevention has led researchers away from exclusive reliance on diagnoses from the *DSM* to define patient or at-risk groups and to focus on both pathogenic processes (eg, deficits in cognitive functioning) and other relevant characteristics (eg, attachment history and personality structure) that might favorably or unfavorably interact with treatment.[75-77] Contemporary outcome research typically reports posttreatment comparisons across groups with at least several covariates and often presents analyses of differential outcome for homogeneous client groups identified by disaggregating procedures. Similarly, outcomes are now measured, not simply at 1 or 2 points, but at numerous points, allowing investigators to assess linear and nonlinear models of improvement in the conditions of clients.[78] Finally, attention to pretreatment variables has also sensitized researchers to the practical problem and potential benefits of differential treatment assignment[79] and prophylactic therapies. These trends encourage researchers to explore interaction effects to account for treatment outcomes.

These trends do not cease when we turn to process research.[80] Quantitative process researchers increasingly investigate dependencies between, and the structure of, serial events within treatments. Sequential or Markov analyses, P-technique, dynamic-factor analyses, analysis of growth curves, and multivariate time-series analyses have been revived or are being newly applied to therapist-client interaction.[81,82] Phase IV researchers are the first to grapple with the complexities of the "talking cure" with methods suited to assess complex qualitative and quantitative changes over time.[13]

Research on process sequences and structures has revealed characteristic patterns of events within sessions and patterns of dominance across successive sessions or over whole treatments.[83,84] In addition, the structures of client, therapist, and client-therapist interactive participation have been characterized across types of therapists and types of clients, and prototypic patterns of interaction or significant change events in successful cases have been confirmed and differentiated from those evident in unsuccessful cases.[85] Thus, models of phases and stages of treatment and averaged growth curves across them have begun to provide the basis by which processive outcomes, or patient progress, can be assessed during the course of treatments. Repeatedly, some facet of the therapeutic relationship has been associated with good processes, and has been related to successful outcomes.[86]

A focus on process has increased the disaffection of researchers with the "*DSM* diagnosis by brand-name treatment" paradigm for psychotherapy research. It is evident that patients do not respond to brand names of treatment, but to technical strategies of intervention and concrete relational processes. Similarly, therapists do not respond to diagnoses, but to the pathogenic relational, cognitive, or emotional processes that impair the patient's ability to function normally.[87] Consequently, researchers are required to specify, through a case formulation, the pathogenic processes responsible for the client's problems and to match, not whole brand-name treatments, but specific types of intervention strategies to them.

The fourth phase has also spawned debates about postpositivist investigative models.[88] Work in this vein emphasizes discovery rather than verification.[89,90] The emphasis directs researchers to identify change episodes within process and to study them through task analysis and other qualitative and quantitative methods to discover mechanisms of change. Sampling methods as used in previous phases are considered counterproductive, as are typical methods of defining and then assessing process and outcome relations.[88] The most important trend, however, is that countercurrent researchers sift through the complexities of interactional and relational meanings.[91,92] Their study, it is argued, will reveal more clearly the change mechanisms operative in treatment.

Phase IV process research challenges some traditional concepts. First, the process-outcome dichotomy implied a qualitative or quantitative disjunction between process events and the event that is measured as an outcome. Clearly, the outcome event may itself be just the last point in the series of processes. Second, the process-outcome dichotomy suggested that phenomena on either side of the divide should somehow be different, and consequently should be measured differently. Obviously, development in a client's relational capacities may be equally relevant to process and outcome and could be measured similarly. Consequently, countercurrent investigations are not easily categorized as process or outcome research. For the countercurrent there are processive outcomes and outcome processes that need meticulous exploration.

In phase IV, then, there is stalwart determination to deal directly with multivariate and interactional complexities that are involved in treatment.[93] These complexities are more likely to be assessed at intake, during treatment, and at outcome. Complex, often nonlinear relations connecting them are viewed through sets of mediators and moderators. In addition, process research has exploded, with the therapeutic relationship and relational processes of meaning forming the central core.[86] Phase IV researchers have provoked several exciting debates revolving around issues of clinical significance, the use of normative growth models in treatment, the study of effectiveness and efficacy, and overall philosophies of science.

COMMENT

The history of psychotherapy research can inform mental health care practice and discussions of mental health care policy. Whereas it is clear that biomedical discoveries, such as the polio vaccine, have led directly to changes in medical practice and policy, and that pharmacological treatments of the severely mentally ill have led directly to changes in medical practice and policy (eg, deinstitutionalization), it is not clear how the demonstrated success of psychosocial treatments will systematically affect therapeutic practices and mental health care policy.[94,95]

That this relationship is unclear does not mean that there is little that the psychotherapy research community can offer. Just the opposite is true. In fact, for a variety of disorders specific psychosocial interventions are "not only better than no treatment but better than credible alternative psychological interventions; and for many disorders, they are as good as or better than effective drug treatments."[95(p118)] Such interventions also interact with medical treatments for physical disorders, increasing survival rates and quality of life, while reducing utilization and medical care costs.[74,96,97] Psychosocial treatments can also correct inaccurate perceptions of health risk, leading to appropriate preventive self-care.[98] In the political context generated by reform of the health care system, practitioners and policy analysts must be better informed about successful psychological treatments and their cost benefits.

Psychotherapy researchers also have developed several critical discourses and findings relevant to practitioners and policymakers alike. For example, interest in clinical significance forces clinical researchers, epidemiologists, and policymakers to reflect on substantive and political issues simultaneously. Decisions must be made about the relative appropriateness of using reference healthy populations and the degree of approximation to their mean that is deemed a criterion of clinical significance. The use of reference populations as healthy must also be carefully considered, symptom complex by symptom complex. For example, public health officials have reported that the United States is experiencing an epidemic of violence. In considering the clinical significance of treatments for aggression and violence in childhood and adolescence, should healthy reference samples be randomly selected from the general population that is in the throes of an epidemic? Furthermore, communities exist in which the incidence of violent acts far exceeds the norm. Should local reference populations then be used? Such knotty scientific and political questions should serve to shape mental health care policy debates.

SOME CURRENT evidence suggests that the positive results achieved in research on efficacy are not similarly achieved in research on effectiveness. A myriad of uncontrollable factors affect the context of service provision that do not affect the context of laboratory research. More research on effectiveness is required to identify the factors that impinge on treatment outcomes. Research on efficacy, however, may have revealed an important fact: treatments succeed better when they are systematically monitored and outcomes are regularly assessed. Governmental agencies that fund systems for the provision of mental health care would be wise to include regulations mandating, and to allocate monies for, ongoing program evaluation at the service site. The relationship between therapists and patients regularly appears in reviews as an important moderator of treatment effects. The finding is important in its own right. It should not be ignored in discussions of general health care policy and in attempts of third-party payers to devise cost-containment programs that minimize "corrective" relationships. Debates about the role of technological efficiency in human relationships have already appeared in discussions of medical care and can be predicted to reappear in our own field. Frankford[99] describes the issues: (1) the perception of the health care crisis and its formulation are "allied with a new and growing scientism—more particularly with a social scientific scientism centered in the tremendous explosion of a new positivist discipline called health services research," and (2) a crisis "perceived in econometric terms generates scientistic responses to the particular ills diagnosed by science" in the first place.[(p774)] He outlines 3 implications: (1) the new outcomes research, originally aligned against biomedical positivism, "strengthens our dependence on that positivism by reinforcing the belief that 'reality' consists only of phenomena that can be quantified and measured"; (2) discourses that are at heart moral and political get displaced "by the language of technique and efficiency"; and (3) the rise of the newly reinforcing movements of scientism in outcomes research and biomedical positivism in medicine "threatens to overwhelm the medical humanities movement, which is an effort internal to medicine that arose in part because of the perception that biomedical positivism was dehumanizing medicine."[(p774)] The dehumanization takes place by reducing patients to objects known by their faceless technological profiles and physicians to technocratic managers intent on normalizing the faceless profiles. Because the therapist-client relationship has been key in psychotherapy processes and outcomes, our field may not be as vulnerable as others to the aforementioned trends. Nevertheless, one of the most important contributions of our field is the demonstration of how, when, and which parameters of relatedness in therapy are clinically important to treatment progress and outcomes.[86,100,101] These parameters may also interact with medical treatments and enhance their potency as they cut their cost.

The interest in matching case-based diagnoses to specific strategies of intervention has coupled with interest in the measurement of multidimensional, averaged growth models of treatment. What this means is that, if not now, in the near future, therapy researchers will be able to better define targets for intervention and criteria for defining functional success. Intervention strategies, not therapy name brands, can be assessed during the course of treatments and altered to optimize patient progress.[102] Results of such research will help formulate "best practice" guidelines in a sensitive and knowledgeable way.

We know that psychotherapy's general success rate for treated groups (62%) has an advantage of 24 percentage points over the success rate of untreated groups (38%), and that these rates compare favorably with success rates for medical interventions.[103] Such results can obviously help psychologists "make the case for psychological services in state houses as well as in Congress,"[(p866)] and affect local and national mental health care policy.[104] It will be pointed out, no doubt, that success rates must be considered in the context of the costs of failure and the benefits of success, in economic and human terms. Here, contemporary researchers can help identify mechanisms that increase success rates and economists can calculate benefits not only to the individual, but also to society. The work ahead entails demonstrating how research-garnered insight into treatment processes and outcomes can be translated into program initiatives that will influence treatment practices and mental health care policies.

We could not outline every way psychotherapy research can affect mental health care policies (eg, we omitted the economics of mental health care and the problem of access). We could not credit all of those who made major or minor contributions. Instead, we sketched psychotherapy research over the past half-century, noting some of its successes. This history showed how research can improve practices, inform policies, and streamline mental health care provision.

Accepted for publication April 27, 1996.

Reprints: Robert L. Russell, PhD, Department of Psychology, Loyola University Chicago, 6525 N Sheridan Rd, Chicago, IL 60626.

REFERENCES

1. Beutler LE, Crago M, eds. *Psychotherapy Research: An International Review of Programmatic Research.* Washington, DC: American Psychological Association; 1987.
2. Freedheim DK, ed. *History of Psvchotherapy: A Century of Change.* Washington, DC: American Psychological Association; 1992.
3. Tannenbaum SJ. Knowing and acting in medical practice: the epistemological politics of outcomes research. *J Health Polit Policy Law.* 1994;19:27-44.
4. Eysenck HJ. The effects of psychotherapy: an evaluation. *J Consult Clin Psychol.* 1952;16:319-324.
5. Eysenck HJ. *Behavior Therapy and the Neuroses.* Elmsford, NY: Pergamon Press Inc; 1960.
6. Levitt EE. The results of psychotherapy with children: an evaluation. *J Consult Clin Psychol.* 1957;21:189-196.
7. Levitt EE. Psychotherapy with children: a further evaluation. *Behav Res Ther.* 1963;1:45-51.
8. Paul GL. *Insight vs Desensitization in Psychotherapy.* Stanford, Calif: Stanford University Press; 1966.
9. Paul GL. Insight vs. desensitization in psychotherapy two years after termination. *J Consult Clin Psychol.* 1967;31:333-348.
10. Castonguay LG, Goldfried MR. Psychotherapy integration: an idea whose time has come. *Appl Prev Psychol.* 1994;3:159-172.
11. Garfield SL, Bergin AE, eds. *Handbook of Psychotherapy and Behavior Change.* 3rd ed. New York, NY: John Wiley & Sons Inc; 1986.
12. VandenBos GR, Cummings NA, DeLeon PH. A century of psychotherapy: economic and environmental influences. In: Freedheim DK, ed. *History of Psychotherapy: A Century of Change.* Washington, DC: American Psychological Association; 1992:65-102.
13. Russell RL, ed. *Reassessing Psychotherapy Research.* New York, NY: Guilford Publications Inc; 1994.
14. Bergin AE. The evaluation of therapeutic outcomes. In: Bergin AE, Garfield SL, eds. *Handbook of Psychotherapy and Behavior Change.* New York, NY: John Wiley & Sons Inc; 1971:217-270.
15. Jones MC. The elimination of children's fears. *J Exp Psychol.* 1924;7:383-390.
16. Skinner BF. *Science and Human Behavior.* New York, NY: Macmillan Publishing Co Inc; 1953.
17. Wolpe J. *Psychotherapy by Reciprocal Inhibition.* Stanford, Calif: Stanford University Press; 1959.
18. Rogers CR. The use of electrically recorded interviews in improving psychotherapeutic techniques. *Am J Orthopsychiatry.* 1942;12:429-434.
19. Frank JD. The Johns Hopkins psychotherapy research project. In: Freedheim DK, ed. *History of Psychotherapy: A Century of Change.* Washington, DC: American Psychological Association; 1992:392-396.
20. Menninger K. Cited by: Wallerstein RS. *Forty-two Lives in Treatment: A Study of Psychoanalysis and Psychotherapy.* New York, NY: Guilford Publications Inc; 1986.
21. Mowrer OH, ed. *Psychotherapy: Theory and Research.* New York, NY: Ronald Press; 1953.
22. Wolff W, Precker JA, eds. *Success in Psychotherapy.* New York, NY: Guilford Publications Inc; 1952.
23. Rogers CR, Dymond RF, eds. *Psychotherapy and Personality Change.* Chicago, Ill: University of Chicago Press; 1954.
24. Luborsky L. A note on Eysenck's article, 'The effects of psychotherapy: an evaluation.' *Br J Psychol.* 1954;45:129-131.
25. Rosenzweig S. A transvaluation of psychotherapy—a reply to Hans Eysenck. *J Abnorm Soc Psychol.* 1954;49:298-304.
26. Gordon T, Grummon DL, Rogers CR, Seeman J. Developing a program of research in psychotherapy. In: Rogers CR, Dymond RF, eds. *Psychotherapy and Personality Change.* Chicago, Ill: University of Chicago Press; 1954:12-34.
27. Hersen M, Michelson L, Bellack AS, eds. *Issues in Psychotherapy Research.* New York, NY: Plenum Press; 1984.
28. Matarazzo JD. Psychotherapeutic processes. *Annu Rev Psychol.* 1965;16:181-224.
29. Dittman A. Psychotherapeutic processes. *Annu Rev Psychol.* 1966;17:51-78.
30. Russell RL. Language in psychotherapy. *Clin Psychol Rev.* 1989;9:505-519.
31. Murray EJ. A content-analysis method for studying psychotherapy. *Psychol Monogr.* 1956;70(Whole No. 420):13.
32. Truax CB. Reinforcement and nonreinforcement in Rogerian psychotherapy. *J Abnorm Psychol.* 1966;71:1-9.
33. Truax CB. Therapist interpersonal reinforcement of client self-exploration and therapeutic outcome in group psychotherapy. *J Counseling Psychol.* 1968;15:225-231.
34. Davison GC. Systematic desensitization as a counterconditioning process. *J Abnorm Psychol.* 1968;73:91-99.
35. Lang PJ, Lazovik AD. Experimental desensitization of a phobia. *J Abnorm Soc Psychol.* 1963;66:519-525.
36. Lang PJ. Fear reduction and fear behavior: problems in treating a construct. In: Shlien JM, Hunt HF, Matarazzo JD, Savage C, eds. *Research in Psychotherapy.* Washington, DC: American Psychological Association; 1968;3:90-102.
37. Glass CR, Arnkoff DB. Behavior therapy. In: Freedheim DK, ed. *History of Psychotherapy: A Century of Change.* Washington, DC: American Psychological Association; 1992:587-628.
38. Rogers CR. The necessary and sufficient conditions of therapeutic personality change. *J Consult Psychol.* 1957;22:95-103.
39. Truax CB, Mitchell KM. Research on certain therapist interpersonal skills in relation to process and outcome. In: Bergin AE, Garfield SL, eds. *Handbook of Psychotherapy and Behavior Change.* New York, NY: John Wiley & Sons Inc; 1971:299-344.
40. Kiesler DJ. Some myths of psychotherapy research and the search for a paradigm. *Psychol Bull.* 1966;65:110-136.
41. Rubinstein EA, Parloff MB, eds. *Research in Psychotherapy.* Washington, DC: American Psychological Association; 1962;1.
42. Shlien JM, Hunt HF, Matarazzo JD, Savage C, eds. *Research in Psychotherapy.* Washington, DC: American Psychological Association; 1968. Vol 3.
43. Strupp HH, Luborsky L, eds. *Research in Psychotherapy.* Washington, DC: American Psychological Association; 1962. Vol 2.
44. Bergin AE, Garfield SL, eds. *Handbook of Psychotherapy and Behavior Change.* New York, NY: John Wiley & Sons Inc; 1971.
45. Meltzoff J, Kornreich M. *Research in Psychotherapy.* New York, NY: Atherton; 1970.
46. Bandura A. Psychotherapy based upon modeling principles. In: Bergin AE, Garfield SL, eds. *Handbook of Psychotherapy and Behavior Change.* New York, NY: John Wiley & Sons Inc; 1971:653-708.
47. Cambell DT, Stanley JC. *Experimental and Quasi-experimental Designs for Research.* Skokie, Ill: Rand-McNally & Co; 1966.
48. Cook TD, Cambell DT. *Quasi-experimentation: Design & Analysis Issues for Field Settings.* Boston, Mass: Houghton Mifflin Co; 1979.
49. Kiesler DJ. *The Process of Psychotherapy: Empirical Foundations and Systems of Analysis.* Hawthorne, NY: Aldine Publishing Co; 1973.
50. Waskow IE, Parloff MB, eds. *Psychotherapy Change Measures.* Rockville, Md: National Institute of Mental Health; 1975.
51. Barrett-Lennard GT. The Relationship Inventory now: issues and advances in theory, method and use. In: Greenberg LS, Pinsof WM, eds. *The Psychotherapeutic Process: A Research Handbook.* New York, NY: Guilford Publications Inc; 1986:439-476.
52. Orlinsky DE, Howard KI. *Varieties of Psychotherapeutic Experience.* New York, NY: Teachers College Press; 1975.
53. Sloane RB, Staples FR, Cristol AH, Yorkston, NJ, Whipple K. *Psychotherapy Versus Behavior Therapy.* Cambridge, Mass: Harvard University Press; 1975.
54. Luborsky L, Singer B, Luborsky L. Comparative studies of psychotherapies: is it true that 'everyone has won and all must have prizes'? *Arch Gen Psychiatry.* 1975;32:995-1008.
55. Elkin IE, Parloff MB, Hadley SW, Autry JH. NIMH Treatment of Depression Collaborative Research Program: background and research plan. *Arch Gen Psychiatry.* 1985;42:305-316.
56. Guerin PJ, Chabot DR. Development of family systems theory. In: Freedheim DK, ed. *History of Psychotherapy: A Century of Change.* Washington, DC: American Psychological Association; 1992:225-260.
57. Pomerleau OR, Rodin J. Behavioral medicine and health psychology. In: Garfield SL, Bergin AE, eds. *Handbook of Psychotherapy and Behavior Change.* 3rd ed. New York, NY: John Wiley & Sons Inc; 1986:483-524.
58. Hersen M, Bellack AS. *Behavioral Assessment: A Practical Handbook.* New York, NY: Pergamon Press; 1976.
59. Arkowitz H. Integrative theories of therapy. In: Freedheim DK, ed. *History of*

Psychotherapy: A Century of Change. Washington DC: American Psychological Association; 1992:261-304.

60. Wolfe BE, Goldfried MR. Research on psychotherapy integration: recommendations and conclusions from a NIMH workshop. *J Consult Clin Psychol.* 1988; 56:448-451.
61. Garfield SL, Bergin AE, eds. *Handbook of Psychotherapy and Behavior Change.* 2nd ed. New York, NY: John Wiley & Sons Inc; 1978.
62. Smith ML, Glass GV. Meta-analysis of psychotherapy outcome studies. *Am Psychol.* 1977;32:752-760.
63. Hersen M, Barlow DH. *Single-Case Experimental Design: Stategies for Studying Behavior Change.* New York, NY: Plenum Press; 1976.
64. Kazdin AE. Methodological and interpretive problems of single-case experimental designs. *J Consult Clin Psychol.* 1978;46:629-642.
65. Bordin ES. The generalizability of the psychoanalytic concept of the working alliance. *Psychother Theory Res Pract.* 1979;16:252-260.
66. Marsden G. Content analysis of therapeutic interviews: 1954-1964. *Psychol Bull.* 1965;63:298-321.
67. Russell RL, Stiles WB. Categories for classifying language in psychotherapy. *Psychol Bull.* 1979;86:404-419.
68. Benjamin LS. Structural analysis of social behavior. *Psychol Rev.* 1974;81: 392-425.
69. Lambert MJ. The individual therapist's contribution to psychotherapy process and outcome. *Clin Psychol Rev.* 1989;9:469-485.
70. Shapiro DA, Harper H, Statup M, Reynolds S, Bird D, Suokas A. The high-water mark of the drug metaphor: a meta-analytic critique of process-outcome research. In: Russell RL, ed. *Reassessing Psychotherapy Research.* New York, NY: Guilford Publications Inc; 1994:1-35.
71. Weisz JR, Weiss B, Donenberg GR. The lab versus the clinic: effects of child and adolescent psychotherapy. *Annu Prog Child Psychiatry Child Dev.* 1993; 441-458.
72. Jacobson NS, Revenstorf D. Statistics for assessing the clinical significance of psychotherapy techniques: issues, problems, and new developments. *Behav Assess.* 1988;10:133-145.
73. Nietzel MT, Russell RL, Hemmings KA, Gretter ML. The clinical significance of psychotherapy for unipolar depression: a meta-analytic approach to social comparison. *J Consult Clin Psychol.* 1987;55:156-161.
74. Rogers JL, Howard KI, Vessey JT. Using significance tests to evaluate equivalence between experimental groups. *Psychol Bull.* 1993;113:553-565.
75. Beutler LE. Differential treatment selection: the role of diagnosis in psychotherapy. *Psychother Theory Res Pract Training.* 1989;26:271-281.
76. Grossarth-Maticek R, Eysenck HJ. Creative novation behavior therapy as a prophylactic treatment for cancer and coronary heart disease, part I: description of treatment. *Behav Res Ther.* 1991;29:1-16.
77. Persons J. The advantages of studying psychological phenomena rather than psychiatric diagnoses. *Am Psychol.* 1986;41:1252-1260.
78. Howard KI, Lueger RJ, Maling MS, Martinovich Z. A phase model of psychotherapy outcome: causal mediation of change. *J Consult Clin Psychol.* 1993;61:678-685.
79. Beutler LE, Clarkin JF. *Systematic Treatment Selection.* New York, NY: Brunner-Mazel Publications; 1990.
80. Greenberg LS, Pinsof WM, eds. *The Psychotherapeutic Process: A Research Handbook.* New York, NY: Guilford Publications Inc; 1986.
81. Russell RL, Trull TJ. Sequential analyses of language variables in psychotherapy process research. *J Consult Clin Psychol.* 1986;54:16-21.
82. Czogalik D, Russell RL. Interactional structures of therapist and client participation in adult psychotherapy: P-techniques and chronography. *J Consult Clin Psychol.* 1995;63:28-35.
83. Wampold BE, Kim K. Sequential analysis applied to counseling process and outcome: a case study revisited. *J Counseling Psychol.* 1989;36:357-364.
84. Wampold BE. Tests of dominance in sequential categorical data. *Psychol Bull.* 1984;96:424-429.
85. Czogalik D, Russell RL. Therapist structures of participation: an application of P-technique and chronographic analysis. *Psychother Res.* 1994;4:77-94.
86. Orlinsky DE, Grawe K, Parks BK. Process and outcome in psychotherapy. In: Bergin AE, Garfield SL, eds. *Handbook of Psychotherapy and Behavior Change.* 4th ed. New York, NY: John Wiley & Sons Inc; 1994:270-376.
87. Shirk S, Russell RL. *Revitalizing Child Psychotherapy: Case Formulations and Treatment Processes.* New York, NY: Guilford Publications Inc. In press.
88. Stiles WB, Shapiro DA, Harper H. Finding the way from process to outcome: blind alleys and unmarked trails. In: Russell RL, ed. *Reassessing Psychotherapy Research.* New York, NY: Plenum Press; 1994:36-64.
89. Orlinsky DA, Russell RL. Tradition and change in psychotherapy research: notes on the fourth generation. In: Russell RL, ed. *Reassessing Psychotherapy Research.* New York, NY: Plenum Press; 1994:185-214.
90. Rice LN, Greenberg LS, eds. *Patterns of Change: Intensive Analysis of Psychotherapy Process.* New York, NY: Guilford Publications Inc; 1984.
91. Hill CE. *Therapist Techniques and Client Outcomes: Eight Cases of Brief Psychotherapy.* Thousand Oaks, Calif: Sage Publications Inc; 1989.
92. Rennie DL. Clients' deference in psychotherapy. *J Counseling Psychol.* 1994; 41:427-437.
93. Elliot R, Anderson C. Simplicity and complexity in psychotherapy research. In: Russell RL, ed. *Reassessing Psychotherapy Research.* New York, NY: Guilford Publications Inc; 1994:65-113.
94. Talley F, Butler S, Strupp HH, eds. *Research Findings and Clinical Practice: Bridging the Chasm.* New York, NY: Basic Books Inc Publishers; 1994.
95. Barlow DH. Psychological interventions in the era of managed competition. *Clin Psychol Sci Pract.* 1994;1:109-122.
96. Meyer TJ, Mark MM. Effects of psychosocial interventions with adult cancer patients: a meta-analysis of randomized experiments. *Health Psychol.* 1995; 14:101-108.
97. Mumford EH, Schlesinger HJ, Glass GV. The effects of psychological intervention on recovering from surgery and heart attacks: an analysis of the literature. *Am J Public Health.* 1982;72:141-151.
98. Kreuter MW, Strecher VJ. Changing inaccurate perception of health risk: results from a randomized trial. *Health Psychol.* 1995;14:56-63.
99. Frankford DM. Scientism and economism in the regulation of health care. *J Health Polit Policy Law.* 1994;19:773-799.
100. Ilardi SS, Craighead WE. The role of nonspecific factors in cognitive-behavior therapy for depression. *Clin Psychol Sci Pract.* 1994;1:138-156.
101. Shirk SR, Saiz C. Clinical, empirical, and developmental perspectives on the therapeutic relationship in child psychotherapy. *Dev Psychopathol.* 1992;4: 713-728.
102. Howard KI, Orlinsky DE, Lueger RJ. The design of clinically relevant outcome research: some considerations and an example. In: Aveline M, Shapiro DA, eds. *Research Foundations for Psychotherapy Practice.* New York, NY: John Wiley & Sons Inc; 1995:3-46.
103. Lipsey MW, Wilson WB. The efficacy of psychological, educational, and behavioral treatment. *Am Psychol.* 1993;48:1181-1209.
104. Frank RG, Sullivan MJ, DeLeon PH. Health care reform in the states. *Am Psychol.* 1994;49:855-867.

Psychotherapy of Depression

Implications for Reform of the Health Care System

John F. Clarkin, PhD; Paul A. Pilkonis, PhD; Kathryn M. Magruder, PhD

This article reviews the empirical evidence supporting the role of psychotherapy and psychosocial interventions in the treatment of patients with depression. Treatment models and the evidence for their effectiveness in the acute- and maintenance-treatment phases are reviewed. Whereas the sophistication of research designs and data analysis for the study of psychotherapy have substantially improved, the review highlights current gaps in our knowledge. Most important for reform of the health care system is the need for studies of efficacy to lead to large-scale investigations of effectiveness. *Arch Gen Psychiatry. 1996;53:717-723*

Depression is a generic mental state with diverse levels of symptom severity and accompanying variation in functional impairment. The diagnostic category of major depression may be composed of multiple disorders with different causes.[1,2] As broadly defined, *depression* is a widespread problem affecting 8% to 18% of the population and twice as many women as men.[3] The incidence of depression is relatively similar throughout the life cycle. The heterogeneity of the construct is, unfortunately, an invitation to conceptual confusion in planning specific treatments for individual patients.

Nonetheless, the treatment of depression must be a central topic in any health care policy. The prevalence of the disorder, including data suggesting an increasing prevalence in younger cohorts,[4] makes it an important public health concern. Depression can be a serious condition, associated with dysfunction in work and family roles, substance abuse, and proneness to suicide. At the same time, it is a disorder for which effective therapies are available, as documented by extensive treatment outcome data for medication therapy and psychotherapy. It is a disorder for which a multisite empirical study has been completed comparing 2 types of psychotherapy with medication therapy.[5] Finally, it is a disorder that has been the focus of a national psychoeducational effort—the Depression Awareness, Recognition, and Treatment program. This review provides evidence supporting the role of psychotherapy in the treatment of depression and identifies some areas for further research that will allow the design of optimally cost-effective treatments.

From the Department of Psychiatry, New York Hospital–Cornell University Medical College Westchester Division, White Plains, NY (Dr Clarkin), the Department of Psychiatry, Western Psychiatric Institute and Clinic, University of Pittsburgh (Pa) School of Medicine (Dr Pilkonis), and the Office of Rural Mental Health, National Institute of Mental Health, Bethesda, Md (Dr Magruder).

EVIDENCE SUPPORTING A ROLE FOR PSYCHOTHERAPY OF DEPRESSION IN THE EMERGING HEALTH CARE SYSTEM

Major advances in the technology of psychotherapy research have occurred in the past 15 years. Manuals describing various psychosocial treatments (ie, behavioral treatment,[6-8] cognitive treatment,[9] interpersonal psychotherapy,[10-12] and short-term dynamic therapies[13,14]) have specified the content and tempo of different therapies for specific patient disorders and conditions and made replication possible. Rating scales for the development of therapist adherence to guidelines in psychosocial treatment manuals and competence are used to document the integrity of treatments.

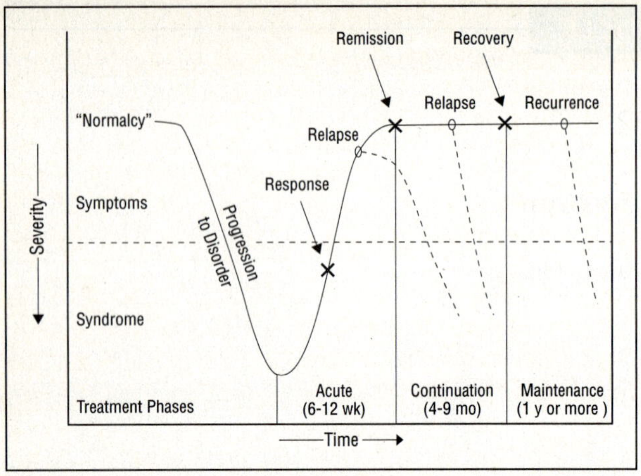

Phases of treatment. Adapted with permission from Kupfer.[15] Copyright 1991, Physicians Postgraduate Press Inc.

There is a growing consensus about terminology for the stages of the disorder[15] and matching treatment phases[16] that helps organize our review (**Figure**). Whereas the model is helpful in clarifying terminology, it focuses entirely on symptoms and neglects functional impairment, and it has limited relevance to patients whose symptomatic course does not conform to typical stages. We rely on a number of excellent literature reviews[17-24] of treatment outcome for summarizing research findings and examining their implications.

Phases of Illness

Acute Phase. Psychosocial treatments for the acute phase of depression have proved effective in comparison with various control conditions.[23,24] Efficacy has been demonstrated with interpersonal, behavioral, and cognitive techniques.[22] The outcomes of interpersonal, cognitive, behavioral, and behavioral-marital therapies are relatively superior to those of short-term dynamic psychotherapy.

The Depression Guideline Panel (DGP)[17] reported a meta-analysis based on 22 acute-phase randomized, controlled trials with cognitive therapy. Compared with medication therapy alone, cognitive therapy had a slight advantage. The Panel, in its own meta-analysis, found that the overall efficacy of behavioral therapy was greater than that of wait-list control conditions and greater than treatment with medication alone. Interpersonal psychotherapy (IPT) has proved more effective than supportive treatment (on demand) and as effective as treatment with amitriptyline hydrochloride alone.[5,25] Brief dynamic psychotherapy has been investigated for acute-phase treatment of depression.[26-32] The DGP[17] reported that the overall efficacy of brief dynamic therapy was somewhat less than that of the other psychotherapeutic techniques and somewhat more than treatment with medication alone.

Much of the research cited was conducted with young to middle-aged adult participants. A recent meta-analysis of 17 studies examined the efficacy of psychosocial treatments for depression among older adults[33] and found that these treatments were reliably more effective than no-treatment comparison conditions. Interpersonal psychotherapy has been adapted for the depressed elderly[34] and depressed adolescents,[35] extending its applicability at both ends of the life cycle. Based on follow-up data, it has been postulated that psychological treatments focused on the development of enduring learning and skills may show superiority over treatments with medication.[36] The prophylactic effects of cognitive therapy after acute-phase treatment have been suggested by many.[9,24,37] Three studies indicate a greater maintenance of improvement in the time after treatment with cognitive therapy than with pharmacotherapy alone[38,39] (noted in Haaga et al[9]). More specifically, patients treated with cognitive therapy showed fewer depressive symptoms[40] or lower relapse rates[39] than did patients treated with acute-phase pharmacotherapy without maintenance medication therapy. Additional studies have found that cognitive therapy, alone or in combination with tricyclic antidepressants, is superior to treatment with medication without subsequent maintenance medication therapy in preventing relapse after the termination of treatment.[38] Pharmacotherapy without maintenance medication therapy has relapse rates in excess of 60%, compared with relapse rates of approximately 30% with cognitive therapy. Methodological limitations complicate the interpretation of these findings, however.[17]

Evidence about the prophylactic value of acute-phase behavioral therapy or IPT is less well studied. One early study found no differences at 1-year follow-up among IPT, amitriptyline, the combination of IPT and amitriptyline, and nonscheduled treatment in relapse rates,[41] but patients who received IPT scored better on measures of social functioning at follow-up, whether they had received medications or not.

Maintenance Phase. Weissman[42] has noted the important role for psychotherapy as an alternative for patients when treatment with medication is not suitable or feasible (eg, during pregnancy, while breast-feeding, before or during major surgery, and among certain elderly) and as an adjunct treatment with medication in the maintenance period when dealing with the social consequences or triggers of depression. A combination of pharmacotherapy and maintenance IPT has been shown to be effective in forestalling recurrence[43] in persons with a history of recurrent depression, especially if the treatment is focused on interpersonal issues.[44]

Treatment

Psychotherapy vs Treatment With Medication. Studies comparing medication therapy with psychotherapy alone have generally found equal efficacy in acute-phase treatment in mild-to-moderate depression.[26,28,45-48] There are no differences in the effectiveness of treatment with tricyclic antidepressants as compared with or combined with cognitive, behavioral, or IPT in the treatment of acute-phase depression. Tricyclic antidepressant medications and psychotherapy are viable and effective treatments for approximately 45% to 85% of depressed outpatients.[23] That treatment with medication and psychotherapy may affect different symptomatic and functional areas at different rates may be relevant to the planning of treatment. For example, data suggest that treatment with amitriptyline improved vegetative symptoms, while IPT improved mood, suicidal ideation, work, and interest earlier.[49,50]

Combination Treatment. The combination of psychosocial and medication therapies is not superior to the use of either modality alone.[23,24] The DGP[17] summarized data about combined acute-phase treatment and found that the efficacy of the combination was roughly equal to treatment with medication alone. However, the null effects between combination treatments and medication alone are statistical comparisons based on outpatient samples. The conclusions drawn from published reviews are often reported as definitive when more data are needed.

The indications for a combination of medication and psychosocial therapies have been reviewed by Conte et al.[51] Miller et al[52] found that treatment outcomes for depressed patients with high levels of cognitive dysfunction were better with medication and cognitive-behavioral therapies than with medication therapy alone. In a sample including patients from primary care and tertiary care settings,[53] the effects of cognitive therapy exceeded those of combined treatment or medication therapy alone in the primary care setting; in the tertiary care setting, combined treatment was more effective than either treatment alone. Combined treatment may have a broader effect than treatment with medication alone,[41,54-56] or result in more rapid improvement than psychotherapy alone[57,58] (cited in Shea et al[24]).

Treatment and Functional Improvement. One review[59] highlighted the lack of information on the treatment of depression and related improvement in functioning. Across 10 studies, work impairment in depressed patients was common, and work indicators demonstrated slower rates of improvement than symptoms. The DGP[17] presumes that the symptomatic treatment of depression with medication will be followed by functional improvement, yet the evidence for this assumption is sparse. Careful examination of the tempo and trajectory of change in depressive symptoms and related psychosocial functioning as related to psychotherapy, medication therapy only, and treatment with medication plus psychotherapy is sorely needed.

RESEARCH ON DEPRESSION

The progression from the status of an "experimental" intervention to one that is part of standard practice is key in the development of any successful treatment. Three research steps are involved in this process: (1) research on treatment efficacy to develop new treatment models; (2) research on treatment effectiveness to test the generalizability of such models in wider ranges of settings, patient populations, and providers; and (3) development and testing of professionally sanctioned minimal standards of care based on research findings.

From Treatment Efficacy to Treatment Effectiveness

The establishment of an *efficacious* treatment as an *effective* treatment is a complex process involving several steps. Efficacy studies are critical to determine whether a treatment has the intended therapeutic effect. Patients are selected according to strict inclusion and exclusion criteria, and therapists are carefully selected and trained to provide prescribed treatment that adheres to the treatment principles and strategies. However, it is also crucial that researchers not stop here if we are to determine the effectiveness of these interventions, that is, their applicability in everyday practice. Effectiveness studies determine the external validity or generalizability of treatments under more ordinary, less pristine conditions. This may mean that the treatment setting is a community clinic, the providers are not specially selected but those normally employed in community clinics, and the patients, who still meet diagnostic criteria, might have comorbid medical or mental disorders. The goal of effectiveness research is to provide information about outcomes of interventions when they are applied to most patients by practicing clinicians in nonresearch settings.

Perhaps the most difficult aspect of establishing the effectiveness of a psychosocial treatment is the fidelity of the treatment provision. Psychosocial treatment providers are prepared in a number of disciplines and have a variety of training experiences. Studies are needed of the variations in and quality of care provided across the disciplines by different provider groups.

There is also a need for descriptive studies of current practice and usual care (eg, type of therapy, intensity, duration, with and without concurrent pharmacotherapy), as well as characterization of the patients treated in these practices in terms of diagnosis, severity, comorbidity (medical and psychiatric), ethnicity, socioeconomic status, and other variables that would relate to choice of treatment approach and to treatment outcomes. Results from such descriptive effectiveness studies can be used to set up randomized trials of promising approaches.

The establishment and use of networks of practitioners as study sites could be particularly informative. Typically, networks are loose coalitions of practitioners who agree to participate in research projects. Membership in the network is voluntary, and the practitioners tend to be of the same discipline. The diversity of the settings in which practitioners work provides a good mix, thus extending generalizability of results. Pediatricians and primary care physicians have already conducted research in their established practice networks, and the American Psychiatric Association is in the process of establishing such a network. Although conducting studies within networks poses problems (eg, the guild orientation of existing networks, the nonrandom, volunteer nature of practicipating providers, and the representativeness of the patient population), the use of networks is an important new approach that may prove useful in establishing the effectiveness of psychotherapeutic approaches.

Approximately half of depressed individuals who are in treatment receive care in the general medical setting.[60] With the current emphasis on managed care and the limited use of specialty providers, a major concern is the transferability of efficacious treatments to the primary care setting. Clearly, there is room for improvement in the primary care setting, as detailed in a recent study[61] that compared the outcomes and costs in the treatment of depression in prepaid general medical practices with those in mental health specialty practices. Care provided in the specialty sector was more appropriate (ie, more counseling and use of appropriate antidepressant medication) than that provided in the prepaid general sector. More appropriate care increased the total cost of care, but it was associated with better functional outcomes. The authors concluded that the trend toward provision of care by general medical providers reduces costs, worsens outcomes, and decreases the value of health care spending as measured by health improvement per dollar.

The DGP[17] practice guidelines for the treatment of depression in primary care assume that physicians will be the basic providers of treatment, and that treatment will emphasize pharmacotherapy. With primary care structured as it is, this is an understandable approach. Primary care physicians have little or no training in the psychosocial treatment of depression. It is not surprising that, despite considerable research, progress has been slow in improving outcomes for depressed patients in the primary care system.

A new model of care that offers great promise for more effective treatment of depression in primary care is the Collaborative Family Health Care (CFHC) model. The CFHC model is based on the premise that the treatment of illness and the nurturance of health are improved through collaboration among physical and mental health professionals, patients and their families, and health care administrators. Proponents of the CFHC model contend that collaborative health care is cost-effective, increases patient and provider satisfaction, and prevents provider burnout. Collaboration maximizes the availability of resources, emphasizes prevention, and transforms the treatment experience for providers and patients. The model rests on 3 key concepts: (1) teams of general and mental health professionals work in concert; (2) the biological, psychological, and social aspects of treatment are given equal importance; and (3) the patient's family is included as a crucial component of treatment. Although this model has not been tested in the psychosocial treatment of depression, results for pharmacotherapy with antidepressant medications are positive.[62]

The effectiveness of psychosocial treatment must be tested in the context of innovative models of primary care provision, such as the CFHC model, because several factors (eg, medical comorbidity, adverse drug reactions, negative interaction with other medications for chronic medical illnesses, advanced age, and pregnancy) contraindicate use of antidepressant medications for many primary care patients, and antidepressant medications may not be the treatment that the patient prefers. Some patients may also need psychotherapy along with antidepressant medication, and this combined treatment may be more effective when provided in the context of a collaborative model in which the team can respond with an integrated treatment approach.

Regardless of the models, settings, or provider types studied, any move from research on efficacy to research on effectiveness must include an expanded range of outcomes beyond just reduction of symptoms. We need broader agreement on instruments to measure psychological functioning (eg, mood, psychotic symptoms, substance abuse, and dangerousness), social functioning (eg, basic needs, community living skills, interpersonal relations, and work or school skills), and physical functioning (eg, physical impairment and self care) of patients with depression.[63] From a pragmatic perspective, improvements in functioning and social role performance are intuitively meaningful outcomes, compelling to patients, therapists, and other audiences because of their "clinical significance." Issues such as quality of life, functional status, cost, use of health services, patient satisfaction, and provider satisfaction must be measured as part of the determination of effectiveness. Other issues to be studied are the relative effectiveness (and cost-effectiveness) of group vs individual psychotherapy, brief treatment (or brief treatment with booster sessions) vs extended treatment, and use of family members as adjunctive therapists.

From Treatment Effectiveness to Minimal Standards of Care

Because data on the effectiveness of psychotherapy as a treatment for depression are sparse at the present time, articulation of the move from those data to minimal standards of care for the individual with depression is difficult. The DGP[17] guidelines are a step in that direction, but they are oriented toward pharmacotherapy in the primary care setting. In the current climate, issues of cost-effectiveness are likely to be paramount in developing minimal standards of care. Although there may be gaps in the findings of research on effectiveness, it would be extremely helpful for the field to have an "alpha" version of minimal standards for use in training programs and to focus the need for future research. This would enable the field to converge around a set of principles that might decrease the variation currently found in practice. As new findings emerge, they can be incorporated into future versions.

Minimal standards of care concerning psychotherapy are intricately intertwined with training standards. Across the diverse mental health disciplines, there should be basic standards to which all psychotherapy practitioners are trained. If the psychotherapy leadership can converge around a set of minimal standards of care, the standards can be incorporated into training programs so third-party payers can be confident in the quality of care that is provided.

The ultimate test of effectiveness of therapy based on minimal standards will be a comparison of outcomes with those of therapy not based on such standards. The test of effectiveness should include multiple practice sites, a wide range of the population, including various ethnic and socioeconomic groups, and a mix of provider disciplines.

A likely step in the progression from studies of effectiveness to minimal standards of care will be a cost-benefit investigation. Data on the relative benefit of brief vs longer treatments, brief treatments with and without booster sessions, group vs individual treatments, and family group treatments are sparse.

The reality of our current health care system is that

a greater number of depressed individuals are seen by general medical providers than by mental health specialists. As primary care physicians experience increased pressure from third-party payers to reduce referrals to specialty care providers and to manage a wider range of relatively common conditions, this state of affairs is likely to continue and suggests the reason behind the choice of depression by the DGP[17] for the formulation of one of the early treatment guidelines. Although there is a work group to revise the DGP treatment guidelines as new data come to light, the danger in the present climate is that the most conservative guidelines (in terms of treatment costs) will be embraced by the managed care companies.

IMPLICATIONS FOR A NATIONAL HEALTH CARE SYSTEM

Likely elements in the emerging health care system that is driven by the insurance industry and managed care organizations will include primary care physicians, ancillary help to the primary care physicians, and treatment in the specialty sector. We would make the following points about the role of psychotherapy in this tiered triage system:

1. Aggregated data may not be sufficient to tailor the treatment to the needs of the individual patient. Ultimately, the aim is to provide optimal care for each individual with depression. The empirical data on psychological treatment and treatment with medication are necessary but of limited value, because they provide mean scores on groups of patients at several points in time. The best care for the individual will involve examination of the antecedents of depression in the individual case, psychosocial treatment that focuses on those antecedent conditions, and continual assessment of the amount and rate of change; if change is insufficient, a different treatment plan is needed. Although not useful in planning for the individual case, group means are most useful in defining the typical course of improvement through treatment. If the individual case is an outlier in this typical course, a change in the treatment plan is indicated.

Regardless of the treatment modalities used, more data-intensive research designs are needed to evaluate therapeutic techniques. With improved designs, use of more powerful tools to model longitudinal data will be possible, rather than relying on group averages and pretreatment-posttreatment analyses. Kraemer and Thiemann[64] provided useful suggestions about the analysis of data from such "intensive designs." In a similar vein, Gibbons et al[65] and Lavori[66] surveyed several competing methods for analyzing longitudinal data, including repeated-measures analysis of variance, multivariate analysis of variance, and random regression models. The last approach is especially useful because it can accommodate most kinds of missing data, irregularly spaced measurements, correlated errors of measurement, time-varying and time-invariant covariates, and individual deviations from the trend of an aggregate response. These models would provide a greater understanding of individual differences in patients and allow inspection of alternative trajectories of change from particular patients or classes of patients. The rate at which different treatments achieve their effects is a considerable concern, especially if we are to investigate modalities of extended care for chronic or recurrent disorders.

2. Research initiatives will be needed to explore the linkage between detection of depression and provision of adequate treatment to the depressed patient. Specific aids, such as physician training and retraining and patient screening questionnaires, are needed to enhance detection by busy physicians. Guidelines for referral by primary care physicians to other levels of care will evolve and be updated with new empirical data and will need amplification (eg, patient vignettes) to be reliably translated into action.

When medication is prescribed by a nonpsychiatric physician or psychiatrist, adherence to a manual that specifies a supportive approach to the patient is probably necessary for effectiveness. It is curious that much attention has been given to therapist adherence to guidelines in psychosocial treatment manuals, while little has been written about the physician approach to prescription and monitoring of medication. Adequate physician adherence to effective clinical management may increase the time and, thus, the cost of "medication-only" treatment.

3. Psychotherapy has a necessary role. For the treatment of depression, psychotherapy has proved efficacious, and the effect sizes for psychotherapy are clinically meaningful. When used alone or in combination with medication therapy, psychotherapy may be a most useful influence on the mediating and moderating variables in depression (eg, "depressogenic" cognitions and inadequate social skills and support) and on the recruitment of family members to support the patient's treatment. Psychotherapy may also be a primary treatment for the substantial number of patients who refuse to take medication (5%-10%), those who discontinue or cannot tolerate medication (10%-15%), or those for whom medication is not appropriate because of pregnancy, major surgery, old age, or other such contraindications.[67] Efforts to find cost-effective ways to provide efficacious psychotherapy for depression are needed.

4. Patient preference should not dictate the treatment, but it must be seriously considered because of its effect on adherence to the treatment prescribed. While initiatives to educate patients about the need for antidepressant medication are used in primary care environments, the effectiveness of this education in enhancing adherence when the treatment regimen is contrary to patient preferences remains to be seen. A recent sophisticated survey of consumer preferences[68] suggests that education geared to fostering medication as a first line of treatment for mild-to-moderate depression may meet substantial opposition. The patient's preferences for a particular treatment should be paramount in the clinician's decision whenever possible. A patient who is disposed to a particular treatment will have higher expectations of success. Patient preference may, at times, collide with the emphasis of managed care on the less costly treatments. Consider, for example, the mild-to-moderately depressed individual who prefers psychotherapy and considers medication "a crutch." The inclination may be to prescribe nothing and tell the patient to return if the symp-

toms continue. A decrement in functioning could then ensue, because early intervention is not used for cost-containment reasons.

5. Many issues must be considered in comparing the treatments for depression and making judgments about the most acceptable and typical treatments for depression. This would include not only differential effectiveness in empirical studies, including symptom change, the clinical importance of the change, and the proportion of patients who change, but also the breadth and durability of the improvements, duration of the treatment, efficiency and costs of administering the treatment, the financial and emotional costs to the patient, and acceptability of the treatment to the patients.[69]

Accepted for publication May 2, 1996.

Reprints: John F. Clarkin, PhD, Department of Psychiatry, New York Hospital-Cornell University Medical Center, Westchester Division, 21 Bloomingdale Rd, White Plains, NY 10605.

REFERENCES

1. Goldin LR, Gershon ES. The genetic epidemiology of major depressive illness. In: Frances AJ, Hales RE, eds. *Psychiatric Update.* Washington, DC: American Psychiatric Press; 1988;7:149-168.
2. Klerman GL, Lavori PW, Rice J, Reich T, Endicott J, Andreasen NC, Keller MB, Hirschfield RMA. Birth cohort trends in rates of major depressive disorder among relatives of patients with affective disorder. *Arch Gen Psychiatry.* 1985;42:689-693.
3. Gotlib IH. Depressive disorders. In: Bellack AS, Hersen M, eds. *Psychopathology in Adulthood.* Boston, Mass: Allyn & Bacon Inc; 1993:179-194.
4. Weissman MM, Bruce ML, Leaf PJ, Florio LP, Holzer C. Affective disorders. In: Robins LN, Regier DA, eds. *Psychiatric Disorders in America.* New York, NY: Free Press; 1991:53-80.
5. Elkin I, Shea TM, Watkins JT, Imber SD, Sotsky SM, Collins JF, Glass DR, Pilkonis PA, Leber WR, Docherty JP, Fiester SJ, Parloff MB. National Institute of Mental Health Treatment of Depression Collaborative Research Program: general effectiveness of treatments. *Arch Gen Psychiatry.* 1989;46:971-982.
6. Lewinsohn PM. The behavioral study and treatment of depression. In: Hersen M, Eisler RM, Miller PM, eds. *Progress in Behavior Modification.* Orlando, Fla: Academic Press Inc; 1975.
7. Lewinsohn PM, Youngren MA, Grosscup S. Depression and reinforcement. In: DePue RA ed. *The Psychobiology of Depressive Disorders.* Orlando, Fla: Academic Press Inc; 1979.
8. Rehm LP. A self-control therapy program for treatment of depression. In: Clarkin JF, Glazer HI, eds. *Depression: Behavioral and Directive Intervention Strategies.* New York, NY: Garland STPM Press; 1981:68-110.
9. Haaga DAF, Dyck MJ, Ernst D. Empirical status of cognitive theory of depression. *Psychol Bull.* 1991;110:215-236.
10. Brown GW, Harris TO. *Social Origins of Depression: A Study of Psychiatric Disorder in Women.* London, England: Tavistock Publishers Ltd; 1978.
11. Pearlin LI, Lieberman MA. Social sources of emotional distress. In: Simmons R, ed. *Research in Community and Mental Health.* Greenwich, Conn: JAI Press Inc; 1979;1:217-248.
12. Weissman MM. Advances in psychiatric epidemiology: rates and risks for major depression. *Am J Public Health.* 1987;77:445-451.
13. Luborsky L. *Principles of Psychoanalytic Psychotherapy: A Manual for Supportive-Expressive Treatment.* New York, NY: Basic Books Inc Publishers; 1984.
14. Strupp HH, Binder JL. *Psychotherapy in a New Key: A Guide to Time-Limited Dynamic Psychotherapy.* New York, NY: Basic Books Inc Publishers; 1984.
15. Kupfer DJ. Long-term treatment of depression. *J Clin Psychiatry.* 1991;52 (suppl):28-34.
16. Frank E, Prien RF, Jarrett JB, Keller MB, Kupfer DJ, Lavori P, Rush AJ, Weissman MM. Conceptualization and rationale for consensus definitions of terms in major depressive disorder: response, remission, recovery, relapse, and recurrence. *Arch Gen Psychiatry.* 1991;48:851-855.
17. Depression Guideline Panel. *Depression in Primary Care, Vol 2: Treatment of Major Depression. Clinical Practice Guideline, Number 5.* Rockville, Md: US Dept of Health and Human Services, Public Health Service, Agency for Health Care Policy and Research; 1993. AHCPR publication 93-0551.
18. Dobson KS. A meta-analysis of the efficacy of cognitive therapy for depression. *J Consult Clin Psychol.* 1989;57:414-419.
19. Emmelkamp PMG. Behavior therapy with adults. In: Bergin AE, Garfield SL, eds. *Handbook of Psychotherapy and Behavior Change.* 4th ed. New York, NY: John Wiley & Sons Inc; 1994:379-427.
20. Free ML, Oei TPS. Biological and psychological processes in the treatment and maintenance of depression. *Clin Psychol Rev.* 1989;9:653-688.
21. Hollon SD, Beck AT. Cognitive and cognitive-behavioral therapies. In: Bergin AE, Garfield SL, eds. *Handbook of Psychotherapy and Behavior Change.* 4th ed. New York, NY: John Wiley & Sons Inc; 1994:428-466.
22. Hollon SD, Najavits L. Review of empirical studies on cognitive therapy. In: Frances AJ, Hales RE, eds. *Review of Psychiatry.* Washington, DC: American Psychiatric Press; 1988;7:643-666.
23. Jarrett RB, Rush AJ. Short-term psychotherapy of depressive disorders: current status and future directions. *Psychiatry.* 1994;57:115-132.
24. Shea MT, Elkin E, Hirschfeld RMA. Psychotherapeutic treatment of depression. In: Frances AJ, Hales RE, eds. *Review of Psychiatry.* Washington DC: American Psychiatric Press: 1988;7:235-255.
25. Weissman MM, Prusoff BA, DiMascio A, Neu C, Goklaney M, Klerman GL. The efficacy of drugs and psychotherapy in the treatment of acute depressive episodes. *Am J Psychiatry.* 1979;136:555-558.
26. Covi L, Lipman RS. Cognitive behavioral group psychotherapy combined with imipramine in major depression. *Psychopharmacol Bull.* 1987;23:173-176.
27. Gallagher DE, Thompson LW. Treatment of major depressive disorder in older adult outpatients with brief psychotherapies. *Psychother Theory Res Pract.* 1982; 19:482-490.
28. Hersen M, Bellack AS, Himmelhoch JM, Thase ME. Effects of social skills training, amitriptyline, and psychotherapy in unipolar depressed women. *Behav Ther.* 1984;15:21-40.
29. Kornblith SJ, Rehm LP, O'Hara MW, Lamparski DM. The contribution of self-reinforcement training and behavioral assignments to the efficacy of self-control therapy for depression. *Cognitive Ther Res.* 1983;7:499-528.
30. McLean PD, Hakstian AR. Clinical depression: comparative efficacy of outpatient treatments. *J Consult Clin Psychol.* 1979;47:818-836.
31. Steuer JL, Mintz J, Hammen CL, Hill MA, Jarvik LF, McCarley T, Motoike P, Rosen R. Cognitive-behavioral and psychodynamic group psychotherapy in treatment of geriatric depression. *J Consult Clin Psychol.* 1984;52:180-189.
32. Thompson LW, Gallagher DE, Breckenridge JS. Comparative effectiveness of psychotherapies for depressed elders. *J Consult Clin Psychol.* 1987;55:385-390.
33. Scogin F, McElreath L. Efficacy of psychosocial treatments for geriatric depression: a quantitative review. *J Consult Clin Psychol.* 1994;62:69-74.
34. Reynolds CF, Frank E, Perel JM, Imber SD, Cornes C, Morycz RK, Mazumdar S, Miller MD, Pollock BG, Rifai AH, Stack JA, George CJ, Houck PR, Kupfer DJ. Combined pharmacotherapy and psychotherapy in the acute and continuation treatment of elderly patients with recurrent major depression: a preliminary report. *Am J Psychiatry.* 1992;149:1687-1692.
35. Mufson L. *Interpersonal Psychotherapy for Depressed Adolescents.* New York, NY: Guilford Press; 1993.
36. Hollon SD, Shelton RC, Loosen PT. Cognitive therapy in relation to pharmacotherapy for depression. *J Consult Clin Psychol.* 1991;59:88-99.
37. Hollon SD, DeRubeis RJ, Seligman MEP. Cognitive therapy and the prevention of depression. *Appl Prev Psychol.* 1992;1:89-95.
38. Blackburn IM, Eunson KM, Bishop S. A two-year naturalistic follow-up of depressed patients treated with cognitive therapy, pharmacotherapy and a combination of both. *J Affect Disord.* 1986;10:67-75.
39. Simons AD, Murphy GE, Levine JL, Wetzel RD. Cognitive therapy and pharmacotherapy for depression: sustained improvement over one year. *Arch Gen Psychiatry.* 1986;43:43-48.
40. Kovacs M, Rush AJ, Beck AT, Hollon SD. Depressed outpatients treated with cognitive therapy or pharmacotherapy: a one-year follow-up. *Arch Gen Psychiatry.* 1981;38:33-41.
41. Weissman MM, Klerman GL, Prusoff BA, Sholomskas D, Padian N. Depressed outpatients: results one year after treatment with drugs and/or interpersonal psychotherapy. *Arch Gen Psychiatry.* 1981;38:51-55.
42. Weissman MM. Psychotherapy in the maintenance treatment of depression. *Br J Psychiatry.* 1994;165(suppl 26):42-50.
43. Frank E, Kupfer DJ, Perel JM, Cornes C, Jarrett DB, Mallinger AG, Thase ME, McEachran AB, Grochocinski VJ. Three-year outcomes for maintenance therapies in recurrent depresssion. *Arch Gen Psychiatry.* 1990;47:1093-1099.
44. Frank E, Kupfer DJ, Wagner EF, McEachran AB, Cornes C. Efficacy of interpersonal psychotherapy as a maintenance treatment of recurrent depression. *Arch Gen Psychiatry.* 1991;48:1053-1059.
45. Beck AT, Hollon SD, Young JE, Bedrosian RC, Budenz D. Treatment of depression with cognitive therapy and amitriptyline. *Arch Gen Psychiatry.* 1985;

42:142-148.
46. Murphy GE, Simons AD, Wetzel RD, Lustman PJ. Cognitive therapy and nortriptyline, singly and together, in the treatment of depression. *Arch Gen Psychiatry.* 1984;41:33-41.
47. Roth D, Bielski R, Jones M, Parker W, Osborn G. A comparison of self-control therapy and combined self-control therapy and antidepressant medication in the treatment of depression. *Behav Ther.* 1982;13:133-144.
48. Rush AJ, Watkins JT. Group versus individual cognitive therapy: a pilot study. *Cognitive Ther Res.* 1981;5:95-103.
49. DiMascio A, Klerman GL, Weissman MM, Prusoff BA, Neu C, Moore P. A control group for psychotherapy research in acute depression: one solution to ethical and methodological issues. *J Psychiatr Res.* 1979;15:189-197.
50. DiMascio A, Weissman, MM, Prusoff BA, Neu C, Zwilling M, Klerman GL. Differential symptom reduction by drugs and psychotherapy in acute depression. *Arch Gen Psychiatry.* 1979;36:1450-1456.
51. Conte HR, Plutchik R, Wild KV, Karasu TB. Combined psychotherapy and pharmacotherapy for depression: a systematic analysis of the evidence. *Arch Gen Psychiatry.* 1986;43:471-479.
52. Miller IW, Norman WH, Keitner GI. Treatment response of high cognitive dysfunction depressed inpatients. *Compre Psychiatry.* 1990;30:62-71.
53. Blackburn IM, Bishop S, Glen AIM, Whalley LJ, Christie JE. The efficacy of cognitive therapy in depression: a treatment trial using cognitive therapy and pharmacotherapy, each alone and in combination. *Br J Psychiatry.* 1981;139:181-189.
54. Friedman AS. Interaction of drug therapy with marital therapy in depressed patients. *Arch Gen Psychiatry.* 1975;32:619-637.
55. Weissman MM. The psychological treatment of depression: evidence for the efficacy of psychotherapy alone, and in comparison with, and in combination with pharmacotherapy. *Arch Gen Psychiatry.* 1979;36:1261-1269.
56. Weissman MM, Kasl SV, Klerman GL. Follow-up of depressed women after maintenance treatment. *Am J Psychiatry.* 1976;133:757-760.
57. Rush AJ, Beck AT, Kovacs M, Weissenburger MA, Hollon SD. Comparison of the effects of cognitive therapy and pharmacotherapy on hopelessness and self-concept. *Am J Psychiatry.* 1982;139:862-866.
58. Wilson PH. Combined pharmacological and behavioural treatment of depression. *Behav Res Ther.* 1982;20:173-184.
59. Mintz J, Mintz LI, Arrunda MJ, Lustman PJ. Treatments of depression and the functional capacity to work. *Arch Gen Psychiatry.* 1992;49:761-768.
60. Narrow WE, Reiger DA, Rae DS, Manderscheid RW, Locke BZ. Use of services by persons with mental and addictive disorders: findings from the National Institute of Mental Health Epidemiologic Catchment Area Program. *Arch Gen Psychiatry.* 1993;50:95-107.
61. Sturm R, Wells KB. How can care for depression become more cost-effective? *JAMA.* 1995;273:51-58.
62. Katon W, Von Korff M, Lin E, Walker E, Simon GE, Bush T, Robinson P, Russo J. Collaborative management to achieve treatment guidelines. *JAMA.* 1995; 273:1026-1031.
63. Uehara ES, Smukler M, Newman FL. Linking resource use to consumer level of need: field test of the level of need-care assessment (LONCA) method. *J Consult Clin Psychol.* 1994;62:695-709.
64. Kraemer HC, Thiemann S. A strategy to use soft data effectively in randomized controlled clinical trials. *J Consult Clin Psychol.* 1989;57:148-154.
65. Gibbons RD, Hedeker D, Elkin I, Waternaux C, Kraemer HC, Greenhouse JB, Shea MT, Imber SD, Sotsky SM, Watkins JT. Some conceptual and statistical issues in analysis of longitudinal psychiatric data. *Arch Gen Psychiatry.* 1993; 50:739-750.
66. Lavori P. ANOVA, MANOVA, my black hen. *Arch Gen Psychiatry.* 1990;47:775-778.
67. Klerman GL. Treatment of recurrent unipolar major depressive disorder. *Arch Gen Psychiatry.* 1990;47:1158-1162.
68. Mental Health: Does therapy help? *Consumer Rep.* 1995;60:734-739.
69. Kazdin AE, Wilson GT. Criteria for evaluating psychotherapy. *Arch Gen Psychiatry.* 1978;35:407-416.

SPECIAL ARTICLE

Advances in the Psychosocial Treatment of Anxiety Disorders

Implications for National Health Care

David H. Barlow, PhD; Cassandra L. Lehman

Recent developments in the psychosocial treatments for anxiety disorders suggest that we have reached an early plateau. Evidence now exists on the effectiveness of psychosocial treatment approaches for every anxiety disorder when compared with no treatment or credible psychosocial placebos. In many cases these procedures have limited clinical effectiveness and much remains to be learned about the disseminability and clinical utility of these approaches in the context of emerging national health care plans. We are just beginning the first generation of multisite studies examining the potentially synergistic effects of proven psychosocial treatments and proven drug treatments. These studies that have substantial significance for national health care are reviewed and some preliminary results are reported.

Arch Gen Psychiatry. 1996;53:727-735

In the quickly developing area of psychotherapy research, progress in the psychosocial treatment of the various anxiety disorders stands out. For almost all anxiety disorders, controlled studies now exist demonstrating the effectiveness of new psychosocial treatments when compared with either no treatment, a well-construed psychosocial "placebo," or even a credible alternative psychotherapeutic intervention. For some disorders treatments are well established; for others treatments are promising but in a preliminary state of development. Furthermore, a variety of questions remain unanswered for most disorders. Among these questions are the precise mechanism of action of these treatments, the interaction of psychosocial treatments with effective pharmacological treatments, and the transportability or user-friendliness of these treatments when integrated into the health care system. While many of these treatments could be characterized as cognitive behavioral, theoretical boundaries are increasingly blurred as elements from interpersonal and more psychodynamic approaches are integrated.

From the Department of Psychology and The Center for Anxiety and Related Disorders, Boston University, Boston, Mass.

In this article we will briefly review the current empirical status of psychosocial treatments for each anxiety disorder in the *DSM-IV* with attention to unanswered questions and current directions in research. Of particular interest are a number of large multisite trials that are currently ongoing and examining the separate and in some cases combined effects of drugs and psychosocial treatments. We will conclude this review by discussing the beginnings of some efforts to make these psychosocial approaches more practical and realistic tools in our emerging system of national health care.

PANIC DISORDER

Panic Disorder With and Without Agoraphobia

Early in the development of brief effective treatments for anxiety disorders, behaviorally oriented psychosocial investigators concentrated on treating phobic situational avoidance behavior with in vivo exposure procedures.[1,2] In an early report appearing in the ARCHIVES,[1] 3 patients with severe agoraphobia benefitted substantially by systematically venturing further from a safe place (the hospital) into

Table 1. Clinical Trials of Cognitive Behavioral Treatments for Panic Disorder and Intent-to-Treat Analysis*

Source, y	Length of Follow-up, mo	Treatment/ No. of Patients/ % Panic Free	Significant Comparison, % Panic Free†	
			Other Treatments	Wait List
Craske et al,[14] 1991‡	24	PCT/15/81	Yes: AR=36	. . .
			Yes: PCT and AR=43	
Clark et al,[15] 1994	12	CT/17/76§	Yes: AR=43§	. . .
			Yes: IMI=48§	
Klosko et al,[16] 1990	PT	PCT/15/87	No: AL=50	Yes: 33
			Yes: PL=36	. . .
Newman et al,[17] 1990	12	CTM/24/87	. . .	. . .
		CTNM/19/87	. . .	
Côté et al,[18] 1992	12	CBTM/13/92	. . .	. . .
		CBTNM/8/100	. . .	
Beck et al,[19] 1992	PT	CT/17/94	Yes: ST=25‖	. . .
Black et al,[20] 1993	PT	CT/25/32	Yes: FL=68	. . .
			No: PL=20	
Margraf and Schneider,[21] 1991	4 wk	CT/22/91	. . .	Yes: 5
Öst et al,[22] 1993	12	CT/19/89§	No: AR=74§	. . .
Telch et al,[23] 1993	PT	PCT/34/85	. . .	Yes: 30
Craske et al,[24] 1995	PT	CBT/16/53	Yes: NPT=8	. . .
Shear et al,[25] 1994	6	CBT/23/45	No: NPT=45	. . .

**AL indicates alprazolam; AR, applied relaxation; CBT, cognitive behavioral therapy; CBTM, cognitive behavioral therapy and medication; CBTNM, cognitive behavioral therapy without medication; CT, cognitive therapy; CTM, cognitive therapy and medication; CTNM, cognitive therapy without medication; FL, fluvoxamine maleate; IMI, imiprimine hydrochloride; NPT, nonprescription treatment; PL, pill placebo; PCT, panic control treatment (exposure and cognitive restructuring); PT, posttreatment; and ST, standard treatment.*

†Yes indicates the comparison was significant; no, comparison not significant; and ellipses, no comparison made.

‡Follow-up study of Barlow et al.[13]

§Percentage of patients who were panic free at follow-up and who had received no additional treatment during the follow-up period.

‖At 8 weeks, which is the end of supportive therapy. At this time, 71% of patients undergoing CT were panic free.

a more crowded downtown area through a series of structured exposure exercises.

By the early 1980s numerous studies conducted by clinicians in various parts of the world had found that exposure-based procedures conducted in vivo (as opposed to in imagination) were consistently effective compared with no treatment or some good placebo.[3-5] Follow-up studies of 4 years or longer revealed maintenance of gains in most cases.[3,6-10] Nevertheless, this treatment approach proved to be far from a panacea since as many as 25% to 40% of patients did not respond in a clinically meaningful fashion, and relatively few of the patients who did respond were "cured."

With changing conceptualizations of panic disorder with agoraphobia,[11,12] psychosocial treatments were developed that were directed more specifically at unexpected panic attacks. In our setting, one such approach called panic control treatment (PCT) (exposure and cognitive restructuring) has been subjected to a number of clinical trials.[13,14] At the same time, Clark and his colleagues[15] at the University of Oxford in England independently developed an approach from a different conceptual point of view that, nevertheless, shares many of the same therapeutic procedures. Both treatment approaches target cognitive, physiological, and behavioral components of panic disorder.

Table 1 presents results from clinical trials or clinical replication series evaluating this treatment approach for panic disorder in terms of panic-free status, the 1 measure common to all studies, and using intent-to-treat analyses, which considers the results in the context of all patients entering the clinical trial, including those who dropped out. In most studies in which comparisons were made, PCT or cognitive therapy was better with approximately 80% panic-free results than no treatment or some credible psychotherapeutic alternative.

Although replications have been reported from a number of different countries and across several different settings (eg, urban vs rural, see Table 1), not every study has reported positive results. For example, intent-to-treat analysis of panic-free status suggests that only approximately 32% of patients described by Black et al[20] were panic free. High attrition and poor results in this study, whether analyzed based on intent-to-treat or completor analyses, may have been due to substantial modifications to the treatment reported by the authors or other variables, which raises concerns regarding the disseminability of these treatments to settings in which expertise did not previously exist, an issue discussed below.

Current Directions

More recent longitudinal analyses suggest that while positive outcomes are maintained at follow-up, when analyzed cross-sectionally some symptom reemergence is common in these chronic disorders during follow-up periods, a result that seems to be true also with pharmacological approaches analyzed in this way.[26] Other recent studies of large groups of patients with panic disorder and no more than mild to moderate agoraphobic avoidance find that pretreatment comorbidity does not predict outcome. Thus, patients who are comorbid experience remission of panic disorder to the same extent as those who are not comorbid. Furthermore, many but not all comorbid disorders also improve at posttreatment.[27]

Efforts to evaluate ways of enhancing the effects of psychosocial treatments of panic disorder with agoraphobia are continuing. Since treatments of agoraphobic avoidance consisting largely of in vivo exposure and treatments of panic disorder focusing on panic attacks evolved relatively independently, experimental efforts are now assessing the benefits of integrating these 2 treatment approaches for the full range of patients with panic disorder with agoraphobia (Page AC, unpublished data, 1994).[8,23,28-30]

The interaction of psychosocial treatments with drug treatments is another area that is currently very active. One important question concerns the possible facilitatory effect of combining these 2 treatments. In the case of in vivo exposure for agoraphobic avoidance behavior, previous studies have suggested that the results of treatment combinations depend on which drug is used. For example, in most studies the use of tricyclic antidepressants such as imipramine seem to facilitate the effects of in vivo exposure.[31] On the other hand, some evidence exists that the concurrent administration of benzodiazepines, particularly high-potency benzodiazepines, may interfere with the effects, particularly the lasting effects, of in vivo exposure or other psychosocial treatments.[3,26,30]

A large 4-site study sponsored by the National Institute of Mental Health evaluating the comparative and combined efficacy cf PCT and imipramine is currently nearing completion. Preliminary results indicate a marked advantage to the combination treatment. Confirmation of this finding will have to await a full analysis of the data. This study should also answer the question regarding the transportability of psychosocial treatments for panic disorder to settings where these treatments have not traditionally been available—a question that is critical for national health care.

In the meantime, other more creative ways to integrate drug and psychosocial treatments are now appearing. Although high-potency benzodiazepines and psychosocial treatments may not combine well when administered concurrently, it may be that a sequential strategy for administration may prove to be beneficial. Recently in 2 separate reports Otto et al[32] and Spiegel et al[33] treated patients with panic disorder who were receiving therapeutic doses of high-potency benzodiazepines with a brief version of PCT that was designed to facilitate discontinuation of the treatment with benzodiazepines without recurrence or relapse of the panic disorder. Using exquisitely slow taper schedules, in some instances as low as 0.125 mg of the drug every 7 days, patients were able to either discontinue the benzodiazepine treatment without relapse to a significantly greater degree with PCT than without[32] or to maintain their drug-free status at a significantly higher rate (up to 6 months after taper) without relapse.[33] Results from Spiegel et al[33] are presented in the **Figure**. This suggests that one might successfully administer a fast-acting, high-potency benzodiazepine on a time-limited basis followed by PCT and discontinuation of treatment with the drug with a successful result.

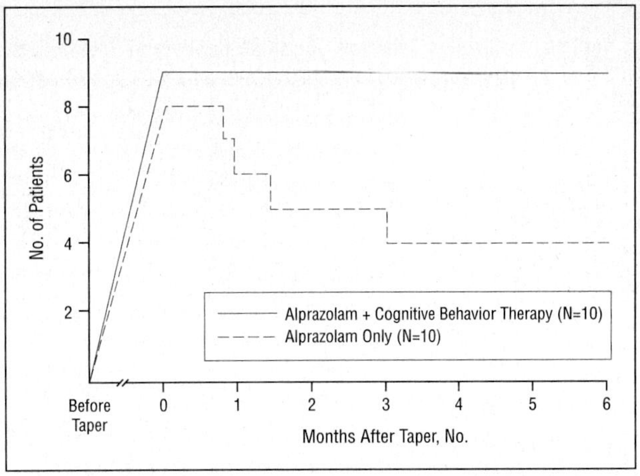

Cumulative number of patients achieving and maintaining drug abstinence in groups receiving alprazolam only and alprazolam plus cognitive behavioral therapy. Significant difference between survival distributions from before taper to 3 months after taper (Lee-Desu statistic=4.197, df=1, *P<.05).*

GENERALIZED ANXIETY DISORDER

Current Approaches

Before considering the evolution of specific brief psychosocial treatments for generalized anxiety disorder (GAD), it is necessary to consider new conceptualizations of the diagnosis itself in *DSM-III-R*[34] and *DSM-IV*.[35] These emphasize chronic and pervasive apprehensive expectation or worry[36] and somatic symptoms reflecting central nervous system tension as well as the empirical basis of changes in the diagnostic criteria.[37-39]

Current psychosocial approaches to GAD combine relaxation or meditation procedures with cognitive therapy for the purpose of bringing the worry process itself under the patient's control. Most of these treatments also include training in coping more effectively with anxiety and the incorporation of problem-solving strategies to address interpersonal sources of anxiety, time management, etc.[40-44] A number of studies have now appeared that suggest the superiority of variations of this new psychosocial approach compared with psychosocial placebos or credible alternative treatments (**Table 2**).[45-48]

In a particularly well-done study, Borkovec and Costello[45] compared the efficacy of applied relaxation in which relaxation procedures were actively used with cognitive behavioral therapy and nondirective therapy in a sample of 55 patients who were carefully diagnosed using the *DSM-III-R*[34] as having GAD. At a 12-month follow-up, 57.9% of patients undergoing cognitive behavioral therapy met rigorous high–end state functioning criteria (close to cured), and this was significantly better than the 33.3% in the applied relaxation condition and the 22.2% in the nondirective condition. Much as with panic disorder, Borkovec et al[55] found that improvement in GAD after treatment was also associated with improvement in any comorbid diagnosis present before treatment.

Current Directions

The studies reviewed above are encouraging since, with this rather difficult disorder, a new generation of brief psychosocial treatments from several different research centers have proven to be more effective than credible alternative psychosocial treatments. However, these studies have yet to be tested beyond the clinics of their originators in any substantial manner. Also, unlike panic disorder reviewed above

Table 2. Controlled Trials of Cognitive Behavioral Treatments for Generalized Anxiety Disorder*†

Source, y	Length of Follow-up, mo	Treatment, No. of Patients	% of Clinical Improvement of Completers (When Available)	Significant Comparison,‡ % of Clinical Improvement: Other Treatments	Significant Comparison,‡ % of Clinical Improvement: Wait List
Barlow et al,[50] 1984	6	CBT, 5		. . .	Yes
Blowers et al,[41] 1987	6	CBT, 20		Yes: ND (some measures)	Yes
Borkovec et al,[51] 1987	6-12	CT+PR, 16		Yes: ND+PR (some measures)	. . .
Butler et al,[52] 1987	6	CBT, 22	58.5		Yes (0)
Borkovec and Mathews,[42] 1988	12	CT+PR, 6		No: SCD+PR	No: ND+PR
Power et al,[53] 1989	PT	CBT, 10		Yes: PL (1 central measure) No: DZ (1 central measure)	. . .
Power et al,[48] 1990	PT	CBT, 21	61.9	No: CBT+DZ=69.8 No: CBT+PL=55.6 Yes: DZ=30.3 Yes: PL=17.5	. . .
Butler et al,[46] 1991	6	CBT, 18	42	Yes: BT=5	Yes
Barlow et al,[40] 1992	24	CBT, 29	55	. . .	Yes (0)
White et al,[54] 1992	6	CBT, 26		No: BT, CT . . .	Yes Yes: APL
Borkovec and Costello,[45] 1993	12	CBT, 18	57.9	Yes: ND=26.7 Yes: AR=37.5	. . .
Durham et al,[47] 1994§	6	CT, 40	>60	Yes: AP <31 Yes: AMT <37	. . .

**AMT indicates anxiety management training; AP, analytic psychotherapy; APL, attention placebo; AR, applied relaxation; BT, behavior therapy; CBT, cognitive behavioral therapy; CT, cognitive therapy; DZ, diazepam; ND, nondirective therapy; PL, pill placebo; PR, progressive relaxation; PT, posttreatment; and SCD, self-control desensitization.*

†Adapted from Borkovec and Whisman.[49]

‡Yes indicates the comparison was significant; no, not significant; and ellipses, no comparison made.

§Intent-to-treat.

and social phobia and obsessive-compulsive disorder (OCD) reviewed below, important multisite studies that look at the separate and combined effects of these approaches with appropriate pharmacological treatments, to our knowledge, have yet to be undertaken.

At our own center we have developed new iteration of our protocol for GAD that is currently undergoing systematic evaluation. In this protocol, termed *worry control treatment*, patients are directly exposed and habituate to the worry process itself and the loss of control associated with this process.[56] The preliminary results of this treatment are encouraging.

OBSESSIVE-COMPULSIVE DISORDER

A New Approach

In this most difficult of all anxiety disorders with very low rates of response to placebo not exceeding 6%,[57] 1 specific psychosocial treatment has emerged with evidence for effectiveness, exposure and response prevention (ERP).[3,58] Other psychosocial approaches, either cognitive behavioral or noncognitive behavioral, have proven to be ineffective. With ERP, first developed clinically in the 1960s[59] and described in some detail by Riggs and Foa,[60] the patient is exposed to triggers for obsessional thoughts, such as contaminating substances, and/or to the intrusive obsessional thoughts themselves while rituals such as washing or checking are prevented. In a more recent innovation,[61] mental rituals such as counting or praying are also identified and prevented. Exposure and response prevention has now been evaluated extensively. A recent review identified 16 studies that administered ERP in an adequate fashion and followed up patients for an average of 29 months, describing in a categorical fashion those who responded to treatment and those who did not (**Table 3**).[62] In 2 of these studies[77,78] and 2 additional studies by Marks and his colleagues,[79,80] some medication was administered acutely but was found to have negligible or short-term effects and was withdrawn with the authors attributing the progress at long-term follow-up to the psychosocial treatment.

Overall the results are encouraging, particularly the finding that therapeutic gains are maintained at follow-up. However, using a convention that is widely adopted in research with this disorder, "responder" in Table 3 is defined as only a 30% or greater reduction in symptoms, suggesting that many patients may remain substantially impaired.

More recently, Hiss et al[81] demonstrated that adding relapse prevention procedures commonly used with addictive disorders[82] to ERP prevented relapse and recurrence over a 6-month period significantly better than an attention placebo control. If these results are replicated, relapse prevention procedures may provide a significant enhancement to ERP.

Current Directions

In view of the severity and substantial impairment associated with OCD, ascertaining possible synergistic effects of psychosocial and drug treatments, particularly clomipramine hydrochloride and some of the newer selective serotonin reuptake inhibitor agents, will be particularly important.

Table 3. Long-term Efficacy of Exposure-Based Treatment for Obsessive-compulsive Disorder*

Source, y	No. of Patients	Length of Follow-up, mo	% of Responders
Meyer et al,[63] 1974	12	6-72	83
Catts and McConaghy,[64] 1975	6	9-24	100
Marks et al,[65] 1975	20	24	75
Boulougouris,[66] 1977	15	34	60
Foa and Goldstein,[67] 1978	19	15	84
Emmelkamp and Rabbie,[68] 1981	22	54	73
Mawson et al,[69] 1982	37	24	83
O'Sullivan et al,[70] 1991	34	72	74
Bolton et al,[71] 1983	12	22	83
Foa et al,[72] 1983	37	12	76
Foa et al,[73] 1984	11	12	80
Hoogduin and Hoogduin,[74] 1984	25	14.5	80
Emmelkamp et al,[75] 1985	42	42	80
Kasvikas and Marks,[76] 1988	39	24	54
Foa et al,[77] 1992	38	16	81
Cottraux et al,[78] 1990	7	6	50
	Total=376	Mean=29.0	Mean=76

**Averages are weighted according to the number of patients in each study. From Foa and Kozak.[62]*

In 1 very important study, Foa and Liebowitz[83] are conducting a multisite investigation comparing clomipramine and behavior therapy in patients with OCD. Patients are assigned to 1 of 4 treatment conditions: behavior therapy, clomipramine, behavior therapy plus clomipramine, or pill placebo. Preliminary results suggest that ERP has more powerful and longer-lasting effects. When completed, the results should allow a definitive evaluation of the comparative efficacy of behavior therapy, clomipramine, and the 2 in combination.

While the Foa and Liebowitz[83] study is important, it is only 1 study, and further replications are needed to develop the most powerful treatment approaches for this very severe condition. As clinical trials accumulate, more information on patient-treatment matching should become available. A disadvantage of ERP is that it is not particularly user-friendly with only a few centers possessing the resources and expertise to carry out the treatment in an appropriate fashion. Evaluations of self-help books have not been encouraging.[80] Nevertheless, further evaluations are necessary, and attempts are being made to disseminate information on appropriate diagnosis and psychosocial treatment of this condition to a larger number of clinicians.

SOCIAL PHOBIA

New Treatment Considerations

Social phobia, by some estimates the most prevalent of all mental disorders,[84] has only recently become a target for serious clinical investigation.[3,85]

There is a developing consensus that a combination of treatments based on exposure to social situations and cognitive therapy may turn out to be the most powerful psychosocial intervention. **Table 4** summarizes the studies to date.

In our former setting, Heimberg et al[89,90] developed a cognitive behavioral group treatment (CBGT) that also consists of structured exposure exercises in the context of group therapy combined with cognitive therapy. In the first study, Heimberg et al[89] contrasted their CBGT to a credible placebo treatment, educational supportive psychotherapy (ES), thus controlling for a variety of nonspecific effects that include attention, treatment credibility, and expectations for treatment outcome. Cognitive behavioral group treatment was superior to ES on several measures at posttreatment, with this difference increasing at 3- and 6-month follow-ups. A 5-year follow-up on a subset of subjects from his original group indicated that individuals receiving CGBT were more likely to maintain their gains and continued to be more improved than comparable subjects in an ES condition.[90]

In 1 additional study comparing CBGT with phenelzine, alprazolam, and pill placebo,[92] subjects in all 4 groups, even those receiving placebo, improved with very few differences among groups. Those authors note that all groups engaged in systematic self-guided exposure exercises to social situations that may have accounted for substantial improvement in the placebo group.

Current Directions

The first phase of an important multisite study directed by Heimberg et al[94] comparing CBGT with phenelzine and both a pill placebo and a psychosocial placebo (ES) is now approaching completion. Results indicate that we have 2 powerful treatments for social phobia with the psychosocial and drug treatments approximately equally effective and both substantially more effective than placebo control conditions. In the second phase of this project, which is just getting under way, these investigators will examine the interaction of drug and psychosocial treatments compared with either one administered separately.

Much as with OCD and GAD, few if any attempts have been made to disseminate this psychosocial treatment to clinicians treating patients with social phobias or otherwise to make the treatment more user-friendly for clinical settings.

SPECIFIC PHOBIA

New Subtyping Scheme and Treatment Considerations

Recent research has led to recognition of the heterogeneity of specific phobia, and this heterogeneity is reflected in a new subtyping scheme in the *DSM-IV*.[35] The identification of blood/injection/injury fear that are characterized by a different physiological response (vasovagal syncope often resulting in fainting) is perhaps the most important development in this regard.

It is possible that some pharmacological approaches may prove to be appropriate for some cases of specific phobia such as situational phobia. Nevertheless, currently the overwhelming evidence is that exposure-based treatments are the treatments of choice for all patients with spe-

Table 4. Controlled Trials of Psychosocial Treatments for Social Phobia*

Source, y	Length of Follow-up, mo	Treatment No. of Patients	% of Clinical Improvement of Completers (When Available)	Significant Comparison,† % of Clinical Improvement: Other Treatments	Wait List
Butler et al,[86] 1984	6	AMT and E, 15		Yes: E	Yes
Mattick and Peters,[87] 1988	3	E and CR, 11	86	Yes: E=52	Yes
Mattick et al,[88] 1989	3	E and CR, 25		Yes: E	Yes
Heimberg et al,[89] 1990	6	CBGT, 20	81	Yes: ES=47	. . .
Heimberg et al,[90] 1993‡	54-75	CBGT, 10		Yes: ES (most measures)	
Hope et al,[91] 1990	6	CBGT, 13		No: E	Yes
Gelernter et al,[92] 1991	2	CBGT, 20		No: PH, AL, PL	. . .
Lucas and Telch,[93] 1993	PT	CBGT, 18	61	Yes: ES=24	
		CBTI	50		. . .
Heimberg et al,[94] 1994	PT	CBGT, 28	75	No: PH=77	
				Yes: PL=41	. . .
				Yes: ES=35	

*AL indicates alprazolam; AMT, anxiety management therapy, CBGT, cognitive behavioral group treatment; CBTI, cognitive behavioral treatment–individual; CR, cognitive restructuring; E, exposure; ES, educational supportive group psychotherapy (placebo treatment); PL, pill placebo; PH, phenelzine sulfate; and PT, posttreatment.

†Yes indicates the comparison was significant; no, not significant; and ellipses, no comparison made.

‡This is a follow-up study to the 1990 Heimberg et al[89] study.

cific phobia, with some strategic differences in the manner of administering the treatment. For example, the very successful treatment of patients with blood/injection/injury phobia involves the usual course of in vivo exposure to increasingly more phobically involved stimuli, with the added requirement that the patient engage in whole-body muscle tension exercises to maintain adequate blood pressure.[95-98] In 1 series of patients with blood/injection/injury phobia, close to 90% were essentially cured after 5 sessions.[98]

Current Directions

A recent innovation is the successful treatment of most patients with a specific phobia, no matter how severe, in 1 session.[99] In this approach, an entire hierarchy of feared stimuli is presented to the patient during a single session, which may take several hours. Of 20 consecutive patients treated in this way, Öst et al[99] report that 90% are either much improved or completely recovered at follow-ups ranging to 4 years. Öst et al[100] replicated this result with patients with blood phobia who were successfully treated in 2 hours.

In view of the prevalence of several specific phobias presenting with clinical levels of impairment (eg, individuals with blood/injection/injury phobia often avoid receiving necessary health and dental care), it should be possible, and would be important, to disseminate this treatment to appropriate health care professionals. This would include the training of nurses and other primary care health care personnel so as to reach a much larger number of individuals with impairing specific phobias who have changed their lifestyle to accommodate their specific phobia.

POSTTRAUMATIC STRESS DISORDER

Treatment Approaches to Date

Adequate clinical trials of psychosocial treatments for posttraumatic stress disorder (PTSD) are only recently emerging. **Table 5** contains a list of currently published clinical trials evaluating psychosocial procedures. Generally, psychosocial treatments for PTSD in these studies have fallen into 2 broad categories: direct exposure in the guise of therapeutic reliving of the traumatic event in imagination (prolonged imaginal exposure) and stress management. The stress management package typically consists of cognitive restructuring along with relaxation and problem-solving strategies that are similar to treatments for GAD but with the addition of anger management. Detailed description of an up-to-date comprehensive psychosocial treatment in the context of rape-induced PTSD dubbed *cognitive processing therapy* (CPT), can be found in an article by Calhoun and Resick.[108]

In a study of 17 women who initally met the criteria for PTSD and received this treatment,[106] none met the criteria for PTSD at posttreatment or at the 6-month follow-up. It is also significant that comorbid mood disorders remitted concurrently without direct therapeutic attention.

Foa et al[104] randomly assigned 45 victims of rape who were diagnosed with PTSD to 1 of 4 conditions: stress inoculation training, prolonged exposure, supportive counseling, and a wait-list control group. Immediately after treatment, stress inoculation training was most effective in reducing PTSD symptoms. However, at a 3.5-month follow-up, exposure-based procedures emerged as the superior treatment since patients in this condition continued to improve. Inportantly, prolonged exposure resulted in significant improvement on measures of numbing and social avoidance.

Other studies[101-103] also found that some variations of these treatments were more effective than wait-list control groups or the standard and customary treatment used in the treatment of Vietnam veterans with PTSD. Clinical trials comparing psychosocial treatments with drug treatments, or combination treatments, to our knowledge, have not yet been reported.

Current Directions

Clinical centers for the care of civilian and war-related traumas are proliferating around the country and exist

Table 5. Controlled Trials of Psychosocial Treatments for Posttraumatic Stress Disorder*

Source, y	Length of Follow-up, mo	Treatment, No. of Patients	% of Completers Without Diagnosis (When Available)	Significant Comparison,† % Without Diagnosis: Other Treatments	Wait List
Keane et al,[101] 1989	PT	IE, 11		. . .	Yes
Cooper and Clum,[102] 1989	PT	ST and IE, 7		Yes: ST	. . .
Boudewyns and Hyer,[103] 1990	PT	DTE, 19		Yes: IT	. . .
Foa et al,[104] 1991	3.5	E, 14		Yes: SIT	Yes
				Yes: SC	
Foa,[105] 1994	3.5	E and SIT, 20	91	Yes: E=29	Yes (0)
				Yes: SIT=42	. . .
	3.5	E and SIT	91‡	No: E=71‡	
				No: SIT=73‡	. . .
Resick and Schnicke,[106] 1992	6	CPT, 17	100		Yes
Foa et al,[107] 1995	5.5	BP, 10	90	Yes: AC=30	

**AC indicates assessment control; BP, brief prevention program; CPT, cognitive processing therapy; DTE, direct therapeutic exposure; E, prolonged exposure; IE, imaginal exposure; IT, individual treatment; PT, posttreatment; SC, supportive counseling; SIT, stress inoculation training; ST, standard treatment.*

†Yes indicates the comparison was significant; no, not significant; and ellipses, no comparison made.

‡Recalculated in terms of at least 50% symptom reduction.

in almost every community. Although it seems that successful psychosocial treatments exist, based on studies reviewed above, we have little or no information on the transportability and user-friendliness of these treatments in veterans centers and rape crisis centers. Additional variables such as social support and a broader consideration of interpersonal factors would also seem to be important treatment considerations worthy of evaluation in view of the buffering effects of social support on symptom expression during and after periods of extreme stress.[3] Clearly, more developmental work is required on this first generation of psychosocial treatments for PTSD. In addition, 1 important preliminary study suggests that a prevention program for recent victims of rape who are at risk of developing PTSD is effective in preventing PTSD.[107]

CONCLUSIONS

It seems clear that we have reached the first plateau in the development of psychosocial treatments for anxiety disorders. Specifically, we now have treatment approaches for almost every anxiety disorder with proven effectiveness when compared not only with no treatment or a wait-list control group but also with credible psychosocial placebos where therapeutic relationships are established and educational and attentional factors are included. These treatment approaches differ from disorder to disorder, but most contain exposure-based procedures, some sort of cognitive therapy or attention to cognitive and emotional factors even if outside of the awareness of the patient, and problem-solving or coping strategies in addition to nonspecific factors. There is also a trend in these treatments to attend more closely to the interpersonal system of the patient and to incorporate these approaches into group-therapy formats.

This is only the first of many plateaus that must be attained. Subsequent steps will have more relevance for health care delivery systems. For example, it is clear from published surveys that these approaches, although successful, have not been widely disseminated to clinicians and therefore are not widely available to patients. This is true even for in vivo exposure-based procedures for agoraphobia, a relatively well-established and straightforward strategy to administer. For example, surveys of patients with panic disorder with agoraphobia in 3 metropolitan areas[109-111] suggested that while many of these patients had received some medication, or perhaps some relaxation strategies, less than 40% and in some cases as few as 15% of the patients had received any exposure-based treatments for their agoraphobic avoidance whatsoever. In an attempt to rectify this situation, clinical investigators are evaluating more user-friendly approaches that are amenable to practice settings that include briefer therapy assisted by structured manuals[112,113] or the inclusion of someone in the patient's own environment, such as a spouse, in assisting with the delivery of treatment.[114,115] For example, Swinson et al[116] administered brief exposure instructions over the phone to patients who had been treated in the emergency department for panic attacks. Subjects receiving these exposure instructions improved significantly over the subsequent 6 months compared with a group of subjects who were simply reassured. Findings such as these may have particular significance for the effective delivery of psychosocial treatments, at least to newly emergent or less severely affected groups of patients. Nevertheless, until additional data are available, serious questions remain concerning the transportability of effective psychosocial treatments to settings where expertise does not currently exist, making efforts to increase user-friendliness and transportability a high priority.

Finally, we are just in the midst of the first generation of multisite studies examining the separate and combined effects of proven psychosocial treatments and proven pharmacological treatments, but these studies will accomplish more than simply providing us with information about the possible synergistic effects of these treatment approaches. These studies should also provide us with information on patient-treatment matching at various sites known for expertise in one approach (eg, pharmacotherapy) vs the other, as well as transportability of specific approaches (ie, psychosocial or drug) into various sites where expertise may not have previously existed in one approach or the other. Finally, these multisite studies provide an invaluable opportunity to examine long-term maintenance of treatment effects. Ultimately, questions regarding long-term maintenance may be among the more important questions in view of the well-known chronicity of anxiety disorders[117] and their substantial impact, not only on the lives of individuals suffering with them but also on the health care system that must care for these individuals over a lifetime.

Accepted for publication April 27, 1996.

Reprints: David H. Barlow, PhD, The Boston Center for Anxiety Disorders and Related Disorders, Boston University, 1 Kenmore Sq, Boston, MA 02215.

REFERENCES

1. Agras S, Leitenberg H, Barlow DH. Social reinforcement in the modification of agoraphobia. *Arch Gen Psychiatry.* 1968;19:423-427.
2. Marks IM. *Fears and Phobias.* London, England: Heineman; 1969.
3. Barlow DH. *Anxiety and Its Disorders: The Nature and Treatment of Anxiety and Panic.* New York, NY: Guilford Press; 1988.
4. Jansson L, Öst L-G. Behavioral treatments for agoraphobia: an evaluative review. *Clin Psychol Rev.* 1982;2:311-336.
5. Mavissakalian M. Antidepressant medications for panic disorder. In: Mavissakalian M, Prien R, eds. *Long-Term Treatments of Anxiety Disorders.* Washington, DC: American Psychiatric Press Inc; 1996:265-284.
6. Burns LE, Thorpe GL, Cavallaro LA. Agoraphobia eight years after behavioral treatment. *Behav Ther.* 1986;17:580-591.
7. Cohen SD, Monteiro W, Marks IM. Two-year follow-up of agoraphobics after exposure and imipramine. *Br J Psychiatry.* 1984;144:276-281.
8. Fava GA, Zielezny M, Savron G, Grandi S. Long-term effects of behavioural treatment for panic disorder with agoraphobia. *Br J Psychiatry.* 1995;166:87-92.
9. Jansson L, Jerremalm A, Öst L-G. Follow-up of agoraphobia patients treated with exposure in vivo or applied relaxation. *Br J Psychiatry.* 1986;149:486-490.
10. Munby J, Johnson DW. Agoraphobia: the long-term follow-up of behavioral treatment. *Br J Psychiatry.* 1980;137:418-427.
11. Klein DF. Importance of psychiatric diagnosis in prediction of clinical drug effects. *Arch Gen Psychiatry.* 1967;16:118-126.
12. Mendel JGC, Klein DF. Anxiety attacks with subsequent agoraphobia. *Compr Psychiatry.* 1969;10:190-195.
13. Barlow DH, Craske MG, Cerny JA, Klosko JS. Behavioral treatment of panic disorder. *Behav Ther.* 1989;20:261-282.
14. Craske MG, Brown TA, Barlow DH. Behavioral treatment of panic: a two-year follow-up. *Behav Ther.* 1991;22:289-304.
15. Clark DM, Salkovskis PM, Hackmann A, Middleton H, Anastasiades P, Gelder M. A comparison of cognitive therapy, applied relaxation and imipramine in the treatment of panic disorder. *Br J Psychiatry.* 1994;164:759-769.
16. Klosko JS, Barlow DH, Tassinari R, Cerny JA. A comparison of alprazolam and behavior therapy in treatment of panic disorder. *J Consult Clin Psychol.* 1990;58:77-84.
17. Newman CF, Beck JS, Beck AT. Efficacy of cognitive therapy in reducing panic attacks and medication. Presented at the 24th Annual Meeting of the Association for Advancement of Behavior Therapy; November 1990; San Francisco, Calif.
18. Côté G, Gauthier J, Laberge B. The impact of medication use on the efficacy of cognitive-behavioral therapy for panic disorder. Presented at the 26th Annual Meeting of the Association for Advancement of Behavior Therapy; November 1992; Boston, Mass.
19. Beck AT, Sokol L, Clark DA, Berchick R, Wright F. A crossover study of focused cognitive therapy for panic disorder. *Am J Psychiatry.* 1992;149:778-783.
20. Black DW, Wesner R, Bowers W, Gabel J. A comparison of fluvoxamine, cognitive therapy, and placebo in the treatment of panic disorder. *Arch Gen Psychiatry.* 1993;50:44-50.
21. Margraf J, Schneider S. Outcome and active ingredients of cognitive-behavioral treatments for panic disorder. Presented at the 25th Annual Meeting of the Association for Advancement of Behavior Therapy; November 1991; New York, NY.
22. Öst L-G, Westling BE, Hellstrom, K. Applied relaxation, exposure in vivo and cognitive methods in the treatment of panic disorder with agoraphobia. *Behav Res Ther.* 1993;31:383.
23. Telch MJ, Lucas JA, Schmidt NB, Hanna HH, Jaimez LaNae T, Lucas RA. Group cognitive-behavioral treatment of panic disorder. *Behav Res Ther.* 1993; 31:279-287.
24. Craske MG, Maidenberg E, Bystritsky A. Brief cognitive-behavioral versus nondirective therapy for panic disorder. *J Behav Ther Exper Psychiatry.* 1995; 26:113-120.
25. Shear MK, Pilkonis PA, Cloitre M, Leon AC. Cognitive behavioral treatment compared with nonprescriptive treatment of panic disorder. *Arch Gen Psychiatry.* 1994;51:395-401.
26. Brown TA, Barlow DH. Long-term outcome in cognitive behavioral treatment of panic disorder. *J Consult Clin Psychol.* 1995;63:754-765.
27. Brown TA, Antony MM, Barlow DH. Diagnostic comorbidity in panic disorder. *J Consult Clin Psychol.* 1995;63:408-418.
28. Michelson L, Marchione K, Greenwald M. Cognitive-behavioral treatments of agoraphobia. Presented at the 23rd Annual Meeting of the Association for the Advancement of Behavior Therapy; November 1989; Washington, DC.
29. van den Hout M, Arntz A, Hoekstra R. Exposure reduced agoraphobia but not panic, and cognitive therapy reduced panic but not agoraphobia. *Behav Res Ther.* 1994;52:447-449.
30. Marks IM, Swinson RP, Basoglu M, Kuch K, Noshirvani H, O'Sullivan G, Lelliott PT, Kirby M, McNamee G, Sengun S, Wickwire K. Alprazolam and exposure alone and combined in panic disorder with agoraphobia: a controlled study in London and Toronto. *Br J Psychiatry.* 1993;162:776-787.
31. Mavissakalian M. Combined behavioral therapy and pharmacotherapy of agoraphobia. *J Psychiatr Res.* 1993;27:179-191.
32. Otto MW, Pollack MH, Sachs GS, Reiter SR, Meltzer-Brody S, Rosenbaum JF. Discontinuation of benzodiazepine treatment. *Am J Psychiatry.* 1993;150: 1485-1490.
33. Spiegel DA, Bruce IJ, Gregg SF, Nuzzarello A. Does cognitive behavior therapy assist slow-taper alprazolam discontinuation in panic disorder? *Am J Psychiatry.* 1994;151:876-881.
34. American Psychiatric Association. *Diagnostic and Statistical Manual of Mental Disorders, Third Edition, Revised.* Washington, DC: American Psychiatric Association; 1987.
35. American Psychiatric Association. *Diagnostic and Statistical Manual of Mental Disorders, Fourth Edition.* Washington, DC: American Psychiatric Press; 1994.
36. Barlow DH, Blanchard EB, Vermilyea JA, Vermilyea BB, Di Nardo PA. Generalized anxiety and generalized anxiety disorder: description and reconceptualization. *Am J Psychiatry.* 1986;143:40-44.
37. Brown TA, Barlow DH, Liebowitz MR. The empirical basis of generalized anxiety disorder. *Am J Psychiatry.* 1994;15:1272-1280.
38. Rapee RM, Barlow DH. *Chronic Anxiety: Generalized Anxiety Disorder and Mixed Anxiety-Depression.* New York, NY: Guilford Publications Inc; 1991.
39. Zinbarg RE, Barlow DH, Liebowitz M, Street L, Broadhead E, Katon W, Roy-Byrne P, Lepine JP, Teherani M, Richard J, Brantley PJ, Kraemer H. The *DSM-IV* field trial for mixed-anxiety depression. *Am J Psychiatry.* 1994;151:1153-1162.
40. Barlow DH, Rapee RM, Brown TA. Behavioral treatment of generalized anxiety disorder. *Behav Ther.* 1992;23:551-570.
41. Blowers C, Cobb J, Mathews A. Generalized anxiety: a controlled treatment study. *Behav Res Ther.* 1987;25:493-502.
42. Borkovec TD, Mathews AM. Treatment of nonphobic anxiety disorders. *J Consult Clin Psychol.* 1988;56:877-884.
43. Durham RC, Turvey AA. Cognitive therapy vs behaviour therapy in the treatment of chronic generalized anxiety. *Behav Res Ther.* 1987;25:229-234.
44. Lindsay, WR, Gamsu CV, McLaughlin E, Hood EM, Espie CA. A controlled trial of treatments for generalized anxiety. *Br J Clin Psychol.* 1987;26:3-15.
45. Borkovec TD, Costello E. Efficacy of applied relaxation and cognitive-behavioral therapy in the treatment of generalized anxiety disorder. *J Consult Clin Psychol.* 1993;61:611-619.
46. Butler G, Fennell M, Robson P, Gelder M. Comparison of behavior therapy and cognitive behavior therapy in the treatment of generalized anxiety disorder. *J Consult Clin Psychol.* 1991;59:167-175.
47. Durham RC, Murphy T, Allan T, Richard K, Treliving LR, Fenton GW. Cognitive therapy, analytic psychotherapy and anxiety management training for generalised anxiety disorder. *Br J Psychiatry.* 1994;165:315-323.
48. Power J, Simpson RJ, Swanson V, Wallace LA, Feistner ATC, Sharp D. A controlled study of cognitive-behaviour therapy, diazepam and placebo alone and in combination for the treatment of generalized anxiety. *J Anxiety Disord.* 1990;4:267-292.
49. Borkovec TD, Whisman MA. Psychosocial treatment for generalized anxiety disorder. In: Mavissakalian M, Prien R, eds. *Anxiety Disorders: Psychological and Pharmacological Treatments.* Washington, DC: American Psychiatric Press Inc; 1996:171-199.
50. Barlow DH, Cohen AS, Waddell M, Vermilyea JA, Klosko JS, Blanchard EB, DiNardo PA. Panic and generalized anxiety disorders: nature and treatment. *Behav Ther.* 1984;15:431-449.
51. Borkovec TD, Mathews AM, Chambers A, Ebrahimi S, Lytle R, Nelson R. The effects of relaxation training with cognitive therapy or nondirective therapy and the role of relaxation-induced anxiety in the treatment of generalized anxiety. *J Consult Clin Psychol.* 1987;55:883-888.
52. Butler G, Cullington A, Hibbert G, Klimes I, Gelder M. Anxiety management for persistent generalized anxiety. *Br J Psychiatry.* 1987;151:535-542.
53. Power KG, Jerrom DW, Simpson RJ, Mitchell MJ, Swanson V. A controlled comparison of cognitive behavior therapy, diazepam and placebo in the management of generalized anxiety. *Behav Psychother.* 1989;17:1-14.
54. White J, Keenan M, Brooks N. Stress control. *Behav Psychol.* 1992;201:97-114.
55. Borkovec TD, Abel JL, Newman H. Effects of psychotherapy on comorbid conditions in generalized anxiety disorder. *J Consult Clin Psychol.* 1995;63:479-483.

56. Brown TA, O'Leary TA, Barlow DH. Cognitive-behavioral treatment of generalized anxiety disorder. In: Barlow DH, ed. *Clinical Handbook of Psychological Disorders.* 2nd ed. New York, NY: Guilford Publication Inc; 1993:137-188.
57. The Clomipramine Collaborative Study Group. Clomipramine in the treatment of patients with obsessive-compulsive disorder. *Arch Gen Psychiatry.* 1991; 48:730-738.
58. Rachman S, Hodgson R. *Obsessions and Compulsions.* Englewood Cliffs, NJ: Prentice Hall; 1980.
59. Meyer V. Modification of expectations in cases with obsessional rituals. *Behav Res Ther.* 1966;4:273-280.
60. Riggs DS, Foa EB. Obsessive compulsive disorder. In: Barlow DH, ed. *Clinical Handbook of Psychological Disorders.* 2nd ed. New York, NY: Guilford Press; 1993:189-239.
61. Salkovskis PM, Westbrook D. Behaviour therapy and obsessional ruminations: can failure be turned into success? *Behav Res Ther.* 1989;27:149-160.
62. Foa EB, Kozak MJ. Psychological treatment for obsessive-compulsive disorder. In: Mavissakalian M, Prien R, eds. *Long-Term Treatments of Anxiety Disorders.* Washington, DC: American Psychiatric Press Inc; 1996:285-309.
63. Meyer V, Levy R, Schnurer A. A behavioral treatment of obsessive-compulsive disorders. In: Beech HR, ed. *Obsessional States.* London, England: Methuen; 1974.
64. Catts S, McConaghy N. Ritual prevention in the treatment of obsessive-compulsive neurosis. *Aust N Z J Psychiatry.* 1975;9:37-41.
65. Marks IM, Hodgson R, Rachman S. Treatment of chronic obsessive-compulsive neurosis by in vivo exposure. *Br J Psychiatry.* 1975;127:349-364.
66. Boulougouris JC. Variables affecting the behavior modification of obsessive-compulsive patients treated by flooding. In: Boulougouris JC, Rabavilas AD, eds. *The Treatment of Phobic and Obsessive-Compulsive Disorders.* Oxford, England: Pergamon Press; 1977:73-84.
67. Foa EB, Goldstein A. Continuous exposure and complete response prevention of obsessive-compulsive neurosis. *Behav Ther.* 1978;9:821-829.
68. Emmelkamp PMG, Rabbie DM. Psychological treatment of obsessive-compulsive disorder. *Biol Psychiatry.* 1981;1095-1098.
69. Mawson D, Marks IM, Ramm L. Clomipramine and exposure for chronic obsessive-compulsive rituals, III: two year follow-up and further findings. *Br J Psychiatry.* 1982;140:11-18.
70. O'Sullivan G, Noshirvani H, Marks I, Monteiro W, Lelliott P. Six-year follow-up after exposure and clomipramine therapy for obsessive-compulsive disorder. *J Clin Psychiatry.* 1991;52:150-155.
71. Bolton D, Collins S, Steinberg D. The treatment of obsessive-compulsive disorder in adolescence: a report of fifteen cases. *Br J Psychiatry.* 1983;142:456-464.
72. Foa EB, Grayson JB, Steketee GS, Doppelt HG, Turner RM, Latimer PR. Success and failure in the behavioral treatment of obsessive-compulsives. *J Consult Clin Psychol.* 1983;51:287-297.
73. Foa EB, Steketee G, Grayson JB, Turner RM, Latimer P. Deliberate exposure and blocking of obsessive-compulsive rituals: immediate and long-term effects. *Behav Ther.* 1984;15:450-472.
74. Hoogduin CAL, Hoogduin WA. The outpatient treatment of patients with an obsessional-compulsive disorder. *Behav Res Ther.* 1984;22:455-459.
75. Emmelkamp PMG, Hoekstra RJ, Visser S. The behavioral treatment of obsessive-compulsive disorder: prediction of outcome at 3.5 years follow-up. In: Pichot P, Brenner A, Wolf R, Thau K, eds. *Psychiatry: The State of the Art.* New York, NY: Plenum Press; 1985:4.
76. Kasvikas Y, Marks I. Clomipramine, self-exposure, and therapist-accompanied exposure in obsessive-compulsive ritualizers: two-year follow up. *J Anxiety Disord.* 1988;2:291-298.
77. Foa EB, Kozak MJ, Steketee GS, McCarty PR. Treatment of depressive and obsessive-compulsive symptoms in OCD by imipramine and behavior therapy. *Br J Psychiatry.* 1992;31:279-292.
78. Cottraux J, Mollard E, Bouvard M, Marks I, Sluys M, Nury AM, Douge R, Cialdella PH. A controlled study of fluvoxamine and exposure in obsessive-compulsive disorder. *Int Clin Psychopharmacol.* 1990;5:299-317.
79. Marks IM, Stern RS, Mawson D, Cobb J, McDonald R. Clomipramine and exposure for obsessive-compulsive rituals, I. *Br J Psychiatry.* 1980;136:1-25.
80. Marks IM, Lelliott P, Basoglu M, Noshirvami H, Monteiro W, Cohen D, Kasvikis Y. Clomipramine self-exposure, and therapist-aided exposure for obsessive-compulsive rituals. *Br J Psychiatry.* 1988;152:522-534.
81. Hiss H, Foa EB, Kozak MJ. Relapse prevention program for treatment of obsessive-compulsive disorder. *J Consult Clin Psychol.* 1994;4:801-808.
82. Marlatt GA, Gordon JR. *Relapse Prevention: Maintenance Strategies in Addictive Behavior Changes.* New York, NY: Guilford Publications Inc; 1985.
83. Foa EB, Liebowitz M. Recent findings on the efficacy of behavior therapy and clomipramine for obsessive-compulsive disorder. Presented at the Psychiatric Research Society Annual Meeting; February 1995; Park City, Utah.
84. Kessler RC, McGonagle KA, Zhao S, Nelson CB, Hughes M, Eshleman S, Wittchen HU, Kendler KS. Lifetime and 12-month prevalence of *DSM-III-R* psychiatric disorders in the United States. *Arch Gen Psychiatry.* 1994;51:8-19.
85. Liebowitz MR, Gorman JM, Fyer AJ, Klein DF. Social phobia: review of a neglected anxiety disorder. *Arch Gen Psychiatry.* 1985;42:729-736.
86. Butler G, Cullington, A, Munby M, Amies P, Gelder M. Exposure and anxiety management in the treatment of social phobia. *J Consult Clin Psychol.* 1984; 52:642-650.
87. Mattick RP, Peters L. Treatment of severe social phobia. *J Consult Clin Psychol.* 1988;56:251-260.
88. Mattick RP, Peters L, Clarke JC. Exposure and cognitive restructing for social phobia: a controlled study. *Behav Ther.* 1989;20:3-23.
89. Heimberg RG, Dodge CS, Hope DA, Kennedy CR, Zollo L, Becker RE. Cognitive-behavioral group treatment of social phobia: comparison to a credible placebo control. *Cognitive Ther Res.* 1990;14:1-23.
90. Heimberg RG, Salzman DG, Holt CS, Blendell KA. Cognitive-behavioral group treatment for social phobia. *Cognitive Ther Res.* 1993;4,325-339.
91. Hope DA, Heimberg RG, Bruch MA. The importance of cognitive intervention in behavioral group therapy for social phobia. Presented at the Tenth National Conference on Phobias and Related Anxiety Disorders; March 1990; Bethesda, Md.
92. Gelernter CS, Uhde TW, Cimbolic P, Arnkoff DB, Vittone BJ, Tancer ME, Bartko JJ. Cognitive-behavioral and pharmacological treatments of social phobia: a controlled study. *Arch Gen Psychiatry.* 1991;48:938-945.
93. Lucas RA, Telch MJ. Group vs individual treatment of social phobia. Presented at the 27th Annual Meeting of the Association for Advancement of Behavior Therapy; November 1993; Atlanta, Ga.
94. Heimberg RG, Juster HR, Brown EJ, Holle C, Makris GS, Leung AW, Schneier FR, Gitow A, Liebowitz MR. Cognitive-behavioral versus pharmacological treatment of social phobia: posttreatment and follow-up effects. Presented at the 28th Annual Meeting of the Association for Advancement of Behavior Therapy; November 1994; San Diego, Calif.
95. Öst L-G, Sterner U. Applied tension, a specific behavioral method for treatment of blood phobia. *Behav Res Ther.* 1987;25:25-29.
96. Öst L-G, Lindahl I-L, Sterner U, Jerremalm A. Exposure in vivo vs applied relaxation in the treatment of blood phobia. *Behav Res Ther.* 1984;22:205-216.
97. Öst L-G, Sterner U, Lindahl IL. Physiological responses in blood phobia. *Behav Res Ther.* 1984;22:109-117.
98. Öst L-G, Sterner U, Fellenius J. Applied tension, applied relaxation, and the combination in the treatment of blood phobia. *Behav Res Ther.* 1989;27:109-121.
99. Öst L-G, Salkovskis PM, Hellström K. One-session therapist-directed exposure vs self-exposure in the treatment of spider phobia. *Behav Ther.* 1991; 22:407-422.
100. Öst L-G, Hellström K, Kaver A. One vs five sessions of exposure in the treatment of injection phobia. *Behav Ther.* 1992;23:263-282.
101. Keane TM, Fairbank JA, Caddell JM, Zimering RT. Implosive (flooding) therapy reduces symptoms of PTSD in Vietnam combat veterans. *Behav Ther.* 1989; 20:245-260.
102. Cooper NA, Clum GA. Imaginal flooding as a supplementary treatment for PTSD in combat veterans: a controlled study. *Behav Ther.* 1989;20:381-391.
103. Boudewyns PA, Hyer L. Physiological response to combat memories and preliminary treatment outcome in Vietnam veteran PTSD patients treated with direct therapeutic exposure. *Behav Ther.* 1990;21:63-87.
104. Foa EB, Rothbaum EO, Riggs D, Murdock T. Treatment of PTSD in rape victims: a comparison between cognitive-behavioral procedures and counseling. *J Consult Clin Psychol.* 1991;59:715-723.
105. Foa, EB. Psychopathology and treatment of PTSD in rape victims. Presented at the annual convention of the American Psychological Society; July 1, 1994; Washington, DC.
106. Resick PA, Schnicke MK. Cognitive processing therapy for sexual assult victims. *J Consult Clin Psychol.* 1992;60:748-756.
107. Foa EB, Hearst-Ikeda D, Perry KJ. Evaluation of a brief cognitive-behavioral program for the prevention of chronic PTSD in recent assault victims. *J Consult Clin Psychol.* 1995;63:948-955.
108. Calhoun KS, Resick PA. Post-traumatic stress disorder. In: Barlow DH, ed. *Clinical Handbook of Psychological Disorders.* 2nd ed. New York, NY: Guilford Publications Inc; 1993:48-98.
109. Breier A, Charney DS, Heninger GR. Agoraphobia with panic attacks: development, diagnostic stability, and course of illness. *Arch Gen Psychiatry.* 1986; 43:1029-1036.
110. Goisman RM, Rogers MP, Steketee GS, Warshaw MG, Cuneo P, Keller MB. Utilization of behavioral methods in a multi-center anxiety disorders study. *J Clin Psychiatry.* 1993;54:213-218.
111. Taylor CB, King R, Margraf J, Ehlers A, Telch M, Roth WT, Agras WS. Use of medication and in vivo exposure in volunteers for panic disorder research. *Am J Psychiatry.* 1989;146:1423-1426.
112. Ghosh A, Marks IM. Self-treatment of agoraphobia by exposure. *Behav Ther.* 1987;18:3-16.
113. Côté G, Gauthier JG, Laberge B, Cormier HJ, Plamondon J. Reduced therapist contact in the cognitive behavioral treatment of panic disorder. *Behav Ther.* 1994;25:123-145.
114. Barlow DH, O'Brien GT, Last CG. Couples treatment of agoraphobia. *Behav Ther.* 1984;15:41-58.
115. Cerny JA, Barlow DH, Craske MG, Himadi WG. Couples treatment of agoraphobia: a two-year follow-up. *Behav Ther.* 1987;18:401-416.
116. Swinson RP, Soulios C, Cox BJ, Kuch K. Brief treatment of emergency room patients with panic attacks. *Am J Psychiatry.* 1992;149:944-946.
117. Keller MB, Hanks DL. Course and outcome in panic disorder. *Prog Neuropsychopharmacol Biol Psychiatry.* 1993;17:551-570.

Alcohol Treatment and Health Care System Reform

Barbara S. McCrady, PhD; James W. Langenbucher, PhD

After reviewing the empirical literature, we suggest that advances in the assessment and treatment of alcohol problems have the following important implications for health care system reform: (1) alcohol use disorders and problems associated with alcohol use are prevalent and are complicated by various comorbid conditions, and they result in large costs to the health care system and to society; (2) alcohol treatment generally results in reduced drinking and more efficient use of health care resources; (3) specific treatments have demonstrated effectiveness; (4) screening and assessment instruments with excellent sensitivity to the heterogeneity of alcohol problems have been developed; (5) evidence that specific treatments have differential effectiveness with different patient groups is accumulating; and (6) good evidence exists for the effectiveness of brief interventions, particularly with less severe and chronic alcohol problems. These findings suggest that alcohol treatment services in a reformed health care system should include (1) universal coverage for alcohol treatment, including full benefits for outpatient care; (2) a rational system of assessment and triage for treatment, including an increased emphasis on screening and brief interventions in primary medical care settings; (3) a full range of treatment services that vary in intensity; and (4) addictions treatment provider incentives and contingencies to provide treatments of proven effectiveness. When fully implemented, an efficient approach to the treatment of alcohol-related problems will result in one of the largest pools of cost savings in a reformed American health care system.

Arch Gen Psychiatry. 1996;53:737-746

Alcoholics consume more than 15% of the national health care budget,[1] seeking attention in medical settings for various secondary health problems.[2] Many illnesses (eg, 13% of breast cancers, 40% of traumatic injuries, 41% of seizures, and 72% of cases of pancreatitis) are due directly to alcohol abuse,[3] rendering alcoholics among the highest cost users of medical care in the country.[4]

Relatively little (ie, approximately 10%) of the total cost of alchoholism to society is spent directly for clinically relevant costs.[1] Proportionally, this is less than 25% of the direct care expenditures encountered elsewhere in mental health. In contrast, most costs associated with alcoholism are experienced indirectly by society. Approximately 34% of the costs are mortality costs (ie, the 100 000 lives annually reduced an average of 28 years by alcohol abuse), and 39% of the costs are morbidity costs (ie, the loss of functional capacity due to the secondary health and social effects of alcoholism). Overall, the impairment in health, the reduction in functional capacity, and the fruitless treatment of "surrogate diagnoses"[5] account for almost 75% of the total costs of alcohol abuse ($100 billion annually)[6] in the United States.

The high costs of alcohol-related problems to society and the lack of resources devoted to their treatment suggest the importance of examining the empirical literature on psychosocial treatments (which is reviewed here) and pharmacological treatments (which is reviewed in an article by Schuckit[7] in the companion issue of the *Journal of Consulting and Clinical Psychology*); examining these treatments will help us make informed recommendations about the role of alcohol-related treatment in a rational

From the Center of Alcohol Studies, Rutgers University, Piscataway, NJ.

health care system. Four research topics are important to health care system reform: the nature and complexity of alcohol-related problems, the identification and diagnosis of alcohol-related problems, the effectiveness of treatments, and the analysis of the socioeconomic effect of treatment. Clear conclusions about the role of alcohol treatment in the health care system emerge.

RESEARCH ON THE NATURE AND COMPLEXITY OF ALCOHOL-RELATED PROBLEMS

Diagnostic clarity is a necessary precondition for health care planning, but planning also must take into account the following factors: (1) mild alcohol-related problems that have important health and social consequences, (2) the complexity of alcohol problems, (3) the high rates of psychiatric comorbidity, and (4) the variable expression of these problems in persons with different sociodemographic profiles.

Epidemiology of Alcohol Use Disorders and Alcohol-Related Problems

Large population-based studies[8-10] have underscored the ubiquitous presence of alcohol-related problems. For example, the Epidemiological Catchment Area study[11] found a lifetime prevalence of alcohol abuse and dependence of 13.7%, the highest of any of the 44 major adult disorders sampled. The emergence of the data on alcohol abuse from the Epidemiological Catchment Area study gave public health workers grounds for serious concern.

Of more importance to health care system reform, however, is the disaggregation of such summary statistics into risk indicators, which can help focus screening and assessment resources, and into comorbid relationships, which can more wisely guide treatment and follow-up. For example, important differences in the epidemiology of alcohol-related problems are found on the basis of sex,[12] race or ethnicity and cultural background,[13] socioeconomic status,[12] age,[14] and place of origin.[11] In addition to risk indicators, work on the concentration of alcohol-related problems in illness groups, psychiatric populations, and even occupational categories can now be used to considerably sharpen the vigilance of health care workers. For example, the role of alcohol in the promotion of liver disease[15] and pancreatitis[16] is perhaps the firmest finding in the pathophysiology of psychiatric disorders. Various other organ-based and systemically based illness categories should also raise the diagnostician's suspicion; these categories include cardiovascular disease, gastrointestinal tract problems, neurologic disorders, and cancers of the gastrointestinal tract and the breast. Psychiatric comorbidities with alcoholism are also well established. Data from the Epidemiological Catchment Area study[11] reveal that almost 50% of all alcoholics have a second psychiatric diagnosis. Data from the Epidemiological Catchment Area study[17] also reveal marked concentrations of alcohol-related risk in a cross-section of American labor; the incidence of a diagnosis of an alcohol use disorder ranges from approximately 1 in 4 construction workers to less than 1 in 100 social workers, laboratory technicians, textile operators, and data entry personnel. The picture that emerges from this research is that alcohol-related problems are intricately bound up in a host of contextual factors.

Diagnosis

One difficulty in developing firm estimates of the prevalence of alcohol abuse and dependence is that, diagnostically, they are "moving targets," subject to different definitions and diagnostic practices during designated periods. In the first 2 editions of the *Diagnostic and Statistical Manual of Mental Disorders* (*DSM* and *DSM-II*),[18,19] alcohol problems were merely named, not described successfully. Reliable rules for diagnosing alcohol problems were not available until the 1970s. In *DSM-III*,[20] alcohol problems were diagnosed at 2 levels: alcohol abuse and alcohol dependence. These levels continue to form the basic structure of our diagnostic codes. In 1987, an updated manual, *DSM-III-R*,[21] incorporated much of the research literature of the late 1970s and the early 1980s; this manual included the concept of the alcohol dependence syndrome,[22] which is a constellation of symptoms that includes narrowing of the drinking repertoire, salience of drinking behavior, tolerance, withdrawal, drinking to relieve withdrawal symptoms, subjective awareness of compulsion to drink, and reinstatement of drinking after abstinence.

In *DSM-IV*,[23] alcohol-related diagnoses were further refined. Alcohol abuse is diagnosed by any of 4 symptoms: hazardous use, interference with role obligations, legal problems caused by drinking, or continued drinking despite social or interpersonal problems. These symptoms have been shown by factor analysis to load on factors not well correlated with dependence severity. Alcohol dependence is diagnosed when any 3 of 7 symptoms are met. The 7 symptoms include tolerance, withdrawal, drinking in larger amounts or over a longer period of time than intended, unsuccessful attempts or a desire to cut down or quit, a great deal of time spent drinking, activities given up or reduced to drink, and continued drinking despite knowledge of negative consequences; these symptoms are based on the alcohol dependence syndrome and are parallel to the diagnostic criteria of the *Draft International Classification of Diseases Related to Health Problems* [*Tenth Edition*] (*ICD-10*).[24] Physiological dependence (tolerance, withdrawal, or both) is emphasized in *DSM-IV* as connoting "a higher risk for immediate general medical problems and a higher relapse rate."[23(p179)] Although the reliability of the 2 categories, alcohol dependence and alcohol abuse, is firmly established, research in the decade ahead must prove the predictive as well as the descriptive value of the *DSM-IV*.[25-28]

Alcohol-Related Problems Below the Diagnostic Threshold

Epidemiological research suggests that a broader population of individuals experience occasional or isolated problems due to alcohol use, although such individuals would not meet the criteria of an alcohol use disorder. The alcohol-related problems perspective[29,30] draws attention to these short-term, milder, and more circumscribed problems. Problem drinkers tend to have shorter drinking histories and fewer physical and social consequences of their drinking, and they tend to have more personal and social resources.[30] A comprehensive system needs to provide services to this population as well as to the population meeting the full diagnostic criteria.

Heterogeneity of Alcohol Use Disorders and Alcohol-Related Problems

Alcohol-related problems are heterogeneous and vary in severity. Several studies have successfully identified homogeneous subtypes within the alcoholic population. Researchers (eg, Babor et al[31]) have noted 2 subtypes: the first is characterized by later onset and is more influenced by environmental factors, and the second is characterized by earlier onset and more antisocial behaviors.

Persons with alcohol-related problems differ in the comorbid psychopathology they experience. Estimates of lifetime drug use disorders comorbid with alcohol dependence are as high as 80%,[32,33] and up to 60% of men who are alcoholics have been reported to manifest anxiety disorders[33] or major depression secondary to alcohol abuse.[34] Estimates of affective disorders among women with alcohol-related problems have been reported at 35%,[33] and estimates of anxiety disorders among these women have been reported at 67%.[33] The reported rates of antisocial personality disorder comorbid with alcohol dependence range from 23%[35] to 53%.[33] Although the prevalence rates of comorbid disorders are high, a portion of these comorbid disorders is transient or substance induced and nonabiding, suggesting that treatment should be focused on the substance use disorder.

Researchers have also noted differences in the expression of alcohol-related problems in persons with different personal characteristics. Drinking patterns, adverse consequences of alcohol use, the social milieu of drinking, and expectancies and beliefs about alcohol all vary systematically by age,[14] race or ethnicity,[36] and sex.[37]

RESEARCH ON IDENTIFICATION AND DIAGNOSIS

Screening and Case Identification

Alcohol-related problems are commonly underdetected by health and mental health professionals.[38] Several methods of case identification and large population screening have been developed. They include the following: questionnaires assessing alcohol-related consequences (eg, the Michigan Alcoholism Screening Test[39]) or problems often associated with alcohol abuse such as trauma[40]; brief interviews (eg, the CAGE questionnaire[41] and the TWEAK test[42]); changes in blood chemistries often associated with heavy alcohol consumption (eg, carbohydrate-deficient transferrin[43] and the aspartate aminotransferase–alanine aminotransferase ratio[44]); and physical examination findings.[45]

The performance of screening measures varies depending on the base population, the screening instrument and the cutoff score employed, and the validation criterion. Despite methodological problems in conducting research on screening instruments, fairly consistent data (which were reviewed by Maisto and Connors[46]) on the CAGE, the Michigan Alcoholism Screening Test, and the TWEAK have emerged. Reported sensitivities range from 0.52 to 1.00, and specificities range from 0.61 to 1.00. These 3 instruments have large amounts of research support across diverse populations, settings, and validation criteria.

Severity of Dependence

The severity of alcoholism has been defined by symptom count, persistence or treatment intractability, complications, quantity or frequency of consumption or both, withdrawal severity, loss of control, and other measures. Many excellent instruments have been developed to reliably and validly assess the severity of alcohol dependence, including the Alcohol Dependence Scale,[47] the Severity of Alcohol Dependence Questionnaire,[48] and the alcohol problems subscale of the Addiction Severity Index.[49]

Diagnosis

Several interviews to diagnose alcohol abuse and alcohol dependence have been developed. The Structured Clinical Interview for *DSM-IV*[50] is a semistructured interview to be used by trained clinicians. Others, including the Psychiatric Research Interview for Substance and Mental Disorders,[51] and the Alcohol Use Disorders and Associated Disabilities Interview Schedule,[52] are still in development. These interviews emphasize a fully prescribed set, sequence, and wording of questions that render highly reliable formal *DSM-IV* or *ICD-10* diagnoses. Thus, although alcohol problems are commonly underdetected and underdiagnosed by health and mental health professionals, appropriate tools are available to facilitate detection and diagnosis. The use of appropriate tools to determine the severity of dependence and to establish formal diagnosis should enhance selection of appropriate treatments and treatment settings.

RESEARCH ON THE EFFECTIVENESS OF TREATMENT

Research on treatments for alcohol problems has progressed from focusing on global effectiveness to testing specific treatment settings and modalities, determining the cost-effectiveness of treatment, and matching treatments to specific patient characteristics.

Treatment Effectiveness

In 1975, Emrick[53] published a review of 384 studies of the relative effectiveness of alcohol treatments. His conclusions were as follows: (1) As a category, treatment was more effective than no treatment; however, treatment primarily reduced alcohol consumption rather than enhanced the rates of total abstinence. (2) No one treatment emerged as more effective than other treatments; however, attempting to evaluate the overall effectiveness of treatment obscures the heterogeneity of treatments and treatment populations. Thus, more contemporary research has examined the effectiveness of specific treatments for specific patient populations.

Specific Treatments

A substantial amount of research supports the effectiveness of specific psychosocial treatment modalities. Illustrative studies and results for each empirically validated treatment modality described below are given in the **Table**.

1. Miller et al[56] reviewed 211 controlled studies that contrasted different treatments. Each study was rated for methodological quality, and outcomes were rated on a 4-point scale (from +2 to −2, with no rating of 0). A positive treatment effect (a rating of +1 or +2) on "at least one alcohol measure for at least one follow-up point"[56(p17)] was noted in 146 (69%) of the 211 studies. Although comparison treatments and follow-up windows varied across studies, the overall finding was that specific treatments can affect drinking, supporting the conclusion drawn by Emrick.[53]

2. Historically, alcohol treatment was provided during an inpatient hospitalization or extended outpatient treatment, but these treatments may be unnecessary for persons with less severe alcohol-related problems. Brief interventions, varying in length from a few minutes to 1 to 3 sessions of assessment and treatment have been proposed as alternatives. Brief interventions use motivational techniques, brief skills training, and advice, and their goals include increased problem recognition and motivation to change, reduced alcohol consumption, and increased treatment seeking. A substantial amount of research supports their effectiveness in producing modest reductions in alcohol consumption, particularly with persons with less severe, chronic, or pervasive alcohol-related problems.[56-58]

3. Positive evidence exists for the effectiveness of treatments derived from classical conditioning models, including aversion therapies[59] that induce nausea aversion, imaginal techniques (covert sensitization[60]), and cue exposure treatment, which is purported to extinguish conditioned responses to preconsumption cues through repeated exposure.[61,62]

4. Specific, focused treatments derived from operant conditioning principles have good support for their effectiveness, particularly the use of behavioral contracting[63] and the community reinforcement approach.[64] Behavioral contracting is used to establish a contingent relationship between a specific client behavior, such as aftercare attendance, and a desired reinforcer. The community reinforcement approach increases clients' access to desired persons, situations, and resources, and makes access contingent on abstinence from alcohol while incorporating additional behavioral treatments derived from a broader social learning framework.

5. Other treatments derived from broader social learning principles, called "broad spectrum behavior therapy," include behavioral self-monitoring, functional analysis of the relationships between environmental antecedent and consequent events and drinking, behavioral self-control training, relaxation training, social skills training, cognitive therapy, systematic desensitization, and training in problem solving. Research evidence strongly supports the effectiveness of some elements of broad spectrum behavior therapy, including social skills training,[65] cognitive therapy,[66] and relapse prevention treatment,[67] while support for other elements is lacking. Patient-treatment matching studies support the particular effectiveness of behavioral approaches with patients who have antisocial personality characteristics.[68] Although no support exists for the effectiveness of self-monitoring, functional analysis, relaxation training, or problem solving as isolated treatments, elements of each are incorporated into social skills training and relapse prevention treatment programs. Research support for behavioral self-control training, which usually includes 6 to 8 sessions of training in self-monitoring drinking and drinking urges, goal setting for rate reduction, and skills to reduce alcohol consumption, is mixed.[56]

6. Substantial support[56] exists for the effectiveness of behavioral marital therapy in the treatment of alcohol problems. Behavioral marital therapy includes the development of behavioral contracts with the marital partner,[69] reciprocity enhancement, and couples communication and problem-solving training.[70,71] Research also supports the importance of family and other social system involvement in initiating treatment[72] and decreasing treatment attrition. Recent studies suggest that the quality of the social support system, the degree of investment that the problem drinker has in the social support system, and the presence of antisocial personality disorder mediate the positive effect of family involvement.[73,74]

7. A meta-analysis of single group evaluation studies[75] concluded that adding attendance at Alcoholics Anonymous (AA) meetings to professional treatment or counseling increases the probability of a positive drinking outcome, participation in AA activities is modestly associated with a better drinking outcome, and a positive relationship exists between AA attendance and improved psychological functioning. However, no randomized clinical trial has found AA to be more effective than a comparison treatment,[76] and 2 trials have reported a better response to comparison treatments than to AA.[77,78]

8. Viewing alcohol-related problems and available treatments as heterogeneous suggests the importance of properly matching clients to treatments. A comprehensive review of patient-treatment matching research[79] found sex, severity of alcohol dependence, family history of drinking problems, antisocial personality characteristics, severity of comorbid psychiatric problems, and social supports to be linked to differential outcomes of different treatments.

9. Research on the selection of nonabstinent drinking goals has generated substantial controversy.[80] In the disease concept of alcoholism, the only appropriate goal of treatment is lifelong abstinence.[81] However, epidemiological and longitudinal data suggest that the course of alcohol problems is variable, and remission or moderate drinking is as likely to occur as progression.[82,83] Long-term follow-ups of clinical samples[83] suggest that moderate drinking is as likely an outcome as total abstinence. Moderate drinking goals help motivate clients to engage in treatment and are most likely to be met when the drinker has few symptoms of alcohol dependence,

believes in controlled drinking as a desirable and possible outcome, is younger, has substantial psychological and social stability, and is a woman.[84]

Treatment Settings

In the 1970s and early 1980s, residential rehabilitation programs proliferated in the United States. Commonly modeled after the treatment program developed at the Hazelden Foundation, Center City, Minn (and hence called "Minnesota Model" programs), most residential rehabilitation programs viewed alcoholism as a chronic, progressive disease and postulated that effective treatment required intensive therapy, removed from the individual's natural environment, to break down denial, enhance commitment to abstinence, and facilitate lifelong involvement with AA.

As residential rehabilitation programs proliferated, questions about the necessity of a set length of treatment and the use of the inpatient setting for rehabilitation were raised because of the results of controlled research. When randomized clinical trials comparing inpatient with day hospital treatment were conducted, no incremental benefit for more intensive treatment for detoxification[85] or rehabilitation was found,[86-88] and substantial cost savings occurred using the day hospital setting.[89] Much of the research comparing treatment settings is limited, however, by the exclusion of persons with comorbid psychopathology, in particular those who abuse other psychoactive substances. Studies comparing rehabilitation in different settings have been limited to socially stable, middle-class populations. Thus, although the data clearly do not support the necessity of residential settings for the detoxification or treatment of persons with uncomplicated alcohol dependence or alcohol abuse, research on the role of these settings for persons with complex problems, including other psychopathology, substance abuse, and social instability, is lacking.

SOCIOECONOMIC ANALYSES OF COST SAVINGS FROM ALCOHOL TREATMENT

The socioeconomic benefits of alcoholism treatment can be found in 3 places.[90] First, savings result when alcoholics return to normal functioning; these savings include increases in employability,[91] improvements in worker behavior,[92,93] and decreases in dependence on institutional assistance.[92,94] Second, savings result from lowered health care costs; research on alcoholics who have received treatment shows that their use of health care after treatment declines dramatically, immediately, and over time converges to almost the level of the normal population.[5,95-99] Third, savings result from the reduced health care costs of family members of treated alcoholics (ie, so-called collateral treatment effects).[100-103] Altogether, reductions in medical care use, encouragement of more appropriate use when services are needed, and reduced overall health care costs by both the treated alcoholics and their family members represent one of the largest sources of potential cost savings in a reformed American health care system.

Global socioeconomic analyses suggest that the provision of any form of alcohol treatment will result in net savings to the health care system and to society. The magnitude of cost savings can be enhanced by the provision of care in less costly treatment settings, such as ambulatory or outpatient detoxification[85] of patients without serious withdrawal histories, the use of partial hospital environments,[86,89] and the provision of lower levels of care generally.

The effectiveness and estimated costs of 33 tested clinical treatments for alcohol-related problems were examined in a comprehensive review.[104] Holder et al[104] found, in general, a negative relationship between the cost of a treatment and the evidence of its effectiveness. Typically in alcoholism treatment, lower cost treatments are at least as effective as higher cost options, at least with patients who are able to manage at these lower care levels.

IMPLICATIONS FOR HEALTH CARE PLANNING

Our review of the research literature on populations with alcohol problems, psychometrically sound assessment devices, effective treatments, and cost analyses has many direct implications for a rational health care system for persons with alcohol-related problems.

Defining the Population

The specialty alcohol health care system should address the needs of a complex and heterogeneous population. The system should be designed to identify and provide assistance to persons whose drinking places them at risk for problems as well as to those with more severe drinking problems; the system must also provide appropriate services for those with complicated medical or psychiatric problems.

Maximizing Access to Services

Barriers to services should be minimized. The current system maximizes barriers to treatment in some ways by providing most treatment within a specialty health care system, by making individuals "admit" to their alcoholism, by touting the superiority of one treatment model and one treatment setting, and by requiring large copayments for outpatient treatment. To maximize access, the following procedures should be implemented: (1) train all primary health care professionals so that they can identify milder alcohol-related problems, as well as diagnosable disorders; (2) train all primary health care professionals so that they can provide brief interventions, and provide appropriate reimbursement for them; (3) develop a range of treatment settings and treatment models; (4) undertake widespread community education that emphasizes the heterogeneity of alcohol-related problems, treatment models, and settings; and (5) provide universal health care coverage for alcohol treatment and full coverage for outpatient treatment.

Flexibility in the Mix of Services Available

Data support the effectiveness of ambulatory treatment for uncomplicated alcohol-related problems. However, alcohol dependence complicated by psychiatric disorders, other

Illustrative Outcomes of Studies of Treatments With Strong Support for Effectiveness*

Type of Treatment	Source, y	No. of Patients	Sex	Description of Treatment	Measure of Alcohol Consumption
Brief and motivational treatments					
Brief interventions	Babor and Grant,[54] 1992	223†	124 M, 99 F	Control (C), 5 min of advice (A), 15 min of brief counseling (B), extended counseling (E) (B+3 FU visits)	Mean drinks per day (MDPD), mean drinks per drinking day (MDPDD)
Motivational enhancement	Miller et al,[55] 1993	42	24 M, 18 F	Motivational enhancement (ME), wait list (WL)	Mean drinks per week (MDPW), peak BAC
Classical conditioning–based treatments					
Covert sensitization	Ashem and Donner,[60] 1968	23	M‡	Covert sensitization (CS), C	Continuous abstinence
Cue exposure treatment	Drummond and Glautier,[61] 1994	36	M	Cue exposure (CE), relaxation (R)	Days to use at different drinking levels. Total drinking score reflects total alcohol consumed
Nausea aversion	Cannon et al,[59] 1981	20	M‡	Nausea aversion (NA), shock aversion (SHA), C	Days abstinent
Conjoint treatments					
Behavioral contracting	Ahles et al,[69] 1983	50	M§	Standard aftercare (SA), aftercare plus contract with significant other; rewards contingent on attendance for first 6 mo of aftercare (SA+)	Total abstinence, days "functioning" (≤2 oz alcohol/d)
Behavioral marital therapy	McCrady et al,[70] 1991	45	33 M, 12 F	Minimal spousal involvement (MSI), alcohol-focused spousal involvement (AFSI), behavioral marital therapy (BMT)	Days abstinent
Operant-based treatments					
Behavioral contracting	Miller,[63] 1975	20	M‖	Usual skid row services (SRS), skid row services available contingent on sobriety (CSRS)	Arrests, employment
Community reinforcement	Azrin et al,[64] 1982	43	36 M, 7 F	Traditional counseling (TC), contract for taking disulfiram (DA), disulfiram contract plus behavior therapy (DA+BT)	Drinking days in past month, MDPDD
Social learning–based treatments					
Cognitive therapy	Oei and Jackson,[66] 1982	32	24 M, 8 F¶	TC, social skills training (SST), cognitive restructuring (CR), SST+CR	Mean ounces of alcohol consumed per week
Relapse prevention	Chaney et al,[67] 1978	40	M§	Relapse prevention coping with high-risk situations (RP), discussion control (DC), no additional treatment control (NTC)	Percentage of abstinent days, percentage of heavy drinking days (10 drinks or more in a day or 7-9 drinks/d for 2 or more days in a row), average length of drinking episode
Social skills training	Monti et al,[65] 1990	69	M§	Communication skills training (CST), CST with family (CSTF), cognitive behavioral mood management training (CBMMT)	Percentage of abstinent days, MDPDD

**FU indicates follow-up; BL, baseline; BAC, breath-alcohol concentration; ANCOVA, analysis of covariance; and r, sample correlation coefficient. Note that the term "significant" was used only when the results differed at the $P<.05$ or better level of significance.*

†United States only.

‡Inpatients.

§Inpatient veterans.

‖Chronic alcohol offenders.

¶All patients (male and female) were inpatients and low in assertiveness.

Times of Measurement	Results

BL, 6-mo FU

Significant time by treatment interactions for males only:

	MDPD		MDPDD	
	BL	6-mo FU	BL	6-mo FU
C	6.4	5.5	9.9	9.9
A	7.4	4.9	11.3	7.8
B	9.6	5.5	13.3	6.6
E	7.5	4.8	11.8	7.9

BL, 6-wk FU, 12-mo FU

Persons who received ME drank significantly less after treatment than persons who were on the WL: 3.7 d/wk vs 5.8 d/wk of drinking.

6-mo FU

Significant difference in probability of continuous abstinence: CS, 40%; C, 0%.

6-mo FU

Persons who underwent CE took significantly more days to their first heavy use (>20 U of alcohol) and had a significantly lower total drinking score than persons who underwent R:

	Days to Heavy Use	Total Drinking Score
CE	110	340
R	64	550

12-mo FU

NA equivalent to C and better than SHA on percentage of abstinent days, using ANCOVA with baseline percentage of abstinent days as a covariate: NA, 309 days; C, 305 days; SHA, 188 days.

6-mo FU, 12-mo FU

Six-month outcomes (contracts still in effect). Significantly higher percentage abstinent and significantly more days functioning for those in the SA+ group vs the SA group.

	Abstinent, %	Functioning, d
SA+	78	162
SA	15	123

Twelve-month abstinent outcomes (contracts no longer in effect). Nonsignificant trend toward more abstinent subjects in SA+ vs SA group: SA+, 40%; SA, 12%.

18-mo FU

Significant difference in linear trends in percentage of days abstinent during the 18 mo: MSI, $r = -0.77$; AFSI, $r = -0.32$; ABMT, $r = 0.78$.

2-mo BL, 2-mo FU

CSRS significantly decreased arrests vs SRS; CSRS significantly increased hours worked per week vs SRS:

	No. of Arrests		Employment, h/wk	
	2-mo BL	2-mo FU	2-mo BL	2-mo FU
CSRS	1.7	0.3	3.2	12.0
SRS	1.4	1.3	4.4	3.2

6-mo FU

DA and DA+BT equivalent, both significantly better than TC on drinking days per month and on MDPDD:

	Drinking Days	MDPDD
DA	7.9	1.7
DA+BT	0.9	0.7
TC	16.9	4.1

3, 6, and 12 mo after discharge

CR and SST+CR are equivalent; both are significantly better than TC and SST at the 12-mo FU on mean ounces of alcohol consumed per week: CR, 9 oz; SST+CR, 4 oz; SST, 16 oz; TC, 33 oz.

12-mo FU

No differences were found between control groups, so the 2 groups were pooled for comparisons: The RP group had fewer drunk days, fewer total drinks, and shorter drinking episodes than the combined control (DC+NTC) group:

	Drunk Days	Total Drinks
RP	11.1	399.8
DC+NTC	64	1593

6-mo FU

CST and CSTF equivalent on MDPDD and significantly less than CBMMT:

	MDPDD	
	BL	6-mo FU
CST	17.39	9.61
CSTF	15.89	7.35
CBMMT	19.48	18.40

substance abuse, severe medical problems, or social deterioration may not be well treated in ambulatory care settings, and more intensive levels of care should also be available. Thus, the specialty care, alcohol health care system should continue to have a range of treatment settings available. Concomitantly, a range of treatment models should be available, particularly those with clear research evidence supporting their effectiveness.

Management of Alcohol-Related Problems in Primary Health Care Settings

Primary health care settings and health care providers (ie, physicians, psychologists, social workers, and nurses) should use screening measures of known sensitivity and specificity to identify persons with alcohol-related problems. Health care providers also should be sensitized to high-risk drinking patterns, and screening devices to identify high-risk patterns need to be developed. Health care settings should provide referral information and brief interventions to motivate patients to change or seek further assistance. Health insurance should cover the costs of screening, brief intervention, and referral in primary health care settings.

Despite the substantial enthusiasm in the alcohol research community for an enhanced role of primary health care providers in identification, brief intervention, and triage, data consistently demonstrate the lack of broad compliance with screening[105] or brief interventions[106] in primary care settings. Barriers to the broad implementation of alcohol screening and brief interventions include the time pressures physicians face in providing care, the increased intrusions of managed-care companies into the physician's practice, and discomfort about raising alcohol-related topics, as well as attitudinal barriers including pessimism about the effectiveness of alcohol treatment and negative judgments about the causes of alcohol-related problems.[105]

Management of Alcohol-Related Problems in the Specialty Alcohol and Mental Health Treatment Network

Assessment and Triage. The development of a system to separate assessment and triage from treatment programs is crucial to the development of an effective alcohol treatment system. Assessment and triage centers should have staff with specific expertise in assessment, detailed knowledge of the treatment effectiveness literature, and knowledge of treatment resources. Assessment should evaluate patients' patterns of alcohol consumption and the consequences of consumption, the severity of dependence, the diagnosis, the concomitant psychiatric, medical, and other substance use disorders, social functioning, the motivation to change, and patients' personal attitudes and beliefs about their drinking. Assessment and triage personnel should recommend an appropriate treatment setting and model, as well as other needed psychological or social services.

Provision of Treatments of Established Effectiveness. The use of unsubstantiated treatments is not unique to the alcohol field,[107] but the gap between science and practice is nonetheless disturbing. Health insurers should support treatment centers and individuals providing treatments with demonstrated effectiveness and those evaluating new treatments and withhold benefits from centers and individuals providing unsubstantiated treatments when alternative treatments of known effectiveness are available. An improved health care system would require that programs incorporate evaluation into their ongoing treatments. Requiring evaluation as a prerequisite for program accreditation or reimbursement could enhance the quality of services provided.

Developing Long-term, Low-Intensity, and Intermittent Treatment. In the treatment of most narcotic addictions, clinical effectiveness is rarely associated with the intrusiveness of treatment. Rather, clinical gains are typically associated with time in treatment,[108] and clinical effectiveness improves linearly after a minimum amount of treatment is provided. Addictive symptoms may recur when treatment is discontinued, but they can be expected to decline gradually over the course of multiple treatment episodes. Because of these suggestive findings, explicitly planning to provide treatment that is low in intensity but that is long-term and may be used intermittently for supportive purposes as a person's drinking gradually diminishes with age would be an important addition to treatment services.

Exploiting Other Natural 'Capture' Sites

Untreated alcoholics occupy 10% to 50% of hospital and emergency room beds; most of them are receiving treatment for the secondary health effects of use. The medical center is a natural capture site for alcohol-related problems. Other sites also offer a population in which the base rate of alcohol-related problems is high. These sites include courthouses, vocational rehabilitation programs, and some industrial settings. Offering effective case identification and referral services in these settings may be a wise long-term decision.

CONCLUSIONS

This review has emphasized the scientific literature, and little attention has been given to the passions and controversies that often dominate the alcohol field. Scientific data, however, have not always shaped public policy, and a marked discrepancy exists between treatments provided most frequently and those with the strongest evidence for effectiveness and cost-effectiveness.[104,109] We recognize that most of the recommendations presented are controversial and will be viewed with equal amounts of enthusiasm and criticism. Despite the controversy inherent in the alcohol field, we believe it is essential that health care planning that deals with alcohol problems should be based on the same standards of evidence applied to other medical and psychological problems.

Health care system reform, whether effected at the national level or at the state and local levels, requires the health professions to respond intelligently to a shrinking pool of resources. Socioeconomic research suggests that resources can be conserved by addressing alcohol-related problems in the health care setting more promptly, intelligently, and reliably. We can begin immediately to reduce health care costs as research on alcoholism treatment is translated into changes in practice behavior. A substantial amount of literature shows the gulf between recommended and actual general medical practice in the treatment of alcohol-related problems, and many physicians and nurses believe that they are neither responsible nor competent to intervene. Health care system reform may be the final stimulus to the remedy of a problem that has, for various reasons, been too long delayed.

Accepted for publication April 22, 1996.

This study was supported in part by grants P50 AA08747 from the National Institute on Alcohol Abuse and Alcoholism (Dr McCrady) and RO1 DA05688 from the National Institute on Drug Abuse, Rockville, Md (Dr Langenbucher).

We thank Dennis Gorman, PhD, for his thoughtful review and feedback on this manuscript.

Reprints: Barbara S. McCrady, PhD, Center of Alcohol Studies, Rutgers University, PO Box 969, Piscataway, NJ 08855-0969.

REFERENCES

1. Rice DP, Kelman S, Miller LS, Dunmeyer S. *The Economic Costs of Alcohol and Drug Abuse and Mental Illness: 1985.* Washington, DC: US Government Printing Office; 1986.
2. Schurman RA, Kramer PD, Mitchell JB. The hidden mental health network: treatment of mental illness by nonpsychiatric physicians. *Arch Gen Psychiatry.* 1985;42:89-94.
3. Merrill J, Fox K, Chang H-H. *The Cost of Substance Abuse to America's Health Care System, Report 1: Medicaid Hospital Costs.* New York, NY: Center on Addiction and Substance Abuse at Columbia University; 1993.
4. Zook CJ, Moore FD. High-cost users of medical care. *N Engl J Med.* 1980; 302:996-1002.
5. Holder HD. Alcoholism treatment and potential health care cost savings. *Med Care.* 1987;25:52-71.
6. Rice D. Unpublished data. In: Horgan C, Marsden ME, Larson MJ, Elliott EA, eds. *Substance Abuse: The Nation's Number One Health Problem. Key Indicators for Policy.* Princeton, NJ: Robert Wood Johnson Foundation; 1994:39.
7. Schuckit MA. Recent developments in the pharmacotherapy of alcohol dependence. *J Consult Clin Psychol.* 1996;64:669-676.
8. Regier DA, Myers JK, Kramer M, Robins LN, Blazer DG, Hough RL, Eaton WW, Locke BZ. The NIMH Epidemiologic Catchment Area program: historical context, major objectives, and study population characteristics. *Arch Gen Psychiatry.* 1984;38:381-389.
9. Knupfer G. The prevalence in various social groups of eight different drinking patterns, from abstaining to frequent drunkenness: analysis of 10 US surveys combined. *Br J Addict.* 1989;84:1305-1318.
10. Fillmore KM, Hartka E, Johnstone BM, Leino EV, Motoyoshi M, Temple M. Preliminary results for a meta-analysis of drinking behavior in multiple longitudinal samples. *Br J Addict.* 1991;86:1203-1210.
11. Helzer JE, Pryzbeck TR. The co-occurrence of alcoholism with other psychiatric disorders in the general population and its impact on treatment. *J Stud Alcohol.* 1988;49:219-224.
12. Helzer JE, Burnam A. Alcohol abuse and dependence. In: Robins LN, Regier DA, eds. *Psychiatric Disorders in America.* New York, NY: Free Press; 1991.
13. Herd DA. A review of drinking patterns and alcohol problems among US blacks. In: Spiegler ED, Tate DA, Aitken A, Christian C, eds. *Alcohol Use Among US Ethnic Minorities.* Rockville, Md: National Institute on Alcohol Abuse and Alcoholism; 1989:3-50. Dept of Health and Human Services publication ADM 89-1435. Research monograph No. 18.
14. Fillmore KM. Prevalence, incidence and chronicity of drinking patterns and problems among man as a function of age: a longitudinal cohort analysis. *Br J Addict.* 1987;82:77-83.
15. Lieber CS, Jones DP, DeCarli LM. Effects of prolonged ethanol intake: production of fatty liver despite adequate diets. *J Clin Invest.* 1966;44:1009-1021.
16. Sarles H. Chronic calcifying pancreatitis: chronic alcohol pancreatitis. *Gastroenterology.* 1974;66:604-616.
17. Mandell W, Eaton WW, Anthony JC, Garrison R. Alcoholism and occupation: a review and analysis of 104 occupations. *Alcohol Clin Exp Res.* 1992;16: 734-746.
18. American Psychiatric Association. *Diagnostic and Statistical Manual of Mental Disorders.* Washington, DC: American Psychiatric Association; 1952.
19. American Psychiatric Association. *Diagnostic and Statistical Manual of Mental Disorders, Second Edition.* Washington, DC: American Psychiatric Association; 1968.
20. American Psychiatric Association. *Diagnostic and Statistical Manual of Mental Disorders, Third Edition.* Washington, DC: American Psychiatric Association; 1980.
21. American Psychiatric Association. *Diagnostic and Statistical Manual of Mental Disorders, Third Edition, Revised.* Washington, DC: American Psychiatric Association; 1987.
22. Edwards G, Gross MM. Alcohol dependence: provisional description of a clinical syndrome. *Br Med J.* 1976;1:1058-1061.
23. American Psychiatric Assoiation. *Diagnostic and Statistical Manual of Mental Disorders, Fourth Edition.* Washington, DC: American Psychiatric Association; 1994.
24. World Health Organization. *Draft International Classification of Diseases and Related Health Problems.* 10th ed. Geneva, Switzerland: World Health Organization; 1992.
25. Blashfield RK, Livesley WJ. Metaphorical analysis of psychiatric classification as a psychological test. *J Abnorm Psychol.* 1991;100:262-270.
26. Klerman GL. Historical perspectives on contemporary schools of psychopathology. In: Millon T, Klerman GL, eds. *Contemporary Directions in Psychopathology: Toward the DSM-IV.* New York, NY: Guilford Press; 1986:5-28.
27. Robins LN, Barrett JE. *The Validity of Psychiatric Diagnosis.* New York, NY: Raven Press; 1989.
28. Spitzer RL, Williams JBW. Having a dream: a research strategy for *DSM-IV. Arch Gen Psychiatry.* 1988;45:871-874.
29. Institute of Medicine. *Broadening the Base of Treatment for Alcohol Problems.* Washington, DC: National Academy of Sciences; 1990.
30. Sobell MB, Sobell LC. *Problem Drinkers: Guided Self-Change Treatment.* New York, NY: Guilford Press; 1993.
31. Babor TF, Hofmann M, DelBoca FK, Hesselbrock V, Meyer RE, Dolinsky ZS, Rounsaville B. Types of alcoholics, I: evidence for an empirically derived typology based on indicators of vulnerability and severity. *Arch Gen Psychiatry.* 1992;49:599-608.
32. Carroll JFX. Treating multiple substance abuse clients. *Recent Dev Alcohol.* 1986;4:85-103.
33. Ross HE, Glaser FB, Germanson T. The prevalence of psychiatric disorders in patients with alcohol and other drug problems. *Arch Gen Psychiatry.* 1988; 45:1023-1031.
34. Hasin DS, Grant BF, Endicott J. Lifetime psychiatric comorbidity in hospitalized alcoholics: subject and family correlates. *Int J Addict.* 1988;23:827-850.
35. Morgenstern J, Langenbucher J. Comorbidity: recent findings and their implications for understanding and treating addictive disorders. Presented at the Annual Meeting of the American Psychological Association; August 13, 1994; Los Angeles, Calif.
36. Neff JA. Race, ethnicity, and drinking patterns: the role of demographic factors, drinking motives, and expectancies. In: Pittman DJ, White HR, eds. *Society, Culture, and Drinking Patterns Reexamined.* New Brunswick, NJ: Rutgers Center of Alcohol Studies; 1991:339-356.
37. Gomberg ESL, Nirenberg TD. *Women and Substance Abuse.* Norwood, NJ: Ablex Publishing; 1993.
38. Moore RD, Bone LR, Geller G, Mamon JA, Stokes EJ, Levine D. Prevalence, detection, and treatment of alcoholism in hospitalized patients. *JAMA.* 1980; 261:403-407.
39. Selzer ML. The Michigan Alcoholism Screening Test: the quest for a new diagnostic instrument. *Am J Psychol.* 1971;127:1653-1658.
40. Skinner HA, Holt S, Roy J, Isreal Y. Identification of alcohol abuse using laboratory tests and a history of trauma. *Ann Intern Med.* 1984;101:847-851.
41. Mayfield D, McLeod G, Hall P. The CAGE questionnaire: validation of a new alcoholism screening instrument. *Am J Psychiatry.* 1974;131:1121-1123.
42. Chan AWK, Pristach EA, Welte JW, Russell M. Use of the TWEAK test in screening for alcoholism/heavy drinking in three populations. *Alcohol Clin Exp Res.* 1993;17:1188-1192.
43. Allen JP, Litten RZ, Anton RF, Cross GM. Carbohydrate-deficient transferrin as a measure of immoderate drinking: remaining issues. *Alcohol Clin Exp Res.* 1994;18:799-814.
44. Irwin M, Baird S, Smith TL, Schuckit M. Use of laboratory tests to monitor heavy drinking by alcoholic men discharged from a treatment program. *Am J Psychiatry.* 1988;154:595-599.
45. Babor TF, Kranzler HR, Lauerman RJ. Early detection of harmful alcohol consumption: comparison of clinical, laboratory, and self-report screening procedures. *Addict Behav.* 1989;14:139-157.
46. Maisto SA, Connors GJ. Contrasting self-report screens for alcohol problems: a review. *Alcohol Clin Exp Res.* 1995;19:1510-1516.
47. Skinner HA, Allen BA. Alcohol dependence syndrome: measurement and validation. *J Abnorm Psychol.* 1982;91:199-209.
48. Stockwell T, Murphy D, Hodgson R. The Severity of Alcohol Dependence Questionnaire: its use, reliability and validity. *Br J Addict.* 1983;78:145-155.
49. McLellan AT, Kushner H, Metzger D, Peters R, Smith I, Grissom G, Pettinati H, Argeriou M. The fifth edition of the Addiction Severity Index. *J Subst Abuse Treat.* 1992;9:199-213.
50. First MB, Gibbon, M, Spitzer RL, Williams JBW. *User's Guide for the Struc-*

tured Clinical Interview for DSM-IV Axis I Disorders (SCID-I, Version 2.0, October 1995 DRAFT Version). New York, NY: Biometrics Research Department, New York State Psychiatric Institute; 1995.
51. Hasin D, Miele G. *Psychiatric Research Interview for Substance and Mental Disorders.* New York, NY: New York State Psychiatric Institute; 1994.
52. Grant BF, Hasin D. *The Alcohol Use Disorders and Associated Disabilities Interview Schedule (AUDADIS).* Rockville, Md: National Institute on Alcohol Abuse and Alcoholism; 1992.
53. Emrick CD. A review of psychologically oriented treatment of alcoholism, II: the relative effectiveness of different treatment approaches and the effectiveness of treatment versus no treatment. *J Stud Alcohol.* 1975;36:88-108.
54. Babor TF, Grant M. *Project on Identification and Management of Alcohol-Related Problems, Report on Phase II: A Randomized Clinical Trial of Brief Interventions in Primary Health Care.* Geneva, Switzerland: World Health Organization; 1992.
55. Miller WR, Benefield G, Tonigan S. Enhancing motivation for change in problem drinking: a controlled comparison of two therapist styles. *J Consult Clin Psychol.* 1993;61:455-461.
56. Miller WR, Brown JM, Simpson TS, Handmaker NS, Bien TH, Luckie LF, Montgomery HA, Hester RK, Tonigan JS. What works?: a methodological analysis of the alcohol treatment outcome literature. In: Hester RK, Miller WR, eds. *Handbook of Alcoholism Treatment Approaches.* 2nd ed. Boston, Mass: Allyn and Bacon; 1995:12-14.
57. Babor TF. Avoiding the horrid and beastly sin of drunkenness: does dissuasion make a difference? *J Consult Clin Psychol.* 1994;62:1127-1140.
58. Bien TH, Miller WR, Tonigan JS. Brief interventions for alcohol problems: a review. *Addiction.* 1993;88:315-336.
59. Cannon DS, Baker TB, Wehl CK. Emetic and electric shock alcohol aversion therapy: six- and 12-month follow-up. *J Consult Clin Psychol.* 1981;49:360-368.
60. Ashem B, Donner L. Covert sensitization with alcoholics: a controlled replication. *Behav Res Ther.* 1968;6:7-12.
61. Drummond DC, Glautier S. A controlled trial of cue exposure treatment in alcohol dependence. *J Consult Clin Psychol.* 1994;62:809-817.
62. Monti PM, Rohsenow DJ, Rubonis AV, Niaura RS, Sirota AD, Colby SM, Goddard P, Abrams DB. Cue exposure with coping skills treatment for male alcoholics: a preliminary investigation. *J Consult Clin Psychol.* 1993;61:1011-1019.
63. Miller PM. A behavioral intervention program for chronic public drunkenness offenders. *Arch Gen Psychiatry.* 1975;32:915-918.
64. Azrin NH, Sisson W, Meyers R, Godley M. Alcoholism treatment by disulfiram and community reinforcement. *J Behav Ther Exp Psychiatry.* 1982;13:105-112.
65. Monti PM, Abrams DB, Binkoff JA, Zwick WR, Liepman MR, Nirenberg TD, Rohsenow DJ. Communication skills training, communication skills training with family and cognitive behavioral mood management training for alcoholics. *J Stud Alcohol.* 1990;51:263-270.
66. Oei TPS, Jackson PR. Social skills and cognitive behavioral approaches to the treatment of problem drinking. *J Stud Alcohol.* 1982;43:532-547.
67. Chaney ER, O'Leary MR, Marlatt GA. Skill training with alcoholics. *J Consult Clin Psychol.* 1978;46:1092-1104.
68. Kadden RM, Cooney NL, Getter H, Litt MD. Matching alcoholics to coping skills or interactional therapies: posttreatment results. *J Consult Clin Psychol.* 1990;57:698-704.
69. Ahles TA, Schlundt DG, Prue DM, Rychtarik RG. Impact of aftercare arrangements on the maintenance of treatment success in abusive drinkers. *Addict Behav.* 1983;8:53-58.
70. McCrady BS, Stout RL, Noel NE, Abrams DB, Nelson HF. Effectiveness of three types of spouse-involved behavioral alcoholism treatment. *Br J Addict.* 1991;86:1415-1424.
71. O'Farrell TJ, Choquette KA, Cutter HSG, Brown ED, McCourt WF. Behavioral marital therapy with and without additional relapse prevention sessions for alcoholics and their wives. *J Stud Alcohol.* 1993;54:652-666.
72. Noel NE, McCrady BS, Stout RL, Fisher-Nelson H. Predictors of attrition from an outpatient alcohol couples treatment program. *J Stud Alcohol.* 1987;48:229-237.
73. Longabaugh R, Beattie M, Noel N, Stout R, Malloy P. The effect of social investment on treatment outcome. *J Stud Alcohol.* 1993;54:465-478.
74. Longabaugh R, Rubin A, Malloy P, Beattie M, Clifford PR, Noel N. Drinking outcomes of alcohol abusers diagnosed as antisocial personality disorder. *Alcohol Clin Exp Res.* 1994;18:778-785.
75. Emrick CD, Tonigan JS, Montgomery H, Little L. Alcoholics Anonymous: what is currently known? In: McCrady BS, Miller WR, eds. *Research on Alcoholics Anonymous: Opportunities and Alternatives.* New Brunswick, NJ: Rutgers Center of Alcohol Studies; 1993:41-78.
76. Ditman KS, Crawford GG, Forgy EW, Moskowitz H, MacAndrew C. A controlled experiment on the use of court probation for drunk arrests. *Am J Psychiatry.* 1967;124:160-163.
77. Brandsma JM, Maultsby MC Jr, Welsh RJ. *Outpatient Treatment of Alcoholism: A Review and Comparative Study.* Baltimore, Md: University Park Press; 1980.
78. Walsh DC, Hingson RW, Merrigan DM, Levenson SM, Cupples LA, Heeren T, Coffman GA, Becker CA, Barker TA, Hamilton SK, McGuire TG, Kelly CA. A randomized trial of treatment options for alcohol-abusing workers. *N Engl J Med.* 1991;325:775-782.
79. Mattson ME, Allen JP, Longabaugh R, Nickless CJ, Connors GJ, Kadden RM. A chronological review of empirical studies matching alcoholic clients to treatment. *J Stud Alcohol.* 1994;12(suppl):16-29.
80. Cook D. Craftsman versus professional: analysis of the controlled drinking controversy. *J Stud Alcohol.* 1985;46:433-442.
81. McCrady BS, Delaney SI. Self-help groups. In: Hester RK, Miller WR, eds. *Handbook of Alcoholism Treatment Approaches: Effective Alternatives.* 2nd ed. Boston, Mass: Allyn and Bacon; 1995:160-175.
82. Fillmore KM. Alcohol use across the life course: a critical review of 70 years of international longitudinal research. Toronto, Canada: Addiction Research Foundation; 1988.
83. Helzer JE, Robbins LN, Taylor JR, Carey K, Miller RH, Combs-Orme T, Farmer A. The extent of long-term moderate drinking among alcoholics discharged from medical and psychiatric facilities. *N Engl J Med.* 1985;312:1678-1682.
84. Rosenberg H. Prediction of controlled drinking by alcoholics and problem drinkers. *Psychol Bull.* 1993;113:129-139.
85. Hayashida M, Alterman AI, McLellan AT, O'Brien CP, Purtill JJ, Volpicelli JR, Raphaelson AH, Hall CP. Comparative effectiveness and costs of inpatient and outpatient detoxification of patients with mild-to-moderate alcohol withdrawal syndrome. *N Engl J Med.* 1988;320:358-365.
86. Longabaugh R, McCrady BS, Fink E, Stout R, McAuley T, McNeill D. Cost-effectiveness of alcoholism treatment in inpatient versus partial hospital settings: six-month outcomes. *J Stud Alcohol.* 1983;44:1049-1071.
87. McLaughlan JFC, Stein RL. Evaluation of a day clinic for alcoholics. *J Stud Alcohol.* 1982;43:261-272.
88. Miller WR, Hester RK. Inpatient alcoholism treatment: who benefits? *Am Psychol.* 1986;41:794-805.
89. McCrady BS, Longabaugh R, Fink E, Stout R, Beattie M, Ruggieri-Authelet A, McNeill D. Cost effectiveness of alcoholism treatment in partial hospital versus inpatient settings after brief inpatient treatment: twelve month outcomes. *J Consult Clin Psychol.* 1986;54:708-713.
90. Langenbucher JW, McCrady BS, Brick J, Esterly R. *Socioeconomic Evaluations of Addictions Treatment.* Washington, DC: White House Printing Office; 1993.
91. National Institute on Alcohol Abuse and Alcoholism. *Benefit–Cost Analysis of Alcoholism Treatment Centers.* Washington, DC: National Institute on Alcohol Abuse and Alcholism; 1976. Publication ADM 281-75-0031.
92. Groeneveld J, Shain M, Brayshaw D, Keaney J, Laird L. Cost effectiveness of EAP: testing assumptions. *Employee Assistance Q.* 1985;1:75-81.
93. Orvis BR, Armor DJ, Williams CE, Barras AJ, Schwarzbach DS. *Effectiveness and Cost of Alcohol Rehabilitation in the United States Air Force.* Santa Monica, Calif: RAND; 1981.
94. Becker FW, Sanders BK. *The Illinois Medicare/Medicaid Alcoholism Services Demonstration: Medicaid Cost Trends and Utilization Patterns—Managerial Report.* Springfield, Ill: Center for Policy Studies and Program Evaluation, Sangamon State University; 1984.
95. Blose JO, Holder HD. The utilization of medical care by treated alcoholics: longitudinal patterns by age, gender, and type of care. *J Subst Abuse.* 1991;3:13-27.
96. Holder HD, Blose JO. Alcoholism treatment and total health care utilization and costs. *JAMA.* 1986;256:1456-1460.
97. Holder HD, Blose JO. Typical patterns and costs of alcoholism treatment across a variety of populations and providers. *Alcohol Clin Exp Res.* 1991;15:190-195.
98. Holder HD, Schachtman RH. Estimating health care savings associated with alcoholism treatment. *Alcohol Clin Exp Res.* 1987;11:66-73.
99. Plotnick DE, Adams KM, Hunter HR, Rowe JC. *Alcoholism Treatment Programs Within Prepaid Group Practice HMO's: A Final Report.* Washington, DC: Group Health Association of America; 1982.
100. Holder HD, Hallan JB. Impact of alcoholism treatment on total health care costs: a six-year study. *Adv Alcohol Subst Abuse.* 1986;6:1-15.
101. National Institute on Alcohol Abuse and Alcoholism. *An Approach to Good Health for Employees and Reduced Health Care Costs for Industry.* Rockville, Md: US Dept of Health and Human Services; 1986.
102. Spear SF, Mason M. Impact of chemical dependency on family health status. *Int J Addict.* 1991;26:179-187.
103. Woodside M, Coughey K, Cohen R. Medical costs of children of alcoholics: pay now or pay later. *J Subst Abuse.* 1993;5:281-287.
104. Holder H, Longabaugh R, Miller WR, Rubonis AV. The cost effectiveness of treatment for alcoholism: a first approximation. *J Stud Alcohol.* 1991;52:517-540.
105. McCrady BS, Richter SS, Morgan TJ, Slade J, Pfeifer C. Involving health care workers in screening for alcohol problems. *J Addict Dis.* In press.
106. Heather N, Campion PD, Neville RG, Maccabe D. Evaluation of a controlled drinking minimal intervention for problem drinkers in general practice (the DRAMS scheme). *J Royal Coll Gen Pract.* 1987;37:358-363.
107. Dawes R. *House of Cards: Psychology and Psychotherapy Built on Myth.* New York, NY: Free Press; 1994.
108. Hser Y-I, Anglin MD, Chou C-P. Evaluation of drug abuse treatment: a repeated measures design assessing methadone maintenance. *Eval Rev.* 1988;12:547-570.
109. Miller WR, Hester RK. The effectiveness of alcoholism treatment methods: what research reveals. In: Miller WR, Heather N, eds. *Treating Addictive Behaviors: Processes of Change.* New York, NY: Plenum Publishing Corp; 1986:121-174.

Psychosocial Treatment for Drug Abuse

Selected Review and Recommendations for National Health Care

Paul Crits-Christoph, PhD; Lynne Siqueland, PhD

Substance abuse and dependence remains an important public health concern because of health-related and other costs to our society. We review selected articles that address questions about the psychosocial treatment of substance abuse disorders; these articles could aid in setting the parameters of a national health care insurance. Data from major program evaluation studies of existing substance abuse treatment programs are presented, followed by reviews of controlled studies of opiate, cocaine, and marijuana abuse and dependence; particular attention is given to studies that have standardized treatment through the use of treatment manuals. Articles about the treatment of substance abuse in adolescents are also reviewed. The existing data suggest that substance abuse treatment should be intensive and should probably involve multiple modalities targeted to various problems encountered in patients with substance use disorders, including comorbid psychiatric problems. However, only a few well-controlled studies have been performed to date; therefore, substantial research is needed before a system truly informed by research can be designed. Suggestions for future research directions are provided. *Arch Gen Psychiatry. 1996;53:749-756*

The 1993 National Institute on Drug Abuse Household Survey reported that an estimated 11.7 million Americans had used an illicit drug during the month before the survey. Although recreational use of cocaine has decreased, no decrease in the number of hard-core, regular cocaine users has yet occurred; the 1993 National Institute on Drug Abuse Household Survey estimated the number of hard-core users to be 476 000. The number of regular marijuana users (ie, once weekly or more) was estimated by the 1993 National Institute on Drug Abuse Household Survey to be 5.1 million.[1] Higher prevalences are noted in samples obtained from clinical settings, prisons, and homeless populations.[2]

The effects of cocaine use beyond the individual user are wide ranging. In New York City, recent cocaine use was detected at autopsy in 18% of persons who were in fatal car accidents and in 20% of persons who committed suicide.[3] Cocaine seems to be related to a risk of suicide, especially among younger African American and Hispanic users.[4] Hard-core drug use also contributes to the spread of the human immunodeficiency virus through sex-for-drugs exchanges and needle sharing.

Treatments for substance abuse are likely to receive considerable attention in the continuing discussions about a national health insurance. A significant amount of federal and private insurance company dollars are already apportioned for the treatment of substance abuse. For example, the cost of treating 150 000 substance abusers in California in 1992 was $200 million.[5] Of course, the cost of substance abuse to society goes beyond the treatment costs and includes the other effects, such as crime, drug enforcement costs, and other health care costs. The total cost of drug use to society was estimated to be $47 billion ($10^9$) during the 1980s (before crack cocaine trafficking).[6] The use of drugs during pregnancy affects medical costs; the average hospital cost of a cocaine-exposed infant is estimated at $13 222 vs the average cost of

From the Department of Psychiatry, University of Pennsylvania, Philadelphia.

$1297 for drug-free infants.[7] The financial benefits of treating 150 000 substance abusers in California has been estimated at $1.5 billion ($10^9$) in savings, mostly as a function of reductions in crime.[5] Thus, improving and evaluating treatments for substance abuse disorders remain a high priority because reductions in substance abuse and associated savings in medical and other costs to society can be realized.

This article reviews selected research articles relevant to the psychosocial treatment of substance abusers, excluding alcohol abuse. Based on these articles, we make recommendations about the type and amount of psychosocial services that might serve as a starting point for a national health care insurance program, and we suggest areas for further research. It is likely that successful treatment of substance abuse will involve a variety of components, including medical care, medications, and practical assistance. This review, however, restricts itself to the narrow perspective of psychosocial interventions, such as cognitive, behavioral, psychodynamic, and family therapies. Because of the limited number of studies available on each type of substance abuse and dependence, it is impossible to conduct a formal meta-analysis. Instead, we present a qualitative review of the existing literature.

DOES PSYCHOSOCIAL TREATMENT FOR SUBSTANCE ABUSE WORK?

Large-scale program evaluation studies surveying thousands of patients have consistently found that psychosocial treatments for substance abuse seem to yield substantial benefits; the standard outpatient treatment involves some form of psychotherapy or counseling, which demonstrates equivalent benefits to therapeutic community treatments and methadone maintenance therapy but superior benefits to detoxification alone or no treatment.[8] However, the Drug Abuse Reporting Program suggested that the advantage of psychosocial treatment vs detoxification alone emerged only after 90 days of treatment.[9] Results from the Treatment Outcome Prospective Study indicate that a notable decrease in regular heroin use was evident for outpatients undergoing methadone therapy and residential patients only after 1 year of treatment and for drug-free clinic outpatients after 6 months of treatment.[10] In addition, patients who complete treatment vs dropouts are more likely to remain drug free; they also have lower relapse rates, less unemployment, and decreased arrests.[11] Another study evaluated 6 programs and concluded that patients improve during treatment but that long-term is better than short-term treatment.[12]

Although these program evaluation studies provide a broad-brush answer to the question of the effectiveness of treatment for substance abuse, the lack of random assignment and the lack of specification and control of the treatment variable in these studies prevent any specific clinical recommendations about how best to treat substance abuse and dependence. To address these questions, we examine controlled efficacy studies, particularly those studies that specify the treatment via the use of treatment manuals. Specification of the treatment through a treatment manual not only allows for clearer clinical recommendations but also minimizes differences between therapists that can hinder the comparison of treatment modalities.[13] Most studies reviewed use the diagnosis of substance dependence as inclusion criteria, unless otherwise noted.

CONTROLLED EFFICACY STUDIES OF OPIATE ABUSE AND DEPENDENCE

Woody et al[14] reviewed 7 studies on the use of psychotherapy for opiate abuse and dependence; they concluded that evidence that psychotherapy was beneficial in the treatment of these patients did exist. One of these earlier studies was a well-controlled study of strategic and structural family therapy comparing paid and unpaid family therapy, paid family participation, and standard methadone therapy in young adult opiate addicts.[15] In paid therapy, patients and family members were paid for attendance at sessions and for drug-free urine samples. Stanton and Todd[15] reported better outcomes using family therapy vs nonfamily therapy on days free of legal and illegal opiates, all illegal drugs, and marijuana. However, Romijn et al[16] failed to replicate these findings; they reported no notable differences between family therapy and standard methadone therapy on any measures of drug use or social functioning. While treatment guidelines and a theoretical model were provided, no formal treatment manual for the Stanton and Todd treatment exists and minimal checks were made on therapist competence and treatment integrity in either the original study or the replication.

Of the other 6 studies reviewed by Woody et al,[14] only 2 involved standardization of the treatment conditions. One study compared supportive-expressive psychodynamic therapy (SE), cognitive therapy (CT), and standard drug counseling (DC) for methadone-treated, opiate-dependent patients.[17,18] Patients in SE and CT also received individual DC. Patients received treatment for a maximum of 6 months, but the average patient attended 10 to 12 sessions of SE or CT and 12 sessions of DC. Outcome evaluations conducted at 7 months after beginning treatment[17,18] and at the 1-year follow-up[19] indicated that SE and CT yielded greater benefits than DC alone on measures of employment, legal problems, psychiatric symptoms, and opiate-positive urine specimens. In a further analysis of data from this study, it was found that patients with high psychiatric severity did better in CT and SE vs DC on psychiatric and drug-use outcomes.[20] Another report from this project indicated that antisocial personality disorder was associated with poorer outcomes (but not when depression was diagnosed).[21] A second evaluation of a manual-guided psychotherapy treatment, however, revealed no notable advantage of methadone plus interpersonal psychotherapy vs low-contact (brief monthly sessions) methadone therapy alone.[22]

Woody et al[23] conducted a partial replication of their 1983 study, comparing SE with DC in psychiatrically symptomatic, opiate-dependent patients in community-based methadone treatment programs. This study was designed to address 2 questions about the 1983 study: (1) Would the findings generalize from a university-affiliated research clinic to typical community-based programs? (2) Were the effects found a result of having 2 "helpers" (a psychotherapist and a drug counselor) compared with only 1 helper (a drug counselor alone)? To address this second question, patients were assigned to either a psychotherapist and a drug counselor or to 2 drug counselors. The results indicated greater benefits for patients who received treatment from a psychotherapist and a drug counselor. Although patients in both treatment conditions had similar overall proportions of opiate-positive urine specimens, the authors reported an increase in opiate-positive urine specimens during the last 12 weeks of the treatment for patients undergoing DC alone but a decrease during this same period for patients undergoing SE and DC. Further, patients in the SE and DC treatment had fewer cocaine-positive urine specimens during treatment and required lower doses of methadone. At the 6-month follow-up, patients who received DC alone had lost some of their gains, while patients who received SE and DC maintained their improvements or continued improving, yielding statistically significant differences that included large effect sizes for drug use and employment outcomes and moderate effect sizes for psychiatric outcomes.

One controlled study has examined the usefulness of an adjunctive treatment attempting to extinguish conditioned responses to drug cues.[24] This study randomized patients to cognitive-behavioral psychotherapy with graduated extinction trials, cognitive-behavioral therapy without extinction trials, and DC without extinction trials. Both conditions with cognitive-behavioral therapy had better outcomes than the DC condition, but no evidence suggested that the extinction procedure added anything to the cognitive-behavioral therapy.

McLellan et al[25] reported the results of randomizing opiate users who are men to minimum methadone maintenance therapy, methadone maintenance therapy plus DC (standard methadone maintenance therapy), or methadone maintenance therapy plus DC and additional psychosocial treatment services (enhanced methadone maintenance therapy), including psychiatric and employment counseling and family therapy. Patients undergoing enhanced methadone maintenance therapy were required to attend at least 1 session with the psychiatrist, the employment counselor, and the family therapist; additional sessions were scheduled at the discretion of the particular professional and the patient. The 6-month outcomes indicated that the patients who received standard methadone maintenance therapy showed faster and greater improvements than did the patients who received minimum methadone maintenance therapy. Further, patients who received the additional psychosocial treatment services showed notably greater improvements than the patients who received only DC in areas of employment, alcohol use, criminal activity, and psychiatric status. Although this study had many advantages vs typical program evaluation studies, including the use of random assignment and a counselor treatment manual, it is impossible to attribute the greater improvements to a specific psychosocial treatment, as a variety of diverse treatment services were implemented.

CONTROLLED EFFICACY STUDIES OF COCAINE ABUSE AND DEPENDENCE

Several studies have examined the relative efficacy of some form of relapse prevention therapy (RPT) for cocaine dependence. Relapse prevention treatments have been adapted from the original work of Marlatt and Gordon[26] and involve various cognitive and behavioral techniques, including the identification of high-risk situations for relapse, the development of coping skills for these situations, the development of a nondrug-using lifestyle, and the cognitive reframing of "slips" as an opportunity to learn (vs viewing the slip as a full relapse or failure).[27]

Carroll et al[28] compared a cognitive-behavioral–based RPT with interpersonal psychotherapy. Forty-two patients were treated once weekly for 12 weeks.[28] Twelve (57%) of the 21 patients treated with RPT were abstinent for longer than 3 weeks during the 12 weeks, while only 7 (33%) of the 21 patients treated with interpersonal psychotherapy met the same criterion; however, this difference was not statistically significant because of the relatively small sample sizes. Patients with high psychiatric severity who received RPT also achieved notably higher rates of abstinence than those who received interpersonal psychotherapy. A study by Carroll et al[29] compared RPT plus desipramine therapy, clinical management plus desipramine therapy, RPT plus placebo, and clinical management plus placebo in the treatment of ambulatory cocaine abusers. All groups showed improvement, but no main effects of medication or psychotherapy and no interaction effect were noted. Further analysis revealed that subjects with a higher baseline severity of cocaine use had better outcomes and retention when they were treated with RPT vs clinical management, while the subjects with a low severity of cocaine use had better outcomes when they were treated with desipramine therapy. Patients with a low severity of cocaine use also showed better outcomes and retention in clinical management vs RPT. In addition, depressed cocaine users treated with RPT remained in treatment notably longer and maintained notably longer periods of consecutive abstinence during treatment than those depressed cocaine users treated with clinical management. Data from the 1-year follow-up revealed a delayed effect for patients treated with RPT (either with desipramine therapy or a placebo) doing notably better than patients treated with supportive clinical management (either with desipramine therapy or a placebo).[30]

Another study, however, found no difference between cocaine users who were treated with RPT and those who were involved with a 12-step support group.[31] A weakness of this study is that *DSM-III-R* criteria for cocaine dependence were not evaluated, and the patients seemed to use cocaine mildly to moderately; 25 (23%) of the patients reported no cocaine use during the month prior to entry into treatment.

Another study compared 3 treatments for outpatient cocaine-dependent patients: (1) family therapy, (2) SE, and (3) paraprofessionally led group therapy.[32,33] Of the patient sample, 88 (72%) of 122 were crack smokers. Attrition was a major problem; only 65 (53%) of the randomized patients attended at least 1 treatment session, and only 27 (22%) of the patients completed at least 6 sessions of treatment. Kang et al[33] did not report comparisons between the treatment conditions; only results across all modalities were reported. Only 14 (25%) of the patients who attended 3 or more sessions were abstinent during treatment. In a follow-up of patients 6 to 12 months after initial contact with the clinic, those authors found that 23 (19%) of the patients reported that they had not used cocaine in the last 3 months. Kang et al concluded that more intensive treatment than once weekly is probably needed. One problem with this study, however, is that no information on the selection, training, and certification of the therapists in the treatment manuals or on the integrity of the delivery of the treatments through the use of adherence or competence ratings was presented.

Hoffman et al[34] reported the results of a study in which the retention rates for 6 treatment conditions were examined. Patients were randomly assigned to either standard group therapy (twice weekly) or intensive group therapy (five times weekly). In addition, patients were further assigned to either no additional services, individual psychotherapy, or individual psychotherapy plus family therapy. The results indicated that retention was best in patients who received intensive individual and group treatment. Patients who received standard group therapy alone attended only 6 sessions on average, while those patients who received intensive group therapy attended from 23 (intensive group alone) to 28 (intensive group plus individual and family therapies) sessions on average.

Higgins et al[35] compared a behavioral treatment (community reinforcement that included behavioral contracting and counseling with a significant other, relapse prevention skills, establishment of alternative recreational activities, and employment, housing, financial, and legal counseling) with standard DC. Treatment was more intensive than in the previous studies: 2 weekly sessions for 12 weeks, followed by 1 weekly session for 12 weeks. Results indicated that 13 (68%) of the patients who received community reinforcement achieved 8 weeks of abstinence and that 8 (42%) of these patients achieved 16 weeks of abstinence; 2 (11%) and 1 (5%) of the patients who received standard DC achieved 8 and 16 weeks of abstinence, respectively. In another study, Higgins et al[36] randomly assigned patients to behavioral treatment with or without an added incentive program involving vouchers that were exchangeable for retail items contingent on cocaine-negative urine samples. Retention was better in patients who had the added incentive of a voucher; 15 (75%) of these patients completed 24 weeks of treatment vs 8 (40%) of these patients who received behavioral treatment alone. Thus, the authors conclude that incentives notably improve outcomes. Higgins et al[37] further report that the best predictor of cocaine abstinence within their contingency-management program is whether a significant other participated. While these findings are encouraging, their generalizability is questionable because all of the patients in the first trial and most of the patients in the second trial were white and none of the patients used crack cocaine. In addition, the reinforcement contingencies used involved incentives (totaling as much as $1000 per patient) and spousal and significant other contracts that are not likely to be practical for many crack cocaine users presenting for treatment in urban settings.

Our review of controlled psychosocial treatment studies of cocaine dependence indicates some promising results for cognitive-behaviorally oriented relapse prevention and community reinforcement approaches. In addition, it seems as if the intensity of the treatment may be important, with 1 standard weekly session being of limited value. However, several limitations of the existing studies are apparent. These include relatively small sample sizes, modest outcomes at best, limited statistical power for testing whether outcome varies by subgroups, which might serve as a basis for matching patients to treatments, no data on the potential mediators of responses to treatment, and little evaluation of the exportability of the treatment models to other sites.

CONTROLLED EFFICACY STUDIES OF MARIJUANA DEPENDENCE

Despite the large number of regular marijuana users compared with users of other illicit drugs, only 1 clinical trial has evaluated manual-guided treatment for marijuana dependence. Stephens et al[38] randomly assigned 212 regular marijuana users to either an RPT modeled after the treatment of Marlatt and Gordon[26] or a nonbehavioral group discussion treatment.[38] Independent ratings of audiotaped therapy sessions verified the fidelity and discriminability of the treatments. Overall, substantial reductions in the frequency of marijuana use and associated problems occurred with both treatments, but no differences between the 2 treatments emerged. Days of marijuana use per month decreased from approximately 27 to approximately 15 days at 12 months after treatment (treatment lasted 12 weeks). The lack of differences between the conditions, however, prevents attribution of any changes to the treatments per se. In addition, the selection of subjects for the study was not based on the diagnosis of a marijuana use disorder from a diagnostic interview.

PSYCHOSOCIAL TREATMENT OF SUBSTANCE ABUSE IN ADOLESCENTS

Several studies have focused on family therapy approaches for the treatment of adolescent drug abusers. These studies did not restrict the samples to a specific type of substance abuse and did not use *DSM-III-R* criteria for defining the sample population. One study compared multidimensional family therapy, multifamily educational therapy, and adolescent group therapy (AGT) for adolescent drug abusers.[39] The results indicated that patients who received multidimensional family therapy decreased their drug use, particularly their use of marijuana, more than patients who received the multifamily educational therapy or AGT after receiving treatment; these patients also had better retention. At follow-up, it was noted that these gains were maintained; however, no notable differences were found between patients who received AGT and those who received the multidimensional family therapy at follow-up. Most adolescents decreased their use of marijuana from daily use to use once or twice weekly.[39,40]

Szapocznik et al[41] have focused on engagement strategies and have found that a strategy based on a structural and strategic systems model leads to 52 (93%) of 56 families engaging in treatment vs 22 (42%) of 52 families engaging, using an engagement-as-usual strategy in Hispanic families with a drug-abusing adolescent. However, no differences in dropout rates between the 2 groups were noted once they were engaged in treatment. Santisteban et al[42] replicated the earlier study and found that the strategic structural systems approach engaged 42 (81%) of families vs 84 (60%) of families in control conditions (family therapy with the usual engagement strategies and group therapy). Szapocznik et al[43,44] have found that 1-person family therapy is as effective as conjoint family therapy on measures of drug use and family functioning and is slightly better than conjoint therapy at sustaining improvement in functioning at follow-up.

Friedman[45] investigated a 6-month course of family therapy vs parent groups in the treatment of adolescent substance abuse. The family therapy treatment followed a manual for "functional" family therapy that uses some of the same techniques used in strategic family therapy (eg, tasks, directions, and problem solving), as well as positive relabeling and communication skill work. The parent group method worked only with the parents (the adolescents received separate individual DC) and was based on a parent effectiveness training method. No notable differences between the 2 treatments on any outcome criteria were found at an evaluation conducted 15 months after the start of treatment.

Joanning et al[46] have reported on the results of a trial comparing family systems therapy (an integration of structural and strategic family therapy models), AGT, and family drug education. Family systems therapy comprised weekly sessions for 7 to 15 weeks (therapists ended early if goals were met); AGT comprised 12 weekly sessions; and family drug education comprised 6 biweekly sessions. At the end of treatment, an estimated 14 (40%) of the adolescents who received family systems therapy were using drugs vs 17 (68%) of the adolescents who received AGT and 19 (66%) of the adolescents who received family drug education. While this study yields promising information on family therapy for adolescent drug abuse, the findings are limited because the investigators excluded adolescents who showed signs of addiction to drugs, thereby limiting the sample to less severe drug use. Moreover, outcome data are only presented for patients who completed treatment.

ATTRITION

As previously mentioned, retention in substance abuse treatment is an important issue, and staying in treatment has been strongly associated with greater improvements. Data on the percentage of patients who dropped out of treatment for each of the studies we have reviewed is given in the **Table**. High dropout rates are apparent even in our sample of relatively recent studies, in which researchers have attempted to provide high-quality therapy using treatment guides or manuals. However, substantial differences in dropout rates across studies and treatment modalities have been noted.[45]

Although retention can be seen as an important outcome measure in its own right, most studies fail to obtain outcome data about the patients who drop out of treatment, thereby potentially introducing biases by comparing treatment conditions using only patients who remained in treatment or using endpoint analyses.[47] Few studies conduct a formal intent-to-treat analysis using all patients randomized to eliminate this potential bias. (The study by Carroll et al[29] is an exception.) Although dropout rates continue to be high in many substance abuse studies, studies of psychosocial interventions with non-substance abuse patients have also tended to report high dropout rates. For example, in a meta-analysis of dropout from psychotherapy, a reported 47% of the patients dropped out.[48] Hollon et al[49] found that 43 (36%) of the patients dropped out before 12 weeks for patients who were receiving CT for depression. When viewed in the context of these dropout rates, the attrition figures shown in the Table for patients receiving psychosocial treatment for substance abuse do not seem to be particularly worse.

RECOMMENDATIONS FOR NATIONAL HEALTH CARE

Although the current environment, in which policy makers are searching for some scientific basis for the decisions that have to be made, encourages a tendency to make the most of available research findings, it is important to acknowledge that research on the efficacy and effectiveness of psychosocial treatment, particularly with substance abuse disorders, is in an early stage of development. Advances in diagnostic methods and procedures for standardizing treatments have increased the possibility that controlled studies can be used for making clinical recommendations and setting policy. The few studies that have been performed to date using these advances, however, suggest that we have farther to go before accurate recommendations can be made. The need to accumulate many studies on 1 substantive topic is particularly salient for psychosocial treatment research, given the limited samples sizes of individual studies and the host of methodological issues that can lead to different findings from study to study.

We must acknowledge that recommendations about the role of psychosocial treatments in national health care policy cannot be made in isolation from other clinical and service delivery issues. Particular issues that must be considered with substance abusers include human immunodeficiency virus testing and counseling, practical assistance regarding employment or housing, regulatory issues regarding drug use, and concurrent medical treatment, including medications. A national health care policy must consider each of these important domains of service delivery, and difficult decisions about where to spend limited funds will need to be made.

Given the above limitations and given that policy recommendations have to start somewhere, what sug-

Attrition Rates in Controlled Treatment Studies of Substance Abuse*

Source, y	% Male	% Minority	Dropout Rate, % (Treatment): Prior to First Session	By 6 Weeks	By 12 Weeks	By 24 Weeks
Opiates						
Woody et al,[17] 1983	100	62	...	20	...	†
Stanton and Todd,[15] 1982	100	42	30	37, 11‡	...	...
Romijn et al,[16] 1990	76	0	...	...	...	13
Rounsaville et al,[22] 1983	61	42	...	40 (IPT), 20 (LC)	...	62 (IPT), 46 (LC)
Cocaine						
Carroll et al,[28] 1991§	74	21	...	29 (RPT), 48 (IPT)	33 (RPT), 62 (IPT)	...
Carroll et al,[29] 1994‖	73	54	...	...	51 (RPT + D), 61 (CM + P), 63 (CM + D), 64 (RPT + P)	...
Kleinman et al,[32] 1990¶	87	84	42	60,# 75**	...	...
Hoffman et al,[34] 1994††	...	91	...	56 (G), ‡‡ 34 (G + I),‡‡ 28 (G + F),‡‡ 34 (G),§§ 35 (G + I),§§ 33 (G + F)§§	86 (G),‡‡ 72 (G + I),‡‡ 70 (G + F),‡‡ 62 (G),§§ 76 (G + I),§§ 69 (G + F)§§	...
Higgins et al,[35] 1993‖‖	¶¶	...	...	5 (CR), 42 (DC)	16 (CR), 74 (DC)	42 (CR), 89 (DC)
Wells et al,[31] 1994	64	16	20 (RPT), 21 (12-S)	...	##	...
Marijuana						
Stephens et al,[38] 1994	...	...	...	...	***	...
Adolescents						
Liddle and Dakof,[39] 1993	70	49	...	...	...	49 (AGT), 30 (MDFT), 35 (MFET)
Friedman,[45] 1989	60	11	7 (FT), 33 (PG)	...	...	...
Joanning et al,[46] 1992	...	32	...	...	...	13 (FST), 53 (AGT), 33 (FDE)

**IPT indicates interpersonal therapy; LC, low contact; RPT, relapse prevention therapy; D, desipramine therapy; CM, clinical management; P, placebo; G, group therapy; I, individual therapy; F, family; CR, community reinforcement; DC, standard drug counseling; 12-S, 12-step social support group; AGT, adolescent group therapy; MDFT, multidimensional family therapy; MFET, multifamily educational therapy; FT, family therapy; PG, parent group; FST, family systems therapy; FDE, family drug education; and ellipses, data not available.*

†*Patients receiving DC averaged 17 sessions; patients receiving supportive-expressive psychodynamic therapy (SE) averaged 12 SE and 12 DC sessions; and patients receiving cognitive therapy (CT) averaged 9.5 CT and 12 DC sessions.*

‡*Indicates 37% of standard methadone maintenance treatment cases, and 11% of FT cases.*

§*N=42.*

‖*N=139.*

¶*N=168; 72% of the patients were crack users.*

#*By week 3.*

***By week 6.*

††*N=303.*

‡‡*Two-week group.*

§§*Five-week group.*

‖‖*Patients studied were primarily white, noncrack users.*

¶¶*Patients were primarily male.*

##*Patients receiving RPT attended an average of 7 of 12 sessions; patients in the 12-S attended an average of 6 of 12 sessions.*

****Of the patients, 69% completed 7 of 10 sessions.*

gestions can we make for the structure of a national health care system for the treatment of substance abuse disorders? Perhaps the central question for designing such a system is the length of treatment that would be covered under a national health insurance. The available data on this question seem quite clear: evaluation studies of existing treatment programs[9,10] and the more promising new treatments evaluated in randomized clinical trials[29] indicate that a 3-month course of outpatient treatment is too brief. Although no studies have systematically varied the length of treatment to answer this question directly, more favorable results have been emerging from studies that use a 6-month duration of treatment.

Insurance providers, whether the government or private insurers, often specify treatment length in numbers of sessions, rather than a designated period. The intensity of treatment is therefore relevant to a concern about total number of sessions covered. In general, treatment once weekly seems to be inadequate,[32] and many treatments are based on at least 2 weekly sessions initially, which sometimes taper to once weekly.[35] Thus, a policy allowing for enough sessions so that intensive treatment can be provided initially (eg, the first 2-3 months), with full treatment to continue for up to 6 months, would be our recommendation.

The intensity of treatment is also an issue regarding multiple services provided for patients with substance abuse disorders. The study by McLellan et al[25] indicates that more services yield greater benefits. Accordingly, a national health insurance for substance abuse disorders ideally should have adequate coverage not only for DC or psychotherapy sessions but additional employment counseling, family therapy, and other services that might be needed.

Regarding the variety of services and treatment modalities that could be offered to patients with substance abuse disorders, it is crucial to acknowledge that a substantial heterogeneity exists among substance abusers in the nature and severity of their addiction-related problems.[50] In particular, the research suggests that patients with substance abuse disorders who also have comorbid psychiatric symptoms or disorders need additional services such as medications or psychotherapy.[17,20,29,30] Thus, the nature and amount of treatment provided might be based on the range of problems encountered for a given patient.

Regarding the specific modalities of treatment, several tentative recommendations can be made. The community reinforcement approach with a subset of patients dependent on cocaine also seems more promising than unfocused, nonspecific DC. For adolescents with substance abuse problems, family therapy seems to be more effective than peer group treatments or family psychoeducational approaches. Although the increasingly popular RPT approach has seemed promising in some studies,[30] other studies have not found it to be uniquely effective, at least for marijuana use.[38] The fact that some studies have found differences between treatment modalities is important to note. Thus, our recommendation for greater intensity of treatment should be qualified by the emerging data that suggest that content of treatment is important (ie, simply increasing the intensity of less effective treatments is not likely to achieve the best results).

FUTURE RESEARCH DIRECTIONS

We can provide a sketch of a variety of research directions that might be useful to pursue to provide further data to shape a national health care plan. One crucial question from a cost perspective is what level of qualifications is needed to produce acceptable results. Although some studies[17,23] have compared professional psychotherapy with DC performed by clinicians with bachelor's or master's degrees, modality has been confounded with the level of previous training or the educational background in these studies. Direct comparisons between certified addiction counselors with bachelor's vs master's degrees or between psychotherapists with master's vs doctoral degrees should be made, in which all therapists are providing the same manual-guided treatment.

Further research on the promising community reinforcement and RPT approaches seems to be warranted. In particular, no studies have yet examined the RPT approach vs family approaches in adolescents. Another approach that warrants further attention is the work on passive cue exposure, as well as active coping techniques combined with cue exposure.[51]

It is likely, however, that there would be a greater yield from examining specific interactions between patient characteristics and treatment modalities rather than just investigating main effects.[52] For example, research that would build on the findings that patients with comorbid psychiatric disorders would be better served by either a different form or intensity of treatment would be useful. Data on such patient-treatment matching would aid in designing the most efficient system. Studies designed to test a priori interaction hypotheses would need relatively large sample sizes. Such a study has recently been completed targeting alcohol abuse and dependence[53] and could serve as a model for studies on drug abuse.

Assessing the short- and long-term costs of treatment programs and specific modalities remains a high priority. The finding that substance abuse treatment actually saves society substantial amounts of money is a powerful argument for providing adequate levels of coverage for the treatment of substance abuse disorders in a national health insurance and for increasing the funding of treatment research that could potentially yield findings that would translate to even greater cost savings.

Although we support a policy of a broad range of research strategies, we would like to emphasize 2 further areas that need attention. The first area is treatment development research. Because existing treatments have shown modest outcomes at best, a need to develop and test newer forms of psychosocial treatment exists. The National Institute on Drug Abuse has established a grant announcement that encourages development research on treatments for substance abuse disorders.[54]

The second area is effectiveness (vs efficacy) research on treatments and the associated dissemination of treatments to the community. It is potentially problematic to move directly from the results of a controlled efficacy trial to the use of techniques in the community without first performing an effectiveness trial and viewing the application of the treatment on a large scale and under the types of conditions found in the community. Novel and more effective ways of actually disseminating treatments and developing and refining training programs also need to be considered.

Accepted for publication April 22, 1996.

This study was supported in part by grants U18-DA07090 from the National Institute on Drug Abuse and P50-MH-45178 from the Clinical Research Center, National Institute of Mental Health, Rockville, Md, and by the National Institute of Mental Health Career Development Award K02-MH00756 (Dr Crits-Christoph).

Reprints: Paul Crits-Christoph, PhD, 3600 Market St, Room 700, Philadelphia, PA 19104.

REFERENCES

1. Substance Abuse and Mental Health Services Administration, Office of Applied Statistics. *National Institute of Drug Abuse Household Survey 1993.* Rockville, Md: National Institute on Drug Abuse, US Department of Health and Human Services; 1994.
2. Regier DA, Farmer ME, Rae DS, Locke BZ, Keith SJ, Judd LL, Goodwin FK. Comorbidity of mental disorders with alcohol and other drug abuse: results from the epidemiologic catchment area (ECA) study. *JAMA.* 1990;264:2511-2518.
3. Marzuk PM, Tardiff K, Leon AC, Stajic M, Morgan EB, Mann JJ. Prevalence of recent cocaine use among motor vehicle fatalities in New York City. *JAMA.* 1990;263:250-256.
4. Marzuk PM, Tardiff K, Leon AC, Stajic M, Morgan EB, Mann JJ. Prevalence of cocaine users among residents of New York City who committed suicide during a one-year period. *Am J Psychiatry.* 1992;149:371-375.
5. Gerstein DR, Johnson RA, Harwood HJ, Fountain D, Suter N, Malloy K. *Evaluating Recovery Services: The California Drug and Alcohol Treatment Assessment General Report.* Sacramento, Calif: California Department of Alcohol and Drug Programs; 1994.
6. Harwood HJ, Napolitano PM, Kristiansen PL, Collins JJ. *Economic Costs to Society of Alcohol and Drug Abuse and Mental Illness: 1980.* Research Triangle Park, NC: Research Triangle Institute; 1984.
7. Calhoun BC, Watson PT. The cost of maternal cocaine abuse, I: perinatal cost. *Obstet Gynecol.* 1991;78:731-734.
8. Simpson DD, Sells SB. Effectiveness of treatment for drug abuse: an overview of the DARP Research Program. *Adv Alcohol Subst Abuse.* 1983;2:7-29.
9. Simpson DD. The relation of time spent in drug abuse treatment to posttreatment outcome. *Am J Psychiatry.* 1981;136:1449-1453.
10. Hubbard RL, Marsden ME, Rachal JV, Harwood HJ, Cavanaugh ER, Ginzburg HM. *Drug Abuse Treatment: A National Study of Effectiveness.* Chapel Hill, NC: University of North Carolina Press; 1989.
11. Stark MJ. Dropping out of substance abuse treatment: a clinically oriented review. *Clin Psychol Rev.* 1992;12:93-116.
12. McLellan AT, Luborsky L, O'Brien CP, Woody GE, Druley KA. Is treatment for substance abuse effective? *JAMA.* 1982;247:1423-1428.
13. Crits-Christoph P, Baranackie K, Kurcias JS, Beck AT, Carroll K, Perry K, Luborsky L, McLellan AT, Woody GE, Thompson L, Gallagher D, Zitrin C. Meta-analysis of therapist effects in psychotherapy outcome studies. *Psychother Res.* 1991;1:81-91.
14. Woody GE, Luborsky L, McLellan AT, O'Brien CP. Individual psychotherapy for substance abuse. In: *Treatments of Psychiatric Disorders: A Task Force Report of the American Psychiatric Association.* Washington, DC: American Psychiatric Association; 1989;2:1417-1429.
15. Stanton MD, Todd TC. *Family Therapy of Drug Abuse and Addiction.* New York, NY: Guilford Press; 1982.
16. Romijn CM, Platt JJ, Schippers GM. Family therapy for Dutch drug abusers: replication of an American study. *Int J Addict.* 1990;25:1127-1149.
17. Woody GE, Luborsky L, McLellan AT, O'Brien CP, Beck AT, Blaine J, Herman I, Hole A. Psychotherapy for opiate addicts: does it help? *Arch Gen Psychiatry.* 1983;40:639-645.
18. Woody GE, Luborsky L, McLellan AT, O'Brien CP. Corrections and revised analyses for psychotherapy in methadone maintenance programs. *Arch Gen Psychiatry.* 1990;47:788-789.
19. Woody GE, McLellan AT, Luborsky L, O'Brien CP. Twelve-month follow-up of psychotherapy for opiate dependence. *Am J Psychiatry.* 1987;144:591-596.
20. Woody GE, McLellan AT, Luborsky L, O'Brien CP, Blaine J, Fox S, Herman I, Beck AT. Psychiatric severity as a predictor of benefits from psychotherapy: the Penn-VA study. *Am J Psychiatry.* 1984;141:1172-1177.
21. Woody GE, McLellan AT, Luborsky L, O'Brien CP. Sociopathy and psychotherapy outcome. *Arch Gen Psychiatry.* 1985;42:1081-1086.
22. Rounsaville BJ, Glazer W, Wilber CH, Weissman MM, Kleber HD. Short-term interpersonal psychotherapy in methadone-maintained opiate addicts. *Arch Gen Psychiatry.* 1983;40:629-636.
23. Woody GE, McLellan AT, Luborsky L, O'Brien CP. Psychotherapy in community methadone programs: a validation study. *Am J Psychiatry.* 1995;192:1302-1308.
24. McLellan AT, Childress AR, Ehrman R, O'Brien CP. Extinguishing conditioned responses during opiate dependence treatment: turning laboratory findings into clinical procedures. *J Subst Abuse Treat.* 1991;3:33-40.
25. McLellan AT, Arndt IO, Metzger DS, Woody GE, O'Brien CP. The effects of psychosocial services in substance abuse treatment. *JAMA.* 1993;269:1953-1959.
26. Marlatt GA, Gordon JR, eds. *Relapse Prevention: Maintenance Strategies in the Treatment of Addictive Behaviors.* New York, NY: Guilford Press; 1985.
27. Rawson RA, Obert JL, McCann MJ, Marinelli-Casey P. Relapse prevention strategies in outpatient substance abuse treatment. *Psychol Addict Behav.* 1993;7:85-95.
28. Carroll KM, Rounsaville BJ, Gawin FH. A comparative trial of psychotherapies for ambulatory cocaine abusers: relapse prevention and interpersonal psychotherapy. *Am J Drug Alcohol Abuse.* 1991;17:229-247.
29. Carroll KM, Rounsaville BJ, Gordon LT, Nich C, Jatlow P, Bisighini RM, Gawin FH. Psychotherapy and pharmacotherapy for ambulatory cocaine abusers. *Arch Gen Psychiatry.* 1994;51:177-187.
30. Carroll KM, Rounsaville BJ, Nich C, Gordon LT, Wirtz PW, Gawin F. One-year follow-up of psychotherapy and pharmacotherapy for cocaine dependence. *Arch Gen Psychiatry.* 1994;51:989-997.
31. Wells EA, Peterson PL, Gainey RR, Hawkins JD, Catalano RF. Outpatient treatment for cocaine abuse: a controlled comparison of relapse prevention and twelve-step approaches. *Am J Drug Abuse.* 1994;20:1-17.
32. Kleinman PH, Woody GE, Todd TC, Millman RB, Kang S, Kemp J, Lipton DS. Crack and cocaine abusers in outpatient psychotherapy. In: Onken LS, Blaine JD, eds. *Psychotherapy and Counseling in the Treatment of Drug Abuse.* Rockville, Md: US Department of Health and Human Services; 1990:24-35. National Institute on Drug Abuse Research Monograph 104.
33. Kang S, Kleinman PH, Woody GE, Millman RB, Todd TC, Kemp J, Lipton DS. Outcomes for cocaine abusers after once-a-week psychosocial therapy. *Am J Psychiatry.* 1991;148:630-635.
34. Hoffman JA, Caudill BD, Koman JJ, Luckey JW, Flynn PM, Hubbard RL. Comparative cocaine abuse treatment strategies: enhancing client retention and treatment exposure. *J Addict Dis.* 1994;13:115-128.
35. Higgins ST, Budney AJ, Bickel WK, Hughes JR, Foeg F, Badger G. Achieving cocaine abstinence with a behavioral approach. *Am J Psychiatry.* 1993;150:763-769.
36. Higgins ST, Budney AJ, Bickel WK, Foerg FE, Donham R, Badger GJ. Incentives improve outcome in outpatient behavioral treatment of cocaine dependence. *Arch Gen Psychiatry.* 1994;51:568-576.
37. Higgins ST, Budney AJ, Bickel WK, Badger GJ. Participation of significant others in outpatient behavioral treatment predicts greater cocaine abstinence. *Am J Drug Alcohol Abuse.* 1994;20:47-56.
38. Stephens RS, Rofman RA, Simpson EE. Treating adult marijuana dependence: a test of the relapse prevention model. *J Consult Clin Psychol.* 1994;62:92-99.
39. Liddle H, Dakof GA. Effectiveness of family therapy versus multi-family therapy and group therapy: results of the adolescents and families project—a randomized clinical trial. Presented at the Society for Psychotherapy Research International Meeting; June 23-26, 1993; Pittsburgh, Pa.
40. Dakof GA, Liddle H. The relationship between family and individual change in family intervention research: panel outcome research in family based interventions with adolescents. Presented at the Society for Psychotherapy Research North American Meeting; February 25-27, 1994; Santa Fe, NM.
41. Szapocznik J, Perez-Vidal A, Brickman AL, Foote FH, Santisteban DA, Harris OE, Kurtines WM. Engaging adolescent drug abusers and their families in treatment: a strategic structural systems approach. *J Consult Clin Psychol.* 1988;56:522-557.
42. Santisteban DA, Szapocznic J, Perez-Vidal A, Kurtines WM, Murray EJ, LaPerriere A. Efficacy of intervention for engaging youth and families into treatment and some variables that may contribute to differential effectiveness. *J Fam Psychol.* 1996;10:35-44.
43. Szapocznik J, Kurtines W, Foote F, Perez-Vidal A, Hervis O. Conjoint versus one person family therapy: some evidence for the effectiveness of conducting family therapy through one person. *J Consult Clin Psychol.* 1983;51:889-899.
44. Szapocznik J, Kurtines WM, Foote F, Perez-Vidal A, Hervis O. Conjoint versus one-person family therapy: further evidence for the effectiveness of conducting family therapy through one person with drug-abusing adolescents. *J Consult Clin Psychol.* 1986;54:395-397.
45. Friedman A. Family therapy vs parent groups: effects on adolescent drug abusers. *Am J Fam Ther.* 1989;17:335-347.
46. Joanning H, Quinn W, Thomas F, Mullen R. Treating adolescent drug abuse: a comparison of family systems therapy, group therapy, and family drug education. *J Marital Fam Ther.* 1992;18:345-356.
47. Lavori PW. Clinical trials in psychiatry: should protocol deviation censor patient data? *Neuropsychopharmacology.* 1992;6:39-48.
48. Wierzbicki M, Pekarik G. A meta-analysis of psychotherapy dropout. *Professional Psychol Res Pract.* 1993;24:190-195.
49. Hollon SD, DeRubeis RJ, Evans MD, Wiemer MJ, Garvey MJ, Grove WM, Tuason VB. Cognitive therapy and pharmacotherapy for depression: singly and in combination. *Arch Gen Psychiatry.* 1992;49:774-781.
50. McLellan AT, Luborsky L, Woody GE, O'Brien CP, Kron R. Are the 'addiction-related' problems of substance abusers really related? *J Nerv Ment Dis.* 1981;169:232-239.
51. Rohsenow DJ, Childress AR, Monti PM, Niaura RS, Abrams DB. Cue reactivity in addictive behaviors: theoretical and treatment implications. *Int J Addict.* 1991;25:957-993.
52. Beutler LE. Have all won and must all have prizes? revisiting Luborsky et al's verdict. *J Consult Clin Psychol.* 1991;59:226-232.
53. Project MATCH Research Group. Project MATCH: rationale and methods for a multi-site clinical trial matching patients to alcoholism treatment. *Alcohol Clin Exp Res.* 1993;17:1130-1145.
54. *Behavioral Therapies Development Program Announcement.* Baltimore, Md: National Institute on Drug Abuse; July 1994. US Dept of Health and Human Services publication PA-94-078.

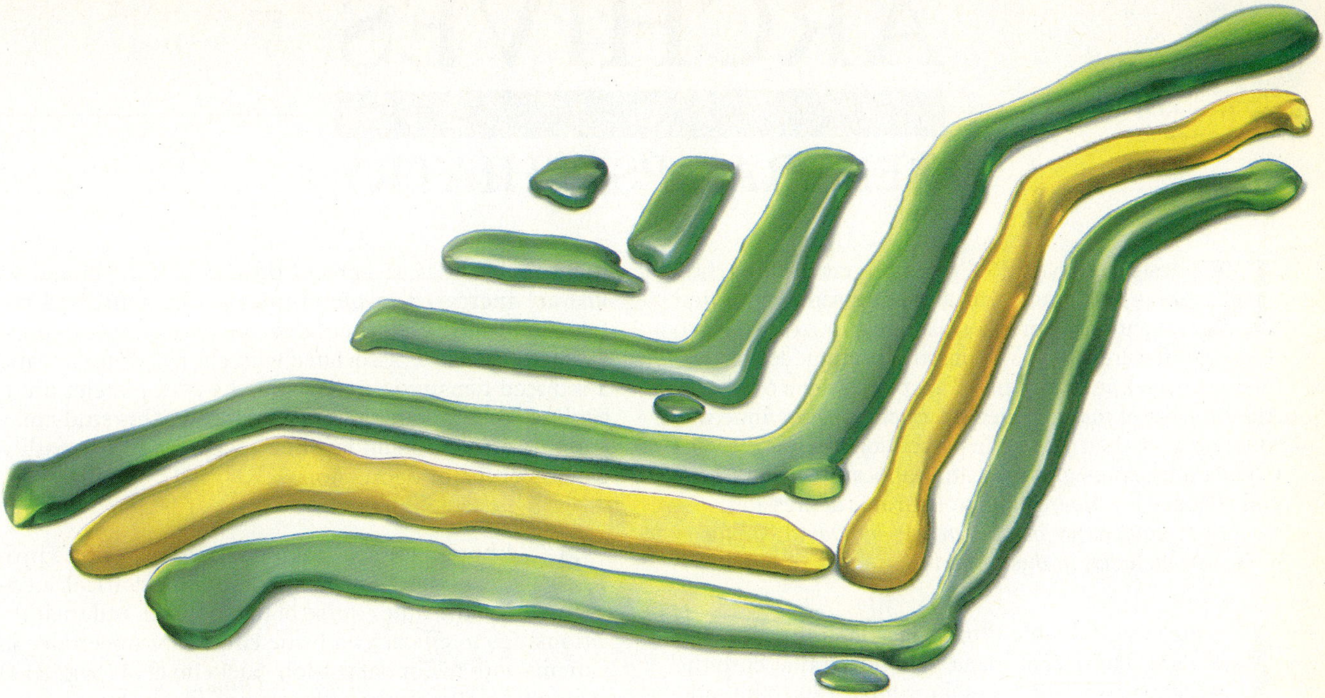

Now, RISPERDAL turns to liquid!

INTRODUCING

ORAL SOLUTION

1 mg/mL

Risperdal®

RISPERIDONE

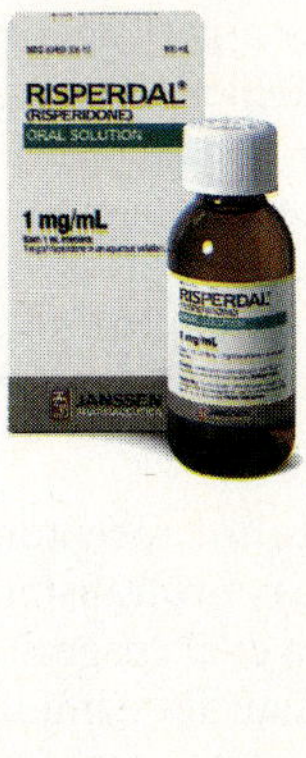

JANSSEN · PHARMACEUTICA · RESEARCH FOUNDATION · SmithKline Beecham Pharmaceuticals

Please see full Prescribing Information.

 JPI-RS-211R August 1996

ARCHIVES OF GENERAL PSYCHIATRY

Kocsis et al (page 769) report the results of the first long-term study of an antidepressant medication for chronic depression. Patients who responded to desipramine were either randomized to continue active treatment with medication or tapered to a placebo after 6 months. After 2 years of maintenance treatment, desipramine was more effective than placebo in prevention of relapse. Maintenance antidepressant medication appears to be indicated and effective for the treatment of chronic depression.

(A Commentary on this article by David Kupfer et al is also included in this issue.)

In the largest double-blind, placebo-controlled trial to date, **Thase et al** (page 777) report that both the selective serotonin reuptake inhibitor sertraline and the tricyclic antidepressant imipramine were comparably effective treatments of dysthymia. Sertraline was much better tolerated, and a greater proportion of patients receiving treatment with imipramine stopped treatment because of adverse events.

Quitkin et al (page 785) reviewed data on 593 patients included in a series of antidepressant studies and attempted to identify the time when patients whose conditions were unimproved while receiving treatment with antidepressants are unlikely to respond and should have their treatment changed. If there was absolutely no change in the patients' by 4 weeks, there was very little chance of their improving. Patients who minimally improve at some point should continue with their treatment for at least 5 weeks and patients whose conditions minimally improve should continue for 6 weeks. At each of these points, patients receiving the drug continued to have a better prognosis than those receiving the placebo.

Using data prospectively collected during the 17-year National Institute of Mental Health Collaborative Program on the Psychobiology of Depression, **Mueller et al** (page 794) report the course of illness in patients who had been sick depressed for 5 years. Slightly over one third recovered from their depression in the next 5 years. The patients who recovered tended to be married and have a briefer illness before they entered the study. Their recovery occurred despite modest levels of drug therapy.

Imidazoline receptors appear to interact with monoamine neurotransmitter systems in the brain. **García-Sevilla et al** (page 803), using immunoblotting techniques to quantitate imidazoline receptor proteins, found that the densities of some of these proteins (35 and 45 kd) are increased in blood platelets of depressed patients and in the brains of suicide victims. Antidepressant treatment was associated with clinical response, and a reduced density of up-regulated 45-kd platelet imidazoline receptors in depressed patients. This study may support a role for imidazoline receptors in the pathogenesis of major depression.

Although electroconvulsive therapy (ECT) produces marked changes in brain electrical activity, the time course of these effects and their relationships to efficacy and side effects are uncertain. In patients with major depression, **Sackeim et al** (page 814) examined global and regional changes in electroencephalographic activity at various time points during and following ECT. Effective forms of ECT were characterized by a marked increase in delta power in prefrontal regions, and this change was associated with the magnitude of symptomatic improvement. These findings suggest that the transient induction of slow-wave activity in prefrontal regions is associated with the antidepressant effects of ECT.

(A Commentary on ECT by Jan Volavka, MD, PhD and Pal Czobar, PhD, is also included in this issue.)

Duval et al (page 833) present the results of a battery of thyroid function tests in depressed inpatients; these tests were carried out at baseline and again after 1 month of antidepressant treatment. They found that changes in thyroid function accompany clinical recovery and are not a direct effect of the antidepressant drug. Thus, serial thyroid function tests may provide the practicing clinician with an objective means of assessing antidepressant treatment response.

Some patients with clinical depression do not respond to standard treatment with tricyclic drugs. Eight controlled studies tested whether these patients' improve when thyroid hormone is added to their tricyclic drug regimen. These studies apparently contradicted each other. However, in a meta-analysis study by **Aronson et al** (page 842), it appeared that thyroid hormone doubles the response rate and improves depression scores. Fewer than 300 patients were studied in total, and the scientific quality of the studies varied. The use of thyroid hormone augmentation should, be reexamined in much larger trials using newer selective serotonin reuptake inhibitor drugs.

Maintenance Therapy for Chronic Depression

A Controlled Clinical Trial of Desipramine

James H. Kocsis, MD; Richard A. Friedman, MD; John C. Markowitz, MD; Andrew C. Leon, PhD; Nina L. Miller, MA; Leah Gniwesch, MA; Michael Parides, MS

Background: Previous studies have shown the efficacy of antidepressants in the treatment of chronic depression. We report the results of a long-term study comparing desipramine hydrochloride and placebo for maintenance therapy of remitted patients with chronic depression.

Methods: Outpatients who met *DSM-III-R* diagnostic criteria for "pure" dysthymia (n=51), dysthymia with current major depression ("double depression") (n=64), or chronic major depression (n=14) were treated on an open basis with desipramine. Full and partial remitters after 10 weeks entered a continuation phase of open treatment with desipramine for 16 weeks. Remitted patients then were randomized to continue desipramine treatment or tapered to placebo treatment for a maintenance phase of up to 2 years. Relapse rates and time to relapse during maintenance therapy were compared between the two treatment groups.

Results: Acute-phase treatment results did not differ significantly according to chronic depression subtype. Remission persisted with a high degree of stability during the continuation phase. Relapse rates during the maintenance phase were 52% for the placebo group and 11% for the active desipramine group (χ^2=8.1, *P*=.004). Most placebo relapses occurred during the first 6 months of maintenance therapy. Active medication was significantly more effective than placebo in that subgroup entering the maintenance phase in full remission and in those patients who fulfilled criteria for a diagnosis of pure dysthymia or double depression on entry to the study.

Conclusion: Long-term maintenance treatment with desipramine appeared to be effective in the prevention or postponement of relapse of depression in patients who responded to desipramine during the acute and continuation phases.

Arch Gen Psychiatry. 1996;53:769-774

PHARMACOTHERAPY of chronic and lifelong depressive states has gained great interest in recent years. Many patients formerly regarded as having personality disorders or neuroses have now been reconceptualized as having affective disorders responsive to medication. Several published short-term, controlled clinical trials have confirmed the efficacy of antidepressant drugs for chronic depression.[1-7] In research settings it has become conventional to subclassify chronic depression according to course and severity using *DSM-III-R*[8] criteria for dysthymia and major depression. Thus, mild depression of insidious onset persisting for longer than 2 years is called "pure dysthymia." Unremitting major depression persisting for at least 2 years is "chronic major depression." Finally, dysthymia punctuated by one or more episodes of major depression is called "double depression."[9] These distinctions now have been further codified in a section on course specifiers for mood disorders in *DSM-IV*. Tricyclic antidepressants,[1-5] selective serotonin reuptake inhibitors,[4,6] serotonin-2 receptor antagonists,[5,7] and a reversible inhibitor of monoamine oxidase[3] have now demonstrated efficacy in the short-term treatment of patients who have diagnoses of double depression,[1] pure dysthymia,[2,4,5,6] or both.[3,7] In general, the response rates have been similar for these two subtypes of chronic depression. Some of these investigations have revealed improvement not only in depressive symptoms, but also in social and vocational functioning.[10,11]

While short-term improvement is important, dysthymia and double depres-

See Methods on next page

From the Department of Psychiatry, New York Hospital–Cornell Medical Center, New York.

METHODS

SUBJECTS

Subjects were selected from responders to advertisements for chronic depression and patients seeking treatment for depression at a psychiatric outpatient clinic. After preliminary telephone screening, potential subjects were given Structured Clinical Interview for *DSM-III-R*[14] interviews by research assistants (N.L.M., L.G.). To be included in the study, patients had to meet *DSM-III-R* criteria for dysthymia with or without current major depression or major depression–chronic subtype and sign an informed consent form. Subjects were excluded if they had a diagnosis of schizophrenia, current substance abuse or dependence, a history of mania or definite hypomania, any severe or chronic medical illness, or medical contraindication to desipramine. All subjects met the *DSM-III-R* criteria for dysthymia and/or major depression of the primary type.

Formal training and testing of Structured Clinical Interview for *DSM-III-R* interviewers for interrater reliability on diagnosis of chronic depression subtypes was conducted as a part of a *DSM-IV* field trial. Details are published elsewhere.[15] Interrater κ statistics were obtained for lifetime dysthymia (0.81), current major depression (0.72), and chronic major depression (0.40). A random subsample of 59 cases also underwent an assessment of personality disorders. They were interviewed by trained raters using the Personality Disorder Examination.[16]

At baseline we also systematically asked about and recorded data on prior psychiatric treatment with medications and psychotherapy.

TREATMENT AND DOSING

Acute Phase

Treatment with desipramine hydrochloride was begun at 25 mg twice a day and was increased according to a set schedule up to 200 mg/d, unless troublesome side effects occurred. Plasma drug concentrations were determined after a stable dose had been achieved for at least 1 week. If the clinical response was deemed unsatisfactory or problematic side effects arose, the doses were adjusted, guided by plasma levels. The recommended range of therapeutic desipramine plasma concentrations was 563 to 1126 nmol/L. Ratings as described below were conducted biweekly for up to 12 weeks. Patients who remitted entered the continuation phase; nonresponders were dropped from the study. An attempt was made to switch to once a day evening dosing by the end of the acute phase. Study therapists were trained in the clinical management of desipramine treatment using the clinical management manual developed by the NIMH Treatment of Depression Collaborative Research Program.[17] Patients were allowed to remain in stable long-term psychotherapy during the study but not to enter into new psychotherapy arrangements. Concomitant use of psychotropic medications was prohibited.

Continuation Phase

The continuation phase lasted 16 weeks. Treatment with desipramine was continued at the final dose achieved during the acute phase. Subjects were seen and rated every 2 weeks. If remission persisted during the continuation phase, they were eligible for the maintenance phase. Patients who relapsed were dropped from the study.

sion by definition are chronic conditions. The patients treated by Kocsis et al[1] and Hellerstein et al[6] reported persistent depressive symptoms of mean durations of 19 and 20 years, respectively. Therefore, the response to longer-term therapy is obviously crucial for these disorders. To date, we know of only a single small pilot study that has examined continuation therapy with a placebo-controlled design.[12] In that study, 12 patients who met *DSM-III* criteria for dysthymic disorder, seven of whom had concurrent major depression, remitted after 6 weeks of phenelzine treatment and were randomly assigned to continue treatment with active medication (n=5) or switch to placebo (n=7). All patients in the placebo group but only one in the phenelzine group relapsed, a statistically significant difference.

See also pages 775 and 777

We have now conducted and herein report the results of the first study, to our knowledge, of long-term maintenance treatment undertaken in patients with chronic depression. The design was similar to that of the National Institute of Mental Health (NIMH) Collaborative Study on Maintenance Pharmacotherapy of Recurrent Depression.[13] It consisted of acute and continuation treatment using desipramine hydrochloride, followed by a maintenance treatment phase during which responders were randomized to either desipramine treatment or placebo. We hypothesized that desipramine would prevent relapse and delay time to relapse in comparison with placebo.

RESULTS

DEMOGRAPHIC AND CLINICAL CHARACTERISTICS

Of 129 subjects entering the study, 51 (40%) met criteria for pure dysthymia, 64 (50%) for double depression, and 14 (10%) for chronic major depression. The ethnic/racial composition of the sample was 88% white, 6% black, 4% Hispanic, and 4% Asian. Other pretreatment demographic and clinical characteristics are shown in Table 1. The typical patient was an employed, well-educated, unmarried woman in her 30s. There were no significant differences on clinical or demographic variables between the double depression and chronic major depression groups except for age at onset. The double depression group reported onset of symptoms at an earlier age. The pure dysthy-

Maintenance Phase

During the first month of maintenance treatment, the patients were given packets containing daily doses of medication. Subjects in the desipramine group continued the same dose throughout. Subjects in the placebo group were tapered by approximately 25% per week over the month and then received identical placebo at the same dose equivalent for the next 23 months or until relapse. Subjects were seen and rated each month during the maintenance phase.

RATINGS AND ASSESSMENTS

The clinician-rated measures of depressive symptoms and severity were the 24-item version of the Hamilton Depression Rating Scale (HAM-D)[18] and the Global Assessment Scale (GAS).[19] Intraclass correlation coefficients computed from conjoint rating sessions were .93 for the HAM-D total score and .89 for the GAS score.

A self-rated measure of social impairment and function, the Social Adjustment Scale–Self-rated[20] was completed at the beginning and end of each phase of the study.

DEFINITIONS OF REMISSION

Full remission was defined as HAM-D scores less than 7 and GAS scores greater than 70 on three consecutive biweekly ratings. Partial remission was defined as at least a 50% reduction from the baseline HAM-D score, HAM-D scores ranging from 7 to 12, and GAS scores of 60 or greater on three successive ratings.

DEFINITION AND MANAGEMENT OF RELAPSE

Suspected relapse occurred when a HAM-D score rose above 12 during the maintenance phase. Clinicians discussed and encouraged compliance and obtained a plasma drug level, which was reviewed by a nonblind observer (J.H.K.) who was not involved in the treatment. The nonblind observer gave instructions or dummy instructions for dosage adjustments. Relapse was defined as HAM-D scores greater than 12 and GAS scores below 60 on three successive ratings over a period of 4 weeks *or* at least one rating meeting these criteria and an urgent need for alternative treatment for a depressive syndrome.

DATA ANALYSIS

Comparisons between those patients receiving desipramine and those receiving placebo on baseline demographic and clinical variables (**Table 1**) were made using χ^2 tests (with Yates' correction where applicable) for qualitative variables and *t* tests or Wilcoxon tests for quantitative variables. These same variables were examined for differences by depressive subtype using χ^2 tests and analysis of variance procedures.

Outcome was considered both as the presence or absence of relapse and as the time to relapse. Relapse rates were compared using the χ^2 test with Yates' correction. Kaplan-Meier estimates of the probability of remaining in remission over the course of the maintenance phase were computed and plotted as survival curves (**Figure**). The log-rank test was used to compare curves between the desipramine and placebo groups, both for the full sample and separately for strata defined by continuation-phase outcome (full or partial remission). In addition, the effect of potential confounding variables on the relation between medication group and relapse was assessed using a Cox proportional-hazards model. All the tests were conducted at the .05 level and were two tailed.

mia group had significantly less pathology on the HAM-D and Social Adjustment Scale–Self-rated than the double depression group.

Fifty-eight subjects had received prior treatment with antidepressant medication, 64 had not, and seven gave no information. Of those who had received prior treatment, 28 had trials that were judged to be adequate (ie, 150 mg/d of imipramine hydrochloride, 20 mg/d of fluoxetine hydrochloride or the equivalent for a period of at least 3 weeks), whereas the remainder had either inadequate or unknown amounts of antidepressant medication. Thus, only 22% of the overall sample had had a previous adequate treatment by history.

Seventy-seven subjects (60% of the sample) reported having received at least weekly psychotherapy for periods longer than 6 months. Twenty-one (16%) had no previous psychotherapy, whereas the remainder had received either brief periods of therapy or therapy of unknown duration.

RESPONSE IN THE ACUTE AND CONTINUATION PHASES

During the acute phase, 105 patients (81%) completed treatment, while 24 (19%) did not. Of the completers, 43 (41%) fully remitted, 23 (22%) partially remitted, and 39 (37%) were nonresponsive. Reasons for dropout included side effects of desipramine (n=11), noncompliance (n=11), and administrative decision (n=2). Rates of response and dropout did not differ significantly across diagnostic subgroups. Response rates based on intention to treat are shown in **Table 2**. Subgroups with and without personality disorders, and with and without anxiety disorders, also did not differ significantly in acute-phase outcomes. The mean (±SD) dosage of desipramine hydrochloride during the acute phase was 227±70 mg/d. The dose range was 50 to 325 mg/d. The mean (±SD) drug plasma concentration was 653±394 nmol/L.

Full (n=43) and partial (n=23) remitters entered the continuation phase. The outcome of this phase is shown in **Table 3**. Six subjects did not complete this phase. Fifty (83%) of the 60 patients who completed the continuation phase did not change in outcome status, whereas three full remitters became partial remitters, seven partial remitters became full remitters, and one partial remitter relapsed. The mean desipramine hydrochloride dosage during the continuation phase was 232±72 mg/d (range, 75 to 350 mg/d). The mean desipramine plasma concentration was 766±409 nmol/L.

Table 1. Pretreatment Demographic and Clinical Characteristics by Chronic Depression Subtype*

Characteristic	Pure Dysthymia (n=51)	Double Depression (n=64)	Chronic Major Depression (n=14)
Age, y (mean±SD)	37±10	37±9	36±11
Female, %	51	61	64
Currently married, %	18	9	14
Age at onset, y (mean±SD)†	14±8	11±6	15±6
HAM-D total score (mean±SD)‡	19±5	24±8	23±6
GAS score (mean±SD)	56±4	55±7	55±6
SAS-SR total score§	2.3±0.4	2.7±0.5	2.5±0.5
Axis II disorder, %‖	48	63	33
Anxiety disorder, %¶	42	21	39

*HAM-D indicates Hamilton Depression Rating Scale; GAS, Global Assessment Scale; and SAS-SR, Social Adjusment Scale–Self-rated.
†F=3.85, P=.02; Duncan's Multiple Range test (pure dysthmia=chronic major depression >double depression).
‡F=8.98, P<.001 (double depression > pure dysthymia).
§F=8.66, P<.001 (double depression > pure dysthymia).
‖Based on pure dysthymia, n=23; double depression, n=27; and chronic major depression, n=9.
¶Based on pure dysthymia, n=36; double depression, n=38; and chronic major depression, n=13.

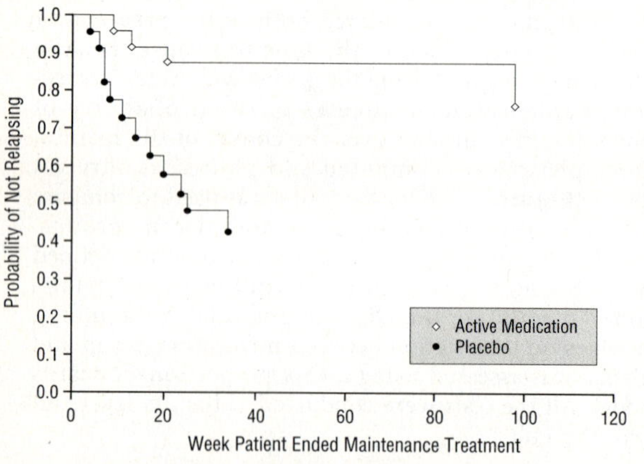

Time to relapse by treatment for all subjects, χ^2 (1 df)=8.43, P=.004.

RESPONSE DURING MAINTENANCE PHASE

Seven eligible patients refused randomization. Three (one in the desipramine group and two in the placebo group) terminated participation in the first month following randomization. Of 53 patients entering maintenance treatment, 28 were randomized to continue desipramine treatment and 25 were randomized to taper to placebo. **Table 4** shows maintenance-phase results for the 50 patients completing at least 1 month, by remitter status and treatment. The relapse rate was significantly higher in the placebo group and significantly greater for placebo both for the overall sample and the full remitter subgroup alone. Figure 1 shows survival curves for the two treatments for all the subjects. Assuming the hazard is proportional, those patients receiving placebo are 3.9 times as likely to relapse as those receiving desipramine, P=.01 based on a normal approximation test (95% confidence interval, 1.4 to 10.9).

The relapse rates did not differ significantly across chronic depressive diagnoses at baseline. Other baseline demographic and clinical variables shown in Table 1 also did not significantly differ between those who entered the maintenance phase and those who did not. Eleven patients randomized to desipramine treatment and 10 assigned to placebo were in stable long-term psychotherapy during the study, a nonsignificant difference. We conducted survival analyses incorporating covariates to assess the effects of potential confounding variables affecting outcome in the maintenance phase. Concomitant psychotherapy, age at onset of depression, HAM-D score at the beginning of maintenance treatment, and dose of desipramine were the variables tested. The increased risk for relapse for patients receiving placebo relative to those receiving desipramine was negligibly affected by each of the covariates.

COMMENT

To our knowledge, this is the first long-term controlled trial of maintenance antidepressant medication therapy for the prevention of relapse of chronic depression. Randomization to receive active medication vs placebo occurred following 26 weeks of treatment and at least 16 weeks of remission. The results showed that desipramine was more effective than placebo in preventing and postponing relapse of depressive symptoms during the maintenance phase in patients who had responded to desipramine during the acute and continuation phases of treatment.

Significant drug-placebo differences also emerged when the analysis was confined to the fully remitted subsample. Differences in maintenance-phase outcome were not due to inequivalence in remitter status at the beginning of maintenance. Similarly, the subtype of chronic depression at the beginning of treatment, ie, pure dysthymia, double depression, or chronic major depression, responded similarly to open desipramine treatment in the acute phase and was equally distributed in groups receiving active drug vs placebo in the maintenance phase. The results suggested that the three subtypes of chronic depression responded similarly to desipramine treatment in the acute, continuation, and maintenance phases. Although the number of patients with chronic major depression was small, the proportion with full remission, partial remission, and nonre-

Table 2. Acute-Phase Outcome by Chronic Depression Subtype

Outcome	Pure Dysthymia (n=51)	Double Depression (n=64)	Chronic Major Depression (n=14)	Total (N=129)
Completed, %	80	84	71	81
Full remission	37	31	29	33
Partial remission	20	16	21	18
Nonresponsive	24	38	21	30
Dropout, %	20	16	29	19

Table 3. Continuation-Phase Outcome by Remission Status After Acute Phase

Outcome	Acute-Phase Full Remitter, No. (n=43)	Acute-Phase Partial Remitter, No. (n=23)
Full remission	37	7
Partial remission	3	13
Nonresponsive	0	1
Dropout	3	2

sponse to acute-phase treatment was similar to the other two groups. Larger samples will be required to confidently define medication response rates in this subgroup.

Some potential limitations of the design and methods of the study deserve comment. Greenhouse et al[21] have suggested a number of possible problems with the classic design of maintenance therapy trials employed in this study. These include the possibility that sudden discontinuation of effective treatment may lead to a drug withdrawal reaction that precipitates an episode of depression. We tapered active drug over a 4-week period. It is possible that a slower taper could lead to a lower relapse rate after drug discontinuation.

A second criticism of this design is that it is likely that the best maintenance therapy is what an individual responds to during acute treatment. This design is biased against maintenance treatments other than desipramine. The alternative design proposed by Greenhouse et al[21] would be to randomize patients to both active drug and placebo in the acute phase and to rerandomize responders in the maintenance phase. However, this would be impractical for disorders such as chronic depression, which have documented low placebo response rates.[1,6]

A third possible limitation in the present study was the absence of independent raters. Ratings were done by study clinicians who may have been able to guess the maintenance treatment based on side effects. This issue has been well reviewed recently by Basoglu et al (personal communication) who pointed out that double-blind procedures do not guarantee rater blindness, but that unblinding need not always affect ratings of outcome. Unfortunately, we do not have data from the current study to address these issues. Assessment of rater guesses and the effect on ratings of outcome was not done. Such assessment is recommended for future studies in this area.

The data collected on prior psychiatric treatment in this sample of chronically depressed patients responsive to desipramine treatment deserve comment. Similar to our previous findings in a separate sample of patients,[1] we found considerable prior exposure to psychotherapy and a rather low prevalence of prior adequate antidepressant medication trials. Thus, although chronically depressed, this was not a treatment refractory group. The selection of psychotherapy as a previous treatment may have reflected biases of either patients or clinicians to view these symptoms as characterologic rather than affective in nature.

Table 4. Maintenance-Phase Results by Remission Status After Continuation Phase

Group	N	% Relapse
Full remission*	40	
Desipramine hydrochloride	22	14
Placebo	18	56
Partial remission	10	
Desipramine	5	20
Placebo	5	40
Total†	**50**	
Desipramine	27	15
Placebo	23	52

*$\chi^2=6.1$, *P*=.01.
†$\chi^2=6.3$, *P*=.01.

Results of the acute and continuation phases of treatment of this study have been previously reported in detail.[22-24] The main conclusions were that (1) response rates have been somewhat lower than those reported in other open and controlled studies of other antidepressant medication in pure dysthymia and double depression; (2) the acute-phase results did not differ significantly according to chronic depression subtype; (3) comorbidity as documented, consisted mainly of anxiety and personality disorders, which did not significantly influence acute-phase treatment response; and (4) remission was stable during the continuation phase. It was interesting that gradual improvement, rather than deterioration, was the most frequent change during continuation. Almost one third of the partial remitters entering the continuation phase fully remitted by the end of that phase.

If the maintenance-phase results are replicated and expanded in larger samples of patients with chronic depression treated with antidepressant medication, a major advance in clinical treatment of chronic depression will have been realized. From a practical standpoint, the 52% relapse rate seen during maintenance with placebo can be used by clinicians to set guidelines for patients who wish to discontinue taking medication after 4 months of remission. Such patients will have about a 50% chance of relapse in the first 6 months after treatment is stopped. Retreatment of the relapses with desipramine has thus far yielded excellent results.[25] From a theoretical standpoint, the sharp distinction between active drug and placebo for prevention of relapse supports the validity of an affective diagnosis and responsiveness to pharmacotherapy.

Future work must also focus on those who do not respond to antidepressant treatment. Studies that compare or cross patients over to other medications, as well as studies of psychotherapy[26,27] alone and in combination with pharmacotherapy, may yield useful strategies for clinicians treating these difficult cases.

Accepted for publication May 31, 1995.

This work was supported by a grant from the National Institute of Mental Health, Rockville, Md (R01-MH37103).

Desipramine (Norpramin) and matching placebo were provided by Marion Merrill Dow Inc, Kansas City, Mo.

Reprint requests to New York Hospital, Box 147, 525 E 68th St, New York, NY 10021 (Dr Kocsis).

REFERENCES

1. Kocsis JH, Frances AJ, Voss CB, Mann JJ, Mason BJ, Sweeney J. Imipramine treatment for chronic depression. *Arch Gen Psychiatry.* 1988;45:253-257.
2. Stewart JW, McGrath PJ, Quitkin FM. Relevance of *DSM-III* depressive subtype and chronicity of antidepressant efficacy in atypical depression. *Arch Gen Psychiatry.* 1989;46:1080-1087.
3. Versiani M. Pharmacotherapy of dsythymia: a controlled study with imipramine, moclobemide or placebo. *Neuropsychopharmacology.* 1994;10(3S):298.
4. Kocsis JH, Thase M, Koran L, Halbreich U, Yonkers K. Pharmacothereapy of pure dysthymia: sertraline vs imipramine and placebo. *Eur Neuropsychopharmacol (Suppl).* 1994;4:204.
5. Bakish D, Lapierre YD, Weinstein R, Klein J, Wiens A, Jones B, Horn E, Browne M, Bourget O, Blanchard A. Ritanserin, imipramine and placebo in the treatment of dysthymic disorder. *J Clin Psychopharmacol.* 1993;13:409-414.
6. Hellerstein D, Yanowitch P, Rosenthal J. A randomized double-blind study of fluoxetine versus placebo in treatment of dysthymia. *Am J Psychiatry.* 1993; 150:1169-1175.
7. Bersani G, Pozzi F, Marini S, Grispini A, Pasini A, Ciani N. 5-HT_2 receptor antagonism in dysthymia disorder: a double-blind placebo controlled study with ritanserin. *Acta Psychiatr Scand.* 1991;83:244-248.
8. American Psychiatric Association. *Diagnostic and Statistical Manual of Mental Disorders, Revised Third Edition.* Washington, DC: American Psychiatric Association; 1987.
9. Keller MB, Shapiro RW. 'Double-depression': superimposition of acute depressive episodes on chronic depressive disorders. *Am J Psychiatry.* 1982;139: 438-442.
10. Kocsis JH, Frances AJ, Voss D, Mason BJ, Mann JJ. Imipramine and social vocational adjustment in chronic depression. *Am J Psychiatry.* 1988;145:997-999.
11. Stewart JW, Quitkin FM, McGrath PJ, Rabkin JG, Markowitz JS, Tricamo E, Klein DF. Social functioning in chronic depression: 6 weeks of antidepressant treatment. *Psychiatry Res.* 1988;25:213-222.
12. Harrison W, Rabkin J, Stewart JW. Phenelzine for chronic depression: a study of continuation treatment. *J Clin Psychiatry.* 1986;47:346-349.
13. Prien RF, Kupfer DJ, Mansky PA, Small JG, Tuason VB, Voss CB, Johnson WE. Drug therapy in the prevention of recurrences in unipolar and bipolar affective disorders. *Arch Gen Psychiatry.* 1984;41:1096.
14. Spitzer RL, Williams JBW. *Structured Clinical Interview for* DSM-III-R*-Patient Version (SCID-P).* New York: Biometrics Research Department, New York State Psychiatric Institute; 1985.
15. Keller MB, Klein DN, Hirschfeld RMA, Kocsis JH, McCullough JP, Miller I, First MB, Holzer CP, Keitner GI, Marin DB, Shea T. *DSM-IV* mood disorders field trial investigation results. *Am J Psychiatry.* 1995;152:843-849.
16. Loranger AW. *Personality Disorder Examination.* White Plains, NY: The New York Hospital–Cornell Medical Center; 1988.
17. Fawcett J, Epstein P, Fiester SJ, Elkin I, Autry JH. Clinical management: imipramine/placebo administration manual. *Psychopharmacol Bull.* 1987;23: 309-324.
18. Hamilton M. A rating scale for depression. *J Neurol Neurosurg Psychiatry.* 1960;25:56-62.
19. Endicott J, Spitzer RL, Fleiss JL, Cohen J. The Global Assessment Scale: a procedure for measuring the overall severity of psychiatric disturbance. *Arch Gen Psychiatry.* 1976;33:767-771.
20. Weissman MM, Prusoff BA, Thompson WD, Harding P, Myers K. Social adjustment by self-report in a community sample and in psychiatric outpatients. *J Nerv Ment Dis.* 1978;166:317-326.
21. Greenhouse JB, Stangl D, Kupfer DJ, Prien RF. Methodologic issues in maintenance therapy clinical trials. *Arch Gen Psychiatry.* 1991;48:313-318.
22. Kocsis JH. Chronic depression-pharmacotherapy studies. In: Akiskal HS, ed. *Chronic Depressions and Their Treatment.* New York, NY: Guilford Press. In press.
23. Marin DB, Kocsis JH, Frances AJ, Parides M. Desipramine for the treatment of 'pure' dysthymia versus 'double' depression. *Am J Psychiatry.* 1994;151:1079-1080.
24. Kocsis JH, Friedman RA, Markowitz JC, Miller N, Gniwesch L, Bram J. Stability of remission during tricyclic antidepressant continuation therapy for dysthymia. *Psychopharmacol Bull.* 1995;31:213-216.
25. Friedman RA, Mitchell J, Kocsis JH. Retreatment of relapse following desipramine discontinuation in dysthymia. *Am J Psychiatry.* 1995;152:926-928.
26. Markowitz JC. Psychotherapy of dysthymia. *Am J Psychiatry.* 1994;151:1114-1121.
27. Markowitz JC. Psychotherapy of the post-dysthymic patient. *J Psychother Pract Res.* 1993;2:157-163.

Conversions From Système International (SI) Units to Traditional Units (Modified From *The SI Manual in Health Care*)

System	Component	SI Reference Interval*	SI Unit	Conversion Factor (Divide by)	Traditional Reference Interval*	Traditional Unit
Plasma	Desipramine, therapeutic	170-700	nmol/L	3.754	50-200	ng/mL

**These reference values are not intended to be definitive since each laboratory determines its own values. They are provided for illustration only.*

COMMENTARY

Maintenance Therapy for Chronic Depression

A Controlled Clinical Trial of Desipramine

In this issue of the Archives, Kocsis et al[1] present the results of their study on maintenance treatment for chronic depression. This study is an important sequel to their equally important earlier demonstration that patients with various forms of chronic depression do, indeed, respond to appropriate pharmacotherapy.[2] With the publication of these results, we now also have evidence that the vast majority of responders to pharmacotherapy remain well when they receive the maintenance pharmacotherapy. These results nicely parallel the earlier findings of Prien et al[3] and Frank et al[4] with respect to maintenance treatment of recurrent depression.

In their present report on maintenance outcomes, Kocsis et al[1] also discuss the "low" response rates to acute-phase pharmacotherapy in this population. There are several plausible explanations for the response rates obtained in the acute phase of their trial. First, Kocsis and colleagues chose the most stringent definition of *full remission,* commonly used in the last decade (ie, Hamilton Depression Rating Scale [HAM-D] score ≤6 and Global Assessment Scale score >70). They also required that the patient maintain this level of remission over the course of six biweekly assessments. What this means is that to be considered a full responder in this trial, patients had to achieve a HAM-D score of 6 or less by week 6 of the acute phase of treatment and maintain it for the subsequent 6 weeks of the acute-phase treatment. In the acute phase of our maintenance therapies in recurrent depression trial,[4] we allowed patients up to 24 weeks to achieve somewhat less stringent remission criteria (HAM-D score ≤7 sustained for 3 weeks) and, indeed, found that only about one third of patients were able to do so in the first 8 weeks of the trial. Although the authors view it as "surprising" that gradual improvement was the most common experience in the continuation phase of treatment, this is really not the case. Given the limited amount of time that patients were allotted to achieve full remission, it seems entirely reasonable that many patients would have continued to improve in the continuation phase of treatment. It is also possible that the "low" response rate may be a result of relatively conservative dosing. The authors note that the average dose of desipramine among patients entering the continuation phase of treatment was 227 (±70) mg, with an average plasma desipramine level of only 174 ng/mL. Interestingly, among patients surviving the continuation phase and entering the maintenance phase of the trial, the average dose of desipramine was 232 (±72) mg and the average plasma desipramine level was 204 (±109) ng/mL. This is at least suggestive of the possibility that response rates might have been higher and better sustained had some of the patients receiving lower doses, and particularly having lower plasma desipramine levels, been maintained on somewhat more aggressive regimen.

The question of whether all patients received fully adequate dosing during acute and continuation phases of treatment may also relate to the authors' finding of better outcomes in those achieving full remission. It may be that the partial responders were, in fact, only partially treated and, thus, were more vulnerable to relapse in the maintenance phase of the trial.

See also pages 769 and 777

At the end of their "Results" section, Kocsis and colleagues[1] provide us with information about the relationship of several covariates of outcome in their maintenance trial. They examine the relationship of concomitant psychotherapy, age at onset of depression, baseline HAM-D score, and desipramine dose to survival time in the maintenance phase of treatment. They note that "the increased risk of relapse for patients receiving placebo . . . was negligibly affected by each variable." It seems likely, however, that power was inadequate for a fair test of the relationship of these covariates to outcome. Furthermore, the issue of dose as a covariate within the actively treated group was not explored. Here power would undoubtedly have been low, but it does raise the important question of whether lower dose was associated with an increased risk of relapse in case of active medication. It also raises the question of whether lower plasma desipramine levels were associated with increased risk of relapse.

One question that the authors do not address is the issue of medication adherence. In our long-term maintenance trial of patients with recurrent unipolar depression, we observed only 12 recurrences in patients receiving active medication.[4] Among those 12 recurrences, we found that seven could be classified as "clearly noncompliant" on the basis of variability in levels of dose ratios over time.[5] In contrast, we found that only 1.5% of the patients surviving the full 3 years of our active-medication trial could be classified as clearly noncompliant.

As Greenhouse et al[6] would predict, most placebo relapses were early in the maintenance-phase treatment. Given the very long-standing illness of many of these patients, we think it reasonable to raise the question of whether this is a function of the study population, of the design of the trial, or some combination of the two. It is also possible that had patients been treated for a somewhat longer time prior to randomization, the placebo relapses might have not occurred so precipitously. In our study of patients with recurrent depression, the average patient had been ill a median of 16 weeks prior to the initiation of the acute-phase treatment and, while the average patient spent approximately the same amount of time as the patients in the trial of Kocsis et al, in the acute-phase treatment, for many patients it took considerably longer to stabilize and, thus, they had longer acute phases of treatment. In addition, their continuation-phase treatment was a total of 20 weeks, compared with the 16 weeks in the trial of Kocsis et al.

One of the most interesting aspects of the findings of Kocsis et al is that there does appear to be a sizable subgroup of patients with very long histories of dysthymia, double depression, or chronic depression who are able to remain well once medication is withdrawn. As the authors themselves note, a large replication trial is indicated before these findings can be considered definitive; however, a particularly important aim of such a replication trial would be to identify that subgroup of chronically depressed individuals who are able to remain well following medication discontinuation.

One final point: As the authors themselves point out, their study does not address the potential role of psychotherapy, particularly any of the depression-specific psychotherapies, in the treatment of the various forms of chronic depression. Future studies in this quite psychosocially impaired population should clearly address the role that psychotherapy may have to play as either a stand-alone or adjunctive treatment for such patients.

David J. Kupfer, MD
Ellen Frank, PhD
Department of Psychiatry
University of Pittsburgh School of Medicine
Western Psychiatric Institute and Clinic
3811 O'Hara St
Pittsburgh, PA 15213

This work was supported by the following National Institute of Mental Health grants: MH-29618 (Drs Frank and Kupfer), MH-49115 (Dr Frank), and MH-30915 (Dr Kupfer).

REFERENCES

1. Kocsis JH, Friedman RA, Markowitz JC, Leon AC, Miller NL, Gniwesch L, Parides M. Maintenance therapy for chronic depression: a controlled clinical trial of desipramine. *Arch Gen Psychiatry.* 1996; 53:769-774.
2. Kocsis JH, Frances AJ, Voss CB, Mann JJ, Mason BJ, Sweeney J. Imipramine treatment for chronic depression. *Arch Gen Psychiatry.* 1988; 45:253-257.
3. Prien RF, Kupfer DJ, Mansky PA, Small JG, Tuason VB, Voss CB, Johnson WE. Drug therapy in the prevention of recurrences in unipolar and bipolar affective disorders: report of the NIMH Collaborative Study Group. *Arch Gen Psychiatry.* 1984;41:1096-1104.
4. Frank E, Kupfer DJ, Perel JM, Cornes CL, Jarrett D, Mallinger A, Thase M, McEachran AB, Grochocinski VJ. Three-year outcomes for maintenance therapies in recurrent depression. *Arch Gen Psychiatry.* 1990;47:1093-1099.
5. Frank E, Perel JM, Malinger AG, Thase ME, Kupfer DJ. Relationship of pharmacologic compliance to long-term prophylaxis in recurrent depression. *Psychopharm Bull.* 1992;28:231-235.
6. Greenhouse JB, Stangl D, Kupfer DJ, Prien RF. Methodologic issues in maintenance therapy clinical trials. *Arch Gen Psychiatry.* 1991;48:313-318.

ORIGINAL ARTICLE

A Placebo-Controlled, Randomized Clinical Trial Comparing Sertraline and Imipramine for the Treatment of Dysthymia

Michael E. Thase, MD; Maurizio Fava, MD; Uriel Halbreich, MD; James H. Kocsis, MD; Lorrin Koran, MD; Jonathan Davidson, MD, Jerrold Rosenbaum, MD, Wilma Harrison, MD

Background: Despite the high prevalence of dysthymia and its associated morbidity, few controlled trials have evaluated the efficacy of antidepressant medication for this disorder. A 12-week, double-blind, placebo-controlled, randomized, multicenter trial was performed to evaluate the safety and efficacy of sertraline hydrochloride and imipramine hydrochloride in treating dysthymia.

Methods: A total of 416 outpatients (271 women and 145 men) aged 25 to 65 years with *DSM-III-R*–defined, early-onset, primary dysthymia without concurrent major depression were randomized to 12 weeks of treatment with sertraline, imipramine, or placebo.

Results: Both active treatments resulted in significantly reduced scores on the 17-item Hamilton Rating Scale for Depression ($P=.04$ and $P=.01$ for sertraline and imipramine vs placebo, respectively), the Montgomery-Asberg Depression Rating Scale ($P=.01$ and $P=.003$ vs placebo, respectively), Hopkins Symptom Checklist ($P<.05$), and the self-rated version of the Inventory of Depressive Symptoms ($P<.05$). With the use of a Clinical Global Impressions improvement score of 1 or 2 (very much or much improved) to define response, response rates were 59% for sertraline, 64% for imipramine, and 44% for placebo ($P=.02$ for sertraline vs placebo and $P<.001$ for imipramine vs placebo). A significantly greater proportion of patients receiving imipramine than those receiving sertraline or placebo discontinued treatment because of adverse events ($P=.001$ and $P<.001$, respectively).

Conclusions: Pharmacotherapy provides considerable relief from the symptoms of dysthymia in patients suffering from this chronic affective disorder, with both sertraline and imipramine being more effective than placebo. The greater tolerability of sertraline is an important consideration because of the chronicity of dysthymia, which may require prolonged treatment with antidepressant medication.

Arch Gen Psychiatry. 1996;53:777-784

From the Department of Psychiatry, University of Pittsburgh (Pa) School of Medicine (Dr Thase); Depression Research Program, Massachusetts General Hospital, Boston (Drs Fava and Rosenbaum); Department of Psychiatry, State University of New York at Buffalo (Dr Halbreich); Department of Psychiatry, New York (NY) Hospital–Cornell Medical Center (Dr Kocsis); Department of Psychiatry, Stanford (Calif) University School of Medicine (Dr Koran); Department of Psychiatry and Behavioral Sciences, Duke University Medical Center, Durham, NC (Dr Davidson); Department of Psychiatry, Columbia University College of Physicians and Surgeons, New York, NY (Dr Harrison); and Pfizer Inc, New York, NY (Dr Harrison).

DYSTHYMIA IS a chronic form of mood disorder that affects 3% to 6% of the adult population of the United States[1,2] and as many as 36% of patients who seek treatment at psychiatric outpatient clinics.[3] The symptoms of dysthymia are less severe than those observed in patients with major depression, and hence dysthymia is often considered to be a disorder of subsyndromal intensity.[4] Nevertheless, patients with this disorder experience considerable social dysfunction and disability,[5,6] including an increased likelihood of not completing high school or college.[7] Dysthymics are also more likely than the general population to use general health services, and they are more likely to take nonspecific psychotropic drugs, such as minor tranquilizers and sedatives.[1]

Patients with dysthymia are also at risk for comorbidity: more than 75% of patients with dysthymia have coexisting psychiatric disorders, including anxiety disorders and substance abuse.[1] Approximately 40% of patients with dysthymia have coexisting major depression—a combination termed *double depression*.[1] Although such patients frequently recover from their major depression, their underlying dysthymia usually remains.[8] Untreated dysthymia rarely improves spontaneously over time,[9] and chronicity is one of the defining characteristics of the disorder.[1]

Dysthymia has historically been underrecognized and undertreated.[10-12] One study of psychiatric outpatients who met the *DSM-III* criteria for dysthymia found that a clinical diagnosis of dysthymia had been considered in less than half, and only 41% had received treatment with an adequate trial of antidepressant medica-

See Patients and Methods on next page

PATIENTS AND METHODS

PATIENTS

Patients were recruited from outpatient psychiatric clinics and through advertisements. Those eligible for study inclusion were psychiatric outpatients between the ages of 25 and 65 years who met *DSM-III-R* criteria for primary dysthymia with early onset (ie, onset occurring before age 21 years). The duration criterion for dysthymia was extended to at least 5 years, during which time patients must not have had a greater than 2-month period free of the symptoms of depression.

Pregnant or nursing women and women of childbearing age who were unwilling to use an effective contraceptive method were excluded. Other exclusion criteria included major medical conditions, bipolar disorder, psychosis, panic disorder, concurrent major depressive disorder, generalized anxiety disorder, history of alcohol or other drug dependency or abuse active within the last 6 months, serious suicidal risk, previous nonresponse to 2 or more adequate antidepressant trials, and use of psychotropic drugs within 2 weeks of enrollment.

STUDY DESIGN

The study was conducted at 17 university-affiliated research clinics in the United States. Eligible patients who gave written informed consent for participation underwent a 1-week single-blind placebo washout phase during which they completed Structured Clinical Interviews for *DSM-III-R* Axis I diagnoses[21] and for *DSM-III-R* personality disorders,[22] the Hamilton Rating Scale for Depression (HAM-D) (29-item version containing supplemental items to assess atypical depressive symptoms),[23] and the Clinical Global Impressions (CGI) scale.[24] The Structured Clinical Interviews and HAM-D ratings were performed by trained raters, and the CGI scale was completed by psychiatrists. Whenever possible, the same rater conducted baseline and follow-up ratings for each patient. Training sessions for raters were conducted before study initiation by means of videotapes, expert trainers, and written manuals. Videotaped patient interviews were independently rated by each study rater. Ratings were compared and discussed in an effort to obtain consistency and agreement in the use of the rating scales across facilities. Physical examinations, laboratory tests, and 12-lead electrocardiograms were also performed.

Patients who did not respond (CGI improvement rating of >2 or a HAM-D 29-item score >12) to placebo during washout were randomized to receive either sertraline, imipramine, or placebo for 12 weeks. Randomization was performed by a computer-generated schedule. The imipramine hydrochloride dose was increased weekly in 50-mg increments from 50 to 300 mg daily unless a therapeutic response was achieved or adverse effects were dose limiting. The sertraline hydrochloride dose was initiated at 50 mg and increased at the physician's discretion in 50-mg increments after 3 weeks at weeks 4, 6, and 7 to a maximum of 200 mg daily.

Efficacy was assessed by the HAM-D (17-item and 29-item) total score and by the change in HAM-D total score from baseline calculated by a week-by-week last observation carried forward method. Additional efficacy measures included the CGI ratings of severity and improvement, the Montgomery-Asberg Depression Rating Scale (MADRS),[25] the Hopkins Symptom Checklist (SCL-90),[26] and the Inventory for Depressive Symptomatology, self-report version (IDS-SR).[27,28] The HAM-D and CGI were repeated at the end of weeks 1 (CGI only), 2, 4, 6, 8, 10, and 12; the CGI was also repeated during an optional visit at week 7 for patients who did not have an adequate response by the end of week 6. The MADRS, Hopkins Symptom Checklist, and IDS-SR were repeated at the end of weeks 8 and 12. Psychosocial functioning was assessed with the Social Adjustment Scale, self-rated version,[29] and the Longitudinal Interval Scale Follow-up

tion.[3] As the persistent impact of the effects of dysthymia on patients' overall health and psychosocial functioning is increasingly acknowledged, so, too, is the importance of treating this disorder. Unfortunately, there has been surprisingly little systematic study of the efficacy of pharmacotherapy on dysthymia without coexisting major depression. Since major depression often spontaneously resolves without improvement of the underlying dysthymia in patients with double depression,[7] the results of treatment studies that include patients with double depression cannot be readily extended to patients with dysthymia alone.

See also pages 769 and 775

While the results of several studies have indicated that pharmacotherapy is effective in dysthymia,[13-18] these trials are limited by a number of factors, including small sample size, heterogeneity of patient sample (ie, no distinction between patients with early-onset and late-onset dysthymia, or patients with primary and secondary dysthymia), inclusion of patients with concomitant major depression, lack of placebo control, and inadequate duration or dosing of therapy.[7,19,20]

This 12-week, multicenter, randomized, placebo-controlled, double-blind, parallel study was designed to evaluate the efficacy and safety of the selective serotonin reuptake inhibitor (SSRI) sertraline hydrochloride and the tricyclic antidepressant imipramine hydrochloride in a large study group of patients with early-onset, primary *DSM-III-R*–defined dysthymia, ie, the most common subform of this disorder.[4] It includes the largest group studied to date of patients with dysthymia who do not have concurrent major depression. This trial therefore extends previous studies by assessing the efficacy of an SSRI and a tricyclic antidepressant in patients with "pure" dysthymia and by evaluating adequate doses of these medications taken for 12 weeks.

RESULTS

PATIENT CHARACTERISTICS

A total of 618 outpatients were screened for inclusion in the study; 202 patients failed to meet eligibility require-

Evaluation.[30] The results of psychosocial functioning are reported elsewhere.[31]

THERAPEUTIC RESPONSE

Treatment Response

Clinical response was defined as a final CGI improvement rating of 1 or 2 (ie, very much or much improved).

Full Remission

In contrast to major depression, for which the MacArthur Foundation Research Network Task Force has provided operational criteria for remission, there are no criteria for defining remission of dysthymia. We prospectively established a criterion for full remission, which required that patients no longer meet *DSM-III-R* criteria for dysthymia *and* achieve a score of 0 on HAM-D item 1 (depressed mood). This criterion was designated because depressive symptoms in dysthymia, although chronic, are usually mild, so it is possible for patients to attain a 50% reduction in total HAM-D score or a HAM-D score of less than 8 and still have dysthymia. These commonly accepted response and remission criteria for major depression were thought to be an insufficient measure of remission from dysthymia. A second remission criterion, a HAM-D cutoff score of 4 or less, was selected by dividing in half the HAM-D cutoff score of less than 8 that was proposed as a remission criterion for major depression by the MacArthur Foundation Research Network Task Force on Recovery, Relapse, and Recurrence.[32]

DATA ANALYSIS

All clinical data were analyzed by means of SAS version 6.08. The intention-to-treat efficacy group (410 patients) consisted of patients who had baseline and at least 1 postrandomization efficacy evaluation while receiving double-blind medication, while the group examined for safety and medication tolerability (412 patients) had at least 1 assessment after receiving double-blind medication.

The treatment groups were examined for homogeneity at baseline with analysis of variance models that included treatment group and center main effects and the treatment group×center interaction effect for continuous data (eg, age, duration of illness, and applicable efficacy assessments). The χ^2 tests for homogeneity at baseline were computed, as appropriate, for demographic characteristics (eg, prevalence of concomitant and previous medication usage, present concurrent medical conditions, and history of illness). Frequency distributions were prepared to characterize the patients with respect to age on entry into the study, age at the first depressive episode, the approximate history of the primary and secondary illnesses, duration of the current episode, and frequency of previous episodes.

An α level of .05 was used in the efficacy analyses to declare significance, and 2-sided statistical tests were performed. The primary measures of efficacy for assessments of continuous data were the changes from baseline to end point (defined as the last observation while receiving double-blind medication). The F ratios from either analysis of variance models or, if assumptions were met, analysis of covariance models, with baseline values serving as the covariates, were used as the omnibus tests of significance to evaluate the between-group and center main effects and the treatment group×center interaction effects. Significant main effects were further explored with unpaired *t* tests. The significance of the within-group changes from baseline was assessed with paired *t* tests.

The significance of the between-group differences in responder and remitter rates (ie, defined with respect to HAM-D, CGI-I, and criteria for dysthymia) was determined with χ^2 tests.

The incidence of adverse events was summarized for the active treatment groups with respect to World Health Organization body-organ system, and the between-group significance in rates was assessed with Fisher 2-sided exact tests.

ments or refused participation. The reasons for screening failure included withdrawal of consent or poor compliance (n=54), medical exclusion (abnormal baseline laboratory results or electrocardiogram, unstable medical illness, or requirement of prohibited medication) (n=52), failure to meet study diagnostic criteria for dysthymia (late onset, <5 years' duration, mild severity) (n=16), and excluded psychiatric disorders (major depression, n=30; severe borderline personality or suicidal ideation, n=3; substance abuse or dependence, n=10; bipolar disorder, n=6; panic disorder, n=6; and other, n=11). Seventeen patients were considered placebo responders at the end of the washout period. Four hundred sixteen patients were randomly assigned to treatment; of these, 412 received double-blind medication. The intent-to-treat analysis consisted of 410 patients who had at least 1 postbaseline evaluation.

A summary of the demographic and diagnostic characteristics of the patients is provided in **Table 1**. Patients in all 3 treatment groups had a duration of illness of approximately 30 years and an age at onset of approximately 12 years. The average duration of the current dysthymic episode for all patients approached 30 years.

There were no significant differences among the 3 treatment groups with respect to gender, age, race, marital or employment status, educational level, duration of dysthymia, or age at onset of dysthymia. The mean baseline scores for the 29-item HAM-D were significantly higher for the imipramine-treated patients than for those who received either sertraline (P=.01) or placebo (P=.03). There were no differences among groups with respect to severity of illness on the CGI at baseline (P>.10).

EFFICACY ANALYSES

Completion of Therapy

Overall, 310 of the patients randomly assigned to treatment completed the 12-week trial. A significantly higher study completion rate was seen for sertraline (84% [113]) than for imipramine (67% [91]) and placebo (76% [106]) (P=.004). Reasons for discontinuation are summarized in **Table 2**. The most common reason for discontinuation among patients who received either sertraline or imipramine was adverse events, whereas the most common reason for discontinuation among patients

Table 1. Demographic and Diagnostic Characteristics of Patients Included in the Intent-to-Treat Analysis

Variable	Sertraline Hydrochloride (n=134)	Imipramine Hydrochloride (n=136)	Placebo (n=140)
Sex, % F	68	66	61
Age, y*	42.6±8.9	41.0±9.1	41.6±9.2
Race, No.			
White	129	130	131
Black	4	3	2
Asian	1	0	1
Other	0	3	6
Duration of illness, y*	30.6±10.4	28.3±10.5	29.4±10.9
Age at onset, y*	12.0±4.8	12.5±4.7	12.3±4.9
Duration of current dysthymic episode, y*	29.9±10.1	28.4±10.5	28.6±11.2
Axis I comorbidity, No. (%)			
Panic disorder†	8 (6)	9 (7)	12 (9)
Social phobia†	13 (10)	13 (10)	16 (11)
Generalized anxiety disorder	13 (10)	21 (16)	11 (8)
Substance abuse†			
Alcohol	29 (22)	25 (18)	32 (23)
Other‡	42 (31)	31 (23)	36 (26)
Axis II comorbidity, No. (%)			
Cluster A	11 (8)	12 (9)	21 (15)
Cluster B	13 (10)	17 (12)	18 (13)
Cluster C	63 (47)	61 (45)	69 (49)

*Mean±SD.
†Lifetime prevalence.
‡Includes abuse of or dependency on cannabis, sedatives, stimulants, opioids, cocaine, or hallucinogens.

Table 2. Reasons for Discontinuation: Intent-to-Treat Analysis*

Reason for Discontinuation	No. (%) Sertraline Hydrochloride (n=134)	Imipramine Hydrochloride (n=136)	Placebo (n=140)	P
Completed study	113 (84)	91 (67)	106 (76)	.004†
Insufficient response	3 (2)	5 (4)	9 (6)	.21
Adverse experience	8 (6)	25 (18)	5 (4)	<.001‡
Unavailable for follow-up	1 (1)	6 (4)	3 (2)	.13
Medical illness or laboratory or ECG abnormality	3 (2)	3 (2)	4 (3)	.93
Other	4 (3)	4 (3)	7 (5)	.60

*ECG indicates electrocardiographic.
†Sertraline >imipramine; sertraline >placebo.
‡Imipramine >sertraline; imipramine >placebo.

who received placebo was insufficient response to treatment.

Efficacy

Table 3 provides the mean baseline scores and mean changes from baseline in the clinician-rated and patient-rated scales. Both active treatments produced significant reductions in both investigator-rated depression scales (HAM-D and MADRS) and the CGI ratings for severity and improvement.

The mean changes (±SDs) from baseline for the 17-item HAM-D scores were −5.6±6.1, −5.9±5.8, and −3.9±5.1 for the sertraline-, imipramine-, and placebo-treated patients, respectively (P=.04 and P=.01 for sertraline and imipramine vs placebo, respectively). There was no significant difference between sertraline and imipramine. A post hoc power analysis indicated that, based on the mean changes from baseline and the SDs, with this sample size, the 2-tailed test at α=.05 had 80% power to detect a difference in mean change from baseline of 2 points between treatment groups. Mean changes for the 29-item HAM-D were −9.2±9.2, −10.2±8.6, and −7.0±8.1 for the sertraline-, imipramine-, and placebo-treated patients, respectively (overall, P=.02); imipramine lowered 29-item HAM-D scores significantly more than placebo did (P=.01), while for sertraline there was a trend (P=.10), but there was no significant difference between the effects of sertraline and those of imipramine (P=.24). Sertraline and imipramine also significantly reduced total MADRS scores relative to placebo (P=.01 and P=.003, respectively). The respective mean decreases (±SDs) from baseline for the sertraline, imipramine, and placebo groups were −9.6±7.9, −9.5±8.4, and −6.7±7.8, respectively. Similarly, both sertraline and imipramine were associated with significantly greater improvement in Global Assessment of Functioning scores than placebo was. The mean increases (±SDs) were 10.7±11.5 for sertraline and 11.8±12.0 for imipramine compared with 7.5±10.2 for placebo (P=.03 for sertraline vs placebo and P=.02 for imipramine vs placebo).

With respect to self-reported symptoms, sertraline and imipramine produced a significantly greater (P<.05) improvement than placebo for the total score and for the depression, hostility, interpersonal sensitivity, and paranoid ideation factors of the Hopkins Symptom Checklist. In addition, imipramine treatment resulted in a significantly greater (P<.05) improvement in the psychoticism factor. Significant improvements for both active treatments compared with placebo were seen on the total IDS-SR scores and several IDS-SR factors. These included mood/cognition and anxiety/hypochondriacal for the 4-factor classifications, and mood/hedonic, self-criticism/guilt, suicidal thoughts/future pessimism, decreased libido, somatic anxiety/arousal, and tense/irritable for the 10-factor classification.

For the efficacy assessments presented, none of the treatment×center interactions was significant (P<.10).

Responder Analysis

Both of the active treatments produced significantly greater responses to treatment than did placebo. The percentages of patients classified as responders by virtue of a CGI improvement score of 2 or less were 59% for sertraline, 64% for imipramine, and 44% for placebo (P=.02 for sertraline vs placebo and P<.001 for imipramine vs placebo). When the more stringent criteria for a full remission were used, both active treatments were also superior to placebo. When the criteria for full remission were no longer meeting *DSM-III-R* criteria for dysthymia *and* a score of 0 on HAM-D item

Table 3. Baseline Scores and Changes From Baseline in Rating Scales*

	Sertraline Hydrochloride (n=134)	Imipramine Hydrochloride (n=136)	Placebo (n=140)	*P*
		Baseline Scores		
Clinician ratings				
HAM-D (17-item)	12.7±4.0	13.4±3.8	12.7±3.9	.11
HAM-D (29-item)	20.5±5.4	22.3±6.4	20.7±6.0	.002
MADRS	18.53±5.8	18.64±5.2	19.00±5.8	.52
Patient self-ratings				
IDS-SR (total)	30.65±10.4	32.15±11.5	29.74±10.8	.04
Mood factor	1.17±0.4	1.18±0.5	1.10±0.5	.22
SCL-90 (total)	148.59±35.7	151.38±42.5	141.94±35.8	.05
Depression factor	2.39±0.7	2.43±0.8	2.23±0.7	.09
Phobic anxiety	1.19±0.3	1.28±0.5	1.19±0.4	.02
Hostility	1.61±0.6	1.63±0.7	1.54±0.5	.21
Paranoid ideation	1.60±0.6	1.64±0.7	1.55±0.5	.17
Anxiety factor	1.68±0.5	1.73±0.6	1.64±0.5	.13
Interpersonal sensitivity	2.05±0.7	2.07±0.7	1.92±0.7	.20
		Changes From Baseline		
Clinician ratings				
HAM-D (17-item)	−5.6±6.1†	−5.9±5.8†	−3.9±5.1	.02
HAM-D (29-item)	−9.2±9.2	−10.2±8.6†	−7.0±8.1	.02
MADRS	−9.6±7.9†	−9.5±8.4†	−6.7±7.8	.01
Patient self-ratings				
IDS-SR (total)	−11.15±12.4†	−11.38±11.9	−7.84±10.7	.06
Mood factor	−0.54±0.6†	−0.53±0.5†	−0.28±0.5	.04
SCL-90 (total)	−26.1±37.0†	−23.5±37.8†	−11.3±34.1	.01
Depression factor	−0.57±0.8†	−0.60±0.8†	−0.25±0.7	.01
Phobic anxiety	−0.06±0.3	−0.10±0.4	−0.03±0.31	.53
Hostility	−0.37±0.6†	−0.22±0.6†	−0.05±0.6	.01
Paranoid ideation	−0.28±0.5†	−0.23±0.6†	−0.09±0.5	.04
Anxiety factor	−0.23±0.5	−0.17±0.6	−0.13±0.5	.30
Interpersonal sensitivity	−0.51±0.64	−0.40±0.61†	−0.16±0.61	<.001

**Values are mean±SD. HAM-D indicates Hamilton Rating Scale for Depression; IDS-SR, Inventory for Depressive Symptomatology, self-report format; MADRS, Montgomery-Asburg Depression Rating Scale; and SCL-90, Hopkins Symptom Checklist.*

†P<.05 vs placebo.

1 (depressed mood), the proportions of patients classified as achieving remission were 50% for sertraline, 44% for imipramine, and 28% for placebo (*P*<.05 for both treatments vs placebo). With the remission criterion of achievement of a score of 4 or less on the HAM-D (17-item), the proportions of patients who achieved remission were 47% for sertraline, 39% for imipramine, and 32% for placebo (*P*=.01 for sertraline vs placebo).

The results in the preceding paragraph are based on an intent-to-treat analysis of the last observation carried forward for all patients. We also compared response rates for patients in the 3 groups who completed 12 weeks of treatment. The remission rates for study completers with the criterion of no longer meeting *DSM-III-R* criteria for dysthymia *and* achieving a score of 0 on HAM-D item 1 (depressed mood) for sertraline, imipramine, and placebo were 54%, 58%, and 33%, respectively (*P*<.001). Response rates for sertraline, imipramine, and placebo were 53%, 56%, and 37%, respectively (*P*<.01) with the criterion of achievement of a final HAM-D score of 4 or less. Again, both active treatments were superior to placebo.

SAFETY

More patients in the imipramine group discontinued treatment because of adverse events than in the sertraline or placebo groups (*P*=.001 and *P*<.001, respectively). The percentages of patients who discontinued treatment were 6% for sertraline, 18% for imipramine, and 4% for placebo. A summary of the most commonly reported treatment-emergent adverse events (>5%) is provided in **Table 4**. The incidences of dry mouth, constipation, dizziness, abnormal vision, and postural hypotension were significantly higher for imipramine, whereas the incidences of diarrhea and insomnia were significantly higher for sertraline (Table 4).

The patients treated with imipramine experienced an increase in standing heart rate (+10.3 beats/min) during double-blind treatment that was significantly greater (*P*<.001) than that for the patients who received sertraline (+0.01 beats/min). The sertraline-treated patients experienced a small increase (+1.52 mm Hg) in supine diastolic blood pressure that was significantly different (*P*=.01) from the slight decrease (−0.01 mm Hg) noted in this measure for the patients who received imipramine.

DOSE

The mean (±SD) dose at time of initial response (CGI improvement score, ≤2) was 89.5±51.5 mg for sertraline hydrochloride and 159.7±8.08 mg for imipramine

Table 4. Most Common Treatment-Emergent Adverse Events*

Adverse Event	Sertraline Hydrochloride No. (%)	Imipramine Hydrochloride No. (%)	Placebo No. (%)	*P*
Autonomic/anticholinergic				
Abnormal vision	7 (5)	19 (14)	4 (3)	<.002†‡
Dry mouth	35 (26)	100 (73)	24 (17)	<.001†‡
Flushing	1 (0.7)	10 (7)	1 (0.7)	.003†‡
Increased sweating	16 (12)	39 (28)	8 (6)	<.001†‡
Micturition disorder	1 (0.7)	15 (11)	1 (0.7)	<.001†‡
Cardiovascular				
Palpitations	6 (4)	12 (9)	3 (2)	.05
Postural hypotension	0 (0)	7 (5)	0 (0)	<.001†‡
Central/peripheral nervous system				
Dizziness	19 (14)	38 (28)	22 (16)	.01†‡
Headache	55 (41)	53 (39)	64 (46)	.48†‡
Paresthesias	6 (4)	8 (6)	4 (3)	.45
Tremor	14 (10)	33 (24)	1 (0.7)	<.001†‡§
Gastrointestinal tract				
Anorexia	16 (12)	15 (11)	4 (3)	.01‡§
Constipation	22 (16)	55 (40)	12 (9)	<.001†‡
Diarrhea	28 (21)	10 (7)	14 (10)	.003§‖
Dyspepsia	17 (13)	17 (12)	9 (6)	.15
Increased appetite	3 (2)	8 (6)	5 (4)	.30
Nausea	37 (27)	35 (26)	28 (20)	.33
Vomiting	6 (4)	10 (7)	2 (1)	.05‡
Psychiatric				
Agitation	13 (10)	11 (8)	3 (2)	.02§
Anxiety	10 (7)	11 (8)	8 (6)	.74
Insomnia	33 (24)	16 (12)	24 (17)	.02‖
Somnolence	31 (23)	44 (32)	17 (12)	<.001‡§
Sexual dysfunction				
Female	5 (5)	8 (9)	1 (1)	.08
Male	14 (33)	10 (22)	7 (13)	.06
Rash	5 (4)	10 (7)	2 (1)	.05‡

**All adverse events with a frequency greater than 5% for either sertraline or imipramine, included if they began or worsened after initiation of treatment irrespective of whether they were considered treatment related.*
†Imipramine >sertraline.
‡Imipramine >placebo.
§Sertraline >placebo.
‖Sertraline >imipramine.

hydrochloride. At initial response, the modal or most frequently administered dose was 50 mg for sertraline hydrochloride and 100 mg for imipramine hydrochloride, while the median dose was 50 mg for sertraline hydrochloride and 150 mg for imipramine hydrochloride. The mean (±SD) final dose was 139.6±58.5 mg and 198.9±91.2 mg for sertraline hydrochloride and imipramine hydrochloride, respectively.

COMMENT

This multicenter placebo-controlled clinical trial in patients with "pure dysthymia" (ie, without concurrent major depression) demonstrates that both sertraline and imipramine are effective in reducing the symptoms of this disorder. The fact that these patients, who had been suffering from dysthymia on average for nearly 30 years, experienced significant relief of symptoms in 12 weeks is a clinically important outcome. Both active treatments produced significantly greater improvement in both clinician- and patient-rated depression scales than placebo and did not differ significantly. Significantly more patients were considered responders to therapy with either sertraline or imipramine than with placebo, whether a response was defined by a CGI improvement score or full symptom remission. In addition, significantly more imipramine-treated patients than sertraline-treated patients discontinued therapy because of adverse events.

Unlike most previous studies of pharmacotherapy in dysthymic patients, the present trial included stringent criteria for a response to therapy, including full remission of dysthymic symptoms. Harrison and Stewart[20] pointed out the limitation of relying solely on arbitrary cutoff scores on depression rating scales to assess treatment response in mildly depressed patients. It is possible for a patient to achieve a 50% reduction on the HAM-D score from a baseline of approximately 15 to 20 and be considered much improved, but at the same time still meet the *DSM-III-R* symptomatic criteria for dysthymia. In the present study, the proportions of patients who achieved a CGI improvement score of 2 or less (a commonly used criterion for a response to treatment[14,15]) were 10% to 15% higher than remission rates.

The present results confirm and extend those of previous studies that demonstrated the efficacy of antidepressants for the treatment of patients with dysthymia. In the first of these, Kocsis et al[33] studied 76 patients with *DSM-III*–defined dysthymic disorder in a 6-week, double-blind, placebo-controlled trial that compared imipramine and placebo. A favorable response was seen in 59% of the imipramine-treated patients and 13% of the placebo-treated patients. More recently, Nardi et al[34] compared the efficacy of imipramine and moclobemide in patients with either "pure dysthymia" or double depression and reported that 54% of the moclobemide-treated patients and 49% of those who received imipramine no longer met the criteria for dysthymia at the end of therapy, in contrast to 24% of the patients who received placebo. The selective serotonin reuptake inhibitor fluoxetine has been found to be effective for the treatment of dysthymia in a small, single-site study.[15] This study compared fluoxetine and placebo in an 8-week trial that included 35 patients who met *DSM-III-R* criteria for dysthymia. A significantly higher percentage of the patients who received fluoxetine (62%) than those who received placebo (19%) responded.

In the present study, we specifically excluded dysthymic patients with coexisting major depression to assess the effect of pharmacotherapy on dysthymic symptoms. As many as 40% of individuals with dysthymia have concurrent major depression,[2] and the extent to which the present results may apply to these patients is not clear. However, nearly 60% of patients with double depression responded to treatment with either sertraline or imipramine in a double-blind multicenter trial,[35] suggesting that pharmacotherapy with sertraline or imipramine is comparably effective in patients with pure dysthymia and double depression.

One caveat is that our study was limited only to patients with primary early-onset dysthymia; it is possible that patients with secondary or late-onset dysthymia may respond differently to pharmacotherapy.

The study was designed to assess the comparative efficacy and safety of maximum tolerated doses of both medications administered for an adequate duration. We believe that the rapid upward dose titration permitted in this study is the primary reason for the high mean final doses of sertraline. A similar pattern of increasing dosage before waiting a sufficient time for the antidepressant effect to occur is also seen in studies of treatment of major depression with other SSRIs because of the well-tolerated side-effect profile of these medications.[36-38] This pattern has also been reported in studies of other antidepressants in dysthymia.[18] Although previous studies have suggested that the same dosages used to treat major depression are necessary in dysthymia,[18,39,40] the considerably lower mean, median, and modal doses of sertraline at initial clinical response suggest that lower doses are probably effective. Further studies will be needed to assess the efficacy of lower doses of SSRIs in the treatment of dysthymia.

The response rate seen in the placebo group was somewhat higher than expected. All study participants made frequent and prolonged study visits to mental health professionals during a 3-month period to complete the many rating scales used to assess both depressive symptoms and psychosocial functioning. Thus, placebo treatment was not the equivalent of no treatment. In addition, a "halo" effect related to participation in a study conducted at major academic institutions may also contribute to explaining the placebo response. There are additional factors that may have been, at least in part, responsible for the relatively high placebo response rate among placebo-treated patients in this study. While dysthymia is a chronic condition, the severity of depression in dysthymic patients waxes and wanes over time, and it is likely that patients will seek treatment when symptoms are most severe. The natural course of dysthymia would thus predict some amelioration of symptoms over the course of the trial in placebo-treated patients. Another factor that may have been involved in the relatively high response rate for placebo-treated patients is that the dysthymic population is quite heterogeneous; patients included in a given treatment group may have varied with respect to 1 or more variables that were not assessed at baseline, but that might have influenced the response to treatment with placebo.

While the present study had a longer duration than most previous trials that have evaluated acute antidepressant treatment in patients with dysthymia, individuals with this condition are highly prone to relapse[7] and are likely to require long-term therapy. The results of the present trial do not address this issue, but available data do suggest that dysthymic patients will maintain response to long-term pharmacotherapy. Kocsis et al[40] reported that dysthymic patients who responded to 6 weeks of treatment with imipramine tended to continue receiving therapy and have a significantly better outcome during a 40-month follow-up period than patients who did not complete or who failed to respond to initial treatment. Long-term studies of the efficacy and tolerability of SSRIs in the treatment of chronic forms of depression are now needed to evaluate the necessity of continuation and maintenance treatment.

Although the 2 active treatments had equivalent efficacy in this study, sertraline was generally better tolerated than imipramine. A significantly higher percentage of imipramine-treated patients discontinued therapy because of adverse events, and many different adverse events occurred with a significantly higher frequency in the imipramine- than the sertraline-treated patients. These findings are consistent with results from previous large-scale trials comparing the safety and efficacy of tricyclic antidepressants and SSRIs in patients with major depression.[41-44] Because the chronicity of dysthymia may require long-term pharmacotherapy, tolerability is an important consideration in selecting an antidepressant for patients with this condition.

Accepted for publication January 18, 1996.

This study was supported in part by a series of grants from Pfizer Inc, New York, NY.

Additional principal investigators and collaborating sites are as follows: Jonathan Cole, MD (McLean Hospi-

tal, Boston, Mass); David Hellerstein, MD (Beth Israel Medical Center, New York, NY); Marc Hertzman (George Washington University, Washington, DC); Martin Keller, MD, and Teri Pearlstein, MD (Brown University, Providence, RI); Frederic Quitkin, MD, and Jonathan Stewart, MD (Columbia University, New York); Delbert Robinson, MD (Hillside Hospital, New York); A. John Rush, MD, and Kimberly Yonkers, MD (University of Texas Southwestern Medical Center, Dallas); Richard Shelton, MD (Vanderbilt University, Nashville, Tenn); Andrea Stone, MD (University of Massachusetts, Worcester); and Sidney Zisook, MD (University of California, San Diego).

Reprints: Michael E. Thase, MD, Western Psychiatric Institute and Clinic, 3811 O'Hare St, Pittsburgh, PA 15213.

REFERENCES

1. Weissman MM, Leaf PJ, Bruce ML, Florio L. The epidemiology of dysthymia in five communities: rates, risks, comorbidity, and treatment. *Am J Psychiatry.* 1988;145:815-819.
2. Kessler RC, McGonagle KA, Zhao S, et al. Lifetime and 12-month prevalence of *DSM-III-R* psychiatric disorders in the United States: results from the National Comorbidity Survey. *Arch Gen Psychiatry.* 1994;51:8-19.
3. Markowitz JC, Moran ME, Kocsis JH, Frances AJ. Prevalence and comorbidity of dysthymic disorder among psychiatric outpatients. *J Affect Disord.* 1992; 24:63-71.
4. Akiskal HS. Dysthymic disorder: psychopathology of proposed chronic depressive subtypes. *Am J Psychiatry.* 1983;140:11-20.
5. Wells KB, Stewart A, Hays RD, et al. The functioning and well-being of depressed patients: results from the Medical Outcomes Study. *JAMA.* 1989;262:914-919.
6. Friedman RA. Social impairment in dysthymia. *Psychiatr Ann.* 1993;23:632-637.
7. Kessler RC, Foster CL, Saunders WB, Stang PE. Social consequences of psychiatric disorders, I: educational attainment. *Am J Psychiatry.* 1995;152:1026-1032.
8. Keller MB, Shapiro RW. 'Double depression': superimposition of acute depressive episodes on chronic depressive disorders. *Am J Psychiatry.* 1982;139: 438-442.
9. Zisook S. Treatment of dysthymia and atypical depression. *J Clin Psychiatry Monogr.* 1992;10:15-23.
10. Keller MB. The difficult depressed patient in perspective. *J Clin Psychiatry.* 1993;54(2 suppl):4-8.
11. Weissman MM, Klerman GL. The chronic depressive in the community: unrecognized and poorly treated. *Compr Psychiatry.* 1977;18:523-532.
12. Harrison WM, Stewart JW. Pharmacotherapy of dysthymic disorder. In: Kocsis JH, Klein DN, eds. *Diagnosis and Treatment of Chronic Depression.* New York, NY: Guilford Press; 1995:124-145.
13. Vallejo J, Gastro C, Catalan R, Salamero M. Double-blind study of imipramine versus phenelzine in melancholias and dysthymic disorders. *Br J Psychiatry.* 1987;151:639-651.
14. Rosenthal J, Hemlock C, Hellerstein DJ, et al. A preliminary study of serotonergic antidepressants in treatment of dysthymia. *Prog Neuropsychopharmacol Biol Psychiatry.* 1992;16:933-941.
15. Hellerstein DJ, Yanowitch P, Rosenthal J, et al. A randomized double-blind study of fluoxetine versus placebo in the treatment of dysthymia. *Am J Psychiatry.* 1993;150:1169-1175.
16. Harrison W, Rabkin J, Stewart JW, et al. Phenelzine for chronic depression: a study of continuation treatment. *J Clin Psychiatry.* 1986;47:346-349.
17. Bersani G, Pozzi F, Marini S, et al. 5-HT_2 receptor antagonism in dysthymia disorder: a double-blind placebo-controlled study with ritanserin. *Acta Psychiatr Scand.* 1991;83:244-248.
18. Bakish D, Lapierre YD, Weinstein R, et al. Ritanserin, imipramine, and placebo in the treatment of dysthymic disorder. *J Clin Psychopharmacol.* 1993;13:409-414.
19. Howland RH. Pharmacotherapy of dysthymia: a review. *J Clin Psychopharmacol.* 1991;11:83-92.
20. Harrison WM, Stewart JW. Pharmacotherapy of dysthymia. *Psychiatr Ann.* 1993; 23:638-648.
21. Spitzer RL, Williams JBW, Gibbon M. *Instruction Manual for the Structured Clinical Interview for* DSM-III-R *(SCID, 4/1/87 Revision).* New York, NY: Biometrics Research Division, New York State Psychiatric Institute; 1987.
22. Spitzer RL, Williams JBW, Gibbon M. *Instruction Manual for the Structured Clinical Interview for* DSM-III-R *Personality Disorders (SCID-II, 10/15/86).* New York, NY: Biometrics Research Division, New York State Psychiatric Institute; 1987.
23. Hamilton M. A rating scale for depression. *J Neurol Neurosurg Psychiatry.* 1960;23:56-62.
24. McGlashan T, ed. *The Documentation of Clinical Psychotropic Drug Trials.* Rockville, Md: National Institute of Mental Health; 1973.
25. Montgomery SA, Asberg M. New depression scale designed to be sensitive to change. *Br J Psychiatry.* 1979;134:382.
26. Derogatis LR, Lipman RS, Rickels K, Ulenthuth EH, Covi L. The Hopkins Symptom Check List (HSCL): a self-report symptom inventory. *Behav Sci.* 1974;19: 1-15.
27. Rush AJ, Giles DE, Schlesser MA, et al. The Inventory for Depressive Symptomatology (IDS): preliminary findings. *Psychiatr Res.* 1986;18:65-87.
28. Rush AJ, Hiser W, Giles DE. A comparison of self-reported vs. clinician-rated symptoms in major depression. *J Clin Psychiatry.* 1987;48:246-248.
29. Weissman MM, Bothwell S. Assessment of social adjustment by patient self-report. *Arch Gen Psychiatry.* 1976;33:1111-1115.
30. Shapiro R, Keller M. *Longitudinal Interval Follow-up Evaluation (LIFE).* Boston, Mass: Lindemann Mental Health Center; 1979.
31. Kocsis JH, et al. Double-blind treatment comparison of sertraline, imipramine, and placebo in the treatment of dysthymia: psychosocial outcomes. *Am J Psychiatry.* In press.
32. Frank E, Prien RF, Jarrett RB, et al. Conceptualization and rationale for consensus definitions of terms in major depressive disorder: remission, recovery, relapse, and recurrence. *Arch Gen Psychiatry* 1991;48:851-855.
33. Kocsis JH, Frances AJ, Voss C. Imipramine for treatment of chronic depression. *Arch Gen Psychiatry.* 1988;45:253-257.
34. Nardi E, Capponi R, Costa DA, et al. Moclobemide compared with imipramine in the treatment of chronic depression (dysthymia *DSM-III-R*): a double-blind placebo controlled trial. *Clin Neuropharmacol.* 1992;15(suppl 1):430A-434A.
35. Keller MB, Harrison W, Fawcett JA, et al. Treatment of chronic depression with sertraline or imipramine: preliminary blinded response rates and high rates of undertreatment in the community. *Psychopharm Bull.* 1995;31:205-212.
36. Feighner JP, Boyer WF. Paroxetine in the treatment of depression: a comparison with imipramine and placebo. *J Clin Psychiatry.* 1992;53(suppl 2):44-47.
37. Bremner JD. Fluoxetine in depressed patients: a comparison with imipramine. *J Clin Psychiatry.* 1994;45:414.
38. Cohn JB, Wilcox C. A comparison of fluoxetine, imipramine, and placebo in patients with major depressive disorder. *J Clin Psychiatry.* 1985;46:26.
39. Stewart JW, McGrath PJ, Quitkin FM. Relevance of *DSM-III* depressive subtype and chronicity to antidepressant efficacy in atypical depression. *Arch Gen Psychiatry.* 1989;46:1080-1087.
40. Kocsis JH, Sutton BM, Frances AJ. Long-term follow-up of chronic depression treated with imipramine. *J Clin Psychiatry.* 1991;52:56-59.
41. Reimherr FW, Byerly WF, Ward MF, et al. Sertraline, a selective inhibitor of serotonin uptake for the treatment of outpatients with major depressive disorder. *Psychopharmacol Bull.* 1988;24:200-205.
42. Chouinard G. A double-blind controlled clinical trial of fluoxetine and amitriptyline in the treatment of outpatients with major depressive disorder. *J Clin Psychiatry.* 1985;46:32-37.
43. Cohn CK, Shrivastava R, Mendels J, et al. Double-blind comparison of sertraline and amitriptyline in elderly depressed patients. *J Clin Psychiatry.* 1990; 51(suppl B):28-33.
44. Bakish D, Lapierre YD, Weinstein R, et al. Ritanserin, imipramine, and placebo in the treatment of dysthymic disorder. *J Clin Psychopharmacol.* 1993;13:409-414.

ORIGINAL ARTICLE

Chronological Milestones to Guide Drug Change

When Should Clinicians Switch Antidepressants?

Frederic M. Quitkin, MD; Patrick J. McGrath, MD; Jonathan W. Stewart, MD; Katja Ocepek-Welikson, MPhil; Bonnie P. Taylor, MA; Edward Nunes, MD; Deborah Deliyannides, MD; Vito Agosti, MSW; Steven J. Donovan, MD; Eva Petkova, PhD; Donald F. Klein, MD

Background: We attempt to identify the time when patients whose conditions are unimproved while receiving antidepressants are unlikely to respond and should have their treatment changed.

Methods: A total of 593 patients were studied. The course of treatment for patients was examined to determine the weeks at which patients who received drug therapy had a better chance of being rated as responders at the study end (week 6) vs patients who received placebo.

Results: At the end of week 3, 19 (32%) of the 59 patients who received drug therapy and 6 (10%) of the 57 patients who received placebo and who never minimally improved were rated as responders at week 6. For those who showed no improvement by week 4, the effects of drug therapy and the placebo were equal. Patients who received drug therapy and whose conditions were unimproved but who had been minimally improved at some point had a superior prognosis with drug therapy vs placebo until week 4. Of those unimproved at week 4 but minimally improved at some point previously, 20 (39%) of the 51 patients who received drug therapy vs 3 (8%) of the 36 patients who received placebo were rated as responders at week 6. Of the 75 patients who minimally improved while receiving drug therapy at the end of week 5, 33 (44%) had a chance of being rated a responder at the end of week 6 vs 9 (26%) of the 35 patients receiving placebo.

Conclusions: Patients tolerant of an adequate dose, whose conditions have never been at least minimally improved by the end of week 4, should have their treatment regimen altered. These patients represented a minority of drug-treated patients in the sample studied (ie, 39/392 [10%]). Patients whose conditions minimally improve at some prior week but not after week 5 should have their treatment changed. Patients whose conditions minimally improve in week 5 should continue treatment until week 6.

Arch Gen Psychiatry. 1996;53:785-792

THE RESPONSE to most antidepressants is approximately 60% to 70%.[1-3] Defining the point at which an unresponsive patient has little chance of benefiting from treatment and should be switched to a new treatment is important. In reviewing the English literature, we could find no controlled study that addressed this question. Several investigators[4-8] suggest that the "onset of action" of antidepressants is rapid and that most patients who will respond demonstrate some change within the first treatment week.

Katz et al[4] and Casper et al[5] have been the strongest adherents to the view that it is possible to rapidly identify patients who will eventually benefit from antidepressants. They contrasted the time course of ultimate responders vs nonresponders to imipramine and amitriptyline treatment; they reported that, after 1 week, change in ". . . depressed mood, anxiety and the physical expression of distress could be detected."[4] They suggested that effect sizes are large and that early change might be readily detected. However, without a placebo control, early improvement attributable to nonspecific effects is difficult to distinguish from true drug effects. Definitive conclusions about the onset of a true drug effect cannot be made in the absence of a placebo group.

Some patients unresponsive to one class of antidepressants will respond to

From the Department of Therapeutics, Columbia University College of Physicians & Surgeons, New York State Psychiatric Institution, New York City.

See Subjects and Methods on next page

SUBJECTS AND METHODS

METHODS

The effect size of antidepressants is approximately 30% to 40%.[1] In placebo-controlled studies, the conditions of approximately 60% to 70% of patients improve while receiving antidepressants, and 30% improve while receiving placebo. Persistent improvement may begin during a 5-week period.[10] If this 30% to 40% difference is distributed across 5 weeks, in some weeks the difference might be 6% to 10% between the drug therapy and the placebo groups. Assessing differences of this size with reasonable confidence requires a large sample size. Ideally, fixed doses would be used so that the effects of time and dose could be disentangled. To be clinically relevant, the point at which the chance of new improvement with placebo and drug therapy is equivalent should be identified so treatment may be changed. Therefore, a placebo group is needed. The costs of such a study would be great, and it is unlikely that this ideal will be met. To approach this question cost-effectively, we examined all studies conducted during a 10-year period in the Depression Evaluation Service, an outpatient research clinic affiliated with Columbia University at the New York State Psychiatric Institute, New York City.[11-18] All studies included a single-blind, 7- to 10-day initial placebo run-in period (IPR) and a 6-week double-blind trial with a fixed flexible dose schedule. The study included 5 drug-placebo contrasts and 3 drug-drug contrasts. The medications used included 3 monoamine oxidase inhibitors (MAOIs) (phenelzine, tranylcypromine, and deprenyl), 3 tricyclic antidepressants (TCAs) (imipramine, desipramine, and amitriptyline), and mianserin. At the end of the 7- to 10-day PR, the clinical status of the patients was reassessed using the CGI (ie, a weekly overall rating of mood change from the treatment baseline). Ratings are made on a 7-point scale (1, very much improved; 2, much improved; 3, minimally improved; and 4-7, unchanged or worse). Patients rated 1 or 2 (ie, at least much better) after the IPR were not enrolled in the double-blind phase. Five hundred ninety-three patients whose conditions were minimally improved, unimproved, or worse continued in a 6-week, double-blind study.

Patients much improved on the CGI (ie, rated 2 on the scale) have a minimum 75% reduction in the intensity and frequency of their depressed mood. This is a good clinical response, and most clinicians would not change treatment for a patient achieving this amount of improvement at any time. All patients who had a rating of 3 on the CGI were considered minimally improved. These patients were noted to have some improvement in their conditions, but most of their depressive affect persisted. Patients were examined weekly and, therefore, could be rated much improved in any week. The basis of comparison for the rating each week was the baseline level of psychopathology. Therefore, a much improved week (or a minimally improved week) could be followed by an unimproved week (because of a symptom exacerbation). Generally, the accepted convention is to categorize patients as responders if they rate as at least much improved (or very much improved, CGI=1) in week 6. Thus, patients could be much improved in any week (ie, weeks 1-5), but if unimproved in week 6, they would not be judged as responders (at study end). Conversely, a patient whose condition was unimproved during weeks 1 to 5 but rated as much improved at week 6 would be judged a responder.

The correlation between the CGI, the Hamilton Depression Rating Scale (HAM-D), and the patient-rated Symptom Checklist–90 was in the 0.7 to 0.8 range at week 6, suggesting that the CGI adequately reflects the severity of the psychopathology. For example, the correlation at 6 weeks on the CGI change scale with the HAM-D summary score was 0.79 (P=.001, n=527) and with the Symptom Checklist–90 Depression Scale was 0.74 (P=.001, n=509).

STATISTICAL ANALYSIS

Inspection of the data suggested that the prognosis of the patients differed depending on whether their conditions were never improved, currently unimproved but minimally improved in the past, or currently minimally improved. Therefore, these groups were analyzed separately.

For question 1, at each week K (K=1 . . . 5) we calculated the probability at week K of being a responder (ie, at the end of the study [week 6]) for 3 groups of patients. The first group was characterized as unimproved in week K and never minimally improved at any time prior to week K. The second group was characterized as unimproved in week K but having been minimally improved at some point prior to week K. The third group was characterized as minimally improved in week K and may or may not have been minimally improved in a prior week. We chose to analyze the data this way because it mimics what occurs clinically. Some patients have a fluctuating course (ie, the second and third groups) and others do not (ie, the first group), and inspection of the data suggested outcome might differ between groups. As a result, the number of patients eligible to answer questions 1b and 1c fluctuates. For example, a patient's condition could be minimally improved in week 2 and then unimproved in week 3. For analysis of the answer to 1b, this patient would be excluded in week 2 but included in week 3. Eligibility would be reversed for such a patient for analysis of the answer to 1c.

We computed the estimated probabilities of response and the confidence intervals for each week for the drug therapy and placebo groups. Odds ratios computed at each week are used to compare the 2 treatment groups. In the formula, A refers to active, and B refers to placebo.

The onset of persistent improvement was studied to estimate the proportion of the effect size observed each week. Standard methods for survival analysis were applied to compare drug therapy with placebo. We illustrate the distribution of the effect size of the drug with incidence curves and hazard functions.

For nominal and ordinal scale data (ie, contrasts of proportions), various nonparametric analyses were performed; all of these analyses were 2-tailed.

another.[9] Therefore, it is relevant to identify the point after which new antidepressant effects are unlikely to occur so that a new treatment could be initiated.

We examine the following question: What are the chances of a patient whose condition is unimproved or minimally improved after the first, second, third, fourth, or fifth week of treatment ultimately benefiting if treatment with antidepressants is continued for 6 weeks?

Table 1. Sample Demographics

Characteristics	No. (%) of Patients Receiving Placebo (n=201)	Drug Therapy (n=392)
Sex		
M	89 (44)	191 (49)
F	112 (56)	201 (51)
Diagnosis (*DSM-III-R*[19])		
Dysthymia	59 (29)	56 (14)
Major depression	91 (45)	223 (57)
Double depression	49 (24)	105 (27)
Depression not otherwise specified	2 (1)	8 (2)
Atypical diagnosis (Columbia criteria[20])	111 (55)	224 (57)
Endogenous diagnosis (RDC criteria[21])	48 (25)*	128 (35)†
Chronicity level‡		
I	26 (14)§	38 (11)‖
II	20 (11)§	41 (12)‖
III	80 (42)§	138 (41)‖
IV	62 (33)§	122 (36)‖

*n=191.
†n=369.
‡Level I indicates depressed less than 10% of adult life; level II, depressed more than 10% but less than 50% of adult life; level III, depressed the overwhelming portion of adult life; and level IV, depressed the overwhelming portion of adult life and has not had a 3-month depression-free period since illness onset.
§n=188.
‖n=339.

This first question is divided into 3 parts because inspection of the data suggested that prognosis differs if a patient's condition was minimally improved at any point during weeks 1 to 5. The questions that we examine in this article are as follows:

1. What are the chances of a patient being rated a responder by week 6 for each of the following categories? (*a*) Previously unimproved and unimproved after week 1, 2, 3, 4, or 5; (*b*) minimally improved in a prior week and unimproved after week 1, 2, 3, 4, or 5; and (*c*) minimally improved after week 1, 2, 3, 4, or 5.

2. Are the observations presented in question 1 consistent across (*a*) diagnoses and (*b*) type of drug?

3. Does failure to use an adequate dose of drug explain the delay in the onset of the drug effect?

4. The Clinical Global Impression Scale (CGI) was used to measure changes in this study. Do other measures of psychopathology support the validity of the CGI?

5. What proportion of the effect size occurs during each week of a 6-week drug trial? This provides a yardstick to help the clinician anticipate the proportion of patients whose conditions should improve each week. The effect size of a drug is the difference in the proportion of patients whose conditions improve while receiving drug therapy vs placebo. Improvement is defined as a rating of at least much improved, which remained constant until the end of the study. A reasonable estimate of the onset of the drug effect is the point of persistent, significant clinical improvement.

RESULTS

In **Table 1**, the demographics of the sample are given. Groups were composed of roughly equal numbers of men and women; the mean age was 38.5 years (range, 18-65 years). Approximately 80% of these patients had either a major depression or a double depression (ie, dysthymia and major depressive disorder), and the remainder had only dysthymia. Approximately 70% of the patients had a predominantly chronic course, having depressive symptoms much of their adult lives.

QUESTION 1a: WHAT ARE THE CHANCES OF A PATIENT BEING RATED A RESPONDER (IE, AT LEAST MUCH IMPROVED) BY WEEK 6 IF UNIMPROVED AFTER WEEK 1, 2, 3, 4, OR 5 AND NEVER EVEN MINIMALLY IMPROVED?

The data given in **Table 2** suggest that a clinically relevant difference in prognosis exists for patients who received drug therapy vs placebo through week 3. The odds ratios for weeks 1 to 3 are significantly different ($P=.006$) from 1 week, but no difference in outcome occurred for weeks 5 to 6. For patients who never demonstrate even minimal improvement, the advantage of continuing the same medication after 4 weeks is dubious.

QUESTION 1b: WHAT ARE THE CHANCES OF A PATIENT BEING RATED A RESPONDER BY WEEK 6 IF THE CONDITION WAS MINIMALLY IMPROVED IN A PRIOR WEEK BUT UNIMPROVED AFTER WEEK 1, 2, 3, 4, or 5?

The data are given in **Table 3**. The conditions of all patients in this analysis were minimally improved in some prior week. However, in the week examined, only patients whose conditions were rated as unimproved were included in the analysis. Some patients exhibit a fluctuating course, exhibiting partial remission and an exacerbation of symptoms (vs baseline). Thus, a subset of patients whose conditions were rated as minimally improved after week 2 and unimproved after week 3 would be included in the analysis during week 3 but not week 2. These data suggest that the prognosis for those patients who received drug therapy vs placebo is superior through week 4 (ie, the odds ratios for weeks 1-4 are significantly different [$P=.003$]). For patients whose conditions were unimproved after week 5 but minimally improved in a prior week, those who received drug therapy have no greater chance of being rated a responder by week 6 than those who received placebo.

QUESTION 1c: IF A PATIENT'S CONDITION IS MINIMALLY IMPROVED IN ANY WEEK OF THE STUDY, WHAT ARE THE CHANCES OF BEING RATED A RESPONDER BY WEEK 6?

Data for patients whose conditions were rated as minimally improved in each week were examined and found to be similar to patients whose conditions were rated as minimally improved in the past but not in the present week with 1 relevant difference (**Table 4**). After week 5, 33 (44%) of the 75 patients who received drug therapy

Table 2. Probability of Responding at Week 6 If Unimproved After Week 1, 2, 3, 4, or 5 and Unimproved in the Past

Treatment	After IPR*	Time After, wk 1	2	3	4	5
Drug therapy						
Unimproved (at each week)	287	175	113	59	39	29
Percentage of those who were unimproved who improved by week 6	60† (171/287)	51 (90/175)	44 (50/113)	32 (19/59)	13 (5/39)	3 (1/29)
Placebo						
Unimproved (at each week)	152	98	72	57	48	41
Percentage of those who were unimproved who improved by week 6	24 (37/152)	20 (20/98)	14 (10/72)	10 (6/57)	6 (3/48)	0 (0/41)
Odds ratio‡,§ (95% confidence interval)	4.5 (2.9-7.0)	4.1 (2.3-7.4)	4.9 (2.3-10.6)	4.0 (1.5-11.2)	2.2 (0.48-10.1)	16.1 (0.02-11 900)
$\beta_{treatment}$/SE§	1.5/0.22	1.4/0.29	1.6/0.39	1.4/5.1	0.79/0.77	2.8/3.3
P of $\beta_{treatment}$§	<.001	<.001	<.001	.007	.30	.40

*IPR indicates initial placebo run-in period.

†For example, 287 patients' conditions were unimproved after the IPR; 171 patients (60%) who received drug therapy eventually improved by week 6.

‡Odds ratio = $\frac{P_A/(1-P_A)}{P_B/(1-P_B)}$, where P_A is the probability of response at week 6 for those receiving active drug therapy, and P_B is the probability of response at week 6 for those receiving placebo.

§The model is: $\log \frac{P}{1-P} = \beta_o + \beta \times \text{treatment}$.

Table 3. Probability of Responding at Week 6 If Unimproved After Week 1, 2, 3, 4, or 5 but Minimally Improved in the Past*

Treatment	After IPR	Time After, wk 1	2	3	4	5
Drug therapy						
Unimproved (at each week)	...	49	55	52	51	37
Percentage of those who were unimproved who improved by week 6	...	63† (31/49)	54 (30/55)	52 (27/52)	39 (20/51)	11 (4/37)
Placebo						
Unimproved (at each week)	...	21	30	31	36	40
Percentage of those who were unimproved who improved by week 6	...	28 (6/21)	7 (2/30)	10 (3/31)	8 (3/36)	2 (1/40)
Odds ratio‡,§ (95% confidence interval)	...	4.3 (1.4-13.3)	16.8 (3.6-79.3)	10.1 (2.7-38.1)	7.1 (1.9-26.8)	4.7 (0.5-46.1)
$\beta_{treatment}$/SE§	...	1.5/0.57	2.8/0.78	2.3/0.67	2.0/0.69	1.6/1.1
P of $\beta_{treatment}$§	...	.01	<.001	<.001	.003	.17

*IPR indicates initial placebo run-in period; ellipses, data not applicable.

†For example, 49 patients' conditions were minimally improved after the IPR and were unimproved in week 1; 31 patients (63%) who received drug therapy eventually improved by week 6.

‡Odds ratio = $\frac{P_A/(1-P_A)}{P_B/(1-P_B)}$, where P_A is the probability of response at week 6 for those receiving active drug therapy, and P_B is the probability of response at week 6 for those receiving placebo.

§The model is: $\log \frac{P}{1-P} = \beta_o + \beta \times \text{treatment}$.

and 9 (26%) of the 35 patients who received placebo were rated as responders after week 6 (odds ratio, 2.3; P=.07). We suggest continuing treatment until week 6, although this is the only trend significant (P=.07), because if the patient's condition is unimproved by week 6 only a 1-week delay in changing treatment exists. Therefore, patients with minimally improved conditions should continue treatment until the sixth week.

QUESTION 2a: ARE THESE OBSERVATIONS CONSISTENT ACROSS DIAGNOSIS?

Dividing the sample into endogenous vs not endogenous, major depressive vs not major depressive, and atypical vs typical[21] did not alter the observations about chance of improvement previously presented. (These data are not given in this article but are available on request from the authors.)

QUESTION 2b: ARE THESE OBSERVATIONS CONSISTENT ACROSS DIFFERENT CLASSES OF DRUGS?

Next, we considered whether the proportion of patients whose conditions were unimproved at week 4 who responded at week 6 differed by classes of medication (ie, TCAs, MAOIs, and mianserin). For patients receiving TCAs, the proportion was 23% (8/35); MAOIs, 36%

Table 4. Probability of Responding at Week 6 If Minimally Improved After Week 1, 2, 3, 4, or 5

Treatment	After IPR*	Time After, wk 1	2	3	4	5
Drug therapy						
Minimally improved (at each week)	105	127	123	129	99	75
Percentage of those who were minimally improved who improved by week 6	77 (81/105)	77† (98/127)	69 (85/123)	60 (77/129)	56 (55/99)	44 (33/75)
Placebo						
Minimally improved (at each week)	49	60	60	50	44	35
Percentage of those who were minimally improved who improved by week 6	43 (21/49)	33 (20/60)	38 (23/60)	30 (15/50)	30 (13/44)	26 (9/35)
Odds ratio‡,§ (95% confidence interval)	4.5 (2.2-9.4)	6.8 (3.4-13.4)	3.6 (1.9-6.9)	3.5 (1.7-7.0)	3.0 (1.4-6.4)	2.3 (0.9-5.6)
$\beta_{treatment}$/SE§	1.5/0.37	1.9/0.35	1.3/0.33	1.2/0.36	1.1/0.39	0.82/0.45
P of $\beta_{treatment}$§	<.001	<.001	<.001	<.001	.005	.07

**IPR indicates initial placebo run-in period.*

†For example, 127 patients' conditions were minimally improved after week 1; 98 patients (77%) who received drug therapy eventually improved by week 6.

‡Odds ratio = $\frac{P_A/(1-P_A)}{P_B/(1-P_B)}$, *where P_A is the probability of response at week 6 for those receiving active drug therapy, and P_B is the probability of response at week 6 for those receiving placebo.*

§The model is: $\log \frac{P}{1-P} = \beta_o + \beta \times \text{treatment}$.

(13/36); and mianserin, 21% (4/19) (χ^2=2.97, 2 *df*, *P*=.30). Thus, a statistically significant difference in response based on class of drug did not exist.

QUESTION 3: DOES FAILURE TO RECEIVE AN ADEQUATE DOSE OF DRUG EXPLAIN THE DELAY IN THE ONSET OF DRUG EFFECT?

To examine the relevance of dose, the proportion of unimproved patients at week 4 who were not receiving an adequate dose was determined. The adequate daily dose was defined as follows: imipramine, ≥200 mg; desipramine, ≥200 mg; amitriptyline, ≥150 mg; phenelzine, ≥60 mg; tranylcypromine, ≥40 mg; deprenyl, ≥40 mg; and mianserin, ≥90 mg. These doses are probably greater than most outpatients receive in the usual clinical setting. Nineteen (25%) of 76 patients who received an adequate dose and whose conditions remained unimproved after week 4 responded after week 6, and 6 (43%) of 14 patients who had not received an adequate dose after week 4 responded by week 6 (χ^2=1.88, 1 *df*, *P*=.29). Of those 14 patients who had not received an adequate dose at week 4, 2 of 6 whose dose was raised and 4 of 8 whose dose was not raised responded at 6 weeks (Fisher exact test; *P*=.94). These data are consistent with the view that a subsequent increase after failure to reach an adequate dose by 4 weeks does not account for all of the improvement from week 4 to week 6.

QUESTION 4: DO OTHER MEASURES OF PSYCHOPATHOLOGY SUPPORT THE VALIDITY OF THE CGI?

Although we previously indicated a high correlation between the CGI and the HAM-D at week 6 (*r*=0.79), this does not precisely demonstrate the validity of the CGI at week 4. The HAM-D was used to help validate the use of the CGI to determine lack of improvement for nonresponders at week 4. The HAM-D at week 4 was compared with the HAM-D at baseline. Ninety patients' conditions were unimproved according to the CGI at week 4. Twenty-five of these patients responded by week 6. Of the 25 responders, 15 had completed the HAM-D at baseline and at 4 weeks (in early studies, the HAM-D was not performed at 4 weeks). In these 15 patients, the HAM-D score at week 4 was greater than or equal to the HAM-D score at baseline for 6 patients and within 20% of the baseline score for another 6 patients, and 3 patients demonstrated more than a 20% but less than a 50% decrease on the HAM-D. Of the nonresponders, 37 had completed the baseline and week 4 HAM-D. The HAM-D score at week 4 was greater than or equal to the baseline HAM-D score for 19 patients, within 20% for 13 patients, and between 20% and 50% lower for 5 patients. These groups were contrasted and found to be nonsignificant (χ^2=0.65, 2 *df*, *P*=.70).

QUESTION 5: WHAT PROPORTION OF THE EFFECT SIZE OCCURS DURING EACH WEEK OF A 6-WEEK TRIAL?

An estimate of the onset of meaningful improvement for an individual patient is the point at which persistent, significant clinical improvement begins. The onset of effect is the week of a rating of much improved or very much improved (ie, CGI=1 or 2), which persisted for the remainder of the study. The data are shown in **Figure 1** and **Table 5** and **Figure 2** and **Table 6**. Because the prognosis may differ for patients whose conditions were minimally improved after the IPR and those whose conditions were unimproved after the IPR, for this analysis they are examined separately.[22] In Figure 1, an incidence table of patients unimproved after IPR is provided, and, in Figure 2, an incidence table of patients minimally improved after IPR is provided; corresponding hazard functions at each week (ie, the instantaneous probability of persistent improvement) for those whose conditions were unchanged or minimally improved after the IPR are also given. For patients whose conditions were unimproved after the IPR, a minimal clinical (but statistically significant) effect at week 2 occurs. However, most of the effect of drug therapy is observed from weeks 3 to 6. Thus, from weeks 3 to 6, the hazard difference between drug therapy and placebo varies from 0.136 to 0.190, and these hazard differences are all significant at $P=.001$ (Table 5). This is evident from examining the point at which no overlap occurs in the upper and lower bounds of the incidence plot contrasting drug therapy and placebo groups (Figure 1).

Data for patients whose conditions were minimally improved after the IPR are given in Table 6. In this group, little difference exists between the patients who received drug therapy vs placebo until week 5. Week 5 is the first point at which the confidence limits of drug therapy and placebo do not overlap (Figure 2), and the hazard estimates of drug therapy and placebo differ notably (Table 6). This difference between the incidence curves (Figures 1 and 2) is due to the improved prognosis of patients whose conditions were minimally improved after the IPR, particularly those minimally improved after IPR and assigned to receive placebo. In fact, examination of the life tables of patients whose conditions were minimally improved after the IPR and assigned to receive placebo and patients whose conditions were unimproved and assigned to receive drug therapy suggests little difference in improvement until weeks 5 and 6.

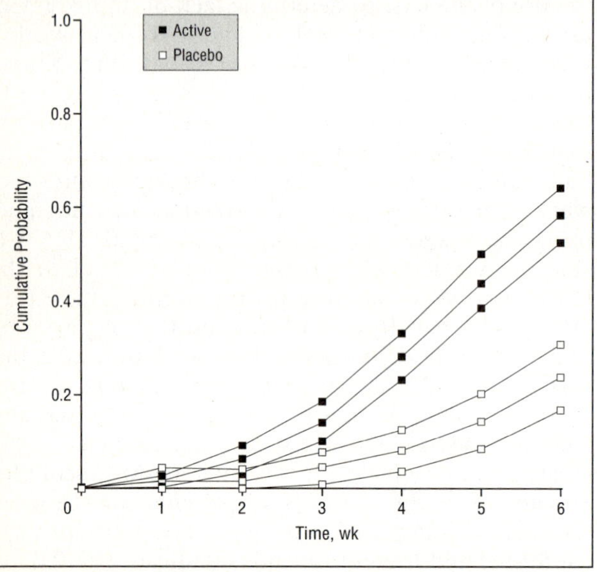

Figure 1. *Incidence plot of the onset of a persistent response (for patients whose conditions were unimproved after the initial placebo run-in period with upper and lower bounds. The hazard estimates that correspond to this figure are provided in Table 5.*

COMMENT

These data are consistent with the observation that a lag in the onset of the effect of antidepressants exists. Patients who did not exhibit even minimal improvement had a superior prognosis while receiving drug therapy until the end of 4 weeks of treatment. Those whose conditions were minimally improved had a superior prognosis vs patients who received placebo until week 6. These observations seemed accurate even for patients who received a dose of drug generally considered adequate by week 4 and consistent across different diagnostic subtypes.

Another salient point must be addressed to place this article in an appropriate clinical context. Selective serotonin reuptake inhibitors (SSRIs) have been available for several years, and, because of their favorable efficacy–side effect ratio, they are widely prescribed. Do milestones identified in this article for the course of older antidepressants apply to SSRIs? A precise answer requires an analysis identical to that performed for MAOIs, TCAs, and mianserin. We were unable to perform such an analysis, but we reviewed studies[22-25] in which the treatment responses of patients who received SSRIs and patients who received TCAs and placebo were compared. In 1 study, following a placebo run in, approximately 700 patients were randomized to receive placebo, imipramine, or fluoxetine for 6 weeks. The mean dose of imipramine was 205 mg/d (range, 50-300 mg/d), and the mean dose of fluoxetine was 70 mg/d (range, 20-80 mg/d). The imipramine dose (205 mg/d) is similar to the 200 mg/d we considered reasonably adequate. Approximately 10 different

Table 5. Hazard Estimates: The Probability of Improving Each Week, Patients Unimproved After IPR*

	Drug Therapy (n=287)		Placebo (n=152)		Drug Therapy vs Placebo	
Time, wk	Improved, No. of Patients	Hazard Estimate (SE)	Improved, No. of Patients	Hazard Estimate (SE)	Hazard Difference (SE)	*P*
0-1	4	0.014 (0.01)	3	0.020 (0.01)	−0.006 (0.02)	.66
1-2	15	0.054 (0.01)	0	0.000 (0.00)	0.054 (0.01)	.001
2-3	23	0.090 (0.02)	4	0.023 (0.01)	0.058 (0.02)	.01
3-4	40	0.178 (0.03)	6	0.042 (0.02)	0.136 (0.03)	.001
4-5	46	0.253 (0.04)	10	0.075 (0.02)	0.178 (0.04)	.001
5-6	42	0.304 (0.05)	14	0.115 (0.03)	0.190 (0.06)	.001

**IPR indicates initial placebo run-in period.*

efficacy measures were examined for each study week. Each drug differed from placebo on various measures from week 2 onward (most after 3 weeks); however, no differences between fluoxetine and imipramine existed, except the HAM-D total score (ie, imipramine superior to fluoxetine) at week 3. During each week of a doxepine-fluoxetine trial and a fluoxetine-amitriptyline trial, minor differences between drugs were noticeable, primarily resulting from the soporific effects of the TCAs. These articles[22-25] suggest that the time course of improvement with fluoxetine and the TCAs is similar. However, it is certainly possible that longer trials for SSRIs would disclose a greater proportion of patients with late onset of improvement. In a preliminary observation, Rosenbaum et al[26] suggest that some late effects of SSRIs may be observed. Therefore, application of the guidelines derived from data about TCAs, MAOIs, and mianserin if applied to SSRIs should be considered preliminary until more data are available. Furthermore, we cannot definitely conclude that in a 6-week trial all improvement while receiving any drug is observed. Although clinical experience suggests that the onset of first improvement is rarely observed after 6 weeks, a definitive answer requires longer controlled trials and not anecdotal observation.

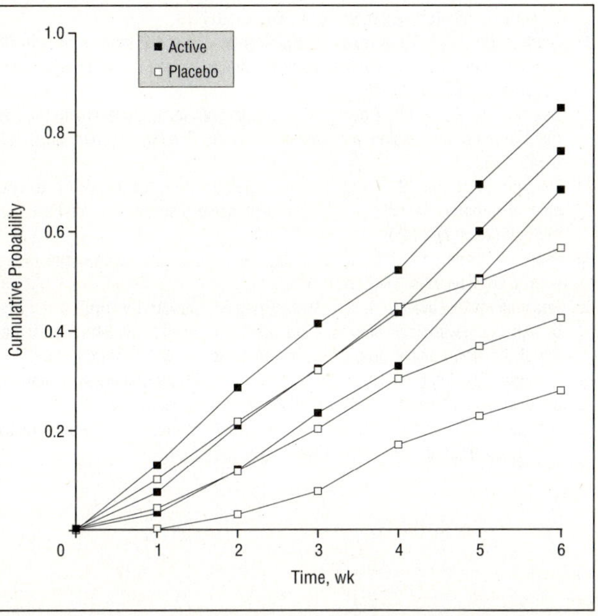

Figure 2. *Incidence plot of the onset of a persistent response (for patients whose conditions were minimally improved after the initial placebo run-in period with upper and lower bounds. The hazard estimates that correspond to this figure are provided in Table 6.*

Several other caveats are relevant. The data given are compromised in several ways. Not all patients were receiving a maximum dose by week 3, different drugs were used, and various ratings were unavailable each study week. Therefore, our recommendation should be considered with the understanding that this data set can only answer the question posed in a less than ideal manner. Supporting the recommendations are the facts that the dose achieved in our patients is generally not exceeded in outpatients and that the different classes of drugs seem to have a similar time course of onset. We know of no other attempt to define chronological milestones, so this article may aid in making clinical decisions until better data are available. The data provided do not support the conclusion, derived from studies lacking a comparison with a placebo group, that most drug effects occur in the first or second week of initiating treatment.[4-8] It is conceivable that the difference in sample characteristics accounts for the discrepancy between studies. However, this seems unlikely because these other studies included primarily inpatients. It is counterintuitive to conclude that more severely ill patients would improve more quickly. It is more likely that the absence of a placebo control prevented an adequate assessment of improvement attributable to nonspecific effects.

The prognosis of patients who received drug therapy and whose conditions were minimally improved at each study week was slightly better vs patients whose conditions were unimproved. This was also true of patients whose conditions were much improved in any week. We chose not to include the data for those patients whose conditions were much improved because the guidelines from those minimally improved are easily applied to those much improved, and the presentation was simplified (data available on request from the authors).

Our data suggest that treatments should be changed at the end of 4 weeks for patients whose conditions never minimally improve, changed at the end of 5 weeks for patients whose conditions were unimproved but minimally improved in a prior week, and continued for at least 6 weeks for patients whose conditions were minimally improved at the end of 5 weeks. At this point, augmen-

Table 6. Hazard Estimates: The Probability of Improving Each Week, Patients Minimally Improved After IPR*

	Drug Therapy (n=105)		Placebo (n=49)		Drug Therapy vs Placebo	
Time, wk	Improved, No. of Patients	Hazard Estimate (SE)	Improved, No. of Patients	Hazard Estimate (SE)	Hazard Difference (SE)	*P*
0-1	8	0.079 (0.03)	2	0.042 (0.03)	0.038 (0.04)	.36
1-2	14	0.156 (0.04)	4	0.089 (0.04)	0.067 (0.06)	.27
2-3	12	0.156 (0.04)	4	0.098 (0.05)	0.058 (0.07)	.38
3-4	11	0.168 (0.05)	5	0.137 (0.06)	0.031 (0.08)	.70
4-5	18	0.353 (0.08)	3	0.092 (0.05)	0.261 (0.10)	.01
5-6	18	0.546 (0.12)	3	0.102 (0.06)	0.444 (0.14)	.001

**IPR indicates initial placebo run-in period.*

tation strategies[1,27,28] or a change to a new drug class should be considered.[9]

Accepted for publication May 15, 1996.

This study was supported by grants MH-39143 and MH-30906 from the National Institute of Mental Health, Bethesda, Md, to the New York State Psychiatric Institute.

We thank Tina Walch, MD, for editorial assistance.

Reprints: Frederic Quitkin, MD, 722 W 168th St, Box 12, New York, NY 10032.

REFERENCES

1. Klein DF, Gittelman-Klein R, Quitkin FM, Rifkin A. *Diagnosis and Drug Treatment of Psychiatric Disorders.* Baltimore, Md: Williams & Wilkins; 1980:276-283.
2. Joyce PR, Paykel ED. Predictors of drug response in depression. *Arch Gen Psychiatry.* 1989;46:88-89.
3. Bielski RJ, Friedel RO. Prediction of tricyclic antidepressant response. *Arch Gen Psychiatry.* 1976;33:1479-1489.
4. Katz MM, Koslow SH, Maas JW, Frazer A, Bowden CL, Casper R, Croughan J, Kocsis J, Redmond E Jr. The timing, specificity and clinical prediction of tricyclic drug effects in depression. *Psychol Med.* 1987;17:297-309.
5. Casper RC, Katz MM, Bowden CL, Davis JM, Koslow SH, Hanin I. The pattern of physical symptom changes in major depressive disorder following treatment with amitriptyline or imipramine. *J Affect Disord.* 1994;31:151-164.
6. Coryell W, Coppen A, Zeigler VE, Biggs JT. Early improvement as a predictor of response to amitriptyline and nortriptyline: a comparison of 2 patient samples. *Psychol Med.* 1982;12:135-139.
7. Stassen HH, Angst J, Delini-Stula A. Severity at baseline and onset of improvement in depression: meta-analysis of imipramine and moclobemide versus placebo. *Eur Psychiatry.* 1994;9:129-136.
8. Katz M, Maas J, Frazer A, Koslow SH. Onset of antidepressant activity, the structure of depression and multiple drug actions. Presented at the American College of Neuropsychopharmacology Meeting; December 4, 1994; San Juan, Puerto Rico.
9. McGrath PJ, Stewart JW, Nunes EV, Ocepek-Welikson K, Rabkin JG, Quitkin KM, Klein DF. A double-blind cross over trial of imipramine and phenelzine for outpatients with treatment refractory depression. *Am J Psychiatry.* 1993;150 (1):118-123.
10. Quitkin FM, Rabkin JG, Markowitz JM, Stewart JW, McGrath PJ, Harrison W. Use of pattern analysis to identify true drug response: a replication. *Arch Gen Psychiatry.* 1987;44:259-264.
11. Stewart J, Quitkin FM, Fyer A, Rifkin A, McGrath P, Liebowitz M, Rosnick L, Klein DF. Efficacy of desipramine in endogenmorphically depressed patients. *J Affect Disord.* 1980;2:165-176.
12. Stewart JW, Quitkin FM, McGrath PJ, Liebowitz MR, Klein DF. Efficacy of desipramine in mildly depressed patients: a double-blind placebo-controlled trial. *Psychopharmacol Bull.* 1981;17:159-161.
13. Quitkin FM, Liebowitz MR, Stewart JW, McGrath PJ, Harrison W, Rabkin JG, Markowitz J, Davies SO. *l*-Deprenyl in atypical depressives. *Arch Gen Psychiatry.* 1984;41:777-781.
14. McGrath PJ, Quitkin FM, Harrison W, Stewart JW. Treatment of melancholia with tranylcypromine. *Am J Psychiatry.* 1984;141:288-289.
15. Liebowitz MR, Quitkin FM, Stewart JW, McGrath PJ, Harrison WM, Markowitz JS, Rabkin JG, Tricamo E, Goetz DM, Klein DF. Antidepressant specificity in atypical depression. *Arch Gen Psychiatry.* 1988;45:129-137.
16. Quitkin FM, McGrath PJ, Stewart JW, Harrison W, Wager SG, Nunes E, Rabkin JG, Tricamo E, Markowitz J, Klein DF. Phenelzine and imipramine in mood reactive depressives: further delineation of the syndrome of atypical depression. *Arch Gen Psychiatry.* 1989;46:787-793.
17. McGrath PJ, Rabkin JG, Stewart JW, Harrison W, Quitkin FM, Markowitz J. Placebo-controlled study of mianserin in depressed outpatients. *Neuropsychobiology.* 1985;14:128-132.
18. Quitkin FM, McGrath PJ, Stewart JW, Harrison W, Tricamo E, Wager SG, Ocepek-Welikson K, Nunes E, Rabkin JG, Klein DF. Atypical depression, panic attacks and response to imipramine and phenelzine: a replication. *Arch Gen Psychiatry.* 1990;47:935-941.
19. American Psychiatric Association. *Diagnostic and Statistical Manual of Mental Disorders, Third Edition, Revised.* Washington, DC: American Psychiatric Association; 1987.
20. Stewart JS, McGrath PJ, Rabkin JG, Quitkin FM. Atypical depression: a valid clinical entity? *Psychiatr Clin North Am.* 1993;16:479-495.
21. Spitzer RL, Endicott J, Robins E. *Research Diagnostic Criteria (RDC) for a Selected Group of Functional Disorders.* 3rd ed. New York, NY: New York State Psychiatric Institute, Biometrics Research; 1977:19.
22. Stark P, Hardison CD. A review of multicenter controlled studies of fluoxetine vs imipramine and placebo in outpatients with major depressive disorder. *J Clin Psychiatry.* 1985;46:53-58.
23. Beasley CM, Sayler ME, Potvin JH. Fluoxetine versus amitriptyline in the treatment of major depression: a multicenter trial. *Int Clin Psychopharmacol.* 1993; 8:143-149.
24. Feighner JP, Cohn JB. Double blind comparative trials of fluoxetine and doxepin in geriatric patients with major depressive disorder. *J Clin Psychiatry.* 1985;46(3, pt 2):20-25.
25. Fabre LF, Crismon L. Efficacy of fluoxetine in outpatients with major depression. *Curr Ther Res.* 1985;37:115-123.
26. Rosenbaum JF, Fava M, Quitkin FM, McGrath PJ, Stewart JW. Time to remission of depression with acute fluoxetine treatment. Presented at the 34th Annual Meeting of the New Clinical Drug Evaluation Unit; June 3, 1994; Marco Island, Fla.
27. Heninger GR, Charnley DS, Steinberg DE. Lithium carbonate augmentation of antidepressant treatment. *Arch Gen Psychiatry.* 1993;40:1335-1342.
28. Prange AJ, Wilson IC, Rabon AM. Enhancement of imipramine antidepressant activity by thyroid. *Am J Psychiatry.* 1969;126:457-469.

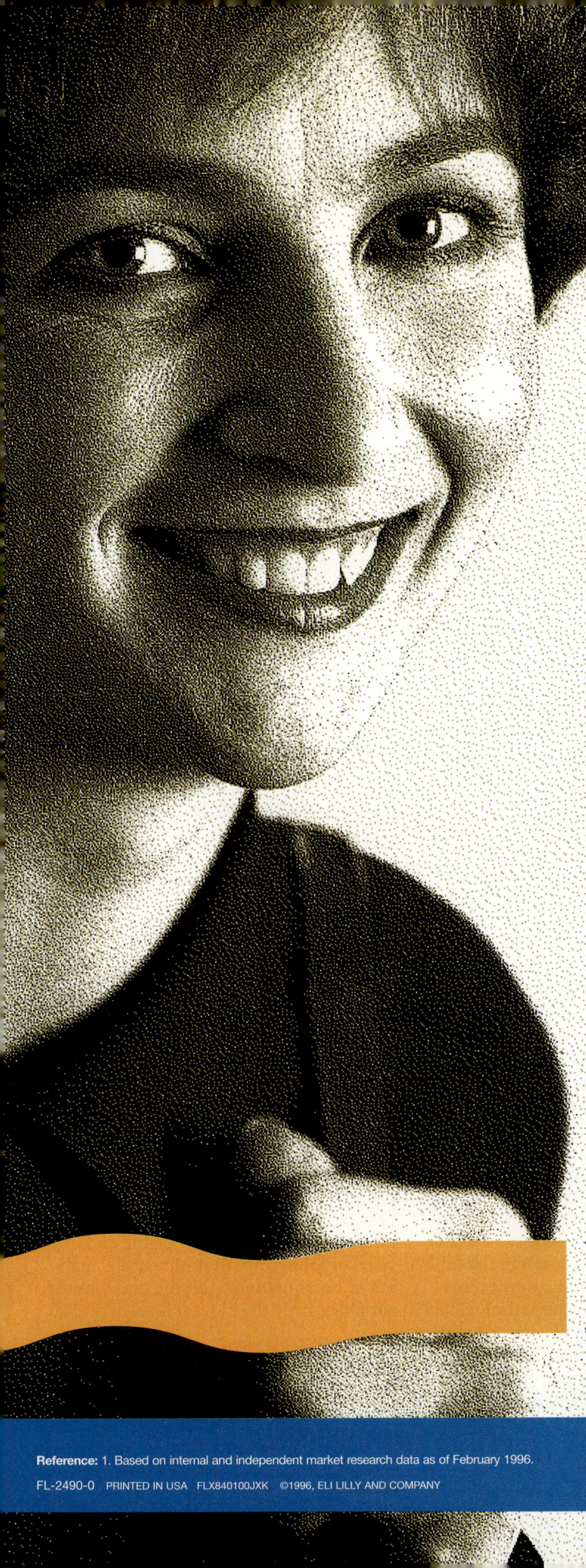

Since 1986, for more than 21 million patients in 90 countries around the world[1]

PROZAC®

fluoxetine hydrochloride

Reference: 1. Based on internal and independent market research data as of February 1996.

Lilly NEUROSCIENCE

Improving lives, restoring hope

ORIGINAL ARTICLE

Recovery After 5 Years of Unremitting Major Depressive Disorder

Timothy I. Mueller, MD; Martin B. Keller, MD; Andrew C. Leon, PhD; David A. Solomon, MD; M. Tracie Shea, PhD; William Coryell, MD; Jean Endicott, PhD

Background: The long-term course of depression in patients who present for treatment carries prognostic and therapeutic implications. This study presents prospective data on the time to recovery from an episode of major depressive disorder of 5 years' duration among patients followed up since 1978 in the National Institutes of Mental Health Collaborative Program on the Psychobiology of Depression.

Methods: Survival analysis was used to examine the 10-year course of the 431 probands with major depressive disorder with a specific focus on the 35 probands who were observed to be continuously ill for the first 5 years. Univariate analytic techniques were used to describe the demographic and clinical variables in the group that recovered and the group that did not. By study design, somatic treatment was assessed but not controlled by the investigators.

Results: By year 10, 93% (Kaplan-Meier estimate) of probands had recovered from their intake episode of major depressive disorder. In those ill for the first 5 years, 38% had recovered within the next 5 years. Shorter duration of illness prior to intake and being married were associated with the group that recovered. Pharmacological treatment dosages averaged 100 mg of imipramine hydrochloride equivalent in the chronically ill group.

Conclusions: Despite lengthy periods of illness, people continued to recover from major depressive disorder for up to 10 years of prospective follow-up. Few demographic and clinical variables distinguished those who recovered from those who did not. Treatment, as observed in this naturalistic study, was at a low level despite lengthy illness.

Arch Gen Psychiatry. 1996;53:794-799

From the National Institutes of Mental Health Collaborative Program on the Psychobiology of Depression–Clinical Studies. A complete listing of the participating investigators is given on page 798.

THE MAJORITY of people who seek treatment for major depressive disorder (MDD) recover from their episode of depression. Since 1978, the National Institutes of Mental Health Collaborative Program on the Psychobiology of Depression (CDS) has monitored the clinical condition of the 955 subjects who sought treatment for a mood disorder at 1 of 5 university medical centers. Keller et al[1] described the 5-year course of illness for the index episode of MDD in 431 subjects. This prospective naturalistic study revealed that 50% of subjects recover within the first 6 months of seeking treatment; there was a small but steady rate of recovery (1%-2% per month) during years 3 to 5 of the follow-up. The strongest predictors of recovery were severity of psychopathological symptoms in the prior week (inverse relation) and length of episode prior to study entry (inverse relation). The finding that 12% of subjects with MDD remain chronically ill after 5 years of prospective follow-up is similar to the 12% to 26% finding in other longitudinal studies of affective disorders.[2-6] These chronically ill patients with depression present a serious public health problem.

Coryell et al[7] examined the course of affective disorder in 129 CDS probands who at intake reported 2 or more years (mean, 6 years) of antecedent illness. These subjects with MDD, mania, or schizoaffective disorder experienced a longer time to recovery than their counterparts, who reported a briefer period of illness prior to intake (mean, 7 months). However, despite lengthy illness there was gradual progress toward recovery, with 77% experiencing at least 8 consecutive weeks of minimal or no symptoms by the end of 5 years of follow-up. In multivariate analyses of baseline demographic and clinical variables, only the highest level of overall

See Subjects and Methods on next page

SUBJECTS AND METHODS

SUBJECTS

Between the years 1978 and 1982, 955 patients who sought psychiatric treatment at 1 of 5 medical centers in the United States (Boston, Mass; Chicago, Ill; Iowa City, Iowa; New York, NY; and St Louis, Mo) were entered into a prospective naturalistic follow-up of patients with affective disorders.[11] This report extends previous analyses on the subgroup of 431 probands with only MDD at intake who had no history of mania, hypomania, schizoaffective disorder, chronic intermittent depressive disorder, or minor depression of at least 2 years' duration. The subset of 35 subjects who were ill for the first 5 years of follow-up and were followed up in years 6 through 10 is the focus of this report. All subjects initially presented for psychiatric care at inpatient or outpatient facilities (75% and 25%, respectively). Because genetic hypotheses were a component of the initial design, a relatively homogeneous sample was recruited such that all subjects were white and English-speaking. The CDS received approval from the institutional review board at each site. All subjects participated after signing informed consent.

ASSESSMENTS

All subjects were assessed at intake with the Schedule for Affective Disorders and Schizophrenia[12] using Research Diagnostic Criteria (RDC).[13] Subjects were interviewed every 6 months for the first 5 years and every year thereafter using the Longitudinal Interval Follow-up Evaluation.[14] This follow-up instrument measures the level of psychopathological symptoms for each RDC major affective disorder on a 6-point scale called the psychiatric status rating (PSR), which has been shown to have good to excellent interrater and test-retest reliability.[14,15] Using chronological anchor points as memory aids for the subject, the rater assigns a PSR for each week from the time of the last interview. Hospital records are routinely secured to corroborate the subject's self-reports. A PSR of 1 or 2 is assigned for those weeks in which there are no or minimal symptoms, respectively. A PSR of 3 or 4 corresponds to partial remission or significant symptoms not meeting full criteria for an RDC disorder, respectively. A PSR of 5 is given for those weeks during which subjects meet full criteria for an RDC disorder, and a 6 when accompanied by psychosis or extreme impairment. Recovery from MDD is defined as beginning with the first of 8 consecutive weeks of no or minimal symptoms (PSR of 1 or 2). The continuous string of PSR scores for MDD lasting up to 520 weeks is the source of data for the analyses of course.

CLINICAL CHARACTERISTICS

We examined demographic and clinical characteristics obtained at intake. These variables were hypothesized to have a relationship to the course of MDD in earlier work.[16] In addition, we updated the Hamilton Depression Rating Scale score (extracted)[12] and the Global Assessment Scale at the 5-year point to reflect the "current" status.

TREATMENT

Treatment was coded weekly using a 5-point summary scale of all antidepressant somatotherapy, including electroconvulsive therapy and pharmacotherapy, called the Composite Antidepressant (CAD) scale (**Table 1**). A CAD score of 0 means that no somatic treatment was provided, and a CAD score of 4 means that treatment equal to 300 mg or more of imipramine hydrochloride equivalent was provided. The study protocol did not influence treatment. Treatment was determined by the patient's private physician.

STATISTICAL METHODS

Outcomes for the analyses were recovery from MDD or end of follow-up (ie, censoring either by unavailability for follow-up or end of the assessment period). Analyses were conducted for the entire group of 431 probands with MDD at baseline and the 35 probands who remained ill for at least 5 years after entry into the study and for whom additional follow-up data were available. Survival analysis was used to analyze time until recovery during the follow-up.[17] The Kaplan-Meier product limit method was used to estimate the cumulative probability of recovery.[18] The interval-specific probabilities of recovery, similar to hazards, represent the proportion of those entering a follow-up interval in an episode of MDD who recovered during the interval.

For the analyses of the demographic variables, χ^2 and Student t tests were used for categorical and continuous variables, respectively. For the analyses of smaller samples, the Fisher exact test was used to compare results on variables with categorical outcomes, and the Mann-Whitney test was used for variables with continuous outcomes with the z statistic to correct for ties. A 2-tailed P value of less than .05 was considered statistically significant.

functioning in the 5 years prior to intake predicted the likelihood of recovery in the follow-up period.

Although other authors have used longitudinal or cross-sectional designs over a long time frame to examine MDD,[6,8-10] this is the first report, to our knowledge, that describes outcomes of a well-characterized sample continuously ill from MDD prospectively followed up for up to 10 years. The purpose of this article is to expand on the earlier reports by presenting the 10-year course of the index episode of illness in the 431 CDS probands with MDD, with a focus on those who stayed ill for at least 5 years. We characterize those continuously ill subjects by examining the course of illness during the subsequent 6 to 10 years of prospective follow-up and describing the demographic and clinical characteristics of those who had a recovery after 5 years and those who did not.

RESULTS

DEMOGRAPHIC AND CLINICAL CHARACTERISTICS

There are few demographic or clinical features that distinguish between those who did and did not recover in the

Table 1. Composite Antidepressant Score

Score	Amounts and Combinations of Somatic Therapies*
0	No treatment
1	Any imipramine hydrochloride, MAOI, or alprazolam or 1 ECT treatment; or ≥1000 mg of tryptophan; but less than amounts for score of 2
2	≥100 mg of imipramine hydrochloride or ≥30 mg of MAOI; any lithium carbonate; or ≥3000 mg of tryptophan; but less than amounts for score of 3
3	≥200 mg of imipramine hydrochloride or ≥60 mg of MAOI or ≥2 ECT treatments; but less than amounts for score of 4
4	≥300 mg of imipramine hydrochloride or ≥75 mg of MAOI or ≥3 ECT treatments

Indicates daily dose of medication and number of electroconvulsive therapy (ECT) treatments per week. MAOI indicates monoamine oxidase inhibitor.

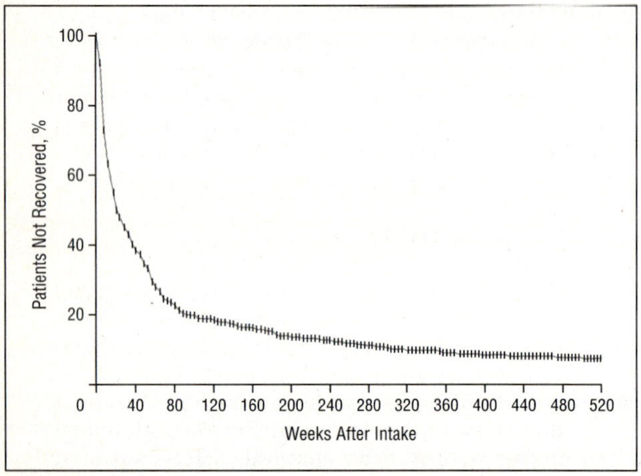

Figure 1. *Survival curve for 431 probands with major depressive disorder at intake.*

first 5 years. The mean (SD) age at intake (38.4 [14.7] years vs 38.3 [13.7] years), proportion of male subjects (39% vs 34%), mean (SD) Global Assessment Scale score at intake (40.8 [10.8] vs 39.4 [11.7]), percentage recruited from the inpatient setting (75% vs 83%), and modal socioeconomic group (Hollingshead-Redlich Scale[19] class III) were similar for the probands who recovered in the first 5 years (n=365) compared with the probands who were ill for at least 5 years (n=35). Thirty-one subjects were unavailable for follow-up while in an episode of MDD and were excluded from these analyses. The recovered vs nonrecovered probands at 5 years did differ by proportion presenting for their first episode of MDD (38% vs 26%, χ^2=6.14, *df*=2; *P*=.05), and Hamilton Depression Rating Scale score at intake (mean [SD]= 25.4 [6.7] vs 28.0 [7.2], *t*= −2.11, *df*=383; *P*=.04). At the Chicago, Iowa City, and New York City sites, about 5% of probands did not recover in the first 5 years, compared with about 15% at the St Louis and Boston sites (χ^2=13.04, *df*=4; *P*=.01).

FULL GROUP WITH MDD AT BASELINE: 10-YEAR COURSE OF RECOVERY

The survival curve of recovery from the index episode for the entire sample of 431 probands with MDD is pre-

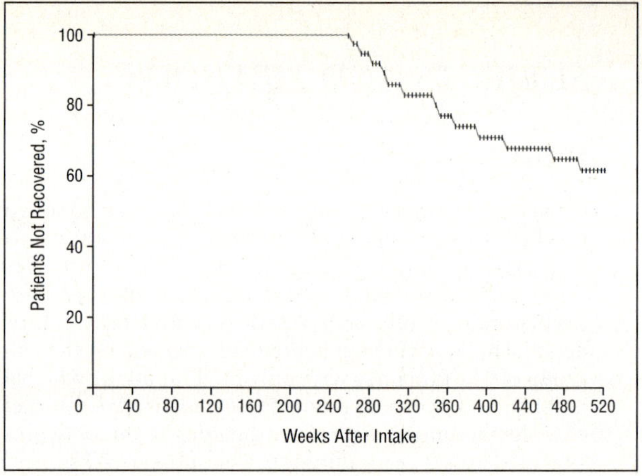

Figure 2. *Survival curve for 35 probands with major depressive disorder at intake who were continuously ill for 5 years.*

sented in **Figure 1**. The probability of recovery within 1 year of baseline was 67%; the probability of recovery within 2 years was 81%; the probability of recovery within 5 and 10 years was 88% and 93%, respectively (Kaplan-Meier estimates).

SUBSET WITH MDD THROUGHOUT FIRST 5 YEARS: COURSE OF RECOVERY

Cumulative and Interval-Specific Probability of Recovery

By design of the grouping strategy, no members of this group recovered from the index episode of MDD in the first 5 years after baseline. **Figure 2** presents the survival curve for this group. The cumulative probability of recovery by the end of the 10th year was 38%. After remaining depressed for the first 5 years after entry into the study, the probability of recovery during the sixth year was 13%; 10% during the seventh year; 8% during the eighth year; 4% during the ninth year; and 9% during the 10th year. Despite this slight variability, the median annual rate of recovery was 9%, a distinct decrease from the first year's rate of 67%.

Clinical Features of Recovered vs Nonrecovered Probands

Univariate analyses of demographic and clinical variables compared the 13 subjects who recovered during years 6 through 10 with the 22 who remained ill for the entire 10 years of observation. **Table 2** presents these clinical and demographic variables, some of which were collected at intake and others that were updated at 5 years. Compared with nonrecovered probands, recovered probands had briefer durations of MDD prior to intake and were less likely to be never married and more likely to be widowed, separated, or divorced. The mean Hamilton Depression Rating Scale score (extracted) updated at the 5-year point approached statistical significance, with the recovered group being less depressed than the nonrecovered group (17.5 vs. 29.3, *z*= −1.93, *P*=.054).

Table 2. Characteristics of Probands With RDC MDD Who Entered Year 6 With No Recovery*

Variables at Intake	Recovered During Years 6-10 (n=13)	Did Not Recover During Years 6-10 (n=22)
Mean (SD) age, y	34.4 (8.7)	40.5 (15.7)
Socioeconomic status, mean (SD) Hollingshead-Redlich Scale [19] score	3.3 (1.1)	3.2 (1.0)
Mean (SD) MDD duration prior to intake, wk†	139 (221)	176 (211)
Mean (SD) GAS score	37 (11.5)	35 (5.4)
Mean (SD) prior No. of MDD episodes	1.5 (1.1)	1.2 (1.1)
% Female	54	73
Marital status, %‡		
Married or living together	46	46
Never married	8	36
Widowed, separated, or divorced	46	18
RDC subtypes of MDD at intake, %		
Endogenous	85	82
Psychotic	15	23
Primary	62	77
Inpatient status, %	8	23
MDD duration >2 y, %	23	41
Variables at week 260		
Mean (SD) Hamilton score§[12]	17.5 (10.9)	29.3 (15.7)
Mean (SD) GAS score	59 (11.4)	48 (16.3)

*RDC indicates Research Diagnostic Criteria[13]; MDD, major depressive disorder; and GAS, Global Assessment Scale.
†z=1.47; P=.01.
‡Fisher exact P=.01.
§z=−1.93; P=.054.

Level of Psychopathological Symptoms

During years 6 through 10, the group mean (SD) of the within-subject mean PSR for the 22 nonrecovered probands is 4.47 (0.74) compared with 2.71 (1.08) for the 13 probands who recovered ($z=-4.13$, $P<.001$). A PSR of 4.47 is just below a level of 5, which corresponds to a level of psychopathological symptoms that would meet full criteria for RDC MDD. A PSR of 2.71, by comparison, is slightly below the level of symptoms defined as no more than moderate impairment but still obvious evidence of MDD, with considerably fewer psychopathological symptoms than those meeting full RDC criteria for MDD. The mean (SD) percentage of time spent at a level of psychopathological symptoms that met full criteria for MDD (PSR of 5 or 6) during years 6 through 10 was 23% (27%) and 54% (37%) for the recovered and nonrecovered probands, respectively (t=2.67, P=.01).

Treatment

The mean (SD) CAD score during years 6 through 10 was 2.3 (0.8) for the recovered group and 2.0 (0.7) for the nonrecovered group ($z=-0.84$, P=.40). During years 6 through 10 the mean (SD) percentage of weekly CAD scores greater than 2 was 34% (44%) and 25% (31%) ($z=-0.09$, P=.93) for the recovered and nonrecovered groups, respectively, and percentage greater than 3 was 11% in both groups (z=0.51, P=.61). We also examined the "adequacy" of antidepressant pharmacotherapy by examining the number of probands who received a minimal (at least 4 consecutive weeks with a CAD score ≥2) and a maximal (at least 4 consecutive weeks with a CAD score ≥4) course of treatment. In the 22 probands who did not recover, 16 (73%) received minimal treatment and 5 (23%) received maximal treatment. This was not different from the 10 (77%) who received minimal treatment and the 3 (23%) who received maximal treatment in the group of 13 probands who recovered in the 6- through 10-year interval. Two of 22 probands who did not recover and 3 of 13 who did recover received no somatic treatment during years 6 through 10 (χ^2=0.41, P=.52).

To evaluate the stability of the pharmacological treatment over years 6 through 10, we examined the within-subject SD of the weekly CAD score. A larger SD of the weekly CAD score corresponds to greater variability in medication doses. Conversely, the smaller this SD, the more "consistent" the medication doses. The mean (SD) of the within-subject SD of the CAD scores is 0.2 (0.2) and 0.5 (0.4) ($z=-2.45$, P=.01) for the recovered and nonrecovered probands, respectively.

COMMENT

A small but significant fraction of people who seek treatment for MDD continue to demonstrate a chronic, unrelenting depression. In the National Institutes of Mental Health CDS, 12% of probands with MDD were ill for 5 years of prospective follow-up, and 7% (Kaplan-Meier estimate) remained ill for the entire 10 years of follow-up. This group differs from the *DSM-IV*[20] category of "chronic" major depression, in that RDC criteria allow incomplete resolution of symptoms during an episode while the *DSM-IV* does not.

The subjects who entered the 6- through 10-year interval ill represent an unusual group of people who have been prospectively observed to be ill for a minimum of 5 years. One might expect that such patients are destined to never recover. Surprisingly, despite 5 years of prospectively observed illness and a mean of approximately 150 weeks of illness prior to intake, these subjects continued to experience a small but consistent rate of recovery of approximately 9% per year on average; 38% of the subjects continuously depressed for the first 5 years recovered during the 6- through 10-year period. This group of subjects was not significantly different on many demographic variables from the probands who experienced a recovery in the first 5 years. Additionally, there were few demographic data that distinguished the chronically depressed subjects who recovered from those who did not. Those who were ill longer prior to intake and were never married experienced a longer time to recovery in years 6 through 10, similar to the first 3 years of follow-up.[16] The small differences in the rates of not recovering in the first 5 years by intake site could reflect intake differences.

Since treatment is not controlled in this naturalistic study, the level of treatment can be seen as either a cause or an effect; eg, high levels of treatment are associated with a worse outcome or sicker subjects get more treatment. In fact, we again found low levels of pharmacological treatment for the sickest subjects *after* they had been ill for 5 years.[1,21] On average, subjects received a daily dose of between 100 and 199 mg of imipramine hydrochloride equivalent. There was no significant difference in the level of pharmacotherapy between those who eventually recovered and those who did not. Additionally, approximately 25% of both recovered and nonrecovered subjects did not receive even a minimal course of antidepressant therapy. The nonrecovered subjects did experience more variation in their daily dose, suggesting attempts to optimize pharmacotherapy; however, the variation was within a narrow range of half a CAD unit or approximately 50 mg of imipramine hydrochloride equivalent. Once again we ask, Why in this modern era do chronically ill subjects receive suboptimal levels of pharmacotherapy? Possible explanations include noncompliance with treatment, adverse effects of long-term administration of medications, discouragement with a chronic illness, and poor access to care.

Coryell and Winokur,[22] in their review of the course of affective disorders, note that previous work suggests that subjects with chronic MDD are characterized as being older, having psychotic features, and having a long history of illness prior to intake. Our data support only the length of illness prior to intake as a characteristic of this group. We excluded probands with schizoaffective disorders but not those with depression with psychotic features and found that psychotic features at intake did not have long-term predictive value. We also did not find age to be predictive. Coryell et al[23,24] found that psychotic features may predict the recurrence of psychotic features on subsequent episodes of MDD but are not associated with differential recovery rates for MDD.

These probands are representative of those with affective disorders who sought treatment at university medical centers. This treatment-seeking selection bias limits the generalizability of our findings. However, despite the differences in methods, these findings on chronicity are similar to those from a community sample. The 16-year follow-up from the Stirling County community sample showed that 75% of a small number of patients with depression had poor outcomes as measured by remaining chronically ill or by experiencing recurrence.[6] This sample also had a low level of treatment. Fewer than 20% saw a psychiatrist and only half told their general physician that they felt depressed.

Results from the Epidemiologic Catchment Area study on health services utilization indicate that people with unipolar major depression accounted for 21% of all visits to ambulatory settings for a mental health disorder.[25] In this study, 54% of people with unipolar major depression had recently sought treatment for their disorder, with the services almost evenly split between specialty mental health and general medical sites.[26] Coryell et al[27] showed that compared with a matched control group of well relatives, CDS probands with MDD experienced significant decrements in function in many life areas, such as educational status, employment, annual income, interpersonal relationships, and overall life satisfaction. It is unknown what the functional consequences and public health impact are of people who are chronically ill with MDD compared with those who successfully recover from their disorder. Fortunately, this group of people who do not recover from MDD appears to be a small fraction of those with MDD for, as we have shown, people with MDD can recover even after lengthy illness.

Accepted for publication March 26, 1996.

This article has been reviewed by the Publication Committee of the Collaborative Depression Study, and has its endorsement. The authors wish to acknowledge the expertise of Mary Duquette and Rita Misek in the preparation of the manuscript and the anonymous reviewers who assisted in its revision.

This study was conducted with the participation of the following investigators: M. B. Keller, MD (Chairperson, Providence, RI); W. Coryell, MD (Co-Chairperson, Iowa City); H. S. Akiskal, MD; J. D Maser, PhD (Washington, DC); P. W. Lavori, PhD; T. I. Mueller, MD; M. T. Shea, PhD (Providence); J. Fawcett, MD; W. A. Scheftner, MD (Chicago); J. Haley (Iowa City); J. Endicott, PhD; A. Leon, PhD; J. Loth, MSW (New York); J. Rice, PhD; T. Reich, MD (St Louis). Other contributors include N. C. Andreasen, MD, PhD; P. J. Clayton, MD; J. Croughan, MD; G. L. Klerman, MD; R. M. A. Hirschfeld, MD; M. M. Katz, PhD; E. Robins, MD; R. L. Spitzer, MD; G. Winokur, MD; and M. A. Young, PhD.

Reprints: Timothy I. Mueller, MD, Department of Psychiatry and Human Behavior, Brown University School of Medicine, Butler Hospital, 345 Blackstone Blvd, Providence, RI 02906.

REFERENCES

1. Keller MB, Lavori PW, Mueller TI, Endicott J, Coryell W, Hirschfeld RMA, Shea T. Time to recovery, chronicity, and levels of psychopathology in major depression: a 5-year prospective follow-up of 431 subjects. *Arch Gen Psychiatry.* 1992;49:809-816.
2. Kerr TA, Roth M, Schapira K, Gurney C. The assessment and prediction of outcome in affective disorders. *Br J Psychiatry.* 1972;121:167-174.
3. Tsuang MT, Woolson RF, Fleming JA. Long-term outcome of major psychoses, I: schizophrenia and affective disorders compared with psychiatrically symptom-free surgical conditions. *Arch Gen Psychiatry.* 1979;36:1295-1301.
4. Rounsaville BJ, Prusoff BA, Padian N. The course of nonbipolar, primary major depression: a prospective 16-month study of ambulatory patients. *J Nerv Ment Dis.* 1980;168:406-411.
5. Angst J. The course of affective disorders. *Psychopathology.* 1987;19:47-52.
6. Murphy JM. Depression in the community: findings from the Stirling County Study. *Can J Psychiatry.* 1990;35:390-396.
7. Coryell W, Endicott J, Keller M. Outcome of patients with chronic affective disorder: a five-year follow-up. *Am J Psychiatry.* 1990;147:1627-1633.
8. Kraepelin E. *Manic-depressive Insanity and Paranoia.* Edinburgh, Scotland: E&S Livingstone; 1921.
9. Winokur G, Morrison J. The Iowa 500: follow-up of 225 depressives. *Br J Psychiatry.* 1973;123:543-548.
10. Zis AP, Goodwin FK. Major affective disorder as a recurrent illness. *Arch Gen Psychiatry.* 1979;36:835-839.
11. Katz M, Klerman GL. Introduction: overview of the clinical studies program. *Am J Psychiatry.* 1979;136:49-51.
12. Endicott J, Spitzer RL. A diagnostic interview: the Schedule for Affective Disorders and Schizophrenia. *Arch Gen Psychiatry.* 1978;35:837-844.
13. Spitzer RL, Endicott J, Robins E. Research Diagnostic Criteria: rationale and reliability. *Arch Gen Psychiatry.* 1978;35:773-782.
14. Keller MB, Lavori PW, Friedman B, Nielsen E, Endicott J, McDonald-Scott P, Andreasen NC. The Longitudinal Interval Follow-up Evaluation: a comprehensive method for assessing outcome in prospective longitudinal studies. *Arch Gen Psychiatry.* 1987;44:540-548.
15. Warshaw MG, Keller MB, Stout RL. Reliability and validity of the Longitudinal Interval Follow-up Evaluation for assessing outcome of anxiety disorders. *J Psychiat Res.* 1994;28:531-545.
16. Keller MB, Shapiro RW, Lavori PW, Wolfe N. Recovery in major depressive disorder: analysis with the life table and regression models. *Arch Gen Psychiatry.* 1982;39:905-910.
17. Kalbfleish JD, Prentice RL. *The Statistical Analysis of Failure-Time Data.* New York, NY: Wiley & Sons Inc; 1980.
18. Kaplan EL, Meier P. Nonparametric estimation from incomplete observations. *J Am Stat Assoc.* 1958;53:457-481.
19. Miller DC. *Handbook of Research and Design and Social Measurement.* 5th ed. Newbury Park, Calif: Sage Publications Inc; 1991:351-359.
20. American Psychiatric Association. *Diagnostic and Statistical Manual of Mental Disorders, Fourth Edition.* Washington, DC: American Psychiatric Association; 1994.
21. Keller MB, Lavori PW, Klerman GL, Andreasen NC, Endicott J, Coryell W, Fawcett J, Rice JP, Hirschfeld RMA. Low levels and lack of predictors of somatotherapy and psychotherapy received by depressed patients. *Arch Gen Psychiatry.* 1986;43:458-466.
22. Coryell W, Winokur G. Course and outcome. In: Paykel ES, ed. *Handbook of Affective Disorders.* 2nd ed. New York, NY: Churchill Livingstone; 1992.
23. Coryell W, Endicott J, Keller M. The importance of psychotic features to major depression: course and outcome during a two-year follow-up. *Acta Psychiatr Scand.* 1987;75:78-85.
24. Coryell W, Winokur G, Shea T, Maser JD, Endicott J, Akiskal HS. The long-term stability of depressive subtypes. *Am J Psychiatry.* 1994;151:199-204.
25. Narrow WE, Regier DA, Rae DS, Manderscheid RW, Locke BZ. Use of services by persons with mental and addictive disorders. *Arch Gen Psychiatry.* 1993;50:95-107.
26. Regier DA, Narrow WE, Rae DS, Manderscheid RW, Locke BZ. The de facto US mental and addictive disorders service system. *Arch Gen Psychiatry.* 1993;50:85-94.
27. Coryell W, Scheftner W, Keller M, Endicott J, Maser J, Klerman GL. The enduring psychosocial consequences of mania and depression. *Am J Psychiatry.* 1993;150:720-726.

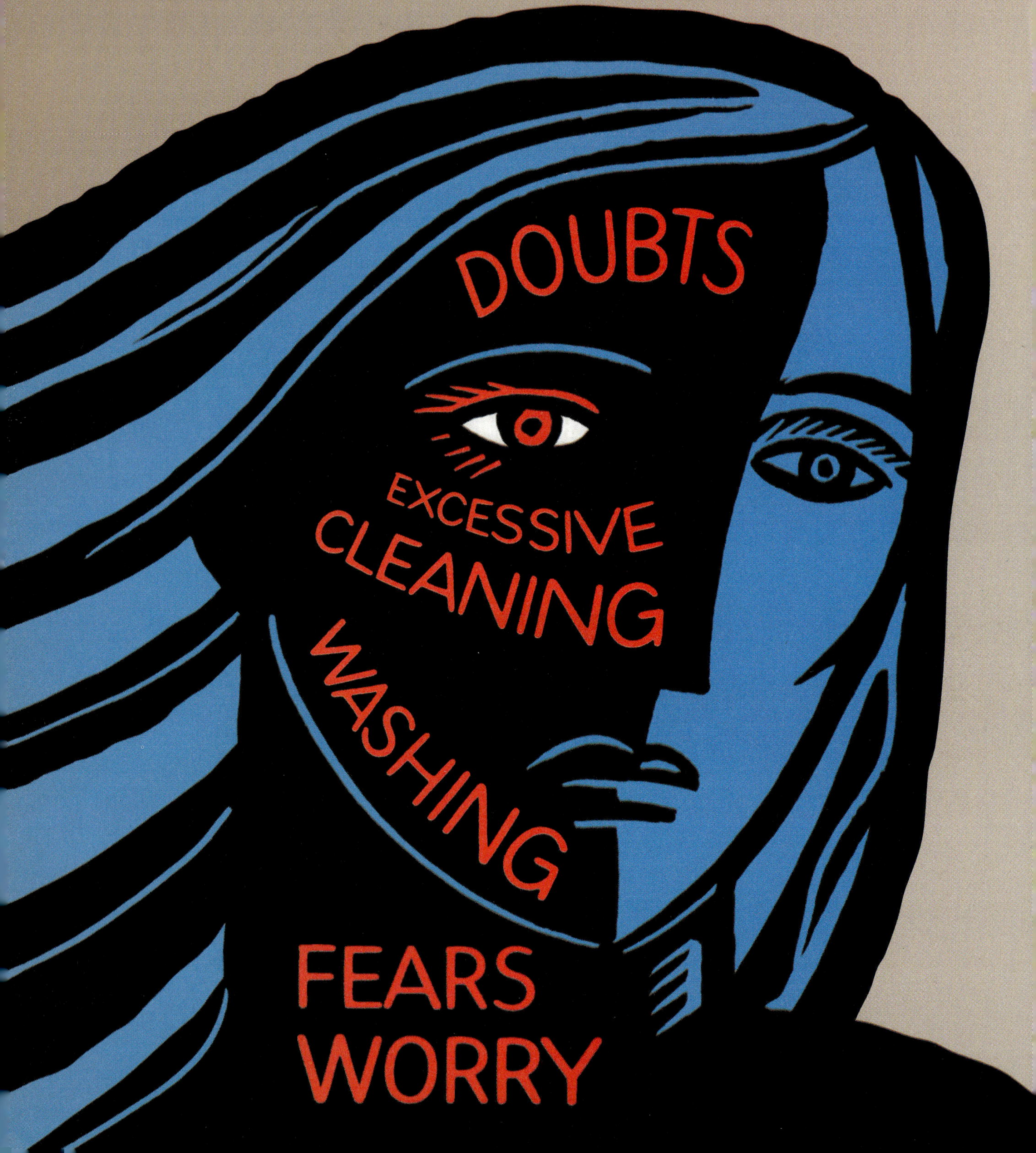
DOUBTS
EXCESSIVE
CLEANING
WASHING
FEARS
WORRY

ORIGINAL ARTICLE

Immunodetection and Quantitation of Imidazoline Receptor Proteins in Platelets of Patients With Major Depression and in Brains of Suicide Victims

Jesús A. García-Sevilla, MD; Pablo V. Escribá, PhD; Magdalena Sastre, PhD; Claude Walzer, PhD; Xavier Busquets, PhD; Galina Jaquet, MD; Donald J. Reis, MD; José Guimón, MD

Background: Imidazoline receptors are a newly discovered family of receptors, some of which, like α_2-adrenoceptors, have a presynaptic inhibitory effect on the release of norepinephrine. The aim of this study was to identify by immunodetection imidazoline receptor proteins in human platelets and the brain to assess their status in depression and suicide.

Methods: Platelets were collected from 26 drug-free depressed patients and 26 controls. Specimens of frontal cortex (Brodmann area 9) were collected from 13 suicide victims and 11 controls. Levels of imidazoline receptor proteins were assessed by immunoblotting techniques. Solubilized imidazoline receptors were separated by gel electrophoresis, transferred to nitrocellulose membranes, labeled with a specific anti–imidazoline receptor antiserum, and quantitated by image analysis.

Results: Platelet and brain membranes expressed similar 45-kd imidazoline receptor proteins, and their mean±SEM immunoreactivities were found to be increased in depressed patients (platelets, 40%±5%) and suicide victims (brain, 51%±14%). Platelets also expressed a 35-kd imidazoline receptor protein that was also found to be up-regulated in depressed patients (21%±4%). In contrast, brain membranes did not express this 35-kd protein but revealed a 29/30-kd imidazoline receptor protein that was found to be down-regulated in suicide victims (19%±3%). In a subset of depressed patients who underwent antidepressant treatment, a change in the immunoreactivity of the up-regulated 45-kd platelet imidazoline receptor protein (−35%±5%), but not of the 35-kd protein, was observed.

Conclusion: The results support a role for the newly discovered imidazoline receptors (mainly the 45-kd receptor expressed in the brain and platelets) in the pathogenesis of depression.

Arch Gen Psychiatry. 1996;53:803-810

MAJOR DEPRESSION has been associated with increased inhibitory α_2-autoreceptor and/or α_2-heteroreceptor activity in the brain that might be related to the deficit in noradrenergic and/or serotonergic function and decreased neurotransmitter release postulated in depression.[1,2] This hypothesis was supported initially by the finding that depressed patients possess supersensitive α_{2A}-adrenoceptors in blood platelets[3-6] and recently by the direct demonstration of increased density and affinity of $\alpha_{2A/C}$-adrenoceptor agonist binding sites in the brains of depressed suicide victims.[1,2,7,8]

However, this α_2-adrenoceptor abnormality in depression was detected mainly by using imidazoline radioligands such as [^{3}H]clonidine/*p*-aminoclonidine, [^{3}H]UK14303 (bromoxidine), and [^{3}H]idazoxan, which, in addition to α_2-adrenoceptors, also bind to distinct membrane proteins called imidazoline receptors.[9-12] Agmatine (decarboxylated arginine) is an endogenous agonist at imidazoline receptors and may act as a new neurotransmitter.[13,14] Imidazoline receptors exist in 2 main types: the clonidine-preferring receptor (I_1 type) and the idazoxan-preferring receptor (I_2 type).[10] In the central nervous system, I_1-imidazoline receptors regulate blood pressure,[11,15-17] probably by inhibiting the release of catecholamines in the brain stem.[17] They also mediate inhibitory effects on norepinephrine release in sympathetic nerve terminals[18,19] and on the secretion

From the Department of Psychiatry, Medical School, University of Geneva, Geneva, Switzerland (Drs García-Sevilla, Walzer, Jaquet, and Guimón); Laboratory of Neuropharmacology, Department of Fundamental Biology and Health Sciences, University of the Balearic Islands, Palma de Mallorca, Spain (Drs García-Sevilla, Escribá, Sastre, and Busquets); and Division of Neurobiology, Department of Neurology and Neuroscience, Cornell University Medical College, New York, NY (Dr Reis).

See Subjects and Methods on next page

SUBJECTS AND METHODS

PATIENT SELECTION

Patients were examined and treated in the Psychiatric Clinic I, Department of Psychiatry, Medical School, University of Geneva, Geneva, Switzerland. This part of the study was approved by the research and ethical review board of the Department of Psychiatry. Twenty-six patients (17 hospitalized patients and 9 outpatients) suffering from recurrent (*DSM-III-R* code 296.3, 18 patients) or single-episode (*DSM-III-R* code 296.2, 8 patients) major depression were selected for the study. The patients were informed of the purpose of the study and gave their written consent to participate. All selected patients were free of other medical illness and were permitted their regular habits but were warned not to use psychotropic drugs, except for moderate doses of prescribed benzodiazepines (mainly flurazepam hydrochloride, 30 mg/d, and lorazepam, 3 mg/d). Depressed patients were free of antidepressant and antipsychotic drugs for a minimum of 2 weeks before the assays (the drug-free period was 2 weeks for 2 patients and ≥8 weeks for 24 patients). The severity of depressive symptoms was assessed by the 17-item Hamilton Rating Scale for Depression (HRSD),[43] which was completed by a research psychiatrist who was blind to the experimental protocol. The mean±SEM global score on the HRSD was 28±1 (range, 20 to 39). Whenever possible, depressed patients were studied again after antidepressant treatment. These patients received the cyclic antidepressant drugs, citalopram hydrochloride, 20 to 40 mg/d (n=7); clomipramine hydrochloride, 100 mg/d (n= 1); or imipramine hydrochloride, 200 mg/d (n=1). The quantitation of platelet imidazoline receptors was repeated 2 to 12 weeks after the onset of treatment. Six patients were considered responders and had their blood sample taken when their mean±SEM score on the HRSD was 8±1 (range, 3-11; range before treatment, 32-22). Two patients were partial responders (HRSD score, 19; scores before treatment, 26 and 28) and had their blood sample taken 9 weeks after the onset of treatment. Another responder did not complete the treatment phase and had the blood sample taken 2 weeks after the onset of treatment (HRSD score, 17; score before treatment, 39).

An equal number of normal volunteers who were matched with the selected patients for sex and as closely as possible for age (±5 years) were also studied. The healthy controls were recruited among hospital employees. Control subjects were interviewed and screened by a research psychiatrist to exclude those with a history of psychiatric disorder or medical illness as well as those with a history of drug or alcohol abuse. Control subjects were drug-free for a minimum of 2 weeks before the assays.

BLOOD SAMPLES

Venous blood was obtained by venipuncture from 26 healthy male (n=10) and female (n=16) volunteers (mean±SEM age, 42±2 years; range, 27-67 years) as well as from 26 drug-free male (n=10) and female (n=16) depressed patients (mean age, 41±2 years; range, 29-64 years). An aliquot of 5 mL of blood from each subject was collected in plastic tubes containing citrate-dextrose solution as an anticoagulant.

Platelets were isolated by centrifugation (350g for 15 minutes) on 5 mL of 1-step Human Platelets Cell Separation Medium (Accurate Chemical & Science Co, Westbury, NY). Then the translucent platelet layer was recovered, mixed with 2 volumes of 0.9% sodium chloride, and recentrifuged (600g for 5 minutes). The pellet of platelets was stored at −80°C until the assays could be performed. Platelet membranes were prepared for immunodetection of imidazoline receptor proteins as described for human brain membranes.[27] The protein content of the samples was measured by the bicinchoninic acid method.[44]

HUMAN BRAIN SAMPLES

Human brains were obtained at autopsy in the Instituto Anatómico Forense, Palma de Mallorca, Spain. This part of the study was approved by the research and ethical review board of the Fondo de Investigaciones Sanitarias, Madrid, Spain. Specimens of the frontal cortex (Brodmann area 9) were collected from 13 suicide victims (9 men and 4 women; mean±SEM age, 54±5 years; mean±SEM postmortem delay, 26±3 hours) and were immediately stored at −80°C. As determined by the medical examiner, the suicide victms died of trauma caused by a fall from a height (n=6), hanging (n=5), carbon monoxide poisoning (n=1), and hydrochloric acid ingestion (n=1). Detailed medical histories of these subjects were not available for this study, except for 4 suicide victims in whom a firm retrospective antemortem clinical diagnosis of major depression could be made (1 suicide victim had 2 previously documented suicide attempts). These patients had probably received antidepressant drugs (amitryptiline hydrochloride, clomipramine hydrochloride, lithium) during their illness, as revealed by prescriptions found in medical histories. The rest of the suicide victims were apparently medication-free, and they were not drug abusers according to family reports.

The control group consisted of similar brain specimens from 11 subjects (7 men and 4 women; mean±SEM age, 53±4 years; mean±SEM postmortem delay, 30±4 hours) without an apparent history of neuropsychiatric disorder or drug abuse who died suddenly of various accidental causes, mainly motor vehicle accidents. Only

of catecholamines in adrenal chromaffin cells.[20] The I_2-imidazoline receptor is mainly localized in glial cells and appears to be associated with the enzyme monoamine oxidase B.[21,22] In the brain, various functional and pathological roles have been assigned to I_2-imidazoline receptors.[22-26]

Recently, various imidazoline receptor proteins have been identified in the brain[27,28] and other tissues,[29-32] which has confirmed the heterogeneity of imidazoline receptors[12,33,34] and the association of some of these proteins with specific receptor types.[33] Human platelets also appear to possess the 2 main types of imidazoline receptors, as identified by imidazoline radioligands.[36-38]

In recent studies, levels of I_1-imidazoline receptors have been found to be increased in platelets of patients with unipolar depression and to be down-regulated after treatment with desipramine hydrochloride.[6,39] In addition, an increased proportion of nonadrenoceptor sites ethanol screening was carried out on blood samples, and ethanol was detected in most suicide victims (n=8) and controls (n=9). The mean age, sex ratio, and postmortem delay (time from death to the storage of the brain specimen) were similar in control subjects and suicide victims (see above). In a given experiment, suicide victims were matched with controls for age, postmortem delay, and, when possible, sex. The specific immunoreactivity of imidazoline receptor proteins was not altered by the postmortem delay (range, 6-48 hours). Tissue storage (time from freezing to immnunoblot analysis; mean±SEM, 22±2 months) did not differ between controls (22±1 months) and suicide victims (23±3 months). Cortical membranes were prepared for immunodetection of imidazoline receptor proteins, as described in detail previously.[27]

IMMUNOBLOT ANALYSIS AND QUANTITATION OF IMIDAZOLINE RECEPTOR PROTEINS AND α-TUBULIN

The levels of imidazoline receptors in platelets and brain membranes were assessed by immunoblotting (Western blotting) using a specific rabbit antiserum raised against the imidazoline receptor, purified from bovine adrenal chromaffin cells.[27,30,45] Briefly,[27,46] solubilized imidazoline receptors were separated by polyacrylamide gel electrophoresis (sodium dodecyl sulfate), transferred to nitrocellulose membranes (Western blotting), labeled with the anti–imidazoline receptor antiserum (1:5000 dilution for 14-16 hours at 4°C), and incubated for 2 hours at room temperature with a blocking solution containing horseradish peroxidase–linked donkey anti–rabbit IgG antiserum (1:5000 dilution). Immunoreactivity was detected using the Enhanced Chemiluminescence Western Blot Detection System (Amersham International, Little Chalfont, England) followed by exposure to film (Amersham ECL Hyperfilm) for 5 to 15 minutes. Films were scanned in an image analyzer (Bio Image, Millipore Corp, Ann Arbor, Mich).[46] α-Tubulin, a cytoskeletal protein used as a loading negative control, was separated and detected as described above using a monoclonal anti–α-tubulin (clone DM 1A) diluted at 1:3000 as the primary antibody. The secondary antibody, horseradish peroxidase–linked sheep anti–mouse IgG, was incubated at 1:5000 dilution as described above.

For the quantitation of platelet imidazoline receptor proteins, 3 to 6 platelet samples from a depressed patient (drug-free and/or after antidepressant treatment) were evaluated using standard curves[46,47] (ie, total protein loaded vs integrated optical density), which consisted of at least 5 points of different protein content (usually 5-50 μg of protein, resulting in a linear relationship) from the same control-matched subject all loaded on the same gel. Moreover, in a given gel, triplicate samples from other controls were similarly evaluated as problem samples to assess the intra-assay (4%) and interassay (8%) coefficients of variation. Given a known amount of membrane protein from a problem sample loaded in the gel well (PR, the real amount), the percentage change with respect to control samples was calculated as the ratio between the amount of protein corresponding to the integrated optical density value of the problem sample interpolated in the control standard curve (PT, the theoretical amount) and PR. Thus, the percentage change is (PT/PR)×100, where this value is 100 for a healthy control sample used as the standard.[46]

For the quantitation of imidazoline receptor proteins in the human brain, a similar procedure was followed that has been described in detail previously.[27,35,46] In brain specimens, the mean intra-assay and interassay coefficients of variation were 6% (same control subject) and 16% (different control subjects). α-Tubulin in platelet and brain membranes was quantitated as described previously.[46]

MATERIALS AND DRUGS

The purification of imidazoline receptors from bovine adrenal chromaffin cells and the production of a specific polyclonal antiserum against these proteins have been described previously.[30,45] The specificity of this antiserum for the detection of imidazoline receptor proteins has also been assessed.[27,45] The isolation and immunodetection of a rat 45-kd peptide strongly supported the relationship of this antiserum with the imidazoline binding site.[48] The polyclonal antiserum does not cross-react with α_2-adrenoceptors. Thus, in membranes from Sf9 (*Spodoptera frugiperda*) cells infected with baculovirus to overexpress the human recombinant α_{2A}-adrenoceptor (Research Biochemicals International, Natick, Mass), the imidazoline receptor antiserum did not recognize the α_{2A}-adrenoceptor (an approximately 70-kd protein), which was readily detected with an antibody against this α_2-adrenoceptor subtype (data not shown). Anti–α-tubulin monoclonal antibody (clone DM 1A) was from Sigma Chemical Co, St Louis, Mo. Secondary antibodies, chemiluminescence reagents, and film for autoradiography were from Amersham International. Other chemicals were from Sigma Chemical Co.

STATISTICS

Results are expressed as mean±SEM. The 1-sample *t* test (identical in its implementation to the paired *t* test) or Student *t* test was used for the statistical evaluations. Pearson correlation coefficients were calculated to test for possible association among variables. The level of significance was $P\leq.05$. All tests were 2-tailed.

(proposed imidazoline receptors) was found in the frontal cortex of depressed suicide victims.[40] Moreover, the brain I_2-imidazoline receptor has been shown to be markedly down-regulated by antidepressant monoamine oxidase inhibitors.[41,42] These preliminary results in depressed patients and suicide victims suggested that enhanced imidazoline receptor activity could be involved, together with supersensitive α_2-adrenoceptors, in the pathogenesis of depression.[40] However, these studies were hampered by the use of imidazoline radioligands that are not fully specific for imidazoline receptors.

The purposes of this study were first to identify, by immunodetection with a specific antibody, imidazoline receptor proteins in human platelets and in the human brain, and then to assess the biological status of platelet and brain imidazoline receptors in major depression and in suicide.

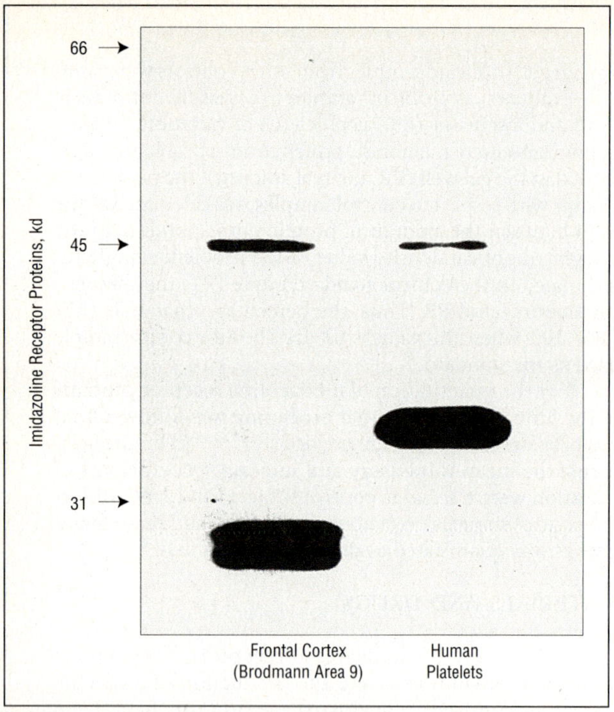

Figure 1. *Immunological detection of imidazoline receptor proteins in the human brain and human platelets. Molecular masses were estimated from referenced standards.*

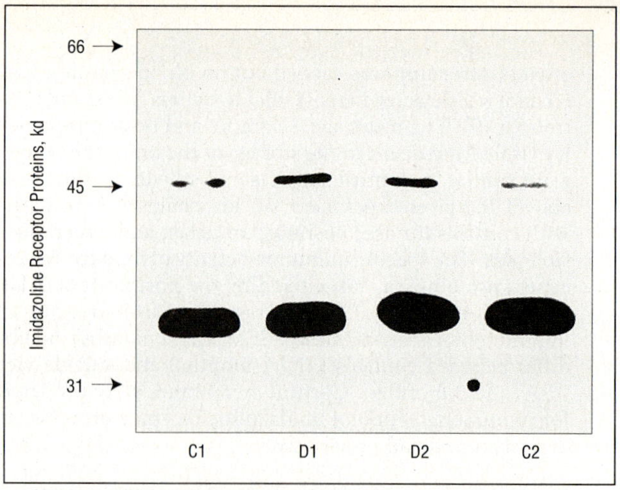

Figure 2. *Representative immunoblots for platelet imidazoline receptor proteins from depressed patients (D1 was a 43-year-old man; D2, a 31-year-old man) and matched healthy controls (C1 was a 47-year-old man; C2, a 33-year-old man). The amounts of total protein loaded per gel well were 16.8 µg (C1), 17.2 µg (D1), 19.5 µg (C2), and 19.1 µg (D2). The 2 bands correspond to the 35-kd and 45-kd proteins. Note that in depressed patients the immunoreactivity of the 45-kd band was markedly increased (D1, 48%; D2, 58%), while the increase in the 35-kd band was more modest (D1, 18%; D2, 18%).*

RESULTS

IMMUNOLOGICAL DETECTION OF IMIDAZOLINE RECEPTOR PROTEINS

Platelet membranes expressed 2 well-defined immunoreactive imidazoline receptor proteins, an intense band of approximately 35 kd and a less intense band of approximately 45 kd (apparent molecular masses). The relative immunoreactivity was 90% to 95% of total immunoreactivity for the 35-kd protein and 5% to 10% for the 45-kd protein (**Figure 1**). The frontal cortex of the human brain also expressed a 45-kd imidazoline receptor protein. In contrast, the platelet 35-kd protein was not expressed in the frontal cortex, which also expressed an intense band of approximately 29/30 kd. The relative immunoreactivity of these brain imidazoline receptors was 85% to 90% of total immunoreactivity for the 29/30-kd protein and 10% to 15% for the 45-kd protein (Figure 1).

In platelets and the brain, the polyclonal antibody used also detected other bands of different molecular masses, but they were not considered for further analysis because they had lesser immunoreactivity and were expressed only in a few subjects and regardless of the clinical status.

DENSITY OF IMIDAZOLINE RECEPTOR PROTEINS IN PLATELETS BEFORE AND AFTER ANTIDEPRESSANT DRUG TREATMENT

In platelet membranes of depressed patients, the total immunoreactivity of imidazoline receptor proteins (the sum of the 2 bands shown in **Figure 2**) was increased (mean±SEM percentage change, 123%±5%; n=26; t=4.79; P<.001) compared with that of age- and sex-matched controls. Specifically, the immunoreactivity of the 35-kd band was increased (percentage change, 121%±4%; n=26; t=5.80; P<.001; range of change, 98%-178%). In addition, the immunoreactivity of the 45-kd band was increased in the platelet membranes of the same depressed patients (percentage change, 140%±5%; n=26; t=8.28; P<.001; range of change, 93%-216%) compared with the same controls (Figure 2). The increase for the 45-kd band was greater than that observed for the 35-kd band (19.5%±5.5%, n=26, t=3.55, P<.005). Moreover, there was no significant correlation between the increases of the 45-kd band and those of the 35-kd band in the same depressed patients (r=0.19, n=26, P>.05), which suggested different expression patterns for the 2 imidazoline receptor proteins. The increases in immunoreactive imidazoline receptor proteins were significant both in patients with a single depressive episode (35-kd band: 116%±4% [mean±SEM], n=8, t=4.00, P<.005; 45-kd band: 157%±4%, n=8, t=14.25, P<.001) and in those with the recurrent type of depression (35-kd band: 122%±5%, n=18, t=4.40, P<.001; 45-kd band: 132%±6%, n=18, t=5.33, P<.001). In the subgroup of patients with a single depressive episode, however, the immunoreactivity of the 45-kd band was greater than that of the 35-kd band (25%, t=3.47, P<.005). The severity of depression on the HRSD did not correlate with the immunoreactivity of platelet imidazoline receptor proteins (r=0.05 and r=−0.12 for the 35-kd and 45-kd bands, respectively). However, the immunoreactivity of the 35-kd band was greater (16%, t=2.74, P<.02) in depressed patients with high suicidal ideation or suicide attempts (score of 2-4 on item 3 of the HRSD; 35-kd band: 127%±5%, n=15) than in those with low suicidal behavior (score of 0 or 1 on the HRSD; 35-kd band: 111%±3%, n=11).

The immunoreactivity of the 45-kd band did not differ in these 2 subgroups of patients (142%±8%, n=15, and 137%±5%, n=11, respectively).

The immunoreactivity of platelet imidazoline receptor proteins was not associated with sex or age. Thus, the increases in depressed men (35-kd band: 115%±2%; 45-kd band: 142%±8%; n=10) were not different than those in depressed women (35-kd band: 123%±6%; 45-kd band: 138%±6%; n=16; $P>.05$). Moreover, the increases in immunoreactivity were not age-related ($r=-0.16$ and $r=-0.13$ for the 35-kd and 45-kd bands, respectively; range of ages, 29-64 years).

In all 9 depressed patients who underwent antidepressant treatment with citalopram hydrochloride (20-40 mg/d for 2 to 12 weeks), clomipramine hydrochloride (100 mg/d for 9 weeks), or imipramine hydrochloride (200 mg/d for 9 weeks), a change in the immunoreactivity of the up-regulated 45-kd imidazoline receptor protein was observed (level before treatment, 151%±9%; level after treatment, 116%±11%; difference, −35%±5%; n=9; $t=6.53$; $P<.001$ by paired t test). In contrast, these treatments did not alter the immunoreactivity of the 35-kd imidazoline receptor protein (level before treatment, 120%±5%; level after treatment, 125%±9%; difference, 5%±8%; n=9; $t=0.60$; $P>.05$ by paired t test).

In a selected group of depressed patients, the level of α-tubulin, used as a negative control, was not changed (drug-free patients: 98%±5%, n=10, $P>.05$; treated patients: 101%±2%, n=4, $P>.05$) compared with the level in matched controls. These negative results discounted possible effects of unspecific variables or unspecific effects of drug treatment on platelet imidazoline receptor proteins.

DENSITY OF IMIDAZOLINE RECEPTOR PROTEINS IN BRAINS OF SUICIDE VICTIMS

In cortical membranes of suicide victims, the total immunoreactivity of imidazoline receptor proteins (the sum of the 2 bands shown in Figure 1) was slightly but significantly decreased (percentage change, 90%±4%; n=13; $t=2.48$; $P<.05$) compared with that of age- and sex-matched controls. This decrease (10%) was caused by the fact that the specific immunoreactivity of the more abundant 29/30-kd band was decreased (percentage change, 81%±3%; n=13; $t=5.84$; $P<.001$; decrease, 19%) (**Figure 3**). In contrast, the immunoreactivity of the 45-kd band was markedly increased in the same cortical membranes of suicide victims (percentage change, 151%±14%; n=13; $t=3.63$; $P<.005$) (Figure 3). The 4 depressed suicide victims had similar immunoreactivity values for the imidazoline receptor proteins (percentage change: 86%±8% for the 29/30-kd band and 159%±25% for the 45-kd band). There was no significant correlation between the increase for the 45-kd band and the decrease for the 29/30-kd band in the frontal cortices of the same suicide victims ($r=0.31$, n=13, $P>.05$).

In a selected group of suicide victims, the levels of α-tubulin were not changed (97%±7%, n=7, $P>.05$) compared with those in matched controls. These negative results discounted possible effects of unspecific variables on brain imidazoline receptor proteins.

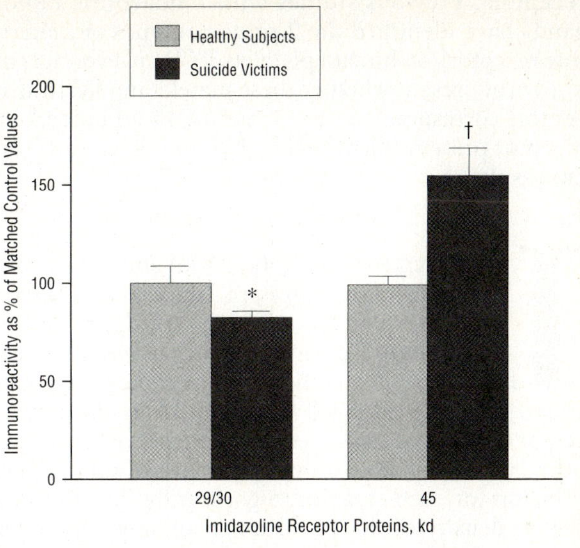

Figure 3. *Imidazoline receptor protein levels in cortical membranes (frontal cortex [Brodmann area 9]) of suicide victims (n=13) as percentages of the levels in matched controls (n=11). T-shaped bars indicate SEMs. Procedures of the immunoblot analysis and quantitation of specific immunoreactivity are described in the "Subjects and Methods" section. Mean±SEM values for healthy subjects evaluated as problem samples were 100%±8% (n=7) for the 29/30-kd protein and 98%±6% (n=6) for the 45-kd protein. Asterisk indicates* $P<.001$; *dagger,* $P<.005$ *(both obtained by 1-sample* t *test).*

COMMENT

This study demonstrates for the first time the presence and heterogeneity of immunoreactive imidazoline receptors (35- and 45-kd proteins) in human platelets, and it documents that levels of these newly discovered receptors are increased in the platelets of depressed patients and, in the case of the 45-kd receptor, in the brains of suicide victims. Moreover, antidepressant treatment was associated with clinical response and reduced density of the up-regulated 45-kd platelet imidazoline receptor in depressed patients. In this context, it is noteworthy that the level of brain 45-kd receptor was increased in suicide victims in spite of the possible negative effect of prior antidepressant treatment. Because imidazoline receptors appear to mediate inhibitory effects on the release of norepinephrine, the results further stress the potential role of imidazoline receptors in the pathogenesis of depression.

Human platelets express 2 distinct imidazoline receptor proteins, a more abundant 35-kd protein and a less abundant 45-kd protein. Significantly, a 45-kd imidazoline receptor protein is also expressed in various regions of the human brain,[27] which suggests that these platelet and brain imidazoline receptors represent the same molecular entity. The platelet 35-kd imidazoline receptor protein, which is not expressed in the human brain or in other tissues (eg, the liver),[27] could represent a new, specific platelet imidazoline receptor. Recently, the isolation, immunodetection, and molecular characterization of a 43/45-kd imidazoline receptor protein from the rat brain[48] and the human brain[49] have been accomplished, demonstrating the unequivocal existence of these receptors. Previous studies with imidazoline radioligands have identified the 2 principal types of imidazoline receptors on human platelets.[36,50] However, it is not known at present whether these platelet imidazoline receptors correspond to the 35- and/or 45-kd imidazoline receptor proteins identified by immunodetection (present results).

LEVELS OF both the 35-kd and 45-kd imidazoline receptor proteins were increased in the platelets of drug-free depressed patients. However, the increase in the level of the 45-kd imidazoline receptor was greater (40%) than that observed for the 35-kd imidazoline receptor (20%), and these increases were not related to each other, which indicated different patterns of abnormal expression for each receptor. Significantly, the abnormal higher density of the 45-kd imidazoline receptor protein in the platelets of depressed patients was also observed in the brains of suicide victims (51%). This increase in the frontal cortex of suicide victims not only stresses further that the platelet and brain 45-kd imidazoline receptor proteins are probably the same molecular entity, but also validates the use of the blood platelet as a model to assess indirectly the biological status of this receptor in the brain during the course of major depression. In contrast, the density of the brain 29/30-kd imidazoline receptor protein (not expressed in platelets) was decreased (19%) in the same suicide victims. Interestingly, the specific binding of $[^3H]$idazoxan to I_2-imidazoline receptors in the frontal cortex of suicide victims was also decreased (40%).[51] In the human brain, the 29/30-kd imidazoline receptor protein has been associated with the I_2-imidazoline receptor labeled by $[^3H]$idazoxan during the process of aging (parallel increases).[35] Together, these data indicate that the brain 29/30-kd imidazoline receptor protein detected by immunoblot is probably related to the I_2-imidazoline receptor characterized with $[^3H]$idazoxan binding, and that the level of this specific type of imidazoline receptor (mainly glial) is decreased in the brains of suicide victims. The possible functional relevance of this finding is at present not known. The association of the human brain 45-kd imidazoline receptor protein with any known pharmacological type of imidazoline receptor remains to be determined ($I_{1/2}$ type).[28,48,49]

Previous studies with $[^3H]$*p*-aminoclonidine, "site-selective" radioligand concentrations for α_2-adrenoceptors (60 pmol/L),[50] and I_1-imidazoline receptors (1.5 nmol/L)[50] and platelet-purified plasma membranes revealed that both receptor sites were upregulated (71% for α_2-adrenoceptors and 73% for I_1-imidazoline receptors) in patients with unipolar depression.[6,52] Recently, by using $[^{125}I]$*p*-iodoclonidine and masking the α_2-adrenoceptors, the platelet I_1-imidazoline receptor has been well characterized.[36] With this approach, the level of platelet I_1-imidazoline receptors also was found to be increased in depressed patients and to be down-regulated by desipramine or fluoxetine treatment.[53] These findings,[6,52,53] together with the up-regulation in the level of the platelet 45-kd imidazoline receptor protein found in depressed patients, which is also down-regulated after antidepressant treatment (present study), suggest that the platelet I_1-imidazoline receptor labeled by $[^{125}I]$*p*-iodoclonidine[53] might be related to the 45-kd imidazoline receptor protein identified in the present study. However, further work is needed to clarify the relationship between platelet imidazoline receptors identified by immunoblot and radioligand binding assays.

Because imidazoline radioligands label both α_2-adrenoceptors and imidazoline receptors,[6,36] it is important to comment on whether previous studies with such radioligands that reported increases in α_2-adrenoceptor levels in the brain[1,2,7] and in platelets[3] in association with depressive disorders quantitated solely α_2-adrenoceptors. The experimental conditions of these studies (use of a catecholamine to define nonspecific binding and/or a high concentration of magnesium chloride to favor the recognition of the high-affinity state of α_2-adrenoceptors) clearly indicated that the specific binding of imidazoline radioligands to brain and platelet membranes was associated with α_2-adrenoceptors.[1,2,36,50] Moreover, the demonstration of an increased density of $[^3H]$epinephrine binding sites[4] together with enhanced epinephrine-induced functional responses[3,5] in platelets of depressed patients made it clear that depression is associated with supersensitive α_{2A}-adrenoceptors.

Finally, the question arises about the role of imidazoline receptors in the catecholamine hypothesis of affective disorders.[54,55] This hypothesis postulates inter alia the existence of a deficit in brain noradrenergic function associated with decreased release of norepinephrine. Recently, peripheral noradrenergic neurons have been shown to possess release-modulating imidazoline receptors that mediate inhibitory effects on the release of norepinephrine.[18,19,56,57] Agmatine, an endogenous agonist at imidazoline receptors,[13,58] also induces inhibitory effects on the release of norepinephrine in the rabbit aorta.[57] In human platelets, agmatine appears to be a rather selective ligand for I_1-imidazoline receptors,[59] and its concentration in plasma (0.45 ng/mL)[58] is comparable to plasma catecholamine levels. Therefore, the results of the present study (increased density of immunoreactive 45-kd imidazoline receptor proteins in the platelets and brains of depressed patients and suicide victims) and the above data suggest that enhanced imidazoline receptor (and α_2-autoreceptor[1,2]) activity could be involved in the pathogenesis of major depression. However, noradrenergic neurons of the rabbit and rat cerebral cortices do not appear to possess inhibitory presynaptic imidazoline receptors regulating the release of norepinephrine.[60] Whether or not this is also true for the noradrenergic axon terminals of the human brain remains to be elucidated.

Imidazoline receptors also have been postulated to modulate the expression (messenger RNA) of the norepinephrine transporter in presynaptic neurons of the rat locus caeruleus,[61] the main brain noradrenergic nucleus that is under the tonic regulation of inhibitory α_2-autoreceptors.[62] The level of α_2-autoreceptors in the locus caeruleus in the human brain has been shown to be markedly increased in suicide victims.[2] Moreover, the brain area where the locus caeruleus is located is also endowed with imidazoline receptors that stimulate the activity of noradrenergic neurons,[63] an effect found to be potentiated after the depletion of serotonin in the brain but not after norepinephrine depletion with reserpine.[63,64] Recently, I_1-imidazoline receptors have been shown to stimulate in vivo and in vitro the expression (messenger RNA) of the catecholamine biosynthetic enzymes tyrosine hydroxylase and phenylethanolamine *N*-methyltransferase in adrenal chromaffin cells.[65] These results further stress the functional interaction between imidazoline receptors and monoamine systems and the possible relevance of this interaction in major depression.

These findings, together with the present results, support a role for the newly discovered imidazoline receptors in the pathogenesis of depression and in the mechanism of action of antidepressant drugs.

Accepted for publication January 30, 1996.

This study was supported by grant 3100-043258.95 (Dr Guimón) from the Fonds National Suisse de la Recherche Scientifique, Bern, Switzerland, and by grant PB94-0002-Mod C (Dr García-Sevilla) from the Dirección General de Investigación Científica y Técnica, Madrid, Spain.

Read in part before the Seventh Congress of Association of European Psychiatrists, Copenhagen, Denmark, September 21, 1994.

The authors thank the staff members of the Psychiatric Clinic I, University Hospitals of Geneva, Geneva, Switzerland, and of the Forensic Anatomical Institute, Palma de Mallorca, Spain, for their cooperation. Dr García-Sevilla is a member of the Institut d'Estudis Catalans.

Reprints: Jesús A. García-Sevilla, MD, Laboratori de Neurofarmacologia, Departament de Biologia Fonamental i Ciències de la Salut, Universitat de les Illes Balears, Cra de Valldemossa, km 7.5, E-07071 Palma de Mallorca, Spain.

REFERENCES

1. González AM, Pascual J, Meana JJ, Barturen F, del Arco C, Pazos A, García-Sevilla JA. Autoradiographic demonstration of increased α_2-adrenoceptor agonist binding sites in the hippocampus and frontal cortex of depressed suicide victims. *J Neurochem.* 1994;63:256-265.
2. Ordway GA, Widdowson PS, Smith KS, Halaris AE. Agonist binding to α_2-adrenoceptors is elevated in the locus coeruleus from suicide victims. *J Neurochem.* 1994;63:617-624.
3. García-Sevilla JA, Guimón J, García-Vallejo P, Fuster MJ. Biochemical and functional evidence of supersensitive platelet α_2-adrenoceptors in major affective disorder: effect of long-term lithium carbonate treatment. *Arch Gen Psychiatry.* 1986;43:51-57.
4. García-Sevilla JA, Udina C, Fuster MJ, Alvárez E, Casas M. Enhanced binding of [^{3}H](-)adrenaline to platelets of depressed patients with melancholia: effect of long-term clomipramine treatment. *Acta Psychiatr Scand.* 1987;75:150-157.
5. Mori H, Koyama T, Yamasuita I. Platelet alpha-2 adrenergic receptor-mediated phosphoinositide responses in endogenous depression. *Life Sci.* 1991;48:741-748.
6. Piletz JE, Halaris A, Saran A, Marler M. Desipramine lowers tritiated para-aminoclonidine binding in platelets of depressed patients. *Arch Gen Psychiatry.* 1991;48:813-820.
7. Meana JJ, Barturen F, García-Sevilla JA. α_2-Adrenoceptors in the brain of suicide victims: increased receptor density associated with major depression. *Biol Psychiatry.* 1992;31:471-490.
8. Sastre M, García-Sevilla JA. α_2-Adrenoceptor subtypes identified by [^{3}H]RX821002 binding in the human brain: the agonist guanoxabenz does not discriminate different forms of the predominant α_{2A}-subtype. *J Neurochem.* 1994;63:1077-1085.
9. Michel MC, Insel PA. Are there multiple imidazoline binding sites? *Trends Pharmacol Sci.* 1989;10:342-344.
10. Michel MC, Ernsberger P. Keeping an eye on the I site: imidazoline-preferring receptors. *Trends Pharmacol Sci.* 1992;13:369-370.
11. Ernsberger PR, Damon TH, Graft LM, Schäffer SG, Christen MO. Moxonidine, a centrally antihypertensive agent, is a selective ligand for I_1-imidazoline sites. *J Pharmacol Exp Ther.* 1993;264:172-182.
12. Miralles A, Olmos G, Sastre M, Barturen F, Martín I, García-Sevilla JA. Discrimination and pharmacological characterization of I_2-imidazoline sites with [^{3}H]idazoxan and alpha-2 adrenoceptors with [^{3}H]RX821002 (2-methoxy idazoxan) in the human and rat brains. *J Pharmacol Exp Ther.* 1993;264:1187-1197.
13. Li G, Regunathan S, Barrow CJ, Eshraghi J, Cooper R, Reis DJ. Agmatine: an endogenous clonidine-displacing substance in the brain. *Science.* 1994;263:966-969.
14. Atlas D. Identifying clonidine-displacing substance. *Science.* 1994;266:462-463.
15. Bousquet P, Feldman J, Schwartz J. Central cardiovascular effects of α-adrenergic drugs: differences between catecholamines and imidazolines. *J Pharmacol Exp Ther.* 1984;230:232-242.
16. Haxhiu MA, Dreshaj J, Schäfer SG, Ernsberger P. Selective antihypertensive action of moxonidine is mediated mainly by I_1-imidazoline receptors in the rostral ventrolateral medulla. *J Cardiovasc Pharmacol.* 1994;24(suppl 1):S1-S8.
17. Tibiriça E, Feldman J, Mermet C, Gomon F, Bousquet P. An imidazoline specific mechanism for the hypotensive effect of clonidine: a study with yohimbine and idazoxan. *J Pharmacol Exp Ther.* 1991;256:606-613.
18. Göthert M, Molderings GJ. Involvement of presynaptic imidazoline receptors in the α_2-adrenoceptor-independent inhibition of noradrenaline release by imidazoline derivatives. *Naunyn Schmiedebergs Arch Pharmacol.* 1991;343:271-282.
19. Molderings GJ, Hentrich F, Göthert M. Pharmacological characterization of the imidazoline receptor which mediates inhibition of noradrenaline in the rabbit pulmonary artery. *Naunyn Schmiedebergs Arch Pharmacol.* 1991;344:630-638.
20. Powis DA, Baker PF. α_2-adrenoceptors do not regulate catecholamine secretion by bovine adrenal medullary cells: a study with clonidine. *Mol Pharmacol.* 1986;29:134-143.
21. Tesson F, Parini A. Identification of an imidazoline-guanidinium receptive site in mitochondria from rabbit cerebral cortex. *Eur J Pharmacol.* 1991;208:81-83.
22. Sastre M, García-Sevilla JA. Opposite age-dependent changes of α_2-adrenoceptors and nonadrenoceptor [^{3}H]idazoxan binding sites (I_2-imidazoline sites) in the human brain: strong correlation of I_2 with monoamine oxidase-B sites. *J Neurochem.* 1993;61:881-889.
23. Regunathan S, Feinstein DL, Reis DJ. Expression of non-adrenergic imidazoline sites in rat cerebral cortical astrocytes. *J Neurosci Res.* 1993;34:681-688.
24. Olmos G, Alemany R, Escribá PV, García-Sevilla JA. The effects of chronic imidazoline drug treatment on glial fibrillary acidic protein concentrations in rat brain. *Br J Pharmacol.* 1994;111:997-1002.
25. Ruiz J, Martín I, Callado LF, Meana JJ, Barturen F, García-Sevilla JA. Non-adrenoceptor [^{3}H]idazoxan binding sites (I_2-imidazoline sites) are increased in postmortem brain from patients with Alzheimer's disease. *Neurosci Lett.* 1993;160:109-112.
26. García-Sevilla JA, Miralles A, Sastre M, Escribá PV, Olmos G, Meana JJ. I_2-imidazoline receptors in the healthy and pathologic human brain. *Ann N Y Acad Sci.* 1995;763:178-193.
27. Escribá PV, Sastre M, Wang H, Regunathan S, Reis DJ, García-Sevilla JA. Immunodetection of putative imidazoline receptor proteins in the human and rat brain and other tissues. *Neurosci Lett.* 1994;178:81-84.
28. Greney H, Bricca G, Dontenwill M, Stutzmann J, Bousquet P, Belcourt A. Characterization of imidazoline binding protein(s) solubilized from human brainstem: studies with [^{3}H]idazoxan and [^{3}H]clonidine. *Neurochem Int.* 1994;25:183-191.
29. Limon I, Coupry I, Lanier SM, Parini A. Purification and characterization of mitochondrial imidazoline-guanidinium receptive sites from rabbit kidney. *J Biol Chem.* 1992;267:21645-21649.
30. Wang H, Regunathan S, Meeley MP, Reis DJ. Isolation and characterization of imidazoline receptor proteins from bovine adrenal chromaffin cells. *Mol Pharmacol.* 1992;42:792-801.
31. Lanier SM, Ivkovic B, Singh I, Neumeyer JL, Bakthavachalam V. Visualization of multiple imidazoline/guanidinium-receptive sites. *J Biol Chem.* 1993;268:16047-16051.
32. Ivkovic B, Bakthavachalam V, Zhang W, Parini A, Diz D, Bosch S, Neumeyer JL, Lanier SM. Development of a high-affinity radioiodinated ligand for iden-

tification of imidazoline/guanidinium receptive sites (IGRS): intratissue distribution of IGRS in liver, forebrain, and kidney. *Mol Pharmacol.* 1994;46:15-23.
33. Diamant S, Eldar-Geva T, Atlas D. Imidazoline binding sites in human placenta: evidence for heterogeneity and a search for physiological function. *Br J Pharmacol.* 1992;106:101-108.
34. Wikberg JES, Uhlén S, Chhajlani V. Evidence that drug binding to non-adrenergic ^{3}H idazoxan binding sites (I-receptors) occurs to interacting or interconvertible affinity forms of the receptor. *Pharmacol Toxicol.* 1992;70:208-219.
35. García-Sevilla JA, Sastre M, Escribá PV. Age-dependent increases of immunoreactive imidazoline receptors in the human brain: possible association of a 29/30 kDa protein with the I_2-imidazoline receptor identified by [^{3}H]idazoxan. *Neurosci Lett.* 1995;184:133-136.
36. Piletz JE, Sletten K. Nonadrenergic imidazoline binding sites on human platelets. *J Pharmacol Exp Ther.* 1993;267:1493-1502.
37. Michel CM, Regan JW, Gerhardt MA, Neubig RR, Insel PA, Motulsky HJ. Nonadrenergic [^{3}H]idazoxan binding sites are physically distinct from α_2-adrenergic receptors. *Mol Pharmacol.* 1990;37:65-68.
38. Zonnenschein R, Diamant S, Atlas D. Imidazoline receptors in rat liver cells: a novel receptor or a subtype of α_2-adrenoceptor? *Eur J Pharmacol.* 1990;190:203-215.
39. Piletz JE, Sletten KR, Halaris AE. Imidazoline-preferring binding sites in human platelets: plasma membrane subtype I_1 is elevated in mood disorders. *Fundam Clin Pharmacol.* 1992;6(suppl 1):49S.
40. Meana JJ, Barturen F, Martín I, García-Sevilla JA. Evidence of increased non-adrenoceptor [^{3}H]idazoxan binding sites in the frontal cortex of depressed suicide victims. *Biol Psychiatry.* 1993;34:498-501.
41. Olmos G, Gabilondo AM, Miralles A, Escribá PV, García-Sevilla JA. Chronic treatment with the monoamine oxidase inhibitors clorgyline and pargyline down-regulates non-adrenoceptor [^{3}H]idazoxan binding sites in the rat brain. *Br J Pharmacol.* 1993;108:597-603.
42. Alemany R, Olmos G, García-Sevilla JA. The effects of phenelzine and other monoamine oxidase inhibitor antidepressants on brain and liver I_2 imidazoline-preferring receptors. *Br J Pharmacol.* 1995;114:837-845.
43. Hamilton M. A rating scale for depression. *J Neurol Neurosurg Psychiatry.* 1960;23:56-62.
44. Smith PK, Krohn RI, Hermanson GT, Mallia AK, Gartner FH. Measurement of protein using bicinchoninic acid. *Anal Biochem.* 1985;150:76-85.
45. Wang H, Regunathan S, Ruggiero DA, Reis DJ. Production and characterization of antibodies specific for imidazoline receptor protein. *Mol Pharmacol.* 1993;43:509-515.
46. Escribá PV, Sastre M, García-Sevilla JA. Increased density of guanine nucleotide-binding proteins in the postmortem brains of heroin addicts. *Arch Gen Psychiatry.* 1994;51:494-501.
47. Gettys TW, Sheriff-Carter K, Moomaw J, Taylor IL, Raymond JR. Characterization and use of crude α-subunit preparations for quantitative immunoblotting of G proteins. *Anal Biochem.* 1994;220:82-91.
48. Escribá PV, Ozaita A, Miralles A, Reis DJ, García-Sevilla JA. Molecular characterization and isolation of a 45-kilodalton imidazoline receptor protein from the rat brain. *Mol Brain Res.* 1995;32:187-196.
49. Greney H, Bennai F, Molines A, Belcourt A, Dontenwill M, Bousquet P. Isolation of a human cerebral imidazoline-specific binding protein. *Eur J Pharmacol.* 1994;265:R1-R2.
50. Piletz JE, Andorn AC, Unnerstall JR, Halaris A. Binding of [^{3}H]-*p*-aminoclonidine to α_2-adrenoceptor states plus a non-adrenergic site on human platelet plasma membranes. *Biochem Pharmacol.* 1991;42:569-584.
51. Sastre M, Escribá PV, Reis DJ, García-Sevilla JA. Decreased number and immunoreactivity of I_2-imidazoline receptors in the frontal cortex of suicide victims. *Ann N Y Acad Sci.* 1995;763:520-522.
52. Piletz JE, Halaris A, Saran A, Marler M. Elevated [^{3}H]-para-amino-clonidine binding to platelet purified plasma membranes from depressed patients. *Neuropsychopharmacology.* 1990;3:201-210.
53. Piletz JE, Halaris A. Involvement of I_1-imidazoline receptors in mood disorders. *Ann N Y Acad Sci.* 1995;763:510-519.
54. Potter WZ, Manji HK. Catecholamines in depression: an update. *Clin Chem.* 1994;40:279-287.
55. Schatzberg AF, Schildkraut JJ. Recent studies on norepinephrine systems in mood disorders. In: Bloom FE, Kupfer DJ, eds. *Psychopharmacology.* 4th ed. New York, NY: Raven Press; 1995:911-920.
56. Fuder H, Schwarz P. Desensitization of inhibitory prejunctional α_2-adrenoceptors and putative imidazoline receptors on rabbit heart sympathetic nerves. *Naunyn Schmiedebergs Arch Pharmacol.* 1993;348:127-133.
57. Molderings GJ, Göthert M. Inhibitory presynaptic imidazoline receptors on sympathetic nerves in the rabbit aorta differ from I_1- and I_2-imidazoline binding sites. *Naunyn Schmiedebergs Arch Pharmacol.* 1995;351:507-516.
58. Raasch W, Regunathan S, Reis DJ. Agmatine, the bacterial amine, is widely distributed in mammalian tissues. *Life Sci.* 1995;56:2319-2330.
59. Piletz JE, Chikkala DN, Ernsberger P. Comparison of the properties of agmatine and endogenous clonidine-displacing substance at imidazoline and alpha-2 adrenergic receptors. *J Pharmacol Exp Ther.* 1995;272:581-587.
60. Göthert M, Molderings GJ, Fink K, Schlicker E. α_2-Adrenoceptor-independent inhibition by imidazolines and guanidines of noradrenaline release from peripheral, but not central noradrenergic neurons. *Ann N Y Acad Sci.* 1995;763:405-419.
61. Shores MM, Szot P, Veith RC. Desipramine-induced increase in norepinephrine transporter mRNA is not mediated via α_2 receptors. *Mol Brain Res.* 1994;27:337-341.
62. Cedarbaum JM, Aghajanian GK. Noradrenergic neurons of the locus caeruleus: inhibition by epinephrine and activation by the α-antagonist piperoxane. *Brain Res.* 1976;112:413-419.
63. Pineda J, Ugedo L, García-Sevilla JA. Stimulatory effects of clonidine, cirazoline and rilmenidine on locus coeruleus noradrenergic neurones: possible involvement of imidazoline-preferring receptors. *Naunyn Schmiedebergs Arch Pharmacol.* 1993;348:134-140.
64. Ruiz-Ortega JA, Ugedo L, Pineda J, García-Sevilla JA. The stimulatory effect of clonidine through imidazoline receptors on locus coeruleus noradrenergic neurones is mediated by excitatory amino acids and modulated by serotonin. *Naunyn Schmiedebergs Arch Pharmacol.* 1995;352:121-126.
65. Evinger MJ, Ernsberger P, Regunathan S, Reis DJ. Regulation of phenylethanolamine *N*-metyhyltransferase gene expression by imidazoline receptors in adrenal chromaffin cells. *J Neurochem.* 1995;65:988-997.

The Effects of Electroconvulsive Therapy on Quantitative Electroencephalograms

Relationship to Clinical Outcome

Harold A. Sackeim, PhD; Bruce Luber, PhD; Gary P. Katzman; James R. Moeller, PhD; Joan Prudic, MD; D. P. Devanand, MD; Mitchell S. Nobler, MD

Background: The efficacy of electroconvulsive therapy (ECT) is determined by stimulus electrical intensity and electrode placement. Three theories offer different accounts for why increasing the stimulus dosage of right unilateral ECT enhances antidepressant effects. This study examined the effects of ECT on interictal quantitative electroencephalograms (EEGs), contrasting these theories in their predictions regarding global, lateralized, and topographic changes in ECT-induced slow-wave activity. The time course of EEG changes and associations with efficacy were also determined.

Methods: Sixty-two inpatients with major depressive disorder were randomized to ECT conditions that differed in stimulus intensity (low vs high dosage) and electrode placement (right unilateral vs bilateral). Resting, eyes closed, 19-lead EEG recordings were obtained at pretreatment, following a single treatment, following an average of 7 treatments, during the week following the ECT course, and after a 2-month follow-up period.

Results: Electroconvulsive therapy produced a marked short-term increase in delta and theta power. At a 2-month follow-up, there were no significant alterations in any frequency band. The ECT treatment conditions differed markedly in efficacy. Global and lateralized EEG effects did not distinguish effective and ineffective forms of treatment. Effective forms of ECT resulted in increased delta power in prefrontal regions, and this change was associated with the magnitude of symptomatic improvement.

Conclusion: The induction of slow-wave activity in prefrontal cortex is linked to the efficacy of ECT.

Arch Gen Psychiatry. 1996;53:814-824

GENERALIZED SEIZURES produce numerous neurobiological changes, making it difficult to isolate the factors mediating the therapeutic effects of electroconvulsive therapy (ECT).[1,2] However, generalized seizures that lack therapeutic properties can be reliably elicited with ECT.[3-5] Contrasting low- and high-efficacy forms of ECT offers a new method to examine mechanisms of action.

Electroconvulsive therapy produces marked changes in interictal brain electrical activity.[6,7] Electroencephalographic (EEG) slowing, reflecting increased power in the delta and theta frequency bands, typically develops progressively during the treatment course and resolves within several weeks.[6-13] Older age and a larger number of treatments may predict greater EEG changes.[6,7,9] Relationships with clinical outcome are uncertain. A few studies claimed that superior clinical outcome was associated with greater global EEG slowing or lateralized effects,[10,14-18] while other studies were negative.[8,13,19-21]

Right unilateral (RUL) ECT is ineffective when electrical dosage is just above the patient's seizure threshold. When dosage is increased, RUL ECT has substantial efficacy.[4-5,22,23] Three theories may account for this phenomenon.[3] First, with RUL ECT, current density is thought to be approximately 3 times greater in the right than left hemisphere.[24] Right unilateral ECT produces greater ictal EEG amplitude and interictal slowing in the right than left hemisphere,[25-27] whereas bilateral (BL) ECT produces either bilaterally increased interictal slow-wave activity or a superimposed asymmetric pattern, with greater left-sided slowing.[8,13,17,18,28-31] By increasing the RUL ECT dosage, current

See Subjects and Methods on next page

From the Department of Biological Psychiatry, New York State Psychiatric Institute (Drs Sackeim, Luber, Moeller, and Prudic and Mr Katzman), and the Department of Psychiatry, College of Physicians and Surgeons, Columbia University (Drs Sackeim, Luber, Moeller, Prudic, Devanand, and Nobler), New York, NY.

SUBJECTS AND METHODS

SUBJECTS

Sixty-two of 96 inpatients who had provided informed consent and participated in a double-blind, randomly assigned ECT trial were included.[5] These patients had EEG assessments at baseline and at 1 or more intervals after the start of ECT. They met the Research Diagnostic Criteria for major depressive disorder, endogenous subtype. Other inclusion/exclusion criteria have been reported.[5] Patients were randomized to treatments that crossed the factors of electrode placement (RUL ECT vs BL ECT) and stimulus intensity (low dosage vs high dosage). **Table 1** presents descriptive features of the treatment groups. Analyses of variance (ANOVAs) (electrode placement by dosage condition) on the continuous variables and log-linear analyses of the dichotomous variables yielded no significant effects, except for the duration of the current episode being shorter in the low-dosage BL ECT group ($P<.05$).

ECT AND CLINICAL OUTCOME

Electroconvulsive therapy methods have been described elsewhere.[5] Other than lorazepam (up to 3 mg/d as needed), there was a minimum psychotropic washout of 5 days before the baseline EEG (mean±SD, 13.7±8.6 days). Seizure threshold was quantified at the first and last treatments of all patients.[46] In the low-dosage groups, stimulus intensity was kept just above seizure threshold throughout treatment. In the high-dosage groups, stimulus intensity was 150% above the initial seizure threshold.

The d'Elia placement[25] was used for RUL ECT, and the bifrontotemporal placement for BL ECT.

Length of the ECT course was determined by a blind evaluation team, who also completed the 24-item Hamilton Rating Scale for Depression (HRSD). Nonresponders received at least 10 treatments. This requirement was reduced to 8 treatments in cases of clinical urgency. Initial responders had at least a 60% reduction in HRSD scores immediately following the ECT course relative to pretreatment, and a maximal post-ECT score of 16. Final responders maintained these gains for 1 week after ECT, while free of psychotropics. Following post-ECT evaluations, 28 (87.5%) of 32 nonresponders received an open course of high-dosage BL ECT; 23 (78.6%) of these 28 patients subsequently met criteria for final response.

Analyses of variance did not yield treatment group differences in the duration of medication washout, dosage of anesthetic medications, seizure duration, or in the number of ECT treatments during the randomized phase (**Table 2**). Dosage of lorazepam in the patients averaged 1.1±1.1 mg/d during the washout period and 1.1±1.0 mg/d during the ECT course, with no treatment group differences. As in the parent study,[5] low-dosage RUL ECT had very weak antidepressant effects. A repeated measures analysis of covariance (ANCOVA) on immediate and 1-week post-ECT HRSD scores, using the pretreatment score as a covariate, yielded main effects of electrode placement ($P=.01$) and dosage condition ($P=.02$) and an interaction ($P<.05$). Post hoc comparisons indicated that, at both time points, the low-dosage RUL ECT group had higher HRSD scores than each of the other groups (P values of $\leq.02$), with no other differences. As seen in Table 2, high-dosage RUL ECT was associated with a strong initial response rate (73.3%) but also with a relatively high rate of rapid relapse.

EEG DATA ACQUISITION

The patients were studied under eyes-closed, supine conditions. Electroencepahalographic measurements lasted at least 5 minutes. Nineteen gold-cup EEG electrodes were placed according to the international "10-20 System," referenced to P_z, with impedances less than 5 kilo-ohms. Horizontal and vertical eye movements were recorded following standard procedures. The electrophysiologic data were amplified with a polygraph (Grass Model 8/24D, Grass Instrument Co, Quincy, Mass), with bandpass filters set at 0.1 to 70 Hz and use of a 60-Hz notch filter. The sampling rate was 100 Hz. The combination of a low-pass filter of 70 Hz and the sampling rate of 100 Hz may have introduced aliasing owing to high-frequency activity, eg, muscle tension.[57] To minimize this and other sources of contamination, both the computer-recorded data and polygraph-paper output were inspected, identifying data containing nonencephalic signal. Artifact rejection was conducted blind to patient information, with the order randomized across patients and assessments. The artifact-free data were subjected to fast Fourier transformation, using 1-second epochs, each overlapping by 0.5 second, and tapered with a Hanning function. Mean absolute power (in squared microvolts per hertz) was computed within 5 frequency bands: delta (0.5-3.5 Hz), theta (3.5-7.5 Hz); alpha (7.5-12.5 Hz); beta 1 (12.5-20.5 Hz), and beta 2 (20.5-32.5 Hz).

Electroencephalographic data were acquired at (1) pre-ECT baseline (n=62), (2) the morning of the second (n=57) and (3) penultimate treatments (n=47), (4) during the week following completion of the randomized ECT course (n=52),

Continued on next page

density in the left hemisphere may approach that of BL ECT, resulting in greater BL seizure generalization, which the first theory posits is necessary for efficacy.[32,33] Thus, this theory predicts that higher-intensity RUL ECT produces less asymmetry in interictal slow-wave activity than low-dosage RUL ECT.

See also page 826

The second theory centers on the view that direct electrical effects or seizure propagation to centrencephalic structures mediate ECT's efficacy.[34-36] At equivalent electrical dosage, BL ECT results in greater current density in subcortical structures than RUL ECT.[24,37] There are indications that higher-intensity stimulation produces greater global (transcortical) EEG slow-wave activity.[8,38-41] Presuming that this transcortical change reflects an effect on subcortical pacemakers,[42] the second theory predicts that increasing the dosage of RUL ECT results in greater diffuse, transcortical EEG slowing. This hypothesis is compatible with evidence that higher stimulus intensity results in a greater acute postictal surge in prolac tin[41,43] and oxytocin,[44] perhaps reflecting the degree of hypothalamic stimulation.

and (5) 2 months after completion of all treatment with ECT (n=34). The second assessment is referred to as post 1 ECT. On average, the third assessment took place prior to the eighth treatment (mean±SD, 8.1±1.8 treatments) and is referred to as post 7 ECT. The fourth assessment occurred on average 4.7±2.0 days following the last treatment in the randomized phase, and is referred to as post ECT course. The treatment groups did not differ in the number of treatments or days between assessments.

DATA ANALYSIS

The EEG data were logarithmically transformed prior to analysis, and all analyses were based on change scores from pretreatment baseline (post-pre). The data analyses examined changes in (1) total global power, (2) global power within the 5 frequency bands, (3) hemispheric asymmetry within the frequency bands, and (4) topographic patterns. The analyses followed a framework in which omnibus repeated measures ANCOVAs established significant between-group effects at specific time points. Follow-up ANCOVAs identified the frequency bands in which the groups differed. Post hoc comparisons were then conducted, with *t* tests based on least-square means. The omnibus tests provided some protection against Type I error. More stringent correction for multiple comparisons to limit Type I error was not used because of the low power resulting from the small size of subgroups. All ANCOVAs used age as a covariate. The ANCOVAs comparing the treatment conditions used electrode placement and dosage condition as between-subject factors. Significance levels in repeated measures ANCOVAs were adjusted with the Huynh-Feldt correction. Two-tailed tests were used throughout, and $\alpha=.05$ was the level for significant effects. Preliminary analyses indicated that gender, unipolar vs bipolar diagnosis, psychotic vs nonpsychotic depression, number of ECT treatments, the interval between last ECT treatment and EEG assessment, absolute electrical charge, seizure duration, and lorazepam dosage had no associations with the EEG measurements.

Total global power was computed as the average power across EEG sites and frequency bands, weighted for band width. One-sample *t* tests established whether total global power had changed across the sample at assessments following baseline. Global power within frequency bands was computed as the average power across sites, independent of band width. Asymmetry in global power was calculated for each frequency band. At each time point, power was averaged across the 8 sites over each hemisphere (ignoring the 2 midline sites) and a laterality index (I_l) was computed, using the following formula:

$$I_l = 100\times\{(R-L)/[(R+L)/2]\}.$$

Repeated measures ANCOVAs were conducted on the change in these asymmetry scores at each time point after baseline, with frequency band as the repeated measures factor.

To screen the time points for more discrete topographic effects, omnibus repeated measures ANCOVAs were conducted separately for each frequency band, with the changes in power relative to baseline at the 18 sites as the repeated measures factor. Significant interaction effects involving treatment conditions and EEG site justified characterization of the topographic alterations. The Scaled Subprofile Model (SSM) was used to separate global and topographic effects[58-61] and was applied the total sample, blind to treatment group and time point. The computations were performed within a frequency band on the change scores at each site. The mean value at each EEG site, determined across the sample, was subtracted from each patient's value at that site. These difference scores produced the approximation to the subject residual profile (SRP), the variability in EEG values that was patient, time point, and EEG site dependent. A principal components analysis was performed on the SRP covariance matrix, extracting a set of unrotated factors. The weights of the EEG sites on each factor described a topographic structure. A patient's loading on a factor quantified the extent to which that topographic pattern was manifested by the patient. These patient loadings are termed *subject scaling factors*. The number of factors retained was determined by requiring that each factor account for at least 5% of the SRP variance, using regression analysis to determine the extent to which the subject scaling factors accounted for variance in global power, and setting an upper limit of 4 patterns. The SSM also has a parameter, the global scaling factor (GSF), that quantifies individual differences in global values, removing the contribution of topographic patterns. Using multiple regression analysis to predict the change in global power within the frequency band on the basis of the subject scaling factors, the GSF corresponded to the residual between predicted and obtained values. Thus, the EEG data were partitioned, so that each patient was scored for manifesting each of a set of profiles, corresponding to changes in specific topographies relative to baseline, as well as for change in region-independent global power. Once these parameters were determined, standard ANCOVA and regression techniques were used to examine treatment group differences and associations with clinical outcome. A more detailed report of the statistical analyses is available on request.

We have offered a third theory.[3,45,46] With BL ECT, current density displays a marked anteroposterior gradient, concentrating anteriorly near the prefrontal pole,[24,37,47,48] and seizures may necessarily initiate in prefrontal regions. In contrast, with RUL ECT, current density is fairly uniform in the anterior two thirds of the stimulated cortex. Brain regions are heterogeneous in seizure threshold, with low thresholds in hippocampal and perirolandic (motor strip) regions.[49-52] Electroconvulsive therapy–induced seizures appear to initiate in the neocortex[29,53,54] and, at low dosage, RUL ECT seizures likely initiate in the motor cortex. At higher RUL stimulus intensity, current density will exceed the threshold of a wider expanse of right hemispheric regions, with prefrontal regions participating in seizure initiation. Therefore, incrementing the electrical dosage of RUL ECT may alter intrahemispheric patterns of seizure discharge before influencing interhemispheric patterns. We have also suggested that interictal EEG slowing and reductions in cerebral blood flow and metabolism result from the inhibitory processes that terminate the sei-

Table 1. Demographic and Clinical Features of the Sample*

Variable	Low-Dosage RUL ECT (n=13)	High-Dosage RUL ECT (n=15)	Low-Dosage BL ECT (n=16)	High-Dosage BL ECT (n=18)
Age, y	56.5±14.5	52.7±14.1	60.2±14.6	53.8±15.3
Sex, % F	69.2	80.0	37.5	66.7
Education, y	13.5±3.4	14.7±3.3	12.8±3.4	13.5±2.3
Socioeconomic status†	2.4±1.1	2.1±1.3	2.4±1.3	2.4±0.9
Bipolar disorder, %	23.1	46.7	25.0	33.3
Psychosis, %	38.5	33.3	31.3	55.6
Pretreatment HRSD score	33.9±9.2	31.2±7.1	32.9±7.3	32.9±7.8
Age at onset, y	37.4±11.4	42.5±16.4	40.4±16.7	41.1±17.2
History of ECT, %	46.2	40.0	56.3	33.3
Duration of episode, wk‡	59.2±32.9	43.7±36.7	29.6±27.2	50.3±36.0
Previous affective episodes, No.§	2.6±2.3	2.5±1.4	3.1±3.0	2.7±3.3
Previous psychiatric hospitalizations, No.§	1.3±1.5	1.9±1.9	2.6±3.4	2.1±2.4

RUL indicates right unilateral; ECT, electroconvulsive therapy; BL, bilateral; and HRSD, Hamilton Rating Scale for Depression. Values other than percentages are mean±SD.
†*Hollingshead Four-Factor Index (where 1 indicates highest socioeconomic status; 5, lowest socioeconomic status).*
‡*Maximum of 104 weeks applied.*
§*Maximum of 10 applied.*

Table 2. Treatment Parameters and Clinical Outcome in the Sample*

Variable	Low-Dosage RUL ECT (n=13)	High-Dosage RUL ECT (n=15)	Low-Dosage BL ECT (n=16)	High-Dosage BL ECT (n=18)
Treatment Parameters				
Duration of medication washout before ECT, d	19.6±8.4	14.3±6.0	18.1±8.5	16.3±7.3
Initial seizure threshold, mC	83.2±31.9	62.5±21.8	179.9±181.0	144.7±70.4
Charge,† mC	94.6±36.4	140.4±47.5	248.0±203.3	317.9±142.8
Charge in high-dosage sessions, mC	. . .	159.4±58.8	. . .	356.1±161.5
Energy,† J	16.8±5.1	25.4±7.6	30.7±23.9	44.2±20.5
Methohexital,† mg	55.3±13.8	52.2±12.4	57.3±21.0	56.8±9.6
Succinylcholine,† mg	38.7±11.0	33.2±10.8	39.3±8.1	43.7±16.2
EEG seizure duration,† s	59.5±23.1	65.5±23.0	63.4±19.6	60.2±16.4
Motor seizure duration,† s	48.9±18.3	48.0±14.2	50.5±17.5	46.0±10.8
ECT treatments, No.	8.9±2.1	9.4±1.7	9.6±2.5	9.3±2.4
Clinical Outcome				
HRSD				
Immediate post ECT course	24.0±13.3	10.6±7.5	11.8±9.7	10.1±9.7
1-week post ECT course	25.1±12.7	14.9±10.4	13.0±9.2	12.9±10.9
Initial responder, %	23.1	73.3	68.8	66.7
Final responder, %	15.4	46.7	68.8	56.6

RUL indicates right unilateral; BL, bilateral; ECT, electroconvulsive therapy; EEG, electroencephalography; HRSD, Hamilton Rating Scale for Depression; and mC, millicoulomb. Values other than percentages are mean±SD.
†*Average per treatment during the randomized phase.*

zure, with their spatial distribution determined more by patterns of seizure onset than propagation.[46,55,56] Consequently, the third theory predicts that interictal physiological asymmetries are not reduced at higher RUL stimulus intensity. Rather, higher-intensity RUL stimulation produces a greater prefrontal ictal discharge, with a larger interictal increase in prefrontal EEG slowing.

In this study, patients with major depression were randomized to ECT conditions that differed in electrode placement and stimulus intensity. Interictal resting EEG was assessed at 5 time points. The first goal was to document the nature and time course of changes in EEG spectral power. The second goal was to contrast the treatment conditions in global, lateralized, and topographic EEG changes, testing the 3 competing theories. The third goal was to relate the EEG changes to clinical outcome.

RESULTS

TREATMENT GROUP COMPARISONS

Total Global Power

Across the sample, there were large increases in total global power at post 7 ECT ($P<.001$) and post ECT course ($P<.001$), with no change at post 1 ECT or 2-month follow-up. The randomized treatment conditions did not differ in the change in total global power at any time point.

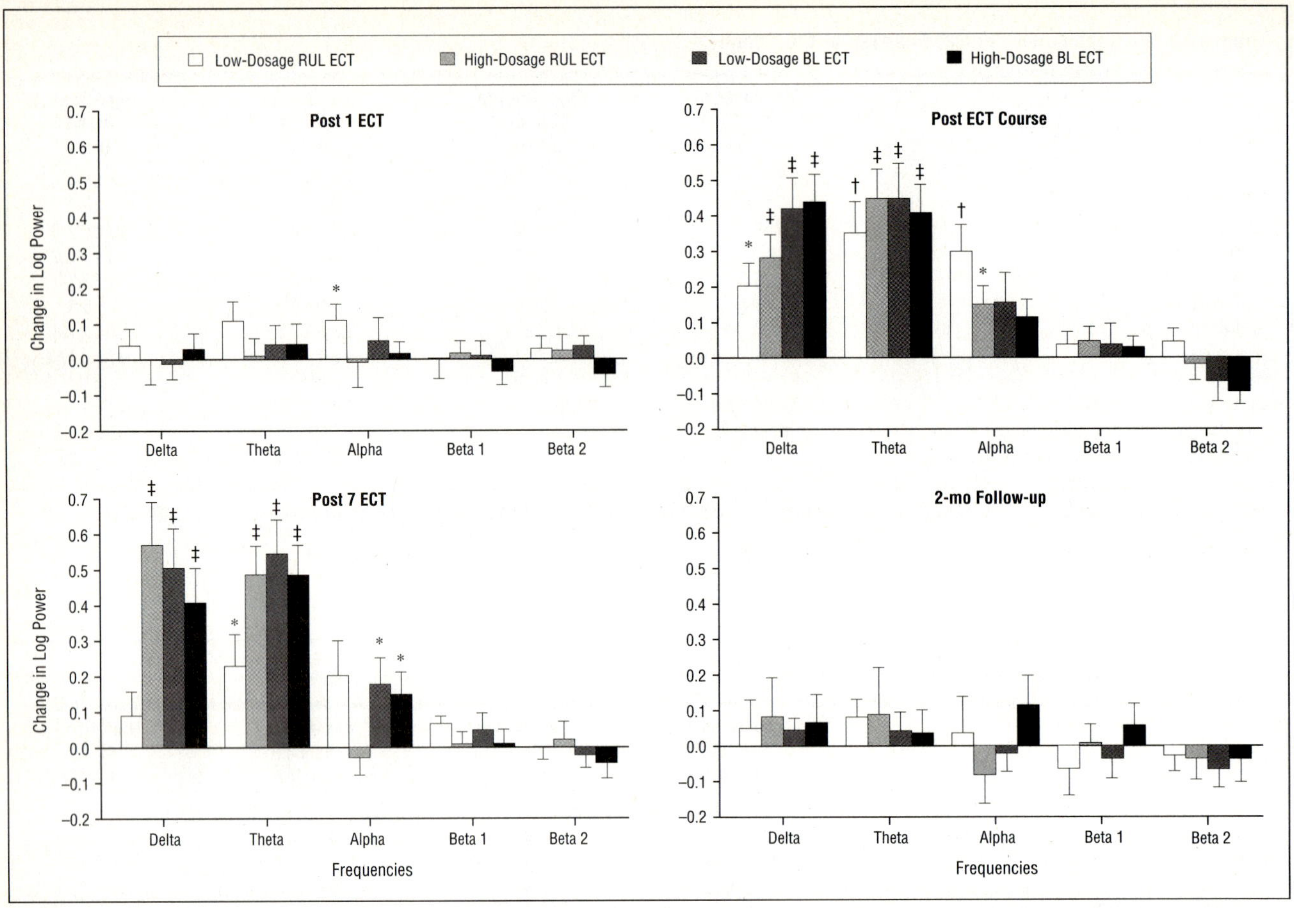

Figure 1. *Mean (±SE) changes in total power within the frequency bands. ECT indicates electroconvulsive therapy; RUL, right unilateral; BL, bilateral; and symbols above the error bars, the significance (by 1-sample* t *test) of the change from baseline for that treatment group as follows: asterisk,* $P<.05$*; dagger,* $P<.01$*; and double dagger,* $P<.001$*. For explanation of post 1 ECT, post 7 ECT, and post ECT course, see the "EEG Data Acquisition" subsection in the "Subjects and Methods" section.*

Total global power at the 2-month follow-up was not influenced by whether patients received a crossover course of high-dosage BL ECT.

Global Power: Frequency Bands

Figure 1 presents the change scores in global power for each frequency band. The omnibus repeated measures ANCOVAs, with frequency band as a within-subject factor, did not yield effects involving treatment group at post 1 ECT or 2-month follow-up. The post 7 ECT analysis yielded significant interactions between dosage condition and frequency ($P=.02$) and among electrode placement, dosage condition, and frequency ($P<.005$). At post ECT course, there was an interaction between electrode placement and frequency ($P=.02$).

At post 7 ECT, low-dosage RUL ECT resulted in less global slowing than each of the other groups (Figure 1). The follow-up ANCOVA on delta power yielded an interaction between electrode placement and dosage condition ($P=.01$). Low-dosage RUL ECT produced a smaller increment in delta power than all other conditions (P values of $<.05$). For theta power, there was a main effect of electrode placement ($P<.05$) and an interaction between electrode placement and dosage condition ($P<.05$). Low-dosage RUL ECT produced less of an increase in theta power than all other conditions ($.07\geq P\geq.01$). There were no effects of treatment condition in the ANCOVAs on the alpha or beta frequencies.

The ANCOVAs for post ECT course yielded only a main effect of electrode placement for delta power ($P<.05$). Bilateral ECT produced a larger global increase than RUL ECT.

Laterality Indexes

The repeated measures ANCOVAs for the post 1 ECT and 2-month follow-up time points yielded no effects. In contrast, there was a significant interaction between electrode placement and frequency band at both post 7 ECT and post ECT course (P values of $<.05$). Follow-up ANCOVAs indicated that at both time points the differences among the treatment conditions in asymmetry pertained only to delta and theta power. In each case, only the main effect of electrode placement was significant ($.05>P\geq.001$). At post 7 ECT and post ECT course, both RUL ECT groups had a greater increase in delta and theta power in the right compared with the left hemisphere (**Figure 2**). This asymmetry in EEG slowing tended to be more pronounced with high-dosage RUL ECT. In contrast, both low- and high-dosage BL ECT resulted in a greater increase in left- than right-sided delta power. Bilateral ECT did not produce an asymmetry in theta power.

Topographic Effects

Repeated measures ANCOVAs were conducted for each frequency band on the changes in power relative to baseline at the 18 EEG sites. The significant interactions with EEG site, indicating differences among the treatment conditions in topographic effects, were restricted to the delta and theta bands at post 7 ECT and post ECT course. All further analyses were limited to these frequencies and time points.

Delta Frequency Band. The SSM was separately applied to the delta and theta frequency bands, submitting to each principal components analysis the change scores at both post 7 ECT and post ECT course (n=99). The principal components analysis for delta power yielded 4 patterns that accounted for 68.6% of the SRP variance. Individual differences in these topographic changes accounted for 50.8% of the variance in the change in global delta power at post 7 ECT and 26.4% at post ECT course. There were no effects of the treatment conditions in the ANCOVAs conducted on the GSF, which is the SSM's estimate of region-independent global effects. This suggested that the pronounced group differences in global delta power were due to contamination of the average global score by topographic effects.

Figure 3 depicts the 4 topographic patterns derived in the SSM delta analysis. **Figure 4** presents the average scores of the treatment conditions in manifesting these topographic changes. At both post 7 ECT and post ECT course, omnibus repeated measures ANCOVAs were conducted with scores of these patterns as the repeated measures factor. These analyses indicated that the treatment conditions differed significantly in manifesting particular topographic changes.

Follow-up ANCOVAs were conducted on the scores for each delta pattern (**Table 3**). The first pattern captured an anteroposterior gradient, reflecting increased delta power in frontal and anterotemporal sites, with no change in posterior cortex (Figure 3). At both time points, this pattern accounted for the largest proportion of the variance in the change in global delta power. At post 7 ECT, the low-dosage RUL ECT group was unique in having low scores for change in this pattern and differed from the high-dosage RUL ECT and low-dosage BL ECT groups ($.08>P>.04$). At post ECT course, this pattern was manifested to a greater extent with BL ECT than RUL ECT, without a dosage effect (Table 3). The high-dosage RUL ECT group appeared to show reduction in this effect relative to post 7 ECT (Figure 4).

The second delta pattern distinguished high-dosage RUL ECT group from the both BL ECT groups. Positive scores reflected increased delta power in specific frontal, central, and particularly temporal sites, greater in the left than right hemisphere. Negative scores reflected bilaterally increased delta power in prefrontal (F_{p1}, F_{p2}) sites, without the bitemporal involvement. At post 7 ECT, the high-dosage RUL ECT group differed from each of the BL ECT groups ($P<.005$). At the post ECT course, expression of this pattern was diminished, and only the high-dosage RUL ECT and low-dosage BL ECT groups differed ($P<.05$). Thus, BL ECT was associated

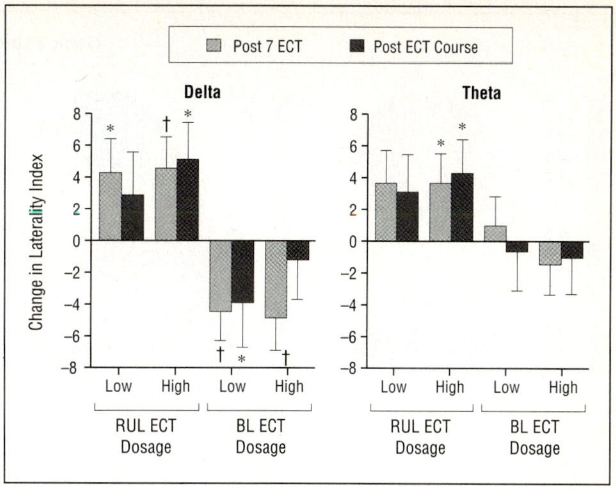

Figure 2. *Mean (±SE) change in asymmetry in power in the delta and theta frequency bands. ECT indicates electroconvulsive therapy; RUL, right unilateral; BL, bilateral; and symbols above the error bars, the significance (by 1-sample* t *test) of the change from baseline for that treatment group as follows: asterisk,* $P<.05$*; dagger,* $P<.01$*. For definition and calculation of* laterality index, *see the "Data Analysis" subsection in the "Subjects and Methods" section.*

with increased delta power in bifrontotemporal regions, greater on the left, while high-dosage RUL ECT produced large delta power increases in prefrontal regions, without the bitemporal involvement. Comparisons of the treatment groups in the delta changes at these specific sites confirmed this interpretation (data not shown).

The third pattern reflected a profile of asymmetry that was sensitive to electrode placement, independent of dosage. Positive scores were associated with increased delta power in left-sided lateral frontal (F_7), temporal, and occipital sites, and relatively reduced delta power in right-sided medial frontal, central, and parietal sites. At post 7 ECT, each BL ECT group tended to differ from each RUL ECT group in manifesting this pattern (*P* values of <.10). There were no effects of treatment condition for the fourth pattern.

Theta Frequency Band. The principal components analysis for theta power yielded 4 patterns that accounted for 71.2% of the SRP variance. These topographic changes accounted for 44.6% of the variance in the change in global theta power at post 7 ECT and 28.3% at post ECT course. At both time points, the first pattern accounted for the major portion of the variation in global theta changes (*P* values of ≤.001). Analyses of covariance revealed no effects of the treatment conditions on the GSF for theta power. Figure 3 also depicts the 4 patterns of theta topographic change. Figure 4 presents the average scores of the treatment conditions for these changes. At both time points, the omnibus repeated measures ANCOVA on the pattern scores produced an interaction between electrode placement and pattern (*P* values of <.01).

Table 3 presents the results of the ANCOVAs conducted on each of the theta pattern scores. Like the first pattern for delta, the first theta pattern captured an anteroposterior dimension, with the greatest theta power increase in frontal regions. However, superimposed on

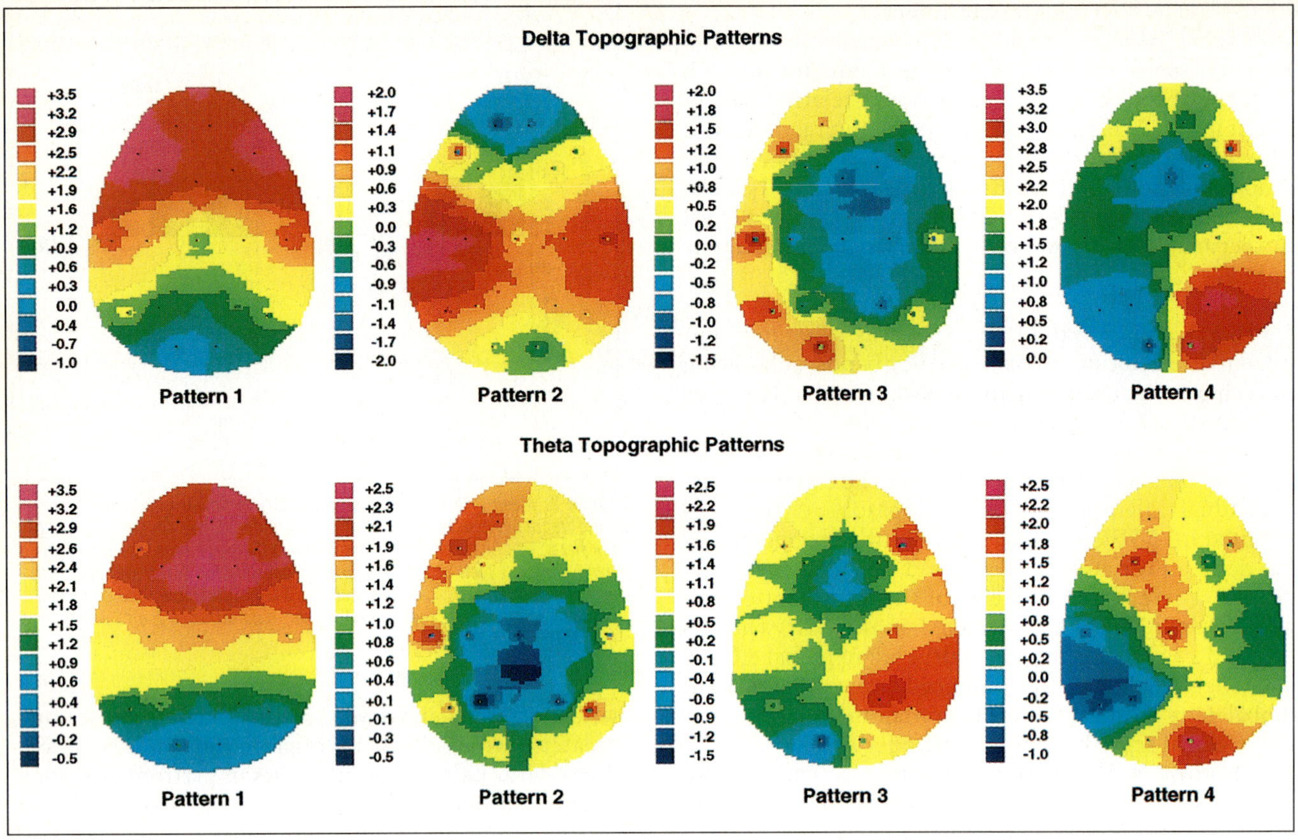

Figure 3. *Color maps of the topographic patterns revealed by the Scaled Subprofile Model[61] for changes in delta and theta power. The color scales differ for each of the maps and denote the weight of the electroencephalographic sites in contributing to the specific pattern.*

this pattern was a dimension of lateralization, with greater right than left theta power increases in frontal and anterotemporal regions and greater left than right increases in posterotemporal and parietal regions. Particularly at post ECT course, BL ECT resulted in greater expression of this pattern than RUL ECT (Figure 4). The second pattern was uniquely expressed by the low-dosage RUL ECT group. Their negative scores on this pattern reflected relatively greater theta increases in central and parietal regions compared with frontal and anterotemporal regions. At post 7 ECT, the low-dosage RUL ECT group tended to differ from the high-dosage RUL ECT group (P=.06) and the low-dosage BL ECT group (P=.02). Only the difference with the low-dosage BL ECT was significant at post ECT course ($P < 0.05$). The third pattern yielded a trend for a main effect of electrode placement only at post 7 ECT. This pattern described another dimension of asymmetry with positive scores reflecting higher right than left theta power increases at all sites other than F_{p1}-F_{p2} and F_3-F_4. The groups did not differ in expression of the fourth pattern at either time point.

CLINICAL OUTCOME

At post 7 ECT and post ECT course, ANCOVAs were conducted on the changes in global delta and theta power and the corresponding GSF values, using electrode placement and response status (responder vs nonresponder) as between-subject factors. Similar repeated measures ANCOVAs were conducted on the changes in topographic profiles to determine whether there were significant interactions between response status and pattern score.

In the ANCOVAs on global values, the only effects involving response status concerned changes in global delta power at post 7 ECT. There were trends for a main effect of response status (P=.09) and for an interaction between electrode placement and response status (P=.05). Nonresponders to RUL ECT tended to have smaller increase in global delta power than each of the other 3 groups ($.10 > P \geq .02$). Since there were no effects for GSF delta power, it is likely that these changes in global delta power related to clinical response were attributable to topographic alterations.

The repeated measures ANCOVAs on the changes in topography scores yielded no effects of response status for the theta frequency band. In contrast, there was a significant interaction between response status and delta topographic pattern at both post 7 ECT ($P < .01$) and post ECT course ($P < .05$). Follow-up ANCOVAs (electrode placement by response status) were conducted on the delta topographic patterns. For the first delta pattern, a main effect of response status was obtained at both post 7 ECT and post ECT course (P values of $< .05$). The increase in delta power in frontal regions was more marked among ECT responders than nonresponders, regardless of electrode placement. No effects of response status were obtained for the second or third delta patterns. At post 7 ECT, there was a trend for an interaction between elec-

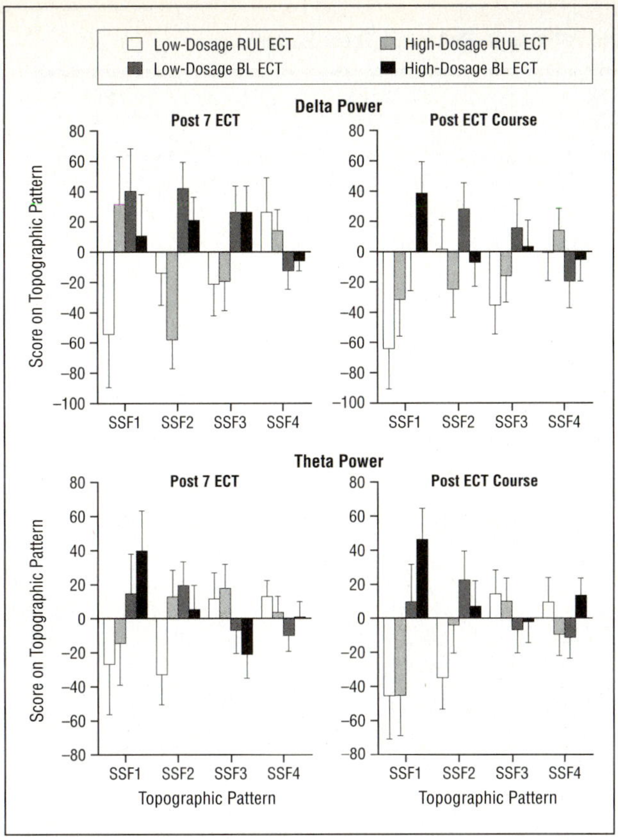

Figure 4. *Mean (±SE) scores for the treatment groups in expressing the topographic patterns that characterized changes in delta and theta power. Groups with no overlap in their associated letters differed in post hoc comparisons of least-squares adjusted means. ECT indicates electroconvulsive therapy; RUL, right unilateral; BL, bilateral; and SSF1 through SSF4, subject scaling factors 1 through 4, respectively. For explanation of post 1 ECT, post 7 ECT, and post ECT course, see the "EEG Data Acquisition" subsection in the "Subjects and Methods" section.*

trode placement and response status for scores on the fourth pattern ($P<.10$). Right unilateral ECT nonresponders had positive scores and differed from each of the other groups (P values of $<.05$). Poor outcome with RUL ECT was associated with a posterior asymmetry, with a greater delta increase in right-side parietal and occipital regions. At post ECT course, there was a trend for a main effect of response status ($P=.07$), without involvement of electrode placement. Again, manifestation of the posterior asymmetry was linked to inferior clinical outcome.

To verify these effects, a simultaneous regression was conducted across the sample predicting the percentage change in HRSD scores 1 week following the completion of ECT relative to baseline on the basis of electrode placement and scores on the 4 delta topographic patterns at post ECT course. Greater symptomatic improvement was associated with positive scores on the first delta pattern ($P<.02$) and poorer outcome with positive scores on the fourth pattern ($P<.01$).

The findings for the first pattern had indicated that positive clinical outcome was associated with greater delta power at frontal sites. As additional verification, the average change in delta power at the 7 prefrontal sites from baseline to post ECT course was computed and normalized by the global delta change. An ANCOVA on these values (response status by electrode placement) produced a main effect of response status ($P=.02$), without any other effects. Regardless of electrode placement, clinical response was associated with increased delta power in prefrontal regions.

COMMENT

SUMMARY OF FINDINGS

We found specificity in the time course of the EEG changes produced by ECT and in the frequency bands affected. Compared with pretreatment, a single treatment had no global, lateralized, or topographic effects on EEG recorded 48 hours later. No changes were discerned in any EEG measurement 8 weeks following completion of ECT. However, there were profound alterations after an average of 7 treatments and again several days following the ECT course. The significant changes were almost exclusively increases in delta and theta power. Extracranial EEG mainly reflects the extracellular current resulting from the summed postsynaptic potentials in pyramidal cells near the cortical surface. The fact that ECT produces marked EEG slowing suggests that synchronization has taken place in the synaptic activity of large neuronal populations, with a reduction in firing rate.[62-64]

MECHANISMS OF THERAPEUTIC ACTION OF ECT

Right unilateral ECT is ineffective when administered with an electrical intensity just above seizure threshold. Increasing the electrical dosage of RUL ECT results in substantial antidepressant effects.[4,5,22,23] The theories that may account for this phenomenon differ in their predictions about the impact of RUL ECT dosage on the laterality of EEG slowing, the magnitude of a diffuse, transcortical increase in slowing, and in the magnitude of change along an anteroposterior cortical gradient.

Laterality

Contrary to the theory predicting that higher-intensity RUL ECT produces less asymmetry in interictal slow-wave activity than low-dosage RUL ECT,[18,32,33] we found that, at the 2 critical time points, both types of RUL ECT produced greater increases of delta and theta power in the right than left hemisphere (Figure 2). Instead, the major differences between these forms of RUL ECT were in the topographic patterns revealed by SSM, particularly at post 7 ECT. High-, relative to low-, dosage RUL ECT produced more prominent increases in delta power in both left and right frontal regions, altering an anteroposterior gradient (Figure 3, delta pattern 1). Further, the second delta pattern distinguished high-dosage RUL ECT from both forms of BL ECT. Bilateral ECT was associated with increased delta power in bitemporal regions, with left-sided accentuation. High-dosage RUL ECT lacked this alteration in temporal sites, but instead produced a more restricted BL prefrontal delta increase. Thus, this

Table 3. Analyses of Covariance on Scores for Change in Topographic Patterns in Delta and Theta Power*

Topographic Patterns	SSF1 F	SSF1 P	SSF2 F	SSF2 P	SSF3 F	SSF3 P	SSF4 F	SSF4 P
Delta Power								
Post 7 ECT†								
EP	0.9	NS	12.5	.001	6.1	.02	2.4	NS
DC	1.0	NS	3.1	.09	0.0	NS	0.0	NS
EP×DC	3.1	.08	0.3	NS	0.0	NS	0.1	NS
Age	0.8	NS	0.0	NS	0.3	NS	0.2	NS
Post ECT course‡								
EP	7.4	.009	1.4	NS	3.2	.08	1.1	NS
DC	2.1	NS	2.5	NS	0.0	NS	0.7	NS
EP×DC	0.0	NS	0.0	NS	0.8	NS	0.0	NS
Age	0.1	NS	0.1	NS	0.1	NS	0.1	NS
Theta Power								
Post 7 ECT†								
EP	3.4	.07	2.4	NS	3.0	.09	2.3	NS
DC	0.7	NS	0.7	NS	0.2	NS	0.1	NS
EP×DC	0.1	NS	4.2	.048	0.6	NS	1.7	NS
Age	0.4	NS	1.9	NS	0.7	NS	1.4	NS
Post ECT course‡								
EP	10.3	.002	3.8	.06	1.0	NS	0.0	NS
DC	0.8	NS	0.1	NS	0.0	NS	0.0	NS
EP×DC	0.8	NS	2.1	NS	0.1	NS	2.7	NS
Age	0.4	NS	1.9	NS	0.3	NS	0.1	NS

*ECT indicates electroconvulsive therapy; EP, electrode placement; DC, dosage condition; SSF1 through SSF4, subject scaling factors 1 through 4, respectively; and NS, not significant.

†For post 7 ECT, df=1, 42.

‡For post ECT course, df=1, 47.

first theory received some support in that high-, relative to low-, dosage RUL ECT produced greater BL prefrontal slowing. However, this effect was specific to prefrontal cortex, and the 2 forms of RUL ECT did not differ in the overall magnitude of asymmetry.

This study confirms previous findings that, despite symmetric electrode placement, BL ECT also produces an asymmetry, reflected in a greater left-sided increase in delta power.[8,13,17,18,28-31] This delta asymmetry was mainly attributable to accentuation in left frontotemporal regions (delta patterns 2 and 3). There is evidence that, with normal aging, left temporal areas are the most common sites for background slow-wave activity.[65,66] In neurological samples, equivalent left and right hemispheric lesions often result in greater impairment in behavioral indexes of left, compared with right, hemispheric function.[67] Thus, relative to homotopic tissue, some left hemispheric regions may have an intrinsically greater vulnerability to a variety of insults, and this may be expressed in the context of BL ECT.

Transcortical Effects

The second theory posited that higher-dosage RUL ECT results in greater current density in deep subcortical regions, that subcortical stimulation is fundamental to antidepressant effects, and that greater stimulation of subcortical pacemakers produces a transcortical increase in slow-wave activity.[34-36,42] In line with this theory, we found that, at post 7 ECT, low-dosage RUL ECT resulted in markedly reduced increases in both delta and theta power across EEG sites (Figure 1). However, with SSM's region-independent measure of global change, there were no differences among the treatment groups at any time point. This indicated that the group differences in apparent transcortical change resulted from differences in topographic effects. The topographic alteration that most strongly determined the mean changes in delta and theta power was the increase in slowing in anterior cortical regions (delta and theta patterns 1). Low-dosage RUL ECT was particularly weak in producing this change. Thus, it appeared that the treatment conditions did not differ in transcortical effects.

This test of the second theory had limitations. Extracranial delta waves are thought to originate from vertically arranged dipoles in cortical layers II, III, and V,[64,68,69] reflecting the firing of GABAergic interneurons inhibiting pyramidal cells[70,71] and/or the summation of long-lasting after-hyperpolarizations, owing to potassium currents in deep cortical pyramidal cells.[72] Reticular thalamic nuclei and thalamocortical circuits modulate cortical delta activity, supporting the importance of subcortical oscillators.[63,64] However, despite widespread cortical projection, it is not known whether alterations of thalamic nuclei necessarily result in diffuse delta increases or whether topographic changes should be expected. Further, corticothalamic circuits play a critical role in modulating delta activity in the thalamus, and ablating cortical areas that project to particular thalamic nuclei can induce spontaneous delta oscillations.[73,74] Thus, it is uncertain that modulation of thalamic pacemakers necessarily produces diffuse increases in delta activity and, even had we obtained such transcortical effects, their origin could be attributed to altered synaptic activity at the cortical level.

Anteroposterior Gradient

We hypothesized that, at low dosage, RUL ECT seizures initiate in perirolandic regions. When stimulus dosage is increased, a broader expanse of right hemispheric regions participate in seizure initiation. This theory assumes that the spatial distribution of reduced functional activity following ECT is largely determined by the topography of seizure onset and that the reduction of functional activity in anterior frontal regions is critical to efficacy.[3,45,46]

The findings were compatible with this theory. Induction of slow-wave activity in frontal regions was the most prominent topographic effect of ECT, but low-dosage RUL ECT was particularly weak in producing this alteration. The EEG changes that were associated with clinical outcome pertained only to the delta band and only to topographic effects. Increased delta power in frontal regions (delta pattern 1) at both post 7 ECT and post ECT course was associated with superior response following ECT, regardless of electrode placement. These findings support the suggestion of Fink and Kahn,[14] linking increased frontal delta activity to positive ECT outcome.

Other imaging studies[56,75,76] have shown that reduced cerebral blood flow and metabolic rate for glucose in prefrontal cortex are the most prominent topographic effects of ECT in the interictal period. We previously reported that the magnitude of CBF reductions in prefrontal cortex, whether assessed in the acute postictal period or during the week following ECT, was strongly related to clinical response.[56] The fact that reduced CBF and increased delta power are both linked to positive outcome suggests that reduced excitatory input or enhanced inhibition in prefrontal regions is associated with efficacy.

An intriguing aspect of these findings is that, with some exceptions,[77,78] the most common baseline abnormality in functional imaging studies of major depression is reduced frontal CBF or metabolism (see Sackeim and Prohovnik[79] for a review). Clinical response to ECT appears to intensify, rather than reverse, these deficits.[56] Similarly, substantial delta activity in the awake adult is usually considered pathologic,[62,63] and the induction of EEG slowing in frontal regions cannot be viewed as reversing a baseline deficit in major depression. Indeed, EEG alterations were not observed at the 2-month follow-up, when the bulk of patients were euthymic. This indicates that frontal delta activity cannot be considered a marker of mood state. Consequently, it is likely that the EEG changes linked to efficacy mark some more fundamental neurobiological processes in the chain leading to therapeutic response.

Accepted for publication May 20, 1996.

This study was supported in part by grants MH35636, MH44779, and MH47739 from the National Institute of Mental Health, Bethesda, Md; by an Established Investigator Award (Dr Sackeim) and a Young Investigator Award (Dr Nobler) from the National Alliance for Research in Schizophrenia and Depression, Chicago, Ill; and by a grant from the Aging and Memory Loss Consortium of the Charles A. Dana Foundation, New York, NY.

We thank Richard Coppola, DSc, and Richard D. Weiner, MD, PhD, who were consultants for this study, and Edward Maclin, PhD, and Eliza A. Coleman, MA, for assistance with data collection.

Reprints: Harold A. Sackeim, PhD, Department of Biological Psychiatry, New York State Psychiatric Institute, 722 W 168th St, New York, NY 10032.

REFERENCES

1. Kety S. Biochemical and neurochemical effects of electroconvulsive shock. In: Fink M, Kety S, McGaugh J, Williams T, eds. *Psychobiology of Convulsive Therapy.* Washington, DC: V. H. Winston & Sons; 1974:285-294.
2. Sackeim HA, Devanand DP, Nobler MS. Electroconvulsive therapy. In: Bloom F, Kupfer D, eds. *Psychopharmacology: The Fourth Generation of Progress.* New York, NY: Raven Press; 1995:1123-1142.
3. Sackeim HA. Central issues regarding the mechanisms of action of electroconvulsive therapy: directions for future research. *Psychopharmacol Bull.* 1994; 30:281-308.
4. Sackeim HA, Decina P, Kanzler M, Kerr B, Malitz S. Effects of electrode placement on the efficacy of titrated, low-dose ECT. *Am J Psychiatry.* 1987;144: 1449-1455.
5. Sackeim HA, Prudic J, Devanand DP, Kiersky JE, Fitzsimons L, Moody BJ, McElhiney MC, Coleman EA, Settembrino JM. Effects of stimulus intensity and electrode placement on the efficacy and cognitive effects of electroconvulsive therapy. *N Engl J Med.* 1993;328:839-846.
6. Abrams R. *Electroconvulsive Therapy.* New York, NY: Oxford University Press; 1992.
7. Weiner RD. EEG related to electroconvulsive therapy. In: Hughes JR, Wilson WP, eds. *EEG and Evoked Potentials in Psychiatry and Behavioral Neurology.* Stoneham, Mass: Butterworth Publishers Inc; 1983:101-126.
8. Weiner RD, Rogers HJ, Davidson JR, Kahn EM. Effects of electroconvulsive therapy upon brain electrical activity. *Ann N Y Acad Sci.* 1986;462:270-281.
9. Pacella BL, Barrera SE, Kalinowsky L. Variations in electroencephalogram associated with electric shock therapy of patients with mental disorders. *Arch Neurol Psychiatry.* 1942;47:367-384.
10. Roth M. Changes in the EEG under barbiturate anesthesia produced by electroconvulsive treatment and their significance for the theory of ECT action. *Electroencephalogr Clin Neurophysiol.* 1951;3:261-280.
11. Weiner RD. The persistence of electroconvulsive therapy-induced changes in the electroencephalogram. *J Nerv Ment Dis.* 1980;168:224-228.
12. Kolbeinsson H, Pëtursson H. Electroencephalographic correlates of electroconvulsive therapy. *Acta Psychiatr Scand.* 1988;78:162-168.
13. Volavka J, Feldstein S, Abrams R, Dornbush R, Fink M. EEG and clinical change after bilateral and unilateral electroconvulsive therapy. *Electroencephalogr Clin Neurophysiol.* 1972;32:631-639.
14. Fink M, Kahn RL. Relation of electroencephalographic delta activity to behavioral response in electroshock: quantitative serial studies. *Arch Neurol Psychiatry.* 1957;78:516-525.
15. Roth M, Kay DW, Shaw J, Green J. Prognosis and pentothal induced electroencephalographic changes in electro-convulsive treatment: an approach to the problem of regulation of convulsive therapy. *Electroencephalogr Clin Neurophysiol.* 1957;9:225-237.
16. Ottosson J-O. Electroconvulsive therapy of endogenous depression: an analysis of the influence of various factors on the efficacy of the therapy. *J Ment Sci.* 1962;108:694-703.
17. Strömgren LS, Juul-Jensen P. EEG in unilateral and bilateral electroconvulsive therapy. *Acta Psychiatr Scand.* 1975;51:340-360.
18. Abrams R, Taylor MA, Volavka J. ECT-induced EEG asymmetry and therapeutic response in melancholia: relation to treatment electrode placement. *Am J Psychiatry.* 1987;144:327-329.
19. Taylor RM, Pacella BL. The significance of abnormal electroencephalograms prior to electroconvulsive therapy. *J Nerv Ment Dis.* 1948;107:220-227.
20. Johnson LC, Ulett GA, Sines JO, Stern JA. Cortical activity and cognitive functioning. *Electroencephalogr Clin Neurophysiol.* 1960;12:861-874.
21. Abrams R, Volavka J, Schrift M. Brief pulse ECT in melancholia: EEG and clinical effects. *J Nerv Ment Dis.* 1992;180:55-57.
22. Abrams R, Swartz CM, Vedak C. Antidepressant effects of high-dose right uni-

lateral electroconvulsive therapy. *Arch Gen Psychiatry.* 1991;48:746-748.

23. Letemendia FJ, Delva NJ, Rodenburg M, Lawson JS, Inglis J, Waldron JJ, Lywood DW. Therapeutic advantage of bifrontal electrode placement in ECT. *Psychol Med.* 1993;23:349-360.
24. Weaver L, Williams R, Rush S. Current density in bilateral and unilateral ECT. *Biol Psychiatry.* 1976;11:303-312.
25. d'Elia G, Perris C. Comparison of electroconvulsive therapy with unilateral and bilateral stimulation. *Acta Psychiatr Scand.* 1970;215:9-29.
26. Kriss A, Halliday AM, Halliday E, Pratt RT. EEG immediately after unilateral ECT. *Acta Psychiatr Scand.* 1978;58:231-244.
27. Staton RD, Hass PJ, Brumback RA. Electroencephalographic recording during bitemporal and unilateral non-dominant hemisphere (Lancaster position) electroconvulsive therapy. *J Clin Psychiatry.* 1981;42:264-269.
28. Martin WL, Ford HF, McDonald EC, Towler ML. Clinical evaluation of unilateral EST. *Am J Psychiatry.* 1965;121:1087-1090.
29. Abrams R, Volavka J, Roubicek J, Dornbush R, Fink M. Lateralized EEG changes after unilateral and bilateral electroconvulsive therapy. *Dis Nerv Syst.* 1970;31 (suppl):28-33.
30. Small JG. EEG and neurophysiological studies of convulsive therapies. In: Fink M, Kety S, McGaugh JW, eds. *Psychobiology of Convulsive Therapy.* Washington, DC: Winston & Sons; 1974:47-64.
31. Marjerrison G, James J, Reichert H. Unilateral and bilateral ECT: EEG findings. *Can Psychiatr Assoc J.* 1975;20:257-266.
32. Abrams R. A hypothesis to explain divergent findings among studies comparing the efficacy of unilateral and bilateral ECT in depression. *Convuls Ther.* 1986;2:253-257.
33. Weiner RD, Coffey CE. Minimizing therapeutic differences between bilateral and unilateral nondominant ECT. *Convuls Ther.* 1986;2:261-265.
34. Abrams R, Taylor MA. Diencephalic stimulation and the effects of ECT in endogenous depression. *Br J Psychiatry.* 1976;129:482-485.
35. Fink M, Ottosson JO. A theory of convulsive therapy in endogenous depression: significance of hypothalamic functions. *Psychiatry Res.* 1980;2:49-61.
36. Fink M, Nemeroff CB. A neuroendocrine view of ECT. *Convuls Ther.* 1989;5:296-304.
37. Rush S, Driscoll D. Current distribution in the brain from surface electrodes. *Anesth Analg.* 1968;47:717-723.
38. Proctor LD, Goodwin JE. Clinical and electro-physiological observations following electroshock. *Am J Psychiatry.* 1945;101:797-800.
39. Fink M, Kahn RL, Green MA. Experimental studies of the electroshock process. *Dis Nerv Syst.* 1958;19:113-118.
40. Ottosson J-O. Experimental studies of the mode of action of electroconvulsive therapy. *Acta Psychiatr Scand Suppl.* 1960;145:1-141.
41. Robin A, Binnie CD, Copas JB. Electrophysiological and hormonal responses to three types of electroconvulsive therapy. *Br J Psychiatry.* 1985;147:707-712.
42. Staton RD, Enderle JD, Gerst JW. The electroencephalographic pattern during electroconvulsive therapy, V: observations on the origins of phase III delta energy and the mechanism of action of ECT. *Clin Electroencephalogr.* 1988;19:176-198.
43. Zis AP, McGarvey KA, Clark CM, Lam RW, Patrick L, Adams SA. Effect of stimulus energy on electroconvulsive therapy-induced prolactin release. *Convuls Ther.* 1993;9:23-27.
44. Riddle WJ, Scott AI, Bennie J, Carroll S, Fink G. Current intensity and oxytocin release after electroconvulsive therapy. *Biol Psychiatry.* 1993;33:839-841.
45. Sackeim HA, Mukherjee S. Neurophysiological variability in the effects of the ECT stimulus. *Convuls Ther.* 1986;2:267-276.
46. Sackeim HA, Long J, Luber B, Moeller JR, Prohovnik I, Devanand DP, Nobler MS. Physical properties and quantification of the ECT stimulus, I: basic principles. *Convuls Ther.* 1994;10:93-123.
47. Lorimer FM, Segal MM, Stein SN. Path of current distribution in brain during electro-convulsive therapy: preliminary report. *Electroencephalogr Clin Neurophysiol.* 1949;1:343-348.
48. Hayes KJ. The current path in ECS. *Arch Neurol Psychiatry.* 1950;63:102-109.
49. Gottesfeld BH, Lesse SM, Herskovitz H. Studies in electroconvulsive shock therapy of varied electrode applications. *J Nerv Ment Dis.* 1944;99:56-64.
50. Penfield W, Jasper H. *Epilepsy and the Functional Anatomy of the Human Brain.* Boston, Mass: Little, Brown & Co Inc; 1954.
51. Ajmone Marsan C. Focal electrical stimulation. In: Purpura DP, Penry JK, Tower DB, Woodbury DM, Walter RD, eds. *Experimental Models of Epilepsy.* New York, NY: Raven Press; 1972:147-172.
52. Prince DA. Neuronal events underlying focal epileptiform potentials. In: Wieser HG, Speckmann EJ, Engel JJ, eds. *The Epileptic Focus.* London, England: John Libbey; 1987:17-26.
53. Miyasaka M. Cortical and subcortical seizure discharge induced by bitemporal electroshock in cats. *Folia Psychiatr Neurol Jpn.* 1959;13:113-123.
54. Chatrian GE, Petersen MC. The convulsive patterns provoked by Indoklon, Metrazol and electroshock: some depth electrographic observations in human patients. *Electroencephalogr Clin Neurophysiol.* 1960;12:715-725.
55. Sackeim HA, Decina P, Prohovnik I, Malitz S, Resor SR. Anticonvulsant and antidepressant properties of electroconvulsive therapy: a proposed mechanism of action. *Biol Psychiatry.* 1983;18:1301-1310.
56. Nobler MS, Sackeim HA, Prohovnik I, Moeller JR, Mukherjee S, Schnur DB, Prudic J, Devanand DP. Regional cerebral blood flow in mood disorders, III: treatment and clinical response. *Arch Gen Psychiatry.* 1994;51:884-897.
57. Dummermuth G, Molinari L. Spectral analysis of EEG background activity. In: Gevins AS, Rémond A. eds. *Methods of Analysis of Brain Electrical and Magnetic Signals: EEG Handbook (Revised Series).* 1987;1:85-99.
58. Moeller J, Strother S, Sidtis J, Rottenberg D. Scaled Subprofile Model: a statistical approach to the analysis of functional patterns in positron emission tomographic data. *J Cereb Blood Flow Metab.* 1987;7:649-658.
59. Moeller JR, Strother SC. A regional covariance approach to the analysis of functional patterns in positron emission tomographic data. *J Cereb Blood Flow Metab.* 1991;11:A121-A135.
60. Sackeim HA, Prohovnik I, Moeller JR, Mayeux R, Stern Y, Devanand DP. Regional cerebral blood flow in mood disorders, II: comparison of major depression and Alzheimer's disease. *J Nucl Med.* 1993;34:1090-1101.
61. Alexander GE, Moeller JR. Application of the Scaled Subprofile Model to functional imaging in neuropsychiatric disorders: a principal components approach to modeling brain function in disease. *Hum Brain Mapping.* 1994;2:79-94.
62. Pedley TA, Traub RD. Physiological basis of EEG. In: Daly DD, Pedley TA, eds. *Current Practice of Clinical Electroencephalography.* 2nd ed. New York, NY: Raven Press; 1990:107-137.
63. Steriade M, Gloor PL, Lopes da Silva FH, Mesulam M-M. Basic mechanisms of cerebral rhythmic activities. *Electroencephalogr Clin Neurophysiol.* 1990; 76:481-508.
64. Steriade M. Cellular substrates of brain rhythms. In: Niedermeyer E, Lopes da Silva FH, eds. *Electroencephalography: Basic Principles, Clinical Applications, and Related Fields.* 3rd ed. Baltimore, Md: Williams & Wilkins; 1994:27-62.
65. Torres F, Faoro A, Lowenson R, Johnson E. The electroencephalogram of elderly subjects revisited. *Electroencephalogr Clin Neurophysiol.* 1983;56:391-398.
66. Breslau J, Starr A, Sicotte N, Higa J, Buchsbaum MS. Topographic EEG changes with normal aging and SDAT. *Electroencephalogr Clin Neurophysiol.* 1989;72:281-289.
67. Semmes J. Hemispheric specialization: a possible clue to mechanism. *Neuropsychologia.* 1968;6:11-26.
68. Calvet J, Calvet MC, Scherer J. Etude stratigraphique corticale de l'activité EEG spontanée. *Electroencephalogr Clin Neurophysiol.* 1964;17:109-125.
69. Petsche H, Pockberger H, Rappelsberger P. On the search for the sources of the electroencephalogram. *Neuroscience.* 1984;11:1-27.
70. Ball CJ, Gloor P, Schaul N. The cortical electromicrophysiology of pathological delta waves in the electroencephalogram of the cat. *Electroencephalogr Clin Neurophysiol.* 1977;43:346-361.
71. Steriade M, Buzsáki G. Parallel activation of thalamic and cortical neurons by brainstem and basal forebrain cholinergic systems. In: Steriade M, Biesold D, eds. *Brain Cholinergic Systems.* New York, NY: Oxford University Press; 1990:3-62.
72. Schwindt PC, Spain WJ, Crill WE. Long-lasting reduction of excitability by a sodium-dependent potassium current in cat neocortical neurons. *J Neurophysiol.* 1989;61:233-244.
73. Steriade M, Curró Dossi R, Nuñez A. Network modulation of a slow intrinsic oscillation of cat thalamocortical neurons implicated in sleep delta waves: cortically induced synchronization and brainstem cholinergic suppression. *J Neurosci.* 1991;11:3200-3217.
74. Curró Dossi R, Nuñez A, Steriade M. Electrophysiology of a slow (0.5-4 Hz) intrinsic oscillation of cat thalamocortical neurones in vivo. *J Physiol (Lond).* 1992;447:215-234.
75. Silfverskiöld P, Gustafson L, Johanson A, Risberg J, Rosen I. Acute and late effects on rCBF, EEG, psychometric testing and clinical outcome. *Ann N Y Acad Sci.* 1986;462:236-248.
76. Volkow ND, Bellar S, Mullani N, Jould L, Dewey S. Effects of electroconvulsive therapy on brain glucose metabolism: a preliminary study. *Convuls Ther.* 1988; 4:199-205.
77. Drevets WC, Videen TO, Price JL, Preskorn SH, Carmichael ST, Raichle ME. A functional anatomical study of unipolar depression. *J Neurosci.* 1992;12:3628-3641.
78. Biver F, Goldman S, Delvenne V, Luxen A, De Maertelaer V, Hubain P, Mendlewicz J, Lotstra F. Frontal and parietal metabolic disturbances in unipolar depression. *Biol Psychiatry.* 1994;36:381-388.
79. Sackeim HA, Prohovnik I. Brain imaging studies in depressive disorders. In: Mann JJ, Kupfer D, eds. *Biology of Depressive Disorders.* New York, NY: Plenum Press; 1993:205-258.

Interictal Electroencephalographic Effects of Electroconvulsive Therapy

Can They Elucidate Mechanism of Action?

Electroconvulsive therapy (ECT) and electroencephalography (EEG) were developed within several years of each other in the early 1930s, and the effects of ECT on the ictal and interictal EEGs were reported soon thereafter. The EEG effects were massive and consistent; it seemed natural to view this EEG change as a concomitant, a precondition, or even an explanation of the clinical effects of ECT. These views were translated into hypotheses that were tested and presented in a large literature that goes back to the 1940s.

See also page 814

At least 3 domains have been studied in the literature involving interictal EEG: the treatment, the EEG, and the clinical outcome. The treatment variables include the position of the ECT electrodes, the stimulus intensity, and the number of treatments given at the time of the EEG. The EEG variables include the topographic distribution over the scalp (the number, location, and connections of the EEG electrodes), the estimates of power in several frequency bands, and an estimate of the average EEG frequency. The outcome variable may be categorical (improved vs not improved), or continuous (relative improvement on a rating scale).

The development of the methods used for the measurement of the EEG and for the statistical evaluation of the large number of variables reflects, to a large extent, the spectacular rise of the researchers' power to compute. For example, in the pioneering work of Fink et al,[1] the EEG activity in 1 frequency band (delta) was measured manually, and the records were globally classified as high, moderate, or low on the delta activity. Later on, the ECT effects on the EEG were assessed by computer; however, only a limited number of EEG scalp locations could be studied because of hardware limitations of the time.[2] Thus, except for limited efforts to assess lateralization, complex analyses of topographic EEG effects could not yet be done.

In the 1990s, the hardware and software available enables the researchers to analyze the EEG simultaneously from essentially any number of recording electrodes that can be fitted on the scalp. Thus, we can finally obtain the data needed to test complex hypotheses regarding the post-ECT changes of the topographic distributions of EEG frequency and power.

Such hypotheses, examined by Sackeim et al and presented in this issue of the ARCHIVES,[3] cannot be adequately tested with traditional statistical methods. There are several reasons why a novel method, the Scaled Subprofile Model (SSM)[4] used by Sackeim et al,[3] is more appropriate. First, very large sets of EEG variables must be acquired for the tests, but practical considerations limit the research to relatively small subject samples. Second, ECT has huge global effects on the EEG; a conventional analysis of covariance may obscure the regionally specific effects that are of particular interest when testing hypotheses regarding the mechanism of ECT action. Third, unlike traditional statistics, the SSM can be used to express the degree to which individual subjects (or groups of subjects receiving different types of ECT) conform to defined EEG regional topographic patterns. Applying the SSM to data from multiple EEG electrodes, Sackeim et al were able to persuasively demonstrate that the effective forms of ECT were associated with an increase of the power in the delta frequency range over prefrontal regions bilaterally.

However, we would like to point out that the SSM does have certain limitations. First, the extracted components are mathematical constructs (descriptors); there is no guarantee that the derived topographical components can be linked to actual physiological generators. For example, we do not know whether a topographical component corresponds to a functional brain circuitry that emits that pattern. Second, we do not know whether these components efficiently represent, or even actually extract, the "signal" that is related to the particular phenomenon we investigate. It is, for example, possible that the signal is in topographical components that were omitted (because of the application of a more or less arbitrary "stopping" or "selection" rule for the components), or it is "spilled over" several components and, thus, may be too weak and masked by variance extraneous to the phenomenon of interest.

The most prominent topographical EEG component identified through the SSM method in the study by Sackeim et al was an anteroposterior gradient factor in delta band activity. Such a topographical component was identified in various frequency bands, including delta, by previous authors using topographical factor analysis[5,6] or dipole source localization.[7] Given the fact that the subject populations in these studies were not receiving ECT and were as diverse as normal adults,[7] normal adolescents,[6] or mentally retarded children,[5] the functional significance of this antero-posterior delta component remains unclear.

The study by Sackeim et al is a significant step in the process of understanding the ECT action: it describes EEG changes better than earlier studies did, but leaves open essential theoretical questions regarding the spatial origin and the mechanism of these changes. High-resolution EEG[8] using dense sensory arrays and coupled with magnetic resonance imaging registration may yield a more precise localization of the sources of electrical potentials recorded on the scalp; using such an approach can further improve our understanding of ECT action. Such methods may clarify whether the therapeutic effect of ECT depends on a focal cortical or subcortical generator or on a distributed action involving several structures.

The interictal slowing analyzed by Sackeim et al may be seen as an aftereffect of seizures that have measurable electrophysiological characteristics, such as intensity, duration, and topographical distribution. Therefore, future researchers may consider the possibility that the study of ictal (rather than the interictal) EEG descriptors may bring them closer to the understanding of the mechanism of ECT action.

Although Sackeim et al do not stress it, one of the most striking and important features of their article is the demonstration of clinical efficacy of the ECT (the data are shown in Tables 1 and 2[3]). If the baseline levels of severity (assessed by the Hamilton Rating Scale for Depression) were representative of the patients' long-term status, these patients had been suffering from severe depressive symptoms for many months during the current episode. Some of the episodes lasted more than a year. Patients receiving the types of ECT that are usual in clinical practice have benefited from the treatments. The efficacy was excellent in terms of the speed of onset and the size of symptom reduction. Even though we may not yet completely understand its mechanism of action, ECT is an indispensable part of our therapeutic armamentarium.

Jan Volavka, MD, PhD
Pal Czobor, PhD
The Nathan S. Kline Institute for Psychiatric Research
140 Old Orangeburg Rd, Bldg 37
Orangeburg, NY 10962

REFERENCES

1. Fink M, Kahn RL, Oaks G. Relation of electroencephalographic delta activity to behavioral response in electroshock. *Arch Neurol Psychiatry.* 1957;78:516-525.
2. Volavka J, Feldstein S, Abrams R, Dornbush R, Fink M. EEG and clinical change after bilateral and unilateral electroconvulsive therapy. *Electroencephalogr Clin Neurophysiol.* 1972;32:631-639.
3. Sackeim HA, Luber B, Katzman GP, Moeller JR, Prudic J, Devanand DP, Nobler MS. The effects of electroconvulsive therapy on quantitative electroencephalograms; relationship to clinical outcome. *Arch Gen Psychiatry.* 1996;53:814-824.
4. Alexander GE, Moeller JR. Application of the Scaled Subprofile Model to functional imaging in neuropsychiatric disorders: a principal component approach to modeling brain function in disease. *Human Brain Mapping.* 1994;2:79-94.
5. Gasser T, Mocks J, Bacher P. Topographic factor analysis of the EEG with applications to development and to mental retardation. *Electroencephalogr Clin Neurophysiol.* 1983;55:445-463.
6. Volkow ND, Gomez-Mont F, Inamdar S, Lamella M, Prichep L, John R. Multivariate analyses of the EEG in normal adolescents. *Biol Psychiatry.* 1987;22:199-204.
7. Michel CM, Lehmann D, Henggeler B, Brandeis D. Localization of the sources of EEG delta, theta, alpha and beta frequency bands using the FFT dipole approximation. *Electroencephalogr Clin Neurophysiol.* 1992;82:38-44.
8. Gevins A, Leong H, Smith ME, Le J, Du R. Mapping cognitive brain function with modern high-resolution electroencephalography. *Trends Neurosci.* 1995;18:429-436.

INTRODUCING

RISPERDAL ON CALL

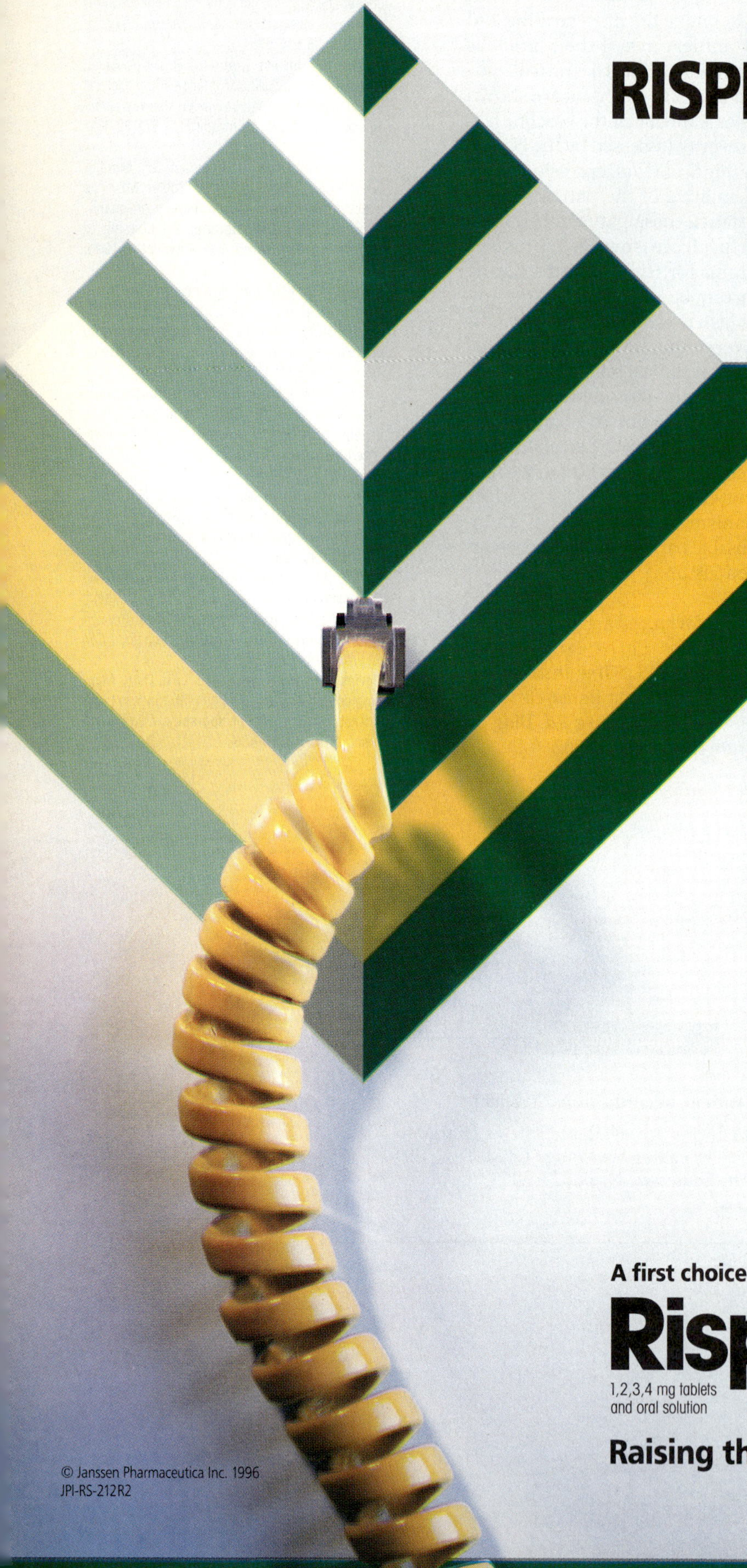

Quick, easy access to the information you want.

Now you can call a toll-free 800 number for instant access to information about RISPERDAL.

Available whenever you need it.

RISPERDAL ON CALL is available 24 hours a day, 7 days a week. You can access it anytime, anywhere—all you need is a touch-tone phone.

The information you need—and more—at your fingertips.

Get product and conversion information, hear physician discussions, or request an important clinical reprint! Just call 1-800-6R-ON-CALL (1-800-676-6225) and follow the voice prompts to your choice of valuable information about RISPERDAL.

What else does RISPERDAL ON CALL offer?

Call 1-800-6R-ON-CALL (1-800-676-6225) today!

A first choice

Risperdal®

RISPERIDONE

1,2,3,4 mg tablets
and oral solution

Raising the standard of care.

ORIGINAL ARTICLE

Effect of Antidepressant Medication on Morning and Evening Thyroid Function Tests During a Major Depressive Episode

Fabrice Duval, MD; Marie-Claude Mokrani, PhD; Marc-Antoine Crocq, MD; Martine Jautz, MAPsych; Paul Bailey, MRCPsych; Than-Son Diep, MD; Jean-Paul Macher, MD

Background: This study sought to determine whether changes in thyroid function that may occur during antidepressant treatment are related to a direct effect of the drug on the thyroid axis or to a change in clinical state.

Methods: Morning and evening thyroid function was evaluated in 30 euthyroid inpatients who met *DSM-IV* criteria for major depressive episode, by determination of free triiodothyronine, free thyroxine, and thyrotropin levels before and after 8 AM and 11 PM protirelin challenges (200 μg intravenously), on the same day. Results at baseline were compared with those after 1 month of antidepressant treatment with either amitriptyline hydrochloride, fluoxetine hydrochloride, or toloxatone.

Results: Clinical efficacy and effects on thyroid function did not differ across the 3 antidepressant drugs. Compared with pretreatment values, significant reductions in basal serum 8 AM free thyroxine, 11 PM free thyroxine, and 8 AM free triiodothyronine levels and increases in 11 PM maximum increment in plasma thyrotropin level and the difference between 11 PM and 8 AM maximum increment in plasma thyrotropin values were observed in responders (n=11) but not in partial responders (n=6) or nonresponders (n=13). Moreover, nonresponders exhibited lower pretreatment 11 PM thyrotropin values (basal and maximal increment above basal) than responders.

Conclusions: The results suggest that (1) changes in thyroid function are related to clinical recovery rather than to a direct effect of the antidepressant drug and (2) patients with the lowest pretreatment evening thyrotropin secretion have the lowest rate of antidepressant response, and this may contribute to treatment resistance.

Arch Gen Psychiatry. 1996;53:833-840

PREVIOUS STUDIES suggest that treatment with antidepressant drugs leads to changes in results of thyroid tests: either decreased peripheral thyroid hormone levels or increased thyrotropin (TSH) levels (basal or after protirelin stimulation).[1-13] However, these results have not always been confirmed,[14-19] owing perhaps to methodological limitations (small sample, variable definitions of depression, hospitalization status, assay sensitivity). Furthermore, it is not known whether the changes in thyroid function are a direct effect of antidepressants on the thyroid axis or a correlate of clinical improvement.

Animal studies[20,21] suggest that long-term antidepressant treatment decreases thyroid function. Data from healthy volunteers do not show a consistent effect of tricyclic antidepressants on TSH secretion.[22,23] In depressed patients, most studies show that treatment with tricyclics,[11,17,24] selective serotonin reuptake inhibitors,[19] or monoamine oxidase inhibitors[25] does not significantly change TSH levels. Moreover, it has been reported,[7,10] although inconsistently,[17] that response to tricyclic antidepressants is associated with decreases within the normal range in levels of thyroxine (T_4) and free thyroxine (FT_4), without changes in triiodothyronine (T_3) or TSH levels. Thus, although not all studies agree, recovery from depression seems associated with reduction or even full correction of thyroid axis abnormalities.[26]

However, in the investigation of the hypothalamic-pituitary-thyroid axis in euthyroid patients by means of the protirelin TSH challenge test, it is useful to consider chronobiological aspects. As currently performed in the morning (at 8 or 9 AM), the protirelin TSH test has modest diagnostic sensitivity (approximately

See Subjects and Methods on next page

From the Centre Hospitalier (Drs Duval, Crocq, Jautz, Diep, and Macher) and the Institute for Research in Neurosciences and Psychiatry (Drs Mokrani and Bailey), Rouffach, France.

30%)[27,28] and thus is of limited use in treatment monitoring. Owing to the circadian activity of the thyrotrophs, which is maximal between 11 PM and 1 AM,[28-35] pituitary TSH secretion is more sensitive to protirelin stimulation in the evening, both in control subjects[28,36] and in depressed patients.[28,37] We recently defined a chronobiological measure of thyroid function: the difference between 11 PM and 8 AM TSH response to protirelin (ΔΔmaxTSH). Reduction of this index was found in 85% of euthyroid inpatients who met *DSM-III-R* criteria for major depressive episode.[37,38]

Furthermore, we also reported, as have others (reviewed by Whybrow and Bauer[39]), a shift to higher morning and evening iodothyronine levels in euthyroid depressed inpatients[38]; this factor may contribute to the blunting of TSH response to protirelin.[40,41]

To our knowledge, this is the first study to examine thyroid hormone levels and protirelin TSH responses at 8 AM and at 11 PM, on the same day, before (medication-free) and after 1 month of antidepressant treatment in a population of inpatients with a major depressive episode.

SUBJECTS AND METHODS

SUBJECTS

After the study was approved by the local ethics committee, 30 inpatients with major depression diagnosed in accordance with *DSM-IV*[42] (11 men and 19 women, aged 19 to 60 years [mean±SD, 39.8±12.9 years; mean age of men, 37.5±11.1 years; mean age of women, 41.1±14.0 years]) gave written informed consent and completed at least 4 weeks of antidepressant treatment. Patients were recruited from the inpatient units of the Psychiatric Hospital of Rouffach, France. Before treatment, patients were free of all drugs for a minimum of 10 days; this washout was supervised in the hospital. Patients were examined with at least 2 unstructured clinical interviews conducted by an experienced research psychiatrist (P.B., T.-S.D., or F.D.) and a structured interview (Schedule for Affective Disorders and Schizophrenia–Lifetime Version[43]) conducted by a separate psychiatrist (M.-A.C.). Moreover, a psychologist made a psychodynamic assessment of each patient by means of a series of psychometric and personality tests.[13,44] The final diagnoses were made by consensus of 2 psychiatrists and a psychologist (M.J.), who were unaware of endocrine results.

Five patients met *DSM-IV* criteria for melancholic subtype. All patients had a history of recurrent major depression (20 with and 10 without full interepisode recovery). Severity of depression was measured with the 17-item Hamilton Rating Scale for Depression (HAM-D)[45]; inclusion in the study required a baseline HAM-D score of 16 or greater (mean±SD, 28.2±5.7).

The control group consisted of 21 hospitalized normal volunteers (9 men and 12 women, aged 19 to 56 years; mean±SD, 36.14±11.1 years; mean age of men, 32.9±9.4 years; mean age of women, 38.6±12.1 years). All were free of concomitant psychiatric and medical illness. None had a personal or family history of major psychiatric illness.

Routine blood tests and physical examination excluded subjects with medical illness. All patients and control subjects had normal basal thyroid hormone values (FT_4, free T_3 [FT_3], and TSH). All subjects were within 15% of ideal body weight. Excluded were subjects with a history of thyroid or other endocrine diseases; those with alcoholism or other drug abuse; those previously treated with lithium salts, carbamazepine, long-acting neuroleptics, monoamine oxidase inhibitors, or electroconvulsive therapy; and women taking oral contraceptives.

All subjects were receiving a caffeine-restricted diet for at least 3 days before testing, and their environment was synchronized, with diurnal activity from 8 AM to 11 PM and nocturnal rest (sleep).

PROCEDURES

We measured TSH, FT_4, and FT_3 levels before and after protirelin was given at 8 AM and 11 PM, on the same day. Previous studies have shown that it is the free fraction of T_4 and T_3 that is considered to be metabolically active[46-48] and that gives direct information about thyroid gland status independent of variations in binding protein concentration.[49-51]

The first protirelin stimulation test was performed at 8 AM. Subjects were in bed, nonsmoking, and fasting from 7 PM on the previous day. An indwelling cannula was inserted at 7 AM into a forearm vein and kept open with an isotonic saline infusion. Protirelin (Protiréline Roche, Produits Roche, Neuilly sur Seine, France), 200 μg, was injected intravenously for 2 minutes at 8 AM. Blood was drawn for assay of plasma TSH, FT_4, and FT_3 15 minutes before protirelin injection (t_{-15}), immediately before injection (t_0), and 15, 30, and 60 minutes after injection (t_{15}, t_{30}, and t_{60}). The challenge was repeated at 11 PM on the same day, with the injection of an additional 200 μg of protirelin intravenously and the same sampling intervals. Subjects were awake before and during the evening sampling and kept without food from 6 PM.

After 1 month of inpatient antidepressant treatment, the same neuroendocrine tests were repeated in all patients.

RESULTS

COMPARISON BETWEEN CONTROL SUBJECTS AND MEDICATION-FREE PATIENTS

Control subjects and untreated patients were comparable for age and sex (**Table 1**). Confirming our previous studies,[28,38] ΔmaxTSH and FT_{4B} values were higher in the evening than in the morning in both control subjects and patients (all $P<.01$ by *t* test). Compared with control subjects, patients demonstrated, both at 8 AM and at 11 PM, significantly higher FT_{4B} and lower TSH_B and ΔmaxTSH values. Moreover, ΔΔmaxTSH values were significantly lower in patients than in control subjects.

In the whole sample, in the control group, and in the depressed group, the effect of age was not significant for the thyroid function tests (TSH_B, ΔmaxTSH, ΔΔmaxTSH, FT_{4B}, and FT_{3B}). This agrees with most studies in depressed patients, which have found that age is not a significant factor in determining blunted response to the protirelin test.[57,58]

Some studies suggest that estrogens can modify hy-

ASSAYS

Blood samples were immediately centrifuged at 3000 rpm and 4°C; serum samples were then stored at −20°C until assay. All hormone concentrations were determined by immunoassay techniques based on enhanced luminescence. Average intra-assay and interassay coefficients of variation were as follows: TSH: 5.1% to 7%; sensitivity, less than 0.04 mU/L (Amerlite TSH-60 Assay, Amersham International plc, Amersham, England); FT_4: 5.1% to 5.3%; sensitivity, 0.5 pmol/L (Amerlite FT_4 Assay, same supplier); and FT_3: 6.0% to 8.0%; sensitivity, less than 0.5 pmol/L (Amerlite FT_3 Assay, same supplier).

ANTIDEPRESSANT TREATMENT

To optimize antidepressant treatment response,[52,53] choice of medication and dosage were determined on a clinical basis (ie, type of depression, history of the disorder, side effect profiles, and, where applicable, previous treatment response and adverse effects [available for 23 patients]).

Three different types of antidepressants were used: (1) the tertiary amine tricyclic antidepressant amitriptyline hydrochloride in 13 patients (daily dose, 204±32 mg; range, 150-300 mg); (2) the selective serotonin reuptake inhibitor fluoxetine hydrochloride in 9 patients (daily dose, 44±9 mg; range, 20-60 mg); and (3) the reversible monoamine oxidase inhibitor–A toloxatone in 8 patients, who all received 1200 mg daily. Antidepressants were given under supervision on the ward, at doses known to be effective.[52] Changes in dose were made according to clinical response, tolerability, and—for amitriptyline only—plasma concentrations (since fluoxetine demonstrated no plasma concentration–response relationships[53]; no data were available for toloxatone). Patients remained hospitalized throughout the duration of the study. Psychotropic drugs other than the study medication were, if possible, avoided. Trimeprazine tartrate (maximum dose, 30 mg orally) was allowed in case of severe sleep disturbance.

CLINICAL RESPONSE

We followed the method of Frank et al[54] in defining response in terms of absolute rather than relative HAM-D scores: response was defined as a final HAM-D score less than 8, nonresponse as a final score greater than 16, and a partial response as a final score between these limits. Raters were always unaware of neuroendocrine results and the medication used.

STATISTICAL ANALYSIS

Baseline TSH (TSH_B), FT_4 (FT_{4B}), and FT_3 (FT_{3B}) values were defined as the mean of the 2 samples before protirelin injection (t_{-15} and t_0). The ΔmaxTSH was defined as the maximum increment above the baseline value after protirelin injection. Since the stimulation of thyroid hormones after protirelin is maximal after the third hour for T_3 and between the fourth and sixth hours for T_4,[55,56] our procedure seems too short (60 minutes) to determine maximum thyroid hormone responses. Therefore, we do not consider 60-minute FT_4 and FT_3 values here (data available on request).

Despite logarithmic or other transformations, the distribution of some data remained nonnormal (Kolmogorov-Smirnov 1-sample test for goodness of fit), and it was necessary to use nonparametric statistical methods. Differences between controls and untreated (drug-free) patients were tested for significance with the Mann-Whitney 2-tailed test (*U* test). Between-group differences after treatment were tested by analysis of variance (Kruskal-Wallis *H* test) and, where the overall effect was significant, by *U* tests, by means of Bonferroni's adjustment for 3 pairwise comparisons. Within-subject differences were evaluated with the Wilcoxon 2-tailed signed-rank test (*t* test). Correlations between quantitative variables were estimated by the Spearman rank coefficient (ρ). Categorical data were analyzed with the Fisher exact test. The level of statistical significance was set at $P=.05$.

pothalamic-pituitary-thyroid axis function by increasing total thyronine levels[59] and TSH response to protirelin.[56,60] Interestingly, the levels of T_3, T_4, and TSH appear relatively constant during the normal menstrual cycle.[59] In our study, the proportion of women in the control group (57%) was comparable with that in the patient group (63%). In the control subjects, but not in depressed patients, women had greater 8 AM and 11 PM ΔmaxTSH than men did ($P<.03$ and $P<.02$, respectively, by *U* test). The ΔΔmaxTSH, TSH_B, FT_{4B}, and FT_{3B} values were not significantly different between men and women, whether they were control subjects or patients. When depressed patients were compared with control subjects of the same sex, 8 AM FT_{4B}, 11 PM FT_{4B}, 8 AM ΔmaxTSH, 11 PM ΔmaxTSH, and ΔΔmaxTSH remained significantly lower in male and female depressed patients (all $P<.05$ by *U* test). Moreover, female depressed patients had lower 8 AM and 11 PM TSH_B levels (all $P<.01$ by *U* test) than female control subjects did.

Receiver operating characteristic (ROC) analysis[61] was used to determine the optimal definition of abnormal TSH response to protirelin, with the following results: (1) 8 AM ΔmaxTSH less than 3.5 mU/L; sensitivity, 37%; specificity, 95%; (2) 11 PM ΔmaxTSH less than 6 mU/L; sensitivity, 57%; specificity, 100%; and (3) ΔΔmaxTSH less than 2.5 mU/L; sensitivity, 87%; specificity, 95%.

EFFECTS OF 1 MONTH OF ANTIDEPRESSANT TREATMENT

After 1 month's treatment, 37% (n=11) of the patients were classified as responders (full recovery), 20% (n=6) as partial responders, and 43% (n=13) as nonresponders (**Table 2**).

Analyses of TSH responses to protirelin after antidepressant treatment (**Figure**) showed that, after treatment, responders had significantly higher responses (8 AM ΔmaxTSH, 11 PM ΔmaxTSH, and ΔΔmaxTSH) than nonresponders. In addition, partial responders had lower posttreatment 11 PM ΔmaxTSH and ΔΔmaxTSH values than did responders. No differences for other thyroid hormone measures were observed across groups after treatment.

Table 1. Demographic Characteristics and Biological Data on Untreated Patients and Normal Controls*

	Control Subjects (n=21)	Depressed Patients (n=30)	*P*
Age, y	36.1±11.1	39.8±12.9	.32
Sex, No. M/F	9/12	11/19	.76
8 AM TSH_B, mU/L	1.27±0.79	0.80±0.48	.03
8 AM ΔmaxTSH, mU/L	7.59±3.52	4.64±2.50	.002
11 PM TSH_B, mU/L	1.02±0.37	0.84±0.92	.006
11 PM ΔmaxTSH, mU/L	11.41±4.44	6.43±3.66	<.001
ΔΔmaxTSH, mU/L	3.84±1.40	1.66±1.67	<.001
8 AM FT_{4B}, pmol/L (ng/dL)	14.6±2.9 (1.1±0.23)	17.8±3.4 (1.4±0.26)	.001
11 PM FT_{4B}, pmol/L (ng/dL)	15.7±3.1 (1.2±0.24)	19.1±3.7 (1.5±0.29)	.001
8 AM FT_{3B}, pmol/L	5.3±1.0	5.6±0.9	.18
11 PM FT_{3B}, pmol/L	5.5±0.9	5.9±1.6	.25

**Values are mean±SD. Analysis was by Mann-Whitney 2-tailed U test, except for sex (analysis by Fisher exact test). TSH_B indicates basal thyrotropin concentration, ΔmaxTSH, peak concentration minus basal thyrotropin concentration; ΔΔmaxTSH, 11 PM minus 8 AM ΔmaxTSH; FT_{4B}, basal free thyroxine concentration; and FT_{3B}, basal free triiodothyronine concentration.*

Full response to antidepressant treatment was associated with significant increments in 11 PM ΔmaxTSH and ΔΔmaxTSH values and significant decrements in 8 AM FT_{4B}, 11 PM FT_{4B}, and 8 AM FT_{3B} values. No such associations were observed in partial responders and nonresponders.

The differences among the 3 groups could not be explained by age, sex distribution, basal HAM-D scores, age at onset of the illness, number of previous episodes, type of depression (ie, with or without melancholic features), or clinical course (ie, with or without full interepisode recovery). However, pretreatment 11 PM TSH values (basal and after protirelin stimulation) were lower in nonresponders than responders.

PROTIRELIN TEST NORMALIZATION AND CLINICAL OUTCOME

The rate of normalization of the protirelin tests after treatment was low (5 of 11 patients for the 8 AM protirelin test and 6 of 17 patients for the 11 PM test) and was not significantly associated with antidepressant response—even though all 3 responders who had pretreatment blunted tests, both at 8 AM and 11 PM, showed normalization of the test.

Among the 26 patients with an initial reduced ΔΔmaxTSH value, 8 showed normalization of the test during treatment. All 8 were treatment responders. Among the 18 patients who did not have a normalized ΔΔmaxTSH test, 6 were partial responders and 12 were nonresponders. Thus, ΔΔmaxTSH normalization was significantly associated with good clinical response to antidepressant treatment ($P<.001$ by Fisher exact test).

RELATIONSHIPS AMONG THYROID AXIS MEASUREMENT CHANGES DURING TREATMENT

There was a significant positive correlation between the increase of ΔΔmaxTSH level (difference between pretreatment and posttreatment ΔΔmaxTSH values) and that of 11 PM ΔmaxTSH ($\rho=0.63$, n=30, $P=.001$). Increase of 11 PM ΔmaxTSH value during treatment was associated with decrease of FT_{4B} value ($\rho=-0.52$, n=30, $P=.01$). There was a positive relationship between decrease of the HAM-D score and decrease of FT_{3B} value (at 8 AM, $\rho=0.43$, n=30, $P=.02$; at 11 PM, $\rho=0.41$, n=30, $P<.03$).

EFFECTS OF THE DIFFERENT ANTIDEPRESSANT DRUGS

The clinical efficacy of the 3 antidepressant drugs was comparable. There were no significant differences in pretreatment or posttreatment measures across the patient groups defined by drug taken. Moreover, no statistically significant changes in results of thyroid function tests were induced by the drugs.

COMMENT

The 3 principal findings of this study are as follows: (1) a chronobiological dysregulation of the hypothalamic-pituitary-thyroid axis occurs in a high proportion of drug-free depressed inpatients; (2) significant changes in thyroid function test results are associated with clinical recovery rather than attributable to a direct effect of the antidepressant drug—for chronobiological reasons, these changes are more obvious in the evening than in the morning; and (3) patients with the lowest pretreatment evening basal and protirelin-stimulated TSH levels have the lowest rate of response to antidepressant treatment.

The different indexes of thyroid axis function that are reported in this study are known to be interrelated. For example, there is a high correlation between protirelin-induced TSH response and basal TSH levels.[38,62] But as can be seen from Tables 1 and 2, the protirelin stimulation test is a more powerful clinical tool than a simple measurement of basal TSH. Moreover, these data show that the 11 PM protirelin test is more powerful than the 8 AM protirelin test, and that the difference in TSH response between these tests is an even more powerful measure. This applies both to distinguishing controls from depressed patients and to distinguishing treatment responders from nonresponders.

This study confirms that protirelin stimulation in the evening produces greater ΔmaxTSH differences between

Table 2. Demographic Characteristics and Biological Data of Depressed Groups Defined by Antidepressant Treatment Response*

	Responder Patients (n=11)	Partial Responder Patients (n=6)	Nonresponder Patients (n=13)
Age, y	38.4±14.1	40.7±11.7	40.5±13.4
Sex, No. M/F	3/8	4/2	4/9
Age at onset, y	31.4±12.4	35.7±11.3	32.3±12.9
No. of previous episodes	2.4±1.0	2.7±1.2	4.0±3.3
HAM-D scores			
Day 0 (range)	28.6±5.5 (19-35)	28.2±6.0 (20-35)	27.8±6.2 (20-37)
Day 28 (range)	6.1±1.5† (3-7)	11.7±1.5‡,§ (10-14)	22.5±5.5‡,§ (20-37)
Δ Scores from baseline	22.5±5.6	16.5±6.1	5.2±6.0‡
% Change in scores from baseline	77.7±9.4	56.9±10.5‖	17.1±18.2‡
Antidepressant drugs, No. AMI/FLU/TOL	5/4/2	4/0/2	4/5/4
8 AM TSH_B, mU/L			
Day 0	1.02±0.54	0.80±0.61	0.62±0.25
Day 28	1.05±0.59	0.68±0.12	0.68±0.32
8 AM ΔmaxTSH, mU/L			
Day 0	5.71±2.79	4.76±2.54	3.68±1.98
Day 28	7.75±3.86	5.12±2.41	4.4±2.30¶
11 PM TSH_B, mU/L			
Day 0	1.28±1.37	0.70±0.48	0.53±0.35¶
Day 28	1.25±0.88	0.86±0.42	0.67±0.49
11 PM ΔmaxTSH, mU/L			
Day 0	8.69±4.21	5.72±3.22	4.85±2.34¶
Day 28	12.19±4.82§	6.00±2.29‖	5.64±2.66‖
ΔΔmaxTSH, mU/L			
Day 0	2.61±2.22	0.96±0.95	1.17±0.97
Day 28	4.20±1.9§	0.87±1.57¶	1.24±1.20‖
8 AM FT_{4B}, pmol/L (ng/dL)			
Day 0	18.9±3.6 (1.5±0.28)	17.5±3.7 (1.4±0.29)	17.1±3.1 (1.3±0.24)
Day 28	14.3±3.6§ (1.1±0.28)	15.9±3.3 (1.2±0.26)	15.4±1.6 (1.2±0.12)
11 PM FT_{4B}, pmol/L (ng/dL)			
Day 0	19.6±3.8 (1.5±0.30)	18.2±3.7 (1.4±0.29)	19.0±4.0 (1.5±0.31)
Day 28	16.0±3.9§ (1.2±0.30)	16.3±2.1 (1.3±0.16)	16.7±2.7 (1.3±0.21)
8 AM FT_{3B}, pmol/L			
Day 0	5.5±0.9	5.9±0.8	5.5±0.9
Day 28	4.8±0.4§	5.5±0.9	5.8±1.1
11 PM FT_{3B}, pmol/L			
Day 0	5.8±1.2	5.8±0.5	6.0±2.2
Day 28	5.1±0.5	5.4±0.4	5.8±0.9

Values are mean±SD. HAM-D indicates Hamilton Rating Scale for Depression; AMI, amitriptyline hydrochloride; FLU, fluoxetine hydrochloride; TOL, toloxatone; TSH_B, basal thyrotropin concentration; ΔmaxTSH, peak concentration minus basal thyrotropin concentration; ΔΔmaxTSH, 11 PM minus 8 AM ΔmaxTSH; FT_{4B}, basal free thyroxine; and FT_{3B}, basal free triiodothyronine.

†$P<.01$ by Wilcoxin 2-tailed signed rank t test, for the difference between values before and after 4 weeks treatment.

‡$P<.001$ by Mann-Whitney 2-tailed U test, adjusted with Bonferroni's method for multiple comparisons, for the difference between partial or nonresponder and responder patients.

§$P<.05$.

‖$P<.01$.

¶$P<.05$.

depressed inpatients and hospitalized control subjects than stimulation in the morning and thus confirms the potential clinical value of the ΔΔmaxTSH test. As previously discussed,[28,38] the ΔΔmaxTSH test, which reflects the normal evening increase in pituitary responsiveness to protirelin, seems to be a chronobiological refinement of the protirelin test. Chronobiological thyroid axis abnormality is also demonstrated by loss of the nocturnal TSH rise in euthyroid drug-free depressed patients.[32,34,63-65]

Low ΔΔmaxTSH values may reflect a down-regulation of pituitary thyrotropin-releasing hormone receptors, possibly because of prolonged hypersecretion of thyrotropin-releasing hormone[27,66]; owing to circadian changes in the sensitivity of target biosystems[67,68] this down-regulation can be more easily demonstrated in the evening. However, the cause of the increased drive in hypothalamic thyrotropin-releasing hormone neurons remains unknown. Moreover, ΔΔmaxTSH takes into account the dynamic and chronobiological characteristics of the negative feedback of thyroid hormones on TSH secretion, since the morning test stimulates secretion of thyroid hormones that may increase the negative feedback in the evening in depressed patients. Indeed, it has been demonstrated that a weak increase in thyroid hormone levels, well within the physiological range, could contribute to the lower protirelin-induced TSH response in depression.[69-71] Therefore, if the negative feedback mechanism is operating in depression—as suggested by some reports,[38,62,72,73] but not all[74]—the increase of basal levels of thyroid hormones, found also in the present study, could be a significant factor in the blunting of TSH response to

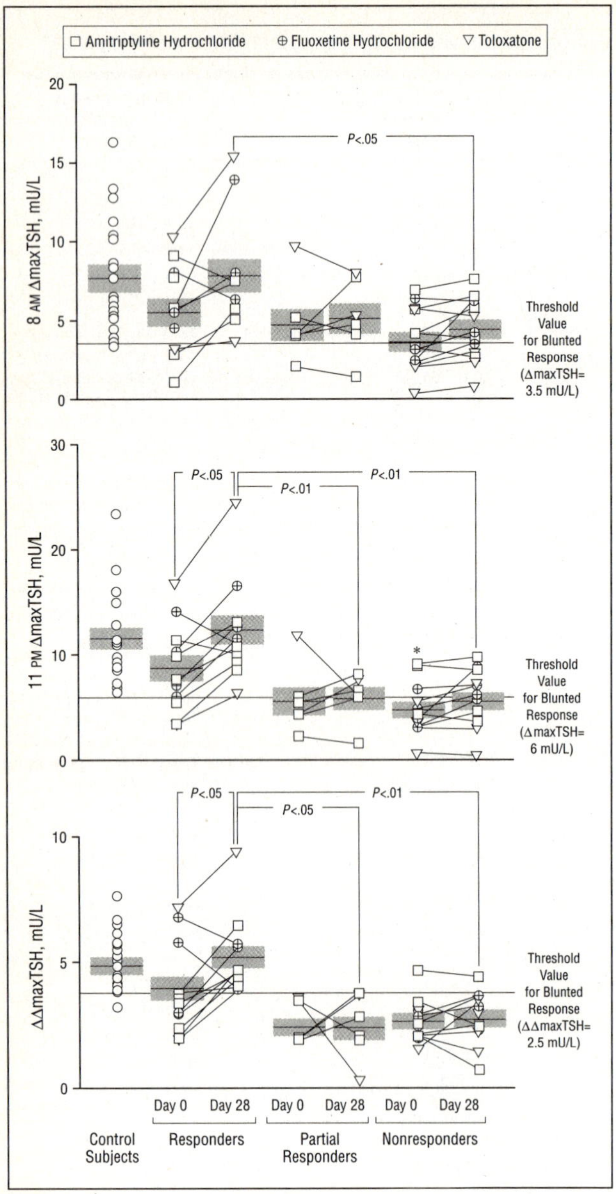

Evolution before and after 1 month of antidepressant treatment of the maximum increment in plasma thyrotropin level above baseline (ΔmaxTSH) after 200 μg of protirelin at 8 AM and 11 PM, and difference between 11 PM and 8 AM ΔmaxTSH (ΔΔmaxTSH) in depressed patients. The ΔmaxTSH and ΔΔmaxTSH values are plotted individually. The solid horizontal lines indicate the group mean; the shaded areas represent ±SEM. Asterisk indicates P<.05 *by Mann-Whitney 2-tailed* U *test adjusted with Bonferroni's method for multiple comparisons, for the difference between nonresponder and responder patients.*

protirelin. Evidence suggests that the increased level of thyroid hormones is not secondary to overproduction of hypophysial TSH. A possible noradrenergic hyperactivity has been evoked by some investigators,[73,75] but other factors, such as sleep disturbance,[40] sleep deprivation,[76,77] or stress,[40,78,79] could contribute to the thyroid hormone increase. Furthermore, increased thyrotropin-releasing hormone secretion could directly increase thyroid hormone release.[80] In this way, the increase in thyroid hormone level could represent a compensatory response to reduce thyrotropin-releasing hormone hypersecretion.

Normalization of ΔΔmaxTSH values after antidepressant treatment was observed in all the responders. In contrast, partial responders and nonresponders showed virtually the same rate of reduced ΔΔmaxTSH values as before treatment. Given the low rate of blunted responses to 8 AM and 11 PM protirelin tests, we failed to find a significant association between normalization of these tests and clinical recovery. However, unlike partial responders and nonresponders, responders exhibited an increase in 11 PM ΔmaxTSH values; a similar tendency at 8 AM was not statistically significant. It should be noted that normalization of ΔΔmaxTSH is not necessarily associated with changes in baseline TSH values. Results obtained from the morning thyroid function tests are consistent with previous reports.[2,4,16,81]

Interestingly, we confirmed the findings of other groups[7,10,82] that antidepressant treatment significantly reduces FT_4 levels in responders; this decrement is not significant in partial responders and nonresponders. Moreover, the decrease in FT_4 correlates with the increase in 11 PM ΔmaxTSH—which is the major determinant of the ΔΔmaxTSH test. Posttreatment plasma FT_3 levels, which correlated with FT_4, showed a decrease in responders only, albeit not significant at 11 PM. The fall in FT_3 appears to be associated with the reduction of depressive symptoms as evaluated by the HAM-D score. This agrees with some[7,83,84] but not all[6,10,25,41] previous studies and may reflect either a chance finding or a weak association.

Joffe and Singer[10] have suggested that the effects of antidepressants include reduced exposure of central neurons to thyroid hormone. Recently, Baumgartner[21] reported that, in rats, desipramine and fluoxetine could enhance tissue uptake of T_4 and type II iodothyronine 5′deiodinase activity, leading to an increase in T_3 tissue concentration. Although we found a small decrease in FT_4 and FT_3 levels after treatment with amitriptyline, fluoxetine, or toloxatone, none of these drugs induced a significant change in peripheral thyroid hormone levels. In this respect, our results are consistent with those of previous studies in humans.[11,14]

In addition, we found that neither basal morning and evening TSH levels (basal and after protirelin stimulation) nor ΔΔmaxTSH values were significantly changed by 4 weeks of treatment with amitriptyline, fluoxetine, or toloxatone. These findings, in conjunction with those of other investigators,[16,19,23,24,85,86] do not support an intrinsic and direct activity of these compounds on thyrotropin-releasing hormone neurons and/or TSH pituitary cells. Furthermore, we failed to confirm differences in the effects of tricyclic antidepressants vs selective serotonin reuptake inhibitors on the thyroid axis.[87] Thus, our findings suggest that the decrease in thyroid function is related to clinical recovery rather than to a pharmacological effect of antidepressants.

The relationship between pretreatment blunted TSH response to morning protirelin injection and subsequent response to antidepressant treatment has been studied, with conflicting results.[4,84,85,87-90] The present study shows that responders have higher evening basal and protirelin-stimulated TSH levels than nonresponders do. This result is consistent with the observation of Loosen[12] that nocturnal TSH concentrations during sleep deprivation are higher in responders than nonresponders. One may therefore hypothesize that patients with the most severely disturbed TSH secretion (basal and after protirelin stimulation) have the worst response to antidepressants and consequently need a different therapeutic strategy. In such cases, adjunctive therapy with thyroid hormones[26,39] might be particularly beneficial to amplify antidepressant effects, since, by increasing the negative feedback on the hypothalamus, thyroid hormones may decrease thyrotropin-releasing hormone overproduction at this level.

Several methodological issues must be considered. First, our 4-week period of investigation may appear short in the evaluation of antidepressant response. Indeed, the response rate might have been increased by a longer duration of the study: 6 weeks is recommended before evaluating antidepressant response.[91] However, it is generally accepted[53] that 1 month of medication is sufficient to show some treatment effect.

Second, although the raters were unaware of the medication used as well as the neuroendocrine results, antidepressant treatment was given in an open-label manner. There is general agreement that no one antidepressant is clearly more effective than another.[52] However, to optimize the response to treatment, we used 3 different classes of compounds by taking into account primarily the specific side effects of each drug, and, when available, previous antidepressant response; most patients (77%) had already been treated with antidepressants—with inconsistent results—at the time of their admission to the hospital. We did not use placebo as a comparative treatment, since the aim of the study was not to demonstrate antidepressant efficacy of the compounds.

Third, because of the modest sample size, it was not possible to analyze statistically the endocrine effects of each drug in relation to its clinical efficacy. For the same reason, failure to find a statistically significant difference must be interpreted with caution, since the power of the study may have been too low to detect such a difference.

In conclusion, the ΔΔmaxTSH test is an improved measure of changes in hypothalamic-pituitary-thyroid axis activity and may be used as a state-related marker of clinical change in hospitalized depressed patients. However, the mechanisms by which ΔΔmax TSH is influenced by antidepressant treatment remain to be elucidated. Further investigations with different classes of antidepressants are suggested.

Accepted for publication May 2, 1996.

Presented in part at the 148th Annual Meeting of the American Psychiatric Association—New Research Program, Miami, Fla, May 23, 1995.

We express our gratitude to Gabrielle Wagner in providing the test kits for hormonal determinations and the support of the physicians and the nurses of Sector VIII, Centre Hospitalier, Rouffach, France.

Corresponding author: Fabrice Duval, MD, Centre Hospitalier, 27 rue du 4ème Spahis Marocain, 68250 Rouffach, France.

REFERENCES

1. Whybrow PC, Coppen A, Prange AJ, Noguerra R, Bailey JE. Thyroid function and the response to lithothyronine in depression. *Arch Gen Psychiatry.* 1972; 26:242-245.
2. Kirkegaard C, Norlem N, Lauridsen UB, Bjørum N, Christiansen C. Protirelin stimulation test and thyroid function during treatment of depression. *Arch Gen Psychiatry.* 1975;32:1115-1118.
3. Kirkegaard C, Bjørum N. TSH response to TRH in endogenous depression. *Lancet.* 1980;8:501-503.
4. Krog-Meyer I, Kirkegaard C, Kijine B, Lumholtz B, Smith E, Lykke Olesen L, Bjørum N. Prediction of relapse with the TRH test and prophylactic amitriptyline in 39 patients with endogenous depression. *Am J Psychiatry.* 1984;141: 945-948.
5. Joffe RT, Roy Byrne PP, Udhe TW, Post RM. Thyroid function and affective illness: a reappraisal. *Biol Psychiatry.* 1984;19:1685-1691.
6. Unden F, Ljuggren JG, Kjellman BF, Beck-Friis J, Wetterberg L. Twenty four-hour serum levels of T_4 and T_3 in relation to decreased TSH serum levels and decreased TSH response to TRH in affective disorders. *Acta Psychiatr Scand.* 1986;73:358-365.
7. Baumgartner A, Gräf KJ, Kürten I, Meinhold H. The hypothalamic-pituitary-thyroid axis in psychiatric patients and healthy subjects, part II: repeated measurements of thyroxine, free thyroxine, triiodothyronine, free triiodothyronine, and reverse triiodothyronine in patients with major depressive disorders and schizophrenia and healthy subjects. *Psychiatry Res.* 1988;24:283-305.
8. Carroll BJ. The dexamethasone suppression test. *Br J Psychiatry.* 1982;140: 292-304.
9. Winokur A, Amsterdam JD, Berwish N, Phillips JL, Maislin G. The relationship between the change in thyrotropin response to TRH and therapeutic response to desipramine in depressed patients. *Biol Psychiatry.* 1989;25:207A. Abstract.
10. Joffe RT, Singer W. Effect of tricyclic antidepressants on thyroid hormone levels in depressed patients. *Pharmacopsychiatry.* 1990;23:67-69.
11. Stein MB, Uhde TW. Thyrotropin and prolactin responses to protirelin (TRH) prior to and during chronic imipramine treatment in patients with panic disorder. *Psychoneuroendocrinology.* 1990;15:381-389.
12. Loosen PT. The thyroid state of depressed patients. *Clin Neuropharmacology.* 1992;15:382A-383A.
13. Duval F, Mokrani MC, Jautz M, Crocq MA, de Andrade E, de Andrade A, Diep TS, Macher JP. Profils biologico-cliniques prédictifs de réponses aux antidépresseurs dans les dépressions majeures. *Psychol Med.* 1993;25:1311-1317.
14. Leichter SB, Kirstein L, Martin ND. Thyroid function and growth hormone secretion in amitriptyline treated depression. *Am J Psychiatry.* 1977;134:1270-1272.
15. Gregoire F, Brauman H, de Bruck R, Corvilain J. Hormone release in depressed patients before and after recovery. *Psychoneuroendocrinology.* 1977; 2:303-312.
16. Langer G, Schoenbeck G, König G. Evidence for neuroendocrine involvement in the therapeutic effects of antidepressant drugs. In: Brambilla F, Racagni G, de Wied D, eds. *Progress in Psychoneuroendocrinology.* New York, NY: Elsevier North Holland Biochemical Press; 1980:197-208.
17. Linnoila M, Gold P, Potter WZ, Wehr TA. Tricyclic antidepressants do not alter the thyroid hormone levels in patients suffering from major affective disorder. *Psychiatry Res.* 1981;4:357-360.
18. Brambilla F, Scarone S, Massironi R, Nobile P, Pugnetti L. Abnormal anterior pituitary responsiveness to hypothalamic hormones in primary affective disorder. *Neuropsychobiology.* 1982;8:269-275.
19. Rosenbaum JF, Fava M, Pava JA, McCarthy MK, Steingard RJ, Bouffides E. Anger attacks in unipolar depression, part 2: neuroendocrine correlates and changes following fluoxetine treatment. *Am J Psychiatry.* 1993;150:1164-1168.
20. Atterwill CK, Catto LC, Heal DJ, Holland CW, Dickens TA, Jones CA. The effects of desipramine (DMI) and electroconvulsive shock (ECS) on the function of the hypothalamo-pituitary-thyroid axis in the rat. *Psychoneuroendocrinology.* 1989;40:339-346.
21. Baumgartner A. The influence of antidepressants (desipramine, fluoxetine), prophylactic drugs (lithium, carbamazepine), and sleep deprivation on thyroid hormone metabolism in rat brain. *Neuropsychopharmacology.* 1994;10:494S. Abstract.
22. Laakmann G, Binz A, Voderholzer U, Daffner C, Müller OA, Neuhauser H, Neulinger E, Wittman M. The influence of psychotropic drugs and releasing hormones on anterior pituitary hormone secretion in healthy subjects and depressed patients. *Pharmacopsychiatry.* 1990;23:18-26.
23. Laakman G. Neuroendocrinological findings in affective disorders after administration of antidepressants. *Adv Biol Psychiatry.* 1980;5:67-84.
24. Hughes D. Clomipramine (Anafranil) and prolactin secretion. *J Int Med Res.* 1973;1:317-320.
25. Joffe RT, Singer W. Effect of phenelzine on thyroid function in depressed patients. *Biol Psychiatry.* 1987;22:1033-1034.
26. Joffe RT, Levitt AJ. The thyroid and depression. In: Joffe RT, Levitt AJ, eds. *The Thyroid Axis and Psychiatric Illness.* Washington, DC: American Psychiatric Press; 1993:195-253.
27. Loosen PT, Prange AJ. Serum thyrotropin response to thyrotropin-releasing hormone in psychiatric patients: a review. *Am J Psychiatry.* 1982;139:405-416.
28. Duval F, Macher JP, Mokrani MC. Difference between evening and morning thyrotropin response to protirelin in major depressive episode. *Arch Gen Psychiatry.* 1990;47:443-448.
29. Vanhaelst L, Van Cauter E, Degaute S, Goldstein J. Circadian variations of serum thyrotropin in man. *J Clin Endocrinol Metab.* 1972;35:479-482.
30. Patel YC, Alford FP, Burger HG. The 24-hour plasma thyrotropin profile. *Clin Sci.* 1972;43:71-77.

31. Weeke A. The 24-hour pattern of serum TSH in patients with endogenous depression. *Acta Psychiatr Scand.* 1980;62:69-74.
32. Kjellman BF, Beck-Friis J, Ljunggren JG, Wetterberg L. Twenty-four serum levels of TSH in affective disorders. *Acta Psychiatr Scand.* 1984;69:491-502.
33. Hugues JN, Reinberg A, Lagoguey M, Modigliani E, Sebaoun J. Les rythmes biologiques de la sécrétion thyréotrope. *Ann Med Interne.* 1983;134:84-94.
34. Souêtre E, Salvati E, Wehr TA, Sack DA, Krebs B, Darcourt G. Twenty-four hour profile of body temperature and plasma TSH in bipolar patients during depression and during remission and in normal controls subjects. *Am J Psychiatry.* 1988;139:282-286.
35. Goichot B, Brandenberger G, Saini J, Wittersheim G, Follenius M. Nyctohemeral patterns of thyroid hormones and their relationship with thyrotropin variations and sleep structure. *J Endocrinol Invest.* 1994;17:181-187.
36. Pérez Lopez FR, Legido A, Abos MD, Lafraga L. Human pituitary chronoendocrinology: repetitive stimulation with LRH/TRH at different times of the day. *Acta Endocrinol.* 1983;102:327-331.
37. Duval F, Mokrani MC, Crocq MA, Rosenberg S, Oliveira Castro J, Valdivieso S, Macher JP. Circadian variations in response to protirelin test in major depresssive episode. *Eur Psychiatry.* 1991;6:79-88.
38. Duval F, Mokrani MC, Crocq MA, Bailey P, Macher JP. Influence of thyroid hormones on morning and evening TSH response to TRH in major depression. *Biol Psychiatry.* 1994;35:926-934.
39. Whybrow PC, Bauer MS. Effects of peripheral thyroid hormones on the central nervous system: relevance to disorders of mood. *Curr Topics Neuroendocrinol.* 1988;8:309-327.
40. Calloway SP, Dolan RJ, Fonagy P, De Souza VF, Wakeling A. Endocrine changes and clinical profiles in depression, II: the thyrotropin-releasing hormone test. *Psychol Med.* 1984;14:759-765.
41. Kirkegaard C, Faber J. Influence of free thyroid hormone levels on the TSH response to TRH in endogenous depression. *Psychoneuroendocrinology.* 1986; 11:491-497.
42. American Psychiatric Association, Committee on Nomenclature and Statistics. *Diagnostic and Statistical Manual of Mental Disorders, Fourth Edition.* Washington, DC: American Psychiatric Association; 1994.
43. Spitzer RL, Endicott J. *Schedule for Affective Disorders and Schizophrenia, Lifetime Version.* New York, NY: Biometrics Research Division, New York State Psychiatric Institute; 1975.
44. Macher JP, Duval F, Crocq MA, Hassler C, Rebourg C, Fleig C, Gindein J, Fleick F. Premiers résultats d'un protocole d'exploration biologico-clinique. *Actual Psychiatr.* 1985;5:67-82.
45. Hamilton MA. A rating scale for depression. *J Neurol Neurosurg Psychiatry.* 1960;23:56-62.
46. Ingbar SH. The thyroid gland. In: Wilson JD, Foster DW, eds. *Williams Textbook of Endocrinology.* Philadelphia, Pa: WB Saunders Co; 1985:682-815.
47. Ekins RP. Methods for measurements of free thyroid hormones. In: Ekins R, Faglia G, Pennisi F, Pinchera A, eds. *Proceedings of the International Symposium on Free Thyroid Hormones, Venice.* Amsterdam, the Netherlands: Excerpta Medica; 1978:72-92.
48. Prange AJ. Markers of hypothalamic-pituitary-thyroid axis dysfunction in depression. In: Racagni G, Brunello N, Fukuda TF, eds. *Biological Psychiatry.* Amsterdam, the Netherlands: Elsevier Science Publishers; 1991;1:84-86.
49. Cahayon P, Castanas E, Guibout M, Codaccioni JL. Assessment and clinical significance of free thyroid hormone radioimmunoassays. In: Ekins R, Faglia G, Pennisi F, Pinchera A, eds. *Proceedings of the International Symposium on Free Thyroid Hormones, Venice.* Amsterdam, the Netherlands: Excerpta Medica; 1978:161-202.
50. Bayer MF, McDougall IR. Radioimmunoassay of free thyroxine in serum, comparison with clinical findings and results of conventional thyroid function tests. *Clin Chem.* 1980;26:1186-1189.
51. Schlienger JL, Sapin R, Demangeat C. La thyroxine libre. *Concours Med.* 1983; 105:5241-5252.
52. Depression Guideline Panel. *Depression in Primary Care, Volume 2: Treatment of Major Depression.* Rockville, Md: US Dept of Health and Human Services, Public Health Service, Agency for Health Care Policy and Research; 1993:35-71. Clinical Practice Guideline Number 5.
53. Burke MJ, Preskorn SH. Short term treatment of mood disorders with standard antidepressants. In: Bloom FE, Kupfer DJ, eds. *Psychopharmacology: The Fourth Generation of Progress.* New York, NY: Raven Press; 1995:1053-1065.
54. Frank E, Prien RF, Jarrett RB, Keller MB, Kupfer DJ, Lavori PW, Rush J, Weissman MM. Conceptualization and rationale for consensus definitions of terms in major depressive disorder. *Arch Gen Psychiatry.* 1991;48:851-855.
55. Weeke J. The response of thyrotropin and triiodothyronine to various doses of thyrotropin releasing hormone in normal man. *Eur J Clin Invest.* 1975;5: 447-453.
56. Burger HG, Patel YC. TSH and TRH: their physiological regulation and the clinical application of TRH. In: Martini L, Besser GM, eds. *Clinical Neuroendocrinology.* New York, NY: Academic Press; 1977:67-131.
57. Gold MS, Pottash AL, Ryan N, Sweeney DR, Davies RK, Martin D. TRH-induced TSH response in unipolar, bipolar, and secondary depression: possible utility in clinical assessment and differential diagnosis. *Psychoneuroendocrinology.* 1980; 5:147-155.
58. Calloway SP, Dolan RJ, Fonagy P, De Souza VF, Wakeling A. Endocrine changes and clinical profiles in depression, II: the thyrotropin-releasing hormone test. *Psychol Med.* 1984;14:759-765.
59. Leibenluft E, Fiero PL, Rubinow DR. Effects of the menstrual cycle on dependent variables in mood disorder research. *Arch Gen Psychiatry.* 1994;51:761-781.
60. Donda A, Reymond F, Rey F, Lemarchand-Beraud T. Sex steroids modulate the pituitary parameters involved in the regulation of TSH secretion in the rat. *Acta Endocrinol.* 1992;122:577-584.
61. Metz CE. Basic principles of ROC analysis. *Semin Nucl Med.* 1978;8:283-298.
62. Maes M, Schotte C, Vandewoude M, Martin M, Blockx P. TSH responses to TRH as a function of basal serum TSH: relevance for unipolar depression in females—a multivariate study. *Pharmacopsychiatry.* 1992;25:136-144.
63. Prange AJ, Garbutt JC, Loosen PT. The hypothalamic-pituitary-thyroid axis in affective disorders. In: Meltzer HY, ed. *Psychopharmacology: The Third Generation of Progress.* New York, NY: Raven Press; 1987:629-636.
64. Weeke A, Weeke J. Disturbed circadian variation of serum thyrotropin in patients with endogenous depression. *Acta Psychiatr Scand.* 1978;57:281-289.
65. Sack DA, James SP, Rosenthal NE, Wehr TA. Deficient nocturnal surge of TSH secretion during sleep deprivation in rapid-cycling bipolar illness. *Psychiatry Res.* 1988;23:179-191.
66. Garbutt JC, Mayo JP, Little KY, Gillette GM, Mason GA, Dew B, Prange AJ. Dose-response studies with protirelin. *Arch Gen Psychiatry.* 1994;51:875-883.
67. Reinberg A, Touitou Y, Gillemant S, Levy F, Lagoguey M. Rythmes circadiens et circannuels des résultats d'épreuves fonctionnelles en endocrinologie. *Ann Endocrinol.* 1982;43:309-335.
68. Reinberg A, Levi F, Smolesky M. Chronopharmacocinétique clinique. *J Pharmacol.* 1984;15:95-124.
69. Snyder PJ, Utiger RD. Inhibition of thyrotropin response to thyrotropin-releasing hormone by small quantities of thyroid hormones. *J Clin Invest.* 1972; 51:2077-2084.
70. Saberi M, Utiger R. Augmentation of thyrotropin responses to thyrotropin-releasing hormone following small decreases in serum thyroid hormone concentration. *J Clin Endocrinol Metab.* 1975;40:435-441.
71. Burger HG, Patel YC. Thyrotropin-releasing hormone—TSH. *Clin Endocrinol Metab.* 1977;6:83-100.
72. Chen CJ, Sikes CR, Dziewanowska ZE, Stokes PE. The influence of blood chemistry on T_4 and FT_4I in major depression. *J Affective Disord.* 1990;20:159-163.
73. Molchan SE, Lawlor BA, Hill JL, Mellow AM, Davis CL, Martinez R, Sunderland T. The TRH stimulation test in Alzheimer's disease and major depression: relationship to clinical and CSF measures. *Biol Psychiatry.* 1991;30:567-576.
74. Loosen PT, Wilson IC, Prange AJ. Endocrine and behavioral changes in depression after thyrotropin releasing hormone (TRH). *J Affective Disord.* 1980; 2:267-278.
75. Nemeroff CB, Evans DL. Thyrotropin-releasing hormone (TRH), the thyroid axis, and affective disorder. *Ann N Y Acad Sci.* 1989;553:304-310.
76. Baumgartner A, Haug HJ. Thyroid hormones during sleep deprivation. *Biol Psychiatry.* 1988;23:537-538.
77. Baumgartner A, Rieman D, Berger M. Neuroendocrinological investigations during sleep deprivation in depression, part II: Longitudinal measurements of thyrotropin, TH, cortisol, prolactin, GH, and LH during sleep and sleep deprivation. *Biol Psychiatry.* 1990;28:569-587.
78. Whybrow PC, Coppen A, Prange AJ, Noguera R, Bailey JE. Thyroid function and the response to liothyronine in depression. *Arch Gen Psychiatry.* 1972; 26:242-245.
79. Morley JE, Schafer RB. Thyroid function screening in new psychiatric admissions. *Arch Intern Med.* 1982;142:591-593.
80. Griffiths EC. Thyrotropin-releasing hormone: endocrine and central effects. *Psychoneuroendocrinology.* 1985;10:225-233.
81. Brady KT, Anton RF. The thyroid axis and desipramine treatment in depression. *Biol Psychiatry.* 1989;25:703-709.
82. Roy-Byrne PP, Joffe RT, Uhde TW, Post RM. Carbamazepine and thyroid function in affectively ill patients. *Arch Gen Psychiatry.* 1984;41:1150-1153.
83. Muller B, Boning GJ. Changes in the pituitary-thyroid axis accompanying major affective disorders. *Acta Psychiatr Scand.* 1988;77:143-150.
84. Kirkegaard C, Bjørum N, Cohn D, Faber J, Lauridsen UB, Nerup J. Studies on the influence of biogenic amines and psychoactive drugs on the prognosis value of the TRH stimulation test in endogenous depression. *Psychoneuroendocrinology.* 1977;2:131-136.
85. Kirkegaard C. The thyrotropin response to thyrotropin-releasing hormone in endogenous depression. *Psychoneuroendocrinology.* 1981;6:189-212.
86. Shelton RC, Winn S, Ekhatore N, Loosen PT. The effects of antidepressants on the thyroid axis in depression. *Biol Psychiatry.* 1993;33:120-126.
87. Brady KT, Lydiard B, Kellner CH, Joffe R, Knight Laird L, Morton WA, Steele TE. A comparison of the effects of imipramine and fluvoxamine on the thyroid axis. *Biol Psychiatry.* 1994;36:778-779.
88. Kirkegaard L, Norlem N, Laridsen UB, Bjørum N. Prognostic value of thyrotropin releasing hormone stimulation test in endogenous depression. *Acta Psychiatr Scand.* 1975;52:170-177.
89. Langer G, Aschauer H, Koinig G, Resch F, Schonbeck G. The TSH response to TRH: a possible predictor of outcome to antidepressant and neuroleptic treatment. *Prog Neuropsychopharmacol Biol Psychiatry.* 1983;7:335-342.
90. Vanelle JM, Poirier MF, Benkelfat C, Galinowski A, Sechter D, Suzini de Luca H, Lôo H. Diagnostic and therapeutic value of testing stimulation of thyroid-stimulating hormone by thyrotropin-releasing hormone in 100 depressed patients. *Acta Psychiatr Scand.* 1990;81:156-161.
91. Nemeroff CB. Augmentation regimens for depression. *J Clin Psychiatry.* 1991; 52:21-27.

ORIGINAL ARTICLE

Triiodothyronine Augmentation in the Treatment of Refractory Depression

A Meta-analysis

Ronnie Aronson, MD; Hilary J. Offman, MD; Russel T. Joffe, MD; C. David Naylor, MD, DPhil

Background: Several trials have addressed the efficacy of liothyronine sodium therapy in euthyroid, nonpsychotic depressed patients refractory to tricyclic antidepressant therapy. We undertook a meta-analysis of these trials.

Methods: The MEDLINE database (1966 to May 1995) and published reference lists were examined for controlled clinical trials of triiodothyronine augmentation in euthyroid patients with refractory depression. Quality assessment and data abstraction were performed independently by two reviewers. Results were aggregated three ways: the relative response rate compared with controls, accepting each trial's definition of clinical response; absolute improvement in response rates; and improvements in depression scores, analyzed as continuous variables without a prespecified threshold for clinical response.

Results: Aggregating eight studies with a total of 292 patients, patients treated with triiodothyronine augmentation were twice as likely to respond as controls (relative response, 2.09; 95% confidence interval [CI], 1.31 to 3.32; $P=.002$). This corresponded to a 23.2% absolute improvement in response rates (95% CI, 4.5% to 41.9%; $P=.02$). Improvements in depression scores were moderately large (standardized effect size, 0.62; $P<.001$). However, study quality was uneven, and results were statistically heterogeneous. Among the four randomized double-blind studies, pooled effects were not significant (relative response, 1.53; 95% CI, 0.70 to 3.35; $P=.29$), but one study with negative results accounted for most of the intertrial heterogeneity in results.

Conclusions: Triiodothyronine augmentation may be an effective empirical method of increasing response rates and decreasing depression severity scores in a subgroup of patients with depression refractory to tricyclic antidepressant therapy, but the total number of patients randomized was small, and additional placebo-controlled data are required for a definitive verdict. Since therapeutic trends now favor other drugs, future trials might usefully examine triiodothyronine augmentation with selective serotonin reuptake inhibitors or compare potentiation strategies, eg, lithium vs triiodothyronine, for managing refractory depression. Such trials would benefit from much larger sample sizes than those reviewed here.

Arch Gen Psychiatry. 1996;53:842-848

From the Departments of Medicine (Drs Aronson and Naylor), Psychiatry (Dr Offman), and Behavioural Science (Dr Naylor) and the Sunnybrook Unit, Clinical Epidemiology and Health Care Research Program (Dr Naylor), University of Toronto (Ontario); Department of Psychiatry, McMaster University, Hamilton, Ontario (Dr Joffe); and the Institute for Clinical Evaluative Sciences, Toronto (Dr Naylor).

DEPRESSION HAS a known lifetime prevalence of 4.4% in the American population.[1] Medical therapies for depression, including tricyclic antidepressants (TCAs), have improved in effectiveness based on advances in diagnosis[2] and pharmacokinetics.[3] However, failure to respond to these medications continues to occur in up to 30% of patients treated in mental health settings,[4] forming a large, persistent clinical problem.

Liothyronine sodium (triiodothyronine [T_3]) was first used empirically in the treatment of depression in 1958.[5,6] Early promise led to the use of low-dose T_3 therapy with TCAs to accelerate the TCA effect. Several placebo-controlled trials[7-10] confirmed a more rapid response in the patients treated with T_3 and TCAs while maintaining a euthyroid state. Several open series[11-15] then studied euthyroid, depressed TCA nonresponders and showed that addition of T_3 could produce response rates of 64% to 90%. A small number of controlled clinical trials ensued. The practice has since become widely reported in reviews[16,17] and textbooks[3,18] and has been extrapolated to other classes of antidepressants[19-21] and psychiatric illnesses.[22-25] More recently, reviews[26-28] of

See Methods on next page

METHODS

LITERATURE SEARCH

An effort was made to identify all comparative clinical trials of adjunctive T_3 therapy in depressed patients refractory to treatment with TCAs alone. A computer-aided search of the National Library of Medicine MEDLINE database for 1966 to May 1995 combined the "exploded" medical subject headings (MeSH) *affective disorders, affective symptoms, depressive disorders,* and *depression,* with *thyroid hormones,* limited to therapeutic use or administration. Further manual search then included review of the reference lists of clinical trials and review articles as well as personal correspondence with research colleagues active in this field.

INCLUSION AND EXCLUSION CRITERIA

We included studies that used accepted criteria for depression, a stated definition of refractory depression, and biochemical evidence of euthyroidism, in which T_3 augmentation was used, along with any form of group comparison. We excluded studies with concomitant therapy known to affect thyroid function, including lithium; studies with insufficient outcome data reported in each group; and multiple reports that involved the same study population. In trials that used multiple treatment arms, if adjunctive T_3 augmentation had been compared with a control group, data from those arms were included. The trials identified for inclusion were reviewed to assess the clinical comparability of study populations, treatment protocols, and outcome measures.

QUALITY ASSESSMENT

Study methods were evaluated independently by two appraisers (R.A. and H.J.O.) using a streamlined version[30] of the Chalmers quality assessment scale.[31] Results were subsequently compared, and differences were settled by consensus. Quality assessments were used in sensitivity analyses to evaluate the effect of study quality on effect size.

DATA ABSTRACTION

Data abstraction was performed using standardized forms to record outcomes, withdrawals, and cointerventions. Outcomes recorded included rates of response as defined by each investigator, change in mean scores on depression inventories, and the statistical analysis used in each study. In one study, control group scores[32] were reported graphically. In one crossover trial,[33] outcome was determined at the point of crossover to create a parallel group design. The duration of treatment prior to crossover and definition of response were consistent with other trial protocols. One study[34] reported response rates only and did not provide mean depression scores.

STATISTICAL ANALYSIS

In meta-analysis, it is assumed that reported study outcomes will differ because of sampling variation alone and that the combination of individual study results will produce a better estimate of the "true" treatment effect. For categorical data, relative risks for each study were pooled using generalized linear mixed modeling methods[35]; this approach generates an estimate of the common relative response rate and was adapted to generate a heterogeneity statistic that tests whether intertrial results differ more than would be expected by chance alone.[36] A mixed model augments the variance of the pooled effect size estimate to reflect the degree of heterogeneity among the separate trial results. The empirical logistic transform was used to force convergence in the heterogeneity test, as two studies had arms with no respondents. We tested the stability of our results using odds ratios rather than relative risks as the measure to summarize the intergroup differences; findings were similar (data available on request from the authors).

The method of DerSimonian and Laird[37] was also used to assess absolute differences in proportions of patients responding in the treatment group vs the control group, with a corresponding heterogeneity statistic. The number of patients who must be treated to produce one additional responder (number needed to treat) was determined by the reciprocal of the pooled absolute difference.

For continuous outcome measures, such as a depression inventory score, the Glass method[38] allows combination of standardized effect sizes (d=[mean decrease in Hamilton Rating Scales for Depression (HRS-D) score in the experimental group minus mean decrease in HRS-D score in the control group]/pooled SD). Standard size-weighting methods were used within a software program to generate pooled effect sizes (True Epistat, Epistat Services Inc, Richardson, Tex) expressed as r values, with R^2 as the percentage of variance in the outcome explained by the effect of treatment, converted to d values using a standard formula.[39] Significance was determined by the weighted mean of the z scores calculated for each study.

Sensitivity analyses were performed to sequentially remove groups of studies with shared methodologic deficiencies[30] to assess their effect on the overall estimate of effect size and on the degree of interstudy heterogeneity.

these studies have cautioned that acceptance of T_3 augmentation in refractory depression is premature. These reviews have correctly noted methodologic deficiencies in studies to date, the small number of randomized controlled trials, and differences in both size and direction of reported treatment effects.

We therefore conducted a meta-analysis of clinical trials investigating T_3 use in euthyroid TCA nonresponders to address these conflicting findings and provide a better estimate of the treatment effect size.[29]

RESULTS

LITERATURE REVIEW

Nine published clinical trials investigating adjunctive T_3 augmentation in depressed TCA nonresponders were identified.[32-34,40-44] One trial[45] was excluded because it was not clearly a comparative trial and provided insufficient outcome data in the treatment groups. Therefore, eight

Table 1. Study Characteristics of Triiodothyronine (T_3) Augmentation Trials*

Study, y	Patients	Initial Therapy	Study Design	Study Therapy
Joffe et al,[44] 1993	33 unipolar outpatients; 22 M, 11 F; mean age, 37.4 y	Imipramine HCl/desipramine HCl, >2.5 mg/kg; plasma levels monitored; duration, 5 wk	Randomized, placebo-controlled, double-blind	Previous TCA dose and T_3, 37.5 μg/d × 14 d, *or* placebo
Joffe and Singer,[43] 1990	38 unipolar outpatients; 24 M, 14 F; mean age, 34.5 y	Imipramine HCl/desipramine HCl, 2.5-3 mg/kg; plasma levels monitored; duration, 4 wk	Randomized, T_4-controlled, double-blind	Previous TCA dose and T_3, 37.5 μg/d × 21 d, *or* T_4, 150 μg/d
Thase et al,[42] 1989	40 unipolar outpatients; 29 M, 11 F; mean age, 42.5 y	Imipramine HCl, MTRD protocol†; plasma levels monitored; duration, 12 wk	Sequential, historical controls, unblinded	Previous imipramine HCl dose and T_3, 25 μg/d × 28 d
Gitlin et al,[33] 1987	16 unipolar outpatients; 7 M, 9 F; mean age, 41 y	Imipramine HCl, up to 300 mg/d; duration, 4 wk	Randomized, placebo-controlled, double-blind, crossover‡	Previous imipramine HCl dose and T_3, 25 μg/d × 14 d, *or* placebo
Goodwin et al,[32] 1982	12 unipolar and bipolar inpatients; 6 M, 6 F; mean age, 38.4 y	Imipramine HCl/desipramine HCl, up to 300 mg/d; duration, 4 wk	Mirror design, placebo-controlled, double-blind	Previous TCA dose and T_3, 25-50 μg/d × 21 d
Steiner et al,[41] 1978	8 F unipolar and bipolar inpatients; mean age, 55.5 y	NR; duration, 6 wk	Randomized, placebo-controlled, double-blind	Impramine HCl, 150 mg/d, and T_3, 25 μg/d × 35 d, *or* placebo
Banki,[40] 1977	49 F unipolar and bipolar inpatients; mean age, 45.5 y	NR; duration, 14 d	Historical controls, unblinded	Amitryptyline HCl, ≤200 mg/d, and T_3, 20-40 μg/d × 7 d
Banki,[34] 1975	96 F unipolar and bipolar inpatients; mean age, 48 y	NR; duration, 10 d	Historical controls, unblinded	Previous TCA dose and T_3, 20-40 μg/d × 10 d

**HCl indicates hydrochloride; TCA, tricyclic antidepressant; T_4, levothyroxine sodium; MTRD, Maintenance Therapies of Recurrent Depression; and NR, not reported.*
†Baseline scores on the Hamilton Rating Scales for Depression were consistent with those of other study populations.
‡Data at crossover were used to preserve comparability in parallel study design.

studies[32-34,40-44] formed the basis of our meta-analysis (**Table 1**).

STUDY QUALITY

Several methodologic limitations that applied to all eight studies were identified (**Table 2**). Incomplete information was given regarding excluded patients, outcome data of withdrawn patients, control group therapeutic protocols, and prospective sample size justification (seven of eight studies). All studies adhered to validated, itemized depression inventories.

Goodwin et al[32] employed a self-controlled design comparing pretreatment and posttreatment scores and did not adhere to their own pretrial definition of response in assessing outcome. Despite these deficiencies, the study was included in the analysis because of two design strengths. The trial was prospective, with pretreatment placebo administration and data collection exceeding the refractory and treatment periods of most other trials. As well, patients, physicians and outcome assessors were blind to the start date of T_3 administration, despite the fact that all patients did eventually receive T_3. Finally, full patient data were provided, allowing extraction of the most conservative outcome data. The effect of this study design was assessed with a sensitivity analysis.

In three trials, historical[34,40] or sequential[42] controls were used and therapy was unblinded. All were prospective and provided descriptions of control selection that adhered to identical criteria. The effect of these trials was also evaluated using a sensitivity analysis.

COMPARABILITY OF TRIALS

Inclusion criteria were very similar in all trials, ie, patients with nonpsychotic, primary depression proven refractory to standard TCA therapy (Table 1). All patients continued TCA therapy and received adjunctive T_3 or placebo. Some minor differences included the choice of published criteria used to define depression, hospitalized patients vs outpatients, and sex distribution. Four studies included patients with bipolar mood disorder,[32,34,40,41] who may respond differently to T_3 augmentation[22,23] and who may have thyroid dysfunction based on prior lithium carbonate therapy. All four studies did document biochemical euthyroidism. Patients drawn by Thase et al[42] from the Maintenance Therapies of Recurrent Depression (MTRD) study had baseline HRS-D scores[46] consistent with scores in other studies. Banki[34,40] used a slightly different definition of refractoriness: shorter duration, 10 days[34] and 14 days[40] vs 4 to 5 weeks in other studies, with a response criterion of 20% change in HRS-D score vs 50% in other studies.

Differences in experimental design other than those mentioned above included minor dose, duration, and timing differences in T_3 administration (Table 1). Once-daily T_3 administration may produce rapid increases in plasma T_3 levels and may have a greater effect than more constant levels. In one study,[43] controls received adjunc-

Table 2. Quality Assessment of Trials of Triiodothyronine Augmentation*

	Joffe et al[44]	Joffe and Singer[43]	Thase et al[42]	Gitlin et al[33]	Goodwin et al[32]	Steiner et al[41]	Banki[40]	Banki[34]
Patient selection								
Defined inclusion and exclusion criteria?	Yes	Yes	Yes	Yes	Yes	Yes	Yes	Yes
Reported No. of patients screened and excluded?	No	No	No	Yes	No	No	No	No
Treatment assignment								
Random assignment?	Yes	Yes	No	Yes	No	Yes	No	No
Provided description of randomization?	Partial	Yes	NA	Partial	NA	Full	NA	NA
Blinding—outcome assessors blind to treatment?	Yes	Yes	No	Yes	Yes	Yes	No	No
Outcome assessment								
Description of criteria for measure?	Yes	Yes	Yes	Yes	Yes	Yes	Yes	Yes
Were criteria objective?	Yes	Yes	Yes	Yes	Yes	Yes	Yes	Yes
Statistical analysis								
Appropriate to study design?	Yes	Yes	Yes	Yes	Yes	No	Yes	Yes
If negative study, power calculation?	...	...	No	No	...	No	...	...

**NA indicates not applicable.*

Table 3. Results of Triiodothyronine (T_3) Augmentation Trials*

		Response Rates, No. (%)		Mean Decrease in HRS-D Score†	
Study, y	Response Criteria	T_3 Group	Control Group	T_3 Group	Control Group
Joffe et al,[44] 1993	≥50% decrease in HRS-D score	10/17 (59)	3/16 (19)	7.7	3.8‡
Joffe and Singer,[43] 1990	≥50% decrease in HRS-D score	9/17 (53)	4/21 (19)	8.8	4.9§
Thase et al,[42] 1989	≥50% decrease in HRS-D score and HRS-D score <10	5/20 (25)	4/20 (20)	3.5	3.0
Gitlin et al,[33] 1987	≥50% decrease in HRS-D score	0/7 (0)	4/9 (44)	5.0	3.0
Goodwin et al,[32] 1982	≥3-point decrease in BHS score	4/12 (33)	0/6 (0)	2.2	0.2‡
Steiner et al,[41] 1978	Moderate increase in CGI Scale score and HRS-D score <10	3/4 (75)	3/4 (75)	17.3	17.5
Banki,[40] 1977	Clinical improvement	22/33 (67)	4/16 (25)	15.0	8.0§
Banki,[34] 1975	Clinical improvement	39/52 (75)	10/44 (23)	NR	NR
Overall	...	**92/162** (57)	**32/136** (24)	...	...

**HRS-D indicates Hamilton Rating Scales for Depression; BHS, Bunney-Hamburg Scale; CGI, Clinical Global Impression; and NR, data not reported.*
†*The BHS score was used for Goodwin et al.*[32]
‡*$P<.05$.*
§*$P<.01$.*

tive levothyroxine sodium (thyroxine [T_4]), which has a much longer half-life (5 to 7 days) than T_3, but since the duration of therapy was short (3 weeks) and the impact on T_3 levels was unclear, this group was considered similar to placebo-controlled groups in other studies. The response rate in this control group was also remarkably consistent with rates in other control groups. The effect of this trial was also assessed by sensitivity analysis. Controls in both reports by Banki[34,40] were treated with increased doses of their previous TCA.

All studies rated depression severity using the HRS-D,[46] except Goodwin et al,[32] who used a modified version of the Bunney-Hamburg Scale.[47] Response (**Table 3**) was defined as a reduction of 50% or greater in HRS-D score in four studies,[33,42-44] as moderate improvement on the Clinical Global Impression scale in one study,[41] as a decrease of three points or more on the Bunney-Hamburg Scale in one study,[32] and clinically in two studies.[34,40]

Some conservative assumptions were made in the analysis of continuous scores. The HRS-D scores reported by Banki[40] included an unspecified measure of variance. We are reporting the most conservative interpretation (SE). Also, in determining the variance of the score decrement in each experimental group, we adopted the most conservative estimate—the SDs of scores from the final assessment. Combining initial and final SDs for each group yielded almost identical effect size results.

POOLED TREATMENT EFFECTS

Augmentation therapy with T_3 had a favorable and statistically significant effect on response rate to TCA therapy and on mean decrease in HRS-D score (**Table 4**). Analysis of data from 292 patients resulted in a doubling in response rates, with a relative response rate of 2.09 (95% confidence interval, 1.31 to 3.32; $P=.002$). The corresponding pooled absolute difference in response rate between treated patients and controls was 23.2% (95% confidence interval, 4.5% to 41.9%; $P=.02$). The number of patients treated to obtain one responder was 4.3. However, there was also significant heterogeneity in response rates among the trials.

Table 4. Results of Pooled Analysis, With Sensitivity Analyses*

Studies	Relative Response: Rate (95% CI)	P	Heterogeneity Test, P	P_t-P_c, % (95% CI)	No. Needed to Treat†	Effect Size: d‡	P	Heterogeneity Test, P
Joffe et al,[44] Thase et al,[42] Steiner et al,[41] Banki,[40] and Banki[34]	2.09 (1.31-3.32)	.002	.04	23.2 (4.5 to 41.9)	4.3	0.62	<.001	.18
Goodwin et al[32]	2.02 (1.23-3.34)	.006	.03	21.1 (−1.1 to 43.3)	4.8	0.56	<.001	.15
Joffe and Singer[43]	1.93 (1.13-3.29)	.02	.02	21.1 (−0.7 to 43.0)	4.8	0.62	<.001	.12
Gitlin et al[33]	2.70 (1.89-3.86)	.006	.45	36.5 (26.7 to 46.4)	2.7	0.64	<.001	.15
Randomized controlled trials only[33,41,43,44]	1.53 (0.70-3.35)	.29	.02	8.6 (−28.7 to 45.8)	12.5	0.60	.001	.28

**CI* indicates confidence interval; P_t, percentage of patients with response in the treatment group; and P_c, percentage of patients with response in the control group.*
†*To obtain one responder.*
‡*Mean decrease in Hamilton Rating Scales for Depression score in the treatment group minus mean decrease in Hamilton Rating Scales for Depression score in the control group, divided by the pooled SD for the treatment and control groups.*

Analyzing response continuously as the measured improvement in depression scores, the pooled standardized effect sizes also showed a statistically significant effect, with an overall combined effect size (*d*) of 0.62 (*P*<.001).

SENSITIVITY ANALYSES

Four sensitivity analyses were performed (Table 4). Eliminating data from Goodwin et al,[32] who had no separate control group, and from Joffe and Singer,[43] who treated controls with T_4, produced minimal change in the relative response rates (2.02 and 1.93, respectively, both statistically significant). However, intertrial heterogeneity of response rates remained significant. We then eliminated the results of Gitlin et al,[33] who had directionally discrepant results and an apparent imbalance in randomization, with higher depression scores in the T_3 group (mean HRS-D score, 22.3, vs 16.9 in controls). This eliminated the statistical heterogeneity in results.

Analysis of data from randomized controlled trials alone[33,41,43,44] produced a lower pooled relative response rate of 1.53 (95% confidence interval, 0.70 to 3.35; *P*=.29). The significant improvement in absolute response rates was also abolished. However, intertrial heterogeneity was significant with either method, owing to dramatic disparities between the two reports by Joffe et al[43,44] and that of Gitlin et al.[33]

Similar analyses were performed for the HRS-D score decrement data (Table 4). These changes were more stable. The sensitivity analyses produced only slight departures from the overall standardized effect size of 0.62 (*P*<.001).

There were not sufficient data provided to include side effects in the formal analysis; however, the five studies[32-34,40,41] that included side effect assessments reported no significant differences compared with controls.

COMMENT

This meta-analysis suggests that T_3 augmentation has a statistically significant effect on both end points, response rate and mean decrease in HRS-D score. The use of response as an end point is arguably the most conservative approach, since its clinical relevance has already been determined by each group of investigators. However, some cautions are warranted. First, the trials reviewed here tended to adopt a definition of clinical response based on a 50% increase in the HRS-D score. This degree of relative change, while suggestive, may not be clinically meaningful for all patients. Also, once we set aside studies that were likely to have overestimated the effects of T_3 augmentation through use of nonconcurrent controls,[34,40,42] only two of the remaining five trials showed clear-cut benefits with T_3 augmentation. Furthermore, when we aggregated the four trials with randomized double-blind design elements, neither the relative nor the absolute improvements in response rates were significant.

On the other hand, just as three trials may have been biased in favor of T_3 augmentation through use of historical controls, one can also postulate reasons why three[33,41,42] of the eight trials did not individually show a significant effect of T_3 therapy. One trial that did not show an effect[41] had only eight subjects and therefore had minimal statistical power to detect a T_3 effect. The other two trials that did not show an effect may have included patients who were more chronically ill (>12 weeks)[42] or who had more severe depression at baseline (see above) in the study arm of patients receiving T_3.[33] It is interesting to note that the report by Gitlin et al[33] was the predominant contributor to the significant heterogeneity noted in the pooling of the categorical variable, response rate. This may be an artifact of the above-noted imbalance in the randomization process in that trial, because the higher baseline HRS-D scores in T_3-treated patients would make them less likely to reach the response threshold despite their greater mean improvement in HRS-D score. Although no categorically defined responses occurred in the T_3 group, the HRS-D improvement was actually greater in the T_3 group than in the control group. Moreover, there was no significant heterogeneity and much less instability in the sensitivity analyses of the pooled effect size estimate when the HRS-D score was analyzed as a continuous-response scale.

Possible mechanisms for thyroid hormone acting in concert with TCAs have been reviewed in detail elsewhere.[48-50] One theory suggests that T_3 acts in euthyroid patients through augmentation of the β-adrenergic system. Alternatively, T_3 may be acting only in "subclinically" hypothyroid patients by supplementing deficiencies in endogenous thyroid hormone levels. The protirelin (thyrotropin-releasing hormone) stimulation test produces an exaggerated thyrotropin response in subclinically hypothyroid patients. Intriguingly, some studies[15,45,51] report relatively lower thyroid levels or relatively higher thyrotropin-releasing hormone responses in those patients who benefit from T_3 augmentation. However, other reports have shown no thyroid function abnormality in depressed patients[14] or elevated thyroid levels (free T_4 indices) in depressed populations.[52-54] Indeed, Loosen[48] estimated an overall incidence of 30% of thyrotropin-releasing hormone response blunting in depression, suggesting subclinical hyperthyroidism. Therefore, both subclinical hyperthyroidism and subclinical hypothyroidism occur in refractory depression and may simply be epiphenomena or random variations within the normal distribution of thyroid hormone levels.

Triiodothyronine might also act by affecting thyroid utilization at critical sites. Joffe[50] and Joffe and Singer[43] have suggested that any relative hyperthyroid state observed in depression may have paradoxical effects at the neuronal level. Neurons derive T_3 largely (approximately 75%) from a local deiodination mechanism, distinct from peripheral deiodination,[55] and this local deiodination could be inhibited by relative increases in systemic T_4 that increase the neuronal, locally derived T_3 supply. According to this theory, T_3 therapy of depression would inhibit thyroidal T_4 production, reducing the substrate available for neuronal T_3 conversion and increasing the rate of local deiodination. However, this is not consistent with the incidence of subclinical hypothyroidism in depression and the higher incidence of depression in frank hypothyroidism. Also, neuronal local deiodination has been shown to function independently of systemic thyroid levels in hypothyroid,[56] uremic,[57] and pregnant[58] rats and may not be affected by systemic T_4 levels.

The physiological role of thyroid hormone in affective illness remains to be clarified. Depressed patients should be studied with standardized protirelin tests to establish true thyroid status and then should be followed up as cohorts with relative hypothyroidism, hyperthyroidism, and euthyroidism to prospectively assess response rates. Deiodinating enzyme inhibitors, such as methimazole, might be studied in depressed patients to separate the effects of T_4 and T_3. Finally, to clarify the importance of the neuron as a separate homeostatic system, further in vitro investigation is necessary to evaluate the effects of systemic T_4 and/or T_3 flux. Studies of neuronal T_3 in a previously used animal model of depression, learned helplessness,[59] might increase our understanding of the process.

In conclusion, T_3 augmentation in TCA nonresponders appears to be an effective, inexpensive, and safe empirical method of producing a response and decreasing depression severity scores in a subgroup of patients with refractory depression. However, only 292 patients in controlled studies were available for meta-analysis, and fewer still in trials with a randomized placebo-controlled design. A definitive verdict demands additional data from placebo-controlled trials; but such TCA and T_3 trials may be difficult, since selective serotonin reuptake inhibitors have gained in popularity and lithium carbonate has been much more widely accepted than T_3 as a potential augmentation tool.[60] Thus, future randomized trials might usefully compare T_3 and lithium as potentiating agents and/or seek to confirm case reports[21] suggesting a potential role for T_3 augmentation in patients refractory to treatment with selective serotonin reuptake inhibitors. We urge much larger sample sizes to avoid the uncertainties that have hitherto arisen in this field because of multiple small and sometimes conflicting studies.

Accepted for publication January 3, 1996.

This study was supported by a grant from the Department of Medicine, University of Toronto (Ontario). Dr Naylor receives personnel support as Career Scientist 02377 of the Ontario Ministry of Health and from the Institute for Clinical Evaluative Sciences in Ontario.

The authors thank Michael J. Gitlin, MD, for his help in providing unpublished data and Judith M. Balogh, MD, FRCPC, for providing an English translation of one clinical trial. We are also grateful to Erluo Chen and Antoni S. H. Basinski for important assistance with the statistical analyses.

Reprints: C. David Naylor, MD, DPhil, ICES-G106, Sunnybrook Health Science Centre, 2075 Bayview Ave, North York, Ontario, Canada M4N 3M5.

REFERENCES

1. Weissman MM, Leaf PJ, Tischler GL, Blazer DG, Karno M, Bruce ML, Florio LP. Affective disorders in five United States communities. *Psychol Med.* 1988;18:141-153.
2. American Psychiatric Association. *Diagnostic and Statistical Manual of Mental Disorders, Third Edition, Revised.* Washington, DC: American Psychiatric Association; 1987.
3. Tasman A, Goldfinger SM, Kaufman CA. *American Psychiatric Press Review of Psychiatry.* Washington, DC: American Psychiatric Press; 1990;9.
4. Roose SP, Glassman AH, Walsh BT, Woodring S. Tricyclic nonresponders: phenomenology and treatment. *Am J Psychiatry.* 1986;143:345-348.
5. Flach FF, Celian CI, Rawson RW. Treatment of psychiatric disorders with triiodothyronine. *Am J Psychiatry.* 1958;114:841-842.
6. Feldmesser-Reiss EE. The application of triiodothyronine in the treatment of mental disorders. *J Nerv Ment Dis.* 1958;127:540-545.
7. Prange AJ Jr, Wilson IC, Rabon AM, Lipton AM. Enhancement of imipramine antidepressant effect by thyroid hormone. *Am J Psychiatry.* 1969;126:457-469.
8. Wilson IC, Prange AJ Jr, McClane TK, Rabon AM, Lipton AM. Thyroid-hormone enhancement of imipramine in non-retarded depressions. *N Engl J Med.* 1979;282:1063-1067.
9. Wheatley D. Potentiation of amitryptyline by thyroid hormone. *Arch Gen Psychiatry.* 1972;26:229-233.
10. Coppen A, Whybrow PC, Noguera R, Maggs R, Prange AJ Jr. The comparative antidepressant value of L-tryptophan and imipramine with and without attempted potentiation by liothyronine. *Arch Gen Psychiatry.* 1972;26:234-241.
11. Tsutsui S, Yamazaki Y, Namba T, Tsushima M. Combined therapy of T3 and antidepressants in depression. *J Int Med Res.* 1979;7:138-146.
12. Ogura C, Okuma T, Uchida Y, Imai S, Yogi H. Combined thyroid (triiodothyronine)-tricyclic antidepressive treatment in depressive states. *Folia Psychiatr Neurol Jpn.* 1974;28:179-186.
13. Earle BV. Thyroid hormone and tricyclic antidepressants in resistant depressions. *Am J Psychiatry.* 1970;126:1667-1669.

14. Schwarcz G, Halaris A, Baxter L, Escobar J, Thompson M, Young M. Normal thyroid function in desipramine nonresponders converted to responders by the addition of L-triiodothyronine. *Am J Psychiatry.* 1984;141:1614-1616.
15. Nakamura T, Nomura J. Comparison of thyroid function between responders and nonresponders to thyroid hormone supplementation in depression. *Jpn J Psychiatry Neurol.* 1992;46:905-909.
16. Nemeroff CB. Augmentation regimens for depression. *J Clin Psychiatry.* 1991; 52(suppl):21-27.
17. Nierenberg AA. What next? a review of pharmacologic strategies for treatment-resistant depression. *Psychopharmacol Bull.* 1990;26:429-460.
18. Extein IL, Gold MS. Thyroid hormone potentiation of tricyclic antidepressants. In: Extein IL, ed. *Treatment of Tricyclic-Resistant Depression.* Washington, DC: American Psychiatric Press; 1989:29-48.
19. Stern RA, Nevels CT, Shelhorse ME, Prohaska ML, Mason GA, Prange AJ Jr. Antidepressant and memory effects of combined thyroid hormone treatment and electroconvulsive therapy: preliminary findings. *Biol Psychiatry.* 1991;30: 623-627.
20. Joffe RT. Triiodothyronine potentiation of the antidepressant effect of phenelzine. *J Clin Psychiatry.* 1988;49:409-410.
21. Joffe RT. Triiodothyronine potentiation of fluoxetine in depressed patients. *Can J Psychiatry.* 1992;37:48-49.
22. Stancer HC, Persad E. Treatment of intractable rapid-cycling manic-depressive disorder with levothyroxine. *Arch Gen Psychiatry.* 1982;39:311-312.
23. Bauer MS, Whybrow PC. Rapid cycling bipolar affective disorder. *Arch Gen Psychiatry.* 1990;47:435-440.
24. Stein MB, Uhde TW. Triiodothyronine potentiation of tricyclic antidepressant treatment in patients with panic disorder. *Biol Psychiatry.* 1990;28:1061-1064.
25. Pigott TA, Pato MT, L'Heureaux F, Hill JL, Grover GN, Bernstein SE, Murphy DL. A controlled comparison of adjuvant lithium carbonate or thyroid hormone in clomipramine-treated patients with obsessive-compulsive disorder. *J Clin Psychopharmacol.* 1991;11:242-248.
26. Stein D, Avni J. Thyroid hormones in the treatment of affective disorders. *Acta Psychiatr Scand.* 1988;77:623-636.
27. Verdoux H, Peyre F, Bourgeois M. Potentiation of antidepressive treatment by thyroid hormone therapy. *Encephale.* 1989;15:517-522.
28. Patten SB, Lupin DA, Boucher SA, Lamarre CJ. Pharmacologic management of refractory depression. *Can Med Assoc J.* 1992;146:483-487.
29. Sacks HS, Berrier J, Reitman D, Ancona-Berk VA, Chalmers TC. Meta-analyses of randomized controlled trials. *N Engl J Med.* 1987;316:450-455.
30. Detsky AS, Naylor CD, O'Rourke K, McGeer AJ, L'Abbe KA. Incorporating variations in the quality of individual randomized trials into meta-analysis. *J Clin Epidemiol.* 1992;45:255-265.
31. Chalmers TC, Smith H Jr, Blackburn B, Silverman B, Schroeder B, Reitman D, Ambroz A. A method for assessing the quality of a randomized control trial. *Control Clin Trials.* 1981;2:31-49.
32. Goodwin FK, Prange AJ, Post RM, Muscettola G, Lipton MA. Potentiation of antidepressant effects by L-triiodothyronine in tricyclic nonresponders. *Am J Psychiatry.* 1982;139:34-38.
33. Gitlin MJ, Weiner H, Fairbanks L, Hershman JM, Friedfeld N. Failure of T3 to potentiate tricyclic antidepressant response. *J Affective Disord.* 1987;13:267-272.
34. Banki C. The use of triiodothyronine in the treatment of depression [in Hungarian]. *Orv Hetil.* 1975;116:2543-2546.
35. Breslow NE, Clayton EG. Approximate inference in generalized linear mixed models. *J Am Stat Assoc.* 1993;88:9-25.
36. Cox DR, Snell EJ. *Analysis of Binary Data.* 2nd ed. London, England: Chapman & Hall Ltd; 1989:60-61.
37. DerSimonian R, Laird N. Meta-analysis in controlled clinical trials. *Control Clin Trials.* 1986;7:177-181.
38. Glass GV. Integrating findings: the meta-analysis of research. In: Shulman LS, ed. *Review of Research in Education.* New York, NY: Peacock Press; 1977: 351-379.
39. Hedges LV, Olkin I. *Statistical Methods for Meta-analysis.* Orlando, Fla: Academic Press Inc; 1985:77.
40. Banki CM. Cerebrospinal fluid amine metabolites after combined amitryptyline-triiodothyronine treatment of depressed women. *Eur J Clin Pharmacol.* 1977; 11:311-315.
41. Steiner M, Radwan M, Elizur A, Blum I, Atsmon A, Davidson S. Failure of L-triiodothyronine to potentiate tricyclic antidepressant response. *Curr Ther Res.* 1978;23:655-659.
42. Thase ME, Kupfer DJ, Jarrett DB. Treatment of imipramine-resistant recurrent depression, I: an open clinical trial of adjunctive L-triiodothyronine. *J Clin Psychiatry.* 1989;50:385-388.
43. Joffe RT, Singer W. A comparison of triiodothyronine and thyroxine in the potentiation of tricyclic antidepressants. *Psychiatry Res.* 1990;32:241-251.
44. Joffe RT, Singer W, Levitt AJ, MacDonald C. A placebo-controlled comparison of lithium and triiodothyronine augmentation of tricyclic antidepressants in unipolar refractory depression. *Arch Gen Psychiatry.* 1993;50:387-393.
45. Targum SD, Greenberg RD, Harmon RL, Kessler K, Salerian AJ, Fram DH. Thyroid hormone and the TSH stimulation test in refractory depression. *J Clin Psychiatry.* 1984;45:345-346.
46. Hamilton M. A rating scale for depression. *J Neurol Neurosurg Psychiatry.* 1960;23:56-62.
47. Bunney WE Jr, Hamburg DA. Methods for reliable longitudinal observation of behavior. *Arch Gen Psychiatry.* 1963;9:280-294.
48. Loosen PT. Hormones of the hypothalamic-pituitary-thyroid axis: a psychoneuroendocrine perspective. *Pharmacopsychiatry.* 1986;19:401-415.
49. Howland RH. Thyroid dysfunction in refractory depression: implications for pathophysiology and treatment. *J Clin Psychiatry.* 1993;54:47-54.
50. Joffe RT. A perspective on the thyroid and depression. *Can J Psychiatry.* 1990; 35:754-758.
51. Baruch P, Jouvent R, Widlocher D. Increased TSH response to TRH in refractory depressed women. *Am J Psychiatry.* 1985;142:145-146.
52. Kirkegaard C, Faber J. Altered serum levels of thyroxine, triiodothyronines and diiodothyronines in endogenous depression. *Acta Endocrinol.* 1981;96:199-207.
53. Whybrow PC, Coppen A, Prange AJ Jr, Noguera R, Bailey JE. Thyroid function and the response to liothyronine in depression. *Arch Gen Psychiatry.* 1972; 26:242-245.
54. Hatotani N, Nomura J, Yamaguchi T, Kitayama I. Clinical and experimental studies of the pathogenesis of depression. *Psychoneuroendocrinology.* 1977;2: 115-130.
55. Crantz FR, Silva JE, Larsen PR. An analysis of the sources and quantity of 3,5,3′′-triiodothyronine specifically bound to nuclear receptors in rat cerebral cortex and cerebellum. *Endocrinology.* 1982;110:367-374.
56. Kaplan MM, Yaskoski KA. Phenolic and tyrosyl ring deiodination of iodothyronines in rat brain homogenates. *J Clin Invest.* 1980;66:551-562.
57. Lim VS, Passo C, Murata Y, Ferrari E, Nakamura H, Refetoff S. Reduced triiodothyronine content in liver but not pituitary of the uremic rat model: demonstration of changes compatible with thyroid hormone deficiency in liver only. *Endocrinology.* 1984;114:280-286.
58. Calvo R, Obregon MJ, Ruiz de Ona C, Ferreiro B, Escobar Del Rey E, Morreale de Escobar G. Thyroid hormone economy in pregnant rats near term: a 'physiological' animal model of nonthyroidal illness? *Endocrinology.* 1990;127:10-16.
59. Martin P, Brochet D, Soubrie P, Simon P. Triiodothyronine-induced reversal of learned helplessness in rats. *Biol Psychiatry.* 1985;20:1023-1025.
60. Nierenberg AA. Treatment choice after one antidepressant fails: a survey of northeastern psychiatrists. *J Clin Psychiatry.* 1991;52:383-385.

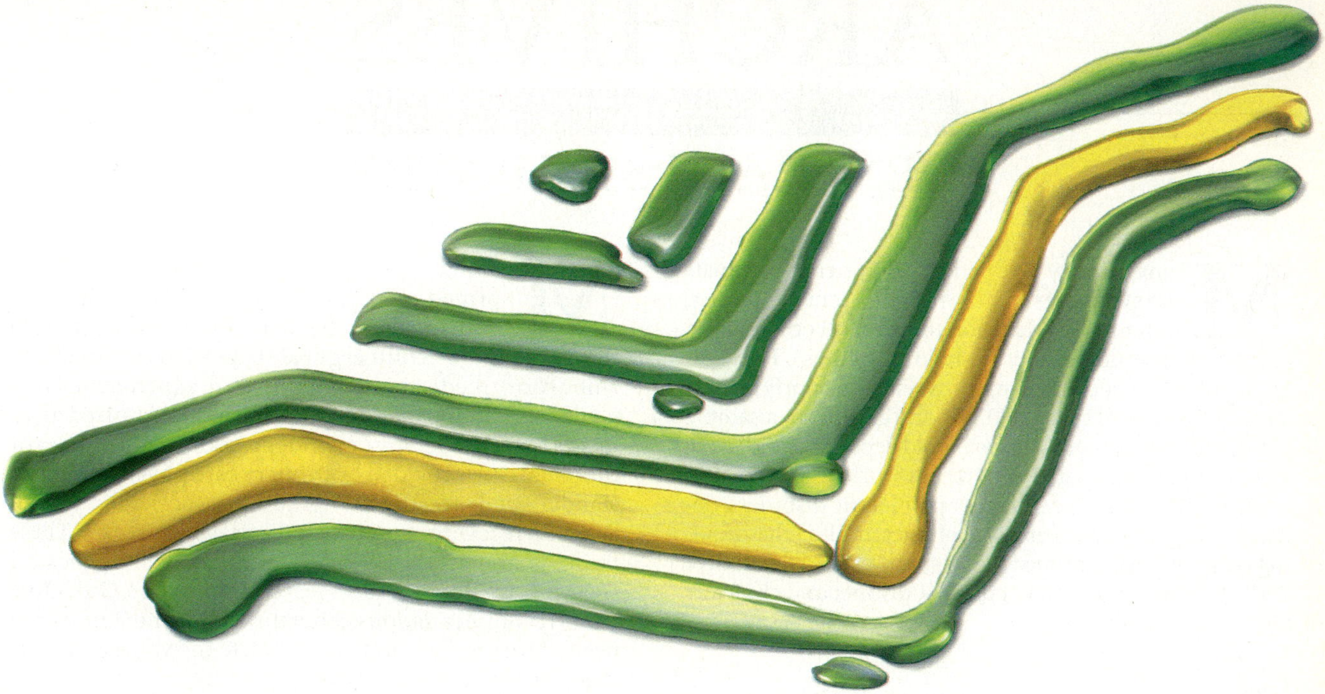

Now, RISPERDAL turns to liquid!

INTRODUCING
ORAL SOLUTION
1 mg/mL
Risperdal®
RISPERIDONE

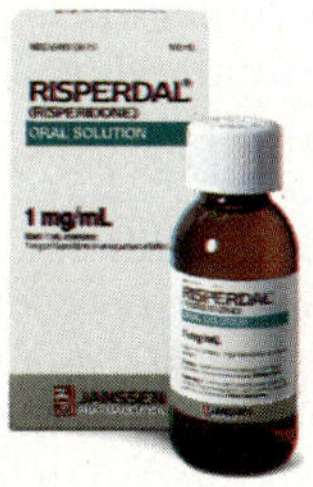

ARCHIVES OF GENERAL PSYCHIATRY

Many primary care patients experience psychiatric symptoms that are not sufficient in number, intensity, or duration to meet full criteria for a psychiatric disorder (ie, subthreshold symptoms). The clinical significance of these symptoms remains poorly understood. **Olfson et al** (page 880) report that within a sample of primary care patients, subthreshold depressive and panic symptoms are associated with recent work loss, even after controlling for the effects of other psychiatric disorders, demographic factors, and perceived physical health. These findings suggest that in primary care, subthreshold depressive and panic symptoms may represent distinct and clinically significant conditions.

Sherbourne et al (page 889) examined the extent to which anxiety disorders that are comorbid with other medical or psychiatric conditions increase the morbidity associated with these conditions. Patients with hypertension, diabetes, and anxiety were as debilitated as patients with depression or heart disease, and this debilitation persisted. The study highlights the clinical and societal importance of identifying comorbid anxiety in these patients.

Thirty-seven percent of the total medical cost to a health maintenance organization (HMO) is consumed by 8% of the patient population. Depression is prevalent among these high users. Among patients with a history of high medical expenditures, **Henk et al** (page 899) found that after adjusting for other variables, those patients who screened positive for depression, on average, accrued $1500 more in total medical expenses during the year the depression screener was administered. This suggests that, in addition to the obvious benefits to the patients, the cost of treating high users' depression could be offset by a decrease in unnecessary medical costs.

Cost-containment policies may affect the distribution and style of counseling or psychotherapy for depression. Using observational data from the Medical Outcomes Study, **Meredith et al** (page 905) describe payment and specialty differences in counseling as it is typically provided. They found large differences in the use of brief counseling for depressed patients of general medical clinicians compared with those of mental health specialists. Prepayment was associated with lower counseling rates than fee-for-service care among general medical patients with depressive symptoms or current depressive disorder. Usual counseling style differed markedly by specialty but only slightly by payment.

Major depression is experienced by 6% to 8% of primary care patients, but few studies have investigated the effectiveness of treatments with this population. **Schulberg et al** (page 913) recruited 276 ambulatory medical patients who were experiencing major depression and randomized them to standardized treatments (psychotherapy or antidepressant medications) or the usual care provided by primary care physicians. Both standardized treatments produced markedly higher 8-month recovery rates than a physician's usual care. These findings support the US Public Health Service Agency for Health Care Policy and Research Depression Guideline Panel recommendations about the nature and duration of needed treatments, and demonstrate the value of adhering to them in routine medical practice.

Unfortunately, few patients with major depression evaluated in a primary care setting receive guideline levels of antidepressant medication or psychotherapy. **Katon et al** (page 924) describe a collaborative model of care that increased education about depression and also integrated mental health professionals into the primary care treatment of depression. When compared with usual care by primary care physicians, this collaborative model increased patient adherence to antidepressant medication, improved patient satisfaction with care of depression, and resulted in more favorable outcomes.

Carve-outs are a rapidly growing feature of managed behavioral health care. Treating mental health and substance abuse care differently from other medical care raises concerns for continuity of care and fairness. **Frank et al** (page 933) explore the efficiency rationale for carve-out arrangements. They note that carve-outs may protect behavioral health coverage from problems in the insurance market. The special circumstances associated with providing mental health care may warrant more risk sharing than is typically found in capitation contracts.

Uncontrolled studies have suggested that enrollment of HMO members with mental illness may be prematurely terminated. However, **McFarland et al** (page 938) found that people with diagnoses of schizophrenia or bipolar disorder who were members of a large HMO remained enrolled longer than members who did not have severe illnesses. Use of public sector community mental health services predicted longer enrollment for the severely mentally ill people, but membership duration was unrelated to the HMO's costs for their care. Collaboration between HMOs and public mental health programs may be beneficial for people with severe mental disorders.

Massachusetts was the first state to shift the administration of Medicaid mental health benefits for all beneficiaries to a behavioral managed care company. **Dickey et al** (page 945) found that after managed care was introduced, the number of beneficiaries treated increased, inpatient admissions and length of stay decreased, and overall expenditures dropped. No cost shifting to the Department of Mental Health was found. Dickey et al recommend studies of the trade-offs between quality of care and costs.

Clozapine is an effective drug for treatment-resistant schizophrenia. The Food and Drug Administration has mandated weekly blood monitoring for patients who are being treated with clozapine because the drug causes agranulocytosis, a potentially fatal reduction in the white blood cell count, in a small number of patients. **Zhang et al** (page 954) report that this monitoring seems to be cost-effective during the first 6 months. Zhang et al suggest that the policy of mandatory weekly blood monitoring after the first 6 months of clozapine treatment should be reexamined.

This special theme issue on managed care also includes a "News & Views" piece on the topic by Harold Pincus, MD, and a "Commentary" on health care reform by Gary Tischler, MD, and Boris Astrachan, MD.

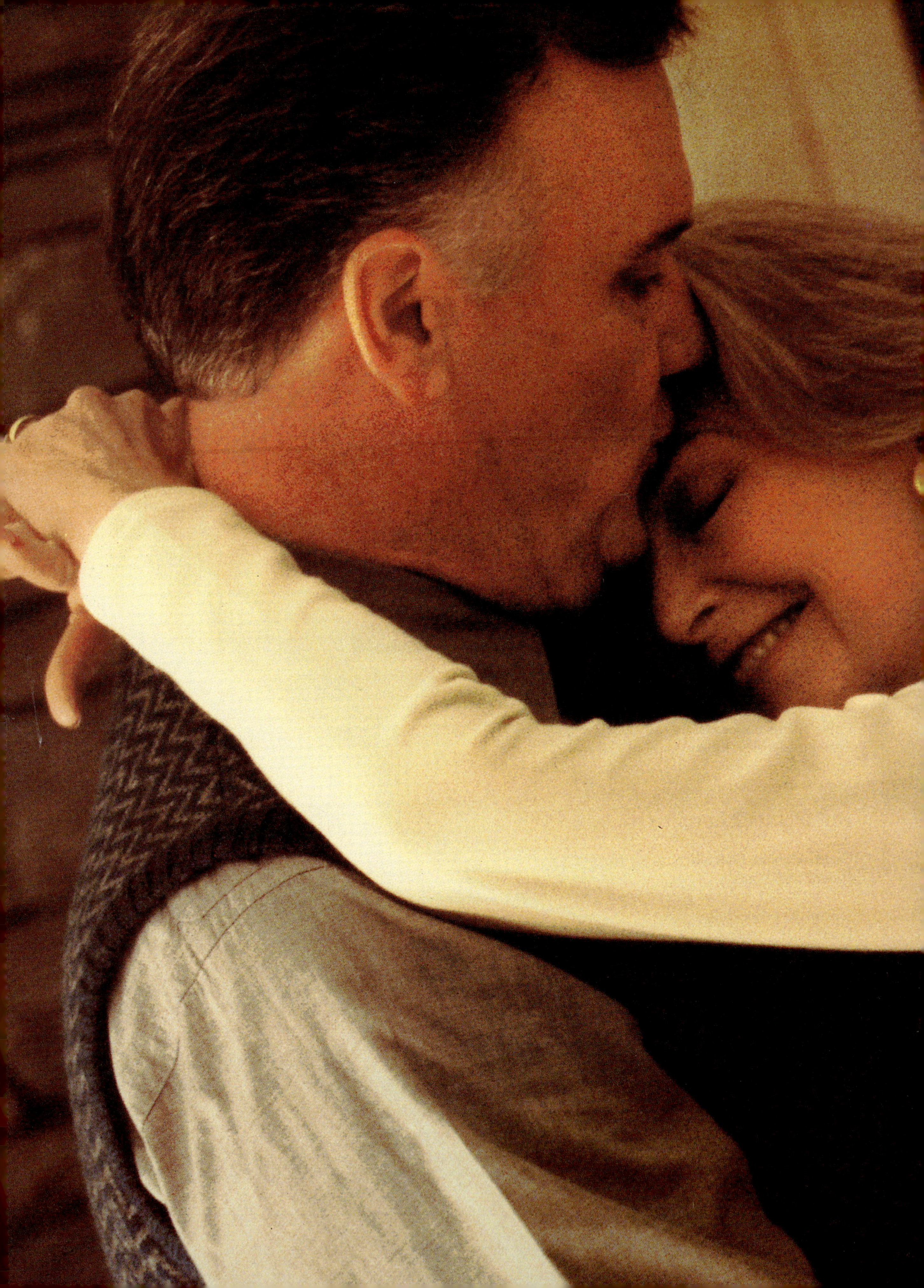

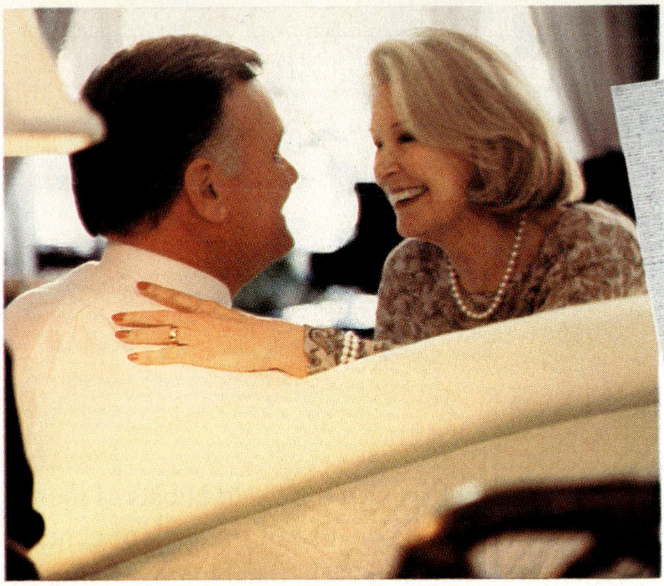

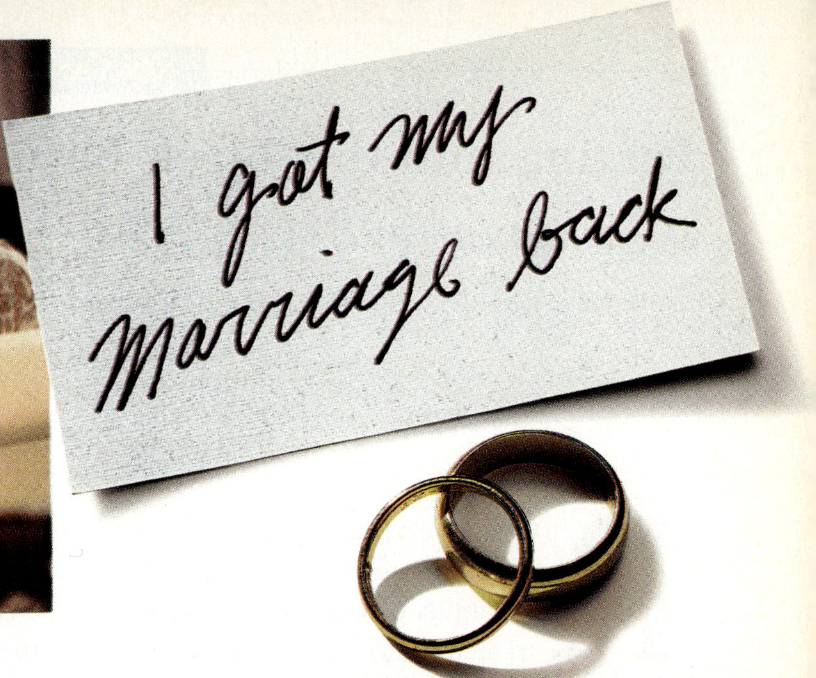

- Efficacy clearly demonstrated in depressed outpatients[1]
- Effective treatment in hospitalized depressed patients with major depressive disorder and melancholia meeting DSM-III-R™ criteria[2]
- No differential response in patients suffering from the symptoms of psychomotor agitation or psychomotor retardation that may accompany depression, based on subgroup analysis of effects on outcome[1]
- EFFEXOR should be taken in two or three divided doses with food

The most common adverse events reported in EFFEXOR clinical trials (incidence >10% and ≥ 2X that of placebo) were nausea, somnolence, dry mouth, dizziness, constipation, nervousness, sweating, asthenia, abnormal ejaculation/orgasm, and anorexia.

Counsel patients that nausea diminishes in most patients.

The effectiveness of EFFEXOR in long-term use (>6 weeks) has not been systematically evaluated in controlled trials.

EFFEXOR is contraindicated in patients taking monoamine oxidase inhibitors (MAOIs). EFFEXOR should not be used in combination with an MAOI or within at least 14 days of discontinuing treatment with an MAOI because of potential for serious adverse reactions. Based on the half-life of EFFEXOR, at least 7 days should be allowed after stopping EFFEXOR before starting an MAOI.

Treatment with EFFEXOR is associated with sustained increases in blood pressure in some patients. The incidence was seen at >5% at dosages above 200 mg/day and appears to be dose dependent. Regular monitoring of blood pressure is recommended.

As with any psychotropic drug, EFFEXOR may impair judgment, thinking, or motor skills; patients should be advised to exercise caution until they have adapted to therapy.

Please see brief summary of Prescribing Information on previous page of this advertisement.

Tablets: 25 mg, 37.5 mg, 50 mg, 75 mg, and 100 mg

VENLAFAXINE HCl

EFFEXOR® MEANS EFFECTIVE

Peering Into the 'Black Box'

Measuring Outcomes of Managed Care

Harold Alan Pincus, MD; Deborah A. Zarin, MD; Joyce C. West, MPP

Research on the impact of managed care on access, quality, outcomes, and costs of mental health and substance abuse services has been limited because of the lack of generalizability of studies, the "black box" focus of much of the research, the dynamic changes in mental health and substance abuse managed care, and the proprietary nature of the health care industry. This article provides a framework for understanding the organizational, financial, and procedural features of health plans and the effect of these features on the characteristics and flow of patients through health plans and the selection and utilization of treatments. The diverse research priorities of key stakeholders, ie, public and private purchasers, managed care organizations, providers, and patients and their families, are described along with a broader societal agenda for delineating the outcomes of health care plans. Critical research and methodologic issues in studying the effects of managed care are outlined, including issues related to identifying and selecting appropriate outcome measures and developing appropriate methods for risk adjustment to adequately control for patient selection bias. This article asserts that government, purchasers, health care plans, providers, consumers, and researchers must collaboratively develop resources and research approaches to fully evaluate the effects of managed care. To realize this objective, auspices with reasonable objectivity are needed along with access to necessary data within the black box of health care systems, a cadre of trained investigators, and sufficient research funding, including the development of an all payers fund to support clinical and health services research.

Arch Gen Psychiatry. 1996;53:870-877

In the rapid evolution of health service delivery systems, the US population is an unwitting participant in a massive, uncontrolled health services research experiment. Between 1992 and 1994, the number of Americans covered by a managed behavioral health care plan increased by 38%, from 78 million to 108 million. With an estimated 58% of the insured population now covered by a managed behavioral health care plan,[1] it is essential for policy and clinical planning to obtain systematic information regarding the impact of these changes on the care of patients. Although the profusion of heterogeneous models of care delivery systems provides unique opportunities for capturing this information, the rapidly changing dynamics of the health care marketplace present enormous challenges for developing well-designed studies that will provide data relevant to the systems that will exist by the time these studies are published. To date, information on the impact of managed care on access, quality, outcomes, and costs has been limited because of

1. the "black box" nature of managed care health services research, in which analyses focus on the overall impact of health care plans (eg, aggregate utilization or costs) with little emphasis on examining the role of specific elements of health care plans in influencing outcomes[2,3];

2. lack of generalizability, in large part because much of the research has

From the Office of Research, American Psychiatric Association, Washington, DC.

comprised studies of specific managed care programs (eg, individual state Medicaid managed care demonstration programs or focused clinical studies of specific medical conditions in one type of plan compared with another)[4-6]; this specificity makes it difficult to "map" the plans and the outcomes onto other contexts;

3. the continuing transmutation of "managed care"; as managed care has evolved from Kaiser-Permanente's 1933 health maintenance organization (HMO) archetype,[7] much of the initial managed care research has become obsolete; HMOs of the 1990s do not resemble HMOs of the 1980s and reflect only a segment of managed care of the 1990s; moreover, managed care of the 1990s is unlikely to be representative of managed care in the future;

4. diverse and often divergent perspectives on what issues are most important to study and with what degree of methodologic rigor; the tendency to focus on one part of the elephant while ignoring others is reinforced by the intensely competitive environment[8]; moreover, the proprietary nature of much of the information inhibits full access not only to the methods of managing care, but also to the quality of the research designs and measures used.[3]

In this article, we provide a commonsense framework for studying the clinical impact of managed care in clinical practice. The framework takes into consideration the various organizational, financial, and procedural features that, in turn, are importantly related to the characteristics and flow of patients and features of treatments. We also summarize the perspectives and activities of different stakeholders, discuss research and methodologic issues in studying the effects of managed care, and examine questions of how and by whom this research can be conducted.

FRAMEWORK FOR EXAMINING THE EFFECTS OF HEALTH CARE PLANS

A framework for facilitating research on the clinical impact of managed care and other service delivery systems would examine the effect(s) of different managed care (and other health insurance) arrangements on broadly defined clinical outcomes. The resultant research would identify the "active ingredients" of managed or other health care plans, the mechanism by which they influence care, and the ultimate effects of those influences.

Existing definitions of *managed care* encompass many organizational and financial characteristics of various systems, and various research agendas have been proposed to examine particular facets of given systems.[2,3,9,10] A review of that literature is beyond the scope of this article; rather, we have sought to identify generic influences on the multiple domains of outcome. Factors influencing outcome are depicted in **Figure 1**. In this diagram, the eligible population is exposed to the health care plan (or black box); the outcomes associated with the exposure can then be determined. The black box has 3 structural elements: organizational and contractual arrangements, financial arrangements, and procedural arrangements. These elements (together or separately) can influence clinical outcomes through 2 mechanisms: (1) affecting the flow and characteristics of patients through the plan and/or (2) affecting the selection and utilization of treatments.

ORGANIZATIONAL AND CONTRACTUAL ELEMENTS

Organizational and contractual elements include contractual arrangements between the plan and other health plans, specific treatment settings, providers, and patients.

The Relationship Between Mental Health and General Medical Systems That Serve the Patient

Systems vary with regard to the relationship between mental health and general medical care (reviewed in general by Pincus[11] and, specifically with regard to managed care, by Trabin and Freeman,[12] Dorwart,[13] Mechanic et al,[2] Weiner and de Lissovoy[10]); the degree of integration or separation of health services

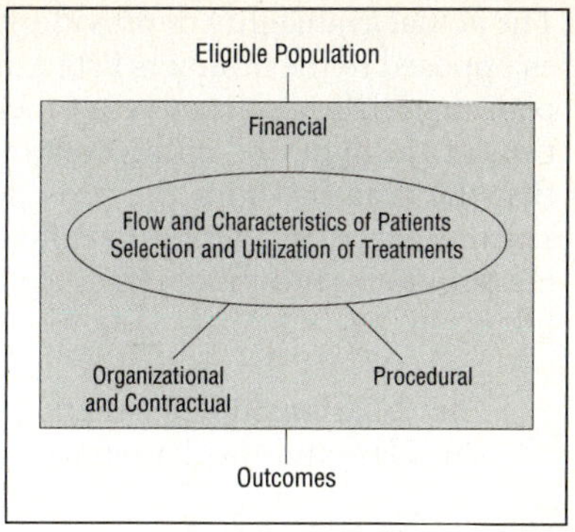

Figure 1. *Examining the "black box" of health care plans.*

that potentially affects clinical care (eg, in such domains as access to specialty mental health care and coordination with general medical care); and costs. When the same system provides both types of services, it is referred to as "integrated."[14] "Carve-out" plans provide mental health services separately from the general health plan that provides the general medical care. "Carve-in" plans maintain separate systems, but within the same corporate infrastructure.[15]

The Relationship Between the Plan and Specific Settings

Some plans are closely affiliated with hospitals, outpatient clinics, and/or other settings. These plans may facilitate access to the settings with which they have close affiliations and discourage or block access to other settings.[16]

The Relationship Between the Plan and the Providers

The numbers and types of providers, as well as the nature of the contractual relationships between the plan and the providers are the principal features of this element. Implicit in this element are the rules for selection, retention, and termination of providers.[9] Within mental health, the ratio of psychiatrists to nonphysician mental health providers and the overall ratio of mental health providers to enrollees vary among plans. In addition, the availability of subspecialists (eg, in addiction psychiatry) and the particular expertise of the plan's providers (eg, in particular forms of psychotherapy) affect the array of services likely to be available to patients.[3,17]

The actual availability of providers, as opposed to the numbers listed in plan materials, also may be a function of the types of arrangements that the plan has with the providers and may affect access to different providers and the services they offer.

The Relationship Between the Plan and the Patients

Different plans have distinctive ways of meeting their obligations to patients concerning choice of provider(s), range of available services, and ease of access to providers and services. Important features include the flexibility in choice of a primary care provider, choice of and access to specialists (eg, presence or absence of a gatekeeper system), and ability to go outside of the plan's provider network entirely (eg, point of service option).

Benefit definitions usually include overall limitations in coverage that typically affect mental health care differently from general medical care (eg, annual limitations in hospital days and outpatient visits in addition to a lifetime limit on total costs).[18] Contractual agreements also may require prior approval for receipt of particularly costly or restricted services (eg, hospitalization).

Although basic services are offered by almost all health plans, variations in the presence and quality of other services influence both the choice of plans by prospective consumers and the range of services received by enrollees. For example, sports medicine facilities, day treatment facilities for persons with severe mental illness, and pharmacy services that include counseling regarding the use of common medications each may appeal to different potential groups of consumers.

FINANCIAL ARRANGEMENTS

Arrangements Between Plans and Providers

The range of payment mechanisms includes fee for service (discounted or not), salaried, capitated, bonuses, withholds, and penalties based on performance.[19] These mechanisms vary with regard to the potential incentives or disincentives that providers may feel with regard to patient care. In addition, arrangements that the plan has with providers concerning the volume of referrals, as well as the criteria for continuation or discontinuation of the contract, may translate into financial pressures that could influence the provider's behavior (eg, plans may exert influence by increasing or decreasing the volume of referrals based on financial or clinical performance criteria).[9,10]

In addition, a variety of arrangements exist at the group level that affect the locus of risk bearing (eg, a group practice that contracts with a managed care organization may have a salaried arrangement, discounted fee-for-service arrangement, or a capitated arrangement). Providers who contract with plans through their groups may be subject to pressures different from those of providers who have individual contracts with plans.[9,10]

Arrangements Between Plans and Patients

The portion of premiums that a given plan requires patients to pay constitutes one form of financial arrangement that is not dependent on individual episodes of care, whereas copayments, deductibles, and other out-of-pocket costs may be required for individual episodes of care or other services (including prescription medications). These costs may vary depending on whether patients see providers within the plan or outside the plan.

PROCEDURAL ARRANGEMENTS

Within the bounds of the contractual agreements between plans and purchasers, a great deal of variation exists in the type and intensity of application of administrative and/or clinical procedures that may affect patients' access to or receipt of services. While these procedures can limit access, they also can expand access to care and improve quality (eg, use of screening tools in primary care).

Procedures That Influence Overall Access to Providers and Treatments

The definition of *medical necessity* frequently forms the basis for decisions regarding access to care.[12,20] In addition, the definition implies acceptable goals of treatment. Plans vary in the degree to which only quite narrow goals (eg, immediate recovery from the acute exacerbation) vs broader goals (eg, optimization of functioning) are considered appropriate.

Although the requirement for precertification for hospitalization is almost ubiquitous, the specific procedures, as well as the scope of other services for which precertification is required (eg, individual psychotherapy), vary widely and influence access.[2,3,10,12] Many plans have specified formularies that restrict the choice of medications. The size and specific content of the formulary will, of course, affect patient care.

Procedures That Influence Access to Specific Providers

Differences exist among plans in the procedures that must be followed before accessing a mental health provider or a specific service. The more steps that are necessary (eg, referral from gatekeeper, prior telephone authorization), the more factors may influence access to care, including the individual incentives or disincentives for providers and patients.

Procedures That Are Designed to Influence Access to Specific Treatments

The term *utilization management* has been used to refer to those procedures that are used by plans to control access to services.[21,22] Common mechanisms include concurrent and retrospective utilization review, high-cost utilization management, and practice guidelines. Garnick et al[23] surveyed 31 mental health and substance abuse managed care utilization review programs in 1990-1991 and found a large variation in the specific utilization review criteria and procedures. Most of the firms reported using explicit clinical criteria to determine whether to authorize an admission or extend days. Many firms would not disclose their criteria; others reported using industrywide length of stay data.

These elements, which are both implicit and explicit, provide a framework for characterizing the various features of managed care and other health care plans that may produce differences in outcomes. The presence of a high copayment (an explicit barrier) and the potential for a loss of confidentiality with one's primary care provider in an integrated system (an implicit barrier) may reduce the overall utilization of mental health services, although the impact of the former is easier to predict than the latter. In either case, the specific mechanisms by which these elements of a managed care plan may influence clinical outcomes are through the flow and characteristics of patients and the selection and utilization of treatments.

THE CHARACTERISTICS AND FLOW OF PATIENTS INTO AND THROUGH THE HEALTH CARE SYSTEM

Variations among health systems will affect the probability of individual patients gaining access to particular providers, settings, and treatments. **Figure 2** schematically illustrates the flow of patients through selected sectors of a health care system. Consideration of the size and composition of these sectors is critical for examining differences in outcomes across health plans. The flow of patients through these sectors may be influenced by the health plan's organizational and contractual, financial, and procedural arrangements such as contractual limitations that exclude preexisting or chronic conditions, gatekeeping arrangements or financial incentives to limit referrals, the use of practice guidelines to promote mental health screening, or review procedures that may raise patients' concerns regarding confidentiality.

Mechanic et al[2] noted that many plans discourage the enrollment of people with severe mental disorders by covering only acute care mental health services and not having an appropriate range of services for those with chronic and severe mental disorders (thereby reducing the number and overall severity within the sector of people with a mental disorder enrolled in the plan).

THE SELECTION AND UTILIZATION OF TREATMENTS

Outcomes are affected not only by the types of patients seen in a health care plan, but by features of treatment as shaped by the policies and practices of a given plan. Such plan-influenced features include not only the modalities (including combinations) of available treatments (eg, medication, psychotherapy) but also their intensity, frequency, and duration. Specific examples of mechanisms that affect the selection and utilization of mental health treatments include organizational factors and contractual factors such as the availability (or unavailability) of specialty treatment providers and settings; financial incentives to limit high-cost treatments; and procedural arrangements, such as utilization management or formulary policies excluding specific medications.

Comparing HMO-enrolled patients with fee-for-service patients, Norquist and Wells[24] found a 40% reduction in use of mental health services by the former, which they attributed to HMO's "less intensive style of care." In the RAND Health Insurance Experiment, which randomly assigned individuals to either prepaid or fee-for-service plans, investigators[25] found that prepaid plan enrollees were likely to have one-third fewer visits than their fee-for-service counterparts and to have received group or family, as opposed to individual, therapy. A first-year evaluation of the Massachusetts mental health and substance abuse managed care program[26] reported a reduction in hospital lengths of stay, and the Medical Outcomes Study[27] found reductions in durations of outpatient treatment for depression among prepaid as opposed to fee-for-service patients. The clinical and other impact of such differential treatment patterns has not been well studied.

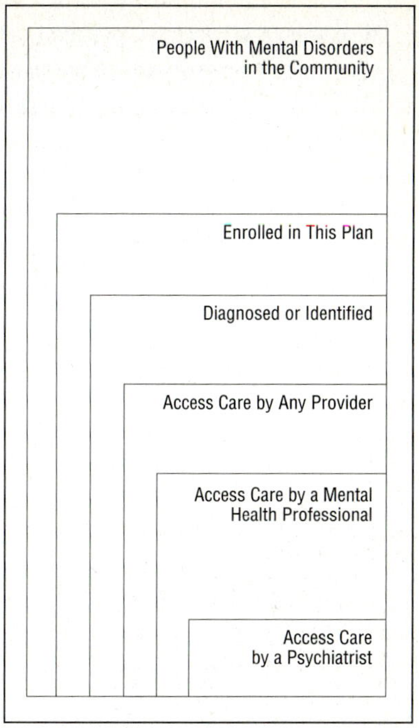

Figure 2. *Issues in measuring access: the flow of patients through a health care plan.*

OUTCOMES FROM DIVERSE PERSPECTIVES: WHO WANTS TO KNOW WHAT?

The effects, or outcomes, of the various processes within the black box of the health care system can be measured across a range of domains (**Table**). For the most part, assessments of managed care selectively reflect the priorities, concerns, and activities of the specific stakeholders in the health care systems: public and private payers, managed care organizations, providers, and patients and their families. Although within each group there is considerable heterogeneity, there also are commonalities (with regard to what is emphasized and what is omitted) that are useful to consider.

Public and Private Purchasers' Perspectives

With managed care, an established mechanism for providing health care in the private sector, the public sector is moving rapidly to apply these approaches for both Medicare and Medicaid populations as well as for services provided under the auspices of state mental health authorities in seeking to ensure the value of their investments, corporate benefits managers, Health Care Financ-

Measuring the Effects of Managed Care: Domains of Measures

Domains of Measures	Examples
Access to care	Proportion of enrollees who utilize mental health services
Use of services	Rates of inpatient, outpatient, or other mental health service utilization
Administrative functioning	Telephone response time, length of time to process claims
Process of care	Adherence to clinical practice guidelines
Consumer satisfaction and choice	Patient and family satisfaction surveys
General mental health status	Global Assessment of Functioning
General health status	Sickness Impact Profile
Functional status (physical, mental, and social functioning)	Medical Outcomes Study SF-36 Health Survey
Quality of life	Lehman Quality of Life Scale
Disorder-specific symptoms and severity	Beck Depression Inventory
Adverse events	Suicide rates or adverse drug reactions
Purchaser health care costs	Short- and long-term health care costs
General medical costs	
Mental health care costs	
Family and patient direct health care costs	Out-of-pocket medical expenses
Family and patient indirect costs	Personal costs such as waiting times, family absenteeism
Employer indirect costs	Worker productivity and absenteeism
Social service costs	Direct costs of social and criminal justice services
Other social costs	Increased crime, domestic violence, and homelessness

ing Administration officials, and state Medicaid and mental health authority directors are all faced with the challenges of monitoring, assessing, and improving the performance of health care plans as well as obtaining reliable, comparable information on the costs and quality of care.[28] In seeking to ensure the value of their investments, purchasers' concerns reflect those of their constituencies (ie, employees or segments of the public for whom they are responsible). Outcomes of interest beyond those related to direct health care costs and the satisfaction and health status of their constituency are related to measures of employee productivity, absenteeism, or broader social contributions of the groups for whom they are responsible.

The Health Employer Data and Information Set (HEDIS)[29] was developed as a tool for large purchasers of health care by the National Committee for Quality Assurance (a nonprofit managed care accrediting organization) and representatives of employers and health plans. The current version (HEDIS 2.5) has more than 60 performance indicators covering quality, access to and satisfaction with care, use of services, finance, and management. Most of the indicators measure administrative performance rather than outcomes of care.[29] The measures specific to mental health are limited to rates of readmission for chemical dependency and rates of follow-up after hospitalization for the treatment of major depressive disorder. A pilot test of the measures showed substantial variation in the indicators across health plans; however, for many of the indicators, it was not clear whether variations among the plans were a reflection of differences in the patient populations or in the quality of care provided.[30] The National Association of State Mental Health Program Directors and the American Behavioral Health Care Association have developed a white paper (unpublished document titled "Public Mental Health Systems, Medicaid Restructuring and Managed Behavioral Healthcare," 1995) advocating standards and policies for best practices for public mental health managed care contracts.

Managed Care Organizations' Perspectives

The questions that most directly confront managed care organizations are those that relate to (1) designing an efficient system (to reduce costs), (2) demonstrating quality (for internal management and marketing purposes), and (3) monitoring the provision of care (to improve quality and cost-effectiveness). Many managed care organizations have developed their own systems for monitoring the care they provide, often as part of continuous quality improvement programs. In this context, the information is fed back not only to managed care administrators but also to providers. Given the intense competition, however, many managed care organizations are reluctant to let outsiders peer into their black box. In addition, managed care organizations may not necessarily use evaluation methods or measures that lend themselves to peer-reviewed research.

The American Managed Behavioral Healthcare Association has, however, recently developed an agreed-on set of performance or "report card" indicators, known as *Performance Measures for Managed Behavioral Healthcare Programs*.[31] The proposed measures assess 3 primary domains relating to access to care, consumer satisfaction, and quality of care for those who utilize a plan's services.

Providers' Perspectives

Individual providers as well as provider groups are under increasing pressure by managed care organizations to reduce costs and utilization. Providers want managed care companies to be judged in terms of the quality of care they are providing, and they want to know which plans are most user-friendly in terms of administrative and clinical practice issues (eg, intrusiveness, rapidity of claims settlements, or availability of treatments).[32] They also want to be evaluated in a fair way (ie, with proper adjustments for the type of patients they see and with an appropriate range of outcome measures). Ideally, such information will be made available in a way that can assist them in improving care, rather than be used in a punitive manner.

A number of provider groups have programs aimed at evaluating and improving the care delivered. The American Psychiatric Association, for example, continues to generate evidence-based practice guidelines that can serve as a basis for developing specific criteria for assessing quality of care.[33-38] In addition to the practice guideline program, the American Psychiatric Association has established a Practice Research Network to serve as a national research infrastructure for the conduct of psychiatric clinical and health services research. The Practice Research Network has received funding from the John D. and Catherine T. MacArthur Foundation to systematically collect and analyze detailed, patient-level data on psychiatric clinical practice patterns and outcomes of care provided by psychiatrists practicing in a broad range of health care settings. This will facilitate comparisons of psychiatric patients, practice patterns, and outcomes of care across health plans.[39]

Patients' and Families' Perspectives

Despite the high prevalence of mental disorders, most members of the public at large do not place the assessment of outcomes for mental disorders among their high-priority questions for evaluating health care plans. Rather, this task has been assumed by patient and family groups, with the support of various government agencies. Patients and families essentially want to keep purchasers, managed care organizations, and providers accountable for providing high-quality care with good results.[40] They want sufficient information to select those plans (or at least influence the selection of plans that purchasers contract with) that provide demonstrably high-quality care with minimal out-of-pocket costs.

The National Alliance for the Mentally Ill and representatives from government, academia, providers, purchasers, consumers, and health plans collaborate through the Outcomes Roundtable project to encourage disorder-specific outcomes assessment of health care plans that emphasize consumer and family perspectives.[41] The federal Center for Mental Health Services through its Mental Health Statistics Improvement Program also has collaborated with consumer and family groups in developing mental health report card indicators that emphasize consumer values and include a broad range of outcome measures.[42]

Broader Societal Perspectives

Importantly, none of these groups represent an overall societal perspective in terms of comprehensively evaluating the full range of costs and outcomes. Each group primarily focuses on the issues facing their specific constituency and the costs they directly incur, eg, private (or even public) purchasers may not have an interest in or responsibility for the impact of health care outcomes on social services or criminal justice costs; carve-out plans may have less interest in general medical offsets than carve-in or integrated plans. It is important that research and policy analyses are geared toward examining the full array of effects of managed care across the broad set of domains noted in the Table. Such an effort is important to place into context specific studies or assessments that selectively examine narrow effects or outcomes of managed care. It is also important for understanding the trade-offs involved in making broader societal decisions that will shape future health care plans.[43,44]

PROBLEMS IN MEASURES AND MEASUREMENT

Selecting Appropriate Measures

As attention to clinical outcomes has expanded, measures for assessing the performance of health care systems also have proliferated. While many measures currently in use, including some adapted from integrated clinical and financial management information systems, have not been subject to formal testing for reliability and validity, efforts are under way to develop a research underpinning for outcome instruments.[45,46] The Center for Mental Health Care Research in Arkansas has developed a number of disorder-specific outcomes modules that are designed to be used in the assessment of outcomes across different types of health plans.[47] The American Psychiatric Association has begun to develop a handbook, *Psychiatric Measures and Outcomes*,[48] to encourage the ongoing, systematic assessment of care with empirically tested measures. The handbook will review measures relevant to psychiatric care, summarizing their psychometric properties and commenting on the advantages and the disadvantages of their use for various applications.

The Problem of Risk Adjustment

Health plan enrollment is not a random process. Such factors as patient age, diagnosis, severity within diagnosis, history (eg, of hospitalizations); general medical and psychiatric comorbidities (eg, personality disorders); and various sociodemographic factors, such as marital and socioeconomic status, extent of social support systems, and patient and family attitudes and preferences, can have direct effects on outcomes irrespective of specific treatment interventions or health care plans.[49-51]

A hypothetical example is seen in 2 health care plans, plan A and plan B, which offer to the same population identical benefits packages, with the singular distinction between the 2 being that plan A's treatment program for schizophrenia is highly specialized, well regarded, and efficient, while plan B's treatment offers no specific program. Plan A would likely attract individuals with schizophrenia, particularly, the more difficult to treat patients, or families who believe that they had members at risk of the illness. As a result, even if plan A were highly efficient in treating high-cost cases of schizophrenia, its mental health costs would be, on average, much higher than plan B's. Moreover, cross-plan comparisons of clinical or functional measures would likely show that plan A enrollees, on average, had worse outcomes than those in plan B, despite plan A's provision of better care for patients with schizophrenia. A fair comparison of the 2 plans would require correcting for case mix in a way that was specific to schizophrenia and could not be easily gamed. Unfortunately, the current technology for making such corrections is limited by inadequacies in the overall database of prognostic factors affecting outcomes. This is true not only for mental disorders but for health conditions generally. Outside of short-term prognostic approaches in critical care medicine (eg, the acute physiology and chronic health evaluation II [APACHE II] system[52]), risk adjustment tools remain at a fairly crude level. Furthermore, there is evidence that generic adjustments are not sufficient.[53] It will be particularly important to develop and apply condition-specific adjustments to achieve accurate representation of outcome.

CONCLUSIONS AND RECOMMENDATIONS

The potential for a relatively large number of factors to exert an influence on clinical outcomes, through a variety of mechanisms, both direct and indirect, makes the researcher's task of describing and comparing health care systems quite complex.[3] Within the mental health field, the problems are compounded by the fact that many disorders, and therefore outcomes, of interest are long-term and require longitudinal studies that are especially costly and difficult. The additional special concerns regarding confidentiality raise other methodologic challenges, including the need to consider out-of-plan care (some of which may be prompted by a concern for confidentiality, implying a likely reluctance to cooperate with some types of research). Finally, the highly competitive market creates an atmosphere in which plans may be reluctant to collaborate or to permit objective study by outside researchers, and may pose questions about the validity of data generated from within.[3]

Despite the complexities involved, it is essential that government, purchasers, health care plans, providers, consumers, and researchers collaboratively develop resources and approaches to move beyond narrow assessments of the temporal epiphenomena of present-day managed care; to examine the mechanisms by which health care systems exert their effects on the health status of individuals and populations; and to extend beyond the narrow interests of individual segments and evaluate the broader effects on society to understand how to improve the system overall.

While the technical barriers are daunting (eg, developing practical and valid measures or improving approaches for risk adjustment), they are not insurmountable. In many ways, more challenging is the question of who will do the research and how will it be supported. The elements for such an effort include auspices with reasonable objectivity, access to necessary data within the black box of health care plans, a cadre of investigators with the essential skills and training, and sufficient funding to conduct the research.

The cooperation of managed care plans and the participation of providers, consumers, and family members are essential. Academic health centers (AHCs) are also critical to such an endeavor. Not only are they the loci of scientific expertise and scholarly objectivity, they also have the role of training and preparing the clinical and health services researchers whose expertise will be needed. Unfortunately, AHCs are at special risk in the newly evolving health care system.[54] Government and private purchasers and payers must consider methods to maintain the academic missions and research infrastructure of AHCs for the development of future investigators and investigations. At the same time, AHCs, in addition to and in the service of making themselves more efficient, must expand their efforts in clinical services and systems research.

The bottom line, however, is the bottom line. Unless there are specific allocations to cover the costs of conducting clinical and health services research, there will no longer be surpluses that can subsidize those efforts. While federal funding and leadership at the National Institute of Mental Health, National Institute on Drug Abuse, National Institute on Alcohol Abuse and Alcoholism, and Agency for Health Care Policy and Research have played a critical role in developing a locus of support for health services and managed care research, the overall level of funding remains quite small. The development of a substantial all payers fund (eg, Harkin Hatfield type legislation[55]) to support clinical and health services research is necessary, not simply to ensure the health of AHCs, but to secure a future of improved health care for all.

Accepted for publication July 2, 1996.

Work on this article was, in part, supported by a grant from the John D. and Catherine T. MacArthur Foundation, New York, NY.

The views of the authors do not necessarily represent the views of the American Psychiatric Association.

Reprints: Harold Alan Pincus, MD, Office of Research, American Psychiatric Association, 1400 K St, NW, Washington, DC 20005.

REFERENCES

1. Oss M. *Managed Behavioral Health Market Share in the United States, 1994.* Gettysburg, Pa: Open Minds; 1995;12.
2. Mechanic D, Schlesinger M, McAlpine DD. Management of mental health and substance abuse services: state of the art and early results. *Milbank Q.* 1995;73:19-55.
3. Wells KB, Astrachan BM, Tischler GL, Unutzer J. Issues and approaches in evaluating managed mental health care. *Milbank Q.* 1995;73:57-75.
4. Wells KB, Hays RD, Burnam A, Rogers W, Greenfield S, Ware JE. Detection of depressive disorder for patients receiving prepaid or fee-for-service care: results from the medical outcomes study. *JAMA.* 1989;262:3298-3302.
5. Lurie N, Moscovice IS, Finch M, Christianson JB, Popkin MK. Does capitation affect the health of the chronically mentally ill? *JAMA.* 1992;267:3300-3304.
6. Christianson JB, Lurie N, Finch M, Moscovice IS, Hartley D. Use of community-based mental health programs by HMOs: evidence from a Medicaid demonstration. *Am J Public Health.* 1992;82:790-806.
7. Flynn DE, McMahon TC, Collins MF. Health maintenance organizations and their implications for psychiatry. *Hosp Community Psychiatry.* 1987;38:255-263.
8. Borenstein DB. A means of rationing psychiatric treatment. *Hosp Community Psychiatry.* 1990;41:1095-1098.
9. Gold M, Nelson L, Lake T, Hurley R, Berenson R. Behind the curve: a critical assessment of how little is known about arrangements between managed care plans and physicians. *Med Care Res Rep.* 1995;52:307-341.
10. Weiner JP, de Lissovoy G. Razing a tower of

Babel: a taxonomy for managed care and health insurance plans. *J Health Polit Policy Law.* 1993; 18:75-103.

11. Pincus HA. Patient-oriented models for linking primary care and mental health care. *Gen Hosp Psychiatry.* 1987;9:95-101.
12. Trabin T, Freeman MA. *Managed Behavioral Healthcare: History, Models, Strategic Challenges and Future Course.* Tiburon, Calif: CentraLink Publishers; 1995.
13. Dorwart RA. Managed mental health care: myths and realities in the 1990s. *Hosp Community Psychiatry.* 1990;10:1087.
14. McFarland BH. Health maintenance organizations and persons with severe mental illness. *Community Ment Health J.* 1994;30:221-242.
15. Frank RG, McGuire TG, Newhouse JP. Risk contracts in managed mental health care. *Health Aff.* 1995;14:50-64.
16. Shortell SM, Gillies RR, Anderson AA. The new world of managed care: creating organized delivery systems. *Health Aff.* 1994;13:5:46-64.
17. Luft HS. How do health-maintenance organizations achieve their 'savings'? *N Engl J Med.* 1978; 298:1336-1343.
18. Grumbach K, Bodenheimer T. Mechanisms for controlling costs. *JAMA.* 1995;273:1223-1230.
19. Gold MR, Hurley R, Lake T, Ensor T, Berenson R. A national survey of the arrangements managed-care plans make with physicians. *N Engl J Med.* 1995;333:1678-1683.
20. Sabin JE, Daniels N. Determining 'medical necessity' in mental health practice. *Hastings Cent Rep.* 1994;24:5-13.
21. Tischler GL. Utilization management and the quality of care. *Hosp Community Psychiatry.* 1990; 41:1099-1102.
22. Hodgkin D. The impact of private utilization management on psychiatric care: a review of the literature. *J Ment Health Admin.* 1991;19:143-157.
23. Garnick DW, Hendricks AM, Dulski JD, Thorpe KE, Horgan C. Characteristics of private-sector managed care for mental health and substance abuse treatment. *Hosp Community Psychiatry.* 1994;45:1201-1205.
24. Norquist GS, Wells KB. How do HMOs reduce outpatient mental health costs? *Am J Psychiatry.* 1991;148:96-101.
25. Manning WG, Wells KB, Benjamin B. *Use of Outpatient Mental Health Care: Trial of a Prepaid Group Practice Versus Fee-for-Service (R-3277-NIMH).* Santa Monica, Calif: RAND; 1986.
26. Callahan JJ, Shepard DS, Beinecke RH, Larson MJ, Cavanaugh D. Mental health/substance abuse treatment in managed care: the Massachusetts Medicaid experience. *Health Aff.* 1995;14:173-184.6
27. Rogers WH, Wells LS, Meredith R, Sturm, Burnam A. Outcomes for adult outpatients with depression under prepaid or fee-for-service financing. *Arch Gen Psychiatry.* 1993;50:517-525.
28. Corrigan JM. How do purchasers develop and use performance measures? *Med Care.* 1995; 33:JS18-JS24.
29. Physician Payment Review Commission. *Prospective Payment Assessment Commission: Joint Report to the Congress on Medicare Managed Care.* Washington, DC: Physician Payment Review Commission; 1995.
30. Epstein A. Performance reports on quality: prototypes, prblems, and prospects. *N Engl J Med.* 1995;333:57-61.
31. American Managed Behavioral Healthcare Association Quality Improvement and Clinical Services Committee. *Performance Measures for Managed Behavioral Healthcare Programs.* Washington, DC: American Managed Behavioral Healthcare Association; 1995.
32. Duval CP. How will physicians respond? *Med Care.* 1995;33:JS31-JS36.
33. American Psychiatric Association. Practice guideline for eating disorders. *Am J Psychiatry.* 1993; 150:212-228.
34. American Psychiatric Association. Practice guideline for major depressive disorder in adults. *Am J Psychiatry.* 1993;150(suppl 4):1-26.
35. American Psychiatric Association. Practice guideline for the treatment of patients with bipolar disorder. *Am J Psychiatry.* 1994;151(suppl12): 1-36.
36. American Psychiatric Association. Practice guideline for treatment of patients with substance use disorders: alcohol, cocaine, opioids. *Am J Psychiatry.* 1995;152(suppl11):1-80.
37. American Psychiatric Association. Practice guideline for psychiatric evaluation of adults. *Am J Psychiatry.* 1995;152(suppl 11):1-80.
38. Zarin DA, Pincus HA, McIntyre JS. Practice guidelines. *Am J Psychiatry.* 1993;150:2.
39. Zarin DA, West JC, Pincus HA, McIntyre JS. The American Psychiatric Association Practice Research Network. In: Sederer LI, Dickey B, eds. *Outcomes Assessment in Clinical Practice.* Baltimore, Md: Williams & Wilkins; 1996:146-156.
40. Ware JE. What information do consumers want and how will they use it? *Med Care.* 1995;33: JS25-JS30.
41. Conference highlights. Conferees agree to include all perspectives in outcomes for mental illness and substance abuse. *Focus.* 1995;7:10.
42. Randal J. Substance Abuse and Mental Health Services Administration launches managed care initiative. *SAMHSA News.* 1995;3:13-14.
43. Krupnick JL, Pincus HA. The cost-effectiveness of psychotherapy: a plan for research. *Am J Psychiatry.* 1992;149:1295-1305.
44. US Congress Office of Technology Assessment. *The Efficacy and Cost Effectiveness of Psychotherapy: The Implications of Cost-Effective Analysis of Medical Technology: Background Paper 3.* Washington, DC: US Government Printing Office; October 1980.
45. Kelley JT. Clinical outcomes measures. *J Clin Outcomes Meas.* 1996;3:59-61.
46. Burlingame GM, Lambert MJ, Reisinger CW, Neff WM, Mosier J. Pragmatics of tracking mental health outcomes in a managed care setting. *J Ment Health Administr.* 1995;22:226-236.
47. Rost K, Smith GR, Burnam MA, Burns BJ. Measuring the outcomes of care for mental health problems. *Med Care.* 1992;30:MS266-MS273.
48. McQueen LE, Rush AJ, Smith GR, Pincus HA. Psychiatric Measures and Outcomes. *Psychiatric Res Rep.* 1996;12:3.
49. Iezzoni LI. Risk adjustment for medical effectiveness research: an overview of conceptual and methodological considerations. *J Invest Med.* 1995;43:136-150.
50. Rost K, Smith GR, Burnam MA, Burns BJ. Measuring the outcomes of care for mental health problems. *Med Care.* 1992;30:MS266-MS273.
51. Maklan CW, Greene R, Cummings MA. Methodological challenges and innovations in patient outcomes research. *Med Care.* 1994;32:JS13-JS21.
52. Knaus WA, Draper EA, Wagner DP, Zimmerman Je. APACHE II: a severity of disease classification system. *Crit Care Med.* 1985;13-818-829.
53. Cleves MA, Golden WE. Assessment of HCFA's 1992 Medicare hospital information report of mortality following admission for hip arthroplasty. *Health Serv Res.* 1996;31:39-46.
54. The academic health care system: preserving the missions as the paradigm shifts. *JAMA.* 1995; 273:549-552.
55. Pincus HA, Ferris S. Taking action. *Psychiatr Res Rep.* 1994;9:2.

1960s:

Conventional antipsychotics radically alter traditional treatment methods

Mass deinstitutionalization

Large-scale shutdown of mental hospitals

Concepts of patient-oriented psychosocial rehabilitation introduced

Discoveries in medicine impact the healthcare system at every level. If the effects of medical breakthroughs are not managed appropriately, the system can sustain significant damage. In the latter half of this century we have seen evidence of this in psychiatry. In the 1960s the introduction of conventional antipsychotics into a weak and rigid system caused severe and long-lasting problems. The advent of atypical agents in the 1990s threatens to do the same. How can we ensure that the existing mental healthcare system is flexible and strong enough to quickly adapt to the changes brought on by the atypicals?

Radical change wrought by conventionals.

The radical changes wrought by haloperidol and other conventional antipsychotics on the mental healthcare system are well documented. Before the introduction of these agents, patients generally experienced limited relief from their episodes of psychosis, and clinicians had few treatment options at their disposal. Conventional antipsychotics offered the first glimmer of hope by providing adequate control of positive symptoms. These agents brought a significant measure of calm and order to previously noisy and chaotic psychiatric wards.

Mass deinstitutionalization recognized as failure.

However, for a variety of social, economic, and political reasons, patients on conventional agents were deinstitutionalized before clinicians could design and implement rehabilitation programs to help them successfully reintegrate into the community. The failure of mass deinstitutionalization is now widely recognized. As all who work with the severely mentally ill know, the effect on many patients and their families has been tragic.

The advent of atypicals: dramatically raising expectations.

Analogous to the introduction of the conventional antipsychotics is the introduction of the atypical agents in the 1990s. Atypical agents, with their control of both positive and negative symptoms, have continued to raise patients' functioning to levels that facilitate reintegration back into the community.

Deficits of system limit potential for recovery.

The ability of the atypicals to restore significant patient functioning has served to highlight the flaws of the system. Often, patients on such therapies begin to outperform all functional expectations before the system is ready to help them develop their newly found skills and abilities.

Compounding the limitations of the mental healthcare system are outdated and misguided community and societal policies, attitudes, and beliefs. These severely restrict the opportunities available to a recovering patient.

System status quo unacceptable.

Clearly, the status quo of the mental healthcare system is unacceptable. Many inside and outside the system are devoted to changing the system, and some progress has been made. However, it is unfair to ask patients, who have already lost significant portions of their lives to mental illness, to wait any longer. Further, dedicated mental healthcare professionals must work within the confines of the system, and they cannot bridge the gaps alone. Finally, families and caregivers often shoulder the burden of providing what the system lacks—too often to the detriment of their own quality of life.

1990s:

Atypical antipsychotics dramatically raise expectations for recovery

Recognition of need to provide support to patient and family

Development of psychosocial rehabilitation programs

Emphasis on permanent reintegration of patients into community

A new approach to managing severe mental illness.

Comprehensive support at multiple levels would benefit patients, their families or caregivers, and professionals. One unique program has recently become available. PATHWAYS TO CHANGE™: managing severe mental illness, is a new comprehensive program of interdisciplinary interventions developed by Janssen Pharmaceutica in conjunction with premier thought leaders in the field. The stated goal of PATHWAYS TO CHANGE™ is to bridge the gaps in the system and raise the standard of care for all persons with severe mental illness.

PATHWAYS TO CHANGE™ is built around a framework known as the systems approach. According to the systems approach, although medication is the cornerstone of successful treatment, therapeutic interventions must occur at multiple levels beyond the adjustment of neuroreceptors for patients to become well, and remain well. Additional interventions must be implemented for patients with severe mental illness, their families and caregivers, the healthcare professionals who treat them, the communities in which they live, and society as a whole.

PATHWAYS TO CHANGE™ interventions.

Consistent with the systems approach model, PATHWAYS TO CHANGE™ interventions address the particular issues at each level that affect patients in their efforts to reach the full potential offered by innovative therapies.

- Following appropriate pharmacotherapy, interventions for patients include support to remain compliant, prevent relapse, maintain continuity of care, and help in their reintegration back into society
- Interventions for families, friends, or caregivers include facilitated access to information, education, and support groups
- Interventions for professionals are designed to help them surmount the challenges of the existing mental healthcare system through programs that enhance patient compliance and aid in patient discharge planning. Other programs will help facilitate case management, provide resources for information, and promote interprofessional collaboration
- Community and societal interventions are geared toward removing any barriers to reintegration. This is accomplished through support of patient advocacy organizations, public awareness, education, and antidiscrimination campaigns. An example of a societal-level intervention is NAMI's recently launched *Open Your Mind* campaign, for which Janssen Pharmaceutica is providing continuing support.

It is only through support provided by these multilevel interventions that the patient with severe and persistent mental illness can successfully reintegrate into the community.

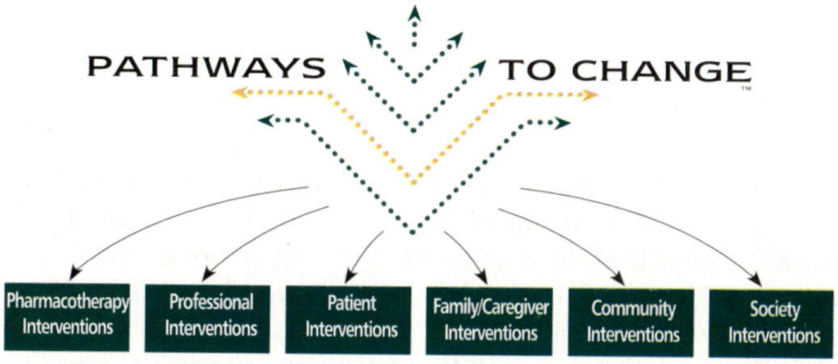

A comprehensive model of interdisciplinary interventions

Meeting the challenges of an evolving system.

We are experiencing an exciting and challenging revolution in the mental healthcare field. The pharmacologic breakthroughs we were waiting for have finally come, offering our patients the first real chance at reclaiming their lives. This revolution, however, is occurring in an atmosphere of cost-containment. We should be ever mindful to take full advantage of programs that provide comprehensive support to reintegrating patients. Indeed, such programs may become our most valuable tools as we meet the challenges of an evolving system.

Subthreshold Psychiatric Symptoms in a Primary Care Group Practice

Mark Olfson, MD, MPH; W. Eugene Broadhead, MD, PhD; Myrna M. Weissman, PhD; Andrew C. Leon, PhD; Leslie Farber, PhD; Christina Hoven, PhD; Roger Kathol, MD

Background: The authors define 6 groups of subthreshold psychiatric symptoms that do not meet the full criteria for a *DSM-IV* Axis I disorder and examine the clinical significance of these symptoms in an outpatient primary care sample.

Methods: The subjects were 1001 adult primary care patients in a large health maintenance organization. Data on sociodemographic characteristics and functional impairment, including scores on the Sheehan Disability Scale, were collected at the time of the medical visit, and a structured diagnostic interview for *DSM-IV* disorders was completed by telephone within 4 days of the visit. Subthreshold symptoms were defined for depressive, anxiety, panic, obsessive-compulsive, drug, and alcohol symptoms.

Results: Subthreshold symptoms were as or more common than their respective Axis I disorders: panic (10.5% vs 4.8%), depression (9.1% vs 7.3%), anxiety (6.6% vs 3.7%), obsessive-compulsive (5.8% vs 1.4%), and alcohol (5.3% vs 5.2%) and other drug (3.7% vs 2.4%) cases. Patients with each of the subthreshold symptoms had significantly higher Sheehan Disability Scale scores (greater impairment) than did patients with no psychiatric symptoms. Many patients (22.6%-53.4%) with subthreshold symptoms also met the full criteria for other Axis I disorders. After adjusting for the confounding effects of other Axis I disorders, other subthreshold symptoms, age, sex, race, marital status, and perceived physical health status, only depressive symptoms, major depressive disorder, and, to a lesser extent, panic symptoms were significantly correlated with the impairment measures.

Conclusions: In these primary care patients, the morbidity of subthreshold symptoms was often explained by confounding mental, physical, or demographic factors. However, depressive symptoms and, to a lesser extent, panic symptoms were disabling even after controlling for these factors. Primary care clinicians who detect subthreshold psychiatric symptoms should consider a broad psychiatric assessment.

Arch Gen Psychiatry. 1996;53:880-886

From the Department of Psychiatry, College of Physicians and Surgeons of Columbia University and New York State Psychiatric Institute, New York (Drs Olfson, Weissman, and Hoven); the Department of Family Medicine, Family Healthcare Centers, Danville, Va (Dr Broadhead); the Department of Psychiatry, Cornell University Medical College, New York, NY (Dr Leon); the Department of Medicine, Kaiser Permanente Medical Center of Oakland, Oakland, Calif (Dr Farber); and the Department of Psychiatry, University of Iowa School of Medicine, Iowa City (Dr Kathol).

CURRENT classification systems of mental disorders have been strongly influenced by descriptions of psychiatric inpatients.[1] The relevance of these definitions has not been established for primary care patients who often present with a different and less severe constellation of psychiatric symptoms.[2,3] In 1 primary care practice, for example, mild depression and mixed anxiety-depression were more common than any specific mental disorder.[4] Such findings have fueled interest in clarifying the clinical status of primary care patients with significant psychiatric symptoms that fall below the threshold criteria for a mental disorder.[5-8]

Subthreshold depressive symptoms have received the greatest attention. Researchers have studied the prevalence,[4,9] family history,[10] course of illness,[11] and extent of impairment associated with subthreshold depressive symptoms. Adults with subthreshold depressive symptoms report more medical comorbidity,[7] days lost from work,[12,13] mental health visits,[12] suicide attempts,[14] and poorer functional status[15] than do individuals without these symptoms. Patients with depressive symptoms that are insufficient to meet the depressive disorder criteria also have poorer social and role functioning than do patients with several common general medical conditions.[16]

Much less is known about subthreshold forms of other mental disorders. However, some data indicate that low-grade

See Materials and Methods on next page

MATERIALS AND METHODS

The data in this report were collected between May and September 1994 at the Department of Medicine, Kaiser Permanente Medical Center, Oakland, Calif, for a study of the Symptom-Driven Diagnostic System for Primary Care.

PROTOCOL

A random sample of patients with prescheduled appointments at the Department of Medicine, Kaiser Permanente Medical Center, were invited to participate in the study. Eligible patients included consecutive new and continuing patients who had appointments set at least 3 days in advance, were between 18 and 70 years of age, could read and write English, and were scheduled for face-to-face contact with their primary care physician. Only patients who signed an informed consent form were enrolled in the study.

A total of 1001 patients participated. This represented 40% of the 2530 patients who were offered participation in a previsit telephone call and 70% of 1435 who initially agreed to participate. Lack of time was the most common reason for declining participation at the previsit call; failure to arrive on time for the appointment and missing the appointment were the most common reasons for not participating at the visit.

Study subjects were compared with a simple random sample of 5005 patients who were drawn from the same population of clinic visits. The study and random sample of patients were similar in regard to age (mean age, 49.2 vs 49.7 years), sex (female, 63.0% vs 58.1%), the number of general medical visits in the past year (4.2 vs 4.2), and the percentage who had ever been seen in the Department of Psychiatry, Kaiser Permanente Medical Center of Oakland (12.1% vs 12.7%).

DEMOGRAPHICS AND ASSESSMENT

Patients who met the prescreening eligibility criteria were invited to report to the clinic 30 minutes prior to their regularly scheduled appointment. At intake, patients completed a history form that included demographic, medical, mental health service, and impairment items. Impairment was measured with the Sheehan Disability Scale (SDS),[29] which was a composite of 3 self-rated 10-point (0=none, 1-3=mild, 4-6=moderate, 7-9=marked, and 10=extreme) Likert response items to assess work, family, and social functioning during the last month. Three impairment items from the Epidemiologic Catchment Area study of the National Institute of Mental Health, Rockville, Md,[30] were used to self-rate "emotional health," "getting along with your partner," and whether patients had missed work because of emotional problems during the last month. A related question queried overall physical health in the past month (excellent, good, fair, or poor).

Patients were also asked if during the last month they had discussed an emotional problem with their physician, talked to a psychiatrist, psychologist, psychotherapist, social worker, family therapist, or drug counselor, or had been to a meeting of Alcoholics Anonymous. A positive response to any of these questions was considered as use of recent mental health care.

TELEPHONE-STRUCTURED INTERVIEW

Within 4 days following the index medical visit, a mental health professional contacted each subject by telephone to administer the Structured Clinical Interview for *DSM-III-R*[31] that was modified to *DSM-IV*[32] criteria. Thirteen mental health professionals (8 psychiatrists and 5 nonphysicians with extensive mental health care experience) were trained to administer the structured interviews. One hundred randomly selected audiotaped interviews were blindly rated by the investigators. Because of low within-rater base rates and nearly complete agreement (all diagnoses in 91.6% of the cases) between raters and reviewers, the Cohen κ statistic was frequently undefined.[33]

Eighty-four percent of the structured interviews were completed within 2 days, and 100% were completed within 4 days following the index medical visit. The structured interview covered MDD, panic disorder, GAD, OCD, and

Continued on next page

symptoms of panic,[17,18] somatization,[19] and alcohol[20,21] and drug[22,23] disorders are associated with significant impairment or medical morbidity.

Psychiatric comorbidity (ie, the existence of multiple mental disorders in the same individual) is common in clinical[24,25] and community[26,27] samples. This phenomenon complicates the attribution of functional impairment to specific mental disorders. The assessment and attribution of functional impairment are important because treatment decisions are commonly based on clinical decisions that concern the "primary" disorder. The potentially confounding effects of comorbid mental disorders have received only scant attention in the developing literature on subthreshold psychiatric symptoms.[28]

We describe the current functioning of a group of primary care patients with psychiatric symptoms who failed to meet the full diagnostic criteria for major depressive disorder (MDD), panic disorder, generalized anxiety disorder (GAD), obsessive-compulsive disorder (OCD), alcohol abuse or dependence, or drug abuse or dependence. We examine the functional impairment associated with these symptoms first without and then with statistical adjustment for possible confounding factors.

RESULTS

Demographic characteristics of the subjects are presented in **Table 1**. The sample was predominantly female, married or living with someone, and between 35 and 65 years of age. The sample was also racially diverse, and most of the subjects had completed at least some college education. A majority of the subjects reported that their total annual family income was between $25 000 and $69 999.

A total of 30.1% (n=301) of the patients met the criteria for subthreshold symptoms. Many of these patients (38.9% [n=117]) also met the criteria for an Axis I mental disorder.

alcohol and substance abuse or dependence. A shorter structured interview based on *DSM* criteria, namely, the Mini-International Neuropsychiatric Interview, was also administered to diagnose current mania, anorexia nervosa, bulimia nervosa, posttraumatic stress disorder, and antisocial personality disorder.[34] Previous research has demonstrated a high concordance between the Mini-International Neuropsychiatric Interview and the Structured Clinical Interview for *DSM-III-R* for these diagnoses (unweighted κ range, 0.67-0.90).[35]

DEFINITIONS OF SUBTHRESHOLD MENTAL SYMPTOMS

Key symptoms from the revised Structured Clinical Interview for *DSM-III-R* were selected from each of 6 mental disorders to define related subthreshold symptoms. Each subthreshold condition was defined to exclude the Axis I disorder from which it was derived.

Subthreshold symptoms were operationally defined as follows:

1. The depressive symptoms required a depressed mood or anhedonia for at least 2 weeks during the last month, but these symptoms excluded patients who met the full criteria for MDD.
2. The panic symptoms required recurrent unexpected discrete episodes of intense fear during the past month, but these symptoms excluded patients who met the full criteria for panic disorder.
3. The anxiety symptoms required excessive anxiety and worry for the past 6 months, but these symptoms excluded patients who met the full criteria for GAD.
4. The OCD symptoms required ever having been either bothered by recurrent or persistent thoughts or engaging in repetitive behaviors that the patient felt driven to perform, but these symptoms excluded patients who met the full criteria for OCD.
5. The alcohol symptoms required 1 or more of the following during the past year: tolerance of alcohol; characteristic withdrawal symptoms from alcohol; taking larger amounts of alcohol over time; unsuccessful attempts to cut down on the consumption of alcohol; spending a lot of time obtaining alcohol; giving up social, work, or leisure activities because of alcohol; and continuing to drink despite knowledge that alcohol was a problem for the patient; however, these symptoms excluded patients who met the full criteria for alcohol abuse or dependence.
6. The drug symptoms were the same as the alcohol symptoms, except that the substance was a drug. Drug classes include stimulants, cannabis, cocaine, hallucinogens, phencyclidine, sedatives or hypnotics, inhalants, opiates, and steroids.

Comparisons were conducted among (1) patients with a mental disorder, (2) patients with related subthreshold symptoms, and (3) patients without mental disorders or subthreshold symptoms (ie, no symptoms).

STATISTICAL METHODS

Between-group comparisons of categoric variables were made with the χ^2 test, except when the expected cell size fell below 5 in which case the Fisher exact test was used. Following significant omnibus χ^2 tests (α=.01, 2-tailed test), data were partitioned, and internal comparisons were made with the χ^2 tests (α=.01, 2-tailed test).

Analysis of variance was used to compare patients with mental disorders, subthreshold symptoms, and no psychiatric symptoms on the SDS within diagnostic categories. Significant omnibus F tests (α=.01) were followed with the Scheffé post hoc test for pairwise comparisons (α=.01).

Multivariate analyses were used to examine associations of each disorder and symptom, with the impairment measures controlling for demographic and clinical factors. The 5 disorders, 5 subthreshold symptoms, patient age, sex, race, marital status, and perceived physical health status were entered as independent variables in logistic regression analyses to examine the strength of associations with the categoric impairment measures. Multiple linear regression was used to examine associations of these independent variables with SDS scores.

DEPRESSIVE SYMPTOMS

The criteria for depressive symptoms were met by 9.1% of the sample. Patients with depressive symptoms (mean age, 45.6 years; SD, 12.3 years) were similar in age to patients with MDD (mean age, 44.4 years; SD, 12.2 years), but they were younger than patients with no symptoms (mean age, 51.4 years; SD, 12.9 years) (F=16.1; df=2, 767; P<.01). Compared with patients who had MDD, patients with depressive symptoms were more likely to be male (24.0% vs 13.7%, χ^2=8.2, df=1, P<.01). Patients with depressive symptoms were less likely than those with no symptoms to report annual family incomes of at least $40 000 (18.2% vs 45.4%, χ^2=23.3, df=1, P<.001). There were no other significant sociodemographic differences among the 3 groups (data not shown).

Patients with depressive symptoms had greater SDS impairment than did patients with no psychiatric symptoms, and they were more likely to report a recent loss of work for mental health reasons, marital distress, and use of mental health services (**Table 2**).

Approximately one third (33.0% [n=30]) of patients with depressive symptoms met the full criteria for another mental disorder. Drug abuse or dependence (n=8) was the most commonly associated disorder. After adjusting for age, sex, race, marital status, perceived physical health status, other mental disorders, and subthreshold symptoms, patients with depressive symptoms were at an estimated 7.7 times increased risk for marital distress and 2.5 times increased risk for a recent loss of work and utilization of mental health services. There was a significant positive association between depressive symptoms and the SDS score after adjusting for the other demographic and clinical variables.

PANIC SYMPTOMS

Approximately one tenth (10.5%) of the sample met the criteria for panic symptoms. A significantly larger proportion of patients with panic symptoms (41.9%) than panic disorder (14.6%) were males (χ^2=11.1, *df*=1, *P*<.001).

Patients with panic symptoms had higher SDS scores than did patients with no symptoms, and they were significantly more likely to report a recent loss of work and utilization of mental health services (Table 2). Many of the patients (41.9% [n=44]) with panic symptoms met the full criteria for another mental disorder. Major depressive disorder (n=11) and alcohol abuse or dependence (n=8) were the most commonly associated disorders. Patients with panic symptoms were more than twice as likely to report recent marital distress and utilization of mental health services (adjusted odds ratios of 2.3 for each, **Table 3**).

ANXIETY SYMPTOMS

Anxiety symptoms were reported by 6.6% of the sample. These patients (mean age, 42.3 years; SD, 11.8 years), and those with GAD (mean age, 41.8 years; SD, 9.7 years) were significantly younger than the patients with no psychiatric symptoms (mean age, 51.4 years; SD, 12.9 years) (F=23.5; *df*=2, 706; *P*<.01). The 3 groups did not otherwise significantly differ with respect to sociodemographic composition (data not shown).

Patients with anxiety symptoms were less impaired than were the patients with GAD, but they were more impaired than those with no symptoms by using the SDS (Table 2). Patients with anxiety symptoms were also significantly more likely than patients with no symptoms to report a recent loss of work, marital distress, and utilization of mental health services (Table 2).

Approximately half of the patients with anxiety symptoms met the full criteria for another mental disorder (48.5% [n=32]). Posttraumatic stress disorder (n=8) and MDD (n=7) were the most commonly associated disorders. No significant associations between anxiety symptoms and the various impairment measures were observed following adjustment for possible confounding factors (Table 3).

OCD SYMPTOMS

The sample included 58 patients (5.8%) who met the criteria for OCD symptoms. Patients with OCD symptoms did not significantly differ either from patients with OCD or those with no symptoms with respect to sociodemographic composition (data not shown). However, patients with OCD symptoms were significantly more impaired than were patients with no symptoms on each of the impairment measures (Table 2).

Most of the patients with OCD symptoms (53.4% [n=31]) met the full criteria for a mental disorder, and many patients (37.9%) met the criteria for more than 1 disorder. Mania (n=8), MDD (n=6), and posttraumatic stress disorder (n=6) were the most commonly associated disorders. After adjusting for the potentially confounding effects of patient age, sex, race, marital status, perceived health status, and other mental conditions, there were no significant correlations between OCD symptoms and each impairment measure (Table 3).

Table 1. Sociodemographic Characteristics of Primary Care Sample*

Characteristic	No. (%) of Sample (N=1001)
Sex	
F	62.7 (628)
M	37.3 (373)
Race	
White	37.1 (371)
Black	47.4 (474)
Other	15.5 (155)
Marital status	
Married	53.5 (535)
Living with someone	7.3 (73)
Never married	14.9 (149)
Separated /divorced	18.8 (188)
Widowed	5.6 (56)
Education	
<8th grade	2.6 (26)
9th-11th grade	6.1 (61)
High school graduate	14.6 (146)
Some college	41.5 (415)
College graduate	35.3 (353)
Income, $	
<15 000	13.6 (126)
<15 000-24 999	16.4 (159)
25 000-39 999	27.5 (267)
40 000-69 999	29.2 (284)
≥70 000	13.9 (135)
Mean (SD) age, y	49.4 (12.8)

**Income data were missing for 30 patients and race was missing for 1 patient.*

DRUG USE SYMPTOMS

Drug use symptoms were reported by 3.7% of the sample. The mean age of patients with drug use symptoms (mean age, 45.5 years; SD, 13.2 years) was between that of patients with drug use disorders (mean age, 40.3 years; SD, 10.9 years) and patients with no psychiatric symptoms (mean age, 51.4 years; SD, 12.9 years) (F=11.9; *df*=2, 664; *P*<.01). A larger proportion of patients with drug use disorders (66.7%) than drug use symptoms (40.5%) were male (χ^2=4.0, *df*=2, *P*<.05).

Patients with drug use symptoms had significantly higher SDS scores than did patients with no psychiatric symptoms (Table 2). Several of the patients with drug use symptoms (37.8% [n=14]) met the criteria for a comorbid mental disorder—most commonly, alcohol abuse or dependence (n=4) or MDD (n=4). The associations between drug use symptoms and SDS scores were not significant after adjustment for patient age, sex, race, marital status, perceived health status, and other mental disorders or symptoms (Table 3).

ALCOHOL USE SYMPTOMS

Alcohol use symptoms were reported by 5.3% of the patients. Compared with patients who had no symptoms, patients with alcohol use symptoms included proportionately more white persons (57.1% vs 36.0%) (χ^2=10.1, *df*=1, *P*<.005), males (57.1% vs 35.3%, *df*=1, χ^2=12.0,

Table 2. Disability in Primary Care Patients With Mental Disorders and Subthreshold Symptoms*

Group No., Description†	SDS Score, Mean (SD)	F (Pairwise Comparison)‡	Loss of Work: % of Patients	Loss of Work: χ^2§ (Comparison)	Marital Distress: % of Patients	Marital Distress: χ^2§ (Comparison)	MH Visit in Past Month: % of Patients	MH Visit in Past Month: χ^2§ (Comparison)
Depression								
1, MDD (n=73)	16.0 (7.9)	207.4	50.7	82.3	33.3	41.1	37.0	64.3
2, Depressive symptoms (n=91)	13.8 (8.5)	(1, 2>3)	40.7	(1, 2>3)	19.7	(1, 2>3)	30.8	(1, 2>3)
Panic								
1, Disorder (n=48)	13.1 (9.8)	73.4	37.5	26.6	21.2	9.6	39.6	50.5
2, Symptoms (n=105)	9.1 (8.2)	(1>2>3)	26.7	(1, 2>3)	11.8	(1>3)	24.8	(1, 2>3)
Anxiety								
1, GAD (n=37)	16.2 (8.4)	112.5	51.4	56.8	15.4	12.6	37.8	35.9
2, Symptoms (n=66)	10.9 (7.5)	(1>2>3)	39.4	(1, 2>3)	20.8	(2>3)	22.7	(1, 2>3)
OCD								
1, Disorder (n=14)	15.6 (10.5)	61.4	35.7	14.7	8.3	12.1	28.6	33.2
2, Symptoms (n=58)	11.1 (9.5)	(1, 2>3)	29.3	(2>3)	22.5	(2>3)	32.8	(2>3)
Drug use								
1, Disorder (n=24)	12.1 (8.3)	33.8	33.3	9.9	6.7		37.5	21.2
2, Symptoms (n=37)	8.4 (7.5)	(1, 2>3)	24.3	(1>3)	11.5	. . .	16.2	(1>3)
Alcohol use								
1, Disorder (n=52)	10.5 (8.4)	35.3	34.6	17.3	7.7		28.8	22.1
2, Symptoms (n=53)	6.8 (6.5)	(1>2>3)	20.8	(1>3)	11.1	. . .	18.9	(1>3)
3, No symptoms (n=606)	3.9 (5.4)	. . .	13.5	. . .	6.8	. . .	9.1	. . .

*SDS indicates Sheehan Disability Scale; MH, mental health; MDD, major depressive disorder; GAD, generalized anxiety disorder; and OCD, obsessive-compulsive disorder.

†See text for definition of mental disorders and subthreshold symptoms. The SDS has a possible score range of 0 to 30, with higher scores representing greater impairment. All comparisons include "no symptoms" as group 3.

‡Omnibus F test was followed by Scheffé post hoc test for pairwise comparisons with .01 significance level.

§Omnibus χ^2 tests ($P<.01$) were followed by χ^2 test on partitioned cells ($P<.01$).

$P<.001$), unmarried persons (64.3% vs 44.7%, $df=1$, $\chi^2=8.2$, $P<.01$), and college graduates (48.2% vs 34.8%, $df=1$, $\chi^2=4.5$, $P<.05$). Patients with alcohol use symptoms had significantly greater SDS impairment than did patients with no symptoms (Tables 2).

Twelve patients with alcohol use symptoms met the full criteria for another mental disorder that was most commonly drug abuse or dependence (n=9). No significant associations between drug use symptoms and impairment measures were observed in the multivariate analyses (Table 3).

COMMENT

More than one quarter of our primary care sample reported psychiatric symptoms that fell below the *DSM-IV* threshold for the diagnosis of MDD, OCD, GAD, panic disorder, drug abuse or dependence, or alcohol abuse or dependence. Patients with each type of subthreshold symptom reported significant impairment in work, family, and social function.

What is the clinical significance of psychiatric symptoms in primary care patients who do not meet the full criteria for a mental disorder? Oftentimes, the answer may involve other comorbid psychiatric disorders and symptoms. We found that patients with subthreshold psychiatric symptoms for 1 disorder commonly met the full diagnostic criteria for another disorder. After adjusting for the confounding effects of other psychiatric disorders and symptoms, as well as patient demographic and health status, most of the subthreshold symptoms were no longer strongly associated with impairment.

Depressive symptoms and, to a lesser extent, panic symptoms were exceptions to this general pattern. Even after controlling for several possible confounding variables, depressive symptoms were significantly correlated with impairment in social, family, and work functioning, and panic symptoms were significantly associated with a loss of work and utilization of mental health services. Among the Axis I disorders, only MDD was significantly associated with impaired functioning after controlling for other factors. These findings support the criterion validity of depressive symptoms, major depression, and panic symptoms as distinct diagnostic entities in primary care.

Prospective epidemiologic[13,36] and clinical[37] research suggests that patients with subthreshold depressive symptoms are at an increased risk for the development of major depression,[14] and are likely to report a history of major depression.[13] However, primary care patients with subthreshold depressive symptoms may represent a highly heterogeneous group. They may include individuals with partially remitted or prodromal major depressive symptoms, a transient adjustment to a stressful life event, symptoms that are secondary to a general medical illness, or a recurrent brief depressive condition.[8,38] Detailed clinical assessments are required to distinguish and characterize these various subgroups.

Few empiric data exist to inform how or whether to treat patients with subthreshold depressive or panic symptoms. For depression, the efficacy of pharmacologic[39] and brief psychotherapeutic[39,40] interventions may be greater in patients with a higher illness severity. At the same time, however, the efficacy of maintenance treatment is well established for patients with histories of major depressive episodes[41] and

Table 3. Associations Among Mental Disorders, Subthreshold Symptoms, and Impairment Measures*

Condition	SDS Score†	Adjusted OR (95% CI) Loss of Work	Marital Distress	MH Visit in Past Month
Depression				
MDD	8.95‡	2.4 (1.4-4.2)	2.6 (1.2-5.7)	2.4 (1.4-4.2)
Symptoms	6.94‡	2.5 (1.2-5.0)	7.7 (3.1-18.9)	2.5 (1.2-5.0)
Panic				
Disorder	1.26	1.5 (0.9-2.6)	0.8 (0.3-2.0)	1.5 (0.9-4.2)
Symptoms	1.06	2.3 (1.1-4.7)	1.0 (0.3-3.1)	2.3 (1.2-3.9)
Anxiety				
GAD	2.24	1.0 (0.5-2.1)	1.1 (0.4-2.7)	1.0 (0.5-2.1)
Symptoms	1.94	1.1 (0.5-2.8)	0.3 (0.1-1.2)	1.1 (0.5-2.8)
OCD				
Disorder	2.79	1.7 (0.9-3.3)	1.6 (0.6-4.1)	1.7 (0.9-2.7)
Symptoms	0.98	0.9 (0.2-3.2)	0.3 (0.0-2.5)	0.9 (0.2-1.7)
Alcohol use				
Disorder	1.74	1.1 (0.5-2.4)	1.2 (0.4-3.9)	1.1 (0.5-2.4)
Symptoms	0.26	1.5 (0.7-3.2)	0.5 (0.1-1.9)	1.5 (0.7-3.2)
Drug use				
Disorder	1.97	0.7 (0.3-1.7)	1.1 (0.3-4.0)	0.7 (0.3-1.7)
Symptoms	0.25	1.6 (0.6-4.5)	0.5 (0.1-5.6)	1.6 (0.6-4.5)

**SDS indicates Sheehan Disability Scale; OR, odds ratio; CI, confidence interval; MH, mental health; MDD, major depressive disorder; GAD, generalized anxiety disorder; and OCD, obsessive-compulsive disorder. See text for definition of mental disorders and subthreshold symptoms. Data are from a multiple regression (SDS score) and logistic regressions (loss of work, marital distress, and MH visit). Results are controlled for patient age, sex, race, marital status, and perceived physical health status.*

†$R^2=0.37$.

‡$P<.01$.

panic disorder,[42] and the availability of antidepressants with few side effects provide a rational basis for revisiting the possibility that some less severely ill depressed patients[43] and patients with subthreshold panic symptoms may benefit from such treatment.

The current findings are constrained by several limitations in the study design. First, collection of the disability data preceded, by up to 4 days, collection of the diagnostic data and psychiatric symptoms. This gap in timing may have attenuated correlations between the diagnostic and disability data. Second, the diagnostic interviews were conducted over the telephone rather than in person. The emerging literature suggests that there is generally good agreement between these 2 modes of interview administration.[44-47] However, illicit drug use may be underreported in telephone interviews.[48] Third, the study was conducted with patients from a large, urban, prepaid internal medicine practice; thus, the findings from this study may not necessarily generalize to primary care patients in other settings or to population-based samples. Fourth, the definition of subthreshold symptoms was relatively broad. While such broad definitions refer to larger numbers of patients, higher levels of impairment would have been found with more narrow definitions of subthreshold symptoms. Fifth, patients were only examined for the most prevalent disorders, but not for the full range of *DSM-IV* disorders. A more comprehensive diagnostic interview would be expected to uncover even higher rates of psychiatric comorbidity. Sixth, a substantial number of patients refused to participate in the study. Although we cannot be certain of the effect of nonresponse on the observed rates of subthreshold psychiatric symptoms, the finding that subjects were similar in demographic composition and prior psychiatric visits to a simple random sample from the primary care population suggests that such nonresponse did not seriously bias the findings.

Primary care patients commonly report psychiatric symptoms that do not reach the diagnostic threshold. The challenge of caring for such patients is complicated by the lack of current consensus concerning their diagnostic status and a dearth of well-established treatment guidelines. Under these conditions, busy primary care clinicians may be tempted to dismiss subthreshold psychiatric symptoms as transient and inconsequential. However, the very patients who exhibit subthreshold symptoms of 1 mental disorder may well meet the criteria for another disorder or exhibit substantial functional impairment. For this reason, clinicians who detect subthreshold symptoms should consider a broader psychiatric assessment.

Accepted for publication April 2, 1996.

Dr Broadhead was the principal investigator (1992-1994) of this project and was succeeded by Dr Kathol in 1995. The Upjohn Company, Kalamazoo, Mich, sponsored and supported the development of the Symptom-Driven Diagnostic System for Primary Care through its Pharmacosurveillance Unit and the work of James A. Coleman, director, and Andreas Pleil, PhD, senior health care economist. Carrie Miller, PhD, was the project manager at the Kaiser Permanente Medical Center. Lena Verdeli, MA, MSc, trained the nurses at the Kaiser Permanente Medical Center. Laura Portera and Joy Pelayo assisted in the data analysis and data management, respectively. Participating physicians at the Kaiser Permanente Medical Center included Harry Fung, MD; Stephen Hawkins, MD; Aguia

Heath, MD; Eric Lipsitt, MD; Julia Morial, MD; Janice Murota, MD; David Popkin, MD; Mark Robinson, MD; Gwynn Simon, MD; Linda Skory, MD; Ronald Yeun, MD; and Juanita Yan, MD. Participating nurses at the Kaiser Permanente Medical Center included Ann Chrisler, RN; Jackie Elshire, RN; Daneen Fortner, RN; Helen Neville, RN; Laura Perry, RN; and Barbara Tompkins, RN.

Corresponding author: Mark Olfson, MD, MPH, Department of Psychiatry, College of Physicians and Surgeons of Columbia University, 722 W 168th St, New York, NY 10032.

REFERENCES

1. Wilson M. *DSM-III* and the transformation of American psychiatry: a history. *Am J Psychiatry.* 1993:150:399-410.
2. Cooper JE. The classification of mental disorders for use in general settings. In: Sartorius N, Goldberg D, de Girolamo G, eds. *Psychological Disorders in General Medical Settings.* Toronto, Ontario: Hogrefe & Huber Publishers; 1990: 49-59.
3. American Psychiatric Association. *Diagnostic and Statistical Manual of Mental Disorders, Fourth Edition, Primary Care Version (*DSM-IV-*PC).* Washington, DC: American Psychiatric Association Press; 1995.
4. Barrett JE, Barrett HA, Oxman TE, Gerber PD. The prevalence of psychiatric disorders in a primary care practice. *Arch Gen Psychiatry.* 1988;45:1100-1106.
5. Jaffe A, Froom J, Galambos N. Minor depression and functional impairment. *Arch Fam Med.* 1994;3:1081-1086.
6. Snaith RP. The concepts of mild depression. *Br J Psychiatry.* 1987;150:387-393.
7. Coulehan JL, Schulberg HC, Block MR, Janosky JE, Arena VC. Depressive symptomatology and medical co-morbidity in a primary care clinic. *Int J Psychiatry Med.* 1990;20:335-347.
8. Sherbourne CD, Wells KB, Hays RD, Rogers W, Burnam MA, Judd LL. Subthreshold depression and depressive disorder: clinical characteristics of general medical and mental health specialty outpatients. *Am J Psychiatry.* 1994; 151:1777-1784.
9. Judd LL, Rapaport MH, Paulus MP, Brown JL. Subsyndromal symptomatic depression: a new mood disorder? *J Clin Psychiatry.* 1994;55:18S-28S.
10. Philipp M. The risk of minor depression in families of probands with major depression: sex differences and familiality. *Eur Arch Psychiatry Clin Neurosci.* 1992;242:89-92.
11. Katon W, Lin E, von Korff M, Bush T, Walker E, Simon G, Robinson P. The predictors of persistence of depression in primary care. *J Affect Disord.* 1994: 31:81-90.
12. Skodol AE, Schwartz S, Dohrenwend BP, Levav I, Shrout PE. Minor depression in a cohort of young adults in Israel. *Arch Gen Psychiatry.* 1994;51:542-551.
13. Broadhead WE, Blazer DG, George LK, Tse CK. Depression, disability days, and days lost from work in a prospective epidemiologic survey. *JAMA.* 1990; 264:2524-2528.
14. Johnson J, Weissman MM, Klerman GL. Service utilization and social morbidity associated with depressive symptoms in the community. *JAMA.* 1992; 267:1478-1483.
15. Berkman LF, Berkman CS, Kasl S, Freeman DH Jr, Leo L, Ostfeld AM, Cornoni-Huntley J, Brody JA. Depressive symptoms in relation to physical health and functioning in the elderly. *Am J Epidemiol.* 1986;124:372-388.
16. Wells KB, Stewart A, Hays RD, Burnam MA, Rogers W, Daniels M, Berry S, Greenfield S, Ware J. The functioning and well-being of depressed patients: results from the Medical Outcomes Study. *JAMA.* 1989;262:914-919.
17. Klerman GL, Weissman MM, Ouellette R, Johnson J, Greenwald S. Panic attacks in the community: social morbidity and health care utilization. *JAMA.* 1991;265:742-746.
18. Leon AC, Portera L, Weissman MM. The social costs of anxiety disorders. *Br J Psychiatry.* 1995;166:19-22.
19. Escobar JI, Golding JM, Hough RL, Karno M, Burnam MA, Wells KB. Somatization in the community: relationship to disability and use of services. *Am J Public Health.* 1987;77:837-840.
20. Webb GR, Redman S, Hennrikus DJ, Kelman GR, Gibberd RW, Sanson-Fisher RW. The relationships between high-risk and problem drinking and the occurrence of work injuries and related absences. *J Stud Alcohol.* 1994;55:434-446.
21. Jenkins R, Harvey S, Butler T, Thomas RL. A six-year longitudinal study of the occupational consequences of drinking over 'safe limits' of alcohol. *Br J Ind Med.* 1992;49:369-374.
22. Calzavara LM, Coates RA, Raboud JM, Farewell WT, Read SE, Shephered FA, Fanning MM, MacFadden D. Ongoing high-risk sexual behaviors in relation to recreational drug use in sexual encounters: analysis of 5 years of data from the Toronto Sexual Contact Study. *Ann Epidemiol.* 1992;3:272-280.
23. Van Trigt L, Kreuger H, Westerman RF, Hull FM. Morbidity at an Amsterdam inner-city clinic in relation to drug use. *Fam Pract.* 1989;6:299-302.
24. Von Korff M, Shapiro S, Burke JD, Teitlebaum M, Skinner EA, German P, Turner RW, Klein L, Burns B. Anxiety and depression in a primary care clinic. *Arch Gen Psychiatry.* 1987;44:152-156.
25. Clayton PJ. The comorbidity factor: establishing the primary diagnosis in patients with mixed symptoms of anxiety and depression. *J Clin Psychiatry.* 1990; 56:15S-22S.
26. Kessler RL, McGonagle KA, Zhao S, Nelson CR, Hughes M, Eshelman S, Wittchen HU, Kendler K. Lifetime and 12-month prevalence of *DSM-III-R* psychiatric disorders in the United States: results from the National Comorbidity Survey. *Arch Gen Psychiatry.* 1994;51:8-19.
27. Regier DA, Farmer ME, Rae DS, Locke BZ, Keith SJ, Judd LL, Goodwin FK. Comorbidity of mental disorders with alcohol and other drug abuse: results from the Epidemiologic Catchment Area (ECA) study. *JAMA.* 1990;264:2511-2518.
28. Liebowitz MR. Mixed anxiety and depression: should it be included in *DSM-IV*? *J Clin Psychiatry.* 1993;54:4S-7S.
29. Leon AC, Shear MK, Portera L, Klerman GL. Assessing impairment in patients with panic disorders: the Sheehan Disability Scale. *Soc Psychiatry Psychiatr Epidemiol.* 1992;27:78-82.
30. Markowitz JS, Weissman MM, Ouellette R, Lish JD, Klerman GL. Quality of life in panic disorder. *Arch Gen Psychiatry.* 1989;46:984-992.
31. Spitzer RL, Williams JBW, Gibbon M, First M. The structured clinical interview for *DSM-III-R* (SCID), I: history, rationale, and description. *Arch Gen Psychiatry.* 1992;49:624-629.
32. American Psychiatric Association. *Diagnostic and Statistical Manual of Mental Disorders, Fourth Edition.* Washington, DC: American Psychiatric Association; 1994.
33. Fleiss JL. *The Design and Analysis of Clinical Experiments.* New York, NY: John Wiley & Sons Inc; 1986.
34. Sheehan D, Janavs J, Knapp E, Sheehan M, Baker R. *Mini-International Neuropsychiatric Interview Clinician Rated, Version 4.0.* Tampa, Fla: University of South Florida College of Medicine; 1992.
35. Sheehan DV, Lecrubiier Y, Janavs J, Weiller, Bonara LI, Keskiner A, Schinka J, Knapp E, Sheehan MF, Dunbar GC. Reliability and validity of the Mini-International Neuropsychiatric Interview (MINI) according to the SCID-P. Presented at the New Clinical Drug Evaluation Unit 35th Annual Meeting; May 31, 1995; Orlando, Fla.
36. Horwath E, Johnson J, Klerman GL, Weissman MM. Depressive symptoms as relative and attributable risk factors for first-onset major depression. *Arch Gen Psychiatry.* 1992;49:817-823.
37. Wells KB, Burnam MA, Rogers W, Hays R, Camp P. The course of depression in adult outpatients. *Arch Gen Psychiatry.* 1992;49:788-794.
38. Angst J. The history and concept of recurrent brief depression. *Eur Arch Psychiatry Clin Neurosci.* 1994;244:171-173.
39. Elkin I, Shea T, Watkins JT, Imber SD, Stotsky SM, Collins JF, Glass DR, Pilkonis PA, Leber WR, Docherty JP, Fiester SJ, Parloff MB. National Institute of Mental Health Treatment of Depression Collaborative Research Program: general effectiveness of treatments. *Arch Gen Psychiatry.* 1989;46:971-982.
40. Paykel ES, Hollyman JA, Freeling P, Sedgwick P. Predictors of therapeutic benefit from amitriptyline in mild depression: a general practice placebo-controlled trial. *J Affect Disord.* 1988;14:83-95.
41. Depression Guideline Panel. *Depression in Primary Care: Treatment of Major Depression: Clinical Practice Guideline.* Rockville, Md: US Dept of Health and Human Services, Public Health Service, Agency for Health Care Policy and Research; April 1993;2. AHCPR publication 93-0551.
42. Boyer W. Serotonin uptake inhibitors are superior to imipramine and alprazolam in alleviating panic attacks: a meta-analysis. *Int Clin Psychopharmacol.* 1995;10:45-49.
43. Stewart JW, Quitkin FM, Klein DF. The pharmacotherapy of minor depression. *Am J Psychother.* 1992;46:23-36.
44. Wells KB, Burnam MA, Leake B, Robins LN. Agreement between face-to-face and telephone-administered versions of the depressive section of the NIMH Diagnostic Interview Schedule. *J Psychiatr Res.* 1988;22:207-220.
45. Paulson SA, Crowe RR, Noyes R, Pfohl B. Reliability of the telephone interview in diagnosing anxiety disorders. *Arch Gen Psychiatry.* 1988;45:62-63.
46. Watson CG, Anderson PE, Thomas D, Nyberg K. Comparison of telephone and face-to-face diagnostic interview schedules. *J Nerv Ment Dis.* 1992;180:534-535.
47. Simon GE, Revicki D, Von Korff ML. Telephone assessment of depression severity. *J Psychiatr Res.* 1993;27:247-252.
48. Gfroerer JC, Hughes AL. The feasibility of collecting drug abuse data by telephone. *Public Health Rep.* 1991;106:384-393.

ORIGINAL ARTICLE

Comorbid Anxiety Disorder and the Functioning and Well-being of Chronically Ill Patients of General Medical Providers

Cathy Donald Sherbourne, PhD; Kenneth B. Wells, MD; Lisa S. Meredith, PhD; Catherine A. Jackson, PhD; Patti Camp, MA

Background: The comorbidity of psychiatric disorders with chronic health conditions has emerged as a topic of considerable clinical and policy interest, in part owing to the evidence that anxiety disorders themselves are associated with morbidity. However, the implications for health-related quality of life that result from anxiety disorders, which are comorbid to chronic medical or psychiatric illness, are not well understood, especially in primary care samples.

Methods: A 2-year observational study of 875 adult patients with hypertension, diabetes, heart disease, and current depressive disorder or subthreshold depression receiving care from general medical providers was conducted. The unique effect of any comorbid anxiety disorder on functioning and well-being (determined with the use of the 36-Item Short-Form Health Survey [SF-36]) was estimated, as well as the differential impact at baseline, 2-year follow-up, and change over time, of any comorbid anxiety disorder for patients with chronic medical conditions or depression.

Results: Patients with comorbid anxiety who received general medical care had lower levels of functioning and well-being than those without comorbid anxiety. These differences were most pronounced in mental health–related quality-of-life measures and when anxiety was comorbid with chronic medical conditions rather than with depression. Hypertensive and diabetic patients with comorbid anxiety were as debilitated as patients with depression or heart disease, and this low health-related quality of life persisted over time. Comorbid anxiety had less of an effect on patients with heart disease who already had a low health-related quality of life.

Conclusion: The finding of substantial differences in the quality of life between hypertensive and diabetic patients with and without comorbid anxiety disorder highlights the clinical and societal importance of identifying comorbid anxiety in these patients.

Arch Gen Psychiatry. 1996;53:889-895

THE COMORBIDITY of psychiatric disorders with chronic health conditions has emerged as a topic of considerable clinical and policy interest. In part, this is owing to the appreciation for how frequently multiple diagnoses occur[1,2] and how their co-occurrence may complicate the course of treatment and impact negatively on health care costs. Anxiety disorders, including panic disorder, phobia, and generalized anxiety disorder (GAD), are associated with a high utilization of health services, increased disability, and poor outcomes,[3-8] which are factors that result in high direct and indirect costs to the individual patient and to society. However, the implications for health-related quality of life (HRQOL) that result from anxiety disorders, which are comorbid to chronic medical or psychiatric illness, are not well understood, especially in primary care samples.

Comparisons of the relative impact of depression and chronic medical conditions on HRQOL found that for most domains of functioning, depression is as much or more debilitating than are the most common chronic conditions.[9] Although the HRQOL of depressed patients tended to improve, they continued to have equivalent or worse functioning and well-being than did patients with chronic medical disease after 2 years.[10] Patients who had depression, but who did not meet diagnostic criteria for major depression or dysthymia, remained essentially unchanged in their

See Patients and Methods on next page

From RAND, Santa Monica, Calif (Drs Sherbourne, Meredith, and Jackson and Ms Camp), and the Department of Psychiatry and Biobehavioral Sciences, University of California, Los Angeles (Dr Wells).

PATIENTS AND METHODS

STUDY DESIGN

The MOS was an observational study of adult outpatients who received care in health maintenance organizations, large multispecialty group practices, and single-specialty group and solo practices in Boston, Mass, Chicago, Ill, and Los Angeles, Calif.[11] Within each system of care, a representative sample of physicians was asked to participate in the study, and their patients were screened for coronary heart disease, hypertension, diabetes, and depression. A detailed description of the sampling strategy has been reported elsewhere.[11,12]

The information that is presented in this article is based on a study of 875 patients who underwent the baseline health examination and completed both the enrollment and the second-year self-administered questionnaires and for whom there were complete data on all outcomes. Informed consent for study participation was gathered at the time of screening and at later stages of the study.

Patients who were excluded from the analyses tended to be older, and they were more likely to be female, nonwhite, and unemployed and to have lower levels of education and income. However, they did not differ in the likelihood of having a comorbid anxiety disorder.

CLINICAL CONDITIONS

The medical tracer condition definitions were based on reports that were made by the patients and physicians of the presence of hypertension, diabetes, and heart disease (ie, congestive heart failure or recent myocardial infarction). Data were collected from the patients and the study clinicians during screening and through a structured medical history interview. There was high agreement between provider and patient reports of myocardial infarction, and there was moderate agreement between provider and patient reports of diabetes or hypertension.[12]

Two definitions of depression are used in this article: (1) current depressive disorder (ie, patients with major depression or dysthymia during the last 12 months and no remission since onset) and (2) subthreshold depression (ie, positive screening test results for depression but not for a current disorder). The presence of current depressive disorder was assessed by using an expanded version of the depression section of the Diagnostic Interview Survey (DIS).[13] The screening-based definition of subthreshold depression[14] differed from the current symptom–based definitions that have been used by other investigators,[15,16] by giving more weight to the duration of depression in the prior year.[17]

ANXIETY DISORDER

We focused on the presence or absence of any current (ie, during the past 12 months) comorbid anxiety disorder (ie, panic disorder, phobia, or GAD). The prevalence of comorbid panic disorder and phobia in these patients was too low to examine their effects separately.[18] We did not assess other anxiety disorders (eg, posttraumatic stress disorder or obsessive-compulsive disorder) because screening versions of the DIS for these conditions had not been developed at the time that the MOS began.

Data on comorbid anxiety disorders were obtained at baseline using a screening version of the DIS. The screening tests for panic disorder and phobia were developed empirically by using data from the St Louis, Mo, site of the Epidemiologic Catchment Area Study[19]; this was done by selecting the best combination of DIS items that predicted a lifetime diagnosis as determined by using the full DIS (L. Robins, PhD, unpublished data, June 1986).

HRQOL over time, with levels of functioning comparable with those of patients with chronic medical conditions.

Anxiety disorder, which is comorbid to other medical or psychiatric conditions, may further increase the morbidity that is associated with these disorders. For example, Wells et al[9] found that the effects of comorbid chronic conditions on HRQOL were additive. In other studies, investigators found that groups of patients with mixed anxiety and depression had even lower levels of mental health than did patients with pure anxiety,[4] and that depressed patients with comorbid panic disorder had poorer role and social functioning than did those without comorbid panic disorder.[7]

With the use of data from the Medical Outcomes Study (MOS), this article presents information on the effects of comorbid anxiety disorder on the functioning and well-being (ie, the HRQOL) of patients with chronic medical conditions or depression who received care from general medical providers and examines the persistence of such effects over time.

RESULTS

DESCRIPTIVE STATISTICS

Baseline characteristics are provided in **Table 1** for the analytic sample. Prevalence estimates for each of the 3 comorbid anxiety disorders, adjusted and weighted to the characteristics of the MOS patient sample, have been presented elsewhere.[18] Comorbid GAD had the highest prevalence in all tracer conditions (range of prevalence, 10.4%-54.1%), followed by phobia (range of prevalence, 4.8%-22.7%) and panic disorder (range of prevalence, 1%-9.4%).

UNIQUE EFFECT OF ANXIETY DISORDER

The **Figure** shows baseline HRQOL for all patients (depressed and medically ill) with and without comorbid anxiety disorder, controlling for demographic characteristics and study condition. Because none of the patients had anxiety disorder alone, these estimates were unique effects. For all measures but pain, patients with

Panic disorder was defined if the patient (1) had a spell or unexpected attack in the last 12 months that caused sudden feelings of being frightened, anxious, or very uneasy in situations when most people would not be afraid; (2) described an attack or spell that interfered with his or her life a lot and could not be attributed to medications, drugs, alcohol, or a physical illness or injury; *and* (3) experienced specific sets of symptoms during 1 of the worst such spells (sensitivity, 0.85; specificity, 1.0).

The screening test for phobia was almost identical to that for the full DIS diagnosis. Phobia was defined if the patient experienced feelings of unreasonable fear of any of 12 things or nondangerous situations that were so strong that people try to avoid them (sensitivity and specificity, 1.0).

Generalized anxiety disorder (validated on the data from the Epidemiologic Catchment Area site at Los Angeles) was defined if the patient (1) felt worried or anxious most of the time for 1 month or more *and* (2) described 2 other symptoms or an unusual amount of trouble with sleeping that could not be attributed to a physical illness, medications, drugs, or alcohol (sensitivity, 1.0; specificity, 0.95).

FUNCTIONING AND WELL-BEING MEASURES

Functioning and well-being were measured by using the 36-Item Short-Form Health Survey (SF-36), as developed by RAND, Santa Monica, Calif; this survey was a self-report HRQOL measure that was adapted from the MOS long-form measures.[20-22] The SF-36 included 8 multi-item measures (with the number of items given in parentheses) as follows: physical functioning (10), role limitations because of physical health problems (4), role limitations because of emotional health problems (3), social functioning (2), freedom from pain (2), energy or fatigue (4), emotional well-being (5), and general health perceptions (5). Internal consistency reliability estimates were 0.78 or greater for every scale. Findings from empiric studies provided support for the construct validity of the measures.[23,24] All outcome measures were scored from 0 (ie, poorest health) to 100 (ie, optimal health) on the scale.

ANALYSIS PLAN

We used multiple linear regression methods to estimate both the main (unique) effect of any comorbid anxiety disorder on HRQOL, as well as the differential impact (eg, interaction effect) for patients with depression or chronic medical conditions who received general medical care. Models controlled for age, gender, ethnicity, education, adjusted family income, site, system of care (ie, prepaid vs fee-for-service care), a count of chronic conditions (ie, difficulty with hearing, persistent cough, sinus congestion, chronic obstructive pulmonary disease, asthma, chronic diarrhea, constipation, diverticulitis, irritable bowel syndrome, arthritis, hip impairments, varicose veins, leg cramps while walking, anemia, and cancer), and the type of study condition (each condition separately and, for interaction models only, interaction with comorbid anxiety disorder). A joint F test of the overall significance of the set of interactions was performed for each outcome.

The predicted level of HRQOL, weighted for sampling probabilities and patient nonresponse, is reported for baseline and follow-up data, by using parameter estimates from the regression models. We also conducted analyses by using change over time as the dependent variable. Difference scores provided conservative tests of the null hypothesis and allowed each individual to serve as her or his own control.[25-27] Inference statistics and SEs were corrected for the clustered sampling design by using an intraclass correlation model.[28] Regression coefficients were considered to be significant at $P \leq .05$ (by the using 1-tailed test). Except as noted, all results were robust across tests of multiple comparisons.[29]

comorbid anxiety disorder had a significantly lower HRQOL than did patients without comorbid anxiety disorder (range of *P* values, .05-.001 [by using the 1-tailed test]). Differences in the HRQOL scores between patients with and without comorbid anxiety disorder ranged from 3.5 for freedom from pain to 24.5 for role limitations that were due to emotional problems. Differences tended to be largest in those scales that reflected primarily mental health rather than physical health concepts (eg, difference: 14.7 for emotional well-being and 5.1 for physical functioning).

DIFFERENTIAL IMPACT ON PHYSICAL HRQOL

Table 2 presents the adjusted baseline and 2-year mean levels of physical HRQOL. For each patient group, levels of HRQOL are given for patients with and without comorbid anxiety disorder. The main effects are indicated by superscript symbols: (1) all of the symbols but the single dagger indicate significant differences between similar patients with and without comorbid anxiety disorder at each time period, while (2) single daggers indicate the significant differences in change in physical health over time between patients with and without comorbid anxiety. Cases in which comorbid anxiety disorder had more of an effect on 1 chronic condition than the others are commented on in the text.

Hypertensive and diabetic patients with comorbid anxiety had significantly worse functioning on most measures of physical HRQOL than those without comorbid anxiety. This was evident at both baseline and the 2-year follow-up, and limitations in the groups of patients with comorbid anxiety tended to persist.

In contrast, there were trends for a better HRQOL in patients with heart disease who had comorbid anxiety as opposed to patients with heart disease who did not have comorbid anxiety. Over time, however, pain increased for patients with heart disease who had comorbid anxiety, and it decreased for patients with heart disease who did not have comorbid anxiety (difference in change between the 2 groups was significant at t=1.65, df=851, P<.05). However, change in HRQOL was similar for patients with heart disease who had and did not have comorbid anxiety otherwise.

Table 1. Demographic Characteristics and Comorbid Anxiety Disorders Among Patients (N=875) Who Received General Medical Care

Variable	No. (%) of Patients*
Characteristic	
Age, y	54.1 (14.7)
Education level, y	12.8 (2.9)
Income level, $	23.5 (15.6)
Male	385 (44)
White	700 (80)
Married	568 (65)
Employed	542 (62)
Disorder	
Subthreshold depression	120 (13.7)†
Subthreshold depression with any anxiety	42 (35.0)‡
Current depression	115 (13.1)
Current depression with any anxiety	77 (67.0)
Hypertension	597 (68.2)
Hypertension with any anxiety	106 (17.8)
Diabetes	229 (26.2)
Diabetes with any anxiety	36 (15.7)
Heart disease	115 (13.1)
Heart disease with any anxiety	16 (13.9)

*Data are given as the number (percentage) of patients for all characteristics and disorders, except for age and levels of education and income, for which the values are given as means (SDs).

†Percentages add to more than 100, since patients can have multiple conditions.

‡Percentage of patients with the condition (ie, subthreshold depression) who have any comorbid anxiety disorder (panic, phobia, or generalized anxiety disorder).

The physical health of depressed patients differed little, depending on the comorbidity status. While a few significant differences are noted in Table 2 for patients with subthreshold depression, such differences were not observed in the multiple-comparison tests across outcomes and, thus, may be owing to chance.

Joint F tests for the significance of interactions between tracer condition and comorbid anxiety disorder at baseline found that there was a differential impact of comorbid anxiety disorder, depending on tracer condition, for role limitations due to physical problems, pain, and general health outcomes. Comorbid anxiety had a differential impact at the 2-year follow-up for the freedom from pain measure only.

DIFFERENTIAL IMPACT ON MENTAL HRQOL

Results for mental HRQOL are given in **Table 3**. Again, the mental health of hypertensive and diabetic patients was significantly lower for those with comorbid anxiety than for those without comorbid anxiety across all 4 measures at both baseline and the 2-year follow-up (range of *P* values, .05-.001). The initial set of limitations persisted for patients with comorbid anxiety.

The mental functioning of patients with heart disease differed little by comorbid anxiety status; however, over time, the scores for patients with comorbid anxiety tended to deteriorate 11 and 14 points in emotional well-being and social functioning, respectively. The emotional well-being and social functioning of patients with heart disease who did not have comorbid anxiety tended to remain the same or improve slightly (difference in change between the 2 groups was significant at $t=1.83$ and $t=2.11$, $df=851$, and $P=.05$ and $P=.03$ for emotional well-being and social functioning, respectively).

The mental health of depressed patients differed little by comorbidity status. For 1 measure, however, those who were currently depressed with anxiety showed fairly low levels of role limitations due to emotional problems that persisted over time (mean values, 47 and 48 at baseline and follow-up, respectively). In contrast, role limitations due to emotional problems improved over time for patients who were currently depressed without anxiety (mean values, 52 and 74 at baseline and follow-up, respectively; the difference in change was significant at $t=1.68$, $df=851$, $P=.05$).

Joint F tests for the significance of interactions between the tracer conditions and comorbid anxiety disorder at baseline supported the differential impact of comorbid anxiety disorder, depending on tracer condition, for emotional well-being, social functioning, and energy or fatigue. Comorbid anxiety also had a differential impact at the 2-year follow-up for emotional well-being but not for the other outcome measures.

COMMENT

Like previously published work, this study found that among patients who receive care from general medical providers, those with comorbid anxiety disorder have lower levels of HRQOL than those without this disorder.[4] Differences tended to be most pronounced in measures that reflected primarily mental health concepts rather than physical health and when anxiety was comorbid with hypertension or diabetes rather than depression. Hypertensive and diabetic patients with anxiety were as debilitated as patients with depression or heart disease, and this debilitation persisted over time. For patients with heart disease, there was a slight trend for physical health to be actually better in patients with comorbid anxiety; however, over time, their emotional well-being and social functioning declined. For these patients, whose physical health is already low, anxiety may serve as a positive coping strategy, which may mobilize them to attune to their physical symptoms to decrease the threat of another myocardial infarction. Because of the small sample of patients with heart disease who had anxiety, these results are tentative.

Comorbid anxiety disorder had little effect on the HRQOL of depressed patients, possibly because of the high comorbidity of both depression and anxiety and the already low HRQOL of depressed patients. Larger samples of depressed patients may be needed to detect significant differences in outcomes between those patients with and without comorbid anxiety disorder. Alternatively, a lack of a differential effect could have been owing to a definitional overlap (ie, the 2 groups of patients shared a substantial overlap in symptoms) that may have complicated our ability to differentiate successfully between them. A less definitional overlap between the chronic medical conditions and anxiety disorder may be 1 rea-

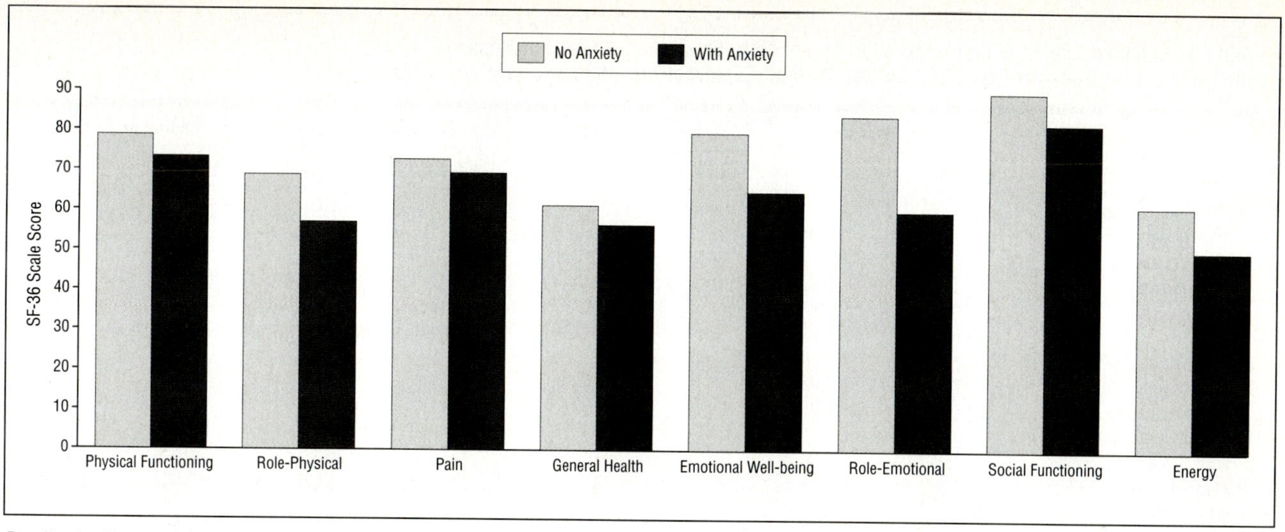

Baseline health-related quality-of-life scores for patients with and without any comorbid anxiety disorder who received general medical care. SF-36 indicates 36-Item Short-Form Health Survey.

Table 2. Adjusted Levels of Physical Functioning, Role-Physical, Pain, and General Health Perceptions for Patients With and Without Comorbid Anxiety Disorders*

Disorder	Physical Functioning		Role-Physical		Freedom From Pain		General Health	
	Baseline	2 y	Baseline	2 y	Baseline	2 y	Baseline	2 y
Subthreshold depression								
With anxiety	66 (9)	64 (10)†	60 (8)	61 (8)	75 (4)	78 (4)‡	58 (6)	59 (7)
Without anxiety	74 (4)	66 (6)	63 (5)	58 (5)	67 (4)	60 (4)	54 (4)	52 (5)
Major depression								
With anxiety	70 (5)	69 (4)	55 (7)	43 (8)	60 (5)	68 (4)	52 (5)	55 (5)
Without anxiety	74 (5)	75 (4)	51 (7)	56 (8)	63 (5)	64 (4)	51 (4)	54 (7)
Hypertension								
With anxiety	74 (4)§	77 (3)†	56 (6)‖	65 (5)¶	65 (4)‖	69 (4)‖	58 (3)§	60 (4)
Without anxiety	81 (2)	79 (2)	72 (2)	77 (2)	75 (2)	79 (2)	64 (2)	64 (6)
Diabetes								
With anxiety	69 (5)‖	65 (5)¶	58 (8)§	43 (8)‡	74 (4)	69 (6)	45 (4)‡	42 (6)¶
Without anxiety	83 (2)	79 (3)	76 (4)	72 (4)	79 (2)	75 (3)	61 (3)	58 (3)
Heart disease								
With anxiety	83 (11)	85 (9)§	60 (14)	67 (16)	90 (5)‡	87 (5)†	68 (11)	60 (9)
Without anxiety	68 (3)	69 (3)	54 (6)	57 (4)	75 (3)	78 (4)	56 (3)	53 (4)

*Data are given as the mean (SE) scale score. A high score on all scales indicates better functioning and well-being. Values are adjusted for comorbidity, sociodemographics, and system of care.

†Indicates that the change in the group with comorbid anxiety is significantly different at $P<.05$ than the change in the group without anxiety.

‡Significantly different from group without anxiety at $P=.005$, by using 1-tailed test.

§Significantly different from group without anxiety at $P=.05$, by using 1-tailed test.

‖Significantly different from group without anxiety at $P=.01$, by using 1-tailed test.

¶Significantly different from group without anxiety at $P=.03$, by using 1-tailed test.

son why we see an additive effect of comorbid anxiety disorder to these conditions. Other anxiety disorders (eg, posttraumatic stress disorder or obsessive-compulsive disorder) might have shown a greater relative HRQOL burden.

Findings for patients with subthreshold depression who have anxiety suggest that this mixed-state *DSM-IV*[30] classification may not have more of a burden in HRQOL than in patients with subthreshold depression alone. These patients, however, were significantly more likely to experience a major depressive episode in the year after baseline than were patients with subthreshold depression alone. Thus, patients with subthreshold depression who have comorbid anxiety may represent a prodromal phase of a major depressive episode rather than a distinct disorder.

Our study has several limitations. First, the screening tests for anxiety disorders, although high in sensitivity and specificity against the full DIS diagnosis, have not been validated against clinical assessments. Still, our analyses that showed that the HRQOL of patients with comorbid anxiety disorder was quite low compared with that of patients without comorbid anxiety suggested that anxiety symptoms, as measured in these screening tests, were clinically important. Data are presently being gathered to understand better the clinical relevance of HRQOL scores themselves. An 18-point difference in role limitations due to physical problems

Table 3. Adjusted Levels of Emotional Well-being, Role-Emotional, Social Functioning, and Energy or Fatigue for Patients With and Without Comorbid Anxiety Disorders*

Disorder	Emotional Well-being		Role-Emotional		Social Functioning		Energy or Fatigue	
	Baseline	2 y	Baseline	2 y	Baseline	2 y	Baseline	2 y
Subthreshold depression								
With anxiety	61 (4)†	57 (5)†	59 (10)	66 (8)	80 (5)	67 (12)	48 (5)	56 (5)
Without anxiety	75 (2)	73 (3)	74 (5)	73 (6)	80 (4)	83 (4)	55 (3)	51 (5)
Major depression								
With anxiety	52 (4)	56 (4)	47 (7)	48 (8)‡§	64 (4)	66 (5)†	47 (4)	52 (4)
Without anxiety	55 (4)	63 (4)	52 (4)	74 (8)	71 (4)	84 (4)	46 (3)	57 (3)
Hypertension								
With anxiety	65 (3)‖	70 (2)‖	55 (9)‖	64 (7)‖	82 (3)‖	86 (4)¶	47 (2)‖	56 (3)†
Without anxiety	82 (1)	83 (1)	88 (2)	90 (2)	93 (1)	92 (1)	64 (2)	66 (1)
Diabetes								
With anxiety	60 (5)‖	56 (4)‖	63 (14)	63 (8)‡	76 (6)‡	70 (7)†	41 (4)‖	45 (5)†
Without anxiety	86 (2)	84 (2)	86 (4)	84 (4)	92 (2)	92 (3)	65 (2)	64 (3)
Heart anxiety								
With anxiety	77 (3)	66 (6)†§	80 (9)	76 (13)	94 (7)	80 (12)§	54 (6)	53 (10)
Without anxiety	82 (2)	83 (2)	77 (4)	89 (4)	82 (4)	89 (3)	54 (2)	55 (3)

Data are given as the mean (SE) scale score. A high score on all scales indicates better functioning and well-being. Values are adjusted for comorbidity, sociodemographics, and system of care.
†*Significantly different from group without anxiety at* P=.005*, by using 1-tailed test.*
‡*Significantly different from group without anxiety at* P=.01*, by using 1-tailed test.*
§*Indicates that the change in the group with comorbid anxiety is significantly different at* P<.05 *than the change in the group without anxiety.*
‖*Significantly different from group without anxiety at* P=.001*, by using 1-tailed test.*
¶*Significantly different from group without anxiety at* P=.05*, by using 1-tailed test.*

was equivalent to the effect of remission in patients with depressive disorder.[31] For persons who scored 69 on the physical functioning scale (as did diabetic patients with anxiety), 24% reported that they could not work because of health problems compared with only 6% of people who scored at level 83.[32] Thus, differences in the HRQOL scores are personally and socially relevant. Other interpretative information can be found elsewhere.[32] Second, information is not presented on patients with anxiety alone—a condition that was not selected for study in the MOS. To strengthen study implications, we bounded the estimated effects of comorbid anxiety disorder between unique effects (that may have overestimated true effects) and incremental effects (that may have underestimated true effects). Third, the extent to which comorbid anxiety disorder in hypertensive and diabetic patients caused decrements in functioning and well-being was unclear from our data, and we do not know if the changes in HRQOL that were observed over time were owing to an exacerbation of the chronic medical condition or the continuing presence of comorbid anxiety. However, sensitivity analyses that controlled for complications in the medical tracer conditions yielded similar results at baseline. Fourth, we were unable to present results separately for panic disorder or phobia because of their low prevalence. Sensitivity tests for patients with GAD only found similar results, suggesting that our findings may be driven primarily by GAD. Since GAD is often considered to be a less serious form of anxiety disorder, the differences in HRQOL that are associated with its occurrence are even more striking.

Finally, one can question whether self-reports of functioning by anxious patients are accurate. As for depressed patients,[33] anxious patients may be unrealistically pessimistic; thus, their self-reports may be biased. Yet, even if anxious patients' assessments are somewhat unrealistic, they are associated with such events as service use.[3,5,8] Reports of HRQOL among depressed patients are related to remission of major depression, supporting the sensitivity of self-reports to clinical change.[31]

Our findings complement those of other investigators who have found that medical disease may be worsened by anxiety.[34] The substantial differences in the quality of life between medically ill patients with and without comorbid anxiety disorder, including the less serious GAD, highlight the importance of identifying comorbid anxiety disorder, especially if treatment of a given disease condition differs, depending on whether anxiety is also present. The recent development of short instruments to recognize and diagnose common mental disorders in primary care should facilitate this process.[35,36] Constraints to the primary care diagnosis of anxiety disorders include time limits and inadequate knowledge of diagnostic criteria. Yet, in the long run, identification and treatment of such patients may reduce unnecessary utilization of health services and improve their HRQOL.

Accepted for publication February 21, 1996.

This study was supported by grant MH 50820-01A1 from the National Institute of Mental Health, Rockville, Md, by grants from the Robert Wood Johnson Foundation, Princeton, NJ, the Henry J. Kaiser Foundation, Menlo Park, Calif, and the Pew Charitable Trusts, Philadelphia, Pa, and by research funds from RAND.

Reprints: Cathy Donald Sherbourne, PhD, RAND, 1700 Main St, PO Box 2138, Santa Monica, CA 90407-2138.

REFERENCES

1. Boyd JH, Burke J, Gruenberg E, Holzer C, Rae D, George L, Karno M, Stoltzman R, McEvoy L, Nestadt G. Exclusion criteria of *DSM-III*: a study of co-occurrence of hierarchy-free syndromes. *Arch Gen Psychiatry.* 1984;41:983-989.
2. Regier D, Burke J, Burke K. Comorbidity of affective and anxiety disorders in the NIMH Epidemiologic Catchment Area Program. In: Maser JD, Cloninger CR, eds. *Comorbidity of Mood and Anxiety Disorders.* Washington, DC: American Psychiatric Press; 1990:chap 6.
3. Boyd JH. Use of mental health services for the treatment of panic disorder. *Am J Psychiatry.* 1986;143:1569-1574.
4. Fifer SK, Mathias SD, Patrick DL, Mazonson PD, Lubeck DP, Buesching DP. Untreated anxiety among adult primary care patients in a health maintenance organization. *Arch Gen Psychiatry.* 1994;51:740-750.
5. Klerman G, Weissman MM, Ouellette R, Johnson J, Greenwald S. Panic attacks in the community: social morbidity and health care utilization. *JAMA.* 1991;265:742-746.
6. Markowitz JS, Weissman MM, Ouellette R, Lish J, Klerman G. Quality of life in panic disorder. *Arch Gen Psychiatry.* 1989;46:984-992.
7. Noyes R. The comorbidity and mortality of panic disorder. *Psychiatr Med.* 1990; 8:41-66.
8. Shapiro S, Skinner EA, Kessler LG, Von Korff M, German P, Tischler G, Leaf P, Benham L, Cother L, Regier D. Utilization of health and mental health services: three Epidemiologic Catchment Area sites. *Arch Gen Psychiatry.* 1984;41:971-978.
9. Wells KB, Stewart A, Hays RD, Burnam A, Rogers W, Daniels M, Berry S, Greenfield S, Ware JE Jr. The functioning and well-being of depressed patients: results from the Medical Outcomes Study. *JAMA.* 1989;262:914-919.
10. Hays RD, Wells KB, Sherbourne CD, Rogers W, Spritzer K. Functioning and well-being outcomes of patients with depression compared with chronic general medical illnesses. *Arch Gen Psychiatry.* 1995;52:11-19.
11. Rogers WH, McGlynn E, Berry S, Nelson E, Perrin E, Zubkoff M, Greenfield S, Wells K, Stewart A, Arnold S, Ware J. Methods of sampling. In: Stewart AL, Ware JE Jr, eds. *Measuring Functional Status and Well-being: The Medical Outcomes Study Approach.* Durham, NC: Duke University Press; 1992:27-47.
12. Wells KB, Rogers W, Burnam MA, Greenfield S, Ware JE Jr. How the medical comorbidity of depressed patients differs across health care setting: results from the Medical Outcomes Study. *Am J Psychiatry.* 1991;148:1688-1696.
13. Burnam MA, Wells KB, Leake B, Landsverk J. Development of a brief screening instrument for detecting depressive disorders. *Med Care.* 1988;26:775-789.
14. Robins LN, Helzer JE, Croughan J, Ratcliff KS. National Institute of Mental Health Diagnostic Interview Schedule. *Arch Gen Psychiatry.* 1981;38:381-389.
15. Broadhead WE, Blazer DG, George LK, Tse CK. Depression, disability days, and days lost from work in a prospective epidemiologic survey. *JAMA.* 1990; 264:2524-2528.
16. Horwath E, Johnson J, Klerman GL, Weissman MM. Depressive symptoms as relative and attributable risk factors for first-onset major depression. *Arch Gen Psychiatry.* 1992;49:817-823.
17. Sherbourne CD, Wells KB, Hays RD, Rogers W, Burnam A, Judd LL. Subthreshold depression and depressive disorder: clinical characteristics of general medical and mental health specialty outpatients. *Am J Psychiatry.* 1994; 151:1777-1784.
18. Sherbourne CD, Jackson CA, Meredith LM, Camp P, Wells KB. Prevalence of comorbid anxiety disorders in general medical and mental health specialty outpatients. *Arch Fam Med.* 1996;5:27-34.
19. Regier DA, Myers JK, Kramer M, Robins L, Blazer D, Hough R, Eaton W, Locke B. The NIMH Epidemiologic Catchment Area Program: historical context, major objectives and study population characteristics. *Arch Gen Psychiatry.* 1984; 41:934-941.
20. Hays RD, Sherbourne CD, Mazel RM. The RAND 36-Item Health Survey 1.0. *Health Econ.* 1993;2:217-227.
21. Ware JE, Sherbourne CD. The MOS 36-Item Short-Form Health Survey (SF-36), I: conceptual framework and item selection. *Med Care.* 1992;30:473-483.
22. Stewart AL, Sherbourne CD, Hays RD, Wells K, Nelson E, Kamberg C, Rogers W, Berry S, Ware J. Summary discussion of MOS measures. In: Stewart AL, Ware JE, eds. *Measuring Functioning and Well-being: The Medical Outcomes Study Approach.* Durham, NC: Duke University Press; 1992:345-371.
23. McHorney CA, Ware JE, Raczek AE. The MOS 36-Item Short-Form Health Survey (SF-36), II: psychometric and clinical tests of validity in measuring physical and mental health constructs. *Med Care.* 1993;31:247-263.
24. McHorney CA, Ware JE, Lu JFR, Sherbourne CD. The MOS 36-Item Short-Form Health Survey (SF-36), III: tests of data quality, scaling assumptions, and validity among diverse patient groups. *Med Care.* 1994;32:40-66.
25. Allison PD. Change scores as dependent variables in regression analysis. *Sociol Methods.* 1990;20:93-114.
26. Overall JE. Contradictions can never a paradox resolve. *Appl Psychol Meas.* 1989;13:426-428.
27. Willett JB. Questions and answers in the measurement of change. In: Rothkopf EZ, ed. *Review of Research in Education, 15.* Washington, DC: American Education Research Association; 1988:345-422.
28. Liang KY, Zeger SL. Longitudinal data analysis using generalized linear models. *Biometrika. 1986;73:13-22.*
29. Computing Resource Center. *Stata Reference Manual: Release 3.* 5th ed. Santa Monica, Calif: Computing Resource Center; 1992.
30. American Psychiatric Association. *Diagnostic and Statistical Manual of Mental Disorders, Fourth Edition.* Washington, DC: American Psychiatric Association; 1994.
31. Wells KB, Sturm R, Sherbourne CD, Meredith LS. *Caring for Depression in America.* Cambridge, Mass: Harvard University Press; 1996.
32. Ware JE Jr, Snow KK, Kosinski M, Gandek B. *SF-36 Health Survey Manual and Interpretation Guide.* Boston, Mass: Health Institute, New England Medical Center; 1993.
33. Beck AT. *Cognitive Therapy and the Emotional Disorders.* New York, NY: International Universities Press Inc; 1976.
34. Lustman PJ. Anxiety disorders in adults with diabetes mellitus. *Psychiatr Clin North Am.* 1988;11:419-432.
35. Spitzer RL, Williams JBW, Kroenke K, Linzer M, de Gruy F, Hahn S, Brody D, Johnson J. Utility of a new procedure for diagnosing mental disorders in primary care: the PRIME-MD 1000 Study. *JAMA.* 1994;272:1749-1756.
36. Weissman MM, Olfson M, Leon AC, Broadhead E, Gilbert T, Higgins E, Barrett J, Blacklow R, Keller M, Hoven C. Brief diagnostic interviews (SDDS-PC) for multiple mental disorders in primary care: a pilot study. *Arch Fam Med.* 1995; 4:220-227.

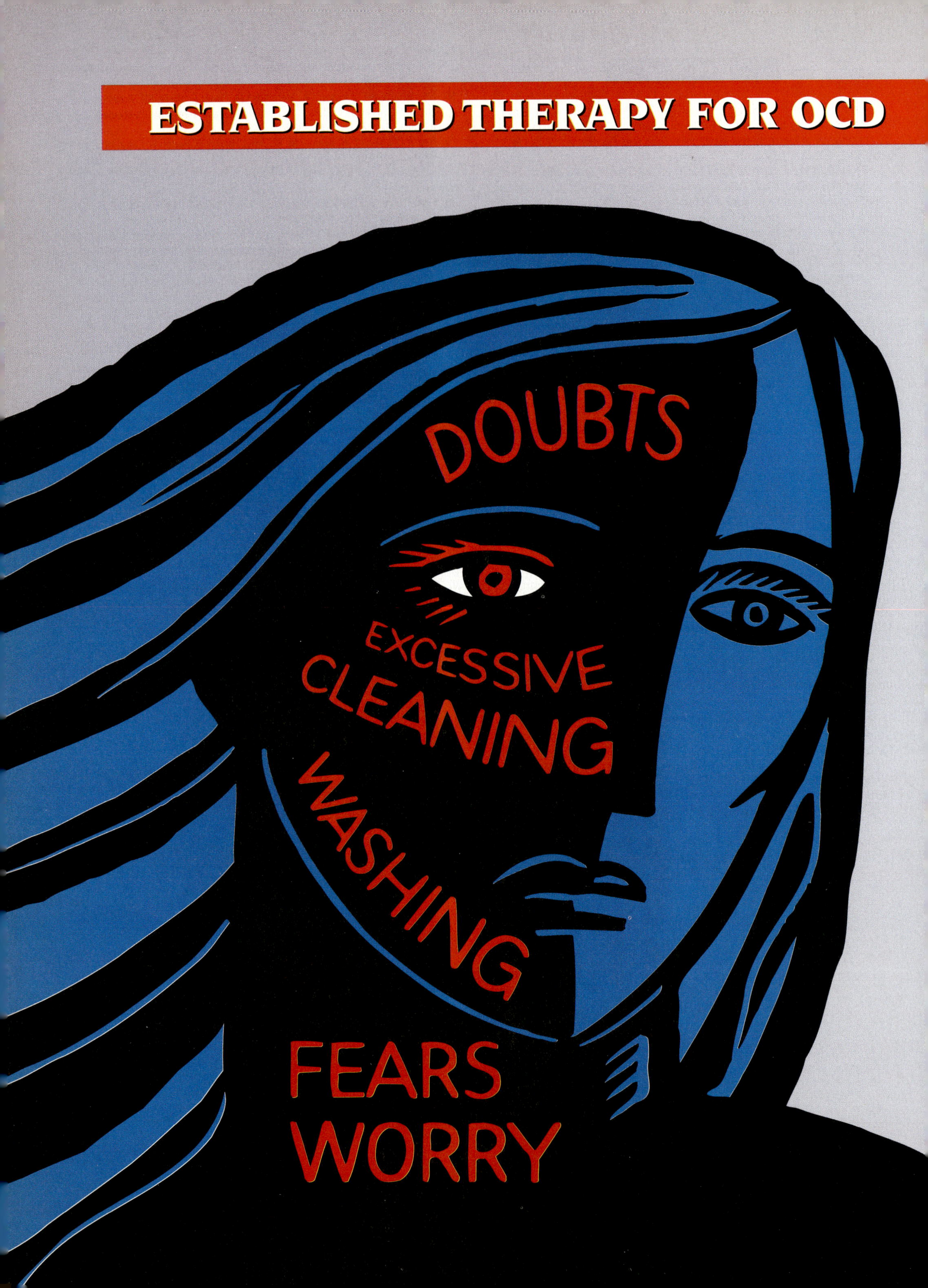
ESTABLISHED THERAPY FOR OCD
DOUBTS
EXCESSIVE
CLEANING
WASHING
FEARS
WORRY

ORIGINAL ARTICLE

Medical Costs Attributed to Depression Among Patients With a History of High Medical Expenses in a Health Maintenance Organization

Henry J. Henk, MS; David J. Katzelnick, MD; Kenneth A. Kobak, PhD; John H. Greist, MD; James W. Jefferson, MD

Background: While previous studies have compared medical utilization between depressed and nondepressed patients, we conducted a study that focused specifically on patients who had a history of high medical expenditures.

Methods: This study was designed to determine whether a positive screen for depression is predictive of continued high medical expenditures. Medical utilization data were obtained on 50 000 patients enrolled in the DeanCare health maintenance organization for 2 consecutive years. Consistent high utilizers were identified based on the medical utilization costs (paid by the health maintenance organization) for those 2 consecutive years, 1992 and 1993. A depression screen based on the Medical Outcomes Survey was mailed to 786 high utilizers. Their costs were determined for 1994. Regression analyses identified 1994 costs associated with depression, adjusting for age, sex, benefits package, and medical comorbidity.

Results: Depressed high utilizers were more likely than nondepressed high utilizers to have higher medical costs in 1994. Among high utilizers, depressed patients' 1994 costs were significantly higher ($5764 vs $4227; $P<.001$), although expenditures for depressed and nondepressed high utilizers were similar for the previous 2 years. The total medical cost associated with depression in 1994, adjusted for age, sex, benefits package, and medical comorbidity, was $1498 per patient.

Conclusions: In the third year (1994), a positive Medical Outcomes Survey screen for depression in high utilizers was associated with $1498 in higher medical costs. The average actual amount spent on depression treatment accounted for only a small portion of total medical costs for depressed high utilizers in the third year.

Arch Gen Psychiatry. 1996;53:899-904

CONCERNS ABOUT increasing costs of medical care have spurred efforts to identify modifiable factors contributing to increased utilization of medical services. Several studies have found depression to be associated with increased utilization of nonpsychiatric health services.[1-6] Identification and treatment of depressed patients with high medical utilization may both alleviate disability and distress from depression and reduce nonpsychiatric medical care costs.

Patients with high medical care use are of interest from both medical and health policy perspectives.[7] Several studies have found that a relatively small percentage of patients account for a disproportionate amount of medical utilization. In a study of a large prepaid health maintenance organization (HMO), 15% of patients accounted for 64% of total health care costs, with patients who had less than the median utilization per year accounting for only 9.5% of total costs.[7] Thirteen percent of members in another HMO accounted for 31% of total physician visits, 35% of hospital admissions, and 30% of outpatient surgical services. Patterns of utilization were related to the degree of psychological distress, especially depression.[8] For inpatient medical treatment, high levels of psychopathology are related to longer stays and higher costs.[1] Manning and Wells[2] found that worse *mental health status* at the time of health insurance enrollment was associated with increased use of both inpatient and outpatient *general medical services* after controlling for physical health status and functioning.

Physical and mental health problems are often concurrent. Regression

See Subjects and Methods on next page

From the Dean Foundation for Health, Research and Education, Madison, Wis.

SUBJECTS AND METHODS

SAMPLE IDENTIFICATION

The data used in this study were collected as part of a pilot study designed to look at disability, depression, and utilization costs among high-utilization primary care patients.[12] The pilot study was approved by both DeanCare HMO and the Dean Foundation Institutional Review Board, Madison, Wis.

Data were obtained for approximately 50 000 patients enrolled in the DeanCare HMO. DeanCare is a group model HMO in Madison, Wis. Patients were included if they were older than 18 years, had drug coverage benefits, and were continuously enrolled for 2 years (October 1991 through September 1993, hereafter described as 1992 and 1993). Medical and pharmaceutical charges paid by the HMO were collected for 3 identical periods, 1992, 1993, and 1994. The first 2 years were used to identify high utilizers, and the third was used as a follow-up year. Patients were identified as high utilizers if their total medical and pharmaceutical costs during *both* of the first 2 years were at or above the median costs for the entire eligible HMO population ($450 for 1992 and $504 for 1993) plus estimated depression treatment costs at DeanCare HMO for 1 year ($1217 for 1992 and $1400 for 1993). This was based on 12 months of antidepressant medication ($750), an initial primary care visit ($125), and 7 follow-up visits ($525). The rationale for using this definition was to identify a population of depressed patients whose utilization was high enough that it was economically possible to see a cost offset by treating their depression in 1 year. Assuming that depressed high utilizers' total medical costs would decrease to the median of the entire HMO population with depression treatment, their pretreatment utilization needed to be at least this amount plus the average cost of treating depression in the HMO ($1400). The thresholds used to identify high utilizers corresponded to the 19th percentile of expenditures in each year. Twenty high utilizers who participated in a depression treatment study in the third year were omitted from the analysis because they did not receive usual care.

CALCULATION OF MEDICAL COSTS

DeanCare HMO captures all submitted claims for every enrollee in 1 of 2 computerized databases (medical and pharmacy). The medical costs referred to in this article are the actual amounts paid by DeanCare. Paid amounts do not include copayments, coinsurance, or deductibles.

DEPRESSION SCREENING

A survey containing the 8-item depression screen from the Medical Outcomes Study (MOS)[13] was mailed to the high utilizers from 2 primary care clinics with an introductory letter from their primary care physician. People who did not return the survey were called and, if reached, administered the survey by telephone. Screening for depression was conducted between the sixth and eighth months of the third year. The MOS depression screen is a brief (8-item) scale consisting of items from the Center for Epidemiologic Studies Depression Scale[14] and the Diagnostic Interview Schedule.[15] It has been shown to have high levels of sensitivity, specificity, and positive predictive value for detecting depressive disorders in patients of both primary care and mental health providers. The MOS depression screen, while not a diagnostic instrument, was used in place of a diagnostic code on claims data for depression because of probable substantial underrecording of depression (eg, in a previously published survey of primary care physicians, 31% of patients who met *DSM-III-R* criteria for major depression received an alternative diagnostic code[16]). The high rate of undiagnosed depression may be attributed to physician hesitancy to document depression formally rather than not recognizing it.[16]

ADJUSTING FOR MEDICAL COMORBIDITY

Other medical illness is a potential confounder of the relationship between depression and medical costs.

analyses may be used to adjust for certain variables, such as age, sex, and concurrent diagnoses. Previous studies have estimated the contribution of comorbid depression to increased medical utilization, adjusting for age, sex, and medical comorbidity.[2,9-11] Members of an HMO with current *DSM-III-R* anxiety or depressive disorder had significantly greater geometric mean (similar to median) costs per 6 months than did a group with neither of these disorders ($973 vs $614; $t[245]=2.96$, $P=.003$).[9] A study of Medi-Cal found total medical costs to be $1043 more per year for depressed patients treated unsuccessfully with an antidepressant than for patients treated successfully.[10]

This report examines a sample of HMO patients with high utilization to determine whether a positive screen for depression is associated with higher total medical utilization during the next year than that in patients with negative screens for depression.

RESULTS

Applying the definition described previously, 786 DeanCare members (9.4%) were identified as high utilizers at the 2 Dean clinics. Sixty-three percent of those eligible completed the survey. High utilizers who completed the survey were significantly older (53.2 vs 49.7 years; $t[784]=3.10$, $P=.002$) than noncompleters. High utilizers who completed the survey had a higher rate of ADGs 10 (chronic medical: stable) and 11 (chronic medical: unstable) and noncompleters had a higher rate of ADGs 20 (dermatologic) and 23 (psychosocial: major); all other comparisons were not significant. No significant difference in sex or third-year cost was found between completers and noncompleters. One hundred fifty (29%) of those high utilizers completing the MOS survey screened positive for depression, 20 of whom were

Identification of medical morbidity was made by means of the ambulatory diagnostic groups (ADGs). Developed at The Johns Hopkins University, Baltimore, Md, ADGs provide a measure of health status and have been used in other studies to control for medical comorbidity.[17-19] This method uses computerized medical records to identify all unique *International Classification of Diseases, Ninth Revision, Clinical Modification* (*ICD-9-CM*) codes attached to ambulatory claims. Each *ICD-9-CM* code denoting a primary diagnosis or subsidiary diagnosis is assigned to one of 34 ADGs. Many different *ICD-9-CM* codes compose each ADG. Therefore, patients being treated for 2 distinctly different diagnoses may fall into 2 separate ADGs or only 1 ADG. For instance, a patient with both thyroiditis, unspecified (*ICD-9-CM* code 245.9) and gangrene (*ICD-9-CM* code 785.4) will fall into only 1 ADG, time limited: major (ADG 3). The severity ratings for the ADGs are limited to categorizing *ICD-9-CM* codes as major, minor, and likely to recur. The ADGs are binary (0, 1) variables, with a 1 indicating that the person met the criteria for that particular diagnostic group. Patients with no diagnoses during the third year were assigned a 0 for all 34 ADG variables. The ADG 23 was excluded from the regression analysis because the MOS screens for many of the *ICD-9-CM* diagnoses included in ADG 23. Unfortunately, ADG 23 is overinclusive and contains diagnoses other than depression: senile dementia, chronic organic brain syndrome, simple type schizophrenia, major depressive disorder—single episode, major depressive disorder—recurrent episode, unspecified psychosis, anxiety state, neurotic depression, acute alcohol intoxication, alcohol dependence, adjustment reaction with mixed disturbance of emotions and conduct, depressive disorder, and unspecified mental retardation.

STATISTICAL ANALYSIS

All statistical tests are considered significant at the .05 level, and all confidence intervals are 95%. Because of the highly skewed distribution of cost data, tests of statistical significance for cost comparisons were based on log-transformed costs. A multivariate regression model was used to estimate the medical costs associated with a positive MOS depression screening while adjusting for age, sex, benefits package, and medical comorbidity. Controlling for these variables was necessary because depression may be correlated with physical health problems that would increase costs. A potentially confounding variable not included in the regression model is the specific Dean clinic to which the patient belonged. This variable was excluded from the models because it did not affect the relationship between depression and medical costs. Other variables, such as race and socioeconomic status, were unavailable.

Regression models were based on log-transformed costs. Without the log transformation, regression estimates would be overly influenced by a few high-cost patients.

RETRANSFORMATION

Although the use of log-transformed costs yields more precisely estimated coefficients, these coefficients are not easily interpretable and may not be sufficient to characterize the impact of depression on the sample if the error is not homoscedastic in depression. The smearing estimator, a nonparametric retransformation method, was used to estimate the cost of depression on the original scale (dollars),[20-22] because the model did not follow the log normal distribution closely enough. The residuals were longer tailed than would be expected with log normal data (by means of a test based on skewness and kurtosis,[23] $P<.001$). The smearing estimate is valid only if the errors are homoscedastic. One cannot reject the assumption that the error is homoscedastic ($t_{488}=0.92$ with $P>.35$). As a result, our estimate of the impact of depression is the exponentiated depression coefficient multiplied by the average cost within the depressed sample, actually $(1-e^{-\beta})\times$(average cost within depressed sample).

treated for depression. In the 180 days surrounding the administration of the MOS depression questionnaire, 35% of patients who were positive for depression on the MOS screen were also given an *ICD-9-CM* diagnosis of major depression, neurotic depression, or bipolar disorder by their physicians. In the same interval, 7% of patients who were negative for depression on the MOS screen were given these *ICD-9-CM* diagnoses. During years 1 and 2, 50% of depressed high utilizers had a physician diagnosis of depression. Forty-nine percent of the depressed high utilizers received antidepressant medication during the 2 years.

Third-year medical costs have a much higher correlation with first- and second-year costs in depressed than in nondepressed high utilizers according to the MOS screen (**Table 1**). By our definition of high utilizer, first- and second-year costs of high utilizers were high, while third-year costs were free to rise or fall. Costs of depressed high utilizers decreased by a mean (±SD) of \$917±\$8705 (14%) in the follow-up year, but nondepressed high utilizer costs decreased by \$2313±\$8540 (35%), with both groups starting with similar second-year costs (**Table 2**). This decrease, in log-transformed costs, was significantly greater for nondepressed high utilizers ($P=.002$). Average costs for depressed high utilizers in the third year were \$1537 higher than for nondepressed high utilizers; average log-transformed third-year costs were significantly higher for depressed high utilizers ($P<.001$). A relatively small proportion (<9%) of third-year medical costs was associated with the direct treatment of depression, such as antidepressant medication, visits to a mental health provider, and psychological testing, even among patients who screened positive on the MOS depression items (**Table 3**).

The previous analyses did not adjust for other

Table 1. Correlation for Utilization Between Years for High Utilizers

Correlation	Depressed (n=130)	Nondepressed (n=362)
Year 1–year 2	0.48*	0.08
Year 1–year 3	0.44*	0.13*
Year 2–year 3	0.39*	0.18*

*Statistically significant ($P<.02$).

Table 2. Average Utilization per Year for High Utilizers Defined as Charges to the HMO*

	Utilization, $ (Mean±SD)	
	Depressed (n=130)	Nondepressed (n=362)
Year 1	5509.50±5426.70	5359.50±5783.30
Year 2	6681.60±8091.30	6540.00±7568.80
Year 3	5764.30†±7260.10	4227.00†±5843.10

*HMO indicates health maintenance organization. There is not a significant difference in log-transformed costs between depressed and nondepressed groups within year 1 or year 2.

†Log transformed costs were significantly different from one another ($t[488]=-3.584$, $P<.001$).

Table 3. Average Medical and Pharmaceutical Costs Derived From Services and Pharmaceuticals Traditionally Attributed to Treatment of Depression*

	Costs, $ (Mean±SD)	
Group	Medical	Pharmacy
Depressed (n=130)	239.05±601.76	279.62±428.23
Nondepressed (n=362)	24.98±136.78	50.85±202.29

*Average medical costs are the total amounts paid by the health maintenance organization for visits to mental health providers and for psychological testing. Average pharmaceutical costs are the total amounts paid by the health maintenance organization for filled prescriptions.

confounding variables. Age, sex, benefits package, and the presence of other medical morbidity might be associated with both higher medical costs and a higher rate of depression. A linear regression model was used to adjust for these potentially confounding variables. The results of the 3 regression models are summarized in **Table 4** and **Table 5**. All models predict total medical costs associated with the variable depression. The first model (model 1) does not adjust for potentially confounding variables. Model 2 adjusts for age, sex, and benefits package and model 3 adjusts for age, sex, benefits package, and medical comorbidity. Table 4 shows the adjusted R^2 (ie, the proportion of the variance in log costs explained by the model) and the overall F test for each of the 3 models. Model 2 accounts for 7.5% of the variance in log total costs. By contrast, adding medical comorbidity (model 3) explained 45% of the variance in log total costs. The added variance explained by incorporating the medical comorbidity (beyond age, sex, and benefits package) is highly significant ($P<.001$).

Adjustment for age, sex, benefits package, and comorbidity identified a 26% higher expenditure for a positive MOS depression screen. That is, if depressed HMO members were relieved of their depression, controlling for age, sex, benefits package, and medical comorbidity, their third-year utilization would decrease 26% ($P=.001$). This translates into an average difference of $1498 in third-year costs (Table 5).

COMMENT

The concept of a mental health cost offset has been elusive. Depression is known to be associated with increased office visits, extra procedures, and overall increased medical utilization.[1,2] From the patient's perspective, depression is associated with decreased quality of life, decreased work productivity, and increased absenteeism.[6,24] Managed care organizations are becoming more focused on quality of care and the importance of treating depression. However, they are concerned that aggressive screening and treatment of depressed patients will increase their total costs. From the economic perspective of managed care organizations, the increased costs of treating depression can be offset only by decreasing other medical utilization. However, the estimated cost per year of appropriately treating depression in primary care ($1400 per year) is greater than the total annual medical expenses of many untreated depressed patients. High utilizers of medical services have a high prevalence of undiagnosed depression. Treatment of depressed high utilizers of medical services has the potential to show a direct cost offset if a substantial percentage of their utilization is secondary to depression. If one takes a longer-term perspective, the benefits of depression treatment may extend into subsequent years where treatment costs are less. This would increase the potential for a cost offset. The inclusion of indirect costs further expands the potential savings of depression treatment.

This study identified a population of patients who were consistent high utilizers for 2 years and found that having a diagnosis of depression in the third year was highly correlated with continued high utilization. This remained true even after adjusting for variables known to be associated with high utilization, such as age, sex, and medical comorbidity. After adjusting for these variables, a positive screen for depression was associated with $1498 of third-year medical costs.

What would have happened if all depressed high utilizers we identified had received effective depression treatment during the third year? Potentially, their utilization pattern would have changed to that seen in the patients who were not depressed in the third year. This would result in an annual savings of as much as $1498, an amount that would pay for their depression treatment.

This study has a number of limitations. First, the diagnosis of depression was made only at a single point in 1994, the third year of data collection. The

Table 4. Percentage of Total Costs Associated With Depression in the Follow-up Year

Model	% of Costs Associated With Depression (95% Confidence Interval)	Log-Transformed Adjusted R^2	*P*, Model Significance
1: Unadjusted	34 (26-41)	0.024	<.001
2: Adjusted for age, gender, and benefit package*	37 (29-44)	0.075	<.001
3: Adjusted for age, gender, benefit package, and comorbidity†	26 (20-33)	0.447	<.001

*Model 2 explains significantly more than model 1 ($F[12,476]=3.297$, $P<.001$).

†Model 3 explains significantly more than model 2 ($F[33,443]=10.420$, $P<.001$).

Table 5. Mean Costs Associated With a Positive Screen for Depression in the Follow-up Year

Model	Average Cost Associated With Depression, $ (95% Confidence Interval)
Unadjusted	1954.86 (1498.72-2363.36)
Adjusted for age and gender	2132.79 (1671.65-2336.29)
Adjusted for age, gender, and comorbidity	1498.72 (1152.86-1902.22)

patients may have been depressed for the entire 3 years of the study or only briefly in the third year when the depression screen was administered. In addition to being depressed in the third year, half of the depressed high utilizers had a physician diagnosis of depression and half filled an antidepressant prescription in the first 2 years. This finding is consistent with a study that found that two thirds of depressed patients with high utilization had a history of depression, usually recurrent.[25]

Second, depression was diagnosed by means of the 8-item MOS screen, a self-administered paper-based depression questionnaire. It has good sensitivity and specificity but is not as reliable as an in-person diagnosis made with a structured clinical interview. In addition, the MOS depression screen provides severity information that is clinically difficult to interpret.

Third, 20 patients were excluded from the study because they were enrolled in an intervention study during the third year. The intervention probably affected the course of their utilization and definitely decreased their level of depression, which is why they were excluded. The 20 patients excluded from the analysis do not differ from the 130 depressed patients in age, sex, ADGs, or year 1 or year 2 utilization (costs). Including these patients in the regression analyses did not affect the relationship between depression and medical costs.

A fourth limitation is that, despite the strong correlation between a diagnosis of depression in the third year and continued high utilization, one cannot assume that there is a causal relationship between the 2 findings. It is possible that a factor not controlled for in the regression analysis caused both depression and continued high utilization. One can conclude, nonetheless, that in this population a diagnosis of depression in the third year is a strong marker for continued high utilization in the third year. It is also possible that some of the high utilizers had continued medical illness in the third year leading to secondary depression and poor quality of life. We tested this hypothesis by looking at the association of specific ADG categories in the third year and a positive MOS depression screen in the third year. Only 2 ADG categories were statistically more prevalent in the depressed group: 23 (includes major depression) and 24 (includes categories of minor depression and psychosocial stresses). No ADG category was statistically more prevalent in the nondepressed group. Therefore, as a group, the data do not support the hypothesis that a higher rate of medical illness in the third year is leading to secondary depression.

Fifth, because some of the diagnostic categories in ADG 23 were not included in the regression model, we may be leaving out diagnoses that are potential confounders of the relationship between depression and total costs. This may cause the depression estimate to be inflated.

Sixth, 37% of high utilizers did not respond to the questionnaire. Although the responders did not differ significantly from the nonresponders in their rate of physician-diagnosed depression, sex, or third-year utilization, other differences between responders and nonresponders may have had an impact on the relationship between depression and medical costs.

The excess medical costs of $1498 per year in depressed high utilizers of medical services suggest that the cost of treating depression for a year could potentially be offset by the decrease in excess medical costs. A randomized controlled study is under way to determine whether treatment of depressed high utilizers will relieve their depression, increase their quality of life, and decrease work absenteeism and their utilization of medical services more than usual care.

Accepted for publication May 15, 1996.

This research was supported in part by a grant from Pfizer Pharmaceuticals, New York, NY.

Presented in part at the National Institute of Mental Health Conference on Mental Health Services, Bethesda, Md, September 11, 1995.

We would like to thank Willard G. Manning, PhD, for providing substantial consultation and assistance with the transformation and retransformation procedures and the regression analyses, Janice Lonowski for coordinating this study, and Sue Dottl for reviewing the manuscript.

Reprints: Henry J. Henk, MS, Dean Foundation for Health, Research and Education, 8000 Excelsior Dr, Madison, WI 53717.

REFERENCES

1. Levenson JL, Hamer RM, Rossiter LF. Psychopathology and pain in medical in-patients predict resource use during hospitalization but not rehospitalization. *J Psychosom Res.* 1992;36:585-592.
2. Manning WG, Wells KB. The effects of psychological distress and psychological well-being on use of medical services. *Med Care.* 1992;30:541-553.
3. Widmer RB, Cadoret RJ. Depression in family practice: changes in pattern of patient visits and complaints during subsequent developing depression. *J Fam Pract.* 1979;9:1017-1021.
4. Katon W, Von Korff M, Lin E, et al. Distressed utilizers of medical care *DSM-III-R* diagnoses and treatment needs. *Gen Hosp Psychiatry.* 1990;12: 355-362.
5. Koenig HG, Shelp F, Goli V, Cohen HJ, Blazer DG. Survival and health care utilization in elderly medical inpatients with major depression. *J Am Geriatr Soc.* 1989;37:599-606.
6. Greenburg PE, Stiglin LE, Finkelstein SN, Berndt ER. The economic burden of depression in 1990. *J Clin Psychiatry.* 1993;54:405-418.
7. Von Korff M, Ormel J, Katon W, Lin EHB. Disability and depression among high utilizers of health care: a longitudinal analysis. *Arch Gen Psychiatry.* 1992; 49:91-100.
8. McFarland BH, Freeborn DK, Mullooly JP, Pope CR. Utilization patterns among long-term enrollees in a prepaid group practice health maintenance organization. *Med Care.* 1985;23:1221-1223.
9. Simon G, Ormel J, VonKorff M, Barlow W. Health care costs associated with depressive and anxiety disorders in primary care. *Am J Psychiatry.* 1995;152: 352-357.
10. McCombs JS, Nichol MB, Stimmel GL, Sclar DA, Beasley CM, Gross LS. The cost of antidepressant drug therapy failure: a study of antidepressant use patterns in a Medicaid population. *J Clin Psychiatry.* 1990;51:60-69.
11. Simon GE, VonKorff M, Barlow W. Health care costs of primary care patients with recognized depression. *Arch Gen Psychiatry.* 1995;52:850-856.
12. Katzelnick DJ, Kobak KA, Greist JH, Jefferson JW. Depression among high utilization primary care patients: effect of identification and treatment on service utilization, disability and quality of life. Read before the National Institute of Mental Health Conference on Mental Health Services, September 11, 1995, Bethesda, Md.
13. Burman MA, Wells KB, Leake B, Landsverk J. Development of a brief screening instrument for detecting depressive disorders. *Med Care.* 1988;26:775-789.
14. Radloff LS. The CES-D scale: a self report depression scale for research on the general population. *Appl Psychol Meas.* 1977;1:385.
15. Robins LN, Helzer JE, Croughan J, Ratcliff KS. National Institute of Mental Health Diagnostic Interview Schedule: its history, characteristics and validity. *Arch Gen Psychiatry.* 1982;38:381-389.
16. Rost K, Smith R, Matthews DB, Guise B. The deliberate misdiagnosis of major depression in primary care. *Arch Fam Med.* 1994;3:333-337.
17. Weiner JP, Starfield BH, Steinwachs DM, Mumford LM. Development and application of a population-oriented measure of ambulatory care case-mix. *Med Care.* 1991;29:452-472.
18. Stardield BH, Weiner JP, Mumford L, Steinwachs DM. Ambulatory care groups: a categorization of diagnosis for research and management. *Health Serv Res.* 1991;26:54-74.
19. Von Korff M, Wagner E, Saunders K. A chronic disease score from automated pharmacy data. *J Clin Epidemiol.* 1992;45:197-203.
20. Duan N, Manning WG, Morris CN, Newhouse JP. A comparison of alternative models for the demand for medical care. *J Bus Econ Stat.* 1983;1:115-126.
21. Duan N, Manning WG, Morris CN, Newhouse JP. Choosing between the sample-selection model and the multi-part model. *J Bus Econ Stat.* 1984;2:283-289.
22. Duan N. Smearing estimate: a nonparametric retransformation method. *J Am Stat Assoc.* 1983;78:605-610.
23. D'Agostino RB. Transformation to normality of the null distribution of g_1. *Biometrika.* 1970;57:679-681.
24. Broadhead WE, Blazer DG, George LK, Tse CK. Depression, disability days, and days lost from work in a prospective epidemiologic survey. *JAMA.* 1990; 264:2524-2538.
25. Katon W, Von Korff M, Lin E, et al. A randomized trial of psychiatric consultation with distressed high utilizers. *Gen Hosp Psychiatry.* 1992;14:86-98.

ORIGINAL ARTICLE

Counseling Typically Provided for Depression

Role of Clinician Specialty and Payment System

Lisa S. Meredith, PhD; Kenneth B. Wells, MD, MPH; Sherrie H. Kaplan, PhD, MPH; Rebecca M. Mazel, MA

Background: To assess how current policy trends may affect the use of counseling for depression, we examined the variation in the *use of counseling* and *usual clinician counseling style* for depression across specialty sectors (psychiatry, psychology, and general medicine) and reimbursement type (fee-for-service or prepaid).

Methods: Three types of observational data from the RAND Medical Outcomes Study: (1) patient-reported demographics, depressive symptoms, clinical status, and perceptions about participation style; (2) clinician reports of counseling during specific patient encounters; and (3) clinician reports of the usual counseling and interpersonal style across patients who were seen in a practice.

Results: While almost all depressed patients who were being treated by mental health specialists received brief counseling for at least 3 minutes, less than half of the depressed patients in the general medical sector received such counseling—even for those patients with a current depressive disorder. Counseling rates were lower under prepaid than fee-for-service care in general medical practices. Psychiatrists relied more on psychodynamic approaches, and psychologists relied more on behavioral therapies relative to each other, but both specialty groups provided longer sessions and used more formal psychotherapeutic techniques (eg, interpretation) than did general medical clinicians. Clinicians who were treating more patients who had prepaid plans reported a lower proclivity for face-to-face counseling, and they spent less time when they were counseling patients compared with clinicians who were treating more patients who had fee-for-service plans; however, these differences were not large.

Conclusion: The use of counseling in the usual care for depression varied by both specialty and payment system, while the usual clinician counseling style differed markedly by specialty, but only slightly by payment system.

Arch Gen Psychiatry. 1996;53:905-912

HEALTH CARE delivery systems are currently implementing cost-containment strategies (eg, gatekeeper policies and prepaid financing) that could affect the use of counseling or psychotherapy for depression—a change that could have important clinical and policy implications. Depression is prevalent and strongly associated with morbidity.[1-4] Reductions in the use of efficacious treatments like psychotherapy for depression[5,6] could worsen patient outcomes, and greater reliance on general medical providers might be especially likely to reduce the use of psychotherapy because of low rates of detection and referral in that sector.[7,8]

The findings from clinical trials in the literature support the efficacy of psychotherapy and "medical counseling" for major depression or general psychological distress.[8] Although evidence has been inconsistent for its efficacy as maintenance therapy (ie, for preventing recurrences),[8,9] some studies have suggested that briefer forms of counseling improve outcomes in general medical depressed[10-12] or psychologically distressed patients.[13] Such findings have been featured prominently in debates over coverage for psychotherapy, but these findings may not generalize to a typical practice because they usually exclude patients with comorbidities, rely on mental health specialty patient samples, use highly structured forms of psychotherapy and standardized clinician training procedures, reimburse counseling through research grants, and rely on selected practice environments (eg, academic centers).[14] Few studies of typically provided counseling are available, and there is no consensus about how to define depression counseling in this context. However, one study[15] examined the usual psychotherapy in mental health specialty practices by using a dose-response model, and another study[16] found that depression counseling, in combination with effective antidepressant use, was associated with better 2-year outcomes across specialty sectors.

See Materials and Methods on next page

From the Social Policy Department, RAND, Santa Monica, Calif (Drs Meredith and Wells and Ms Mazel); the Department of Psychiatry and Biobehavioral Sciences, UCLA Neuropsychiatric Institute and Hospital, UCLA School of Medicine, Los Angeles, Calif (Dr Wells); and The Health Institute, New England Medical Center, Boston, Mass (Dr Kaplan).

MATERIALS AND METHODS

DATA AND SAMPLE

The data are from the RAND Medical Outcomes Study, an observational study of care for adult patients in health maintenance organizations, large multispecialty groups, and solo practices in Los Angeles, Calif; Boston, Mass; and Chicago, Ill. Across systems of care, a sample of 523 clinicians was selected from the specialties of family medicine, general internal medicine, cardiology, endocrinology, psychiatry, and clinical psychology, and from masters-level therapists in group practices. Participation rates for eligible clinicians ranged from moderate to high.[35,36] A consecutive sample of 22 399 adults who were visiting study providers during an average 9-day period was obtained, and both patients and clinicians completed postvisit screening questionnaires. Additional study details have been reported elsewhere.[37,38]

Analyses were restricted to enrolled clinicians who completed a Clinician Background Questionnaire (n=470) that was administered during fall 1986 and to their depressed patients (described in the "Data Analysis" subsection). The average age of the clinicians was 40 years (55% were 40 years of age or younger), 22% were women, and 12% were nonwhite. There were 349 general medical clinicians, 76 psychiatrists, 74 psychologists, and 24 master's-level therapists; 38 clinicians reported that they received psychoanalytic training. About 20 of the depressed patients were sampled from a psychoanalyst's office. Clinician and patient characteristics are shown in **Table 1** by specialty. The means for the binary variables are interpreted as percentages.

STUDY DEFINITION AND MEASURES OF COUNSELING FOR DEPRESSION

We defined *counseling* as a face-to-face interaction between the clinician and patient that lasted for 3 minutes or more that was designed to have a therapeutic effect for depression, including psychoanalysis. We selected a broad definition of counseling to permit a comparison of specialty and generalist care.[21] Clinicians were asked in single items to report whether they had provided counseling for depression or for other emotional or family problems during each patient visit.

We defined the *usual clinician counseling style* as seven domains of clinician-perceived counseling and interpersonal style. These domains were measured by a battery of counseling items that were included in a self-administered questionnaire that was completed by clinicians before the period of screening patients. **Table 2** describes each of the counseling measures and provides scoring information and descriptive statistics. Multi-item scales were first validated by using an a priori rationale and the criteria of multitrait-scaling methods. Measures were then derived by averaging responses across items and rescaling the average to a range from 0 to 100. A high score on these scales reflects a *stronger counseling orientation*. Internal consistencies all exceeded minimum standards of internal consistency for group comparisons.[39]

DATA ANALYSIS

We used multiple regression analyses (ordinary least squares regression for continuous measures and logistic regression for discrete measures). Payment and specialty differences in the use of counseling during the visit and perceptions of interpersonal style were analyzed with the patient as the unit of analysis and controlled for geographical site, payment, specialty, payment by specialty interaction, patient demographics (gender, age, education, and income), for casemix (using a global measure of psychological sickness),[16] and for the clustered sampling design.[40,41] To rule out differences in counseling because of detection, we also adjusted for a clinician's detection of depression,[8] which was highly correlated with counseling (0.7 for all clinicians) since it preceded the diagnosis. We present adjusted counseling rates for three samples of depressed patients in the RAND Medical Outcomes Study: (1) all patients from the cross-sectional screener sample (n=3456) who exceeded an established cutoff-point on an eight-item brief self-report depression symptom scale[42] that was completed at the time of the office visit; (2) a subset of those patients who exceeded the initial screener cutoff-point and who were eligible for the longitudinal panel (n=976); and (3) a subset of patients who had a baseline assessment (n=733) who also met Diagnostic Interview Schedule criteria for current major depression or dysthymia[43,44] and, therefore, might benefit most from counseling.

Payment and specialty differences in the usual counseling and interpersonal style were analyzed in clinician-level models that controlled for site, payment (ie, whether more than 50% of patients had prepaid plans), specialty, average patient demographics (gender, age, and race) for the clinician's practice, and individual clinician demographics (gender, age, and race). We also assessed clinicians' academic training (MD or PhD degree or master's level). For comparing clinician specialties, we included both system (health maintenance organization, large multispecialty groups, and solo practices) and payment (prepaid or fee-for-service) type as covariates in the regression models. For comparisons that involved system and payment, we included only one or the other (system or payment). We also examined the sensitivity of our findings to adjustments for clinical characteristics of their patients: (1) the average probability of having a current depressive disorder as assessed by the brief eight-item depression screener (described above) and (2) the mean score on general health perceptions. These were derived by aggregating patient-level responses across all patients for a given clinician. Since our conclusions were insensitive to this adjustment, we present results that were unadjusted for patient sickness. To illustrate differences in style, we generated means for payment and specialty groups (but not for master's-level therapists because of the low number) based on parameters of the regression models.

Construct and predictive validity of clinicians' usual counseling and interpersonal style measures was analyzed at the patient level through estimating relationships with selected clinical quality-of-care measures (provision of counseling during the screening visit, detection of depression,[8] and effective antidepressant use[16]). These models controlled for the same set of covariates that were described for the counseling use analysis. To illustrate results, we generated the adjusted means for quality-of-care measures at low and high values of clinician style scores.

Table 1. Patient, Clinician, and Practice Characteristics of Depressed Patients by Specialty*

Characteristic	Clinician Specialty: General Medical	Mental Health Specialties: Psychiatry	Psychology
Patient demographics			
No.	2460	553	478
% Female	71.6 (45.1)	67.5 (46.9)	67.8 (46.8)
% Nonwhite	28.0 (44.4)	12.4 (32.6)	11.6 (31.9)
Mean age, y	46.5 (17.2)	40.5 (12.0)	38.2 (11.3)
Clinician demographics			
No.	349	76	74
% Female	18.3 (38.7)	15.7 (36.6)	22.0 (41.8)
% Nonwhite	14.6 (35.4)	10.5 (30.9)	2.7 (16.3)
Mean age, y	39.6 (6.6)	40.6 (4.7)	41.9 (5.6)
Practice characteristics			
Mean % of patients with prepaid coverage	44.1 (39.9)	30.2 (36.2)	40.3 (41.4)
Mean No. of outpatient visits/wk	74.4 (48.9)	33.4 (13.5)	29.4 (12.0)
Practice casemix (among all patients)			
Mean probability of depressed patients	6.6 (5.0)	25.9 (11.8)	19.3 (8.9)
Mean % of patients detected	34.7 (47.6)	86.8 (33.9)	84.1 (36.6)
Mean current health perception†	63.4 (10.4)	67.6 (12.6)	74.3 (8.5)

*The SDs are given in parentheses.
†Scored from 0 to 100 points, where a high score indicated better health perceptions.

Studies of specialty variation in counseling have found relatively higher rates of formal psychotherapy among mental health specialists; in the general medical sector, such studies have found more reliance on medical counseling,[17,18] which is briefer than formal psychotherapy and consists primarily of advice and education.[19,20] Studies of psychotherapy processes in mental health specialty practices have identified discrete domains of interpersonal care, including egalitarian participation and decision-making styles.[21,22] These domains were redefined as generic aspects of interpersonal process in health care encounters and in studies of care for chronic medical conditions (eg, diabetes); however, to our knowledge, specialty sectors have not been compared on these domains.[23]

The literature on variation by payment system includes early studies that suggested that the demand for mental health visits (mostly psychotherapy) is responsive to a variation in the generosity of fee-for-service insurance coverage.[24] Furthermore, one study[25] found that the response of mental health utilization to insurance generosity was similar for patients with and without a psychiatric diagnosis. Other studies[26-28] have found similar probabilities of mental health use in prepaid plans, relative to comparable fee-for-service plans, but lower costs for prepayment, owing to lower visit intensity, substitution of nonphysicians for physicians, and greater reliance on group rather than individual therapy. Lower counseling rates for general medically depressed patients who had prepaid plans compared with those for such patients who had fee-for-service plans were found, but the differences could have been owing to patient sickness.[7]

This article estimates the use of depression counseling by specialty and payment system and the style of that counseling, by using concepts from studies of psychotherapy, interpersonal style of health care, preventive counseling,[23,29,30] social cognitive theory,[31,32] and treatment style.[33,34] We do not directly examine counseling outcomes.

We made the following hypotheses: (1) similarly depressed patients would have lower rates of counseling in the general medical than in the mental health specialty sector, (2) prepayment would be associated with lower counseling rates within the general medical sector only, (3) general medical clinicians would use less intensive and more advice-oriented depression counseling compared with that used by mental health specialists, and (4) prepayment would be associated with a stronger orientation, relative to fee-for-service care, toward advice-oriented rather than psychodynamically oriented counseling.

RESULTS

PAYMENT AND SPECIALTY DIFFERENCES IN THE EXTENT OF COUNSELING

We found large differences by specialty in the adjusted percentage of patients who were counseled ($P<.05$); there were significantly more depressed patients who were likely to be counseled in the mental health specialty sector. A priori pairwise comparisons, for significant overall specialty effects, indicated that differences between general medical clinicians and either psychiatrists or psychologists reached statistical significance and that the use of counseling was similarly high for patients who were seen by psychologists and psychiatrists. Among general medical clinicians, only one third or less, and among mental health specialists, only one half or less, of depressed patients were counseled for depression or other psychosocial problems. However, there were no significant differences by specialty in patients' perceptions of their clinicians' usual participation style (**Table 3**).

We found significant payment differences in the percentage of patients who were receiving emotional or family counseling in two of the three samples ($P<.05$ in each), and these effects were entirely owing to payment differences within the general medical sector. Within that sector, prepayment was associated with significantly lower counseling rates—11 percentage points lower than fee-for-service plans compared with only five percentage points lower in the mental health sector (a 30% difference). Payment was also significantly associated with patients' perceptions of egalitarian participation style ($P<.05$), especially within the general medical sector. Patients who were seen by general medical clinicians with fee-for-service arrangements rated the care that they received from their usual clinician as significantly more egalitarian (by five to seven points on a 0- to 100-point scale) compared with that of similar general medical patients with prepaid coverage. This pattern was similar for all three subsamples, including patients with a current depressive disorder.

Table 2. Description and Properties of Counseling and Interpersonal Style Measures*

Measure	Definition or Item Content	Scoring	κ	α	Mean	SD
Patient-level measures						
Detection of depression	Clinician reported counseling the patient for 3 min or more about depression during the visit	0/1, where a "1" indicates that the patient was counseled	1	...	40.5	49.1
Counseled for depression	Clinician reported counseling the patient for 3 min or more about depression during the visit	0/1, where a "1" indicates that the patient was counseled	1	...	40.5	49.1
Counseled for other emotional or family problem	Clinician reported counseling the patient for 3 min or more about other emotional or family problems during the visit	0/1, where a "1" indicates that the patient was counseled	1	...	56.1	49.6
Egalitarian participation style	Extent to which the patient felt that the physician or other health care professional just seen: Would involve the patient in choosing between treatments; would gladly answer questions about treatment; makes an effort to give the patient control over his or her own treatment; asks the patient to take responsibility for his or her own treatment	0- to 100-point scale, where a high score indicates a more egalitarian participation style	4	.71	84.1	15.8
Clinician-level measures						
Usual clinician counseling style						
Initiation	Whether and extent to which clinician usually raises issue for discussion with patients: Marital or family problems; depression; sexual functioning; coping with physical illness or symptoms	0- to 100-point scale, where a high score indicates more counseling initiative taken by the clinician as opposed to the patient	4	.75	45.1	15.1
Perceived skill	Perceptions of skill in counseling patients: Marital or family problems; depression; sexual functioning; coping with physical illness or symptoms	0- to 100-point scale, where a high score indicates higher perceptions of skill	4	.82	48.4	17.4
Intensity (duration)	Amount of time taken to deal with emotional issues or patients' personal problems	0/1, where a "1" indicates that the clinician usually counseled for more than 10 min	1	...	62.2	48.5
Preference for depression counseling	Likelihood of providing ongoing (≥3 visits), face-to-face counseling to treat moderate-to-severe depression: Depression, no major medical illness; depression and recent myocardial infarction; depression and hypertension; depression and diabetes	0- to 100-point scale, where a high score indicates a clinician's stronger preference for usually counseling depressed patients	4	.97	67.4	35.8
Technique	Usual technique used in face-to-face counseling of patients for personal, emotional, or family problems	0/1, where a "1" indicates that a clinician usually used the technique (each technique scored as a separate measure)				
	Education or advice		1	...	90.8	28.9
	Interpretations or confrontations		1	...	65.6	47.6
	Counseling family members		1	...	57.4	49.5
	Behavioral treatments (eg, relaxation)		1	...	41.7	49.4
	Psychodynamic therapy		1	...	33.6	47.3
Usual clinician interpersonal style						
Egalitarian participation	Extent to which clinician conveys a sense of dominance, directiveness, judgmentalness, and superiority to patients: Good physicians use their authority to shape patient behavior; treatment recommendations presented with authority are more likely to be accepted by patients; competent professionals who maintain an air of authority usually obtain the best results in treating patients; sometimes it is best to pressure patients to get them to do what is best for them	0- to 100-point scale, where a high score indicates a more egalitarian style	4	.62	48.7	15.6
Share treatment decisions	Tendency for clinician to share treatment decisions with the patient: I prefer that patients leave treatment decisions up to me; if I make patients feel that they are making treatment choices themselves, their disease management is better; it's best to let patients participate in decisions whenever choices between treatment options are available; most patients cannot make intelligent choices about care	0- to 100-point scale, where a high score indicates a stronger tendency to share treatment decisions	4	.64	77.2	14.2

**Means for binary measures are interpreted as percentages.*

Table 3. Counseling and Interpersonal Care Delivered to Depressed Patients by Clinician Specialty and Practice Payment Status*

Patient-Level Measure	General Medical FFS	General Medical PP	Psychiatry FFS	Psychiatry PP	Psychology FFS	Psychology PP
Screener sample: depressive symptoms or disorder (n=3456)						
Depression counseling, %†‡	33.0	27.9	51.3	63.2	45.0	49.9
Psychosocial counseling, %†‡§	49.5	42.1	93.2	90.3	94.1	95.9
Egalitarian participation style (0-100 points)§	86.8	82.0	85.7	84.7	87.7	84.7
Longitudinal panel: depressive symptoms or disorder (n=976)						
Depression counseling, %†	41.1	28.8	56.8	74.3	52.9	47.2
Psychosocial counseling, %†	51.7	42.9	91.1	86.8	96.0	98.5
Egalitarian participation style (0-100 points)§	87.4	81.6	86.6	85.6	85.8	84.1
Baseline sample: current depressive disorder (n=733)						
Depression counseling, %†	47.4	37.8	63.3	66.7	64.0	65.8
Psychosocial counseling, %†§	61.4	50.2	97.5	95.4	95.7	88.7
Egalitarian participation style (0-100 points)§	89.2	82.3	85.5	84.0	87.8	82.6

Averages are based on regression analyses (logistic for counseling measures and ordinary least squares for participation style), which controlled for study site, clinician specialty, patient payment status, patient demographic characteristics, patient casemix, and clinician detection of depression. FFS indicates fee-for-service; PP, prepaid.

†*Main effect of specialty is statistically significant (P<.05).*

‡*Interaction between specialty and payment is statistically significant (P<.05).*

§*Main effect of payment is statistically significant (P<.05).*

Table 4. Clinician Usual Style of Care by Clinician Specialty and Practice Payment Status (n=470)*

Clinician-Level Measure†	Clinician Specialty: General Medical	Mental Health Specialties: Psychiatry	Mental Health Specialties: Psychology	Payment Status: <50% PP	Payment Status: ≥50% PP
Usual counseling style					
Initiation	44.0	49.8	45.1	44.6	45.6
Perceived skill	40.1‡§	64.7	64.0	49.1	47.0
Intensity, % counseling for ≥10 min	36.1‡§‖	74.8	81.1	51.2¶	47.9
Preference for depression counseling	51.8‡§	92.7	94.1	69.8¶	62.9
Usual interpersonal style					
Egalitarian participation#	56.2	56.7	55.4	56.0	56.2
Share treatment decisions	74.7‡§	80.7	82.3	76.2	76.7

**PP indicates prepaid.*

†*Unless noted otherwise, all measures were scaled from 0 to 100 points in the direction indicated by their name. Averages are based on ordinary least squares regression that controlled for study site, clinician specialty, patient payment status, and clinician demographics.*

‡*Mean for general medical is significantly different from mean for psychiatry at P<.05.*

§*Mean for general medical is significantly different from mean for psychology at P<.05.*

‖*Mean for psychiatry is significantly different from mean for psychology at P<.05.*

¶*Mean for payment is significantly different at P<.05.*

#*Means in a given row for a given effect (eg, specialty and payment) sharing the same superscript are not significantly different at P<.05.*

PAYMENT AND SPECIALTY DIFFERENCES IN USUAL CLINICIAN COUNSELING STYLE

Clinicians who treated primarily patients who had prepaid plans were significantly less likely to report usually spending more than 10 minutes of an office visit dealing with personal or emotional problems than were those clinicians who were treating primarily patients who had fee-for-service coverage, and they reported lower preferences for personally counseling depressed patients (**Table 4**). For intensity, this finding was primarily owing to differences within the general medical sector: the specialty by payment interaction term was statistically significant (F [2, 246]=7.25, P<.001). Nearly all clinicians who treated a greater proportion of patients who had prepaid plans provided education or advice for psychosocial problems (95.5%) compared with slightly lower rates for clinicians who treated primarily patients who had fee-for-service plans (87.1%). Other aspects of the usual counseling style were unrelated to the predominant form of payment at the practice level. Specialty by payment interaction terms for other counseling domains had lower levels of significance and would not survive a multiple-comparison test.

We found significant differences by specialty for all counseling style measures (eg, perceived skill, intensity, preference, and technique [Table 4 and **Figure**]), except for initiative. Psychologists and psychiatrists reported similar counseling styles across all measures. Compared with general medical clinicians, reports of perceived skill by mental health specialists were 24 to 25 points higher (on a 0- to 100-point distribution) for psychosocial counseling. Compared with general medical clinicians, mental health specialists were 66% more likely to report that they usually spent more than 10 minutes of an office visit dealing

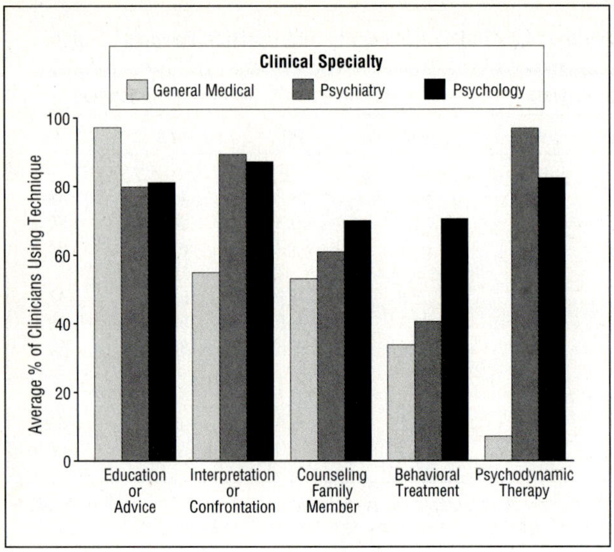

Adjusted percentage of clinicians who used face-to-face counseling techniques in the last month.

with their patients' personal or emotional problems, that they had stronger preferences for personally counseling depressed patients (scoring 41 to 42 points higher on a 0- to 100-point scale), and that they were more likely to share treatment decisions with their patients (scoring five to seven points higher).

The Figure shows the profiles of therapeutic techniques that were used for counseling patients' personal, emotional, or family problems by specialty of clinician. Compared with mental health specialists, general medical clinicians relied more on education and advice ($P<.01$) but less on interpretation and confrontation and family member counseling ($P<.01$). Compared with psychiatrists, psychologists provided significantly more behavioral treatment ($P<.001$); compared with psychologists, psychiatrists provided significantly more psychodynamically oriented therapy ($P<.001$), and general medical clinicians provided significantly less of both therapies than did mental health specialists ($P<.001$).

Counseling style for the 24 master's-level clinicians (eg, mental health nurses, psychiatric social workers, and nurse practitioners) was between that of mental health specialists and general medical clinicians. Compared with other mental health specialists, these clinicians reported a significantly lower skill at counseling for psychosocial problems, had lower preferences for providing face-to-face counseling, and were less likely to share treatment decisions.

CLINICIANS' USUAL COUNSELING STYLE AND SUBSEQUENT CLINICAL TREATMENT

Table 5 presents the average (adjusted) percentage of patients who received clinical treatments of depression during the screening visit for low (25th percentile on the 0- to 100-point scale) or high (75th percentile on the 0- to 100-point scale) values on the usual clinician counseling style measures for their own clinician (collected before that visit). The actual differences between high and low values on the continuous measures ranged from 21% to 41%, depending on the counseling style measure. Patients who were seen by clinicians who reported a greater tendency to initiate counseling were significantly more likely to have their depression detected, relative to other patients (a 26% difference in counseling initiation scores was equivalent to a 5% difference in detection rates). Patients who were seen by clinicians with a higher perceived skill in psychosocial counseling were significantly more likely to have their depression detected and to receive psychosocial counseling (a 41% difference in perceived skill was associated with a 10% difference in detection or counseling). Patients who were seen by clinicians who typically provided less than 10 minutes of psychosocial counseling compared with those who counseled for 10 minutes or more were only one third as likely to use an effective antidepressant medication. Patients who were seen by clinicians who reported a low preference for face-to-face counseling compared with clinicians who reported a high preference (a 28% difference) were less likely to have their depression detected (12%) or to receive counseling for depression (10%) or other psychosocial problems (15%). Patients who were seen by clinicians who scored high on egalitarian participation compared with those who scored low on the scale (a 21% difference) were also significantly more likely to have their depression detected (12%) or receive depression counseling (25%). The measure of shared decision making was not associated with clinical treatment measures.

COMMENT

We found low to moderate rates for brief counseling (of at least 3 minutes) among general medical clinicians compared with those among mental health specialists; within this sector, prepayment was associated with lower counseling rates for all patients with depressive symptoms and for the subset of patients with a current depressive disorder, for whom specific forms of psychotherapy were efficacious.[3] Recent work[5] has shown that even these brief counseling measures are markers for a course of therapy that may be associated (especially in combination with use of antidepressants) with substantial improvement in functioning outcomes, as well as increased treatment costs. Thus, shifts of depressed patients to general medical care under gatekeeping policies could affect the probability of their receiving counseling, especially under prepayment. In contrast, access of depressed patients to at least some counseling is similarly high in mental health specialty care, regardless of payment.

But, is the "counseling" provided similar across different types of health care settings? We found large differences by specialty in the usual clinician counseling style. Compared with general medical clinicians, psychologists and psychiatrists were more confident in their skill, provided longer sessions, had stronger preferences for face-to-face counseling, were more willing to share treatment decisions with their patients, and had a more psychodynamic counseling style. Counseling among psychiatrists was characterized by a psychodynamic style that consisted of psychotherapy and interpretation or confrontation, and counseling among psychologists was characterized by these features plus behavioral treatment. These differences in counseling were consistent with expecta-

Table 5. Associations Between Clinician Usual Counseling and Interpersonal Style and Clinical Treatment Delivered to Depressed Patients During the Screening Visit

Clinician Usual Counseling Style	% of Patients Receiving Clinical Treatment During Screening Visit			
	Detection of Depression	Depression Counseling	Psychosocial Counseling	Effective Use of Antidepressant Medication
Initiation*				
25th percentile (score of 38)	47.9†	39.0	54.7	12.1
75th percentile (score of 56)	52.8	41.5	59.3	12.3
Perceived skill*				
25th percentile (score of 38)	46.7‡	37.2	55.0†	13.5
75th percentile (score of 62)	57.0	44.3	64.7	11.3
Intensity				
Counseled, <10 min	48.3	36.8	57.3	5.8§
Counseled, ≥10 min	51.5	42.0	56.1	14.8
Preference for counseling depression*				
25th percentile (score of 56)	46.2§	36.1‡	55.4‡	13.1
75th percentile (score of 100)	58.5	46.4	62.1	10.1
Egalitarian participation style*				
25th percentile (score of 38)	49.1†	37.9†	55.4	12.4
75th percentile (score of 58)	51.5	43.1	58.0	11.7

*Scored on a 0- to 100-point scale.
†$P<.10$.
‡$P<.05$.
§$P<.01$.

tions based on training and theoretical orientation. Clinicians with more patients who had fee-for-service plans spent more time with their patients and had stronger preferences for personally counseling them than those with more patients who had prepaid plans, especially within general medicine. A study of primary care physicians found that those clinicians who practiced in fee-for-service systems were more likely to counsel their patients on psychosocial risk factors than were physicians who practiced in health maintenance organization systems.[45] However, differences by payment in the present study are small relative to the very large and consistent specialty differences.

Do these components of the usual counseling style matter in terms of health outcomes? Our study was not designed to answer this question. In preliminary analyses, we found no consistent significant associations of style measures with functioning outcomes, but statistical power was low. Other studies have found only weak evidence for differences in depression outcomes by the type of brief psychotherapy,[8] and some have argued that all psychosocial therapies have common elements (eg, empathy).[9] Therefore, whether some counseling for depression occurs may be more important than style.

However, counseling style could indirectly affect outcomes through changing the probability of treatment. For example, we found that a clinician's self-reported usual style of care predicted subsequent detection and counseling for depression. The value of usual counseling measures as screening tools for physician groups with a high or low proclivity to treat depression should be explored in future research. For example, the finding that clinicians who spend more time counseling their depressed patients also have a higher rate of effective antidepressant medication use could mean that these clinicians provide more education about proper medication use.

Our study has important limitations. It was conducted in selected health care delivery systems and geographical areas, and findings may not generalize beyond these settings. Data were collected between 1986 and 1989, and the usual care practices could differ now; in particular, fee-for-service care has become more managed and may currently be similar to prepaid systems. Despite these limitations, we doubt that overall styles of counseling have changed, except that medical visits may have become even briefer and mental health specialty referral less frequent.

Our health services approach to measuring counseling was cruder than in clinical research because of the limited resources and focus on typical care. We may have been more likely to capture broader stylistic differences by specialty and not merely distinctions in formal counseling style that could occur among mental health specialties, particularly by payment. Descriptive data from the RAND Medical Outcomes Study illustrate this point by using patient reports at baseline (among the enrolled sample) of the type of therapy received by payment. While most patients who were seen by mental health specialists received individual therapy (79%), 5% received group therapy, 5% received family therapy, 1% received other therapy, and 10% reported receiving no therapy. Most group therapy patients had less severe forms of depression and prepaid insurance, but precision was poor for formal comparisons. Thus, there could be other differences in the type of psychotherapy by payment that we did not detect. However, the literature supports the efficacy of group as well as individual brief psychotherapies[3]; thus, this could be a style rather than a quality-of-care difference. Despite the crudeness of our counseling measures, their ease of administration may make them useful for studying the "usual" patient-clinician encounters across specialty sectors.

Policies that shift patients more into prepaid care

and into general medical care could affect the distribution and style of counseling for depression as well as costs of care and, possibly, its quality if counseling for depression as typically provided improves outcomes. A new generation of health services studies on the cost-effectiveness of psychotherapy is needed to address this issue fully. We have taken only the first steps by demonstrating variation in counseling for policy-relevant groups and outlining one approach for conceptualizing counseling style in typical practice.

Accepted for publication October 4, 1995.

This research was supported by grants from the National Institute of Mental Health, Bethesda, Md; the Agency for Health Care Policy and Research, Rockville, Md; the Henry J. Kaiser Family Foundation, Menlo Park, Calif; the Robert Wood Johnson Foundation, Princeton, NJ; the Pew Charitable Trusts, Philadelphia, Pa; the Sepulveda (Calif) Veterans Affairs Center for the Study of Healthcare Provider Behavior; and RAND, Santa Monica, Calif.

Presented in part at the meetings of the Society of Behavioral Medicine and the American Public Health Association, San Francisco, Calif, March and October 1993.

Recruitment of clinicians was accomplished through the cooperation and assistance of the American College of Physicians, Philadelphia, Pa; the American Academy of Family Physicians, Kansas City, Mo; the American Academy of Pediatrics, Elk Grove Village, Ill; the American Psychiatric Association, Washington, DC; and the American Psychological Association, Washington, DC, and their local chapters in Medical Outcomes Study sites.

Corresponding author: Lisa S. Meredith, PhD, Social Policy Department, RAND, 1700 Main St, Santa Monica, CA 90407-2138.

REFERENCES

1. Regier DA, Narrow WE, Rae DS, Manderscheid RW, Locke BZ, Goodwin FK. The de facto US mental and addictive disorders service system: Epidemiologic Catchment Area prospective 1-year prevalence rates of disorders and services. *Arch Gen Psychiatry.* 1993;50:85-94.
2. Regier DA, Boyd JH, Burke JD Jr, Rae DS, Meyers JK, Kramer M, Robins LN, George LK, Karno M, Locke BZ. One-month prevalence of mental disorders in the United States. *Arch Gen Psychiatry.* 1988;45:977-986.
3. Wells KB, Stewart AL, Hays RD, Burnam MA, Rogers W, Daniels M, Berry S, Greenfield S, Ware JE. The functioning and well-being of depressed patients: results from the Medical Outcomes Study. *JAMA.* 1989;262:914-919.
4. Hays RD, Wells KB, Sherbourne CD, Rogers W, Spritzer K. Functioning and well-being outcomes of patients with depression compared with chronic general medical illnesses. *Arch Gen Psychiatry.* 1995;52:11-19.
5. Klerman GL, Weissman MM. *New Applications of Interpersonal Psychotherapy.* Washington, DC: American Psychiatric Press Inc; 1993.
6. Depression Guideline Panel. *Depression in Primary Care: Detection, Diagnosis, and Treatment: Quick Reference Guide for Clinicians: No 5.* Rockville, Md: US Dept of Health and Human Services, Public Health Service, Agency for Health Care Policy and Research; 1993. AHCPR publication 93-0552.
7. Rogers WH, Wells KB, Meredith LS, Sturm R, Burnam MA. Outcomes for adult depressed outpatients under prepaid and fee-for-service financing. *Arch Gen Psychiatry.* 1993;50:517-525.
8. Wells KB, Hays RD, Burnam MA, Rogers W, Greenfield S, Ware JE Jr. Detection of depressive disorder for patients receiving prepaid or fee-for-service care: results from the Medical Outcomes Study. *JAMA.* 1989;262:3298-3302.
9. Frank E, Kupfer DJ, Perel JM, Cornes C, Jarrett DB, Mallinger AG, Thase ME, McEachran AB, Grochocinski VJ. Three-year outcomes for maintenance therapies in recurrent depression. *Arch Gen Psychiatry.* 1990;47:1093-1099.
10. Brodaty H, Andrews G. Brief psychotherapy in family practice: a controlled prospective intervention trial. *Br J Psychiatry.* 1983;143:11-19.
11. Peiffer SI. Brief office counseling and the primary care physician. *South Med J.* 1986;79:721-722.
12. Mynors-Wallis LM, Gath DH, Lloyd-Thomas AR, Tomlinson D. Randomised controlled trial comparing problem-solving treatment with amitriptyline and placebo for major depression in primary care. *BMJ.* 1995;310:441-445.
13. Klerman GL. Evaluating the efficacy of psychotherapy for depression: the USA experience. *Eur Arch Psychiatry Clin Neurosci.* 1989;238:240-246.
14. Wells KB, Rogers W, Burnam MA, Greenfield S, Ware JE Jr. How the medical comorbidity of depressed patients differs across health care settings: results from the Medical Outcomes Study. *Am J Psychiatry.* 1991;148:1688-1696.
15. Howard KI, Kopta SM, Krause MS, Orlinsky DE. The dose-effect relationship in psychotherapy. *Am Psychol.* 1986;41:159-164.
16. Sturm R, Wells KB. How can care for depression become more cost-effective? *JAMA.* 1995;273:51-58.
17. Olfson M, Pincus HA. Outpatient psychotherapy in the United States. I: volume, costs, and user characteristics. *Am J Psychiatry.* 1994;151:1281-1288.
18. Olfson M, Pincus HA. Outpatient psychotherapy in the United States. II: patterns of utilization. *Am J Psychiatry.* 1994;151:1289-1294.
19. Schurman RA, Mitchell JB, Kramer PD. When doctors listen: counseling patterns of nonpsychiatrist physicians. *Am J Psychiatry.* 1985;142:934-938.
20. Verhaak PFM, Wennink HJ. What does a doctor do with psychosocial problems in primary care? *Int J Psychiatry Med.* 1990;20:151-162.
21. Hall JA, Roter DL, Katz NR. Meta-analysis of correlates of provider behavior in medical encounters. *Med Care.* 1988;26:657-675.
22. Inui TS, Carter WB. Problems and prospects for health services research on provider-patient communication. *Med Care.* 1985;23:521-538.
23. Greenfield S, Kaplan SH, Ware JE, Yano EM, Frank HJL. Patients' participation in medical care. *J Gen Intern Med.* 1988;3:448-457.
24. Manning WG, Wells KB. Preliminary results of a controlled trial of the effect of prepaid group practice on the outpatient use of mental health services. *J Hum Res.* 1986;21:293-320.
25. Landerman LR, Burns BJ, Swartz MS, Wagner HR, George LK. The relationship between insurance coverage and psychiatric disorder in predicting use of mental health services. *Am J Psychiatry.* 1994;12:1785-1790.
26. Diehr P, Price K, Williams SJ, Martin DP. Use of outpatient somatic health services by patients who use or need mental health services in three provider plans. *J Med Syst.* 1985;9:389-400.
27. Diehr P, Williams SJ, Martin DP. Ambulatory mental health services utilization in three provider plans. *Med Care.* 1984;22:1-13.
28. Wells KB, Manning WG, Benjamin B. Use of outpatient mental health service in HMO and fee-for-service plans: results from a randomized controlled trial. *Health Serv Res.* 1986;21:453-474.
29. Wells KB, Ware JE Jr, Lewis CE. Physicians' practices in counseling patients about health habits. *Med Care.* 1984;22:240-246.
30. Wells KB, Ware JE Jr, Lewis CE. Physicians' attitudes in counseling patients about smoking. *Med Care.* 1984;22:360-365.
31. Bandura A. *Social Learning Theory.* Englewood Cliffs, NJ: Prentice-Hall International Inc; 1977.
32. Bandura A. *Social Foundations of Thought and Action.* Englewood Cliffs, NJ: Prentice-Hall International Inc; 1986.
33. Meredith LS, Wells KB, Camp P. Clinician specialty and treatment style for depressed outpatients with and without medical comorbidity. *Arch Fam Med.* 1994;3:1065-1072.
34. Kaplan SH, Greenfield S, Ware JE Jr. Assessing the effects of physician-patient interactions on the outcome of chronic disease. *Med Care.* 1989;27:S110-S127.
35. Berk ML, Meyers S. Reasons for nonresponse on the physicians practice survey. In: *Proceedings of the Social Statistics Section.* Alexandria, Va: American Statistical Association; 1980:202-204.
36. Gunn WJ, Rhodes IN. Physician response to a telephone survey: effects of monetary incentives on response level. *Public Opin Q.* 1981;45:109-115.
37. Tarlov A, Ware JE Jr, Greenfield S, Nelson EC, Perrin E, Zubkoff M. The Medical Outcomes Study: an application of methods for monitoring the results of medical care. *JAMA.* 1989;262:925-930.
38. Rogers W, McGlynn E, Berry SH, Nelson EC, Perrin E, Zubkoff M, Greenfield S, Wells KB, Stewart AL, Arnold SB, Ware JE. Creation of data bases on the health of individuals: methods of sampling. In: Stewart AL, Ware JE Jr, eds. *Measuring Functioning and Well-being: The Medical Outcomes Study Approach.* Durham, NC: Duke University Press; 1992:27-47.
39. Cronbach LJ. Coefficient alpha and the internal structure of tests. *Psychometrika.* 1951;16:297-334.
40. Huber PJ. The behavior of maximum likelihood estimates under nonstandard conditions. In: *Fifth Berkeley Symposium on Mathematical Statistics and Probability, 1965.* Berkeley, Calif: University of California; 1967;1:221-233.
41. Liang K-Y, Zeger SL. Longitudinal data analysis using generalized linear models. *Biometrika.* 1986;73:13-22.
42. Burnam MA, Wells KB, Leake B, Landsverk J. Development of a brief screening instrument for detecting depressive disorders. *Med Care.* 1988;26:775-789.
43. Robbins JM, Kirmayer LJ, Cathebras P, Yaffe MJ, Dworkind M. Physician characteristics and the recognition of depression and anxiety in primary care. *Med Care.* 1994;32:795-812.
44. Wells KB, Burnam MA, Leake B, Robins LN. Agreement between face-to-face and telephone-administered versions of the depression section of the NIMH Diagnostic Interview Schedule. *J Psychiatr Res.* 1988;22:207-220.
45. Scutchfield FD, de Moor C. Preventive attitudes, beliefs, and practices of physicians in fee-for-service and health maintenance organization settings. *West J Med.* 1989;150:221-225.

Treating Major Depression in Primary Care Practice

Eight-Month Clinical Outcomes

Herbert C. Schulberg, PhD; Marian R. Block, MD; Michael J. Madonia, MSW; C. Paul Scott, MD; Eric Rodriguez, MD; Stanley D. Imber, PhD; James Perel, PhD; Judith Lave, PhD; Patricia R. Houck, MS; John L. Coulehan, MD

Background: We studied whether standardized treatments of major depression whose efficacy was established with psychiatric patients are equally effective when provided to primary care patients, and whether standardized treatments are more effective than a primary care physician's usual care.

Methods: A randomized controlled trial was conducted, in which primary care patients meeting *DSM-III-R* criteria for a current major depression were assigned to nortriptyline (n=91) or interpersonal psychotherapy (n=93) provided within well-structured parameters, or a physician's usual care (n=92). The main outcome measures were degree and rate of improvement in severity of depressive symptoms and proportion of patients recovered at 8 months.

Results: Severity of depressive symptoms was reduced more rapidly and more effectively among patients randomized to pharmacotherapy or psychotherapy than among patients assigned to a physician's usual care. Among treatment completers, approximately 70% of patients participating in the full pharmacotherapy or psychotherapy protocol but only 20% of usual care patients were judged as recovered at 8 months.

Conclusions: Pharmacotherapy and psychotherapy effectively treat major depression among primary care patients when provided within specific parameters and for the full acute and continuation phases. Treatment principles recommended by the Depression Guideline Panel of the Agency for Health Care Policy and Research are supported.

Arch Gen Psychiatry. 1996;53:913-919

MAJOR DEPRESSION in primary care practice has notable health policy implications since the disorder's point prevalence approximates 6% to 8%,[1] it generates significant health care costs,[2] and it produces profound social and vocational disability.[3] The RAND Medical Outcomes Study[4] and the PRIME-MD 1000 Study[5] concluded that the debilitating effects of depression equal or surpass those of many chronic physical illnesses. Nevertheless, both primary care physicians and their patients focus on physical illnesses and frequently minimize the manifestations of affective illness.[6]

Educational interventions to improve the primary care physician's recognition and treatment of major depression have highlighted the dearth of evidence regarding effectiveness of treatments for major depression in primary care patients. Since the nature and course of major depression experienced by patients presenting in the general medical sector may differ from that experienced by patients presenting in psychiatric facilities,[7] the primary care practice recommendations formulated by the Depression Guideline Panel of the US Public Health Service Agency for Health Care Policy and Research (AHCPR)[8] on the basis of research conducted with psychiatric patients rest on a limited database.[9] The AHCPR Panel,[9] therefore, recommended randomized controlled trials investigating the effectiveness of treatments for major depression transferred from the psychiatric to the general medical sector.

When we[7] reviewed prior pharmacotherapy studies conducted with primary care patients, we found few reports with satisfactory internal and external validity. Even fewer studies of psychological treatments alone had been conducted with depressed primary care patients through the late 1980s.[10]

See Patients and Methods on next page

From the Departments of Psychiatry and Medicine, University of Pittsburgh School of Medicine (Drs Schulberg, Block, Scott, Rodriguez, Imber, Perel, and Lave and Ms Houck); Department of Family Medicine, The Western Pennsylvania Hospital, Pittsburgh (Dr Block and Mr Madonia); St Margaret Memorial Hospital Family Practice Residency, Pittsburgh (Dr Scott); and Department of Preventive Medicine, State University of New York at Stony Brook, School of Medicine (Dr Coulehan).

PATIENTS AND METHODS

The study was conducted at 4 academically affiliated ambulatory health centers, using a protocol approved by the University of Pittsburgh Biomedical Institutional Review Board. Faculty physicians and residents with faculty supervision provide care in these centers for largely lower socioeconomic class urban populations on a fee-for-service basis.

PATIENTS

Potential subjects were patients aged 18 to 64 years who presented in study site waiting rooms. A research associate sought informed consent for a 3-phase assessment of eligibility for the clinical trial. From March 1991 through December 1993, 7652 patients completed the Center for Epidemiologic Studies–Depression scale,[14] which measures mood state and neurovegetative symptoms during the preceding week. Of these 7652 patients, 1492 scored at or above the positivity criterion of 22 and were not presently being treated for a mood disorder. These high-scoring patients were asked to continue with the second assessment, in which a research associate administered the Diagnostic Interview Schedule's Depression section.[15] The *DSM-III-R* criteria[16] for a current major depression were met by 678 (64%) of the 1059 patients responding to the Diagnostic Interview Schedule Depression section assessment.

Members of this subgroup were asked to meet with a consultation-liaison psychiatrist at the health center to establish protocol eligibility. Of the 678 referred patients, 275 (41%) refused and 403 (59%) completed this third assessment. Psychiatrists judged 283 (70%) of the evaluated patients clinically eligible and 120 (30%) clinically ineligible within protocol criteria (see Schulberg et al[17]), requiring both a *DSM-III-R* diagnosis of current major depression and a minimum 17-item Hamilton Rating Scale–Depression (HRS-D) score of 13, as well as no psychiatric or medical conditions precluding a randomized treatment assignment. Of these 283 protocol-eligible patients, 276 (98%) agreed to a randomized treatment assignment. This total met the sample size determined a priori as needed to detect with 90% power at the .05 significance level the hypothesized 33% difference in the proportion of patients who recover when receiving a standardized treatment (66%) and UC (33%).

INTERVENTIONS

Pharmacotherapy

The investigators in 1989 considered nortriptyline hydrochloride the best antidepressant to prescribe medical patients with a major depression because (1) its efficacy and therapeutic dosage range had been demonstrated with psychiatric patients[8]; (2) it could be monitored with blood level tests and have dosages customized; and (3) it achieves therapeutic effects at lower dosage levels and with fewer anticholingeric side effects and less orthostatic hypotension[18] than other tricyclic drugs could produce. Patients were treated in their own ambulatory health center site at no cost by board-certified family practitioners or general internists trained in pharmacotherapy protocol procedures through a written manual[19,20] and didactic sessions. Patients treated with nortriptyline continued to receive needed medical services from their own primary care physicians.

During the acute phase of treatment, clinicians established "target" symptoms, assessed suicidality, and addressed resistance to taking the antidepressant medication.[21] Patients were seen weekly or biweekly as the initial nortriptyline dose of 25 mg was increased in 25-mg increments to a therapeutic dosage within the range of 190 to 270 nmol/L, as determined by serum levels and symptoms checked at brief follow-up visits. Potential side effects of the nortriptyline were reviewed at each visit and rated on a Side Effects Scale.[22]

The acute phase of treatment was considered complete when the patient was assessed as having reached a "point of stability." The criteria for this determination were intended to resemble those applied by physicians in routine practice: (1) clinical improvement in the patient's symptoms; (2) a nortriptyline blood level within the 190- to 570-nmol/L therapeutic window on 3 consecutive tests; and (3) the physician considered monthly follow-up visits sufficient. Furthermore, the investigators knew that the patient's Beck Depression Inventory[23] score at the point of stability was reduced by 33% to 50% over baseline, although not necessarily achieving full recovery. If the patient's symptoms failed to improve within approximately 6 weeks, his or her Beck Depression Inventory score was 20 or greater, and an independent psychiatrist-consultant judged the patient a nonresponder to nortriptyline, the patient was dropped from the protocol and referred to his or her primary care physician for alternative treatments in accord with usual health center practices.

Patients completing the acute phase of treatment entered the continuation phase of treatment receiving the same nortriptyline regimen at which they had achieved a steady therapeutic serum level, and were seen for 6 monthly visits. Patients whose Beck Depression Inventory score deteriorated during this phase to its baseline level and were judged as relapsed by an independent psychiatrist were referred to their primary care physician for treatment within standard health center procedures. Patients remaining well throughout the 6-month continuation phase then had their medication tapered over a period of several weeks.

Psychotherapy

Since depressed medical outpatients are frequently stressed by troublesome interpersonal relationships, we selected

With the aim of advising primary care physicians about beneficial treatments for major depression, we conducted a randomized controlled trial of depression-specific therapies within the conceptual and methodologic framework of effectiveness research.[11,12] Thus, this study considered a "physician's usual care" rather than a placebo the proper comparison condition for standardized treatments, and it included other design features intended to balance internal and external validity.[13]

This article presents findings about the effectiveness of standardized pharmacologic and psychotherapeutic treatments for major depression when provided to primary care patients. Eight-month clinical out-interpersonal psychotherapy (IPT) as the psychological treatment. It has well-documented efficacy with depressed psychiatric patients[24,25] and has been adapted for treatment of primary care and other populations.[26,27] However, IPT's effectiveness had yet to be investigated with adult primary care patients experiencing a *DSM-III-R* major depression.

Psychiatrists and clinical psychologists already skilled in psychotherapeutic procedures served as the IPT therapists. They were trained in standardized IPT, and the progress of their patients was monitored through consultative meetings and a review of audiotaped sessions. The acute phase of IPT consisted of approximately 16 weekly sessions conducted at the health center. If a patient's Beck Depression Inventory score did not drop by 33% to 50% over an 8- to 10-week period and an independent psychiatrist-consultant judged the patient a nonresponder, the patient was referred to his or her health center primary care physician for nonprotocol treatment; IPT's acute phase was followed by 4 monthly continuation-phase sessions to preserve therapeutic gains. Similarly to patients treated with nortriptyline, IPT patients continued to receive any needed medical services from their primary care physician.

Usual Care

The various procedures of wide-ranging type and duration commonly used by primary care physicians to treat depression constitute UC. As such, it reflects the physician's clinical judgment about how best to treat a mood disorder and the severity level at which such treatment is required.[13] During the study's early weeks, UC patients were instructed to inform their physicians of their mood disorder and to discuss treatment for it. However, it soon became evident that patients were not communicating with their physicians and/or were not receiving requested help. We, therefore, considered it ethically and clinically necessary during the remainder of the study to inform each UC physician about the patient's psychiatric diagnosis so as to ensure his or her awareness of it.

Physicians whose patients had been randomized to UC were free to provide them any clinically appropriate intervention and to consult with the mental health specialists routinely available at their health centers or with primary care colleagues. When scheduled protocol follow-up assessments determined that a UC patient's clinical state had worsened or suicidal ideation existed, the researchers immediately conveyed such information to the patient's physician.

BACKGROUND AND OUTCOME ASSESSMENT

The sociodemographic characteristics of study patients measured at baseline (M0) are listed in **Table 1**. Clinical characteristics measured at M0 included the severity of the patient's depression, level of overall functioning as measured by the Global Assessment Scale,[28] and history of prior outpatient and inpatient psychiatric treatment. Assessments were also conducted at baseline to determine whether patients had ever experienced other *DSM-III-R* psychiatric (Axis I) and personality (Axis II) disorders, and the severity of present comorbid physical illnesses as measured by the Duke Severity of Illness Checklist.[29]

Response of depressive symptoms to interventions was assessed at months 1 (M1), 2 (M2), 3 (M3), 4 (M4), 6 (M6), and 8 (M8). Clinical evaluators, blinded to a patient's treatment assignment and trained to achieve interrater reliabilities exceeding 0.90, administered the 17-item HRS-D[30] to assess severity of a patient's depression.

ANALYSES

Outcome analyses were conducted on 2 samples: (1) the intent-to-treat sample of 276 patients randomized to a protocol intervention, including those who failed to appear for an initial meeting with the therapist to whom they had been assigned; and (2) the treatment-completer sample of 150 patients who completed both the acute and continuation phases of the protocol. All UC patients were considered treatment completers, given its varying nature, except those (n=11) who asked not to be contacted for follow-up assessments.

Clinical outcome was determined through a mixed model (random effects) repeated-measures analysis of variance (ANOVA) comparing mean scores on the HRS-D across groups and at successive time points.[31] When significant at the .05 level with the Wald χ^2 statistic, these ANOVA analyses were followed by post hoc group *t* tests at each assessment point to compare specific group differences significant at the .01 level. Distribution of 8-month clinical outcomes (asymptomatic, partially symptomatic, and symptomatic) based on actual and imputed (as described below) HRS-D scores was tested with the Kruskal-Wallis statistic for categorical data.[32] Using actual and imputed data, odds ratios were calculated for the 8-month outcome classified as recovered/not recovered (HRS-D score, $\leq 7/\geq 8$).

The mixed model repeated-measures ANOVA, with group and time as fixed effects and intercept as a random effect, was fitted separately for the intent-to-treat (n=276) and the treatment-completer (n=150) groups.[33] The models assume compound symmetry, ie, the same correlation between repeated observations and individual specific intercepts. The individual specific intercepts and fixed group and time parameters were used to impute missing HRS-D data points for months M1 through M8. The extent of missing data was similar across the 3 intent-to-treat randomized groups: 31% of IPT, 36% of UC, and 42% of nortriptyline patients were missing 3 or more of the 6 post-baseline data points. The rate of such missing data among treatment completers was 3% for IPT, 0% for nortriptyline, and 27% for UC patients.

comes are compared with those achieved by physicians providing usual care (UC) to similarly depressed patients in their practices. Thus, this study is the first, to our knowledge, that investigated clinical outcomes of depressed ambulatory medical patients treated within principles that the AHCPR guidelines[8] consider necessary to achieve full recovery.

RESULTS

PATIENT CHARACTERISTICS

The 3 treatment groups did not differ on the characteristics measured at baseline (Table 1). All were experiencing more severe affective and functional distress than

Table 1. Baseline Characteristics of Patients Randomized for Treatment of Major Depression*

Characteristics	IPT (n=93)	NT (n=91)	UC (n=92)	Statistic†	*P*
Sociodemographic					
Mean (SD) age, y	37.1 (11.4)	38.6 (11.6)	38.6 (12.4)	.63	.54
% Female	82.8	80.2	87.0	1.52	.47
% White	53.8	59.3	53.3	.84	.67
Married, %	26.9	35.2	27.2	1.94	.38
Educational level of HS or greater, %	82.8	79.1	84.8	1.03	.60
Employed, %	42.9	44.4	40.7	.27	.87
Clinical					
Severity of depression scores, mean (SD)					
CES-D	36.7 (8.8)	37.3 (9.4)	38.0 (8.4)	.48	.62
HRS-D	22.3 (4.6)	23.7 (5.3)	23.4 (5.3)	1.86	.16
BDI	25.0 (9.4)	25.5 (11.4)	27.3 (9.7)	1.15	.32
Other scale scores, mean (SD)					
GAS	50.7 (6.8)	50.6 (7.4)	48.8 (6.9)	1.84	.16
DUSOI	34.8 (16.1)	33.3 (15.0)	34.4 (15.4)	.22	.81
Prior psychiatric treatment, %					
Outpatient	48.1	46.2	44.9	.16	.92
Inpatient	23.4	20.6	22.1	.16	.92
Lifetime other *DSM-III-R* disorder, %					
Axis I	69.9	75.3	79.7	2.11	.35
Axis II	67.6	65.7	76.2	1.93	.38

**IPT indicates interpersonal psychotherapy; NT, nortriptyline hydrochloride; UC, usual care; HS, high school; CES-D, Center for Epidemiologic Studies–Depression scale; HRS-D, 17-item Hamilton Rating Scale–Depression; BDI, Beck Depression Inventory; GAS, Global Assessment Scale; and DUSOI, Duke Severity of Illness Checklist.*

†F for continuous and χ^2 for dichotomous variables.

is thought to typify major depression in primary care practice.[34] However, the cohort includes the very patients for whom an active intervention is recommended by the AHCPR Depression Guideline Panel.[8]

ATTRITION

The treatment history of patients randomized to pharmacotherapy (nortriptyline) and psychotherapy (IPT) is detailed in **Table 2**. Some patients chose to leave the protocol before meeting even once with the clinician, others during treatment's acute or continuation phase. Still other patients were dropped when judged by their clinicians to be treatment nonresponders. Consequently, only 33% of the pharmacotherapy sample completed the full drug regimen recommended by the AHCPR guidelines[8] and only 42% of the patients randomized to psychotherapy participated fully in the IPT protocol.

Attrition patterns of pharmacotherapy and psychotherapy patients did not differ during each treatment's acute phase (χ^2=0.36, *df*=1, *P*=.55) but significantly fewer nortriptyline than IPT patients completed the protocol's continuation phase (χ^2=6.2, *df*=1, *P*=.01). Treatment completers and dropouts were compared on their demographic and clinical characteristics. Only age significantly distinguished IPT completers from dropouts; the former were 42.9 and the latter 32.9 years old (F=20.7, *df*=1, *P*=.001). Among patients randomized to the nortriptyline treatment, whites (43%) completed the full protocol significantly more often than nonwhites (19%) (χ^2=5.6, *df*=1, *P*=.02). Compared with dropouts, nortriptyline treatment completers also had significantly lower HRS-D scores (24.4 vs 22.1) at baseline (F=3.8, *df*=1, *P*=.05), and only 52% met lifetime criteria for an Axis II disorder vs 76% among dropouts (χ^2=4.3, *df*=1; *P*=.04). Attrition patterns for the 2 standardized treatments were not compared with that for UC because the latter has no defined phases and is wide ranging in frequency and duration.

PATTERNS OF UC

A review of health center records for UC patients and their responses to a health services utilization questionnaire determined that 63% were but 37% were not provided some mental health treatment within 2 months of being randomized to UC. The patients who were and were not so treated during this initial period did not differ on 6 sociodemographic characteristics, 12 measures of current and lifetime clinical status, and physician experience level (house staff or attending).

Primary care physicians prescribed an antidepressant for 45% of the UC patients within 2 months of randomization during the period March 1991 through February 1994. Forty-one percent of the individual prescriptions were for nortriptyline, a high percentage likely resulting from health center physicians' awareness that this medication was being provided to study patients. Health center records indicated that 90% of the patients prescribed antidepressant medications received the minimally adequate dosages recommended by the AHCPR guidelines,[8] eg, 10 mg/d of fluoxetine for a minimum of 4 weeks. However, treatment with the medications typically was discontinued after 3 to 4 months; only 43% of UC patients were prescribed an antidepressant for the approximately 35-week period followed in standardized pharmacotherapy.

Table 2. Treatment History of Patients Randomized to Pharmacotherapy and Psychotherapy*

Treatment Phase	Pharmacotherapy	Psychotherapy
Acute phase		
Failed to appear	13 (14.3)	13 (14.0)
Dropout		
Patient initiated	17 (18.7)	25 (26.9)
Clinician initiated	11 (12.1)	8 (8.6)
Completed treatment	50 (54.9)	47 (50.5)
Total	**91 (100.0)**	**93 (100.0)**
Continuation phase		
Dropout		
Patient initiated	15 (30.0)	5 (10.6)
Clinician initiated	5 (10.0)	3 (6.4)
Completed treatment	30 (60.0)	39 (83.0)
Total	**50 (100.0)**	**47 (100.0)**

*Values are expressed as number (percentage) of patients.

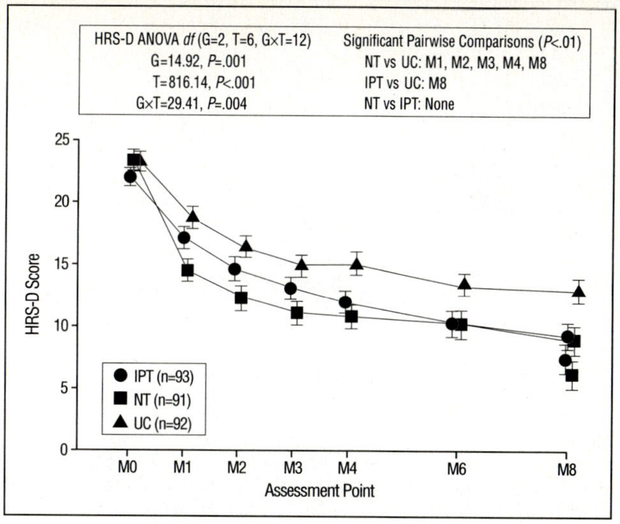

Figure 1. *Course of depressive severity from baseline (M0) to month 8 (M8) among intent-to-treat cohorts who were randomized to interpersonal psychotherapy (IPT), nortriptyline hydrochloride (NT), or usual care (UC). HRS-D indicates 17-item Hamilton Rating Scale–Depression; ANOVA, analysis of variance; G, group; and T, time.*

SEVERITY ANALYSES

Both standardized treatments were more clinically and rapidly effective than UC in reducing depressive severity. As **Figure 1** indicates for the full randomized cohort (intent-to-treat), the 3 treatment groups had equivalent baseline (M0) HRS-D scores of approximately 23. At 8 months, however, the UC patients scored 13.1 (SE, 0.9); the IPT patients, 9.3 (SE, 0.9); and the NT patients, 9.0 (SE, 1.0). The ANOVA indicates statistically significant main effects for group and time, as well as for group × time. Post hoc group t test comparisons set at $P \leq .01$ to minimize chance findings revealed no significant differences in HRS-D scores between the 2 standardized treatments at any time point.

Outcomes were also examined for the smaller sample of patients who completed both the acute and continuation phases of treatment (treatment-completer analyses). Data for all 81 UC patients participating in follow-up assessments are included in these analyses since no HRS-D differences were found at 8 months between those patients who did (n=53) and did not (n=28) receive a mental health treatment within 2 months following randomization. **Figure 2** again reveals statistically significant ANOVA main effects on the HRS-D for group and time, as well as for the interaction of group and time. The latter finding emphasizes the particularly rapid improvement associated with pharmacotherapy. The significant differences in depressive severity between nortriptyline and UC patients pertained at assessments M1 through M8. However, the differences significant at M1 and M2 between patients participating in the nortriptyline therapy and IPT were no longer found at M3 and at subsequent assessments.

RECOVERY ANALYSES

Another test of treatment effectiveness is whether patients meet a predefined level of clinical recovery at a specified point in time. For this analysis, we applied the classification suggested by Frank et al[35] to 8-month HRS-D scores (see **Figure 3**). Statistically significant differences were

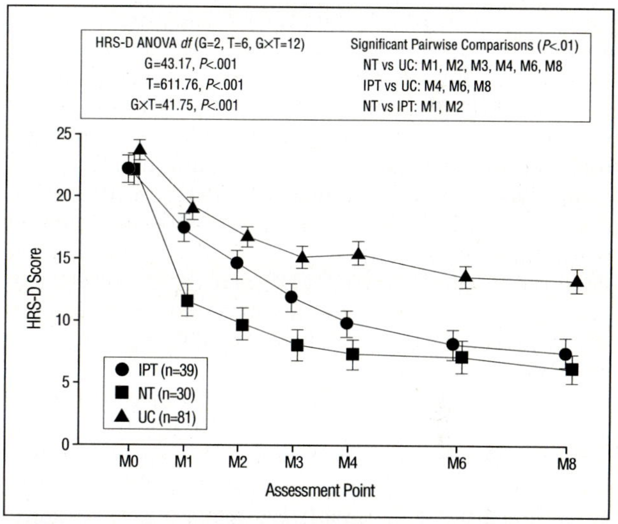

Figure 2. *Course of depressive severity from baseline (M0) to month 8 (M8) among treatment-completer cohorts who were provided interpersonal psychotherapy (IPT), nortriptyline hydrochloride (NT), or usual care (UC). HRS-D indicates 17-item Hamilton Rating Scale–Depression; ANOVA, analysis of variance; G, group; and T, time.*

found among the 3 treatment groups for both the intent-to-treat (χ^2=26.67, df=4, $P<.001$) and treatment-completer samples (χ^2=35.56, df=4, $P<.001$). In the former analysis, almost half of all patients randomized to either of the standardized treatments were asymptomatic at 8 months while less than one fifth of the UC patients improved to this degree (Figure 3). Among the treatment-completer subsamples, approximately 70% of patients completing either standardized treatment exhibited few or no remaining depressive symptoms at 8 months compared with only one fifth of the UC patients (**Figure 4**). The odds ratio of being asymptomatic for depression at 8 months for the intent-to-treat pharmacotherapy vs UC samples is 4.13 (95% confidence interval, 2.12-8.06) and for the intent-to-treat psychotherapy vs UC samples it is 3.79 (95% confidence interval, 1.95-7.39).

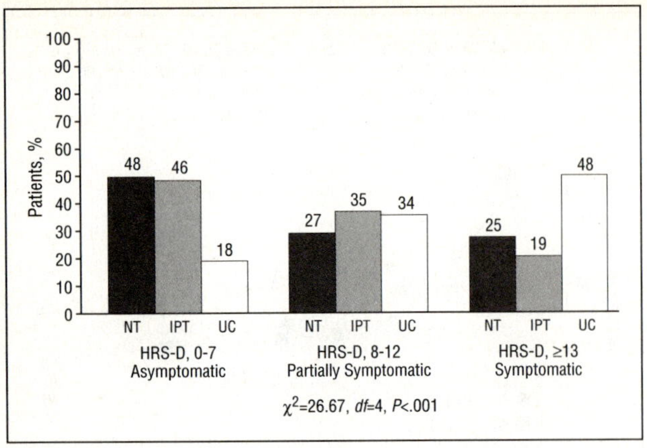

Figure 3. *Status of depressive symptoms at 8 months among intent-to-treat cohorts who were randomized to nortriptyline hydrochloride (NT) (n=91), interpersonal psychotherapy (IPT) (n=91), or usual care (UC) (n=92). HRS-D indicates 17-item Hamilton Rating Scale–Depression.*

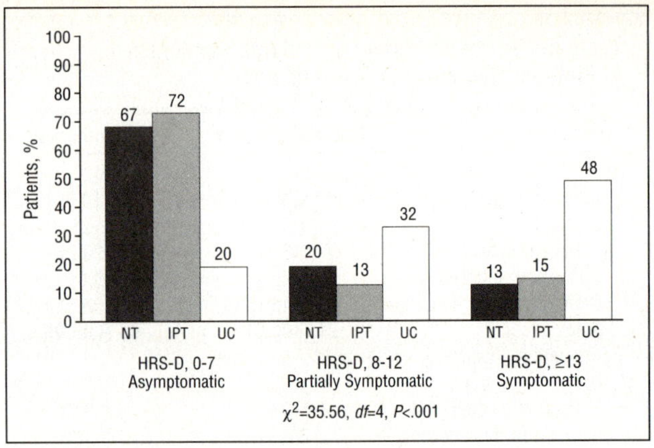

Figure 4. *Status of depressive symptoms at 8 months among treatment-completer cohorts who were provided nortriptyline hydrochloride (NT) (n=30), interpersonal psychotherapy (IPT) (n=39), or usual care (UC) (n=81). HRS-D indicates 17-item Hamilton Rating Scale–Depression.*

COMMENT

Our randomized controlled trial determined that standardized pharmacotherapy and psychotherapy are significantly more effective than a primary care physician's UC in resolving episodes of major depression. Thus, our findings provide empiric support for the recommendation of the AHCPR Depression Guideline Panel[8] that depressed patients be provided both acute and continuation phase treatments of specified dosages and durations. The outcome differences between standardized treatments and UC observed in this study are particularly striking given that researchers informed primary care physicians that patients randomized to them for UC were experiencing a major depression. Given these findings, did the study's recruitment and treatment methodology affect the nature and generalizability of its results?

Our study's 3-phased recruitment strategy generated a considerable number of patient refusals, which raises concerns as to whether selection bias possibly confounded clinical outcomes. We, therefore, compared psychiatric evaluation participants and nonparticipants on available measures. More women than men refused the evaluation (42% vs 25%, χ^2=9.4, *df*=1, *P*=.002), and the nonparticipants were younger than participants (32.9 vs 38.1 years, F=29.5, *df*=1, *P*=.001). The 2 groups did not differ with respect to race, marital and educational status, or depressive severity when screened with the Center for Epidemiologic Studies–Depression scale. However, significantly more of the participants than nonparticipants acknowledged prior visits to a mental health specialist (55% vs 43%, χ^2=6.2, *df*=1, *P*=.01).

Another factor possibly affecting the generalizability of findings to routine practice is the differing nature of this protocol's expectations of subjects compared with the practical and motivational demands imposed on subjects in psychiatric clinical trials. Thus, while our subjects were identified through a more comprehensive case-finding effort than is typical for psychiatric studies, it also likely identified subjects with lesser motivation to be treated for depression. The fact that 14% of patients accepting randomization to either pharmacotherapy or psychotherapy failed to keep their initial treatment appointment (Table 2) also underscores the AHCPR Depression Guideline Panel[8] recommendation that patient preference be considered when selecting a treatment.

Another unique feature of this protocol is that subjects were required to participate in the continuation phase as well as acute phase of treatment to be deemed treatment completers. Since only 33% and 42% of patients randomized to pharmacotherapy and psychotherapy, respectively, were so classified, does this reflect difficulties specific to this protocol, or does it reflect what can be expected in routine general medical practice when primary care physicians seek patient compliance with the full course of treatment? We believe that the study's adherence patterns resemble those likely to be found in routine practice where compliance declines steadily over time.[36-38] Among the patients likely to drop out prematurely, some will feel well and not consider extended treatment beneficial; others will feel no improvement and seek alternative treatments. The adherence problem encountered with depressed patients is not exceptional and resembles that facing primary care physicians treating patients with other chronic illnesses such as hypertension.[39]

Despite the greater effectiveness of standardized treatments compared with a physician's UC, depressive symptoms did diminish among patients receiving the nonstandardized intervention. The group's baseline HRS-D score of 23.4 (SE, 0.8) dropped to 15.3 (SE, 0.9) and 13.1 (SE, 0.9) at the 4- and 8-month assessments, respectively (Figure 1). The UC patients possibly improved because of (1) the primary care physician's proper and persistent treatment of the depression; (2) depression's natural course, in which partial remission but not full recovery is common[40,41]; or (3) a positive response to the care and attention experienced in periodic meetings with the study's blinded clinical evaluators for follow-up assessments. Of particular interest is why UC patients who were and were not provided a mental health treatment exhibited similar 8-month outcomes, a finding akin to that obtained by Scott and Freeman.[42]

We conclude that pharmacotherapy and psychotherapy consistent with the AHCPR guidelines[8] are markedly superior to a physician's UC in resolving an episode of major depression. Even after discounting the significant attrition likely to be experienced with a standardized treatment of extended duration, it remains the intervention of choice compared with a physician's UC. Validity of the study's findings is bolstered by their close resemblance to those obtained with psychiatric patients in the National Institute of Mental Health Treatment of Depression Collaborative Research Program,[25] ie, both medical and psychiatric patients completing treatment improve more rapidly with medication than with psychotherapy. As in the NIMH study,[43] however, the clinical differences are no longer significant when assessed 4, 6, and 8 months after the start of treatment (Figure 2). Thus, patients unwilling or unable to take an antidepressant drug can be informed that they have an equal probability of recovering from the depression whether treated pharmacologically or psychotherapeutically, even though clinical progress will likely be slower with the latter intervention. Additionally, clinicians and managed care reviewers should refrain from declaring depressed patients treated with psychotherapy as nonresponders until they have received an adequate "dose" of it, which, as Figure 2 and a study by Shapiro et al[44] indicate, is in the range of 12 to 16 sessions.

What are the health policy implications of these results? Some contend that services provided by primary care physicians cost less than those provided by mental health specialists but that the generalist's treatment may not be equally effective.[45] While our findings about the outcome of UC could be interpreted as confirming this assertion, we also found that motivated internists and family physicians can be trained in standardized pharmacotherapy to achieve the same clinical outcomes as have been reported for psychiatrists.[8] Since as many depressed persons seek help from generalist physicians as specialists,[46] the question requiring further research is whether primary care physicians can follow treatment principles recommended by the AHCPR Depression Guideline Panel.[8]

Accepted for publication April 1, 1996.

Corresponding author: Herbert C. Schulberg, PhD, Western Psychiatric Institute and Clinic, 3811 O'Hara St, Pittsburgh, PA 15213.

REFERENCES

1. Katon W, Schulberg H. Epidemiology of depression in primary care. *Gen Hosp Psychiatry.* 1992;14:237-242.
2. Simon G, Von Korff M, Barlow W. Health care costs of primary care patients with recognized depression. *Arch Gen Psychiatry.* 1995;52:850-856.
3. Broadhead E, Blazer D, George L, Tse C. Depression, disability days, and days lost from work in a prospective epidemiologic survey. *JAMA.* 1990;264:2524-2528.
4. Wells K, Stewart A, Hays R, Burnam A, Rogers W, Daniels M, Berry S, Greenfield S, Ware J. The functioning and well-being of depressed patients. *JAMA.* 1989; 252.914-919.
5. Spitzer R, Kroenke K, Linzer M, Hahn S, Williams J, deGruy F, Brody D, Davies M. Health-related quality of life in primary care patients with mental disorders. *JAMA.* 1995;274:1511-1517.
6. Eisenberg L. Treating depression and anxiety in primary care. *N Engl J Med.* 1992;326:1080-1084.
7. Schulberg H, Coulehan J, Block M, Scott C, Imber S, Perel J. Strategies for evaluating treatments for major depression in primary care patients. *Gen Hosp Psychiatry.* 1991;13:9-18.
8. Depression Guideline Panel. *Clinical Practice Guideline Number 5: Depression in Primary Care, 2: Treatment of Major Depression.* Rockville, Md: US Dept of Health and Human Services, Public Health Service, Agency for Health Care Policy and Research; 1993. AHCPR publication 93-0551.
9. Munoz R, Hollon S, McGrath E, Rehm L, VandeBos G. On the AHCPR Depression in Primary Care Guidelines. *Am Psychol.* 1994;49:42-61.
10. Brown C, Schulberg H. The efficacy of psychosocial treatments in primary care: a review of randomized clinical trials. *Gen Hosp Psychiatry.* 1995;17:414-424.
11. Clarke G. Improving the transition from basic efficacy research to effectiveness studies. *J Consult Clin Psychol.* 1995;63:718-725.
12. Katon W, Von Korff M, Lin E, Walker E, Simon G, Bush T, Robinson P, Russo J. Collaborative management to achieve treatment guidelines. *JAMA.* 1995; 273:1026-1031.
13. Schulberg H, Coulehan J, Block M, Lave J, Rodriguez E, Scott C, Madonia M, Imber S, Perel J. Clinical trials of primary care treatments for major depression: issues in design, recruitment, and treatment. *Int J Psychiatry Med.* 1993;23:29-42.
14. Radloff L. The CES-D scale: a self-report depression scale for research in the general population. *Appl Psychol Measur.* 1977;1:385-401.
15. Robins L, Helzer J, Croughan J, Ratcliff K. National Institute of Mental Health Diagnostic Interview Schedule. *Arch Gen Psychiatry.* 1981;38:381-389.
16. American Psychiatric Association. *Diagnostic and Statistical Manual of Mental Disorders, Third Edition, Revised.* Washington, DC: American Psychiatric Association;1987.
17. Schulberg H, Madonia M, Block M, Coulehan J, Scott C, Rodriguez E, Black A. Major depression in primary care practice. *Psychosomatics.* 1995;36:129-137.
18. Roose S, Glassman A, Siris S, Walsh T, Bruno R, Wright L. Comparison of imipramine- and nortriptyline-induced orthostatic hypotension: a meaningful difference. *J Clin Psychopharmacol.* 1981;1:316-319.
19. Fawcett J, Epstein P, Fiester S, Elkin I, Autry J. Clinical management: imipramine/placebo administration manual. *Psychopharmacol Bull.* 1987;23:309-324.
20. Reynolds C, Frank E, Perel J, Imber S, Cornes C, Morycz R, Mazumdar S, Miller M, Pollock B. Riffai H, Stack J, George C, Houck P, Kupfer, D. Combined pharmacotherapy and psychotherapy in the acute and continuation treatment of elderly patients with recurrent major depression: preliminary report. *Am J Psychiatry.* 1992;149:1687-1692.
21. Schulberg H, Block M, Madonia M, Rodriguez E, Scott C, Lave J. Applicability of clinical guideline pharmacotherapy for major depression in primary care settings. *Arch Fam Med.* 1995;4:106-112.
22. Kupfer D, Perel J, Frank E. Adequate treatment with imipramine in continuation treatment. *J Clin Psychiatry.* 1989;50:250-255.
23. Beck A, Ward C, Mendelson M, Mock J, Erbaugh J. An inventory for measuring depression. *Arch Gen Psychiatry.* 1961;4:53-63.
24. Klerman G, Weissman M, Rounsaville B, Chevron E. *Interpersonal Psychotherapy of Depression.* New York, NY: Basic Books; 1984.
25. Elkin I, Shea T, Watkins J, Imber S, Sotsky S, Collins J, Glass D, Pilkonis P, Leber W, Docherty J, Fiester S, Parloff M, for National Institute of Mental Health Treatment of Depression Collaborative Research Program. General effectiveness of treatments. *Arch Gen Psychiatry.* 1989;46:971-982.
26. Klerman G, Budman S, Berwick D, Weissman M, Damico-White J, Demby A, Feldstein M. Efficacy of a brief psychosocial intervention for symptoms of stress and distress among patients in primary care. *Med Care.* 1987;25:1078-1088.
27. Klerman G, Weissman M, eds. *New Applications of Interpersonal Psychotherapy.* Washington, DC: American Psychiatric Press, 1993.
28. Endicott J. Spitzer R, Fleiss J, Cohen J. The Global Assessment Scale: a procedure for measuring the overall severity of psychiatric disturbance. *Arch Gen Psychiatry.* 1976;33:766-771.
29. Parkerson G, Broadhead W, Tse C. The Duke Severity of Illness Checklist (DUSOI) for measurement of severity and comorbidity. *J Clin Epidemiol.* 1993;46:379-393.
30. Hamilton M. The Hamilton Rating Scale for Depression. In: Sartorius N, Banto T, eds. *Assessment of Depression.* New York, NY: Springer-Verlag NY Inc; 1986.
31. Dixon W, Merdian K. *ANOVA and Regression With BMDP5V.* Los Angeles, Calif: Dixon Statistical Association; 1992.
32. Mehta C, Patel N. *Stat Xact Turbo: Statistical Software for Exact Nonparametric Inference: User Manual.* Cambridge, Mass: Cytel Software Corp; 1992.
33. Gibbons R, Hedeker D, Elkin I, Waternaux C, Kraemer H, Greenhouse J, Shea T, Imber S, Sotsky S, Watkins J. Some conceptual and statistical issues in analysis of longitudinal psychiatric data. *Arch Gen Psychiatry.* 1993;50:739-750.
34. Coyne J, Fechner-Bates S, Schwenk T. Prevalence, nature, and comorbidity of depressive disorders in primary care. *Gen Hosp Psychiatry.* 1994;16:267-276.
35. Frank E, Prien R, Jarrett R, Keller M, Kupfer D, Lavori P, Rush A, Weissman M. Conceptualization and rationale for consensus definitions of terms in major depressive disorder. *Arch Gen Psychiatry.* 1991;48:851-855.
36. Myers E, Branthwaithe A. Out-patient compliance with antidepressant medication. *Br J Psychiatry.* 1992;160:83-86.
37. Katon W, Von Korff M, Lin E, Bush T, Ormel J. Adequacy and duration of antidepressant treatment in primary care. *Med Care.* 1992;30:67-76.
38. Simon G, Von Korff M, Wagner E, Barlow W. Patterns of antidepressant use in community practice. *Gen Hosp Psychiatry.* 1993;15:399-408.
39. Clark L. Improving compliance and increasing control of hypertension: needs of special hypertensive populations. *Am Heart J.* 1991;121:664-669.
40. Wells K, Burnam M, Rogers W, Hays R, Camp P. The course of depression in adult outpatients. *Arch Gen Psychiatry.* 1992;49:788-794.
41. Ormel J, Oldehinkel T, Brilman E, Vanden Brink W. Outcome of depression and anxiety in primary care. *Arch Gen Psychiatry.* 1993;50:759-766.
42. Scott I, Freeman C. Edinburgh primary care depression study: treatment outcome, patient satisfaction, and cost after 16 weeks. *BMJ.* 1992;304:883-887.
43. Watkins J, Leber W, Imber S, Collins J, Elkin I, Pilkonis P, Sotsky S, Shea M, Glass D. Temporal course of change in depression. *J Consult Clin Psychol.* 1993;61:858-864.
44. Shapiro D, Barkham M, Rees A, Hardy G, Reynolds S, Startup M. Effects of treatment duration and severity of depression on the effectiveness of cognitive-behavioral and psychodynamic-interpersonal psychotherapy. *J Consult Clin Psychol.* 1994;62:522-534.
45. Sturm R, Wells K. How can care for depression become more cost-effective? *JAMA.* 1995;273:51-58.
46. Narrow W, Regier D, Rae D, Manderscheid R, Locke B. Use of services by persons with mental and addictive disorders. *Arch Gen Psychiatry.* 1993;50:95-107.

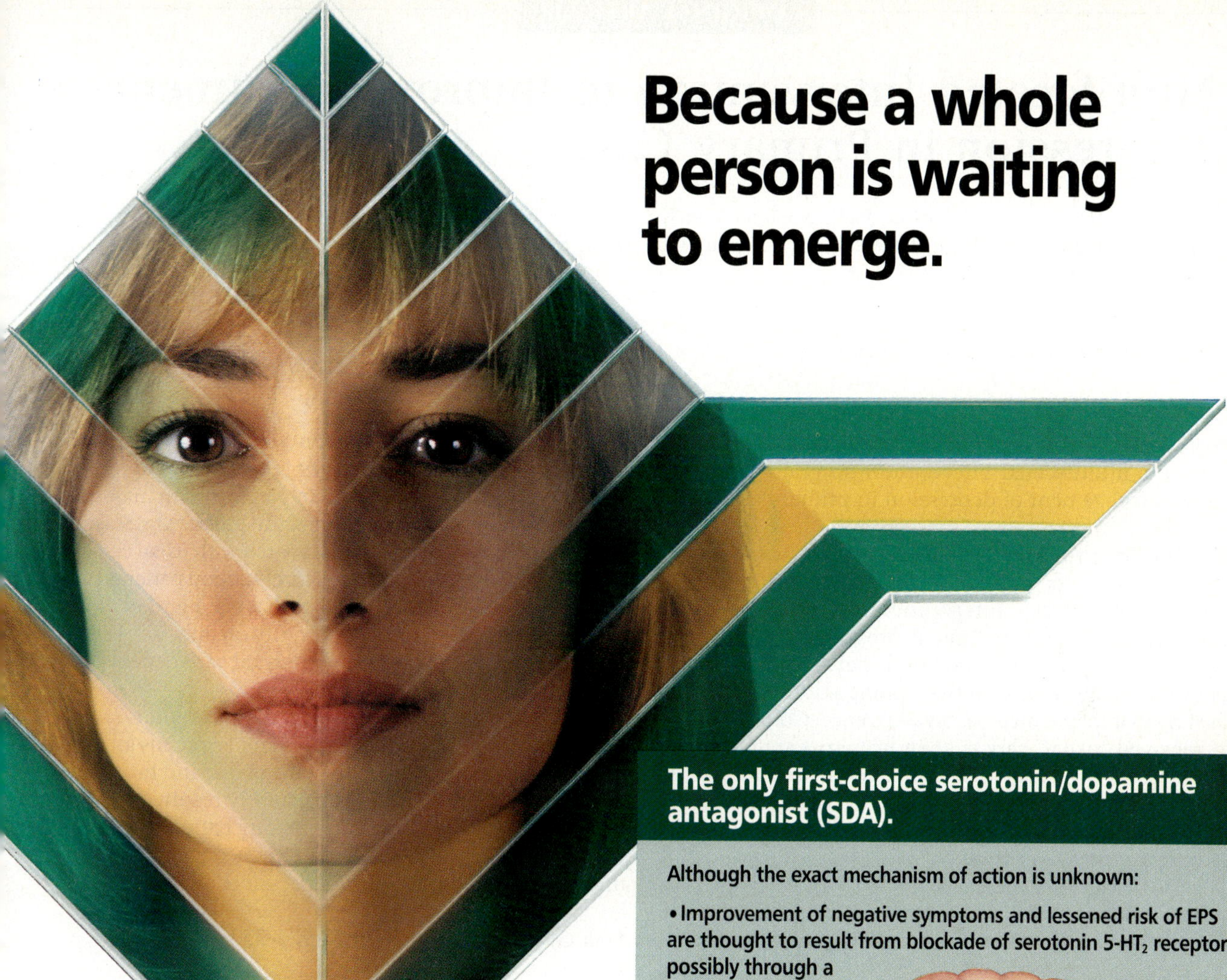

Because a whole person is waiting to emerge.

The only first-choice serotonin/dopamine antagonist (SDA).

Although the exact mechanism of action is unknown:

- Improvement of negative symptoms and lessened risk of EPS are thought to result from blockade of serotonin 5-HT_2 receptors, possibly through a modulatory effect on dopamine D_2 activity in the frontal cortex and the basal ganglia.*
- Improvement of positive symptoms is thought to result from blockade of dopamine D_2 receptors in the limbic system.*

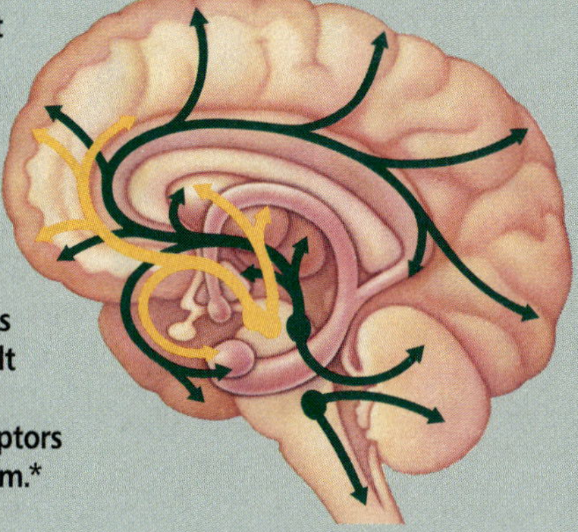

Dopaminergic system   Serotoninergic system

A first choice

Risperdal®
RISPERIDONE
1,2,3,4 mg tablets
oral solution 1 mg/mL

Raising the standard of care.

*Ereshefsky L, Lacombe S. Pharmacological profile of risperidone. *Can J Psychiatry.* 1993;38(Suppl 3):S80-S88.

Please see the brief summary of Prescribing Information adjacent to this ad.

 JPI-RS-123DR2

JANSSEN · PHARMACEUTICA · RESEARCH FOUNDATION ·

SB SmithKline Beecham Pharmaceuticals

ORIGINAL ARTICLE

A Multifaceted Intervention to Improve Treatment of Depression in Primary Care

Wayne Katon, MD; Patricia Robinson, PhD; Michael Von Korff, ScD; Elizabeth Lin, MD, MPH; Terry Bush, PhD; Evette Ludman, PhD; Gregory Simon, MD, MPH; Edward Walker, MD

Background: This research study evaluates the effectiveness of a multifaceted intervention program to improve the management of depression in primary care.

Methods: One hundred fifty-three primary care patients with current depression were entered into a randomized controlled trial. Intervention patients received a structured depression treatment program in the primary care setting that included both behavioral treatment to increase use of adaptive coping strategies and counseling to improve medication adherence. Control patients received "usual" care by their primary care physicians. Outcome measures included adherence to antidepressant medication, satisfaction with care of depression and with antidepressant treatment, and reduction of depressive symptoms over time.

Results: At 4-month follow-up, significantly more intervention patients with major and minor depression than usual care patients adhered to antidepressant medication and rated the quality of care they received for depression as good to excellent. Intervention patients with major depression demonstrated a significantly greater decrease in depression severity over time compared with usual care patients on all 4 outcome analyses. Intervention patients with minor depression were found to have a significant decrease over time in depression severity on only 1 of 4 study outcome analyses compared with usual care patients.

Conclusion: A multifaceted primary care intervention improved adherence to antidepressant regimens and satisfaction with care in patients with major and minor depression. The intervention consistently resulted in more favorable depression outcomes among patients with major depression, while outcome effects were ambiguous among patients with minor depression.

Arch Gen Psychiatry. 1996;53:924-932

MAJOR AND minor depressive disorders are among the most common illnesses seen by primary care physicians, with a prevalence rate of each of these affective disorders estimated at 6% to 10% of the population.[1-3] Patients with major and minor depression tend to have high medical costs,[4] multiple unexplained symptoms (eg, fatigue, pain complaints),[5] and greater social and vocational disability than patients with medical illnesses such as hypertension or arthritis.[2,6]

While randomized trials in specialty settings have shown the efficacy of antidepressant medications and specific psychotherapies in the treatment of major depression,[7] epidemiologic studies of community and primary care populations have demonstrated that only about 1 in 3 people with major depression receive these treatments.[8,9] Primary care practice represents a potential setting in which to substantially increase the percentage of people with major depression who receive effective treatments and to test these treatments in patients with minor depression. Almost 50% of patients who are treated for major and minor depression are seen exclusively in primary care, with another 20% to 30% treated in both specialty and primary care settings.[10]

Unfortunately, primary care studies have demonstrated that as many as 50% of patients with either major or minor depression do not receive an accurate diagnosis.[3-8] Even when accurate diagnosis does occur and treatment with antidepressant medication is started, approximately one third of patients discontinue treatment with medications during the

See Patients and Methods on next page

From the Departments of Psychiatry and Behavioral Sciences (Drs Katon and Walker), University of Washington Medical School, and the Center for Health Studies (Drs Robinson, Von Korff, Lin, Bush, Ludman, and Simon), Group Health Cooperative of Puget Sound, Seattle.

PATIENTS AND METHODS

STUDY SETTING

The setting for this study was a large primary care clinic, the Northgate Medical Center of Group Health Cooperative of Puget Sound (GHC), an HMO serving over 380 000 persons in western Washington. This primary care clinic is staffed by 22 board-certified family physicians and provides health care to approximately 22 000 adult patients.

ELIGIBILITY FOR RANDOMIZATION

Patients who were diagnosed by primary care physicians as meeting criteria for definite or probable major depression and who had agreed to initiate antidepressant therapy were eligible for this study. They were asked to talk with the research assistant about a new program to improve treatment of depression within the primary care clinic. The research assistant described the program and screened the referred patients for eligibility. Inclusion criteria included (1) a 20-item depression symptom checklist (SCL-20) (adapted from the SCL-90[19]) screening score of 0.75 or greater, (2) age 18 to 80 years, and (3) willingness to take antidepressant medication. Exclusion criteria included (1) current alcohol abuse (screening score of 2 or more on the CAGE questionnaire [alcoholism screening questionnaire containing 4 structured questions]),[20] (2) current psychotic symptoms or serious suicidal ideation or plan, (3) dementia, (4) pregnancy, (5) terminal illness, (6) limited command of English, and (7) plan to withdraw from the Group Health insurance plan within the next 12 months. The recruitment procedure and the study protocol were approved by the institutional review boards of the University of Washington and the GHC.

USUAL CARE

Eligible patients were asked for informed consent to participate in a randomized trial of "an intervention designed to improve the care of depression." Consenting patients were randomly assigned to either a collaborative model of care, provided by both the primary care physician and 1 of the 2 study psychologists (P.R. or E. Ludman, PhD) or to "usual care" by the primary care physician. Patients who were randomized to the usual care arm received treatment for depression from their primary care physician in the GHC. In most cases, usual care for depression, given by the GHC family physicians, involves prescription of an antidepressant medication, 2 to 3 visits over the first 3 months of treatment, and the option to refer to GHC mental health services.

INTERVENTION

Patient

A multifaceted intervention was developed that targeted the patient, the physician, and the process of care. The research assistant scheduled the first study visit with the psychologist. Prior to the first study visit, the intervention patients were provided a brief booklet on the biology of depression and how antidepressant medications work, as well as a second brief booklet on simple cognitive behavioral techniques for managing depression. A 20-minute videotape was also given to patients to take home and view with their spouses; by way of 4 physician-patient vignettes, this videotape covered material similar to that provided in the written materials.

Physician

Primary care physicians participated in a didactic on antidepressant and behavioral treatment of depression prior to the randomized trial. Case-by-case consultation concerning depressed patients in the randomized trial also provided ongoing feedback and interaction between the 2 study psychologists (P.R., E. Ludman, PhD) and the primary care physicians.

Process of Care

A highly structured, primary care depression treatment program that was described in a 125-page manual was developed. The program included both behavioral treatment, targeted at teaching cognitive behavioral skills to manage depression, and counseling to improve medication adherence. Patients scheduled between 4 and 6 contacts with a psychologist who worked in the primary care setting. Total direct treatment time ranged from 2.5 to 3.5 hours of contact with the psychologist (a 1-hour initial evaluation and planning meeting, and 3 to 5 subsequent half-hour contacts). The direct contact phase of treatment started within 1 week of patient referral and ended 3 to 6 weeks after the initial visit. The psychologists also conducted telephone contacts with patients 2, 4, 12, and 24 weeks after completion of the direct contact phase of treatment.

The brief psychotherapy was solution focused,[21] multimodal,[22] and incorporated widely accepted therapeutic techniques that were based on the social cognitive theory of Bandura,[23] and the social learning theory models of Lewinsohn et al,[24,25] Beck and coworkers,[26,27] and Hayes.[28] The content of the first 4 sessions involved education, skills training, and homework assignments or behavioral experiments designed to improve mood and facilitate generalization of skills to daily life. Intervention patients were provided a book entitled *I Can If I Want To*, which explained cognitive behavioral methods of managing depression.[22] Optional sessions (5 and 6) often involved skill training in assertion, problem-solving communications in conflictual situations, and relaxation training.

At each visit, patients completed a Beck Depression Inventory (short form)[29] and a quick checklist for *DSM-III-R*[30] major depressive symptoms. The therapists also screened patients for potential side effects to antidepressant medication and checked antidepressant medication dosage and patient adherence. This information was reviewed by the psychiatrist (W.K.) in a weekly team meeting. The psychiatrist tracked each patient's progress (Beck Depression Inventory scores, medication dosage, side effects) on a typewritten form and recommended changes in dosage or type of medication based on the clinical progress of the patient. The psychologist then brought recommendations regarding timely medication changes to the primary care provider, who then made the medication adjustment. The protocol included the option of referral of nonresponding patients for a direct visit with the liaison psychiatrist.

Continued on next page

Primary care physicians received a handwritten consultation note the same day as each in-person visit. During the last in-person session, the therapist and patient developed a relapse prevention plan that addressed both antidepressant medication use and continued practice of behavioral skills and activities. A copy of this plan was put in each patient's medical chart.

The psychologists were doctorally trained therapists with prior experience delivering cognitive and behavioral treatments. Training was provided by the senior psychologist (P.R.) and consisted of 20 hours of training and weekly clinical supervision for the 1-year study period. Audiotapes of 9% of the total psychologist visits were reviewed to assess therapist adherence to the 125-page treatment manual. Treatment integrity was assessed on a Likert scale of 1 to 3 (low to high adherence) on 12 to 13 session-specific items (eg, presented model, checked for homework completion, presented theory of short-term change). The possible scores ranged from 13 to 39 for session 1 and 12 to 36 for all other sessions. The therapist adherence mean score for session 1 was 39 for both therapists. Mean scores for subsequent sessions ranged from 34 to 36, suggesting continuing adherence to the treatment protocol. Patients attended a mean (±SD) of 5.2±1.7 visits and received a mean (±SD) of 3.4±1.3 telephone follow-up calls. In addition, 6 patients (7.8%) saw the consultant psychiatrist for 1 to 3 visits.

STUDY MEASURES

Patients' depression and satisfaction with care were assessed at 1, 4, and 7 months after randomization by telephone interviewers who were blinded to the patients' randomization status. The telephone interview included the 20 depression items from the SCL-90, which are scored on a 0 to 4 measure of severity. We report the average item score (range, 0-4.0). The SCL-90 has been used in numerous studies of medical patients and has been found to have high reliability and validity.[19]

The Inventory for Depressive Symptomatology (IDS)[31] (clinician rated) is a 28-item scale, measuring depressive symptoms on a 0 to 3 severity index (range, 0-84). It has been demonstrated to have high reliability and validity. The IDS was structured with skip patterns to allow it to be conducted by nonclinicians by telephone, and a computer program was written by the study team to allow rating of *DSM-III-R* criteria[30] for major and minor depression.

In a test-retest design with 57 patients, a κ value of 0.52 was found for the diagnosis of major depression based on a comparison of this structured interview with the Structured Clinical Interview for *DSM-III-R* Diagnosis[32] depression module. In each case of disagreement, patients fell 1 symptom short on the IDS for the *DSM-III-R* requirement of at least 5 symptoms (the IDS was slightly more conservative in diagnosing major depression).

Patients were classified as having minor depression if (1) they had 2 to 4 symptoms of major depression nearly every day for 2 weeks or more, or (2) they were diagnosed by the primary care physician as being in need of antidepressant medication, despite having fewer than 2 major depressive symptoms on the IDS (19 [21.6%] of the 88 patients with minor depression). Patients were classified as having major depression if they had either a depressed mood or diminished pleasure in activities, plus at least 4 of the *DSM III-R* major depressive symptoms. A question about the number of depressive episodes experienced by patients over their lifetime that lasted 2 weeks or more and were accompanied by symptoms such as trouble sleeping, low energy, and trouble concentrating was added from the *Diagnostic Interview Schedule Version III-A*.[33]

At 4-month follow-up, satisfaction with management of depression was rated on 5-point ordinal scales that rated treatment from poor to excellent. Perceived helpfulness of antidepressant medications was rated on a 4-point ordinal scale from helping "not at all" to helping a "great deal."

The NEO Personality Inventory (NEO) is a 5-factor inventory, covering 60 items (12 items for each factor).[34] The individual items are scored on a 0- to 4-point index, scaled from strongly disagree to strongly agree. Seven items from the neuroticism scale were used in this study (range, 0-28) because these 7 items have been found to predict persistence of depressive symptoms in a primary care population even when controlling for depression severity.[35]

Adherence to antidepressant medication was assessed at 1-, 4- and 7-month follow-up by telephone interview. Patients were asked if they were still taking an antidepressant medication and were considered adherent if they reported having taken this medication at least 25 of the last 30 days.

Telephone interviewers received 3 hours of training prior to the first follow-up interview, plus individual practice sessions with the supervisor (a master's level clinician with extensive training in structured interviews) lasting 1 to 3 hours. Each interviewer was tested against either the supervisor or project director during a practice interview, as well as during a study interview, with reliability exceeding 80% for each interview question.

Both adherence to antidepressant medications and medical comorbidity were also assessed using the HMO's computerized prescription refill records. Dosage and duration of antidepressant medication was measured using the HMO's computerized records of prescriptions filled and refilled.[14] Refill records were processed to determine which patients continued treatment with antidepressants for at least 30 days and used medication at or above the lowest dosage level in the range of therapeutic doses recommended by the Agency for Health Care Policy and Research (AHCPR) guidelines.[7,14] The range of therapeutic dosages recommended in the AHCPR guidelines were 75 to 300 mg for amitriptyline hydrochloride, imipramine hydrochloride, doxepin hydrochloride, desipramine hydrochloride, and trazodone hydrochloride; 40 to 200 mg for nortriptyline hydrochloride; and 10 to 40 mg for fluoxetine hydrochloride. A similar analysis estimated adherence to this minimum therapeutic dosage level over 90 days.

To check reliability between automated and self-reported adherence to medication over time, comparisons were made between self-reported and automated pharmacy data. κ Statistics indicated excellent and significant reliability between the 2 sources of data. At the 1-month telephone interview, self-reported use of medications for 25 or more days in the prior month compared with duration of antidepressant prescription for 25 or more days derived from automated data revealed a κ of 0.83, an SE of 0.12, and a *P* value of .001. At the 4-month telephone interview, self-reported use of medications in the prior 4 months compared with 116 or more days of antidepressant use, derived from automated data, revealed a κ of 0.90, an SE of 0.13, and a *P* value of <.001.

The Chronic Disease Score (CDS) is a measure of chronic medical illness that is derived from the patient's use of prescription medications over a 6-month period.[36] This method rates each patient according to the number of medications typically used to treat chronic medical conditions such as heart disease and diabetes. Psychotropic medications and medications used primarily for symptom management (eg, analgesics) are not included in the index. The CDS has been found to have high stability over a 1-year period, to have a high correlation with physician ratings of severity of medical illness, and to predict hospitalization and mortality in the year following assessment after controlling for age, sex, and health care visits.[36]

STATISTICAL ANALYSES

Eligible patients were stratified into moderate and severe depression groups based on their SCL-20 depression score (moderate, 0.75 to <1.75; severe, 1.75 to 4.0). Within each stratum, patients were randomized to the intervention or the usual care group in blocks. Within each block, the randomization sequence was computer generated. Randomization was blocked so that assignment to the intervention and control groups was equalized after every eighth assignment. Patients were stratified in data analysis by an algorithm diagnosis of either major or minor depression, based on the IDS data. The IDS diagnoses were not available at the time of randomization. Analyses were stratified by major and minor depression status rather than symptom severity because prior research has demonstrated efficacy of antidepressant treatment for major depression, but not minor depression.[7]

χ^2 Analyses with correction for continuity were used to examine treatment group differences (intervention vs control) at 4-month follow-up on adherence to antidepressant medication, satisfaction with treatment for depression, satisfaction with help from antidepressant medication, and the percentage of patients who improved 50% or more on the SCL-20 depression items and IDS. The Wilcoxon 2-sample test was used for the nonparametric analyses of skewed utilization data (α of $P<.05$ was used for significance). Treatment group differences on the 2 depression outcome variables (SCL-20 depression items and IDS) were assessed using a mixed modeling technique for repeated measures (Proc Mixed procedure in SAS[37]) to test whether there was a difference in the extent of improvement between intervention and control patients over time, after adjusting for key clinical and demographic variables. Mixed models provide solutions to the commonly observed problems of missing data, serial correlation, and time varying covariates, and they accommodate systematic person-specific deviations from the average time trend.[38] This method allowed us to analyze an additional 13 cases in the minor depression group and an additional 15 cases in the major depression group that would have been deleted with traditional repeated measures analyses because 1 of the observation points at 1, 4, or 7 months was missing. We used a compound symmetry structure, which assumes equal correlations between time points, and adjusted for the covariates time, sex, and randomization group as class variables and age, neuroticism, and CDS as continuous variables.[37] For significant interaction effects, univariate tests were examined to determine where the groups differed in their rates of change.

first month of treatment, and only 40% reach adequate dosage and duration of treatment.[11-15] Recent data also suggest that patients with minor depression are frequently treated with antidepressant agents by primary care physicians, despite lack of controlled trials demonstrating efficacy of these medications in this less severe affective illness.[16]

Even fewer primary care patients with major or minor depression receive specific psychotherapies that have proven efficacy in randomized trials.[7,8] These research-tested therapies are usually provided in 12 to 20 sessions, but more recent research has suggested that 6 sessions of problem-focused therapy is as effective as antidepressant medication in patients with major depression in primary care.[17,18] Even by this less intensive psychotherapy standard, only one third of patients with major or minor depression in studies in a large health maintenance organization (HMO) were referred to specialty mental health services, and only one sixth received 5 or more psychotherapy visits.[16] Mental health services that are integrated into primary care could potentially help primary care physicians improve patient adherence to antidepressant medications as well as facilitate access to psychotherapies that have proven efficacy.

We recently reported the effects on the process and outcomes of care of a brief multifaceted depression intervention in primary care that was tested in a randomized controlled trial. Collaborative care was shown to improve the outcomes of patients with major depression but not minor depression.[16] This model emphasized patient education and collaborative management by the primary care physician and an on-site consulting psychiatrist. In this second study, we hope to adapt the collaborative care model to permit its implementation by a nonpsychiatrist provider and to integrate behavioral treatment of depression into the delivery model. In this second depression intervention program, 2 psychologists (P.R., E. Ludman, PhD) working within the primary care clinic provided brief behavioral treatment to increase the use of adaptive coping strategies, as well as counseling, to improve medication adherence. Supervision of pharmacological management by the psychologists was provided by a study psychiatrist (W.K.). Using a randomized design, we examine whether this program (1) increased the quality of acute-phase pharmacotherapy of depression to guideline standards, (2) was acceptable to primary care physicians and patients, and (3) improved clinical outcomes for both major and minor depression.

Demographic and Clinical Characteristics of Depressives

Characteristics*	Major Depression Group (n=65) Intervention (n=31)	Major Depression Group (n=65) Usual Care (n=34)	Minor Depression Group (n=88) Intervention (n=46)	Minor Depression Group (n=88) Usual Care (n=42)
Mean (±SD) age, y	43.1±9.3	44.8±15.9	49.2±13.9	47.2±13.8
Median (range)†	43 (22-58)	40 (23-74)	45 (22-82)	47 (21-76)
Female, %	77.4	73.5	71.7	73.8
White, %	77.4	91.2	91.3	85.7
≥1 y of college, %	90.3	70.6†	87.0	81.0
Married or cohabitating, %	48.4	32.3	52.2	47.6
Employed full-time or part-time, %	87.1	73.5	73.3	76.2
Chronic disease (mean±SD)‡ (range)	1.19±1.6 (0-5)	1.1±2.0 (0-7)	1.5±2.6 (0-12)	1.2±2.3 (0-10)
NEO neuroticism (mean±SD) (range)	18.1±6.15 (1-28)	15.7±6.7 (4-27)	14.8±6.1 (1-28)	15.6±5.1 (6-26)
IDS (28-item) (mean±SD) (range)	46.8±10.8 (29-64)	46.0±8.8 (33-65)	27.3±7.4 (10-42)	28.2±11.3 (8-51)
SCL-20 depression (mean±SD) (range)	2.46±0.53 (1.3-3.35)	2.35±0.51 (1.25-3.4)	1.77±0.49 (0.8-3.0)	1.62±0.54 (0.80-3.0)
Recurrent major depression (≥2 episodes)	59.1	65.4	66.7	64.9

**NEO indicates NEO Personality Inventory; IDS, Inventory of Depressive Symptomatology; SCL-20, 20-item depression symptom checklist.*

†P<.05. (Although the t *test was significant, the Cochran-Mantel-Haenszel test comparing the differences in 6 levels of education [grade 2, junior high, high school, some college, college graduate, graduate school] was not significant [χ^2 (4)=6.23,* P*=.18].) Possible ranges: chronic disease, 0-35; NEO Personality Inventory score, 0-28; IDS, 0-84; SCL, 0.75-4.0 (0-0.74 were ineligible scores).*

‡Median scores on chronic disease are not useful because over half of the patients with major and minor depression have no chronic medical illnesses and score 0.

RESULTS

Two hundred seventeen patients were referred to the study by the primary care physicians over a 1-year period. One hundred fifty-three patients (70.5%) were successfully randomized to the study. Thirty patients (13.8%) refused enrollment (7 were not interested in involvement, 7 did not attend the baseline interview, 9 were too busy, 3 preferred treatment by the primary care physician alone, 2 no longer thought they were depressed, 1 was too medically ill, and 1 could not be contacted after referral). Patients refusing enrollment did not differ from patients agreeing to be randomized on age (47.9±16.9 vs 46.4±13.6 [mean±SD], t=0.41, P=.68) or sex (83.3% female vs 73.9% female, $\chi^2(1)=1.2$, P=.27). A total of 34 (15.7%) patients were ineligible, including 7 (3.2%) who scored below the SCL-20 depression criteria of 0.75; 4 (1.8%) who spoke limited English; 3 (1.4%) who refused medication; 3 (1.4%) who were CAGE-positive; 3 (1.4%) who were too medically ill; 3 (1.4%) who were in an ongoing substance abuse program; 3 (1.4%) who were inappropriately referred; 3 (1.4%) who had been in a previous study of depression in primary care; 2 (0.9%) who already had a spouse in the current depression treatment trial; 1 (0.5%) who was too young; 1 (0.5%) who lived too far away to participate; and 1 (0.5%) who was being treated in a different primary care clinic. Adherence to antidepressants, 50% or more reduction in depressive symptoms, and satisfaction with treatment are reported for the sample of 153 patients randomly assigned to the intervention or usual care groups.

Of the 153 patients randomized, 140 (91.5%) completed the 1-month follow-up, 128 (83.7%) completed the 4-month follow-up, and 117 (76.5%) completed the 7-month follow-up. One hundred thirteen patients (73.8%) completed all 3 follow-ups and 141 (92.2%) completed at least 2 of the 3 follow-ups. Sixty (77.9%) of the 77 intervention patients vs 53 (69.7%) of the 76 control patients completed all 3 follow-ups ($\chi^2(1)=1.33$, P=.25). There were no statistically significant differences on any demographic or clinical variable between the 40 patients who missed completing at least 1 follow-up and the 113 patients who completed all 3 follow-ups. The mixed model technique for repeated measures was completed on the 141 patients who completed at least 2 of the 3 follow-up interviews.

PATIENT CHARACTERISTICS

There were 65 patients with major depression and 88 patients with minor depression enrolled in the trial. There were no significant differences between intervention and control patients in either depression subgroup in any demographic or clinical variable (**Table**).

TREATMENT ADHERENCE TO INTEGRATED PROGRAM

Of the 77 patients who were randomized to the intervention, 57 (74%) completed 6 sessions, 7 (9.1%) completed 5 sessions, 4 (5.2%) completed 4 sessions, 2 (2.6%) completed 3 sessions, 1 (1.3%) completed 2 sessions, and 1 (1.3%) completed 1 session. Five patients (6.5%) declined participation in the intervention after randomization and before the initial visit. The criteria for treatment completion were attendance at 4 planned sessions, and 88.3% of those patients randomized to intervention and 94.4% of patients who actually started the program completed the program. All intervention patients were included in the outcome analyses, whether they completed the integrated program or not, following the intention-to-treat principle of analysis of randomized trial data.

MEDICATION ADHERENCE: MAJOR DEPRESSION GROUP

Based on the telphone interview data, intervention patients were significantly more likely to adhere to antidepressant medication for 25 days or more in the last 1-month period at 4-month follow-up compared with usual care patients (89% vs 62%, $\chi^2(1)=5.35$, $P=.02$). Similar trends were seen at 1-month (85% vs 63%, $\chi^2(1)=3.50$, $P=.06$) and 7-month follow-up (79% vs 54%, $\chi^2(1)=3.37$, $P=.07$).

Based on automated prescription data on refills among patients with major depression, differences between intervention patients and usual care patients in the percentage who received a dosage of antidepressant medication for at least 30 days at or above the lowest dosage level recommended by AHCPR guidelines (66.7% vs 57.6%, $\chi^2(1)=0.55$, $P<.46$) or for at least 90 days were not statistically significant (62.1% vs 54.6, $\chi^2(1)=0.36$, $P=.55$).

MEDICATION ADHERENCE: MINOR DEPRESSION GROUP

Based on the telephone interview data, intervention patients were significantly more likely than usual care patients to report adherence to antidepressants in 25 of the last 30 days at the 4-month (74% vs 44%, $\chi^2(1)=6.98$, $P=.01$) and 7-month follow-up (65% vs 41%, $\chi^2(1)=4.05$, $P=.04$), with similar trends at 1-month follow-up (81% vs 67%, $\chi^2(1)=2.33$, $P=.13$). Based on automated prescription data on refills, intervention patients with minor depression were significantly more likely than usual care patients to receive a dosage of antidepressant medication for at least 30 days at or above the lowest dosage level recommended by AHCPR guidelines (84.8% vs 53.9%, $\chi^2(1)=9.73$, $P<.002$) with similar trends for at least 90 days (69.6% vs 39.5%, $\chi^2(1)=3.08$, $P=.08$).

SATISFACTION WITH TREATMENT

At 4-month follow-up, significantly more intervention patients with major depression rated the quality of care they received for depression as good to excellent compared with usual care patients (88.5% vs 56.0%, $\chi^2(1)=6.7$, $P<.009$). At 4-month follow-up, there was a nonsignificant trend toward an increased percentage of intervention patients with major depression rating antidepressant medication as helping somewhat to a great deal when compared with usual care patients (80% vs 58.3%, $\chi^2(1)=2.7$, $P<.10$).

At 4-month follow-up, intervention patients with minor depression were significantly more likely than usual care patients to rate the quality of care they received for depression as good to excellent (97.1% vs 71.4%, $\chi^2(1)=8.7$, $P=.003$). At 4-month follow-up, no significant differences were seen between intervention and usual care patients with minor depression on their rating of the antidepressant medication as helping somewhat to a great deal (94.6% vs 88.6%, $\chi^2(1)=0.85$, $P=.36$).

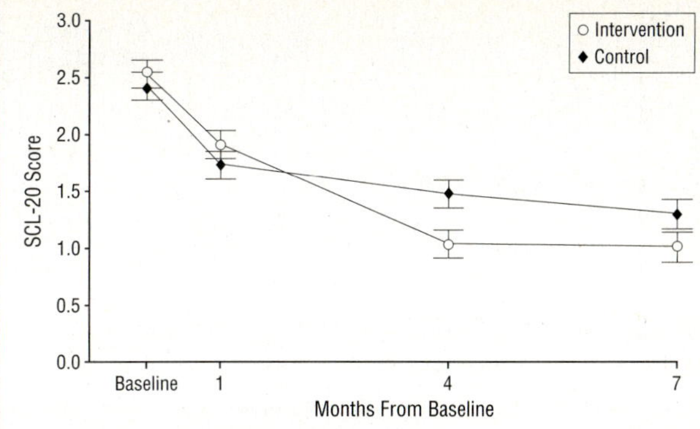

Figure 1. *Patients with major depression adjusted for age, sex, neuroticism, and chronic disease. SCL-20 indicates 20-item depression symptom checklist score.*

CHANGES IN OUTCOME

Both intervention and control groups tended to report substantial improvement from baseline to 1-, 4-, and 7-month follow-up. Among control patients with major depression, 23.1% met criteria for major depression and 30.8% met criteria for minor depression, respectively, at 4-month follow-up vs 7.4% and 33.8% of intervention patients. Among control patients with minor depression, 33.3% met criteria for minor depression (2-4 symptoms) at 4-month follow-up vs 25.6% of intervention patients.

Significantly more intervention patients with major depression showed 50% or more improvement on the SCL-20 depression items compared with usual care patients (70.4% vs 42.3%, $\chi^2(1)=4.3$, $P=.04$). When age, sex, NEO score, and CDS were used as covariates, this difference remained significant ($\chi^2(1)=5.0$, $P=.02$). On the IDS, 74.1% of intervention patients showed 50% or more improvement compared with 42.3% of usual care patients ($\chi^2(1)=5.5$, $P=.02$). When age, sex, NEO score, and CDS were used as covariates, the intervention and control differences on the IDS remained significant ($\chi^2(1)=4.7$, $P=.03$). As shown in **Figure 1**, the Proc Mixed analyses for patients with major depression found a significant group-by-time interaction on the SCL-20 depression item score ($F(3,206)=5.56$, $P=.001$). This difference in change over time between intervention and usual care groups was due to significant differences in the rate of change in severity from baseline to 4-month follow-up ($F(1,206)=3.07$, $P=.002$) and baseline to 7-month follow-up ($F(1,206)=2.12$, $P=.04$). Proc Mixed analyses for patients with major depression found a similar significant group-by-time interaction on the IDS ($F(3,206)=2.96$, $P=.03$). This was due to intervention effects in change from baseline to 4-month follow-up ($F(1,206)=2.81$, $P=.005$).

There were no significant differences between intervention patients and usual care patients with minor depression in the percentage of patients who improved 50% or more at 4-month follow-up on either the SCL-20 depression item score (66.7% vs 52.8%, $\chi^2(1)=1.5$, $P=.22$) or the IDS (51.3% vs 52.8%, $\chi^2(1)=.02$, $P=.90$). This comparison remained nonsignificant for the SCL-20 depres-

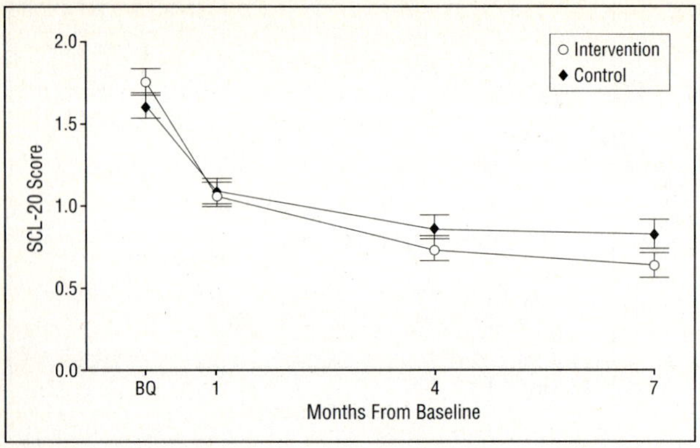

Figure 2. *Patients with minor depression adjusted for age, sex, neuroticism, and chronic disease. SCL-20 indicates 20-item depression symptom checklist score.*

sion item score and IDS when age, sex, NEO score, and CDS were used as covariates (SCL=$\chi^2(1)=2.7$, $P=.10$; IDS=$\chi^2(1)=.01$, $P=.91$). As shown in **Figure 2**, the Proc Mixed analyses for patients with minor depression found a significant group-by-time interaction on the SCL-20 depression item score ($F(3,296)=3.10$, $P=.03$). This difference in change over time between intervention and usual care groups was due to significant differences in rate of change in severity from baseline to 4-month follow-up ($F(1,296)=2.25$, $P=.03$) and baseline to 7-month follow-up ($F(1,296)=2.85$, $P=.005$). Proc Mixed analyses for patients with minor depression found no significant group-by-time interaction on the IDS ($F(1,296)=0.46$, $P=.71$). We conducted a separate analysis excluding patients from the minor depression sample who had fewer than 2 *DSM III-R* major depressive symptoms at baseline (19 patients were excluded). Estimated effects were similar but not significant for the SCL-20 depression item score or IDS using Proc Mixed analyses.

HEALTH CARE VISITS (EXCLUDING PSYCHOLOGIST INTERVENTION VISITS)

In the first 12 weeks of treatment, usual care patients had 2.9±1.4 visits with their primary care physician vs 3.1±1.7 visits in intervention patients ($t=1.02$, $P=.30$). In the 6-month period beginning with the primary care referral visit, usual care patients received a mean of 4.1±2.0 visits with their primary care physician compared with 4.6±2.6 visits in intervention patients ($t=1.3$, $P=.19$).

In the first 12-week period, beginning with the primary care referral, 20% of intervention patients vs 29% of usual care patients were seen by a GHC mental health specialist (outside the primary care clinic) ($\chi^2(1)=1.6$, $P=.21$). In the 6-month period, beginning with the primary care referral, 24% of intervention patients vs 33% of usual care patients were seen by a GHC mental health specialist ($\chi^2(1)=1.5$, $P=.21$).

COMMENT

A multifaceted primary care intervention providing increased patient education, brief cognitive behavioral therapy, surveillance of medication adherence, and an on-site integrated role for the psychologist and psychiatrist in primary care significantly improved the process of care for depression. At most follow-up points, significantly more intervention patients compared with usual care patients with both major and minor depression were likely to be adhering to antidepressant medication. When dosage as well as duration of therapy were taken into account, this treatment program led to improvements in patient adherence to a dosage of antidepressant medication that was at or above the lowest dosage in the range recommended in the AHCPR guidelines[7] for patients with minor depression (with similar nonsignificant trends in intervention patients with major depression). Satisfaction with care of depression in intervention patients with minor and major depression was also increased compared with controls. Of greatest significance, the intervention was associated with improvement in all clinical outcomes for major depression. The outcome results for minor depression were ambiguous, with a suggestion of effectiveness in 1 outcome analysis of 4.

Limitations of the study include the following: (1) our patient population was predominantly white and middle class, and the success of the intervention may or may not generalize to other socioeconomic or ethnic groups; (2) the research was completed in a large HMO clinic staffed by family physicians, and the intervention model used in the study may be more difficult to integrate into fee-for-service care or smaller clinic settings; (3) since referral to the study was dependent on the accuracy of primary care physician diagnosis, the study results may not generalize to the estimated 40% to 50% of patients with depression who do not receive an accurate diagnosis in primary care; (4) the multifaceted nature of the intervention did not allow us to determine the specific active components of the program that were most helpful. However, the medical literature has demonstrated that programs that have been successful in improving patient outcomes target multiple levels, including patient, physician, and process aspects of care.[39] A final limitation is that usual care patients may have benefited from the training that primary care physicians received in the study (spillover effect). However, if a training effect had taken place, it would have reduced the magnitude of intervention and control differences in outcomes.

The multifaceted intervention used in this study was well accepted by both patient and primary care physicians. Only 13.8% of the primary care patients who were referred to the study refused to participate, and intervention patients with both major and minor depression were significantly more likely than usual care patients to rate the care they received for depression as good to excellent. Moreover, almost 90% of patients randomized to the intervention completed at least 4 sessions with a psychologist. In a poststudy questionnaire, 65% of primary care physicians stated that the intervention had increased their satisfaction in treating depression a great deal, and 100% preferred the on-site program for the treatment of depression to referral of depressed patients to specialty care.

Owing to the economic pressures of health care reform, the productivity of primary care physicians is an issue of growing significance, and often these physicians have fewer support staff (nurses, medical assistants) because of budget cuts. Concurrently, the widespread use of guidelines that are aimed at improving quality of care has placed additional demands on primary care physicians to "do more with less" (enhance clinical outcomes with fewer resources). The intervention used in the current study may provide a model of how mental health professionals can assist the primary care physician in educating patients, monitoring and reinforcing adherence, and helping patients with behavioral and lifestyle changes that may be beneficial to their clinical outcome. Care extenders, such as nurses or psychologists, have been successful in improving the quality of treatment of other medical disorders such as arthritis[40] and hypertension.[41]

The findings in this study are consistent with a recent review by Brown and Schulberg[42] of psychosocial treatments that have been most successful in randomized controlled trials in primary care. They found that all studies that used "manualized" treatments on homogeneous populations (ie, major depression or generalized anxiety disorder) showed significantly greater reductions in psychological symptoms than the usual care provided by the primary care physician. Our study took this methodology a step further by attempting to potentiate the ability of the primary care physician to provide guideline-level pharmacotherapy for depression, combined with brief behavioral treatment by a psychologist in the primary care clinic.

Over half the patients who were referred to a psychologist in this study met criteria for minor depression. Primary care physicians frequently treat patients with minor depression with antidepressant medication,[16,35] but to our knowledge there are no controlled trials demonstrating efficacy of antidepressant medication in these patients.[7] A problem in attempting to treat this subgroup of patients is that it is difficult for specific interventions to improve on the rate of recovery in usual care. As shown in Figure 2, both intervention and usual care groups with minor depression tend to improve rapidly over a 1-month period. This high rate of recovery in usual care patients with minor depression occurred despite the fact that they were often treated with below-guideline levels of antidepressant medication. This suggests a high rate of spontaneous remission of symptoms in patients with minor depression, a high placebo response to supportive visits and low-dosage antidepressant medication, or that low-dosage medication may be as effective as higher-dosage antidepressant treatment. To test active treatments against placebo, future studies of these patients may benefit from including a 4-week "watchful waiting phase" prior to randomization to exclude patients who recover quickly without a specific treatment.

The intervention in this study is a second model of integrating mental health professionals into the primary care treatment of depression, tested in a randomized trial that significantly improved adherence to antidepressant medications, satisfaction with care, and outcomes of patients with major depression.[16] Taken together, these 2 studies suggest that integration of a range of specialty mental health providers into primary care practice can improve outcomes and patient satisfaction for treatment of major depression when used with a structured approach to providing patient care.

Accepted for publication February 5, 1996.

This study was supported by National Institute of Mental Health, Health Services Division, Rockville, Md, grant MH4-1739 (Dr Katon).

The study would not have been possible without the support of the physicians and staff of the GHC. We would like to thank Stephanie Hauge, MA, for her role in recruiting and enrolling patients, Kathleen Saunders, JD, for her expertise with automated data systems, and Laura J. Ichikawa, MS, for assisting in statistical analysis.

Reprints: Wayne Katon, MD, Department of Psychiatry and Behavioral Sciences, Box 356560, University of Washington Medical School, Seattle, WA 98195-6560.

REFERENCES

1. Katon W, Schulberg H. Epidemiology of depression in primary care. *Gen Hosp Psychiatry.* 1992;14:237-247.
2. Ormel J, Von Korff M, Ustun TB, Pini S, Korten A, Oldehinkel T. Common mental disorders and disability across cultures: results from the WHO Collaborate Study on psychological problems in general health care. *JAMA.* 1994;272:1741-1748.
3. Ormel J, Oldehinkel T, Brilman E, vanden Brink W. Outcome of depression and anxiety in primary care: a three-wave 3½-year study of psychopathology and disability. *Arch Gen Psychiatry.* 1993;50:759-766.
4. Simon GE, Ormel J, Von Korff M, Barlow W. Health care costs associated with depressive and anxiety disorders in primary care. *Am J Psychiatry.* 1995;152:352-357.
5. Simon GE, Von Korff M. Somatization and psychiatric disorder in the NIMH Epidemiologic Catchment Area Study. *Am J Psychiatry.* 1991;148:1494-1500.
6. Wells KB, Stewart A, Hays RD, Burnam MA, Rogers W, Daniels M, Berry S, Greenfield S, Ware J. The functioning and well-being of depressed patients: results from the Medical Outcomes Study. *JAMA.* 1989;262:914-919.
7. Public Health Service Agency for Health Care Policy and Research. *Depression in Primary Care: Treatment of Major Depression.* Rockville, Md: US Dept of Health and Human Services; 1993:2. AHCPR publication 93-051.
8. Eisenberg L. Treating depression and anxiety in primary care: closing the gap between knowledge and practice. *N Engl J Med.* 1992;326:1080-1084.
9. US Dept of Health and Human Services. *Healthy People 2000: National Health Promotion and Disease Prevention Objectives.* Washington, DC: US Government Printing Office; 1979:207-224. DHHS publication (PHS)91-50212.
10. Narrow WE, Regier DA, Rae DS, Manderscheid RW, Locke BZ. Use of services by persons with mental and addictive disorders: findings from the National Institute of Mental Health Epidemiologic Catchment Area Study. *Arch Gen Psychiatry.* 1993;50:95-107.
11. Public Health Service Agency for Health Care Policy and Research. *Depression in Primary Care: Detection and Diagnosis.* Rockville, Md: US Dept of Health and Human Services; 1993. AHCPR publication 93-0551.
12. Katon W, Von Korff M, Lin E, Bush T, Ormel J. Adequacy and duration of antidepressant treatment in primary care. *Med Care.* 1992;30:67-76.
13. Wells KB, Katon W, Rogers B, Camp P. Use of minor tranquilizers and antidepressant medications by depressed outpatients: results from the Medical Outcomes Study. *Am J Psychiatry.* 1994;151:694-700.
14. Simon G, Von Korff, Wagner EH, Barlow W. Patterns of antidepressant use in community practice. *Gen Hosp Psychiatry.* 1993;15:399-408.
15. Lin E, Von Korff M, Katon W, Bush T, Simon GE, Walker E, Robinson P. Primary care physician role in adherence to antidepressant therapy. *Med Care.* 1995;33:67-74.
16. Katon W, Von Korff M, Lin E, Walker E, Simon G, Bush T, Robinson P, Russo J. Collaborative management to achieve treatment guidelines: impact on depression in primary care. *JAMA.* 1995;273:1026-1031.
17. Mynors-Wallis LM, Gath DH, Lloyd-Thomas AR, Tomlinson D. Randomized

controlled trial comparing problem solving treatment with amitriptyline and placebo for major depression in primary care. *BMJ.* 1995;310:441-446.

18. Schulberg HC, Coulehan JL, Block MR, Lave J, Rodriquez E, Scott CP, Madonia JS, Imber S, Perel J. Clinical trials of primary care treatment for major depression: issues in design, recruitment and treatment. *Int J Psychiatry Med.* 1993;23:29-42.
19. Derogatis LR, Rickels K, Uhlenhuth EH, Covi L. The Hopkins Symptom Checklist: a measure of primary symptom dimensions. In: Pichot P, ed. *Psychological Measurements in Psychopharmacology: Problems in Pharmacopsychiatry.* Basel, Switzerland: Kargerman; 1974.
20. Mayfield D, McLeod G, Hall P. The CAGE Questionnaire: validation of a new alcoholism screening instrument. *Am J Psychiatry.* 1974;131:1121-1123.
21. de Shazer S, Berg-Insoo K, Lipchik E, Nunnally E, Molnar A, Gingrich W, Weiner-Davis M. Brief therapy: focused solution development. *Fam Process.* 1986;25:207-221.
22. Lazarus A, Fay A. *I Can If I Want To.* New York, NY: Quill William Morrow; 1975.
23. Bandura A. Self-efficacy: toward a unifying theory of behavioral change. *Psychol Rev.* 1977;84:191-215.
24. Lewinsohn PM, Antonuccio DO, Breckenridge JS, Teri L. *The Coping With Depression Course: A Psychoeducational Intervention for Unipolar Depression.* Eugene, Ore: Castalia Publishing Co; 1984.
25. Lewinsohn PM, Hoberman HM, Teri L, Hautzinger M. An integrative theory of unipolar depression. In: Reiss S, Bootzin RR, eds. *Theoretical Issues in Behavioral Therapy.* New York, NY: Academic Press Inc; 1985:313-359.
26. Rush AJ, Beck AT, Kovacs M, Hollon S. Comparative efficacy of cognitive therapy and pharmacotherapy in the treatment of depressed outpatients. *Cognitive Ther Res.* 1977;1:17-37.
27. Beck AT. Cognitive therapy: past, present and future. *J Consult Clin Psychol.* 1993;61:194-198.
28. Hayes SC. A contextual approach to therapeutic change. In: Jacobson N, ed. *Psychotherapists in Clinical Practice: Cognitive and Behavioral Perspectives.* New York, NY: Guilford Press; 1987:327-387.
29. Beck AT, Beck RW. Screening depressed patients in family practice: a rapid technique. *Postgrad Med.* 1972;52:81-85.
30. American Psychiatric Association. *American Psychiatric Association Diagnostic and Statistical Manual of Mental Disorders, Third Edition, Revised.* Washington, DC: American Psychiatric Association Press; 1987.
31. Rush AJ, Giles DE, Schlesser MA, Fulton CL, Weissenburger J, Burns C. The Inventory for Depressive Symptomatology: preliminary findings. *Psychiatry Res.* 1986;18:65-87.
32. Williams JB, Gibbon M, First MB, Spitzer R, Davies M, Borus J, Howes MJ, Kane J, Pope HG, Rounsaville B, Wittchen H-U. The Structured Clinical Interview for *DSM-III-R* (SCID), II: multisite test-retest reliability. *Arch Gen Psychiatry.* 1992;49:630-636.
33. Robins LN, Helzer JE. *Diagnostic Interview Schedule (DIS), Version III-A.* St Louis, Mo: Dept of Psychiatry, Washington University School of Medicine; 1985.
34. Costa PT, McCrae RR. *The NEO Personality Inventory Manual.* Odessa, Fla: Psychological Assessment Resources; 1985.
35. Katon W, Lin E, Von Korff M, Bush T, Walker E, Simon G, Robinson P. The predictors of persistence of depression in primary care. *J Affect Disord.* 1994;31:81-90.
36. Von Korff M, Wagner EH, Saunders K. A chronic disease score from automated pharmacy data. *J Clin Epidemiol.* 1992;45:197-203.
37. *SAS/Statistics Software: Changes and Enhancements.* Cary, NC: SAS Institute Inc; 1994. SAS Technical Report. Release 6.10.
38. Gibbons RD, Hedeker D, Elkin I, Waternaux C, Kraemer HC, Greenhouse JB, Shea MT, Imber SD, Sotsky SM, Watkins JT. Some conceptual and statistical issues in analysis of longitudinal psychiatric data. *Arch Gen Psychiatry.* 1993;50:739-750.
39. Starfield B. *Primary Care: Concept, Evaluation and Policy.* New York, NY: Oxford University Press Inc; 1992.
40. Lorig K, Holman H. Arthritis self-managed studies: a twelve-year review. *Health Educ.* 1993;20:17-28.
41. Bass MJ, McWhinney IR, Donner A. Do family physicians need medical assistants to detect and manage hypertension? *Can Med Assoc J.* 1986;134:1247-1255.
42. Brown C, Schulberg HC. The efficacy of psychosocial treatments in primary care: a review of randomized clinical trials. *Gen Hosp Psychiatry.* 1995;17:414-424.

Some Economics of Mental Health 'Carve-Outs'

Richard G. Frank, PhD; Haiden A. Huskamp; Thomas G. McGuire, PhD; Joseph P. Newhouse, PhD

We discuss the rationale for benefit carve-out contracts in general and for mental health and substance abuse in particular. We focus on the control of adverse selection as a principal explanation and find that this is consistent with the widespread use of sole-source contracting with periodic rebidding. We also find that some degree of risk sharing is common; we interpret this as a method of balancing cost-containment incentives with incentives to maintain access and quality on unmeasured dimensions.

Arch Gen Psychiatry. 1996;53:933-937

How employers and public purchasers structure their health insurance plans has changed in recent years. Traditionally, the purchaser, usually an employer, contracted with a single insurance plan to cover a full range of health risks. Increasingly, however, purchasers of health insurance are offering beneficiaries a range of plans. Purchasers may also "carve out" certain benefits, which means that they are separating the health insurance function by disease or service category and contracting separately for the management of those risks. This article addresses the issue of why a health buyer might break up health insurance risks in this way, emphasizing carve-out contracts in the area of mental health and substance abuse (MHSA).

At present, mental health carve-out contracts are a rapidly growing feature of health insurance. According to Oss,[1] approximately 53 million people are enrolled in carve-out programs of all types. Between 20 and 25 million people are enrolled in so-called risk-based carve-out contracts (whereby the carve-out vendor assumes some or all of the financial risk for claims), which account for about 60% of the total revenue of firms that manage MHSA benefits. Carve-outs are more common among larger firms than smaller firms. Umland[2] reports that 35% of employers with 5000 or more employees were contracting with a specialty MHSA carve-out vendor compared with a rate of about 3% for firms with fewer than 500 employees.

The setting for the problem that we analyze is an employer or public agency such as Medicaid that pays for health insurance for a large number of enrollees. Enrollees have a choice of competing managed care plans such as health maintenance organizations that offer a standardized benefit package. The employer must decide if some part of the health insurance risk should be carved out of the general contract and administered separately. If a carve-out approach is chosen, the employer must then choose whether to allow various vendors to compete for employees' business or to let a single contract cover all employees.

THE RATIONALE FOR CARVE-OUTS IN MHSA

Most employer-provided health insurance covers MHSA treatment. Virtually all private plans, however, put special limits on coverage for these conditions.[3] Typically, a private plan requires higher copayments for MHSA care than for general medical services, limits the number

From the Departments of Health Care Policy (Drs Frank and Newhouse and Ms Huskamp), and Health Policy and Management (Dr Newhouse), Harvard School of Public Health; Department of Economics, Boston University, Boston, Mass (Dr McGuire); and Kennedy School of Government, Cambridge, Mass (Dr Newhouse).

of covered MHSA office visits, limits MHSA-covered hospital days to 30 or 60 per year, and often imposes annual or lifetime limits on plan costs for MHSA care as well. Coverage for medical services is typically not subject to these limits. In spite of less favorable coverage, costs of MHSA treatment have averaged around 8% to 12% of an employers' health benefit costs and have been a special concern for employers in recent years. The presence of a public safety net permits employers to avoid paying for very expensive mental health treatment. Beyond this, there are other reasons for limited coverage that relate to the case for using carve-out contracts. One reason for special limits is that the utilization of MHSA services is more responsive to insurance coverage and payment features than other areas of health care.[4,5] For example, the RAND Health Insurance Experiment showed that utilization of mental health services is twice as responsive to cost-sharing provisions as is utilization of general medical services. This response in terms of utilization to insurance coverage is called *moral hazard*. A second reason for special limits is that a health plan offering more generous coverage may draw an adverse selection of the insured population. An employer or public agency might carve out MHSA care for 1 or both of 2 main reasons: (1) better management of market failures resulting from moral hazard and (2) better management of adverse selection. We take up these 2 reasons in turn.

Management of Moral Hazard

Firms engaged in managing MHSA benefits argue that they can do a better job of managing the moral hazard associated with mental health services and thus managing the cost of care. By assembling networks of specialty providers who are willing to accept lower prices and by using techniques including care management and utilization review, firms in the "behavioral health" field promise to make care more cost-effective and to generally save employers money while preserving access to necessary services. In one spectacular example, the Massachusetts State government began contracting with a carve-out firm to provide MHSA benefits to almost 200 000 state and local employees in a public insurance group in Massachusetts in July 1993. Based on preliminary research, benefit payouts were reduced by 40%, with no detectable decrease in the rate at which people enter treatment. Other case studies showing favorable results are reported in business publications or unpublished reports.

Nevertheless, is it necessary to carve out the mental health benefit and to separate the risk of mental disorders from risk of other health care costs to apply the technology of moral hazard management used by carve-out firms? The carve-out firms, some of which have now been acquired by large insurers, may have special expertise, and there may be some network economies associated with running a managed care plan in a region. Yet these advantages by themselves do not necessitate an employer's use of a carve-out contract. The employer could instead contract with a single insurer, who would be responsible for all risks including MHSA, as was traditionally done. That single insurer could also hire a specialized management firm, and some do, to manage the risk internally without a formal carve-out. In other words, because all insurers have an incentive to control cost, an employer need not necessarily use a carve-out to have access to the management techniques possessed by the specialized MHSA benefit management firms.

Management of Adverse Selection

A second reason to carve out a MHSA benefit derives from an employer's concern with the consequences of adverse selection. Adverse selection occurs because insurance plans operating in competitive markets have a strong financial incentive to avoid the most costly and difficult-to-treat enrollees by making health plans unattractive to certain subpopulations such as the severely mentally ill. In fact, insurers have historically competed for "good risks" by offering insurance coverage that strictly limited coverage for the treatment of mental illness.[5] Adverse selection is thus an important explanation for the limited coverage of mental health care.

Many MHSA problems are persistent and, therefore, predictable to an individual seeking insurance coverage, so individuals who predict that they will need MHSA treatment will seek a plan with generous coverage of these services. Furthermore, mental health expenditures (in comparison with other areas of spending) are relatively highly correlated with future total health expenditures, implying that competing health plans would like to avoid persons using mental health services. During the 1960s and 1970s, the Federal Employees Health Benefit Program (FEHBP) was an example of how concerns about selection drove competing insurers to lower benefits for MHSA services, as plans with generous MHSA benefits attracted those who wished to use such a benefit. A comparison of the much smaller response to price in the RAND Health Insurance Experiment with those derived from the FEHBP strongly suggests adverse selection in the FEHBP. Mental health use in the "high option" FEHBP can be 2 or 3 times higher than in the low option, even though coverage differences are quite small.[6] Whereas the RAND Health Insurance Experiment randomized the underlying risk among plans, the more generous FEHBP plans differentially attracted the poorer risks, thereby making it appear that generous coverage induced high utilization.

Adverse selection has also played a role in public regulation of insurance benefits for MHSA care over the past few decades. Concern for the effects of competition among insurers to avoid the mentally ill was the principal justification for state regulations, stipulating minimum coverage for mental health care adopted by 22 states during the 1970s and 1980s. However, when costs are controlled by managed care, regulation of the terms of coverage is not sufficient to ensure that competition for good risks does not undermine the actual availability of benefits. A managed care organization could, for example, state in its benefit booklet that up to 20 outpatient visits per person per year are covered, but make it very difficult for an enrollee to begin or continue receiving care by using a restrictive case management process or a limited panel of MHSA providers. Thus, the administrative mechanisms that can effectively control moral hazard can also be used to gain favorable risk selection by a managed care organization. By carving out the mental health benefit, an employer eliminates the incentive to "overmanage" mental health costs to attract good risks.

Mandated Minimums

A third, and probably less important, reason why buyers may carve out MHSA is to guarantee that a proportion of total benefit dollars be designated for MHSA treatment. In the context of managed care, a carve-out program can serve a function similar to a minimum-benefit mandate in a fee-for-service world. A carve-out "sets aside" a designated level of funding for MHSA services in a separate contract. This, however, could also be achieved without a carve-out if a health plan set an internal subbudget and enforced this arrangement.

EVIDENCE ON THE EXPLANATIONS

The foregoing theoretical discussion has emphasized the management of adverse selection as a key factor in a decision to carve out MHSA benefits. Empirical support for this view comes from analyzing the decisions of large purchasers. If selection is a concern, one would tend to observe a single MHSA carve-out firm that served all members of the group rather than several carve-out firms competing for individual members of the group. If, on the other hand, management of moral hazard were a primary concern, one might see one firm or several firms serving the group.

As of summer 1995, approximately 19 states had received approval for waivers from Medicaid program regulations to develop managed care plans. Eleven of these states chose a carve-out plan for mental health. In 10 of the 11 states adopting carve-out programs for mental health and/or substance abuse care, all competition for enrollees between carve-out plans has been eliminated. By contrast, in most of the states with a carve-out program there is competition between general health plans. In 5 of the 10 cases, a single vendor was selected to serve the entire state Medicaid population. In the other 5 states, several managed care organizations were given exclusive contracts to cover a particular geographic area within the state. The actions taken by the great majority of states are consistent with a desire to prevent competing for good risks or adverse selection.

Recent experience with private health plans also suggest that use of carve-outs relates to concerns about selection. The state of Ohio's health plan for state employees recently created a carve-out program for MHSA that is common to all health plan choices. Thus, enrollees choosing health maintenance organizations, preferred provider organizations, and more conventional indemnity plans are all covered by a single carve-out plan for MHSA. Several large self-insured firms such as IBM and Pacific Gas and Electric have adopted similar approaches to that found in the Ohio State employees' plan. All of these experiences offer support for a linkage between organizational design of MHSA benefits and adverse selection concerns.

Further support for the selection explanation comes from data we collected. These data come from the Requests for Proposals (RFPs) for carve-out programs that a large behavioral health care company received over the past several years, as well as data on the contracts between a large insurer and various behavioral health care firms that manage the MHSA benefit for regional populations. Of the 74 contracts and RFPs that we examined, in every case a single vendor supplied MHSA carve-out services to all eligible enrollees (in a few cases, enrollees of health maintenance organizations were not eligible for the carve-out program). In no case did a private employer set up competition between organizations for MHSA risks. We did find some contrary behavior among some public buyers. Franklin County (Columbus, Ohio) has proposed paying any 1 of 5 community mental health centers a capitation rate (including some risk adjustment) for enrolling a Medicaid-eligible individual. In creating the TennCare program, the state of Tennessee initially created 3 competing MHSA carve-out programs that operated statewide. The state of Connecticut is also an exception; it recently offered multiple choices of managed health plans to its Medicaid recipients. Each plan in Connecticut has an MHSA carve-in.

One possible reason for the discrepancy in public and private buying patterns just noted is that private employers and public buyers may have different goals, particularly with respect to the public mental health system. For a private employer, being "fair" to the local mental health providers or supporting the local public system are low priorities at best. The goals of a public buyer, however, may include strengthening the local public system (perhaps by promoting quality competition among local organizations), structuring the supply of services to distribute public funds in a "fair" way (for example, by ensuring that each existing public provider has a chance to serve the buyer's enrollees), or providing choice of providers for enrollees. These goals could lead a public buyer to use the competing contractor approach, but this approach to structuring the market may come at substantial cost by creating incentives for adverse selection.

COST-SHARING FEATURES AND INCENTIVES IN THE CONTRACT

The parties to an MHSA carve-out contract have differing objectives. The vendor is concerned primarily with maximizing profit (or minimizing costs in the case of a nonprofit vendor), whereas the buyer cares about minimizing payments to the vendor and guaranteeing a particular level of access to care and quality of services for its enrollees. Because the vendor has an information advantage over the buyer regarding the costs of managing the benefit (or managerial effort) and because the quality of care being delivered is poorly measured, it is difficult for the buyer to monitor the vendor's performance. The "quality" measures that can be written into a contract at this point are very primitive. As a result, the buyer seeks to write a contract that aligns the vendor's objectives with its own. To do so, the buyer employs 2 mechanisms: competition for the contract and risk sharing within the contract period.[7]

Competition for the Contract

The contract award process is competitive. First, an employer's staff or a benefit consultant typically develops purchasing specifications and a list of qualified potential bidders. Then the purchaser issues an RFP to potential bidders that usually includes information on the benefit structure, financial risk-sharing arrangements, historical utilization and expenditure data, and quality standards. The bidders' proposals consist of a technical component that describes the delivery of clinical services and the management process and also a cost-reimbursement component. Larger purchasers may make site visits to a set of finalists and subsequently sign a contract based on final negotiated costs and technical specifications. Most contracts are 2 or 3 years in duration. Typically between 4 and 10 firms bid for contracts for larger population groups, where a rather generous health plan has been in place. Thus, vendors compete for the contract. The purpose of competition is to keep the contract cost down and to seek commitments from vendors on specifications (such as network size) that can be written into a contract. To enhance the competition, at the end of the 2- or 3-year periods buyers procure a new contract so that the current contractor must compete with other vendors to secure the new contract. Buyers, including public employee programs such as the Ohio State employees health plan, have commonly switched managed care vendors after the initial carve-out contract expires. Thus, even in cases where a single contract is let, competition serves to drive down costs.

Risk Sharing

Through the contract's risk-sharing arrangement, the buyer seeks to balance the vendor's incentives to reduce costs with those aimed at maintaining adequate levels of access and quality. The extreme risk-sharing arrangement is pure capitation, whereby a vendor receives a specified dollar amount per enrollee per period and is at full financial risk for that enrollee's claims. The use of some risk sharing is becoming more common, however. In a typical arrangement, risk corridors are defined around a per person expenditure target t. For example, a common risk corridor will be defined as $\pm 10\%$ of t. If claims costs fall below 90% of t, the difference between the target and the actual amounts will be fully recovered by the buyer, whereas claims costs above 110% of t will be absorbed by the buyer (ie, all financial risk below $0.9t$ and above $1.1t$ is kept by the buyer). For the "at risk" portion of the payment schedule, between 90% and 110% of t, contracts will specify a risk-sharing rate such as 50% between the buyer and the vendor.

Why is a risk-sharing contract in the buyer's interest? One possible reason is that the contractor may be small relative to the buyer and less able and willing to bear large financial risk (and thus require a higher fee to take on large amounts of risk). So, although risk sharing dulls the vendor's incentives to reduce cost, it may lower the payment the buyer must make to the contractor for bearing financial risk. Indeed, many MHSA carve-out firms are small in relation to the buyers. In its first contract, Options Mental Health, Norfolk, Va, accepted a segment of the risk of MHSA claims from the Commonwealth of Massachusetts. The largest behavioral health care companies have revenues on the order of $300 million (with value added or profit less than 10% of this), while the annual budget of the Commonwealth is approximately $5 billion.[1] Extensive cost sharing of financial risks by the Commonwealth may enable vendors to make a lower bid on the cost target by reducing the "cost of risk."

A second reason stems from the possibility that managed MHSA plans will respond to capitation contracts by reducing utilization and quality of care to unacceptable levels in ways that are not easily monitored by the buyer. Capitation offers the managed care organization no payments for providing extra services. A common concern is that such incentives will encourage managed care organizations to place too much weight on profits compared with access and quality. Because individuals with mental and addictive disorders often function poorly as consumers and because quality of care indicators in the MHSA area remain crude, there are few other mechanisms that can be used to attenuate the incentives for managed MHSA care vendors to stint in ways that cannot be detected.

The data that we collected on RFPs and contracts in behavioral health care illustrate a range of risk-sharing features. These data come from RFPs contained in the marketing department of a large behavioral health care firm in March 1995. This firm had been in operation for several years and had a nearly complete collection of the major RFPs from private employers in the early 1990s. Public system RFPs, eg, Medicaid, are not included in these data, although state government as private insurer RFPs are. In less than a fifth of the RFPs (9 of 50), the employer specified that it sought a full-capitation contract in which the vendor would be paid a per person per month payment for MHSA costs and would bear all the risk. More frequently (16 of 50), the employer explicitly stated it did not want a full-risk contract with a vendor. In the most common case (25 of 50), the employer did not specify the terms of the financial risk sharing to be proposed by the vendor. Nonetheless, vendors sometimes proposed risk-sharing contracts even when they were not invited by an employer. Thus, an RFP that reads like a full-capitation request can result in a contract with risk sharing.

CONCLUSIONS

Our analysis leads to 2 initial conclusions concerning carve-out contracts for managed behavioral health care. The first relates to competition for "good risks." We believe that adverse selection has long undermined the insurance market for MHSA coverage, resulting in inefficient forms of insurance. The era of managed care and capitation has heightened the incentives for health plans to avoid "bad risks." Buyers of health care can limit these incentives by carving out the MHSA benefit to a single vendor. The second relates to achieving the objective of minimizing cost for a given level of access and quality. Buyers rely on periodic competition for the contract to do so. Additionally, they rely on risk-sharing arrangements that attenuate the incentive to undertreat MHSA patients while preserving an incentive to reduce costs. Thus, they seek to balance cost containment with access and quality of care objectives.

Accepted for publication June 21, 1996.

Research for this article was supported by Cooperative Agreement 18-C-90314/1-01 from the Health Care Financing Administration, Baltimore, Md, and grant K05-MH001263 from the National Institute of Mental Health, Rockville, Md.

Reprints: Richard Frank, PhD, Department of Health Care Policy, Harvard University, Parcel B, First Floor, 25 Shattuck St, Boston, MA 002115.

REFERENCES

1. Oss M. *Managed Behavioral Health Market Share in the United States.* Gettysburg, Pa: Open Minds; June 1994.
2. Umland B. Behavioral healthcare benefit strategies of self-insured employers. *Behav Healthcare Tomorrow.* November/December 1995:65-70.
3. Frank RG, McGuire TG. Health care reform and financing of mental health services. In: Manderscheid R, Sonnenschein M, eds. *Mental Health, United States, 1994.* Washington, DC: US Government Printing Office; 1994:8-21.
4. Manning WG. *Effects of Mental Health Insurance: Evidence From The Health Insurance Experiment.* Santa Monica, Calif: RAND; 1989. RAND publication R-3815 NIMH/HCFA.
5. McGuire TG. *Financing Psychotherapy: Costs Effects and Public Policy.* Cambridge, Mass: Ballinger; 1981.
6. Padget D Patrick C, Burns B, Schlesinger H, Cohen J. The effect of insurance benefit changes and use of child adolescent outpatient mental health services. *Med Care.* 1993;31:2, 96-110.
7. Frank RG, McGuire TG, Newhouse JP. Risk contracts in managed mental health care. *Health Affairs.* 1995;14:3, 50-64.

ORIGINAL ARTICLE

Enrollment Duration, Service Use, and Costs of Care for Severely Mentally Ill Members of a Health Maintenance Organization

Bentson H. McFarland, MD, PhD; Richard E. Johnson, PhD; Mark C. Hornbrook, PhD

Background: The rapid growth of prepaid health care and the increasing enrollment of Medicaid clients in health maintenance organizations (HMOs) raise concerns about the adequacy of services for persons with severe mental illness in capitated health plans. Uncontrolled studies have suggested that enrollment of HMO members with mental illness may be prematurely terminated.

Methods: We identified 250 adult Kaiser Permanente Northwest Region (Portland, Ore) members who were enrolled during 1986 or 1987 and had chart diagnoses of schizophrenia or bipolar disorder. Severely mentally ill subjects were matched by age and sex with control HMO members with and without diabetes mellitus. Records of the HMO and the state mental health agency were reviewed to determine HMO enrollment duration, private and public service utilization, and HMO costs of care during the 4-year follow-up period.

Results: The severely mentally ill subjects had 42 months of HMO enrollment during the follow-up period compared with 37 months for the controls without diabetes mellitus and 47 months for the patients with diabetes mellitus ($P<.001$). When HMO enrollment prior to the study was taken into account, the severely mentally ill subjects and those with diabetes mellitus had similar membership duration. Among the severely mentally ill subjects, community mental health service use was related to longer duration of HMO enrollment ($P<.05$) but HMO costs of care per member per month were not related to retention. The severely mentally ill subjects were high users of mental health services but their use of general medical care was similar to that of the controls without diabetes mellitus.

Conclusions: This controlled study found no evidence for early termination of HMO members with costly mental illness. Use of community mental health care was associated with longer duration of HMO enrollment.

Arch Gen Psychiatry. 1996;53:938-944

THE DRAMATIC growth in health maintenance organization (HMO) enrollment has heightened concern about the adequacy of treatment available for persons with severe mental illness in prepaid systems.[1,2] This topic is of particular interest to the dozens of states[3,4] that are now in the process of replacing fee-for-service with capitated health care systems for Medicaid clients, many of whom have severe mental disorders.[5] Indeed, Mechanic[6] has suggested that public mental health programs should be gradually integrated into the larger, prepaid health care system while bearing in mind the many challenges involved.[7] Conversely, Scheffler et al[8] have recommended that programs for persons with severe mental illness remain "carved out" of general health care. Furthermore, editorial writers have claimed that traditional HMOs "disenroll individuals who develop serious mental disorders"[9] and have stated that "HMOs have routinely excluded any coverage of chronic mental illness."[10] On the other hand, HMOs have also been described in which persons with severe mental illness "receive relative priority."[11] Inconveniently, there have been few empirical data with which to inform this debate.[1,2]

One of the few pertinent studies is the 1987 Minnesota project, which included a comparison of health status for chronically mentally ill Medicaid clients who had been randomized to fee-for-service vs prepaid (HMO) health care.[2,12-14] Unfortunately, the project ended prematurely after only a year of operation. Few if any differences were found for chronically mentally ill persons, although the subset of this group with schizophrenia may have

From the Kaiser Permanente Center for Health Research (Drs McFarland, Johnson, and Hornbrook) and Oregon Health Sciences University (Dr McFarland), Portland.

See Methods on next page

METHODS

STUDY SITE

The study was conducted in the Northwest Region of Kaiser Permanente, a nonprofit, prepaid, group-practice HMO that currently serves some 385 000 members in greater Portland, Ore. The HMO has been in operation for over 50 years, provides comprehensive medical benefits, and includes a specialty mental health department presently consisting of about 20 psychiatrists and 80 other mental health professionals.[18] The HMO's mental health and substance abuse benefits conform to those mandated by Oregon law. Since 1987, Oregon insurers have been required to cover up to $2000 of outpatient and up to $8500 of inpatient, residential, or day treatment mental health and/or substance abuse services every 24 months for adult beneficiaries. The HMO allows substitution of inpatient for outpatient benefits. However, the total adult mental health and/or substance abuse benefit is a maximum of $10 500 per 24 months. In addition, the vast majority of HMO members have a pharmacy benefit. A 1995 survey of the membership showed that 84% of enrollees obtain all of their prescriptions and 12% obtain some or most of their prescriptions (including those written by non-HMO clinicians) at the HMO's pharmacies. The HMO maintains a membership information processing system that records eligibility for services based on monthly premium payments. Administrative personnel attempt to contact individuals whose premiums are unpaid. For purposes of this study, disenrollment was defined to have occurred at the beginning of a 90-day or longer period of ineligibility. The project was reviewed and approved by the Kaiser Permanente Northwest Region Committee for the Protection of Human Subjects on February 16, 1995.

SELECTION OF SUBJECTS

The years 1986 and 1987 were chosen as a baseline period so that this project could be compared with earlier work.[2,12-16] Because the HMO's outpatient charts were not computerized at the time, severely mentally ill subjects were selected from the 2334 persons who received an antipsychotic drug (excluding prochlorperazine and thiethylperazine, which are used in the HMO only for treatment of nausea and vomiting) or lithium from an HMO pharmacy during 1986 or 1987; individuals in the original group who also received anticancer drugs or drugs used in the treatment of acquired immunodeficiency syndrome were excluded. To minimize the numbers of subjects who might have conditions such as Alzheimer disease, the study focused on the 733 potential subjects who were between ages 10 and 46 years in 1986. Of this group, 526 had mental health department charts (indicating they had had at least 1 contact with an HMO mental health specialist at some time). Individuals were then randomly selected from these 526 persons for mental health chart abstraction. Subjects who carried chart diagnoses of bipolar disorder (including mania, manic-depression, and hypomania) or schizophrenia (including schizophreniform disorder and schizoaffective disorder) in the mental health record were retained in the study. Mental health chart abstraction proceeded through 440 charts until 250 subjects meeting these inclusion criteria were located. Persons who were excluded at this stage typically had diagnoses of substance abuse (primarily amphetamines, cocaine, and/or alcohol) or psychotic depression. Since this study was designed to be descriptive in nature, the sample size of 250 was selected so that the SEs of the mean of annualized utilization estimates (measured in office visits per person per year) would be less than 10% of the estimated mean value. As in other record review projects, diagnoses were assigned based on the majority of those found in the subjects' mental health charts.[19,20] This group of subjects was labeled "cohort 1."

CONTROL MEMBERS WITH AND WITHOUT DIABETES MELLITUS

The severely mentally ill subjects in cohort 1 were then matched with other HMO members. The "pharmacy" controls were taken from the population of HMO members who used the system's outpatient pharmacies during 1986 or 1987 (and had not received an antipsychotic drug or lithium). This group included some two thirds of the HMO's membership. The "membership" controls were selected from the HMO's enrolled population during 1986 and 1987, which averaged about 290 000 persons on any given day at that time. Subjects were matched for sex, year of birth, and "coverage status" (ie, whether the subject was a subscriber or a dependent of the subscriber). For studies of the

Continued on next page

been adversely affected by assignment to the independent practice association model HMOs that participated in the project.[2,14]

Somewhat related to this issue is the RAND observational Medical Outcomes Study,[15,16] which raised the possibility that during 1986 through 1988 psychiatric patients with major depressive disorder in prepaid health care may have switched insurance coverage (ie, terminated HMO enrollment) sooner than their counterparts in the fee-for-service sector. It was suggested that the limited mental health services provided to these subjects (referred to as HMO "skimping") may have contributed to their departure from the HMO.[16,17] However, the Medical Outcomes Study lacked a control group within the HMO.

To address these issues, we conducted a multiyear longitudinal cohort study of HMO members with severe mental illnesses such as schizophrenia or bipolar disorder. Based on the existing literature,[9,15] we hypothesized that the severely mentally ill HMO members would disenroll earlier than matched control subjects. We further hypothesized that severely mentally ill members with higher costs to the HMO would disenroll earlier than their lower-cost counterparts.[9,10] We also wished to learn if there was a relation between HMO members' use of public mental health services and their duration of enrollment.

RESULTS

DEMOGRAPHICS

In cohort 1 there were equal numbers of males and females. Subjects in cohort 1 were (on average) 32 years old in 1986, with an age range from 13 to 45 years and an SD of 8 years. The ethnicity distribution was 80% white, 5% African Amerienrollment duration of cohort 1, the subjects were also matched for sex and year of birth (within 5 years) with 234 people selected from the 2140 individuals who were HMO members during 1986 or 1987 and who had been discharged by a general medical-surgical unit (in 1986 or 1987) with a diagnosis of diabetes mellitus.

SERVICE UTILIZATION

Cohort 1 subjects' HMO service utilization data were obtained from 1986 through 1990 record reviews and computerized databases. In addition, the names and dates of birth for all subjects without diabetes mellitus in cohort 1 were matched against state mental health agency computerized utilization data. The state agency provided information about subjects' use of community mental health programs and the state mental hospitals from 1986 through 1990. While there were extensive data on state hospital usage (including dates of admission and discharge, diagnoses, and so forth) the community mental health data were limited to enrolled vs not enrolled during particular time periods. The Chronic Disease Score[21,22] (based on nonpsychotropic drug dispensing) was used to gauge the severity of physical illnesses in subjects from cohort 1 without diabetes mellitus.

COSTS

The HMO's accounting data and Medicare cost reports became available in 1987 and were used to calculate cost coefficients for each unit of service (eg, outpatient visit to a provider, day in a medical-surgical unit, and so on). The cost coefficients were then multiplied by units of service for cohort 1 to determine the cost (in 1990 dollars) for each type of care.[23,24] Billing records were used to determine the costs (in 1990 dollars) of services purchased by the HMO (eg, general hospital inpatient psychiatric care) for members of cohort 1. Public sector costs were not available.

SECULAR TRENDS IN ENROLLMENT DURATION

To address possible secular trends in enrollment duration, a second group of severely mentally ill subjects (labeled "cohort 2") was chosen from the HMO members discharged from a general hospital during 1990 through 1992 with diagnoses of schizophrenia or bipolar disorder. These people were matched for age and sex with HMO controls with and without diabetes mellitus as described for cohort 1. The enrollment duration study focused on the 165 female and 116 male (average age, 31 years in 1990) severely mentally ill subjects in cohort 2 who were between the ages of 10 and 46 years at the time of the index hospital discharge, of whom there were 139 with a diagnosis of schizophrenia and 5 who also had a diagnosis of diabetes mellitus. Follow-up for cohort 2 started with the index hospital discharge and ended December 31, 1995.

STATISTICAL ANALYSIS

Service utilization and cost data for cohort 1 are reported on a per member per month of enrollment basis. In 2-way analyses of variance (ANOVA), data were transformed as needed so that the residuals were roughly normally distributed. For example, the total cost per person per month was transformed by adding 1 to the cost numerator, dividing by the months of enrollment denominator, and then taking the logarithm of that ratio. To account for multiple comparisons, the studentized range test was used to compare the cohort 1 severely mentally ill subjects' utilization and costs with those of the controls.[25] Enrollment duration comparisons used the log-rank test and the Cox proportional hazards model stratified to account for the matching.[26] Changes in coverage status (subscriber vs dependent) were examined using the Miettinen method.[27]

Cox proportional hazards models were used to examine factors associated with retention of cohort 1 severely mentally ill subjects in the HMO during the follow-up period from 1986 through 1990.[26] Blocks of potential predictors were planned for stepwise inclusion in the proportional hazards models. These potential predictor variables were demographics (age, sex, schizophrenia vs bipolar disorder); enrollment status at the start of the study (subscriber vs dependent, Medicare vs no Medicare, Medicaid vs no Medicaid, years of HMO enrollment prior to the start of the study); and utilization (state hospital admission at any time while an HMO member during the study period, use of community mental health services while an HMO member at any time during the study period, total HMO costs of care per member per month, and HMO mental health costs of care per member per month).

can, 2% Asian American, 2% Hispanic, and 12% unknown. There were no differences in the distributions of known ethnicity between the severely mentally ill subjects and the controls. Some 30% of the 250 severely mentally ill persons in cohort 1 (for whom data were available) had never married. In contrast only 12% of the controls (for whom data were available) had never married. At the beginning of the study about half (53%) of the 750 subjects without diabetes in cohort 1 were subscribers, while 44% were dependents and the remaining few were nonmembers. Only 12% of the cohort 1 severely mentally ill subjects changed coverage status from dependent to subscriber during the 4-year follow-up period, compared with 22% of the controls without diabetes mellitus (relative risk, 0.53; 95% confidence interval, 0.30-0.92). The severely mentally ill subjects in cohort 1 were much more likely to have Medicare coverage than the controls without diabetes mellitus (10% vs 0.2%, $P<.001$ by Fisher exact test). There was no difference in the prevalence of Medicaid coverage (5% vs 4%).

The 250 severely mentally ill subjects in cohort 1 had lengthy histories of mental illness. At the time of their first HMO mental health department contact, the vast majority (73%) reported having had at least 1 previous psychiatric hospitalization, with 40% of severely mentally ill subjects reporting 3 or more admissions. Many (41%) were known to have been admitted to a state mental hospital in Oregon. The majority (57%) had had contact with the HMO's emergency psychiatric service at some time during their enrollment.

DIAGNOSES

The diagnostic algorithm showed that 79 (32%) of the 250 severely mentally ill subjects in cohort 1 had chart diagnoses

Table 1. Service Utilization*

Service	Severely Mentally Ill Subjects (n=250)	Pharmacy Controls (n=250)	Membership Controls (n=250)
Inpatient admissions			
Medical-surgical	11 (27)	15 (48)	5.9 (18)
Psychiatry	31 (66)	0	0.096 (1.5)
State hospital	6.1 (32)	0.88 (11)	0.068 (1.1)
Outpatient visits			
General medical	770 (1010)	770 (1130)	610 (920)
Mental health	460 (560)	8.7 (46)	18 (140)
Substance abuse	27 (110)	7.3 (64)	4.9 (32)
Used community mental health program, No. (%)	101 (40)	12 (5)	12 (5)

**Services per 1000 member-months of health maintenance organization enrollment. All data are presented as mean (SD) unless otherwise indicated. Data were collected from 1986 through 1990.*

of schizophrenia, 98 (39%) had bipolar disorder, and the remaining subjects had multiple diagnoses. As expected, 92% of the 98 persons with bipolar disorder had received prescriptions for lithium, while 93% of the 79 subjects with schizophrenia had been dispensed antipsychotic drugs. Some 30% of the bipolar subjects had received antipsychotic drugs as well as lithium.

SERVICE USE

Health care utilization data for the 1986 through 1990 study period are presented in **Table 1**. Not surprisingly, the severely mentally ill HMO members utilized greater amounts of services than did the controls without diabetes mellitus. As expected, the severely mentally ill subjects had greater per member per month use of mental health [$F(2,498)=120.1$, $P<.001$] and substance abuse outpatient services [$F(2,498)=6.5$, $P<.003$] as well as greater use of general hospital psychiatric inpatient services [$F(2,498)=86.3$, $P<.001$]. During the study period, 88 (35%) of the severely mentally ill subjects in cohort 1 had 274 general hospital psychiatric admissions while the pharmacy controls had none and the membership controls had 1.

Interestingly, there were no statistically significant differences among the 3 groups without diabetes mellitus in the per member per month use of general medical outpatient services. However, differences were observed with respect to use of general medical-surgical inpatient care [$F(2,498)=4.5$, $P=.01$]. The studentized range test indicated that the severely mentally ill subjects' use of general medical-surgical inpatient care was equivalent to that of the pharmacy controls.

The Chronic Disease Score (based on pharmacy data other than psychotropic drugs for the 665 subjects without diabetes mellitus enrolled in 1986) showed that the severely mentally ill subjects had the highest score (mean=0.48, SD=1.18), followed by the pharmacy controls (mean=0.31, SD=0.92), who were in turn followed by the membership controls (mean=0.15, SD=0.65). These differences are highly statistically significant (2-way ANOVA $F[2,418]=7.9$, $P<.001$). Because the Chronic Disease Score was not normally distributed, we also examined the percentage of each group with a nonzero score (47 [20%] of 231 severely mentally ill subjects, 34 [15%] of 225 pharmacy controls, and 16 [8%] of 209 membership controls). These frequency differences were also highly statistically significant ($\chi^2=14.3$, $df=2$, $P<.001$).

During their HMO enrollment in the follow-up period, 30 (12%) of the severely mentally ill subjects in cohort 1 were admitted to a state mental hospital compared with 3 (1%) of the pharmacy controls and 1 (0.4%) of the membership controls ($\chi^2=48.5$, $df=2$, $P<.001$). Similarly, 101 (41%) of the severely mentally ill subjects in cohort 1 used community mental health services during the follow-up period compared with 12 each (5%) among the pharmacy and membership controls ($\chi^2=152.7$, $df=2$, $P<.001$).

COSTS

Table 2 and **Table 3** show the HMO costs of care per member per month for the subjects without diabetes mellitus in cohort 1. The vast majority (98% of the severely mentally ill subjects, 95% of the pharmacy controls, and 87% of the membership controls) incurred HMO costs. The severely mentally ill subjects had substantially higher HMO costs of care per member per month of enrollment than did the controls without diabetes mellitus. The average cost for the subjects with severe mental illness was $380 (median of $203) per member per month vs an average of $149 (median of $33) for the pharmacy controls and $90 (median of $23) for the membership control subjects [2-way ANOVA on the transformed total cost $F(2,419)=81.4$, $P<.001$]. The studentized range test showed that the 3 groups were all statistically significantly different from one another at the $P=.05$ level.

Looking in more detail at costs per member per month for the severely mentally ill subjects showed that the median combined mental health cost (inpatient, outpatient, and pharmaceutical) was $99 with the median, excluding psychotropic pharmaceuticals, at $74. Median outpatient mental health cost was $48. The 90th percentile figures were $798 per member per month for total costs, $544 for all mental health costs, $492 for mental health costs excepting psychotropic medications, $284 for inpatient care, and $214 for outpatient mental health costs.

ENROLLMENT DURATION

The Kaplan-Meier product-limit estimates in the **Figure** show the retention of cohort 1 subjects in the HMO from the start of time under observation (in 1986 and 1987) until disenrollment or the end of follow-up on December 31, 1990. Mean enrollment duration for cohort 1 is shown in **Table 4**. The enrollment durations of the cohort 1 groups differ significantly (log-rank $\chi^2=40.7$, $df=3$, $P<.001$). The stratified Cox model showed that the most powerful predictor of enrollment duration was not being in the membership control group ($\chi^2=25.1$, $df=1$, $P<.001$), with the next most powerful predictor being years of HMO enrollment prior to entering the study ($\chi^2=17.8$, $df=1$, $P<.001$). Once prior years of HMO enrollment had been taken into account, there were no statistically significant enrollment

Table 2. Costs of Care, 1987 Through 1990

Service	Mean (SD) Cost per Member per Month, 1990 $		
	Severely Mentally Ill Subjects (n=225)	Pharmacy Controls (n=223)	Membership Controls (n=218)
Inpatient			
Medical-surgical	59 (182)	77 (531)	35 (147)
Psychiatry	118 (317)	0	0.4 (6)
Substance abuse	2 (12)	0.1 (1)	0
Outpatient			
General medical	59 (69)	55 (83)	43 (67)
Mental health	94 (138)	4 (24)	3 (19)
Substance abuse	7 (32)	2 (16)	1 (8)
Pharmaceutical			
General medical	14 (25)	9 (19)	6 (11)
Psychiatric	28 (39)	0.4 (2)	1 (5)
Substance abuse	0.0004 (0.005)	0.03 (0.4)	0
Total	**380** (473)	**149** (592)	**90** (194)

Table 3. Subjects With Nonzero Costs*

	Severely Mentally Ill Subjects (n=225)	Pharmacy Controls (n=223)	Membership Controls (n=218)
Inpatient			
Medical-surgical	76 (34)	49 (22)	34 (16)
Psychiatry	88 (39)	0	1 (1)
Substance abuse	4 (2)	2 (1)	0
Outpatient			
General medical	212 (94)	208 (93)	183 (84)
Mental health	192 (85)	13 (6)	17 (8)
Substance abuse	36 (16)	7 (3)	8 (4)
Pharmaceutical			
General medical	205 (91)	198 (89)	159 (73)
Psychiatric	205 (91)	44 (20)	35 (16)
Substance abuse	1 (1)	1 (1)	0
Total	220 (98)	212 (95)	189 (87)

**All data are presented as number (percent).*

differences among those subjects with diabetes mellitus, severe mental illness, and pharmacy controls in cohort 1. Table 4 also shows that the enrollment duration of cohort 2 subjects was similar to that of cohort 1.

RETENTION

Among the severely mentally ill cohort 1 subjects, stepwise Cox proportional hazards modeling showed that the factors related to longer duration of enrollment in the HMO were years of HMO enrollment prior to the start of the study period (χ^2=7.6, *df*=1, *P*<.006); age (χ^2=5.6, *df*=1, *P*<.02); and community mental health service use (χ^2=3.9, *df*=1, *P*<.05).

Costs of care (total costs per member per month or mental health costs per member per month) for cohort 1 were not significantly related to retention based on the Cox proportional hazards modeling. Other factors not significantly related to cohort 1 enrollment duration in the proportional hazards models included sex, schizophrenia vs bipolar disorder, subscriber status, or use of the state hospital.

COMMENT

Results from this study need to be interpreted in light of its design. The project was not a randomized trial nor did it include a comparison group of subjects outside the HMO. Since the study was designed to take advantage of existing data, subjects were not interviewed and clinical outcomes were not measured. Consequently, there could well have been important but unrecorded differences among the groups. Furthermore, subjects' reasons for disenrollment and for use of public mental health services were not available.

The project examined "prevalent" cases of people with severe mental illness who were using HMO services. At the time of this study it was not possible to identify HMO members with newly emerging (ie, "incident") psychosis. Certainly, the "careers" of severely mentally ill persons who do not receive treatment may well be different from those of the subjects described here. For example, persons who become psychotic and refuse HMO mental health services might be unable to maintain enrollment and quickly leave the organization. Indeed, earlier work has shown that the treated prevalence of schizophrenia within this HMO is less than what would be expected from Epidemiologic Catchment Area data, although the treated prevalence of bipolar disorder is comparable to the national estimate.[18] Very recent improvements in the HMO's automated data systems may provide an opportunity to conduct an incidence study focusing on people with newly emerging psychosis.

Another issue is the degree of severity of the subjects' mental disorders. For example, some 67% of the cohort 1 severely mentally ill subjects were self-reported to be employed at the time of their first HMO mental health clinic visit. Interestingly, the Epidemiologic Catchment Area project found that 43% of the persons identified in that study as having schizophrenia were employed.[28] The severely mentally ill HMO members may be that subset of persons with conditions like schizophrenia, who have a relatively good prognosis.[29-37]

Nonetheless, the frequent use of emergency and inpatient psychiatric services for this population suggests that many of these individuals were, indeed, severely disabled. Furthermore, the Chronic Disease Score indicated that the severely mentally ill persons appeared to have had physical as well as mental health problems. These individuals were also much more likely to have Medicare coverage than the controls without diabetes mellitus. Presumably, the severely mentally ill subjects became eligible for Medicare coverage by virtue of qualifying for Social Security Disability Insurance due to their mental illness.[38] The relatively low rate of Medicaid participation by the severely mentally ill subjects in cohort 1 may well have been due to state policies at the time of the study, which, in effect, deemed persons receiving Social Security Disability Insurance to be "too wealthy" for Medicaid.

Relatively few of the severely mentally ill subjects in cohort 1 (compared with the controls without diabetes mellitus) changed coverage status from dependent to sub-

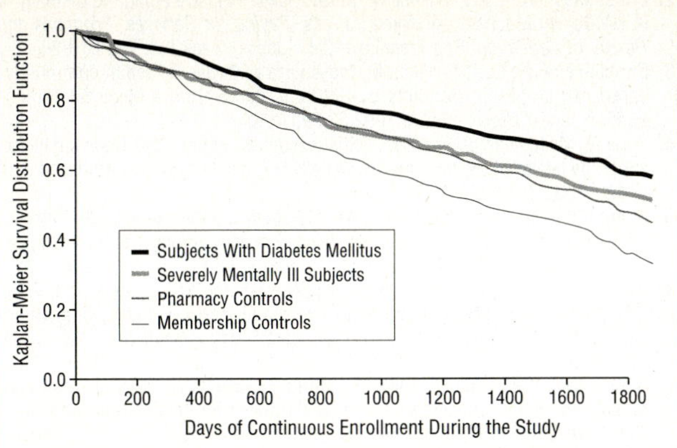

Kaplan-Meier survival curve of enrollment duration.

Table 4. Duration of Enrollment in Days*

	Cohort 1 (1986-1990)	Cohort 2 (1990-1995)
Subjects with diabetes mellitus	1424 (39)	1437 (40)
Severely mentally ill subjects	1263 (45)	1298 (48)
Pharmacy controls	1236 (45)	...
Membership controls	1023 (47)	...

**Data from Kaplan-Meier survival distribution function. Data are given as mean (SE); ellipses indicate not applicable.*

scriber during the 4-year follow-up period. One explanation for these findings is that the severely mentally ill subjects who entered the study as dependents were not as likely as their matched controls to obtain competitive employment (and thereby become subscribers in their own right). Indeed, naturalistic follow-up studies of patients with mania suggest that significant disability would be expected for at least some of those severely mentally ill HMO subjects who had bipolar disorder.[39,40]

Its limitations notwithstanding, this study showed that HMO members with severe mental illness had enrollment duration longer than that of controls without diabetes mellitus but somewhat shorter than that of members with diabetes mellitus. Furthermore, costs to the HMO were unrelated to duration of enrollment. To the authors' knowledge, cohort 1 has been followed up longer than any group of mainstream managed care beneficiaries with severe mental illness. This study is also one of the few that measured both private and public mental health service use.[13] In contrast to the Medical Outcomes Study,[15-17] this project involved a variety of HMO control subjects.

It is worthwhile examining the factors that did and did not explain the severely mentally ill subjects' retention within the HMO. There was no support for the contention that HMO members were "disenrolled" due to severe mental illness.[9] Of course, as expected in a "prevalence" study, subjects with very brief periods of enrollment were unlikely to be included in the sample. Consequently, length of HMO eligibility prior to the study was a good predictor of enrollment duration during follow-up. Indeed, when length of enrollment before the study period was included in the Cox proportional hazards analysis, the severely mentally ill subjects had retention times longer than the membership controls but equivalent to that of the diabetic subjects and the pharmacy controls.

We were also unable to find evidence that this HMO "routinely excluded any coverage of chronic mental illness."[10] Indeed, the severely mentally ill subjects in cohort 1 were provided amounts of service that generated costs to the HMO several times that of the membership controls. This cost difference was accounted for chiefly by mental health care. Based on the HMO's cost data, it appears that 36% of the severely mentally ill subjects in cohort 1 exceeded the state-mandated outpatient mental health benefit of $2000 per 24 months. Psychiatric inpatient costs were generally less than the state-mandated $8500 per 24 months, but 9% of severely mentally ill cohort 1 subjects did exceed the benefit limit. Looking at combined inpatient and outpatient mental health costs showed that 12% of severely mentally ill cohort 1 subjects exceeded the $10 500 per 24 months limit. Of course, one could challenge the accuracy of the cost data. However, it should be noted that some of the costs (eg, general hospital inpatient psychiatric services) represent payments from the HMO to its vendors. In any event, it seems clear that coverage was provided to HMO members who were severely mentally ill. Furthermore, HMO costs were not related to enrollment duration.

An important issue is the HMO's policies toward serving persons with severe mental illness. As with many HMOs, this organization's mental health services were theoretically limited to treatment of conditions that, in the judgment of the attending physician, were subject to significant improvement through relatively short-term therapy.[41] In practice, as demonstrated by these results, mental health services were provided to persons with chronic conditions. Since this approach to persons with severe mental illness may not be found in other HMOs, these results may have limited generalizability.[42-44]

Indeed, the distinctions among HMOs[44] may explain the apparent discrepancy between the retention data from this project and the implication from the Medical Outcomes Study[15] that severely mentally ill subjects would have a shorter enrollment than healthier members. It should be noted that the Medical Outcomes Study was conducted in several prepaid settings (including a traditional staff model HMO), with the poorest outcomes for depressed psychiatric patients observed in independent practice associations.[17] Differences between the independent practice association approach to severe mental illness and that provided by traditional HMOs could be responsible for the disparate outcomes observed in the 2 studies. As Judith L. Feldman, MD, remarked: "When you've seen one HMO you've seen one HMO" (oral communication, 1988).

The integrated service delivery system provided by traditional HMOs may be of particular value for severely mentally ill members who have physical as well as mental health problems, as suggested by our data. It is interesting to note that the costs of general medical-surgical care for severely mentally ill subjects were similar to those of the pharmacy controls even though the Chronic Disease Score suggested that the former had more physical illness than the latter. An integrated system might be more efficient than a mental health "carve-out" for people with both physical and severe mental health problems. On the other hand, while the data from cohort 2 suggest that this HMO is continuing to serve severely mentally ill members, the now fiercely competitive health care environment[45] makes one wonder if any HMO will be able to provide the level of mental health service described here.

It should pointed out that the HMO was by no means the sole provider of mental health care to these individuals. Nearly half of the severely mentally ill subjects in cohort 1 also used community mental health services. Furthermore, the use of community mental health care was associated with longer duration of HMO enrollment. While this observational study cannot determine causality, it is conceivable that the subjects who maintained their HMO membership were able to optimize use of both private and public services. One might imagine that the HMO's expertise in areas such as psychopharmacology, emergency psychiatric services, and inpatient psychiatric care could complement the public mental health sector's capabilities in fields such as rehabilitation and vocational training. Unfortunately, shrinkage of public sector mental health funds combined with private sector competition may leave persons with severe mental illness struggling to find appropriate care.[46] Nonetheless, there may be considerable value in studying ways HMOs and community mental health agencies can work together to offer an efficiently integrated package of services that will benefit people with severe mental illness.[6]

Accepted for publication June 21, 1996.

Supported in part by grants P50 MH43458, R01 MH45015, and K02 MH01238 from the National Institute of Mental Health, Bethesda, Md, .

Presented in part at the 147th Annual Meeting of the American Psychiatric Association, Philadelphia, Pa, May 25, 1994, and at the 123rd Annual Meeting of the American Public Health Association, San Diego, Calif, November 1, 1995.

Reprints: Bentson H. McFarland, MD, PhD, Center for Health Research, Kaiser Permanente, Northwest Region, 3800 N Kaiser Center Dr, Portland, OR 97227.

REFERENCES

1. McFarland BH. Health maintenance organizations and persons with severe mental illness. *Community Ment Health J.* 1994;30:221-242.
2. Christianson JB, Osher FC. Health maintenance organizations, health care reform, and persons with serious mental illness. *Hosp Community Psychiatry.* 1994;45:898-905.
3. General Accounting Office. *Medicaid Expansions.* Gaithersburg, Md: US General Accounting Office; 1993. Report HRD-91-78.
4. General Accounting Office. *Medicaid Section 1115 Waivers.* Washington, DC: US General Accounting Office; 1995. Report HEHS-96-44.
5. Taube CA, Goldman HH, Salkever D. Medicaid coverage for mental illness: balancing access and costs. *Health Aff (Millwood).* 1990;9:5-18.
6. Mechanic D. Integrating mental health into a general health care system. *Hosp Community Psychiatry.* 1994;45:893-897.
7. Mechanic D, Schlesinger M, McAlpine DD. Management of mental health and substance abuse services: state of the art and early results. *Milbank Q.* 1995; 73:19-55.
8. Scheffler R, Grogan C, Cuffel B, Penner S. A specialized mental health plan for persons with severe mental illness under managed competition. *Hosp Community Psychiatry.* 1993;44:937-942.
9. Sharfstein SS. Capitation versus decapitation in mental health care. *Hosp Community Psychiatry.* 1994;45:1065.
10. Schlesinger M. Perspectives: ethical issues in policy advocacy. *Health Aff (Millwood).* 1995;14:23-29.
11. Sabin J. Perspectives: organized psychiatry and managed care: quality improvement or holy war? *Health Aff (Millwood).* 1995;14:32-33.
12. Christianson JB, Lurie N, Finch M, Moscovice I. Mainstreaming the mentally ill in HMOs. In: Mechanic D, Aiken LJ, eds. *Paying for Services: Promises and Pitfalls of Capitation.* San Francisco, Calif: Jossey-Bass Inc; 1989:19-28.
13. Christianson JB, Lurie N, Finch M, Moscovice I, Hartley D. Use of community-based mental health programs by HMOs: evidence from a Medicaid demonstration. *Am J Public Health.* 1992;82:790-796.
14. Lurie N, Moscovice IS, Finch M, Christianson JB, Popkin MK. Does capitation affect the health of the chronically mentally ill? results from a randomized trial. *JAMA.* 1992;267:3300-3304.
15. Sturm R, McGlynn EA, Meredith LS, Wells KB, Manning WG, Rogers WH. Switches between prepaid and fee-for-service health systems among depressed outpatients: results from the Medical Outcomes Study. *Med Care.* 1994;32:917-929.
16. Sturm R, Jackson CA, Meredith LS, Yip W, Manning WG, Rogers WH, Wells KB. Mental health care utilization in prepaid and fee-for-service plans among depressed patients in the Medical Outcomes Study. *Health Serv Res.* 1995; 30:319-340.
17. Rogers WH, Wells KB, Meredith LS, Sturm R, Burnam A. Outcomes for adult outpatients with depression under prepaid or fee-for-service financing. *Arch Gen Psychiatry.* 1993;50:517-525.
18. Johnson RE, McFarland BH. Treated prevalence rates of severe mental illness among HMO members. *Hosp Community Psychiatry.* 1994;45:919-924.
19. Lurie N, Popkin M, Dysken M, Moscovice I, Finch M. Accuracy of diagnoses of schizophrenia in Medicaid claims. *Hosp Community Psychiatry.* 1992;43:69-71.
20. Glazer WM, Pino CD, Quinlan D. The reassessment of chronic patients previously diagnosed as schizophrenic. *J Clin Psychiatry.* 1987;48:430-434.
21. VonKorff M, Wagner EH, Saunders K. A chronic disease score from automated pharmacy data. *J Clin Epidemiol.* 1992;45:197-203.
22. Johnson RE, Hornbrook MC, Nichols GA. Replicating the Chronic Disease Score (CDS) from automated pharmacy data. *J Clin Epidemiol.* 1994;47:1191-1199.
23. Mullooly JP, Bennett MD, Hornbrook MC, Barker WH, Williams WW, Patriarca PA, Rhodes PH. Influenza vaccination program for elderly persons: cost-effectiveness in a health maintenance organization. *Ann Intern Med.* 1994;121: 947-952.
24. Hornbrook MC, Goodman MJ. Assessing relative health plan risk with the RAND-36 health survey. *Inquiry.* 1995;32:56-74.
25. Armitage P, Berry G. *Statistical Methods in Medical Research.* 2nd ed. Oxford, England: Blackwell; 1987.
26. Collet D. *Modelling Survival Data in Medical Research.* London, England: Chapman & Hall; 1994.
27. Miettinen O. Estimation of the relative risk from individually matched series. *Biometrics.* 1970;26:75-86.
28. Keith SJ, Regier DA, Rae DS. Schizophrenic disorders. In: Robins LN, Regier DA, eds. *Psychiatric Disorders in America: The Epidemiologic Catchment Area Project.* New York, NY: Free Press; 1991:33-52.
29. Breier A, Schreiber JL, Dyer J, Pickar D. National Institute of Mental Health longitudinal study of chronic schizophrenia. *Arch Gen Psychiatry.* 1991;48: 239-246.
30. Breier A, Schreiber JL, Pickar D, Dyer J. Long-term outcome in chronic schizophrenia. *Arch Gen Psychiatry.* 1992;49:503.
31. Harding CM, Strauss JS. Editorial. How serious is schizophrenia? comments on prognosis. *Biol Psychiatry.* 1984;19:1597-1600.
32. Harding CM, Zubin J, Strauss JS. Chronicity in schizophrenia: fact, partial fact, or artifact? *Hosp Community Psychiatry.* 1987;38:477-486.
33. Harding CM, Brooks GW, Ashikaga T, Strauss JS, Breier A. The Vermont longitudinal study of persons with severe mental illness, I: methodology, study sample, and overall status 32 years later. *Am J Psychiatry.* 1987;144:718-726.
34. Harding CM, Brooks GW, Ashikaga T, Strauss JS, Breier A. The Vermont longitudinal study of persons with severe mental illness, II: long-term outcome of subjects who retrospectively met *DSM-III* criteria for schizophrenia. *Am J Psychiatry.* 1987;144:727-735.
35. Marengo J, Harrow M, Sands J, Galloway C. European versus US data on the course of schizophrenia. *Am J Psychiatry.* 1991;148:606-611.
36. McGlashan TH. A selective review of recent North American long-term follow-up studies of schizophrenia. *Schizophr Bull.* 1988;14:515-542.
37. Schwartz F, Terkelsen KG, Smith TE. Long-term outcome in chronic schizophrenia. *Arch Gen Psychiatry.* 1992;49:502.
38. McFarland BH. Commentary. In: Backlar P, ed. *The Family Face of Schizophrenia.* New York, NY: Tarcher/Putman; 1994.
39. Harrow M, Goldberg JF, Grossman LS, Meltzer HY. Outcome in manic disorders: a naturalistic follow-up study. *Arch Gen Psychiatry.* 1990;47:665-671.
40. Maj M, Pirozzi R, Kemali D. Long-term outcome of lithium prophylaxis in bipolar patients. *Arch Gen Psychiatry.* 1991;48:772.
41. Lubotsky-Levin B, Glasser JH. Comparing mental health benefits, patterns, and costs. In: Feldman JL, Fitzpatrick RJ, eds. *Managed Mental Health Care.* Washington, DC: American Psychiatric Press; 1992.
42. Fink PJ, Dubin WR. No free lunch: limitations on psychiatric care in HMOs. *Hosp Community Psychiatry.* 1991;42:363-365.
43. Westermeyer J. Problems with managed psychiatric care without a psychiatrist-manager. *Hosp Community Psychiatry.* 1991;42:1221-1224.
44. Moldawsky RJ. In defense of HMOs. *Hosp Community Psychiatry.* 1992;43: 81-82.
45. Jellinek MS, Nurcombe B. Two wrongs don't make a right: managed care, mental health, and the marketplace. *JAMA.* 1993;270:1737-1739.
46. McFarland BH. Ending the millennium: commentary on HMOs and the seriously mentally ill: a view from the trenches. *Community Ment Health J.* In press.

ORIGINAL ARTICLE

Managing the Care of Schizophrenia

Lessons From a 4-Year Massachusetts Medicaid Study

Barbara Dickey, PhD; Sharon-Lise T. Normand, PhD; Edward C. Norton, PhD; Hocine Azeni, MA; William Fisher, PhD; Frederic Altaffer, PhD

Background: In 1992, Massachusetts launched a statewide managed care plan for all Medicaid beneficiaries.

Methods: This retrospective, multiyear, cross-sectional study used administrative data from the Massachusetts Division of Medical Assistance and Department of Mental Health, consisting of claims for 16 400 disabled adult patients insured by Medicaid in Massachusetts between July 1, 1990, and June 30, 1994. The main outcome measures include annual rates of hospitalization, emergency department utilization, and follow-up care 30 days after discharge; length of inpatient stay; and per-person inpatient and outpatient expenditures.

Results: Between 1991 and 1994, the likelihood of an inpatient admission decreased from 29% to 24% and was accompanied by a slight reduction in length of stay (median number of bed-days per admission dropped by 3.3 days). There was a slight decrease in the number of patients who sought care in general hospital emergency department utilization. However, there was a small increase in the fraction of patients readmitted within 30 days of discharge. Medicaid and Department of Mental Health expenditures for mental health per treated beneficiary decreased slightly, from $11 060 to $10 640, during the 4-year study period.

Conclusion: Although per-person expenditures dropped and most patient patterns of care remained the same, longer-term study is recommended to assess whether the trends can be maintained.

Arch Gen Psychiatry. 1996;53:945-952

From the Departments of Psychiatry (Dr Dickey) and Health Care Policy (Dr Normand), Harvard Medical School, Boston, Mass; Mental Health Services Research, McLean Hospital, Belmont, Mass (Dr Dickey and Mr Azeni); Department of Biostatistics, Harvard School of Public Health, Boston (Dr Normand); Center for Economics Research, Research Triangle Institute, Research Triangle Park, NC (Dr Norton); Center for Psychosocial and Forensic Services Research, University of Massachusetts Medical School, Worcester (Dr Fisher); and Mentor Inc, Boston (Dr Altaffer).

THE TREATMENT of schizophrenia remains a major clinical challenge to health care providers.[1] The behavioral problems and thought disorders that are characteristic of schizophrenia make management complex and expensive. For example, in the United States, even though slightly more than 1% of adults have the disorder, treatment expenditures account for more than 2.5% of all health care expenditures.[2,3] It is not unusual for those with schizophrenia to have disabilities that lead to loss of employment and private health insurance. When this occurs, government becomes the primary health care insurer. Almost two thirds of all the expenditures for schizophrenia treatment come from federal, state, and local government sources.[2]

With so much government money at stake, it is not surprising that reforms are rapidly changing the provision of government services to the mentally ill. All but 6 states are pursuing managed care for Medicaid beneficiaries, including those with severe mental illness, such as schizophrenia. In some states, Medicaid managed care plans tap into existing health maintenance organization networks.[4] In other states, Medicaid contracts with mental health managed behavioral care companies to provide administrative functions and direct beneficiaries to a local provider network.

There are 2 fundamental issues in the evaluation of managed care for the severely mentally ill. First, can managed care succeed in providing quality care to psychiatrically disabled patients, especially those diagnosed as having schizophrenia?[5-8] These individuals are at high risk for catastrophic psychiatric and medical care but seldom are able to navigate effectively within the health care system and often lack advocates on their behalf. Even though providers surveyed in Massachusetts have reported that quality has not

See Patients and Methods on next page

PATIENTS AND METHODS

THE MASSACHUSETTS MANAGED MENTAL HEALTH PROGRAM

In 1992, Massachusetts received a 1915b waiver from the Health Care Financing Administration. Under this plan, all beneficiaries were asked either to enroll in a local health maintenance organization or to select a Medicaid-approved primary care clinician. Virtually all psychiatrically disabled beneficiaries chose a primary care clinician. Medicaid contracted with a single proprietary vendor, Mental Health Management of America, a division of First Mental Health, Boston, Mass, to manage the provision of mental health benefits. The vendor had 4 specific cost-containment strategies: (1) negotiation of reimbursement rates with a network of providers who would be paid on a fee-for-service basis, (2) implementation of an aggressive utilization management plan, (3) development of community-based alternatives to hospitalization, and (4) collaboration with the DMH to fund emergency service teams to screen patients for appropriateness of inpatient admission, with a view toward diverting many of them to alternative treatment sites.

Under the terms of the contract with Medicaid, the vendor was required to make available to recipients all the mental health and substance abuse benefits: acute inpatient treatment, crisis stabilization, outpatient evaluation and treatment, psychiatric day treatment, residential detoxification, and methadone treatment. The vendor was directed to add diversionary services, including acute residential treatment programs, family stabilization teams, and partial hospitalization programs. The contract further specified that the vendor would be responsible for the centralized functions of utilization review, claims processing, systems support, and provider relations, and for decentralized regionally based case management and network management. The contract with the vendor excluded payment for long-term nursing home care, mental health services provided by the DMH, and any medical treatment or outpatient pharmacy. In addition, it did not include members of health maintenance organizations and those who had Medicaid as a second payer. Disabled beneficiaries were covered at a higher rate than other beneficiaries, and providers were reimbursed by the vendor on a fee-for-service basis.

DATA SOURCES

We used administrative data obtained from Medicaid and the DMH. Together, these files provided information regarding patient sociodemographic status, reimbursed inpatient and outpatient care, discharge diagnoses, and timing of services.

DEFINITION OF CROSS-SECTIONAL COHORTS

We created 4 separate cohorts, 1 for each fiscal year of the study, that together described treatment spanning the period from July 1, 1990 (the start of fiscal year 1991) through June 30, 1994 (the end of fiscal year 1994). The members of each cohort consisted of all adult Massachusetts Medicaid beneficiaries, aged 18 to 64 years, who were disabled and treated, either as inpatients or outpatients, for schizophrenia (*International Classification of Diseases, Ninth Revision, Clinical Modification,* primary diagnostic code of 295) at least once during the fiscal year. The cross-sectional cohorts were created by assigning patients with a schizophrenia claim to the fiscal year in which the claim was submitted; for this reason, it was possible for patients to appear in more than 1 cohort.

With the use of the patient's unique Medicaid identification number, patient-level files for each fiscal year were constructed by identifying paid claims for all psychiatric and substance abuse care (claims with a primary diagnostic code of 290-315), medical care (claims with any primary diagnostic code excluding V codes and 290-315 or any claim with a mental health *Current Procedure Terminology* procedure code), and other services, such as pharmacy, transportation, and dental care. Finally, to ensure that we had a complete record of service use for each patient, we merged state hospital admissions from the DMH inpatient files with the administrative Medicaid information by means of unique patient identification numbers.

SOCIODEMOGRAPHIC AND COMORBIDITY DATA

We used Medicaid membership files to identify the date of birth, sex, race, and residence ZIP code for each patient in our study cohort. To measure the degree of substance abuse in our sample, we assumed that if a patient was ever diagnosed as a substance abuser (primary or secondary diagnostic *International Classification of Diseases, Ninth Revision, Clinical Modification* code of 291, 292, 303.00, 303.90, 304, or 305) in a given year, then the patient had a drug or other alcohol abuse problem in the given year.

ADMISSION TYPE

During the study, the DMH had contracted with a few general hospitals for inpatient beds to replace some of the beds in state hospitals closed as part of a larger deinstitutionalization plan. Thus, DMH-funded admissions occurred in both state and general hospitals. To differentiate between beds funded by Medicaid and those funded by the DMH, we classified each mental health inpatient admission as either a DMH admission or a Medicaid admission. The admission policy for Medicaid recipients to a DMH bed required that beds be available to forensic patients and to patients with behavioral management requirements that could not be met in general hospital psychiatric units or in freestanding psychiatric facilities otherwise reimbursed by Medicaid.

been compromised,[9] both critics and advocates would like to have more evidence before accepting this conclusion.

The second issue is whether managed care actually reduces costs or shifts costs onto families, other state agencies, or medical care providers. When there are strong financial incentives to reduce acute hospital admissions, managed care plans will be financially motivated to divert beneficiaries to the long-term care system run by the state mental health agency. Individuals with schizophrenia are likely to be eligible for both Medicaid benefits and a state-funded long-term care system of community and hospital-based services. Shifting costs to the state mental health agency may result in greater profits for managed care plans but may not improve continuity

EVALUATION OF ACCESS TO CARE

We defined access to care in each year as the number of Medicaid beneficiaries with a primary diagnosis of schizophrenia who had at least 1 Medicaid-paid claim. We also examined the number of incident patients in each year. We classified a patient as incident if there was no mental health claim with a primary diagnosis of schizophrenia for the patient in the previous year(s). Because we did not have Medicaid data before 1991, we were unable to identify new patients in 1991 and consequently may also have overestimated the number of incident patients in the remaining years.

MENTAL HEALTH INPATIENT UTILIZATION

We defined mental health inpatient utilization as hospital admissions with primary mental health discharge diagnoses corresponding to schizophrenia, or any other psychiatric and substance abuse disorder. Because we hypothesized that hospital admissions would drop as a result of the screening and diversion programs of the managed care plan, we examined the distribution of mental health inpatient admissions in each year. We also estimated the likelihood of having any mental health inpatient admission by the percentage of patients who had at least 1 such admission in a given year. Finally, for those patients who had at least 1 mental health inpatient admission in a given year, we examined the number of bed-days per admission.

CONTINUITY OF CARE

To describe follow-up care after discharge, we first defined inpatient transfers as admissions to another hospital within 24 hours after a discharge and then linked information from the transfers to form a complete inpatient episode of care for each patient in our cohorts. We then categorized each discharge into 1 of 4 mutually exclusive categories: discharges for which there was no outpatient or inpatient contact within 30 days, discharges for which there was outpatient contact within 30 days, discharges resulting in rehospitalization within 30 days, and discharges for which both an outpatient contact and a rehospitalization within 30 days resulted. Outpatient contact included a visit to any hospital outpatient department or to a clinic; a visit to a physician office; or the provision of any 1 of a set of mental health services, such as psychological testing, case management, or day treatment.

Because we believed that, ideally, continuous patient care should be rendered from 1 provider, we also calculated the number of unique hospitals to which patients with more than 1 hospitalization were admitted. Finally, we estimated the distribution in each year of general hospital emergency department visits. We did not calculate the distribution for state hospitals because they do not have emergency departments.

ASSESSMENT OF EXPENDITURES

We derived costs for Medicaid services from the paid claims that indicated the amount reimbursed. Although we could not determine whether paid claims overestimated or underestimated the true cost of treatment, these costs represented public expenditures through this entitlement program. Because the DMH operates on a fixed budget and records only use of services, we estimated costs for inpatient care by means of the per diem for state hospitals calculated by the DMH. These estimated per diem costs are based on accounting costs, calculated by dividing total annual inpatient expenditures, including capital costs, by the number of actual patient bed-days in each facility annually. Hospital-specific per diem costs were used to estimate the episode costs for each person admitted to a DMH facility by multiplying the calculated per diem by the number of days in the episode.

Inpatient mental health expenditures (psychiatric or substance abuse care) were dichotomized into Medicaid and DMH admissions to examine the extent of cost shifting between these 2 government agencies. All inpatient expenses are clustered together so that room and board, ancillaries, and physician fees are included.

Outpatient mental health expenditures included hospital outpatient department or clinic services, physician services, and other mental health services provided in freestanding mental health agencies.

Non–mental health expenditures were composed of medical care, pharmacy, transportation, and dental care. Claims for the last 3 categories did not report diagnoses, and consequently we were unable to distinguish mental health–related from non–mental health–related expenditures.

We aggregated the inpatient and outpatient mental health expenditures and then added all categories for total expenditures. Within each category of expenditures we report the number and percentage of persons with any expenditures, the average expenditure per person with any expenditure, and the total expenditure. For inpatient care we also report expenditure per admission.

STATISTICAL ANALYSES

We computed simple univariate summary statistics by year. For continuous-valued variables, we calculated sample means and SDs; we also constructed box plots[12] to display the center and spread of the distributions of the observations. Inpatient utilization was stratified by admission type (DMH or Medicaid). All expenditure figures are reported in 1994 dollars by adjusting expenditures in 1991, 1992, and 1993 for inflation by means of the gross domestic product deflator.[13]

of care; moreover, the societal costs may be higher. To date, there are no studies of how the reduction in mental health expenditures for acute care might shift costs to long-term care.

Evaluations of managed care plans are in an early stage of development, and little descriptive information is available to provide benchmarks against which to compare different approaches to cost containment.[10] Earlier reports[9,11] of the Massachusetts plan studied only the first year after implementation. In addition, these studies were limited to claims for mental health treatment.

We developed a database on adult Medicaid beneficiaries with schizophrenia to examine access to care, use of services, and treatment costs associated

Table 1. Demographic Characteristics of Cross-sectional Cohorts*

	All Patients, No. (%)				Incident Patients, No. (%)		
	FY 1991 (N=6614)‡	FY 1992 (N=7295)‡	FY 1993† (N=10 685)‡	FY 1994† (N=7541)‡	FY 1992 (N=2528)§	FY 1993 (N=5484)§	FY 1994 (N=1774)§
Age, y							
18-21	172 (2.6)	184 (2.5)	331 (3.1)	179 (2.4)	118 (4.7)	246 (4.5)	104 (5.9)
22-39	3234 (48.9)	3503 (48.0)	4843 (45.3)	3538 (46.9)	1302 (51.5)	2480 (45.2)	934 (52.6)
40-64	3208 (48.5)	3608 (49.5)	5511 (51.6)	3824 (50.7)	1108 (43.8)	2758 (50.3)	736 (41.5)
Mean±SD	41±12	41±12	41±12	41±11	39±12	40±12	38±11
Female	3182 (48.1)	3486 (47.8)	5808 (54.4)	3470 (46.0)	1201 (47.5)	3291 (60.0)	764 (43.1)
Race							
African American	618 (9.3)	699 (9.6)	891 (8.3)	772 (10.2)	260 (10.3)	430 (7.8)	187 (10.5)
American Indian	3 (0.0)	3 (0.0)	9 (0.1)	4 (0.1)	1 (0.0)	5 (0.1)	0 (0.0)
Asian American	19 (0.3)	25 (0.3)	28 (0.3)	22 (0.3)	14 (0.6)	15 (0.3)	12 (0.7)
Hispanic	86 (1.3)	125 (1.7)	188 (1.8)	102 (1.4)	76 (3.0)	126 (2.3)	38 (2.1)
White	5865 (88.7)	6413 (87.9)	9537 (89.3)	6464 (85.7)	2164 (85.6)	4891 (89.2)	1377 (77.6)
Unknown	23 (0.3)	30 (0.4)	32 (0.3)	177 (2.3)	13 (0.5)	17 (0.3)	160 (9.0)
Substance abuse	636 (9.6)	775 (10.6)	3108 (29.1)	1023 (13.6)	355 (14.0)	1875 (34.2)	324 (18.3)

**Patients are disabled Massachusetts Medicaid beneficiaries treated for schizophrenia. FY indicates fiscal year.*
†Managed care plan years.
‡Number of treated beneficiaries.
§Number of new treated beneficiaries.

with schizophrenia before and after the introduction of managed care. Because care for our disabled population is not limited to services reimbursed by Medicaid alone, the data are drawn from 2 state agencies: the Division of Medical Assistance (Medicaid) and the Department of Mental Health (DMH). Data cover 2 years of the plan after implementation and include nonpsychiatric medical care, pharmacy, transportation, and dental care. These additional data are important to include because they account for roughly 40% of the total expenditures. We also examined incident patients, those not treated for schizophrenia before managed care was introduced.

RESULTS

DESCRIPTION OF THE CROSS-SECTIONAL COHORTS

Between July 1, 1990, and June 30, 1994, we observed 16 400 disabled adults who contributed a total of 32 135 annual observations. Despite changes in the number of treated beneficiaries during the 4-year period, we found that the sociodemographic characteristics remained virtually unchanged (**Table 1**): approximately half the beneficiaries were female and the majority were white, with a mean age of 41 years. Eleven percent were ethnic or racial minorities. Comorbid substance abuse increased as a proportion of the total study population. This increase might be a coding artifact resulting from changes in diagnostic practice or an increased awareness of substance abuse. Reimbursement of the treatment of substance abuse received much attention from providers because of the emphasis placed by the managed care vendor on outpatient rather than inpatient detoxification. It is also possible, given increases in the level of alcohol and other drug dependence in the general population, that there is increasing substance abuse among many of these patients, and the increase is being documented by providers.

ACCESS TO CARE

The number of Medicaid beneficiaries with schizophrenia being treated increased from 6614 in 1991 to 7541 in 1994 (Table 1). However, in 1993, the year managed care was introduced in Massachusetts, the number of treated beneficiaries increased by more than 3000 from the previous year. This 1993 increase occurred despite a decrease in the number of providers. The increases might be an epidemiological phenomenon, but the stable demographic characteristics suggest that is not the source of the increase. More likely, the increase can be attributed to the advocacy work of the mental health provider community and family members who wanted to ensure that those who met the eligibility criteria were actually enrolled in Medicaid. In fact, the incident patients in 1993 were more likely to be older, white, female, and substance abusers than new patients in the remaining years (Table 1). The most striking demographic change for new schizophrenia patients was the higher percentage, in all years, of substance abusers.

MENTAL HEALTH INPATIENT UTILIZATION

The percentage of patients who had at least 1 inpatient admission dropped by 4 percentage points during the study period, from 29.8% in 1991 to 25.4% in 1994 (**Table 2**). The decrease in the likelihood of a mental health admission during the study period was larger for DMH admissions than for Medicaid admissions (Table 2). Even though the probability of an admission decreased, the total number of DMH admissions remained almost the same in all 4 years. Medicaid admissions dropped 65% in 1993 but returned to the

Table 2. Mental Health Inpatient Utilization* for Disabled Patients With Schizophrenia

	FY 1991	FY 1992	FY 1993†	FY 1994†
No. of treated beneficiaries	6614	7295	10685	7541
Total No. of admissions	3937	4624	2486	3870
Distribution of hospital admissions, No. (%)‡				
0	4690 (70.9)	5120 (70.2)	9146 (85.6)	5623 (74.6)
1	991 (15.0)	1120 (15.4)	1001 (9.4)	1085 (14.4)
2	459 (6.9)	471 (6.5)	318 (3.0)	388 (5.1)
3	198 (3.0)	252 (3.5)	114 (1.1)	202 (2.7)
4	125 (1.9)	148 (2.0)	58 (0.5)	108 (1.4)
≥5	151 (2.3)	184 (2.5)	48 (0.4)	135 (1.8)
≥1 inpatient admission, No. (%)‡				
All admissions	1924 (29.1)	2175 (29.8)	1539 (14.4)	1918 (25.4)
DMH admissions	1082 (16.4)	1098 (15.1)	1038 (9.7)	915 (12.1)
Medicaid admissions	1170 (17.1)	1466 (20.1)	608 (5.7)	1232 (16.3)

*Hospital admissions for treatment of mental illnesses or substance abuse.
†Managed care plan years.
‡Percentage was calculated with number of treated beneficiaries used as the denominator. FY indicates fiscal year; DMH, Department of Mental Health.

pre–managed care level by 1994. For those admitted, the median number of bed-days per admission decreased by about 3.3 days; there was a drop of 2.5 days for Medicaid admissions and of 3 days for DMH admissions (**Figure 1**).

CONTINUITY OF CARE

We found little evidence of change in continuity of care. Rapid readmissions were up slightly, from 22.1% in 1991 to 24.2% in 1994 (**Table 3**), but there was essentially no change in the absence of outpatient follow-up contact, with the proportion of discharges without any follow-up contact remaining at 29%. (We were unable to identify in these data follow-up that may have occurred through DMH-funded community support services.) For patients with multiple admissions, there was an increase in the percentage who were admitted to more than 1 hospital (Table 3) but no increase in the percentage of patients who used emergency departments.

MENTAL HEALTH EXPENDITURES

Inpatient

Medicaid inpatient expenditures dropped dramatically in 1993, in the first year of managed care, but rose the following year (**Table 4**). The savings in Medicaid inpatient expenditures were largely offset, however, by increased expenditures on DMH hospital admissions. The annual Medicaid per-inpatient costs dropped below pre–managed care levels, while DMH per-inpatient costs were higher after implementation of the managed care program.

Outpatient

Both total expenditures and per–treated beneficiary expenditures rose from their pre–managed care levels. The large increase in the number of beneficiaries in 1993 led to a dip in per–treated outpatient expenditures, but by

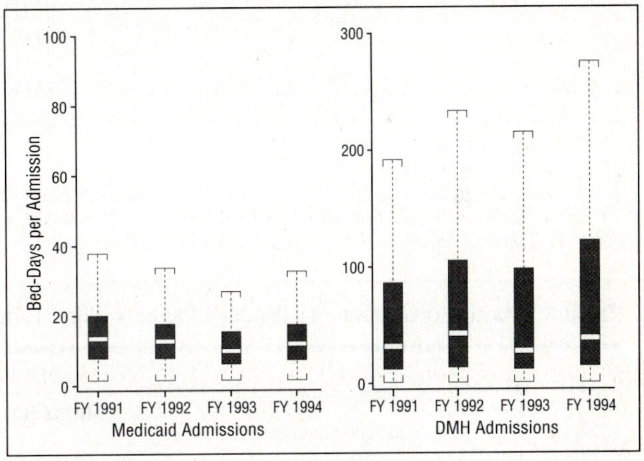

Figure 1. *Distribution of bed-days per admission among adult (aged 18-64 years) Massachusetts Medicaid beneficiaries treated for schizophrenia from July 1, 1990, through June 30, 1994. The horizontal line in the interior of the box is located at the median of the data, the height of each box is the interquartile distance, and the dotted lines extend a distance of 1.5 times the interquartile distance. FY indicates fiscal year; DMH, Department of Mental Health.*

1994 this effect had disappeared. Given the large reductions in inpatient treatment, it was expected that outpatient treatment would expand, although these increases suggest only a modest cost shifting from inpatient to outpatient treatment.

NON–MENTAL HEALTH EXPENDITURES

Total expenditures of inpatient and outpatient medical and surgical care rose with the influx of new beneficiaries in 1993 (and then dropped as the number declined in 1994), but the per-person treated costs were about the same across all 4 study years. These data do not provide evidence that mental health treatment was shifted to the non–mental health sector. Other non–mental health expenditures include transportation and dental costs, which remained essentially the same during the study period. Pharmacy costs doubled both in total expenditures and per person treated.

Table 3. Continuity of Care for Disabled Patients With Schizophrenia*

	No. (%)			
	FY 1991	FY 1992	FY 1993†	FY 1994†
Follow-up care within 30 d of a discharge				
None	1077 (29.2)	1199 (27.3)	932 (38.0)	1117 (29.7)
Outpatient contact	1797 (48.7)	2178 (49.7)	1159 (47.2)	1729 (46.0)
Rehospitalization	142 (3.8)	127 (2.9)	124 (5.1)	215 (5.7)
Rehospitalization and outpatient contact	677 (18.3)	880 (20.1)	238 (9.7)	696 (18.5)
Total No. of Discharges	**3693 (100.0)**	**4384 (100.0)**	**2453 (100.0)**	**3757 (100.0)**
Distribution of unique hospitals‡				
1 Hospital	361 (38.7)	342 (32.4)	227 (42.2)	298 (35.8)
2 Hospitals	364 (39.0)	431 (40.9)	213 (39.6)	381 (45.7)
3 Hospitals	145 (15.5)	171 (16.2)	64 (11.9)	113 (13.6)
4 Hospitals	42 (4.5)	71 (6.7)	24 (4.5)	29 (3.5)
≥5 Hospitals	21 (2.3)	40 (3.8)	10 (1.9)	12 (1.4)
Total No. of Patients With ≥2 Hospitalizations	**933 (100.0)**	**1055 (100.0)**	**538 (100.0)**	**833 (100.0)**
Emergency department visits				
0	5626 (85.1)	6219 (85.3)	9894 (92.6)	6653 (88.2)
1	545 (8.2)	577 (7.9)	562 (5.3)	435 (5.8)
2	192 (2.9)	221 (3.0)	140 (1.3)	210 (2.8)
3	92 (1.4)	97 (1.3)	44 (0.4)	82 (1.1)
4	44 (0.7)	69 (0.9)	22 (0.2)	43 (0.6)
≥5	115 (1.7)	112 (1.5)	23 (0.2)	118 (1.6)
Total	**6614 (100.0)**	**7295 (100.0)**	**10 685 (100.0)**	**7541 (100.0)**

**FY indicates fiscal year.*
†Managed care plan years.
‡Distribution of patients with 2 or more hospitalizations categorized by the number of unique hospitals to which they were admitted during the fiscal year. In FY 1991, 38.7% of the 933 patients who had at least 2 hospitalizations went to a single hospital, 39.0% were admitted to 2 distinct hospitals, 15.5% were admitted to 3 distinct hospitals, 4.5% were admitted to 4 distinct hospitals, and the remainder (2.3%) were admitted to 5 or more distinct hospitals.

Table 4. Annual Expenditures for Disabled Patients With Schizophrenia*

	FY 1991	FY 1992	FY 1993†	FY 1994†
	Mental Health Expenditures‡			
Medicaid mental health inpatient admissions				
No. of inpatients	1170	1466	608	1232
Average annual expenditure per inpatient, $	16 916	17 722	10 205	13 673
Total annual expenditure, ×$1000	19 791	25 980	6205	16 845
DMH mental health inpatient admissions				
No. of DMH inpatients	1082	1098	1038	915
Average annual expenditure per DMH inpatient, $	40 323	44 773	57 898	54 997
Total annual expenditure, ×$1000	43 629	49 161	60 098	50 322
Outpatient mental health care				
No. who are outpatients	6517	7191	10 685	7541
Average annual expenditure per recipient, $	1525	1574	1246	1752
Total annual expenditure, ×$1000	9938	11 319	13 108	12 774
	Non–Mental Health Expenditures			
Inpatient or outpatient non–mental health care				
No. who received non–mental health care	5736	6386	9541	6325
Average annual expenditure per recipient, $	6478	7389	6928	7672
Total annual expenditure, ×$1000	37 157	47 054	66 102	48 527
Pharmacy				
No. who use pharmacy	6239	6964	10 142	6980
Average annual expenditure per recipient, $	897	1087	1331	1634
Total annual expenditure, ×$1000	5598	7573	13 503	11 407
Transportation or dental care				
No. who use transportation or dental care	3896	4115	6521	4225
Average annual expenditure per recipient, $	425	450	441	441
Total annual expenditure, ×$1000	1654	1852	2875	1865
	Total Expenditures			
No. of patients	6614	7295	10 685	7541
Average annual expenditure per patient, $	17 806	19 594	15 151	18 796
Total annual expenditure, ×$1000	**117 767**	**142 940**	**161 891**	**141 740**

**FY indicates fiscal year; DMH, Department of Mental Health.*
†Managed care plan years.
‡All expenditures have been converted to 1994 dollars by means of the gross domestic product deflator. The cumulative inflation rates from 1991 until 1994 were 7.1%, 4.1%, and 2.1%, respectively.

TOTAL EXPENDITURES

The total Medicaid and DMH expenditures for mental health per treated beneficiary fell slightly from $11 090 to $10 600 during the 4-year study period. When all other Medicaid reimbursed care is added to mental health care, there is a slight increase in the total per-person expenditures (Table 4). The total dollar expenditures fluctuated with the number of treated beneficiaries across the study years, but it was decreasing, not increasing, at the end of the study period. The total Medicaid and DMH dollar expenditure for mental health care after managed care reversed the upward trend and stabilized at about $80 million in 1993 and 1994 (**Figure 2**).

COMMENT

Using a unique database of patient-level mental health treatments constructed from 2 sources, Medicaid and the DMH, we found that managed care was associated with some gains in continuity of care but a slight increase in rapid readmissions. Furthermore, there were reductions in mental health expenditures at the per-person level, primarily because fewer inpatient bed-days were reimbursed by Medicaid. The use of DMH inpatient beds for these beneficiaries remained about the same. Total mental health expenditures during the 4-year study period were contained, despite a growth in the number of treated beneficiaries.

There are several general conclusions from this study. First, because our measures of access and continuity of care are based on administrative data, they are limited in their scope and sensitivity. Furthermore, we have no way of knowing whether the pre–managed care levels were appropriate. Finally, for those with chronic illnesses, examination of short-term results is not an adequate indicator of the value of managed care. Information regarding the appropriateness of processes of care, such as the adequacy of discharge planning, or knowledge regarding patient well-being is crucial in judging the adequacy of quality. Because there is no clear evidence about the effectiveness of managed care plans to provide services needed by the most seriously mentally ill, we believe that continued research is essential to document the benefits or risks to clients.

Second, although we established that there were cost savings under managed care, we cannot be certain of the actual magnitude of the savings. Our assessment before and after managed care allows only 2 types of comparisons. The first type simply focuses on levels and directions of trends observed before and after implementation. The second approach compares observed postintervention levels with the levels that would have been expected in the absence of the intervention.[14] From the perspective of the first approach, the vendor appears to have achieved a net reduction in expenditures and service use. The reduction in Medicaid inpatient expenditures was a function of 3 factors: the negotiated rates with the network hospitals, the reduced number of admissions, and the reduction in the total number of bed-days.

Third, the introduction of this managed care plan

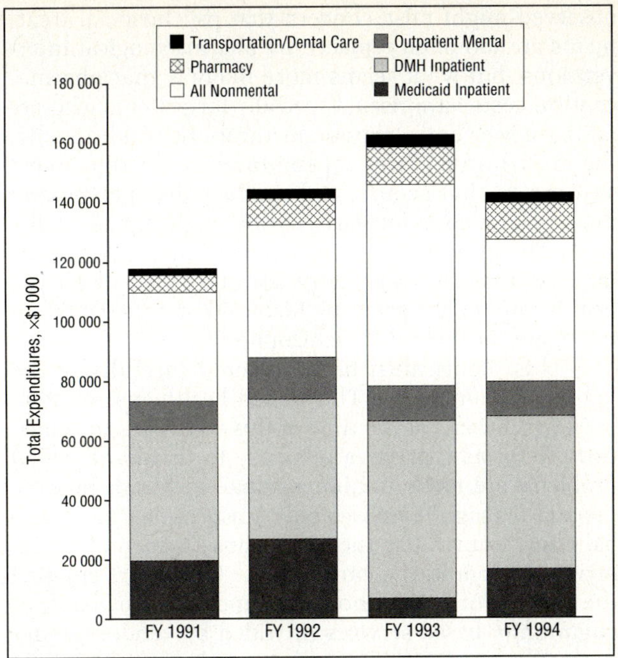

Figure 2. *Total expenditures for disabled schizophrenic patients by type of care among adult (aged 18-64 years) Massachusetts Medicaid beneficiaries treated for schizophrenia from July 1, 1990, through June 30, 1994. All expenditures have been converted to 1994 dollars by means of the gross domestic product deflator and are reported in thousands of dollars. Totals are reported in Table 4. FY indicates fiscal year; DMH, Department of Mental Health.*

resulted in an unanticipated increase in the number of beneficiaries treated for schizophrenia. In this study we observed an increase in additional patients in 1993 who had a profound effect on the system, at least in the first year. The increase in treated patients in 1993, which shrank in 1994, tells us less about access to care and more about diagnostic variability in mental health. Rather than roughly 3000 members losing their coverage, as it appears, we found that they remained enrolled and were being treated for other mental illnesses. The marked increase in the number of beneficiaries in 1993 is real, regardless of diagnostic category. However, it creates a denominator problem: comparing percentages across years may be misleading, and per-person mean costs may be lower because individuals who need less intensive treatment are added to the membership. For example, the proportion of treated beneficiaries who had 1 or more admissions to a DMH inpatient bed during a year appears to drop from 15% to 10%, but the actual number of admissions did not change. This suggests that many of the new patients were among those less seriously ill. Trends such as these have been exhibited in a range of evaluations in a number of divergent fields.[15,16] Their ubiquitous character suggests the need for caution on the part of administrators and providers who would attempt to learn in the first few months after implementation what the ultimate effects of managed care will be on savings or service use.

Our final conclusion relates to cost shifting. We did find some evidence of cost shifting in this study. For example, one striking finding is the doubling of pharmacy costs. The increases in pharmacy costs observed might raise concern that psychosocial treatments are too often replaced by pharmacological interventions, but what seems more likely is that pharmaceutical costs have risen, especially for patients who are taking newer antipsychotic medications. Additionally, the growth in medical expenditures might signal cost shifting to that sector, and the fact that per-person medical care costs increase slightly might signal such a shift. The growth in medical expenditures are important because they compose about a third of all the health care dollars spent by Medicaid and the DMH on treatment for those with schizophrenia.

This report must be considered carefully in the light of its limitations. The mental health environment in Massachusetts at the time of this study was in transition. Reforms that are a response to fiscal and social problems are rarely unidimensional. In Massachusetts, prepaid managed care was only 1 aspect of a more global effort to privatize the Massachusetts mental health service system in the early 1990s. This effort entailed the closing of 3 state hospitals and the expansion of community-based services provided by vendors under contract to the DMH. The current study design does not rule out secular trends.

Although this study raises many questions, it also provides preliminary findings about the relationship of managed care with service use and with expenditures for seriously mentally ill adults with schizophrenia. Future studies of managed care will need to continue to explore the trade-off between quality of care and costs, cost shifting between government agencies, and the difference between short-term and long-term effects.

Accepted for publication June 21, 1996.

This research was supported by grant RO1-MH54076 from the National Institute of Mental Health, Rockville, Md.

We thank the Massachusetts Department of Mental Health and the Division of Medical Assistance for providing data and technical support. Thanks also to Richard Lindrooth, Research Triangle Institute, Research Triangle Park, NC, for providing technical assistance.

Reprints: Barbara Dickey, PhD, McLean Hospital, Administrative Building, 115 Mill St, Belmont, MA 02178-9106.

REFERENCES

1. Lehman AF, Carpenter WT, Goldman HH, Steinwalchs DM. Treatment outcomes in schizophrenia: implications for practice, policy, and research. *Schizophr Bull.* 1995;21:669-675.
2. Rupp A, Keith SJ. The costs of schizophrenia. *Psychiatr Clin North Am.* 1993;16:413-423.
3. Regier DA, Narrow WE, Rae DS, Manderscheid RW, Locke BZ, Goodwin FK. The de facto US mental and addictive disorders service system. *Arch Gen Psychiatry.* 1993;50:85-94.
4. Hurley RE, Freund DA, Paul JE. *Managed Care in Medicaid: Lessons for Policy and Program Design.* Ann Arbor, Mich: Health Administration Press; 1993.
5. Sharfstein SS. Utilization management: managed or mangled psychiatric care? *Am J Psychiatry.* 1990;147:965-966.
6. Tischler GL. Utilization management of mental health services by private third parties. *Am J Psychiatry.* 1990;147:967-973.
7. Schlesinger M. On the limits of expanding health care reform: chronic care in prepaid settings. *Milbank Q.* 1986;64:189-215.
8. Schlesinger M. Striking a balance: capitation, the mentally ill, and public policy. In: Mechanic D, Aiken LH, eds. *Paying for Services: Promises and Pitfalls of Capitation, New Directions for Mental Health Services.* San Francisco, Calif: Jossey-Bass Inc; 1989;43:97-115.
9. Callahan JJ, Shepard DS, Beinecke RH, Larson MJ, Cavanaugh C. *Evaluation of the Massachusetts Medicaid Mental Health/Substance Abuse Program.* Waltham, Mass: Brandeis University; January 1994.
10. Wells KB, Astrchan BM, Tischler GL, Unutzer J. Issues and approaches in evaluating managed mental health care. *Milbank Q.* 1995;73:57-75.
11. Dickey B, Norton EC, Normand SL, Azeni H, Fisher W, Altaffer F. Massachusetts Medicaid managed health care reform: treatment for the psychiatrically disabled. *Adv Health Econ.* 1995;15:99-116.
12. Statistical Sciences Inc. *S-PLUS: User's Manual.* Seattle, Wash: Statistical Sciences Inc; 1991;1:5-51.
13. US Dept of Commerce. *Survey of Current Business.* Washington, DC: US Dept of Commerce; 1995.
14. Cook TD, Campbell CT. *Quasi-Experimentation: Design and Analysis for Field Settings.* Chicago, Ill: Rand McNally; 1979.
15. Rossi PH, Freeman HE. *Evaluation: A Systematic Approach.* 5th ed. Newbury Park, Calif: Sage Publications; 1993.
16. McCleary R, Hay RA. *Applied Time Series Analysis for the Social Sciences.* Beverly Hills, Calif: Sage Publications; 1980.

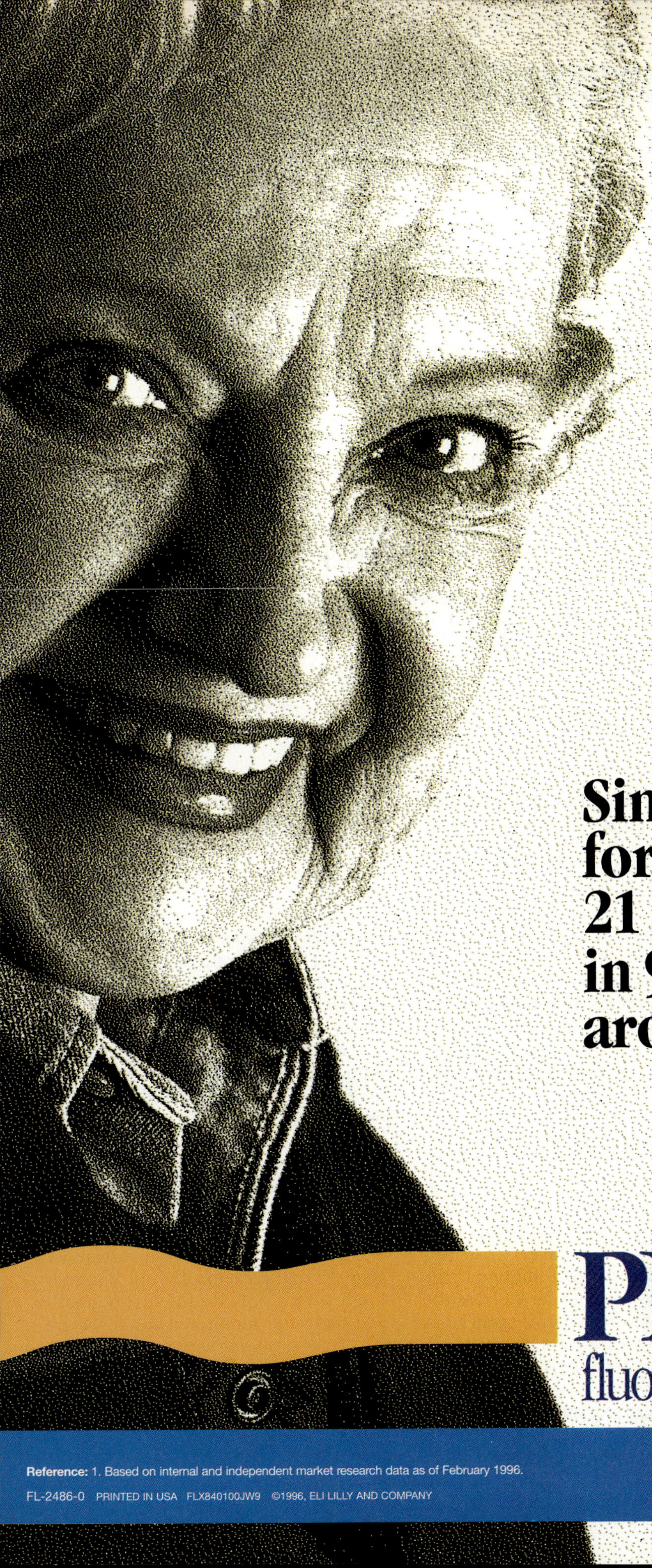

ORIGINAL ARTICLE

Cost-effectiveness of Clozapine Monitoring After the First 6 Months

Mingliang Zhang, PhD; Richard R. Owen, MD; Sandra K. Pope, MPH; G. Richard Smith, MD

Background: Clozapine is effective in treating patients with schizophrenia who do not respond to conventional neuroleptic drugs. The drug is unique in that it is available only with a US Food and Drug Administration–mandated system for weekly monitoring of patients' white blood cell counts. No study has been conducted to evaluate the cost-effectiveness of this mandatory monitoring system.

Methods: A benchmark case was established by utilizing cumulative incidence rates of agranulocytosis from a recent study with a large sample of clozapine-treated patients. We assumed a 20% mortality among patients with agranulocytosis, $30.61 in monitoring costs each week, and 14.4 years of remaining life expectancy after detection of agranulocytosis. Based on these benchmark assumptions, cost-effectiveness ratios in dollars per quality-adjusted life-year were calculated for the first, second, and third 6-month periods during which a patient was receiving clozapine. Sensitivity analyses were performed with more conservative assumptions in 5 alternative scenarios.

Results: In the benchmark case, costs per quality-adjusted life-year gained were $61 694, $925 418, and $420 644 for the first, second, and third 6-month periods of clozapine treatment, respectively. In the alternative scenarios, these costs ranged from $7923 to $46 056 for the first 6-month period and from $54 025 to $690 850 for the second and third 6-month periods.

Conclusions: While the costs of monitoring patients with schizophrenia in the first 6-month period of clozapine treatment seem to be justifiable, monitoring thereafter may not be cost-effective because of the very low incidence of agranulocytosis in the later periods.

Arch Gen Psychiatry. 1996;53:954-958

CLOZAPINE IS an atypical antipsychotic agent that is effective in treating patients with schizophrenia who do not respond to conventional neuroleptic drugs. Although the drug was discovered 30 years ago,[1] it was unavailable in the United States until 1990 because of the risk of agranulocytosis,[2-4] a serious and potentially fatal side effect characterized by few or no granulocytes in the peripheral blood.[2] Clozapine was approved by the Food and Drug Administration with a unique mandatory requirement that patients taking clozapine be monitored weekly to ensure that their white blood cell (WBC) counts are above 3.0×10^9/L.[5]

Studies have shown that clozapine treatment is not only clinically effective,[6-11] but also cost-effective.[7,11-13] In fact, some studies show that, in addition to the clinical benefits patients derive from the treatment, the total direct treatment costs for clozapine-treated patients are reduced because of fewer rehospitalizations.[14]

At the time of marketing, the drug and WBC monitoring components were "bundled," ie, the drug was provided only through a system that combined distribution and monitoring, the Clozaril Patient Monitoring System. The manufacturer would not disclose the charges for each component of the "bundle" of drug and monitoring service. Because of the outcry about the expense and its restrictiveness, the system was changed in 1991 so that individual physicians, pharmacies, and laboratories could form independent monitoring systems. Although the whole package (drug and WBC monitoring) has been found to be cost-effective, this does not necessarily mean that the drug and the monitoring are cost-effective when considered separately. Several authors have expressed concern about the expense of WBC monitoring.[15,16] The manufacturer (Sandoz Pharmaceuticals Corp, Hanover, NJ) contends that weekly WBC monitoring is necessary,[17] whereas some researchers suggest that patients should be monitored weekly only for the first 6 months and thereafter monitored at a lower fre-

See Materials and Methods on next page

From the Veterans Affairs Health Services Research and Development Field Program, Veterans Affairs Medical Center, Little Rock, Ark (Drs Zhang, Owen, and Smith); and Centers for Mental Healthcare Research (Drs Zhang, Owen, and Smith) and Center for Outcomes Research and Effectiveness (Drs Zhang, Owen, and Smith and Ms Pope), Department of Psychiatry, University of Arkansas for Medical Sciences, Little Rock.

MATERIALS AND METHODS

One simple strategy to evaluate the cost-effectiveness of clozapine monitoring would be to examine the costs per life saved, since the purpose of monitoring is to save lives. However, this method would assign equal weights to saving the life of a person with a remaining life expectancy of 20 years and a person with a remaining life expectancy of only 10 years. A modification to this approach would calculate costs per life-year saved, instead of costs per life saved. This modification is still limited because it does not adjust for quality of life in these remaining life years. For example, to a patient with schizophrenia who responds to clozapine but not to conventional neuroleptic drugs, 1 year of life without clozapine has lower quality than 1 year of life with clozapine. Therefore, the patient's remaining life-years when clozapine treatment is terminated should be adjusted for quality. Researchers apply a quality index, known as utility in cost-utility analyses,[19,20] to adjust for quality of life in each life-year. The *cost-effectiveness ratio* is costs per quality-adjusted life-year (QALY). We used this method in our study.

Charges from local laboratories for WBC tests and information from published literature on the incidence of agranulocytosis and mortality rates from agranulocytosis among clozapine-treated patients were used to create a benchmark case, which we believe is the most likely scenario for the costs and benefits of monitoring. We then conducted sensitivity analyses by changing the assumptions made in the benchmark case to evaluate cost-effectiveness in alternative (more conservative) scenarios. We examined cost-effectiveness ratios for the first, second, and third 6-month periods of clozapine treatment. The benchmark assumptions are as follows.

COSTS OF WBC MONITORING

The 2 components in monitoring costs are: the costs of WBC tests and the costs to the patient of obtaining the tests. The costs of WBC tests include technician time to draw the blood sample, the costs of WBC count determination itself, and physician time to read results. To determine the costs of a test, one of us (R.R.O.) called 4 local laboratories about their charges for WBC tests. Costs (approximated by charges) per test varied substantially among these 4 laboratories: $11, $12, $23.25, and $36.20. Given the large variation of costs, we use the average cost, $20.61, for our benchmark case. According to Meltzer and Cola,[12] average monitoring costs are $1000 a year, or $19.23 per test, which is comparable with our benchmark assumption. Patient costs include the patient's time traveling to and from the laboratory, a family member's or caregiver's traveling time if accompanying the patient, and transportation costs. Given the variation in travel modalities, distance to the laboratory, time spent waiting for and receiving the blood drawing, and parking fees, we assume that all these costs to the patient are $10 per week (each test). Therefore, the total monitoring costs for each test are $30.61 ($20.61+$10) in the benchmark case.

Realizing the existence of large variations in laboratory charges and the arbitrariness of our assumption about patient costs, we examined an alternative scenario that used the lowest ($11) of the 4 laboratory charges and assumed only $5 for patient costs, for a total monitoring cost of $16 for each test (scenario A).

INCIDENCE OF AGRANULOCYTOSIS AMONG PATIENTS TAKING CLOZAPINE

The true incidence is unknown, and estimates vary depending on the sample size of the study and other patient factors.[4,5] According to Baldessarini and Frankenburg,[1] weekly WBC monitoring detected 47 agranulocytosis cases among 7500 patients taking clozapine in the United States, a crude incidence of 0.63%. More recently, Alvir et al[5] analyzed data on 11 555 patients treated with clozapine and monitored weekly, finding 73 cases of agranulocytosis, a crude incidence of the same magnitude (0.63%). We used the data of Alvir et al[5,21] as the basis for the incidence. We believe that the rate in their study is the most reliable one available since their study had the largest sample to date. Alvir and Lieberman[21] reported that the cumulative incidence of agranulocytosis after 6, 12, and 18 months of clozapine treatment was 0.75%, 0.80%, and 0.91%, respectively. These cumulative rates are adjusted for censoring of observations by survival analysis. Using these rates, we can derive the incidence for the second 6-month period by subtracting the 6-month cumulative rate from the 12-month cumulative rate, or 0.05% (0.8%−0.75%). Similarly, the incidence for the third 6-month period is the

Continued on next page

quency because agranulocytosis is rare after the first 6 months.[5] A practice similar to the latter suggestion has already been adopted in several European countries.[5,18] To date, no study has been conducted to evaluate the cost-effectiveness of *monitoring* patients who are taking clozapine after the initial 6 months; this study is designed to fulfill this need.

For those patients who do develop agranulocytosis, the benefit of WBC monitoring is potentially lifesaving. (We use the term *benefit* as a synonym for effectiveness, although we do not perform a cost-benefit analysis in this study.) The unanswered question is whether repeated weekly WBC monitoring past the initial 6 months of treatment for tens of thousands of patients is cost-effective. In this study, we compared the costs of weekly WBC monitoring for all patients receiving clozapine with the benefits for patients whose agranulocytosis is detected by the weekly monitoring. We focused our analysis on patients with schizophrenia, the largest group receiving clozapine treatment.[5]

RESULTS

The costs and benefits of WBC monitoring of patients with schizophrenia taking clozapine, based on the assumptions of the benchmark case, are calculated in **Table 1** for the first, second, and third 6-month periods. In a 6-month monitoring period, each patient needs 26 tests at a cost of $30.61 each; the total cost is $795.90 per patient ($30.61×26 tests). To calculate the benefit of monitoring for each patient, we first calculate the probability of death without monitoring by multiplying the agranulocytosis incidence (0.75%, 0.05%, and 0.11% for the first, second, and third 6-month periods, respecdifference between the 18-month and 12-month cumulative rates, or 0.11% (0.91%−0.80%).

MORTALITY RATE AMONG PATIENTS WITH AGRANULOCYTOSIS

To determine how many patients with agranulocytosis would die if the monitoring system did not exist, we examined cases of agranulocytosis in Europe detected before the WBC monitoring requirement. The mortality was as high as 35% among these patients with agranulocytosis.[1] However, this rate is likely to be a high estimate for current medical practice for several reasons. (1) Before the mid-1970s, an increased risk of clozapine-associated agranulocytosis was not suspected[4]; therefore, patients with early cases sometimes continued taking clozapine for days or weeks after agranulocytosis was discovered, possibly increasing mortality.[2] (2) In current practice, even if continuous monitoring were not required, heightened awareness of the agranulocytosis risk could facilitate detection of new cases. (3) The use of granulocyte colony-stimulating factor has been reported to speed recovery from agranulocytosis and could reduce morbidity and mortality in clozapine-induced agranulocytosis, regardless of whether WBC monitoring is required.[22,23]

Additionally, not all deaths can be prevented even if agranulocytosis is detected by monitoring, and we are interested in the differential effects of WBC monitoring. For example, even with the current monitoring system, 2 of the 73 patients with agranulocytosis in the study by Alvir et al[5] died. For these reasons, we assumed a 20% mortality in our benchmark case. However, we will also examine a scenario where the mortality is assumed to be 35% (scenario B).

QALYs

To estimate the potential QALYs saved because of WBC monitoring during clozapine treatment, we estimate equivalently the QALYs lost if a patient dies of agranulocytosis as a result of not being monitored. Three pieces of information are crucial to the estimate of QALYs: the average patient's age at onset of agranulocytosis when taking clozapine, the patient's remaining life expectancy once agranulocytosis is detected and treatment is terminated, and the patient's quality of life in these remaining years. The age at onset of agranulocytosis depends on the age of the patient starting clozapine treatment; agranulocytosis tends to occur in older patients. In the study by Alvir et al,[5] patients with agranulocytosis had an average age of 45.6 years, approximately 10 years older than other patients taking clozapine. For these analyses, we used 45.6 years as the age at onset in our benchmark case. However, we will examine an alternative scenario with age at onset at 35 years (scenario C).

Life expectancy of patients with schizophrenia is shorter than that of the general population because they are more prone to high-risk behaviors, such as suicide.[24-26] According to a study by Newman and Bland,[24] life expectancy is about 20% shorter for patients with schizophrenia. Therefore, if the general population's life expectancy is 75 years, then patients with schizophrenia have a life expectancy of 60 years. We assumed in the benchmark case that a patient with agranulocytosis detected during clozapine treatment is expected to live for an additional 14.4 calendar years (60 years of life expectancy−45.6 years average age at onset of agranulocytosis). Equivalently, a patient taking clozapine who dies of agranulocytosis that was undetected because of a lack of WBC monitoring would lose 14.4 calendar years of life. In scenario C, this loss would be 25 calendar years.

Davies and Drummond[13] reported a gain of 0.4 year of mild or no disability for each year of clozapine treatment, based on posttreatment Brief Psychiatric Rating Scale scores. If we assume that such patients treated with clozapine have 1 QALY for each calendar year, then a patient whose clozapine treatment is terminated has at most 0.6 QALY for each subsequent year (1 QALY−0.4 QALY). In our benchmark case, we used 0.6 QALY for each calendar year to adjust for quality of life for those patients whose clozapine treatment is terminated because of monitoring. Because this estimate was based on a single study that used only the Brief Psychiatric Rating Scale to define disability, we examined a more conservative scenario (scenario D) that uses 0.8 QALY for each year after a patient's clozapine treatment is terminated (note that the maximum is 1.0 QALY). In the benchmark case, the total QALYs a patient with agranulocytosis gains, if his or her life is saved because of WBC monitoring, is 8.6 QALYs (0.6×14.4 years of remaining life expectancy) and 11.5 QALYs (0.8×14.4) in scenario D.

tively) by the estimated mortality of patients with agranulocytosis (20%). For example, without monitoring, a patient's probability of death from agranulocytosis in the first 6-month period is estimated to be 0.15% (0.75%×20%). We then calculate the QALYs per patient that would have been lost without monitoring by multiplying the probability of death by 8.6 QALYs. For the first 6-month period, 12.9×10^{-3} QALYs (8.6 QALYs×0.15%) would have been lost for each patient without monitoring. Alternatively phrased, monitoring potentially saves 12.9×10^{-3} QALYs for each patient in the first 6-month period.

The cost-effectiveness ratio, dollars per QALY, is calculated by dividing the total costs of monitoring by the total QALYs saved for each patient, as presented in the bottom row in Table 1. For the first 6-month period, the cost-effectiveness ratio is \$61 694 (795.86/$[12.90\times10^{-3}]$) per QALY. The cost-effectiveness ratios for the second and third 6-month periods are similarly calculated in the last 2 columns of Table 1. While the costs of monitoring stay the same for every 6-month period, the benefit drops dramatically after the first 6-month period because of the low risk of agranulocytosis in later periods. As a result, the cost-effectiveness ratios in the later periods are much higher than in the first 6-month period: \$925 418 and \$420 644 per QALY in the second and third 6-month periods, respectively.

In **Table 2**, we present cost-effectiveness ratios of WBC monitoring for the first, second, and third 6-month periods in the alternative scenarios. Although lower than in the benchmark case, the ratios are still very high for the second and third 6-month periods. Even in the most conservative scenario (scenarios A, B, C, and D combined), costs per QALY gained are still \$118 857 and \$54 025 for the second and third 6-month periods, respectively.

Table 1. Costs and QALYs for 1 Patient Taking Clozapine and Undergoing Weekly WBC Monitoring: The Benchmark Case*

	1st 6 mo	2nd 6 mo	3rd 6 mo
Costs			
a. No. of tests	26	26	26
b. Costs/test, $	30.61	30.61	30.61
c. Total costs (a×b), $	795.86	795.86	795.86
Benefits (effectiveness)			
d. Incidence of agranulocytosis, %	0.75	0.05	0.11
e. Mortality of agranulocytosis, %	20	20	20
f. Mortality without monitoring (d×e), %	0.15	0.01	0.022
g. QALYs lost because of death	8.6	8.6	8.6
h. QALYs lost without (or gained because of) monitoring (f×g)	12.90×10^{-3}	0.86×10^{-3}	1.892×10^{-3}
Cost-effectiveness ratio			
Costs/QALY (c/h), $	61 694	925 418	420 644

*QALYs indicates quality-adjusted life-years; WBC, white blood cell.

Table 2. Costs per QALY for 1 Patient Taking Clozapine and Undergoing Weekly WBC Monitoring: Alternative Scenarios*

	Cost/QALY, $		
Scenarios	1st 6 mo	2nd 6 mo	3rd 6 mo
A	32 248	483 720	219 873
B	35 254	528 810	240 368
C	35 371	530 573	241 169
D	46 056	690 850	314 023
E	7923	118 857	54 025

*QALY indicates quality-adjusted life-year: WBC, white blood cells. Basic assumptions of benchmark case: (1) Cost per test, $30.61; (2) mortality rate among agranulocytosis patients, 20%; (3) age at onset of agranulocytosis, 45.6 years; and (4) each year without clozapine, 0.6 QALYs. Alternative scenarios: A, assume $16/test, other benchmark assumptions do not change; B, assume a 35% mortality rate among agranulocytosis patients, other benchmark assumptions do not change; C, assume age at onset of agranulocytosis at 35 years, ie, a loss of 15 QALYs (0.6×25) because of death without monitoring, other benchmark assumptions do not change; D, assume 0.8 QALYs for every calendar year (instead of 0.6 QALYs), other benchmark assumptions do not change; and E, scenarios A, B, C, and D combined.

COMMENT

Several economic evaluation techniques exist: cost-benefit analysis, cost-effectiveness analysis, and cost-utility analysis. In a cost-benefit analysis, all of the benefits (effectiveness) are converted into monetary values by such approaches as the willingness-to-pay approach or the human capital approach. A treatment program is deemed cost-beneficial if the benefits in dollars are greater than its costs. If this technique applied in our study, we would need to assign monetary values to lives (or life-years) saved because of WBC monitoring. However, valuing life in monetary terms is complicated and controversial. A cost-effectiveness analysis avoids the difficulty of assigning dollar values to human life. Instead, it examines the costs per unit of change in outcomes. A cost-utility analysis is a special case of cost-effectiveness analysis where the outcomes are measured by QALYs, although some authors distinguish the 2 as separate approaches.[27] Our study is essentially a cost-utility analysis, since we use QALYs to measure the outcomes (benefits). Detailed discussions on the advantages and disadvantages of these different economic evaluation techniques can be found elsewhere.[27]

Given the assumptions made in the benchmark case, the costs of monitoring patients with schizophrenia taking clozapine in terms of QALYs saved are tremendous, especially after the first 6 months of treatment. This is because agranulocytosis occurs rarely after the first 6 months. With the same monitoring frequency as in the first 6 months, the mandatory monitoring requirement in the later months may be questioned on the basis of cost-effectiveness.

Patrick and Erickson[28] (their Tables 2.2, 2.3, and 2.4) surveyed studies on costs per QALY for 23 different treatment programs. After adjusting for medical inflation,[29] we find that 10 of these programs cost less than $5000 per QALY; another 6 of them cost less than $20 000 per QALY; and only 2 of the programs cost more than $100 000 per QALY. In our benchmark case, the costs per QALY in the second and third 6-month periods range from $0.5 million to $1 million and are higher than those of any of the 23 treatment programs surveyed. Even in the most conservative scenario, the costs are more than $54 000 per QALY and are comparable with the costliest programs. We contend that monitoring patients after 6 months of clozapine treatment is not cost-effective when compared with other treatment programs for various medical conditions.

The limitations in this cost-effectiveness analysis include the assumptions that had to be made to obtain a benchmark case. However, these assumptions were based on data from the literature. To test the sensitivity of our conclusions to these assumptions, more conservative assumptions were used in alternative scenarios.

We assumed that preventing patients from dying of agranulocytosis is the sole benefit of monitoring. Another possible benefit of monitoring is preventing future excess treatment costs by early detection of agranulocytosis. In other words, precautions may be taken when a patient's agranulocytosis is detected by monitoring, so that future excess hospitalizations can be prevented. However, this benefit has little effect on our results. For example, suppose a patient with agranulocytosis costs $10 000 more in hospitalization when not monitored than when monitored. This translates to a savings of $5 per patient because of monitoring in the second 6-month period (0.05%×$10 000) and a savings of $11 in the third 6-month period (0.11%×$10 000). Since the monitoring costs for a 6-month period are relatively high, subtracting these savings from the monitoring costs has minimal effect on the cost-effectiveness ratios.

Another potential benefit may be derived from a patient's weekly contact with a health professional because of WBC monitoring, if such regular contact is therapeutic. However, we have no data to quantify this benefit. Regular contact with health professionals is likely to benefit most patients with schizophrenia, regardless of whether they take clozapine. Even if the benefit of regular contact is specific to those patients taking clozapine, such contact could be provided through other means, instead of weekly WBC monitoring.

Weekly monitoring also reduces the benefits for those patients who have low WBC counts detected, but who would not ultimately develop agranulocytosis. If their clozapine treatment is discontinued as a result, these patients would no longer benefit from clozapine treatment. This effect would increase the cost/QALY ratios. However, the proportion of patients in this category is so small that the impact on our cost-effectiveness ratios will be minimal.

A patient's future QALYs saved from monitoring were not discounted in our analyses. The total QALYs saved with discounting will be lower than our current numbers imply; the cost-effectiveness ratios will be greater. This in turn will reinforce our conclusions.

We do not have data to conduct a cost-effectiveness analysis beyond 18 months. However, it is generally agreed that agranulocytosis is rare in the later months of the treatment. According to Alvir et al,[5] only 1 (1.4%) of the 73 patients with agranulocytosis was detected after 12 months of clozapine treatment. However, because of mandatory requirements, some patients may be monitored for years. We contend that monitoring patients after 18 months is probably even less cost-effective than the numbers indicated in Tables 1 and 2.

Several options exist for changing monitoring requirements for patients with schizophrenia who are taking clozapine. The first is to do no monitoring after the first 6-month period. Another option would be to monitor patients biweekly after the first 6-month period. With this second method, the costs will be reduced by half. However, the benefits may drop as well if not all the agranulocytosis cases are detected in biweekly intervals. Therefore, the cost-effectiveness ratios are probably higher than half of those values in Tables 1 and 2. Even if all the potential agranulocytosis cases can be detected in biweekly intervals, the costs per QALY (half of those in Tables 1 and 2) are still hardly justifiable, compared with other treatment programs.

One may argue that clozapine monitoring protects the manufacturer-provider from product liability and malpractice suits resulting from an adverse event. However, the risk of these suits is diminished if patients are monitored in the first 6 months of clozapine treatment, since most of the agranulocytosis cases occur in this period. In addition, if tort reform imposes a cap on jury awards for pain and suffering, the manufacturer's and provider's liability will be limited in that the economic loss for most patients with schizophrenia is relatively small because of their high likelihood of disability and unemployment.

In summary, as a society, difficult choices have to be made because resources are scarce. Priorities for health care financing have to be established. The cost-effectiveness of WBC monitoring during the first 6 months of clozapine treatment is comparable with that of some commonly available procedures and treatments. However, the money spent on monitoring patients with schizophrenia *after* the first 6-month period of clozapine treatment to achieve 1 QALY may achieve more QALYs if it were spent on alternative treatments.

Accepted for publication January 18, 1996.

This study was supported by grant HFP 90-019 from the Department of Veterans Affairs, Washington, DC, and grant MH4819 from the National Institute of Mental Health, Bethesda, Md. Dr Owen is a Research Associate awardee of the Veterans Affairs Health Services Research and Development Services (RCD 94-311), and Dr Smith is a Research Scientist Development awardee of the National Institute of Mental Health (MH00843).

Reprints: Mingliang Zhang, PhD, 5800 W 10th St, Suite 605, Little Rock, AR 72204.

REFERENCES

1. Baldessarini RJ, Frankenburg FR. Clozapine: a novel antipsychotic agent. *N Engl J Med.* 1991;324:746-754.
2. Amsler HA, Teerenhovi L, Barth E, Harjula K, Vuopio P. Agranulocytosis in patients treated with clozapine: a study of the Finnish epidemic. *Acta Psychiatr Scand.* 1977;56:241-248.
3. Idanpaan-Heikkila J, Alhava E, Olkinuora M, Palva IP. Agranulocytosis during treatment with clozapine. *Eur J Clin Pharmacol.* 1977;11:193-198.
4. Anderman B, Griffith RW. Clozapine-induced agranulocytosis: a situation report up to August 1976. *Eur J Clin Pharmacol.* 1977;11:199-201.
5. Alvir JMJ, Lieberman JA, Safferman AZ, Schwimmer JL, Schaaf JA. Clozapine-induced agranulocytosis: incidence and risk factors in the United States. *N Engl J Med.* 1993;329:162-167.
6. Meltzer HY, Okayli G. Reduction of suicidality during clozapine treatment of neuroleptic-resistant schizophrenia: impact on risk-benefit assessment. *Am J Psychiatry.* 1995;152:183-190.
7. Honigfeld G, Patin J. A two-year clinical and economic follow-up of patients on clozapine. *Hosp Community Psychiatry.* 1990;41:882-885.
8. Maier GJ, Miller RD, Roach L. The real cost of clozapine: a patient buys freedom. *Hosp Community Psychiatry.* 1992;43:177-178.
9. Meltzer HY, Burnett S, Bastani B, Ramirez LF. Effects of six months of clozapine treatment on the quality of life of chronic schizophrenic patients. *Hosp Community Psychiatry.* 1990;41:892-897.
10. Naber D, Hippius H. The European experience with use of clozapine. *Hosp Community Psychiatry.* 1990;41:886-891.
11. Revicki DA, Luce BR, Weschler JM, Brown RE, Adler MA. Cost-effectiveness of clozapine for treatment-resistant schizophrenic patients. *Hosp Community Psychiatry.* 1990;41:850-854.
12. Meltzer HY, Cola PA. The pharmacoeconomics of clozapine: a review. *J Clin Psychiatry.* 1994;55(suppl B):161-165.
13. Davies LM, Drummond MF. Assessment of costs and benefits of drug therapy for treatment-resistant schizophrenia in the United Kingdom. *Br J Psychiatry.* 1993;162:38-42.
14. Meltzer HY, Cola P, Way L, Thompson PA, Bastani B, Davies MA, Snitz B. Cost effectiveness of clozapine in neuroleptic-resistant schizophrenia. *Am J Psychiatry.* 1993;150:1630-1638.
15. Lehmann LS, Rodriguez L. Clozapine and the mandatory monitoring system. *N Engl J Med.* 1991;324:490.
16. Salzman C. Mandatory monitoring for side effects: the 'bundling' of clozapine. *N Engl J Med.* 1990;323:827-829.
17. Westlin WF. Comments by a Sandoz official. *Hosp Community Psychiatry.* 1990; 41:874-876.
18. Kleinerman MJ. Controversy grows over monitoring system for new schizophrenia drug. *JAMA.* 1990;264:2488.
19. Torrance GW. Measurement of health state utilities for economic appraisal: a review. *J Health Econ.* 1986;5:1-30.
20. Feeny DH, Torrance GW. Incorporating utility-based quality-of-life assessment measures in clinical trials: two examples. *Med Care.* 1989;27:S190-S204.
21. Alvir JMJ, Lieberman JA. Agranulocytosis: incidence and risk factors. *J Clin Psychiatry.* 1994;55(suppl B):137-138.
22. Gerson SL. G-CSF and the management of clozapine-induced agranulocytosis. *J Clin Psychiatry.* 1994;55:139-142.
23. Gullion G, Yeh HS. Treatment of clozapine-induced agranulocytosis with recombinant granulocyte colony-stimulating factor. *J Clin Psychiatry.* 1994;55: 401-405.
24. Newman SC, Bland RC. Mortality in a cohort of patients with schizophrenia: a record linkage study. *Can J Psychiatry.* 1991;36:239-245.
25. Black DW, Fisher R. Mortality in *DSM-IIIR* schizophrenia. *Schizophr Res.* 1992; 7:109-116.
26. Mortensen PB, Juel K. Mortality and causes of death in schizophrenic patients in Denmark. *Acta Psychiatr Scand.* 1990;81:372-377.
27. Drummond MF, Stoddart GL, Torrance GW. *Methods for the Economic Evaluation of Health Care Programmes.* New York, NY: Oxford University Press; 1987.
28. Patrick DL, Erickson P. *Health Status and Health Policy: Quality of Life in Health Care Evaluation and Resource Allocation.* New York, NY: Oxford University Press; 1993.
29. US Dept of Commerce. *Statistical Abstract of the United States 1994.* 114th ed. Washington, DC: Economics and Statistics Administration; 1994.

COMMENTARY

A Funny Thing Happened on the Way to Reform

Out at Free Enterprise, where the Needies fight
The Greedies for the great Grail of the World
And always lose, we can help balance up
The scales of earthly good; not much, but some;
And for a wonder, though it hurt at first,
It will feel good because our kindness did it.

Howard Nemerov, Trying Conclusions: New and Selected Poems, 1961-1991. *Chicago, Ill: The University of Chicago Press; 1991.*

TWO YEARS ago, we were eagerly awaiting major changes in the financing, organization, and delivery of health care. But a funny thing happened on the way to reform. America's corporate class discovered that it had the will, the ways, and the means to reshape the health care establishment. They seized the moment and effected a far more dramatic "takeover" than the consolidations and mergers we read about in the business sections of our daily newspapers. The values of the marketplace and the world of commerce became the catalysts of change. Corporate policy now dominates where public policy once ruled. The advocates of managed competition vanquished the champions of health rights. Marketspeak has become the lingua franca capturing the cost of caring for the ill in a simple phrase, "the medical loss ratio."

As we stand on the threshold of the 21st century, much of what we once identified as social goods are now regarded as commodities. Economic issues dominate where social issues once held sway. In a world where human service agencies are regarded as market entities, the health care sector is little more than a microcosm of a larger universe that is being battered by change. The changes reflect a profound redefinition of the social contract that provides the foundation on which the human service system within the United States rests. Efforts to transform human services and recast the health care system into an aggressive market force have distorted our sense of proportion and made it increasingly difficult to balance universal need against individual wants.

As 2 individuals who have devoted most of their careers to building and stabilizing organizations, we have expended considerable effort in designing institutions and creating institutional climates that allow work to be accomplished well. Labor of this nature requires that one be sensitive to and realistic about the nature of the world outside of the organization and the profession. It is the larger world that defines practice and establishes the parameters within which change and adaptation occur. That being the case, we find it puzzling that physicians pay so little attention to how changes in the larger work world affect their lives. In the pages to follow, we advance the premise that managed care and managed competition are but reflections of changes occurring in the work world at large, and then we consider their implications before concluding with what we believe the response of leadership ought to be.

CHANGES IN THE WORLD OF WORK

The chaos that many psychiatrists and physicians experience is not dissimilar to that confounding professionals and managers in other fields. At the heart of the matter is the impact of a sophisticated information technology on organizing work and providing access to profit. Information technology enhances productivity, fosters greater accountability, and facilitates control by management. Emphasis has shifted from individual labor and craft to team production methods, and the organization of work is guided by access to information in real time. In the process, there has been a devaluation of the worker as professional, artisan, or craftsman. The technology also has eased the task of "outsourcing"—a large entity subcontracting work out to small or medium-sized concerns—and expedited the substitution of less skilled workers for more highly trained ones.

The application of information technology in these ways is but one reflection of an evolving monotheism: market worship. When unrestrained, market worship feeds on gain and competition. As corporations move into a growing global economy, they are able to purchase services and goods all over the world and to negotiate intensely over price. Through fits of reengineering and tides of consolidation, the worshipers leave in their wake extraordinary savings often gained at the cost of deep layoffs. Savings can then be reinvested or pushed into profit.

Several articles in *The New York Times* entitled "The Downsizing of America"[1-7] described the multiple individual dislocations accompanying this massive restructuring of work, and the resultant loss of trust in the workplace and the community. Attention has also focused on an economic seesaw tilted toward income inequality and the concentration of wealth, what Head[8] has described as the "huge transfer of wealth from skilled, middle-class American workers to the owners of capital assets and to a new technological aristocracy." The share of total income and stock holdings has become more concentrated in the top 5% of households at the same time that the gap between executive and worker compensation has widened. While a greening of the wealthy is occurring, average working people require 2 incomes to get by. "We shall beat our swords into plowshares and our spears into pruning hooks" has become "we shall plow our profits to shareholders and pound wages into the ground."

A PARALLEL UNIVERSE: THE HEALTH CARE ENTERPRISE

Health care has proved to be far from immune to the influence of the information revolution and a resurgent mercantilism. Information technology has become deeply imbricated into the management structure of the health care enterprise. We now rely on information systems to record and monitor care, generate bills, and schedule patient flow. Data are generated that allow comparisons of program and provider efficiency and regulation of work and productivity. Managed care activities and the position of third parties as care managers are strengthened by the ready availability of information, which facilitates the monitoring and oversight of practice. Algorithms and decision trees provide digital wisdom in the form of practice guidelines and disease management profiles that create a facade of empiricism based on normative judgments.

Nor is health care free from the effects of market worship. Under the guise of managed competition, wealth is diverted from the health care enterprise to the owners of capital assets and to the new managerial elites. The consolidations of industry are mirrored in the health care arena's merger and acquisition frenzy and "partnering" to realize the advantages and pleasures of horizontal or vertical integration. Industry's reengineering is health care's "operations improvement." Whether regarded as "downsizing" or "right sizing," both are activities where jobs are lost, more skilled technical employees are replaced by "team players" supported by sophisticated information systems, and the endless quest for productivity increments, dollar savings, and profitability is reinforced. Thus are the issues in the larger world of work replicated in the work world of health care.

MANAGED MENTAL HEALTH CARE: LESSONS LEARNED AND QUESTIONS RAISED

The introduction of information technology, managed care, and managed competition are not onerous changes in and of themselves. There is nothing intrinsically wrong in wanting to limit cost, to increase efficiency, or to enhance accountability. As the articles in this issue of the ARCHIVES suggest, the effects of change are frequently complex, often inconsistent, at times paradoxical, but usually measurable, and always enlightening.

One series of studies in the current issue of the ARCHIVES[9-11] tells an interesting and instructive story about the interaction of primary and behavioral health care within a managed care context. The story begins by placing the magnitude of the problem in an epidemiological, clinical, and economic framework by documenting the prevalence of mental disorders and subthreshold conditions in a variety of primary care settings, its impact on health status, impairment, and disability, and the added costs that undiagnosed and untreated mental disorders bring to the primary care endeavor. At the same time, it alerts us to important differences in practice patterns among professions that hold import for decisions concerning the organization and staffing of behavioral health care services within a managed care context.[12]

A theme running through several articles in this issue is the ubiquity of depression and the extent to which it is often undiagnosed and/or inadequately treated.[9,11,13,14] The studies add to our appreciation of the effectiveness of diagnostic and therapeutic interventions, but leave us perplexed at the desultory pace of knowledge transfer. As we review these articles that seek ways to enhance the detection of mental disorders in primary care settings and "fold" behavioral interventions into the therapeutic armamentarium of primary care physicians, we can only wonder about next steps. If our ultimate goal is to expedite the translation of lessons learned and relearned into practice patterns, what exactly is it that requires "fixing"? Is the flaw in how we organize and finance care (the system), where we provide care (the setting), how we deliver care (the physician-patient relationship), the protagonists themselves, or the interaction among these factors?

A second series of articles in this issue of the ARCHIVES[15-17] tell a cautionary tale. They suggest that there is still much to learn about the utility and benefits of "carve-in" vs "carve-out" approaches for dealing with special-needs populations. Managed mental health care carve-outs are big business. As states move to managed medicaid, they are becoming even bigger business. The data from Massachusetts documented significant savings in overall mental health care costs with managed care.[17] When one focuses more narrowly and looks at a specific disorder, in this case schizophrenia, a mixed picture emerges. Although modest cost savings and a decrease in the number of patients hospitalized are reported, the number of individuals without follow-up care after an inpatient episode is higher, as are inpatient readmission rates. This finding reminds us of the different origins of public and private sector case management.[18,19] The former originated as a valuable treatment adjunct aimed at coordinating the care provided to patients with serious and persistent mental illness; the latter originated as an administrative procedure intended to enhance productivity and contain costs. Thus, the approaches differ in their essential foci, resource acquisition vs efficiency.

The finding that treating patients with serious and persistent mental illness in health maintenance organizations[16] imposes significant expenditures in a risk-sharing situation while still requiring access to state and community mental health services leads us to contemplate a host of other issues such as the role of government as purchaser vs provider, the efficacy of the private vs public sector as provider of last resort, and the impact of for-profit vs not-for-profit status on service delivery. It should not be forgotten that the public sector, historically responsible for serving the patients with serious and persistent mental illness and forced to live within limited budgets, has pioneered clinical innovations that include inpatient diversion programs, assertive community treatment, and aggressive case management.

In a somewhat different vein, the imponderables associated with standardizing care are illustrated by a study by Zhang et al[20] of cost benefit in extending routine monitoring for agranulocytosis in patients with schizophrenia treated with clozapine (Clozaril).[20] While the example is of a psychotropic medication, the findings speak very much to the importance of considering standards from a longitudinal, not cross-sectional, perspective. As knowledge accumulates, changes in practice should occur. As practices change, the standards by which they are judged must change as well. The study also points to the limitations of standardization and the importance of disclosure in evaluating and interpreting practice guidelines and assessing standard setting processes. Parenthetically, it is intriguing that a protocol established by a pharmaceutical firm as part of a marketing strategy for a useful but somewhat dangerous drug became standardized and largely superseded the normative judgment of clinicians.

The cautionary tale in the second series of studies relates to the question of whether an unregulated market provides a suitable environment for dealing with a population of unremitting need and with potentially catastrophic associated costs. The answer is still, at best, a "yes/no/maybe" matter. It is a question that requires further evaluation from perspectives that take into account more than simple efficiencies and productivity.[21]

THE ROOTS OF MANAGED CARE AND MANAGED COMPETITION

Whether or not managed care and managed competition prove to be transient phenomena, they have altered the world of work by introducing new principles and novel technologies into medical practice. But what catalyzed these changes?

During the quarter century following World War II, health care and mental health care policies were geared toward correcting inequalities in the nation's health care system. As government became more expansive and struggled with identifying an appropriate role in providing for services, policy formulation was largely guided by the premise in Aristotle's *Politics* that

> health of mind and body is so fundamental to the good life that if a person has any right as a citizen, then he has an absolute moral right to such a measure of good health as society and society alone is able to provide. . . .

The view of health as a basic human right proved to be a concept of enormous subjective force. Availability and accessibility became the sine qua non of a health care policy that gave priority on the basis of need—not personal circumstance or income. In pursuit of these goals, the rate setting structure that was put in place facilitated the recovery of financing, construction, and acquisition costs. A direct effect of this policy was to encourage hospitals and the health care industry to improve their capital plant and to invest in technological innovation. Federal initiatives in the areas of education and training and of research and development increased the size of the manpower pool, encouraged the growth of the medical specialties and subspecialties, and gave a powerful impetus to high-tech medicine. At the service delivery level, the passage of the Medicare and Medicaid acts in 1963 established a cost-based pattern of reimbursement. To obtain the support of organized medicine, the Medicare and Medicaid amendments to the Social Security Act emphasized direct payment for service. As major private insurers came to accept the principles of cost-based reimbursement and fee-for-service compensation, the health care system in this country was reshaped.

The sum of these changes was a huge increase in the capacity of the health care sector, a surge in demand, and the corollary, rising costs. Between the late 1940s and the present, the health care sector's share of the gross domestic product increased almost 3-fold, from 5% to 14%. Today, we spend more of our gross domestic product on health care than any other nation. As a nation, we spend more on health care than we do on defense.

Many factors have been implicated as catalysts of what some uncharitably view as the unholy triad of health profligacy: capacity, demand, and expense.[22,23] Hospitals and practitioners increased in number. The nursing home industry mushroomed. There was an explosion in the development of medical devices and pharmaceuticals. In all of this, the monetarization of health care was central. The unregulated fee-for-service and cost reimbursement approaches used to finance health care lacked the constraints that could discipline spending. Thus, they contributed further to monetarizing practice.

Interestingly, the usual market relationships did not seem to apply to health care. Take, for example, the relationship between income and productivity. In the face of "excess" numbers of subspecialists, hours worked went down but income remained stable or increased. Patient expectations undoubtedly played a role in the market aberrations. Patients had come to expect patterns of practice that emphasize specialty care and access to the most sophisticated and current diagnostic and therapeutic procedures and therapies available. The aging of the population, the flowering of high technology, administrative procedures, defensive medical practice secondary to the malpractice threat, the surge in wages, and cost shifting among patients and providers all contributed to burgeoning costs. The fallout was a rise in health care expenditures that, until recently, exceeded the annual growth of expenditures for other goods and services by more than 2%.

Because health care expenditures are factored into the costs of any product that our nation sells, it became axiomatic for much of the business community to view the seemingly uncontrollable growth of the health care sector as compromising the nation's competitive position by sapping its economic vitality and jeopardizing its balance of trade. Government, on the other hand, became increasingly preoccupied at the extent to which the health care expenditures had come to command a disproportionate share of resources at the expense of other social goods, ie, education, social welfare, or corrections. Additionally, a growing alienation between "we the people" and our leaders has fostered a distrust of and frustration with government that complicates statecraft to a point where it becomes increasingly difficult to balance the needs of the many against the needs of the few.

THE IMPLICATIONS OF CHANGE

We have moved from an era that seemed more predictable from the perspective of security of employment and earnings to a time of economic anxiety and uncertainty. Forces such as unions and regulatory authorities that previously contested social inequity and economic inequality have been weakened and are far less robust in their pursuit of a universal as opposed to individual good. Social issues have taken a backseat to monetary issues. The public has become cautious about pursuing a course of action that may significantly disadvantage them economically.

The ideological positions of groups that Reinhardt[24] dubbed "pure egalitarians" and "food people" conditions the debate over health care reform. By defining the extremes, the pure egalitarians and food people establish the boundaries of the discussion. Pure egalitarians are the most catholic of the health rights advocates. For them, health care is a social good supported by each according to his or her means, and available to each according to his or her needs. As such, financing is through mandatory contributions that are based on the ability to pay, and availability is on equal terms to all members of society.

Food people, on the other hand, are the most orthodox market worshipers—priests of the marketplace. For them, health care is a commodity not unlike a television set or a car. Beyond a threshold of care provided the poor and near poor, the right and obligation to dictate the timeliness, choose the quantity, and decide on the quality of services they desire are individual matters. Choice is constrained only by the resources people have available to them.

The professions' role in the debate has been muted. In part, this is a function of the corporatization of health care; in part, of the dramatic shift in the perception of medicine as profession.[22,25-27] Starr[26] identified the well-established beginnings of corporatization in 1982. The monetarization of medicine spurred the formation of physician groups and networks that functioned more easily as corporate entities. Additionally, the for-profit sector saw opportunity in the health care arena as the capacity of medicine to generate profit increased. Where there is profit to be made, those who have mastered the art will seek to gain. Companies that can efficiently run hotel services, feed hundreds of individuals, and oversee complex financial empires seemed ideally suited for administering hospitals, nursing homes, or managed care firms. As the corporatization of health care and the commercialization of medicine became dominating principles, entities once regarded as services having economic components came to be seen primarily as businesses.

Accompanying monitarization and corporatization were trends toward specialization, high-tech medicine, and health care of a more impersonal nature. These changes recast the image of physicians. Today, we are less likely to be depicted as masterful artisans or skilled scientists. The more likely caricature will be of a mundane technocrat, or worse, an avaricious philistine. An accusation of cupidity carries with it the implication that physicians speak mostly out of self-interest. To the extent that our pronouncements are viewed as self-serving, our interests are suspect. For many, a profession's primary investment is seen as protecting the status quo within a field and maintaining an established standard of living for its members. The perception carries with it a healthy skepticism about the capacity of a profession to act as a change agent committed to modifying the service delivery system in ways that could potentially diminish its station.

The muted voice of the professions also bespeaks a heightened tension between physicians and managers. As the practice of medicine moves into organized settings and institutions, physicians are more likely to be regarded as employees. We practice within hierarchical settings where efficiency is maximized through the concentration of expertise, skill, and authority in the hands of senior managers. Managers rather than peers define the scope of work. The setting itself limits autonomy and minimizes collegiality. By accentuating gatekeeping rather than care-giving functions, downplaying health care advocacy responsibilities, and imposing guidelines with no appreciation of the verity, "a cookbook is not a cook," the managerial mentality seeks to deprofessionalize medicine and transform physicians into medical mercenaries.

RESPONSE FROM LEADERSHIP

Today, the physician no longer occupies center stage as the arbiter of health care. The nature of Aesculapian authority, which grants the healer the right to probe human minds and bodies in ways permitted to no one else, has been modified by the changing roles of professionals, the growth of the market economy, and the development of an increasingly informed populace. Today's consumers and purchasers are more inclined to question the care provided and are more insistent that the effects live up to the claims. Changing economic circumstances and shifting public attitudes now support a host of initiatives that are aimed at altering traditional patterns of care, increasing cost consciousness, and redefining the nature of the relationship among patients, providers, and purchasers. To the extent that control over the substance of its work is the defining characteristic of a profession, as Freidson[28] argues, then the threat of one's work being other-directed rather than self-directed challenges the profession's integrity and threatens its unique occupational status. In meeting this challenge, it is imperative that we speak, not out of guild or personal interest, but in support of change that is aimed at meeting the basic health care needs of all Americans. If medicine is to play a meaningful role in the debate, it must challenge the notion of health care as a market-driven commodity and offer in its stead an alternative vision.

The first step in articulating the vision is a return to the Aristotelian view of societal obligation and of health care as a social good. Some would have us believe that universal health care and prodigality are one and the same. That need not be the case. Advocating the right to that measure of health that society and society alone can provide is neither inconsistent nor incompatible with applying lessons learned from managed care and managed competition to achieve productivity gains and introduce pricing restraint. Indeed, care management as the arbiter of need and ombudsman of quality could very well be the centerpiece of an emergent health status–driven as opposed to market-driven vision.

Disclosure and an informed populace and consumer are also essential in expounding an alternative vision. Maintaining the public trust demands that patients be informed of any limits imposed on benefits and services, on provider selection, and on access to the information necessary for them to make informed choices about available diagnostic and treatment options. It is public interest, not proprietary interests, that should determine provider and purchaser access to the who and how of criteria and standard development, to the actual criteria and standards, and to the rules governing how they will be used in making decisions that pertain to patients, procedures, practice settings, and providers. Public interest also demands that the patient and the purchaser have access to data on patterns of care, treatment outcomes, and patient satisfaction.

As information is shared, one must guard against standardization of practice becoming an end in and of itself. Current conceptions of acceptable care are limited by extant knowledge. In the 18th century, for example, adequate psychiatric practice involved bleeding and purging, spinning patients rapidly in revolving chairs, and alternating hot and cold baths. As knowledge accumulates and practices change, standards by which care is judged must also change. Hence, it is imperative that the vision must strive to preserve innovation. This involves strengthening the biomedical research infrastructure and enlarging the talent pool on which it relies. It also entails ensuring that the criteria and standards used in care management are regarded merely as a framework for examining practices, and not as dogma reifying today's practices at the cost of tomorrow's innovations. The constituency in support of innovation is broad. As Ginsberg[29] points out, Americans and American medicine are committed to translating advances in medical knowledge and techniques into improved diagnostic, therapeutic, and rehabilitative procedures.

At the heart of the matter, however, is the need to reaffirm the social contract between government and the people. We are neither, as the Roman elite would have had it, a citizenry easily bought off by "bread and circus" nor a herd that sees *Soylent Green* as an apocalyptic alternative. The reaffirmation may very well require that federal and state governments use their statutory authority to support the right of all citizens to satisfactory health care. Governmental oversight can be vital in ensuring the availability, accessibility, appropriateness, and adequacy of care, while its regulatory prerogatives can be employed to put in place relevant disclosure and unbiased appeal processes. Equitable pricing by both the providers of health care and the suppliers of services and goods to the health care industry can be achieved through the prudent exercise of the massive purchasing power of federal, state, and local governments. In all of this, we would hope that the effort is guided by an appreciation of the complexity of the problem tempered by reason and compassion.

Gary L. Tischler, MD
Boris M. Astrachan, MD
Department of Psychiatry
University of Illinois
912 S Wood St
Chicago, IL 60612

REFERENCES

1. Uchitelle L, Kleinfield NR. On the battlefield of business: millions of casualties. *The New York Times.* March 3, 1996;145(50335):1, 14-17.
2. Kleinfield NR. The company as family: no more. *The New York Times.* March 4, 1996;145(50356): 1, A8-A10.
3. Bragg R. Big holes where the dignity used to be. *The New York Times.* March 5, 1996;145 (50357):1, A8-A10.
4. Rimer S. A hometown feels less like home. *The New York Times.* March 6, 1996;145(50358):1, A8-A10.
5. Johnson K. In the class of 70: wounded winners. *The New York Times.* March 7, 1996;145 (50359):1, A12-A14.
6. Kolbert E. Clymer A. The politics of layoffs: in search of a message. *The New York Times.* March 8, 1996;145(50360):1, A12-A13.
7. Saeger DE, Lorh S. A search of answers to avoid the layoffs. *The New York Times.* March 9, 1996; 145(50361):1, 10-11.
8. Head S. The new ruthless economy. *The New York Review of Books.* February 29, I996;43:47-52.
9. Olfson M, Broadhead WE, Weissman, MM, Leon AC, Farber L, Hoven C, Kathol R. Subthreshold psychiatric symptoms in a primary care group practice. *Arch Gen Psychiatry.* 1996;53:880-886.
10. Sherbourne CD, Wells KB, Meredith LS, Jackson CA, Camp P. Comorbid anxiety disorder and the functioning and well-being of chronically ill patients of general medical providers. *Arch Gen Psychiatry.* 1996;53:889-895.
11. Henk HJ, Katzelnick DJ, Kobak KA, Greist JH, Jefferson JW. Medical costs attributed to depression among patients with a history of high medical expenses in a health maintenance organization. *Arch Gen Psychiatry.* 1996;53:899-904.
12. Meredith LS, Wells KB, Kaplan SH, Mazel RM. Counseling typically provided for depression: role of clinician specialty and payment system. *Arch Gen Psychiatry.* 1996;53:905-912.
13. Schulberg HC, Block MR, Madonia MJ. Scott CP, Rodriguez E, Imber SD, Perel J, Lave J. Houck PR, Coulehan JL. Treating major depression in primary care practice: eight-month clinical outcomes. *Arch Gen Psychiatry.* 1996;53:913-919.
14. Katon W, Robinson P, Von Korff M, Lin E, Bush T, Ludman E, Simon G, Walker E. A multifaceted intervention to improve treatment of depression in primary care. *Arch Gen Psychiatry.* 1996;53:924-932.
15. Frank RG. Huskamp HA, McGuire TG, Newhouse JP. Some economics of mental health 'carve-outs.' *Arch Gen Psychiatry.* 1996;53:933-937.
16. McFarland BH, Johnson RE, Hornbrook MC. Enrollment duration, service use, and costs of care for severely mentally ill members of a health maintenance organization. *Arch Gen Psychiatry.* 1996;53:938-944.
17. Dickey B, Normand S-LT, Norton EC, Azeni H, Fisher M, Altaffer F. Managing the care of schizophrenia: lessons from a 4-year Massachusetts Medicaid study. *Arch Gen Psychiatry.* 1996;53: 945-952.
18. Unutzer J, Tischler GL. The many faces of managed care. In: Moscarelli M, Rupp A, Sartorius N, eds. *Handbook of Mental Health Economics and Health Policy.* London, England: John Wiley & Sons Inc; 1996;1:42:493-502.
19. Sledge WH, Astrachan B, Thompson K, Rakfeldt J, Leaf P. Case management in psychiatry: an analysis of tasks. *Am J Psychiatry.* 1995;152: 9:1259-1265.
20. Zhang M, Owen RR, Pope SK, Smith GR. Cost-effectiveness of clozapine monitoring after the first 6 months. *Arch Gen Psychiatry.* 1996;53: 954-958.
21. Tischler GL. Utilization management and the quality of care. *Hosp Community Psychiatry.* 1990; 41:10:1099-1102.
22. Docherty JP. Myths and mystification of managed care. *J Ment Health Administration.* 1990; 17:138-144.
23. Tischler GL. Utilization management of mental health services by private third parties. *Am J Psychiatry.* 1990;147:8:967-973.
24. Reinhardt UE. Turning our gaze from bread and circus games. *Health Aff.* 1994;14:1:33-36.
25. Tenery RM. Socialized care wrong? 'corporatized' not much better. *American Medical News.* April 1, 1996;39(13):17.
26. Starr P. *The Social Transformation of American Medicine.* New York, NY: Basic Books Inc Publishers; 1982.
27. Stevens R. *In Sickness and In Wealth: American Hospitals in the Twentieth Century.* New York, NY: Basic Books Inc Publishers; 1989.
28. Freidson E. *Profession of Medicine: A Study of the Sociology of Applied Knowledge.* New York, NY: Dodd Mead & Co; 1970.
29. Ginsberg E. High-tech medicine and rising health care costs. *JAMA.* 1990;263:1820-1822.

TPH Replication Study: Not!

We reported a population association between a tryptophan hydroxylase (*TPH*) intron 7 polymorphism with suicidal behavior in Finnish alcoholic offenders and with cerebral spinal fluid 5-hydroxyindoleacetic acid concentration in impulsive offenders.[1] Abbar et al[2] found no association between a different *TPH* polymorphism and suicidal behavior in a clinically and ethnically divergent sample. Our *TPH* association was presented as a preliminary result requiring replication. However, the study by Abbar et al[2] has little relevance to the validity of the association we observed. They used a different, unpublished *TPH* marker to genotype both women and men who were undergoing psychiatric care and who had a dissimilar and mixed diagnostic profile and a different ethnic background. Therefore, the assertion by Abbar et al of a "discrepancy" between their and our results has no basis.

The *Ava* II restriction fragment length polymorphism used by Abbar et al[2] is distinct from the intron 7 marker (D.A.N., unpublished data, 1996), and the strength of the linkage disequilibrium with the intron 7 polymorphism is unknown. When Abbar et al report their typing method, the disequilibrium can be determined.

According to Abbar et al,[2] of the 62 patients who attempted suicide, only 17 had alcohol abuse or dependence; only 8 had antisocial personality disorder. Most of the patients (42 of the 62) had a mood disorder. Our sample comprised 20 control subjects and 70 patients. All of the patients were alcoholic, 28 had antisocial personality disorder, 27 had intermittent explosive disorder, and 1 had conduct disorder.[1] Genetic influences on suicidal behavior may not perfectly overlap between alcoholic, antisocial patients and depressed patients. Data from the Abbar et al article indicated that the patients who attempted suicide and who had antisocial personality disorder diagnosed had an increased frequency of the more common *Ava* II allele, which was contrary to the other diagnostic groups. This may be analogous to our original observation.

We compared alcoholic Finnish offenders who had a history of suicide attempts with alcoholic offenders without such a history. However, Abbar et al[2] reanalyzed our data using our CEPH (Centre d'Etude du Polymorphisme Humain) and Swedish control subjects, although they warn, "Stratification bias has been seen when the selection of patients and controls was inappropriate." Stratification bias may have resulted from their inappropriate comparison.

Because of founder effects and genetic drift, Finns are genetically distinct. Certain allele frequencies in Finns differ from other populations. As correctly understood by Abbar et al,[2] the intron 7 allele frequencies in the other populations we evaluated are similar in Finns. However, this tells us nothing about the frequencies of unknown variants. A functional variant or variants would have to exist at or close to the *TPH* gene if the intron 7 marker association is valid because the intron 7 polymorphism is unlikely to alter function (D.A.N., unpublished data, 1996). It would be erroneous to assume that the frequency of an unknown variant or its linkage disequilibrium relationships are conserved across populations.

Abbar et al[2] believe that our data indicate that offenders with the *TPH U* allele are protected against suicidal behavior. This significant difference was the reason we originally reported the association of the *L* allele with suicidal behavior in alcohol offenders ($P=.02$).[1] Abbar et al[2] believe that we are incorrect in stating that the *U* allele was associated with suicidal behavior:

Population Association Between Tryptophan Hydroxylase Genotype and History of Suicide Attempts

	History of Suicide Attempts					
	Impulsive		Nonimpulsive		All Violent Offenders	
Variable	With, No. (%)	Without, No.	With, No. (%)	Without, No.	With, No. (%)	Without, No.
Genotype*						
UU	2 (22)	7	0 (0)	3	2 (17)	10
UL	18 (58)	13	1 (20)	4	19 (53)	17
LL	11 (69)	5	4 (67)	2	15 (65)	7
P†	.07		.09		.02	
Total	**31**	**25**	**5**	**9**	**36**	**34**
U allele frequency	0.35	0.54	0.10	0.56	0.32	0.54

*Genotype was determined as described by Nielsen et al.[3]
†Probabilities were calculated with the Pearson χ^2 test.

"... violent offenders who have a *TPH U* allele are protected against suicidal behaviors." They also note, "If confirmed, this may indicate that *TPH* is a protective gene against suicidal behaviors." We are confused by the discussion by Abbar et al of "protective" vs "nonprotective." A gene could be described as protective or as nonprotective. However, if one allele of a gene is described as protective, then the other allele (by symmetry) is nonprotective. Thus, the assertions that the *U* allele is protective and that the *L* allele is nonprotective are equivalent, and nothing can be disagreed with or corrected.

We thank Abbar et al[2] for identifying an error in our Table 2. All of the data in this table are correct; however, the calculated *U* allele frequencies were transposed. We apologize for this error and for any resulting inconvenience. The *U* allele frequencies were reported correctly throughout the text. Our conclusions were based on the actual data and not on the transposed allele frequencies in this table, as suggested.[2] A corrected version of the table is included for clarification (**Table**).

Again, we apologize for the transposed *U* allele frequencies in the published version of Table 2. We thank Abbar et al[2] for acknowledging that our data showed that alcoholic offenders with the *TPH U* allele may be protected against suicidal behavior. We reiterate that the article by Abbar et al was not a replication study for the *TPH* intron 7 association with suicidal behavior in Finnish alcoholic offenders, despite assertions to the contrary.

David A. Nielsen, PhD
David Goldman, MD
Laboratory of Neurogenetics
Division of Intramural Clinical and Biological Research
National Institute on Alcohol Abuse and Alcoholism
Flow Building, Room 2
12501 Washington Ave
Rockville, MD 20852

Matti Virkkunen, MD
Riitta Tokola, MD
Helsinki, Finland

Robert Rawlings, MS
Markku Linnoila, MD, PhD
Bethesda, Md

1. Nielsen DA, Goldman D, Virkkunen M, Tokola R, Rawlings R, Linnoila M. Suicidality and 5-hydroxyindoleacetic acid concentration associated with a tryptophan hydroxylase polymorphism. *Arch Gen Psychiatry*. 1994;51:34-38.
2. Abbar A, Courtet P, Amadéo S, Caer Y, Mallet J, Baldy-Moulinier M, Castelnau D, Malafosse A. Suicidal behavior and the tryptophan hydroxylase gene. *Arch Gen Psychiatry*. 1995;52:846-849.
3. Nielsen DA, Dean M, Goldman D. Genetic mapping of the human tryptophan hydroxylase gene on chromosome 11 using an intronic conformational polymorphism. *Am J Hum Genet*. 1992;51:1366-1371.

Physician Recruitment

Psychiatry
Multiple Specialties/Group Practice
Locum Tenens Wanted
Graduate Training/Residencies/Fellowships
Chiefs/Department Heads/Directors
Academic/Faculty
CME Corner
Courses/Symposia/Seminars
Practices For Sale
Notices

1996 Professional Opportunity Rates

Regular	1x 1.60/wd	*3x 1.45/wd
Bold	1x 1.75/wd	*3x 1.60/wd

*In order to receive the 3 time frequency price, the request must be made upon initial placement. The minimum charge is 20 words. A word consists of one or more letters surrounded by space on each side.

For information on display advertising and our network buys contact an account representative.

Policy

Orders for classified advertising must be submitted in writing. Although the American Medical Association believes the classified advertisements in these pages to be from reputable sources, the Association does not investigate the offers made and assumes no liability concerning them. Acceptance of advertising is restricted to professional opportunities, practices for sale, and medical office space available. The Association reserves the right to decline, withdraw, or edit advertisements at its discretion. Every care is taken to avoid mistakes but responsibility cannot be accepted by the Association for clerical or printer's errors.

Reply Box Service

Confidential box numbers are available for an additional $20 per issue, plus the words: Box ____, c/o AGNP.

When responding to a box number, please send to Archives of General Psychiatry, Box ____, c/o AGNP, 515 N State St, Chicago, IL 60610.

Cancellations/Changes

Cancellations/changes must be received in writing ar least 25 days prior to the date of the issue. In order to expedite, please fax to 312-464-5909 to the attention of your account representative.

General Information

To contact a Physician Recruitment Advertising account representative, call 312-464-2475/2490/2491/4485 or **800-AMA-2260**. Or fax your insertion order to **312-464-5909**. Mail your materials to **AMA Physician Recruitment Advertising, 12th Floor, 515 N State St, Chicago, IL 60610.**

Psychiatry

WISCONSIN, LA CROSSE: Franciscan Skemp Healthcare, Mayo Health System, an integrated delivery network with more than 130-physicians at eleven sites and serving a primary care population base of 350,000, seeks a BC residency trained psychiatrist to serve as Clinical Director of Behavioral Health Services. Responsibilities include providing clinical direction for all behavioral health services, working collaboratively on strategic planning and operations and developing and improving managed care expertise in behavioral health. General psychiatric clinical positions are also available and would include a mix of inpatient and outpatient care. Outpatient behavioral health services are offered at several sites and include chemical dependency care and eating disorders clinic. Inpatient services are available at the main campus in La Crosse and include psychiatric, chemical dependency, adolescent care. Various residential services are available. La Crosse, 52,000 population, located in scenic Mississippi River bluff country, offers numerous year-round outdoor activities, ideal family-oriented environment and excellent public and private schools. Healthcare and higher education are our two largest industries. Contact Tim Skinner, or Bonnie Nulf, Franciscan Skemp Healthcare, 700 West Avenue South, La Crosse, WI 54601, 800-269-1986 or 608-791-9844; fax 608-791-9898.

NEAR TWIN CITIES: Community psychiatry with emphasis on child and adolescent populations. Practice offers highly qualified colleagues, a multidisciplined approach, beautiful facilities, competitive salary, and benefit programs. Community offers impressive growth, good school choices, convenient access to the Twin Cities, many nearby lakes, and safe neighborhoods. Contact Verne Meyer, 1-800-967-2711, fax 320-587-7252 or delacore.hutchtel.net.

TEXAS, the SOUTHEAST, and the SUNBELT STATES- There are Excellent Private Practice Opportunities Available in Family Practice/General Practice (both Solo and Group Openings). Major Cities and Rural Communities Are Available.

Call 1-800-284-4560/Houston 713-493-2797

Or send CV to:
P.O. Box 42314
Houston, TX 77242-2314
FAX 713-493-2234

Reuben Bronstein & Associates

Locum Tenens Wanted

HKA LOCUM TENENS is looking for quality multiple specialty physicians to do Locum Tenens. We have opportunities coast-to-coast. We furnish Occurence Malpractice Insurance (no tail necessary). Please call **HKA LOCUM TENENS at (800)226-6347, Extension AM7.1.**

© 1995 MAILSTAR

For more **Professional Opportunities** please refer to the Physician Recruitment sections in ***JAMA*** and ***AMNews.***

Graduate Training/Residencies/Fellowships

FELLOWSHIP IN SLEEP DISORDERS MEDICINE: Mayo Clinic, Rochester, Minnesota, offers a one-year fellowship in sleep disorders medicine. Open to physicians who have finished an approved training program in pulmonary medicine, neurology, or psychiatry. Clinical experience in all aspects of adult sleep disorders medicine is provided, as well as ample time for research. Our center sees about 2,000 new patients per year. Stipend $31,000-$35,000, depending on training. For information, call Peter J. Hauri, PhD 507-266-6885. To apply, contact Ms Renee Ziemer Mayo Graduate School of Medicine, Siebens 5, 200 First Street, SW, Rochester, MN 55905, 507-284-3126. Deadline for completed application December 20th of each year.

Academic/Faculty

FACULTY POSITION IN PSYCHIATRIC NEUROIMAGING RESEARCH: The University of North Carolina School of Medicine at Chapel Hill is seeking candidates for a tenured (or tenure track) faculty position to provide leadership in neuroimaging research for the Department of Psychiatry and the Mental Health and Neuroscience Clinical Research Center. Candidates should have an MD or PHD, postdoctoral training in psychiatry or psychology together with expertise in morphologic/morphometric and/or functional magnetic resonance imaging and spectroscopy and a documented record of accomplishment in the area of psychosis and/or affective disorders research. The successful candidate will work in collaboration with a team of MHCRC investigators from both the University of North Carolina and Duke University, and will be expected to obtain support to develop his or her independent research as well. Faculty appointment and salary will be commensurate with the candidate's level of experience and accomplishment. Interested applicants should send a curriculum vitae, statement of research interests and three letters of reference to Jeffrey A. Lieberman, MD, Vice Chairman, Department of Psychiatry, Chair of Search Committee, Campus Box #7160, University of North Carolina School of Medicine, Chapel Hill, NC 27599-7160. The search will be continued until the successful candidate is found.

Announcement

Conference on Alcohol and Family Violence

The fourth annual conference of Physicians for a Violence-free Society, "Alcohol: Fuel for Family Violence?" will be held February 7 through 9, 1997, in San Francisco, Calif. Physicians, nurses, other health care providers, social workers, counselors, substance-abuse professionals, and policy makers will attend. The conference program will explore the complex relationship between family violence and alcohol abuse. Continuing medical education credit is available.

For information and registration, write JoAnn Dwyer, LMSW–ACP, Physicians for a Violence-free Society, PO Box 35528, Dallas, TX 75235-0528; or call (214) 590-8807; fax (214) 590-4079.

THIS MONTH IN ARCHIVES OF GENERAL PSYCHIATRY

Genetic factors play a significant etiologic role in autism, but how autism is inherited is still unanswered. **Hallmayer et al** (page 985) studied 38 families with at least 2 siblings with autism and tested the possibility that a gene that causes susceptibility to autism is located on the X chromosome. Although the study excluded any moderate to strong gene effect on the X chromosome, smaller gene effects could not be excluded.

Brain serotonin function may be altered in some patients with autistic disorder. **McDougle et al** (page 993) determined in autistic adults that rapidly lowered levels of tryptophan, an esential amino acid and precursor of serotonin, resulted in a significant increase in behaviors characteristic of autism, including whirling, hand flapping, pacing, banging and hitting self, rocking, and toe walking. The patients are also less calm and happy and more anxious following depletion. Future studies might include the acute tryptophan depletion test in children and adolescents with autism to study the influence of brain development on serotonin function.

In the first double-blind study of autistic adults to date, **McDougle et al** (page 1001) report that fluvoxamine maleate was more effective than placebo in reducing repetitive thoughts and behavior and aggression, as well as improving some aspects of social behavior, particularly language usage. The drug was well tolerated, with mild sedation and nausea described in only a few patients. Controlled studies of fluvoxamine and other selective serotonin uptake inhibitors are needed to determine the safety and effectiveness of these drugs in children and adolescents with this disorder.

Shafii et al (page 1009) found that levels of nocturnal serum melatonin in depressed youth was significantly higher than in healthy controls. Depressed youth without psychosis had much higher melatonin levels than the controls, whereas those with psychosis had lower levels. Dysregulation of the pineal gland involving increased or decreased levels of nocturnal serum melatonin might be related to various subtypes of depression among children and adolescents.

Kendler et al (page 1022) found that using a computer algorithm and a senior clinician to assess nonaffective psychosis in the National Comorbidity Survey resulted in estimated lifetime prevalences of 2.2% and 0.7%, respectively. The clinician diagnosis of nonaffective psychosis was significantly associated with low income; unemployment; a marital status of single, divorced, or separated; and urban residence. Estimates of the prevalence of psychosis in community samples are strongly influenced by the method of assessment and diagnosis.

Can the origins of adult mental disorders be identified early in life in some persons? **Caspi et al** (page 1033) found that children who were undercontrolled at age 3 years were more likely at age 21 years to be diagnosed with antisocial personality and to be involved in crime; whereas inhibited children were more likely to be depressed as young adults. Both groups were more likely to attempt suicide compared with other children, and boys in both groups were more likely to develop problems. Early appearing behavioral styles may be persisting risk factors for some forms of psychopathologic functioning.

It is known that cigarette smoking is more common among those with depression and, conversely, that depression is more frequent among smokers. This raises the interesting question of what leads to associations between cigarette smoking and depression. **Fergusson et al** (page 1043) explore this issue using data gathered in a 16-year study of the development of depression and cigarette smoking in a large sample of young people in New Zealand. Their principal conclusion is that much of the correlation between cigarette smoking and depression arises because the risk factors associated with cigarette smoking overlap with those associated with depression.

Fletcher et al (page 1051) evaluated memory and attentional skills in younger and older groups of chronic cannabis users and nonusers in Costa Rica. Testing when the subjects were free of the acute effects of cannabis revealed poorer performance on measures of working memory and attentional skills only in the older chronic users. This field study cannot rule out all competing causes of the decrements in cognitive skills reported here, but the results do show an association between long-term use of cannabis and impairment of cognitive skills.

A "Commenary" on recent advances in autism research by P. Anne McBride, MD, George M. Anderson, PhD, and Theodore Shapiro, MD, is also included in this issue.

1960s: Conventional antipsychotics radically alter traditional treatment methods

Mass deinstitutionalization

Large-scale shutdown of mental hospitals

Concepts of patient-oriented psychosocial rehabilitation introduced

Discoveries in medicine impact the healthcare system at every level. If the effects of medical breakthroughs are not managed appropriately, the system can sustain significant damage. In the latter half of this century we have seen evidence of this in psychiatry. In the 1960s the introduction of conventional antipsychotics into a weak and rigid system caused severe and long-lasting problems. The advent of atypical agents in the 1990s threatens to do the same. How can we ensure that the existing mental healthcare system is flexible and strong enough to quickly adapt to the changes brought on by the atypicals?

Radical change wrought by conventionals.

The radical changes wrought by haloperidol and other conventional antipsychotics on the mental healthcare system are well documented. Before the introduction of these agents, patients generally experienced limited relief from their episodes of psychosis, and clinicians had few treatment options at their disposal. Conventional antipsychotics offered the first glimmer of hope by providing adequate control of positive symptoms. These agents brought a significant measure of calm and order to previously noisy and chaotic psychiatric wards.

Mass deinstitutionalization recognized as failure.

However, for a variety of social, economic, and political reasons, patients on conventional agents were deinstitutionalized before clinicians could design and implement rehabilitation programs to help them successfully reintegrate into the community. The failure of mass deinstitutionalization is now widely recognized. As all who work with the severely mentally ill know, the effect on many patients and their families has been tragic.

The advent of atypicals: dramatically raising expectations.

Analogous to the introduction of the conventional antipsychotics is the introduction of the atypical agents in the 1990s. Atypical agents, with their control of both positive and negative symptoms, have continued to raise patients' functioning to levels that facilitate reintegration back into the community.

Deficits of system limit potential for recovery.

The ability of the atypicals to restore significant patient functioning has served to highlight the flaws of the system. Often, patients on such therapies begin to outperform all functional expectations before the system is ready to help them develop their newly found skills and abilities.

Compounding the limitations of the mental healthcare system are outdated and misguided community and societal policies, attitudes, and beliefs. These severely restrict the opportunities available to a recovering patient.

System status quo unacceptable.

Clearly, the status quo of the mental healthcare system is unacceptable. Many inside and outside the system are devoted to changing the system, and some progress has been made. However, it is unfair to ask patients, who have already lost significant portions of their lives to mental illness, to wait any longer. Further, dedicated mental healthcare professionals must work within the confines of the system, and they cannot bridge the gaps alone. Finally, families and caregivers often shoulder the burden of providing what the system lacks—too often to the detriment of their own quality of life.

1990s:

Atypical antipsychotics dramatically raise expectations for recovery

Recognition of need to provide support to patient and family

Development of psychosocial rehabilitation programs

Emphasis on permanent reintegration of patients into community

A new approach to managing severe mental illness.

Comprehensive support at multiple levels would benefit patients, their families or caregivers, and professionals. One unique program has recently become available. PATHWAYS TO CHANGE™: managing severe mental illness, is a new comprehensive program of interdisciplinary interventions developed by Janssen Pharmaceutica in conjunction with premier thought leaders in the field. The stated goal of PATHWAYS TO CHANGE™ is to bridge the gaps in the system and raise the standard of care for all persons with severe mental illness.

PATHWAYS TO CHANGE™ is built around a framework known as the systems approach. According to the systems approach, although medication is the cornerstone of successful treatment, therapeutic interventions must occur at multiple levels beyond the adjustment of neuroreceptors for patients to become well, and remain well. Additional interventions must be implemented for patients with severe mental illness, their families and caregivers, the healthcare professionals who treat them, the communities in which they live, and society as a whole.

PATHWAYS TO CHANGE™ interventions.

Consistent with the systems approach model, PATHWAYS TO CHANGE™ interventions address the particular issues at each level that affect patients in their efforts to reach the full potential offered by innovative therapies.

- Following appropriate pharmacotherapy, interventions for patients include support to remain compliant, prevent relapse, maintain continuity of care, and help in their reintegration back into society
- Interventions for families, friends, or caregivers include facilitated access to information, education, and support groups
- Interventions for professionals are designed to help them surmount the challenges of the existing mental healthcare system through programs that enhance patient compliance and aid in patient discharge planning. Other programs will help facilitate case management, provide resources for information, and promote interprofessional collaboration
- Community and societal interventions are geared toward removing any barriers to reintegration. This is accomplished through support of patient advocacy organizations, public awareness, education, and antidiscrimination campaigns. An example of a societal-level intervention is NAMI's recently launched *Open Your Mind* campaign, for which Janssen Pharmaceutica is providing continuing support

It is only through support provided by these multilevel interventions that the patient with severe and persistent mental illness can successfully reintegrate into the community.

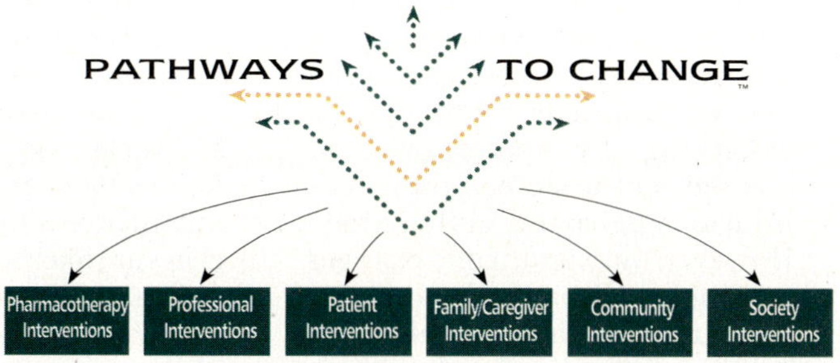

A comprehensive model of interdisciplinary interventions

Meeting the challenges of an evolving system.

We are experiencing an exciting and challenging revolution in the mental healthcare field. The pharmacologic breakthroughs we were waiting for have finally come, offering our patients the first real chance at reclaiming their lives. This revolution, however, is occurring in an atmosphere of cost-containment. We should be ever mindful to take full advantage of programs that provide comprehensive support to reintegrating patients. Indeed, such programs may become our most valuable tools as we meet the challenges of an evolving system.

JANSSEN · PHARMACEUTICA · RESEARCH FOUNDATION ·

JPI-RS-283 Printed in U.S.A. October 1996

COMMENTARY

Autism Research

Bringing Together Approaches to Pull Apart the Disorder

In this issue, 3 articles[1-3] present important results and extend the continuing effort to understand the biological bases of autistic disorder. The problems in this quest are not unique to autism but appear in only slightly altered form in investigations of every neuropsychiatric disorder. All of the authors have wrestled with the universal issues of syndrome definition, multiple symptom domains, clinical heterogeneity, neurochemical and pharmacological specificity, and the interpretation of behavioral responses seen during challenge and treatment protocols. These issues raise basic questions about how to approach a characterization of the etiology and pathophysiology of autism, as well as how to integrate data from diverse levels of inquiry including molecular genetics, developmental neurobiology, neuropathology, neurochemistry, neuropsychology, and clinical pharmacology. Strategies for future research will be considered following a review of the specific aims, methods, and findings of the 3 studies.

See also pages 985, 993, and 1001

The double-blind, placebo-controlled fluvoxamine trial reported by McDougle and colleagues[2] was an attempt to find a more effective, better-tolerated, and safer treatment for autism. The work was prompted by the promising results of pilot studies assessing the benefit of potent selective and nonselective serotonin reuptake inhibitors in the management of autistic individuals.[4,5] Consistent with these previous studies, fluvoxamine was found to reduce perseverative symptoms and aggression and to improve language use and general functioning. The authors emphasize that the results pertain only to adults and that they have observed untoward behavioral effects (irritability, agitation) in some children treated with serotonin reuptake inhibitors. The work follows a long-standing interest in a possible role for serotonin in autism, and is closely related to a second study[3] from the same group evaluating the behavioral effects of a reduction in the availability of the serotonin precursor tryptophan.

Autistic individuals who participated in the tryptophan depletion study received a tryptophan-free amino acid drink and a sham drink administered on consecutive weeks according to a double-blind, randomized, crossover design. Consumption of the tryptophan-free cocktail resulted in a reduction of the mean plasma tryptophan level to 14% of the baseline level. In a majority of subjects, tryptophan depletion was associated with a global worsening of symptoms, with increased motor stereotypies, self-injurious behavior, and anxiety. However, no significant changes were noted in social relatedness or repetitive thoughts and behaviors. Behavioral deterioration did not occur following administration of the sham drink, which actually resulted in a doubling of the mean plasma tryptophan level. McDougle and colleagues conclude that an acute reduction in tryptophan availability may exacerbate maladaptive behavior in some autistic adults, and that their findings provide further evidence of dysregulated serotonin function in autism. Critical to their argument is the assumption that the active treatment resulted in a decrease in brain tryptophan similar to that measured for plasma tryptophan, with at least some corresponding change in central serotonin synthesis and function.[6]

The third report, by Hallmayer and coworkers,[1] is an examination of the possible involvement of the X chromosome in autism. It is the first reported application of the sib-pair approach to the search for genetic influences in the disorder. The sib-pair approach is most easily conceptualized when affected brother-brother sibling pairs are studied for possible X-linked inheritance of a trait. For a given locus on the X chromosome, a male offspring can inherit either 1 of 2 possible alleles (or gene markers) from his mother's 2 X chromosomes. By chance, brothers would be expected to share X chromosome genes half of the time. If the rate of brother-brother sharing of markers is much above this chance rate, it indicates that that region of the chromosome may contain a susceptibility gene.

As discussed in the report, the sib-pair approach is particularly useful in situations where the mode of inheritance is unclear and multiple genes are likely to influence the syndrome under study. The greater the difference in risk for the disorder to siblings of probands compared with the general population, the greater the power of the method. The estimated 75-fold greater risk for autism among siblings of autistic probands is relatively large, making the approach especially powerful. A choice was made to focus on the X chromosome because of the male excess (3- to 4-fold) in autism. The results indicate that most of the X chromosome can be excluded from exerting more than a very slight effect on risk. However, the investigators did identify 1 region that might explain up to a 4-fold increase in risk to siblings of autistic individuals. Although the authors interpret these results as providing limited evidence for a gene of "minor" effect on the X chromosome, 3 or 4 such genes (each explaining up to a 4-fold increase in risk) could explain much or all of the estimated 75-fold increased risk.

The fluvoxamine treatment and tryptophan depletion studies are related to a long line of research on possible serotonergic alterations in autism. Many studies have found elevated levels of platelet serotonin in autistic patients[7,8] Two neuroendocrine challenge studies have suggested that central serotonergic responsivity may be reduced in autism.[9,10] Reports of differences in cerebrospinal fluid 5-hydroxyindoleacetic acid levels and the presence of autoantibodies to the serotonin-1_A receptor have not been replicated. In a more speculative fashion, the rich serotonergic enervation of the limbic cortex[11] and the neurotrophic effects of serotonin[12,13] have also suggested a potential role for the neurotransmitter in this developmental disorder, with its central aspect of altered social relatedness.

As pointed out by McDougle and coauthors,[2,3] there is ample evidence that serotonin is involved in the mediation of a range of behaviors and psychological processes, including mood, anxiety, obsessive-compulsive symptoms, aggression, impulsivity, sleep, and social interaction and affiliation.[14,15] It is striking that most, if not all, of these behavioral domains can be altered in autism. Thus, it is not surprising that serotonergic agents influence symptom expression in autistic patients. However, it is unclear to what extent serotonin is involved in the etiology or pathophysiology of the altered behavior. This is the case whether the behavior occurs as part of the autistic syndrome or in relative isolation, as in obsessive-compulsive disorder or an impulse-control disorder. A fundamental problem is determining whether a drug or challenge agent is affecting a primary or causal lesion, influencing part of the downstream pathophysiology, or serving to elicit (or inhibit) counterbalancing but unrelated processes. The problem is doubly complex: even in the unlikely event that an agent has direct effects on only 1 neurotransmitter system, the close interrelationships between neurotransmitters ensures that additional systems will be affected.[16,17]

In a related vein, serotonin reuptake inhibitors do not stand alone in their apparent ameliorating effects on autistic symptoms. Several controlled trials have shown benefit of dopamine antagonists, particularly haloperidol, in reducing social withdrawal, motor stereotypies, and maladaptive behaviors such as hyperactivity, aggression, and self-injurious acts.[18,19] The response rates seen for haloperidol are typically around 50%,[19] similar to the 53% positive response rate reported in this issue[2] for fluvoxamine. Furthermore, a considerable degree of variability is seen in the responses of autistic individuals to psychotropic medication, whether we consider effects on core autistic symptoms or associated behavioral problems. Clinical experience dictates that where 1 medication is unhelpful or produces untoward effects, another may bring significant symptomatic relief. Indeed, responses to classes of psychotropic medication may prove useful in defining subgroups of autistic individuals. Finally, caution is warranted in interpreting the results of early trials of promising medications. Witness the disappointment that followed initial enthusiasm for the indirect serotonin agonist fenfluramine, as reports of low success rates[20-22] and possible neurotoxicity[23,24] emerged. McDougle and colleagues underscore the need for controlled trials of fluvoxamine and other serotonin reuptake inhibitors in autistic children and adolescents; hopefully, additional studies in patients of all ages will firmly establish fluvoxamine as a safe and effective treatment.

The measurement of behavior in several different domains or along different dimensions is critical to the careful assessment of drug response or challenge effects in autism. It also raises the central question of whether the symptom domains of autism represent separate functional deficits. Reports of an increased prevalence of cognitive and social deficits, either alone or in combination, in the nonautistic relatives of autistic probands[25,26] suggest that the components can be considered individually. The increasing likelihood that multiple genes are involved in most cases of autism[26-29] provides additional support for thinking of autism as a multidimensional spectrum disorder.[30-33] Although there is some indication that the multiple symptom domains may arise from distinct deficits in brain functioning, the nature of their correspondence to basic etiologic alterations is not at all clear. One could hope, perhaps, that a one-to-one relationship might persist through the levels of symptomatology, pathophysiology, and etiology. However, the tendency for the symptom domains to cluster indicates some degree of interaction between components. And, as is the case in various neurological disorders, it is possible for multiple deficits (behavioral and neuropsychological) to arise from a single etiologic alteration. In turn, this alteration or abnormality could arise either from a single gene or through the interplay of several genes. Determining the levels and extent of the possible interactions poses a fundamental, complex, and critical problem.

More generally, arguments for a dimensional approach in studying the biology of psychiatric disorders have been made from clinical, neurobiological, and genetic perspectives. Van Praag[34] has emphasized the problems with an overly categorical approach to viewing clinical phenomena in studies of the neurochemistry of depression and related disorders. Quite similar conclusions are drawn by Cloninger[35] and others[36] when considering reasons for the difficulty in elucidating the genetics of schizophrenia and personality disorders. The earlier seminal studies of Rosenthal et al[37] would not have provided as compelling evidence of a hereditary contribution to schizophrenia if "schizophrenia spectrum disorders" had not been considered in addition to classic cases of the disorder. The dimensional approach permits simplification and quantification through the analysis of dissected components; it also can lead to more precise phenotypic subtyping.

Though the separate domains of autistic symptoms have been the object of considerable research, studies evaluating neurochemical markers, genetic linkage, and clinical interventions have made insufficient use of the dimensional approach. The approach addresses the ubiquitous problems of heterogeneity and polygenetics. Practically, it means more patients need to be studied more carefully. For instance, although several researchers have alluded to the presence of elevated levels of platelet (or whole blood) serotonin in a "subgroup" of autistic patients, no one has studied a large enough group to permit a definition of what sort of modality actually exists in the population. Similarly, the limited number of studies seeking behavioral correlates of platelet serotonin have been carried out in relatively small groups of subjects, usually without much regard for possible race, sex, or age effects. In the molecular realm, the power of genetic methods capable of examining continuous behavioral or cognitive traits is quite promising. For developmental disorders, this promise has been realized by the successful mapping of a quantitative trait locus for dyslexia to chromosome 6, using a sib-pair approach.[38] Even more encouraging, in terms of possible parallels to autism, is the recent identification of susceptibility loci for 2 distinct components of dyslexia (phonological segregation and single word reading) on separate chromosomes.[39] Finally, the application of a more dimensional and component approach to both the genetics and the neurobiology of autism should be facilitated by the continued refinement of comprehensive and systematic behavioral assessment instruments.[40-42]

Individually, the 3 studies help to establish a new medication for treating autistic patients, suggest that serotonin may be especially important in the mediation of autistic symptoms, and indicate that a gene of minor influence in autism may possibly reside on the X chromosome. Collectively, they serve to emphasize the complexity of the problem of understanding the biological bases of autism. On the phenomenological level, one has the difficult problem of trying to disentangle the domains of behavior. Progress in this area will continue to come from careful description and metrification, and from thorough consideration of the interactions between domains. Similarly, at the biological level, the challenge is to isolate and analyze the various levels and systems involved in possible brain abnormalities, while appreciating their connectivity.

Advances in the psychological and biological spheres probably depend on a thorough integration of the 2 areas. Practically, this is brought about by the simultaneous and reciprocal application of the multiple perspectives and methods available. While this plea for integration has been made often and at times eloquently, its realization is no simple matter.[43-48] However, as these 3 articles and some of the aforementioned examples demonstrate, there is good reason to think that meaningful integration can be accomplished. It is also promising that now, more than ever, autism research is informed by and in turn informs research across all of biological, molecular, and clinical psychiatry. Thus, we should expect significant advances in our understanding and treatment of autism in the foreseeable future.

P. Anne McBride, MD
Department of Psychiatry
Cornell University Medical College
525 E 68th St, Box 147
New York, NY 10021

George M. Anderson, PhD
Yale Child Study Center
New Haven, Conn

Theodore Shapiro, MD
Cornell University Medical College
New York

REFERENCES

1. Hallmayer J, Hebert JM, Spiker D, Lotspeich L, McMahon WM, Petersen PB, Nicholas P, Pingree C, Lin AA, Cavalli-Sforza LL, Risch N, Ciaranello RD. Autism and the X chromosome: multipoint sib-pair analysis. *Arch Gen Psychiatry.* 1996;53:985-989.
2. McDougle CJ, Naylor ST, Cohen DJ, Volkmar FR, Heninger GR, Price LH. A double-blind, placebo-controlled study of fluvoxamine in adults with autistic disorder. *Arch Gen Psychiatry.* 1996;53:1001-1008.
3. McDougle CJ, Naylor ST, Cohen DJ, Aghajanian GK, Heninger GR, Price LH. Effects of tryptophan depletion in drug-free adults with autistic disorder. *Arch Gen Psychiatry.* 1996;53:993-1000.
4. Cook EH, Rowlett R, Jaselskis C, Leventhal BL. Fluoxetine treatment of children and adults with autistic disorder and mental retardation. *J Am Acad Child Adolesc Psychiatry.* 1992;31:739-745.
5. Gordon CT, State RC, Nelson JE, Hamburger SD, Rapoport JL. A double-blind comparison of clomipramine, desipramine, and placebo in the treatment of autistic disorder. *Arch Gen Psychiatry.* 1993;50:441-447.
6. Young SN. The 1989 Borden Award Lecture: some effects of dietary components (amino acids, carbohydrate, folic acid) on brain serotonin synthesis, mood, and behavior. *Can J Physiol Pharmacol.* 1991;69:893-903.
7. Cook EH. Autism: review of neurochemical investigation. *Synapse.* 1990;6:292-308.
8. Anderson GM, Horne WC, Chatterjee D, Cohen DJ. The hyperserotonemia of autism. *Ann N Y Acad Sci.* 1990;600:331-342.
9. McBride PA, Anderson GM, Hertzig ME, Sweeney JA, Kream J, Cohen DJ, Mann JJ. Serotonergic responsivity in male young adults with autistic disorder: results of a pilot study. *Arch Gen Psychiatry.* 1989;46:213-221.
10. Hoshino Y, Tachibana R, Watanabe M, Murata S, Yokoyama F, Kaneko M, Yashima Y, Kumoshiro H. Serotonin metabolism and hypothalamic-pituitary function in children with infantile autism and minimal brain dysfunction. *Jpn J Psychiatry Neurol.* 1984;26:937-945.
11. Bachevalier J. Medial temporal lobe structures and autism: a review of clinical and experimental findings. *Neuropsychologia.* 1994;32:627-648.
12. Moiseiwitsch JR, Lauder JM. Serotonin regulates mouse cranial neural crest migration. *Proc Natl Acad Sci U S A.* 1995;92:7182-7186.
13. Whitaker-Azmitia PM, Azmitia EC. Astroglial 5-HT1a receptors and s-100 beta in development of plasticity. *Perspect Dev Neurobiol.* 1994;2:233-238.
14. Whitaker-Azmitia PM, Peroutka SJ, eds. *The Neuropharmacology of Serotonin.* New York, NY: New York Academy of Sciences; 1990:418-586.
15. Saxena PR. Serotonin receptors: subtypes, functional responses and therapeutic relevance. *Pharmacol Therapeutics.* 1995;66:339-368.
16. Chesselet MF. Presynaptic regulation of neurotransmitter release in the brain: facts and hypothesis. *Neuroscience.* 1984;12:347-375.
17. Zoli M, Agnati LF, Hedlund PB, Li XM, Ferre S, Fuxe K. Receptor-receptor interactions as an integrative mechanism in nerve cells. *Mol Neurobiol.* 1993;7:293-334.

18. Anderson LT, Campbell M, Adams P, Small AM, Perry R, Shell J. The effects of haloperidol on discrimination learning and behavioral symptoms in autistic children. *J Autism Dev Disord.* 1989;19:227-239.
19. Perry R, Campbell M, Adams P, Lynch N, Spencer EK, Curren EL, Overall JE. Long-term efficacy of haloperidol in autistic children: continuous versus discontinuous administration. *J Am Acad Child Adolesc Psychiatry.* 1989;28:87-92.
20. Stern LM, Walker MK, Sawyer MG, Oades RD, Badcock NR, Spence JG. A controlled crossover trial of fenfluramine in autism. *J Child Psychol Psychiatry.* 1990;31:569-585.
21. Campbell M, Adams P, Small AM, Curren EL, Overall JE, Anderson LT, Lynch N, Perry R. Efficacy and safety of fenfluramine in autistic children. *J Am Acad Child Adolesc Psychiatry.* 1988; 27:434-439.
22. Leventhal BL, Cook EH, Morfold M, Ravitz AJ, Heller W, Freedman DX. Clinical and neurochemical effects of fenfluramine in children with autism. *J Neuropsychiatry Clin Neurosci.* 1993;5: 307-315.
23. Ricaurte GA, Molliver ME, Martello MB, Katz JL, Wilson MA, Martello AL. Dexfenfluramine neurotoxicity in brains of non-human primates. *Lancet.* 1991;338:1487-1488.
24. Gualtieri CT. Fenfluramine and autism: careful reappraisal is in order. *J Pediatr.* 1986;108:417-419.
25. Folstein SE, Rutter ML. Autism: familial aggregation and genetic implications. *J Autism Dev Disord.* 1988;18:3-30.
26. Bailey A, Le Couteur A, Gottesman I, Bolton P, Simonoff E, Yuzda E, Rutter M. Autism as a strongly genetic disorder: evidence from a British twin study. *Psychol Med.* 1995;25:63-77.
27. Jorde LB, Hasstedt SJ, Ritvo ER, Mason-Brothers A, Freeman BJ, Pingree C, McMahon WM, Petersen B, Jenson WR, Moll A. Complex segregation analysis of autism. *Am J Hum Genet.* 1991;49:932-938.
28. Bolton P, Macdonald H, Pickles A, Rios P, Goode S, Crowson M, Baily A, Rutter M. A case-control family history study of autism. *J Child Psychol Psychiatry.* 1994;35:877-900.
29. Smalley SL, Asarnow RF, Spence MA. Autism and genetics: a decade of research. *Arch Gen Psychiatry.* 1988;45:953-961.
30. Gillberg CL. Autism and autistic-like conditions: subclasses among disorders of empathy. *J Child Psychol Psychiatry.* 1992;33:813-842.
31. Goodman R. Infantile autism: a syndrome of multiple primary deficits? *J Autism Dev Disord.* 1989; 19:409-424.
32. Wing L, Wing JK. Multiple impairments in early childhood autism. *J Autism Child Schizophr.* 1971; 1:256-266.
33. Szatmari P. The validity of autistic spectrum disorders: a literature review. *J Autism Dev Disord.* 1992;583-600.
34. Van Praag HM. Diagnosis, the rate-limiting factor of biological depression research. *Neuropsychobiology.* 1993;28:197-206.
35. Cloninger CR. Turning point in the design of linkage studies of schizophrenia. *Am J Med Genet.* 1994;54:83-92.
36. Tuinier S, Verhoeven WM. Dimensional classification and behavioral pharmacology of personality disorders: a review and hypothesis. *Eur Neuropsychopharmacol.* 1995;5:135-146.
37. Rosenthal D, Wender PH, Kety SS, Welner J, Schulsinger F. The adopted-away offspring of schizophrenics. *Am J Psychiatry.* 1971;128:307-311.
38. Cardon LR, Smith SD, Fulker DW, Kimberling WJ, Pennington BF, DeFries JC. Quantitative trait locus for reading disability on chromosome 6. *Science.* 1994;266:276-279.
39. Grigorenko EL, Wood FB, Meyer MS, Hart LA, Speed WC, Shuster A, Pauls DL. Susceptibility loci for distinct components of developmental dyslexia on chromosomes 6 and 15. *Am J Hum Genet.* In press.
40. Hameury L, Roux S, Barthelemy C, Adrien JL, Desombre H, Sauvage D, Garreau B, Lelord G. Quantified multidimensional assessment of autism and other pervasive developmental disorders: application for bioclinical research. *Eur Child Adolesc Psychiatry.* 1995;4:123-135.
41. Le Couteur A, Rutter M, Lord C, Rios P, Robertson S, Holdgrafer M, McLennan J. Autism Diagnostic Interview: a standardized investigator-based instrument. *J Autism Dev Disord.* 1989; 19:363-387.
42. Lord C, Rutter M, Goode S, Heemsbergen J, Jordan H, Mawhood L, Schopler E. Autism Diagnostic Observation Schedule: a standardized observation of communicative and social behavior. *J Autism Dev Disord.* 1989;19:185-212.
43. Bailey A, Phillips W, Rutter M. Autism: towards an integration of clinical, genetic, neuropsychological, and neurobiological perspectives. *J Child Psychol Psychiatry.* 1996;37:89-126.
44. Ciaranello AL, Ciaranello RD. The neurobiology of infantile autism. *Annu Rev Neurosci.* 1995; 18:101-128.
45. Cohen, DJ, Volkmar F, Anderson G, Klin A. Integrating biological and behavioral perspectives in the study and care of autistic individuals: the future. *Isr Psychiatry Relat Sci.* 1993; 30:15-32.
46. Courchesne E, Townsend J, Chase C. Neurodevelopmental principles guide research on developmental psychopathologies. In: Cicchetti D, Cohen DJ, eds. *Manual of Developmental Psychopathology.* New York, NY: John Wiley & Sons Inc; 1995:195-226.
47. Denckla MB. New diagnostic criteria for autism and related behavioral disorders: guidelines for research protocols. *J Am Acad Child Adolesc Psychiatry.* 1986;25:221-224.
48. Oades RD, Eggers C. Childhood autism: an appeal for an integrative and psychobiological approach. *Eur Child Adolesc Psychiatry.* 1994;3: 159-175.

INDEX TO ADVERTISERS

Janssen Pharmaceuticals

Risperdal Oral Solution *1058*

Pathways *978-979, 1032*

Risperdal *1015-1020*

Eli Lilly & Co.

Prozac 1996 . . . . *971*

Ortho-McNeil Pharmaceutical, Inc

Haldol Decanoate . . . . *Cover 2-969*

PHYSICIAN RECRUITMENT *1071-1072*

Roche Laboratories

Klonopin *1041-1042*

SmithKline Beecham

Paxil *978-979*

Solvay Pharmaceuticals

Lithobid *1049-1050*

Luvox *990-992*

U.S. Pharmaceuticals, Pfizer Inc.

Aricept *973*

Zoloft . . . . *984A-B, 1008A-B, Cover 3-Cover 4*

While every precaution is taken to ensure accuracy, we cannot guarantee against the possibility of an occasional change or omission in the preparation of this index.

ORIGINAL ARTICLE

Autism and the X Chromosome

Multipoint Sib-Pair Analysis

Joachim Hallmayer, MD; Joan M. Hebert, MA; Donna Spiker, PhD; Linda Lotspeich, MD; William M. McMahon, MD; P. Brent Petersen, MD; Peter Nicholas, LCSW; Carmen Pingree, MS; Alice A. Lin, MS; Luca L. Cavalli-Sforza, MD; Neil Risch, PhD; Roland D. Ciaranello, MD†

Background: Genetic factors undoubtedly play a major etiologic role in autism, but how it is inherited remains unanswered. The increased incidence in males suggests possible involvement of the X chromosome.

Methods: Using data from 38 multiplex families with autism (2 or more autistic siblings), we performed a multipoint sib-pair linkage analysis between autism and 35 microsatellite markers located on the X chromosome. The model included a single parameter, the risk ratio λ_{XS} (ie, ratio of risk to siblings compared with the population prevalence), owing to an X-linked gene. Different λ_{XS} values were assumed and regions of exclusion were established.

Results: The entire X chromosome could be excluded for a λ_{XS} value of 4. The ability to exclude an X-linked gene decreased with smaller λ_{XS} values, and some positive evidence was obtained with smaller values. A maximum lod score of 1.24 was obtained at locus *DXS424* with a λ_{XS} value of 1.5.

Conclusions: We were able to exclude any moderate to strong gene effect causing autism on the X chromosome. Smaller gene effects ($\lambda_{XS}<4$) could not be excluded, in particular, a gene of small effect located between *DXS453* and *DXS1001*.

Arch Gen Psychiatry. 1996;53:985-989

THERE IS general agreement that genetic factors play a major role in the predisposition to autism. Studies show that the recurrence risk for autism among siblings is at least 75 times higher than among the general population,[1] and that the concordance rate for monozygotic (MZ) twins is much higher than for dizygotic (DZ) twins.[2-5] However, the question of how autism is inherited remains unanswered. Polygenic,[6,7] autosomal recessive,[3] and X-linked[8,9] models have been proposed. None explains the empirical data of autism entirely.[10]

One difficulty in explaining the mode of inheritance is the significant sex differences found in the frequency of autism. Males with autism outnumber females by about 3 or 4 to 1.[11] Similar sex differences have been found in families with more than 1 child with autism.[12] Although X-linked recessive inheritance may explain such a male excess, the same sample of multiplex families has also shown that at least some families are incompatible with an X-linked mode of inheritance.[13]

A major difficulty in the interpretation of data on the mode of inheritance concerns the precise definition of the autism phenotype. So far, there is no agreement about how an autistic phenotype in parents of autistic children might be defined and diagnosed. Studies that have investigated the parents of autistic probands have shown higher rates of communication and social deficits compared with control groups.[1,14] Other work suggests increased affective disorders in first-degree relatives of probands with autism.[15,16] However, no consensus exists about the type and severity of symptoms or behaviors that should define the autistic phenotype in a parent. Because most of these symptoms may be common in a large population-based sample of adults, such phenotypic expression in parents may not represent the genetic liability sought in genetic studies.

The most straightforward method for identifying the genetic basis of diseases inherited in a mendelian fashion where the

See Materials and Methods on next page

From the Department of Psychiatry and Behavioral Sciences, Nancy Pritzker Laboratory of Developmental and Molecular Neurobiology, and the Autism Genetics Program (Drs Hallmayer, Spiker, Lotspeich, and Ciaranello and Ms Hebert), and the Department of Genetics (Ms Lin and Drs Cavalli-Sforza and Risch), Stanford University, Stanford, Calif; and the Department of Psychiatry, University of Utah (Dr McMahon), and Children's Behavior Therapy Unit (Dr Petersen, Mr Nicholas, and Ms Pingree), Salt Lake City. Dr Hallmayer is now affiliated with Graylands Hospital, University of Western Australia, Perth.

†Dr Ciaranello died on December 15, 1994.

MATERIALS AND METHODS

MULTIPLEX FAMILIES

Families were recruited if they had a minimum of 2 children with clinical records indicating a diagnosis of autism.[12] Two standardized instruments were then used for gathering diagnostic information: the Autism Diagnostic Interview (ADI)[20,21] and the Autism Diagnostic Observation Schedule.[22] To be classified as autistic, the child must have scores above the prespecified cutoff points in the 4 areas of the ADI that correspond to a diagnosis of autism in the *International Classification of Disease, 10th Revision*[23] diagnostic system. Children were considered unaffected if their scores were below the cutoff points in all 4 areas of the ADI, and children were classified as "unknown" if their scores were above the cutoff point in 1, 2, or 3 areas of the ADI. All evaluations were videotaped, and interrater reliability was routinely checked; κ coefficients were greater than 0.90 for the comparison of affected vs unaffected children. More details on the diagnostic protocol can be found elsewhere.[12]

Altogether, 38 families were available for the study. One family had 5 affected children; 1 had 4; 3 had 3; and 33 had 2. Most families were white (n=34); 2 were black and 2 were Asian. Altogether, these sibships contained 84 children who fulfilled the criteria for autism. The ratio of boys to girls was 2.5 for the affected subjects, 1.5 for the unaffected subjects, and 0.6 for the subjects considered unknown. The mean age of the autistic children was 14.9 years (SD=9.3). The 75th and 25th percentiles were 20.2 and 6.7 years, respectively.

Nonverbal (performance) IQ scores were available for 62 subjects, with full-scale IQ scores available for another 16 subjects. (The 6 subjects with missing IQ data ranged in age from 3½ to 6½ years.) For the 78 subjects with available IQ data, 43 (55%) had IQ scores in the mentally retarded range (<70), while 35 (45%) had IQ scores greater 70. Twenty-two (28%) of the 78 subjects had IQ scores of 50 or less.

On the ADI, 61 subjects (73%) were classified as verbal for scoring the communication domain items (had at least 3-word phrase speech), while the other 23 (27%) were classified as nonverbal for scoring the communication domain items. For the verbal subjects, the median ADI language score was 22 (maximum possible score, 30), while for the nonverbal subjects, it was 14 (maximum possible score, 16). For the total sample, the median ADI social total score was 34.5 (maximum possible score, 42), and the median ADI rituals score was 8 (maximum possible score, 12). These ADI scores suggest that most children in this sample were moderately to severely impaired.

GENOTYPING

In general, polymerase chain reactions were carried out in 25-μL volume containing 50 to 100 ng of human genomic DNA as template, 200-μmol/L deoxyadenosine triphosphate, deoxyguanosine triphosphate, and deoxythymidine triphosphate, 20-μmol/L deoxycytidine triphosphate plus 1 μCi of α-phosphorus 32–labeled deoxycytidine triphosphate (New England Nuclear, Boston, Mass), 12.5 pmol of each primer, 50-mmol/L potassium chloride, 10-mmol/L TRIS, 1.25-mmol/L magnesium chloride, and 1 U of Taq polymerase (Pharmacia, Uppsala, Sweden). Samples were overlaid with mineral oil and amplified after an initial denaturation step of 2 to 4 minutes at 94°C in 25 temperature cycles consisting of 1 minute at 94°C, 1 minute at 55°C, and 1 minute at 72°C. Minor modifications were made to the reaction conditions for the following primer pairs: *DXS737, DXS1105, DXS228, DXS1106, DXS456,*

causative genes are as yet unidentified is genetic linkage analysis. The extension of this method to diseases that have a more complex mode of inheritance is problematic and has led to contradictory results in the effort to map susceptibility genes for psychiatric diseases.[17] A robust method for mapping susceptibility loci for complex diseases is the analysis of only affected sib pairs. Affected sib-pair analysis is based on excess sharing of markers linked to a disease susceptibility locus (identity by descent). The detection of linkage does not

See also pages 980, 993, and 1001

require assumptions about the mode of inheritance. Since the affection status of the parent is not considered in these analyses, the strategy of using only affected sib pairs allows researchers to restrict the assignment of an affected phenotype to a narrow definition that has high reliability.

Risch[18,19] has shown that the power to detect linkage by using affected sib pairs is only dependent on the risk ratio λ_{XS} (ie, ratio of risk to siblings compared with the population prevalence) and no other genetic model parameter. Studies for autism generally agree that the sibling recurrence risk for autism is about 3%, while the prevalence of the disease in the general population is estimated to be 1 in 2500, corresponding to a large λ_{XS} value of 75.[10] It is difficult to determine how much of this overall λ_{XS} value can be attributed to one gene. Recent systematic twin studies have estimated a concordance rate of 75% for MZ twins and 0% for DZ twins.[4,5] The latter rate is unlikely to be real, but rather owing to small sample size. It is not statistically different from 3%, the recurrence risk for sibs who have the same degree of genetic relatedness. Thus, for modeling purposes, we assume a DZ concordance rate of 3%, giving an MZ to DZ concordance ratio of 75/3-25. The very high ratio of MZ to DZ concordance cannot be explained by 1 or 2 loci.[18] Even under the assumption of a recessive model, at least several interacting loci are required. Any single recessive gene could contribute at most 4-fold to the ratio of MZ to DZ risk; a nonrecessive gene would contribute less. The observed ratio suggests that at least 3 loci are involved, and probably more, with no single gene having a very large effect.

In the present study, we used 38 families, each with at least 2 siblings with autism, to test the possibility that a gene that causes susceptibility to autism is located on the X chromosome.

DXS990, DXS538, DXS1126, and *DXS15.* More major modifications were made for these primer pairs: *DXS1060, DXS1226, DXS1195, DXS1227, DXS1220, DXS1059, DXS292,* and *FRAXA.* Precise reaction conditions are available from the authors. One microliter of the amplified product was mixed with formamide sample buffer and analyzed on a 6% denaturing polyacrylamide sequencing gel. Samples were electrophoresed at 55 W for 2 to 3 hours, dried without fixation, and exposed for 2 hours to overnight at −70°C using intensifying screens. Genotype assignments were done by researchers who were unaware of the affection status of the children.

Thirty-five X-linked microsatellite markers (**Table**) were amplified. The first round of amplification was carried out with 33 markers in 33 families. Three microsatellites (*DXS548, DXS1126,* and *DXS1195*) were typed in only a subset of families. Since 2 markers (*DXS424* and *DXS737*) gave slightly positive results, we tested an additional set of 5 families for markers *DXS737, DXS424, DXS1105,* and *DXS1001.* Two additional microsatellites (*DXS1220* and *DXS1059*) were typed in families in whom the results from flanking markers were either discordant or in whom at least 1 of the flanking markers was uninformative. Parents were genotyped, and thus identity by descent for the marker loci could be calculated directly without marker allele frequencies. Hence, the results are independent of allele frequency specification. The markers span a region of 178 centimorgans (cM) covering the entire human X chromosome, except for the pseudoautosomal region (Table).

MULTIPOINT SIB-PAIR ANALYSIS

Multipoint sib-pair analysis can increase the power to detect linkage and to locate a disease locus,[18] as well as allow for exclusion mapping.[19] This method is easily extended to an X-linked locus, where sharing of maternal alleles identical by descent (IBD) is examined. For an X-linked locus, λ_{XS} may differ for male-male, male-female, and female-female sib pairs. However, under the assumption of X-linked recessive inheritance, the probabilities of sharing a maternal allele are the same for each type of pair. This sharing probability is $1-(1/\lambda_{XS})$, where λ_{XS} is defined in terms of recurrence in brothers of male probands and sisters of male probands (or the reverse), for male-male and male-female pairs. For female-female pairs, the formula is somewhat more complicated. A complete multipoint lod score at a given map location is calculated allowing for interference, assuming the Kosambi mapping function.

For each sib pair, a lod score is calculated at any given map location. It is defined as the log 10 of the ratio between the likelihood of the observed identity by descent data for the various markers, given a value of λ_{XS} greater than 1, and the likelihood of the observed identity by descent data given a λ_{XS} value of 1 (no effect). The total lod score is the individual lod scores summed over all the sib pairs.

Because the parents are typed, identity by descent information at a given location is obtained by finding the nearest flanking markers to that location that give unambiguous IBD information.[19,24] This analysis provides maximal use of information from multiple markers compared with interval mapping methods, which are based only on immediately flanking markers.[25,26]

Multipoint calculations were carried out for λ_{XS} values of 4, 3, 2, and 1.5. These values were chosen to represent a range of plausible gene effects from moderate to minor. It was unnecessary to test larger effects because essentially complete exclusion was obtained at a λ_{XS} value of 4. All calculations were carried out using the computer program ASPEX, a multipoint exclusion mapping program.[19]

To test for this possible susceptibility gene, we used multipoint sib pair analysis.[18,19] The model incorporates a single parameter, λ_{XS}, which is the sibling risk ratio owing to a recessive gene located on the X chromosome. We tested different λ_{XS} values and established regions of exclusion.

RESULTS

The Table presents the identity by descent-sharing data for the 35 X-linked loci studied. Most markers showed no substantial excess of identity by descent. However, a number of markers in the region between *DXS453* and *DXS424* showed some evidence of increased allele sharing. The greatest excess is for marker *DXS424,* with 25 of 34 alleles shared.

Distances between markers are taken from Figure 1 of Fain et al.[27] The **Figure** displays the results of multipoint analysis. None of the lod scores reached the positive significance level. There were some positive lod scores observed, in particular around *DXS424,* where the maximum lod score of 1.24 was obtained for a λ_{XS} value of 1.5. Another lower peak (0.93) was observed at *DXYS1X.* Overall, the power of the sample given this λ_{XS} value was low. Only a small portion of the X chromosome could be excluded (31 cM of 188 cM). The areas of exclusion included the fragile X region. Assuming a gene effect that would account for a risk ratio to siblings of 2 resulted in exclusion of more than half of the chromosome (108 cM). An area of 179 cM could be excluded assuming a λ_{XS} value of 3; and a λ_{XS} value of 4 resulted in the exclusion of the entire chromosome, except for a small 3.5-cM region that was close to the exclusion level.

COMMENT

Compared with other psychiatric diseases, there have been few attempts to locate a gene involved in susceptibility to autism. In the only published study to date,[28] 27 multiplex families and 7 families with 1 autistic child were tested for linkage using serum and red blood cell markers. The 30 markers tested mapped to 9 different chromosomes. The assumed model was autosomal recessive with complete penetrance. No significant linkages were detected.

Our study was based on multiplex sibships recruited and evaluated during the last 5 years.[12] We applied an affected sib-pair approach. This approach requires neither a definition of the affection status of parents nor any specification of the mode of inheritance. To mini-

Schematic Map of 35 Markers Typed on the X Chromosome and Their Allelic Identity by Descent for Sibling Pairs With Autism

		Allelic Identity by Descent	
Map Location, cM*	Locus	Shared	Nonshared
9.9†	*DXS1233*	16	19
11.7	*DXS1060*	20	16
16.0	*KAL*	18	19
19.9	*DXS1043*	13	10
29.9	*DXS1195*	7	7
38.2	*DXS1226*	18	22
42.7	*DXS989*	13	22
50.1	*DXS997*	17	24
58.0	*DXS538*	19	23
61.8	*DXS1058*	14	18
69.6	*DXS228*	11	12
69.7	*MAOA*	20	23
78.4	*DXS1003*	19	20
82.8	*DXS1126*	4	0
86.9	*DXS991*	22	17
93.6	*DXS453*	23	14
99.6	*DXYS1X*	10	8
103.7	*DXS990*	16	8
107.4	*COL4A5*	17	10
109.9	*DXS1106*	21	18
116.9	*DXS1105*	18	9
117.0	*DXS456*	14	6
118.9	*DXS1059*	12	7
123.7	*DXS1220*	11	11
126.2	*DXS424*	25	9
133.7	*DXS1001*	17	19
144.0	*DXS737*	14	7
147.0	*HPRT*	23	21
151.5	*DXS692*	7	9
152.8	*DXS984*	14	14
156.3	*DXS1227*	12	18
168.2	*DXS292*	5	11
175.4	*DXS548*	15	13
175.7	*FRAX*	15	22
187.9	*DXS15*	16	26

**Distances are measured according to the map by Fain et al.[27]*
†Approximately 4 cM distal to the pseudoautosomal region.

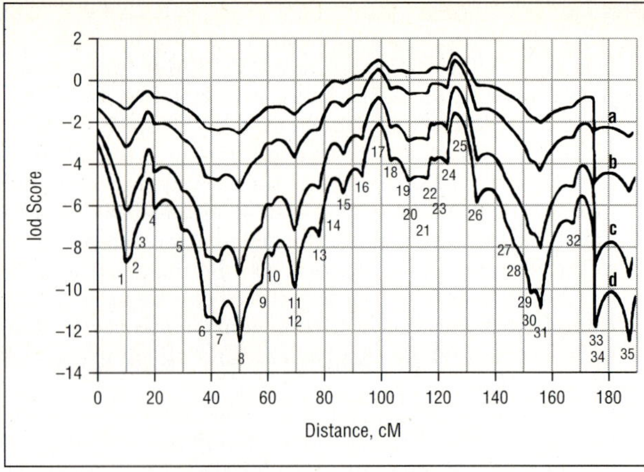

Results of sib-pair multipoint analysis between 35 markers and autism: (1) DXS1233, *(2)* DXS1060, *(3)* KAL, *(4)* DXS1043, *(5)* DXS1195, *(6)* DXS1226, *(7)* DXS989, *(8)* DXS997, *(9)* DXS538, *(10)* DXS1058, *(11)* DXS288, *(12)* MAOA, *(13)* DXS1003, *(14)* DXS1126, *(15)* DXS991, *(16)* DXS453, *(17)* DXYS1X, *(18)* DXS990, *(19)* Col4A5, *(20)* DXS1106, *(21)* DXS1105, *(22)* DXS456, *(23)* DXS1059, *(24)* DXS1220, *(25)* DXS424, *(26)* DXS1001, *(27)* DXS737, *(28)* HPRT, *(29)* DXS692, *(30)* DXS984, *(31)* DXS1227, *(32)* DXS292, *(33)* DXS548, *(34)* FRAX, *and (35)* DXS15. *Distances between markers are shown in Figure 1 of Fain et al.[27] For curve a, λ_{XS}=1.5; curve b, λ_{XS}=2.0; curve c, λ_{XS}=3.0; and curve d, λ_{XS}=4.0.*

mize ambiguity, we took the conservative approach of excluding individuals who showed some symptoms characteristic of autism but did not reach the cutoff points set for diagnosis of autism (as measured by the ADI).

Recently, we excluded the fragile X location based on linkage analysis with several markers in the region.[29] The present study extends this analysis to the entire X chromosome (except for the pseudoautosomal region).

Based on the ratio of the expected proportion of affected sib pairs sharing 0 or 1 allele (IBD) for male-male and male-female pairs or 1 or 2 alleles (IBD) for female-female pairs, we estimated the maximum contribution of a single locus located on the X chromosome to the total λ_{XS}.[30] We were able to exclude the entire X chromosome for λ_{XS} values of 4 or greater. Since the total λ_{XS} value in autism is around 75, these data indicate that the recurrence risk observed in siblings cannot be largely attributed to a major gene located on the X chromosome. For smaller gene effects (λ_{XS}=1.5), only small portions (about 17%) of the X chromosome could be excluded. Furthermore, for this value of λ_{XS}, a positive lod score of 1.24 at *DXS424* was obtained. Thus, an X-linked susceptibility gene of weak effect in this region is still possible.

In our linkage analyses, we assumed that the amount of sharing of maternal alleles for affected sib pairs is the same for all sex combinations for the pairs. The degree to which this is true depends on the exact genetic model. For an X-linked recessive model, the expected sharing is the same for all types of pairs. A recessive model also gives the highest sex ratio (male to female). An additive model gives an equal prevalence for boys and girls (ie, sex ratio of 1), but then the expected sharing is somewhat greater for male-male pairs than male-female or female-female pairs. Thus, if the elevated sex ratio in autism is due to an X-linked locus, it is likely that the sharing of maternal alleles would be similar by sex of sib pairs. If the increased sex ratio is not due to X linkage, there may be excess sharing for male-male pairs, but most likely not dramatically so. Hence, although our assumption of equal sharing for all types of sib pairs implies a recessive model, it is likely that little difference would result from using other types of plausible models.

One possibility is that a subset of familial autism is caused by a gene located on the X chromosome, whereas other cases are caused by autosomal genes, environmental influences, or their interactions. Assuming a proportion (α) of families are X linked and the remaining $(1-\alpha)$ are unlinked, the expected amount of allele sharing for an X-linked locus would be $\alpha+[(1-\alpha)/2]=(1+\alpha)/2$. In terms of λ_{XS}, the expected allele sharing would be $1-(1/2\lambda_{XS})$. Equating these 2 formulas gives $\alpha=1-(1/\lambda_{XS})$. Thus, because we were able to exclude the hypothesis λ_{XS}=4 from the X chromosome, we equivalently can exclude the hypothesis $\alpha=1-1/4=3/4$ of all families are simply X linked. Because λ_{XS}=2 was excluded from more than half of the X chromosome, the hypothesis that $\alpha=1-1/2=1/2$

of all families are X-linked can be excluded from the same chromosomal regions.

We have provided evidence that no gene with a large impact on susceptibility resides on the X chromosome. However, we do have some limited evidence that a gene of minor effect may exist there. Further analysis with additional multiplex families examining the same X chromosomal region will be required to either further support the existence of such a locus or exclude this region entirely.

Accepted for publication April 23, 1996.

Supported by grant MH39437 from the National Institute of Mental Health (NIMH), Rockville, Md, and by grants from the Scottish Rite, the Spunk Fund, Inc, the Solomon and Rebecca Baker Fund, and the endowment fund of the Nancy Pritzker Laboratory, Stanford, Calif, and by grant HG00348 from the National Institutes of Health, Bethesda, Md (Dr Risch). Drs Hallmayer and Lotspeich are the recipients of Young Investigator Awards from the National Alliance for Research in Schizophrenia and Affective Disorders; Dr Ciaranello was the recipient of Career Scientist Award MH00219 from the NIMH; and Dr McMahon is the recipient of Child Mental Health Academic Award MH00980-03 from the NIMH.

We dedicate this article to the memory of Dr Ciaranello, whose vision and passion to locate a gene underlying autistic disorders is still alive in his colleagues who are carrying on this work.

We wish to express our gratitude to the families who have participated in this research.

Reprints: Donna Spiker, PhD, Stanford Autism Genetics Program, Department of Psychiatry and Behavioral Sciences, Mail Code 5540, Stanford University School of Medicine, Stanford, CA 94305.

REFERENCES

1. Bolton P, Macdonald H, Pickles A, Rios P, Goode S, Crowson M, Bailey A, Rutter M. A case-control family history study of autism. *J Child Psychol Psychiatry.* 1994;35:877-900.
2. Folstein SE, Rutter M. Infantile autism: a genetic study in 21 twin pairs. *J Child Psychol Psychiatry.* 1977;18:297-321.
3. Ritvo ER, Freeman BJ, Mason-Brothers A, Mo A, Ritvo AM. Concordance for the syndrome of autism in 40 pairs of afflicted twins. *Am J Psychiatry.* 1985; 142:64-77.
4. Steffenburg S, Gillberg C, Hellgren L, Andersson L, Gillberg IC, Jakobsson G, Bohman M. A twin study of autism in Denmark, Finland, Iceland, Norway and Sweden. *J Child Psychol Psychiatry.* 1989;30:405-416.
5. Bailey A, LeCouteur A, Gottesman I, Bolton P, Simonoff E, Yuzda E, Rutter M. Autism as a strongly genetic disorder: evidence from a British twin study. *Psychol Med.* 1995;25:63-77.
6. Jorde LB, Hasstedt SJ, Ritvo ER, Mason-Brothers A, Freeman BJ, Pingree C, McMahon WM, Petersen B, Jenson WR, Mo A. Complex segregation analysis of autism. *Am J Hum Genet.* 1991;49:932-938.
7. Tsai L, Stewart MA, August G. Implications of sex differences in the familial transmission of infantile autism. *J Autism Dev Disord.* 1981;11:165-173.
8. Gurling H. Candidate genes and favored loci: strategies for molecular genetic research into schizophrenia, manic depression, autism, alcoholism, and Alzheimer disease. *Psychiatric Dev.* 1986;4:289-309.
9. Szatmari P, Jones MB. IQ and the genetics of autism. *J Child Psychol Psychiatry.* 1991;32:897-908.
10. Smalley SL. Genetic influences in autism. *Psychiatr Clin North Am.* 1991;1: 125-139.
11. Lord C, Schopler E, Revecki D. Sex differences in autism. *J Autism Dev Disord.* 1982;12:317-330.
12. Spiker D, Lotspeich L, Kraemer HC, Hallmayer J, McMahon W, Petersen PB, Nicholas P, Pingree C, Wiese-Slater S, Chiotti C, Wong DL, Dimiceli S, Ritvo E, Cavalli-Sforza LL, Ciaranello RD. Genetics of autism: characteristics of affected and unaffected children from 37 multiplex families. *Am J Med Genet.* 1994;54:27-35.
13. Hallmayer J, Spiker D, Lotspeich L, McMahon WM, Petersen PB, Nicholas P, Pingree C, Ciaranello R. Male-to-male transmission in extended pedigrees with multiple cases of autism. *Am J Med Genet.* 1996;67:13-18.
14. Piven J, Wzorek M, Landa R, Lainhart J, Bolton P, Chase GA, Folstein S. Personality characteristics of the parents of autistic individuals. *Psychol Med.* 1994; 24:783-795.
15. Gold N. Depression and social adjustment in siblings of boys with autism. *J Autism Dev Disord.* 1993;23:147-163.
16. Piven J, Gayle J, Chase GA, Fink B, Landa R, Wzorek MM, Folstein SE. A family history study of neuropsychiatric disorders in the adult siblings of autistic individuals. *J Am Acad Child Adoles Psychiatry.* 1990;29:177-183.
17. Risch N. Genetic linkage and complex diseases, with specific reference to psychiatric disorders. *Genet Epidemiol.* 1990;7:3-16.
18. Risch N. Linkage studies for genetically complex traits, II: the power of affected sib pairs. *Am J Hum Genet.* 1990;46:229-241.
19. Risch N. Exclusion mapping for complex diseases. *Am J Hum Genet.* 1993; 53(suppl):A185. Abstract.
20. Le Couteur A, Rutter M, Lord C, Rios P, Robertson S, Holdgrafer M, McLennan J. Autism Diagnostic Interview: a standardized investigator-based instrument. *J Autism Dev Disord.* 1989;19:363-387.
21. Lord C, Rutter M, Le Couteur A. Autism Diagnostic Interview–Revised: a revised version of a diagnostic interview for caregivers of individuals with possible pervasive developmental disorders. *J Autism Dev Disord.* 1994;24: 659-685.
22. Lord C, Rutter M, Goode S, Heemsbergen J, Jordan H, Mawhood L, Schopler E. Autism Diagnostic Observation Schedule: a standardized observation of communicative and social behavior. *J Autism Dev Disord.* 1989;19:185-212.
23. World Health Organization. *International Statistical Classification of Diseases, 10th Revision (ICD-10): Classification of Mental and Behavioural Disorders: Clinical Description and Diagnostic Guidelines.* Geneva, Switzerland: World Health Organization; 1992.
24. Schwab SG, Albus M, Hallmayer J, Honig S, Boormann M, Lichtermann D, Ebstein RP, Ackerheil M, Lerer B, Risch N, Maier W, Wildenauer DB. Evaluation of a susceptibility gene for schizophrenia on chromosome 6p: multipoint affected sib pair linkage analysis. *Nat Genet.* 1995;11:325-327.
25. Olson JM. Multipoint linkage analysis using sib pairs: an interval mapping approach using dichotomous outcomes. *Am J Hum Genet.* 1995;56:788-798.
26. Hauser ER, Boehnke M, Guo S-W, Risch N. Affected sib pair interval mapping and exclusion for complex genetic traits: sampling considerations. *Genet Epidemiol.* 1996;13:117-137.
27. Fain PR, Kort EN, Chance PF, Nguyen K, Redd DF, Econs MJ, Barker DF. A 2D crossover-based map of the human X chromosome as a model for map integration. *Nat Genet.* 1995;9:261-266.
28. Spence MA, Ritvo ER, Marazita ML, Funderburk SJ, Sparkes RS, Freeman BJ. Gene mapping studies with the syndrome of autism. *Behav Genet.* 1985;15: 1-13.
29. Hallmayer J, Pintado E, Lotspeich L, Spiker D, McMahon W, Petersen PB, Nicholas P, Pingree C, Kraemer HC, Wong DL, Hebert J, Lin A, Cavalli-Sforza LL, Ciaranello R. Molecular analysis and test of linkage between the *FMR-1* gene and infantile autism in multiplex families. *Am J Hum Genet.* 1994;55:951-959.
30. Risch N. Assessing the role of HLA-linked and unlinked determinants of disease. *Am J Hum Genet.* 1987;40:1-14.

ESTABLISHED THERAPY FOR OCD

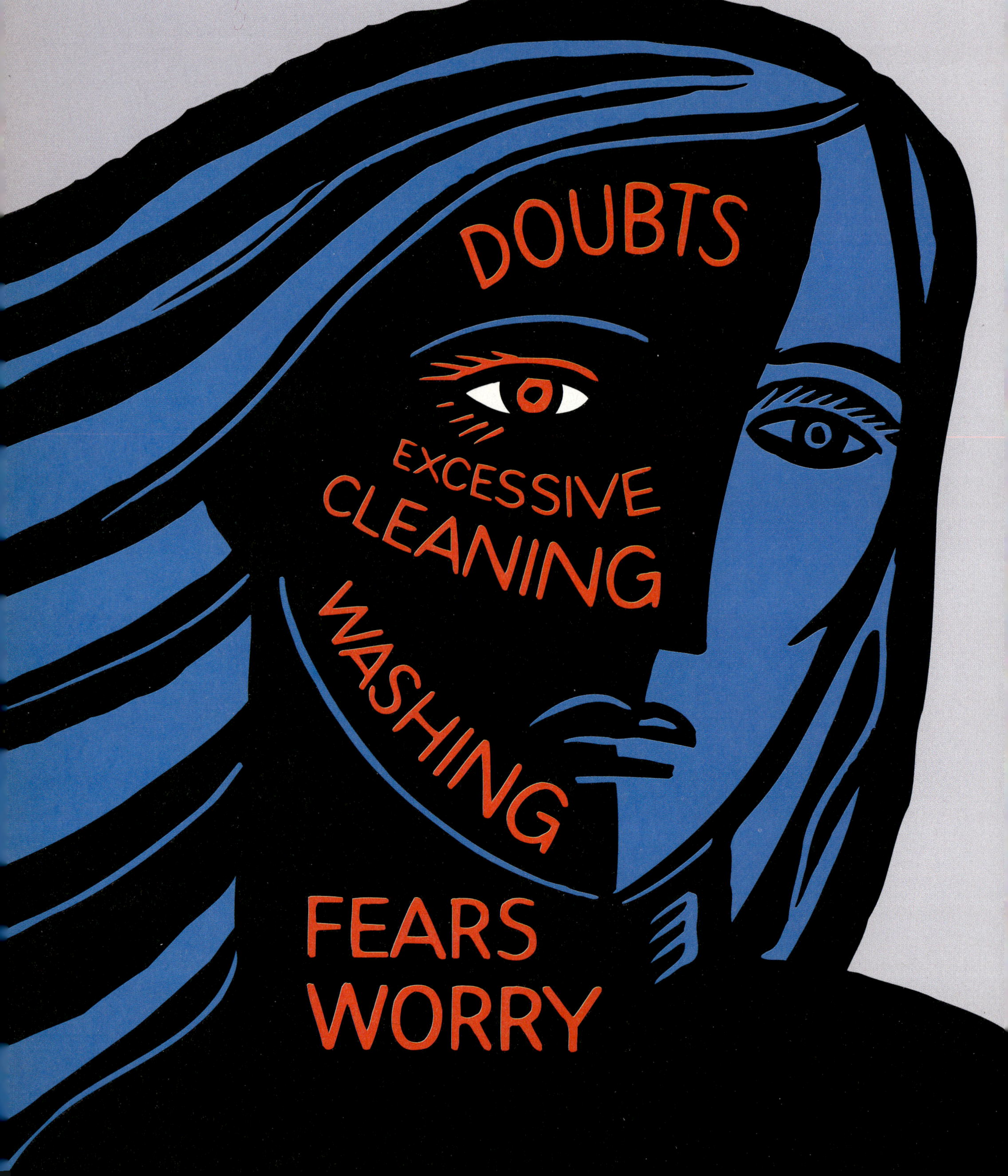

Effects of Tryptophan Depletion in Drug-Free Adults With Autistic Disorder

Christopher J. McDougle, MD; Susan T. Naylor, RN, MSN; Donald J. Cohen, MD; George K. Aghajanian, MD; George R. Heninger, MD; Lawrence H. Price, MD

Background: The primary objective of this study was to investigate the behavioral and biochemical responses to acute tryptophan depletion in drug-free adult patients with autistic disorder.

Methods: Twenty drug-free adults with autistic disorder (16 men and 4 women) (mean [±SD] age, 30.5±8.5 years) underwent short-term tryptophan depletion in a double-blind, placebo-controlled, randomized crossover design. Patients received a 24-hour, low-tryptophan diet followed the next morning by an amino acid drink. Behavioral ratings were obtained on the morning of the amino acid drink (baseline) and 180, 300, and 420 minutes after the drink. Plasma free and total tryptophan levels were obtained at baseline and 5 hours after the drink. The active and sham testing sessions were separated by 7 days.

Results: Eleven (65%) of the 17 patients who completed both test days showed a significant global worsening of behavioral symptoms with short-term tryptophan depletion, but none of the 17 patients showed any significant change in clinical status from baseline after sham depletion ($P=.001$). Tryptophan depletion led to a significant increase in behaviors such as whirling, flapping, pacing, banging and hitting self, rocking, and toe walking ($P<.05$). In addition, patients were significantly less calm and happy and more anxious. No significant change was observed in social relatedness or repetitive thoughts and behavior. Plasma total and free tryptophan levels were reduced 86% and 69%, respectively, 5 hours after the tryptophan-deficient amino acid drink. Patients who had a significant global exacerbation of symptoms had significantly higher baseline plasma total tryptophan levels ($P<.001$) and Autism Behavior Checklist scores ($P=.005$) than did patients who showed no significant change in symptoms after tryptophan depletion.

Conclusions: The results of this study are consistent with previous research that has implicated a dysregulation in serotonin function in some patients with autism. These data suggest that the short-term reduction of serotonin precursor availability may exacerbate some symptoms characteristic of autism in some patients. Continued investigation into the role of serotonin in the pathogenesis and treatment of autistic disorder is warranted.

Arch Gen Psychiatry. 1996;53:993-1000

From the Clinical Neuroscience Research Unit, Abraham Ribicoff Research Facilities, Connecticut Mental Health Center (Drs McDougle, Aghajanian, Heninger, and Price and Ms Naylor), and the Department of Psychiatry (Drs McDougle, Cohen, Aghajanian, Heninger, and Price and Ms Naylor) and the Child Study Center (Drs McDougle and Cohen), Yale University School of Medicine, New Haven, Conn.

SEROTONIN (5-hydroxytryptamine [5-HT]) has been the subject of biological research in autistic disorder for the past 35 years. Initial interest in the 5-HT system arose from the finding that 6 of 23 children with autism had elevated levels of peripheral whole blood serotonin (WBS) compared with the reference range for normal subjects.[1] Although this "hyperserotonemia" has been replicated in subsequent studies of children with autism,[2] it also has been identified in neuropsychiatric populations with disorders other than autism.[3] Despite the hyperserotonemia observed in a subgroup of patients, cerebrospinal fluid (CSF) levels of the primary central metabolite of 5-HT, 5-hydroxyindoleacetic acid (5-HIAA), have been found to be lower than[4] or no different from[5] matched control subjects.

Based in large part on this elevated peripheral biological marker, researchers began treating patients who have autism with the indirect 5-HT receptor agonist fenfluramine hydrochloride, which reliably reduces WBS levels. After an initial report in 1982 describing its positive effects in 3 hyperserotonemic boys with autism,[6] controlled studies have shown fenfluramine to be ineffective for treating

See Patients and Methods on next page

PATIENTS AND METHODS

PATIENTS

Twenty consecutive adults who were admitted to the program with autistic disorder (4 women and 16 men; 8 inpatients and 12 outpatients; mean [±SD] age, 30.5±8.5 years; age range, 20-53 years) and their parents or legal guardians gave voluntary, written informed consent (or assent for those patients who were limited due to cognitive level) to participate in the study, which had been approved by the Human Investigation Committee of the Yale University School of Medicine, New Haven, Conn. All patients currently met *Diagnostic and Statistical Manual of Mental Disorders, Revised Third Edition*[46] and *International Classification of Diseases, 10th Revision*[47] criteria for autistic disorder. The patients were referred by group homes for persons with autism, family members, community-based psychiatrists, and chapters of the Autism Society of America throughout New England.

Each patient's symptoms were at least "moderate" in severity, as defined by the global severity of illness rating on the Clinical Global Impression Scale.[48] The Autism Diagnostic Interview[49] and the Autism Diagnostic Observation Schedule[50] were completed by trained professionals (C.J.M. and S.T.N.) to aid in diagnoses and to provide additional measures of severity of the condition. The Autism Behavior Checklist (ABC)[51] was completed with each patient's parent or legal guardian to determine the patient's level of autistic behavior. Previous studies have shown that an ABC score of more than 78 typically differentiates persons diagnosed as having autism from persons who are severely mentally retarded, deaf or blind, severely emotionally disturbed, or normal.[51] The Wechsler Adult Intelligence Scale–Revised[52] was administered to determine each verbal patient's full-scale IQ. The Leiter International Performance Scale[53] was administered to the patient who was nonverbal. All patients received a complete physical and neurological evaluation, electrocardiography, urinalysis, and laboratory tests of renal, hepatic, hematopoietic, and thyroid function. All female patients received a serum pregnancy test. Patients for whom an identified cause of autism had been determined (eg, fragile X syndrome, inborn error of metabolism, birth trauma, maternal viral infection during pregnancy), those with seizure disorders, and women with positive pregnancy test results were excluded from the study. All patients had been drug-free for at least 5 weeks before testing. Patient characteristics are given in the **Table**.

METHODS

Each test day lasted from about 8 AM until 5 PM and occurred in a quiet, well-lit hospital room with 1 bed and a window to the outside. Patients were free to walk in the room during the testing. All test days were conducted in the same environment for each patient. The study used a double-blind, placebo-controlled, randomized crossover design. The short-term TRYP depletion test consisted of a 24-hour, 160 mg/d low-TRYP diet (9660 kJ, 7% protein, 27% fat, 64% carbohydrate) with placebo capsules given with each meal, followed the next morning by a TRYP-free, 15-amino acid drink, as described by Young et al.[40] Sham testing consisted of a 24-hour, 160 mg/d low-TRYP diet supplemented with capsules containing 500 mg of TRYP given with each meal, followed the next morning by a 16-amino acid drink containing 2.3 g of TRYP. Patients returned to normal dietary intake at 5 PM on the day of each testing session. The active and sham testing sessions were separated by 7 days. The composition of the diet and the amino acid drink used on our unit have been previously described.[38] Three of the 20 patients were unable to complete the study because they became nauseous and vomited the amino acid drink; patient 19 had received the depletion drink and patients 18 and 20 had received the sham drink. No other significant adverse effects occurred during the study.

behavioral symptoms in most patients with autism.[7-10] This lack of efficacy has been observed despite robust fenfluramine-induced reductions in WBS. In addition to reducing peripheral WBS, however, fenfluramine also lowers CSF concentrations of 5-HIAA.[11] Moreover, fenfluramine has been reported to produce irreversible changes in 5-HT neurons in certain regions of the brain in rats, guinea pigs, and rhesus monkeys.[12] The fenfluramine-induced reduction in brain 5-HT may be related to its lack of efficacy and to the symptom exacerbation that occurs in some patients with autism.[13]

See also pages 980, 985, and 1001

More recent data indicate that central 5-HT function may be reduced in some patients with autism. Results from 2 neuroendocrine challenge studies involving a small number of children[14] and adults[15] with autism suggest that central 5-HT responsivity may be decreased. In addition, preliminary reports indicate that potent 5-HT uptake inhibitors, such as clomipramine hydrochloride,[16,17] fluoxetine hydrochloride,[18-22] and fluvoxamine maleate,[23-24] which reliably increase brain 5-HT neurotransmission, may improve social relatedness and reduce aggression and interfering repetitive thoughts and behavior in some patients with autism.

The synthesis of 5-HT depends on dietary intake of its precursor, the essential amino acid tryptophan (TRYP).[25,26] Data suggest that dietary TRYP depletion may specifically reduce brain 5-HT function.[27-30] Increases[31,32] and decreases[29,30,32] in dietary TRYP intake lead to corresponding changes in brain TRYP and 5-HT levels in laboratory animals. Dietary TRYP depletion also alters behavioral indexes of 5-HT function—increasing pain sensitivity,[33,34] acoustic startle,[35] and muricidal behavior[36]—and reduces rapid eye movement sleep.[30] Most of these effects are reversed by TRYP repletion, probably through alterations in central 5-HT function. In lieu of dietary TRYP depletion, administration of TRYP-free amino acid mixtures to vervet monkeys similarly decreases plasma levels of TRYP and CSF levels of TRYP and 5-HIAA, with no change in CSF levels of tyrosine, homovanillic acid, or 3-methoxy-4-hydroxyphenylethylene glycol.[29] The mechanism of this effect is believed to

BEHAVIORAL RATINGS

Behavioral ratings were completed by an experienced research nurse (S.T.N.) who was unaware of the challenge type assignment. Two members of the primary caregiving team (eg, group home staff, parent or sibling, workshop staff) who worked most closely with the patient on a daily basis participated in the detailed assessment of behavioral symptoms at baseline and throughout each test day. Ratings consisted of an 11-point clinician-rated global severity change scale (−5 indicates very bad, could not be worse; 0, unchanged; 5, much improvement, could not be better)[45]; the Ritvo-Freeman Real-Life Rating Scale, a clinician-rated in vivo observational measure of signs and symptoms characteristic of autism, including subscale 1: sensory motor behaviors (eg, whirling, flapping, pacing, banging or hitting self, rocking), subscale 2: social relationship to people (eg, ignores interaction attempt, isolates self), subscale 3: affectual reactions (eg, abrupt change in affect, crying), subscale 4: sensory responses (eg, covering ears or eyes, sniffing self or objects), and subscale 5: language (eg, immediate and/or delayed echolalia, noncommunicative vocalizations)[54]; 15-point clinician-rated severity scales for repetitive thoughts and repetitive behavior (range, 0 [no symptoms] to 14 [extreme])[39]; and 18 100-mm clinician-rated visual analog scale items (agitated, angry, anxious, calm, depressed, drowsy, energetic, eye contact, fearful, happy, hungry, initiates social interaction, irritable, mellow, nervous, sad, talkative, and tired). All scales were administered at baseline (15 minutes before the amino acid drink) and 180, 300 (point of maximal decrease in plasma free and total TRYP levels), and 420 minutes after the drink.

BIOCHEMICAL MEASURES

Plasma free and total TRYP levels were obtained at baseline and at 300 minutes after the amino acid drink. Total plasma TRYP was assayed by high-performance liquid chromatography with fluorometric detection. Free plasma TRYP was assayed by obtaining the ultrafiltrate of plasma from cellulose-based filters (30 000 molecular weight cutoff) (1000 g) at room temperature and subjecting the ultrafiltrate to the high-performance liquid chromatography with fluorometric detection method.[55]

DATA ANALYSIS

Changes in behavioral ratings were analyzed by analysis of variance (ANOVA) with repeated measures. Main effects of challenge type (sham vs depletion) and time (changes over the times sampled) were determined, as was the interaction of challenge type × time (indicating the overall effect of the TRYP depletion during the study). The reported P values for all ANOVAs used the Huynh-Feldt correction factor when the sphericity assumption was not met. This correction factor decreases the degrees of freedom used in the ANOVA to reflect lack of homogeneity in the variance of measures across time. For clarity, uncorrected df are presented. Paired Student t tests were used to determine significant changes in free and total TRYP blood levels (baseline to +300 minutes). Unpaired Student t tests were used to compare baseline free and total TRYP blood levels and to determine significant changes in these measures after depletion between patients who had a global symptom exacerbation and those who showed no significant change in behavior after TRYP depletion. Global symptom exacerbation or improvement was categorically defined as a 2-point or greater decrease or increase, respectively, in the clinician-rated global severity change scale score. Fisher exact test was used to determine the relationships between ABC score (≤78 vs >78) and full-scale IQ (≤70 vs >70) with global symptom exacerbation or improvement after TRYP depletion. Data are presented as mean(±SD) except where otherwise indicated, and results are reported as significant when $P<.05$ (2-tailed). Only patients who completed both test days (N=17) were included in the data analysis.

involve induction of hepatic protein synthesis with subsequent depletion of available plasma TRYP.[37] The onset of action of these TRYP-free amino acid mixtures in laboratory animals is rapid, with maximal reductions of plasma TRYP and brain 5-HT occurring within 2 hours of ingestion.[29,30] In humans, the maximal reduction of plasma free and total TRYP levels occurs 5 hours after ingestion of the amino acid mixture.[38]

The short-term TRYP depletion paradigm has been used to investigate the mechanism of action of psychotherapeutic agents. Rapid TRYP depletion resulted in a depressive relapse in 66% of antidepressant-remitted patients with major depression, primarily those maintained on 5-HT uptake inhibitors,[38] and in an exacerbation of depressive but not obsessive-compulsive symptoms in patients with obsessive-compulsive disorder (OCD) stabilized on 5-HT uptake inhibitors.[39]

Other studies have investigated the effects of short-term TRYP depletion in normal subjects[40,41] and drug-free patients with major depression,[42] OCD,[43] and panic disorder.[44] In healthy men, short-term TRYP depletion led to a mild impairment in attentive performance and "an increase in depressive affect which was certainly not of a clinical nature."[40] In our studies of drug-free patients with major depression,[42] OCD,[43] and panic disorder,[44] we have observed no significant change in symptoms at the point of maximal depletion of plasma TRYP. Although some physical symptoms, including drowsiness and faintness[39] and mild headache, nausea, and sweating,[38] have been associated with short-term TRYP depletion, these effects have been reported on the active depletion and sham testing days. Smith et al[41] determined in their study of healthy men that the change in depressive affect results from central processes rather than from cognitive processing of peripheral sensations or mental states such as fatigue.

We recently reported that short-term TRYP depletion led to a marked worsening of anxiety, irritability, agitation, mood, and perseveration in a drug-free woman with autistic disorder.[45] The purpose of the current double-blind, placebo-controlled investigation was to extend these studies of short-term TRYP depletion to a larger group of unmedicated patients with autistic disorder. Based on the hypothesis that central 5-HT function may be reduced in some patients with autism, it was posited that

Clinical Characteristics of Patients With Autistic Disorder (N=20)

Patient No.	Age, y	Sex	Full-Scale IQ*	ABC Score†
Global Exacerbation of Symptoms Following Acute Tryptophan Depletion				
1	29	M	97	70
2	23	F	75	84
3	24	M	56	90
4	40	F	106	98
5	36	M	115	98
6	33	M	112	99
7	23	M	32	99
8	25	M	114	118
9	31	M	96	123
10	36	M	91	124
11	26	M	96	147
No Change in Symptoms Following Acute Tryptophan Depletion				
12	33	M	114	61
13	27	M	79	74
14	53	M	45	74
15	22	M	86	75
16	22	M	105	77
17	45	M	107	124
Patients Who Did Not Complete Both Test Days				
18	27	F	108	63
19	35	F	84	104
20	20	M	98	106
All Patients				
Mean	30.5	...	90.8	95.4
SD	8.5	...	23.5	23.5

*All patients received the Wechsler Adult Intelligence Scale–Revised except patient 7 (nonverbal), who received the Leiter International Performance Scale.

†ABC indicates Autism Behavior Checklist.

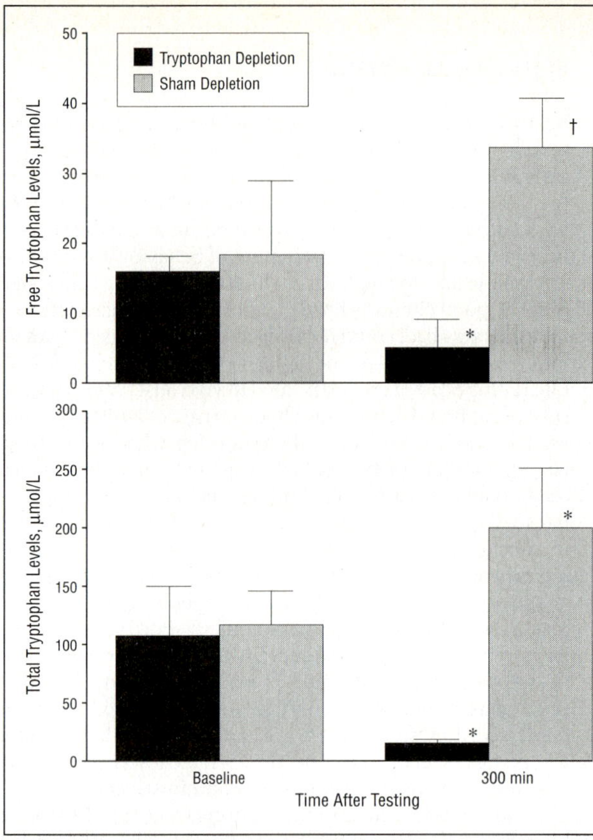

Figure 1. *Mean (±SD) free (top) and total (bottom) plasma tryptophan levels at baseline and the +300-minute period (5 hours after the drink) during sham depletion and tryptophan depletion. Asterisk indicates* P<.001 *compared with baseline (2-tailed paired* t *test); dagger,* P<.003 *compared with baseline (2-tailed paired* t *test).*

short-term TRYP depletion would result in an exacerbation of the agitation and aggression, impaired social relatedness, and repetitive thoughts and behavior characteristic of some patients with autism.

RESULTS

BIOCHEMICAL EFFECTS

During sham testing, plasma free and total TRYP levels increased in all patients (**Figure 1**), as would be expected with normal food intake. Free TRYP level was 18.2±10.7 µmol/L at baseline and increased to 33.6±7.0 µmol/L 5 hours after the TRYP-supplemented drink (*P*<.003). Total TRYP level was 115.0±29.9 µmol/L at baseline and increased to 199.0±53.5 µmol/L 5 hours after the TRYP supplemented drink (*P*<.001).

Short-term TRYP depletion markedly decreased plasma free and total TRYP levels (Figure 1). Baseline plasma free TRYP values were 16.0±2.1 µmol/L and decreased to 5.0±4.4 µmol/L 5 hours after the TRYP-free amino acid drink (*P*<.001). Plasma total TRYP values were 105.1±43.7 µmol/L at baseline and decreased to 14.7±4.5 µmol/L 5 hours after the TRYP-free drink (*P*<.001).

BEHAVIORAL EFFECTS

Clinician-Rated Global Severity Change Scale

The ANOVA assessing the change in clinician-rated global severity disclosed a significant main effect of challenge type (F=9.54; *df*=1,16; *P*<.007), time (F=4.00; *df*=2,32; *P*<.03), and challenge type × time (worse with short-term TRYP depletion) (F=4.31; *df*=2,32; *P*<.03). Eleven (65%) of the 17 patients who completed both test days showed a significant global worsening of behavioral symptoms with short-term TRYP depletion; none of the 17 patients showed any significant change in clinical status from baseline after sham depletion (*P*=.001, Fisher exact test) (**Figure 2**). Patients with ABC scores higher than 78 were significantly more likely to have an exacerbation of symptoms (10 of 11 patients) than were patients whose ABC scores were 78 or lower (1 of 6 patients) (*P*=.005, Fisher exact test) (Table). Patients who had a significant global exacerbation of symptoms also had significantly higher baseline plasma total TRYP levels than did those who showed no significant change in symptoms (115.9±17.1 vs 85.2±8.9 µmol/L) (*t*=4.07; *df*=15; *P*<.001, unpaired *t* test) (**Figure 3**). No difference was found in baseline plasma free TRYP levels between patients who had symptom exacerbation and those who showed no change (16.1±5.2 vs 15.4±3.0 µmol/L). Patients who showed a significant global exacerbation of

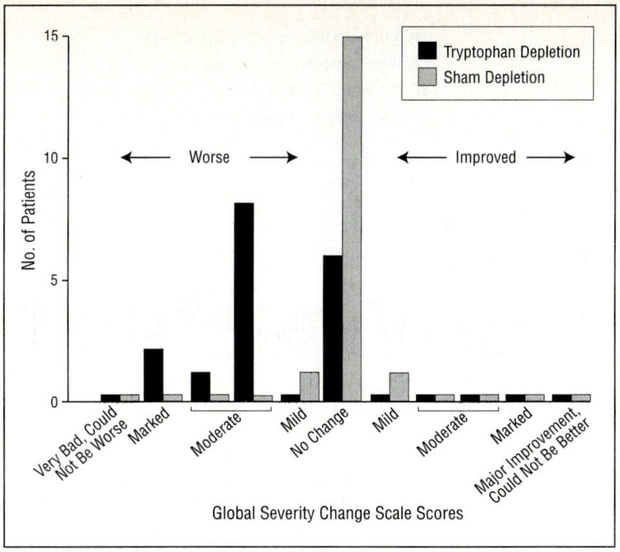

Figure 2. *Clinician-rated global severity change scale scores at the +300-minute period (5 hours after the drink) after tryptophan depletion (11 of 17 patients significantly worse) and sham depletion (none of 17 patients significantly worse) for 17 patients with autism (P=.001, Fisher exact test).*

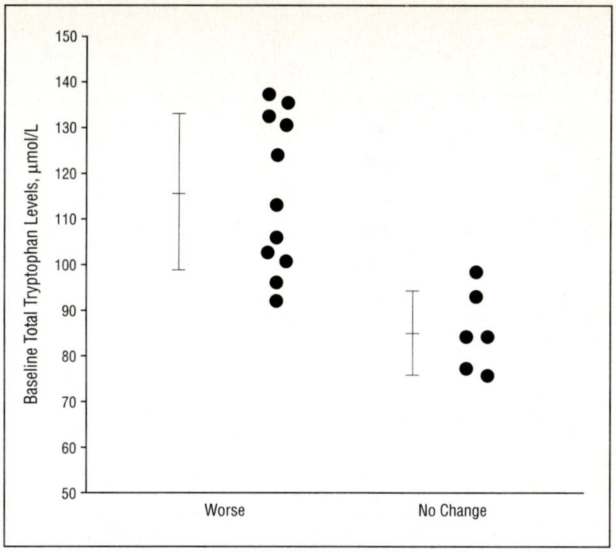

Figure 3. *Baseline plasma total tryptophan levels for 11 of 17 patients with autism who had a global exacerbation of symptoms ("worse") after short-term tryptophan depletion vs 6 of 17 patients who showed no change ("no change") (115.9±17.1 vs 85.2±8.9 μmol/L) (t=4.07; df=15; P<.001, unpaired t test).*

symptoms had a significantly greater decrease in plasma total TRYP levels (115.9±17.1 to 16.7±7.4 μmol/L) compared with those who showed no change (85.2±8.9 to 11.0±3.4 μmol/L) ($t=-3.35$; $df=15$); ($P<.004$). The percent change in plasma total TRYP levels, however, was not significantly different between the 2 groups. This finding probably is a result of the significant difference identified in baseline plasma total TRYP levels. No significant difference was found in change scores of plasma free TRYP levels between patients who showed a symptom exacerbation (16.1±5.2 to 5.9±8.1 μmol/L) compared with those who had no change after depletion (15.4±3.0 to 2.3±0.5 μmol/L) ($t=0.46$; $df=15$). Full-scale IQ was unrelated to change in clinician-rated global severity scale measures.

Ritvo-Freeman Real-Life Rating Scale

Baseline scores on the Ritvo-Freeman Real-Life Rating Scale did not differ significantly between test days. The ANOVA assessing the change in sensory motor behaviors (subscale 1) during short-term TRYP depletion and sham testing disclosed a significant challenge type × time interaction (increased with short-term TRYP depletion) ($F=2.69$; $df=3,48$; $P<.05$). The sensory motor behaviors that were assessed included whirling, flapping, pacing, banging and hitting self, rocking, and toe walking.[54] The individual scores for each patient at the 5-hour period for the depletion and sham testing days are shown in **Figure 4**. The ANOVAs assessing the challenge type × time interactions for subscales 2 to 5 were not significant.

Clinician-Rated Repetitive Thoughts and Repetitive Behavior Severity Scales

No significant differences were seen in baseline scores on these measures between test days. The ANOVAs assessing the change in repetitive thoughts and repetitive behavior during short-term TRYP depletion and sham testing disclosed no significant challenge type × time interactions (**Figure 5**).

Clinician-Rated Visual Analog Scales

No significant differences were found in baseline measures of these variables between test days. Significant main effects of time and challenge type × time for the 18 clinician-rated visual analog scales were as follows: anxious, significant main effect of time (increased) ($F=8.22$; $df=3,48$; $P<.001$) and a trend toward a significant challenge type × time interaction (increased with short-term TRYP depletion) ($F=2.20$; $df=3,48$; $P<.10$); calm, significant challenge type × time interaction (decreased with short-term TRYP depletion) ($F=4.12$; $df=3,48$; $P<.01$); happy, significant challenge type × time interaction (decreased with short-term TRYP depletion) ($F=3.45$; $df=3,48$; $P<.03$); hungry, significant main effect of time (increased) ($F=9.93$; $df=3,48$; $P<.001$); and tired, significant main effect of time (increased) ($F=3.77$; $df=3,48$; $P<.02$).

COMMENT

Short-term TRYP depletion resulted in a clinically and statistically significant global exacerbation of behavioral symptoms in 11 (65%) of the 17 drug-free patients with autism, as measured on the clinician-rated global severity change scale, but sham testing produced no significant change in symptoms. Patients with ABC scores higher than 78, consistent with higher levels of autistic behavior, were significantly more likely to have a global exacerbation of symptoms after TRYP depletion than were patients with ABC scores of 78 or lower. Patients who had a global exacerbation of symptoms after TRYP deple-

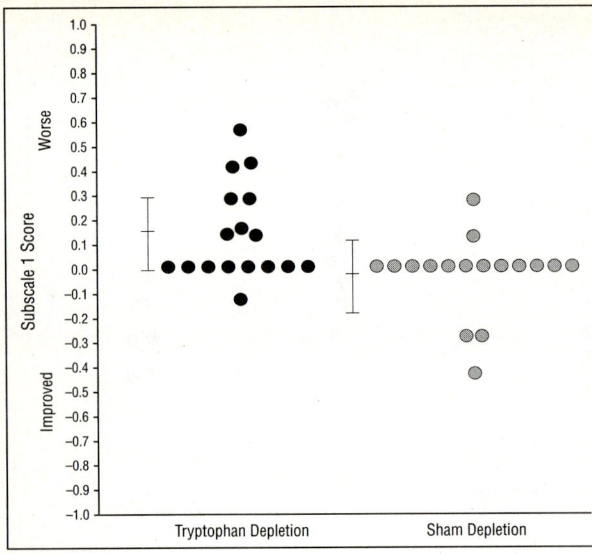

Figure 4. *Ritvo-Freeman Real-Life Rating Scale scores. Subscale 1 (whirling, flapping, pacing, banging and hitting self, rocking, and toe walking) at the +300-minute period (5 hours after the drink) after tryptophan depletion and sham depletion for 17 patients with autism.*

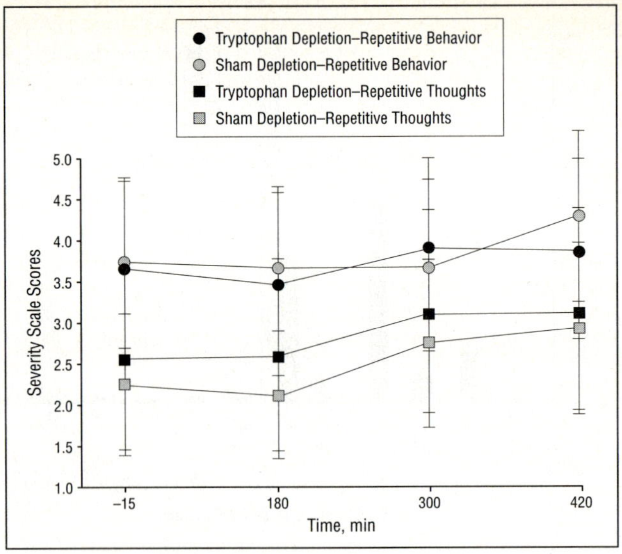

Figure 5. *Mean (±SEM) clinician-rated repetitive thoughts and repetitive behavior severity scale scores over time (minutes) for 17 patients with autism receiving tryptophan depletion and sham depletion.*

tion also had significantly higher baseline plasma total TRYP levels than did those who showed no significant change in symptoms after the drink. Global symptom exacerbation was unrelated to full-scale IQ. Short-term TRYP depletion led to a significant increase in a number of behaviors characteristic of autism, including whirling, flapping, pacing, banging and hitting self, rocking, and toe walking. In addition, patients were significantly less calm and happy and more anxious after short-term TRYP depletion compared with sham testing. These behavioral changes occurred in the context of significantly reduced plasma free (69%) and total (86%) TRYP, and, presumably, brain 5-HT levels. Significant changes in social relationship to people, affectual reactions, sensory responses, and language, as measured by subscales 2 to 5 of the Ritvo-Freeman Real-Life Rating Scale were not observed with short-term TRYP depletion. Similarly, no change occurred in the severity of repetitive thoughts and behavior.

Indirect evidence from related areas of preclinical and clinical research supports a role for central 5-HT in the neuromodulation of some of the clinical characteristics of autism, including aggression, social dysfunction, and repetitive thoughts and behavior. For example, CSF levels of 5-HIAA have been reported to be reduced in children with conduct and other aggressive behavioral disorders.[56,57] Moreover, the selective 5-HT uptake inhibitors fluvoxamine,[24] fluoxetine,[58] and sertraline hydrochloride[59] and the nonselective 5-HT uptake inhibitor clomipramine,[60] which increase synaptic 5-HT in the brain, have been reported to reduce aggression and self-injurious behavior in patients with autism and other developmental disabilities.

Many consider the core disturbance in autistic disorder to be impaired reciprocal verbal and nonverbal social interaction.[61] Central 5-HT has been found to contribute to the regulation of social behavior and social hierarchies in animals. For example, administration of the TRYP hydroxylase enzyme inhibitor *p*-chlorophenylalanine to vervet monkeys resulted in decreased grooming, approaching, resting, and eating behavior, and increased locomotion, being solitary, being vigilant, and avoidance. Fluoxetine, TRYP, and the 5-HT receptor agonist quipazine had the opposite effect.[62] In a recently published study in adolescent male rhesus monkeys living in naturalistic settings, those with low CSF 5-HIAA concentrations showed less social competence and emigrated from their social groups at a younger age than did males with higher concentrations of CSF 5-HIAA.[63] No measurable change in social relatedness was detected in the adult patients with autism after short-term TRYP depletion in our study. However, our measures for detecting and quantifying subtle changes in human social behavior may be insensitive and inaccurate.

Based primarily on drug treatment response data,[64] brain 5-HT has also been hypothesized to be involved in modulating the repetitive thoughts and behavior characteristic of OCD.[65] We have shown that short-term TRYP depletion has no significant effect on repetitive thoughts and behavior in drug-free patients with OCD.[43] Similarly, we observed no change in these phenomena in the patients with autism who completed our study. Although the repetitive thoughts and behavior of adults with OCD and autistic disorder have been shown to improve with 5-HT uptake inhibitor treatment, this response often takes 8 to 12 weeks.[24,64,66] Short-term changes in 5-HT precursor availability do not seem to alter the severity of repetitive thoughts and behavior in either diagnostic group.

Potent 5-HT uptake inhibitors, which increase central 5-HT neurotransmission, have been reported to improve some symptoms of autism.[16-24] In the first published controlled study of a potent 5-HT uptake inhibitor, Gordon et al[17] found clomipramine treatment for 5 weeks superior to that of the selective norepinephrine uptake inhibitor desipramine hydrochloride and placebo in randomized, crossover studies in children with autism. The core symptoms of autism and obsessive-compulsive symptoms were improved. In the first controlled study of a selective 5-HT uptake inhibitor, McDougle et al[24] reported that fluvoxamine was superior to placebo in reducing repetitive thoughts and behavior, maladaptive behavior and aggression, and in improving social relatedness, especially language usage, in adults with autism. Although caution should be exercised in drawing conclusions about underlying neurochemical dysregulation based on drug response data, these findings, considered with the results of the current study, support the hypothesis that central 5-HT function may be reduced in some patients with autism.

The short-term depletion of TRYP, and presumably brain 5-HT, resulted in a significant worsening of behavioral symptoms in 65% of patients with autistic disorder who participated in this controlled study. However, short-term TRYP depletion may have affected neuropeptides, second messenger systems, receptor synthesis, or some other nonspecific aspect of brain function. Moreover, it is possible that TRYP depletion and the consequent reduction of 5-HT may have altered some critical balance between 5-HT and other neurotransmitter systems (eg, dopamine and norepinephrine). Previous studies have described a lack of change in behavioral symptoms after TRYP depletion in drug-free patients with depression,[42] OCD,[43] and panic disorder.[44] The significant worsening of symptoms in most unmedicated adults with autism, therefore, suggests that these patients may be vulnerable to short-term alterations in central 5-HT neurotransmission, and that a dysregulation in brain 5-HT function may be more integral to the symptom manifestation of autism. Clearly, however, the results of this study require replication before definitive statements can be made in this regard.

Future studies might include using the short-term TRYP depletion paradigm to study children and adolescents with autism to provide a comparison group for assessing the influence of brain developmental changes on 5-HT function. It would be important to obtain baseline levels of WBS in subsequent studies to determine the relation between peripheral hyperserotonemia and TRYP depletion–induced symptom exacerbation. McBride et al[15] found a negative correlation between fenfluramine-induced prolactin release and baseline WBS content in their patients with autism. That baseline levels of plasma total TRYP were higher in patients with autism who showed symptom exacerbation with short-term TRYP depletion compared with those who remained clinically unchanged may be important in this light. In summary, the results of this study indicate that continued investigation into the role of 5-HT in the pathogenesis and treatment of autistic disorder may prove fruitful.

Accepted for publication October 26, 1995.

This work was supported by a National Alliance for Research on Schizophrenia and Depression Young Investigator Award (Dr McDougle), the State of Connecticut Department of Mental Health and Addiction Services, the Korczak Foundation for Autism and Related Disorders, and grants M01 RR06022-33, P50 MH30929-18, HD 03008-27, and P01 MH25642 from the National Institutes of Health, Bethesda, Md.

We thank the clinical and pharmacy staff of the Clinical Neuroscience Research Unit for their valuable assistance, Elizabeth Kyle for preparing the manuscript, Sally J. Vegso, MS, for the statistical analyses, and Elizabeth M. Ruff for the graphics work.

Reprints: Christopher J. McDougle, MD, Connecticut Mental Health Center, 34 Park St, Room 333B, New Haven, CT 06519.

REFERENCES

1. Schain RJ, Freedman DX. Studies on 5-hydroxyindole metabolism in autistic and other mentally retarded children. *J Pediatr.* 1961;58:315-320.
2. Anderson GM, Freedman DX, Cohen DJ, Volkmar FR, Hoder EL, McPhedran P, Minderaa RB, Hansen CR, Young JG. Whole blood serotonin in autistic and normal subjects. *J Child Psychol Psychiatry.* 1987;28:885-900.
3. Hanley HG, Stahl SM, Freedman DX. Hyperserotonemia and amine metabolites in autistic and retarded children. *Arch Gen Psychiatry.* 1977;34:521-531.
4. Cohen DJ, Shaywitz BA, Johnson WT, Bowers MB. Biogenic amines in autistic and atypical children: cerebrospinal fluid measures of homovanillic acid and 5-hydroxyindoleacetic acid. *Arch Gen Psychiatry.* 1974;31:845-853.
5. Narayan M, Srinath S, Anderson GM, Meundi DB. Cerebrospinal fluid levels of homovanillic acid and 5-hydroxyindoleacetic acid in autism. *Biol Psychiatry.* 1993;33:630-635.
6. Geller E, Ritvo ER, Freeman BJ, Yuwiler A. Preliminary observations on the effect of fenfluramine on blood serotonin and symptoms in three autistic boys. *N Engl J Med.* 1982;307:165-169.
7. Campbell M. Fenfluramine treatment of autism. *J Child Psychol Psychiatry.* 1988;29:1-10.
8. Ekman G, Miranda-Linné F, Gillberg C, Garle M, Wetterberg L. Fenfluramine treatment of twenty children with autism. *J Autism Dev Disord.* 1989;19:511-532.
9. Sherman J, Factor DC, Swinson R, Darjes RW. The effects of fenfluramine (hydrochloride) on the behaviors of fifteen autistic children. *J Autism Dev Disord.* 1989;19:533-543.
10. Duker PC, Welles K, Seys D, Rensen H, Vis A. Brief report: effects of fenfluramine on communicative, stereotypic, and inappropriate behaviors of autistic-type mentally handicapped individuals. *J Autism Dev Disord.* 1991;21:355-363.
11. Chase TM, Shoulson I. Behavioral and biochemical effects of fenfluramine in patients with neurologic disease. *Postgrad Med J.* 1975;51:105-109.
12. Schuster CR, Lewis M, Seiden LS. Fenfluramine: neurotoxicity. *Psychopharmacol Bull.* 1986;22:148-151.
13. Volkmar FR, Paul R, Cohen DJ, Shaywitz BA. Irritability in autistic children treated with fenfluramine. *N Engl J Med.* 1983;309:187.
14. Hoshino Y, Tachibana JR, Watanabe M, Murata S, Yokoyama F, Kaneko M, Yashima Y, Kumoshiro H. Serotonin metabolism and hypothalamic-pituitary function in children with infantile autism and minimal brain dysfunction. *Jpn J Psychiatry Neurol.* 1984;26:937-945.
15. McBride PA, Anderson GM, Hertzig ME, Sweeney JA, Kream J, Cohen DJ, Mann JJ. Serotonergic responsivity in male young adults with autistic disorder: results of a pilot study. *Arch Gen Psychiatry.* 1989;46:213-221.
16. McDougle CJ, Price LH, Volkmar FR, Goodman WK, Ward-O'Brien D, Nielsen J, Bregman J, Cohen DJ. Clomipramine in autism: preliminary evidence of efficacy. *J Am Acad Child Adolesc Psychiatry.* 1992;31:746-750.
17. Gordon CT, State RC, Nelson JE, Hamburger SD, Rapoport JL. A double-blind comparison of clomipramine, desipramine, and placebo in the treatment of autistic disorder. *Arch Gen Psychiatry.* 1993;50:441-447.
18. Cook EH, Rowlett R, Jaselskis C, Leventhal BL. Fluoxetine treatment of children and adults with autistic disorder and mental retardation. *J Am Acad Child Adolesc Psychiatry.* 1992;31:739-745.
19. Mehlinger R, Scheftner WA, Poznanski E. Fluoxetine and autism. *J Am Acad Child Adolesc Psychiatry.* 1990;29:985.
20. Hamdan-Allen G. Brief report: trichotillomania in an autistic male. *J Autism Dev Disord.* 1991;21:79-82.
21. Todd RD. Fluoxetine in autism. *Am J Psychiatry.* 1991;148:1089.
22. Ghaziuddin M, Tsai L, Ghaziuddin N. Fluoxetine in autism with depression. *J Am Acad Child Adolesc Psychiatry.* 1991;30:3.
23. McDougle CJ, Price LH, Goodman WK. Fluvoxamine treatment of coincident autistic disorder and obsessive-compulsive disorder: a case report. *J Autism*

Dev Disord. 1990;20:537-543.
24. McDougle CJ, Naylor ST, Cohen DJ, Volkmar FR, Heninger GR, Price LH. A double-blind, placebo-controlled study of fluvoxamine in adults with autistic disorder. *Arch Gen Psychiatry.* 1996;53:1001-1008.
25. Rose WC, Haines WJ, Warner DT. The amino acid requirements of man. *J Biol Chem.* 1954;206:421-430.
26. Gal EM, Dreses PA. Studies on the metabolism of 5-hydroxytryptamine (serotonin), II: effect of tryptophan deficiency in rats. *Proc Soc Exp Biol Med.* 1962;110:368-371.
27. Fernstrom JD. Effects of the diet on brain neurotransmitters. *Metabolism.* 1977; 26:207-223.
28. Curzon G. Influence of plasma tryptophan on brain 5HT synthesis and serotonergic activity. In: Haber G, Gabay S, eds. *Serotonin: Current Aspects of Neurochemistry and Function.* New York, NY: Plenum Publishing Corp; 1981: 207-219.
29. Young SN, Ervin FR, Phil RO, Finn P. Biochemical aspects of tryptophan depletion in primates. *Psychopharmacology (Berl).* 1989;95:508-511.
30. Moja EA, Cipollo P, Castoldi D, Tofanetti O. Dose-response decrease in plasma tryptophan and in brain tryptophan and serotonin after tryptophan-free amino acid mixtures in rats. *Life Sci.* 1989;44:971-976.
31. Moir ATB, Eccleston D. The effects of precursor loading in the cerebral metabolism of 5-hydroxyindoles. *J Neurochem.* 1968;15:1093-1108.
32. Fernstrom JD, Hirsch MJ. Rapid repletion of brain serotonin in malnourished corn-fed rats following L-tryptophan injection. *Life Sci.* 1975;17:455-464.
33. Lytle LD, Messing RB, Fisher L, Phebus L. Effects of long-term corn consumption on brain serotonin and the response to electric shock. *Science.* 1975; 190:692-694.
34. Messing RB, Fisher LA, Phebus L, Lytle LD. Interaction of diet and drugs in the regulation of brain 5-hydroxyindoles and the response to painful electric shock. *Life Sci.* 1976;18:707-714.
35. Walters JK, Davis M, Sheard MH. Tryptophan-free diet: effects on the acoustic startle reflex in rats. *Psychopharmacology.* 1979;62:103-109.
36. Gibbons JL, Barr GA, Bridger WH, Leibowitz SF. Manipulations of dietary tryptophan: effects on mouse killing and brain serotonin in the rat. *Brain Res.* 1979; 169:139-153.
37. Harper AE, Benevenga NJ, Wohlhueter RM. Effects of ingestion of disproportionate amounts of amino acids. *Physiol Rev.* 1970;50:428-548.
38. Delgado PL, Charney DS, Price LH, Aghajanian GK, Landis H, Heninger GR. Serotonin function and the mechanism of antidepressant action: reversal of antidepressant induced remission by rapid depletion of plasma tryptophan. *Arch Gen Psychiatry.* 1990;47:411-418.
39. Barr LC, Goodman WK, McDougle CJ, Delgado PL, Heninger GR, Charney DS, Price LH. Tryptophan depletion in patients with obsessive-compulsive disorder who respond to serotonin reuptake inhibitors. *Arch Gen Psychiatry.* 1994; 51:309-317.
40. Young SN, Smith SE, Pihl RD, Ervin FR. Tryptophan depletion causes a rapid lowering of mood in normal males. *Psychopharmacology (Berl).* 1985;87:173-177.
41. Smith SE, Pihl RO, Young SW, Ervin FR. A test of possible cognitive and environmental influences on the mood-lowering effect of tryptophan depletion in normal males. *Psychopharmacology.* 1987;91:451-457.
42. Delgado PL, Price LH, Miller HL, Salomon RM, Aghajanian GK, Heninger GR, Charney DS. Serotonin and the neurobiology of depression: effects of tryptophan depletion in drug-free depressed patients. *Arch Gen Psychiatry.* 1994; 51:865-874.
43. Barr LC, Goodman WK, Delgado PL, McDougle CJ, Price LH. Effects of tryptophan depletion in drug-free obsessive compulsive disorder patients. *Biol Psychiatry.* In press.
44. Goddard AW, Sholomskas DE, Augeri FM, Walton KE, Charney DS, Heninger GR, Goodman WK, Price LH. Effects of tryptophan depletion in panic disorder. *Biol Psychiatry.* 1994;36:775-777.
45. McDougle CJ, Naylor ST, Goodman WK, Volkmar FR, Cohen DJ, Price LH. Acute tryptophan depletion in autistic disorder: a controlled case study. *Biol Psychiatry.* 1993;33:547-550.
46. American Psychiatric Association. *Diagnostic and Statistical Manual of Mental Disorders, Third Edition, Revised.* Washington, DC: American Psychiatric Association; 1987.
47. World Health Organization. *International Statistical Classification of Diseases, 10th Revision (ICD-10).* Geneva, Switzerland: World Health Organization; 1992.
48. Guy W. *ECDEU Assessment Manual for Psychopharmacology.* Washington, DC: US Dept of Health, Education, and Welfare; 1976. Publication 76-338.
49. Le Couteur A, Rutter M, Lord C, Rios P, Robertson S, Holdgrafer M, McLennan J. Autism Diagnostic Interview: a standardized investigator-based instrument. *J Autism Dev Disord.* 1989;19:363-387.
50. Lord C, Rutter M, Goode S, Heemsbergen J, Jordan H, Mawhood L, Schopler E. Autism Diagnostic Observation Schedule: a standardized observation of communicative and social behavior. *J Autism Dev Disord.* 1989;19:185-212.
51. Krug DA, Arick JR, Almond PJ. *Autism Screening Instrument for Education Planning.* Portland, Ore: ASIEP Educational Co; 1980.
52. Wechsler D. *Manual for the Wechsler Adult Intelligence Scale–Revised.* San Antonio, Tex: The Psychological Corp; 1981.
53. Leiter RG. *Leiter International Performance Scale.* Chicago, Ill: Stoelting Co; 1948.
54. Freeman BJ, Ritvo ER, Yokota A, Ritvo A. A scale for rating symptoms of patients with the syndrome of autism in real life settings. *J Am Acad Child Adolesc Psychiatry.* 1986;25:130-136.
55. Anderson GM, Young JG, Cohen DJ, Schlicht KR, Patel N. Liquid-chromatographic determination of serotonin and tryptophan in whole blood and plasma. *Clin Chem.* 1981;27:775-776.
56. Kruesi MJ, Rapoport JL, Hamburger S, Hibbs E, Potter WZ, Lenane M, Brown GL. Cerebrospinal fluid monoamine metabolites, aggression, and impulsivity in disruptive behavior disorders of children and adolescents. *Arch Gen Psychiatry.* 1990;47:419-426.
57. Kruesi MJ, Hibbs ED, Zahn TP, Keysor CS, Hamburger SD, Bartko JJ, Rapoport JL. A 2-year prospective follow-up study of children and adolescents with disruptive behavior disorders: prediction by cerebrospinal fluid 5-hydroxyindoleacetic acid, homovanillic acid, and autonomic measures? *Arch Gen Psychiatry.* 1992;49:429-435.
58. Markowitz PI. Effect of fluoxetine on self-injurious behavior in the developmentally disabled: a preliminary study. *J Clin Psychopharmacol.* 1992;12:27-31.
59. Kelley LA, Hellings JA, Gabrielli WF, Kilgore E. Sertraline response in mentally retarded adults. Presented at the American Psychiatric Association 146th Annual Meeting; May 22-27, 1993; San Francisco, Calif.
60. Garber HJ, McGonigle JJ, Slomka GT, Monteverde E. Clomipramine treatment of stereotypic behaviors and self-injury in patients with developmental disabilities. *J Am Acad Child Adolesc Psychiatry.* 1992;31:1157-1160.
61. Volkmar FR. Social development. In: Cohen D, Donnellan A, eds. *Handbook of Autism and Pervasive Developmental Disorders.* New York, NY: John Wiley & Sons Inc; 1987:41-60.
62. Raleigh MJ, Brammer GL, Yuwiler A, Flannery JW, McGuire MT, Geller E. Serotonergic influences on the social behavior of vervet monkeys (*Cercopithecus aethiops sabaeus*). *Exp Neurol.* 1980;68:322-324.
63. Mehlman PT, Higley JD, Faucher I, Lilly AA, Taub DM, Vickers J, Suomi SJ, Linnoila M. Correlation of CSF 5-HIAA concentration with sociality and the timing of emigration in free-ranging primates. *Am J Psychiatry.* 1995;152:907-913.
64. Goodman WK, Price LH, Rasmussen SA, Delgado PL, Heninger GR, Charney DS. Efficacy of fluvoxamine in obsessive-compulsive disorder: a double-blind comparison with placebo. *Arch Gen Psychiatry.* 1989;46:36-43.
65. Insel TR, Mueller EA, Alterman A, Linnoila M, Murphy DL. Obsessive-compulsive disorder and serotonin: is there a connection? *Biol Psychiatry.* 1985; 20:1174-1188.
66. McDougle CJ, Kresch L, Goodman WK, Naylor ST, Volkmar FR, Cohen DJ, Price LH. Repetitive thoughts and behaviors in adults with autistic disorder and obsessive compulsive disorder: a case-controlled study. *Am J Psychiatry.* 1995;152:772-777.

ORIGINAL ARTICLE

A Double-blind, Placebo-Controlled Study of Fluvoxamine in Adults With Autistic Disorder

Christopher J. McDougle, MD; Susan T. Naylor, RN, MSN; Donald J. Cohen, MD; Fred R. Volkmar, MD; George R. Heninger, MD; Lawrence H. Price, MD

Background: Autistic disorder is characterized by a fundamental disturbance in social interaction, impairments in communication, and a markedly restricted repertoire of activities and interests. Abnormalities in the serotonin neurotransmitter system have been identified in some persons with autism. No consistently effective and safe drugs have been developed for treating the symptoms of autism.

Methods: Thirty adults with autistic disorder completed a 12-week double-blind, placebo-controlled trial of the potent and selective serotonin uptake inhibitor fluvoxamine maleate. Behavioral ratings were obtained at baseline and after 4, 8, and 12 weeks of treatment.

Results: Eight (53%) of 15 patients in the fluvoxamine-treated group were categorized as responders compared with none of 15 in the placebo group (P=.001). Fluvoxamine was superior to placebo in reducing repetitive thoughts and behavior (P<.001), maladaptive behavior (P<.001), and aggression (P<.03), and in improving some aspects of social relatedness (P<.04), especially language usage (P<.008). Treatment response was not correlated with age, level of autistic behavior, or full-scale IQ. Other than mild sedation and nausea in a few patients, fluvoxamine was well tolerated. No dyskinesias, adverse cardiovascular events, or seizures occurred.

Conclusions: Fluvoxamine is more effective than placebo in the short-term treatment of the symptoms of autistic disorder in adults. Controlled studies of fluvoxamine and other potent and selective serotonin uptake inhibitors seem warranted in children and adolescents with autism.

Arch Gen Psychiatry. 1996;53:1001-1008

AUTISTIC DISORDER is a lifelong neuropsychiatric syndrome of childhood onset first described by Kanner in 1943.[1] Core clinical characteristics include a fundamental disturbance in social interaction, impairments in communication, and a markedly restricted repertoire of activities and interests.[2] Associated features that are often present include aggression toward people and the environment, self-injury, and repetitive thoughts and behavior.[3]

Although typically considered a "childhood" disorder, most persons with autism experience notable functional impairment throughout their lives. Follow-up studies of children with autism have found that only 5% to 10% become independent as adults, 25% progress but still require supervision, and the remainder continue to be severely impaired and in need of a high level of institutionalized care.[4] Thus, the syndrome represents a substantial public health problem with tragic cost to the individual, the family, and the community.

Although little is definitively known about the pathogenesis of autism,[5] abnormalities in the serotonin (5-hydroxytryptamine [5-HT]) neurotransmitter system have been identified in a subgroup of patients. Schain and Freedman[6] first reported elevated levels of whole-blood 5-HT in the peripheral vascular system of children with autism in 1961. Others have replicated this finding in groups of children with autism compared with normal control subjects.[7] Antibodies against human brain 5-HT receptors were identified in the blood and cerebrospinal fluid of a child with autism,[8] although subsequent studies found no difference in the degree of immunoglobulin inhibition of binding of the 5-HT1A agonist [^{3}H]-8-hydroxy-N,N-

From the Clinical Neuroscience Research Unit, Abraham Ribicoff Research Facilities, Connecticut Mental Health Center (Drs McDougle, Heninger, and Price and Ms Naylor), and the Department of Psychiatry (Drs McDougle, Cohen, Heninger, and Price and Ms Naylor) and the Child Study Center (Drs McDougle, Cohen, and Volkmar), Yale University School of Medicine, New Haven, Conn.

See Patients and Methods on next page

PATIENTS AND METHODS

PATIENTS

Thirty adults who were diagnosed as having autistic disorder and their parent or legal guardian provided written informed consent (or assent for patients with cognitive limitations) for participation in this study, which had been approved by the Human Investigation Committee of Yale University School of Medicine, New Haven, Conn. Diagnoses were based on *Diagnostic and Statistical Manual of Mental Disorders, Revised Third Edition (DSM-III-R)*[36] and *International Classification of Diseases, 10th Revision*[37] criteria for autistic disorder. The sample consisted of 27 men and 3 women aged 18 to 53 years (mean[±SD] age, 30.1±7.7 years) who were referred by group homes for patients with autism, community-based psychiatrists, chapters of the Autism Society of America throughout New England, and family members. Nine patients were treated on the inpatient division of the Clinical Neuroscience Research Unit of the Connecticut Mental Health Center, New Haven, and 21 participated as outpatients in the Adult Pervasive Developmental Disorders Clinic of the Clinical Neuroscience Research Unit. The study was conducted between September 1, 1990, and December 31, 1993.

Each patient's symptoms were at least "moderate" in severity, as defined by global severity of illness rating on the Clinical Global Impression (CGI) Scale.[38] The Autism Diagnostic Interview[39] and the Autism Diagnostic Observation Schedule[40] criteria were completed by trained professionals (C.J.M. and S.T.N.) to aid in diagnosis and to provide additional measures of severity of the condition. The Autism Behavior Checklist[41] was completed with the parent or legal guardian of each patient to determine the patient's level of autistic behavior. Full-scale IQ was measured with the Wechsler Adult Intelligence Scale-Revised[42] in the 26 verbal patients, and the Leiter International Performance Scale[43] was used to assess IQ in the 4 nonverbal patients. Patients were psychotropic drug-free for at least 6 weeks before the start of the trial. Screening procedures included a medical history, physical and neurological examinations, complete blood count with differential; electrolytes, fasting glucose, serum urea nitrogen, creatinine, liver and thyroid function tests; urinalysis; electrocardiogram; and serum pregnancy test in women. Patients were excluded if they met *DSM-III-R* criteria for schizophrenia or had psychotic symptoms, if they had abused illicit substances within the previous 6 months, or if a notable medical condition, including seizure disorder, was identified. Women with positive serum pregnancy test results were excluded. One male patient had fragile X syndrome; none of the other patients had a diagnosed genetic, metabolic, or neurological cause for their syndrome.

STUDY DRUG ASSIGNMENT AND TREATMENT

After 2 visits during which baseline behavioral ratings were obtained, patients were randomized to 12 weeks of double-blind treatment with fluvoxamine or placebo (lactose) in identical-looking capsules. To ensure compliance, the medication was administered by parents or other primary caretakers. Fluvoxamine or placebo was started at 50 mg every night. The dosage could then be increased by 50 mg daily every 3 or 4 days to a maximum dosage of 300 mg/d, as tolerated, if maximal clinical response was not obtained. Thus, the maximum dosage of fluvoxamine was attained within 3 weeks, and patients received this dose for at least 9 weeks. Fluvoxamine blood levels were not obtained, because previous studies have shown no correlation between blood level and clinical response.[44] The prescribing psychiatrist (C.J.M.), the nurse (S.T.N.) who performed the behavioral ratings, the patients, and all family and other members of the patients' treatment teams were unaware of drug assignment.

dipropyl-2-aminotetralin to 5-HT1A receptors between patients with autism and control subjects.[9,10] Blunted neuroendocrine responses to pharmacological probes of the 5-HT system have been observed in children with autism[11] and adults[12] compared with normal control subjects. Finally, short-term dietary depletion of the 5-HT precursor tryptophan has been associated with an exacerbation of behavioral symptoms in drug-free adults with autism.[13]

See also pages 980, 985, and 993

To date, consistently effective and safe pharmacological treatments for persons with autistic disorder are limited.[14] Haloperidol, a dopamine receptor antagonist, has been found more effective than placebo in decreasing hyperactivity, temper tantrums, irritability, stereotypies, and withdrawal in children with autism.[15] However, haloperidol-related dyskinesias (withdrawal and tardive) have been identified in up to 29% of children with autism.[16] Despite initial enthusiasm for fenfluramine hydrochloride,[17] a drug with multiple effects on 5-HT neuronal function, the efficacy and safety of this drug as a treatment for autism is now being reconsidered.[18] Controlled studies by Campbell et al[19] and others[20-22] have found fenfluramine no better than placebo in reducing interfering behavioral symptoms in children with autism. Furthermore, fenfluramine administration may result in potentially irreversible changes in 5-HT neurons.[23] Although results from open-label studies of the opiate receptor antagonist naltrexone suggested that social withdrawal and stereotypies were reduced and verbal production was increased,[24] a double-blind study in 41 children with autism found the drug useful only for hyperactivity.[25] Moreover, naltrexone had no therapeutic effects on autistic symptoms or self-injurious behavior and increased the incidence of stereotypic behavior in adults with autism.[26]

Preliminary findings suggest that drugs that facilitate 5-HT neurotransmission may reduce certain symptoms in some patients with autism. McDougle et al[27] reported that the selective 5-HT uptake inhibitor fluvoxamine maleate reduced interfering repetitive thoughts

RATING SCALES

Each patient, along with the members of the treatment team (eg, group home staff, parent or sibling, workshop staff), participated in a detailed assessment of behavioral symptoms at baseline and again at the end of weeks 4, 8, and 12. The same informants and the patient were present for each of the rating sessions. Repetitive thoughts and behavior were rated with a modified version of the Yale-Brown Obsessive Compulsive Scale (Y-BOCS),[45] a 10-item, semistructured, clinician-rated questionnaire that is valid and reliable for assessing the severity of obsessive-compulsive symptoms in patients with obsessive-compulsive disorder (OCD). Each item on the Y-BOCS is scored on a 5-point scale, from 0, indicating least symptomatic, to 4, indicating most symptomatic, so that the total Y-BOCS score (sum of items 1-10) ranges from 0 to 40. The first 5 items of the Y-BOCS are designed to assess the severity of repetitive thoughts; the last 5 items determine the severity of repetitive behavior. Because 4 of the patients were nonverbal and thus unable to provide information about repetitive thoughts, their maximum Y-BOCS score was 20. Based on previous findings,[46] the ego-dystonicity diagnostic criterion for OCD was eliminated in rating the repetitive thoughts and behavior of the patients with autism. Aggression was rated with a modified version of the Brown Aggression Scale, a 9-category instrument that assesses different aspects of aggressive behavior.[47] Patients could receive a score from 0, indicating nonoccurrence, to 4, indicating many, numerous, or multiple aggressive events on each of the 9 categories (range for total score, 0-36). The Ritvo-Freeman Real-Life Rating Scale[48] served as an in vivo observational measure of various symptoms of autism, including sensory-motor behaviors, social relationship to people, affectual reactions, sensory responses, and language. Each of the 5 subscales contains several items that are scored on a 4-point scale, with 0 indicating never; 1, rarely; 2, frequently; and 3, almost always. These 5 subscale scores were totaled to yield a Ritvo-Freeman Scale overall score (range for total score, −0.4175 to 6.89). The Vineland Adaptive Behavior Scale[49] maladaptive behavior subscales (parts 1 and 2) also were administered at each assessment timepoint. Finally, the CGI global improvement item (7, indicating very much worse, to 1, indicating very much improved) was recorded at each rating session after the baseline period.

STATISTICAL ANALYSIS

Baseline ratings were obtained from the mean scores of the 2 initial behavioral assessments. An analysis of variance (ANOVA) with repeated measures was calculated for all 12 weeks of fluvoxamine or placebo treatment to assess the significance of main effects of drug, time, and drug × time interactions. The reported *P* values for all ANOVAs used the Huynh-Feldt correction factor. This correction factor decreases the *df* used in the ANOVA to reflect lack of homogeneity in the variance of measures across timepoints; for clarity, uncorrected *df* are given. Paired Student *t* tests were calculated to evaluate change from baseline within treatment groups. Analysis of covariance (ANCOVA), using the baseline score as a covariate, was used to determine when significant drug-placebo differences took place.

Fisher exact test was used to compare the 2 groups for rate of responders vs nonresponders. Response was determined by scores obtained at the end of the last week of treatment on the CGI. Patients with CGI scores of much improved or very much improved were categorized as responders. Pearson correlations were used to evaluate the relations between treatment response and age, level of autistic behavior as determined with the Autism Behavior Checklist, and full-scale IQ. Data are given as mean (±SD), unless otherwise indicated, and results are reported as significant when $P<.05$ (2-tailed).

and behavior and aggression and improved social relatedness in a 30-year-old man with autism. Cook et al[28] and others[29-32] found the selective 5-HT uptake inhibitor fluoxetine hydrochloride useful for reducing ritualistic behavior and aggression and improving social function in children and adults with autism. McDougle et al[33] described symptomatic improvement with the nonselective 5-HT uptake inhibitor clomipramine hydrochloride in young adults with autism. In a controlled study, Gordon et al[34] found clomipramine more effective than desipramine hydrochloride, a potent inhibitor of norepinephrine uptake, and placebo, in children with autism. However, clomipramine resulted in prolongation of the corrected QT interval, severe tachycardia (resting heart rate up to 160-170 beats/min), and a grand mal seizure, respectively, in 3 of the children. Because of the risks of tardive and withdrawal dyskinesias with haloperidol,[16] neurotoxic effects with fenfluramine,[23] the lack of robust effects with naltrexone,[25,26] and the potential for cardiac toxic effects, sudden death, and seizures with tricyclics such as clomipramine,[34,35] safer and more effective drug treatments for the symptoms of autism are needed.

To our knowledge, our study of fluvoxamine is the first controlled investigation of selective 5-HT uptake inhibitor treatment in children or adults with autistic disorder. It was hypothesized that fluvoxamine would be more effective than placebo in reducing interfering repetitive thoughts and behavior and aggression, in improving social relatedness, and would be safer and better tolerated than other currently available drug treatments for autism.

RESULTS

All 30 patients completed the 12-week study and were thus included in the efficacy analysis. Fifteen patients were randomized to fluvoxamine and 15 received placebo. There was no significant difference in dosage between patients randomized to fluvoxamine maleate (276.7±41.7 mg/d) vs placebo (283.3±36.2 mg/d) (**Table**).

The clinical characteristics of the fluvoxamine and placebo groups are given in the Table. The fluvoxamine group (age, 30.1±7.1 years) consisted of 2 women and

Clinical Characteristics of Autistic Patients (N=30)

Patient No.	Age, y	Sex	Full-scale IQ*	ABC Score†	Dose, mg/d
			Fluvoxamine Group		
1	27	M	79	74	200
2	31	M	71	63	300
3	22	M	86	75	300
4	33	M	112	99	300
5	34	M	110	100	200
6	20	M	98	106	250
7‡	31	M	68	93	300
8	29	F	55	109	300
9	31	M	96	123	300
10	33	M	114	61	300
11	45	M	107	124	300
12	43	F	45	117	300
13	25	M	108	56	300
14	24	M	56	90	200
15	23	M	32	99	300
Mean	30.1	...	82.5	92.6	276.7
SD	7.1	...	26.8	22.3	41.7
			Placebo Group		
16	36	M	91	124	200
17	29	M	97	70	300
18	29	M	74	99	300
19	25	M	56	112	300
20	22	M	25	128	300
21	25	M	114	118	300
22	36	M	115	98	300
23	26	M	114	106	300
24	18	M	88	64	250
25	27	M	30	93	300
26	26	M	96	147	300
27	35	M	82	47	300
28	37	M	25	93	300
29	53	M	45	74	300
30	27	F	108	63	200
Mean	30.1	...	77.3	95.7	283.3
SD	8.4	...	33.1	27.9	36.2
			All Patients		
Mean	30.1	...	79.9	94.2	280.0
SD	7.7	...	29.7	24.9	38.5

**All patients received the Wechsler Adult Intelligence Scale–Revised except patients 15, 20, 25, and 28 (nonverbal), who received the Leiter International Performance Scale.*

†ABC indicates Autism Behavior Checklist.

‡Patient 7 has fragile X syndrome.

13 men; the placebo group (age, 30.1±8.4 years) consisted of 1 woman and 14 men. No significant differences were seen in age, sex distribution, Autism Behavior Checklist scores, or full-scale IQ scores between the 2 groups.

GLOBAL TREATMENT RESPONSE

Ratings on the CGI showed fluvoxamine superior to placebo ($F=21.12$; $df=3,84$; $P<.001$). In comparing fluvoxamine and placebo on global improvement, fluvoxamine showed significant superiority beginning at week 4 ($t=3.0$; $df=28$; $P<.006$) and continuing at weeks 8 ($t=4.6$; $df=28$; $P<.001$) and 12 ($t=5.3$; $df=28$; $P<.001$) (**Figure 1**). In the fluvoxamine group, the global improvement measure first became significant after 4 weeks ($t=2.7$; $df=14$; $P<.02$) and remained highly significant at weeks 8 ($t=4.5$; $df=14$; $P<.001$) and 12 ($t=5.1$; $df=14$; $P<.001$). No significant change in the CGI score was identified with placebo (Figure 1).

Eight (53%) of 15 of the fluvoxamine-treated patients were categorized as responders compared with none of 15 in the placebo group ($P=.001$, Fisher exact test). Treatment response was not correlated with age, level of autistic behavior, or full-scale IQ.

RESPONSE OF REPETITIVE THOUGHTS AND BEHAVIOR

As measured by reduction in total Y-BOCS scores, fluvoxamine was superior to placebo in the treatment of repetitive thoughts and behavior ($F=11.48$; $df=3,84$; $P<.001$). Baseline Y-BOCS scores did not differ significantly between the fluvoxamine (21.4±7.3) and placebo (21.5±6.8) groups. In the comparison of fluvoxamine and placebo on total repetitive thoughts and

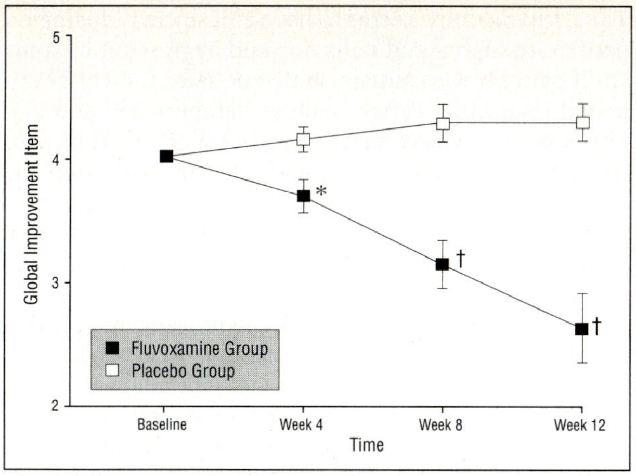

Figure 1. *Global improvement in patients with autism who were given fluvoxamine or placebo for 12 weeks, as measured on the Clinical Global Impression Scale global improvement item. Asterisk indicates* P<.006, *change from beginning of treatment trial, fluvoxamine vs placebo, Student* t *test; dagger,* P<.001, *change from beginning of treatment trial, fluvoxamine vs placebo, Student* t *test. Variance bars represent SE.*

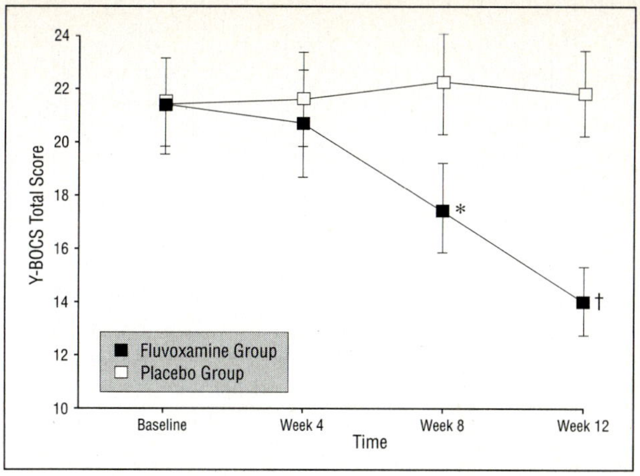

Figure 2. *Change in severity of repetitive thoughts and behavior in patients with autism who were given fluvoxamine or placebo for 12 weeks, as measured on the Yale-Brown Obsessive Compulsive Scale (Y-BOCS), ranging from 0, no symptoms; to 40, most severe symptoms. Asterisk indicates* P<.01, *change from baseline, fluvoxamine vs placebo, analysis of covariance; dagger,* P<.001, *change from baseline, fluvoxamine vs placebo, analysis of covariance. Variance bars represent SE.*

behavior, fluvoxamine produced significant reductions in Y-BOCS scores beginning at week 8 (F=7.67; *df*=1,27; *P*<.01) and continuing at week 12 (F=13.62; *df*=1,27; *P*<.001) (**Figure 2**).

In the fluvoxamine group, the reduction in Y-BOCS scores first became significant at week 8 of treatment (*t*=2.4; *df*=14; *P*<.03). By week 12, the reduction in Y-BOCS scores became highly significant (*t*=3.6; *df*=14; *P*<.003), representing a 36% decrease from baseline (21.4±7.3 to 13.7±9.1). In contrast, no significant change occurred with placebo (21.5±6.8 [baseline] to 21.9±6.7 [end of week 12]) (Figure 2).

Fluvoxamine was more effective than placebo in reducing Y-BOCS subscale scores for repetitive thoughts (F=6.02; *df*=3,84; *P*<.003) and repetitive behavior (F=10.04; *df*=3,84; *P*<.001). Baseline repetitive thoughts (9.6±4.9 vs 8.4±6.5) and behavior (11.8±4.5 vs 13.1±3.0) did not differ significantly between the fluvoxamine and placebo groups. In comparing the therapeutic effect of fluvoxamine and placebo on repetitive thoughts, fluvoxamine produced a significant reduction beginning at week 8 (F=5.76; *df*=1,27; *P*<.02) and continuing at week 12 (F=6.36; *df*=1,27; *P*<.02). For repetitive behavior, fluvoxamine proved to be significantly better than placebo beginning at week 8 (F=5.99; *df*=1,27; *P*<.02) and continuing at week 12 (F=18.19; *df*=1,27; *P*<.001).

RESPONSE OF MALADAPTIVE BEHAVIOR

As measured by the total score on the Vineland maladaptive behavior subscales (parts 1 and 2), fluvoxamine was more effective than placebo (F=12.15; *df*=3,84; *P*<.001). No significant difference was seen in Vineland maladaptive behavior subscale scores between the 2 groups at baseline (19.5±6.8 vs 22.3±8.1). In comparing the reduction in maladaptive behaviors, fluvoxamine was significantly better than placebo beginning at week 4 (F=4.33; *df*=1,27; *P*<.05) and continuing through weeks 8 (F=19.42; *df*=1,27; *P*<.001) and 12 (F=19.47; *df*=1,27; *P*<.001).

RESPONSE OF AGGRESSIVE SYMPTOMS

As measured by total score on the Brown Aggression Scale, fluvoxamine was superior to placebo in reducing aggression (F=4.57; *df*=3,84; *P*<.03). No significant difference was found in Brown Aggression Scale scores between the fluvoxamine and placebo groups at baseline (9.3±10.8 vs 12.3±12.3). In comparing fluvoxamine and placebo, fluvoxamine was superior to placebo beginning at week 4 (F=4.78; *df*=1,27; *P*<.04). After 8 (F=7.63; *df*=1,27; *P*<.01) and 12 (F=6.40; *df*=1,27; *P*<.02) weeks, fluvoxamine was significantly better than placebo in the reduction of aggression.

In the fluvoxamine group, the reduction in aggression first became significant after 8 weeks (*t*=2.3; *df*=14; *P*<.04), although a trend toward a significant reduction began at week 4 (*t*=1.8; *df*=14; *P*<.10). After 12 weeks, a significant reduction in aggression continued in the fluvoxamine group (*t*=2.0; *df*=14; *P*<.02). At no time after baseline was there a significant reduction in aggression with placebo.

RESPONSE ON RITVO-FREEMAN REAL-LIFE RATING SCALE

Overall Score

Fluvoxamine was superior to placebo in improving the behavioral symptoms of autistic disorder as measured by the Ritvo-Freeman Scale overall score (F=3.1; *df*=3,84; *P*<.04). In comparing fluvoxamine and placebo, fluvoxamine was superior to placebo beginning after 8 weeks (F=5.03; *df*=1,27; *P*<.03) and continuing after 12 weeks (F=5.02; *df*=1,27; *P*<.03).

Subscales 1 to 5

The drug × time interactions for subscales 1 to 4 were not significantly different. Fluvoxamine was superior to

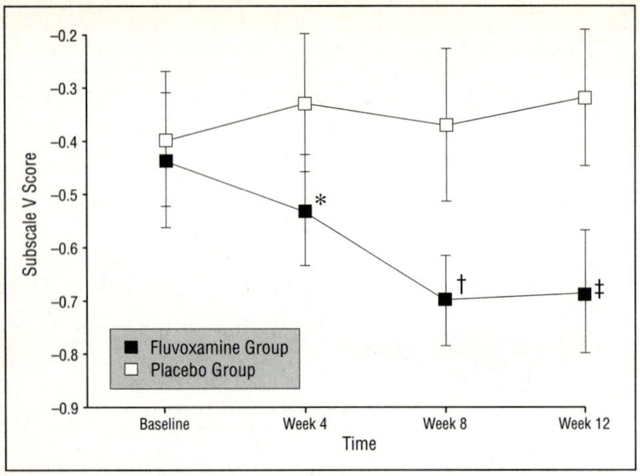

Figure 3. *Change in Ritvo-Freeman Real-Life Rating Scale subscale 5 (language) scores in patients with autism who were given fluvoxamine or placebo for 12 weeks. Asterisk indicates* P<.03, *change from baseline, fluvoxamine vs placebo, analysis of covariance; dagger,* P<.01, *change from baseline, fluvoxamine vs placebo, analysis of covariance; double dagger,* P<.003, *change from baseline, fluvoxamine vs placebo, analysis of covariance. Variance bars represent SE.*

placebo in improving language usage (subscale 5) in adults with autism ($F=4.8$; $df=3,84$; $P<.008$). In comparing the fluvoxamine and placebo groups, fluvoxamine was superior beginning at week 4 ($F=5.14$; $df=1,27$; $P<.03$) and continuing at weeks 8 ($F=7.40$; $df=1,27$; $P<.01$) and 12 ($F=10.95$; $df=1,27$; $P<.003$) (**Figure 3**).

ADVERSE EFFECTS

Fluvoxamine was well tolerated, with no medically significant adverse events. Four patients reported nausea (3 in the treatment group and 1 in the placebo group) during the first 2 weeks, but they experienced tolerance and were able to continue. Three patients experienced moderate sedation (2 in the treatment group and 1 in the placebo group), which also resolved. No anticholinergic adverse effects developed and no significant changes in pulse or sitting and standing blood pressure occurred. No laboratory or electrocardiographic changes could be attributed to fluvoxamine, and no seizures or dyskinesias were observed.

COMMENT

Fluvoxamine was significantly better than placebo for reducing behavioral symptoms of adults with autistic disorder. Using a conservative measure of meaningful clinical change (much improved or very much improved on the global improvement item of the CGI), 8 (53%) of 15 patients randomly assigned to fluvoxamine were rated as responders after 12 weeks of treatment, compared with none of 15 patients given placebo. Fluvoxamine was more effective than placebo in reducing interfering repetitive thoughts and behavior, aggression, and impaired social relatedness, especially abnormal language usage, in patients with autism. Other than mild sedation and gastrointestinal distress in a few patients, fluvoxamine was well tolerated. No dyskinesias, adverse cardiovascular events, or seizures occurred. Thus, fluvoxamine seems to have efficacy in reducing repetitive thoughts and behavior and aggression in some adult patients with autism, and to be safer and better tolerated than other drugs, such as haloperidol[15] and clomipramine,[34] which have been found effective in controlled studies in children with autism. Although the treatment trial was only 12 weeks, the lack of seizures with fluvoxamine is noteworthy, as almost one third of patients with autism have seizures,[50] and haloperidol and clomipramine can lower the seizure threshold.

In addition to the statistically significant changes that occurred in behavioral rating scale measures in this study, clinically meaningful improvement in adaptive function also was observed. For example, 2 fluvoxamine responders were able to move from group home settings to their own supervised apartments. Another patient obtained and has maintained full-time employment without the supervision of a job coach. Finally, one young man experienced a significant reduction in his intense preoccupation with motorcycle magazines and recently flew across the country in an airplane to participate in his cousin's wedding.

Repetitive thoughts and behavior are integral clinical features of autism[1-3] and OCD.[2] In a case-controlled study, we found that age- and sex-matched adults with autistic disorder and OCD could be readily distinguished based on their current types of repetitive thoughts and behaviors.[46] It was hypothesized that the significant difference in cognitive ability between the 2 groups may account for some of the disparity in symptom manifestation.[46] Despite these phenomenological differences, fluvoxamine has now been shown to be significantly better than placebo in reducing repetitive thoughts and behavior in adults with autism and OCD.[51] As has been shown in OCD,[52] the potent blockade of central 5-HT neuronal uptake may be an important component of the mechanism of action of drugs that preferentially reduce the repetitive thoughts and behavior of patients with autism. Consistent with this, a controlled study found the nonselective but potent 5-HT uptake inhibitor clomipramine better than the potent norepinephrine uptake inhibitor desipramine in reducing repetitive thoughts and behavior in children with autism.[34]

That the aggressive behavior of patients with autism was reduced by fluvoxamine is consistent with a growing body of evidence that altered 5-HT function may contribute to aggressive and impulsive behavior. Cerebrospinal fluid levels of 5-hydroxyindoleacetic acid, the principal central metabolite of 5-HT, have been shown to be significantly reduced in children with conduct and other aggressive behavioral disorders,[53,54] in humans who show impulsive vs nonimpulsive violent behavior,[55] and in aggressive and impulsive free-ranging male rhesus monkeys.[56] Decreased central 5-HT turnover, as reflected by reduced cerebrospinal fluid levels of 5-hydroxyindoleacetic acid, has been reported in some groups of children with autism,[57] but not others.[58] The selective 5-HT uptake inhibitors fluoxetine[59] and sertraline,[60] and the nonselective 5-HT uptake inhibitor clomipramine,[61] also have been found effective in reducing aggressive and self-injurious behavior in patients with developmental disabilities. Although fluvoxamine-induced irritability, agitation, and aggression were not observed in the adults with autism in our study, we have observed such untoward effects in some patients with autism treated with 5-HT uptake inhibitors, especially children.

Impaired social interaction and communication often is considered to be the core disturbance in autistic disorder.[62] Thus, the improvement in some aspects of social relatedness and language usage in the fluvoxamine-treated adults with autism in this study is especially noteworthy. As reflected by the significant improvement in subscale 5 (language) of the Ritvo-Freeman Real-Life Rating Scale, the patients showed increased communicative use of language, initiated or responded more frequently to communication, initiated more appropriate verbal communication, and showed less noncommunicative use of immediate and delayed echolalia. The observed improvement in social and language dysfunction may have been secondary to the overall reduction in repetitive behavior, including repetitive verbalization and echolalia. It is unlikely that fluvoxamine treatment fundamentally changed the course of atypical social and language development characteristic of autism. A large body of preclinical evidence suggests that 5-HT is critically involved in social function. For example, in vervet monkeys placed in extended isolation, whole-blood 5-HT levels rise and the animals' behavior resembles that of subordinate members of their social group.[63] In related monkey studies, administration of the 5-HT precursor tryptophan, the 5-HT receptor agonist quipazine maleate, and the 5-HT uptake inhibitor fluoxetine, all of which increase central 5-HT neurotransmission, resulted in dose-dependent increases in approaching, grooming, resting, and eating, and decreases in locomoting, avoiding, being vigilant, and being solitary.[64]

In summary, the potent and selective 5-HT uptake inhibitor fluvoxamine was significantly more effective than placebo in reducing interfering repetitive thoughts and behavior, and aggression, and in improving some aspects of social relatedness and language use in adults with autistic disorder. Fluvoxamine was well tolerated, with only minor side effects, including mild dyspepsia and sedation. Because of the potential for efficacy and the apparent improved tolerability and safety in comparison with drugs used previously to treat autism, controlled studies of fluvoxamine and other potent and selective serotonin uptake inhibitors seem warranted in children and adolescents with autism.

Accepted for publication January 3, 1996.

This work was supported by a National Alliance for Research on Schizophrenia and Depression Young Investigator Award (Dr McDougle), the State of Connecticut Department of Mental Health and Addiction Services, The Korczak Foundation for Autism and Related Disorders, and grants M01 RR06022-33, P50 MH30929-18, HD 03008-27, and P01 MH25642 from the National Institutes of Health, Bethesda, Md.

Fluvoxamine and financial support were provided by Solvay Pharmaceuticals, Marietta, Ga.

We thank the clinical and pharmacy staff of the Clinical Neuroscience Research Unit for their valuable assistance, Elizabeth Kyle, AS, for preparing the manuscript, Sally Vegso, MS, for the statistical analyses, and Elizabeth Ruff for the graphics work.

Reprints: Christopher J. McDougle, MD, Connecticut Mental Health Center, 34 Park St, Room 333B, New Haven, CT 06519.

REFERENCES

1. Kanner L. Autistic disturbances of affective contact. *J Nerv Child.* 1943;2:217-250.
2. American Psychiatric Association. *Diagnostic and Statistical Manual of Mental Disorders, Fourth Edition.* Washington, DC: American Psychiatric Association; 1994.
3. Rapin I. Introduction and overview. In: Bauman ML, Kemper TL, eds. *The Neurobiology of Autism.* Baltimore, Md: The Johns Hopkins University Press; 1994: 1-17.
4. Wing L. *Diagnosis and Treatment of Autism.* New York, NY: Plenum Publishing Corp; 1989.
5. Rubenstein JLR, Lotspeich L, Ciaranello RD. The neurobiology of developmental disorders. In: Lahey BB, Kazdin AE, eds. *Advances in Clinical Child Psychology.* New York, NY: Plenum Publishing Corp; 1990;13:1-52.
6. Schain RJ, Freedman DX. Studies on 5-hydroxyindole metabolism in autistic and other mentally retarded children. *J Pediatr.* 1961;58:315-320.
7. Anderson GM, Freedman DX, Cohen DJ, Volkmar FR, Hoder EL, McPhedran P, Minderaa RB, Hansen CR, Young JG. Whole blood serotonin in autistic and normal subjects. *J Child Psychol Psychiatry.* 1987;28:885-900.
8. Todd RD, Ciaranello RD. Demonstration of inter- and intraspecies differences in serotonin binding sites by antibodies from an autistic child. *Proc Natl Acad Sci U S A.* 1985;82:612-616.
9. Yuwiler A, Shih JC, Chen C-H, Ritvo ER, Hanna G, Ellison GW, King BH. Hyperserotoninemia and antiserotonin antibodies in autism and other disorders. *J Autism Dev Disord.* 1992;22:33-45.
10. Cook EH Jr, Perry BD, Dawson G, Wainwright MS, Leventhal BL. Receptor inhibition by immunoglobulins: specific inhibition by autistic children, their relatives, and control subjects. *J Autism Dev Disord.* 1993;23:67-78.
11. Hoshino Y, Tachibana JR, Watanabe M, Murata S, Yokoyama F, Kaneko M, Yashima Y, Kumoshiro H. Serotonin metabolism and hypothalamic-pituitary function in children with infantile autism and minimal brain dysfunction. *Jpn J Psychiatry Neurol.* 1984;26:937-945.
12. McBride PA, Anderson GM, Hertzig ME, Sweeney JA, Kream J, Cohen DJ, Mann JJ. Serotonergic responsivity in male young adults with autistic disorder: results of a pilot study. *Arch Gen Psychiatry.* 1989;46:213-221.
13. McDougle CJ, Naylor ST, Cohen DJ, Aghajanian GK, Heninger GR, Price LH. Effects of tryptophan depletion in drug-free adults with autistic disorder. *Arch Gen Psychiatry.* 1996;53:993-1000.
14. McDougle CJ, Price LH, Volkmar FR. Recent advances in the pharmacotherapy of autism and related conditions. In: Volkmar FR, ed. *Psychoses and Pervasive Developmental Disorders.* Philadelphia, Pa: WB Saunders Co; 1994; 3:71-89.
15. Campbell M, Anderson LT, Meier M, Cohen IL, Small AM, Samit C, Sachar EJ. A comparison of haloperidol and behavior therapy and their interaction in autistic children. *J Am Acad Child Adolesc Psychiatry.* 1978;17:640-655.
16. Campbell M, Adams P, Perry R, Spencer EK, Overall JE. Tardive and withdrawal dyskinesia in autistic children: a prospective study. *Psychopharmacol Bull.* 1988;24:251-255.
17. Geller E, Ritvo E, Freeman B, Yuwiler A. Preliminary observations on the effect of fenfluramine on blood serotonin and symptoms in three autistic boys. *N Engl J Med.* 1982;307:165-169.
18. Campbell M. Fenfluramine treatment of autism. *J Child Psychol Psychiatry.* 1988;29:1-10.
19. Campbell M, Adams P, Small AM, Curren EL, Overall J, Anderson LT, Lynch N, Perry R. Efficacy and safety of fenfluramine in autistic children. *J Am Acad Child Adolesc Psychiatry.* 1988;27:434-439.
20. Ekman G, Miranda-Linné F, Gillberg C, Garle M, Wetterberg L. Fenfluramine treatment of twenty children with autism. *J Autism Dev Disord.* 1989;19:511-532.
21. Sherman J, Factor D, Swinson R, Darjes R. The effects of fenfluramine (hydrochloride) on the behaviors of fifteen autistic children. *J Autism Dev Disord.* 1989;19:533-543.
22. Duker P, Welles K, Seys D, Rensen H, Vis A. Brief report: effects of fenfluramine on communicative, stereotypic, and inappropriate behaviors of autistic-type mentally handicapped individuals. *J Autism Dev Disord.* 1991;21:355-363.

23. Schuster C, Lewis M, Seiden L. Fenfluramine: neurotoxicity. *Psychopharmacol Bull.* 1986;22:148-151.
24. Campbell M, Overall JE, Small AM, Sokol MS, Spencer EK, Adams P, Foltz RL, Monti KM, Perry R, Nobler M, Roberts E. Naltrexone in autistic children: an acute open dose range tolerance trial. *J Am Acad Child Adolesc Psychiatry.* 1989;28:200-206.
25. Campbell M, Anderson LT, Small AM, Adams P, Gonzalez NM, Ernst M. Naltrexone in autistic children: behavioral symptoms and attentional learning. *J Am Acad Child Adolesc Psychiatry.* 1993;32:1283-1291.
26. Willemsen-Swinkels SHN, Buitelaar JK, Nijhof GJ, van Engeland H. Failure of naltrexone hydrochloride to reduce self-injurious and autistic behavior in mentally retarded adults: double-blind, placebo-controlled studies. *Arch Gen Psychiatry.* 1995;52:766-773.
27. McDougle CJ, Price LH, Goodman WK. Fluvoxamine treatment of coincident autistic disorder and obsessive-compulsive disorder: a case report. *J Autism Dev Disord.* 1990;20:537-543.
28. Cook EH, Rowlett R, Jaselskis C, Leventhal BL. Fluoxetine treatment of children and adults with autistic disorder and mental retardation. *J Am Acad Child Adolesc Psychiatry.* 1992;31:739-745.
29. Mehlinger R, Scheftner WA, Poznanski E. Fluoxetine and autism. *J Am Acad Child Adolesc Psychiatry.* 1990;29:985.
30. Hamdan-Allen G. Brief report: trichotillomania in an autistic male. *J Autism Dev Disord.* 1991;21:79-82.
31. Todd RD. Fluoxetine in autism. *Am J Psychiatry.* 1991;148:1089.
32. Ghaziuddin M, Tsai L, Ghaziuddin N. Fluoxetine in autism with depression. *J Am Acad Child Adolesc Psychiatry.* 1991;30:3.
33. McDougle CJ, Price LH, Volkmar FR, Goodman WK, Ward-O'Brien D, Nielsen J, Bregman J, Cohen DJ. Clomipramine in autism: preliminary evidence of efficacy. *J Am Acad Child Adolesc Psychiatry.* 1992;31:746-750.
34. Gordon CT, State RC, Nelson JE, Hamburger SD, Rapoport JL. A double-blind comparison of clomipramine, desipramine, and placebo in the treatment of autistic disorder. *Arch Gen Psychiatry.* 1993;50:441-447.
35. Riddle MA, Geller B, Ryan N. Another sudden death in a child treated with desipramine. *J Am Acad Child Adolesc Psychiatry.* 1993;32:792-797.
36. American Psychiatric Association. *Diagnostic and Statistical Manual of Mental Disorders, Third Edition, Revised.* Washington, DC: American Psychiatric Association; 1987.
37. World Health Organization. *International Statistical Classification of Diseases, 10th Revision (ICD-10).* Geneva, Switzerland: World Health Organization; 1992.
38. Guy W. *ECDEU Assessment Manual for Psychopharmacology.* Washington, DC: National Institute of Mental Health, US Dept of Health, Education and Welfare; 1976. Publication 76-338.
39. Le Couteur A, Rutter M, Lord C, Rios P, Robertson S, Holdgrafer M, McLennan J. Autism Diagnostic Interview: a standardized investigator-based instrument. *J Autism Dev Disord.* 1989;19:363-387.
40. Lord C, Rutter M, Goode S, Heemsbergen J, Jordan H, Mawhood L, Schopler E. Autism Diagnostic Observation Schedule: a standardized observation of communicative and social behavior. *J Autism Dev Disord.* 1989;19:185-212.
41. Krug DA, Arick JR, Almond PJ. *Autism Screening Instrument for Education Planning.* Portland, Ore: ASIEP Educational Co; 1980.
42. Wechsler D. *Manual for the Wechsler Adult Intelligence Scale—Revised.* San Antonio, Tex: The Psychological Corp; 1981.
43. Leiter RG. *Leiter International Performance Scale.* Chicago, Ill: Stoelting Co; 1948.
44. van Harten J. Clinical pharmacokinetics of selective serotonin reuptake inhibitors. *Clin Pharmacokinet.* 1993;24:203-220.
45. Goodman WK, Price LH, Rasmussen SA, Mazure C, Fleischmann R, Hill C, Heninger GR, Charney DS. The Yale-Brown Obsessive Compulsive Scale (Y-BOCS), I: development, use, and reliability. *Arch Gen Psychiatry.* 1989;46:1006-1011.
46. McDougle CJ, Kresch L, Goodman WK, Naylor ST, Volkmar FR, Cohen DJ, Price LH. A case-controlled study of repetitive thoughts and behavior in adults with autistic disorder and obsessive-compulsive disorder. *Am J Psychiatry.* 1995;152:772-777.
47. Brown GL, Goodwin FK, Ballenger JC, Goyer PF, Major LF. Aggression in humans correlates with cerebrospinal fluid amine metabolites. *Psychiatr Res.* 1979;1:131-139.
48. Freeman BJ, Ritvo ER, Yokota A, Ritvo A. A scale for rating symptoms of patients with the syndrome of autism in real life settings. *J Am Acad Child Adolesc Psychiatry.* 1986;25:130-136.
49. Sparrow SS, Balla DA, Cicchetti DV. *Vineland Adaptive Behavior Scales.* Circle Pines, Minn: American Guidance Service; 1984.
50. Volkmar FR, Nelson DS. Seizure disorders in autism. *J Am Acad Child Adolesc Psychiatry.* 1990;1:127-129.
51. Goodman WK, Price LH, Rasmussen SA, Delgado PL, Heninger GR, Charney DS. Efficacy of fluvoxamine in obsessive-compulsive disorder: a double-blind comparison with placebo. *Arch Gen Psychiatry.* 1989;46:36-43.
52. Goodman WK, Price LH, Delgado PL, Palumbo J, Krystal JH, Nagy LM, Rasmussen SA, Heninger GR, Charney DS. Specificity of serotonin reuptake inhibitors in the treatment of obsessive compulsive disorder: comparison of fluvoxamine and desipramine. *Arch Gen Psychiatry.* 1990;47:577-585.
53. Kruesi MJ, Rapoport JL, Hamburger S, Hibbs E, Potter WZ, Lenane M, Brown GL. Cerebrospinal fluid monoamine metabolites, aggression, and impulsivity in disruptive behavior disorders of children and adolescents. *Arch Gen Psychiatry.* 1990;47:419-426.
54. Kruesi MJ, Hibbs ED, Zahn TP, Keysor CS, Hamburger SD, Bartko JJ, Rapoport JL. A 2-year prospective follow-up study of children and adolescents with disruptive behavior disorders: prediction by cerebrospinal fluid 5-hydroxyindoleacetic acid, homovanillic acid, and autonomic measures? *Arch Gen Psychiatry.* 1992;49:429-435.
55. Linnoila M, Virkkunen M, Scheinin M, Nuutila A, Rimon R, Goodwin FK. Low cerebrospinal fluid 5-hydroxyindoleacetic acid concentration differentiates impulsive from nonimpulsive violent behavior. *Life Sci.* 1983;33:2609-2614.
56. Mehlman PT, Higley JD, Faucher I, Lilly AA, Taub DM, Vickers J, Suomi SJ, Linnoila M. Low CSF 5-HIAA concentrations and severe aggression and impaired impulse control in nonhuman primates. *Am J Psychiatry.* 1994;151:1485-1491.
57. Cohen DJ, Shaywitz BA, Johnson WT, Bowers MB. Biogenic amines in autistic and atypical children: cerebrospinal fluid measures of homovanillic acid and 5-hydroxyindoleacetic acid. *Arch Gen Psychiatry.* 1974;31:845-853.
58. Narayan M, Srinath S, Anderson GM, Meundi DB. Cerebrospinal fluid levels of homovanillic acid and 5-hydroxyindoleacetic acid in autism. *Biol Psychiatry.* 1993;33:630-635.
59. Markowitz PI. Effect of fluoxetine on self-injurious behavior in the developmentally disabled: a preliminary study. *J Clin Psychopharmacol.* 1992;12:27-31.
60. Kelley LA, Hellings JA, Gabrielli WF, Kilgore E. Sertraline response in mentally retarded adults. Presented at the American Psychiatric Association 146th Annual Meeting; May 22-27, 1993; San Francisco, Calif.
61. Garber HJ, McGonigle JJ, Slomka GT, Monteverde E. Clomipramine treatment of stereotypic behaviors and self-injury in patients with developmental disabilities. *J Am Acad Child Adolesc Psychiatry.* 1992;31:1157-1160.
62. Volkmar FR. Social development. In: Cohen D, Donnellan A, eds. *Handbook of Autism and Pervasive Developmental Disorders.* New York, NY: John Wiley & Sons Inc; 1987:41-60.
63. Brammer GL, Raleigh MJ, McGuire MT. Physiological and behavioral relationships in individually-housed male vervet monkeys. *Am J Primatol.* 1984;6:400.
64. Raleigh MJ, Brammer GL, Yuwiler A, Flannery JW, McGuire MT, Geller E. Serotonergic influences on the social behavior of vervet monkeys (*Cercopithecus aethiops sabaeus*). *Exp Neurol.* 1980;68:322-324.

Nocturnal Serum Melatonin Profile in Major Depression in Children and Adolescents

Mohammad Shafii, MD; Duncan R. MacMillan, MD; Mary P. Key, MS, MT; Ann McCue Derrick, RN, MS; Nancy Kaufman, MS; Irwin D. Nahinsky, PhD

Background: In major depression, biological rhythm disturbances in sleep, appetite, and mood suggest dysregulation in neuroendocrine functions, possibly in the pineal gland. In this study, pineal gland function was examined by measuring nocturnal serum melatonin levels during both wakefulness and sleep in depressed children and adolescents.

Methods: Twenty-two youths aged 8 to 17 years primarily with major depression were compared with 19 controls. Blood samples were drawn every half hour from 6 PM to 7 AM. Nocturnal serum melatonin levels were measured by radioimmunoassay.

Results: The overall nocturnal serum melatonin profile from 6 PM to 7 AM was significantly higher (mean±SD, 0.18±0.14 nmol/L) in the depressed group than in the controls [mean±SD, 0.15±0.10 nmol/L, $F(1,26)=4.37$, $P<.05$]. In dim light, when the subjects were awake, no difference existed between the 2 groups. After lights-out, from 10 PM to 7 AM, the melatonin profile rose in both groups; however, the depressed group had a significantly higher increase (mean±SD, 0.24±0.14 nmol/L) than the controls [mean±SD, 0.18±0.07 nmol/L, $F(1,26)=4.93$, mean square error=0.11, $P=.04$]. Post hoc analysis showed a significantly higher melatonin profile in depressed subjects without psychosis (n=15) than in depressed subjects with psychosis (n=7) or in the controls.

Conclusion: Measuring the overall nocturnal serum melatonin profile during darkness may help to differentiate children and adolescents with major depression without psychosis from those with psychosis and from controls.

Arch Gen Psychiatry. 1996;53:1009-1013

MOOD DISORDERS such as major depression and dysthymia are serious, episodic, chronic, and debilitating disorders in youth.[1-9] Symptoms of major depression, such as mood, appetite, and sleep disturbances, suggest circadian rhythm disturbances. Because the pineal gland and its hormone, melatonin, contribute to the regulation and entrainment of circadian rhythms to a 24-hour cycle, the study of the pineal gland in depressive disorders may be fertile ground for such investigation.[10,11]

In healthy individuals, nocturnal serum melatonin levels begin to increase 2 hours before bedtime but surge a half hour following lights-out during sleep. Most melatonin is secreted during the dark cycle of the night, from 11 PM to 3 AM, with a 2 AM peak.[12,13] In more than 20 studies on melatonin in adult depression, a number showed a decrease in the nocturnal serum or urine melatonin levels or a phase-shift in the melatonin peak,[14-19] a few showed no difference,[20-23] and 2 showed an increase.[24,25]

To our knowledge, only 3 studies reported on melatonin levels in major depression in youth. Cavallo et al[26] found that the nocturnal serum melatonin level was lower in 9 depressed boys aged 7 to 13 years with mixed diagnoses than in a control group of 10 boys who were of normal height, genetically short, or had delayed pubescence. We measured bedtime and overnight urine melatonin levels in 96 psychiatric inpatients aged 6 to 16 years[27,28] and found that in patients with primary major depression, the overnight urine melatonin level was significantly higher than in patients with secondary depression or in the nondepressed psychiatric controls. Watterman et al[29] reported no difference between the level of 6-hy-

See Subjects and Methods on next page

From the Departments of Psychiatry and Behavioral Sciences (Dr Shafii and Mss McCue Derrick and Kaufman), Pediatrics (Dr MacMillan and Ms Key), and Psychology (Dr Nahinsky), University of Louisville School of Medicine, Louisville, Ky.

SUBJECTS AND METHODS

Children and adolescents aged 8 to 17 years with depressive symptoms who were either inpatients or outpatients and healthy controls were asked to participate in this study with the University of Louisville Human Studies Committee's approval. Assent or informed consent of subjects and a parent or guardian were obtained. Subjects were divided into 2 groups.

SUBJECTS

Depressed Group

Of the 22 patients in this group, 18 were diagnosed with major depression, 1 with severe dysthymia, and 3 with bipolar disorder, depressive phase. Most of the subjects had comorbid diagnoses such as anxiety, conduct and/or oppositional disorder, attention-deficit disorder, or posttraumatic stress disorder.

We included the 1 case of severe dysthymia and the 3 cases of bipolar disorder, depressive phase, with the 18 cases of major depression because longitudinal follow-up of mood disorders in children and adolescents shows overlap and movement between these diagnostic entities. Many dysthymic youth go on to have major depressive episodes, and many youth with major depression, particularly those with psychosis, subsequently develop bipolar disorders.[1,2,30-33]

Control Group

The control group consisted of healthy children and adolescents with no present or past personal or family history of psychiatric disorder, alcohol or other drug abuse, or antisocial behavior in siblings, parents, aunts or uncles, or grandparents. Some of the control subjects were the children of support staff or the nursing staff and others were friends or neighbors of the depressed subjects or controls.

METHODS

Subjects, controls, and parents were interviewed by a member of our research team and the principal investigator. In addition to a clinical interview, the Diagnostic Interview for Children and Adolescents–Revised[34,35] was used, along with the Child Behavioral Checklist, Youth Self-Report[36]; Children's Depression Inventory[37]; Children's Depression Rating Scale[38]; and Depression Self-Rating Scale.[39] Height and weight were measured and stages of pubertal development were obtained using the Tanner stages.[40] From girls, information regarding menarche and date of most recent menstrual period was obtained. None of the subjects had seasonal affective disorder.

Blood samples were drawn from the psychiatric inpatients after the first night of hospitalization. This allowed time to explain the study and receive informed consent. The inpatients went to their rooms after dinner, between 5:30 and 6 PM. The outpatient subjects and the controls, after having dinner, went to the sleep laboratory at the hospital between 5:30 and 6 PM to spend the night. A pediatric nurse introduced a 22-gauge streamline soft venous catheter into a vein. The room lights were dimmed to 50 lux or less (just barely enough light to read) until bedtime at 10 PM. The first blood specimen was collected at 6 PM. Subjects were able to watch television. From 6 PM to 7 AM, intermittent blood sampling was performed every half hour. A blood sample of 3 mL was drawn to have 1 mL of serum for the melatonin assay.

droxymelatonin sulfate in the overnight urine of youth with major depression and that of controls. This study differs from the 2 mentioned above in that the metabolite of melatonin, rather than the parent compound, was measured. Also, urine was collected 12 hours after the administration of insulin as part of a growth hormone challenge study, which might have affected the results.

In the present study, we hypothesized that a dysregulation of the pineal gland in the form of an increase of serum melatonin exists in youth with major depression.[27,28] Recognizing the limitations of previous studies, including ours, we incorporated the following into the research design: a healthy control group; a drug-naive or drug-free period 2 weeks prior to study; extensive diagnostic structured interviews and rating scales; intermittent rather than continuous blood sampling; and dim light during wakefulness to assess dim-light melatonin onset.[11,19]

RESULTS

The depressed group consisted of 9 boys and 13 girls (15 white and 7 African American) and the control group, 11 boys and 8 girls (19 white). Tanner stages 1 and 2 were defined as prepubescence and stages 3 through 5 as pubescence. In both groups, the ratio of pubescent adolescents to prepubescent children was slightly more than 2:1. Concerning the seasonal effect on melatonin levels, depressed subjects were recruited during a depressive episode when they came to the clinic, usually in the spring or fall, whereas control subjects were recruited when they were most available, usually the spring and summer, so there was an uneven distribution of subjects and controls regarding the season of the year. However, in our earlier study,[27,28] neither race nor season affected melatonin levels.

The depressed group weighed significantly more than the control group. A MANOVA was performed on the variables of height and weight in both groups using sex and Tanner stages as independent variables. Both height (r=0.09, P<.01) and weight (r=0.17, P<.01) correlated significantly with serum melatonin levels. Therefore, height and weight variables were used as covariates in subsequent analyses to test effects of the independent variables on serum melatonin levels. The overall serum melatonin level in the depressed group (mean±SD, 0.18±0.14 nmol/L) was significantly higher than in the control group [mean±SD, 0.15±0.10 nmol/L, $F(1,26)=4.37$, mean square error=0.12, P<.05]. Sex, stages of pubescence, and season had no significant effect.

When we eliminated the 1 case of severe dysthy-

Altogether, 27 blood samples were drawn, for a total of 81 mL. All room light was turned off at 10 PM. By collecting samples intermittently from 6 PM onward in dim light or dark conditions, we were able to look for dim-light melatonin onset and possible phase-advanced melatonin secretions. In addition, we examined the patterns of secretion and the peak of melatonin levels throughout the night. The samples were stored at 4°C until transported to the laboratory and were coded to ensure blindness with respect to time of collection and source. Aliquots from coded samples of all subjects were stored frozen at −20°C until assayed. Of a possible 1107 blood samples, 1099 (99.3%) were collected. The other 8 samples (missing data points) were not collected because of vein collapse, infiltration, or other factors.

Melatonin Determinations

Serum melatonin levels were measured using a single-antibody radioimmunoassay, which employed a rabbit antiserum (KALAB, Danville, Calif) and a tritiated melatonin tracer (New England Nuclear, Boston, Mass).[12-14] Samples were extracted with methylene chloride, evaporated to dryness at 37°C, resuspended in assay buffer, and stored at either 4°C if assayed the following day or –20°C if assayed later than the next day. Radioimmunoassays of the extracts were performed to measure melatonin concentrations against a standard curve of known melatonin standard concentrations. Unknown sample extract or assay standard, tracer, and antiserum were mixed together and incubated. After incubation, the bound fraction (that containing the sample melatonin extracts or standards and tracer melatonin bound to antibody) was precipitated with saturated ammonium sulfate and counted in 10 mL of scintillation cocktail in a scintillation counter. Disintegrations per minute of standard divided by disintegrations per minute of the total bound fraction were calculated and plotted on semilogarithmic paper. The disintegrations per minute of unknown divided by disintegrations per minute of the total bound fraction were calculated and results for the unknown samples were read from the curve. Some investigators report melatonin values in nanomoles per liter, some in picograms per milliliter, and some in nanograms per liter. The conversion formula is as follows: picograms per milliliter equals nanograms per liter equals the nanomoles per liter value ×232.26 (molecular weight of melatonin).

Quality Control

The sensitivity of the assay is 0.01 nmol/L and cross-reactivity for most related compounds such as serotonin and 5-hydroxyindoleacetic acid is greater than 1 million to 10 million pg/mL. Within- and between-assay coefficient variations have been less than 5% and 7%, respectively, throughout the anticipated range of melatonin values. Quality control was assured through the use of multiple internal controls for each assay and through regular participation in the College of American Pathologists surveys. The Pediatric Endocrine Laboratory of the University of Louisville is fully licensed to perform a wide range of radioimmunoassay procedures.

Statistical Analysis

The Statistical Package for the Social Sciences (SPSS)[41] was used for analysis of data. The multiple analysis of variance (MANOVA) with multiple covariance analysis to correct for height and weight was used at an α level of .05 (2-tailed test). In addition, orthogonal polynomial trend analyses were employed to test for various trends.

mia and the 3 cases of bipolar disorder in the depressive phase, there was no change in the results, which continued to be significant [mean±SD, 0.18±0.15, $F(1,39)=4.34$, mean square error=0.030, $P<.05$].

Figure 1 reveals a generally negatively accelerated trend for melatonin levels for both groups from 6 PM to 7 AM, with a pronounced divergence of the 2 groups after 10 PM, the lights-out time. From 10:30 PM to 7 AM when the lights were out and the subjects and controls were, for the most part, asleep, the melatonin levels in the depressed group (mean±SD, 0.24±0.14 nmol/L) were significantly higher than in the control group [mean±SD, 0.18±0.07 nmol/L, $F(1,26)=4.93$, mean square error=0.11, $P=.04$]. After the lights were out, and eliminating the 4 cases mentioned previously, the mean levels of the depressed group were slightly lower (0.22 nmol/L). The difference continued to be statistically significant. While the lights were on from 6 to 10 PM, there were no differences between the depressed group (mean, 0.08 nmol/L) and the controls (mean, 0.07 nmol/L). These evening levels were somewhat higher than those reported elsewhere, which could possibly be related to the specificity of this radioimmunoassay for melatonin.

There was a significant straight-line relationship between time and melatonin level, overlaid with an appreciable curvilinear trend ($P<.001$).

In post hoc analysis, the depressed group was separated into depressed with psychosis (n=7, mean±SD melatonin level, 0.11±0.11) and depressed without psychosis (n=15, mean±SD melatonin level, 0.19±0.15) (**Figure 2**). The group with psychotic depression had melatonin levels with a trend toward a lower mean compared with controls. The group with nonpsychotic depression continued to show the high melatonin levels seen earlier, with some increase. The estimations of the total melatonin concentrations during the night, or the total area under the curves, are as follows: the depressed group with psychosis, 2.97 nmol/L; the depressed group without psychosis, 5.24 nmol/L; and the control group, 3.94 nmol/L. These differences were significant, especially during the time when the lights were out (MANOVA, $P<.01$ and $P<.001$).

COMMENT

Inherent in the clinical definition of major depression are the symptoms of circadian rhythm disturbances. The suprachiasmatic nuclei of the hypothalamus are the generators of circadian rhythms of slightly more than 24 hours. The pineal gland and melatonin regulate suprachiasmatic nuclei through their receptor sites, entraining circadian rhythms to a 24-hour cycle.[11] Nocturnal

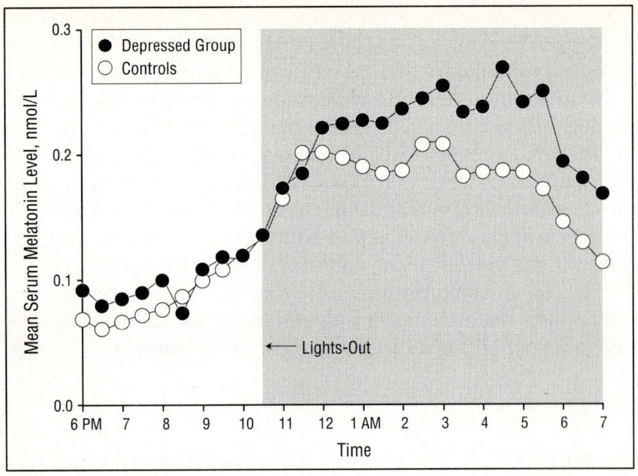

Figure 1. *Nocturnal serum melatonin profile in depressed children and adolescents and healthy controls.*

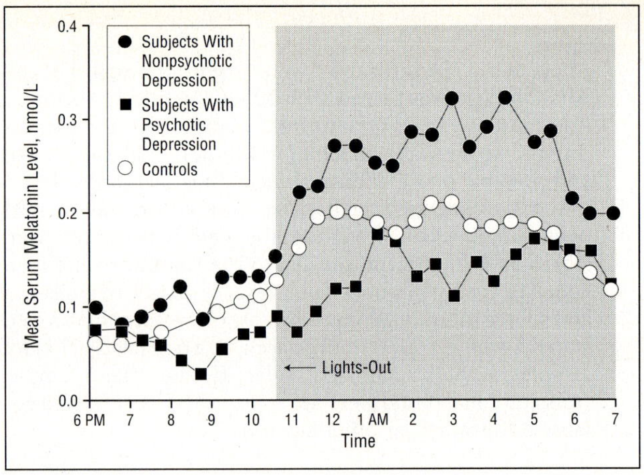

Figure 2. *Nocturnal serum melatonin profile in subjects with nonpsychotic depression, psychotic depression, and healthy controls.*

darkness, primarily between 11 PM and 3 AM, affects the retina, stimulating the β-adrenergic neurons and the suprachiasmatic nuclei, and results in the synthesis of melatonin from serotonin in the pinealocytes of the pineal gland. We measured the nocturnal serum melatonin levels in children and adolescents with major depression and in a healthy control group.

In a study of 22 children and adolescents primarily with major depression, the nocturnal serum melatonin level was significantly higher compared with 19 healthy controls. In post hoc analysis, the depressed patients without psychosis had a much higher nocturnal serum melatonin level than the controls. In contrast, the depressed patients with psychosis had a somewhat lower nocturnal serum melatonin level than the controls.

Our findings are compatible with those of Lewy et al,[42] who found that the plasma melatonin levels in adult patients with manic-depressive illness were lower in the psychotic depressive phase and higher in the manic phase. Recently, Wahlund et al[43] also found that the mean melatonin peak level in depressed adults with psychosis was significantly lower than in those without psychosis.

Interestingly, individuals, whether children, adolescents, or adults, who were depressed with psychosis had lower serum melatonin levels. One wonders if this is just a coincidental finding, whether melatonin may have antipsychotic properties, or, perhaps, whether higher levels of melatonin protect a depressed patient from psychotic symptoms.

Our study had the following limitations: a small number of subjects, mixed diagnostic groups, and comorbid diagnoses. The depressed group, as a whole, weighed more than the controls. Higher levels of melatonin in the depressed group could be related to weight rather than depression. However, Young et al[44] found that there was a reverse relationship between weight, body mass, and serum melatonin levels. If weight had a major effect, the depressed group should have had lower rather than higher melatonin levels.

Looking at the effect of weight on the nocturnal melatonin levels in the 2 subtypes of depression, we found that the mean weight of the depressed group with psychosis was 56.4 kg, and of the depressed group without psychosis, 59.4 kg (SD, ±14.7). There was no significant difference between these 2 groups regarding weight and weight had no effect on their nocturnal melatonin levels.

In most adult studies of major depression, the nocturnal serum melatonin level was lower than in healthy controls, although some studies found no difference and 2 found higher levels. How can these differences be reconciled with each other and with our findings?

During the last 2 decades, the significant advancement in research in child and adolescent depression is related to the use of research diagnostic criteria and depressive rating scales. The criteria for depressive disorders in children and adolescents is basically the same as the criteria for adults. However, biological research findings in depressive disorders in children and adolescents have differed from the findings in adults. For example, in adult major depression, changes in electroencephalographic patterns during sleep, such as an increase of rapid eye movement sleep and a decrease or absence of deep non–rapid eye movement sleep (stages III and IV) are not found in children and adolescents with major depression.

Also, in children and adolescents, in contrast to adults, tricyclic antidepressants are not effective in the treatment of major depression. Is childhood and adolescent major depression biologically different from adult depression even though phenomenologically the same? Or perhaps, childhood and adolescent major depression is similar to that of the 20% to 30% of adults with major depression who are not responsive to tricyclic antidepressants.

Similarity of symptoms within a diagnostic category does not necessarily mean that the underlying biological mechanisms are the same. This is now apparent in, for example, endocrine disorders such as diabetes mellitus or hyperparathyroidism.

Clinical diagnosis of major depression based only on phenomenological symptoms is broad and covers various known and probably unknown subtypes of major depression, whether in adults, children, or adolescents. More attention needs to be given to the diverse biological findings in major depression to decipher biological subtypes of this disorder. Dysregulation of the pineal gland in the form of increased or decreased nocturnal serum melatonin levels might be related to various subtypes of major depression, rather than invalidity or lack of replicability of various studies.

Accepted for publication March 26, 1996.

This study was funded in part by grant 92-24 from the Alliant Community Trust Fund, Louisville.

This article was presented at a symposium, "Melatonin in Psychiatric and Neoplastic Disorders," at the 1995 American Psychiatric Association Annual Meeting, Miami, Fla, May 24, 1995.

We wish to thank Sharon Lee Shafii, RN, for her significant editorial contribution; Amy Willard; Sandra Elam, MD (Director), Kathy Smith, RN (Team Leader), and the staff of the Ackerly Psychiatry Inpatient Service, Kosair Children's Hospital; Kathy Porter, RN, Suzanne Layman, RNC, CPN, and Robert Tillett, Jr, MD, Director, Sleep Center, Alliant Medical Pavilion; and Allan Tasman, MD, Professor and Chair, Department of Psychiatry and Behavioral Sciences, University of Louisville.

Reprints: Mohammad Shafii, MD, Professor of Psychiatry, Bingham Child Guidance Center, 200 E Chestnut St, Louisville, KY 40202.

REFERENCES

1. Kovacs M, Feinberg TL, Crouse-Novak MA, Paulauskas SL, Finkelstein R. Depressive disorders in childhood, I: a longitudinal prospective study of characteristics and recovery. *Arch Gen Psychiatry.* 1984;41:229-237.
2. Kovacs M, Akiskal HS, Gatsonis C, Parrone PL. Childhood-onset dysthymic disorder. *Arch Gen Psychiatry.* 1994;51:365-374.
3. Harrington R, Fudge H, Rutter M, Pickles A, Hill J. Adult outcomes of childhood and adolescent depression, I: psychiatric status. *Arch Gen Psychiatry.* 1990;47:465-473.
4. Shafii M, Shafii SL. Clinical manifestations and developmental psychopathology of depression in children and adolescents. In: Shafii M, Shafii SL, eds. *Clinical Guide to Depression in Children and Adolescents.* Washington, DC: American Psychiatric Press; 1992:3-42.
5. Rohde P, Lewinsohn PM, Seeley JR. Are adolescents changed by an episode of major depression? *J Am Acad Child Adolesc Psychiatry.* 1994;33:1289-1298.
6. Shafii M, Carrigan S, Whittinghill JR, Derrick AM. Psychological autopsy of completed suicide in children and adolescents: a comparative study. *Am J Psychiatry.* 1985;142:1061-1064.
7. Shafii M, Steltz-Lenarsky J, Derrick AM, Beckner C, Whittinghill JR. Comorbidity of mental disorders in the post-mortem diagnosis of completed suicide in children and adolescents. *J Affect Disord.* 1988;15:227-233.
8. Kashani JH, McGee RO, Clarkson S, Anderson JC, Walton LA, Williams S, Silva PA, Robins AJ, Cytryn L, McKnew DH. Depression in a sample of 9-year-old children: prevalence and associated characteristics. *Arch Gen Psychiatry.* 1983; 40:1217-1223.
9. Kashani JH, Carlson GA, Beck NC, Hoeper EW, Corcoran CM, McAllister JA. Depression, depressive symptoms, and depressed mood among a community sample of adolescents. *Am J Psychiatry.* 1987;144:931-932.
10. Wetterberg L, Beck-Friis J, Kjellman BF. Melatonin as a marker for a subgroup of depression in adults. In: Shafii M, Shafii SL, eds. *Biological Rhythms, Mood Disorders, Light Therapy, and the Pineal Gland.* Washington, DC: American Psychiatric Press; 1990:69-95.
11. Lewy AJ, Sack RL, Singer CM. Bright light, melatonin, and winter depression: the phase-shift hypothesis. In: Shafii M, Shafii SL, eds. *Biological Rhythms, Mood Disorders, Light Therapy, and the Pineal Gland.* Washington, DC: American Psychiatric Press; 1990:141-173.
12. Wetterberg L: Melatonin in humans: physiological and clinical studies. *J Neural Transm.* 1978;13(suppl):289-310.
13. Wetterberg L. Clinical importance of melatonin. *Prog Brain Res.* 1979;52:539-547.
14. Wetterberg L, Beck-Friis J, Aperia B, Petterson U. Melatonin/cortisol ratio in depression. *Lancet.* 1979;2:1361.
15. Brown RP, Kocsis JH, Caroff S, Amsterdam J, Winokur A, Stokes PE, Frazer A. Differences in nocturnal melatonin secretion between melancholic depressed patients and control subjects. *Am J Psychiatry.* 1985;142:811-816.
16. Brown RP, Kocsis JH, Caroff S, Amsterdam J, Winokur A, Stokes P, Frazer A. Depressed mood and reality disturbance correlate with decreased nocturnal melatonin in depressed patients. *Acta Psychiatr Scand.* 1987;76:272-275.
17. Kennedy SH, Garfinkel PE, Parienti V, Costa D, Brown GM. Changes in melatonin levels but not cortisol levels are associated with depression in patients with eating disorders. *Arch Gen Psychiatry.* 1989;46:73-78.
18. Lewy AJ, Wehr TA, Goodwin FK, Newsome DA, Markey SP. Light suppresses melatonin secretion in humans. *Science.* 1980;210:1267-1269.
19. Lewy AJ, Sack RL, Singer CM. Immediate and delayed effects of bright light on human melatonin production: shifting 'dawn' and 'dusk' shifts the dim light melatonin onset (DLMO). *Ann N Y Acad Sci.* 1985;452:253-259.
20. Jimerson DC, Lynch HJ, Post RM, Wurtman R. Urinary melatonin rhythms during sleep deprivation in depressed patients and normals. *Life Sci.* 1977; 20:1501-1508.
21. Mendlewicz J, Linkowski P, Branchey L. Abnormal 24 hour pattern of melatonin secretion in depression. *Lancet.* 1979;2:1262.
22. Boyce PM. 2-sulphatoxy melatonin in melancholia. *Am J Psychiatry.* 1985; 142:125-127.
23. Thompson C, Franey C, Arendt J, Checkley S. A comparison of melatonin secretion in normal subjects and depressed patients. *Br J Psychiatry.* 1988;152: 260-266.
24. Stewart JW, Halbreich U. Plasma melatonin levels in depressed patients before and after treatment with antidepressant medication. *Biol Psychiatry.* 1989; 25:33-38.
25. Rubin RT, Heist EK, McGeoy SS, Hanada K, Lesser IM. Neuroendocrine aspects of primary endogenous depression. *Arch Gen Psychiatry.* 1992;49:558-567.
26. Cavallo A, Holt KG, Hejazi MS, Richards GE, Meter WJ. Melatonin circadian rhythm in childhood depression. *J Am Acad Child Adolesc Psychiatry.* 1987; 26:395-399.
27. Shafii M, Foster MB, Greenberg RA, Derrick AM, Key MP. Urinary melatonin in depressed children and adolescents. In: 1988 CME Syllabus & Proceedings Summary, 141st Annual Meeting of the American Psychiatric Association; May 1988; Montreal, Quebec. Abstract.
28. Shafii M, Foster MB, Greenberg RA, Derrick AM, Key MP. The pineal gland and depressive disorders in children and adolescents. In: Shafii M, Shafii SL, eds. *Biological Rhythms, Mood Disorders, Light Therapy, and the Pineal Gland.* Washington, DC: American Psychiatric Press; 1990:97-116.
29. Watterman GS, Ryan ND, Perel JM, Dahl RE, Birmaher B, Williamson DE, Thomas CR, Puig-Antich J. Nocturnal urinary excretion of 6-hydroxymelatonin sulfate in prepubertal major depressive disorder. *Biol Psychiatry.* 1992;31:582-590.
30. Carlson GA, Strober M. Manic-depressive illness in early adolescence: a study of clinical and diagnostic characteristics in six cases. *J Am Acad Child Adolesc Psychiatry.* 1978;17:138-153.
31. Strober M, Carlson G. Bipolar illness in adolescents: clinical, genetic and pharmacologic predictors in a three- to four-year prospective follow-up. *Arch Gen Psychiatry.* 1982;39:549-555.
32. Strober M. Bipolar disorders: natural history, genetic studies, and follow-up. In: Shafii M, Shafii SL, eds. *Clinical Guide to Depression in Children and Adolescents.* Washington, DC: American Psychiatric Press; 1992:251-268.
33. Weissman MM, Warner V, Wickramaratne P, Prusoff BA. Early-onset major depression in parents and their children. *J Affect Disord.* 1988;15:269-277.
34. Welner Z, Reich W, Herjanic B, Jung KG, Amado H. Reliability, validity, and parent-child agreement studies of the Diagnostic Interview for Children and Adolescents (DICA). *J Am Acad Child Adolesc Psychiatry.* 1987;26:649-653.
35. Reich W, Shayka JJ, Taibleson C. *Diagnostic Interview for Children and Adolescents.* St Louis, Mo: Washington University; 1991.
36. Achenbach TM, Edelbrock CS. The Child Behavior Profile, II: boys aged 6-11 and 12-16. *J Consult Clin Psychol.* 1979;47:223-233.
37. Kovacs M. Rating scales to assess depression in school-aged children. *Acta Paedopsychiatry.* 1981;46:305-325.
38. Poznanski EO, Grossman JA, Buchsbaum Y, Banegas M. Preliminary studies of the reliability and validity of the Children's Depression Rating Scale. *J Am Acad Child Adolesc Psychiatry.* 1984;23:191-197.
39. Birleson P. The validity of depressive disorder in childhood and the development of a self-rating scale: a research report. *J Child Psychol Psychiatry.* 1981; 22:73-88.
40. Tanner JM. *Growth at Adolescence.* 2nd ed. Oxford, England: Blackwell Scientific Publishers; 1962.
41. SPSS (Statistical Package for the Social Sciences) DATA ENTRY II. Chicago, Ill: SPSS Inc; 1987.
42. Lewy AJ, Wehr TA, Gold PW, Goodwin FK. Plasma melatonin in manic-depressive illness. In: Usdin E, Kopin JJ, Barchas J, eds. *Catecholamines: Basic and Clinical Frontiers.* New York, NY: Pergamon Press; 1979:1173-1175.
43. Wahlund B, Sääf J, Wetterberg L. Classification of patients with affective disorders using platelet monoamine oxidase activity, serum melatonin and post-dexamethasone cortisol. *Acta Psychiatr Scand.* 1995;91:313-321.
44. Young IM, Francis PL, Leone AM, Stovell P, Silman RE. Constant pineal output and increasing body mass account for declining melatonin levels during human growth and sexual maturation. *J Pineal Res.* 1988;5:71-85.

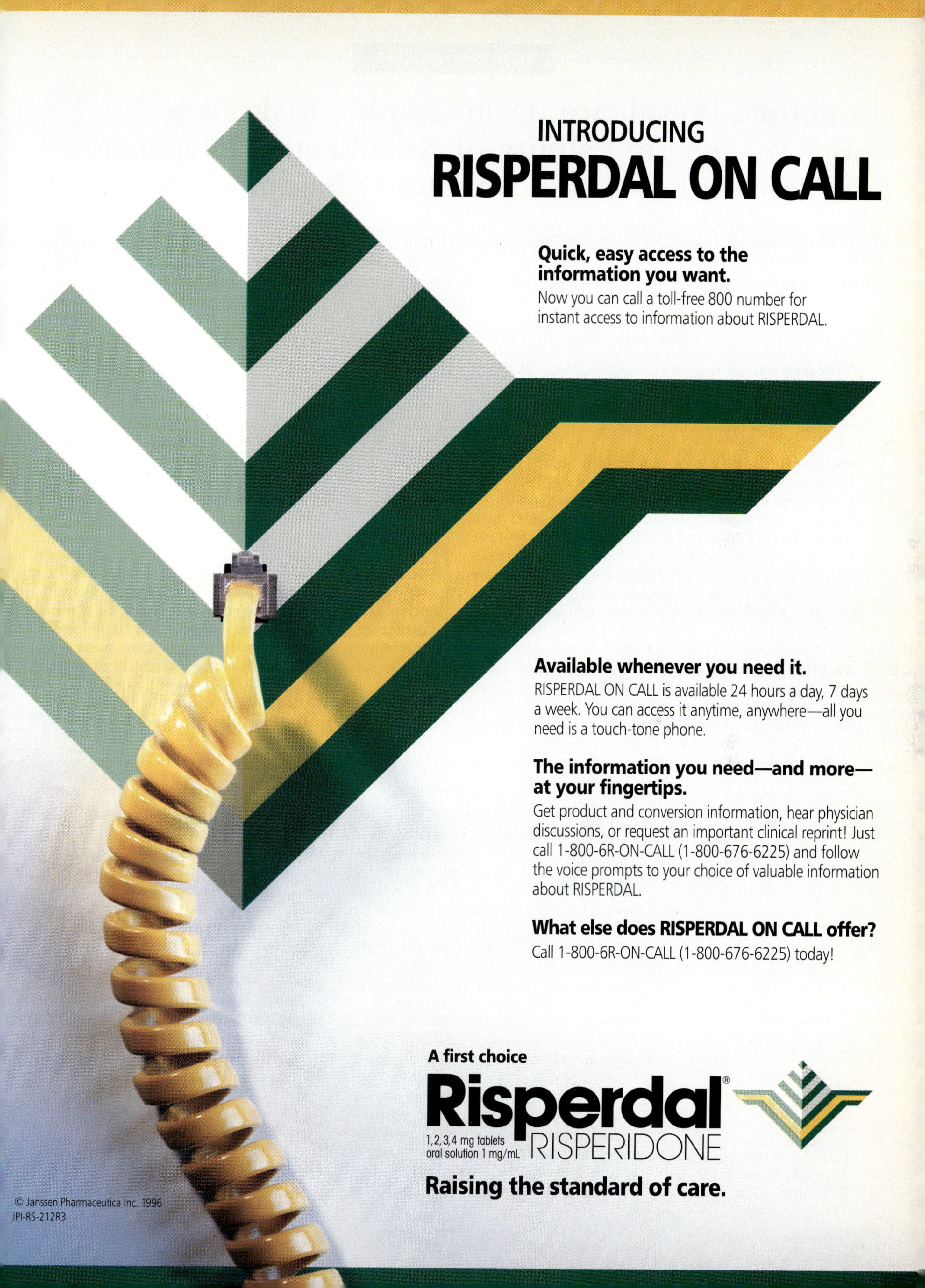
INTRODUCING
RISPERDAL ON CALL
Quick, easy access to the information you want.
Now you can call a toll-free 800 number for instant access to information about RISPERDAL.
Available whenever you need it.
RISPERDAL ON CALL is available 24 hours a day, 7 days a week. You can access it anytime, anywhere—all you need is a touch-tone phone.
The information you need—and more—at your fingertips.
Get product and conversion information, hear physician discussions, or request an important clinical reprint! Just call 1-800-6R-ON-CALL (1-800-676-6225) and follow the voice prompts to your choice of valuable information about RISPERDAL.
What else does RISPERDAL ON CALL offer?
Call 1-800-6R-ON-CALL (1-800-676-6225) today!
A first choice
Risperdal®
1,2,3,4 mg tablets
oral solution 1 mg/mL
RISPERIDONE
Raising the standard of care.
© Janssen Pharmaceutica Inc. 1996
JPI-RS-212R3

Lifetime Prevalence, Demographic Risk Factors, and Diagnostic Validity of Nonaffective Psychosis as Assessed in a US Community Sample

The National Comorbidity Survey

Kenneth S. Kendler, MD; Timothy J. Gallagher, PhD; Jamie M. Abelson, MSW; Ronald C. Kessler, PhD

Background: We seek to estimate lifetime prevalence and demographic correlates of nonaffective psychosis in the US population assessed by a computer-analyzed structured interview and a senior clinician.

Methods: In the National Comorbidity Survey, a probability subsample of 5877 respondents were administered a screen for psychotic symptoms. Based on the response to this screening, detailed follow-up interviews were conducted by mental health professionals (n=454). The initial screen and clinical reinterview were reviewed by a senior clinician. Results are presented for narrowly (schizophrenia or schizophreniform disorder) and broadly (all nonaffective psychoses) defined psychotic illness.

Results: One or more psychosis screening questions were endorsed by 28.4% of individuals. By computer algorithm, lifetime prevalences of narrowly and broadly defined psychotic illness were 1.3% and 2.2%, respectively. Of those assigned a narrow diagnosis by the computer, the senior clinician assigned narrow and broad diagnoses to 10% and 37%, respectively. By clinician diagnosis, lifetime prevalence rates of narrowly and broadly defined psychosis were 0.2% and 0.7%, respectively. A clinician diagnosis of nonaffective psychosis was significantly associated with low income; unemployment; a marital status of single, divorced, or separated; and urban residence. Clinician confirmation of a computer diagnosis was predicted by hospitalization, neuroleptic treatment, duration of illness, enduring impairment, and thought disorder.

Conclusions: Lifetime prevalence estimates of psychosis in community samples are strongly influenced by methods of assessment and diagnosis. Although results using computer algorithms were similar in the National Comorbidity Survey and Epidemiologic Catchment Area studies, diagnoses so obtained agreed poorly with clinical diagnoses. Accurate assessment of psychotic illness in epidemiologic samples may require collection of extensive contextual information for clinician review.

Arch Gen Psychiatry. 1996;53:1022-1031

From the Departments of Psychiatry and Human Genetics, Medical College of Virginia/Virginia Commonwealth University, Richmond, Va (Dr Kendler); the Department of Psychiatry, Washington University School of Medicine, St Louis, Mo (Dr Gallagher); and the Institute for Social Research, University of Michigan, Ann Arbor (Ms Abelson and Dr Kessler).

ALTHOUGH epidemiologic investigations of psychotic illness have been conducted for many years,[1-5] the interpretation of results continues to be beset by methodological problems.[6] In the general population, psychotic symptoms are rare and their evaluation is problematic, requiring the elimination of respondent misunderstanding, schizotypal traits, drug-induced states, and culturally sanctioned magical or religious beliefs. These epidemiologic studies have relied largely on 2 sources of diagnostic information: psychiatric hospital records and interviews. While hospital records contain information about contemporaneously recorded psychotic symptoms and signs, unless specifically designed for research, they usually vary so widely in detail and accuracy that applying diagnostic criteria to them is problematic. Depending on the organization of psychiatric care, maintenance of medical records, and consent requirements, such records may be difficult to obtain. Furthermore, hospital records produce estimates of *treated* prevalence. In western countries, 15% to 20% of subjects with schizophrenia in the general population (and probably more with milder psychotic illnesses) have had no prior contact with mental health professionals.[7]

With personal interviews, it is possible to estimate total rather than treated

See Subjects and Methods on next page

SUBJECTS AND METHODS

SAMPLE

The NCS, a nationwide survey of the US population ages 15 through 54 years, is based on a stratified, multistage area probability sample of the noninstitutionalized civilian population in the 48 coterminous states.[17] The NCS included a nonresponse survey, carried out in a sample of initial nonrespondents who were offered a substantial financial incentive to complete a short form of the diagnostic interview. The survey data were weighted to compensate for this nonresponse. The data were also weighted to adjust for variation in probabilities of selection within households, for differential selection of new households, and for the underrepresentation of difficult-to-reach households. These weighted data, finally, were poststratified by means of an iterative procedure to approximate the national population distributions of the cross-classification of age, sex, race or ethnicity, marital status, education, living arrangements, region, and urbanicity as defined by the 1989 US National Health Interview Survey.[19]

The NCS used a 2-phase sample design, in the first phase of which the part I diagnostic interview was administered to all 8098 respondents. In the second phase, a part II risk factor interview, including a screen for psychotic symptoms, was administered to a probability subsample of 5877 respondents consisting of (*a*) all part I respondents aged 15 to 24 years, (*b*) all older part I respondents who were positive on initial questions in 1 or more diagnostic sections of the CIDI (possible cases), and (*c*) a 1-in-6 random subsample of all remaining part I respondents. All analyses using the part II data were weighted to reflect probability of selection.

INITIAL DIAGNOSTIC ASSESSMENT

The instrument used in the initial assessment, administered by the highly experienced field staff of the Survey Research Center at the University of Michigan, was a modified University of Michigan version of the CIDI[18] (UM-CIDI). Diagnoses were generated by the use of the CIDI diagnostic program.[20] Interviewers completed a 7-day training program for the NCS.

The UM-CIDI contained the 13 probes to screen for psychotic symptoms from the original CIDI plus follow-up questions about treatment, impairment, and possible organic causes. In addition, the UM-CIDI had interviewers rate the presence of 4 "signs" of psychosis contained in the original CIDI: neologisms, thought disorder, flat affect, and "behaves as if hallucinating." While the original CIDI provided only a small space for the interviewer to record examples of psychotic symptoms, the UM-CIDI provided an entire page for each psychotic symptom on which the interviewer was to record verbatim responses to probes about the nature and/or causes of the putative psychotic symptom. The UM-CIDI contains an original CIDI item in which the interviewer assesses whether the putative psychotic symptom was "realistic."

REINTERVIEW

We developed a new instrument ("Section K Telephone Reinterview") to conduct clinical reinterviews with individuals who screened positive for psychosis in the CIDI. While this interview maintained the structure of the original CIDI, it added numerous additional probes for each stem question, inquiring in detail about the putative psychotic symptoms.

To generate a computer diagnosis of psychotic disorders, we applied the CIDI computer algorithm to the reinterview, using only those items derived from the original CIDI. To score a psychotic symptom as present, this algorithm requires that (1) the interviewer rate the symptom as "not realistic"; (2) the symptom be accompanied by either treatment seeking or major impairment ("interfere with life or activities a lot"); and (3) the symptom not be due to illness or injury, medications, drugs or alcohol. In addition to diagnoses of schizophrenia and schizophreniform disorder, we generated computer diagnoses for NAP, which equaled *DSM-III-R*[21] categories of schizophrenia, schizophreniform disorder, schizoaffective disorder, delusional disorder, or psychosis not otherwise specified.

In the NCS 1868 individuals responded yes to at least 1 of the 13 stem questions for psychotic symptoms in the

Continued on next page

prevalence. Pioneered in early Scandinavian studies[8,9] where personal assessments were performed by psychiatrists, this approach was also used in the Epidemiologic Catchment Area (ECA) study,[10] in which lay interviewers administered the Diagnostic Interview Schedule (DIS),[11] which contains sections assessing schizophrenia and schizophreniform disorder.

Personal interviews, however, also have limitations as assessment tools for psychotic illness. They may generate false negatives due to inadequate probing or denial of prior psychotic symptoms.[12-14] Through misinterpretation, lay interviewers may assign false-positive diagnoses of psychosis.[12,14-16]

Herein, we present results on lifetime prevalence (LTP), psychosocial correlates, and patterns of comorbidity of nonaffective psychosis (NAP) from the National Comorbidity Survey (NCS).[17] A unique feature of this study was a 5-tiered approach to assessing psychotic symptoms. First, lay interviewers administered a revised version of the Composite International Diagnostic Interview (CIDI),[18] including a section screening for psychotic symptoms. Second, interviews containing possible psychotic symptoms were sorted into varying categories of the assessed probability of true psychotic illness. Third, a small proportion of subjects from the low-probability and all subjects from the high-probability classes were recontacted by experienced mental health professionals and administered the psychosis section of the CIDI plus extensive additional probes. Fourth, the CIDI computer algorithm was applied to the completed follow-up interviews, generating computer diagnoses of psychotic disorder. Fifth, a senior psychiatric diagnostician (K.S.K.) reviewed all available information and made best estimate clinical diagnoses.

lay-administered UM-CIDI. After weighting, 28.4%±1.3% (mean±SE) of the US population was estimated to endorse 1 or more probes for psychosis. We developed a 7-category classification for these interviews in which individuals who responded to more than 1 psychotic probe were assigned the highest score for any item they endorsed. These categories (and the number of individuals so classified) were (1) misunderstood (n=143), (2) realistic (n=418), (3) "light" (n=431, unusual experiences, usually occurring rarely, that raised no suspicion of psychosis), (4) need more information (n=313, insufficient information to form any clear judgment but available information raises little question of true psychosis), (5) possible (n=406, at least a suspicion of psychosis), (6) drug related (n=117, possible or probable psychotic symptoms that occurred only in relation to drug use), and (7) probable or definite (n=40).

Individuals who classified the CIDI interviews and conducted reinterviews had either a Master's or Doctoral degree in a mental health–related field or a Bachelor's degree and at least 4 years of clinical experience. They were trained and supervised by one of us (J.M.A.), a clinical social worker with extensive experience in the evaluation of psychotic patients. Difficulties were discussed with one of us (K.S.K.).

We did not reinterview those classified as "misunderstood" or "realistic," as we were confident that they did not have a psychotic disorder. We reinterviewed 38 individuals with "light" symptoms and 38 "needing more information." As we rated none of these 76 respondents as having true psychotic symptoms, we did not reinterview other individuals in these categories.

We attempted to reinterview all individuals classified as categories 5, 6, or 7, with 1 exception: a subsample of subjects who had been previously recontacted for a validation study of major depression were not recontacted for this study because of concerns about respondent burden. The numbers of individuals whom we tried to reinterview, could not contact, refused, and successfully reinterviewed were for category 5: 368, 83, 9, and 276, respectively; for category 6: 115, 42, 1, and 72, respectively; and for category 7: 38, 7, 1, and 30, respectively.

Reinterviewers were provided, for each respondent, information concerning religion, employment, education, CIDI diagnoses of major depression, mania or generalized anxiety disorder, and previous responses to the CIDI Psychotic Disorders probes. They were instructed to probe items initially responded to positively plus any additional relevant items. The reinterview lasted an average of 24 minutes (range, 5-120 minutes), and editing time averaged 40 minutes.

The diagnostic arbiter (K.S.K.) in this study has had extensive experience diagnosing psychotic disorders in nonclinical populations with high reliability.[22-26] Blind to prior classification, he reviewed interviews, associated demographic information, reinterviews, and relevant sections of the original CIDI for 172 individuals: 30 randomly selected from the group classified as "easy," all 138 from the group classified as "difficult," and 4 "probable or definite" CIDI cases not successfully reinterviewed. The 30 "easy" and 138 "difficult" cases were also rewieved by the second diagnostician (J.M.A.). For NAP, raw and chance-corrected agreements (κ)[27] between the 2 diagnosticians were 0.93 and 0.82, respectively.

ANALYSIS PROCEDURES

The data analyzed in this report were obtained from a stratified multistage sample and were subsequently weighted to adjust for differential probabilities of selection and nonresponse. Poststratification to the total US population in the target age range was also made. As a result of this complex sample design and weighting, estimates of SEs based on the usual assumptions of equal-probability simple random sampling are biased. More complex analysis methods are needed to obtain appropriate SEs. Estimates of SEs of proportions were obtained using the Taylor series linearization method.[28] The PSRATIO program in OSIRIS[29] was used to make these calculations. Estimates of standard errors of logistic regression coefficients were obtained using the method of balanced repeated replication (BRR).[30,31] This procedure began by generating 44 balanced subsamples of the survey data. The LOGISTIC program in SAS[32] was used to make individual calculations for each of these 44 replicate subsamples. A SAS BRR macro[30-32] was used to compute estimates of the SEs of model coefficients from the distribution of the coefficients in the 44 replicates.

RESULTS

CIDI DIAGNOSIS: SCHIZOPHRENIA OR SCHIZOPHRENIFORM DISORDER

We present LTP and demographic correlates for narrow psychotic illness (schizophrenia or schizophreniform disorder) and broad psychotic illness (all NAP). Applying the CIDI diagnostic program[20] to follow-up interviews, LTP was estimated at 1.3%±0.2% for narrowly defined psychotic illness and 1.1%±0.2% for schizophrenia alone. Descriptive data on the sociodemographic distributions of these computer-based diagnoses are seen in **Table 1**. The associations are presented as odds ratios (ORs) estimated from logistic regression equations in each of which dummy variables defining categories of a single sociodemographic variable were used to predict 1 of the 2 diagnostic measures. The ORs are reported in relation to an omitted category of each sociodemographic variable that has an implicit OR of 1.0. Because of the small number of affected individuals, confidence intervals (CIs) are presented at the 90% level. In addition, likelihood-ratio χ^2 tests are provided (with significance noted at 10% level, 2-tailed) to evaluate the significance of the overall association. The latter tests are useful in evaluating joint significance in cases where the sociodemographic variable has 3 or more categories.

The overall χ^2 test showed significant associations of CIDI diagnoses with income, employment, religion, region, and "area raised." An increased probability of computer-diagnosed narrowly defined psychotic illness was associated with unemployment, non-Catholic religious affiliation, living in the West, and being raised in a nonrural area. The association with income was complex with

Table 1. Demographic Correlates of the CIDI Computer Diagnosis of Narrowly Defined Psychosis and the Clinician Diagnosis of NAP in the National Comorbidity Survey*

	CIDI Narrow Psychosis†								Clinician NAP							
			Cases			Noncases					Cases			Noncases		
Variable Categories	OR	90% CI	%	SE	n	%	SE	n	OR	90% CI	%	SE	n	%	SE	n
Age, y			χ^2_3= 0.39								χ^2_3=3.02					
15-24	0.82	0.32-2.13	22.9	8.1	17	25.9	1.0	1504	2.17	1.15-4.10‡	36.2	8.1	15	25.8	1.0	1507
25-34	1.04	0.39-2.73	34.3	7.1	25	30.9	1.0	1793	1.49	0.73-3.01	29.7	7.1	12	30.9	1.0	1806
35-44	0.88	0.38-2.08	25.9	6.7	19	27.4	1.0	1589	1.35	0.63-2.88	23.9	6.7	10	27.4	0.9	1598
45-54	1.00	...	16.9	2.9	12	15.8	0.9	917	1.00	...	10.3	2.9	4	15.9	0.9	926
15-54, linear	1.02	0.99-1.04	...	...	...	...	...	...	0.98	0.95-1.01	...	...	...	...	...	...
Sex			χ^2_1= 0.90								χ^2_1=0.94					
Male	1.00	...	42.1	8.0	31	47.9	1.4	2781	1.00	...	39.9	8.0	16	47.9	1.4	2796
Female	1.26	0.78-2.05	57.9	8.0	43	52.1	1.4	3023	1.39	0.79-2.44	60.1	8.0	24	52.1	1.4	3041
Race or ethnicity			χ^2_3= 1.55								χ^2_3=2.75					
White	1.00	...	71.7	8.6	53	76.4	2.4	4433	1.00	...	64.7	8.6	26	76.4	2.4	4459
Black	1.34	0.69-2.61	14.3	5.6	11	11.4	1.1	659	1.92	0.93-3.98	18.5	5.6	7	11.3	1.1	662
Hispanic	1.02	0.34-3.02	8.6	5.2	6	9.0	1.9	522	1.51	0.47-4.85	11.5	5.2	5	8.9	1.9	523
Other	1.77	0.69-4.54	5.5	3.4	4	3.3	0.6	190	1.92	0.36-10.42	5.4	3.4	2	3.3	0.6	192
Education, y			χ^2_3= 5.03								χ^2_3=3.68					
0-11	2.24	1.02-4.93‡	25.9	5.9	19	23.2	1.4	1346	2.32	1.04-5.20‡	34.6	5.9	14	23.2	1.4	1351
12	2.23	0.99-5.04	40.7	7.5	30	36.7	1.3	2127	1.58	0.63-3.93	37.3	7.5	15	36.7	1.3	2142
13-15	2.24	0.98-5.13	24.2	5.4	18	21.7	1.0	1259	1.16	0.46-2.88	16.2	5.4	7	21.8	1.0	1271
16+	1.00	...	9.2	4.8	7	18.5	1.3	1071	1.00	...	11.8	4.8	5	18.4	1.3	1073
0-16+, linear	0.92	0.83-1.03	...	...	...	...	...	...	0.91	0.78-1.06	...	...	...	...	...	...
Household income, ×$1000/y			χ^2_2= 9.54§								χ^2_2=4.99§					
0-19	1.47	0.89-2.41	40.6	9.1	30	27.7	1.8	1609	2.18	1.11-4.29‡	44.6	9.1	18	27.8	1.8	1621
20-34	0.47	0.24-0.94‡	11.3	5.7	8	24.0	1.2	1393	1.12	0.60-2.09	19.8	5.7	8	23.9	1.2	1394
35+	1.00	...	48.1	7.1	36	48.3	2.0	2801	1.00	...	35.7	7.1	14	48.4	2.0	2822
0-120+, linear	0.95	0.91-0.99‡	...	...	...	...	...	...	0.92	0.87-0.98‡	...	...	...	...	...	...
Marital status			χ^2_2= 0.63								χ^2_2=5.78§					
Married	1.00	...	64.2	7.4	47	62.1	1.0	3605	1.00	...	45.3	7.4	18	62.3	1.0	3634
Separated, widowed, or divorced	1.19	0.63-2.24	11.8	4.8	9	9.6	0.6	559	2.72	1.42-5.21‡	18.9	4.8	8	9.6	0.6	560
Never married	0.82	0.42-1.58	23.9	7.3	18	28.2	0.9	1639	1.75	0.98-3.11	35.8	7.3	14	28.1	0.9	1642
Employment			χ^2_3= 20.10§								χ^2_3=11.13§					
Working	1.00	...	55.8	6.8	41	60.9	1.4	3537	1.00	...	52.9	6.8	21	60.9	1.4	3557
Student	0.62	0.29-1.30	10.3	5.1	8	18.4	1.0	1067	0.81	0.34-1.92	12.9	5.1	5	18.3	1.0	1069
Homemaker	0.79	0.27-2.35	9.1	4.0	7	12.7	1.1	735	0.80	0.34-1.86	8.7	4.0	4	12.6	1.1	738
Other	3.58	2.09-6.14‡	24.8	6.9	18	8.0	0.9	464	3.84	2.06-7.18‡	25.6	6.9	10	8.1	0.9	472
Religion			χ^2_3= 16.50§								χ^2_3=1.66					
Protestant	2.15	1.09-4.26‡	53.9	6.9	40	52.4	1.8	3041	0.86	0.41-1.79	44.9	6.9	18	52.5	1.8	3063
No preference	3.13	1.31-7.48‡	13.9	5.4	10	9.3	0.7	541	1.54	0.56-4.23	14.3	5.4	6	9.4	0.7	546
Other	5.29	2.30-12.15‡	17.0	4.0	12	6.8	0.6	397	1.38	0.43-4.49	9.4	4.0	4	6.9	0.6	406
Catholic	1.00	...	15.2	7.8	11	31.4	1.9	1824	1.00	...	31.4	7.9	13	31.2	1.9	1822
Household composition			χ^2_3= 2.07								χ^2_3=5.88					
Lives alone	0.84	0.28-2.54	4.9	3.1	4	5.6	0.5	323	2.37	0.77-7.31	9.6	3.1	4	5.5	0.5	323
Lives with parent	0.72	0.37-1.41	15.7	5.5	12	11.9	0.8	689	1.55	0.69-3.49	22.3	5.5	9	11.9	0.8	692
Lives with other	1.31	0.68-2.53	15.2	6.8	11	21.2	0.9	1229	2.62	1.15-5.94‡	22.8	6.8	9	21.1	0.9	1231
Lives with spouse	1.00	...	64.2	7.4	47	61.4	1.0	3561	1.00	...	45.3	7.4	18	61.5	1.0	3591
Region			χ^2_3= 9.32§								χ^2_3=4.63					
Northeast	0.51	0.21-1.25	17.6	7.4	13	20.3	2.2	1177	0.60	0.27-1.33	20.4	7.4	8	20.2	2.2	1181
Midwest	0.36	0.12-1.05	15.6	9.1	11	25.4	2.6	1472	0.46	0.12-1.67	19.5	9.1	8	25.3	2.6	1475
South	0.56	0.24-1.29	32.4	7.1	24	34.2	2.1	1983	0.45	0.22-0.93‡	25.9	7.1	10	34.2	2.1	1997
West	1.00	...	34.4	7.9	25	20.2	1.2	1171	1.00	...	34.2	7.9	14	20.3	1.2	1183
Urban/city			χ^2_2 = 2.56								χ^2_2=12.32§					
Large metropolitan area	1.69	0.83-3.46	53.9	7.7	40	46.8	3.5	2715	5.81	3.17-10.63‡	72.5	7.7	29	46.7	3.5	2725
Small metropolitan area	1.45	0.72-2.95	31.4	7.6	23	31.7	4.2	1839	2.57	1.14-5.77‡	21.8	7.6	9	31.8	4.2	1853
Rural	1.00	...	14.7	2.0	11	21.5	2.9	1250	1.00	...	5.8	2.0	2	21.6	2.9	1258
Area raised			χ^2_4= 8.82§								χ^2_4=6.65					
City	3.13	1.68-5.83‡	37.8	5.5	28	25.9	1.4	1504	5.03	2.09-12.11‡	40.3	5.5	16	25.9	1.4	1515
Suburb	1.94	0.78-4.85	14.4	4.2	11	15.9	1.1	925	2.13	0.70-6.53	10.5	4.2	4	15.9	1.1	931
Midsize town	1.63	0.63-4.20	8.7	6.3	6	11.4	0.9	662	4.24	1.18-15.22‡	14.8	6.3	6	11.3	0.9	662
Small town	2.39	1.18-4.83‡	28.0	5.8	21	25.1	1.1	1459	3.09	1.19-8.02‡	23.9	5.8	10	25.2	1.1	1470
Rural	1.00	...	11.1	5.2	8	21.6	1.4	1254	1.00	...	10.4	5.2	4	21.6	1.4	1258

*CIDI indicates Composite International Diagnostic Interview; NAP, nonaffective psychosis; OR, odds ratio; CI, confidence interval; and subscript in χ^2, the degrees of freedom.

†Schizophrenia or schizophreniform disorder.

‡Unity is outside 90% CI of OR.

§χ^2 is significant at the .10 level.

the lowest risk found in the middle-income range. However, when coded as a linear variable, income was significantly and inversely related to risk for a computer-diagnosed narrowly defined psychotic illness. Although the overall χ^2 test for education was not significant, a significantly increased risk of computer-diagnosed narrowly defined psychotic illness was associated with having less than a high school education.

CIDI DIAGNOSIS: NAP

The LTP of broadly defined NAP, diagnosed by computer algorithm from the follow-up interview, was 2.2%±0.3%. A CIDI diagnosis of NAP was significantly associated with income, employment, religion, region, and area raised. Demographic correlates of NAP differ from those for the more narrow diagnoses in having a different relationship with income (the significant effect now being an elevated risk associated with the lowest income) and having a lower risk associated with both Catholic and Protestant religious affiliations. In addition, a significantly increased risk is found for broadly defined psychosis in Hispanics.

CLINICIAN DIAGNOSIS

Based on clinician diagnoses, LTP was estimated at 0.16%±0.06% for narrowly defined psychotic illness and 0.15%±0.05% for schizophrenia alone. These disorders were too infrequently diagnosed (a total of 9 cases) to permit meaningful risk factor analyses. In a number of cases, the diagnostician (K.S.K.) was confident about the presence of NAP, but information was lacking to enable a more specific *DSM-III-R* diagnosis to be given with certainty. In further analyses of clinician-defined psychotic illness, we focused on the broader category of NAP, with an estimated LTP of 0.7%±0.1%.

Crude ORs for the demographic correlates of clinician NAP diagnoses are seen in Table 1. On the basis of an overall χ^2 test, the risk of illness was significantly associated with income, marital status, employment, and urbanicity. Specifically, an increased risk of a clinician NAP diagnosis was associated with unemployment; residing in a metropolitan area; low income levels; and a marital status of separated, widowed, or divorced. In the absence of an overall significant χ^2 test, significant associations were also noted with young age, less than a high school education, living with nonrelatives, residing outside the south, or being raised in a city or town.

The wide age range of the NCS respondents complicates the interpretation of the association between marital status and psychopathology. When we examine the clinician diagnosis of NAP only in individuals aged 30 years or older, the OR is somewhat greater among those who are single (OR=3.84; 90% CI, 1.00 to 14.80) than among those separated, widowed, or divorced (OR=3.47; 90% CI, 1.88 to 6.38). This difference is more marked in those aged 35 years or older: OR=10.20 (90% CI, 2.17 to 47.86) for single individuals and OR=5.62 (90% CI, 2.37 to 13.33) for separated, widowed, or divorced.

Since both childhood and current residence are significantly associated with risk for clinician-defined NAP, we attempted to clarify the nature of these relationships by examining a combined model. In this model, current residence in a metropolitan or other urban area was associated with significantly greater risk than residence in rural areas (OR=5.90; 90% CI, 2.95 to 11.77 and OR=2.54; 90% CI, 1.08 to 5.96, respectively). However, compared with being raised in a rural area, neither being raised in a city (OR=1.25; 90% CI, 0.75 to 2.08) nor in a suburb (OR=0.52; 90% CI, 0.21 to 1.25) was significantly associated with the risk for psychosis controlling for current urbanicity.

Table 2. Patterns of Lifetime Comorbidity for Clinician Diagnosis of NAP*

	Prevalences of Other Disorders Among Respondents With NAP, %	OR	95% CI
Affective disorders			
Major depression	66.6	9.4	5.2-16.7†
Dysthymia	28.3	5.4	2.8-10.4†
Mania	20.9	15.7	6.6-37.2†
Any	73.4	10.7	5.6-21.8†
Anxiety disorders			
Generalized anxiety disorder	30.9	8.0	3.8-16.8†
Agoraphobia	27.5	5.1	2.4-10.6†
Simple phobia	30.8	3.4	1.8-6.3†
Social phobia	39.5	4.1	1.9-9.0†
Panic disorder	25.5	9.1	4.0-21.1†
Posttraumatic stress disorder	28.9	4.9	2.2-10.7†
Any	71.4	5.9	2.4-14.6†
Substance use disorder			
Alcohol dependence	43.2	4.4	2.4-8.1†
Drug dependence	37.7	7.1	3.6-14.0†
Alcohol abuse or dependence	57.0	4.2	2.2-8.2†
Drug abuse or dependence	44.8	6.2	3.1-12.5†
Any	58.5	3.7	1.8-7.3†

**NAP indicates nonaffective psychosis; OR, odds ratio; and CI, confidence interval.*

†Unity is outside 95% CI.

Individuals receiving a clinician diagnosis of NAP were at significantly increased risk for a wide range of CIDI diagnoses assigned *without* diagnostic hierarchies, including all anxiety disorders, alcohol and drug abuse and dependence, and affective disorders (**Table 2**). Only 7% of NAP cases did *not* receive at least 1 additional psychiatric diagnosis.

THE RELATIONSHIP BETWEEN CIDI AND CLINICIAN DIAGNOSES

Only 10.5% of weighted cases assigned a CIDI computer diagnosis of narrowly defined psychosis were so diagnosed by K.S.K., an additional 26.1% being diagnosed as another NAP. Of cases diagnosed as NAP by the CIDI computer algorithm, 28.4% were so diagnosed by the senior clinician (K.S.K.). Of the cases diagnosed by the CIDI as being broad but not narrowly defined psychosis, none and 9.8% were judged by K.S.K. to have narrowly and broadly defined psychosis, respectively.

We examined whether information recorded in the CIDI reinterview could predict a clinician diagnosis of NAP among those cases diagnosed by the CIDI computer algorithm as (1) narrowly or (2) broadly defined psychosis. Individual psychotic symptoms recorded on the CIDI did not strongly predict clinician diagnosis of psychosis (**Table 3**); however, they were more predictive in cases with a narrow than with a broad CIDI di-

Table 3. Prediction of a Clinical Diagnosis of NAP From Variables Coded on the CIDI Interview Among Subjects With a CIDI Diagnosis of Narrowly or Broadly Defined Psychosis*

	Predicting a Clinical Diagnosis of NAP Among Subjects With a CIDI Computer Diagnosis of			
	Schizophrenia or Schizophreniform Disorder		NAP	
Predictor Variable	OR	95% CI	OR	95% CI
K1, Spying or following	2.10	0.65-6.80	2.40	0.77-7.45
K2, Experimenting, poisoning	0.68	0.19-2.43	0.89	0.28-2.75
K3, Reading mind	0.90	0.07-12.25	0.79	0.14-4.58
K4, Others hear your thoughts	0.52	0.06-4.41	0.39	0.07-2.01
K5, Hear others' thoughts	0.90	0.15-5.34	0.91	0.20-4.21
K6, Under control of force	1.68	0.40-7.14	1.00	0.27-3.67
K7, Thoughts into mind	4.29	1.07-17.17†	3.07	0.79-11.85
K8, Sent messages	3.24	1.12-9.41†	1.85	0.29-11.71
K9, Hypnotized, lasers, x-rays	2.49	0.26-24.24	3.50	0.35-34.75
K10, Visions	6.26	1.40-27.96†	3.56	0.54-23.37
K11, Voices	3.76	0.91-15.49	2.07	0.56-7.71
K12, Strange smells	1.02	0.11-9.42	0.55	0.09-3.26
K13, Unusual feelings	2.10	0.52-8.47	0.85	0.21-3.54
No. of symptoms				
Low	1.00	...	1.00	...
Medium	6.86	0.88-53.55	2.12	0.14-32.47
High	14.79	1.64-133.64†	4.19	0.29-60.45
Delusions and hallucinations	1.00	...	1.00	...
Delusions only	0.02	0.00-0.13†	0.39	0.00-85.57
Hallucinations only	0.20	0.03-1.24	0.25	0.04-1.48
Thought disorder	...	...	4.86	1.01-23.40†
Flat affect	1.54	0.30-7.84	2.30	0.47-11.39
Impairment during symptoms	1.13	0.74-1.72	1.27	0.83-1.94
Enduring impairment	1.96	1.09-3.52†	2.16	1.13-4.15†
Duration	1.13	1.00-1.28†	1.14	1.03-1.26†
Neuroleptic treatment	2.80	0.89-8.82	4.27	1.26-14.53†
Seeking help	0.89	0.34-2.29	1.02	0.46-2.27
Hospitalization	7.02	1.43-34.35†	8.99	2.20-36.71†
Age at onset	0.93	0.86-1.01	0.96	0.90-1.02

**CIDI indicates Composite International Diagnostic Interview; NAP, nonaffective psychosis; OR, odds ratio; and CI, confidence interval.*
†Unity is outside 95% CI.

agnosis. Endorsement of 4 items assessing common persecutory delusions (K2) and various aspects of "thought transfer" (K3-5) predicted a *decreased* probability of a clinician diagnosis of psychosis. Given a CIDI diagnosis of narrowly defined psychosis, items assessing auditory and visual hallucinations, delusions of thought insertion (K7), and ideas of reference from the television or radio (K8) were significantly associated with an *increased* probability of a clinician diagnosis of psychosis.

Could the total number or kind of endorsed psychotic symptoms predict clinician diagnosis? In those with a narrow computer-CIDI diagnosis, the clinician diagnosis of psychosis was significantly predicted both by total number of endorsed psychotic symptom items and by the combination of delusions and hallucinations. Subjects who endorsed only items reflecting delusions were particularly *unlikely* to be confirmed as psychotic by the clinician.

Of the 4 "signs" of psychosis rated by interviewers, 2 (neologisms and "behaves as if hallucinating") were too rare to analyze. While flat affect did not predict clinician diagnosis, an interviewer rating of "thought disorder" did significantly predict the clinician diagnosis of NAP in those with a CIDI broad diagnosis.

In cases with a CIDI diagnosis of either narrowly or broadly defined psychosis, several other clinical characteristics of the respondents significantly predicted a clinician diagnosis of psychosis, including respondent reports of enduring impairment, duration of their psychotic symptoms, treatment with neuroleptic drugs, or hospitalization.

Among respondents diagnosed by the CIDI-computer algorithm with narrowly defined psychosis, we created a summary variable of the 8 significant predictors of clinician diagnosis seen in Table 3. Using weighted data, individuals with between 0 and 3, 4, or 5 or more of these 8 variables were diagnosed by K.S.K. as psychotic 20.0%, 84.4%, and 79.1% of the time, respectively. However, of the cases that were diagnosed by K.S.K. as psychotic, only 40.5% had 5 or more "predictor" variables.

COMMENT

CIDI DIAGNOSES

In a representative sample of the US population, we found, by applying a computer algorithm for *DSM-III-R* diagnoses to CIDI questions from our follow-up interview, an LTP of schizophrenia of 1.1%. Despite methodologic differences in the various studies, the diagnostic algorithms for psychotic disorders in the UM-CIDI and DIS are sufficiently similar to warrant comparing our results with those obtained with the DIS in epidemiologic samples. The standardized LTP of schizophrenia in the ECA study was similar, ie, 1.3.[5] Other studies using the DIS in general population samples report a range of LTPs of schizophrenia from 0.3% to 1.6%.[33-38]

Demographic predictors of a computerized diagnosis of schizophrenia were generally similar in the NCS and ECA studies.[5] Both found higher rates of disorder significantly associated with low socioeconomic status, younger age, unemployment, and a marital status of single, divorced, or separated. Both studies found a nonsignificant 30% to 35% higher rate of illness in female individuals. However, the ECA study reported significantly lower rates of disorder in Hispanics, while we found no significant differences across race or ethnicity, but a trend toward *higher* prevalences in nonwhite individuals.

How do the prevalence estimates for schizophrenia found by the CIDI in the NCS compare with those obtained using hospital diagnoses or examinations by psychiatrists? In a review of prevalence studies of schizophrenia, Torrey[3] finds that, although nearly all studies used a diagnostic approach to schizophrenia broader than *DSM-III-R*, only 1 of 17 found an LTP of schizophrenia exceeding 1%. Including studies reporting shorter prevalence periods, 4 of 76 reported prevalences of schizophrenia that were 1% or greater. Only 2 studies of selected small populations with suspected high LTPs[39,40] produced estimates substantially in excess of those estimated from the CIDI interviews in the NCS. The LTP of schizophrenia from the NCS, generated by a computer analysis of the CIDI, is toward the very upper end, if not outside the range, of prevalence estimates found by more traditional methods. If this difference in LTP estimates does not reflect true population differences or cohort effects, then the higher rate of schizophrenia and associated disorders found by the CIDI is likely to result from either false negatives using other methods or false positives from the CIDI. The diagnostic follow-up procedure built into the NCS permits us to directly evaluate this issue.

COMPARISON OF CIDI AND CLINICIAN DIAGNOSES

Built into the NCS study of psychosis was a follow-up interview, conducted by mental health professionals, which contained the psychosis section from the CIDI and extensive additional probes to assess psychotic symptoms. Clinical diagnoses based on this interview suggested that a large proportion of the CIDI diagnoses of psychosis were false positives.

In 2 prior large-scale studies where clinicians reevaluated epidemiologic samples of individuals who received diagnoses of schizophrenia by the DIS, the DIS diagnoses were confirmed only 22%[14] and 16% of the time.[41] In a study examining psychiatric outpatients and community subjects,[16] clinicians confirmed 30.2% of cases diagnosed as schizophrenic by the DIS. A lay-administered psychosis screening questionnaire was predicted, in the general population, to produce a true-positive rate of 17%.[42]

Our results, consistent with previous findings, suggest that standard structured psychiatric interviews, analyzed by computer, are a questionable method of case-detection for psychotic illnesses in the general population and generate an unacceptably high proportion of false positives. Given the rarity of psychotic illness in the general population, the false-positive rate will be low only if the method of assessment has a higher specificity than can be achieved with the current methods.

We attempted to understand the high false-positive rates generated by the CIDI-computer algorithm. Among the criteria for a "psychotic" symptom in the CIDI is the interviewer judgment that it is not "plausible" or "realistic." This is too low a threshold. A number of beliefs or hallucinatorylike experiences judged by the clinician as nonpsychotic were assessed by the interviewers as unrealistic. Examples would include subcultural beliefs (eg, witchcraft), schizotypal symptoms (eg, isolated ideas of reference), or brief hallucinatory experiences (eg, seeing a ghost or a recently deceased relative). In addition, interviewers sometimes coded as unrealistic responses we considered likely to reflect real experiences.

PREDICTION OF CLINICAL DIAGNOSIS FROM THE CIDI INTERVIEW

Given the poor agreement between CIDI-computer and clinician diagnoses, could other information in the CIDI better predict clinical assessment? In general, clinical correlates were stronger predictors than were psychotic symptoms themselves. A clinician diagnosis of psychosis was strongly predicted by a history of psychiatric hospitalization or neuroleptic drug treatment. A similar pattern was seen in the follow-up of the Baltimore ECA sample.[43] Other clinical correlates, including duration and enduring impairment, also predicted clinician diagnoses.

There was a wide variability in the relationship between endorsement of individual psychotic symptoms and the final clinician diagnosis. In particular, endorsement of items assessing common persecutory themes and "thought transfer"–like experiences were associated with a lower probability of a clinician diagnosis of psychosis. In general population samples, these items appear to perform particularly poorly at assessing true psychotic symptomatology, probably because the questions are frequently misunderstood by respondents and answers are often misinterpreted by interviewers. Diagnoses based on interviews with individuals who endorsed only delusions had an especially low rate of validation by the clinician, suggesting that assessment of delusions by structured interview is particularly difficult and likely to lead to false-positive diagnoses.

We then tried to develop a scale from the 8 items that significantly predicted a clinician diagnosis of psychosis among those with a CIDI-computer diagnosis of narrowly defined psychotic illness. If rigorous criteria were used, it was possible to define a group of psychotic subjects with a relatively low rate of false positives. However, such criteria would end up missing over 50% of cases considered psychotic by the senior clinician. Based on these results, it is difficult to be optimistic about the development of a structured interview assessment for the general population to be used by lay interviewers that has high both sensitivity and specificity for the assessment of psychotic illness.

CLINICAL DIAGNOSIS

We also examined LTP and sociodemographic correlates of NAP, as assessed by the senior clinician's diagnosis. This diagnostic assessment, which is likely, in our judgment, to be more valid than CIDI-computer diagnoses, produced an estimated LTP of NAP of 0.7%±0.1%. This figure is toward the upper end of the range of LTPs reported in Torrey's[3] detailed review. This is to be expected, because the diagnosis of NAP is broader than most definitions of schizophrenia used in previous epidemiologic surveys.

One of the major disappointments in this study was our inability to confidently report LTP for schizophrenia in the NCS using clinician diagnoses. While we were able to assign this diagnosis in a small number of cases, there were a significant number of individuals who were clearly psychotic and may have had schizophrenia, but whom we could not assign diagnoses with confidence with the available information. Therefore, our LTP estimates for schizophrenia by clinician diagnosis should be interpreted only as a plausible lower limit.

Consistent with nearly all prior studies,[4] we found psychotic illness to occur disproportionately among the disadvantaged (as assessed by income, education, or employment) and among those who were single or divorced. Our results, however, do not address the question of the causal relationship between psychotic illness and these measures. Somewhat less anticipated was the strong relationship found between psychotic illness and both current and childhood residence. Limited previous evidence[44,45] has suggested a positive association between rates of psychosis and residence in and, more rarely, having been raised in an urban area. Our results, however, are most consistent with the hypothesis that rates of psychosis are lower among those raised in and/or currently residing in rural areas.

We attempted to gain insight into the possible causal relationship between place of residence and risk of psychosis by jointly examining current and childhood residence. When both sets of variables were examined in a single model, the results indicated that the effect resulted entirely from current residence. These findings would suggest that the association most plausibly results from in-migration of individuals prone to psychosis from rural to more urban areas. We also examined 2 further models that included either current residence (destination) or childhood residence (origination) and a variable that reflected "movement" in either a more or a less urban direction. The "destination-movement" model again suggested that the association with psychosis resulted entirely from the place of current residence. However, the "origination-movement" model produced more complex results, suggesting a significant association with risk of psychosis for both urban childhood environment and movement into a more urban area.

Because of their greater probable validity, we examined patterns of comorbidity only, using NAP as assessed by the senior diagnostician. Consistent with many prior clinical reports,[46-48] as well as results from the ECA study,[49] we found high rates of comorbidity; when diagnoses were made without hierarchies, individuals with NAP were at substantially increased risk for anxiety disorders, affective disorders, and substance use disorders.

LIMITATIONS

This article should be interpreted in the context of 4 potential methodologic limitations, all of which would tend to produce an *underestimate* of the LTP of psychotic illness in the NCS.

First, our LTP estimates may be underestimated because participants in the NCS were selected from residential units. Using 1990 US Census rates,[50] and estimates of the LTP of psychotic illness in various nonresidential populations,[5,51] we calculated that the bias introduced by excluding nonresidential populations was modest: their inclusion increased the LTP of clinical NAP by no more than 0.1%.

Second, we reinterviewed only 10% of the individuals classified as "light" or "needs more information." Although none of these was found to have true psychosis, the upper 95% CI on this estimate is 3.8%. Although unlikely, such a "worst-case" scenario would substantially increase our LTP estimates for NAP from 0.7 to around 1.2%.

Third, the NCS was unable to interview 18% of the predesignated respondents, usually because they refused.[17] In a follow-up survey of a probability subsample of these nonrespondents, we obtained screening information from slightly less than half of those contacted. By comparing this and other information (eg, small-area Census data, household observations) obtained from initial nonrespondents with the information obtained from NCS respondents, we generated a probability-of-nonresponse score for each respondent in the main survey.[52] An increased rate of NAP was found among respondents with high scores on this measure. Based on these results, a nonresponse weight was developed and applied to the entire NCS sample to adjust for biases in LTP estimates owing to nonresponse. If we markedly underestimated the prevalence of NAP in the initial nonrespondents whom we could not interview, then our LTP estimates of NAP may be considerably too low.

Fourth, we initially conducted follow-up interviews only with individuals who responded positively to 1 or more psychotic symptoms in their initial CIDI interview. What proportion of individuals with psychotic illness would deny all of the 13 specific probes in the CIDI? While we are unaware of any definitive answer to this question, the proportion may not be trivial.[13,43] In an attempt to explore this issue, we reviewed the interviews of all 56 respondents who denied psychotic symptoms but were rated, by the lay interviewer, as having 1 or more of the "signs" of psychosis. Of these individuals, we were confident that 42 did not have NAP. We attempted to conduct a follow-up interview with the remaining 14 respondents, but we succeeded only in 4. Of these, none had a history of psychosis. While far from ideal, these results do not suggest that we are missing large numbers of psychotic individuals by our CIDI screen.

IMPLICATIONS

A substantial proportion of the general population respond positively to questions assessing a history of psychotic experiences.[42,53-55] Rigorously studying the epidemiology of psychosis requires the accurate identification of the large proportion of such responses that are false positives. The CIDI interview, in our hands, did not succeed at this task. Although further efforts at developing standardized assessments might be successful, including more intensive training courses for lay interviewers, our current recommendation for population-based studies of psychotic illness is either to have experienced clinicians as interviewers or, more realistically, to collect extensive contextual information about putative psychotic symptoms to be reviewed by a senior diagnostician.

Accepted for publication January 3, 1996.

The NCS is a collaborative epidemiologic investigation of the prevalence, causes, and consequences of psychiatric morbidity and comorbidity in the United States. The NCS is supported by the National Institute of Mental Health (grants MH46376 and MH49098), with supplemental support from the National Institute of Drug Abuse (through a supplement to MH46376) and the W. T. Grant Foundation (grant 90135190). Ronald C. Kessler, MD, is the Principal Investigator. Collaborating NCS sites and investigators are: The Addiction Research Foundation, Toronto, Ontario (Robin Room, PhD); Duke University Medical Center, Durham, NC (Dan Blazer, MD, PhD, and Marvin Swartz, MD); The Johns Hopkins University, Baltimore, Md (James Anthony, PhD, William Eaton, PhD, and Philip Leaf, PhD); the Max-Planck Institute of Psychiatry, Munich, Germany (Hans-Ulrich Wittchen, PhD); the Medical College of Virginia, Richmond (Kenneth S. Kendler, MD); the University of Michigan, Ann Arbor (Lloyd Johnston, PhD, and Ronald C. Kessler, PhD); New York University, New York (Patrick Shrout, PhD), State University of New York at Stony Brook (Evelyn Bromet, PhD); The University of Toronto (R. Jay Turner, PhD); and Washington University School of Medicine, St Louis, Mo (Linda Cottler, PhD). Preparation of this report was also supported by Research Scientist Development Awards to Drs Kendler (grant MH01277) and Kessler (grant MH00507).

We thank Kate McGonagle, PhD, Barbara Salem, MSW, and the staff and interviewers for their work on this project.

A complete list of NCS publications can be obtained from the NCS Study Coordinator, Room 1006, Institute for Social Research, the University of Michigan, Box 1248, Ann Arbor, MI 48106-1248. A complete list of NCS publications, study documentation, and interview schedules can be obtained directly from the NCS Homepage by using the URL; http://www.umich.edu/~ncsum/. Appendix materials for the present paper can be found in document P13.WP within this file. A public use NCS data file can also be reached through: gopher.icpsr.umich.edu.

Reprints: Kenneth S. Kendler, Department of Psychiatry, Medical College of Virginia, Box 980710, Richmond, VA 23298-0710.

REFERENCES

1. Mishler EG, Scotch NA. Sociocultural factors in the epidemiology of schizophrenia: a review. *Psychiatry.* 1963;26:315.
2. Eaton WW. Epidemiology of schizophrenia. *Epidemiol Rev.* 1985;7:105-126.
3. Torrey EF. Prevalence studies in schizophrenia. *Br J Psychiatry.* 1987;150: 598-608.
4. Eaton WW, Day R, Kramer M. The use of epidemiology for risk factor research in schizophrenia: an overview and methodologic critique. In: Tsuang MT, Simpson JC, volume eds, and Nasrallah HA, series ed: *Handbook of Schizophrenia, 3: Nosology, Epidemiology and Genetics.* Amsterdam, the Netherlands: Elsevier Science Publishers BV; 1988:169-204.
5. Keith SJ, Regier DA, Rae DS. Schizophrenic disorders. In: Robins LN, Regier DA, eds. *Psychiatric Disorders in America: The Epidemiologic Catchment Area Study.* New York, NY: The Free Press; 1991:33-52.
6. Bromet E, Davies M, Schulz SC. Basic principles of epidemiologic research in schizophrenia. In: Tsuang MT, Simpson JC, volume eds, and Nasrallah HA, series ed. *Handbook of Schizophrenia, 3: Nosology, Epidemiology and Genetics.* Amsterdam, the Netherlands: Elsevier Science Publishers BV; 1988:151-168.
7. Link B, Dohrenwend BP. Formulation of hypotheses about the ratio of untreated to treated cases in the true prevalence studies of functional psychiatric disorders in adults in the United States. In: Dohrenwend BP, Dohrenwend BS, Gould MS, Link B, Neugebauer R, Wunsch-Hitzig R, eds. *Mental Illness in the United States: Epidemiological Estimates.* New York, NY: Praeger Publishers; 1980:133-149.
8. Sjögren T. Genetic-statistical and psychiatric investigations of a West Swedish population. *Acta Psychiatr Neurol Suppl.* 1948;52.
9. Larsson T, Sjögren T. A methodologic, psychiatric and statistical study of a large Swedish rural population. *Acta Psychiatr Neurol Scand Suppl.* 1954;89.
10. Robins LN, Regier DA, eds. *Psychiatric Disorders in America.* New York, NY: The Free Press; 1991.
11. Robins LN, Helzer JE. *Diagnostic Interview Schedule (DIS): Version III-A.* St Louis, Mo: Washington University School of Medicine; 1985.
12. Spengler PA, Wittchen H-U. Procedural validity of standardized symptom questions for the assessment of psychotic symptoms: a comparison of the DIS with two clinical methods. *Compr Psychiatry.* 1988;29:309-322.
13. Pulver AE, Carpenter WT, Jr. Lifetime psychotic symptoms assessed with the DIS. *Schizophr Bull.* 1983;9:377-382.
14. Helzer JE, Robins LN, McEvoy LT, Spitznagel E. A comparison of clinical and diagnostic interview schedule diagnoses. *Arch Gen Psychiatry.* 1985;42:657-666.
15. Wittchen H-U, Semler G, Von Zerssen D. A comparison of two diagnostic methods: clinical *ICD* diagnoses vs *DSM-III* and Research Diagnostic Criteria using the Diagnostic Interview Schedule (Version 2). *Arch Gen Psychiatry.* 1985;42: 677-684.
16. Canino GJ, Bird HR, Shrout PE, Rubio-Stipec M, Bravo M, Martinez R, Sesman M, Guzman A, Guevara LM, Costas H. The Spanish diagnostic interview schedule: reliability and concordance with clinical diagnoses in Puerto Rico. *Arch Gen Psychiatry.* 1987;44:720-726.
17. Kessler RC, McGonagle KA, Zhao S, Nelson CB, Hughes M, Eshleman S, Wittchen H-U, Kendler KS. Lifetime and 12-month prevalence of *DSM-III-R* psychiatric disorders in the United States: results from the National Comorbidity Survey. *Arch Gen Psychiatry.* 1994;51:8-10.
18. World Health Organization: *Composite International Diagnostic Interview (CIDI, Version 1.0).* Geneva, Switzerland: World Health Organization; 1990.
19. US Department of Health and Human Services. *National Health Interview Survey, 1989* [computer file]. Hyattsville, Md: National Center for Health Statistics; 1992.
20. World Health Organization. *Composite International Diagnostic Interview Computer Programs (Version 1.1).* Geneva, Switzerland: World Health Organization; 1990.
21. American Psychiatric Association. *Diagnostic and Statistical Manual of Mental Disorders, Third Edition, Revised.* Washington, DC: American Psychiatric Association; 1987.
22. Kendler KS, Gruenberg AM. An independent analysis of the Copenhagen sample of the Danish Adoption Study of Schizophrenia, VI: the relationship between psychiatric disorders as defined by *DSM-III* in the relatives and adoptees. *Arch Gen Psychiatry.* 1984;41:555-564.

23. Kendler KS, Gruenberg AM, Tsuang MT. Psychiatric illness in first-degree relatives of schizophrenic and surgical control patients: a family study using *DSM-III* criteria. *Arch Gen Psychiatry.* 1985;42:770-779.
24. Kendler KS, McGuire M, Gruenberg AM, O'Hare A, Spellman M, Walsh D. The Roscommon Family Study, I: methods, diagnosis of probands and risk of schizophrenia in relatives. *Arch Gen Psychiatry.* 1993;50:527-540.
25. Su Y, Burke J, O'Neill FA, Murphy B, Nie L, Kipps B, Bray J, Shinkwin R, Ni Nuallain M, MacLean CJ, Walsh D, Diehl SR, Kendler KS. Exclusion of linkage between schizophrenia and the D_2 dopamine receptor gene region of chromosome 11q in 112 Irish multiplex families. *Arch Gen Psychiatry.* 1993;50:205-211.
26. Kendler KS, Gruenberg AM, Kinney DK. Independent diagnoses of adoptees and relatives as defined by *DSM-III* in the provincial and national samples of the Danish Adoption Study of Schizophrenia. *Arch Gen Psychiatry.* 1994;51:456-468.
27. Cohen J. A coefficient of agreement for nominal scales. *Educ Psychol Meas.* 1960;20:37-46.
28. Woodruff RS, Causey BD. Computerized method for approximating the variance of a complicated estimate. *J Am Stat Assoc.* 1976;71:315-321.
29. University of Michigan. *OSIRIS VII.* Ann Arbor, Mich: Institute for Social Research, The University of Michigan; 1981.
30. Kish L, Frankel MR. Balanced repeated replications for standard errors. *J Am Stat Assoc.* 1970;65:1071-1094.
31. Koch GG, Lemeshow S. An application of multivariate analysis to complex sample survey data. *J Am Stat Assoc.* 1972;67:780-782.
32. SAS Institute. *SAS/STAT User's Guide, Version 6, Fourth Edition.* Cary, NC: SAS Institute Inc; 1990;1, 2.
33. Hwu H-G, Yeh E-K, Chang L-Y. Prevalence of psychiatric disorders in Taiwan defined by the Chinese Diagnostic Interview Schedule. *Acta Psychiatr Scand.* 1989;79:136-147.
34. Wells JS, Bushnell JA, Hornblow AR, Joyce PR, Oakley-Browne MA. Christchurch psychiatric epidemiology study, I: Methodology and lifetime prevalence for specific psychiatric disorders. *Aust N Z J Psychiatry.* 1989;23:315-326.
35. Wittchen H-U, Essau CA, Von Zerssen D, Krieg J-C, Zaudig M. Lifetime and six-month prevalence of mental disorders in the Munich Follow-up Study. *Eur Arch Psychiatry Clin Neurosci.* 1992;241:247-258.
36. Lee CK, Kwak YS, Yamamoto J, Rhee H, Kim YS, Han JH, Choi JO, Lee YH. Psychiatric epidemiology in Korea, I: gender and age differences in Seoul. *J Nerv Ment Dis.* 1990;178:242-246.
37. Bland RC, Orn H, Newman SC. Lifetime prevalence of psychiatric disorders in Edmonton. *Acta Psychiatr Scand Suppl.* 1988;338:24-32.
38. Canino GJ, Bird HR, Shrout PE, Rubio-Stipec M, Bravo M, Martinez R, Sesman M, Guevara LM. The prevalence of specific psychiatric disorders in Puerto Rico. *Arch Gen Psychiatry.* 1987;44:727-735.
39. Book JA. A genetic and neuropsychiatric investigation of a North-Swedish population with special regard to schizophrenia and mental deficiency. *Acta Genet Stat Med.* 1953;4:1-100.
40. Torrey EF, McGuire M, O'Hare A, Walsh D, Spellman MP. Endemic psychosis in Western Ireland. *Am J Psychiatry.* 1984;141:966-970.
41. Anthony JC, Folstein M, Romanoski AJ, Von Korff MR, Nestadt GR, Chahal R, Merchant A, Brown CH, Shapiro S, Kramer M, Gruenberg EM. Comparison of the lay Diagnostic Interview Schedule and a standardized psychiatric diagnosis: experience in eastern Baltimore. *Arch Gen Psychiatry.* 1985;42:667-675.
42. Bebbington P, Nayani T. The Psychosis Screening Questionnaire. *Int J Meth Psychiatr Res.* 1995;5:11-19.
43. Eaton WW, Romanoski A, Anthony JC, Nestadt G. Screening for psychosis in the general population with a self-report interview. *J Nerv Ment Dis.* 1991;179:689-693.
44. Lewis G, David A, Andreasson S, Allebeck P. Schizophrenia and city life. *Lancet.* 1992;340:137-140.
45. Freeman H. Schizophrenia and city residence. *Br J Psychiatry.* 1994;164(suppl 23):39-50.
46. Freed EX. Alcoholism and schizophrenia: the search for perspectives. *J Stud Alcohol.* 1975;36:853-881.
47. Johnson DAW. Studies of depressive symptoms in schizophrenia, I: The prevalence of depression and its possible causes. *Br J Psychiatry.* 1981;139:89-101.
48. Tsuang MT, Simpson JC, Kronfol Z. Subtypes of drug abuse with psychosis: demographic characteristics, clinical features, and family history. *Arch Gen Psychiatry.* 1982;39:141-147.
49. Boyd JH, Burke JD, Gruenberg E, Holzer CE,III, Rae DS, George LK, Karno M, Stoltzman R, McEvoy L, Nestadt G. Exclusion criteria of *DSM-III:* a study of co-occurrence of hierarchy-free syndromes. *Arch Gen Psychiatry.* 1984;41:983-989.
50. US Bureau of the Census. *Statistical Abstract of the United States, 1994.* 114th ed. Washington, DC: US Government Printing Office; 1994.
51. Fischer PJ, Breakey WR. The epidemiology of alcohol, drug, and mental disorders among homeless persons. *Am Psychol.* 1991;46:1115-1128.
52. Kessler RC, Little RJA, Groves RM. Advances in strategies for minimizing and adjusting for survey nonresponse. *Epidemiol Rev.* 1995;17:192-204.
53. Rees WD. The bereaved and their hallucinations, in Schoenberg B, Gerber I, Wiener A, Kutscher AH, Peretz D, Carr AC, eds: *Bereavement: Its Psychosocial Aspects.* New York, NY: Columbia University Press; 1975.
54. The Roper Organization. *Unusual Personal Experiences: An Analysis of the Data From Three National Surveys.* Las Vegas, Nev: Bigelow Holding Corp; 1992.
55. Ross CA, Joshi S. Schneiderian symptoms and childhood trauma in the general population. *Compr Psychiatry.* 1992;33:269-273.

Behavioral Observations at Age 3 Years Predict Adult Psychiatric Disorders

Longitudinal Evidence From a Birth Cohort

Avshalom Caspi, PhD; Terrie E. Moffitt, PhD; Denise L. Newman, PhD; Phil A. Silva, PhD

Background: This study provides, to our knowledge, the first empirical test of whether behavioral differences among children in the first 3 years of life are linked to specific adult psychiatric disorders: anxiety and mood disorders, antisocial personality disorder, recidivistic and violent crime, alcoholism, and suicidal behavior.

Methods: In a longitudinal-epidemiological study, 3-year-old children were classified into groups based on examiner observations of their behavior. At age 21 years, they were reassessed for psychopathologic functioning using standardized interviews based on *DSM-III-R* criteria.

Results: Although effect sizes were small, *undercontrolled* (includes children who are impulsive, restless, and distractible) and *inhibited* (includes children who are shy, fearful, and easily upset) children differed significantly from comparison children in young adulthood. Undercontrolled 3-year-olds were more likely at 21 years to meet diagnostic criteria for antisocial personality disorder and to be involved in crime. Inhibited 3-year-olds were more likely at 21 years to meet diagnostic criteria for depression. Both groups were more likely to attempt suicide, and boys in both groups had alcohol-related problems. Controls for family social class did not change the findings.

Conclusion: Some forms of adult psychopathologic abnormality are meaningfully linked, albeit weakly, to behavioral differences observed among children in the third year of life.

Arch Gen Psychiatry. 1996;53:1033-1039

DEVELOPMENTAL theories hypothesize that the origins of many adult mental disorders can be identified in behavioral characteristics that appear already in the first few years of life.[1,2] A scientific test of this hypothesis is difficult because it requires costly longitudinal studies from birth to adulthood. Thus, empirical evidence about continuities from behavioral characteristics in early childhood—from the first 3 years of life—to psychopathologic abnormality in adulthood is practically nonexistent.[3] Several longitudinal studies have linked behavioral characteristics in late childhood to adult adjustment problems.[4-8] Other longitudinal studies, involving preschool samples followed up into adolescence, have linked behavioral characteristics in early childhood to adjustment problems in early-adolescence[9] and mid-adolescence.[10] As part of a longitudinal investigation of a large representative sample of children studied from age 3 to 21 years, this article provides, to our knowledge, the first empirical test of whether behavioral differences in early childhood are differentially linked to specific adult psychiatric disorders: anxiety, depression, mania, antisocial personality disorder, recidivistic and violent crime, alcoholism, and suicidal behavior.

The predictor variables for this study were introduced previously.[11] We reported that, on the basis of behavioral observations at age 3 years, children in our study could be reliably classified into 1 of 5 distinct groups. The first 3—labeled *undercontrolled*, *inhibited*, and *well-adjusted*—resemble groups identified by Chess and Thomas[12] in their pioneering studies of child temperament. The undercontrolled type, resembling the Chess-Thomas *difficult* type, includes children who are impulsive, restless, and distractible. The inhibited type, resembling the Chess-Thomas *slow-to-warm-up* type, includes children who are shy, fearful, and easily upset. The well-adjusted type, resembling the Chess-Thomas *easy* type, includes children who are capable of self-control when it is demanded of them, are adequately self-confident, and do not

From the Department of Psychology, University of Wisconsin, Madison (Drs Caspi, Moffitt, and Newman); and Dunedin Multidisciplinary Health and Development Unit, University of Otago Medical School, Dunedin, New Zealand (Dr Silva).

See Subjects and Methods on next page

SUBJECTS AND METHODS

SAMPLE

Participants are members of the Dunedin Multidisciplinary Health and Development Study. Silva[26] has described the study's history. It is a longitudinal investigation of a complete cohort born between April 1, 1972, and March 31, 1973, in Dunedin, a city of approximately 120 000 on New Zealand's South Island. Perinatal data were obtained at delivery, and when the children were traced for follow-up at age 3 years, 91% of the eligible births participated in the assessment, providing a base sample of 1037 (52% male) for longitudinal study. The children's fathers were representative of the social class distribution in the general population of similar age in New Zealand. The study members were of predominantly European ancestry. Fewer than 7% identified themselves as Maori or Polynesian, which matches the ethnic distribution of the South Island.

The Dunedin cohort has been reassessed at ages 3, 5, 7, 9, 11, 13, 15, 18, and 21 years. The basic procedure involves bringing participants to the research unit within 60 days of their birthday for a full day of individual data collection. The various research topics are presented as standardized modules, each administered by a different trained examiner in counterbalanced order (eg, physical examination, mental health interview, delinquency interview, injury risk assessment). At each assessment, interview data are supplemented by a search of official records and questionnaires are mailed to informants who know each study member well.

Assessment of Behavior Styles in 3-Year-Olds

At age 3 years, children participated in a 90-minute testing session involving cognitive and motor tasks. Each child was tested by 1 of 10 examiners who had no knowledge of the child's behavioral history. Following the testing, the examiner rated the child's behavior on 22 behavioral characteristics, based on scales derived from the Collaborative Study on Cerebral Palsy, Mental Retardation, and Other Neurological Disorders of Infancy and Childhood.[27] Factor- and cluster-analyses of the examiners' behavioral ratings revealed 5 reliable, homogeneous, and mutually exclusive clusters of children at age 3.[11,27] Undercontrolled children (n=106, 62% male) were described as irritable, impulsive, and impersistent; they had difficulty sitting still, were rough and uncontrolled in their behavior, and labile in their emotional responses. Inhibited children (n=80, 40% male) were socially reticent (fearful and limited communication), inhibited in the testing situation, upset by strangers, and had difficulty concentrating on tasks. The behavior of well-adjusted children (n=405, 48% male) was rated by examiners as within normal limits for their age. Confident children (n=281, 52% male) were zealous, eager to explore the testing materials, and adjusted to the testing situation quickly. Reserved children (n=151, 48% male) were timid and somewhat uncomfortable in the testing session; however, unlike inhibited children, their response disposition was not extreme, and their caution did not interfere with their task orientation.

Assessment of Mental Health Problems at Age 21 Years: Psychiatric Diagnosis

The Diagnostic Interview Schedule (DIS), developed by the National Institute of Mental Health for the Epidemiological Catchment Area program,[28] was used to obtain diagnoses of mental disorder in the last 12 months. The Dunedin version of the DIS was modified to use only those items that were criteria for *DSM-III-R*[29] classifications, to omit lifetime prevalence questions, and to score items as 0, no; 1, sometimes; and 2, yes, definitely. In identifying disorder, only scores of 2 were used to indicate a symptom (commensurate with a 5 in the original DIS). Diagnoses were determined by computer-assisted algorithms that followed explicit criteria specified by *DSM-III-R*. The measurement and prevalence of mental disorders in the Dunedin study is reported elsewhere.[30]

For this study, we examined the following groupings of psychiatric disorder: (1) anxiety disorders (n=195) consisting of generalized anxiety disorder, obsessive-compulsive disorder, panic disorder, agoraphobia, social phobia, simple phobia, or any combination of these disorders; (2) depressive disorders (n=172) consisting of major depressive episode, dysthymia, or both; (3) manic episode (n=19), consisting of study members who experienced a manic episode in the past 12 months; (4) antisocial personality disorder (n=31); and (5) alcohol dependence (n=94).

Clinical Significance of Impairment Associated With Mental-Health Problems

Using a reporting period of the past 12 months, we assessed 6 indexes of impairment associated with mental health problems. These included reports of treatment seeking for psychiatric symptoms, hospitalizations for psychiatric symptoms, use of psychotropic medication, reports of suicide attempts, and court convictions for criminal offenses exclusive of traffic violations. In addition, respondents who reported symptoms in any of the modules of the DIS reported whether they experienced functional interference in work and daily activities associated with those symptoms. We created an overall impairment scale by summing these 6 indexes of impairment.

Informant Index of Mental Health

This index was based on the endorsement of symptoms of mental-health problems in a mailed questionnaire completed

become unduly upset when confronting new people and situations. Typological research has identified these 3 types of children using different sources of information (eg, parent reports or observations), different statistical methods (eg, inverse factor analysis or cluster analysis), in different parts of the world (eg, United States, the Netherlands or New Zealand), and in different age groups (eg, early childhood or early adolescence),[13] suggesting that these 3 types are the best candidates for inclusion in a generalizable classification of temperament. We also found 2 types of children not anticipated by Chess and Thomas: the *confident* type that included children who at 3 years were zealous and friendly and the *reserved* type that included children who at 3 years were slightly cautious.

We previously reported that these behavior styles at age 3 years predict personality traits at age 18 years,[11] adding to a growing body of longitudinal research about by a significant other nominated by the study member as someone who knew them well. Of the 961 participants at age 21 years, 914 (95.1%)-nominated informants returned valid questionnaires. The questionnaire asked the informant to rate the study member on a series of positive and negative attributes. Thirteen of the items represented signs of mental disorders for each of the major categories of the DIS, worded in a general manner such as "Feeling depressed, miserable, sad or unhappy," or "Problems related to the use of alcohol."[30] Informants rated items as 0, does not apply; 1, applies somewhat; and 2, definitely applies.

Measures of Criminality

Computerized records of participants' cumulative court convictions at all courts in New Zealand and Australia were obtained by searching the central computer systems of the New Zealand police. Conviction records excluded traffic offenses, with the exception of driving under the influence of alcohol or criminally negligent driving. Informed consent for the search was obtained at age 21 years. For this study, we examined 2 variables. The criminal recidivism group (n=80) included individuals who had been convicted of 2 or more criminal offenses. The violent offender group (n=44) included individuals who had been convicted of at least 1 of the following offenses: inciting violence, cruelty to an animal, using an attack dog on a person, possession of an offensive weapon, threatening a police officer, rape, manual assault, assault on a police officer, assault with a deadly weapon, manslaughter, and aggravated robbery.

Suicidality

As part of the mental-health interview, participants were asked about suicide attempts they had made during the past 12 months. Attempts were counted whether or not they had required medical attention.

Attrition

At age 21 years, mental-health interviews were missing for 76 members (7.3%) of the original sample of 1037; 17 persons died since age 3 years, 9 persons were not located, 19 refused to participate, and 31 were interviewed by telephone, but were not asked questions about mental health. The 76 nonrespondents did not differ from the 21-year-old participants on family social class ($t[939]=1.35$, $P=.18$), race (χ^2 [1]=.41, $P=.52$), or sex (χ^2 [1]=1.26, $P=.26$). Missing data were not disproportionately concentrated among any of the 5 temperament groups (χ^2 [4]=6.25, $P=.18$). These results suggest that our findings are not compromised by attrition bias.

STATISTICAL ANALYSIS

Contingency tables and analyses of variance (ANOVA) were used to test the hypothesis that undercontrolled and inhibited 3-year-olds would have more mental health problems at age 21 years than other types of children. In addition, multivariate logistic regressions were used to examine specific continuity between behavior styles at age 3 years and particular types of adult psychiatric disorders at 21 years. Each regression equation contained a dummy variable representing undercontrolled children and a dummy variable representing inhibited children. The contrast or reference group in each regression equation was the well-adjusted group. After entering these 2 main effects and the main effect of sex, we added 2 interaction terms to test whether the association between undercontrolled and inhibited behavior at age 3 years and specific disorders at 21 years differed for male subjects and female subjects. We examined whether a model with sex interaction terms yielded significant improvements in the fit of the model to the data than a model with main effects only. In presenting the results, we report odds ratios (ORs) and the *P* values associated with the regression coefficients for the undercontrolled and inhibited dummy variables. The ORs indicate the factor by which the odds of a specific outcome occurring increased for undercontrolled and inhibited children relative to well-adjusted children. When there was no significant sex-by-temperament interaction effect, we report combined results for male and female subjects because this model constitutes a better form for the estimation of relative risk for undercontrolled and inhibited children. When there was a significant interaction at $P<.05$, results are reported separately by sex. To establish that the associations between behavior styles at age 3 years and adult disorders are independent of the family circumstances in which the study members grew up, we included a measure of family social class[31] as a covariate in all regression models. All reported ORs are adjusted for family social class. All significance tests are 2 tailed.

In performing the regression analyses we had to choose between a reference group of well-adjusted children or a reference group combining well-adjusted, reserved, and confident children. We performed the analyses using both options and the statistical and substantive findings did not change significantly. We report analyses using well-adjusted children as the reference group because, as noted in the introduction, this group provides an interpretive fit with previous studies about the structure of temperament. In contrast, the generality of additional types, such as the reserved and confident groups, has yet to be replicated in other samples to test whether they constitute independent types or whether they can be subsumed within the 3 replicable types.

the coherence of personality development beginning in early childhood.[14,15] At 18 years, undercontrolled children described themselves as danger-seeking, impulsive, prone to respond with strong negative emotions to everyday events, and enmeshed in adversarial relationships. At 18 years, inhibited children described themselves as overcontrolled, harm-avoidant, and nonassertive. The behavior style of well-adjusted 3-year-olds was still discernible at 18 years, when, statistically, they defined normal, average young adults. The confident and reserved children resembled the well-adjusted children in their personality profile at age 18 years.

This article extends the study of development and tests 2 hypotheses about links between behavior styles at age 3 years and psychopathologic abnormality at 21 years. First, we tested whether undercontrolled and inhibited children are more likely to have psychiatric problems than other children. This hypothesis follows Thomas et al[16] who re-

Behavior Styles at 3 Years of Age and *DSM-III-R* Diagnoses, Level of Impairment Associated With Psychiatric Symptoms, and Informant-Observed Problems at 21 Years of Age

Outcome at Age 21 Years	Sample Base Rate at Age 21 Years	Behavior Styles at Age 3 Years*: Well-adjusted (n=375)	Undercontrolled (n=94)	Inhibited (n=73)	Reserved (n=142)	Confident (n=268)	χ^2 or F (*P*)
Any disorder, %	40	38†	46	53‡§	37†	42	χ^2=8.5 (.07)
Multiple disorders, %	19	15†‖	27‡	29‡¶	21	18†	χ^2=12.4 (.01)
Mean (SD) impairment scale	0.76 (0.98)	0.65 (0.83)†‖¶	0.99 (1.27)‡§	0.93 (1.12)‡	0.70 (0.94)‖	0.81 (1.01)‡	F=3.14 (.01)
Mean (SD) informant scale	3.90 (3.67)	3.75 (3.37)‖	4.82 (4.12)‡¶	4.69 (4.11)¶	3.87 (3.67)	3.58 (3.74)†‖	F=2.76 (.03)

**Although 961 sample members participated in the mental health interview at 21 years of age, a few were missing complete information across all the Diagnostic Interval Schedule modules; hence N=952.*
†*P<.05, pairwise contrast with the inhibited group.*
‡*P<.05, pairwise contrast with the well-adjusted group.*
§*P<.05, pairwise contrast with the reserved group.*
‖*P<.05, pairwise contrast with the undercontrolled group.*
¶*P<.05, pairwise contrast with the confident group.*

ported that of the 141 children in their study, difficult and slow-to-warm-up children required more psychiatric attention by early adolescence than easy children. Second, we tested whether behavioral characteristics of 3-year-olds provide discriminant validity in predicting specific psychiatric outcomes in adulthood.[17] We expected that inhibited children would be at risk for anxiety disorders and for depressive disorders. We expected that undercontrolled children would be at risk for antisocial personality disorder and criminal behavior. Regarding alcohol-related problems and suicidal behavior, we expected that both undercontrolled and inhibited children would be at increased risk, although for different reasons. Research suggests that undercontrolled children may be attracted to the "good time" they associate with alcohol's disinhibiting effects, whereas inhibited children may use alcohol as a "self-medicating" strategy, to escape dysphoria.[18] This hypothesis is consistent with the notion that there may be at least 2 distinct temperamental-developmental pathways to adult alcohol problems.[19,20] Similarly, research has shown that impulsive behavior and depressive disorders are independently linked to suicide attempts, suggesting that undercontrolled and inhibited childhood behaviors may also represent distinct risks for suicidal behavior in later life.[21,22]

The current study offers several advantages for testing these hypotheses. First, it combines long-term follow-up with an epidemiological sampling frame. We can thus capture the full range of population variation on measures of toddler behavior and adult psychopathologic abnormality. Previous shorter-term studies have examined small or homogeneous samples, or clinic-referred samples, and the generalizability of results from such studies may be compromised by their selectivity.[23] Second, the current study uses a well-established diagnostic interview enabling us to differentiate between adult psychiatric outcomes. Previous shorter-term studies have focused on nonspecific measures of psychopathologic functioning or on global measures of maladjustment, which may obscure meaningful differences in the developmental importance of distinct behavior styles.[24] Third, the current study uses multiple data sources to test longitudinal predictions. Studies that rely on a single data source to measure both predictor and outcome variables cannot separate true prediction from confounded method variance. The only unconfounded strategy is to gather data from different sources at different ages.[25] We use behavioral observations at age 3 years to predict outcomes at age 21 years, measured via self-reports, informant reports, and official records.

With independent data sources, we offer the first test in an epidemiological sample of the hypothesis that behavior in early childhood is linked to adult psychopathologic functioning. Our study constitutes a rigorous test in that it spans 18 years, uses independent data sources, and seeks to predict specific psychiatric disorders at age 21 years from behavioral observations made by an examiner after only 90 minutes of interaction with each child at age 3 years. Because the time span is long and the behavioral observations brief, this test provides a conservative estimate of the extent to which individual differences in early childhood influence adult mental health, and we expected modest effect sizes.

RESULTS

ARE UNDERCONTROLLED AND INHIBITED CHILDREN MORE LIKELY TO HAVE PSYCHIATRIC PROBLEMS?

The **Table** gives the association between behavior styles at age 3 years and mental health problems at age 21 years. As shown in the Table, the 1-year prevalence rate of psychiatric disorder, assessed by diagnostic interview at age 21 years, was 40%. This estimate is consistent with prevalence data for this age group in the National Comorbidity Survey,[32] in which the 12-month prevalence rate of any psychiatric disorders among 15- to 24-year-olds was 37%.

The Table also shows that, as predicted, undercontrolled and inhibited children were the most likely to have a psychiatric disorder, and were also the most severely impaired by their condition. The likelihood of any psychiatric disorder at 21 years was weakly linked to behavior styles at age 3 years (χ^2 [4]=8.5, *P*=.07). As expected, undercontrolled (46%) and inhibited (53%) children were the most likely to be diagnosed with a psychiatric disorder. The likelihood of multiple disorders at 21 years was significantly linked to behavior styles at age

3 years, (χ^2 [4]=12.4, P=.01). Undercontrolled (27%) and inhibited (29%) children were significantly more likely to suffer from multiple disorders. An ANOVA of the impairment scale at age 21 years, with the behavior styles at age 3 years as the independent factor, also revealed a significant effect [F (4,947)=3.14, P=.01]. Undercontrolled and inhibited children were the most impaired. Finally, an ANOVA of the informant reports of mental health problems at age 21 years, with the behavior styles at age 3 years as the independent factor, revealed a significant effect [F (4,878)=2.76, P=.03]. According to informants, undercontrolled and inhibited children had the most mental health problems at age 21 years, corroborating the results based on clinical interviews with the sample members themselves.

In summary, across 18 years and across 3 different data sources—observer ratings, diagnostic interviews, and informant reports—the results provide support for the hypothesis that undercontrolled and inhibited children are at increased risk of psychiatric problems. By contrast, well-adjusted, reserved, and confident children were not distinguishable and had better mental health outcomes at age 21 years.

DO BEHAVIOR STYLES AT AGE 3 YEARS PREDICT SPECIFIC ADULT PSYCHIATRIC OUTCOMES?

Anxiety Disorders

Figure 1 shows the association between behavior styles at age 3 years and anxiety disorders at 21 years. The Figure shows the 1-year prevalence rates (ie, cohort base rates) of specific disorders in the Dunedin sample as a whole, and the rates for well-adjusted, undercontrolled, and inhibited children. Because the sample is an unselected birth cohort, the sample rates may be treated as estimates of population rates among young adults in New Zealand.

Figure 1 shows that behavior styles at age 3 years could not significantly distinguish persons at risk for developing an anxiety disorder. However, before concluding that behavior styles do not constitute risk for anxiety disorders we conducted 3 additional tests. First, we tested the possibility that behavior styles at age 3 years could distinguish persons at risk for developing 2 or more anxiety disorders, but this test was not significant. Second, we tested whether behavior styles at age 3 years could predict specific subtypes of anxiety disorders (eg, social phobia, agoraphobia, or obsessive-compulsive disorder), but these tests were not significant. Third, because categorical data are less sensitive than continuous measures, we examined scores on an anxiety symptom scale, consisting of 19 items from the DIS. An ANOVA of the number of anxiety symptoms at age 21 years did not show the predicted relation between inhibited behavior at age 3 years and anxiety at age 21 years. Rather, there was weak indication that, relative to well-adjusted children (mean±SD, 2.6±5.2), undercontrolled (mean±SD, 3.9±6.9) and inhibited (mean±SD, 3.6±6.7) children had slightly elevated anxious symptomatology [F (2,538)=2.54, P=.08]. This association was not conditioned by sex [F (2,538)=0.66, insignificant].

Mood Disorders

The center panel in Figure 1 shows the link between behavior styles at age 3 years and depressive disorders at 21 years. As predicted, inhibited children were significantly more likely to be diagnosed with depression at age 21 years (OR=2.2, P<.01, 95% confidence interval [CI]=1.2-3.9). Undercontrolled children were not significantly more likely to be diagnosed with depression. Although manic episodes could not be predicted from behavior styles at age 3 years, none of the inhibited children experienced mania, which is characterized by symptoms of increased activity, inflated self-esteem, and impulsive behaviors. Thus, inhibition showed predictive specificity within the family of mood disorders. There were no significant interaction effects between behavior style and sex in predicting mood disorders.

Antisocial Behavior and Criminality

Figure 2 shows the association between behavior styles at age 3 years and antisocial outcomes at age 21 years. As predicted, undercontrolled children were significantly overrepresented in every outcome examined. They were 2.9 times as likely to be diagnosed with antisocial personality disorder (P<.05, 95% CI, 1.1-8.1), 2.2 times as likely to be recidivistic offenders (P<.05, 95% CI, 1.1-4.7), and 4.5 times as likely to be convicted for a violent offense (P<.01, 95% CI, 1.8-10.9). There were no sex interaction effects.

Unexpectedly, inhibited children were also significantly more likely to be convicted for a violent offense (OR=2.9, P<.05, 95% CI, 1.0-8.4). However, this association was moderated by an interaction effect; inhibited boys (OR=5.7, 95% CI, 1.6-20.1), but not girls (OR=0.84, 95% CI, 0.09-7.9), were more likely to have been convicted for a violent offense.

Alcohol-Related Problems

Figure 3 shows the association between behavior styles at age 3 years and alcohol dependence at age 21 years. Undercontrolled children were 2.2 times as likely to be diagnosed with alcohol dependence (P<.05, 95% CI, 1.1-4.4). However, this association was moderated by an interaction effect; undercontrolled boys (OR=2.7, 95% CI, 1.2-6.2), but not girls (OR=0.53, 95% CI, 0.06-4.4), were more likely to have alcohol dependence. As predicted, inhibited children also had elevated rates of alcoholism, but this result did not attain statistical significance (OR=1.8, P=.15, 95% CI, 0.80-4.1).

To further explore the relation between childhood behavior styles and alcohol-related problems, we examined scores on an alcohol abuse symptom scale, consisting of 23 items from the DIS. An ANOVA of the number of alcohol symptoms at age 21 years, with behavior styles at age 3 years as the independent factor, revealed a significant effect [F (2,531)=6.72, P=.01]. Both undercontrolled and inhibited children had significantly more alcohol-related problems. However, this main effect was moderated by an interaction effect with sex [F (2,531)=5.80, P=.01]. As shown in **Figure 4**, both undercontrolled and inhibited boys, but not girls, had significantly more alcohol-related problems. Thus, whereas inhibited boys did not meet the

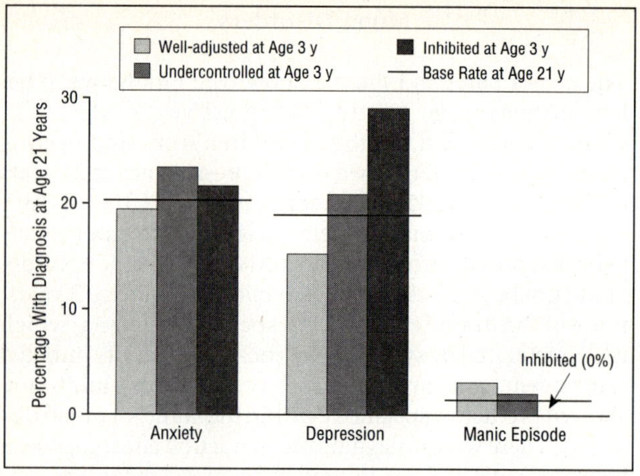

Figure 1. *The association between behavior styles at age 3 years and adult anxiety and mood disorders.*

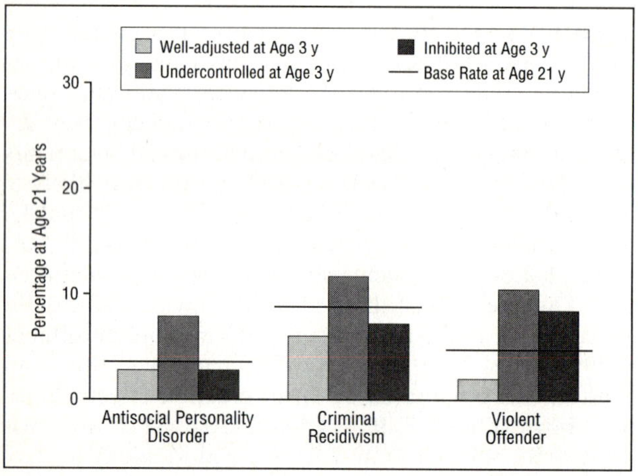

Figure 2. *The association between behavior styles at age 3 years and adult criminal behavior.*

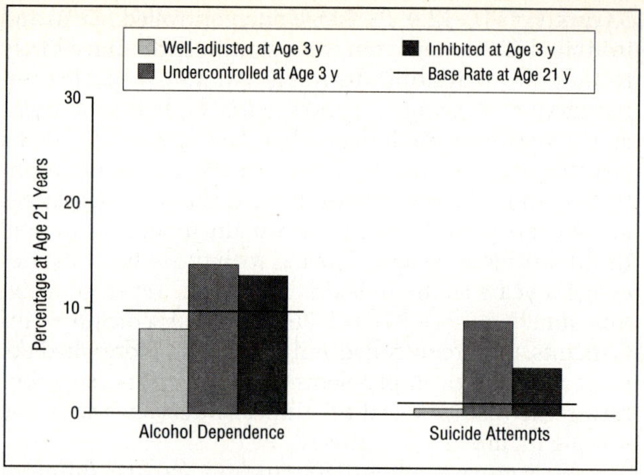

Figure 3. *The association between behavior styles at age 3 years and adult alcohol dependence and suicide attempts.*

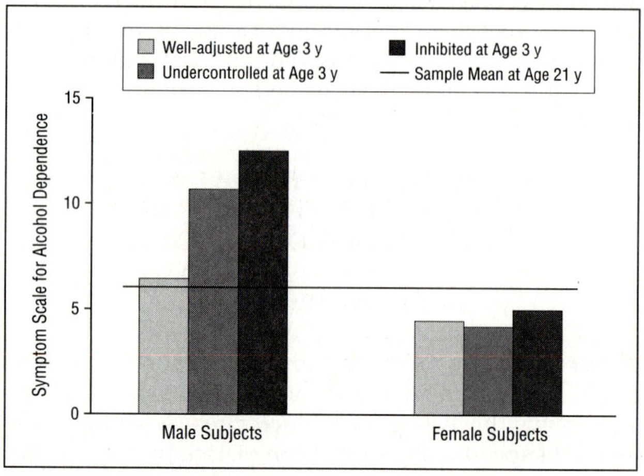

Figure 4. *Scores on Diagnostic Interview Schedule alcohol abuse symptom scale at age 21 years as a function of behavior styles at age 3 years and sex.*

DSM-III-R diagnostic cut-off for alcohol dependence, they did experience more problems associated with alcohol.

Suicide Attempts

Figure 3 shows the association between behavior styles at age 3 years and suicide attempts at 21 years. Suicide attempts were significantly more concentrated among undercontrolled and inhibited children; undercontrolled children were 16.8 times ($P<.01$, 95% CI, 3.5-81.7) and inhibited children were 6.5 times as likely ($P<.05$, 95% CI, 1.1-39.8) to report attempting suicide. There were no sex interaction effects.

COMMENT

Results from the Dunedin study suggest that behavior styles observed in the third year of life are significantly related to mental-health problems at age 21 years. These relations were obtained even with adjustments for social class characteristics. The empirical connections represent small effect sizes, but they span 18 years and distinct data sources, from observer ratings after a 90-minute exposure to the child at age 3 years to mental health information gathered from clinical interviews with the sample members at 21 years. Although small cell sizes in some analyses may render some statistical estimates unstable, the patterns of associations reported were corroborated across independent data sources such as clinical interviews, informant reports, and official records. Still, the present results should be regarded with caution until they are replicated in other samples.

The results provide evidence that specific behavior styles in early childhood are connected to specific psychiatric problems in adulthood. Undercontrolled children were characterized by an impulsive, undercontrolled behavior style at age 3 years. At 21 years, they were more likely to meet the criteria for antisocial personality disorder and to be involved in criminal activities. Inhibited children were shy, fearful, and easily upset in novel settings at age 3 years. At 21 years, they were significantly more likely to meet diagnostic criteria for depression.

There were also similarities between the undercontrolled and inhibited groups, suggesting that children with different behavior styles may be at general risk for similar adult outcomes. Both groups were significantly more likely to attempt suicide, and both groups of boys were more likely to report alcohol-related problems. The latter finding is consistent with causative accounts that posit 2 pathways to alcohol-related problems: one associated with undersocialized behavior, the other with neurotic-depressive behavior.[19] That the relation between both behavior styles and alcohol-related problems was confined to boys is consistent with evidence that enduring, heritable behavior traits may play a more important role in alcohol-related problems among males than females.[33]

There was 1 unexpected finding and 1 negative finding in our study. The unexpected finding was that inhibited boys, like undercontrolled children, were more likely to have been convicted for a violent offense. However, they were not more likely to be recidivistic offenders; they appeared in court records only once. Nor did they meet the diagnostic criteria for antisocial personality disorder. This suggests that inhibited boys who had been convicted for violence may have committed a single offense that was uncharacteristic of their usual behavior. The negative finding was that inhibited children were not, as predicted, at increased risk for anxiety disorders. This finding is inconsistent with shorter-term studies linking behavioral inhibition to anxiety problems.[34,35] However, those studies relied on very small samples and found differences only for specific subsets of extremely inhibited children, for example, children who showed a stable pattern of inhibition at 4 assessment ages or children with a family history of psychiatric disorder. It is thus possible that inhibited childhood behavior is a risk factor for anxiety disorders among a specific segment of children who have a family history of anxiety or who experience chronic family stress.[36]

Although specific episodes of psychiatric disorders may be transient, documentation of a link between behavior styles in early childhood and psychopathologic abnormality in adulthood, paired with knowledge about the consistency of personality from childhood through adulthood,[37] suggests that, in the absence of significant characterological change, early-appearing behavioral differences may act as a persisting risk factor for some forms of psychiatric disorders.

Accepted for publication April 22, 1996.

This research was supported by grants MH-49414 (Dr Caspi) and MH-45070 (Dr Moffitt) from the National Institute of Mental Health, Bethesda, Md; the William T. Grant Foundation, New York, NY; and the William Freeman Vilas Trust, University of Wisconsin, Madison. The Dunedin Multidisciplinary Health and Development Research Unit is supported by the Health Research Council of New Zealand.

We thank the Dunedin Unit investigators and staff, the New Zealand Police, and the study members and their families.

Reprints: Avshalom Caspi, PhD, Department of Psychology, 1202 W Johnson St, University of Wisconsin, Madison, WI 53706.

REFERENCES

1. Goldsmith HH, Buss AH, Plomin R, Rothbart M, Thomas A, Chess S, Hinde RA, McCall RB. Roundtable: what is temperament? four approaches. *Child Dev.* 1987;58:505-529.
2. Rothbart M, Ahadi S. Temperament and the development of personality. *J Abnormal Psychol.* 1994;103:55-66.
3. Halverson CF, Kohnstamm GA, Martin RP, eds. *The Developing Structure of Temperament and Personality From Infancy to Adulthood.* Hillsdale, NJ: Lawrence Erlbaum Associates; 1994.
4. Caspi A, Bem DJ, Elder GH. Continuities and consequences of interactional styles across the life course. *J Pers.* 1989;57:375-406.
5. Huesmann LR, Eron LD, Lefkowitz MM, Walder LO. Stability of aggression over time and generations. *Dev Psychol.* 1984;20:1120-1134.
6. Magnusson D. *Individual Development From an Interactional Perspective.* Hillsdale, NJ: Lawrence Erlbaum Associates; 1988.
7. Pulkkinen L. The role of impulse control in the development of antisocial and prosocial behavior. In: Olweus D, Block J, Radke-Yarrow M. eds. *Development of Antisocial and Prosocial Behavior.* New York, NY: Academic Press Inc; 1986:149-175.
8. Robins L. *Deviant Children Grown Up.* Baltimore, Md: Williams & Wilkins; 1966.
9. Tremblay RE, Pihl RO, Vitaro F, Dobkin PL. Predicting early onset of male antisocial behavior from preschool behavior. *Arch Gen Psychiatry.* 1994;51:732-739.
10. Block J, Block JH, Keyes S. Longitudinally foretelling drug usage in adolescence: early childhood personality and environmental precursors. *Child Dev.* 1988;59:336-355.
11. Caspi A, Silva PA. Temperamental qualities at age 3 predict personality traits in young adulthood: longitudinal evidence from a birth cohort. *Child Dev.* 1995;66:486-498.
12. Chess S, Thomas A. *Origins and Evolution of Behavior Disorders.* Cambridge, Mass: Harvard University Press; 1987.
13. Robins RW, John OP, Caspi A, Moffitt TE, Stouthamer-Loeber M. Resilient, overcontrolled, and undercontrolled children: three replicable personality types. *J Pers Soc Psychol.* 1996;70:157-171.
14. Block J. Studying personality the long way. In: Funder D, Parke RD, Tomlinson-Keasey C, Widaman K, eds. *Studying Lives Through Time: Personality and Development.* Washington, DC: American Psychological Association; 1993:9-41.
15. Kagan J. *Galen's Prophecy.* New York, NY: Basic Books Inc Publishers; 1994.
16. Thomas A, Chess S, Birch HG. The origins of personality. *Sci Am.* 1970;223:102-109.
17. Bates JE, Wachs TD, Emde RN. Toward practical uses for biological concepts of temperament. In: Bates JE, Wachs TD, eds. *Temperament: Individual Differences at the Interface of Biology and Behavior.* Washington, DC: American Psychological Association; 1994:275-306.
18. Weinberger DA, Bartholomew K. Social-emotional adjustment and patterns of alcohol use among young adults. *J Pers.* 1996;64:495-527.
19. Cloninger CR. Neurogenetic adaptive mechanisms in alcoholism. *Science.* 1987; 36:410-416.
20. Zucker RA, Fitzgerald HE, Moses HD. Emergence of alcohol problems and the several alcoholisms. In: Cicchetti D, Cohen DJ, eds. *Developmental Psychopathology.* New York, NY: John Wiley & Sons Inc; 1995:677-711.
21. Andrews JA, Lewinsohn PM. Suicidal attempts among older adolescents: prevalence and co-occurrence with psychiatric disorders. *J Am Acad Child Adolesc Psychiatry.* 1992;31:655-662.
22. Virkkunen M, De Jong J, Bartko J, Linnoila M. Psychobiological concomitants of history of suicide attempts among violent offenders and impulsive fire setters. *Arch Gen Psychiatry.* 1989;46:604-606.
23. Cohen P, Cohen J. The clinician's illusion. *Arch Gen Psychiatry.* 1984;41:1178-1182.
24. McDevitt SC. Continuity and discontinuity of temperament in infancy and early childhood: a psychometric perspective. In: Plomin R, Dunn J, eds, *The Study of Temperament: Changes, Continuities, and Challenges.* Hillsdale, NJ: Lawrence Erlbaum Associates; 1986:27-39.
25. Bank L, Patterson GR. The use of structural equation modeling in data from different types of assessments. In: Rosen JC, McReynolds P. eds, *Advances in Psychological Assessment.* New York, NY: Plenum Press; 1992:41-74.
26. Silva PA. The Dunedin Multidisciplinary Health and Development study: a fifteen-year longitudinal study. *Pediatr Perit Epidemiol.* 1990;4:96-127.
27. Caspi A, Henry B, McGee R, Moffitt TE, Silva PA. Temperamental origins of child and adolescent behavior problems: from age three to age fifteen. *Child Dev.* 1990;66:55-68.
28. Robins LN, Regier DA. eds. *Psychiatric Disorders in America.* New York, NY: Free Press; 1991.
29. American Psychiatric Association. *Diagnostic and Statistical Manual of Mental Disorders, Third Edition, Revised.* Washington, DC: American Psychiatric Association; 1987.
30. Newman DL, Moffitt TE, Caspi A, Magdol L, Silva PA, Stanton W. Psychiatric disorder in a birth cohort of young adults: Prevalence, comorbidity, clinical significance, and new case incidence from age 11 to 21. *J Consult Clin Psychol.* 1996;105:299-312.
31. Elley WB, Irving, JB. The Elley-Irving Socio-Economic Index 1981 census revision. *N Z J Educ Stud.* 1985;20:115-128.
32. Kessler RC, McGonagle KA, Zhao S, Nelson CB, Hughes M, Eshleman S, Wittchen HU, Kendler KS. Lifetime and 12-month prevalence of *DSM-III-R* psychiatric disorders in the United States: results from the National Comborbidity Study. *Arch Gen Psychiatry.* 1994;51:8-19.
33. McGue M, Pickens RW, Svikis DS. Sex and age effects on the inheritance of alcohol problems: a twin study. *J Abnorm Psychol.* 1992;101:3-17.
34. Biederman J, Rosenbaum JF, Hirshfeld DR, Faraone SV, Bolduc EA, Gersten M, Meminger SR, Kagan J, Snidman N, Reznick S.. Psychiatric correlates of behavioral inhibition in young children of parents with and without psychiatric disorders. *Arch Gen Psychiatry.* 1990;47:21-26.
35. Hirshfeld DR, Rosenbaum JF, Biederman J, Bolduc EA, Faraone, SV, Snidman N, Reznick JS, Kagan J. Stable behavioral inhibition and its association with anxiety disorder. *J Am Acad Child Adolesc Psychiatry.* 1992;31:103-111.
36. Bernstein GA, Borchardt CM. Anxiety disorders of childhood and adolescence: a critical review. *J Am Acad Child Adolesc Psychiatry.* 1991;30:519-532.
37. Caspi A, Bem DJ. Personality continuity and change across the life course. In: Pervin L, ed. *Handbook of Personality: Theory and Research.* New York, NY: Guilford Press; 1990:549-575.

Comorbidity Between Depressive Disorders and Nicotine Dependence in a Cohort of 16-Year-Olds

David M. Fergusson, PhD; Michael T. Lynskey, MSc; L. John Horwood, MSc

Background: There has been growing interest in the associations between cigarette smoking and symptoms of depression. This study documents the comorbidity between depression and nicotine dependence in a birth cohort of 16-year-olds and examines the extent to which comorbidity between depression and nicotine dependence could be explained by risk factors associated with both outcomes.

Methods: Data were gathered during the course of a 16-year longitudinal study of a birth cohort of 947 New Zealand children for (1) depressive disorders and nicotine dependence at age 16 years; and (2) prospectively measured risk factors including family social position, family history of criminality, parental smoking, life events, parental attachment, conduct problems, self-esteem, and affiliations with delinquent peers.

Results: There was evidence of moderate to strong comorbidity between depression and nicotine dependence at age 16 years; teenagers with a depressive disorder had odds of nicotine dependence that were 4.6 times those of teenagers without depressive disorder. Analyses using logistic regression and log-linear modeling methods revealed that a substantial component of the comorbidity between depression and nicotine dependence was explained by common or correlated risk factors associated with both outcomes. After adjustment for common or correlated risk factors, the adjusted odds ratio between depression and nicotine dependence was 2.3.

Conclusions: Comorbidities between depression and nicotine dependence seem to be well established by the age of 16 years. Much of this comorbidity can be explained by common or correlated risk factors associated with depression or nicotine dependence.

Arch Gen Psychiatry. 1996;53:1043-1047

THERE HAS been growing interest in the associations between cigarette smoking and symptoms of depression. Studies[1-5] have shown that rates of depressive symptoms or depressive disorders are higher among smokers or those with nicotine dependence. For example, Breslau et al[2] reported odds ratios between depression and mild and moderate criteria of nicotine dependence that ranged from 2.1 to 5.7 in a sample of 1007 young adults in the United States. Romans et al[5] reported that for a sample of 272 New Zealand women 20 years or older, 63.2% of those who showed psychiatric morbidity were smokers compared with only 22.7% of those who did not show psychiatric morbidity. In general, 2 explanations have been offered for the comorbidity between depressive disorders and nicotine dependence.

First, the comorbidity between these disorders may arise from the influence of a range of social, familial, and individual risk factors that predispose the individual to depression and nicotine dependence. Some evidence supports this proposition to the extent that there have been many factors, including measurements of social background, family substance use practices, and early behavioral tendencies that have been shown to be associated with increased risks of depressive disorders[6-8] and nicotine dependence.[9-11]

This conclusion is supported, to some extent, by the findings of Kendler et al[4] who examined the comorbidity of depression and cigarette smoking in a sample of 1566 female twins. Their findings suggested that the comorbidity between cigarette smoking and depression arose from common familial factors that were associated with increased risks of both outcomes. They concluded that "the association between smoking and

From the Department of Psychological Medicine, Christchurch School of Medicine, Christchurch, New Zealand.

See Subjects and Methods on next page

SUBJECTS AND METHODS

DATA COLLECTION

Data were collected during the course of the Christchurch Child Development Study.[16] The Christchurch Health and Development Study is a longitudinal study of a birth cohort of 1265 children born in the Christchurch, New Zealand, urban region during mid-1977. These children have been studied at birth, 4 months, 1 year, and annual intervals to the age of 16 years. The data analyzed in this study were measured in the following ways.

Depressive Disorders (15-16 Years)

When the subjects were aged 16 years, they and their parents were questioned about symptoms of depression (MD or dysthymia) in the subject during the last year. These symptoms were measured by self-report using an abbreviated version of the Diagnostic Interview Schedule for Children[17] and additional items designed to meet *DSM-III-R*[18] criteria that were not covered in the original version of this instrument. Parental reports were obtained using measurements derived from the parent version of the Diagnostic Interview Schedule for Children supplemented by items from the Diagnostic Interview Schedule.[19] Subjects were classified as experiencing a depressive disorder if they met *DSM-III-R* criteria for major depression or dysthymia on the basis of either parental or self-report.

Nicotine Dependence

At age 16 years, subjects were questioned about their frequency of cigarette smoking. Teenagers who reported smoking were then asked a series of questions about nicotine dependence. These questions concerned failure to quit or reduce smoking, irritability when cigarettes were unavailable, difficulties in going a day without a cigarette, morning cough, needing a cigarette first thing in the morning, continued smoking despite medical advice, and stealing money or using savings to obtain cigarettes. On the basis of self-report, the subject was classified as meeting *DSM-III-R* criteria if he or she (1) smoked at least 5 cigarettes per day and (2) reported 2 or more additional symptoms of nicotine dependence. These criteria broadly correspond to the criterion of mild nicotine dependence used by Breslau et al.[2]

Common Social and Contextual Factors

There have been many factors including social, familial, individual, and peer risk factors that have been identified in the literature as being associated with increased risks of depressive disorders and nicotine dependence.[6-10] To adjust the associations between depressive disorders and nicotine dependence for the effects of common risk factors, a range of prospectively measured social, familial, individual, and peer factors were included in the analyses.

Family Social Position

This was a composite measure of the family's social background based on information about parental education, family occupational status, maternal age, parental ethnicity, and family type (1-parent or 2-parent family). The index ranks the sample from children with a highly advantaged profile to those with a highly disadvantaged profile and has been shown to be predictive of a wide range of health, social, and behavioral outcomes in this cohort.[20]

Family Criminality

At age 15 years, the subject's parents were asked if they or the subject's siblings had a record of criminal offending. This measure was based on parental self-definition of criminal behavior.

Parental Smoking

When the subjects were 11 years old, their parents were asked a series of questions concerning the extent to which they smoked cigarettes.

Family Life Events

Each year from 11 to 14 years, parents were questioned about life events occurring in the previous year using a 49-item life event inventory, based on the inventory developed by Henderson et al.[21] To produce a global measurement of the extent of family exposure to adverse life events, reports of life events during the 4-year period were summed to produce an overall measurement of exposure to life events.

Parental Attachment

Parental attachment was assessed at age 15 years using the parental attachment scale developed by Armsden and Greenberg.[22] The full parental attachment scale was used in this analysis, and this scale was found to have good reliability (α=.87).

major depression (MD) arises largely from familial factors, which are probably genetic, that predispose to both smoking and MD."[4(p36)]

A second explanation derives from the self-medication theory of substance use.[12-15] It could be proposed that rates of smoking are higher among those with depressive disorders because smoking may be one means of alleviating depression and associated stresses.

An important issue in understanding this association concerns the age at which comorbidities between depression and nicotine dependence develop. Most studies[1-5] examining this issue have been based on adult populations with respondents being 20 years or older. These studies do not make it possible to determine the age at which clear comorbidity between depression and nicotine dependence is established. However, it seems possible that this comorbidity may be established during adolescence because it has been well documented that rates of depressive disorders[6-8] and cigarette smoking [9,10] increase rapidly from 14 to 18 years of age.

Conduct Problems (12 Years)

Problems with conduct were assessed using parent and teacher reports of disordered conduct or oppositional behaviors based on items derived from the Rutter[23] and Conners[24,25] parent and teacher questionnaires. These measurements were combined to produce an overall measurement of the extent to which the subject was reported to show disordered conduct or oppositional behaviors.[26] The reliability of this scale was $\alpha=.93$.

Self-esteem

Self-esteem was assessed at age 15 years using the Coopersmith Self-Esteem Inventory.[27] The full-scale score was used in this analysis and was found to have good reliability ($\alpha=.86$).

Affiliations With Delinquent Peers (15 Years)

To measure the extent to which the subject affiliated with delinquent or substance using peers at age 15 years, a general index of peer affiliations was constructed. This index was based on self-reports of the extent to which the subject's best friend and other friends used tobacco, alcohol, and cannabis; truanted; or broke the law. These items were summed to produce a scale measurement of the extent to which the subject reported affiliations with delinquent or substance using peers.[28] The resulting scale was of moderate internal consistency ($\alpha=.78$).

A series of additional measurements of social, familial, and individual characteristics was also considered for inclusion in the analyses. These measurements included measurements of family and childhood adversity, neuroticism, early smoking experimentation, and parental substance use behaviors. In these preliminary analyses, a series of logistic regression equations was fitted that included the aforementioned factors. In all cases, the additional predictors above made nonsignificant net contributions to either depression or nicotine dependence when allowance was made for the factors described earlier.

SAMPLE SIZE

The analyses reported herein were based on a sample of 947 respondents for whom there were complete data for depressive disorders and nicotine dependence at age 16 years. This sample represented 74.9% of the initial cohort of children and 85.3% of the subjects who were alive and resided in New Zealand at the age of 16 years. To examine the effects of sample losses on the representativeness of the sample, comparisons were made of the sociodemographic characteristics of the 947 subjects included in the analysis with the remaining 318 subjects excluded from the analyses. This suggested that losses to follow-up during the course of the study were not associated with child ethnicity, sex, maternal age, or family size. There were, however, small but statistically detectable tendencies ($P<.01$) for the sample to underrepresent children from families in which mothers lacked formal educational qualifications, families of low-socioeconomic status, and single-parent families. However, previous analyses that have incorporated statistical corrections for nonrandom sample loss suggest that these losses have a negligible effect on study validity.[29,30]

STATISTICAL ANALYSIS: 3 STAGES

1. The comorbidities between nicotine dependence and depression were described by estimating the odds ratios and 95% confidence intervals between dichotomously scored measurements of nicotine dependence and depression, and testing these associations using the χ^2 test of independence (**Table 1**). Separate estimates were presented for male and female subjects. The homogeneity of associations between nicotine dependence and depression for male and female subjects was tested by log-linear modeling techniques.[31]

2. The similarity of the risk factors for depression and nicotine dependence was examined using logistic regression methods[31] to identify significant childhood and family predictors of the outcomes (**Table 2**). The extent of correlation between risk factors for nicotine dependence and risk factors for depression was assessed by using the logistic regression results to estimate composite risk factor scores representing the individuals' risks of nicotine dependence and risks of depression given childhood, family, and related factors and by estimating the correlation between these risk scores.

3. Finally, the joint relationships between (1) risk factors for nicotine dependence, (2) risk factors for depression, (3) nicotine dependence at age 16 years, and (4) depression at age 16 years were modeled using log-linear modeling[31] to estimate the linkages between these factors (**Figure**). Log-linear modeling methods were applied to a $4\times4\times2\times2$ table of risk factors for depression, risk factors for nicotine dependence, nicotine dependence, and depression at age 16 years. Model fitting employed forward and backward selection procedures to identify the best-fitting and most parsimonious model. From the fitted log-linear model parameters, an estimate of the odds ratio between nicotine dependence and depression adjusted for common/correlated risk factors was obtained.[31]

All statistical tests are 2 tailed and based on $\alpha=.05$.

This article reports on the results of a study of the comorbidity between depressive disorders and nicotine dependence in a birth cohort of New Zealand children studied to the age of 16 years. The aims of this study are (1) to document the extent of comorbidity between depression and nicotine dependence at ages 15 to 16 years and (2) to determine the extent to which any comorbidity between depression and nicotine dependence could be explained by a series of risk factors assessed by the age of 15 years.

RESULTS

THE ASSOCIATION BETWEEN NICOTINE DEPENDENCE AND DEPRESSION AT AGE 16 YEARS

Table 1 shows the relationship between depression and nicotine dependence for male and female subjects. Significant associations between nicotine dependence and

Table 1. Rate of Nicotine Dependence Among Sample Members Meeting Criteria for a Depressive Disorder and Remaining Sample Members

Variable	Depressive Disorder	No Depressive Disorder	Odds Ratio (95% CI)*
Total sample, No. (%)			
Nicotine dependent	90 (20.0)	857 (5.1)	4.6 (2.5-8.4)
Male subjects, No. (%)			
Nicotine dependent	26 (23.1)	447 (5.2)	5.5 (2.0-15.1)
Female subjects, No. (%)			
Nicotine dependent	64 (18.9)	410 (5.1)	4.3 (2.0-9.2)

*CI indicates confidence interval; N, sample size.

Table 2. Logistic Regressions of Odds of Depressive Disorder and Nicotine Dependence at Age 16 Years on (Prospectively Measured) Risk Factors

	Depressive Disorder			Nicotine Dependence		
Risk Factor	β	SE	P	β	SE	P
Family social position	.23	0.11	<.05	−.03	0.14	>.80
Family history of criminality	.86	0.33	<.05	.33	0.46	>.40
Parental smoking	.54	0.31	<.10	.15	0.36	>.60
Life events (11-14 y)	.04	0.02	<.05	−.01	0.02	>.50
Parental attachment (15 y)	−.03	0.02	<.05	.00	0.01	>.90
Conduct problems (12 y)	.00	0.01	>.70	.04	0.01	<.005
Self-esteem (15 y)	−.08	0.02	<.005	−.06	0.03	<.05
Affiliations with delinquent peers	.13	0.06	<.05	.48	0.07	<.001
Sex	.75	0.32	<.05	.31	0.39	>.40

affective disorder were present for both. Tests of the equality of odds ratios for male and female subjects based on log-linear modeling methods showed that the association between nicotine dependence and depression did not vary significantly with sex.

Risk Factors for Nicotine Dependence and Depression

To examine the similarity of risk factors for nicotine dependence and depression, logistic regression models were fitted to the data. The results of this analysis are summarized in Table 2 that shows estimates of the logistic regression coefficients and SE for each outcome. Table 2 suggests relatively little overlap between the risk factors for each outcome. However, risk factors that were common to both outcomes were affiliation with delinquent peers and lower self-esteem. Subsequent analysis suggested the presence of a substantial correlation between the risk factors for the 2 conditions. To assess this correlation, risk factor scores for each outcome were estimated by solving the logistic regression model for each subject using the regression coefficients for risk factors that were significantly related to each outcome. These risk factor scores gave estimates of the individual's risks for depression and nicotine dependence conditional on the risk factors given in Table 2. The resulting risk factor scores were highly correlated (r=0.64).

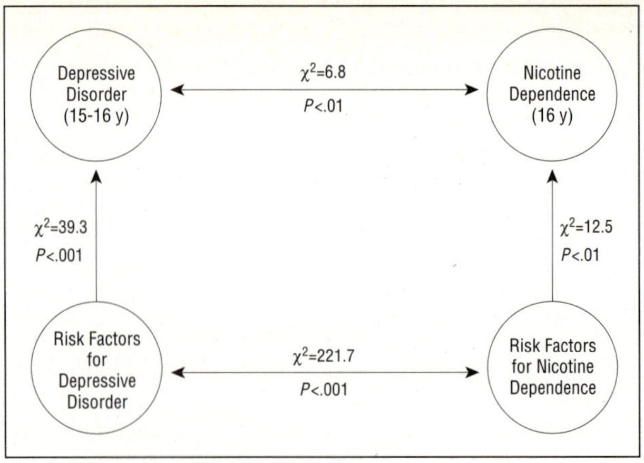

Fitted log-linear model of risk factors for depressive disorder, risk factors for nicotine dependence, depressive disorder (15-16 years), and nicotine dependence (16 years). Logistic regressions χ^2 goodness-of-fit of model=14.5, df=39, $P>.90$.

Modeling the Relationship Among Nicotine Dependence, Depression, and Risk Factors

To describe the relationships among the risk factors in Table 2, nicotine dependence, and major depression at age 16 years, methods of log-linear modeling were used. In this analysis, the individual's risk of nicotine dependence or depression, conditional on childhood factors was represented by the risk factor scores described earlier. A 4×4×2×2 contingency table was formed using the 2 risk factor scores classified into quartiles and the dichotomous measurements of nicotine dependence and depression. This table was then analyzed using log-linear modeling methods to find the best-fitting and most parsimonious model to describe the data. The final fitted model is shown in the Figure. The Figure also shows the statistically significant linkages between the 4 measurements (risk factors for nicotine dependence, risk factors for depression, depressive disorder, and nicotine dependence at age 16 years) using the log-likelihood ratio χ^2 estimate. The Figure shows (1) risk factors for depression and risk factors of nicotine dependence were strongly associated with each other; (2) each risk factor set was predictive of its respective outcome; and (3) when the common influences of the correlated risk factors were taken into account, a small but significant association was noted (logistic regressions χ^2=6.8, P<.01) between nicotine dependence and depression.

From the log-linear model, it was possible to estimate the extent to which the common and correlated effects of risk factors explained the comorbidity between nicotine dependence and depression. This analysis showed that after adjustment for common or correlated risk factors, the odds ratio between nicotine dependence and depression was reduced from 4.6 (95% confidence interval [CI]=2.5-8.4) to 2.3 (95% CI=1.2-4.4).

SUPPLEMENTARY ANALYSES

Analyses were conducted to determine whether these conclusions differed (1) when the sample was stratified by sex; (2) when depressive disorders were defined on the basis of self-report only; and (3) when the data were analyzed using continuous measures of outcomes and methods of structural equation modeling. These analyses showed that (1) the aforementioned conclusions held for male and female subjects; (2) the same conclusions were reached when depression was defined on the basis of self-reported data only; and (3) the analysis of continuous measures of tobacco use and symptoms of depression using methods of structural equation modeling produced the same general conclusions.

COMMENT

There was evidence of clear comorbidity between depressive disorders and nicotine dependence in this cohort of 16-year-olds; subjects with depression had odds of nicotine dependence that were more than 4.5 times the odds for those without depression. This relationship was similar for male and female subjects. These results suggest that comorbidities between nicotine dependence and depression are well established by the age of 16 years.

Examination of the risk factors associated with vulnerability to depressive disorders by age 16 years and the risk factors associated with nicotine dependence at this age suggested the presence of some overlap and considerable correlation between the risk factors for depression and the risk factors for nicotine dependence. When the effects of common or correlated risk factors were considered using methods of log-linear modeling, the extent of comorbidity between depressive disorders and nicotine dependence was reduced substantially. However, even after this adjustment there was a small to moderate (odds ratio=2.3) association between depressive disorders and nicotine dependence.

These findings are generally consistent with the conclusions drawn by Kendler et al[4] that the association between nicotine dependence and depression is largely or wholly noncausal and likely to reflect antecedent factors that are associated with both conditions. However, Kendler et al[4] concluded that the factors leading to this comorbidity were likely to be genetic, whereas the present analysis suggests that a substantial component of the association is explained by common or correlated social and childhood factors. It is difficult to reconcile these findings in the absence of a more general model that shows the linkages between genetic factors, life-course factors, and the onset of nicotine dependence and depression. One explanation that reconciles these conclusions is the suggestion that the risk factors identified in this analysis may describe some of the common pathways by which genetic predispositions to nicotine dependence and depression are expressed. Irrespective of the extent to which the comorbidity between nicotine dependence and depression arises because of the effects of common genetic or common environmental factors, both studies make it clear that a substantial amount of this comorbidity is likely to arise from familial, social, and other processes that are antecedent to the onset of nicotine dependence or depression. The results of this study show that these processes operate in such a way that the comorbidity between nicotine dependence and depression is well established by midadolescence.

Accepted for publication March 26, 1996.

This research was funded by grants from the Health Research Council of New Zealand, Auckland, The National Child Health Research Foundation, Wellington, and the Canterbury Medical Research Foundation, Christchurch, New Zealand.

Corresponding author: David M. Fergusson, PhD, Christchurch Health and Development Study, Christchurch School of Medicine, PO Box 4345, Christchurch, New Zealand.

REFERENCES

1. Anda RF, Williamson DF, Escobedo LG, Mast EE, Giovino GA, Remington PL. Depression and the dynamics of smoking. *JAMA.* 1990;264:1541-1545.
2. Breslau N, Kilbey MM, Andreski P. Nicotine dependence, major depression, and anxiety in young adults. *Arch Gen Psychiatry.* 1991;48:1069-1074.
3. Glassman AH, Helzer JE, Covey LS, Cottler LB, Stetner F, Tipp JE, Johnson J. Smoking, smoking cessation, and major depression. *JAMA.* 1990;264:1546-1549.
4. Kendler KS, Neale MC, MacLean CJ, Heath AC, Eaves LJ, Kessler RC. Smoking and major depression: a causal analysis. *Arch Gen Psychiatry.* 1993;50:36-43.
5. Romans SE, McNoe BM, Herbison GP, Walton VA, Mullen PE. Cigarette smoking and psychiatric morbidity in women. *Aust N Z J Psychiatry.* 1993;27:399-404.
6. Angold A. Childhood and adolescent depression, I: epidemiological and aetiological aspects. *Br J Psychiatry.* 1988;152:601-617.
7. Fleming JE, Offord DR. Epidemiology of childhood depressive disorders: a critical review. *J Am Acad Child Adolesc Psychiatry.* 1990;29:571-580.
8. Rutter M, Izard CE, Read PB. *Depression in Young People: Developmental and Clinical Perspectives.* New York, NY: Guilford Press; 1986.
9. Conrad KM, Flay BR, Hill D. Why children start smoking cigarettes: predictors of onset. *Br J Addict.* 1992;87:1711-1724.
10. Miller SK, Slap G. Adolescent smoking: a review of prevalence and prevention. *J Adolesc Health Care.* 1989;10:129-135.
11. Breslau N, Kilbey M, Andreski P. Nicotine dependence and major depression: new evidence from a prospective investigation. *Arch Gen Psychiatry.* 1993;50:31-35.
12. Glass RM. Blue mood, blackened lungs. *JAMA.* 1990;264:1583-1584.
13. Khantzian EJ. The self-medication hypothesis of addictive disorders: focus on heroin and cocaine dependence. *Am J Psychiatry.* 1985;142:1259-1264.
14. Neighbors B, Kempton T, Forehand R. Co-occurrence of substance abuse with conduct, anxiety, and depression disorders in juvenile delinquents. *Addict Behav.* 1992;17:379-386.
15. Covey LS, Tam D. Depressive mood, the single-parent home and adolescent cigarette smoking. *Am J Public Health.* 1990;80:1330-1333.
16. Fergusson DM, Horwood LJ, Shannon FT, Lawton JM. The Christchurch Child Development Study: a review of epidemiological findings. *Paediatr Perinat Epidemiol.* 1989;3:302-325.
17. Costello A, Edelbrock C, Kalas R, Kessler M, Klaric SA. *Diagnostic Interview Schedule for Children (DISC).* Bethesda, Md: National Institute of Mental Health; 1982.
18. American Psychiatric Association. *Diagnostic and Statistical Manual of Mental Disorders, Third Edition, Revised.* Washington, DC: American Psychiatric Association; 1987.
19. Robins L, Helzer JE, Croughan J, Ratcliff KS. National Institute of Mental Health Diagnostic Interview Schedule: its history, characteristics, and validity. *Arch Gen Psychiatry.* 1981;38:381-389.
20. Fergusson DM, Horwood LJ, Lawton JM. Vulnerability to childhood problems and family social background. *J Child Psychol Psychiatry.* 1990;31:1145-1160.
21. Henderson A, Byrne D, Duncan-Jones P. *Neurosis and the Social Environment.* Sydney, Australia: Academic Press; 1981.
22. Armsden GC, Greenberg MT. The inventory of parent and peer attachment: individual differences and their relationship to psychological well-being in adolescence. *J Youth Adolesc.* 1987;16:427-454.
23. Rutter M, Tizard J, Whitmore K. *Education, Health and Behaviour.* London, England: Longman Publishing; 1970.
24. Conners CK. A teacher rating scale for use in drug studies with children. *Am J Psychiatry.* 1969;126:884-888.
25. Conners CK. Symptom patterns in hyperkinetic, neurotic and normal children. *Child Dev.* 1970;41:667-682.
26. Fergusson DM, Horwood LJ, Lloyd M. Confirmatory factor models of attention deficit and conduct disorder. *J Child Psychol Psychiatry.* 1991;32:257-274.
27. Coopersmith S. *SEI–Self-Esteem Inventories.* Palo Alto, Calif: Consulting Psychologists Press; 1981.
28. Fergusson DM, Horwood LJ. The role of adolescent peer affiliations in the continuity between childhood behavioral adjustment and juvenile offending. *J Abnorm Child Psychol.* 1996;24:205-221.
29. Fergusson DM, Lynskey MT, Horwood LJ. The role of peer affiliations, family and individual factors in continuities in cigarette smoking between childhood and adolescence. *Addiction.* 1995;90:647-660.
30. Fergusson DM, Horwood LJ, Lynskey MT. Maternal depressive symptoms and depressive symptoms in adolescence. *J Child Psychol Psychiatry.* 1995;36:1161-1178.
31. Agresti A. *Categorical Data Analysis.* New York, NY: John Wiley & Sons Inc; 1990.

ORIGINAL ARTICLE

Cognitive Correlates of Long-term Cannabis Use in Costa Rican Men

Jack M. Fletcher, PhD; J. Bryan Page, PhD; David J. Francis, PhD; Kimberly Copeland, MA; Mary J. Naus, PhD; Chester M. Davis, PhD; Robin Morris, PhD; Dina Krauskopf, MA; Paul Satz, PhD

Background: Cognitive correlates of long-term cannabis use have been elusive. We tested the hypothesis that long-term cannabis use is associated with deficits in short-term memory, working memory, and attention in a literate, westernized culture (Costa Rica) in which the effects of cannabis use can be isolated.

Methods: Two cohorts of long-term cannabis users and nonusers were studied. Within each cohort, users and nonusers were comparable in age and socioeconomic status. Polydrug users and users who tested positive for the use of cannabis at the time of cognitive assessment after a 72-hour abstention period were excluded. The older cohort (whose age was ~45 years) had consumed cannabis for an average of 34 years, and comprised 17 users and 30 nonusers, who had been recruited in San José, Costa Rica, and had been observed since 1973. The younger cohort (whose age was ~28 years) had consumed cannabis for an average of 8 years, and comprised 37 users and 49 nonusers. Short-term memory, working memory, and attentional skills were measured in each subject.

Results: Older long-term users performed worse than older nonusers on 2 short-term memory tests involving learning lists of words. In addition, older long-term users performed worse than older nonusers on selective and divided attention tasks associated with working memory. No notable differences were apparent between younger users and nonusers.

Conclusion: Long-term cannabis use was associated with disruption of short-term memory, working memory, and attentional skills in older long-term cannabis users.

Arch Gen Psychiatry. 1996;53:1051-1057

From the Departments of Pediatrics (Dr Fletcher) and Psychiatry and Behavioral Sciences (Drs Fletcher and Davis), University of Texas–Houston Medical School; Department of Psychiatry, University of Miami (Fla) School of Medicine (Dr Page); Department of Psychology, University of Houston (Drs Francis and Naus and Ms Copeland); Department of Psychology, Georgia State University, Atlanta (Dr Morris); Department of Psychology, University of Costa Rica, San José (Dr Krauskopf); and the Neuropsychiatric Institute, University of California, Los Angeles (Dr Satz).

WITH THE exception of anecdotal reports and clinical observations,[1,2] the adverse effects of long-term cannabis use on cognitive skills have not been clearly demonstrated. Most studies of nonintoxicated North American users have found polydrug use and low levels of chronicity among these users.[3-6] These studies have generated null results, with the exception of 1 study that found deficiencies in memory retrieval processes.[7] The subjects in this study also used drugs other than cannabis and were not assayed for abstinence. Although cross-cultural studies of Egyptian[8] and Indian[9,10] cannabis users have been interpreted as showing adverse cognitive effects, sampling and other methodological problems limit these studies.[11,12] Cross-cultural studies that were designed better yielded mostly null results for cognitive correlates of long-term cannabis use.[13,14]

The most recent cross-cultural study was conducted in San José, Costa Rica, from 1985 to 1986.[15] Anthropological and neuropsychological studies of 27 long-term, frequent cannabis users and 30 nonusers were conducted; these studies were derived from a case-control study of 41 users and 41 nonusers, who were evaluated in San José from 1973 to 1975.[14] These subjects were originally matched for age, occupational status, education, marital status, and consumption of alcohol and tobacco. No consistent differences were found between users and nonusers on sociocultural variables other than those associated with a lifestyle involving cannabis use (eg, occasional imprisonment and solitary living arrangements). The biomedical and neuropsychological tests yielded uniformly null results. However,

See Subjects and Methods on next page

SUBJECTS AND METHODS

SUBJECTS

Data collection took place in San José during a 15-month period beginning in January 1990. The cohort originally studied in 1973 was the product of a street recruitment approach, where field-workers observed potential subjects in the everyday context of their lives in the neighborhoods of San José. Observing and informally interviewing people in their natural habitats led to the identification of networks of social relations among people in the neighborhoods. This allowed identification of cannabis users through other users of cannabis and identification of nonusers from the same neighborhoods.[14]

A sample of younger, shorter-term users and comparable nonusers was recruited in 1990. To remain consistent with the accrual of the older cohort, no new subjects with a history or evidence of psychiatric or neurological disorders or a history of habitual use of drugs other than cannabis and alcohol were recruited. Specifically, no subjects who had ever abused inhalants or who reported use of cocaine or other drugs (eg, lysergic acid diethylamide, heroin, and other opiates) more than twice in their lives were included. Any subject with a history of treatment for alcohol abuse, evidence of alcoholic dementia, or a history of delirium tremens was eliminated.

The study was approved by the University of Texas–Houston Health Science Center Committee for the Protection of Human Subjects and by the Costa Rican government. Separate consents were obtained for the cognitive tests, the drug assays, and the interviews. Subjects were informed that their self-reports would be discussed with family members and friends.

Older Cohort

The 41 users and 41 nonusers in the 1973 cohort were selected from a base sample of 84 long-term users and 156 nonusers. Long-term use was originally defined as the use of cannabis 3 times weekly for at least 10 years. The user and nonuser groups were matched in 1973 for age, sex (all men), occupation, education, marital status, and consumption of alcohol and tobacco.[14] In 1973, the user group had consumed a daily average of 9.6 cannabis cigarettes (the fundamental unit of consumption and sale) for an average of 16.9 years, representing an average exposure to approximately 80 mg of Δ^9-tetrahydrocannabinol daily.[14] For this follow-up, we were able to identify 69 of these subjects, 56 of whom were tested for the study. Thirteen of the original 82 subjects were unavailable for follow-up since 1985.[15] Sixty of the 69 remaining potential subjects were available. Of the 56 subjects who gave consent, 6 users did not abstain for the required 72 hours and 3 users tested positive for cocaine use, leaving 30 nonusers and 17 abstaining users. None of these subjects reported even experimental use of other drugs, which was verified through the social networks. To evaluate possible selective attrition from the original sample in 1973, participants and nonparticipants were compared; they did not differ significantly ($P>.10$) in medical status, consumption of alcohol and tobacco, chronicity of cannabis use, and sociocultural variables.[15]

At this follow-up, the user group had been consuming cannabis for an average of 34 years (a median of 5.2 marijuana cigarettes per day, 2-7 times weekly). Use had decreased from the levels in the 1973 and 1985 studies because of the greater potency and the increased cost of cannabis. Two users had ceased consumption for more than 8 years prior to this study. To avoid biasing the comparisons in favor of rejecting the null hypothesis, these 2 subjects were included in the user group for the cognitive studies but were excluded from the computations of use. For this follow-up, the subjects remained healthy; we observed no evidence of interim major medical problems (eg, head injuries) that might influence the results. The comparability of alcohol abuse was of particular importance. Alcohol abuse was defined by subject acknowledgement of any 1 of the following 3 conditions: (1) drinking 4 to 5 drinks daily, (2) experiencing "blackouts," or (3) drinking in the morning. Approximately two thirds of the older cohort abused alcohol according to these criteria, but the percentages were comparable between groups (**Table**). None of the subjects identified themselves as alcohol abusers nor did any subject or informant report treatment for alcohol abuse.

Younger Cohort

The younger cohort (n=123) was identified and screened by the same methods used to identify the older cohort for this study. To be identified as a user, the subject had to consume cannabis at least twice weekly for 5 years but for no longer than 12 years. Of the 123 cases, a final sample of 49 nonusers and 37 abstaining users was established. Twenty-five users tested positive for use of cannabis at the time of testing, and 12 subjects tested positive for cocaine use; all of these subjects were excluded from the study. The remaining 37 abstaining users had consumed marijuana for an average of approximately 8 years (a median of 3.8 cigarettes per day, 2-7 times weekly).

As the data in the Table indicate, users and nonusers in both cohorts were comparable for age and intellectual level[17] ($P>.10$), but younger users smoked more tobacco ($F[1,183]=15.86$, $P<.001$), were more likely to abuse alcohol ($\chi^2[1,N=85]=17.80$, $P<.001$), and had lower levels of education ($\chi^2[2,N=85]=7.44$, $P<.03$) vs younger nonusers. No comparisons involving the older cohort achieved statistical significance ($P>.10$).

The frequency of polydrug use in the younger cohort, as noted by the number of subjects who tested positive for cocaine use, reflects clear differences between the younger and older cohorts. Initiation to cannabis generally occurred during adolescence for both cohorts but tended to be earlier for the older users (≈15 years) than for the younger users (≈16.5 years). Drug use has greater social consequences (eg, harsher legal penalties and peer rejection) in current Costa Rican society vs the society of 1973, which is reflected by these cohort differences. The lack of comparability between the younger groups leads to the expectation that the younger users will perform worse than the younger nonusers on the cognitive tasks but for reasons other than the use of cannabis. This difference would tend to mitigate against the hypothesized pattern of results, in which differences were predicted only between the older groups.

DRUG ASSAYS

Each subject provided a urine sample to be assayed for use of cannabis and other drugs 72 hours prior to and at the time of the cognitive assessment. Subjects were instructed to abstain from the use of cannabis and other drugs for the interval between the 2 samples. Subjects were informed that reimbursement for participation was contingent on no evidence of drug use on the second urine sample, which encouraged abstention.

The initial assay was a toxicological screen (EMIT system, Syva, San José, Calif); Δ^9-tetrahydrocannabinol and other drugs, including cocaine, opiates, amphetamine, and benzodiazepines, were identified by this screen. In addition, a semiquantitative immunoassay of Δ^9-tetrahydrocannabinol and its metabolites was performed based on the enzyme-multiplied immunoassay technique. Finally, Δ^9-tetrahydrocannabinol was measured by a high-performance thin-layer chromatographic procedure that included in situ densitometric scanning for detection. Urine was measured by comparison with a standard curve prepared by adding 50, 100, and 300 ng of Δ^9-tetrahydrocannabinol carbolic acid per milliliter to drug-free urine. Any subject who had a Δ^9-tetrahydrocannabinol concentration greater than 80 ng/mL on the chromatographic test was excluded. The high-performance thin-layer chromatographic assay is sensitive to 25 ng/mL.

As expected, Δ^9-tetrahydrocannabinol concentrations differed between the 2 assays. The average Δ^9-tetrahydrocannabinol concentrations 72 hours before testing were variable but quite high in the user groups (older cohort=238.5±476.3 ng/mL, younger cohort=129.1±272.5 ng/mL). The variability reflects the period and amount of cannabis consumed in the days prior to the test, for which the subjects received no warning. At the time of testing, the concentrations were well below the 50-ng/mL cutoff used to indicate positive results for cannabis use (older users=9.7±16.6 ng/mL, younger users=8.6±22.3 ng/mL).

PROCEDURES

The cognitive studies were conducted in the field office in San José. The evaluation required 4 to 5 hours, depending on whether the intelligence test was administered (only to the younger cohort). Two technicians, who were "blind" to the subjects' identities as users or nonusers, administered the tests in Spanish. Only the field-workers and an office manager knew the group identity of the subjects.

All subjects were systematically interviewed, and self-reports were verified by asking other members of the network about the respondent. The interviews included a sociocultural survey of life history and social, educational, and occupational functioning and questions about psychiatric and medical histories and drug-use patterns. The interviews were conducted in the neighborhoods in an open-ended fashion to encourage the respondent to talk freely and openly with the interviewer, who took notes and then completed a schedule outlining the variables coded for this study.

TASKS

In a series of experiments, separate components of memory and attention were evaluated. Four memory tests were selected, based on a modification of the 3-store model originally proposed by Atkinson and Shiffrin,[18] and used extensively in studies of acute and carryover effects of cannabis.[19,20] A 12-trial Spanish word version of the selective reminding task was used.[21] In addition, a free recall paradigm that instructed the subject to rehearse aloud between trials was employed.[22] Three 3-trial conditions of implicit organization (ie, unrelated/unblocked words, related/unblocked words, and related/blocked words) for 16 words were included in this task. A sorting task was used to evaluate free recall and control processes in short-term memory.[23] Finally, episodic memory was evaluated using a task in which stories were read to the subjects, who were asked to tell everything they could remember about the stories immediately after the reading and 90 minutes later. Probe questions were asked to separate memory for facts and inferences.[24]

The 8 attention tasks evaluated preparedness, selection, and allocation components of attention based on views of attention as a central, limited capacity that can be flexibly shifted or allocated.[25-27] Preparedness was measured with a computer-based, reaction-time procedure.[26] Selection was evaluated using measures of focused and sustained attention. The focused attention tasks included 4 cancellation tasks that required the subject to identify random and organized verbal and nonverbal stimuli under timed conditions[28] and a visual search task that required the subject to search 4 quadrants of 16 letters each for a target letter appearing in only 1 target.[26] For sustained attention, 2 "X-A" versions of the continuous performance test were used.[29] One version had a short interstimulus interval (1 millisecond), and the other version was a vigilance paradigm because of a longer interstimulus interval (1 minute).

To measure allocation, competition paradigms based on dual-task performance were employed.[30] For each task, the subject was asked to depress a manual finger tapper as fast as possible for 15 (task 1) or 60 (task 2) seconds with the right and then the left hand. The subject was then asked to name as many objects as possible in 15 seconds from a specific semantic category (task 1) or complete 1 trial of a free recall memory task not previously employed (task 2). Finally, the subject was asked to tap as fast as possible for the specified period while simultaneously performing the cognitive task. These divided attention tasks permit an evaluation of the allocation of attentional resources by measuring the reduction in performance using dual- vs single-task conditions.[26] The ability to flexibly shift and allocate attentional focus was measured with the Wisconsin Card Sorting Test.[27]

STATISTICAL ANALYSIS

The data were analyzed using a multivariate approach to repeated-measures analysis of variance with 2 between-subject factors, group (2 levels, user and nonuser) and cohort (2 levels, older and younger), and 1 or 2 within-subject factors, which represented subcomponents of a task, the presence of multiple trials, or both. We hypothesized that interactions of group by cohort would emerge, indicating poorer performance by older users vs older nonusers and no significant differences ($P<.05$) between the younger user groups. Significant group by cohort interactions ($P<.05$) were evaluated by testing for group differences within cohorts. To control the level of α, the follow-ups were adjusted using the Bonferroni inequality to control α at a family-wise level of $P=.05$. We considered each task to represent a separate experiment, so the focus was on maintaining Type I errors at $\alpha=.05$ for each task.

Sociodemographic and Drug-Use Variables by Group (Users and Nonusers) and Cohort (Older and Younger)

	Group			
	Older		Younger	
Variable	Users	Nonusers	Users	Nonusers
Age, y				
Mean	45.31	45.64	29.29	27.28
SD	1.53	1.15	1.04	0.90
Educational level, %*				
Primary or less	47	63	62	33
Secondary	47	33	32	52
High school or university	6	4	5	15
Alcohol abuse, %*				
No	25	33	22	67
Yes	75	67	78	33
Tobacco use (pack-years)*				
Mean	30.43	29.89	14.41	7.80
SD	7.80	1.59	1.38	1.21
Full scale intelligence quotient†				
Mean	110.33	115.50	113.78	115.33
SD	10.54	8.06	11.82	11.59

*$P<.05$ for comparison of younger users and nonusers.
†Spanish version of the Wechsler Adult Intelligence Scale.[17]

when restudied in 1985 and 1986, users performed worse than nonusers on cognitive measures of short-term memory and attention. The users also showed a decline in the level of mental effort at work, the quality of their occupational status, and a continued trend toward more solitary living arrangements.[15]

Problems interpreting these results remained. The cognitive measures that detected poorer performance by the users in the 1985 study were not part of the initial assessment, and comparisons between the studies begun in 1973 and 1985 yielded little evidence for deterioration of cognitive skills in the users during the intervening 12 years. The degree of chronicity required to establish adverse cognitive effects also remained unclear. Most notably, the absence of drug assays made it unclear whether the cognitive deficits observed in the 1985 study were attributable to the long-term use of cannabis, to subacute intoxication, or to carryover effects, which are observed from approximately 24 to 72 hours after consumption and which reflect the amount of time required for cannabis metabolites to fully metabolize out of the body.[16]

This investigation assessed the cognitive functioning of the long-term users and nonusers, who have been observed since 1973. In addition, a second cohort comprising younger, shorter-term users and comparable nonusers was evaluated to determine whether cognitive problems could be observed in these users. We hypothesized that only the older long-term users (vs comparable nonusers) would show poor performance on cognitive tasks related to memory and attention, which could not be attributed to acute or carryover effects of cannabis.

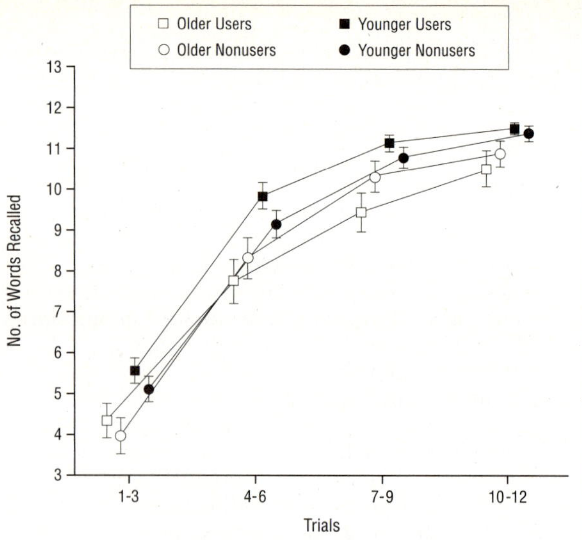

Figure 1. *Long-term storage scores on the verbal selective reminding test by group, cohort, and trials, indicating a poorer performance by the older user group. Bars indicate SE.*

RESULTS

MEMORY TASKS

The 2 more complex tasks involving the learning of a list of words (verbal selective reminding and free recall) yielded significant group by cohort interactions that showed poorer performance by the older user groups. These results differed from the story recall task, which, consistent with our previous studies,[12,14] did not differentiate users group in either the younger or older cohorts.

Analysis of the sorting task showed no group by cohort interaction, but the group by trials interaction was significant ($F[2,113]=4.17$, $P<.05$). Analysis of the group effect at each level of trials did not achieve the critical level of α ($P>.0167$).

For the verbal selective reminding test, **Figure 1** displays the significant group by cohort by trials interaction for the long-term storage variable ($F[3,127]=3.83$, $P<.01$). Follow-ups of the group by trials interaction within each cohort at the critical level of α ($P<.025$) were significant only for the older cohort ($F[3,43]=3.74$, $P<.018$). As Figure 1 shows, older users encoded words at a slower rate than older nonusers; no differences between groups were observed in the younger cohort. No significant differences ($P>.05$) were found between the older users and nonusers on consistent, long-term retrieval, although a trend of poorer performance by the older users was apparent.

The most difficult task, free recall, also showed a group by cohort by trials interaction ($F[2,124]=4.44$, $P<.01$) and a group by list interaction ($F[2,124]=3.63$). For the first interaction, analysis of the group by trials interaction within cohorts was performed at $P<.025$. This test was significant only for the older cohort ($F[2,40]=5.94$, $P<.006$). **Figure 2** shows that the older users recalled words at a slower rate than the older non-

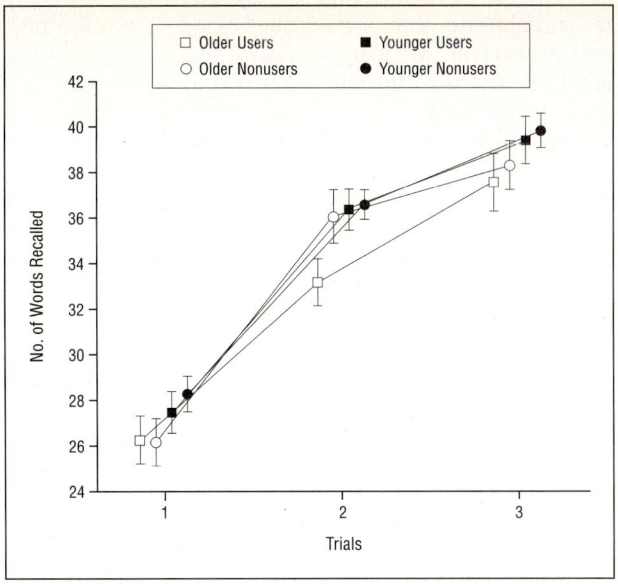

Figure 2. *Percentage of words recalled on the free recall task by group, cohort, and trials, indicating a poorer performance by the older user group. Bars indicate SE.*

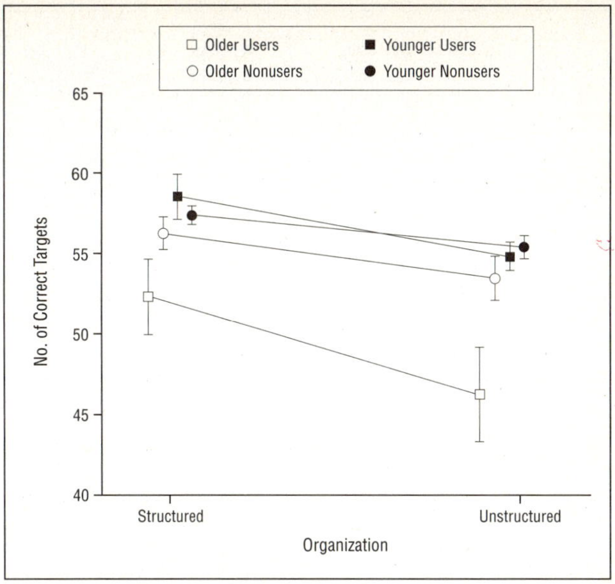

Figure 3. *Number of correctly identified targets on the cancellation tests by group, cohort, and organization, indicating a poorer performance by the older user group. The magnitude of the group difference is larger for unstructured material. Bars indicate SE.*

users, and no significant differences ($P>.05$) between the younger groups are shown. Follow-up of the group by list interaction (ie, no interaction with cohort) did not meet the critical level of α.

ATTENTION TASKS

Analysis of the attention tasks showed significant group by cohort interactions ($P<.05$) on measures of selective and divided attention; performance was always poorer in the older user group. No effects involving group were significant ($P>.05$) for the reaction time measure, visual search, continuous performance tests, or the Wisconsin Card Sorting Test. These results suggest that differences in the cognitive functioning of long-term cannabis users and nonusers are most apparent on more difficult attention tasks, which place time pressure on subjects to respond quickly. Hence, tasks that do not manipulate symbolic material (reaction time), that are self-paced (eg, continuous performance tests and the Wisconsin Card Sorting Test), or that proceed for longer durations of time (eg, the continuous performance test, the visual search, the vigilance test, and the finger tapping–free recall test) are not associated with cannabis use.

Group differences reflecting long-term cannabis use were most striking for the cancellation (selective attention) and competition (allocation) tasks. For correct responses on the cancellation tasks, the group by organization ($F[1,118]=8.08$, $P<.01$) and the cohort by organization ($F[1,118]=3.78$, $P<.05$) interactions were significant. The 3-way interaction of group, cohort, and organization was not significant ($F[1,118]=1.25$, $P<.27$). However, given the hypotheses and the significance of both 2-way interactions, the group by organization interaction within each cohort ($P<.025$) was examined in the follow-up. **Figure 3** shows that the older user group identified relatively fewer targets on the unstructured task ($F[1,35]=6.03$, $P<.023$) than the structured task ($F[1,35]<1$).

For the competition tasks, a significant 3-way interaction of group, cohort, and condition (**Figure 4**) was found ($F[1,129]=11.68$, $P<.01$). Analysis of the group by condition interaction within each cohort was significant only for the older cohort ($F[1,45]=12.21$, $P<.002$). The older users showed a greater decrement in finger tapping using the dual-task conditions vs the single-task condition. When subjects show a decrement in performance on 1 task, performance on the other task is maintained. We found this to be true in this study, as analysis of the verbal retrieval data showed no effects of group or cohort ($F<1$). The second competition task, which involved a longer period of finger tapping and a free recall task, did not yield effects involving group.

COMMENT

Costa Rica was originally selected as a setting for the evaluation of the effects of long-term cannabis use because long-term, frequent users who did not use drugs other than cannabis, alcohol, and tobacco could be identified. The setting also provided access to nonusers who were from similar sociodemographic backgrounds and who consumed alcohol and tobacco at levels comparable with the users. The older groups were originally matched on multiple sociodemographic and drug-use variables.[14] In this follow-up, the older users and nonusers did not engage in polydrug use and remained comparable in their consumption of alcohol and tobacco.

The results demonstrated that only the older long-term users of cannabis performed worse on measures of selective attention, divided attention, and short-term memory vs comparable nonusers. The most robust effects occurred on the cancellation and competition tasks. On the cancellation tasks, the older users consistently

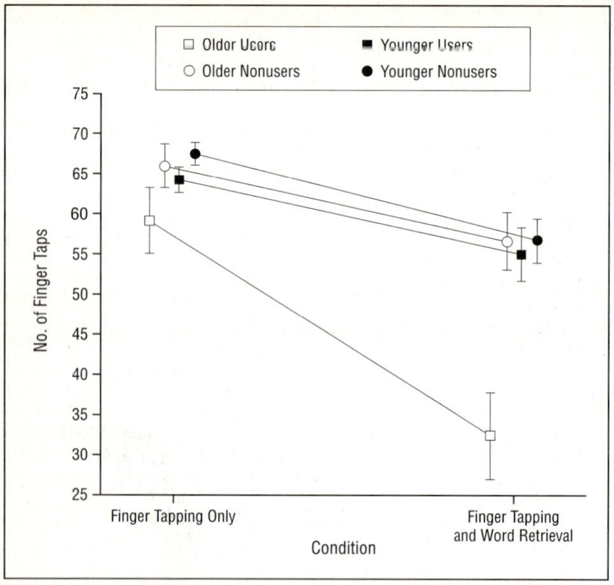

Figure 4. *Speed of finger tapping on the competition task using single- and dual-task conditions. The older user group had poorer performance and larger differences between the single- and dual-task conditions. Bars indicate SE.*

demonstrated an inability to rapidly select relevant information, particularly on the most complex tasks, which involved unstructured, nonverbal material. Poorer performance by long-term users on cancellation tasks was also reported in the studies conducted in Egypt[8] and India[9,10] and in our 1985 follow-up.[15] When divided attention was assessed with shorter trials of finger tapping and verbal retrieval, the ability of the older long-term user group to perform 2 tasks simultaneously was diminished vs the older nonuser group.

On the 2 more complex short-term memory tasks, the older user group showed more difficulty learning and retaining information across trials. These effects were not apparent for material that was contextually related (story recall) or on less complex serial recall tasks (sorting). The only North American study to use selective reminding procedures also found poorer performance in a sample of long-term users.[7]

The short-term memory deficiencies are consistent with studies that show disruption of learning and memory (ie, delayed-match-to-sample tasks) in rats due to acute administration of Δ^9-tetrahydrocannabinol.[31] These acute effects are similar to those observed in rats with damage to the hippocampus.[31,32] In humans, impairment on tasks such as the selective reminding tests has been observed in subjects who have undergone hippocampectomy for epilepsy.[32] In the rat, the hippocampus is rich in cannabinoid receptors.[33] Hence, the poorer performance of the older users may reflect impairment in brain systems associated with short-term memory.

The deficiencies on the selective and divided attention tasks may be related to deficiencies in the working memory, a component of the memory system providing a central source of control and allocation of memory and attentional resources.[34] Working memory is mediated by anterior regions of the brain, specifically, the prefrontal cortex.[35] The forebrain is also rich in cannabinoid receptors.[33] The divided attention task is a prototypic working memory task because of the requirement to allocate attentional resources. Although the cancellation tasks could be interpreted to represent the operation of an attention system in posterior brain regions,[27,28] the fact that decrements occurred only on unstructured material is commonly interpreted as an inability to allocate resources from the working memory system.[26,28] Although these parallels between animal and human studies are speculative, the results show impairments in 2 components of the memory system responsible for short-term memory that are consistent with animal studies of the brain metabolism of Δ^9-tetrahydrocannabinol.

This study also has several limitations. A field study of this sort cannot have a statistical design that permits causal inferences. The results are correlational and show an association between long-term cannabis use and performance. Despite the careful approach to sampling, it is always possible that unmeasured factors led to the differences between the older groups. Although no evidence of selective attrition was noted, it is possible that results would be different if all members of the original cohort could be studied. Until recently, North Americans typically did not use cannabis to the degree apparent in these cohorts of Costa Rican users, so the results may not generalize to other cultures. Nevertheless, the consumption patterns are surprisingly similar to those reported in the North American study by Block and Ghoneim.[7] The tasks that yielded group differences did not exist when the 1973 study was completed. This study would have been strengthened with prospective evaluation of these cognitive skills. It is also possible that the associations of cognitive performance and cannabis reflect the use of cannabis and alcohol, tobacco, or both; this pattern of joint use is invariably associated with cannabis use. Finally, the absence of differences between the younger groups may reflect a variety of factors, including higher educational levels, later average initial exposure to cannabis, and less chronicity.

It is also apparent that the deficiencies observed in this study and in the study by Block and Ghoneim[7] are subtle. The older long-term users are largely functional and employable, and they do not demonstrate the types of dementia and amnesic syndromes associated with alcohol use of comparable magnitude. The health of the subjects continues to be adequate over time,[15] and no evidence exists for the severity of health risks associated with use of other drugs, such as alcohol. Nevertheless, the risks of long-term use of even smaller amounts of cannabis are likely magnified in a more technological society, particularly given the possibility of carryover effects. Certain occupations may carry particular risk because of safety issues and effects on productivity and learning. The development of reliable methods for quick and efficient detection of cannabis use is needed. Furthermore, the findings suggest a need to focus efforts on the prevention of cannabis use through balanced educational programs for children and their parents. It is clear that the younger cohort and, to a lesser extent, the older cohort began to move toward polydrug use, a pattern consistent with studies of North American subjects.[36] This pattern underscores the need for preventive efforts to reduce the risk of consumption of drugs by young people.

Accepted for publication March 26, 1996.

This study was supported by grant 1 R01 DA06555 from the National Institute on Drug Abuse, Baltimore, Md.

We thank Pilar Zúniga Alfaro and Esmeralda Arce Arias for evaluating the subjects; Manuel Monestel Ramirez, Rigoberto Astorga Morales, and Silvia León Cubero for completing the fieldwork; and officials in the Ministry of Health of the Costa Rican government for their continued facilitation of this research.

Reprints: Jack M. Fletcher, PhD, Department of Pediatrics, University of Texas–Houston Medical School, MSB7.142, 6431 Fannin, Houston, TX 77030.

REFERENCES

1. Adamec C, Pihl RO, Leiter L. An analysis of the subjective marijuana experience. *Int J Addict.* 1976;11:295-307.
2. McGlothlin L, West LJ. The marijuana problem: an overview. *Am J Psychiatry.* 1968;125:126-134.
3. Hollister LE. Marijuana in man: three years later. *Science.* 1971;172:21-29.
4. Schaeffer J, Andrysiak T, Ungerleider JT. Cognition and long-term use of cannabis (ganga). *Science.* 1981;213:465-466.
5. Wert RC, Raulin ML. The chronic cerebral effects of cannabis use, II: psychological findings and conclusions. *Int J Addict.* 1985;605:629-642.
6. Grant I, Rochford J, Fleming T, Stunkard H. A neuropsychological assessment of the effects of moderate marijuana use. *J Nerv Ment Dis.* 1973;156:278-280.
7. Block RL, Ghoneim RL. Effects of chronic marijuana use of human cognition. *Psychopharmacology.* 1993;110:219-228.
8. Souief MI. Chronic cannabis users: further analysis of objective test results. *Bull Narc.* 1975;27:1-26.
9. Wig NN, Varma VK. Patterns of long-term heavy cannabis use in North India and its effects of cognitive functions: a preliminary report. *Drug Alcohol Depend.* 1977;2:211-219.
10. Varma UK, Malhotra AK, Dang R, Das K, Nehra R. Cannabis and cognitive functions: a prospective study. *Drug Alcohol Depend.* 1988;21:147-152.
11. Fletcher JM, Satz P. A methodological commentary on the Egyptian study of chronic hashish use. *Bull Narc.* 1977;29:29-34.
12. Peterson RC, ed. *Marijuana and Health.* Washington, DC: National Institute on Drug Abuse; 1977.
13. Fletcher JM, Satz P, Carter WE. Chronic cannabis use: recent cross-cultural evidence from Costa Rica and other cultures. *Contemp Drug Probl.* 1978;7:3-30.
14. Carter WE, Coggins W, Doughty P, eds. *Cannabis in Costa Rica.* Philadelphia, Pa: Institute for the Study of Human Issues; 1980.
15. Page JB, Fletcher JM, True WR. Psychosociocultural perspectives on chronic cannabis use: the Costa Rican follow-up. *J Psychoactive Drugs.* 1988;23:57-65.
16. Yesavage J, Leirer VU, Denari M, and Hollister LE. Carry-over effects of marihuana intoxication on aircraft pilot performance: a preliminary report. *Am J Psychiatry.* 1985;1423:1325-1329.
17. Wechsler D. *Escala Intelligencia de Wechsler Adultos.* New York, NY: Psychological Corp; 1967.
18. Atkinson RC, Shiffrin RM. Human memory: a proposed system and its control processes. In: Spence KW, Spence JT, eds. *The Psychology of Learning and Motivation.* New York, NY: Academic Press; 1968;2:89-195.
19. Miller L, Cornett T, McFarland D. Marijuana: an analysis of storage and retrieval deficits in memory with the technique of restricted reminding. *Pharmacol Biochem Behav.* 1977;8:327-332.
20. Tinklenberg JR, Darley C. A model of marijuana's cognitive effects. In: Braude MC, Szara S, eds. *The Pharmacology of Marijuana.* New York, NY: Raven Press; 1976:45-65.
21. Buschke H. Spontaneous remembering after recall failure. *Science.* 1974;184:579-581.
22. Best DL, Ornstein PA. Children's generation and communication of memoric organizatorial strategies. *Dev Psychol.* 1986;22:845-853.
23. Ornstein P, Naus MJ. Rehearsal processes in children's memory. In: Ornstein PA, ed. *Memory Development in Children.* Hillsdale, NJ: Lawrence Erlbaum Associates; 1978:69-99.
24. Paris SG, Lindauer BK. The role of inference in children's comprehension and memory for sentences. *Cogn Psychol.* 1976;8:217-227.
25. Posner M, Boies SJ. Components of attention. *Psychol Rev.* 1971;78:391-408.
26. Cooley EL, Morris RD. Attention in children: a neuropsychologically based model for assessment. *Dev Neuropsychol.* 1990;6:239-274.
27. Mirsky AF, Anthony BJ, Duncan CC, Ahearn MB, Kellam SG. Analysis of the elements of attention: a neuropsychological approach. *Neuropsychol Rev.* 1991;2:109-145.
28. Mesulam MM. Attention, confusional states, and neglect. In: Mesulam MM, ed. *Principles of Behavioral Neurology.* Philadelphia, Pa: FA Davis Co Publishers; 1985:1075-1168.
29. Rosvold HE, Mirsky AF, Sarason J, Bronsome ED, Beck LH. A continuous performance test of brain damage. *J Consult Psychol.* 1956;20:343-350.
30. Hiscock M. Verbal manual time sharing in children as a function of task priority. *Brain Cogn.* 1982;1:119-131.
31. Heyser CJ, Hampson RE, Deadwyler SA. Effects of delta-9-tetrahydrocannabinol on delayed match to sample performance in rats: alterations in short-term memory associated with changes in task specific timing of hippocampal cells. *J Pharmacol Exp Ther.* 1993;271:294-307.
32. Squire LR. *Memory and Brain.* New York, NY: Oxford University Press Inc; 1987:202-240.
33. Herkenham M, Lynn AB, Johnson MR, Melvin LS, de Costa BR, Rice KC. Characterization and localization of cannabinoid receptors in rat brain: a quantitative in vitro autoradiographic study. *J Neurosci.* 1991;11:563-583.
34. Baddely AD. Working memory. *Science.* 1992;255:556-559.
35. Goldman-Rakic PS, Friedman HR. The circuitry of working memory revealed by anatomy and metabolic imaging. In: Levin HS, Eisenberg HM, Benton AL, eds. *Frontal Lobe Function and Dysfunction.* New York, NY: Oxford University Press Inc; 1991:72-91.
36. Wesson DW, Carlin AS, Adams KM, Beschner G. *Polydrug Abuse: The Results of a National Collaborative Study.* New York, NY: Academic Press; 1978.

Announcement

Free Patient Record Forms Available

Patient record forms are available free of charge to ARCHIVES readers by calling or writing FORMEDIC, 12D Worlds Fair Dr, Somerset, NJ 08873-9863, telephone (908) 469-7031.

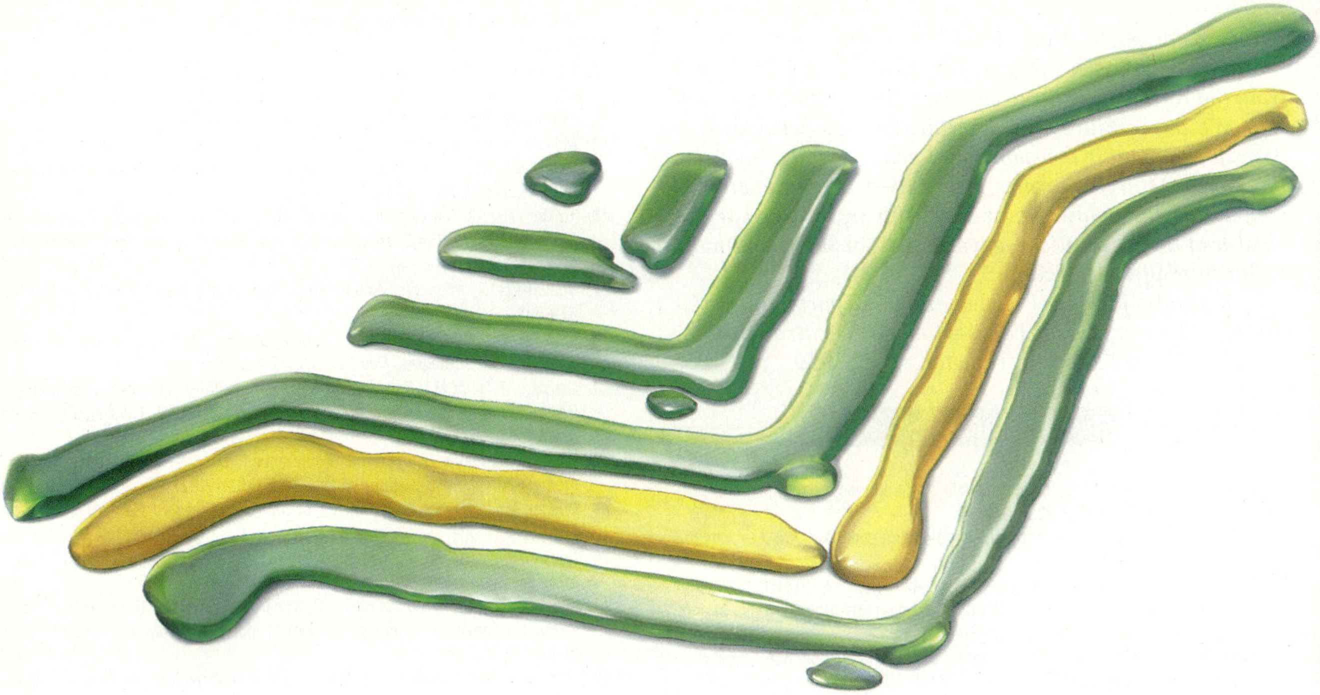

Is Research in Normal and Ill Children Involving Radiation Exposure Ethical?

Zametkin et al[1] break new ground in the understanding of attention deficit hyperactivity disorder (ADHD) with positron emission tomography (PET) findings in adolescents with ADHD. Their research also reports PET results in healthy adolescents, raising important considerations regarding the use of normal controls in the pediatric age group. Clearly, the brain of a fetus, infant, older child, or adolescent is different from that of an adult and may require the development of normative information for this age group. The issue of consent in healthy children is quite complicated and varies within the differing pediatric age groups.

Do standards of consent for children exist that can adequately meet the growing complexity of research in children? The Code of Federal Regulations regarding the protection of human subjects[2] was produced in 1983 and is quite general, especially in regard to pediatric research. In reporting their own consent process for research in healthy children at the Children's Memorial Hospital in Chicago, Gidding et al[3] analyze the risk in terms of age and hazard. Examples of easily acceptable (minimal risk) research are routine office procedures in children younger than 8 years, blood draw and immunization in 8- to 12-year-old children, and tilt-table testing in children 13 years and older. Invasive diagnostic testing is considered to be of moderate risk; chemotherapy and extracorporeal membrane oxygenation, of high risk. The latter two categories require the investigators to strongly defend their rationale for requiring this research in healthy children. These limited examples clearly do not cover the range of research currently needed in children.

For studies using radiation, is sufficient information available to determine the maximum safe radiation dose in healthy research subjects of adolescent or younger ages? Sedation, an additional risk in younger children undergoing neuroimaging, represents another blockade to the study of healthy children. Given that research in children will always be more difficult than that in adults, has the time arrived for updated and more specific federal guidelines for research in healthy children? Has communication between the medical and governmental communities to date been sufficient to guarantee the protection of this population?

Lt Col Charles T. Morton, MC, USAF
Department of the Air Force
Wilford Hall Medical Center (AETC)
2200 Bergquist Dr
Suite 1
Lackland AFB, TX 78236-5300

The views expressed in this article are those of the author and do not reflect the official policy of the Department of Defense or other departments of the US government.

1. Zametkin AJ, Liebnauer LL, Fitzgerald GA, King AC, Minkunas DV, Herscovitch P, Yamada EM, Cohen RM. Brain metabolism in teenagers with attention-deficit hyperactivity disorder. *Arch Gen Psychiatry*. 1993;50:333-340.
2. US Department of Health and Human Services. Protection of human subjects (45 CFR 46). *Federal Register*. March 8, 1983;48:9814-9820.
3. Gidding SS, Camp D, Flanagan MH, Kowalski JA, Lingl LL, Silverman BL, Langman CB. A policy regarding research in healthy children. *J Pediatr*. 1993;123:852-855.

In reply

The letter by Dr Morton, addresses a concern to us all—the safety and well-being of human subjects in research studies, and in particular healthy pediatric populations. Zametkin and colleagues[1] present a PET study of adolescents with ADHD and matched normal controls. That study was an attempt to further understand brain systems underlying a disorder that affects a significant number of children each year. The exposure of these minors to radiation was held to minimal levels. Given that ADHD is a significant and important psychiatric disorder to study, afflicting thousands of children each year, this study seemed warranted.

Nevertheless, we share Dr Morton's concerns about the use of any invasive procedure in pediatric populations. In this regard, we are encouraged by the fact that an alternative, noninvasive approach to functional neuroimaging in developmental populations is now available. This is functional magnetic resonance imaging (fMRI), which can be used to examine brain state changes in awake, behaving subjects much as PET is able to do.[2-4] This technique is based on the observation that hemoglobin becomes highly paramagnetic in its deoxygenated state. Thus, deoxygenated hemoglobin can be used as a naturally occurring contrast agent, with highly oxygenated areas producing a larger magnetic resonance (MR) signal than less oxygenated regions. Furthermore, because it uses MRI as the imaging modality, and does not require the use of ionizing radiation or any exogenously administered contrast agents, it has no known risks or complications, beyond the potential discomfort of remaining immobile in the scanner during the imaging session. Thus, it is well suited for use in developmental populations.

We have recently used fMRI to study the activation of prefrontal cortex in healthy 9- to 11-year-olds.[5] This brain region and related circuitry have been implicated in a number of developmental psychiatric disorders, including ADHD. Using a procedure that is considered to be safe and that is commonly used in pediatric populations, we can obtain normative data that will help us better interpret findings from pathological populations.

It is important to periodically raise the questions that

Dr Morton has, to keep us all aware of the balance between the significance of our work and the safety of our human subjects. Such questioning is a critical force in helping to accelerate the development of new, safer methods for studying the brain, such as fMRI.

B. J. Casey, PhD
Jonathan D. Cohen, MD, PhD
Department of Psychiatry
University of Pittsburgh Medical Center
Pittsburgh, Pa 15213

1. Zametkin AJ, Liebnauer LL, Fitzgerald GA, King AC, Minkunas DV, Herscovitch P, Yamada EM, Cohen RM. Brain metabolism in teenagers with attention-deficit hyperactivity disorder. *Arch Gen Psychiatry*. 1993;50:333-340.
2. Kwong KK, Belliveau JW, Chesler DA, Goldberg IE, Weisskoff RM, Poncelet P, Kennedy DN, Hoppel BE, Turner R, Cheng HM, Brady TJ, Rosen BR. Dynamic magnetic resonance of human brain activity during primary sensory stimulation. *Proc Natl Acad Sci U S A*. 1992;89:5675-5679.
3. Ogawa S, Lee TS, Nayak AS, Glynn P. Oxygenation-sensitive contrast in magnetic resonance image of rodent brain at high magnetic fields. *Magn Reson Med*. 1990;26:68-78.
4. Turner R, Le Bihan D, Moonen CTW, Despres D, Frank J. Echo-planar time course MRI of cat brain oxygenation changes. *Magn Reson Med*. 1991;22:159-166.
5. Casey BJ, Cohen JD, Jezzard P, Turner R, Noll DC, Trainor R, Giedd J, Pannier L, Kaysen D, Rapoport JL. Activation of prefrontal cortex in children during a non-spatial working memory task with functional MRI. *Neuroimage*. 1995;2:221-229.

In reply

The letter from Dr Morton in this issue of the ARCHIVES *is a thoughtful and well-tempered query about research performed in our laboratory. We appreciate the comments of Dr Morton because they focus on the importance of facilitating research in minors. Clinical research studies remain an obligatory step in improving the treatment of these patients. However, because of the intendant difficulties of research that has included minors, many investigators have been reluctant to consider clinical studies that have as their objective an improved understanding of those brain abnormalities that lead to serious brain disorders that afflict pediatric populations.*

During the early 1990s, our laboratory received permission to study a limited number of "normal," healthy control subjects, aged 12 to 18 years, as part of a clinical research protocol that involved administering a radioactive tracer for measuring functional brain activity by PET. The study, despite our best efforts to minimize the amount of tracer required, still resulted in an exposure of approximately 500 mrem to each subject's bladder, although considerably less to all other organs. The protocol was reviewed and approved by the National Institute of Mental Health (NIMH) Human Subject Protection Committee and the National Institutes of Health (NIH) Radiation Research Safety Committee. Among the members of the latter committee were radiation health physicists.

In more recent deliberations of the NIMH Institutional Review Board (IRB) regarding newer protocols involving PET and normal minors, a special session of the IRB was convened that was attended by invited experts, including the director of the National Institute of Child Health and Human Development. This meeting and subsequent meetings of the NIMH Human Subject Protection Committee judiciously evaluated the risk involved and the importance of the information to be gained in full cognizance of the Code of Federal Regulations (CFR).[1]

In preparation for these deliberations we carefully reviewed the following questions: (1) What is the actual biological risk in minors from the radiation doses in the range of 100 to 500 mrem? Current NIH and occupational guidelines[2] call for restricting the exposure of minors participating in research to no more than one tenth of the 3 rem (3000 mrem) per quarter and 5 rem (5000 mrem) per year of adults. (2) Who developed, framed, and translated the current CFR? When were these regulations developed and was any consideration given to the issues of age? Were considerations of the participation of normal minors addressed? (3) What are the risks that normal children and adolescents face in day-to-day life? (4) Can answers to the causes of severe brain diseases be found without radiation exposure? (5) Has research involving ionizing radiation been conducted in the United States on normal minors before? Let us address each of these questions briefly because space does not permit extensive answers.

1. If one reviews a summary of the considerable world literature[3] on radiation exposure to minors and the effects of low-level exposure over a 20- to 30-year period, the conclusion one draws is that if any risk really exists, it is extremely small. An illuminating report on low-level ionization radiation exposure in Scientific American *stated that "the evidence assembled so far indicates that the hazard, if it is real, is too small to be detectable."[4]*

2. Among the multiple authors of the CFR, several were personally interviewed by a member of our team (A.J.Z.). It is clear that no attempt was made to distinguish older minors from younger minors and that the intent of the document pertains to "children" (<8 years), not adolescents.

The discussion pertaining to research in normal controls in the development of the CFR was very limited and not a major focus of the code. Thus, we agree with Dr Morton that it is time to update regulations in this area by involving clinical scientists who use radiation for research or therapeutic purposes.

3. Another related issue is determining what constitutes minimal risks in different age groups. Sufficient to say, having carefully examined the day-to-day lifestyle of the 20th-century teenager, we argued that the radiation exposure risk of our studies paled in comparison not only to the risk for normal teenage behavior, but also to many routine (but medically necessary) medical procedures (third molar extraction [wisdom teeth], for example).

4. Can research in minors be performed without exposure to radiation or without normal controls? The answer of course is yes. However, at the time that these studies were initiated, PET offered many considerable advantages over fMRI or MRI spectroscopy that we believe still remains true. Thus, PET holds a unique place and tremendous promise for studying the large array of chemical processes in the living human brain. While the use of normal subjects could be avoided by using multiple patient groups for comparison, if even one group is "abnormal" the ultimate comparison with "healthy normals" is crucial.

5. Finally there are at least 6 studies, 3 of which are summarized by Freeman,[5] involving large numbers of nor-

mal healthy children conducted in the United States in which ionizing radiation was used in nonmedically indicated research studies. The question of normal minors participating in research involving ionizing radiation was recently debated in IRB A Review of Human Subject Research,[5] *a journal devoted to the discussion of difficult ethical issues in clinical research.*

In summary, we strongly believe that research involving ionizing radiation can involve normal controls with the following caveats: (1) the scientific questions are carefully formulated, well designed, and address important medical questions; (2) the local IRBs are well informed about the level of risk (in most cases a function of dose), and the final decisions are left to the local IRBs. We do believe the time is right for federal regulations to be updated to reflect current research methods concerning issues of older and younger minors and normal controls vs patients with an illness. Guidelines will facilitate the process whereby IRBs must make ethical and safe decisions about the participation of minors in research.

The current system has served us well, although outdated in several respects, and in the interim forced us and our IRB to carefully analyze the risk to benefit ratios for our studies.

As Nobel laureate, Rosalyn Yalow, MD, so aptly stated: "We live in a world in which perception of risk is too often confused with real risk. In no field is unjustified risk-related fear more pervasive than in the area of unreasonable concern with hazards of low levels of ionizing radiation."[6]

Alan J. Zametkin, MD
David J. Schwartz
Monique Ernst, MD, PhD
Robert M. Cohen, MD, PhD
Section on Clinical Brain Imaging
Bldg 10, Room 4N317
National Institute of Mental Health
900 Rockville Pike
Bethesda, MD 20892

1. Title 45 CFR, part 4b. 1991:15-16.
2. Radiation Safety Branch. *The National Institutes of Health Radiation Safety Guide.* Washington, DC: US Dept of Health, Education, and Welfare; 1979: 19. DHEW publication NIH79-18.
3. Subcommittee on Risks of Low-Level Ionizing Radiation. *Low-Level Radiation Effects: A Fact Book.* New York, NY: The Society of Nuclear Medicine Inc; 1983.
4. Upton AC. The biological effects of low-level ionizing radiation. *Sci Am.* 1982; 246:2:41.
5. Freeman WL. Research with radiation and healthy children: greater than minimal risk. *IRB Rev Hum Subject Res.* September/October 1994;16:1-5.
6. Gilsanz V, Roe TF, Goodman W. Does radiation in healthy children pose greater than minimal risk? *IRB Rev Hum Subject Res.* September/October 1994;16:6.

Parenthood, Completed Suicide, and Mental Disorders

A study by Hoyer and Lund,[1] which was published in the ARCHIVES, reported a negative association between rates of suicide and number of children among women in Norway, suggesting that parenthood might have a protecting effect against suicide. The authors discuss the question of whether this protection is due to having children per se or by possible selection factors related to mental disorders. Ideally, differences in suicide risk related to parenthood could be estimated by controlling for specific mental disorders, but no such data have yet been reported.

Subjects and Methods. In the National Suicide Prevention Project in Finland,[2] all suicides (N=1397) committed in Finland between April 1, 1987, and March 31, 1988, were analyzed using the method of psychological autopsy. On the basis of the interviews of next of kin, 57% (651/1141) of suicide victims were reported to have had children. Those victims who had children were significantly older (median age, 48 years) than those victims who had no children (median age, 32 years) (median 2-sample test, $S=136.00$, $z=-12.39$, $P<.001$). As expected, marital status and parenthood were closely interrelated; of those who had children, 94% (611/651) were or had at some time been married, whereas, of those who had no children, 88% (430/490) were never married ($\chi^2=769$, $df=1$, $P<.001$). A difference existed between the sexes in parenthood, as 54% (478/885) of men vs 68% (173/256) of women were reported to have had children ($\chi^2=14.92$, $df=1$, $P<.001$). When age was controlled for, the difference remained significant (Mantel-Haenszel $\chi^2=6.00$, $df=1$, $P=.01$).

The mental disorders of suicide victims in Finland, according to *DSM-III-R*[3] criteria, were examined in a diagnostic study of a random sample of 229 suicide cases.[4] Within this sample, the distribution of mental disorders among those who had children can be compared with those who had no children. This comparison revealed notable differences between the 2 groups. Depressive disorders and, specifically, major depression were more prevalent among those who were parents than those who were not parents: depressive disorders, 77% (87/113) vs 60% (43/72) ($\chi^2=6.28$, $df=1$, $P=.01$); major depression, 39% (45/114) vs 24% (17/72) ($\chi^2=4.99$, $df=1$, $P=.02$). Schizophrenia was more common among those who had no children vs those who had children: 14% (10/72) vs 3% (3/113) ($\chi^2=8.49$, $df=1$, $P=.004$).

The Hoyer and Lund[1] study comprised only women. Among Finnish suicide victims who were women, major depression was markedly more common among those women who had children (62% [18/29]) than those who had no children (31% [5/16]) ($\chi^2=3.92$, $df=1$, $P=.05$). No other statistically significant differences between the groups of women were found. Among men, those with children were less likely to have had schizophrenia than those who had no children: 2% (2/84) vs 16% (9/56) ($\chi^2=8.70$, $df=1$, $P=.003$).

Most of the differences in mental disorders between the groups seemed to be age related. When age was controlled by dichotomizing the sample (median cutoff point, 43 years), only the differences in the prevalence of schizophrenia remained statistically significant (Mantel-Haenszel χ^2 for all=4.80, $df=1$, $P=.03$; Mantel-Haenszel χ^2 for men=4.41, $df=1$, $P=.04$).

Comment. Comparable prevalence rates for *DSM-III-R*[3] mental disorders in the general population in Finland are unavailable; possible differences in suicide risk related to parenthood between persons with similar specific mental disorders cannot, therefore, be estimated. However, an epidemiological survey in Finland using the Present State Examination method (ie, the Mini-Finland Health Survey) found notable age-adjusted differences in mental disorders according to marital status.[5] Our findings suggest differences in characteristics, including age and distribution of mental disorders, between those suicide victims who have children and those who have no children. Although many of the differences in mental disorders between these groups seem to be related to differences in age distribution, schizophrenia is likely to be more common among victims with no children, independent of age. Future studies should account for these differences as possible confounding factors when estimating the effects of parenthood on suicide risk. Furthermore, some difference exists between the sexes in parenthood among suicide victims, and the possible protective role of having children may vary between men and women.

Erkki T. Isometsä, MD
Martti E. Heikkinen, MD
Markus M. Henriksson, MD
Hillevi M. Aro, MD, PhD
Mauri J. Marttunen, MD
Jouko K. Lönnqvist, MD, PhD
National Public Health Institute
Department of Mental Health
Mannerheimintie 166
SF-00300 Helsinki
Finland

1. Hoyer G, Lund E. Suicide among women related to number of children in marriage. *Arch Gen Psychiatry*. 1993;50:134-137.
2. Lönnqvist J. National Suicide Prevention Project in Finland: a research phase of the project. *Psychiatr Fenn.* 1988;19:125-132.
3. American Psychiatric Association. *Diagnostic and Statistical Manual of Mental Disorders, Third Edition, Revised.* Washington, DC: American Psychiatric Association; 1987.
4. Henriksson MM, Aro HM, Marttunen MJ, Heikkinen ME, Isometsä EI, Kuoppasalmi KI, Lönnqvist JK. Mental disorders and comorbidity in suicide. *Am J Psychiatry*. 1993;150:935-940.
5. Lehtinen V, Lindholm T, Veijola J, Väisänen E. The prevalence of PSE-CATEGO disorders in a Finnish adult population cohort. *Soc Psychiatry Psychiatr Epidemiol.* 1990;25:187-192.

Schizophrenia and Temporal Lobe Epilepsy

In the April 1994 issue of the ARCHIVES, Gold et al[1] report the results of an important study in which they directly compared the neuropsychological performance of a group of patients with long-term intractable temporal lobe epilepsy (TLE) with that of a group of patients with severe chronic schizophrenia (SCZ). Studies that directly compare patients with SCZ with patients with a well-defined neurologic illness on detailed neuropsychological tasks are needed to elucidate the neurologic substrate of SCZ. However, the interpretations by Gold et al of the results of their study and the far-reaching conclusions drawn about the neurology of SCZ are debatable.

In chronic neuropsychiatric conditions, confounding factors such as the effects of institutionalization, medication, and deterioration in psychosocial skills can significantly affect neuropsychological performance. Therefore, the difference in the neuropsychological performance between patients with chronic SCZ and patients with chronic, poorly controlled epilepsy probably reflects the difference in psychosocial handicaps resulting from these 2 different diseases and not necessarily a difference in the neurologic features of the 2 conditions.

Gold et al report decreased attention in patients with SCZ compared with patients with TLE as the main finding of their study. However, they provide no measures of the mental state of the patients at the time of testing. Psychotic symptoms could have significantly impaired the performance of the group with SCZ on measures of attention and concentration. For the group with TLE, too, information about psychopathologic features or seizure status at the time of testing (ie, ictal, postictal, or preictal) is not provided, and it is unknown whether the patients with TLE were more in touch with reality and more cooperative than the patients with SCZ. It is possible that seizure activity itself (ie, functional impairment) and not the underlying structural lesion may cause SCZ-like symptoms.[2] Therefore, it is important to know the seizure status of the patients with TLE at the time of testing.

The group with SCZ, despite poor attention, may have performed better than the group with TLE on the linguistic and memory tasks because the latter had never adequately acquired these skills (because of the early onset of a chronic illness) and not because different brain regions are involved in the 2 conditions. If a control group was also tested, it would have perhaps been shown that linguistic and memory deficits were present in the group with SCZ. Anand et al[3] have reported that, by using fine-grained neurolinguistic tasks, severe deficits, particularly in semantic language, are present in patients with early psychosis compared with healthy control subjects.

In their discussion, Gold et al assert that because their study does not support a temporal lobe disturbance in patients with SCZ, the disturbance, therefore, must be in the frontal lobes. Not temporal does not automatically mean frontal. Many other regions of the brain may be responsible (eg, the basal ganglia or the brain as a whole may be impaired). It should also be noted that a frontal lobe impairment is similar to the negative symptoms of SCZ. To explain the positive symptoms, an impairment in the executive functions of the frontal lobes over temporal lobe function, leading to the dysfunction of the latter, has been hypothesized.[4] If Gold et al have entirely excluded a temporal lobe dysfunction by their findings, it is difficult to understand how the positive symptoms of SCZ can arise from the sole dysfunction of the frontal lobes. It is TLE that is most frequently associated with the positive symptoms of SCZ,[5] while such a phenomenon is rarely encountered in patients with frontal lobe seizures.[6] Structural lesions of the temporal lobe are sometimes associated with psychotic states,[7] while those of the frontal lobes are usually associated with a deficit state more akin to the negative symptoms of SCZ.

In summary, it would have been better if Gold et al had chosen a group of early schizophrenics for their study and measured the severity and nature of the psychopathologic features at the time of neuropsychological testing. This group could then be compared, on standard and more fine-grained neuropsychological tasks, with patients suffering from a recent onset of TLE or frontal lobe seizures. A control group with a nonneurologic, nonpsychotic illness would have further strengthened the results. A comparison of the 2 groups using neuroimaging studies, such as the magnetic resonance imaging or the positron emission topography scan, could further provide data about the structural and functional neurologic comparison between the 2 groups.

Amit Anand, MD
Department of Psychiatry
Yale University School of Medicine
West Haven VA Medical Center
950 Campbell Ave
West Haven, CT 06516

1. Gold JM, Hermann BP, Randolph C, Wyler AR, Goldberg TE, Weinberger DR. Schizophrenia and temporal lobe epilepsy: a neuropsychological analysis. *Arch Gen Psychiatry*. 1994;51:265-272.
2. Mace CJ. Epilepsy and schizoprenia. *Br J Psychiatry*. 1993;163:439-445.
3. Anand A, Wales RJ, Jackson HJ, Copolov DL. Linguistic impairment in early psychosis. *J Nerv Ment Dis*. 1994;182:488-493.
4. Morice R. Beyond language: speculations on the pre-frontal cortex and schizophrenia. *Aust N Z J Psychiatry*. 1986;20:7-10.
5. Trimble MR. First-rank symptoms of Schneider: a new perspective. *Br J Psychiatry*. 1990;156:195-200.
6. Delgado-Escueta AV, Swartz BE, Walsh GO, Chauvel P, Bancaud J, Broglin D. Frontal lobe seizures and epilepsies in neurobehavioral disorder. In: Smith D, Treiman D, Trimble M, eds. *Advances in Neurology*. New York, NY: Raven Press; 1991:55:317-339.
7. Stevens JR. Psychosis and the temporal lobe. In: Smith D, Treiman D, Trimble M, eds. *Advances in Neurology*. New York, NY: Raven Press; 1991:55:79-96.

The study by Gold et al[1] of the neuropsychological performance of patients with severe chronic SCZ in comparison with patients with unilateral TLE is a thoughtful approach to understanding the cognitive dysfunction in SCZ. Unfortunately, several problems with their study are important to document. The authors stress the analogy of these 2 disorders for their early developmental origin. However, examination of the epilepsy cohorts reveals a mean age of onset of 11.1 years (left temporal lobe) and 13.8 years (right temporal lobe) with a broad SD. A recent study by Roberts et al[2] demonstrated that the psychopathogic comparison of TLE and psychotic disorder was of maximal validity when the first seizure occurred before 6 years of age. Considering the group with SCZ, Gold et al present few data regarding the histories of the patients, although they acknowledge a bias toward poor prognosis. Calculation reveals a mean schizophrenic illness duration of 12 years. This chronicity could explain some of the abnormalities found in this group, such as motor slowing, which has been shown to be a deficit predominating in patients with SCZ who were previously treated rather than in those with first-episode SCZ.[3] In the study by Gold et al, the use of patients with first-episode SCZ would have eliminated the influence of pharmacotherapy and disease progression while maintaining the validity of a study designed to examine disorders with similar temporal lobe pathologic features acquired in early life.

Although Gold et al make a case for the development of neuropsychological scales derived from patients with SCZ (or their equivalent), they do not mention the problem of inferring localized anatomical abnormalities from neuropsychological tests.[4] In addition, they omit details concerning the theory of temporal lobe–prefrontal area connectivity,[5] which may help explain findings of frontal lobe abnormalities in patients with TLE.[6] This omission may be of interest because it suggests that the documented impairments in abstraction of the group with SCZ are not necessarily incompatible with the pathologic features affecting the temporal lobe.[7] Another point of note is the absence of a control group in this study. Whereas with a control group, localized cognitive dysfunction would be clear even if it occurred in all patients groups (as is compatible with the hypothesis of a common pathologic feature), without a control group it is only possible to highlight abnormalities of the group with SCZ in comparison with either the left or right TLE cohort.

Finally, despite the many historical comparisons between TLE and SCZ, it could be argued that little evidence suggests that SCZ is a disorder with pure unilateral brain damage, and, as a result, the use of unilateral TLE as a neuropsychological model of SCZ may be of limited benefit.

Alexander J. Mitchell, MB, BS
Department of Clinical Neurology, Ward 6
Royal Victoria Infirmary
Queen Victoria Road
Newcastle upon Tyne NE1 4LP
England

1. Gold JM, Hermann BP, Randolph C, Wyler AR, Goldberg TE, Weinberger DR. Schizophrenia and temporal lobe epilepsy: a neuropsychological analysis. *Arch Gen Psychiatry*. 1994;51:265-272.
2. Roberts GW, Done DJ, Brunton C, Crow TJ. A 'mock-up' of schizophrenia: temporal lobe epilepsy and schizophrenia-like psychosis. *Biol Psychiatry*. 1990; 28:127-143.
3. Saykin AJ, Shtasel DL, Gur RL, Kester DB, Mozley LH, Stafiniak P, Gur RC. Neuropsychological deficits in neuroleptic naive patients with first-episode schizophrenia. *Arch Gen Psychiatry*. 1994;51:124-131.
4. Anderson SW, Damasio H, Jones RD, Tranel D. Wisconsin Card Sorting Test performance as a measure of frontal lobe damage. *J Clin Exp Neuropsychol*. 1991;13:909-922.
5. Weinberger DR. Anteromedial temporal-prefrontal connectivity: a functional neuroanatomical network implicated in schizophrenia. In: Carroll BJ, Barrett JE, eds. *Psychopathology and the Brain*. New York, NY: Raven Press; 1991.
6. Hermann BP, Wyler AR, Richley ET. Wisconsin Card Sorting Test performance in patients with complex partial seizures of temporal lobe origin. *J Clin Exp Neuropsychol*. 1988;10:467-476.
7. Nestor PG, Shentoni ME, McCarley RW, Haimson J, Smith RS, O'Donnell B, Kimble M, Kikinis R, Jolesz FA. Neuropsychological correlates of MRI temporal lobe abnormalities in schizophrenia. *Am J Psychiatry*. 1993;150:1849-1855.

In reply

RESPONSE TO DR ANAND

Dr Anand suggests the possibility that the group differences we reported might be the result of numerous confounding variables, such as medication effects, the effect of institutionalization, deterioration in psychosocial skills, or the effect of psychotic symptoms. Although these variables are important, we do not think that our results are likely due to such confounding variables for several reasons. We do not see any basis for concluding that psychosocial handicaps, shared to varying degrees by all the patients in the study, can provide a principled account for differences in group performance profile. It would seem most likely to us that the cohort with severe chronic SCZ has experienced even more severe handicaps than the patients with TLE but still managed to perform better than the patients with epilepsy on several measures. Similarly, the English-language literature about medication effects in patients with SCZ does not support the conclusion that large negative effects are to be anticipated.[1] Indeed, recent studies of clozapine demonstrating dramatic symptomatic benefits concomitant with minimal cognitive benefits would seem to be the best demonstration of the fundamental dissociation between cognitive impairment and symptomatic state in patients with SCZ.[2-4] In terms of seizure status, all testing was conducted when it was deemed to be clinically appropriate and valid. No testing was conducted when patients showed any effects of seizure activity. Published data from the EpiCare Center, Memphis, Tenn, showing the stability of most cognitive results after successful temporal lobe surgery, should be seen as evidence that the baseline presurgery data that we reported are likely representative of the true abilities of the patients rather than artifactual reflections of postictal confusion.[5]

We agree with Dr Anand that the linguistic differences we observed are likely explained, in large part, by the early age of onset in the temporal lobe group, as we stated in the original article.[6] We certainly did not state, or mean to imply, that all language functions are normal in patients with SCZ. However, little doubt exists that the performance of the group with SCZ on the language functions assessed by the Wechsler Adult Intelligence Scale–Revised verbal comprehension factor are far closer to the normal population mean than the attentional functions assessed by the freedom from distractibility factor. This does not exclude linguistic abnormalities assessed by other methods.

We did not claim that our study "does not support a temporal lobe disturbance in patients with SCZ. . . ." In our conclusion, we simply stated that "temporal lobe dysfunction does not provide by itself an adequate account of the cognitive abnormality of schizophrenia."[6(p271)] We completely agree with the statement by Dr Anand that "not temporal does not automatically mean frontal." We thought the results were suggestive of frontal dysfunction based on the literature examining the neuropsychological effects of focal frontal damage. It is certainly possible that other types of injury (eg, injury to the basal ganglia) can produce similar impairments. We have addressed this issue in a study comparing patients with frontal lobe epilepsy with patients with SCZ, in which we found that both groups did, in fact, share similar impairments of attention, the deficit that we thought could not be explained on the basis of a temporal lobe abnormality.[7]

Although we agree that future studies employing patients with first-episode SCZ, more detailed cognitive measures, and neuroimaging data might provide fresh insight about these questions, it is important to acknowledge the inherent limitations of this type of comparative approach. By definition, the pathologic features of the different patient groups are different, even if they involve the same brain areas. Thus, the data are probably best considered as providing constraints and limitations on models of the pathologic features of the brain in patients with SCZ, constraints that are difficult to achieve with studies only comparing the neuropsychological performance of patients with normal control subjects. However, such constraints may be useful in the development of more specific cognitive-anatomical hypotheses that can be investigated with more direct, experimental methods.

RESPONSE TO DR MITCHELL

Dr Mitchell notes that the age of onset of our patients with TLE is somewhat older than that reported by Roberts et al[8] as being associated with psychosis. We dated onset conservatively from the onset of chronic seizures; initial seizures often predated the onset of chronic seizures by many years. Thus, the "onset" of temporal lobe disturbance in our sample may be substantially "younger" than it seems. Having noted this, we do agree that the study of patients with early onset of seizures may be of particular interest in relationship to SCZ.

Dr Mitchell notes the issue of how the study of patients with first-episode SCZ might have altered our conclusions. We differ from Dr Mitchell in evaluating the importance of the differences between patients with first-episode SCZ and those with chronic SCZ in the article by Saykin et al,[9] which he cited. The group profiles are quite parallel, and the differences in the first-episode group compared with normal control values in the visual-motor factor seem to be greater than 1.5 z. Two of the measures in this scale were among our most discriminating variables. As noted in response to Dr Anand, we are not convinced that reliable evidence exists that neuroleptics impair the neuropsychological performance of patients with SCZ, and we are unaware of any widely recognized evidence of disease progression in cognition in patients with SCZ that accounts for the group differences we reported.

The statement by Dr Mitchell that "they do not mention the problem of inferring localized anatomical abnormalities from neuropsychological tests" is surprising, as we discussed the issue at some length.[6(p266)] Indeed, we were drawn to an explicit comparative study approach as a means of addressing the issue. We agree with Dr Mitchell that the connectivity of temporal-frontal regions makes the interpretation of behavioral findings complex. However, we do think it is fair to conclude that patients with SCZ demonstrate numerous impairments different from those found in patients with unilateral TLE. Thus, we agree with Dr Mitchell that unilateral TLE, by itself, does not provide a useful model of SCZ, as we stated in our original article.[6] Given our interest in testing the limits of a temporal lobe model, we did not study a normal control group. The fact that patients with SCZ demonstrate a range of impairments compared with normal controls is well documented, as are the abnormalities noted in patients with TLE. The use of standardized tests should make it pos-

sible for interested readers to estimate the extent of impairment among the groups.

James M. Gold, PhD
Maryland Psychiatric Research Center
PO Box 21247
Baltimore, MD 21228
Bruce P. Hermann, PhD
Madison, Wis
Daniel R. Weinberger, MD
Washington, DC

1. Cassens G, Inglis AK, Appelbaum PS, Guntheil TG. Neuroleptics: effects on neuropsychological function in chronic schizophrenic patients. *Schizophr Bull.* 1990;16:477-499.
2. Goldberg TE, Greenberg RD, Griffin SJ, Gold J, Pickar D, Kleinman J, Weinberger D. The effect of clozapine on cognition and psychiatric symptoms in patients with schizophrenia. *Br J Psychiatry.* 1993;163:43-48.
3. Buchanan RW, Holstein C, Breier A. The comparative efficacy and long-term effect of clozapine treatment on neuropsychological test performance. *Biol Psychiatry.* 1994;36:717-725.
4. Haggar C, Buckley P, Kenney JT, Friedman L, Ubogy D, Meltzer HY. Improvement in cognitive functions and psychiatric symptoms in treatment-refractory schizophrenic patients receiving clozapine. *Biol Psychiatry.* 1993;34:702-712.
5. Hermann BP, Wyler AR. Neuropsychological outcome of anterior temporal lobectomy. *J Epilepsy.* 1988;1:35-45.
6. Gold JM, Hermann BP, Randolph C, Wyler AR, Goldberg TE, Weinberger DR. Schizophrenia and temporal lobe epilepsy: a neuropsychological analysis. *Arch Gen Psychiatry.* 1994;51:265-272.
7. Gold J, Hermann B, Randolph C, Chelune G, Trenerry M, Loring D, Goldberg T, Weinberger D. Frontal dysfunction in schizophrenia. *Soc Neurosci.* 1994;20:1260. Abstract.
8. Roberts GW, Done DJ, Brunton C, Crow TJ. A 'mock-up' of schizophrenia: temporal lobe epilepsy and schizophrenia-like psychosis. *Biol Psychiatry.* 1990; 28:127-143.
9. Saykin AJ, Shtasel DL, Gur RL, Kester DB, Mozley LH, Stafiniak P, Gur RC. Neuropsychological deficits in neuroleptic naive patients with first-episode schizophrenia. *Arch Gen Psychiatry.* 1994;51:124-131.

Alterations of Membrane Phospholipid Metabolism in Patients With Schizophrenia Assessed by Phosphorus Magnetic Resonance Spectroscopy

Stanley et al[1] used phosphorus 31 magnetic resonance spectroscopy to evaluate high-energy phosphate metabolism in the prefrontal cortex of patients with schizophrenia and control subjects. Stanley et al and Pettegrew et al[2] have documented changes in the membrane phospholipid metabolism of patients with schizophrenia, and they have suggested that these changes may, in part, be involved in the pathophysiology of schizophrenic illnesses. They found that the levels of phosphomonoesters (PMEs) (ie, the precursors of phospholipid biosynthesis) and orthophosphates were reduced and that the levels of phosphodiesters (PDEs) (ie, phospholipid degradation products) and intracellular magnesium were elevated in the prefrontal cortex of patients with schizophrenia who were and were not taking medication. They suggested that the reduction of PMEs could be due to the decreased biosynthesis or the altered degradation of PMEs and that the increase of PDEs may be due to the increase of phospholipase A_1 or A_2 or the decrease of phosphodiesterase activity. Furthermore, they suggested that an elevated intracellular magnesium level could alter the function of phosphate-transferring enzymes (directly or indirectly). We suggest that explanations based on the altered enzyme activities in these brain regions of patients with schizophrenia may be an oversimplification and that an additional hypothesis can be offered based on in vitro studies. Our findings about the metabolic compartmentation of the biosynthetic pathway for phosphatidylcholine (PC), the major membrane phospholipid in the human brain (quantitatively, >50% of all phospholipid mass in the brain), suggest a more likely explanation for these observations.

Several studies have shown that the regulation of PC metabolism in various mammalian cultured cell types is similar, implying that studies of PC metabolism in cultured rat brain cells may approximate the metabolism in the human brain.[3] We studied the uptake and incorporation of radiolabeled, membrane-impermeant substrates of PC biosynthesis in intact, electropermeabilized cultured glioma cells.[4,5] This pathway involves the following sequence:

$$\text{Choline} \rightarrow \text{Phosphocholine} \rightarrow \text{Cytidinediphosphate Choline} \rightarrow \text{PC}$$

These permeabilized cells were shown to be metabolically viable and to perform phospholipid metabolism at almost the levels of nonpermeabilized control cells. We found that exogenous precursors of PC biosynthesis (ie, choline, phosphocholine, and cytidinediphosphate choline labeled with radioactive carbon) did not mix freely with the endogenous pools of these substrates and were not incorporated into PC, despite concurrent hemicholinium-3-sensitive, transporter-mediated exogenous tritiated choline uptake and incorporation into the phospholipid. When the level of intracellular calcium (Ca^{2+}) was reduced to less than 200 nmol/L with egtazic acid (a Ca^{2+} chelator), however, phosphorylated precursors rapidly mixed with endogenous pools and were incorporated into PC. These results suggested that the biosynthetic intermediates of this pathway are not freely diffusible in cells but rather are "channeled" sequentially between enzymes in the pathway, implying metabolic compartmentation and regulation by intracellular Ca^{2+}. This functional organization may lead to enhanced catalytic efficiency for the enzymes in this pathway.

Because of these observations, an alternative biochemical explanation could be suggested for the findings of Stanley et al and other groups dealing with altered PME and PDE levels in patients with schizophrenia. If the metabolic compartmentation of PC biosynthesis was disturbed in the brain regions of these patients, then PME levels could be reduced and PDE levels might be secondarily elevated by the enhanced phospholipid catabolism in an attempt to produce additional choline to sustain PC biosynthesis. The reduced orthophosphate levels (in view of normal adenosine triphosphate levels) could result from decreased phospholipid synthesis. Elevations of intracellular magnesium levels would also be expected to coincide with changes in intracellular Ca^{2+} levels inversely (via a magnesium-induced *N*-methyl-D-aspartate receptor blockade), which would be consonant with changes in Ca^{2+} levels that are likely to disrupt the functional organization of PC synthesis.

We would be interested to know if the level of intracellular Ca^{2+} was altered in these studies.[1,2] Furthermore, cytidinediphosphate choline and cytidinediphosphate ethanolamine, PDEs that are involved in the biosynthesis of phospholipids, would be expected to be reduced based on the interpretation of Stanley et al and this hypothesis. Studies of phospholipid metabolism in the brains of patients with schizophrenia have demonstrated a reduced PC mass in cell membranes, elevated phospholipase A_2 levels, and an altered phospholipid fatty acid composition,[6] which may normalize after neuroleptic treatment. Detailed studies using ^{31}P magnetic resonance spectroscopy and in vitro methods would be useful to test our hypothesis that alterations in the coordinate regulation of PC biosynthesis via functional organization may be involved in the pathobiology of schizophrenia and, in part, may account for the pleiotropic effects on PMEs and PDEs described in the study by Stanley et al and in other ^{31}P magnetic resonance spectroscopy studies.

Tony P. George, MD
Department of Psychiatry
Yale University School of Medicine
Neuropsychopharmacology Research Unit, Room B-254
Sterling Hall of Medicine
333 Cedar St
New Haven, CT 06520-8066
Matthew W. Spence, MD, PhD
Alberta Heritage Foundation for Medical Research
Edmonton, Alberta

1. Stanley JA, Williamson PC, Drost DJ, Carr TJ, Rylett RJ, Malla A, Thompson RT. An in vivo study of the prefrontal cortex of schizophrenic patients at different stages of illness via phosphorus magnetic resonance spectroscopy. *Arch Gen Psychiatry*. 1995;52:399-406.
2. Pettegrew JW, Keshavan MS, Panchaligam K, Strychor S, Kaplan DB, Tretta MG, Allen M. Alterations in brain high-energy phosphate and membrane phospholipid metabolism in first-episode, drug-naive schizophrenics. *Arch Gen Psychiatry*. 1991;48:563-568.
3. Morash SC, Cook HW, Spence MW. Phosphatidylcholine metabolism in cultured cells: catabolism via glycerophosphocholine. *Biochim Biophys Acta*. 1988;961:194-202.
4. George TP, Morash SC, Cook HW, Byers DM, St Claire Palmer FB, Spence MW. Phosphatidylcholine biosynthesis in cultured glioma cells: evidence for channeling of intermediates. *Biochim Biophys Acta*. 1989;1004:283-291.
5. George TP, Cook HW, Byers DM, St Claire Palmer FB, Spence MW. Channeling of intermediates in the CDP-choline pathway of phosphatidylcholine biosynthesis is dependent on intracellular Ca^{2+}. *J Biol Chem*. 1991;266:12 419-12 423.
6. Gattaz WF, Hubner CV, Nevalainen TJ, Thuren T, Kinnunen PK. Increased serum phospholipase A_2 activity in schizophrenia: a replication study. *Biol Psychiatry*. 1990;28:495-501.

Rapid Eye Movement Density Among Adolescents With Major Depressive Disorder Revisited

In the context of a follow-up study investigating the clinical continuity of major depressive disorder (MDD) and biological markers from prepuberty and adolescence to young adulthood, we are performing new analyses on polysomnographic data previously reported by Goetz et al[1] in the ARCHIVES. During this process, we noted a finding that we did not originally report; this finding replicates some recent articles regarding rapid eye movement (REM) density during the first REM period.

Goetz et al[1] described the sleep of 49 adolescents, mostly outpatients (86%), in whom MDD (ie, 25 adolescents with endogenous MDD [MDD-E] and 24 adolescents with nonendogenous MDD [MDD-NE]) was diagnosed and 40 adolescents without a history of a psychiatric disorder. Findings included increased sleep latency, increased awake time, and decreased sleep efficiency among adolescents with depression vs adolescent controls. No unconfounded REM sleep differences between the adolescents with depression and adolescent controls were reported. For data analysis and group comparisons, a repeated measures analysis of variance (RM-ANOVA) was employed. We were interested in addressing across-night effects that could be due to adaptation, the presence of an intravenous catheter, or both. Significant across-night effects were reported for awake time ($P<.03$), sleep efficiency ($P<.02$), stage 4 minutes ($P<.04$), stage REM minutes ($P<.03$), and total REM activity ($P<.02$). We also reported a significant group and night interaction for full-night REM density ($P<.02$) in which the group with MDD-E exhibited a variant pattern across nights vs the group with MDD-NE and the control group.

The English literature reporting associations between REM sleep measures and MDD among younger cohorts (ie, prepubertal, adolescent, and young adult cohorts) is divided. Puig-Antich et al[2] reported no REM sleep differences between a group of prepubertal children with MDD (ie, MDD-E and MDD-NE) and 2 groups of control children who did not have MDD. Although not a focus of that article, it was noted that REM densities for the first REM period during the second night of sleep differed significantly (ANOVA, $P<.006$). The 2 groups with MDD were at either end of the continuum; the densities of the group with MDD-NE were the highest (mean±SD, 3.07±1.01), and the densities of the group with MDD-E were the lowest (2.02±0.82). The densities of the 2 non-MDD control groups were intermediary. Dahl et al[3] also reported no notable sleep differences between prepubertal children with MDD and control children. Lahmeyer et al[4] and Kutcher et al[5] reported a shorter REM latency and increased REM density in older adolescents with MDD vs adolescent controls, and Emslie et al[6] reported shortened REM latency among hospitalized children (age, 8-13 years) with MDD compared with age-matched control subjects. Kutcher et al[5] reported a shorter REM latency among young adults with MDD than young adult controls. However, Appelboom-Fondu et al,[7] Taub et al,[8] Hawkins et al,[9] Kempenaers et al,[10] and Kupfer et al[11] found no differences in REM sleep between adolescents and young adults with MDD and adolescent and young adult controls. However, individual REM period parameters were not reported in most of these articles because these parameters were not yet under regular scrutiny.

Dahl et al[12] and Goetz et al[13] reported no sleep differences between adolescents and young adults with MDD and adolescent and young adult controls; however, in both articles, a subgroup analysis revealed notably increased REM density among adolescents with MDD who were suicidal. Lauer et al[14] suggested that REM density rather than REM latency may better differentiate younger cohorts with MDD from age-matched controls. In 2 recent articles, Dahl et al[15] first reported that the cholinergic REM induction test resulted in a shorter REM latency among children with MDD than control children. Second, Dahl et al[16] showed that adherence to a uniformly imposed sleep-awake schedule (among adolescents with MDD and control adolescents) prior to obtaining laboratory sleep measures yielded longer sleep latency and shorter REM latency among the adolescents with MDD.

The first night in the sleep laboratory is usually considered a night of adaptation and is generally excluded from analysis. Furthermore, any night involving an invasive intervention (ie, an indwelling catheter) can affect sleep characteristics and should also be excluded from analysis, unless the focus is on night effects. During the mid-1980s, individual REM period parameters, such as REM density, were not routinely analyzed and reported; however, in light of recent articles, these measures are undergoing routine scrutiny.

During the reanalysis of this polysomnographic data, we learned that we may have made a Type II error having used the RM-ANOVA analytic scheme. Thus, we report the results of a reanalysis of the data originally reported by Goetz et al[1] with some modifications. Because the RM-ANOVA revealed notable adaptation and catheter night effects, we focus on only night 2 sleep data. This resulted in the inclusion of 3 additional subjects with MDD (who were missing either night 1 or 3 data). We also analyzed for group effects in 2 ways: (1) by maintaining the endogenous and nonendogenous subgroupings and (2) by grouping all subjects with MDD.

This reanalysis of only night 2 sleep parameters yielded results identical to the earlier article, in which the 3-night RM-ANOVA was used; the exceptions were new findings for REM density and REM density during the first REM period. The full-night mean (SD) REM densities were 3.11 (0.80), 3.01 (0.80), and 2.75 (0.78) for the subjects with MDD-E, the subjects with MDD-NE, and the control subjects, respectively; no notable differences were found. However, when the 2 groups with MDD were grouped, the full-night REM densities were marginally higher among the group with MDD (n=47) than the control group (n=37): 3.06 ± 0.79 vs 2.75 ± 0.78 ($t=1.83$, $df=82$, $P<.07$). Rapid eye movement densities during the first REM period differed marginally for the 3-group analysis: subjects with MDD-E (n=27), 2.32 (0.98); subjects with MDD-NE (n=25), 2.40 (1.01); and control subjects (n=38), 1.93 (0.76) ($f=2.83$, $df=2,89$, $P<.07$). For the 2-group analysis, the combined groups with MDD exhibited a significantly higher REM density during the first REM period than the control group: 2.36 ± 0.98 vs 1.93 ± 0.76 ($t=2.27$, $df=88$, $P<.03$).

This reanalysis is based on a single night of sleep data, the second consecutive night of sleep during a 3-night series. In this context, the stability of the finding may be questioned, and the data may be subject to the effects of differential "first night" effects. This remains a caveat, although in the report by Goetz et al[1] the REM densities did not differ between the groups across nights 1 and 2.

This reanalysis highlights 2 issues. While the endogenous-nonendogenous subtyping is no longer heuristic, it would seem from the study by Puig-Antich et al[2] and this reanalysis that this subtyping may be important in prepuberty, as these MDD subtypes were so different from each other in REM density during the first REM period. However, these subtypes were similar in adolescents. This is another indication that maturation must play a role in the association between sleep abnormalities and the depressive syndrome. Furthermore, it would seem that our earlier analytic method resulted in a Type II error, and this reanalysis stands as a replication of recent articles in which an association between MDD and REM density during the first REM period was found. We concur with Lauer et al[14] and Reynolds and Kupfer[17] that REM density during the first REM period may be a better candidate as a biological marker than is REM latency, particularly among younger cohorts.

Raymond R. Goetz, PhD
Susan I. Wolk, MD
Jeremy D. Coplan, MD
Myrna M. Weissman, PhD
Columbia University College of Physicians and Surgeons
New York State Psychiatric Institute
722 W 168th St
New York, NY 10032
Ronald E. Dahl, MD
Neal D. Ryan, MD
Pittsburgh, Pa

This study was supported by grant MH-50666 (Dr Weissman) and Clinical Research Center grant MH-43878 (Dr Shaffer) from the National Institutes of Mental Health, Bethesda, Md.

1. Goetz RR, Puig-Antich J, Ryan N, Rabinovich H, Ambrosini P, Nelson B, Kawiec V. Electroencephalographic sleep of adolescents with major depression and normal controls. *Arch Gen Psychiatry.* 1987;44:61-68.
2. Puig-Antich J, Goetz R, Hanlon C, Tabrizi MA, Davies M, Weitzman ED. Sleep architecture and REM sleep measures in prepubertal children with major depression. *Arch Gen Psychiatry.* 1982;39:932-939.
3. Dahl RE, Ryan ND, Birmaher B, Al-Shabbout M, Williamson D, Neidig M, Nelson B, Puig-Antich J. Electroencephalographic sleep measures in prepubertal depression. *Psychiatry Res.* 1991;38:201-214.
4. Lahmeyer HW, Poznanski EO, Bellur SN. EEG sleep in depressed adolescents. *Am J Psychiatry.* 1983;140:1150-1153.
5. Kutcher S, Williamson P, Marton P, Szalai J. REM latency in endogenously depressed adolescents. *Br J Psychiatry.* 1992;161:399-402.
6. Emslie GJ, Rush JA, Weinberg WA, Rintelmann JW, Roffwarg HP. Children with major depression show reduced rapid eye movement latencies. *Arch Gen Psychiatry.* 1990;47:119-124.
7. Appelboom-Fondu J, Kerkofs M, Mendlewicz J. Depression in adolescents and young adults: polysomnographic and neuroendocrine aspects. *J Affect Disord.* 1988;14:35-40.
8. Taub JM, Hawkins DR, Van de Castle RL. Electrographic analysis of the sleep cycle in young depressed patients. *Biol Psychol.* 1978;7:203-214.
9. Hawkins DR, Taub JM, Van de Castle RL. Extended sleep (hypersomnia) in young depressed patients. *Am J Psychiatry.* 1985;142:905-910.
10. Kempenaers C, Kerkhofs M, Linkowski P, Mendlewicz J. Sleep EEG variables in young schizophrenic and depressed patients. *Biol Psychiatry.* 1988; 24:828-833.
11. Kupfer DJ, Frank E, Ehlers CL. EEG sleep in young depressives: first and second night effects. *Biol Psychiatry.* 1989;25:87-97.
12. Dahl RE, Puig-Antich J, Ryan ND, Nelson B, Dachille S, Cunningham SL, Trubnick I, Klepper TP. EEG sleep in adolescents with major depression: the role of suicidality and inpatient status. *J Affect Disord.* 1990;19:63-75.
13. Goetz RR, Puig-Antich J, Dahl RE, Ryan ND, Asnis GM, Rabinovich H, Nelson B. EEG sleep of young adults with major depression: a controlled study. *J Affect Disord.* 1991;22:91-100.
14. Lauer CJ, Riemann D, Wiegand M, Berger M. From early to late adulthood: changes in EEG sleep of depressed patients and healthy volunteers. *Biol Psychiatry.* 1991;29:979-993.
15. Dahl RE, Ryan ND, Perel J, Birmaher B, Al-Shabbout M, Nelson B, Puig-Antich J. Cholinergic REM induction test with arecoline in depressed children. *Psychiatry Res.* 1993;51:269-282.
16. Dahl RE, Ryan ND, Matly MK, Birmaher B, Al-Shabbout M, Williamson DE, Kupfer DJ. Sleep onset abnormalities in depressed adolescents. *Biol Psychiatry.* 1996;39:400-410.
17. Reynolds CF, Kupfer DJ. Sleep research in affective illness: state of the art circa 1987. *Sleep.* 1987;10:199-215.

REVIEWERS FOR 1996

The constituency of the ARCHIVES comprises a "university" of often interchangeable writers and readers, students, knowledgeable practitioners, and scholars of medicine and the sciences underlying the field of psychiatry. The editors are deeply grateful to the many colleagues listed below for their generous assistance in editorial critique and review. The donation of their special expertise is a necessary contribution on which intellectual standards in the field heavily depend.

Larry Abel
James Abelson
Robert Abrams
Gerard Addonizio
Daniel Aeschbach
W. Stewart Agras
Hagop S. Akiskal
Anne Marie Albano
Marilyn Albert
Georgios Alexopoulos
John S. Allen
Christer Allgulander
Margaret Altemus
Lori Altshuler
Jose Alvir
Jay Amsterdam
Connie Anders
George Anderson
Douglas H. Anglin
Adrian Angold
Burton Angrist
Jules Angst
Lawrence Annable
James C. Anthony
Ray Anton
William Apfeldorf
Paul Appelbaum
Stephan Arndt
Stephen Arnold
Robert Asarnow
Marie Asberg
Wesson Ashford
Boris Astrachan
Thomas Babor
Lee Baer
James C. Ballenger
Russell A. Barkley
David Barlow
Miron Baron
Herbert Barry III
John J. Bartko
Lance Bauer
Mark Bauer
Andrew Baum
Lewis Baxter
Mace Beckson
Allan Beigel
Morris Bell
Alan S. Bellack
Laura Bellodi
Ruth Benca
Elisa Benedek
Francine Benes
Chawki Benkelfat
Neal Benowitz
Sarah Berga
Lisa Berkman
Karen Faith Berman
Paul C. Bermanzohn
Wade Berrettini
Joseph Biederman
Robert Bilder
Eric Bing
Hector Bird
Donald Black
Jack Blaine
R. Clifford Blair
Randy Blakely
Jack Blanchard
Dan G. Blazer
Susan Blumenthal
Michael Borenstein
Gilbert Botvin
Constance M. Bowe
David Braff
Devra L. Braun
Xandra O. Breakefield
Alan Breier
Hans Breiter
David Brent
Naomi Breslau
Timothy D. Brewerton
W. E. Broadhead
Jonathan Brodie
Scott E. Brodie
Evelyn Bromet
David Brook
Judith S. Brook
Fred Brookstein
C. Hendricks Brown
George W. Brown
Gregory M. Brown
Tim Brown
Walter Armin Brown
Pollock Bruce
Gerard E. Bruder
Robert W. Buchanan
Kathy Bucholz
Monte Buchsbaum
Jan Buitelaar
William E. Bunney
Jack D. Burke
Greg Burkhardt
Audrey Burnam
Barbara J. Burns
Nelson Butters
Daniel Buysse
Alexander Bystritsky
John Cacciola
Remi Cadoret
Eric Caine
Oliver G. Cameron
Tyrone D. Cannon
Dennis Cantwell
Gabrielle Carlson
Bernard J. Carroll
Kathleen M. Carroll
Cameron Carter
Rosland Cartwright
Daniel E. Casey
Ned Cassem
Verne Caviness
Aravinda Chakravarti
Dennis S. Charney
Ching-Piao Chien
Anna R. Childress
John Clarkin
Paula Clayton
Brett Clementz
Emil Coccaro
C. Edward Coffey
Donald Cohen
Jonathan Cohen
Robert Cohen
Steve Cole
D. Jackson Coleman
David E. Comings
Robert Conley
Edwin H. Cook
Judith Cook
Jody Corey-Bloom
William Coryell
Jane Costello
Eric Courchesne
Rex Cowdry
P. J. Cowen
Paul Crits-Christoph
Tim Crow
Raymond Crowe
Thomas Crowley
John Csernansky
Jeffrey Cummings
Charles Czeisler
Pal Czobar
Mary F. Dallman
Michael Daniels
Anthony David
Jonathan Davidson
Lucy Davidson
Michael Davidson
Kenneth Davis
Michael Davis
Nancy Day
Claude De Montigny
Lynn DeLisi
Gustav Degreef
Pedro Delgado
Kevin Delucchi
William C. Dement
Edward Demet
Elena Khalsa-Dennison
D. P. Devanand
Darryl Devine
Mary Amanda Dew
Barbara Dickey
Steve Dinwiddie
Lisa Dixon
Bruce Dobkin
John Docherty
Nancy Docherty
Bruce Dohrenwend
R. J. Dolan
Robert Dorwart
Alan Douglass

Wayne Drevets
Sean Drummond
David Dunner
Renee Dupont
Mary Durham
Maureen Durkin
Felton Earls
Charmane Eastman
William Eaton
Lindon Eaves
Craig Edelbrock
Cindy L. Ehlers
Burr Eichelman
Everett H. Ellinwood
Graham J. Emslie
Jean Endicott
Mary Jane R. England
Sherrie Epstein
Javier Escobar
Susan Essock
Christopher Evans
Dwight Evans
John L. Fahey
Christopher Fairburn
Stephen Faraone
Lars Farde
Kym Faull
Jan Fawcett
Michael Feil
George Fein
Michael Fendrich
Wayne S. Fenton
David M. Fergusson
John D. Fernstrom
Steven Ferris
Max Fink
Joseph J. Fins
Marion Fischman
Barbara Fish
Baruch Fishman
Michael Flaum
Stephen Fleck
Jack M. Fletcher
Kenneth Fletcher
Edna B. Foa
Marshal F. Folstein
Judith Ford
Gary Foster
Allen Frances
Richard Frank
Jean Frazier
Robert Freedman
Arnold J. Friedhoff
David Friedman
Lee Friedman
Richard A. Friedman
C. D. Frith
Paul Fudala
David Fulker
Ray Fuller
Joaquin M. Fuster
Abby Fyer
Kenneth D. Gadow
Guillaume Galbaud du Fort
Rohan Ganguli
Linda Ganzini
Jordan Garber
Charles Gardner
Tom Garrick
Marjorie Garvey
Constatine Gatsonis
Frank Gawin
Alan Gelenberg
Joel Gelernter
Elliot Gershon
Robert D. Gibbons
Jay Giedd
Donna Giles
Christopher Gillberg
J. Christian Gillin
Michael Gitlin
Alexander Glassman
William Glazer
James Gold
Phillip W. Gold
Terry E. Goldberg
Jacqueline M. Golding
David Goldman
Howard Goldman
Patricia Goldman-Rakic
Jill Goldstein
Michael Goldstein
Rise B. Goldstein
Wayne Goodman
Donald Goodwin
David Gorelick
Jack Gorman
Irving Gottesman
Allan Gottschalk
Madelyn Gould
Igor Grant
John Greden
Michael Green
Benjamin D. Greenberg
David Greenblatt
Shelly Greenfield
Laurence Greenhill
Joel Greenhouse
Steven Greenwald
Tom Greider
John H. Greist
Christine Grella
Michael Grundman
John G. Gunderson
Raquel Gur
Thomas Gutheil
Donald Guthrie
Barry Guze
Samuel Guze
Harry E. Gwirtsman
Gretchen Haas
Henry Haigler
Angelos Halaris
Uriel Halbreich
Katherine Halmi
Stephan B. Hamann
Martin Harrow
John A. Harvey
Ruth S. Hassanein
Richard Hauger
Daniel Healey
Robert Heaton
Stephan Heckers
Don Hedecker
Larry Hedges
Martti Heikkinen
Gary Heiman
John E. Helzer
Herbert Hendin
Robert Hendren
Hugh Hendrie
George Heninger
Henry Henk
Jack E. Henningfield
Markus Henriksson
Margaret Hertzig
Victor Hesselbrock
J. D. Higley
Elizabeth Hill
Robert Hirschfeld
Susan Hodge
Rudolf Hoehn-Saric
Myron Hofer
Gerard E. Hogarty
Ann Hohmann
Henry Holcomb
Theodore Holford
Jimmie C. Holland
Eric Hollander
Florian Holsboer
Philip Holzman
James Hudson
John Hughes
Carroll W. Hughs
Steven W. Hurt
William G. Iacono
Thomas R. Insel
Goran B. Isacsson
Erkki Isometsa
Barry L. Jacobs
Jerome H. Jaffe
Kay Jamison
David M. Janowsky
Lissy Jarvik
Daniel C. Javitt
Peter Jensen
Terry Jernigan
Dilip Jeste
Tong Joh
Michael R. Johnson
Robin Johnson
Allison Jones
Edward Jones
Reese Jones
Jeffrey N. Joyce
Peter R. Joyce
Lewis L. Judd
Charles Kaelber
Bruce Kagan
Jerome Kagan
Tatsu Kakuma
Anthony Kales
Kyle Kampman
Denise Kandel
John Kane
Hooshang Kangarloo
Tzu-Cheg Kao
Bert Kaplan
Byram Karasu
Marvin Karno
Wayne Katon
Charles Kaufman
Walter Kaye
Jurgen Kayser
Sheppard Kellam
Kelly Kelleher
Adrienne Keller
Martin Keller
Steven Keller
John Kelsoe
Kenneth Kendler
Cille Kennedy
James Kennedy
John Kennedy
Robert S. Kern
P. A. Kernan
Andrew Kertesz
David A. Kessler
Ronald Kessler
Terrence Ketter
Kenneth Kidd
Joel Killen
Kathleen Kim
L. Erlenmeyer-Kimling
Daniel Kindlon
Dennis K. Kinney
Herbert D. Kleber
Rachel G. Klein
Arthur Kleinman
Joel Kleinman
C. J. Klett
James H. Kocsis
Paul Koegel
Alex Kopelowicz
Lorrin Koran
Ania Korszun
Thomas Kosten
Maria Kovacs
Rachel Kramer
Henry Richard Kranzler
Daniel F. Kripke
Ziad Kronfol
Marcus Kruesi
John Krystal
Michael J. Kuhar
Walter Kukull
Sanjiv Kumra
Samuel Kuperman

Y. Kyroda
Asenath LaRue
Ben Lahey
H. Richard Lamb
Douglas R. Langbehn
Philip Lavori
James Leckman
Julian Leff
Tony Lehman
Andrew Leon
Francois Lesperance
Bennett Leventhal
Harvey S. Levin
Louise Levine
Robert A. Levine
Seymour Levine
Douglas F. Levinson
Deborah Levy
David Lewis
Alfred Lewy
Robert Liberman
Jeffrey A. Lieberman
Michael Liebowitz
Greg Light
Marsha Linehan
Walter Ling
Markku Linnoila
Don H. Linszen
Deborah Lipschitz
Jouko Lonnquist
Peter T. Loosen
Armand Loranger
Lester Luborsky
Christopher Lucas
Daniel Luchins
R. Bruce Lydiard
Jeffrey M. Lyness
Eleanor Maccoby
Michael Maes
Kathy Magruder
Alain Malafosse
Kevin Malone
Husseini K. Manji
J. John Mann
Willard Manning
Salvatore Mannuzza
Joseph Marcus
Stephen Marder
Jeffrey Steven Markowitz
John Markowitz
Isaac Marks
Frederick Marsteller
Peter Martin
Mauri Marttunen
Barbara Mason
Aleksander Mathe
Roy J. Mathew
Karen Mathews
Steven Matthysse
Matig Mavissakalian
Jeffrey Max
P. Anne McBride
Robert W. McCarley
Joan McCord
James T. McCracken
Christopher J. McDougle
Susan L. McElroy
Bruce S. McEwen
Thomas P. McGlashan
Patrick McGrath
Peter McGuffin
Michael McGuire
James McKay
William McKinney
A. Thomas McLellan
James Meador-Woodruff
Sarnoff Mednick
Paul E. Meehl
Nancy Mello
Herbert Y. Meltzer
David B. Menkes
Kathleen Merikangas
Roger Meyer
Dieter Meyerhoff
Barnett Meyers
Enrico Mezzacappa
Robert Michels
Andrew Miller
Betty Miller
Frank T. Miller
Robert B. Millman
Mark Mintin
Jim Mintz
James E. Mitchell
Steven Moldin
Margaret Moline
John Monahan
Barry Morenz
Randi Morgan
Hal Morgenstern
Eve K. Moscicki
James M. Mountz
Timothy I. Mueller
Laura Mufson
Kevin Muldoon
M. F. Muldoon
Declan Murphy
Dennis Murphy
George Murphy
Jane Murphy
Robin M. Murray
Bengt Muthen
Henry A. Nasrallah
J. Craig Nelson
Charles Nemeroff
David A. Nielsen
Eric A. Nofzinger
Thomas Nordahl
Carol North
Russell Noyes
Keith Nuechterlein
Edward Nunes
John I. Nurnberger
David Nutt
Svante Nyberg
Eadbhard O'Callaghan
Stephanie O'Malley
Daniel Offer
David R. Offord
Mark Olfson
John W. Olney
J. Ormel
Edward Ornitz
Jurg Ott
Michael Otto
John E. Overall
Andrew J. Pakstis
Carmine H. Pariante
Gordon Parker
Robert Pasnau
Gavril Pasternak
Paresh Patel
Steven M. Paul
David Pauls
Godfrey D. Pearlson
Giampaolo Perna
Stephen J. Peroutka
Helen Pettinati
Jay Pettegrew
Frederick Petty
Cynthia Pfeffer
Adolf Pfefferbaum
David Pickar
Roy Pickens
Carl F. Pieper
Teresa Pigott
Kathleen Pike
Paul Pilkonis
Harold Pincus
Roger Pitman
Robert Plutchik
Russell Poland
John Polich
Simcha Pollack
Harrison G. Pope
Michael Popkin
Joel Posener
Michael Posner
Robert Post
Steve Potkin
Arthur Prange
Sheldon H. Preskorn
Lawrence H. Price
Jim W. Prichard
Robert Pynoos
Bruce Quinn
Frederic Quitkin
Bruce S. Rabin
Peter Rabins
Judith Rabkin
George K. Radda
Marcus E. Raichle
Adrian Raine
Michael J. Raleigh
Stanley Rapoport
Allen Raskin
Scott Rauch
Rebecca Rausch
D. Eugene Redmond
Darrel Regier
Theodore Reich
David Reiss
Martin Reite
Charles F. Reynolds
Howard Rhoades
George Ricaurte
John P. Rice
Charles Rich
John Richters
Arthur Rifkin
Craig Risch
Neil Risch
Rosalinda Roberts
Marjorie Robertson
Lee Robins
Delbert Robinson
Donald Robinson
Robert Robinson
Joseph Rochford
Howard P. Roffwarg
William Rogers
Dan Rojas
Steven Romano
Jed Rose
Jerrold Rosenbaum
James E. Rosenberg
Stanley D. Rosenberg
Norman E. Rosenthal
Christopher Ross
Kevin Roth
Thomas Roth
Walton Roth
John Rotrosen
Bruce Rounsaville
Alec Roy
Peter Roy-Byrne
John Rubenstein
Donald Rubin
Robert Rubin
Mathew Rudorfer
Judith Rumsey
Agnes Rupp
A. John Rush
Andrew T. Russell
Megan Rutherford
Michael Rutter
Neal D. Ryan
Harold Sackeim
Bruce Sales
Khalil Saliba
Carl Salzman
Elaine Sanders-Bush
James Sands
Michael Sanfilipo
Robert Sapolsky
Paul Satz
Cary Savage
Andrew Saykin

Lawrence Scahill
Richard Scheffler
Susan Schenk
Joseph Schildkraut
Thomas E. Schlaepfer
Nina Schooler
Marc Schuckit
Herbert Schulberg
Susan K. Schultz
S. Charles Schulz
Jeffrey Schwartz
Goran Sedvall
Mary Seeman
Phillip Seeman
Steven P. Segal
William Seiple
Edward M. Sellers
Edward C. Senay
Walt Senterfitt
David Servan-Schreiber
Erich Seifritz
Sally Severino
Richard I. Shader
David Shaffer
David Shapiro
Theodore Shapiro
Steven S. Sharfstein
Katherine Shear
David V. Sheehan
Martha Shenton
James Shore
Patrick E. Shrout
Carol Siegel
Larry Siever
Soren Sigvordsson
David Silbersweig
Gregory Simon
George Simpson
John Simpson
Samuel G. Siris
Andrew E. Skodol
William Sledge
G. Richard Smith
Gwen Smith
William Sobel
Paul H. Soloff
David Solomon
Susan Solomon
Steven Southwick
Sydney Spector
M. Anne Spence
David Spiegel
Lisa A. Spielman
Robert L. Spitzer
Herbert Spohn
Larry R. Squire
Stephen M. Stahl
Jeff A. Stanley
Larry Stark
Marvin Stein
Emily Stern
Yaakov Stern
Janice R. Stevens
Mark A. Stewart
David Stoff
Peter Stokes
Robert Stout
John Strauss
Michael Strober
Albert J. Stunkard
Roland Sturm
Maria Sullivan
Patrick Sullivan
Suzanne Sunday
Virgnia Susman
Ezra Susser
Victor W. Swayze
Susan Swedo
John Sweeney
Charles Swenson
Neil Swerdlow
Martin Szuba
Nori Takei
Hadassah Tamir
Carol Tamminga
Jody Tanabe
Peter E. Tanguay
Kenneth Tardiff
Pierre Tariot
C. Barr Taylor
Eric Taylor
Laurence Tecott
Linda Teri
Michael Terman
Leonore Terr
Gunvant Thaker
Leon Thal
Michael E. Thase
Haraldur Thorsteinsson
Allen Tien
Allan J. Tobin
John Travers
John Q. Trojanowski
Ming T. Tsuang
Gary Tucker
L. Lee Tynes
Thomas Uhde
E. H. Uhlenhuth
George Vaillant
Wilfred Van Gorp
Daniel Van Kammen
Jim van Os
Herman Van Praag
Bessel A. Van der Kolk
Frank C. Verhulst
Milton Viederman
Veronica Vieland
Benedetto Vitiello
Gerald Vogel
Jan Volavka
Nora Volkow
B. T. Volpe
Joseph R. Volpicelli
Antonia Vossen
Dale Walker
B. Timothy Walsh
Herbert Ward
Virginia Warner
Christine Waternaux
Stephen G. Waxman
Susan Waxman
Michael Weale
Tom Wehr
Thomas Weickert
Daniel Weinberger
Robert Weinreb
Sheldon Weintraub
Sheila Weiss
Michael Welch
Elizabeth J. Weller
Charles Wells
Kenneth Wells
K. M. A. Welsh
Paul H. Wender
Joseph Westermeyer
Peter Whybrow
Cynthia Wible
Priya Wickmaratne
Thomas A. Widiger
Janet B. W. Williams
G. Terrence Wilson
Ronald M. Winchel
Marilyn Winkleby
Andrew Winokur
George Winokur
Anna Wirz-Justice
Sandra Witelson
Hans-Ulrich Wittchen
Deane Wolcott
Adam Wolkin
Owen Wolkowitz
Ben Wolozin
Cheryl Wong
Dean F. Wong
Dona Wong
Catherine Woodman
Peter Woodruff
George Woody
Robert F. Woolson
Richard J. Wurtman
Richard Jed Wyatt
Joel Yager
Joe Yamamoto
Jerome A. Yesavage
Elizabeth Young
Robert Young
Robert Yu
Stuart Yudofsky
Theodore Zahn
Alan Zametkin
Vincent Zarcone
Mark Zimmerman
Robert Zipursky
Athanasios Zis
George Zubenko
Stephen R. Zukin

Announcement

Archives of General Psychiatry notes with great sadness the death of George Winokur, MD, on October 12, 1996. Dr Winokur had been an ARCHIVES Editorial Board member since 1975. His obituary will be published in a forthcoming issue of this journal.

EDITORIAL

Quality of Care

A Call for Papers for the Annual Coordinated Theme Issues of the AMA Journals

Of the many elemental management objectives of American health system reform, 3 have always stood out: control of cost, promotion of quality, and access for all to basic medical care. Many of us hoped to achieve all 3 of these major objectives in a comprehensive, organized, and timely way while preserving necessary patient and physician autonomy, promoting prevention, and emphasizing primary care, among other factors.[1]

Alas, such was not to be. What has happened? Cost control has been achieved in many sectors in large part because of the managed care revolution. Access has worsened. And quality is now under attack.[2,3]

The *JAMA* Editorial Board and senior staff and the editors of the *Archives* Journals have completed their annual Delphi process to identify and rank the most important topics for our journals to address in the upcoming year. Near the top was quality of care. Since quality cuts across all disciplines, we voted unanimously to dedicate substantial numbers of pages of all 12 of our publications (*JAMA*, 10 *Archives* Journals, and *American Medical News*) to the subject of quality of care in theme issues to be published late in 1997.

Some say that quality cannot be studied, cannot even be defined; they say that quality is in the eye of the beholder. However, the American Society for Quality Control disagrees, defining quality as "the totality of features and characteristics of a product or service that bears on its ability to satisfy given needs."[4] We agree with their definition, but in medicine we also need to address whose needs are being satisfied. We suggest that quality can only exist when information on medical options is freely communicated and the patient's own preferences determine the choice of appropriate care.

We suggest that interested authors consider the following principles of accountability to the public for health quality[5] as they prepare their report of studies and proposals for manuscripts for this special publishing event. (See reference 5 for expansions and explanations of these principles.)

- *The quality measures must be powerful enough to provide direction to the new American health system.*
- *The measures must anticipate the behavioral changes they induce.*
- *Patients' opinions and preferences should come first.*
- *It's time for outcomes accountability.*
- *The influence of health plans on the measures chosen should be minimized.*

So have at it, critics and gurus alike. Quality of health care in our country is everybody's concern and everybody's business. Some say that the managed care revolution will compromise, erode, and even threaten to destroy high-quality care. Others say the managed care revolution will promote quality of care as well as cost containment. Let us receive your best efforts—research articles, review articles, special communications, opinion pieces—for our consideration in our 12 publications. Since *JAMA* and *American Medical News* are weeklies and the *Archives* Journals are monthlies (except *Archives of Internal Medicine*, which is biweekly), there are no deadlines for the receipt of these articles about quality. However, in order to be given the best consideration for our publication at this common time in late 1997, manuscripts should be received at the appropriate editorial offices by March 1, 1997. Good luck, and we look forward to hearing from you.

George D. Lundberg, MD
John E. Wennberg, MD

This editorial is reprinted with permission from JAMA *(1996; 276:1514).*

REFERENCES

1. Lundberg GD. The failure of organized health system reform—now what? *JAMA.* 1995;273:1539-1541.
2. Angell M, Kassirer JP. Quality and the medical marketplace—following elephants. *N Engl J Med.* 1996;335:883-885.
3. Blumenthal D. Quality of care—what is it? *N Engl J Med.* 1996;335:891-894.
4. Lundberg GD. The 'new' AMA—a rededication to excellence. *JAMA.* 1986;256: 1038-1040.
5. Ellwood P, Lundberg GD. Managed care: a work in progress. *JAMA.* 1996; 276:1083-1086.

1960s:

Conventional antipsychotics radically alter traditional treatment methods

Mass deinstitutionalization

Large-scale shutdown of mental hospitals

Concepts of patient-oriented psychosocial rehabilitation introduced

Discoveries in medicine impact the healthcare system at every level. If the effects of medical breakthroughs are not managed appropriately, the system can sustain significant damage. In the latter half of this century we have seen evidence of this in psychiatry. In the 1960s the introduction of conventional anti-psychotics into a weak and rigid system caused severe and long-lasting problems. The advent of atypical agents in the 1990s threatens to do the same. How can we ensure that the existing mental healthcare system is flexible and strong enough to quickly adapt to the changes brought on by the atypicals?

Radical change wrought by conventionals.

The radical changes wrought by haloperidol and other conventional antipsychotics on the mental healthcare system are well documented. Before the introduction of these agents, patients generally experienced limited relief from their episodes of psychosis, and clinicians had few treatment options at their disposal. Conventional antipsychotics offered the first glimmer of hope by providing adequate control of positive symptoms. These agents brought a significant measure of calm and order to previously noisy and chaotic psychiatric wards.

Mass deinstitutionalization recognized as failure.

However, for a variety of social, economic, and political reasons, patients on conventional agents were deinstitutionalized before clinicians could design and implement rehabilitation programs to help them successfully reintegrate into the community. The failure of mass deinstitutionalization is now widely recognized. As all who work with the severely mentally ill know, the effect on many patients and their families has been tragic.

The advent of atypicals: dramatically raising expectations.

Analogous to the introduction of the conventional antipsychotics is the introduction of the atypical agents in the 1990s. Atypical agents, with their control of both positive and negative symptoms, have continued to raise patients' functioning to levels that facilitate reintegration back into the community.

Deficits of system limit potential for recovery.

The ability of the atypicals to restore significant patient functioning has served to highlight the flaws of the system. Often, patients on such therapies begin to outperform all functional expectations before the system is ready to help them develop their newly found skills and abilities.

Compounding the limitations of the mental healthcare system are outdated and misguided community and societal policies, attitudes, and beliefs. These severely restrict the opportunities available to a recovering patient.

System status quo unacceptable.

Clearly, the status quo of the mental healthcare system is unacceptable. Many inside and outside the system are devoted to changing the system, and some progress has been made. However, it is unfair to ask patients, who have already lost significant portions of their lives to mental illness, to wait any longer. Further, dedicated mental healthcare professionals must work within the confines of the system, and they cannot bridge the gaps alone. Finally, families and caregivers often shoulder the burden of providing what the system lacks—too often to the detriment of their own quality of life.

1990s:

Atypical antipsychotics dramatically raise expectations for recovery

Recognition of need to provide support to patient and family

Development of psychosocial rehabilitation programs

Emphasis on permanent reintegration of patients into community

A new approach to managing severe mental illness.

Comprehensive support at multiple levels would benefit patients, their families or caregivers, and professionals. One unique program has recently become available. PATHWAYS TO CHANGE™: managing severe mental illness, is a new comprehensive program of interdisciplinary interventions developed by Janssen Pharmaceutica in conjunction with premier thought leaders in the field. The stated goal of PATHWAYS TO CHANGE™ is to bridge the gaps in the system and raise the standard of care for all persons with severe mental illness.

PATHWAYS TO CHANGE™ is built around a framework known as the systems approach. According to the systems approach, although medication is the cornerstone of successful treatment, therapeutic interventions must occur at multiple levels beyond the adjustment of neuroreceptors for patients to become well, and remain well. Additional interventions must be implemented for patients with severe mental illness, their families and caregivers, the healthcare professionals who treat them, the communities in which they live, and society as a whole.

PATHWAYS TO CHANGE™ interventions.

Consistent with the systems approach model, PATHWAYS TO CHANGE™ interventions address the particular issues at each level that affect patients in their efforts to reach the full potential offered by innovative therapies.

- Following appropriate pharmacotherapy, interventions for patients include support to remain compliant, prevent relapse, maintain continuity of care, and help in their reintegration back into society
- Interventions for families, friends, or caregivers include facilitated access to information, education, and support groups
- Interventions for professionals are designed to help them surmount the challenges of the existing mental healthcare system through programs that enhance patient compliance and aid in patient discharge planning. Other programs will help facilitate case management, provide resources for information, and promote interprofessional collaboration
- Community and societal interventions are geared toward removing any barriers to reintegration. This is accomplished through support of patient advocacy organizations, public awareness, education, and antidiscrimination campaigns. An example of a societal-level intervention is NAMI's recently launched *Open Your Mind* campaign, for which Janssen Pharmaceutica is providing continuing support

It is only through support provided by these multilevel interventions that the patient with severe and persistent mental illness can successfully reintegrate into the community.

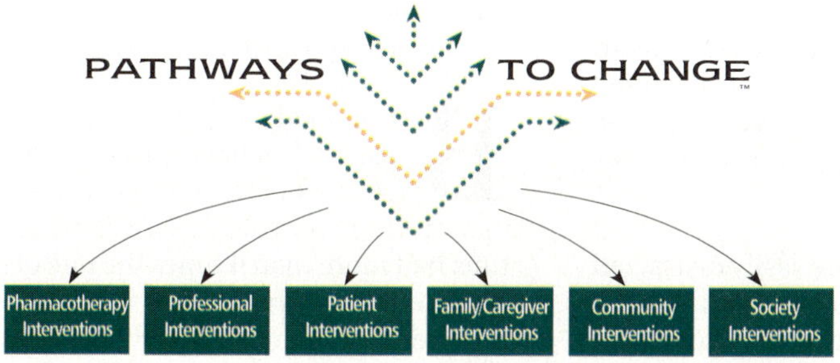

A comprehensive model of interdisciplinary interventions

Meeting the challenges of an evolving system.

We are experiencing an exciting and challenging revolution in the mental healthcare field. The pharmacologic breakthroughs we were waiting for have finally come, offering our patients the first real chance at reclaiming their lives. This revolution, however, is occurring in an atmosphere of cost-containment. We should be ever mindful to take full advantage of programs that provide comprehensive support to reintegrating patients. Indeed, such programs may become our most valuable tools as we meet the challenges of an evolving system.

JANSSEN · PHARMACEUTICA · RESEARCH FOUNDATION ·

JPI-RS-283 Printed in U.S.A. October 1996

ARCHIVES OF GENERAL PSYCHIATRY

Childhood-onset schizophrenia is a rare but severe form of the disorder that is often treatment refractory. In the first controlled trial of an atypical neuroleptic in very early-onset schizophrenia (psychotic symptoms documented before age 12 years), **Kumra et al** (page 1090) found clozapine to be clearly superior to haloperidol on all measures of psychosis and overall functioning. However, neutropenia and seizures were major concerns.

High expressed emotion (EE) predicts schizophrenic relapse. However, the determinants of EE have not been explored. **King** and **Dixon** (page 1098) tested a model suggesting that aspects of family dynamics underlie two components of EE and that these family variables influence symptoms—type and social adjustment in schizophrenic young adults. They found that family dynamics were unassociated with EE and that family adaptability was negatively associated with social adjustment. Higher levels of emotional overinvolvement were associated with better social adjustment 9 months later.

Studies of schizophrenia have identified many cognitive disturbances. **Servan-Schreiber et al** (page 1105) developed a computer simulation model of the brain mechanisms that may account for these disturbances, and tested this in a new behavioral study. They examined the performance of schizophrenic patients in a cognitive task that requires memory of previous events to guide behavior. Unmedicated schizophrenic patients, but not control subjects, had difficulty guiding their behavior based on such memory.

Many schizophrenic patients are easily distracted by irrelevant sensory information in their environment, a phenomenon that may be related to more complex symptoms such as auditory hallucinations. **Freedman et al** (page 1114) used electrophysiological methods to demonstrate diminished inhibition of the brain's response to repeated sounds in schizophrenia. Averaged evoked potentials recorded from patients and normal subjects, as well as single neuron activity recorded from laboratory animals, point to the loss of an inhibitory mechanism in the hippocampus, which could underlie the patients' distractibility.

Heinz et al (page 1123) found reduced sensitivity of central dopamine receptors, low levels of anxiety and depression, and a trend toward high novelty seeking in patients with alcoholism who had poor treatment outcome. High levels of novelty seeking and low harm avoidance were correlated with reduced control of alcohol intake, which interacted with dopamine receptor sensitivity. This study identifies behavioral correlates of increased relapse risk that may be targeted in future treatment programs.

The Great Smoky Mountains Study is a longitudinal epidemiologic study of youth aged 9 to 13 living in the southern Appalachians that focuses on the development of psychiatric disorders and the need for mental health services. **Costello et al** (page 1129) found that the 3-month prevalence of any *DSM-III-R* psychiatric disorder was 20.3% in this population. Poverty was prevalent (26%) and was the strongest demographic correlate of diagnosis. This study shows that child psychiatric disorders are as common in this rural area as in many urban areas.

In a separate paper from the same study, **Costello et al** (page 1137) examined serious emotional disturbance (SED), defined as a psychiatric diagnosis causing impaired functioning in 1 or more areas. Federal and state funding for mentally ill children is increasingly being restricted to those with SED. The authors found SED in 4% to 8% of children aged 9 to 13 years. Three of 5 children with SED (62.3%) reported no recent mental health care from any professional provider. Plans to target mental health care resources to children with SED need to ensure access to those resources.

Brent et al (page 1145) studied the extent to which suicidal behavior runs in the families of adolescent suicide victims compared with adolescent community controls. Relatives of adolescent suicide victims had more than 4 times the rate of suicide attempts and completions of the control relatives, even after considering the higher rates of psychiatric disorders in the relatives of the suicide victims. These findings suggest that liability to suicidal behavior may be familially transmitted independently of psychopathology.

The influence of psychosocial factors on suicide often is conjectured to be merely an epiphenomenon of psychiatric illness. **Gould et al** (page 1155) examined environmental, social, and familial characteristics of 120 child and teen suicides and a similar number of controls. Notable risks for suicide were derived from schoolwork problems, a family history of suicidal behavior, stressful life events, and poor father-child communication. Psychosocial factors increased suicide risk beyond the risk attributable to psychiatric illness, and such factors are a necessary part of a suicide risk assessment in teenagers.

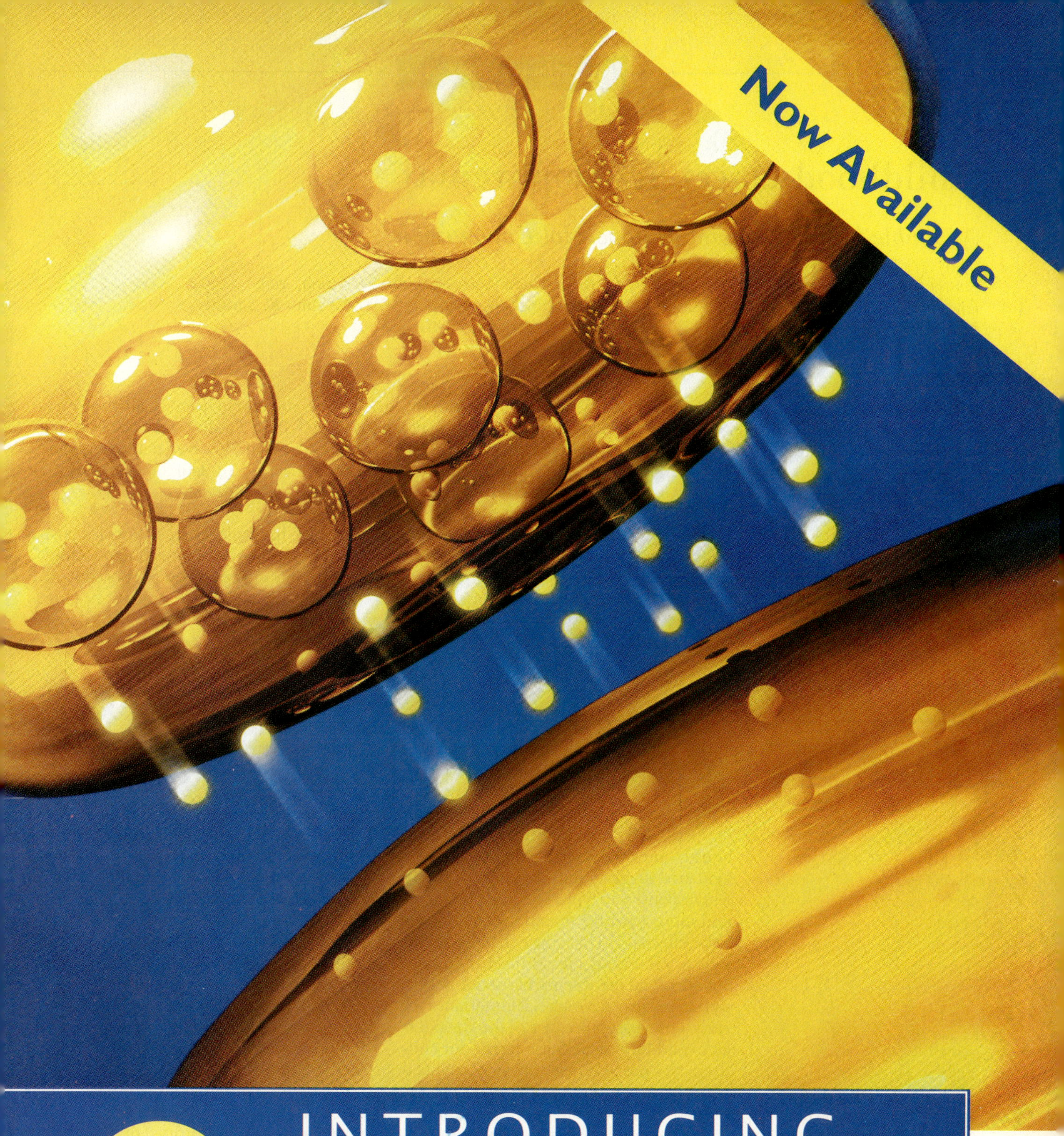
Now Available

Childhood-Onset Schizophrenia

A Double-blind Clozapine-Haloperidol Comparison

Sanjiv Kumra, MD; Jean A. Frazier, MD; Leslie K. Jacobsen, MD; Kathleen McKenna, MD; Charles T. Gordon, MD; Marge C. Lenane, MSW; Susan D. Hamburger, MA, MS; Amy K. Smith; Kathleen E. Albus; Javad Alaghband-Rad, MD; Judith L. Rapoport, MD

Background: Childhood-onset schizophrenia is a rare but severe form of the disorder that is often treatment-refractory. In this study, the efficacy and adverse effects of clozapine and haloperidol were compared for children and adolescents with early-onset schizophrenia.

Methods: Twenty-one patients (mean [±SD] age, 14.0±2.3 years) with onset of *Diagnostic and Statistical Manual of Mental Disorders, Revised Third Edition*–defined schizophrenia that began by age 12 years and who had been nonresponsive to typical neuroleptics participated in the study. Patients were randomized to a 6-week double-blind parallel comparison of clozapine (mean [±SD] final dose, 176±149 mg/d), or haloperidol, (16±8 mg/d).

Results: Clozapine was superior to haloperidol on all measures of psychosis (P=.04-.002). Positive and negative symptoms of schizophrenia improved. However, neutropenia and seizures were major concerns. To date, one third of the group has discontinued using clozapine.

Conclusions: Clozapine has striking superiority for positive and negative symptoms in treatment-refractory childhood-onset schizophrenia. However, due to possibly increased toxic effects in this pediatric population, close monitoring for adverse events is essential.

Arch Gen Psychiatry. 1996;53:1090-1097

From the Child Psychiatry Branch, National Institute of Mental Health, Bethesda, Md (Drs Kumra, Jacobsen, Alaghband-Rad, and Rapoport and Mss Lenane, Hamburger, Smith, and Albus); Harvard University School of Medicine, Boston, Mass (Dr Frazier); Northwestern University School of Medicine, Chicago, Ill (Dr McKenna); and University of Maryland School of Medicine, Baltimore (Dr Gordon).

CHILDHOOD-ONSET schizophrenia is a chronic disorder accompanied by a significant deterioration in adaptive functioning from already-impaired premorbid levels.[1-5] Some evidence suggests that these children are less responsive to typical neuroleptic agents and more sensitive to extrapyramidal adverse effects.[3,6-8] Thus, the enhanced therapeutic effects of clozapine for nonresponders and the absence of risk for tardive dyskinesia may have special importance for early-onset cases. Because of the considerable morbidity this illness carries for children, the possible usefulness of atypical neuroleptics for childhood-onset schizophrenia is of great interest.

Research in this field has been limited. Only 2 controlled trials of typical neuroleptics have been done in children with schizophrenia. The first, by Pool et al,[9] supported a modest but significant superiority of loxiapine (Loxitane) and haloperidol (Haldol) over placebo for 75 adolescents with schizophrenia. More recently, a placebo-controlled trial of haloperidol in children with schizophrenia found haloperidol superior to placebo on several measures.[10,11]

No controlled trials of atypical neuroleptics have been done in children or adolescents. Two large open-label, retrospective medical chart studies indicated that two thirds to three fourths of adolescents with treatment-refractory schizophrenia showed some degree of clinical improvement, and that 11% of adolescents showed a complete remission of symptoms during clozapine treatment. Clozapine seemed helpful for positive and negative symptoms, although, as with adult patients, certain negative symptoms such as anergy, mutism, and thought-blocking were less responsive to treatment.[12] About one fourth of these adolescent patients discontinued taking clozapine due to insufficient antipsychotic efficacy, deterioration of symptoms, or severe adverse effects.[13,14] These findings were limited by diagnostic heterogeneity, administration of clozapine with additional psychotropic drugs, inclusion of some

See Subjects and Methods on next page

SUBJECTS AND METHODS

STUDY DESIGN

Children and adolescents aged 6 to 18 years who had been diagnosed as having schizophrenia were sought by national recruitment through professional and patient advocacy organizations. Subjects were screened by at least 2 child psychiatrists (S.K., J.A.F., L.K.J., K.M., C.T.G., J.A.-R., or J.L.R.) at the Clinical Center of the National Institutes of Health, Bethesda, Md.[16]

Inclusion criteria were diagnosis of schizophrenia defined by the *Diagnostic and Statistical Manual of Mental Disorders, Revised Third Edition*,[17] with documented psychotic symptoms by age 12 years; intolerance, nonresponse, or both to at least 2 different neuroleptic drugs; and a full-scale IQ of 70 or higher. Exclusionary criteria were neurologic or medical disease. During a screening evaluation, children and families were interviewed for historical data, including a detailed developmental history. Diagnosis was determined using previous records and clinical and structured interviews, which included the Schedule for Affective Disorders and Schizophrenia for School-Age Children–Epidemiologic Version[18] and the Diagnostic Interview for Children and Adolescents–Revised.[19]

The protocol was approved by the Institutional Review Board at the NIMH, and each parent and child gave informed consent or assent before the child was entered into the study.

The study sample consisted of 21 patients (11 boys and 10 girls). Five of the 10 patients given clozapine and 6 of the 11 patients given haloperidol were boys. The group had considerable previous hospitalization and neuroleptic exposure (**Table 1**). On average, patients were receiving mean (±SD) 2.1±1.8 medications at the time of admission to the study. Most of the patients had received high doses of standard neuroleptics, risperidone, and several augmenting agents, including mood stabilizers and antidepressants. Almost all of the patients were pubertal at the time of the study. Other demographic and past psychiatric characteristics of the 2 groups are given in Table 1.

The mean (±SD) full-scale IQ, based on the best premorbid IQ or testing done at the NIMH, for the subjects who were testable (n=18) was 79±12. Many of the children were acutely ill at the time of testing, so these data are an underestimation of their true abilities based on earlier educational and developmental history. Three subjects could not be tested adequately due to the severity of their illness and inability to comply, although all had shown normal educational and developmental achievement before onset of psychosis.

PROCEDURE

On admission to the hospital, all medications were tapered during a 2-week period, followed by a 4-week drug-free interval as tolerated. A neurologic examination, medical and developmental evaluation, and psychometric testing and structured psychiatric interviews were carried out. Laboratory measures included an electroencephalogram (EEG), electrocardiogram, magnetic resonance imaging of the cerebrum, complete blood cell count, thyroid functions, liver chemistries, human immunodeficiency virus serologic tests, hepatitis screen, platelet serotonin levels, prolactin, lead levels, rapid plasma reagin, sedimentation rate, creatine kinase, toxicology screen, pregnancy test, and 24-hour urine collection for catecholamine metabolites. A lumbar puncture was performed and cerebrospinal fluid collected for analysis of monoamines and metabolites, antinuclear antibodies, and herpes simplex titers.

The 21 patients entering the double-blind study were

Continued on next page

adult patients, lack of a control group, and lack of standardized ratings.

A systematic, prospective, open trial of clozapine in 11 treatment-refractory adolescents with childhood-onset schizophrenia carried out at the National Institute of Mental Health (NIMH) rated the conditions of 75% of patients as improved compared with their condition on admission medication. Clozapine improved positive and negative symptoms, although sedation, hypersalivation, and weight gain were troublesome.[15]

To our knowledge, our study is the first double-blind study of clozapine for treatment-refractory children and adolescents with early-onset schizophrenia. We hypothesized that clozapine would be superior to haloperidol for this group. The adverse effects of both drugs also were compared.

RESULTS

Twenty-one patients enrolled in the study, of whom 20 completed the 4-week washout-baseline phase of the study; 1 patient required randomization to blinded medication after 1 week of the taper period due to clinical deterioration. Ten patients were randomly assigned to clozapine, 11 to haloperidol. The 2 medication groups did not differ significantly with respect to any demographic variables (Table 1). No significant differences were seen between clozapine and haloperidol baseline ratings, with the exception that the Bunney-Hamburg Rating Scale total score baseline variance was greater for the haloperidol group than for the clozapine group ($P<.03$) (Table 2).

Four patients did not complete the 6-week double-blind medication trial due to serious adverse events. Three patients discontinued taking medication during the fourth week of medication (2 receiving clozapine and 1 receiving haloperidol), and an additional patient interrupted clozapine treatment during week 5. For each of these patients, the final scores for the Bunney-Hamburg Psychosis Rating Scale, BPRS, and the Subjective Treatment Emergent Symptoms Scale were carried forward in the analysis of the data.

For the 21 patients, the mean (±SD) dose of medication at the last treatment week for haloperidol was 16±8 mg/d (range, 7-27 mg/d), or 0.29±0.19 mg/kg per day (range, 0.08-0.69 mg/kg per day) and clozapine, 176±149 mg/d (range, 25-525 mg/d) or 3.07±2.59 mg/kg per day (range, 0.34-7.53 mg/kg per day). The dose of medica-randomly assigned to a 6-week parallel treatment trial of clozapine (up to 525 mg/d) or haloperidol (up to 27 mg/d), as clinically indicated. Randomization was done by the National Institute of Health pharmacy using a table of random numbers. In addition to coded antipsychotic medication, patients prophylactically received benztropine mesylate tablets up to 6 mg/d (haloperidol group) or identical placebo tablets (clozapine group) to enhance the double-blind study. Dosing was done by the treating physician; physicians and nurses were unaware of the treatment assignment of each patient. A doctor of pharmacy with specialty training in psychiatry was aware of the treatment assignment and served as the clinical monitor for the study.

Clozapine doses were prescribed by the treating physician at 6.25 to 25 mg/d or haloperidol at 0.25 to 1.0 mg/d depending on the patient's weight. The smallest individual pill strength for clozapine was 6.25 mg and for haloperidol, 0.25 mg. Doses could be increased every 3 to 4 days by 1 to 2 times the starting dose on an individual basis.

EVALUATION OF EFFICACY

Weekly behavioral ratings were completed by a psychiatrist (S.K., J.A.F., L.K.J., C.T.G., or K.M.) during the course of the double-blind treatment (**Table 2**), using the Brief Psychiatric Rating Scale (BPRS)[20] and the Bunney-Hamburg Psychosis Rating Scale.[21] During weeks 1 and 4 of the drug-free baseline period and weeks 2 and 6 of the medication phase, additional rating instruments were completed, including the Children's Global Assessment Scale,[22] the Clinical Global Impressions (CGI) Scale,[23] the BPRS for Children (BPRS-C),[24] the Scale for the Assessment of Positive Symptoms,[25] and the Scale for the Assessment of Negative Symptoms.[26]

The 11 patients who were initially randomly assigned to haloperidol treatment subsequently received an open trial of clozapine and were rated in a similar fashion. Data for the CGI Scale and serious adverse effects for these patients is reported herein. All patients were contacted by telephone at regular intervals after discharge from the hospital and were seen in person after 2 years for a follow-up evaluation.

EVALUATION OF ADVERSE EFFECTS AND VITAL SIGNS

Adverse effects were evaluated weekly by the Subjective Treatment Emergent Symptoms Scale,[27] which was modified to include adverse events known to be associated with clozapine.[28] Extrapyramidal symptoms and involuntary movements were rated on the Abnormal Involuntary Movement Scale[29] and the Simpson-Angus Neurological Rating Scale.[30] In addition, weekly complete blood cell counts with differential, liver function tests, an encephalogram, and an electrocardiogram were done at baseline and at week 6.

DATA ANALYSIS

Analysis of covariance, using baseline measures as the covariate, was used to examine the differences between drug treatments at week 6 for all efficacy variables, using an SAS analysis of covariance program.[31] An "intent-to-treat" analysis was carried out for all patients who had a baseline assessment and at least 1 assessment after randomization, with the last observation carried forward, on the BPRS, Bunney-Hamburg Psychosis Rating Scale, and the Subjective Treatment Emergent Symptoms Scale. Incidents of adverse reactions were compared across groups using the χ^2 statistic. A *t* test was used to compare demographic data, baseline ratings, week 6 CGI Scale, and vital sign variables. Analysis of variance was used to compare the variances for all efficacy variables at baseline. All *P* values are 2-tailed, and statistical significance was set at the 5% level ($P<.05$).

tion at the last treatment week for the 7 patients receiving clozapine who successfully completed the treatment trial was 239±134 mg/d (range, 125-525 mg/d). Adverse effects that limited dose increase for both medication groups included tachycardia and sedation.

CLINICAL RESPONSE

In spite of small numbers, several end-point measures showed significant differences favoring clozapine. For the 4 overall indexes of improvement, clozapine was superior to haloperidol (Table 2 and **Table 3**). Clozapine also significantly decreased positive and negative symptoms of schizophrenia as measured on the Scale for the Assessment of Positive Symptoms and the Scale for the Assessment of Negative Symptoms. Cluster analysis of the BPRS-C (Table 3) disclosed a marked improvement in depression, social withdrawal, and thinking disturbance and a trend toward improvement in behavioral problems for the clozapine group.

The CGI Scale was also used to analyze the complete sample of patients in the study (open and double-blind trials of clozapine, n=21) for global improvement after 6 weeks of treatment with clozapine. This index uses a 7-point scale from 1, indicating very much improved, to 7, indicating very much worse to assess how much patients have benefited from a clozapine trial compared with their clinical condition at admission to the project. Of the 21 patients who had an open or blinded clozapine trial, the conditions of 2 (9.5%) were rated as very much improved, 11 (52.4%) as much improved, 7 (33%) as minimally improved, and 1 (4.8%) as worse.

EVALUATION OF ADVERSE EFFECTS AND VITAL SIGNS

Adverse reactions seen during the double-blind medication phase of the trial are given in **Table 4**; only the adverse effects that differed between the 2 drugs ($P<.05$) are reported. The adverse effect profiles of the 2 medications were similar except that drowsiness ($P<.04$) and salivation ($P<.02$) were greater with clozapine, while haloperidol produced more insomnia ($P<.03$). Weight, pulse, temperature, and blood pressure did not differ. Presumably, the extrapyramidal adverse effects of haloperidol were masked by the prophylactic benztropine. On the Simpson-Angus Neurological Rating Scale, only salivation was seen to increase, and only for the clozapine group. Similarly, the total score on the Abnormal Involuntary Movement Scale did not change for either group from baseline to the end of the medication phase of the trial.

More serious adverse events, however, were causes for concern throughout the trial (Table 3). Although no cases of agranulocytosis occurred, hematopoietic toxic effects were a major issue for clozapine. Five patients who received clozapine experienced a drop in the absolute neutrophil count below 1500 mm^3; for 3 of these patients, the white blood cell count normalized spontaneously. Two patients had to be dropped from the double-blind protocol at week 4 after neutropenia recurred with rechallenge. Although 1 of these patients was of Ashkenazi Jewish descent, the human lymphocyte antigen phenotype did not match the phenotypes that are known to be associated with an increased risk of clozapine-induced agranulocytosis.[32] Both of these patients were taking concomitant antibiotic medications during the medication phase of the study; 1 had been receiving amoxicillin before the first drop in absolute neutrophil count, and the other was receiving penicillin during the first rechallenge.

Two patients in the double-blind clozapine trial had clinically significant seizure activity: the first experienced myoclonus at the end of week 4 while receiving 400 mg/d of clozapine, followed by a tonic-clonic seizure the next day. Clozapine dosage was reduced and 3 different anticonvulsants were tried sequentially. No further seizures occurred, but the EEG continued to show epileptiform spikes, and use of clozapine was discontinued. A second patient experienced bifrontal and posterior delta-frequency slowing on the EEG at week 5. Three weeks after discharge from the hospital, this patient experienced tonic-clonic seizures while receiving 275 mg/d of clozapine. Clozapine dosage was lowered and valproate sodium was given, but the patient continued to have petit mal seizures, so use of clozapine was discontinued. Neither patient had preexisting epilepsy.

Of the 11 patients who received an open trial of clozapine, 3 required prophylactic anticonvulsant treatment. In each case, the child experienced EEG abnormalities in association with clinical deterioration (ie, increased aggression, psychosis, or irritability). After the clozapine dose was lowered and valproate was added, symptoms improved for 2 patients. The third patient, however, experienced facial myoclonus with associated cortical spikes on EEG and clinical deterioration, necessitating discontinuation of clozapine treatment.

Other adverse effects during clozapine treatment included one instance of 2- to 3-fold elevation in hepatic enzymes that was judged clinically significant. Two patients experienced a sinus tachycardia while receiving clozapine (heart rate >100 bpm) documented by electrocardiogram. Most patients tolerated the increase in heart rate, but 1 patient required the addition of atenolol during the open trial of clozapine.

One patient was dropped from the study in the fifth week of haloperidol treatment because of early signs of neuroleptic malignant syndrome. During a 48-hour period, liver transaminase levels were elevated (aspartate transaminase, 1083 U/L; alanine transaminase, 313 U/L; lactic dehydrogenase, 4030 U/L); the creatine kinase level rose to 83 000 U/L, and, when fractionated, was found

Table 1. Patient Characteristics for Clozapine-Haloperidol Comparison Trial*

	Treatment Group	
Characteristic	**Clozapine**	**Haloperidol**
Schizophrenia subtype		
Disorganized	5	5
Undifferentiated	5	5
Paranoid	0	1
Sex		
Male	5	6
Female	5	5
Age, y		
At time of NIMH study	14.40 (2.95)	13.73 (1.62)
At onset of psychosis	9.60 (2.22)	10.36 (1.36)
At first hospitalization	11.50 (3.17)	11.67 (2.00)
Duration of illness, y	4.75 (1.93)	3.42 (1.64)
Months of hospitalization	12.80 (16.91)	6.05 (7.38)
Months of neuroleptic treatment	28.70 (16.54)	17.73 (13.45)
Tanner stage	4.05 (1.12)	3.55 (1.13)

Values are given as number of patients and mean (±SD). No significant statistical differences were seen between groups. NIMH indicates National Institute of Mental Health.

Table 2. Clinical Ratings for Children and Adolescents With Childhood-Onset Schizophrenia at Baseline and During Clozapine and Haloperidol Treatment*

	Baseline		Week 6		ANCOVA		
Measure	**Clozapine (n=10)**	**Haloperidol (n=11)**	**Clozapine (n=10)**	**Haloperidol (n=11)**	**F**	***df***	***P***
Brief Psychiatric Rating Scale	83.7 (14.0)	84.7 (17.6)	52.5 (12.6)	64.7 (18.1)	5.1	2,20	.04†
Bunney-Hamburg Rating Scale	19.4 (2.8)	20.1 (6.0)	11.7 (3.3)	15.3 (3.8)	6.1	2,20	.02†
Scale for the Assessment of Negative Symptoms	77.9 (36.0)	83.0 (26.1)	46.0 (30.3)	72.2 (24.7)	13.4	2,16	.002†
Scale for the Assessment of Positive Symptoms	53.9 (25.8)	59.0 (24.9)	19.1 (11.7)	35.9 (15.6)	10.0	2,16	.01†
Children's Global Assessment Scale	26.3 (11.9)	23.2 (12.5)	44.9 (9.5)	27.9 (12.1)	9.2	2,16	.01‡
Abnormal Involuntary Movement Scale	14.7 (15.5)	14.0 (5.8)	12.1 (4.8)	12.2 (3.5)	0.01	2,15	.91
Simpson-Angus Neurological Rating Scale	12.1 (1.7)	11.9 (2.1)	12.0 (1.6)	13.9 (3.5)	1.6	2,15	.23

Except where indicated, values are given as mean (±SD). No significant differences were found between the 2 medication groups, except for the Bunney-Hamburg Rating Scale, for which the variance for the haloperidol group is greater than the clozapine group. ANCOVA indicates analysis of covariance.

†*Week 6 clozapine <week 6 haloperidol.*

‡*Week 6 clozapine >week 6 haloperidol.*

Table 3. Test Results for Children and Adolescents With Childhood-Onset Schizophrenia: Change Score From Weeks 0 to 6 of Medication Trial*

Measure	Treatment Group		t	P	Comments
	Clozapine (n=6)	Haloperidol (n=10)			
Brief Psychiatric Rating Scale					
Depression†	2.50 (2.59)	−0.60 (2.17)	2.58	.02	C>H
Thinking disturbance†	6.00 (2.45)	3.00 (2.83)	2.15	.05	C>H
Withdrawal†	4.50 (2.81)	1.00 (2.71)	2.47	.03	C>H
Anxiety	5.00 (2.53)	4.30 (3.50)	0.43	.68	C=H
Behavior problems	4.17 (3.49)	0.80 (3.22)	1.96	.07	C=H
Motor agitation	2.50 (1.64)	3.30 (3.02)	−0.59	.56	C=H
Organicity	2.00 (1.41)	0.60 (3.92)	1.02	.33	C=H
Total†	**26.67** (9.07)	**12.40** (12.08)	2.49	.03	C>H
Clinical Global Improvement Index‡	2.00 (0.58)	3.30 (1.49)	−2.50	0.03	C>H

**C indicates clozapine group; H, haloperidol group. Except where indicated, values are given as mean (±SD).*
†Baseline scores were subtracted from week 6 scores of medication trial.
‡For clozapine group, n=7.

to be 100% muscle; blood pressure was labile; confusion increased; no other neurologic symptoms were observed. With haloperidol discontinuation and supportive measures, vital signs and laboratory values normalized within a few days.

COMMENT

To our knowledge, this is the first controlled study of clozapine for children and adolescents with schizophrenia. Compared with patients who have later-onset schizophrenia, these patients have more severe premorbid abnormalities in language and motor development, premorbid psychiatric disorders, lower performance IQ, and a more severe and chronic course.[4,5,33] All had been nonresponsive to at least 2 typical neuroleptics.

Consistent with the greater disease severity experienced by this group, the level of baseline psychopathologic characteristics was higher than that previously reported for adult subjects of inpatient studies. For example, the mean (±SD) baseline BPRS total score in the present study was 84.2±15.6, whereas the mean baseline BPRS total scores in the studies by Kane et al[28] and Pickar et al[34] were 61±12 and 62±16, respectively.

The results of our study indicate that clozapine is superior to haloperidol for positive and negative symptoms in this population. In addition, we believe that clozapine was effective for primary negative symptoms, because our group had a low baseline level of extrapyramidal symptoms, yet we still observed a striking improvement in negative symptoms as measured by the Scale for the Assessment of Negative Symptoms. Our findings are consistent with the adult literature and the open and retrospective reports on clozapine for adolescents with treatment-refractory schizophrenia.[13,14,28,34-39] We believe that our sample is representative of treatment-refractory childhood schizophrenia reported in the literature.[3,33,36,39-41] The superiority of clozapine in this clinical trial is especially impressive in view of the small sample and severity of this group's illness.

Two children experienced a true awakening from their thought disorder and psychotic symptoms. One of these children, who had delusions, auditory hallucinations, multilated himself, and had other severe negative symptoms, had a complete remission of psychosis and behavioral problems after receiving clozapine and conversed in sentences for the first time in years. He now lives with his family, attends a day program regularly, and has been able to maintain friendships. Last year he successfully participated in 2 chess tournaments and enjoys taking nature walks.

For most children and adolescents in the study, clozapine improved interpersonal functioning and enabled a return to a less restrictive setting. Based on our continued monthly telephone contacts and interim history at 2-year follow-up, we believe that for some patients, maximal clozapine effects may not be seen until after 6 to 9 months of treatment, as reported for adults.[38,42,43] One child entered the project catatonic, internally preoccupied, and requiring constant highly skilled supervision to remain safe. She gradually responded to clozapine during the course of a year and became more spontaneously verbal, attended school regularly, and went shopping and on passes outside her residential treatment center to visit her mother.

Children and adolescents treated with clozapine need to be carefully monitored. We have continued to follow up the patients in this study. Thirteen patients have continued taking clozapine therapy for an additional mean (±SD) 30±15 months after completion of the study. Clozapine therapy has been stopped in 8 of our 21 patients because of seizures (n=3), hematological abnormalities (n=2), or treatment nonresponse (n=3). Two large, open, retrospective series of adolescents with schizophrenia report a dropout rate of 5% to 17% because of similar adverse events.[13,14] Whether our 38% dropout rate is a chance event or reflects the younger mean age of our sample with associated greater susceptibility to toxic effects of the drugs cannot be determined.

To date, 5 (24%) of the 21 patients enrolled in this study have experienced mild to moderate neutropenia. In adult patients, a cumulative risk of 1.5% to 2.0% of neutropenias has been estimated.[44] The risk for agranulocytosis has been reported to be higher in patients younger than 21 years compared with those between 21 and 40 years

Table 4. Most Frequent Side Effects and Adverse Reactions of Children and Adolescents With Childhood-Onset Schizophrenia During the 6-Week Double-blind Clozapine-Haloperidol Comparison Study*

Variable	Treatment Group: Clozapine (n=10)	Treatment Group: Haloperidol (n=11)	*P*	Comments
No. (%) of side effects				
Drowsiness	9 (90)	3 (27)	.04	C>H
Insomnia	0 (0)	4 (36)	.03	H>C
Salivation	7 (70)	2 (18)	.02	C>H
No. (%) of adverse reactions				
Tachycardia (resting heart rate of ≥100 bpm)	7 (70)	5 (45)	.26	
Drop in absolute neutrophil count	4 (40)	0 (0)	.02	C>H
Neuroleptic malignant syndrome	0 (0)	1 (9)	.33	
Seizures	1 (10)	0 (0)	.28	
Mean (±SD) vital signs†				
Weight change, kg	0.90 (6.47)	0.94 (2.89)	.986	
Blood pressure change, mm Hg				
Systolic	−1.6 (12.9)	3.27 (17.6)	.487	
Diastolic	−4.4 (14.3)	−7.00 (13.3)	.671	

*Only side effects in which P≤.05 are included from the Subjective Treatment Emergent Symptoms Scale (modified version). All 21 subjects were included in the analysis of side effects and adverse events. C indicates clozapine group; H, haloperidol group.

†Last week receiving drug minus baseline.

old.[32] The pharmacokinetics of clozapine metabolism also may be different for children compared with adults and may explain the differential incidence of toxic effects. When children metabolize clozapine, higher concentrations are produced of the metabolite *N*-desmethylclozapine, which has been associated with hematopoietic toxicity.[45,46]

As reported for adults,[47] 2 of our patients who were rechallenged with clozapine experienced a recurrence of neutropenia, which tended to happen more rapidly with rechallenge. Both patients were treated with concomitant penicillin or penicillin-related antibiotics during the course of clozapine treatment. One patient had received antibiotics before the first drop in the absolute neutrophil count, and the second patient received antibiotics during the first rechallenge. This suggests a possible drug interaction between clozapine and certain antibiotics, as has been previously suggested[48] and that caution must be used when treating patients receiving clozapine with other medications that can cause neutropenia.

Children and adolescents with schizophrenia treated with clozapine need to be carefully monitored for seizures. In a review by Freedman et al,[49] 3 (4%) of 80 clozapine-treated adolescents had seizures, while 32 (60%) of 53 patients experienced mild to marked epileptiform changes on EEG. To date, 6 (29%) of the 21 children in our sample required the addition of an anticonvulsant agent; 2 of these patients experienced tonic-clonic seizures. Devinsky and Pacia[50] reported that 1.3% of adult patients treated with clozapine had generalized tonic-clonic seizures during the first 6 months of therapy, and that myoclonic movements could progress to tonic-clonic seizures.[51,52]

Three patients in our study were given anticonvulsants after they became more irritable and aggressive and experienced epileptiform changes on EEG. These patients responded behaviorally to a lower dose of clozapine and the addition of valproate. Thus, in children, the EEG may be a sensitive indicator of clozapine toxicity as previously reported in adult studies.[53] In our study, none of the patients had a history of epilepsy. The rate of titration of clozapine in our study was comparable with the open and retrospective reports of clozapine for adolescents with treatment-refractory schizophrenia.[13,14,36,37,39,40]

The third major adverse effect of clozapine in our sample was weight gain. Adult patients treated with clozapine experience a significant weight gain during short- and long-term treatment with clozapine.[54,55] Our trial was too short to detect such a change, because weight gain was reported to be evident during weeks 8 to 16 of the clozapine trial.[54] Although our sample is small, the 2 best responders in the double-blind clozapine trial were the patients who had gained the most weight during the trial, consistent with similar reports in adults of an association between weight gain and improvement in BPRS score.[54]

Children and adolescents may be sensitive to the adverse effects of neuroleptics.[8,56,57] Supporting this hypothesis is evidence from open clinical trials with pediatric populations receiving risperidone (daily dose, 2-6 mg), which found that the incidence of serious adverse effects, including extrapyramidal side effects, weight gain, and galactorrhea, is high.[58]

Although the mean dose in this study for the haloperidol group is high compared with other reports (range, 1.80-9.8 mg/d),[9-11] our sample was unique in that all patients were treatment-refractory to typical neuroleptics, including haloperidol. The mean drug doses are not equivalent (by adult equivalence standards) because of an increased rate of tachycardia and serious adverse effects in the clozapine group, which lowered the overall mean dose of clozapine, and clinical nonresponse for positive symptoms in the haloperidol group, which resulted in a higher mean dose. The relatively high mean haloperidol dose could have mitigated the improvement in negative symptoms in the haloperidol group, but did not result in an increase in extrapyramidal adverse effects.

In summary, the superior efficacy of clozapine for the treatment of childhood-onset schizophrenia has considerable clinical importance. Childhood-onset schizophrenia is still poorly understood, but data from clinical phenomenology, smooth-pursuit eye movements, autonomic activity, and anatomic brain imaging suggest continuity with later-onset schizophrenia.[59-61] For children and adolescents with schizophrenia, the onset of their illness occurs during a period in which social and cognitive development is unfinished, resulting in more severe social disability.[62,63] The enhanced therapeutic effects for some and the beneficial adverse effect profile of clozapine has led to meaningful improvements in the course of their illnesses and long-term outcome.[64] Because children with schizophrenia who are receiving long-term treatment with typical neuroleptics risk up to a 4% chance of experiencing tardive dyskinesia,[65,66] the absence of tardive dyskinesia during clozapine treatment is a major advance.[67,68] For these reasons, the judicious use of clozapine for selected severely ill children and adolescents with schizophrenia is warranted. Ideally, benefits seen with clozapine treatment in children with schizophrenia will be maintained in the presence of even greater safety with some of the newer atypical antipsychotic drugs. Currently, the NIMH Childhood-Onset Schizophrenia Project is conducting clinical trials with these agents to test this hope.

Accepted for publication June 21, 1996.

We thank Eric Goldstein, PharmD; Sandoz Pharmaceuticals Corp, Hanover, NJ; and Pharmaceutical Developmental Services Clinical Section at the National Institutes of Health, Bethesda, Md, for their assistance in the provision of the blinded medications used in this study. We also thank Barbara Karp, MD, Dale Grothe, PharmD, David Pickar, MD, and Alan Breier, MD, for their support of and consultation to this project and the nurses of the Child Psychiatry Branch Inpatient Unit at the National Institutes of Health who cared for the patients in this study.

Reprints: Sanjiv Kumra, MD, FRCP(C), Child Psychiatry Branch, NIMH, Bldg 10, Room 6N240, 9000 Rockville Pike, Bethesda, MD 20892.

REFERENCES

1. McClellan J, Werry J. Practice parameters for the assessment and treatment of children and adolescents with schizophrenia. *J Am Acad Child Adolesc Psychiatry.* 1994;33:616-635.
2. Asarnow J, Tompson M, Goldstein M. Childhood-onset schizophrenia: a follow-up study. *Schizophr Bull.* 1994;20:599-617.
3. Green W, Gayol M, Hardesty A, Bassiri M. Schizophrenia with childhood onset: a phenomenological study of 38 cases. *J Am Acad Child Adolesc Psychiatry.* 1992;31:968-976.
4. Alaghaband-Rad J, McKenna K, Gordon C, Albus K, Hamburger S, Rumsey J, Frazier J, Lenane M, Rapoport J. Childhood-onset schizophrenia: the severity of premorbid course. *J Am Acad Child Adolesc Psychiatry.* 1995;34:1273-1283.
5. Gordon C, Frazier J, McKenna K, Giedd J, Zametkin A, Zahn T, Hommer D, Hong W, Kaysen D, Albus K, Rapoport J. Childhood-onset schizophrenia: an NIMH study in progress. *Schizophr Bull.* 1994;20:697-712.
6. Campbell M, Spencer E. Psychopharmacology in child and adolescent psychiatry: a review of the past five years. *J Am Acad Child Adolesc Psychiatry.* 1988;27:269-279.
7. Realmuto GM, Erickson WD, Yellin AM, Hopwood JH, Greenberg LM. Clinical comparison of thiothixene and thioridazine in schizophrenic adolescents. *Am J Psychiatry.* 1984;141:440-442.
8. Keepers G, Clappison V, Casey D. Initial anticholinergic prophylaxis for acute neuroleptic induced extrapyramidal syndromes. *Arch Gen Psychiatry.* 1983; 40:1113-1117.
9. Pool D, Bloom W, Mielke DH, Roniger JJ, Gallant DM. A controlled evaluation of loxitane in 75 adolescent schizophrenic patients. *Curr Ther Res.* 1976;19: 99-104.
10. Spencer EK, Kafantaris V, Padron-Gayol MV, Rosenberg CR, Campbell M. Haloperidol in schizophrenic children: early findings from a study in progress. *Psychopharmacol Bull.* 1992;28:183-186.
11. Spencer EK, Campbell M. Children with schizophrenia: diagnosis, phenomenology, and pharmacotherapy. *Schizophr Bull.* 1994;20:713-725.
12. Carpenter WT, Conley RR, Buchanan RW, Breier A, Tamminga CA. Patient response and resource management: another view of clozapine treatment of schizophrenia. *Am J Psychiatry.* 1995;152:827-832.
13. Schmidt M, Trott G, Blanz B, Nissen G. Clozapine medication in adolescents. In: Stefanis C, Rabavilas A, Soldatos C, eds. *Psychiatry: A World Perspective.* Proceedings of the VIII World Congress of Psychiatry. Belle Mead, NJ: Excerpta Medica-Princeton; 1989;1:1100-1104.
14. Remschmidt H, Schulz E, Martin M. An open trial of clozapine in 36 adolescents with schizophrenia. *J Child Adolesc Psychopharmacol.* 1994;4:31-41.
15. Frazier JA, Gordon CT, McKenna K, Lenane MC, Jih D, Rapoport JL. An open trial of clozapine in 11 adolescents with childhood-onset schizophrenia. *J Am Acad Child Adolesc Psychiatry.* 1994;33:658-663.
16. McKenna K, Gordon C, Lenane M, Kaysen D, Fahey K, Rapoport J. Looking for childhood-onset schizophrenia: the first 71 cases screened. *J Am Acad Child Adolesc Psychiatry.* 1994;33:636-644.
17. American Psychiatric Association. *Diagnostic and Statistical Manual of Mental Disorders, Revised Third Edition.* Washington, DC: American Psychiatric Association; 1987.
18. Orvaschell H, Tabrizi M, Chambers W. *Schedule for Affective Disorders and Schizophrenia for School-Age Children-Epidemiologic Version (Kiddie-SADS-E).* Philadelphia: Medical College of Pennsylvania, Eastern Pennsylvania Psychiatric Institute; 1987.
19. Reich W, Welner Z. *DICA-RC (DSM-III-R Version).* St Louis, Mo: Washington University; 1988.
20. Overall JE, Gorham DE. The Brief Psychiatric Rating Scale. *Psychol Rep.* 1961; 10:799-812.
21. Bunney WE, Hamburg DA. Methods for reliable longitudinal observation of behavior. *Arch Gen Psychiatry.* 1963;9:280-294.
22. Shaffer D, Gould MS, Brasic J, Ambrosini P, Fisher P, Bird H, Aluwahlia S. A Children's Global Assessment Scale (CGAS). *Arch Gen Psychiatry.* 1983;40: 1228-1231.
23. Guy W. *ECDEU Assessment Manual for Psychopharmacology.* Rockville, Md: US Dept of Health and Human Services; 1976.
24. Overall J, Pfefferbaum B. A Brief Psychiatric Rating Scale for Children. *Innovations.* 1984;3:264.
25. Andreasen NC. *The Scale for the Assessment of Positive Symptoms, (SAPS).* Iowa City: The University of Iowa; 1984.
26. Andreasen NC. *The Scale for the Assessment of Negative Symptoms (SANS).* Iowa City: The University of Iowa; 1983.
27. Campbell M, Palig M. Subjective Treatment Emergent Symptoms Scale (STESS). *Psychopharmacol Bull.* 1985;21:1063-1082.
28. Kane J, Honigfeld G, Singer J, Meltzer H. Clozapine for the treatment-resistant schizophrenia: a double-blind comparison with chlorpromazine. *Arch Gen Psychiatry.* 1988;45:789-796.
29. Rapoport J, Connors C, Reatig N. Rating scales and assessment instruments for use in pediatric psychopharmacology research. *Psychopharm Bull.* 1985; 21:713-1111.
30. Simpson G, Angus J. A rating scale for extrapyramidal side effects. *Acta Psychiatr Scand.* 1970;(suppl 212):9-11.
31. SAS Institute. *SAS Language and Procedures: Usage, Version 6, First Edition.* Cary, NC: SAS Institute Inc; 1989.
32. Alvir JM, Lieberman JA, Safferman AZ, Schwimmer JL, Schaaf JA. Clozapine-induced agranulocytosis. *N Engl J Med.* 1993;329:162-167.
33. Yang PC, Liu CY, Chiang SQ, Chen JY, Lin TS. Comparison of adult manifestations of schizophrenia with onset before and after 15 years of age. *Acta Psychiatr Scand.* 1995;91:209-212.
34. Pickar D, Owen RR, Litman RE, Konicki E, Gutierrez R, Rapoport MH. Clinical and biologic response to clozapine in patients with schizophrenia: crossover comparison with fluphenazine. *Arch Gen Psychiatry.* 1992;49:345-353.
35. Breier A, Buchanan RW, Kirkpatrick B, Davis OR, Irish D, Summerfelt A, Car-

penter WT. Effects of clozapine on positive and negative symptoms in outpatients with schizophrenia. *Am J Psychiatry.* 1994;151:20-26.
36. Jacobsen L, Walker M, Edwards J, Chappell P, Woolston J. Clozapine in the treatment of a young adolescent with schizophrenia. *J Am Acad Child Adolesc Psychiatry.* 1994;33:645-650.
37. Birmaher B, Baker R, Kapur S, Quintana H, Ganguli R. Clozapine for the treatment of adolescents with schizophrenia. *J Am Acad Child Adolesc Psychiatry.* 1991;31:160-164.
38. Meltzer HY. Treatment of the neuroleptic nonresponsive schizophrenic patient. *Schizophr Bull.* 1992;18:515-542.
39. Mozes T, Toren P, Chernauzen N, Mester R, Yoran-Hagesh R, Blumensohn R, Weizman A. Clozapine treatment in very early onset schizophrenia. *J Am Acad Child Adolesc Psychiatry.* 1994;33:65-70.
40. Towbin KE, Dykens EM, Pugliese RG. Case study: clozapine for early developmental delays with childhood-onset schizophrenia: protocol and 15-month outcome. *J Am Acad Child Adolesc Psychiatry.* 1994;33:651-658.
41. Remschmidt HE, Schulz E, Martin M, Warnke A, Trott G. Childhood-onset schizophrenia: history of the concept and recent studies. *Schizophr Bull.* 1994;20:727-745.
42. Meltzer HY. Clozapine: is another view valid? *Am J Psychiatry.* 1995;152:821-825.
43. Kane JM, Schooler N, Marder S, Wirshing W, Ames D, Umbricht D, Safferman A, Baker R, Ganguli R. Efficacy of clozapine vs haloperidol in a long-term clinical trial. *Schizophr Res.* 1996;18:127. Abstract.
44. Gerson SL. Clozapine: deciphering the risks. *N Engl J Med.* 1993;329:204-205.
45. Piscitelli SC, Frazier JA, McKenna K, Albus KE, Grothe DR, Gordon CT, Rapoport JL. Plasma clozapine and haloperidol concentrations in adolescents with childhood-onset schizophrenia: association with response. *J Clin Psychiatry.* 1994;55:94-97.
46. Gerson SL, Arce C, Meltzer HY. *N*-desmethyclozapine: a clozapine metabolite that suppresses hemapoiesis. *Br J Haemotol.* 1994;85:123-125.
47. Safferman A, Lieberman J, Alvir J, Howard A. Rechallenge in clozapine-induced agranulocytosis. *Lancet.* 1992;339:1296-1297.
48. Krassner M. *Sandoz Pharmaceuticals Corporation Brochure on Possible Drug Interactions With Clozapine.* East Hanover, NJ: Pharmaceutical Safety Division, Sandoz Pharmaceuticals Corp; 1995.
49. Freedman J, Wirshing W, Russell A, Bray M, Unutzer J. Absence status seizures during successful long-term clozapine treatment of an adolescent with schizophrenia. *J Child Adolesc Psychopharmacol.* 1994;4:53-62.
50. Devinsky O, Pacia S. Seizures during clozapine therapy. *J Clin Psychiatry.* 1994;55:153-156.
51. Devinsky O, Honigfeld G, Patin J. Clozapine-related seizures. *Neurology.* 1991;41:369-371.
52. Pacia SV, Devinsky O. Clozapine-related seizures: experience with 5629 patients. *Neurology.* 1994;44:2247-2249.
53. Welch J, Manschreck T, Redmond D. Clozapine-induced seizures and EEG changes. *J Neuropsychiatry Clin Neurosci.* 1994;6:250-256.
54. Leadbetter R, Shutty M, Pavalonis D, Vieweg V, Higgins P, Downs M. Clozapine-induced weight gain: prevalence and clinical relevance. *Am J Psychiatry.* 1992;149:68-72.
55. Umbricht D, Pollack S, Kane J. Clozapine and weight gain. *J Clin Psychiatry.* 1994;55(suppl B, part 9):157-160.
56. Campbell A, Baldessarini RJ, Teicher MH. Decreasing sensitivity to neuroleptic agents in developing rats: evidence for a pharmacodynamic factor. *Psychopharmacology.* 1988;94:46-51.
57. Baldessarini RJ, Teicher MH. Dosing of antipsychotic agents in pediatric populations. *J Child Adolesc Psychopharmacol.* 1995;5:1-4.
58. Mandoki M. Risperidone treatment of children and adolescents: increased risk of extrapyramidal side effects? *J Child Adolesc Psychopharmacol.* 1995;5:49-67.
59. Zahn T, Jacobsen L, Gordon C, McKenna K, Frazier JA, Rapoport J. Autonomic nervous system markers of psychopathology in childhood-onset schizophrenia. *Arch Gen Psychiatry.* In press.
60. Jacobsen L, Hong W, Hommer D, Frazier J, Giedd J, Gordon C, Karp B, McKenna K, Rapoport J. Smooth pursuit eye movements in childhood-onset schizophrenia: comparison with ADHD and normal controls. *Biol Psychiatry.* In press.
61. Frazier J, Giedd J, Hamburger S, Albus K, Kaysen D, Vaituzis A, Rajapaske J, Lenane H, McKenna K, Jacobsen L, Gordon C, Breier A, Rapoport J. Brain anatomic magnetic resonance imaging in childhood-onset schizophrenia. *Arch Gen Psychiatry.* 1996;53:617-624.
62. Hafner H, Nowotny B. Epidemiology of early-onset schizophrenia. *Eur Arch Psychiatry Clin Neurosci.* 1995;245:80-92.
63. Benes M, Turtle M, Khan Y, Farol P. Myelination of a key relay zone in the hippocampal formation occurs in the human brain during childhood, adolescence, and adulthood. *Arch Gen Psychiatry.* 1994;51:477-484.
64. Breier A, Schreiber J, Dyer J, Pickar D. National Institute of Mental Health Longitudinal Study of Chronic Schizophrenia: prognosis and predictors of outcome. *Arch Gen Psychiatry.* 1991;48:239-246.
65. Levkovitch Y, Kronenberg J, Kayser N, Zvyvagelski M, Gaoni B, Gadoth N. Clozapine for tardive dyskinesia in adolescents. *Brain Dev.* 1995;17:213-215.
66. Gualtieri C, Quade D, Hicks R, Mayo J, Schroeder S. Tardive dyskinesia and other clinical consequences of neuroleptic treatment in children and adolescents. *Am J Psychiatry.* 1984;141:20-23.
67. Casey D. Clozapine: neuroleptic-induced EPS and tardive dyskinesia. *Psychopharmacology (Berl).* 1989;99(suppl):47-53.
68. Kane J, Woerner M, Pollack S, Safferman A, Lieberman J. Does clozapine cause tardive dyskinesia? *J Clin Psychiatry.* 1993;54:327-330.

Correction

Error in Table 3. In the article titled "Relapse Prevention by Acamprosate: Results From a Placebo-Controlled Study on Alcohol Dependence," published in the August ARCHIVES (1996;53:673-680), on page 677, in Table 3, the mean±SD *DSM-III-R* score in the acamprosate group should have been stated as "7.78±1.28." The journal regrets the error.

ORIGINAL ARTICLE

The Influence of Expressed Emotion, Family Dynamics, and Symptom Type on the Social Adjustment of Schizophrenic Young Adults

Suzanne King, PhD; Mike J. Dixon, PhD

Background: The goal of this study was to test a path analytic model that reflects the hypothesis that family cohesion and family adaptability underlie family members' expressed emotion (critical comments and emotional overinvolvement), that these family variables underlie the preponderance of positive symptoms in a patient with schizophrenia 9 months after relatives are interviewed, and that all of these variables influence the patient's social adjustment at follow-up.

Methods: The subjects were 69 patients who met the *DSM-III-R* criteria for schizophrenia and 108 of their relatives. Relatives were assessed with the Camberwell Family Interview and the Family Adaptability and Cohesion Evaluation Scales III. Patients were interviewed 9 months later with the Brief Psychiatric Rating Scale and the Social Adjustment Scale II.

Results: Significant amounts of variance were explained by the model for three of the five social adjustment components. Neither family cohesion nor adaptability was associated with either critical comments or emotional overinvolvement. Family cohesion was negatively associated and emotional overinvolvement was positively associated with a preponderance of positive symptoms. Greater family adaptability was associated with lower social adjustment scores, and greater emotional overinvolvement was associated with higher social adjustment. Cohesion had a significant positive indirect effect on social adjustment through its association with symptom type.

Conclusions: Critics of expressed emotion will be pleased to see that one component of high expressed emotion (emotional overinvolvement) is actually associated with a better social outcome in patients. Proponents of the expressed emotion concept will be pleased to see the applicability of expressed emotion to other facets of schizophrenic outcome. The results highlight the importance of using the expressed emotion scales in their continuous rather than dichotomized state and of analyzing critical comments and emotional overinvolvement separately.

Arch Gen Psychiatry. 1996;53:1098-1104

From the Department of Psychiatry, McGill University, Montreal, Quebec, and Psychosocial Research Unit, Douglas Hospital Research Centre, Verdun, Quebec.

EXPRESSED EMOTION (EE) research has brought the family to the forefront of psychosocial investigations of schizophrenia. Studies by Brown et al[1-3] and others[4-12] have demonstrated that patients living in households in which one or more family members either are highly critical of the patient or are emotionally overinvolved in the patient's life (high EE households) have a risk of relapse within 9 months of hospital discharge three to four times greater than that of patients living in low EE homes.[13]

Expressed emotion is based on responses made during the Camberwell Family Interview (CFI).[14,15] One-to-one, tape-recorded, private interviews are conducted with family members and are coded using five scales. Three scales determine a family's EE status: critical comments (CC) is a frequency count of comments made to the interviewer that criticize the patient and that go beyond a simple description of negative behaviors; emotional overinvolvement (EOI) reflects self-sacrifice, overprotection, intrusiveness, and overdramatization beyond what is considered normal; hostility reflects a generalized critical attitude toward and/or a frank rejection of the patient.

The criterion for labeling a household as high EE is that combination of CFI scales that discriminates best between those patients who relapse within 9 months of hospital discharge and those who do not. Thus, traditionally, an individual high EE relative is one who makes

See Subjects and Methods on next page

SUBJECTS AND METHODS

SUBJECTS

Patients were required to meet the following criteria: (1) between 17 and 35 years of age, (2) out of hospital and considered stabilized by their treating psychiatrist, (3) living with a close relative, and (4) a *DSM-III-R* diagnosis of schizophrenia without evidence of organicity, significant intellectual handicap, or primary diagnosis of substance abuse. The age range was selected to create a relatively homogeneous sample of families in the stressful "launching" stage[31] and with respect to length of illness.

These criteria were met by 119 patients. Each patient was approached by an interviewer during an ordinary outpatient clinic visit. Following a description of the project, the patient was invited to sign an informed consent form, including consent to contact the patient's relatives. Thirty-one (26%) of the 119 potential subjects refused to participate.

Of the 88 initial acceptors, six subsequently refused an interview and one moved out of the province. Another 12 were eliminated when the relatives either refused to be involved in the study (n=11) or died (n=1). The final sample included 69 patients and 108 relatives.

SAMPLE DESCRIPTION

The 69 patients ranged in age from 19 to 36 years (mean, 28.7 years; SD, 4.4 years) at the beginning of the study, with zero to seven previous hospitalizations (mean, 2.2; SD, 1.8). The sample included 51 men (74%) and 18 women. The sample was primarily white (87% [n=60]), with seven black and two Asian subjects. The majority of patients (88% [n=61]) had never been married, with only four subjects (6%) currently married.

The 108 relatives in the 69 households were well distributed among the five Hollingshead classes, with 65% (n=71) in the lower and lower-middle classes (IV and V) and 4% (n=4) in the upper class (I). The 108 relatives included 52 mothers, 32 fathers, 16 siblings, three spouses, and five others (stepparents, in-laws, etc).

ASSESSMENT OF RELATIVES

The expressed emotion status of each relative was assessed with the CFI administered individually and, when two relatives were included for a given patient, by different interviewers.

Relatives were administered the Family Adaptability and Cohesion Evaluation Scale III (FACES III).[32] The Cohesion Scale includes 10 items indicating the perception of closeness felt among family members as well as their tendency to spend time together. The Adaptability Scale includes 10 items reflecting the family's propensity to change (eg, "Different people act as leaders in our family"). All 20 items use a four-point response scale, with "all of the time," "most of the time," "some of the time," and "none of the time" as options. The manual reports internal consistency estimates of 0.77 for cohesion and 0.62 for adaptability and indicates that the two scales are independent. FACES III discriminates between families with and without a variety of social and psychological problems.[33]

ASSESSMENT OF PATIENTS

Nine months after relatives' interviews, patients were interviewed with the Social Adjustment Scale II (SAS II),[34] which reflects functioning in several roles, including work (as worker, student or homemaker), household member, external family member, and social-leisure. The interview also yields a global score reflecting general social adjustment. Ratings range from low (a score of 1) to high (a score of 7) levels of functioning.

The patient's symptom severity was assessed using the 24-item University of California, Los Angeles, version of the Brief Psychiatric Rating Scale (BPRS).[35,36] Based on a factor analysis of the BPRS,[37,38] a positive symptom cluster score was computed as the sum of ratings for hallucinations, unusual thought content (including delusions), and conceptual disorganization. The negative symptom cluster score was the sum of ratings for motor retardation, blunted affect, and emotional withdrawal. A symptom type score was computed by subtracting the negative symptom score from the positive symptom score, creating a continuous variable ranging from −21 to +21.

Continued on next page

six or more CC or has a rating of 3 or more on EOI. Some also consider any rating of hostility an indication of high EE. If any of the relatives interviewed are rated high in EE, then the entire household bears the high EE label.

Hooley[16,17] and others[18-20] have remarked that although this dichotomized household EE variable has proven predictive validity, how it develops and predicts later relapse remain uncertain. Family systems theory, as operationalized by the Circumplex Model of Marital and Family Systems,[21] may provide some clues to the development of EE. The model comprises two axes. The cohesion axis reflects the degree to which members feel close to one another and prefer to spend time together. It ranges from "disengagement" to "enmeshment." Adaptability reflects the propensity of the family to change rules and routines in response to developmental and transitory events and ranges from "rigidity" to "chaos." Theoretically, a family and its members function at their best when scores are in the middle of both axes.

Extreme family cohesiveness may give rise to the intrusive behaviors that are reflected in EOI. Similarly, rigidity (low family adaptability) may explain the propensity to criticize schizophrenic behaviors that disrupt established family routines.

As for how EE might predict relapse, a patient with schizophrenia may respond to household EE by adjusting the nature of his or her symptom profile. The balance between positive and negative symptom severity might reflect a patient's location along a continuum between residual schizophrenia and florid exacerbation. Alternatively, the family's EE may be a response to rather than a cause of a pattern of symptoms that leads to relapse.[22,23]

Certain aspects of the EE method may obscure the relationship between the family and the course of schizo-

The CFI, SAS II, and BPRS interviewers were all trained to interrater reliabilities of 0.8 or better and were monitered regularly to ensure that high interrater reliabilities were maintained throughout the study.

Using an approximation of the criteria used by Goldstein et al,[39] a relapse was considered to have occurred during the 9-month follow-up period if the patient was admitted to a psychiatric facility or made an emergency visit to a clinic or psychiatric facility resulting in retention for observation or if prescribed antipsychotic dosages were increased by 50% or more.

THE MODEL

Path analysis can be a first step in testing plausible models of underlying causal relationships. As an extension of multiple linear regression, path analysis estimates the amount of variance in the dependent variable explained by the independent variables collectively and allows associations within the model to be decomposed into their various direct and indirect effects. As such, a single model may have multiple endogenous, or dependent, variables.

The **Figure** shows the model of the hypothesized causal relationships that were studied in this investigation. The causal order has been influenced by both theoretical and empirical factors. Since the outcome variables (symptom type and five measures of social adjustment) were measured 9 months later than the independent variables, there is a temporal component to the model. Within the family therapy literature, the dynamics of the family organization are thought to produce dysfunctional communication patterns in the family that, in turn, produce bizarre thoughts and behavior in the offspring, resulting in repetitive failures in most aspects of life.[40] Thus, variables reflecting family dynamics have been specified as influencing EE, which influences variables describing functioning in the schizophrenic young adult 9 months after the relatives are interviewed. Because different components of social adjustment are differentially influenced by positive and negative symptoms,[30] symptom type has been represented as influencing the level of social adjustment at follow-up. Expressed emotion is purported to influence symptom type because intervention studies have demonstrated that schizophrenic relapse is more likely when a family's EE rating changes from high to low.[41] Because relapse is associated more with positive than negative symptom syndromes,[30] this model tested the hypothesis that the effect of EE on outcome is mediated by symptom type.

DATA ANALYTIC PROCEDURES

Preliminary Analysis

After edit-checking of the data, interrater reliabilities (intraclass correlations) were computed for the CFI. Internal consistency estimates (Cronbach's α)[42] were then computed for the two FACES III scales. The Pearson correlation between the two scales was also calculated.

Before conducting the path analyses that were central to this investigation, we attempted to replicate the results of earlier EE studies by conducting a χ^2 analysis of the association between EE status (high vs low) and relapse.

Next, we tested the assumption of linear association between the two variables involved in each of the 13 paths of the model. These trend analyses were done by regressing a dependent variable on a single independent variable, then on the independent variable and its square. If the addition of the polynomial term was not associated with a significant increase in the coefficient of determination (R^2), then the relationship was taken to be linear in nature.

Finally, to determine the appropriateness of using household average scores for the family variables, Pearson correlations between the two family members were computed for CC, EOI, cohesion, and adaptability using data from all two-relative families.

Path Analyses

Next, five models were tested, one for each of the five estimates of social adjustment: general social adjustment, adjustment as household member, social adjustment with external family members, adjustment in the work role, and adjustment in social and leisure activities. The LISREL 8 program[43] was used to conduct all of the path analyses. This program tests the significance of all direct, indirect, and total effects within a model. Each analysis was conducted (1) using household average scores for the family variables and (2) using the dichotomized household EE variable (high vs low) instead of the CC and EOI scales in their continuous form. An a priori α level of .05 was set for all tests of significance in the path analyses.

phrenia. First, dichotomizing CFI scales when, presumably, they reflect continuous underlying psychological constructs discards variance that is potentially useful.[24] Second, there is no unifying construct that warrants combining the CC and EOI ratings into a single scale, and, indeed, at least one study has demonstrated the utility of considering the scales separately.[25] Finally, classifying families into only two groups (high EE vs low EE) ignores the diversity of family environments, which could be reflected by using the CFI scales independently in their continuous form.

Other problems arise from choosing relapse as the sole outcome variable in EE research. Because high EE has been associated with relapse, the implicit conclusion is that high EE is patently "pernicious."[26] However, relapse is incapable of reflecting the diversity of functioning levels of patients with schizophrenia and, as noted by Falloon,[27(p474)] "has drawn attention to relatively infrequent, often brief, management crises and away from the long-term course of schizophrenia." It is possible that high EE may be related to better outcome in other areas of functioning despite the association with relapse. Some recommend using social adjustment as an outcome measure since it reflects the patient's relationship with the social environment.[12,28,29] Any study of the relationship between EE and social adjustment ought to consider the patient's symptom profile, since different aspects of social adjustment are differentially related to positive and negative symptoms in patients with schizophrenia.[30]

The goal of the current study was to better understand the development of EE and the relationship between EE and social adjustment. Specifically, we wished to understand whether family adaptability and cohesion underlie CC and EOI, whether EE can explain variance in social adjustment 9 months after relatives are interviewed, and whether any relationship between EE and social adjustment is mediated by the relative severity of positive and negative symptoms in the patient. By using the CFI scales in their original, continuous forms, we hoped to increase our explanation of variance compared with what might be explained using the dichotomized EE variable. These goals were addressed using path analysis.

RESULTS

RELIABILITIES

By the end of the study, intraclass correlations among raters for the CFI were .89 for CC and .80 for EOI. Raters achieved perfect agreement in ratings of hostility.

Internal consistency estimates for the FACES III scales were close to those reported in the manual; in our sample, Cronbach's α values of .74 and .63 were computed for cohesion and adaptability, respectively. The two scales were more highly correlated in our sample (r=.28) than in the standardization sample reported in the manual (r=.03), however.

REPLICATION OF RELAPSE PREDICTION

During the 9-month follow-up period, 26 of the 71 patients for whom we had clinical data met our criteria for relapse, yielding an overall relapse rate of 37%. Nearly 61% (n=42) of households were categorized as high EE. Five (17%) of the 29 patients in low EE households relapsed, compared with 21 (50%) of the 42 patients in high EE homes (χ^2=7.9, df=1, P=.005). These relapse rates resemble those found in studies that began their 9-month follow-up at hospital discharge.[16]

TESTS OF LINEARITY

Trend analyses were conducted[44] for each pair of variables associated with each of the 13 paths in the model. As none of the polynomial terms was significant, the results indicated that all significant relationships among variables were linear and not curvilinear in nature, a consistent finding reported in the literature on FACES III in recent years.[45]

PATH ANALYSES

The results of the five path analyses are presented in the **Table**. Standardized direct effect path coefficients (analogous to regression coefficients) are presented to allow comparisons of coefficients within equations; the unstandardized, or metric, coefficients are also presented for comparisons of results across samples[44] in the event of future replication.

FAMILY DYNAMICS AND EE

One percent of the variance in CC and 5% of variance in EOI could be explained by adaptability and cohesion together. These results suggest that family dynamics, as conceptualized by the Circumplex Model of Marital and Family Systems, do not underlie expressed emotion. The FACES III and CFI scores appear to be statistically independent, however, and thus do not pose multicollinearity problems for the rest of the model.

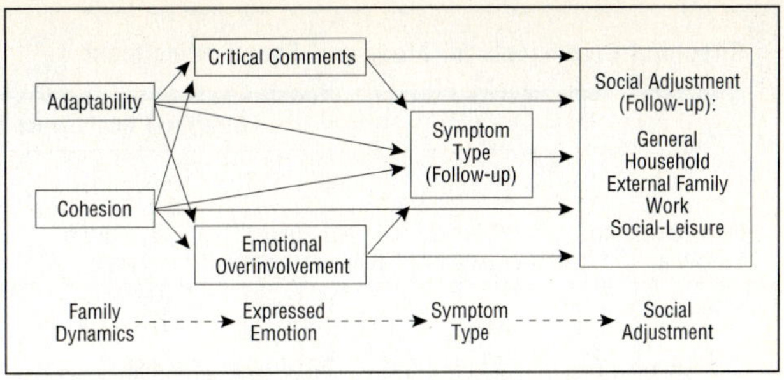

A causal model of social adjustment in schizophrenic young adults, reflecting the hypothesis that two components of family dynamics underlie two components of expressed emotion and that all four family variables predict symptom type and social adjustment in the patient 9 months after relatives are interviewed.

EXPLANATION OF SYMPTOM TYPE

Twenty-eight percent of the variance in symptom type was explained by the four family variables taken together. Two variables had significant path coefficients. First, the higher the family's cohesion rating, the greater the preponderance of negative vs positive symptoms in the patient 9 months later. Second, greater emotional overinvolvement was associated with a more positive symptom type.

EXPLANATION OF SOCIAL ADJUSTMENT

General Social Adjustment

Our model explained a significant amount (16%) of the variance in the SAS II general score. As for family dynamics, only adaptability had a significant direct effect on general adjustment: when the other variables in the model were held constant, higher family adaptability ratings were associated with poorer social adjustment. There was no association between either CC or EOI and general social adjustment when the other variables in the model were held constant. As for symptom type, better general scores were associated with a preponderance of negative symptoms, all else being equal.

Household Member

Twenty percent of the variance in the ability of the patient to get along with other members of the household was explained by the model. Neither of the family dynamics variables had a significant direct effect on functioning in the role of household member. Emotional overinvolvement was the only EE variable to have an effect, with better functioning in the family member role associated with higher EOI score. Better functioning in the role of household member was associated with a more negative symptom type.

Structural Coefficients for Models of Social Adjustment

Predetermined Variables	Critical Comments	Emotional Overinvolvement	Symptom Type	General	Household Member	External Family	Work	Social Leisure
	Structural Coefficients by Dependent Variable, Standardized (Metric) [SE]			Social Adjustment Scale II*				
Adaptability	−.07 (−.05) [.09]	.18 (.05) [.03]	−.01 (−.01) [.08]	−.31† (−.06†) [.02]	−.18 (−.05) [.03]	−.26‡ (−.06‡) [.03]	−.20 (−.07) [.04]	−.27‡ (−.08‡) [.04]
Cohesion	−.07 (−.04) [.09]	.07 (.02) [.03]	−.47§ (−.31§) [.07]	−.13 (−.02) [.02]	−.01 (−.00) [.04]	−.07 (−.02) [.03]	.10 (.03) [.04]	−.13 (−.04) [.04]
Critical comments			.15 (.15) [.11]	−.12 (−.03) [.03]	.08 (.03) [.05]	.02 (.01) [.04]	.04 (.02) [.06]	−.15 (−.06) [.05]
Emotional overinvolvement			.22‡ (.65‡) [.31]	.16 (.12) [.09]	.39§ (.45§) [.13]	.28‡ (.28‡) [.12]	−.12 (−.15) [.17]	.12 (.13) [.14]
Symptom type				−.27‡ (−.07‡) [.04]	−.33‡ (−.13‡) [.05]	−.36† (−.12†) [.05]	−.00 (−.00) [.06]	−.23 (−.09) [.06]
R^2	.01	.05	.28§	.16‡	.20†	.18‡	.06	.14
Residual	>.99	.96	.72	.84	.80	.82	.94	.87

*χ^2=.10, df=1, P=.76.
†P<.01.
‡P<.05.
§P<.001.

External Family

A significant amount (18%) of the variance in the ability of patients with schizophrenia to get along with family members who live outside their household was explained by the model. The higher the rating of family adaptability, the poorer the patient's relationships with the external family 9 months later. While CC appeared to be unrelated to this role, better SAS II scores were associated with higher EOI ratings when the other variables in the model were controlled for. Again, a preponderance of negative symptoms was associated with better adjustment in this role.

Work

The model explained a nonsignificant proportion of variance in this SAS II scale.

Social-Leisure

The model explained 14% of the variance in patients' social-leisure adjustment. Again, better adjustment in this role was associated with lower adaptability ratings (*P*<.05). Neither CC, EOI, nor symptom type contributed significantly to the model.

INDIRECT EFFECTS

To determine whether the relationship between family variables and social adjustment was mediated by symptom type, the indirect effects were considered. While cohesion did not have a significant direct effect on any of the five SAS II scales, it did have a sizable indirect effect (evidently through symptom type) on the general (*P*=.06) and external family (*P*=.02) scores; thus, the higher the rating of family cohesion, the greater the preponderance of negative symptoms in the patient 9 months later; the more negative the symptom type, the better the patient's functioning on the general, household, and external family scales. As such, the indirect effect of cohesion on social adjustment was positive, with higher cohesion ratings ultimately associated with better social adjustment.

As for expressed emotion, the indirect effects of EOI on the general (*t*=−1.45, *P*=.15), household (*t*=−1.63, *P*=.11), and external family (*t*=−1.68, *P*=.10) scores were at the trend level. In short, higher EOI scores tended to be associated with a preponderance of positive symptoms 9 months later (*P*=.07), and the more positive the symptom type, the poorer the patient's social adjustment in terms of the general, household member, and external family member roles. Thus, while EOI had a significant positive direct effect on some aspects of social adjustment, its indirect effect tended to be negative. The negative indirect effects are sufficiently weaker than the positive direct effects, however, such that the resulting total effects of EOI on the household (b, 0.36; SE, 0.14; *P*<.01) and external family (b, 0.20; SE, 0.12; *P*=.10) scores are still positive.

USING THE HOUSEHOLD EE SCORE

To compare our results with those of studies that used traditional EE scores, a second set of analyses was conducted using the dichotomized household EE variable. Making this substitution, the model tended to explain less variance than when CC and EOI were used: the new model explained 16.4% of the variance in the general score (*P*=.04), 12.8% of the variance in the household score (*P*=.09), 10.7% of the variance in the external family score (*P*=.08), 6.2% of the variance in the work score (*P*=.31), and 14.6% of the variance in the social-leisure score (*P*=.09). In none of these equations was the direct effect for EE statistically significant.

COMMENT

This study was influenced in part by the vulnerability-stress model,[46,47] which postulates that personal and environmental vulnerability and protective factors combine and interact with intermediate cognitive and physiological states in influencing various aspects of outcome. Given that the current study addresses only a small piece of the larger interdisciplinary puzzle, the 14% to 20% of variance explained by a model showcasing family factors alone can be considered meaningful.[44]

The model presented in the Figure represents the hypothesis that family factors influence patient variables measured 9 months later. The causal relationships at work in the real world are probably considerably more complex than our model, and we recognize that interpretations of the results could be made that consider alternative causal directions as well.

The two components of family dynamics studied have interesting associations with symptom type and social adjustment. First, greater family cohesion was associated with a preponderance of negative symptoms. As the cohesion scale reflects a sense of closeness and a tendency to do things together as a family, it may be that patients with schizophrenia react to this social pressure by retreating into negative symptoms. At the same time, higher levels of family cohesion may reduce fears of abandonment and alleviate the positive symptoms that may be brought on by real or imagined pending loss.[48]

Adaptability had a negative association with general social adjustment and with the role of external family member. This may reflect a need of individuals with schizophrenia for a highly structured environment, an observation made in qualitative research.[49,50] Expectations may also be at work: when a family considers itself to be highly adaptable, there may be a tendency to make allowances for the schizophrenic member; patients may respond to the lowered expectations by not making the effort required to be more active in social endeavors.

While adaptability and cohesion were useful in our models of symptom type and social adjustment, they do not appear to underlie EE. These results fail to support the hypothesis that dysfunctional family dynamics result in extreme family communications.[51] This negative finding may have been caused by our choice of measurement tools. FACES III has been criticized for its failure to demonstrate the predicted curvilinear relationship with outcome.[45,52-55] While one possible explanation is that the scale itself is unable to measure extremes of the two scales (eg, the enmeshed family), a rival explanation is that the theory is faulty, that extreme levels of family cohesion are more conducive to individual and family functioning than are moderate levels.

Although the origins of EE remain elusive, the relationships of CC and EOI to social adjustment seem clear. It appears that CC, which has been considered the most crucial EE scale for predicting relapse,[48] does not have significant linear or curvilinear associations with social adjustment.

Unlike CC, EOI is related to social adjustment but in an unexpected direction: the self-sacrificing, overprotective, and intrusive behaviors considered in the EOI rating appear to be conducive to the social functioning of the patient with schizophrenia, particularly as it relates to the family. This suggests that the attitudes and behaviors that have been assumed to be noxious to patients appear not to be interpreted negatively by the patients themselves, who, during the SAS II interview, report their relationships with these relatives to be free of tension. Thus, the results of our study support the hypothesis of Hooley[16,17] that patients in high EE homes may achieve higher levels of functioning despite their greater propensity to relapse.

A better understanding of the relationship between the family and social adjustment is achieved when the SAS II scales are grouped into those that reflect adjustment within and outside of the family context. The two SAS II family scores, household member and external family, were significantly associated with EOI. The two SAS II global scores that reflect social functioning outside of the family context, work and social-leisure, were most sensitive to family adaptability. Because the social norms in force outside of the family are less forgiving, a more rigid family environment may assist the patient in making the transition to the outside world. Within the family context, however, the emotional climate is an important predictor of harmony. Interestingly, the SAS II external family score, which is subject to both intrafamilial and extrafamilial forces, was associated equally with adaptability and EOI.

Our findings contradict those of earlier studies of EE and social adjustment, which concluded that low EE was associated with better social adjustment than high EE.[8,56,57] An important methodological difference between those studies and ours is that we conducted the CFIs when the patient was out of the hospital.

The extent to which the statistically significant results we report are also clinically meaningful can only be judged on the basis of appropriate clinical trials of psychosocial interventions that include a variety of outcome measures. Nonetheless, we believe that the results of this study demonstrate that a given variable may appear to be a risk factor when one aspect of outcome is considered and a protective factor for other outcome variables. Among our own results, for example, EOI has been shown to be a strong predictor of relapse[58] as well as being positively related to social adjustment.

In conclusion, we have demonstrated that simplifying the relationship between the family and schizophrenic outcome by describing families with a single dichotomous variable and by using the relapse-nonrelapse dichotomy to describe the wide range of functioning in individuals with a diagnosis of schizophrenia may hide the complexity inherent in families. By expanding our measurement of the family at one end of the equation and of schizophrenic outcome at the other end, we have shown that at least one part of what goes into making a high EE home and into predicting relapse may also contribute to better social functioning between relapses.

Accepted for publication January 3, 1996.

This research was supported by grant NHRDP 6605-3327-63 from Health and Welfare Canada, Ottawa, Ontario (Dr King); by Quebec Health Research Fellowship FRSQ 910107-103 (Dr King); and by a postdoctoral fellowship from the Alzheimer Society of Canada, Toronto, Ontario (Dr Dixon).

The authors thank the many dedicated interviewers and research assistants who made this project possible: Solange Marchildon, PhD, Johanne Tardif, MSc, Hannah Hershman, MEd, Marie-Clause LaMarche, MSc, Louise Labelle, MSc, Teeya Blatt, MSc, and Zeycan Yegin, MA. Many thanks to Serge Charlebois for secretarial assistance.

Reprint requests to Douglas Hospital Research Centre, 6875 Lasalle Blvd, Verdun, Quebec, Canada H4H 1R3 (Dr King).

REFERENCES

1. Brown GW, Carstairs GM, Topping G. Post-hospital adjustment of chronic mental patients. *Lancet.* 1958;11:685-689.
2. Brown GW. Experiences of discharged chronic schizophrenic patients in various types of living group. *Milbank Mem Fund Q.* 1959;37:105-131.
3. Brown GW, Monck EM, Carstairs GM, Wing JK. Influence of family life on the course of schizophrenic illness. *Br J Prev Soc Med.* 1962;16:55-68.
4. Vaughn CE, Leff JP. The influence of family and social factors on the course of psychiatric illness: a comparison of schizophrenic and depressed neurotic patients. *Br J Psychiatry.* 1976;129:125-137.
5. Barrelet L, Pellizzer G, Ammann L. Family expressed emotion and outcome of schizophrenics: a study in a French cultural environment. *Arch Suisses Neurol Psychiatrie.* 1988;139:27-34.
6. Bertrando P, Beltz J, Bressi C, Clerici M, Farma T, Invernizzi G, Cazzullo CL. Expressed emotion and schizophrenia in Italy: a study of an urban population. *Br J Psychiatry.* 1992;161:223-229.
7. Cazzullo CL, Bressi C, Bertrando P, Clerici M, Maffei C. Schizophrénie et expression émotionnelle familiale: étude d'une population italienne. *Encephale.* 1989;15:1-6.
8. Hogarty GE, McEvoy JP, Munetz M, DiBarry AL, Bartone P, Cather R, Coley SJ, Ulrich RF, Carter M, Madonia MJ. Dose of fluphenazine, familial expressed emotion, and outcome in schizophrenia: results of a 2-year controlled study. *Arch Gen Psychiatry.* 1988;45:797-805.
9. Jenkins JH, Karno M, de la Selva A, Santana F. Expressed emotion in cross-cultural context: familial responses to schizophrenic illness among Mexican Americans. In: Goldstein MJ, Hand I, Hahlweg K, eds. *Treatment of Schizophrenia: Family Assessment and Intervention.* Berlin, Germany: Springer-Verlag; 1986:35-49.
10. Leff J, Sartorius N, Korten A, Ernberg G. The International Pilot Study of Schizophrenia: 5-year follow-up findings. *Psychol Med.* 1992;22:131-145.
11. McCreadie RG. The Nithsdale Schizophrenia Survey, I: psychiatric and social handicaps. *Br J Psychiatry.* 1982;140:582-586.
12. Vaughn CE, Snyder KS, Jones S, Freeman WB, Falloon IRH. Family factors in schizophrenic relapse: replication in California of British research on expressed emotion. *Arch Gen Psychiatry.* 1984;41:1169-1177.
13. Parker G, Hadzi-Pavlovic D. Expressed emotion as a predictor of schizophrenic relapse: an analysis of aggregated data. *Psychol Med.* 1990;20:961-965.
14. Brown GW, Rutter M. The measurement of family activities and relationships: a methodological study. *Hum Relat.* 1966;19:241-263.
15. Vaughn C, Leff J. The measurement of expressed emotion in the families of psychiatric patients. *Br J Soc Clin Psychol.* 1976;15:157-165.
16. Hooley JM. An introduction to EE measurement and research. In: Goldstein MJ, Hand I, Hahlweg K, eds. *Treatment of Schizophrenia: Family Assessment and Intervention.* Berlin, Germany: Springer-Verlag; 1986:25-34.
17. Hooley JM. Expressed emotion: a review of the critical literature. *Clin Psychol Rev.* 1985;5:119-139.
18. Jenkins JH. Anthropology, expressed emotion, and schizophrenia. *Ethos.* 1991; 19:387-431.
19. Kanter J, Lamb HR, Loeper C. Expressed emotion in families: a critical review. *Hosp Community Psychiatry.* 1987;38:374-380.
20. Koenigsberg HW, Handley R. Expressed emotion: from predictive index to clinical construct. *Am J Psychiatry.* 1986;143:1361-1373.
21. Olson DH, Russell CS, Sprenkle DH. Circumplex Model of Marital and Family Systems, II: empirical studies and clinical intervention. In: Vincent J, ed. *Advances in Family Intervention, Assessment and Theory.* Greenwich, Conn: JAI Press Inc; 1979:128-176.
22. Jenkins JH, Karno M. The meaning of expressed emotion: theoretical issues raised by cross-cultural research. *Am J Psychiatry.* 1992;149:9-21.
23. Mintz LI, Nuechterlein KH, Goldstein MJ, Mintz J, Snyder KS. The initial onset of schizophrenia and family expressed emotion: some methodological considerations. *Br J Psychiatry.* 1989;154:212-217.
24. Kerlinger FN. *Foundations of Behavioral Research.* 2nd ed. New York, NY: Holt Rinehart & Winston; 1973.
25. Miklowitz DJ, Strachan AM, Goldstein MJ, Doane JA, Snyder KS, Hogarty GE, Falloon IRH. Expressed emotion and communication deviance in the families of schizophrenics. *J Abnorm Psychol.* 1986;95:60-66.
26. Goldstein MJ, Hand I, Hahlweg K, eds. *Treatment of Schizophrenia: Family Assessment and Intervention.* Berlin, Germany: Springer-Verlag; 1986.
27. Falloon IRH. Relapse in schizophrenia: a review of the concept and its definitions. *Psychol Med.* 1983;13:469-477.
28. Carpenter WT, Kirkpatrick B. The heterogeneity of the long-term course of schizophrenia. *Schizophr Bull.* 1988;14:645-652.
29. Strauss JS, Carpenter WT Jr. Prediction of outcome in schizophrenia, III: 5-year outcome and its predictors. *Arch Gen Psychiatry.* 1977;34:159-163.
30. Pogue-Geile MF, Harrow M. Negative and positive symptoms in schizophrenia and depression: a followup. *Schizophr Bull.* 1984;10:371-387.
31. Olson DH, McCubbin HI, Barnes HL, Larsen AS, Muxen MJ, Wilson MA. *Families: What Makes Them Work.* Beverly Hills, Calif: Sage Publications Inc; 1983.
32. Olson DH, Portner J, Lavee Y. *FACES III: Family Adaptability and Cohesion Evaluation Scales.* Minneapolis: University of Minnesota; 1985.
33. Clarke J. *The Family Types of Schizophrenics, Neurotics and 'Normals.'* Minneapolis: University of Minnesota; 1984. Thesis.
34. Schooler N, Hogarty G, Weissman MM. Social Adjustment Scale II (SAS II). In: Hargreaves WA, Attkisson CC, Sorenson JE, eds. *Resource Materials for Community Mental Health Program Evaluators.* Washington, DC: US Dept of Health, Education, and Welfare; 1979:290-330. Publication ADM 79-328.
35. Overall G, Gorham D. The Brief Psychiatric Rating Scale. *Psychol Rep.* 1962; 10:799-812.
36. Lukoff D, Liberman RP, Nuechterlein KH. Symptom monitoring in the rehabilitation of schizophrenic patients. *Schizophr Bull.* 1986;12:578-593.
37. Overall JE, Hollister LE, Pichot P. Major psychiatric disorders: a four-dimensional model. *Arch Gen Psychiatry.* 1967;16:146-151.
38. Breier A, Wolkowitz OM, Doran AR, Roy A, Boronow J, Hommer DW, Pickar D. Neuroleptic responsivity of negative and positive symptoms in schizophrenia. *Am J Psychiatry.* 1987;144:1549-1555.
39. Goldstein MJ, Rodnick EH, Evans JR, May PRA, Steinberg MR. Drug and family therapy in the aftercare of acute schizophrenics. *Arch Gen Psychiatry.* 1978; 35:1169-1177.
40. Haley J. *Leaving Home: The Therapy of Disturbed Young People.* New York, NY: McGraw-Hill International Book Co; 1980.
41. Leff J, Kuipers L, Berkowitz R, Sturgeon D. A controlled trial of social intervention in the families of schizophrenic patients. *Br J Psychiatry.* 1982;141: 121-134.
42. Cronbach LJ. Coefficient alpha and the internal structure of tests. *Psychometrika.* 1951;16:297-334.
43. Joreskog K, Sorbom D. *LISREL 8.* Chicago, Ill: Scientific Software International; 1993.
44. Pedhazur EJ. *Multiple Regression in Behavioral Research.* 2nd ed. New York, NY: Holt Rinehart & Winston; 1982.
45. Olson DH. Three-dimensional (3-D) circumplex model and revised scoring of FACES III. *Fam Proc.* 1991;30:74-79.
46. Nuechterlein KH, Dawson ME. A heuristic vulnerability/stress model of schizophrenic episodes. *Schizophr Bull.* 1984;10:300-312.
47. Zubin J, Spring B. Vulnerability: a new view of schizophrenia. *J Abnorm Psychol.* 1977;86:103-126.
48. Hogarty GE, Anderson CM, Reiss DJ, Kornblith SJ, Greenwald DP, Javna CD, Madonia MJ. Family psychoeducation, social skills training, and maintenance chemotherapy in the aftercare treatment of schizophrenia. *Arch Gen Psychiatry.* 1986;43:633-642.
49. Corin EE. Facts and meaning in psychiatry: an anthropological approach to the lifeworld of schizophrenics. *Cult Med Psychiatry.* 1990;14:153-188.
50. Corin E, Lauzon G. Positive withdrawal and the quest for meaning: the reconstruction of experience among schizophrenics. *Psychiatry.* 1992;55:266-281.
51. Haley J. *Leaving Home: The Therapy of Disturbed Young People.* New York, NY: McGraw-Hill International Book Co; 1980:26-46.
52. Anderson SA, Gavazzi SM. A test of the Olson Circumplex Model: examining its curvilinear assumption and the presence of extreme types. *Fam Proc.* 1990; 29:309-324.
53. Pratt DM, Hanson JC. A test of the curvilinear hypothesis with FACES II and III. *J Marital Fam Ther.* 1987;13:387-392.
54. King S. Sex differences in a causal model of career maturity. *J Counseling Dev.* 1989;68:208-215.
55. King S. Background and family variables in a causal model of career maturity: comparing hearing and hearing-impaired adolescents. *Career Dev Q.* 1990;38: 240-260.
56. Barrowclough C, Tarrier N. Social functioning in schizophrenic patients. *Soc Psychiatry Psychiatr Epidemiol.* 1990;25:125-129.
57. Mavreas VG, Tomaras V, Karydi V, Economou M, Stephens CN. Expressed emotion in families of chronic schizophrenics and its association with clinical measures. *Soc Psychiatry Psychiatr Epidemiol.* 1992;27:4-9.
58. King S. *Testing a Causal Model of Functioning in Schizophrenic Young Adults: The Influence of Expressed Emotion and Family Dynamics.* Ottawa, Ontario: Health and Welfare Canada; 1993. Publication NHRDP 6605-3327-63.

ORIGINAL ARTICLE

Schizophrenic Deficits in the Processing of Context

A Test of a Theoretical Model

David Servan-Schreiber, MD, PhD; Jonathan D. Cohen, MD, PhD; Sandra Steingard, MD

Background: Schizophrenic patients show various deficits in cognitive functions that have been difficult to understand in terms of a common unifying hypothesis. Previously described neural network models of cognitive tasks suggest that several schizophrenic performance deficits may be related to a single function—an impairment in maintaining contextual information over time and in using that information to inhibit inappropriate responses.

Methods: We tested first-episode schizophrenic patients and patients later in the course of their illness on a new variant of the Continuous Performance Test designed specifically to elicit deficits in the processing of contextual information.

Results: Unmedicated schizophrenic patients showed a deterioration of their signal detection performance that followed the pattern predicted by the context hypothesis, ie, they responded inappropriately when correct responding required the maintenance of context information over time to inhibit the expression of a habitual response. This deficit correlated with positive symptoms. The results also suggested that the deficit may be worse in unmedicated patients who have had a longer course of illness. Medicated patients showed a more diffuse performance deficit.

Conclusions: These results support the view that a single deficit in the processing of context information may underlie various cognitive impairments observed in schizophrenia. They also suggest that such an impairment is associated with positive rather than negative symptoms, and that it may worsen with the course of the illness as in the kraepelinian view of schizophrenia.

Arch Gen Psychiatry. 1996;53:1105-1112

From the Department of Psychiatry, University of Pittsburgh (Drs Servan-Schreiber, Cohen, and Steingard), and the Department of Psychology, Carnegie Mellon University (Dr Cohen), Pittsburgh, Pa. Dr Steingard is now with the Howard Center for Human Services, Burlington, Vt.

SCHIZOPHRENIC PATIENTS show deficits in laboratory tasks that probe cognitive functions ranging from attention to language, memory, and problem-solving. There is no clear understanding of what cognitive processes may be disturbed to produce such disparate deficits. In previous work, we addressed this problem by constructing computer simulation models that specify the information-processing mechanisms underlying normal performance in some cognitive tasks.[1,2] This suggested that several schizophrenic deficits could be related to a disturbance in a single mechanism with pervasive implications for cognition: the representation and maintenance of context information.[3]

Context information is information that has to be held actively in mind in such a form that it can be used to mediate an appropriate behavioral response. For example, in the sentence "In order to keep chickens, you need a pen," the phrase "in order to keep chickens" provides context that constrains the word "pen" to its weaker meaning—"fenced enclosure" rather than to its more common meaning—"writing implement." Context information can be the result of processing a sequence of previous stimuli, a specific previous stimulus, or even a set of task instructions. By this definition, context information is relevant to but does not necessarily form part of the content of the actual response. This distinguishes the role of context from that of short-term memory (ie, storing the identity of recently presented stimuli). We assume that context information is relevant to the performance of almost all cognitive tasks—even simple perceptual tasks—to the extent that subjects must keep in mind at least a set of task instructions that are necessary to identify relevant stimuli and me-

See Subjects and Methods on next page

SUBJECTS AND METHODS

SUBJECTS

Four groups of subjects were studied: unmedicated, first-episode schizophrenic patients (n=11); unmedicated, multiepisode schizophrenic patients (n=6); medicated schizophrenic patients (n=21); and psychiatrically hospitalized patient controls (n=11). All were inpatients who were moderately to severely ill (mean [±SD] Brief Psychiatric Rating Scale [BPRS] score, 34.5±8.23). The BPRS is a 16-item scale, scaling 1 to 7 for each item.[17] Diagnoses were made by a staff psychiatrist, and confirmed by trained research personnel using the Structured Clinical Interview for *DSM-III-R*[18] for schizophrenic patients and the Schedule for Affective Disorders and Schizophrenia[19] for mood-disorder patients.

Unmedicated first-episode schizophrenic subjects all were admitted for the first time, without any history of neuroleptic medication. They had a mean duration of prodromal symptoms of 134 weeks (n=6; prodromal data was unavailable for 5 patients). In all cases, the diagnosis of schizophrenia was confirmed 6 months later. Unmedicated multiepisode schizophrenic subjects were all newly admitted patients who had a documented history of noncompliance with medication for 1 month or more before admission to the hospital. They were tested before receiving neuroleptic medication. Medicated schizophrenic subjects were recently admitted despite outpatient treatment with standard doses of neuroleptic medication and were tested while continuing to receive the same medication. Two of the medicated schizophrenic patients were first-episode right-handed male subjects who had started to receive medication before admission to the hospital. They were included with the medicated schizophrenic group of 19 multiepisode patients because they did not differ in age, education, or any experimental variables (ie, they fell within 1 SD of the mean of the remainder of the medicated subjects on all measures). Controls were inpatients on the mood disorders unit of Western Psychiatric Institute and Clinic, Pittsburgh, Pa. All were diagnosed as having major depressive disorder, and none experienced psychotic symptoms.

Subjects were screened for the following exclusion criteria: alcohol or substance abuse, any substance use within 2 weeks before the study, neurologic illness, or history of head trauma with loss of consciousness. The BPRS was administered within 1 week of admission to the study. Ratings were completed by trained members of the research team who were unaware of the task performance of subjects. The positive symptoms subscale of the BPRS consisted of the sum of 3 items: conceptual disorganization, hallucinatory behavior, and unusual thought content.

No statistically reliable difference was seen between the medicated and unmedicated schizophrenic patients and the patient controls in age, sex, education level, or total BPRS score. However, there were reliably more left-handed medicated patients than unmedicated patients or patient controls by χ^2 analysis, and more left-handed multiepisode schizophrenic patients than first-episode schizophrenic patients or patient controls. These demographic data are given in the **Table**.

PROCEDURE

All subjects provided informed consent in accordance with the university institutional review board. They were tested within 10 days of their admission to the hospital using a modified version of the A-X CPT.[20,21] Sequences of letters were presented one at a time in the center of a visual display, and subjects were instructed to respond whenever the letter X ("target") followed the letter A ("cue"). In this task, the cue provided the context within which to evaluate the target. The remaining letters of the alphabet were used as distractors, with the exception of the letter K, which was excluded because it looks like the letter X. Letters were presented on a computer screen, nondegraded, in Helvetica font, in white against a black background, and subtended a visual angle of 3°. Subjects responded by pressing a button with a finger of their dominant hand. Stimuli appeared for 250 milliseconds, and subjects had a total of 1 second from stimulus onset in which to respond. Feedback was provided in the form of a beep for hits (ie, correct button presses), a buzz for false alarms or misses, and no sound for a correct rejection. This feedback was important to signal to the subjects whether they had responded within the 1-second window (because a failure to respond

diate appropriate responses to them. However, context information is more important to some tasks than others. In particular, it is expected to play an important role when subjects have to maintain information over time and when they have to inhibit an otherwise habitual response. Conversely, it is expected to be least relevant to tasks that do not involve a delay, or do not require subjects to inhibit their natural tendencies.

We have proposed that a disturbance of context can account not only for a general cognitive impairment but also for the specific pattern of schizophrenic deficits observed across various cognitive tasks.[3] We constructed computer simulation models of 3 tasks that are considered to tap different cognitive processes: the Stroop task (selective attention), the identical pairs version of the Continuous Performance Test (CPT) (vigilance and signal-detection ability), and a lexical disambiguation task (language processing). Models of all 3 tasks used a similar architecture (**Figure 1**). We showed that, in simulations of all 3 tasks, a single disturbance to the module supporting context produced changes in performance that matched those observed in schizophrenia.

Furthermore, our models specify mechanisms related to 2 cognitive functions thought to be impaired in schizophrenia: working memory[4-6] and behavioral inhibition.[7-15] Working memory refers to the ability to keep information actively in mind and manipulate it in ways required by a given task. Behavioral inhibition refers to the ability to inhibit a habitual, but inappropriate, response.

Our models show that both the active maintenance of task-relevant information and the inhibition of task-irrelevant information can be carried out by the module responsible for representing and maintaining context. Thus, memory and inhibition reflect the operation of a single underlying mechanism—the context module—

within that time was regarded as a miss). The task was run on an Apple Macintosh computer, using PsyScope software.[22] Testing was done in an isolated room in the inpatient unit after a brief practice period.

The standard procedure for the A-X CPT was modified in 2 ways. First, the frequency of cue-target sequences (A-X) was increased so that these occurred 80% of the time. A randomly chosen noncue letter preceded the target (eg, B-X) in another 10% of trials, and the cue was followed by a distractor (eg, A-Y) in the remaining 10% of trials. Increasing the frequency of cue-target sequences served to engage subjects more actively in the task and to introduce a strong tendency to respond to occurrences of the letter X. This, in turn, forced subjects to rely on the previous letter in the noncue followed by target condition (eg, B-X), as context to inhibit the habitual tendency to respond to X. We predicted that a deficit in this inhibitory function would lead schizophrenic patients to generate a greater number of false alarms to such sequences, which we refer to as "BX errors."

The second modification involved varying the interstimulus interval (ISI) to test subjects' ability to maintain context information over time. We used 2 ISIs: 750 milliseconds and 5 seconds. Each subject was tested in 2 blocks of the task, 1 with the short ISI (750 milliseconds), and 1 with the long ISI (5 seconds). The order was counterbalanced across subjects. A total of 450 stimuli were presented in the short ISI condition and 150 were given in the long ISI condition, to control for time on task. In each case, the proportion of target and nontarget events remained the same (A-X, 80%; B-X, 10%; A-Y, 10%). Subjects had only 1 second to respond, independently of ISI, to prevent differences in speed-accuracy trade-offs between groups from affecting hits and misses differentially across conditions.

We predicted that the performance of control subjects would improve in the 5-second ISI condition, consistent with previous observations that subjects typically perform better in slower-paced tasks.[23] We predicted the reverse for schizophrenic patients: an impairment in the maintenance of context (memory function) would lead to a worsening of performance at the longer delay. More specifically, we predicted an increase in the number of BX errors at the long ISI (evidence that a failure to maintain context [memory] results in an accompanying failure to suppress a strong response tendency [inhibition]).

Finally, we predicted that patients with a recent onset of schizophrenia would have a selective impairment at long delays, but that patients tested at a later stage of illness would fail to withhold responses even at short delays (evidence of a failure to represent as well as maintain context information).

DATA ANALYSIS

Hit and false-alarm rates for each subject were used to compute measures of response criterion[24] and sensitivity (d').[25] C, which is computed as $-0.5(Z_{\text{hits}}+Z_{\text{false alarms}})$, is a measure of criterion recommended for tests in which discrimination varies as a function of group. The d' was computed in the standard manner (using all false alarms—BX and AY), and separately using just the BX false alarms. The latter, by directly comparing performance in the AX and BX conditions, provides a measure of the sensitivity of target detection to the nature of the previous stimulus. This was used as a measure of sensitivity to context (hereafter referred to as "d'-context"). For all computations, in cases of a perfect hit rate (1.0) or false-alarm rate (0.0), a small constant correction (0.001) was made to allow estimation of the signal detection indices.[26,27] This leads to a maximum possible d' value of 6.2 for perfect scores. To verify the assumptions of signal detection theory, the correlations between d' and C were computed within each group, after excluding subjects who made no false alarms (this latter group artificially divides the sample into 2 clusters). After application of the Bonferonni correction for number of significance tests, none of the 6 possible correlations were significant at the .05 level (actual $\alpha=.01$).

We performed a separate repeated-measures analysis of variance (ANOVA) for each of the dependent variables of interest (number of AY false alarms, number of BX false alarms, d', and d'-context). Each ANOVA used group (schizophrenic-medicated, schizophrenic-unmedicated, patient controls) as a between-subject factor, and ISI (short, long) as a within-subject factor. Specific contrasts were evaluated with Student *t* tests. Unless specifically mentioned, 2-tailed tests were applied. One-tailed *t* tests were used to evaluate the specific a priori predictions that motivated the study.

under different task conditions. Under conditions of response competition, when a strong response tendency must be overcome for appropriate behavior (eg, accessing the weaker, but contextually appropriate meaning of "pen"), the context module can be seen as playing an inhibitory role. In contrast, when a delay occurs between information relevant to a response and the execution of that response, the context module can be seen as playing a memory role by actively maintaining that information over time and supporting it against the cumulative effects of noise. According to this view, the role of the context module should be most important when there is both a need to maintain information over time and a need to use that information to inhibit a habitual response.

Our models also suggest that memory and inhibition are differentially sensitive to disturbances of the context module. With mild to moderate disturbances, a deficit appears only when a delay occurs between the context and a response. This is because, with partial degradation of the context information, sufficient information may remain at short or no delays to mediate a contextually appropriate response (eg, inhibit a habitual, but irrelevant response). At longer delays, however, representations succumb to the cumulative effects of noise, and a failure to inhibit the inappropriate response may be observed. Thus, the models predict that mild to moderate disturbances in patients with schizophrenia should manifest primarily at long delays, which might be viewed as a "memory" deficit. With sufficiently severe disturbances of the context mechanism, degraded context representations should produce disturbances even at brief delays, which might be viewed as an "inhibition" deficit.

Assuming a kraepelinian view of schizophrenia, this may relate directly to the course of the illness, with a memory deficit early on, and, as the illness progresses, a

Demographic Data and Brief Psychiatric Rating Scale (BPRS) Scores of Subjects

	Subjects With Schizophrenia			
Characteristic	First Episode, Unmedicated	Multiepisode, Unmedicated	Medicated	Controls
No. of patients	11	6	21	11
Age, y	25.7	26.3	32.2	36.6
Education, y	13.4	11.0	12.4	14.3
Gender, M/F	6/5	4/2	16/5	3/8
Handedness, R/L	10/1	6/0	17/4	10/1
BPRS score	36.6	37.0	33.6	30.7*

Score was not available for 2 of the control subjects.

gradual reduction in the delay that can be tolerated. Eventually, late in the illness, a deficit would be observed even without a delay and may be perceived clinically as a "failure of inhibition." In both cases, the same mechanism is impaired, although to a different degree.

To test these predictions, we developed a variant of the CPT, a task that has been used widely in schizophrenia research.[16] This variant forces subjects to maintain context information over a delay and to use that information to inhibit a habitual but inappropriate response.

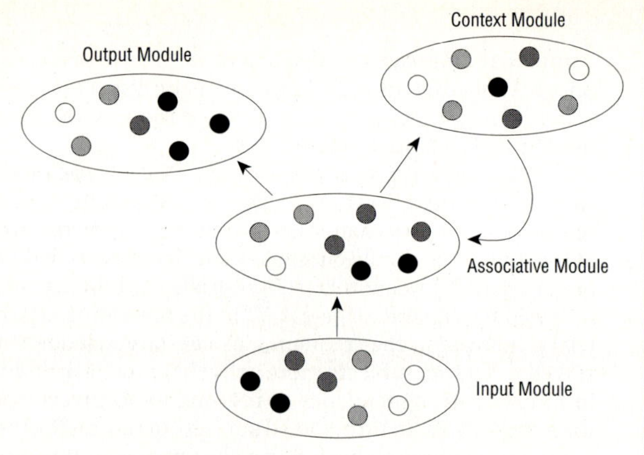

Figure 1. *Schematic representation of the neural network model used to simulate contextual influences on response selection.[3] Several modules consist of individual "neural assemblies" that each have a different level of activation. Neural assemblies receive and send activation from and to other modules. The input module is for representing externally presented stimuli, the output module for producing a response, and the associative module for relating stimuli to appropriate responses. The context module can modulate the flow of information through the associative module. Bidirectional connections between the associative and context modules allow stimuli presented to the network to contribute to the construction of context representations, which in turn can influence the processing (and interpretation) of subsequently presented stimuli.*

RESULTS

Medicated and unmedicated schizophrenic patients showed generally poorer performance compared with patient controls (**Figure 2**, top left) (main effect of group, *P*<.001; planned comparisons, *P*<.02 for overall d′ in controls vs each group of schizophrenics). The predicted difference in the effect of ISI on performance in the 3 groups was marginally significant in the ANOVA (group×ISI interaction, *P*=.06). Planned comparisons confirmed the hypotheses. Control subjects showed an improvement in overall performance in the long compared with the short ISI condition (planned comparison for d′, *P*<.01). The unmedicated schizophrenic patients showed no change in overall performance (*P*=.32). Unexpectedly, however, the medicated patients showed an improvement in performance similar to that of controls at the long ISI (*P*<.01).

The measure of sensitivity to context (d′-context) provided more direct and specific support for our predictions (Figure 2, top right). There was a main effect of group (*P*<.01) and a significant interaction between group and ISI (*P*=.02). The performance of controls on this measure was unaffected by ISI (*P*=.45), nor was the performance of medicated schizophrenic patients (*P*=.33). However, as predicted, unmedicated patients were specifically impaired at the longer ISI (*P*=.005).

Significant predicted differences also were observed in specific types of errors across ISI. (The improvement in the overall performance [d′] of controls and medicated schizophrenic patients at the long ISI means that any increases in specific types of errors at the long ISI for unmedicated patients cannot be attributed to a greater overall difficulty of the task in this condition.)

Unmedicated schizophrenic patients showed an increase in BX false alarms at the long ISI, but controls and medicated patients showed no such increase (Figure 2, lower left) (group×ISI interaction, *P*=.08; planned contrast for unmedicated patients, *P*=.04, 1-tailed). Finally, for AY false alarms, only a main effect of ISI was seen (*P*<.001) (Figure 2, lower right). Such errors were less common at the long ISI for both groups of schizophrenic patients and for controls (*P*<.01 for each group).

To test our predictions related to the course of illness, we compared the d′-context of first-episode with multiepisode schizophrenic patients (unmedicated only) and controls. A group×ISI ANOVA with repeated measures disclosed an expected main effect of ISI (*P*<.05, performance across groups was worse at the long ISI), and a main effect of group (*P*<.01, control subjects did better overall). However, only a trend was seen toward a group×ISI interaction (*P*=.15). First-episode patients did not differ from controls at the short ISI, but a trend existed toward a difference at the long ISI (*P*<.10 after Bonferonni correction for 6 comparisons, actual α=.008). In contrast, multiepisode patients differed from controls at the short and long ISI (*P*<.05 after same Bonferonni correction). Furthermore, a separate ANOVA conducted on only first-episode and multiepisode patients disclosed that, while multiepisode patients showed overall worse performance, there was no group×ISI interaction (*P*=.58). This indicates that the performance of both types of patients followed the same pattern of degradation with delay.

These findings provide tentative support for our prediction of poorer performance at the long delay compared with the short delay (ie, memory deficit) at all stages of illness, combined with an additional deficit specific to later stages of the illness that affects short delays (ie, inhibition deficit). Age did not confound findings re-

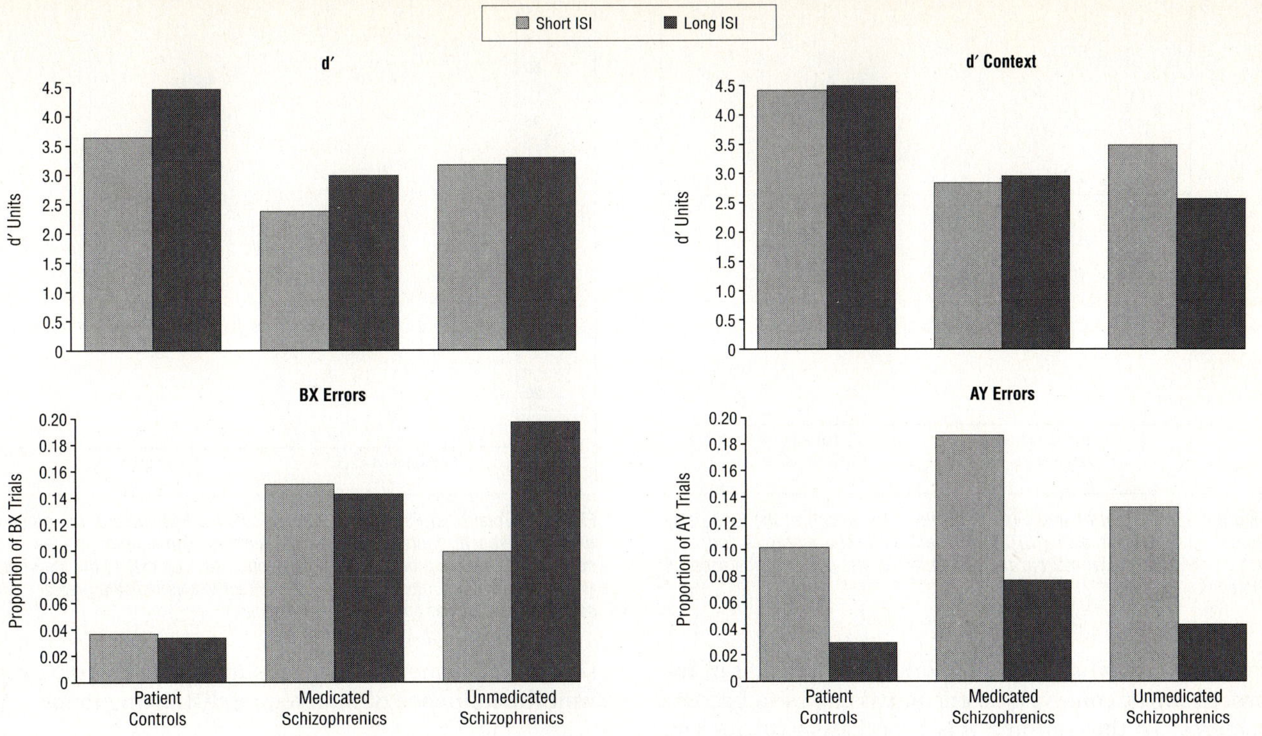

Figure 2. *Performance of patient controls and unmedicated and medicated schizophrenic patients in the modified A-X Continuous Performance Test. The d′ and d′-context are indices of signal detection performance. "AY" and "BX" errors refer to the 2 different types of false alarms that can be committed in this version of the task. ISI indicates interstimulus interval.*

lated to first vs multiepisode status, because no effect of age group (above or below the median of 31 years) was seen on performance at either ISI.

We also evaluated our d′-context measure in relation to clinical symptoms using BPRS scores. Because none of the controls performed below d′-context of 2.5, and many of the unmedicated schizophrenic patients did (**Figure 3**), we divided the patients into 2 groups, those who performed in the same range as controls (d′-context ≥2.5) and those who did not (d′-context <2.5). This division of unmedicated schizophrenic patients into high and low sensitivity to context disclosed a strong association with clinical symptoms. The point-biserial correlation between high and low sensitivity to context and BPRS was 0.66 ($P<.01$) (**Figure 4**). Most of this association was accounted for by positive symptoms ($r=0.60$, $P<.01$) rather than negative symptoms ($r=0.23$, $P=.38$) or other symptoms. No such correlation existed between sensitivity to context and BPRS at the short ISI ($r=0.30$, $P=.28$). Furthermore, medicated schizophrenic patients—who had a similar degree of clinical impairment (Table)—also did not show such an association (point biserial correlation with BPRS total, $r=0.12$, $P=.62$, for the long ISI).

COMMENT

This study was motivated by a set of computer simulation models of the biological mechanisms underlying cognitive deficits associated with schizophrenia.[3] It was designed to test 2 specific predictions made in a previous report[3(63,65)]: the performance of schizophrenic patients on a CPT task should be sensitive to the delay between the presentation of contextual information (the cue) and an ambiguous stimulus (the target), and schizophrenic patients should show a specific inability to use contextual information to inhibit the habitual response to an ambiguous stimulus. Both predictions were confirmed. Our results suggest that the deficit is modified by neuroleptic medications and the course of illness, and is associated with specific clinical symptoms of schizophrenia.

PROCESSING OF CONTEXT: SPECIFIC VS GENERALIZED DEFICIT?

Impaired CPT performance typically has been attributed to a nonspecific "diffuse loss of attention"[28] rather than to a deficit in a circumscribed cognitive mechanism. A general attention deficit is unlikely to be an explanation for our present findings, because unmedicated schizophrenic patients responded to potential targets (X not preceded by A), but not to nontargets (Y), more often than did patient controls and medicated schizophrenic patients. This shows that they were engaged in the task and attentive to the nature of the stimuli.

Deficits in the processing of context have pervasive effects on cognition and may account for performance deficits in a wide array of cognitive tasks. Even "sensory-processing" tasks may be affected by the inability to maintain expectations about the experimental stimuli and to maintain a preparatory response set (ie, context). One

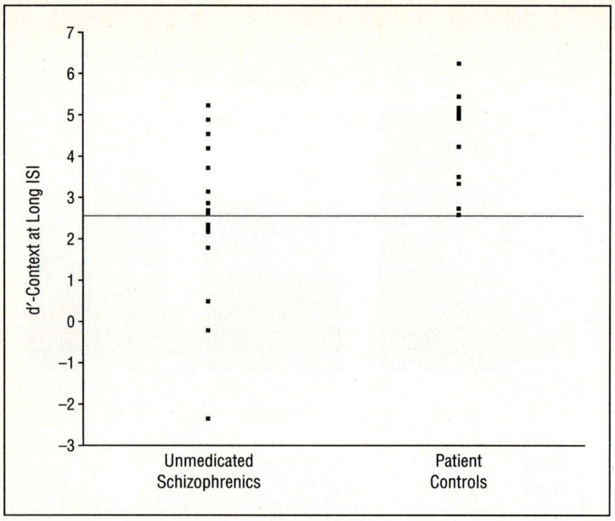

Figure 3. *Scatterplot of sensitivity to context (d′-context) at the long delay (long interstimulus interval [ISI]) for unmedicated schizophrenics and patient controls. Horizontal bar represents the lowest performance score in the control group.*

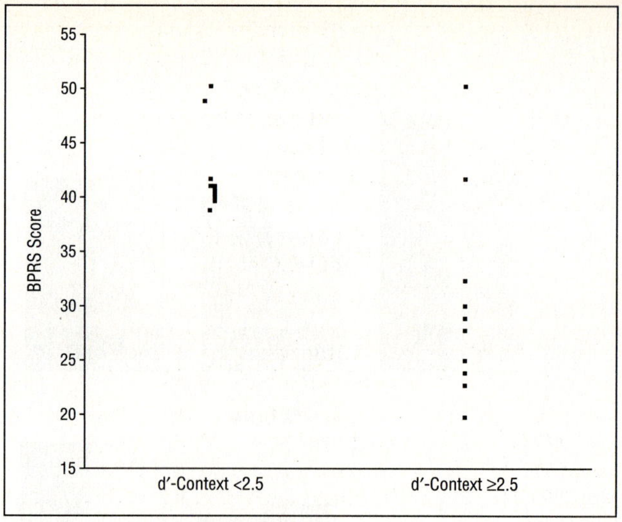

Figure 4. *Total Brief Psychiatric Rating Scale (BPRS) score in the group of unmedicated schizophrenic patients divided into high scorers and low scorers as a function of sensitivity to context (d′-context) at the long delay (long interstimulus interval) (larger d′-context values indicate greater sensitivity to context and better performance).*

then may ask whether the hypothesis of a deficit in the processing of context is so encompassing as to become vacuous. To the contrary, this hypothesis explains and refines the more general concept of a "diffuse loss of attention" associated with schizophrenia since Emil Kraepelin. Although a context deficit produces a general impairment of all cognitive processing, it is not akin to "neglect" of external stimuli. Rather, it induces specific types of errors that can be predicted from a knowledge of a subject's habitual response tendencies and the requirement to maintain information across delays. Furthermore, a deficit in the processing of context does not produce a "generalized deficit" in the sense of Chapman and Chapman,[29] in which differences in the severity of the impairment are due only to a difference in difficulty or other psychometric properties of the task. We designed this version of the CPT precisely to reveal a specific deficit (inability to use context at long delays to inhibit habitual responses) within a more general deficit (impaired signal detection performance). In this task, the long and short delay conditions had the same overall level of difficulty and similar psychometric properties (data not shown). Nevertheless, schizophrenic patients showed a specific impairment in the long delay condition, which puts the highest demands on the processing of context, compared with the short delay condition, which challenged subjects' ability to keep up with a more rapid pace.[30]

Finally, "memory for context" is not equivalent to short-term memory. We view it as a component of the more general construct of working memory. Previous studies have indicated that schizophrenic patients do not show deficits on short-term memory tasks such as digit span,[5,30,31] even when they show deficits in working memory.[5] Although some tasks have been purported to elicit deficits of short-term memory in schizophrenics, these involve supraspan conditions (ie, remembering more than 7 digits) or distractions. Such tasks require the use of encoding strategies that rely on the representation and maintenance of context information rather than simply short-term memory to manage supraspan items or to prevent the influence of intervening distracting items.

INHIBITION AND MEMORY FUNCTIONS IN SCHIZOPHRENIC DEFICITS

Various studies have attributed cognitive deficits in schizophrenia to deficits in working memory[4,5] or in inhibition,[8,9] 2 functions that have been thought to involve distinct subsystems of the prefrontal cortex (PFC).[32] Our models have shown how active maintenance and inhibition can be ascribed to a single processing mechanism, operating under different task conditions. Roberts et al[33] provided empirical support for this view by showing that increasing memory load produces failures of inhibition in an antisaccade task. This suggests that both functions rely on a single resource-limited mechanism. Our present findings are consistent with this view and show that a failure of this mechanism can manifest as what seems to be a memory deficit or an inhibition deficit, depending on the nature of the task.

SENSITIVITY TO CONTEXT AND DEVELOPMENTAL COURSE OF THE ILLNESS

Our models suggest that when the initial representation of context is only moderately disturbed, performance at short delays is unaffected, yet the cumulative effects of noise over time produce a deficit at longer delays.[3] In this study, this was the pattern found in the unmedicated first-episode schizophrenic patients at the short ISI (near-normal performance) compared with the long ISI (impaired performance).

However, further deterioration of the initial representation of context—as might be expected from a progression of the illness—results in a deficit even at short delays. This is the pattern of deficit that was shown by multiepisode schizophrenic patients.

In traditional terms, first-episode schizophrenic patients showed a memory disturbance (deficits only after a delay). In comparison, multiepisode patients showed an inhibition disturbance (ie, a failure to override inappropriate responses without a significant delay). Only a longitudinal study could show a progression of deficits from a memory impairment to a memory and inhibition impairment.

SENSITIVITY TO CONTEXT AND CLINICAL SYMPTOMS

One of our more surprising results concerned the correlation between sensitivity to context and clinical symptoms. Several investigators, including ourselves, have hypothesized a relation between cognitive dysfunction and negative symptoms of schizophrenia.[3,6,34-42] However, sensitivity to context correlated with positive symptoms of the illness but not with negative symptoms. The hypothetical link between negative symptoms, hypofrontality, and impaired performance on working memory tasks in schizophrenic patients has not received strong support from empirical studies.[35,43,44]

An association between positive symptoms and attentional disturbance also has often been proposed,[45] and several studies have documented such a relation.[43,46-51] A common interpretation is that positive symptoms distract subjects during the laboratory task. Indeed, a disturbance in the processing of context would be expected to lead to distractibility (the traditional "failure to maintain set"). This is supported in our study by the correlation between positive symptoms and poor performance on the d′-context measure in unmedicated patients.

SENSITIVITY TO CONTEXT AND NEUROLEPTIC MEDICATIONS

The performance of medicated patients (as measured by d′-context) was inferior to that of patient controls ($P<.05$ with Bonferonni correction), but was not influenced by ISI. In contrast, unmedicated patients (first and multiepisode patients) showed an impairment in d′-context at the long ISI compared with the short ISI. It is as though the neuroleptics, while inducing a general degradation in performance, protected the medicated patients from the degrading effects of noise at the long ISI. Earle-Boyer et al[52] reported a similar finding. The different patterns of performance shown by the medicated and unmedicated patients exemplifies the difference in effects produced by a "generalized deficit" in the sense of Chapman and Chapman[29] (overall worsening of performance with medication) on the one hand, and a "specific deficit" on the other hand (differential impairment in the long vs short delay conditions due to an impairment in the processing of context).

LIMITATION OF THE STUDY

Based on our models and a large body of indirect evidence, we have previously argued that PFC houses the mechanism responsible for processing context, and that schizophrenic deficits on the CPT are related to a disturbance of dopamine function in PFC.[3] The present study does not directly address this relation. Recent functional imaging studies have shown the role of PFC in a version of the CPT that relies on mechanisms similar to the ones described in this article.[53,54] However, whether CPT deficits are related to a disturbance of dopamine in PFC remains a question for future research.

Accepted for publication March 26, 1996.

This work was supported by grants MH47073, MH47566, and MH45156 from the National Institute of Mental Health, National Institutes of Health, Bethesda, Md (Drs Servan-Schreiber and Cohen).

We thank Nina Schooler, PhD, John Sweeney, PhD, and Cameron Carter, MD, for their valuable comments and advice during all phases of this study. We also thank Dr Schooler, John Gurkliss, MD, Matcheri Keshavan, MD, Vijoy Abraham, and Gretchen Haas, PhD, for their substantial contributions to the conduct of this study, without whom it could not have been done. Olga Tereshko edited the manuscript several times and gave it its final form.

Corresponding author: Jonathan D. Cohen, MD, PhD, Department of Psychology, Carnegie Mellon University, Schenley Park, Pittsburgh, PA 15213.

REFERENCES

1. Cohen JD, Dunbar K, McClelland JL. On the control of automatic processes: a parallel distributed processing account of the Stroop effect. *Psychol Rev.* 1990; 97:332-361.
2. Cohen JD, Servan-Schreiber D, McClelland JL. A parallel distributed processing approach to automaticity. *Am J Psychol.* 1992;105:239-269.
3. Cohen JD, Servan-Schreiber D. Context, cortex and dopamine: a connectionist approach to behavior and biology in schizophrenia. *Psychol Rev.* 1992;99:45-77.
4. Goldman-Rakic PS. Prefrontal cortical dysfunction in schizophrenia: the relevance of working memory. In: Carroll BJ, Barrett JE, eds. *Psychopathology and the Brain.* New York, NY: Raven Press: 1991:1-23.
5. Park S, Holzman PS. Schizophrenics show spatial working memory deficits. *Arch Gen Psychiatry.* 1992;49:975-982.
6. Weinberger DR, Berman KF, Zec RF. Physiological dysfunction of dorsolateral prefrontal cortex in schizophrenia: I, regional cerebral blood flow evidence. *Arch Gen Psychiatry.* 1986;43:114-125.
7. Storms LH, Broen WE. A theory of schizophrenic behavioral disorganization. *Arch Gen Psychiatry.* 1969;20:129-144.
8. Maher B. The language of schizophrenia: a review and interpretation. *Br J Psychiatry.* 1972;120:3-17.
9. Manschreck T, Maher BA, Milavetz JJ, Ames D, Weisstein CC, Schneyer ML. Semantic priming in thought-disordered schizophrenic patients. *Schizophr Res.* 1988;1:61-66.
10. Chapman LJ, Chapman JP, Miller GA. A theory of verbal behavior in schizophrenia. In: Maher BA, ed. *Progress in Experimental Personality Research.* Orlando, Fla: Academic Press Inc; 1964:135-167.
11. Wapner S, Krus DM. Effects of lysergic acid diethylamide, and differences between normals and schizophrenics, on the Stroop Color-Word Test. *J Neuropsychiatry.* 1960;2:76-81.
12. Abramczyk RR, Jordan DE, Hegel M. 'Reverse' Stroop effect in the performance of schizophrenics. *Percept Mot Skills.* 1983;56:99-106.
13. Wysocki JJ, Sweet JI. Identification of brain-damaged, schizophrenic, and normal medical patients using a brief neuropsychological screening battery. *Int J Clin Neuropsychol.* 1985;7:40-44.
14. Carter CS, Robertson LC, Nordahl TE, O'Shora-Celaya LJ, Chaderjian MC. Abnormal processing of irrelevant information in schizophrenia: the role of illness subtype. *Psychiatry Res.* 1993;48:17-26.
15. Cohen JD, Carter CS. Stroop facilitation and interference: same or different mechanisms? Presented as a poster abstract at the Second Annual Meeting of the Cognitive Neuroscience Society; March 17, 1996; San Francisco, Calif.
16. Rosvold HE, Mirsky AF, Sarason I, Bransome ED, Beck LH. A continuous per-

formance test of brain damage. *J Consult Clin Psychol.* 1956;20:343-350.
17. Overall JE, Gorham DR. The Brief Psychiatric Rating Scale. *Psychol Rep.* 1962; 10:799-803.
18. Spitzer RL, Williams JB. *Structured Clinical Interview for DSM-III-R.* New York, NY: New York State Psychiatric Institute; 1987.
19. Endicott J, Spitzer RL. A diagnostic interview: the schedule for affective disorders and schizophrenia. *Arch Gen Psychiatry.* 1978;35:837-844.
20. Wohlberg GW, Kornetsky C. Sustained attention in remitted schizophrenics. *Arch Gen Psychiatry.* 1973;28:533-537.
21. Nuechterlein KH. Vigilance in schizophrenia and related disorders. In: Steinhauer SR, Gruzelier JH, Zubin J, eds. *Handbook of Schizophrenia: Neuropsychology, Psychophysiology, and Information Processing.* Amsterdam, the Netherlands: Elsevier Science Publishers; 1991;5:397-433.
22. Cohen JD, MacWhinney B, Flatt M, Provost J. A new graphic interactive environment for designing psychology experiments. *Behav Res Methods Instruments Comput.* 1993;25:257-271.
23. Parasuraman R. Memory load and event rate control sensitivity decrements in sustained attention. *Science.* 1979;205:924-927.
24. Snodgrass JG, Corwin J. Pragmatics of measuring recognition memory: applications to dementia and amnesia. *J Exp Psychol Gen.* 1988;17:34-50.
25. Green DM, Swets JA. *Signal Detection Theory and Psychophysics.* Melbourne, Fla: Krieger Publishing Co; 1966.
26. McNicol D. *A Primer on Signal Detection Theory.* London, England: George Allen & Unwin Publishers Ltd; 1972.
27. Nuechterlein KH. Signal detection in viligance tasks and behavioral attributes among offspring of schizophrenic mothers and among hyperactive children. *J Abnorm Psychol.* 1983;92:4-8.
28. Cornblatt BA, Lenzenweger MF, Erlenmeyer-Kimling L. The Continuous Performance Test, Identical Pairs Version: II, contrasting attentional profiles in schizophrenic and depressed patients. *Psychiatry Res.* 1989;29:65-85.
29. Chapman LJ, Chapman JP. The measurement of differential deficit. *J Psychiatr Res.* 1978;14:303-311.
30. Oltmanns TF, Neale JM. Schizophrenia performance when distractors are present: attentional deficit or differential task difficulty? *J Abnorm Psychol.* 1975; 84:205-209.
31. Larsen SF, Fromholt P. Mnemonic organization and free recall in schizophrenia. *J Abnorm Psychol.* 1976;85:61-65.
32. Fuster JM. *The Prefrontal Cortex.* New York, NY: Raven Press; 1980.
33. Roberts RJ Jr, Hager LD, Heron C. Prefrontal cognitive processes: working memory and inhibition in the antisaccade task. *J Exp Psychol Gen.* 1994;123: 374-393.
34. Nuechterlein KH, Edell WS, Norris M, Dawson ME. Attentional vulnerability indicators, thought disorder and negative symptoms. *Schizophr Bull.* 1986;12: 408-426.
35. Andreasen NC, Rezai K, Alliger R, Swayze VW, Flaum M, Kirchner P, Chen G, O'Leary DS. Hypofrontality in neuroleptic-naive patients and in patients with chronic schizophrenia. *Arch Gen Psychiatry.* 1992;49:943-958.
36. Ingvar DH. Abnormal distribution of cerebral activity in chronic schizophrenia: a neurophysiological interpretation. In: Baxter CF, Melnechuk T, eds. *Perspectives in Schizophrenia Research.* New York, NY: Raven Press; 1980:107-125.
37. Buchsbaum MS, Ingvar DH, Kessler R, Waters RN, Cappelletto J, Van Kammen DP, King AC, Johnson JL, Manning RG, Flynn RW, Mann LS, Bunney WE Jr, Sokoloff L. Cerebral glucography with positron tomography. *Arch Gen Psychiatry.* 1982;39:251-259.
38. Levin S. Frontal lobe dysfunctions in schizophrenia: II, impairments of psychological and brain functions. *J Psychol Res.* 1984;18:57-82.
39. Wolkin A, Jaeger J, Brodie JD, Wolf AP, Fowler J, Rotrusen J, Gomez-Mont F, Cancro R. Persistence of cerebral metabolic abnormalities in chronic schizophrenia as determined by positron emission tomography. *Am J Psychiatry.* 1985;142:564-571.
40. Andreasen NC. Neural mechanisms of negative symptoms. *Br J Psychiatry.* 1989;155(suppl 7):93-98.
41. Berman KF, Torrey F, Daniel DG, Weinberger DR. Regional cerebral blood flow in monozygotic twins discordant and concordant for schizophrenia. *Arch Gen Psychiatry.* 1992;49:927-934.
42. Wolkin A, Sanfilip M, Wolf AP, Angrist B, Brodie JD, Rotresen J. Negative symptoms and hypofrontality in chronic schizophrenia. *Arch Gen Psychiatry.* 1992; 49:959-965.
43. Siegal BV, Buchsbaum MS, Bunney WE, Gottschalk L, Haier RJ, Lohr JB, Lottenberg S, Najafi A, Nuechterlein K, Potkin SG. Cortical-striatal-thalamic circuits and brain glucose metabolic activity in 70 unmedicated male schizophrenic patients. *Am J Psychiatry.* 1993;150:1325-1336.
44. Strauss ME. Relations of symptoms to cognitive deficits in schizophrenia. *Schizophr Bulletin.* 1993;19:215-231.
45. McGhie A, Chapman J. Disorders of attention and perception in early schizophrenia. *Br J Med Psychol.* 1961;34:103-116.
46. Nuechterlein KH, Dawson ME, Gitlan M, Ventura J, Goldstein MJ, Snyder KS, Yee CM, Mintz J. Developmental processes in schizophrenic disorders: longitudinal studies of vulnerability and stress. *Schizophr Bull.* 1992;18:387-425.
47. Lawson JS, McGhie A, Chapman J. Distractibility in schizophrenic and organic cerebral disease. *Br J Psychiatry.* 1967;113:527-535.
48. Oltmanns TF. Selective attention in schizophrenic and manic psychoses: the effect of distraction on information processing. *J Abnorm Psychol.* 1978;87: 212-225.
49. Bilder RM, Mukherjee S, Rieder RO, Pandurangi AK. Symptomatic and neuropsychological components of defect states. *Schizophr Bull.* 1985;11:409-419.
50. Walker E, Harvey P. Positive and negative symptoms in schizophrenia: attentional performance correlates. *Psychopathology.* 1986;19:294-302.
51. Harvey P, Pedley M. Auditory and visual distractibility in schizophrenia: clinical and medication status correlations. *Schizophr Res.* 1989;2:294-300.
52. Earle-Boyer EA, Serper MR, Davidson M, Harvey P. Continuous performance tests in schizophrenic patients: stimulus and medication effects on performance. *Psychiatry Res.* 1991;37:47-56.
53. Cohen JD, Forman SD, Braver TS, Casey BJ, Servan-Schreiber D, Noll DC. Activation of prefrontal cortex in a nonspatial working memory task with functional MRI. *Hum Brain Mapping.* 1994;1:293-304.
54. Cohen JD, Ganguli R, Carter C, Brar J, Nichols T, DeLeo M, Mintor A. Hypofrontality and working memory dysfunction in schizophrenia. *Biol Psychiatry.* 1995;37:143A. Abstract.

INTRODUCING

RISPERDAL ON CALL

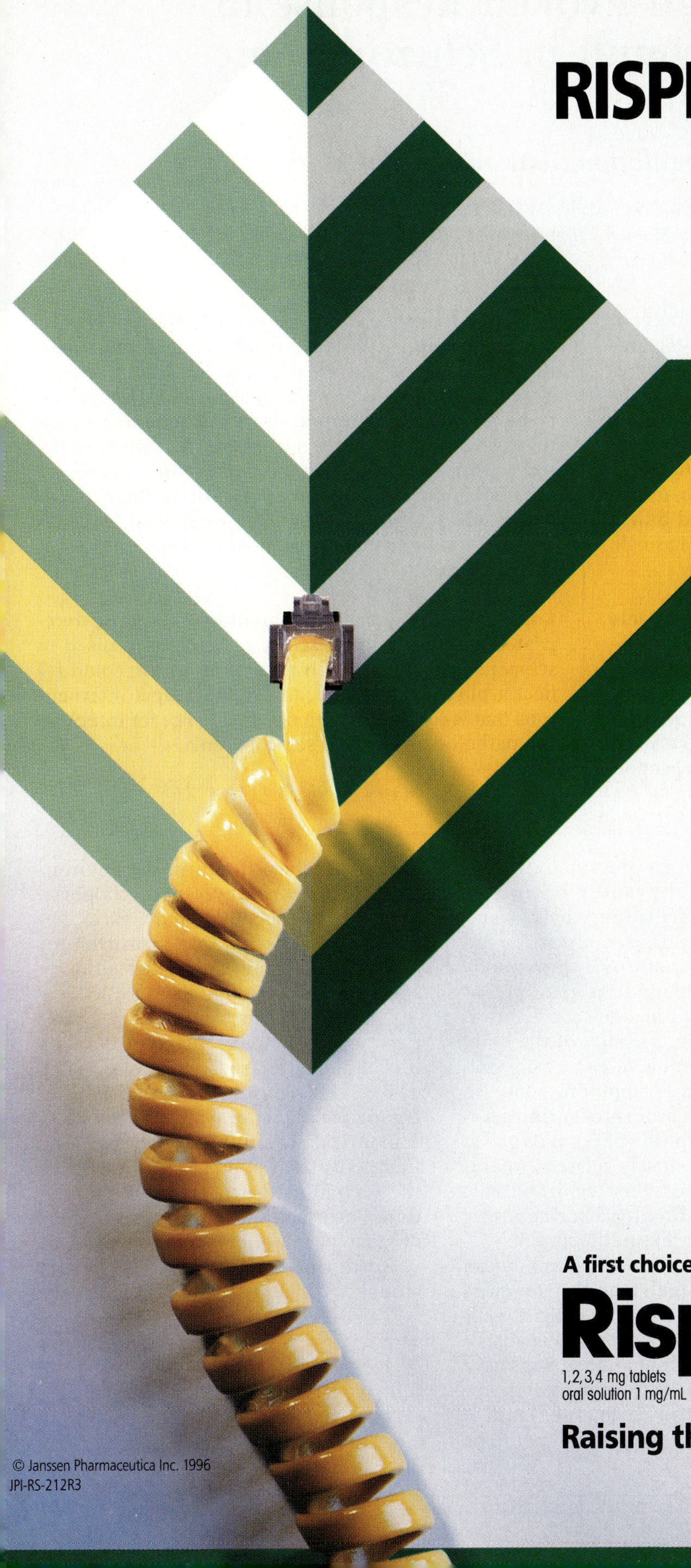

Quick, easy access to the information you want.

Now you can call a toll-free 800 number for instant access to information about RISPERDAL.

Available whenever you need it.

RISPERDAL ON CALL is available 24 hours a day, 7 days a week. You can access it anytime, anywhere—all you need is a touch-tone phone.

The information you need—and more—at your fingertips.

Get product and conversion information, hear physician discussions, or request an important clinical reprint! Just call 1-800-6R-ON-CALL (1-800-676-6225) and follow the voice prompts to your choice of valuable information about RISPERDAL.

What else does RISPERDAL ON CALL offer?

Call 1-800-6R-ON-CALL (1-800-676-6225) today!

A first choice

Risperdal®

RISPERIDONE

1,2,3,4 mg tablets
oral solution 1 mg/mL

Raising the standard of care.

ORIGINAL ARTICLE

Inhibitory Gating of an Evoked Response to Repeated Auditory Stimuli in Schizophrenic and Normal Subjects

Human Recordings, Computer Simulation, and an Animal Model

Robert Freedman, MD; Lawrence E. Adler, MD; Marina Myles-Worsley, PhD; Herbert T. Nagamoto, MD; Christine Miller, PhD; Michael Kisley, MS; Kara McRae; Ellen Cawthra, RN; Merilyne Waldo, PhD

Background: Altered sensory response is a prominent feature of schizophrenia. Inhibitory gating mechanisms, shown by diminished P50 evoked responses to repeated auditory stimuli, seem to be deficient in schizophrenic persons. These inhibitory mechanisms usually are studied by averaging the electroencephalographic responses to many presentations of pairs of stimuli. Although averaging increases signal-to-noise ratio, it may obscure trial-to-trial differences. We compared differences between schizophrenic and normal persons in single trials and averages of P50 response.

Methods: Recordings from 10 schizophrenic patients and 10 normal subjects were analyzed using conventional averaging and single-trial measurements. A computer simulation of both methods examined their ability to extract evoked responses from background activity. Related single-neuron activity in the hippocampus in an animal model also was studied, because neuronal action potentials can be reliably identified in single trials.

Results: Averaged evoked potentials showed significant suppression of the P50 response to the second stimulus of the pair in normal patients, but not in schizophrenic patients. Single-trial analysis did not detect a response above background activity. Computer simulations gave similar results, suggesting that failure to detect suppression in single trials comes from inadequate differentiation of signal from noise. Recordings in animals confirmed almost complete suppression of the response of hippocampal pyramidal neurons to the second stimulus.

Conclusions: The normal inhibition of response to repeated auditory stimuli seems to be compromised in schizophrenia. This loss of inhibitory gating could reflect a physiological deficit of hippocampal interneurons that is consonant with other evidence for interneuron pathologic defects in schizophrenia.

Arch Gen Psychiatry. 1996;53:1114-1121

Neurophysiological characterization of schizophrenia has emphasized alterations in response to sensory stimuli as possible indicators of pathophysiological neuronal defects.[1,2] Unfortunately, the inaccessibility of the brain limits studies of human sensory physiology to observations of motor responses to stimuli[3,4] or to recordings of surface electroencephalographic (EEG) activity.[5-10] Nevertheless, 2 closely related conclusions have emerged. First, schizophrenic persons have difficulty discriminating and/or responding to specific stimuli.[3,5,9,10] Second, they have diminished inhibition of response to stimuli that do not require their attention.[4,6-8] Based on patients' self-reports of these phenomena, Venables[11] proposed that schizophrenic persons have a fundamental defect in involuntary attention that normally enables the brain to focus on objects of interest and not to be drawn to other stimuli in the environment.[12] Summarizing recent psychophysiological evidence, Braff and Geyer[13] hypothesized a deficit in a sensorimotor gating mechanism that regulates the response to sensory stimuli.

Various forms of inhibitory synaptic transmission are obvious candidate mechanisms for sensory gating. They can be shown using the conditioning-testing paradigm, in which responses to 2 identical stimuli are compared. The first activates a population of neurons; the second activates the same population, but usually with diminished effect because of inhibitory mechanisms activated during the response to the first stimulus.[14] The first stimulus thus con-

From the Department of Psychiatry, Denver Veterans Administration Medical Center and University of Colorado Health Sciences Center, Denver, Colo (Drs Freedman, Adler, Nagamoto, Miller, and Waldo and Mss McRae and Cawthra and Mr Kisley); and the Department of Psychiatry, University of Utah School of Medicine, Salt Lake City (Dr Myles-Worsley).

See Subjects and Methods on next page

SUBJECTS AND METHODS

SUBJECTS

Ten patients, 6 men and 4 women (mean [±SD] age, 46.0±14.2 years), were diagnosed as having schizophrenia by Research Diagnostic Criteria[34] after a Schedule for Affective Disorders and Schizophrenia[35] interview and review of medical records. All 10 patients met criteria for chronic schizophrenia; 4 were paranoid and 6 were mixed type. One of the schizophrenic patients, whose recording is shown in **Figure 1**, had never been treated with medication. The others were taking typical neuroleptic medications (200-1300 chlorpromazine equivalents), which increase the amplitude of the conditioning wave but do not alter the inhibitory gating of the P50 response.[36,37] The schizophrenic subjects were compared with normal subjects who were sex- and age-matched within 4 years (45.8±14.3 years), had no personal history of mental illness or substance abuse and no family history of schizophrenia. These subjects were also compared with a larger group of 36 schizophrenic subjects and 43 normal subjects who met the same diagnostic criteria; their recordings had been analyzed using conventional averaging.[38] All subjects gave informed consent to the procedure.

ELECTROPHYSIOLOGICAL RECORDING

The patient lay prone, with the head and neck supported to reduce neck muscle response to the sound. The stimuli were clicks of approximately 1-millisecond duration generated by a 0.04-millisecond square wave. At the subject's ear, the mean sound intensity was 75-dB sound pressure level. The clicks were presented in pairs, with 0.5-second intrapair interval and 10 seconds between pairs. The subjects were awake, with eyes fixed on a distant point. The EEG was monitored and, if signs of drowsiness were observed (eg, initiation of alpha or other slow waves), recording was interrupted and the subject reminded to stay awake.

Electroencephalographic activity was recorded from the vertex, referenced to the left ear. Electrode resistance was less than 10 kΩ. Electro-oculographic activity was recorded between the superior orbit and lateral canthus. Activity was recorded with a bandpass of 1 to 300 Hz and digitized at 1000 Hz for acquisition by computer. The computer recorded activity for 100 milliseconds before the conditioning stimulus, and 500-millisecond intervals following the conditioning stimulus and the test stimulus. Trials were rejected if EEG or electro-oculographic channel voltage exceeded plus or minus 35 μV. Three sets of 32 artifact-free trials were recorded for each subject. For 2 schizophrenic subjects, only 2 sets of 32 artifact-free trials could be obtained.

EVOKED POTENTIAL AVERAGING

A single average was compiled from the 3 sets of 32 trials and filtered digitally to exclude activity below 10 and above 100 Hz.[39] Responses from 2 subjects are shown in Figure 1. A computer algorithm selected a wave in 3 windows: prestimulus, conditioning, and test. The conditioning P50 response, the most positive peak 40 to 80 milliseconds poststimulus, was measured relative to the preceding negative trough. The test P50 response was at the same latency plus or minus 10 milliseconds from the test stimulus. The prestimulus was selected from the period before the first stimulus, 40 to 80 milliseconds after initiation of recording. If no wave was found in the prestimulus or test window, the value was recorded as 0.

ANALYSIS OF SINGLE TRIALS

The first 40 trials used in the previous analysis were analyzed for each subject.[24] Each trial was filtered and waves selected as described. Because the premise of single-trial averaging is that significant variance in latency may exist, the window for the test response was set at 40 to

Continued on next page

ditions inhibitory mechanisms, whose strength is tested by the second stimulus. Suppression of the auditory evoked P50 response in normal persons has long been known;[15-20] more recently, loss of suppression of the P50 response[21-25] and other evoked responses[8,26,27] also has been reported in schizophrenic persons.

Like most evoked potentials, the amplitude of the P50 wave is less than background EEG activity.[28] Therefore, a number of responses are averaged: evoked activity that occurs at a constant or almost constant time after the stimulus sums linearly; other randomly occurring waves tend to cancel out, summing as the square root of the amplitude.[29] The sum is divided by the number of trials to obtain an average. Eighty to 100 pairs are typically used to record P50 responses, so that about one tenth of the noise remains in the average. In a background EEG of 20 μV, P50 waves exceeding 2 μV would thus be detectable. However, averaging also may conceal important variance in the data. The assumption of constant signal and random noise often has been questioned.[2,29,30] For example, diminished amplitude could represent a diminished amplitude for each single test response, increased variance in the latency of the waves, or fewer large responses. Differences in resting EEG also might contribute to differences in the measurement of evoked activity.[31-33]

Strategies have been devised to extract evoked responses from single EEG recordings. All rely on conventional averaging to determine response values that are then used to identify single evoked responses. Although sophisticated techniques have been devised, Lopes de Silva,[29] in his authoritative textbook on electroencephalography, recommends simply identifying a wave of the same polarity in the latency range normally expected for the evoked response. A series of individual trials are added together, all shifted in time to align waves to the latency of the averaged response. The newly developed average will have a significantly larger evoked response. Presumably, the enhancement

80 milliseconds after the test stimulus, regardless of the latency of the conditioning response. For display, individual trials were aligned for each subject so that the largest wave within each window occurred at the latency of the conditioning response in the conventional average. The aligned trials were summed, and the sum divided by the number of trials. Reported amplitudes are the mean obtained from the analysis of each trial; percentage ratios were calculated from these means.

Preplanned comparisons of conditioning to prestimulus and test response amplitude for each averaging method and a comparison of the P50 ratios generated by the 2 methods were made using the Student *t* test (2-tailed, α=.05).

COMPUTER SIMULATION

A computer simulation was performed to determine the effects on each peak-detection technique of changing various values in the P50 wave and the background EEG. Three 130-member arrays were modeled, each epochs of 130 milliseconds, simulating prestimulus, conditioning, and test periods, including background EEG activity (12.5-Hz alpha, 20-Hz $beta_1$, and 40-Hz $beta_2$) and auditory evoked response. Forty trials were generated and analyzed as conventional averages and single trials. For the averaging algorithm, the P50 peak and preceding trough latencies were determined from the average waveform. In each trial used to form the average, the change in amplitude between these 2 timepoints was determined and used to calculate the SE of the P50 amplitude. For the single-trials strategy, the amplitudes of each trial were used to calculate the mean and SE.

All values were varied independently, holding other values constant: the amplitude of each of the 3 sine waves and of the P50 wave, the phase of each wave, and the SD of the latency of the P50 wave.

ANIMAL ELECTROPHYSIOLOGY

Three male Sprague-Dawley rats were anesthetized with chloral hydrate (400 mg/kg, intraperitoneal) and placed in a stereotaxic frame with hollow ear bars for delivery of auditory stimuli. A microelectrode was lowered into the CA3 pyramidal layer of the hippocampus. The location was confirmed by the appearance of action potentials from a layer of pyramidal neurons and by the ability to elicit an antidromic neuronal population discharge by stimulation of the hippocampal commissure, which in rats consists principally of CA3 pyramidal neuron axons projecting across the midline to the contralateral hippocampus. The microelectrode recorded auditory evoked potentials and action potential from individual neurons. Action potentials from a single neuron were maximized by using a hydraulic micromanipulator to position the electrode close to that neuron. Pyramidal neurons were identified from the oscilloscope display by their action potential shape, which includes several smaller wavelets and a duration of the principal component of the action potential more than 0.6 milliseconds and an amplitude more than 250 μV. A Schmitt trigger circuit discriminated the action potential from other electrical activity and generated a logic pulse for subsequent computer analysis. For each neuron recorded, 40 stimulus pairs were given, and a peristimulus time histogram of the response was compiled, analogous to the auditory average evoked response. The single-trial responses were also recorded.

From a 100-millisecond period in the histogram before the conditioning stimulus, the spontaneous discharge rate was measured in 10-millisecond bins (intervals). Activity that exceeded the mean plus 3 SDs was identified as an excitatory response; activity that was less than the mean minus 3 SDs was identified as an inhibitory response. For the 5 cells recorded in 3 animals, 3 had periods following the conditioning stimulus that met these criteria, 2 excitatory and 1 inhibitory. In these, the identical time interval was analyzed in the test response. For the 2 excited cells, individual trials were examined to determine the latency of the first action potential in each excitatory response. Results were compared with those from an additional 30 CA3 pyramidal neurons recorded in 26 animals, of which 21 had excitatory responses to tone.[40]

represents the elimination of latency shifts. However, because the nearest wave may not be the evoked response but rather a background wave, temporal alignment, while seeming to increase the amplitude of the response, might simply enhance noise at the expense of the true signal.[2]

We tried to determine what conventional averaging and the sum of waves from single trials each disclose about the P50 response to paired stimuli. We performed (1) a comparison of the ability of the 2 techniques to distinguish signal from noise in actual recordings, (2) a computer-based simulation to determine the importance of background EEG amplitude and latency variance with each technique, and (3) recordings from a putative source of the P50 wave, the pyramidal neurons of the hippocampus, in an animal model to determine how the neurons themselves respond to paired stimuli. Action potentials from single neurons have a high signal strength, so they can be detected reliably without averaging.

RESULTS

EVOKED RESPONSES FROM SCHIZOPHRENIC AND NORMAL SUBJECTS

The average evoked response recorded from normal subjects (**Figure 2**) showed a conditioning P50 response that was significantly larger than the prestimulus activity (t=7.46, df=18, P<.001). The test response was only 20% of the conditioning response (t=7.16, df=18, P<.001) and was not significantly different from the prestimulus activity. Schizophrenic subjects had a conditioning wave of similar amplitude, also significantly different from prestimulus activity (t=5.12, df=18, P<.001). However, for schizophrenic subjects, the test response was 80% of the conditioning response and significantly larger than the prestimulus activity (t=4.56, df=18, P<.001). Schizophrenic subjects had ratios of the amplitude of the test response to the conditioning response significantly larger than normal subjects (t=8.07, df=18, P<.001). These ra-

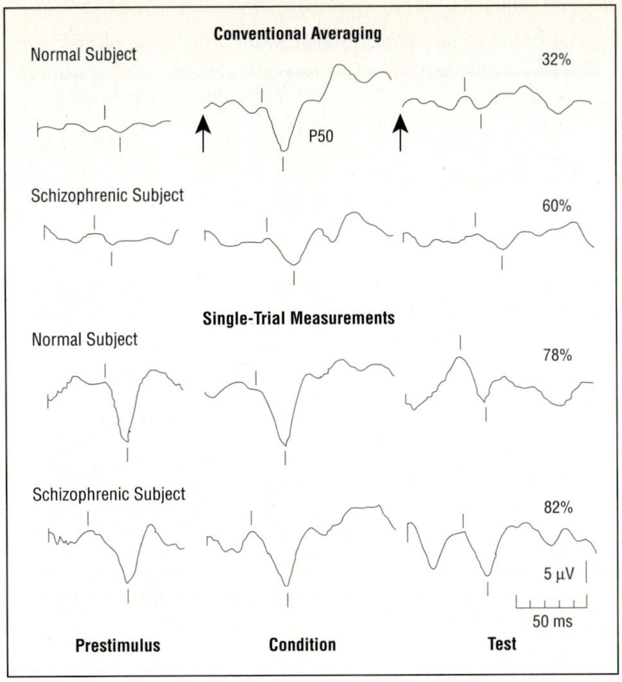

Figure 1. *Comparison of conventional averaging (top) with the mean of single-trial measurements (bottom) for a normal subject and a never-medicated schizophrenic patient for the P50 response to paired auditory stimuli (arrows). The percentages at right are the ratio of the test to the conditioning-response amplitude. The conditioning P50 response is indicated by the most positive peak 40 to 80 milliseconds poststimulus (tic below each tracing) measured relative to the preceding negative trough (tic above the tracing).*

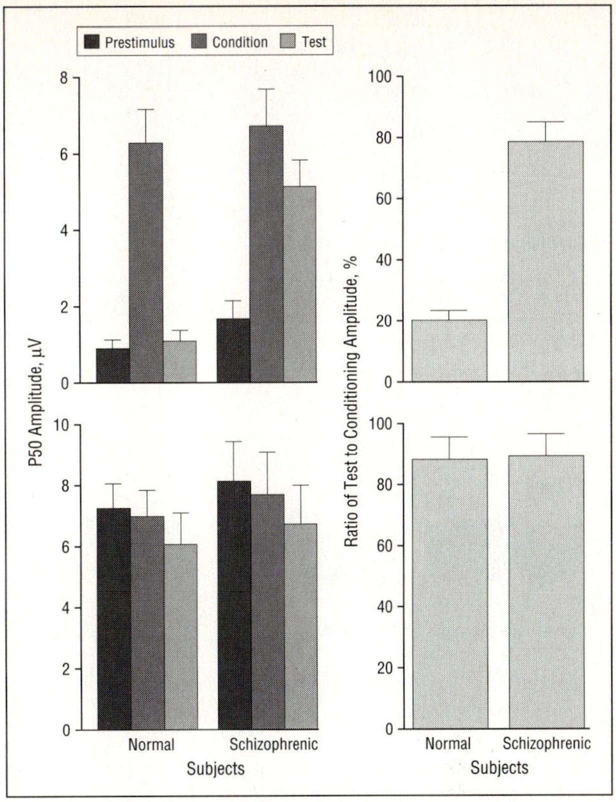

Figure 2. *Mean and SE of measurements of the P50 response obtained with conventional averaging (top) and single-trial measurement from 10 normal and 10 schizophrenic subjects (bottom).*

tios were similar to those from the larger group of schizophrenic ([mean±SD] 100.1%±31.8%, n=36) and normal subjects (17.8%±17.0%, n=43).

In the single-trial recordings from the normal and schizophrenic subjects (Figure 1, top, and Figure 2, top), selection of the largest wave in each 40- to 80-millisecond interval resulted in almost identical waves being detected in the prestimulus, conditioning, and testing periods. Thus, the conditioning wave was no longer significantly larger than the prestimulus activity for either group of subjects, and the ratio of the test to the conditioning amplitude approached 100%.

COMPUTER SIMULATION OF EVOKED RESPONSES

The results with simulated waves were similar to those observed in recordings from human subjects. The computer simulation allowed comparison of the measurement of the P50 amplitude either by conventional averaging or by selection of individual waves, with the amplitude of the P50 wave that was initially added to the background EEG as an input to the simulation. This input P50 amplitude represents the true response of the brain to the auditory stimulus. The 2 measurement methods differed in their ability to measure the true P50 amplitude accurately when the P50 was embedded in background EEG. Conventional averaging detected a conditioning response larger than the prestimulus activity and suppression of the test response. Selection of individual waves generated responses with almost identical amplitude in the prestimulus, condition, and test periods (**Figure 3**). A comparison of results for a range of P50 amplitudes showed that the selection of individual waves did not measure the amplitude of the input P50, but the signal detected in even a single 40-trial average approximated the amplitude of the input wave (**Figure 4**).

Further simulations were performed varying other values, including the overall amplitude of the EEG, the relative amplitudes of alpha, $beta_1$, and $beta_2$, and the SD of the latency of P50. For each set of values, the measurements obtained from both techniques were compared for a conditioning signal (input P50=10 μV) and for no signal (P50=0 μV). The results of the averaging technique were unaffected by increases in the background EEG amplitude, but the single-trial method included noise in the estimate of P50 amplitude, producing larger waves as the background activity increased, whether or not a P50 signal existed in the input (**Table**). When individual components of the EEG were considered, alpha was associated with the greatest decrease in P50 amplitude for both techniques. $Beta_1$ gave the greatest apparent output in the absence of a P50 signal in the single-trial method, but $beta_2$ gave the noisiest signal for the averaging method. As expected, increase in the SD of the latency did not affect the results of the single-trial method, because single trials are selected regardless of latency, but did decrease the P50 amplitude measured by averaging. However, in no case did selection of individual trials produce a more accurate measurement of P50 than conventional averaging.

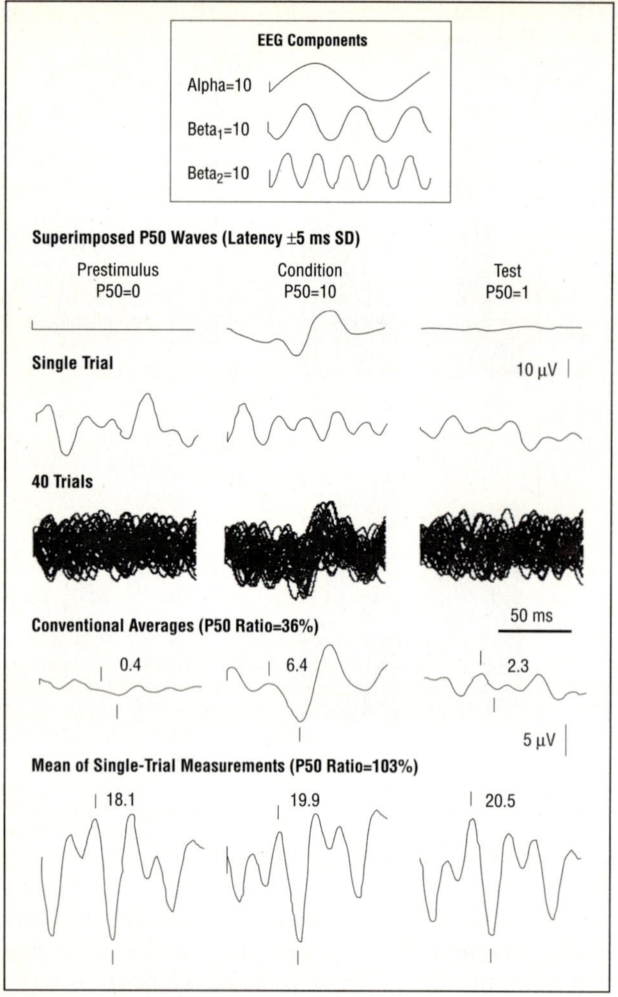

Figure 3. *Computer simulation of P50 detection. Prestimulus, condition, and test responses were added to a background electroencephalogram (EEG) consisting of alpha, beta$_1$, and beta$_2$. Resultant single trials, 40 superimposed trials, conventional averages, and single-trial measurements are shown. See legend to Figure 1 for explanation of tic marks.*

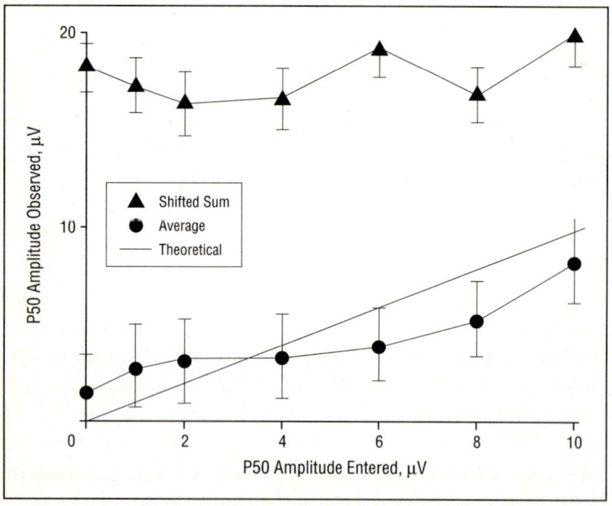

Figure 4. *Simulated measurement of P50 by conventional averaging and single-trial measurement. The theoretical line represents measurement of a signal equal to the P50 added to the background electroencephalogram. Mean and SE from a 40-trial simulation with each technique are shown.*

Simulation of the Measurement of the Amplitude of P50*

	P50 Amplitude Measured, μV			
	Averaging		Single Trials	
P50 Input Amplitude, μV	**0**	**10**	**0**	**10**
Amplitude of the EEG for each component, μV				
2.5	0.2	7.5	4.4	9.5
5	0	7.7	8.6	11.4
10	1.3	8.3	18.1	20.0
Influence of single EEG components (10 μV)				
Alpha	0	4.8	6.3	8.8
Beta$_1$	0.2	8.6	15.2	15.4
Beta$_2$	2.4	5.8	12.0	14.3
SD of the latency of P50, ms				
2.5	1.8	9.0	17.6	20.0
5	1.3	8.3	18.1	20.0
10	1.3	4.3	17.2	21.2

**Each value was obtained from a 40-trial simulation. EEG indicates electroencephalogram.*

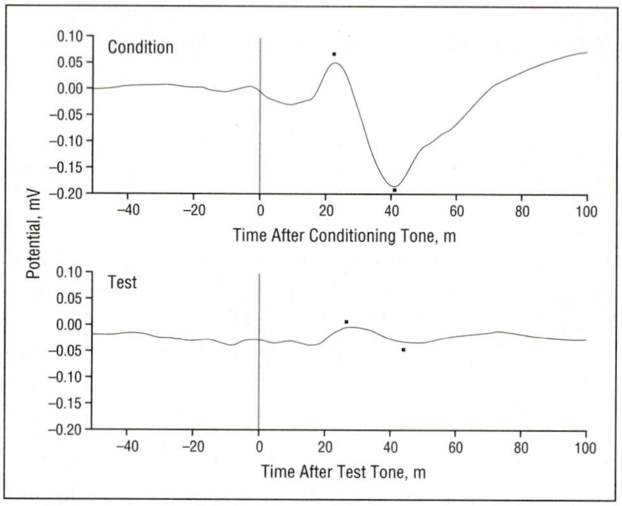

Figure 5. *Grand average of the P20/N40 response to condition and test stimuli recorded in the hippocampal CA3 pyramidal layer from 3 rats. The ratio of test to conditioning amplitude is 12%.*

EVOKED RESPONSES AND SINGLE-NEURON RECORDINGS FROM AN ANIMAL MODEL

Microelectrode recordings of auditory evoked activity from the CA3 pyramidal cell layer of the rat hippocampus disclosed a P20/N40 waveform that was inhibited in the test response, as has been observed with human P50 (**Figure 5**). Recordings from individual neurons showed excitatory responses beginning 10 to 30 milliseconds after the tone, coincident with the P20 portion of the evoked response, and inhibitory response 40 to 60 milliseconds after the tone, coincident with the N40 portion (**Figure 6**). The difference in discharge rate during the excitatory and inhibitory responses was significantly different from the prestimulus discharge rates (cell 1, t=4.31, df=9, P<.005; cell 2, t=10.84, df=9, P<.001; cell 3, t=3.25, df=9, P<.01). In all 3 cases, no significant response to the test stimulus was observed. The SD of the latency of

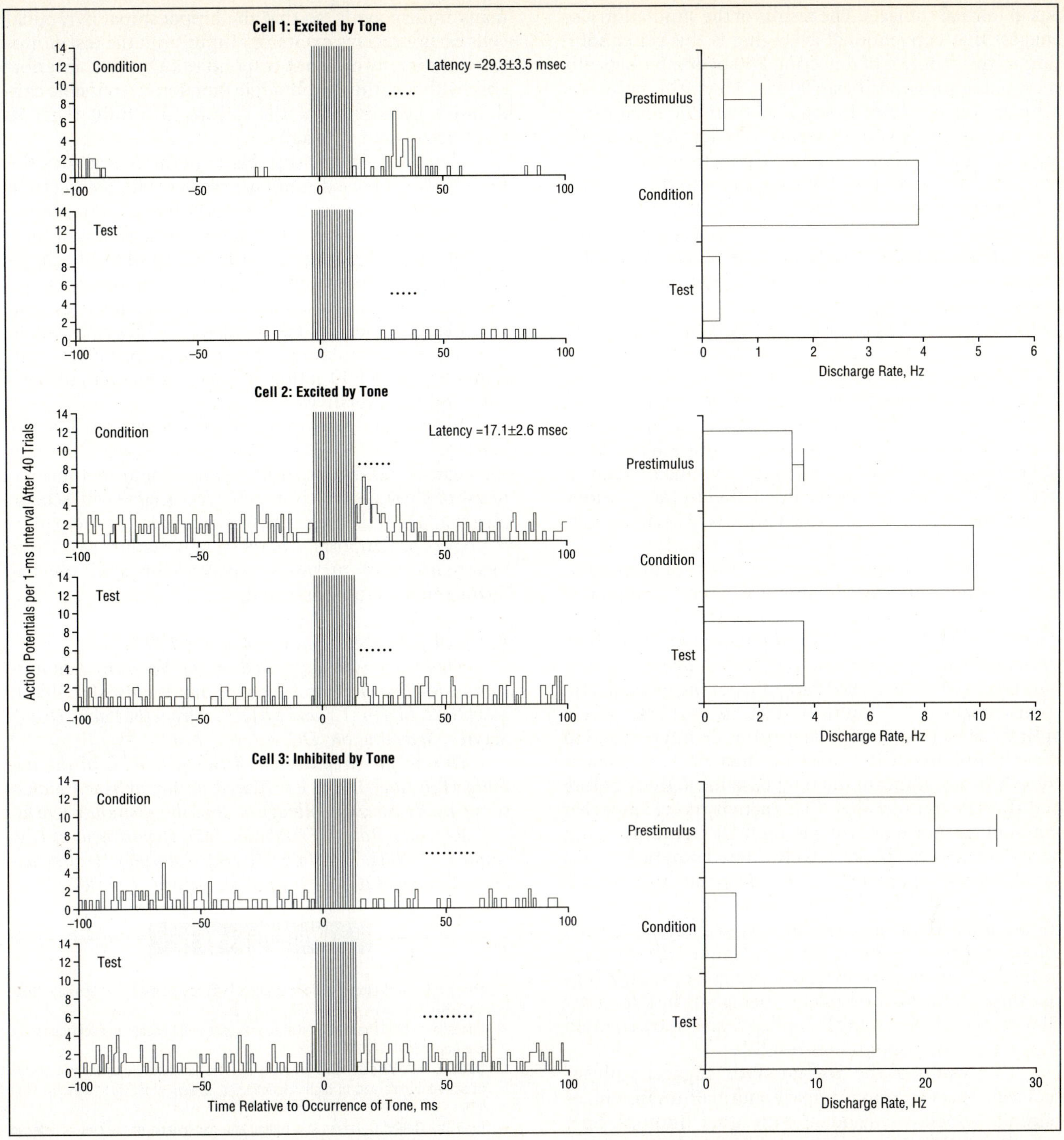

Figure 6. *Left, Peristimulus histograms from rat hippocampal neurons. Vertical lines indicate the 10-millisecond tones. Dotted lines above the conditioning response indicate the interval in which cell discharge exceeded (cells 1 or 2) or was lower (cell 3) than the mean baseline rate ±2 SDs. The same interval is marked in the test response for comparison. Right, Baseline discharge rates and SD and discharge during these intervals are shown in the bar graphs. For the excited cells, the mean (±SD) of latency to the first action potential in each trial are indicated.*

the initial action potential in the excitatory responses was less than 5 milliseconds. For the population of 21 pyramidal cells that responded to tone, the conditioning stimulus increased the discharge rate for each cell by at least 3 SDs more than its prestimulus rate. The mean peak increase, from 4.2 to 16.8 Hz, occurred 16 milliseconds after the conditioning tone. None of the cells discharged significantly more than the prestimulus rate within the first 50 milliseconds after the test stimulus.

COMMENT

We found that single-trial analysis of the EEG after auditory stimulation does not disclose new information about differences in the suppression of P50 in the conditioning-testing paradigm between schizophrenic and normal subjects. Rather, it extracts a noisy signal that leads to the erroneous conclusion that no such suppression exists in normal subjects. The results of the simulation also suggest that conventional averaging is the better solution to the problem of detecting P50 over a biologically reasonable range of these values. Thus, the failure of schizophrenic persons to suppress their P50 response to repeated auditory stimuli seems to reflect a true difference in their psychophysiologic characteristics.

Despite the results of this inquiry into the merits of averaging as opposed to single-trial analysis, it is unsatisfying to be unable to detect human auditory response except through the averaging method. Magnetoencephalography has detected a P50 dipole in the superior temporal gyrus, but this technique also relies on averaging to extract signal from noise.[41] Depth recording in neurosurgical patients has disclosed a deeper additional site for P50, beyond the range of magnetoencephalography, in the hippocampus.[42] The 2 sites are not incompatible, because the superior temporal gyrus is the major source of sensory input to the hippocampus through a relay in the entorhinal cortex.[43] In laboratory animals, neurons in these structures can be recorded directly, as was done in this study, to determine the neuronal activity underlying the generation of the evoked potential.

We have confirmed that the response of hippocampal neurons to the second sound is almost completely suppressed, as measured by their action-potential discharge. From the single-neuron recordings, there is no evidence that the suppression of the test evoked potentials is caused by increased variability of the neuronal response to the test stimulus. In fact, the test response is entirely absent. Although the neurons do not respond to the test stimulus, cells 2 and 3, like many pyramidal neurons, have a significant ongoing baseline activity before and after the test stimulus.[40] This activity is evidence that much of the noise in evoked-potential recording is not an artifact that can be selectively filtered out; rather, it is the discharge, spontaneous or in response to other afferent stimuli, of the same neurons whose response to the auditory stimuli generates the evoked potential. Such single-neuron recordings cannot generally be performed in humans; however, recordings from single hippocampal neurons in a patient being studied for possible temporal lobectomy for epilepsy also showed rapid suppression of response to sound.[44]

The results of the present study suggest a physiological aspect to hippocampal abnormalities in schizophrenia, which is consonant with other findings. Specifically, a disorder involving inhibitory interneurons could prevent the habituation of auditory evoked responses such as P50. Histochemical evidence suggests that there are decreased numbers of inhibitory interneurons that contain nicotinamide-adenine dinucleotide phosphate-diaphorase.[45] A subgroup of interneurons has a particularly high expression of the α7-nicotinic cholinergic receptor,[46] which pharmacological studies have shown to be critical for auditory sensory gating.[47] During the conditioning response, the interneurons are activated by these nicotinic receptors as a result of the activation of cholinergic input to the hippocampus. The interneurons then release γ-aminobutyric acid (GABA), which may activate presynaptic $GABA_B$ receptors to prevent the subsequent release of neurotransmitters such as glutamate for many milliseconds, so that the hippocampal pyramidal cells do not receive excitatory input from the test stimulus and therefore do not respond to it.[48] Thus, interference with nicotinic cholinergic function is a possible candidate mechanism for the failure to inhibit the P50 response in schizophrenia.

Evidence supporting this hypothesis includes the finding of decreased numbers of nicotinic receptors in hippocampus in postmortem brain tissue from schizophrenic persons[49] and a preliminary suggestion of linkage for the P50 gating deficit in the families of schizophrenic persons at the chromosomal site of the α_7-nicotinic receptor.[50,51] Whether the heavy smoking found in schizophrenic persons is related to abnormalities in this receptor is unknown, but nicotine produces transient reversal of P50 gating deficits in schizophrenic persons and their relatives.[52,53]

Elementary neurophysiological measures, like the behavior of the P50 evoked response to repeated stimuli, thus can be used to identify putative neuronal mechanisms of physiological dysfunction associated with schizophrenia. The full range of consequences for the pathobiology of schizophrenia of the possible failure to activate interneurons by nicotinic receptors or other mechanisms remains to be assessed.

Accepted for publication October 26, 1995.

This work was supported by the Veterans Administration Medical Research Service and grants MH 38321, MH42642, MH44212, and MH00728 from the Public Health Service, Washington, DC.

During the preparation of this article, 2 of the authors (R.F. and L.E.A.) reviewed an unpublished manuscript by Yi Jin and colleagues describing similar work.

Reprints: Robert Freedman, MD, Department of Psychiatry, C-2681-71, University of Colorado Health Sciences Center, 4200 E Ninth Ave, Denver, CO 80262.

REFERENCES

1. Shagass C. An electrophysiological view of schizophrenia. *Biol Psychiatry.* 1976; 11:3-30.
2. Buchsbaum MS. The middle evoked response components and schizophrenia. *Schizophr Bull.* 1977;3:93-104.
3. De Amicis LA, Wagstaff DA, Cromwell RL. Reaction time crossover as a marker of schizophrenia and of higher functioning. *J Nerv Ment Dis.* 1986;174:177-179.
4. Braff DL, Grillon C, Geyer MA. Gating and habituation of the startle reflex in schizophrenic patients. *Arch Gen Psychiatry.* 1992;49:206-215.
5. Roth WT, Cannon EH. Some features of the auditory evoked response in schizophrenics. *Arch Gen Psychiatry.* 1972;26:466-471.
6. Landau SC, Buchsbaum MS, Carpenter W, Strauss J, Sacks M. Schizophrenia and stimulus intensity control. *Arch Gen Psychiatry.* 1975;32:1239-1245.
7. Shagass C, Roemer RA, Straumanis JJ, Amadeo M. Temporal variability of somatosensory, visual and auditory evoked potentials in schizophrenia. *Arch Gen Psychiatry.* 1979;36:1341-1348.
8. Adler LE, Pachtman E, Franks R, Pecevich M, Waldo MC, Freedman R. Neurophysiological evidence for a defect in neuronal mechanisms involved in sensory gating in schizophrenia. *Biol Psychiatry.* 1982;17:639-654.
9. Morstyn R, Duffy FH, McCarley RW. Altered P300 topography in schizophrenia. *Arch Gen Psychiatry.* 1983;40:729-734.
10. Javitt DC, Doneshka P, Zylberman I, Ritter W, Vaughan HG Jr. Impairment of early cortical processing in schizophrenia: an even-related potential confirmation study. *Biol Psychiatry.* 1993;33:513-519.
11. Venables P. Input dysfunction in schizophrenia. *Prog Exp Pers Psychopathol Res.* 1964;1:1-47.

12. McGhie A, Chapman JS. Disorders of attention and perception in early schizophrenia. *Br J Med Psychol.* 1961;34:103-116.
13. Braff DL, Geyer MA. Sensorimotor gating and schizophrenia: human and animal model studies. *Arch Gen Psychiatry.* 1990;47:181-188.
14. Eccles JC. *The Inhibitory Pathways of the Central Nervous System.* Springfield, Ill: Charles C Thomas Publisher; 1969.
15. Roth WT, Kopell BS. The auditory evoked response to repeated stimuli during a vigilance task. *Psychophysiology.* 1969;6:301-309.
16. Fruhstorfer H, Soveri P, Jarvilehto T. Short-term habituation of the auditory evoked response in man. *Electroencephalogr Clin Neurophysiol.* 1970;28:153-159.
17. Chapman CR, Colpitts YH, Mayeno JK, Baglioardi GJ. Rate of stimulus repetition changes evoked potential amplitude: dental and auditory modalities compared. *Exp Brain Res.* 1981;43:246-252.
18. Papanicolau AC, Loring DW, Eisenberg HM. Age-related differences in recovery cycle of auditory evoked potentials. *Neurobiol Aging.* 1984;5:291-295.
19. Jerger K, Biggins C, Fein G. P50 suppression is not affected by attentional manipulations. *Biol Psychiatry.* 1992;31:365-377.
20. Guterman Y, Josiassen RC, Bashore TR Jr. Attentional influence on the P50 component of the auditory event-related brain potential. *Int J Psychophysiol.* 1992;12:197-209.
21. Boutros NN, Zouridakis G, Overall J. Replication and extension of P50 findings in schizophrenia. *Clin Electroencephalogr.* 1991;22:40-45.
22. Erwin RJ, Mawhinney HM, Gur RC, Gur RE. Midlatency evoked responses in schizophrenia. *Biol Psychiatry.* 1991;30:430-442.
23. Judd LJ, McAdams L, Budnick B, Braff DL. Sensory gating deficits in schizophrenia: new results. *Am J Psychiatry.* 1992;149:488-493.
24. Jin Y, Potkin SG, Wu J, Dang C, Sandman C. Single-trial P50 in normal and schizophrenic subjects. *Biol Psychiatry.* 1994;35:631. Abstract.
25. Kathmann N, Engel RR. Sensory gating in normal subjects and schizophrenic patients: a failure to find strong P50 suppression in normal subjects. *Biol Psychiatry.* 1990;27:1216-1226.
26. Roth WT, Horvath TB, Pfefferbaum A, Kopell BS. Event-related potentials in schizophrenic patients. *Electroencephalogr Clin Neurophysiol.* 1980;48:127-139.
27. Mukundan CR. Middle latency components of evoked responses in schizophrenic patients. *Biol Psychiatry.* 1986;21:1097-1100.
28. Niedermeyer E. The normal EEG of the waking adult. In: Niedermeyer E, Lopes de Silva FH, eds. *Electroencephalography: Basic Principles, Clinical Applications, and Related Fields.* Baltimore, Md: Williams & Wilkins; 1993:91-117.
29. Lopes de Silva FH. Event-related potentials: methodology and quantification. In: Niedermeyer E, Lopes de Silva FH, eds. *Electroencephalography: Basic Principles, Clinical Applications, and Related Fields.* Baltimore, Md: Williams & Wilkins; 1993:763-772.
30. Callaway E, Jones RT, Donchin E. Auditory evoked potential variability in schizophrenia. *Electroencephalogr Clin Neurophysiol.* 1970;29:421-428.
31. Sugerman AA, Goldstein L. The EEG in schizophrenia. *Am J Psychiatry.* 1972; 128:1466-1467.
32. Lund TR, Sponheim SR, Iacono W, Clementz B. Internal consistency reliability of resting EEG power spectra in schizophrenic and normal subjects. *Psychophysiology.* 1995;32:66-71.
33. Itil TM, Saletu B, Davis S. EEG findings in chronic schizophrenics based on digital computer period analysis and analog power spectra. *Biol Psychiatry.* 1972;5:1-13.
34. Spitzer RL, Endicott J, Robins E. Research diagnostic criteria. *Arch Gen Psychiatry.* 1978;35:773-782.
35. Endicott J, Spitzer RL. A diagnostic interview: the schedule for affective disorders and schizophrenia. *Arch Gen Psychiatry.* 1978;35:837-844.
36. Straumanis JJ, Shagass C, Romer RA. Influence of antipsychotic and antidepressant drugs on evoked potential correlates of psychosis. *Biol Psychiatry.* 1982;17:1101-1122.
37. Freedman R, Adler LE, Waldo MC, Pachtman E, Franks RD. Neurophysiological evidence for a defect in inhibitory pathways in schizophrenia: comparison of medicated and drug-free patients. *Biol Psychiatry.* 1983;18:537-551.
38. Waldo MC, Cawthra E, Adler LE, Dubester S, Staunton M, Nagamoto H, Baker N, Madison A, Simon J, Scherzinger A, Drebing C, Gerhardt G, Freedman R. Auditory sensory gating, hippocampal volume, and catecholamine metabolism in schizophrenics and their siblings. *Schizophr Res.* 1994;12:93-106.
39. Coppola R. Isolating low-frequency activity in EEG spectrum analysis. *Electroencephalogr Clin Neurophysiol.* 1979;21:101-105.
40. Miller CL, Freedman R. The activity of hippocampal interneurons and pyramidal cells during the response of the hippocampus to repeated stimuli. *Neuroscience.* 1995;69:371-381.
41. Reite M, Teale P, Zimmerman J, Davis K, Whalen J. Source location of a 50-msec latency auditory evoked field component. *Electroencephalogr Clin Neurophysiol.* 1988;70:490-498.
42. Goff WR, Williamson PD, VanGilder JC, Allison T, Fisher TC. Neural origins of long-latency evoked potentials recorded from the depth and from the cortical surface of the brain in man. *Prog Clin Neurophysiol.* 1980;7:126-145.
43. Amaral DG, Insausti R, Cowan M. Evidence for a direct projection from the superior temporal gyrus to the entorhinal cortex in the monkey. *Brain Res.* 1983;275:263-277.
44. Wilson CL, Babb TL, Halgren E, Wang ML, Crandall PH. Habituation of human limbic neuronal response to sensory stimulation. *Exp Neurol.* 1984;84:77-97.
45. Akbarian S, Vinuela A, Kim JJ, Potkin SG, Bunney WE Jr, Jones EG. Distorted distribution of nicotinamide-adenine dinucleotide phosphate-diaphorase neurons in temporal lobe of schizophrenics implies anomalous cortical development. *Arch Gen Psychiatry.* 1993;50:178-187.
46. Freedman R, Wetmore C, Stromberg I, Leonard S, Olson L. Alpha-bungarotoxin binding to hippocampal interneurons: immunocytochemical characterization and effects on growth factor expression. *J Neurosci.* 1993;13: 1965-1975.
47. Luntz-Leybman V, Bickford P, Freedman R. Cholinergic gating of response to auditory stimuli in rat hippocampus. *Brain Res.* 1992;587:130-136.
48. Hershman K, Freedman R, Bickford PC. $GABA_B$ antagonists diminish the inhibitory gating of auditory response in the rat hippocampus. *Neurosci Lett.* 1993;190:133-136.
49. Freedman R, Hall M, Adler LE, Leonard S. Evidence in postmortem brain tissue for decreased numbers of hippocampal nicotinic receptors in schizophrenia. *Biol Psychiatry.* 1995;38:22-33.
50. Coon H, Plaetke R, Holik J, Hoff M, Myles-Worsley M, Freedman R, Byerley W. Use of a neurophysiological trait in linkage analysis of schizophrenia. *Biol Psychiatry.* 1993;34:277-289.
51. Freedman R, Adler LE, Bickford P, Byerley W, Coon H, Cullum CM, Griffth J, Harris JG, Leonard S, Miller C, Myles-Worsley M, Nagamoto HT, Rose G, Waldo M. Schizophrenia and nicotinic receptors. *Harvard Rev Psychiatry.* 1994;2: 179-192.
52. Adler LE, Hoffer LJ, Griffith J, Waldo MC, Freedman R. Normalization by nicotine of deficient auditory sensory gating in the relatives of schizophrenics. *Biol Psychiatry.* 1992;32:607-616.
53. Adler LE, Hoffer LD, Wiser A, Freedman R. Normalization of auditory physiology by cigarette smoking in schizophrenic patients. *Am J Psychiatry.* 1993; 150:1856-1861.

INDEX TO ADVERTISERS

Glaxo Wellcome, Inc.
Wellbutrin SR *1077, 1089*

Janssen Pharmaceuticals
Person-to-Person *1144*
Pathways *1086-1087*
Risperdal *1112A-F, 1113*

Ortho-McNeil Pharmaceutical, Inc
Haldol Decanoate . . . . *Cover 2-1073*

Roche Laboratories
Klonopin *1079-1080*

SmithKline Beecham
Paxil *1163-1164*

U.S. Pharmaceuticals, Pfizer Inc.
Aricept *1075*
Zoloft . . . . *1104A-B, 1136A-B, Cover 3-Cover 4*

W.B. Saunders Company
Book/Pub *1153*

While every precaution is taken to ensure accuracy, we cannot guarantee against the possibility of an occasional change or omission in the preparation of this index.

ORIGINAL ARTICLE

Psychopathological and Behavioral Correlates of Dopaminergic Sensitivity in Alcohol-Dependent Patients

Andreas Heinz, MD; Peter Dufeu, Dipl Psych; Silke Kuhn, Dipl Psych; Michael Dettling, MD; Klaus Gräf, MD; Irene Kürten, MTA; Hans Rommelspacher, MD; Lutz G. Schmidt, MD

Objectives: To explore 2 facets of dopamine receptor sensitivity in alcoholics: (1) whether reduced sensitivity of central dopamine receptors is correlated with anxiety, depression, or novelty seeking and (2) whether this reduction is associated with poor treatment outcome.

Method: Sixty-four alcohol-dependent patients were assessed according to their clinical outcome, sensitivity of central dopamine receptors (apomorphine-induced growth hormone secretion), mood states, and personality traits before and after detoxification.

Results: Patients with poor treatment outcome displayed a blunted growth hormone response before, but not after, detoxification. Growth hormone response was not significantly correlated with novelty seeking. Relapsing patients tended to be less depressed than patients who remained abstinent during observation.

Conclusion: This study did not support the hypothesis that reduced sensitivity of dopamine receptors is associated with anxiety, depressed mood, or high novelty seeking in alcoholism.

Arch Gen Psychiatry. 1996;53:1123-1128

ALCOHOL-INDUCED stimulation of central dopamine (DA) receptors has been suggested to play a major role in the development of alcohol addiction by causing an individual to experience pleasure or satisfaction, thus reinforcing drug consumption.[1-3] In animal experiments, stimulation of central DA neurons increases forward locomotion and exploratory behavior.[4,5] Cloninger[6] compared exploratory behavior in rodents with a personality trait in humans that he called *novelty seeking* (NS). He hypothesized that alcohol-seeking behavior is a special kind of exploratory behavior, which is increased in humans who show a greater DA response to alcohol.[7] This hypothesis was based on a study by Schuckit et al,[8] who found an increased sensitivity of prolactin response to alcohol in young men with a high risk of developing alcohol dependence. Cloninger[7] suggested that spontaneous alcohol-seeking behavior leads to an inability to abstain from alcohol, and that this behavior is especially pronounced in a subgroup of alcoholics with early disease onset and impulsive and risk-taking behavior.

Balldin et al[9-11] proposed a different hypothesis after finding reduced sensitivity of postsynaptic DA receptors, as assessed by stimulation of growth hormone (GH) release with the D1 and D2 receptor agonist apomorphine hydrochloride in some long-term alcoholics. They suggested that a hyposensitive, "weak" DA system needs external stimulation by alcohol-induced DA release. We recently reported that hyposensitivity of central DA receptors before detoxification depends on the amount of long-term alcohol consumption and is associated with early relapse in alcoholics.[12] Reduced activity of central DA transmission may be an underlying cause of anhedonia, depression, and dysphoria in alcoholics.[13,14] Anhedonia and depression may, in turn, increase relapse risk in alcoholics.[15-18] We therefore hypothesized that, in alcoholics with a poor treatment outcome, reduced sensitivity of central DA receptors is associated with depressed mood and anxiety. With respect to Cloninger's Tridimensional Personality Questionnaire (TPQ),[6] we tested the hypothesis that relapsing patients display

See Subjects and Methods on next page

From the Department of Psychiatry, Freie Universität Berlin (Germany).

SUBJECTS AND METHODS

SUBJECTS

Alcohol-dependent patients who applied for detoxification treatment in our outpatient unit were diagnosed according to the criteria of the *International Classification of Diseases, 10th Revision*.[19] Psychiatric history and psychopathological variables were assessed by means of the substance abuse section of the Composite International Diagnostic Interview[20] and the Brief Psychiatric Rating Scale.[21] Ninety-eight of 276 patients who were consecutively admitted to the outpatient unit were willing to participate in the clinical study. Patients who used any drug other than alcohol and who had metabolic, endocrine, or primary neuropsychiatric disorders were excluded. Moreover, patients who had abstained from alcohol for more than a day were excluded, as animal studies have evidenced that DA receptor densities increase within 5 days of abstinence.[22] Only patients with a body mass index between 20 and 30 kg/m^2 were tested. Altogether, 64 patients were included in the study.

METHODS OF ASSESSMENT

Personality traits were measured on the TPQ[6] before detoxification and at the end of the observation period. Patients with low harm avoidance (HA) (scores not higher than the mean HA score of all patients) and high NS (scores higher than half the SD above the mean NS score of all patients) were considered to be type 2 alcoholics. These cutoff points were based on the recommendation of C. Robert Cloninger, MD (oral communication, November 19, 1992).

On the day of admission to the hospital, short-term and long-term alcohol consumption was assessed by clinical interview and biochemical tests for blood alcohol concentration and carbohydrate-deficient transferrin.[23] Withdrawal symptoms were treated with clomethiazole if the patient's score on the Clinical Institute Withdrawal Assessment for Alcohol Scale (modified according to Sullivan et al[24]) was higher than 12, since this substance is not known to interfere with dopaminergic functions.[25] Patients remained on the ward for 3 weeks. After detoxification, the patients' psychiatric histories were taken in clinical interviews. The patients assessed their mood states regularly (weekly during the first 2 months, then monthly) by means of the Self-rating Anxiety Scale[26] and the Self-rating Depression Scale.[27]

After release from the hospital, the patients were observed at our follow-up outpatient unit for 6 months. During this time they were seen on a weekly basis for the first 2 months and then biweekly until the end of observation. In addition, blood alcohol concentrations and carbohydrate-deficient transferrin levels in serum were assessed to validate the patients' self-reports for the previous weeks. At the end of the observation period, relatives were contacted to verify the patients' abstinence. Relapse was defined as a minimum consumption of 50 g of alcohol (about 1 L of beer or 1 bottle of wine). However, all patients who relapsed started to consume alcohol on a regular basis once their first relapse had occurred.

HORMONAL TEST PROCEDURE

All patients were tested before detoxification (on the day of admission, day 1) and after detoxification (7 days later, day 8). Patients were admitted at 8 AM to the detoxification unit. The times of last alcohol consumption and blood alcohol concentrations were recorded. Patients received a light lunch at noon. At 2:30 PM they were asked to lie in a supine position and a cannula was inserted in a brachial vein. A blood sample was drawn for baseline value (5 mL). At 2:45 PM, apomorphine hydrochloride (0.01 mg/kg of body weight) was injected subcutaneously. Nineteen patients (2 women and 17 men) served as placebo controls in a double-blind design and were given saline instead of apomorphine subcutaneously. Blood samples were collected at 30-minute intervals (+30, +60, +90, and +120 minutes). The samples were kept on ice and centrifuged within 3 hours; the serum samples were stored at −20°C. Serum GH concentrations were assessed by immunoradiometric assay kits (Medgenix Diagnostics S.A., Fleurus, Belgium). The lower limit of sensitivity was 0.5 μg/L. The intra-assay coefficients of variation were 6.5% at a GH level of 6 μg/L and 14.0% at a GH level of 1 μg/L; the interassay coefficients of variation were 7.8% and 18.3%, respectively. If necessary, the first dose of clomethiazole was given after the last blood sample was drawn.

Ten paid, age-matched nonalcoholics (2 women and 8 men), who had no history of substance abuse and who were sober when tested, served as healthy controls. Apomorphine-induced GH secretion of the subjects was tested according to the same time and test protocol.

The study was approved by the Ethics Committee of the Universitäts-Klinikum Rudolf Virchow, Berlin, Germany. Written informed consent was obtained from all subjects.

STATISTICAL ANALYSES

As the apomorphine-induced GH responses (net response at 60 minutes minus baseline) did not appear to be normally distributed, the data were log transformed. The net GH response at 60 minutes was chosen because it renders our results comparable with those of previous reports.[9-11] Analyses of the area under the curve confirmed the choice of this value. Multivariate analysis of variance procedures were applied to compare the between-group differences in mean values for GH response and the scores on the Self-rating Anxiety Scale and Self-rating Depression Scale. At defined measuring times (days 1 and 8), group differences in GH response were assessed by the Student-Newman-Keuls test. Other variables were compared across groups by the Student t test, Mann-Whitney test, or χ^2 test.

Correlations among the normally distributed Self-rating Anxiety Scale, Self-rating Depression Scale, and TPQ data were assessed by Pearson correlation coefficient; all other correlations were assessed by Spearman correlation coefficient. As multiple testing was done to generate a hypothesis for correlations among personality traits, long-term alcohol intake, and GH secretion, Bonferroni's correction was applied to adjust the α value. Accordingly, only results with an α error less than .003 were regarded as significant.

Table 1. Clinical Data of Patients*

	Abstinent (n=19)	Relapsed (n=26)	Placebo Controls (n=19)
Sex, No. M/F	17/2	23/3	17/2
Mean±SD age, y	44±10	44±8	47±9
Mean daily consumption, g	236±163	217±167	287±162
Age at onset of craving, y	33±10	34±9	34±10
Age at onset of reduced control of drinking, y	36±17	35±8	36±12
Age at onset of withdrawal syndrome, y	38±10	36±7	38±10
No. of previous detoxifications	2±2	3±2	4±4
No. of fulfilled ICD-10 criteria	6±2	6±1	7±1†
No. of patients with alcohol-dependent fathers	2	12‡	6
Cloninger type 2 alcoholics, No.	6	8	5
Secondary complications (loss of work; reduced social activities; neglect of work, school, or children; fights; problems driving motor vehicle), No.	17	22	15
Sentences for criminal acts, No.	4	10	5
No. of patients with steatosis hepatitis	13	16	15
Laboratory findings (day of admission)			
Alanine aminotransferase, U/L	50±42	27±16	39±39
γ-Glutamyl transpeptidase, U/L	186±254	123±202	169±235
Albumin, g/L	50±6	49±5	47±4
Acute drinking status on day of admission			
Blood alcohol, g/L	1.1±1.0	1.0±1.1	0.3±0.8§
Carbohydrate-deficient transferrin, mg/L	26.3±26.1	21.9±16.1	13.4±10.1
Severity of withdrawal symptoms, total CIWA score	43.8±46.3	41.2±55.0	35.5±37.0
Total dose of clomethiazole, mg	864±1199	590±1230	160±2359

*Abstinent indicates patients who remained abstinent after detoxification (6-month observation period); relapsed, patients who relapsed within 6 months after detoxification; and placebo controls, patients challenged with saline. Comparisons between groups were nonsignificant except where indicated. ICD-10 indicates International Classification of Diseases, Tenth Revision; CIWA, Clinical Institute Withdrawal Assessment.

†$P<.05$ vs relapsed group, Student t test.

‡$P<.05$ vs abstinent group, χ^2 test.

§$P<.05$ vs abstinent group, Student t test.

high NS and that NS is significantly correlated with the sensitivity of DA receptors.[7]

RESULTS

TREATMENT OUTCOME

Nineteen patients served as placebo controls, while 45 patients underwent apomorphine challenge. Twenty-six of the apomorphine-challenged patients relapsed (3 women and 23 men), while 19 patients remained abstinent (2 women and 17 men) for 6 months. The 2 patient groups did not differ in duration of alcohol dependence, mean alcohol consumption, frequency of social complications, or liver abnormalities (**Table 1**). All relapsing patients resumed regular alcohol consumption once their first relapse had occurred. Most of them subsequently dropped out of the study; only 5 were available for follow-up at the end of the 6-month observation period.

DOPAMINERGIC SENSITIVITY

To determine age-related effects, the groups were subdivided according to the mean age (older vs younger than mean age). Neither gender- nor age-related differences appeared in apomorphine-induced GH response, nor was there a significant correlation between age and GH response in any patient group. The baseline GH values did not differ significantly between relapsers and abstainers before or after detoxification (**Table 2**).

The repeated-measures multivariate analysis of variance showed a significant group effect (apomorphine-challenged controls, relapsing and abstinent patients; $F=18.5$, $df=3$, $P<.001$), time effect (day 1 vs day 8; $F=5.5$, $df=1$, $P=.02$), and group×time interaction for GH secretion (net response at 60 minutes). Before detoxification (day 1), apomorphine-stimulated GH secretion was significantly lower in subsequent relapsers than in either abstinent patients or controls, respectively (Student-Newman-Keuls test, $P<.05$). After detoxification, GH response increased in most subsequent relapsers. At day 8, the relapsers, abstainers, and healthy controls no longer differed significantly from each other (**Figure 1** and Table 2). These findings were confirmed when the area under the curve instead of the net GH response at 60 minutes was assessed. Again, a significant group difference between subsequent relapsers and abstainers was found on day 1 (analysis of variance, $F=4.53$, $df=1$, $P=.02$) but not on day 8.

Significantly more relapsing patients than abstinent patients had alcohol-dependent fathers ($\chi^2=5.42$, $P=.02$; Table 1). However, GH response did not differ between patients with a family history of alcoholism and those without it at any assessment time. In the 19 patients who were challenged with placebo (saline) in-

Table 2. Growth Hormone Response and Personality Traits in Relapsing and Abstinent Patients at Different Assessment Points*

	Relapsed (n=26)	Abstinent (n=19)	Difference, *P*
Growth hormone, μg/L			
Baseline (range)			
Day 1	0.6 (0.5-2.1)	0.5 (0.4-1.3)	.63 (NS)†
Day 8	0.5 (0.5-1.1)	0.5 (0.4-1.1)	.96 (NS)†
Net response at 60 min (range)			
Day 1	0.7 (−0.3-4.5)	8.6 (0.9-19.0)	.03†
Day 8	7.7 (2.5-21.1)	9.6 (2.5-22.9)	.62 (NS)†
Tridimensional Personality Questionnaire (mean±SD)			
Novelty seeking			
Day 1	17.23±5.90	16.72±5.23	.78 (NS)‡
Month 6	14.00±4.36	15.20±5.90	. . . §
Harm avoidance			
Day 1	14.90±8.06	18.00±6.99	.21 (NS)‡
Month 6	9.33±3.06	15.19±8.52	. . . §
Reward dependence			
Day 1	18.05±4.40	16.61±5.05	.35 (NS)‡
Month 6	10.00±5.00	15.33±5.72	. . . §

*Growth hormone was measured as baseline and net response after apomorphine challenge (median with first and third quartiles in parentheses). NS indicates not significant.

†Mann-Whitney test.

‡Student t test.

§No statistical test performed; only 5 relapsing patients could be assessed at month 6.

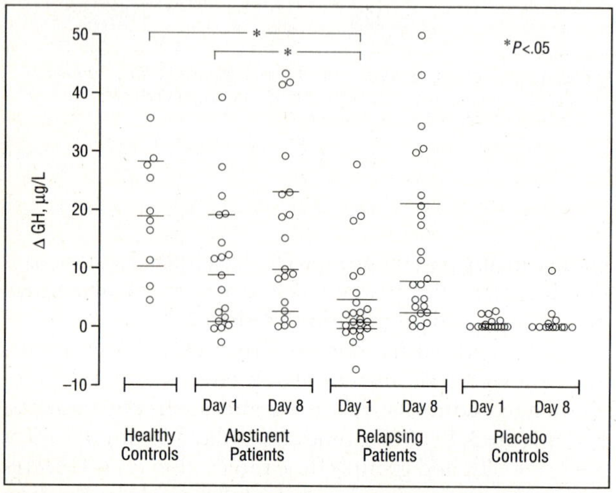

Figure 1. *Apomorphine-induced growth hormone (GH) response in healthy controls (n=10) and both relapsing (n=26) and abstinent (n=19) patients on the day of admission to the hospital (day 1) and after 8 days of abstinence (day 8). Placebo controls were 19 patients given saline solution. Median and first and third quartiles are shown.*

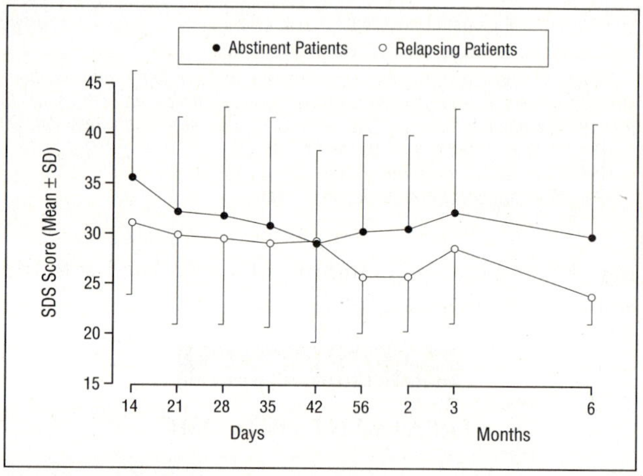

Figure 2. *Self-rating Depression Scale (SDS) after detoxification.*

stead of apomorphine, GH release did not show a significant increase over baseline values, regardless of whether the patients were assessed before or after detoxification (Student *t* test, *t*=1.24, *P*=.23; Figure 1).

An acute effect of alcohol consumption was observed only in patients who remained abstinent during observation. In this group, patients who had consumed alcohol on the day of admission displayed a significantly lower GH response than patients who had had their last drink the day before (Student *t* test, *t*=−2.64, *P*=.02). Relapsers showed a blunted GH response, irrespective of whether or not they had consumed alcohol on the day of admission.

DEPRESSION AND ANXIETY

A comparison of self-rated depression (the Self-rating Depression Scale) in all patients over the observation period showed no significant group effect but a significant effect of time (multivariate analysis of variance, F=4.24, *df*=4, *P*=.003; **Figure 2**) as well as a significant group×time interaction (F=3.96, *df*=4, *P*=.01). After 14 days and 2 months of abstinence, there were trends toward a difference between relapsing and abstinent patients (Student *t* test, *t*=1.55/1.68, *P*=.10). Only a significant effect of time was found for self-rated anxiety as assessed on the Self-rating Anxiety Scale (F=2.62, *df*=4, *P*=.04; **Figure 3**).

THE TPQ

No significant differences in HA, NS, or reward dependence (RD) were observed between relapsing and absti-

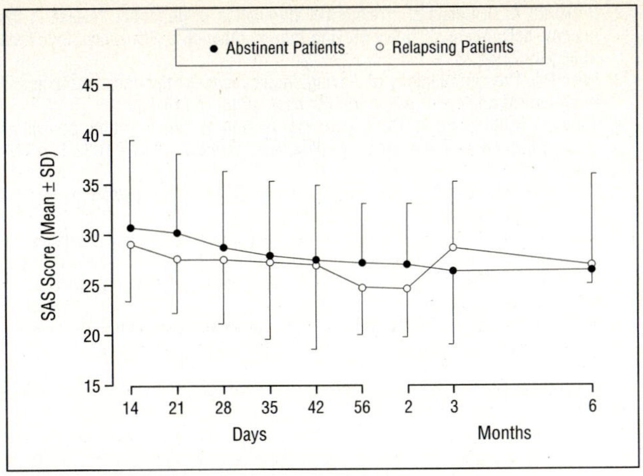

Figure 3. *Self-rating Anxiety Scale (SAS) after detoxification.*

Table 3. Correlations Between Long-term Alcohol Consumption and Both Log-Transformed Growth Hormone Response and Personality Traits (Spearman Correlation Coefficient)

	Long-term Alcohol Consumption	
	In Relapsers	In Abstinent Patients
Novelty seeking in relapsers	*r*=0.667*	NS†
Fear of uncertainty (harm avoidance, subscore 2)	NS	*r*=−0.639‡
Growth hormone response	*r*=0.433§	NS

*P<.001.
†*NS indicates not significant.*
‡P=.01.
§P=.02.

nent patients (Table 2). The frequency of type 2 alcoholics was not increased in relapsers compared with abstinent patients (Table 1). No difference in NS, HA, or RD between patients with and without alcoholic fathers was noted.

Comparison of HA scores before detoxification and at the end of the observation period for all 24 patients (5 relapsers and 19 abstinent patients) available for follow-up after 6 months showed a significant decrease (17.86±7.53 vs 14.56±8.48; t=3.26, P=.003). Separate assessment of the 19 abstainers showed no significant change in NS or RD during the 6-month follow-up period (Table 2).

CORRELATIONS

Depressed Mood, Anxiety, and HA

Significant correlations between HA before detoxification and self-rated depression and anxiety after 14 and 21 days of abstinence were observed in all patients (Pearson correlation coefficient, r=0.37 to 0.45, P=.01, respectively). To avoid excessive multiple testing, further correlations were not assessed.

Personality Traits, Long-term Alcohol Consumption, and GH Response

No significant correlations were found between NS or HA (total scores and subscores) and DA receptor sensitivity (log-transformed GH response), either before or after detoxification in both relapsing and abstinent patients. The most relevant test of the hypothesis that NS is related to DA receptor sensitivity was the correlation between "exploratory excitability" (NS, subscore 1) and GH response on day 1. This correlation did not prove to be significant (r=−0.28, P=.20).

In abstinent patients, a negative correlation was found between "fear of uncertainty" (HA, subscore 2) and long-term alcohol consumption in the month before admission to the hospital (Spearman r=−0.64, P=.01; **Table 3**). However, when the Bonferroni correction was applied, the result was not statistically significant. Relapsing patients showed a significant correlation between NS and long-term alcohol consumption (Spearman r=0.67, P<.001) and a trend toward a correlation between long-term alcohol consumption and GH response (Table 3).

COMMENT

In patients who relapsed within the 6-month observation period, apomorphine-induced GH release before detoxification was significantly lower than in abstinent patients and healthy controls. Our previous finding that reduced DA sensitivity in alcoholics is associated with poor treatment outcome is thus confirmed in this sample of patients.[12] After detoxification, there was no longer a significant difference in DA receptor sensitivity between subsequent relapsers and abstainers. However, some subsequent relapsers displayed blunted GH response even after 8 days of abstinence (Figure 1). Interestingly, George et al[28] found increased levels of homovanillic acid after detoxification in some subsequent relapsers. The reason for this increase in the DA metabolite is unclear. However, increased central release of DA may well induce a down-regulation of DA receptors.[22,29] In placebo controls, we found comparatively low levels of GH secretion before and after detoxification, indicating that GH secretion after apomorphine application actually represents DA receptor function and not nonspecific stress effects. Because Schuckit et al[8] found an increased sensitivity of prolactin response in young men at risk, differences in GH response between patients with and without alcoholic fathers were assessed; however, no significant difference in GH response or any of the personality traits was found.

Contrary to our hypothesis, hyposensitivity of central DA receptors was not associated with depression or anxiety. Instead, relapsing patients showed a trend toward lower anxiety and depression scores than those of abstinent patients. This finding is opposed to several reports of an increased relapse rate in depressed patients.[15-18] It is noteworthy, however, that most of these studies[15-17] evaluated the effect of depression as an independent diagnosis, while in our study mood states were assessed and patients with primary psychiatric diseases other than alcoholism were excluded. In a meta-analysis of 8 studies that included evaluation of the influence of mood states on relapse rate, Hartka et al[30] reported an inverse correlation between depressed mood and relapse rate during the first 2 years after detoxification. The positive correlations between HA and depression and anxiety in our study may explain this finding. Cautious behavior, as indicated by high HA, may help anxious and depressed patients to avoid situations where they might be tempted to resume drinking. This interpretation is further supported by the finding of a nonsignificant negative correlation between long-term alcohol consumption and "fear of uncertainty" (HA, subscore 2) in abstinent patients before detoxification. A similar effect of anxiety on relapse risk has been reported by Powell et al[31] in opiate addicts.

It has been previously observed that HA and depression covary positively in healthy controls.[32] Our study confirms this finding and shows that HA is not a stable personality trait, but in fact decreased significantly in all patients during observation. Assessment of abstinent patients showed that RD and NS did not change significantly during the observation period, indicating that the TPQ is a resilient measure of personality traits.

Although Cloninger[6,7] assumed that NS is influenced by central DA transmission, and although we have found reduced dopaminergic sensitivity in relapsing patients, in this study we did not find any difference between the NS scores of the abstinent and relapsing patients before or after detoxification. Moreover, NS was not significantly correlated to GH release. It is therefore unlikely that NS is directly influenced by the sensitivity of central DA receptors. However, there was a positive correlation between NS and long-term alcohol consumption in the relapsers. In these patients, low levels of anxiety and depression correlated with low HA, and a tendency toward NS may reduce control of alcohol intake, thus explaining the high relapse risk in these patients.

Altogether, this study did not support the hypothesis that alcoholics with poor treatment outcome and decreased sensitivity of central DA receptors suffer from depressed mood and anxiety. This study also failed to find a significant correlation between DA sensitivity and NS in alcohol-dependent patients. Instead, reduced sensitivity of central DA receptors in relapsing patients seemed related to long-term alcohol consumption and disappeared within 8 days of abstinence. High levels of NS and low levels of depression and HA were associated with reduced control of alcohol intake. Thus, rather than directly influencing mood states or personality traits, DA sensitivity seems to represent the effect of alcohol-consuming behavior interacting with anxiety, depression, and risk-taking behavior.

Accepted for publication January 18, 1996.

This study was supported by grants Az: He 916/7-1 and He 2597/1-1 from Deutsche Forschungsgemeinschaft, Bonn, Germany.

Corresponding author: Andreas Heinz, MD, Clinical Brain Disorders Branch, National Institute of Mental Health Neuroscience Center at St Elizabeths, 2700 Martin Luther King Jr Ave SE, Washington, DC 20032.

REFERENCES

1. Mereu G, Fadda F, Gessa GL. Ethanol stimulates the firing rate of nigral dopaminergic neurons in unanesthetized rats. *Brain Res.* 1984;292:63-69.
2. Imperato A, Di Chiara G. Preferential stimulation of dopamine release in the nucleus accumbens of freely moving rats by ethanol. *J Pharmacol Exp Ther.* 1986;239:219-228.
3. Wise RA. The neurobiology of craving: implications for the understanding and treatment of addiction. *J Abnorm Psychol.* 1988;97:118-132.
4. Tabakoff B, Kiianmaa K. Does tolerance develop to the activating, as well as the depressant, effects of ethanol? *Pharmacol Biochem Behav.* 1982;17:1073-1076.
5. Wise RA, Bozarth MA. A psychomotor stimulant theory of addiction. *Psychol Rev.* 1987;94:469-492.
6. Cloninger CR. A systematic method for clinical description and classification of personality variants: a proposal. *Arch Gen Psychiatry.* 1987;44:573-588.
7. Cloninger CR. Neurogenetic adaptive mechanisms in alcoholism. *Science.* 1987;236:410-416.
8. Schuckit MA, Parker DC, Rossman LR. Ethanol-related prolactin responses and risk for alcoholism. *Biol Psychiatry.* 1983;18:1153-1159.
9. Balldin J, Alling C, Gottfries CG, Lindtstedt G, Langström G. Changes in dopamine receptor sensitivity in humans after heavy ethanol intake. *Psychopharmacology.* 1985;86:142-146.
10. Balldin JI, Berggren UC, Lindstedt G. Neuroendocrine evidence for reduced dopamine receptor sensitivity in alcoholism. *Alcohol Clin Exp Res.* 1992;16:71-74.
11. Balldin J, Berggren U, Lindstedt G, Sundkler A. Further neuroendocrine evidence for reduced D2 dopamine receptor function in alcoholism. *Drug Alcohol Depend.* 1993;32:159-162.
12. Heinz A, Dettling M, Kuhn S, Gräf KJ, Kürten I, Rommelspacher H, Schmidt LG. Blunted growth hormone response is associated with early relapse in alcohol-dependent patients. *Alcohol Exp Clin Res.* 1995;19:62-65.
13. Rossetti ZL, Melis F, Carboni S, Diana M, Gessa GL. Alcohol withdrawal in rats is associated with a marked decrease in extraneuronal dopamine. *Alcohol Clin Exp Res.* 1992;16:529-532.
14. Heinz A, Schmidt LG, Reischies FM. Anhedonia in schizophrenic, depressed, or alcohol-dependent patients: neurobiological correlates. *Pharmacopsychiatry.* 1994;27(suppl):7-10.
15. Aneshensel CS, Huba GJ. Depression, alcohol use, and smoking over one year: a four-wave longitudinal causal model. *J Abnorm Psychol.* 1983;92:134-150.
16. Rounsaville BJ, Dolinsky ZS, Babor TF, Meyer RE. Psychopathology as a predictor of treatment outcome in alcoholics. *Arch Gen Psychiatry.* 1987;44:505-513.
17. O'Sullivan K, Rynne C, Miller J, O'Sullivan S, Fitzpatrick V, Hux M, Cooney J, Clare A. A follow-up study on alcoholics with and without co-existing affective disorder. *Br J Psychiatry.* 1988;152:813-819.
18. Glenn SW, Parsons OA. Prediction of resumption of drinking in posttreatment alcoholics. *Int J Addict.* 1991;26:237-254.
19. World Health Organization. *International Classification of Diseases, 10th Revision.* Göttingen, Germany: Huber; 1991.
20. Robins LN, Wing J, Wittchen HU, Helzer JE, Babor TF, Burke J, Farmer A, Jablenski A, Pickens R, Regier DA. The Composite International Diagnostic Interview: an epidemiological instrument suitable for use in conjunction with different diagnostic systems and in different cultures. *Arch Gen Psychiatry.* 1988;45:1069-1077.
21. Overall JE, Gorham DR. The Brief Psychiatric Rating Scale. *Psychol Rep.* 1962;10:799-812.
22. Rommelspacher H, Raeder C, Kaulen P, Brüning G. Adaptive changes of dopamine-D2 receptors in rat brain following ethanol withdrawal: a quantitative autoradiographic investigation. *Alcohol.* 1992;9:355-362.
23. Stibler H, Borg S, Joustra M. Micro anion exchange chromatography of carbohydrate-deficient transferrin in serum in relation to alcohol consumption. *Alcohol Clin Exp Res.* 1986;10:535-544.
24. Sullivan JT, Sykora K, Schneiderman J, Narkanjo CA, Sellers EM. Assessment of alcohol withdrawal: the revised Clinical Institute Withdrawal Assessment for Alcohol Scale (CIWA-Ar). *Br J Addict.* 1989;84:1353-1357.
25. Majumdar SK. The influence of chlormethiazole on the neuroendocrine system in chronic alcoholics. *Acta Psychiatr Scand Suppl.* 1986;329:69-72.
26. Zung WWK. A rating instrument for anxiety disorders. *Psychosomatics.* 1971;12:371-379.
27. Zung WWK. A Self-rating Depression Scale. *Arch Gen Psychiatry.* 1965;12:63-70.
28. George DT, Lindquist T, Rawlings RR, Eckhardt MJ, Moss H, Mathis C, Martin PR, Linnoila M. Pharmacologic maintenance of abstinence in patients with alcoholism: no efficacy of 5-hydroxytryptophan or levodopa. *Clin Pharmacol Ther.* 1992;52:553-560.
29. Dettling M, Heinz A, Dufeu P, Rommelspacher H, Gräf KJ, Schmidt LG. Dopaminergic responsivity in alcoholism: trait-, state- or residual marker? *Am J Psychiatry.* 1995;152:1317-1321.
30. Hartka E, Johnstone B, Leino EV, Motoyoshi M, Temple MT, Fillmore KM. The collaborative alcohol-related longitudinal project: a meta-analysis of depressive symptomatology and alcohol consumption over time. *Br J Addict.* 1991;86:1283-1298.
31. Powell J, Dawe S, Richards D, Gossop M, Marks I, Strang J, Gray J. Can opiate addicts tell us about their relapse risk? Subjective predictors of clinical prognosis. *Addict Behav.* 1993;18:473-490.
32. Svrakic DM, Przybeck TR, Cloninger CR. Mood states and personality traits. *J Affective Disord.* 1992;24:217-226.

ORIGINAL ARTICLE

The Great Smoky Mountains Study of Youth

Goals, Design, Methods, and the Prevalence of DSM-III-R *Disorders*

E. Jane Costello, PhD; Adrian Angold, MRCPsych; Barbara J. Burns, PhD; Dalene K. Stangl, PhD; Dan L. Tweed, PhD; Alaattin Erkanli, PhD; Carol M. Worthman, PhD

Background: The Great Smoky Mountains Study of youth focuses on the relationship between the development of psychiatric disorder and the need for and use of mental health services.

Methods: A multistage, overlapping cohorts design was used, in which 4500 of the 11 758 children aged 9, 11, and 13 years in an 11-county area of the southeastern United States were randomly selected for screening for psychiatric symptoms. Children who scored in the top 25% on the screening questionnaire, together with a 1 in 10 random sample of the rest, were recruited for 4 waves of intensive, annual interviews (n=1015 at wave 1). In a parallel study, all American Indian children aged 9, 11, and 13 years were recruited (N=323 at wave 1).

Results: The 3-month prevalence (±SE) of any *DSM-III-R* axis I disorder in the main sample, weighted to reflect population prevalence rates, was 20.3%±1.7%. The most common diagnoses were anxiety disorders (5.7%±1.0%), enuresis (5.1%±1.0%), tic disorders (4.2%±0.9%), conduct disorder (3.3%±0.6%), oppositional defiant disorder (2.7%±0.4%), and hyperactivity (1.9%±0.4%).

Conclusions: The prevalence of psychiatric disorder in this rural sample was similar to rates reported in other recent studies. Poverty was the strongest demographic correlate of diagnosis, in both urban and rural children.

Arch Gen Psychiatry. 1996;53:1129-1136

From the Developmental Epidemiology Program, Duke University Medical Center, Durham, NC (Drs Costello, Angold, Burns, Stangl, Tweed, and Erkanli); and the Department of Anthropology, Emory University, Atlanta, Ga (Dr Worthman).

THE GREAT Smoky Mountains Study (GSMS) was designed to examine the development of, need for, and use of mental health services in children and adolescents in an area of the southeastern United States. The study addresses the extent of met and unmet need for mental health care; the role played by education, primary care, child welfare, and juvenile justice in the provision of mental health care for children; the interrelationship of diagnosis and functional impairment; individual, family, and community predictors of need for mental health care; the impact of different service delivery systems in urban and rural communities; and the interplay of individual development and the development of need for and use of services.

In this and companion articles[1-3] we present the baseline findings on these topics from the first wave of data collection. Analyses across later waves of data collection will address the developmental goals of the study. This article presents the sampling design and procedures common to the entire study, the baseline estimates of rates of psychiatric disorder in 9-, 11-, and 13-year-olds, and the impact of sex, race, income, and rural or urban residence on those rates.

RESULTS

PREVALENCE OF PSYCHIATRIC DISORDERS

Table 2 shows the 3-month weighted prevalence estimates and SEs in wave 1, for *DSM-III-R* diagnoses and combinations of diagnoses, for boys, girls, and both. Diagnoses in parentheses are rare disorders that yielded fewer than 5 cases in the interviewed sample.

See also page 1137

The weighted 3-month population prevalence rate (±SE) was 20.3%±1.7%. The CAPA makes several diagnoses not commonly included in other community

See Subjects and Methods on next page

SUBJECTS AND METHODS

SETTING

The southern Appalachian mountain region of North Carolina was chosen as the study site for the following reasons. (1) This sparsely populated area, with its 180 000 inhabitants spread over 12 194 km^2, is representative of an understudied section of the United States: the rural areas of the south and southeast. (2) Almost all children attend public schools, which means that school records could be used to provide the initial sampling frame for the study. (3) Half the population live in the only sizable town in the area, while the rest live in the rural areas, providing the opportunity to compare psychiatric disorder and service provision in rural and urban settings. (4) The area contains the Qualla Boundary, a federal reservation that is home to the 8000-strong Eastern Band of the Cherokee Nation, a community with different traditions of dealing with mental illness and its own mental health service system.

SAMPLING

Like several epidemiologic studies,[4-6] the GSMS used a screening-stratified sampling design to maximize 3 study goals within a reasonable budget: (1) to understand the developmental pathways of a large sample of children with a high need for mental health care (*case finding*); (2) to estimate the prevalence of disorders and risk factors in the population (*prevalence estimation*); and (3) to map the identified cases onto the general population (*generalizability*). A household sample would meet goal 2 but would need to be large (and expensive) to generate enough cases to meet goals 1 and 3. Recruiting from service settings might achieve goal 1, but generalizability would be hard to achieve because of referral bias and the fact that many children are seen in multiple service sectors.

The screening questionnaire was designed to identify children with a high probability of mental health service use, ie, children with psychiatric symptoms. All children with scores above a cutoff point defined from pilot testing were recruited for the main study. In addition, a 1 in 10 random sample of the remainder were also recruited. Weights inversely proportional to probability of selection were attached to each subject's data, so that estimates of population prevalence could be made.[7] All prevalence estimates and statistical testing was carried out by means of SUDAAN,[8] a SAS-based software package for survey data analysis, which adjusts estimates and variances for the design characteristics.

Power calculations for a range of exposure levels and outcome prevalence indicated that a household sample of 4000 would generate enough cases of the more common child psychiatric disorders (>1% prevalence) to permit, for example, tests of sex-by-age differences in rates.

Screening Sample

Children aged 9, 11, and 13 years at baseline were selected. Nine years was selected as the lowest age for 3 main reasons: (1) rates of professional mental health service use are low in younger children[9]; (2) psychiatric epidemiologic methods for evaluating younger children are not well developed[10,11]; and (3) we are interested in the impact of puberty on the onset of some psychiatric disorders. By the end of 4 annual interviews, the 9-year-olds will be 12 years old, and the 11-year-olds, 14 years old. This "overlapping cohorts"[12] design permits us to assess and, if necessary, control for cohort effects, while examining children across an 8-year age range (9-16 years) within 4 years.

A multistep probability sampling procedure was used. The 12 000 children aged 9, 11, and 13 years in the public school's database were arranged by households and were selected with probability proportional to the total number of age-eligible children in the household. An age category (9, 11, or 13 years) was drawn from each selected household, with the probability of selection being proportional to the number of children in the age group for that household. Within the selected age category, 1 child was selected on an equiprobability basis to generate a total screening sample of 4500 children (1570 were 9-year-olds, 1590 were 11-year-olds, and 1340 were 13-year-olds). The parent or guardian of each child completed a brief screening questionnaire about the index child. If the parent could not be reached by telephone, contact was made by mail or, if necessary, by home visits.

The screening measure consisted of the "externalizing" broad-band scale items from the Child Behavior Checklist.[13,14] The substance abuse question in the Child Behavior Checklist was expanded to cover specific substances (tobacco, cannabis, inhalants, etc), for a total of 57 questions. Previous studies have attested to the Child Behavior Checklist's reliability and ability to identify child mental health services users.[13,15] We used only parent-reported items for 3 reasons. (1) Pilot testing showed that screening 2 or more people (eg, a parent and the child) greatly increased refusals and incomplete data without much improvement in case identification. (2) Evidence from previous studies suggested that parental reports of behavioral problems best predict most types of psychiatric symptoms and service use.[14-16] (3) It was important to keep the screen as short as possible. A potential disadvantage of this approach was that it did not screen for anxiety, depression, and other nonexternalizing disorders. However, there is evidence that parents are often poor reporters of children's anxiety and depression, and that there is a considerable amount of comorbidity with behavioral problems.[5,15-17] Thus, a screen for behavioral symptoms was likely also to identify children with emotional problems.

American Indian Participants

American Indian children were not included in the random selection process because of our interest in oversampling this group. We were given permission by the Board of Education on the Qualla Boundary to recruit all 9-, 11-, and 13-year-olds attending reservation schools, and extended the study to include all American Indian children attending public schools, to obtain a 100% sample of age-appropriate enrolled members of any American Indian tribe. Because extra funding is available for American Indian students in public schools under Public Law 874, or Title V of the Indian Education Act, records of ethnicity are carefully maintained by the schools. A total of 450 American Indian children were identified in either public or reservation schools. Apart from the sampling procedures, data collection and methods were identical for all ethnic groups.

Results from the American Indian children will be reported in a separate article.

MEASURES

Table 1 shows the measures, their content area, the informant, and the occasions on which they are used.[18-30] The measures of each area are reviewed briefly below; further details may be obtained from the first author (E.J.C.).

Construct 1: Risk for Mental Health Service Use

Diagnoses and Symptoms. The Child and Adolescent Psychiatric Assessment (CAPA)[18,19] is an interview that elicits information about symptoms that contribute to a wide range of diagnoses. The CAPA combines the characteristics of an "interviewer-based" and a "respondent-based" interview.[18] Like respondent-based interviews, the CAPA uses a highly structured protocol, with required questions and probes. However, as in an interviewer-based interview, the onus throughout is on the interviewer to ensure that subjects (1) understand the question being asked, (2) provide clear information on behavior or feelings relevant to the symptom, and (3) have the symptom at a prespecified level of severity as defined in an extensive glossary. Diagnoses are generated by computer algorithms. Separate algorithms are available for child and parent reports and "combined reports," where a symptom is regarded as being present if either the parent or the child reports it.

The *DSM-III-R*[20] was the taxonomy used for wave 1; subsequent waves will be analyzed by means of both *DSM-III-R*[20] and *DSM-IV*.[21] A test-retest reliability study of a clinical sample aged 10 to 17 years[19] found $\kappa=0.52$ for oppositional disorder, $\kappa=0.61$ for conduct disorder, $\kappa=0.95$ for substance abuse, $\kappa=0.52$ for separation anxiety, $\kappa=0.77$ for overanxious disorder, $\kappa=0.65$ for dysthymia, and $\kappa=0.85$ for major depression.

Level of Functioning. The functional impairment or incapacities section of the CAPA, which follows the section on symptoms, relates the symptoms to the child's ability to function at a developmentally appropriate level in relationships with family, peers, and teachers, in activities at school, at home, and in the community. A test-retest study of the incapacities section with 77 children showed an intraclass correlation of 0.76.[19]

Four other measures of functioning were collected. Interviewers completed the Children's Global Assessment Scale,[22] for which the interviewer gives the child a single score ranging from 0 to 100, and the Child and Adolescent Functional Assessment Scale,[23] which rates the child on role performance at school, ability to think clearly, behavior toward self and others, mood and emotional state, and caregiver's resources, needs, and level of social support. Both of these scales show reasonable reliability in clinic populations.[22,23] Parent and child completed the Social Interactions Survey,[24] which assesses the child's ability to relate well to peers, parents, teachers, and other adults. The Social Interactions Survey consists of 12 vignettes describing a social situation (eg, rejection by peers). The subject marks on a 0- to 100-point scale the extent to which the vignette describes the child in question. One-week retest reliability on a sample of 32 children aged 9 to 12 years yielded intraclass correlation coefficients of 0.86 for peer relationships and 0.85 for adult relationships. In the second and third waves of the study, 3 teachers for each child completed the Teacher Report Form,[25] a version for teachers of the Child Behavior Checklist that includes information on the child's academic and social functioning at school.

Construct 2: Service Use, Access, and Barriers to Care

The Child and Adolescent Services Assessment (CASA)[26] is an interview about use of specialty mental health providers, pediatricians, other medical care providers, school counselors, probation officers, Department of Social Services staff, self-help groups, spiritual advisors, family, and friends. The CASA has 3 parts. First, a screen assesses the use of a list of providers. For each provider actually seen by the index child, probes are used to determine the onset, frequency, and duration of contacts, services provided, cost, who paid, and the recipient's level of perceived benefit. The CASA then asks about barriers to using services for mental health care: time, distance, lack of transportation, cost, lack of a common language, and fear that the child will be taken away or that parental rights will be lost. Reliability studies on the CASA[26] show that it has high retest reliability ($\kappa>0.80$) for the more intensive services, such as inpatient hospitalization, good reliability ($\kappa>0.60$) for less intensive professional mental health services, such as outpatient treatment and school services, and moderate to low reliability for nonprofessional services, such as consulting ministers and friends. A comparison of CASA parent reports of mental health service use with the records of local mental health agencies for 160 high-intensity service users showed complete agreement for inpatient services, 91% agreement for outpatient services, and 79% agreement overall.[26]

Construct 3: Family Resources

Information is collected on family income, parental occupation and educational status, and health and mental health insurance.

Construct 4: Family Functioning, Psychiatric Symptoms, and Family Burden

The CAPA includes a section on the quality of family relationships (parent-child and parent-parent relationships, parenting style, etc). Retest reliability is good (eg, intraclass correlation of 0.76 for the family relationships scale). A brief section also reviews the psychiatric problems of the index child's parents or primary caretakers. Questions cover history of treatment for psychiatric or substance abuse problems, and criminal convictions. Kappa statistics for individual items are all 0.60 or better.

The caregiver completes the Child and Adolescent Burden Assessment,[2] a section in CAPA, for children with any identified psychiatric problems. This instrument covers such issues as the economic burden of having a child with mental health problems, the impact on family finances and relationships, restrictions on activities, including ability to work, parental psychological distress, and stigma.

Continued on next page

Construct 5: Child's Physical Health and Development

Each child is weighed and measured, and blood samples are assayed for luteinizing hormone, follicle-stimulating hormone, testosterone, dehydroepiandrosterone, and androstenedione in boys and girls, and estradiol in girls, by means of fluorometric immunoassay methods developed by Worthman and Stallings.[27] Children also complete a self-report measure of Tanner staging,[28] which provides a good approximation to physical examination for pubertal development, and answer a series of questions on self-perception of developmental status relative to other children and satisfaction with developmental status. In the second and third waves of data collection, parents complete the Childhood (Medical) Conditions section of the National Health Interview Survey Supplement Booklet,[29] which collects basic information about the child's physical health history.

Construct 6: Adversity and Traumatic Events

The CAPA includes an extensive review of long-term adversity, such as poverty and living in an unsafe neighborhood, and life events that could contribute to posttraumatic stress disorder and other disorders.

Construct 7: Community Resources

The network of services available in the area has been studied by members of the group (E.J.C., A.A., and B.J.B.) as part of another study in the same community, and a detailed analysis of the service system for children and adolescents is available.[30]

INTERVIEWERS AND INTERVIEWER TRAINING

Interviewers are residents of the area in which the study is taking place. Some, but not all, of the interviewers for the American Indian sample are American Indians. All interviewers have at least bachelor's-level degrees and receive 1 month of training. After training, quality control is maintained through postinterview reviews of each schedule, weekly staff meetings to review audiotapes of randomly selected field interviews, and regular refresher sessions with one of us (A.A.).

PROCEDURES FOR THE FIRST WAVE

Children were screened and interviewed as close as possible to the birthday on which they became 9, 11, or 13 years old. Families recruited for the interview stage of the study were visited at home by 2 interviewers. After the informed consent and physical procedures, parent and child were interviewed in separate rooms. Each parent and child was paid $10 after the interview was completed.

Figure 1 shows the completion rates for various stages of sample recruitment for the main study. Of the 4500 names selected, 433 were eliminated, either because the family had moved out of the study area or because errors in the database misclassified the child's age. It proved impossible to complete 56 of the 1071 interviews scheduled for the main sample within the window of 6 months from the child's birthday, because of severe weather in the mountains. These families remain in the study and form part of the wave 2 data collection but are treated as having missing data for wave 1. The racial composition of the main sample at wave 1 was as follows: African American, 79; Hispanic, 6; Asian American, 3; mixed race, 11; and white, 916. There were also 323 American Indians in the companion study.

The availability of screening data made it possible to check on potential differences between the interviewed sample and (1) the families who were selected for the main study but refused to participate and (2) families who agreed to participate but could not be interviewed at wave 1. Comparisons were made, by χ^2 or t tests, on age, sex, income, rural or urban residence, mean within-group screen score, percentage scoring in the high-risk range, percentage of children below grade for age, and the percentage who had sought help because of the child's emotional or behavioral problems. There were no statistically significant differences on any individual variable or combination of variables, with $P<.1$ used as the criterion. We conclude that the results of the study are unlikely to be seriously biased by nonresponse.

FOLLOW-UP TELEPHONE CONTACTS AND INTERVIEWS

After the wave 1 interviews, families are contacted by telephone every 3 months. They report on any service use during the intervening period, as well as any change of address, school, or family structure. Thereafter, the parent and child are reinterviewed annually by means of a protocol almost identical to that used in wave 1.

studies, and some of these, notably tic disorders and enuresis, occurred at a fairly high rate. We calculated an overall prevalence rate for a set of "core" diagnoses made in several other studies (Table 2). Also, while strictly diagnosed *DSM-III-R* depressive disorders were rare, there was a substantial group of children (28 of the interviewed sample) who had the core symptoms of mood disorder and anhedonia but did not quite reach the criterion either for duration (for dysthymia) or for number of other symptoms (for major depression). It seemed appropriate to include this markedly symptomatic group, and they are designated in Table 2 under "depression not otherwise specified" and included in the overall and core prevalence rates.

There were 307 children with a *DSM-III-R* diagnosis in the sample, whereas a prevalence rate of 20.3% would yield 206 cases from a random population sample of 1015. Thus, the screening process yielded a sample containing 49% more cases. We discuss the cost-efficiency of 2-stage sampling in detail in another article.[31]

COMORBIDITY

Comorbidity was not uncommon in the sample: 100 of the 307 children with a diagnosis had more than 1. Some children had more than 1 diagnosis within 1 category (eg, more than 1 anxiety disorder), while others had, for

Table 1. Content Areas and Instruments

Construct	Instruments	Informants	Occasions
1a. Psychiatric symptoms, *DSM-III-R*[20] and *DSM-IV*[21] psychiatric diagnoses	Child and Adolescent Psychiatric Assessment (CAPA)[18,19]	Parent, child	Annual interviews
1b. Level of functioning	CAPA impairment scales,[18,19] Child and Adolescent Functional Assessment Scale (CAFAS),[23] Children's Global Assessment Scale (CGAS),[22] Social Competence scales of the Teacher Report Form (TRF),[25] Social Interactions Survey[24]	Parent, child, teachers; CGAS and CAFAS are based on interviewer's judgment after full CAPA assessment	Annual interviews (TRF from wave 2)
2. Service use, access and barriers to care	Child and Adolescent Services Assessment[26]	Parent, child	Annual interviews, 3-monthly telephone checks
3a. Family impact of child's psychopathology	Child and Adolescent Burden Assessment[2]	Parent	Annual interviews, 3-monthly telephone checks
3b. Family structure, functioning, history of psychiatric treatment, arrests, substance abuse problems, suicides	CAPA[18,19]	Parent, child*	Annual interviews
4. Family resources	CAPA[18,19]	Parent, child	Annual interviews
5. Child's physical health and development	(*a*) Measurement of height and weight[27] (*b*) Hormone assay[27] (*c*) Tanner staging[28] (*d*) National Health Interview Survey (NHIS)[29]	(*a*) Child (direct measurement) (*b*) Child (direct measurement) (*c*) Child (d) Parent	Annual interviews (National Health Interview Survey from wave 2)
6. Adversity and traumatic events	CAPA, including Traumatic Life Events section[18,19]	Parent, child	Annual interviews
7. Service system characteristics	Network interview[30]	Providers	Year 4

**Structure and functioning only.*

example, both an emotional and a behavioral disorder. **Figure 2** shows the numbers of children interviewed with various types of comorbidity, while the percentages are weighted to reflect the population rates. Overall, 1.5% of the population had both an emotional and a behavioral disorder. Comorbidity was more commonly associated with some diagnoses than others. Only 21% (weighted) of children with an "other" disorder (mainly tics and enuresis) had an emotional or behavioral disorder, whereas 53% of children with depression (including depression not otherwise specified) were comorbid, as were 38% of children with a behavioral disorder and 28% of those with an anxiety disorder.

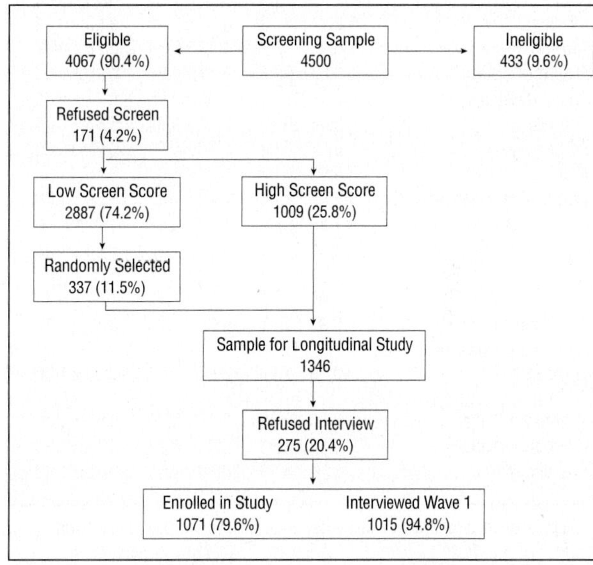

Figure 1. *Sampling design for the Great Smoky Mountains Study.*

DEMOGRAPHIC CORRELATES OF DIAGNOSIS

The relationship between diagnosis and sex, age, race, income, and urban or rural location was examined by logistic regression. Since rates of disorder were similar in 11- and 13-year-olds, and somewhat higher in 9-year-olds, a dichotomous variable (9 vs 11+13 years) was used in the logistic regressions. Income was dichotomized as being above or below the federal poverty line, and race as African American vs other. SUDAAN[8] was used to generate the odds ratios (ORs), confidence intervals (CIs), and probabilities. All ORs control for the other demographic correlates.

Sex

Boys were at higher risk for any psychiatric disorder (24.9%±2.6% [SE] vs 15.5%±2.2%; OR, 1.8; 95% CI, 1.3-2.5; *P*<.001). This was mainly the result of their higher rates of behavioral disorders (9.5% vs 3.5%; OR, 2.9; 95% CI, 1.6-5.1; *P*<.001) and enuresis (7.7% vs 2.5%; OR, 2.8; 95% CI, 1.4-5.6; *P*=.003). Comorbidity of emotional and behavioral disorders was almost 3 times as common in boys as in girls (2.2% vs 0.8%; OR, 2.7; 95% CI, 0.9-7.7; *P*=.06).

Age

Rates of separation anxiety, tics, and enuresis fell significantly between 9 and 11 years of age, but there were no other significant age differences.

Table 2. Three-Month Prevalence of CAPA/*DSM-III-R* Diagnoses*

Diagnosis	Prevalence, % (±SE) Female	Male	Total
Separation anxiety	4.30±1.20	2.70±0.91	3.49±0.75
Overanxious disorder	1.90±0.89	0.88±0.24	1.38±0.46
Generalized anxiety disorder	2.40±1.08	0.95±0.57	1.67±0.61
Simple phobia	0.42±0.17	0.13±0.09	0.27±0.10
(Agoraphobia)	0	0.13±0.09	0.07±0.05
(Panic disorder)	0	0.07±0.07	0.03±0.03
(Avoidant disorder)	0.07±0.07	0	0.03±0.03
Social anxiety	0.83±0.63	0.33±0.15	0.58±0.32
(Elective mutism)	0	0	0
Obsessive-compulsive disorder	0.14±0.10	0.20±0.12	0.17±0.08
(Posttraumatic stress disorder)	0.05±1.60	0	0.02±0.96
(Anorexia nervosa)	0	0	0
(Bulimia)	0.07±0.07	0.14±0.10	0.10±0.06
(Major depression)	0.07±0.07	0	0.03±0.03
(Dysthymia)	0.07±0.07	0.20±0.12	0.13±0.07
Depression not otherwise specified	1.22±0.65	1.68±0.66	1.45±0.46
(Hypomania)	0.07±0.07	0.13±0.09	0.10±0.06
(Manic episode)	0	0	0
Conduct disorder	1.13±0.28	5.43±1.23	3.32±0.64
Oppositional defiant disorder	2.33±0.70	3.16±0.47	2.75±0.41
ADHD†	0.95±0.26	2.90±0.73	1.94±0.39
(Substance abuse/dependence)	0.13±0.09	0.07±0.07	0.10±0.06
Motor tic	2.71±1.12	4.32±1.48	3.53±0.94
(Vocal tic)	0.20±0.11	1.28±0.64	0.75±0.33
(Tourette disorder)	0.07±0.07	0.13±0.09	0.10±0.06
Trichotillomania	0	0.34±0.15	0.17±0.08
Enuresis	2.48±0.85	7.66±1.74	5.11±0.99
Encopresis	0.07±0.07	1.36±0.59	0.72±0.30
(Schizophrenia)	0.13±0.09	0.07±0.07	0.10±0.06
Any anxiety disorder‡	6.96±1.60	4.46±1.09	5.69±0.96
Any depressive disorder	1.36±0.65	1.68±0.66	1.52±0.46
Any emotional disorder	8.05±1.71	5.67±1.26	6.84±1.05
Any behavioral disorder	3.50±0.76	9.53±1.44	6.56±0.81
Any tic disorder	2.90±1.13	5.47±1.49	4.20±0.94
Any other disorder§	5.87±1.41	14.96±2.28	10.48±1.37
Any emotional or behavioral disorder	10.79±1.83	13.04±1.77	11.93±1.26
Comorbid emotional and behavioral diagnoses	0.75±0.35	2.16±0.75	1.47±0.45
Any core disorder‖	10.86±1.83	13.31±1.78	12.10±1.26
Any disorder	15.54±2.23	24.88±2.62	20.25±1.72

**Diagnoses in parentheses had fewer than 5 cases in the interviewed sample. CAPA indicates Child and Adolescent Psychiatric Assessment; ADHD, attention-deficit hyperactivity disorder.*

†Based on parent report only.

‡*Separation anxiety, overanxious disorder, generalized anxiety disorder, simple phobia, agoraphobia, panic disorder, avoidant disorder, social anxiety.*

§*Encopresis, enuresis, tics, Tourette disorder, obsessive-compulsive disorder, bulimia, trichotillomania.*

‖*Any emotional or behavioral disorder, schizophrenia, obsessive-compulsive disorder, anorexia, bulimia, Tourette disorder, trichotillomania, posttraumatic stress disorder, elective mutism, encopresis.*

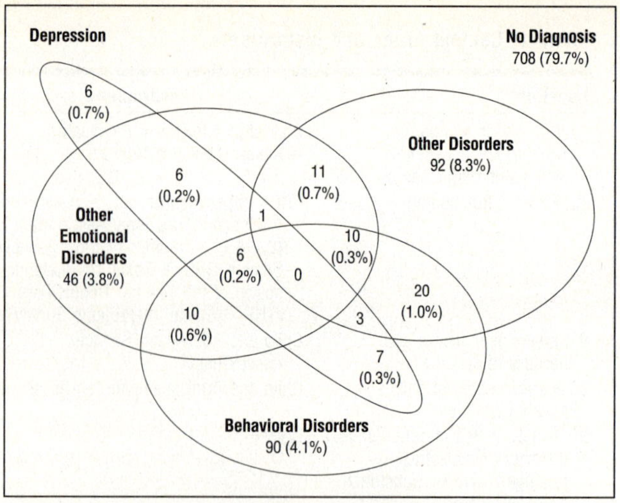

Figure 2. *Comorbidity among diagnostic areas, showing number of interviewed children with diagnoses and weighted 3-month prevalence rates (in parentheses). Associations between diagnostic categories, with odds ratio, 95% confidence intervals, and associated* P *values, are as follows: depressive/anxiety disorders, 4.9, 1.5 to 16.5, and .01; depressive/behavioral disorders, 6.6, 2.1 to 20.5, and .001; depressive/other disorders (chiefly enuresis and tic disorders; see Table 2), 0.8, 0.2 to 3.8, and .79; anxiety/behavioral disorders, 3.2, 1.5 to 6.7, and .002; anxiety/other disorders, 1.1, 0.8 to 3.5, and .146; and behavioral/other disorders, 2.6, 1.3 to 4.8, and .004.*

Race

The only comparison examined here was between African American children, who made up 8.1% of the sample, and white children. African American children were more likely to have functional enuresis, but rates of all other disorders, and of comorbidity, were similar.

Income

The children from the poorest families were at increased risk of any disorder (33.4%±3.9% vs 15.9%±1.7%; OR, 3.2; 95% CI, 2.3-4.4; $P<.001$) and of every type of diagnosis except for tic disorders. The highest risk was for behavioral disorders (11.0% vs 4.4%; OR, 2.7; 95% CI, 1.6-4.4; $P<.001$). Poor children had comorbid emotional and behavioral conditions at 3 times the rate of other children (6.5% vs 2.0%; OR, 3.3; 95% CI, 1.7-6.6; $P<.001$).

Place of Residence

Any differences between urban and rural children became nonsignificant when poverty was included in the model.

COMMENT

LIMITATIONS

Limitations of the present study include the following: (1) Information is available for only 3 groups of children recruited at ages 9, 11, and 13 years. (2) This is a southern, rural, predominantly white sample, containing almost no Hispanic or Asian-American children. (3) Wave 1 of the GSMS collected information only from the index child and 1 parent. Other research has shown that parents often have different views of the same child, as do teachers and others in the child's immediate circle.[16] In the second and subsequent waves, questionnaire information is being collected from 3 teachers for each child, as well as from treatment settings. (4) The CAPA provides prevalence estimates only for the 3 months preceding the interview. However, data on service use is collected every 3 months between interviews, so complete longitudinal data will be available. (5) By screening for behavioral but not emotional or other problems, we may have increased the SEs of the estimates of depression, anxiety, tics, enuresis, etc; however, the screen-low group was large enough (N=260) to prevent any significant distortion of the prevalence estimates.

PREVALENCE

The most important conclusion to be drawn from the data presented herein is that rates and correlates of childhood psychiatric disorder were similar in this remote, rural area of the United States to those found in studies in urban areas.[32-34] Poverty does not have to be accompanied by urban pressures to be associated with psychiatric symptoms.

In a previous publication,[35] we summarized rates of child psychiatric disorders reported by several recent epidemiologic studies, finding that they fell within a fairly narrow range (17.6%-22.0%). The overall prevalence rates of disorder and comorbidity found in the GSMS sample fell within the expected range.[6,32-34,36-39]

From a public health point of view, the high rate of comorbidity illustrated in Figure 2 is a cause for concern. The Dunedin, New Zealand, longitudinal study has documented a high rate of learning difficulties and other problems in adolescents who had some types of psychiatric comorbidity in childhood.[37,40] Studies of adults have shown that those with multiple disorders in the course of a lifetime are at higher risk of having "severe" disorders (psychoses or disorders requiring hospitalization or causing severe role impairment)[41] and of substance abuse.[42,43] This study replicated others in finding that depression, in particular, is highly likely to be accompanied by other disorders.[44]

CORRELATES OF PSYCHIATRIC DISORDER

In general, the patterns linking rates of psychiatric disorder to differences in sex, age, race, and place of residence support those previously reported.[6,32,36,45] Thus, we found more behavioral disorders in boys than in girls, decreasing rates of separation anxiety, tics, and enuresis with age, and an increased risk in children from impoverished families. On the other hand, rates of disorder were high only in children living in the direst poverty; children from families with even a modestly higher income, up to twice the federal poverty level, had rates of psychiatric disorders no higher than those of children from the highest income groups. Once we controlled for poverty, however, we did not find the higher rates of disorder in urban children that others have reported.[32-34,46] Nor were African-American children at higher risk for anything other than enuresis, controlling for poverty and urban residence.

Adults in the southern United States appear to report fewer mental health problems than those in other areas of the country. In the National Comorbidity Survey of adults, Kessler et al[41] found marked regional differences in lifetime prevalence rates, with lower rates of all but affective disorders in the southern United States, although the odds ratios comparing other regions with the south did not reach significance. The North Carolina site of the adult Epidemiologic Catchment Area Study had the lowest rates of affective disorders, substance use or abuse, and antisocial personality disorders, but ranked highest in rates of somatization, panic, generalized anxiety, and obsessive-compulsive disorders. As George et al[47] pointed out, caution must be used in drawing inferences about the south on the basis of a single, highly urbanized site. Sampling procedures used in the National Comorbidity Study, on the other hand, were designed to yield regional estimates and probably provide the best basis for regional comparisons. The Isle of Wight–Inner City comparison by Rutter and colleagues[46] found twice as much psychopathology in urban youth, but they ascribed the difference to the higher rates of poverty and life stresses in the urban sample. A cautious inference from this study is that the lower rate in the south has more to do with poverty than with latitude or urbanization.

Accepted for publication February 5, 1996.

This project was supported by grant MH48085 from the National Institute of Mental Health, Bethesda, Md. Additional support was provided through a project grant (Dr Worthman) and Faculty Scholar awards (Drs Costello, Angold, and Worthman) from the William T. Grant Foundation and a Center grant from the Leon Lowenstein Foundation, New York, NY (Dr Angold). We gratefully acknowledge support of the psychometric studies of the Child and Adolescent Psychiatric Assessment from the William T. Grant Foundation.

The field work for this study was supervised by Teresa Sweeney. Stephen Messer, PhD, and Willie Ashley, PhD, assisted with clinical supervision and interviewing. Joe Morrissey, PhD, developed the institutional survey. Ralph Folsom, PhD, of Research Triangle Institute, Research Triangle Park, NC, assisted with the multistage sampling design. We wish to acknowledge with gratitude the help of the superintendents of schools in the 11-county area of the study, Jonathan L. Taylor, the Principal Chief of the Eastern Band of the Cherokee Nation, James L. Sanders, MSW, the Bureau of Indian Affairs Director of Social Services on the Qualla Boundary, and Joyce Dugan, the Director of Education. The cooperation of the entire community of western North Carolina is warmly appreciated.

Reprints: E. Jane Costello, PhD, Developmental Epidemiology Program, Duke University Medical Center, Box 3454, Durham NC 27710.

REFERENCES

1. Costello EJ, Angold A, Burns BJ, Erkanli A, Stangl DK, Tweed DL. The Great Smoky Mountains Study of youth: functional impairment and severe emotional disturbance. *Arch Gen Psychiatry.* 1996;53:1137-1143.
2. Angold A, Messer SC, Stangl D, Farmer EMZ, Costello EJ, Burns BJ. Perceived parental burden and service use for child and adolescent psychiatric disorders. *Am J Public Health.* In press.
3. Burns BJ, Costello EJ, Angold A, Tweed D, Stangl D, Farmer EMZ, Erkanli A.

Children's mental health service use across service sectors. *Health Affairs.* 1995; 14:147-159.
4. Dohrenwend BP, Levav I, Schrout PE, Schwartz S, Naveh G, Link BG, Skodol AE, Stueve A. Socioeconomic status and psychiatric disorders: the causation-selection issue. *Science.* 1992;255:946-952.
5. Rutter M, Tizard J, Whitmore K. *Education, Health, and Behaviour.* London, England: Longman; 1970.
6. Bird HR, Canino G, Rubio-Stipec M, Gould MS, Ribera J, Sesman M, Woodbury M, Huertas-Goldman S, Pagan A, Sanchez-Lacay A, Moscoso M. Estimates of the prevalence of childhood maladjustment in a community survey in Puerto Rico: the use of combined measures. *Arch Gen Psychiatry.* 1988;45: 1120-1126.
7. Shrout PE, Newman SC. Design of two-phase prevalence surveys of rare disorders. *Biometrics.* 1989;45:549-555.
8. Shah BV, Folsom RE, LaVange LM, Wheeless SC, Boyle KE, Williams RL. *SUDAAN Software for the Statistical Analysis of Correlated Data: Statistical Methods and Mathematical Algorithms Used in SUDAAN.* Research Triangle Park, NC: Research Triangle Institute; 1995.
9. US Congress, Office of Technology Assessment. Mental health problems: prevention and services. In: *Adolescent Health, Volume II: Background and the Effectiveness of Selected Prevention and Treatment Services.* Washington, DC: Office of Technology Assessment; 1991:433-496.
10. Costello AJ, Edelbrock CS, Dulcan MK, Kalas R, Klaric SH. *Development and Testing of the NIMH Diagnostic Interview Schedule for Children in a Clinic Population: Final Report (Contract No. RFP-DB-81-0027).* Rockville, Md: Center for Epidemiologic Studies–National Institute of Mental Health; 1984.
11. Breton JJ, Bergeron L, Valle JP, Lepine S, Houde L, Gaudet N. Do children aged 9 through 11 years understand the DISC version 2.25 questions? *J Am Acad Child Adolesc Psychiatry.* 1995;34:946-956.
12. Schaie KW. A general model for the study of developmental problems. *Psychol Bull.* 1965;64:92-107.
13. Achenbach TM, Edelbrock CS. Behavorial problems and competencies reported by parents of normal and disturbed children aged four through sixteen. *Monogr Soc Res Child Dev.* 1981;46(1, No. 188):1-82.
14. Achenbach TM, Edelbrock C. *Manual for the Child Behavior Checklist and Child Behavior Profile.* Burlington, Vt: University of Vermont; 1983.
15. Bird HR, Gould MS, Rubio-Stipec M, Staghezza BM, Canino G. Screening for childhood psychopathology in the community using the Child Behavior Checklist. *J Am Acad Child Adolesc Psychiatry.* 1991;30:116-123.
16. Achenbach TM, McConaughy SH, Howell CT. Child/adolescent behavioral and emotional problems: implications of cross-informant correlations for situational specificity. *Psychol Bull.* 1987;101:213-232.
17. McConaughy SH, Achenbach TM. Comorbidity of empirically based syndromes in matched general population and clinical samples. *J Child Psychol Psychiatry.* 1994;35:1141-1157.
18. Angold A, Prendergast M, Cox A, Harrington R, Simonoff E, Rutter M. The Child and Adolescent Psychiatric Assessment (CAPA). *Psychol Med.* 1995;25: 739-753.
19. Angold A, Costello EJ. A test-retest reliability study of child-reported psychiatric symptoms and diagnoses using the Child and Adolescent Psychiatric Assessment (CAPA-C). *Psychol Med.* 1995;25:755-762.
20. American Psychiatric Association Committee on Nomenclature and Statistics. *Diagnostic and Statistical Manual of Mental Disorders, Revised Third Edition.* Washington, DC: American Psychiatric Association; 1987.
21. American Psychiatric Association Committee on Nomenclature and Statistics. *Diagnostic and Statistical Manual of Mental Disorders, Fourth Edition.* Washington, DC: American Psychiatric Association; 1994.
22. Shaffer D, Gould MS, Brasic J, Ambrosini PJ, Fisher PW, Bird HR, Aluwahlia S. A Children's Global Assessment Scale (CGAS). *Arch Gen Psychiatry.* 1983; 40:1228-1231.
23. Hodges K, Bickman L, Ring-Kurtz S, Rieter M. Multidimensional measure of level of functioning for children and adolescents. In: Algarian A, Friedman R, eds. *A System of Care for Children's Mental Health: Expanding the Research Base.* Tampa, Fla: Research Training Center for Children's Mental Health; 1991: 149-154.
24. DeRosier ME. Actual and perceived peer relationships: implications for children's academic, behavioral, and emotional adjustment problems. Presented at the Society for Research in Child Development Biennial Meeting; March 30, 1995; Indianapolis, Ind.
25. Achenbach TM, Edelbrock CS. *Manual for the Teacher's Report Form and Teacher Version of the Child Behavior Profile.* Burlington, Vt: Department of Psychiatry, University of Vermont; 1986.
26. Farmer EMZ, Angold A, Burns BJ, Costello EJ. Reliability of self-reported service use: test-retest consistency of children's responses to the Child and Adolescent Services Assessment (CASA). *J Child Fam Stud.* 1994;3:307-325.
27. Worthman CM, Stallings JF. Measurement of gonadotropins in dried blood spots. *Clin Chem.* 1994;40:448-453.
28. Dorn LD, Susman EJ, Nottelmann ED, Inoff-Germain ED, Chrousos GP. Perceptions of puberty: adolescent, parent, and health care personnel. *Dev Psychopathol.* 1990;26:322-329.
29. Public Health Service. *National Health Interview Survey: Supplement Booklet.* Washington, DC: US Dept of Commerce Bureau of the Census; 1988.
30. Morrissey JP. An interorganizational network approach to evaluating children's mental health service systems. In: Bickman L, Rog D, eds. *Evaluating Children's Mental Health Services: Methodological Issues.* San Francisco, Calif: Jossey Bass; 1992:85-98.
31. Erkanli A, Soyer R, Angold A. Optimal bayesian two-phase designs for prevalence estimation. *J Stat Plann Inference.* In press.
32. Reinherz HZ, Giaconia RM, Lefkowitz ES, Pakiz B, Frost AK. Prevalence of psychiatric disorders in a community population of older adolescents. *J Am Acad Child Adolesc Psychiatry.* 1993;32:369-377.
33. Offord DR, Boyle MH, Szatmari P, Rae-Grant NI, Links PS, Cadman DT, Byles JA, Crawford JW, Munroe-Blum H, Byrne C, Thomas H, Woodward CA. Ontario Child Health Study, II: six-month prevalence of disorder and rates of service utilization. *Arch Gen Psychiatry.* 1987;44:832-836.
34. Rutter M, Yule B, Quinton D, Rowlands O, Yule W, Berger M. Attainment and adjustment in two geographical areas, II: some factors accounting for area differences. *Br J Psychiatry.* 1974;125:520-533.
35. Costello EJ. Developments in child psychiatric epidemiology. *J Am Acad Child Adolesc Psychiatry.* 1989;28:836-841.
36. Cohen P, Cohen J, Kasen S, Velez CN, Hartmark C, Johnson J, Rojas M, Brook J, Streuning EL. An epidemiological study of disorders in late childhood and adolescence, 1: age- and gender-specific prevalence. *J Child Psychol Psychiatry.* 1993;34:851-867.
37. Anderson JC, Williams S, McGee R, Silva PA. Cognitive and social correlates of *DSM-III* disorders in preadolescent children. *J Am Acad Child Adolesc Psychiatry.* 1989;28:842-846.
38. McGee R, Feehan M, Williams S, Partridge F, Silva PA, Kelly J. *DSM-III* disorders in a large sample of adolescents. *J Am Acad Child Adolesc Psychiatry.* 1990;29:611-619.
39. Graham P, Rutter M. Psychiatric disorders in the young adolescent: a follow-up study. *Proc R Soc Med.* 1973;66:1226-1229.
40. Moffitt TE. Juvenile delinquency and attention deficit disorder: boys developmental trajectories from age 3 to age 15. *Child Dev.* 1990;61:893-910.
41. Kessler RC, McGonagle KA, Zhao S, Nelson CB, Hughes M, Eshleman S, Wittchen HU, Kendler KS. Lifetime and 12-month prevalence of *DSM-III-R* psychiatric disorders in the United States: results from the National Comorbidity Study. *Arch Gen Psychiatry.* 1994;51:8-19.
42. Regier DA, Farmer ME, Rae DS, Locke BZ, Keith SJ, Judd LL, Goodwin FK. Comorbidity of mental disorders with alcohol and other drug abuse: results from the Epidemiologic Catchment Area (ECA) study. *JAMA.* 1990;264:2511-2518.
43. Helzer JE, Burnam A, McEvoy LT. Alcohol abuse and dependence: a diagnosis of alcoholism. In: Robins LN, Regier DA, eds. *Psychiatric Disorders in America: The Epidemiologic Catchment Area Study.* New York, NY: Free Press; 1991: 81-115.
44. Angold A, Costello EJ. Depressive comorbidity in children and adolescents: empirical, theoretical, and methodological issues. *Am J Psychiatry.* 1993;150: 1779-1791.
45. Lewinsohn PM, Hops H, Roberts RE, Seeley JR, Andrews JA. Adolescent psychopathology, I: prevalence and incidence of depression and other *DSM-III-R* disorders in high school students. *J Abnorm Psychol.* 1993;102:133-144.
46. Rutter M, Yule B, Quinton D, Rowlands O, Yule W, Berger M. Attainment and adjustment in two geographical areas, III: some factors accounting for area differences. *Br J Psychiatry.* 1975;126:520-533.
47. George LK, Landerman R, Blazer DG, Anthony JC. Cognitive impairment. In: Robins LK, Regier DA, Robins LN, eds. *Psychiatric Disorders in America: The Epidemiologic Catchment Area Study.* New York, NY: Free Press; 1991:291-327.

ORIGINAL ARTICLE

The Great Smoky Mountains Study of Youth

Functional Impairment and Serious Emotional Disturbance

E. Jane Costello, PhD; Adrian Angold, MRCPsych; Barbara J. Burns, PhD; Alaattin Erkanli, PhD; Dalene K. Stangl, PhD; Dan L. Tweed, PhD

Background: Federal regulations require states to estimate the prevalence and incidence of serious emotional disturbance (SED) in children, defined as a *DSM-III-R* diagnosis in the presence of impaired functioning in 1 or more areas. We reviewed the published data on SED and examined rates and correlates of SED in an ongoing epidemiologic study of children.

Methods: Rates of *DSM-III-R* disorders, functional impairment, and their co-occurrence (SED) were examined in a representative population sample of 9-, 11-, and 13-year-olds from a predominantly rural area of North Carolina. Three measures of functional impairment were used, and their interrelationship and impact on rates of SED were examined.

Results: Serious emotional disturbance was identified in 4% to 8% of the study population, depending on the measure of impairment; the rate of *DSM-III-R* disorder ignoring impairment was 20.3%. One quarter of children identified as having SED on any measure were identified by all 3, and one half by 2 or more. Behavioral disorders, emotional disorders, and comorbidity were associated with a significant increase in the likelihood of SED; enuresis and tic disorders in the absence of comorbidity were not. Diagnosis and impairment made independent contributions to the increase in service use seen in children with SED. Poverty greatly increased the likelihood of SED.

Conclusions: Specific areas of functional impairment should be examined when SED is assessed and treatment is planned. Plans to target mental health care resources to children with SED need to be accompanied by efforts to ensure access to those resources.

Arch Gen Psychiatry. 1996;53:1137-1143

IN BOTH MANAGED care and traditional service settings, payers have been trying to ensure that services are provided only to children who most need them. Some insurance companies have gone in the direction of reducing the range of *DSM-IV*[1] diagnoses for which treatment is reimbursed. Another direction is that taken by Congress in the 1992 reauthorization bill for the Alcohol, Drug Abuse, and Mental Health Administration, which allocates funds to states for provision of community mental health services to children with "serious emotional disturbance" (SED). Children with SED are defined as persons aged from birth to 18 years, who currently or at any time during the past year have had a diagnosable mental, behavioral, or emotional disorder of sufficient duration to meet the diagnostic criteria specified within *DSM-III-R* (or comparable criteria), that resulted in functional impairment that substantially interferes with or limits the child's role or functioning in family, school, or community activities.[2] This definition of SED excludes children whose disorders result in distress but not impairment, and underlines the need to distinguish between these 2 types of suffering.

Legislation is far ahead of the research literature in concluding that the children most in need of federal funding for mental health services are those with both a diagnosis and functional impairment. In addition, research has not provided estimates of how many children will be identified by means of the new federal criteria for SED. Policy decisions need a consensus on what types of functioning are likely to be impaired in the presence of child psychiatric disorder, and what constitutes impairment that "substantially interferes" with a child's functioning.

See Subjects and Methods on next page

From the Developmental Epidemiology Program, Duke University Medical Center, Durham, NC.

SUBJECTS AND METHODS

MEASUREMENT OF FUNCTIONAL IMPAIRMENT FOR SED

Studying SED requires measures of both child psychiatric disorders and functional impairment. Considerable advances have been made in the first area, in both taxonomy and assessment. At present, however, we lack either an agreed taxonomy of impairment or a choice of measures of the construct. In the past, impairment has been given operational form in 3 general frameworks. (1) *Need for help:* Children can be defined as impaired if they are seen as unable to function adequately without professional help. This definition has resulted in estimates of rates of SED ranging from 2%[3] to 19%,[4] depending on who made the judgment of need: psychiatrist, parent, teacher, or some combination. (2) *Global impairment: DSM-IV* provides a 100-point scale to measure "the clinician's judgment of the individual's overall level of functioning."[1(p30)] A Children's Global Assessment Scale (CGAS)[5] is also available. Taking a score of 60 or less as an index of impairment, rates of SED in 4 recent community studies ranged from 3.2% to 19.6%,[6] suggesting that the CGAS may be influenced by community norms and attitudes to children. (3) *Specific impairment:* The federal definition of functional impairment refers to difficulties that substantially interfere with or limit role functioning in one or more major life activities including basic daily living skills (eg, eating, bathing, dressing); instrumental living skills (eg, maintaining a household, managing money, getting around the community, taking prescribed medication); and functioning in social, family, and vocational/educational contexts.[2] A review of published studies (E.J.C. and D.L.T., unpublished report to the Center for Mental Health Services, Washington, DC, 1994) shows that rates of SED associated with specific areas of functioning vary widely, depending on the area and the diagnosis under study. The Ontario Child Health Study[7,8] is the only study to permit the calculation of rates of SED for specific types of impairment; these are in the range of 1% to 2% for any combination of a single diagnosis and either "problems getting along" or "poor school performance," but it is not possible to calculate a cumulative prevalence rate from this study.

An opportunity to examine the effect of definitions of impairment on rates of SED arises in an ongoing epidemiologic study that used several measures of impairment in conjunction with a highly structured psychiatric assessment.

METHODS

The Great Smoky Mountains Study is a longitudinal study of the development of psychiatric disorder and need for mental health services in rural and urban youth. The details of the study design and instruments used can be found in a separate article.[9] Briefly, a representative sample of 4500 children aged 9, 11, and 13 years old, recruited from 11 counties in western North Carolina, was selected using a household equal probability design. Stratification on risk for mental health service use reduced the sample size to 1015. High risk was defined as a score in the range expected to be in the top quartile of parental responses to the Child Behavior Checklist externalizing scale.[10] A 1 in 10 random sample of children who scored below the cutoff point made up the low-risk group. Weights inversely proportional to the probability of selection were included in the data analyses to obtain population prevalence estimates. The refusal rate was 20%.

Child and parent were interviewed separately by highly trained lay interviewers, using the third edition of the Child and Adolescent Psychiatric Assessment (CAPA),[11] which generates *DSM-III-R* diagnoses and measures of impairment, the Child and Adolescent Services Assessment,[12] and measures of some demographic characteristics, family burden, maternal depression, family psychiatric history, and the child's physical health and development. Families were contacted by telephone every 3 months and reinterviewed annually. The data presented herein are based on the first wave of interviews.

ASSESSMENT OF FUNCTIONAL IMPAIRMENT

Disability or impairment was assessed by means of the CAPA incapacities (impairment) scale and the Child and Adolescent Functional Assessment Scale (CAFAS).[11,13] Both of these can be used to produce both domain-specific scales and a global measure of level of functioning. In addition, the study used the CGAS,[5] described above, which provides a global impairment score. Interviewers scored the CGAS after the psychiatric and CAPA impairment assessments were completed.

Distress and Functional Impairment in the CAPA

In studies that use the CAPA, the concept of "present distress" is built into the process of determining whether individual symptoms are present.[11] Interviewers are trained to determine whether the symptom is present at the level of intensity defined as "clinically significant" in an extensive glossary. For most symptoms of emotional (internalizing) disorders, the phenomena are required to be *unpleasant* to the subject, to be *intrusive* into other activities or thoughts, and to occur during *more than 1 activity*. In

RESULTS

Table 3 shows the rates of SED obtained with each of the 3 measures of impairment. The CAPA and CAFAS identified similar rates of SED, beginning at 6.8% and 7.6%, respectively.

Rates of SED with the CGAS were lower, beginning at 4.2% with a CGAS score of 70 or less and falling to 0.5% with a CGAS score of 50 or less.

The **Figure** shows the extent to which the 3 measures of impairment identified the same children with SED. The Figure applies to SED with a highest level of functioning of 70 on the CGAS, 10 on the CAFAS, or 2

See also page 1129

on the CAPA. Of the 11% of children identified as having SED by 1 or more measure, 53.6% were identified by 2 or 3 measures and 24.5% by all 3. Agreement between measures according to Cohen's κ as the coefficient of addition, the computer scoring algorithms include duration requirements for many emotional symptoms; for example, many are required to last on average for at least 1 hour per day, for a defined period of weeks or months, to count toward the diagnosis.

In the area of disruptive behavior or externalizing disorders, the notion of distress is extended to include probable distress to others caused by the behavior. For example, disobedience is noted as present only when it occurs in relation to more than 1 activity, and if adults cannot always get the child to conform by normal means, such as remonstration. Symptoms that are qualitatively abnormal, such as psychotic hallucinations or euphoric mood states, are carefully defined in the glossary to reduce confusion with normal phenomena, such as hypnopompic hallucinations or happiness after an athletic triumph. Interviewers record detailed descriptions of all such phenomena for review by a clinician. Lay interviewers have been shown to be capable of attaining good levels of test-retest reliability by these methods.[14] The CAPA does not collect information for diagnoses that require a physical or psychological examination as part of the diagnostic process: autism and other pervasive developmental disorders, organic mental disorders, and somatoform disorders.

CAPA Incapacity Ratings

The functional impairment or incapacities section of the CAPA, which follows the symptom review, requires the interviewer to rate the child's ability to function at a developmentally appropriate level in relationships with family, peers, and teachers, and also covers activities at school, home, and in the community, school expulsion or suspension, jobs, and spare time activities. The term *incapacity* is used to avoid confusion with the definitions of "impairments, disabilities, and handicaps" used in the World Health Organization's classification.[15] When incapacity in a particular area is identified, the respondent is asked to attribute it to 1 or more of the symptom areas examined earlier (eg, social withdrawal attributed to depression). **Table 1** contains a list of the areas assessed. A test-retest study of the incapacities section of the child's CAPA showed an intraclass correlation of 0.76.[14]

The CAFAS

This measure, developed for use by child mental health and welfare professionals,[13] rates the child's functioning and need for services in the areas of role performance, thinking, behavior toward self and others, moods and emotions, substance use, and availability of resources from the family or caregiver (**Table 2**). The CAFAS does not collect the information to make the ratings, but provides a format for systematically recording information about the level of functioning. The goal of the CAFAS is to concentrate on impairment associated with a symptom area, rather than the symptoms themselves, but the distinction is sometimes hard to make. As the examples in Table 2 show, 3 of the CAFAS scales overlap to a considerable extent with psychiatric symptoms: moods and emotions (includes irritability, fears and phobias, and depression), thinking (includes hallucinations, disorientation, and obsessions), and substance use. Two scales assess the availability of resources for adequate functioning in the immediate environment—the caregiver and the family—rather than the child's functioning itself. The 2 remaining scales—behavior toward others and self and role performance—focus more clearly on the child's own functioning and meet federal criteria for functioning impairment. It is not always possible to identify exactly the area of poor functioning by means of the CAFAS, as several types of behavior may be included under 1 heading; for example, school problems, running away from home, being on probation, and failure to comply with rules and expectations within the home would all receive a rating of 20 ("major/persistent disruption") on the Role Performance scale. The maximum (worst) score on these 2 scales of the CAFAS is 60. Test-retest data on the CAFAS are currently being collected (K. Hodges, PhD, oral communication, May 31, 1995). The CAFAS was included in the study because it is increasingly being used by social service agencies to evaluate children's service needs, because it is one of the few current instruments to make a serious attempt to do so for children with psychiatric disorders, and because its use could well be recommended or mandated by state or federal agencies for assessing SED.

DATA ANALYSIS

In the analyses presented herein, a symptom or impairment was considered to be present if either parent or child reported it. This approach most closely mirrors clinical practice. In the figure and tables, the numbers of subjects reported are numbers of children in the interviewed sample, while the rates and statistical tests are weighted by the design characteristics. Psychiatric disorder is counted as present if 1 or more *DSM-III-R* diagnoses was made. Data in Table 2 are given for all the CAFAS scales, but only the "role performance" and "behavior to others/self" scales were used in the analyses presented in **Table 3**, **Table 4**, and **Table 5**. Weighted prevalence estimates and statistical tests were calculated by means of the SUDAAN package for OS/2.[16] Rates of SED are based on the presence of both a *DSM-III-R*[17] diagnosis and impairment as defined in the text. To assess the effects of impairment and diagnosis on professional mental health, education, child welfare, juvenile justice, primary medical care, and informal service use, we fit a categorical linear model with generalized logits.

agreement was as follows: CGAS with CAPA, κ=0.45; CGAS with CAFAS, κ=0.64; CAPA with CAFAS, κ=0.68.

Tables 1 and 2 show the rates of SED associated with different types of impairment measured by the CAFAS and CAPA. (Since the CGAS assesses only global impairment, it is not included herein.) With the CAPA, SED was most commonly associated with withdrawn relationships with parents (2.4%) and discordant relationships with teachers (2.3%) and parents (2.2%). Serious emotional disturbance associated with school expulsion or suspension was the other type to be seen in more than 2.0% of children. With the CAFAS, poor relationships and rule infractions were most commonly associated with SED.

RELATIONSHIP BETWEEN TYPE OF DIAGNOSIS AND SED

Table 4 shows rates of SED by type of diagnosis. Logistic regression was used to examine the increase in like-

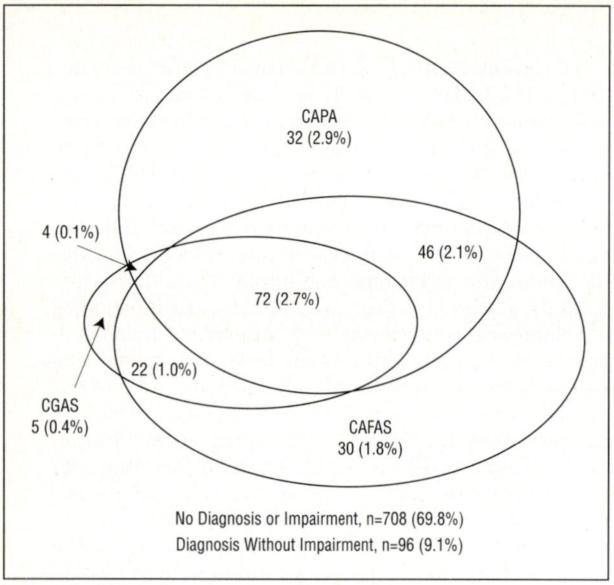

Agreement among rates of serious emotional disturbance by means of 3 measures of impairment. CAPA indicates Child and Adolescent Psychiatric Assessment; CAFAS, Child and Adolescent Functional Assessment Scale; and CGAS, Children's Global Assessment Scale.

Table 1. Prevalence of SED by Areas of Functioning Assessed in the Child and Adolescent Psychiatric Assessment in Children With a Diagnosis*

Area and Type of Functional Impairment	Prevalence of SED, %†		
	Withdrawal	Discord	Other
Parental relationship‡	2.35	2.21	. . .
Relationships with siblings			
In home	1.06	1.26	. . .
Out of home	0.17	0.04	. . .
Self-care	. . .	. . .	0.20
Chores	. . .	. . .	0.74
Homework	. . .	. . .	1.46
Leaving the house	. . .	. . .	0.54
School performance	. . .	. . .	1.27
School suspension or expulsion	. . .	. . .	2.04
Relationships with teachers	1.29	2.27	. . .
Peer relationships at school	0.82	0.81	. . .
Spare-time activities	. . .	. . .	0.54
Relations with adults	1.05	0.47	. . .
Relations with peers	0.03	0.14	. . .
Employment	0.47	1.08	. . .
Any incapacity	. . .	. . .	6.8

*SED indicates serious emotional disturbance.
†An SED associated with each type of impairment.
‡Assessed for biological parents, and other parental figures if the child lives with them.

Table 2. Prevalence of SED by Areas of Functioning Assessed Using the Child and Adolescent Functional Assessment Scale in Children With a Diagnosis*

Area and Type of Functional Impairment	Prevalence of SED, %†
Role performance‡ (eg, disobedient at home, expelled, incarcerated)	5.6
Thinking (eg, thought distortions, hallucinations, persistent bizarre or destructive fantasies)	1.5
Behavior toward others and/or staff‡ (eg, promiscuity, fighting, inability to sustain close relationships)	6.0
Mood and/or emotions (eg, marked mood changes, school nonattendance because of fears and phobias, incapacitating depression)	5.3
Substance use	0.4
Caregiver resources: basic needs (eg, risk to health or safety of child because of inability to meet basic needs)	1.4
Caregiver resources: family and/or social support (eg, family setting potentially dangerous to child, hostile, rejecting, or abusive)	2.4
Any impairment	10.7
Any impairment on Role Performance and Behavior Scale	7.6

*SED indicates serious emotional disorder.
†An SED associated with each type of impairment.
‡Scales included in analyses in text.

Table 3. Rates of SED Using Different Measures and Levels of Impairment*

CGAS		CAFAS		CAPA	
Score	No. (%)	Score	No. (%)	Score	No. (%)
70	103 (4.2)	10	170 (7.6)	2	139 (6.8)
60	45 (1.8)	20	97 (3.8)	4	89 (4.1)
50	15 (0.5)	30	35 (1.2)	6	50 (2.0)
40	7 (0.2)	40	12 (0.4)	8	36 (1.5)
30	5 (0.2)	50	2 (0.1)	10	20 (1.0)
20	5 (0.2)	60	0 (0.0)	12	12 (0.7)

Level refers to the number and weighted proportion (percent) of the sample with a DSM-III-R diagnosis and this score or worse on the measure of impairment. SED indicates serious emotional disturbance; CGAS, Children's Global Assessment Scale; CAFAS, Child and Adolescent Functional Assessment Scale; and CAPA, Child and Adolescent Psychiatric Assessment.

lihood of a given diagnosis, controlling for the presence of other disorders. Only diagnoses present in at least 1% of children are reported: depression, anxiety, conduct, oppositional, attention-deficit hyperactivity and tic disorders, and enuresis. Of course, rates of SED depend in part on the prevalence of the disorder, but the odds ratios presented show that, irrespective of rates of diagnosis, a much higher proportion of children with behavioral disorders and depression were judged to be impaired than were children with tics or enuresis. The association between anxiety disorders and impairment was also statistically significant, but smaller. In the light of the recent debate about attention-deficit hyperactivity disorder and eligibility for Supplemental Security Income, it is worth noting that 73% of children with attention-deficit hyperactivity disorder were impaired. The presence of SED was also much more likely if children had diagnoses in more than 1 area. A comparison of the 3 measures of impairment showed that there was a significant ($P<.001$) association between each type of diagnosis and each of the 3 measures of impairment, with 1 exception: the association between the CGAS and enuresis and tic disorders was not significant.

Table 4. Rates of SED Associated With Different Diagnostic Groups*

Diagnostic Group	Prevalence of SED, %	Prevalence of Diagnosis Without Impairment, %	Subjects With Diagnosis Who Have SED, %	Odds Ratio (95% CI)	χ^2 Test of Association (*P*)
Any diagnosis	11.1	9.1	54.9	4.1 (3.0-5.6)	81.1 (<.001)
ADHD	1.41	0.52	73.1	9.4 (4.0-21.7)	27.3 (<.001)
Oppositional defiant disorder	2.51	0.24	91.3	36.4 (15.7-84.2)	70.5 (<.001)
Conduct disorder	2.86	0.77	78.8	13.6 (7.2-25.7)	64.5 (<.001)
Anxiety disorder	2.61	3.09	45.8	2.8 (1.7-4.7)	15.6 (<.001)
Depressive disorder	1.11	0.40	73.4	9.0 (3.5-23.2)	20.9 (<.001)
Enuresis or encopresis	3.87	1.87	32.6	1.5 (0.9-2.7)	2.3 (1.25)
Tic disorder	1.29	2.91	32.6	1.4 (0.7-2.7)	1.0 (.31)
More than 1 diagnostic group	2.29	0.86	72.6	9.0 (4.6-17.6)	42.2 (<.001)

**SED indicates serious emotional disturbance; CI, confidence intervals; and ADHD, attention-deficit hyperactivity disorder. SED is determined by a* DSM-III-R *diagnosis and impairment using 1 or more of 3 criteria: Children's Global Assessment Scale score of no more than 70; Child and Adolescent Functional Assessment Scale score of at least 10; and Child and Adolescent Psychiatric Assessment impairment score of at least 2. Estimates are weighted.*

SED AND NEED FOR MENTAL HEALTH SERVICES

Table 5 shows the association between SED and various definitions of need for mental health services: need for help with emotional or behavioral problems, as reported by the child or parent, and need reflected in mental health care recently received in 1 of 5 settings. Each of the service settings was regressed on diagnosis and impairment by means of an interactive model (impairment, diagnosis, and impairment × diagnosis). In no case was the interaction term significant, supporting an additive model to predict service use.

Since the service setting variables are multiple observations from the same subject, we also used a polytomous regression model to take the correlation among the service settings into account, and to guard against inflated *P* values. As in the logistic fits described in Table 5, we first considered a saturated model including the interaction term impairment × diagnosis. As there was no interaction effect, we dropped this term and fit a main-effect additive model. We found that there was a small effect (χ^2=38.14, *P*=.08) of impairment, while there was a strong effect of diagnosis (χ^2=62.0, *P*<.001). Since the residual χ^2 was also small (16.48, *P*=.94), the polytomous additive model fit the data well.

Perhaps more striking than the fact that children with SED were more likely to receive some services is that 3 (60%) of 5 children with SED in this sample reported no recent mental health care from any professional in any setting, and 4 (80%) of 5 reported no recent care in a professional mental health setting. A comparison of the CAFAS, CAPA, and CGAS for assessing impairment (details may be obtained from the first author) found that all 3 predicted self- or parent-reported need for help. The CAPA definition of SED was associated with high rates of professional mental health service use and of involvement with child welfare. Associations between the other 2 definitions of SED and the specific types of service use did not reach statistical significance.

SOCIODEMOGRAPHIC CORRELATES OF SED

In a logistic regression that included sex, race, age, urban or rural residence, family income, and history of repeated school grades, children living in poverty (herein defined as below the federal poverty line) were at significantly greater risk of having SED (odds ratio, 2.4; 95% confidence interval, 1.4-3.0). We examined the correlates of SED associated with specific disorder in a polytomous logistic regression. Poverty increased the likelihood of SED in children with behavioral disorders, tics, and enuresis, controlling for comorbidity. The same pattern of association was observed between poverty and SED by means of the CAPA and the CAFAS, but not the CGAS.

COMMENT

The relationship between functional impairment and child psychiatric disorder has implications for clinical services, epidemiology, and public policy.

CLINICAL ISSUES

Careful ascertainment of which areas of performance show impairment is clearly important for treatment planning. There is a lack of research data on the implications for choice of treatment of different patterns of distress and impairment associated with various diagnoses. Treatment specificity could be improved by careful evaluation of changes in both symptomatic distress and functional impairment over time, with and without treatment.

EPIDEMIOLOGICAL ISSUES

Epidemiologists and clinicians have devoted immense effort to improving the quality and consistency of assessment procedures for child psychopathology. Paradoxically, it is partly this improvement that has brought into the spotlight the need for standardized measures of impairment. The *Diagnostic and Statistical Manual* is primarily a clinical document, written for

Table 5. Likelihood of Reporting Need for Help and Service Use Given Diagnosis and/or Impairment

	Diagnosis		Impairment		
Need or Service (Prevalence, %)	**Odds Ratio**	**95% Confidence Interval (*P*)**	**Odds Ratio**	**95% Confidence Interval (*P*)**	**Model χ^2 (*df*=2) (*P*)**
"Needs help" (10.7)	3.7	2.3-5.7 (<.001)	7.5	4.7-12.0 (<.001)	148.3 (<.001)
Service setting					
Professional mental health (4.0)	2.9	1.5-5.7 (.002)	5.3	2.6-10.9 (<.001)	45.2 (<.001)
Education (13.1)	2.4	1.6-3.7 (<.001)	2.1	1.4-3.1 (<.001)	42.0 (<.001)
Child welfare (0.8)	5.0	1.0-25.7 (.05)	16.5	1.4-192.4 (.03)	18.7 (<.001)
Juvenile justice (0.7)	1.0	0.2-4.8 (.94)	16.6	1.9-141.3 (.01)	10.6 (.005)
Primary medical care (1.9)	3.3	1.3-8.5 (.02)	1.6	0.6-4.2 (.34)	8.7 (.01)
Any professional service (16.0)	2.5	1.7-3.6 (<.001)	2.7	1.9-3.9 (<.001)	66.6 (<.001)
Informal (4.7)	2.1	1.1-4.0 (.02)	1.8	1.0-3.4 (.06)	11.9 (.003)

use in settings where individuals present themselves for treatment, ie, there is the a priori assumption of distress and possibly of reduced functioning as an aspect of the presenting symptoms; it was not necessary to write this explicitly into the criteria for each disorder. Assessment instruments designed around the *DSM* have sometimes ignored this, omitting any specific attempts to assess either distress or impairment. In clinical settings this may not be a problem. In general population studies, however, it has become increasingly clear in the past 15 years that if the *DSM* criteria are applied strictly, but without taking distress and impairment into account, rates of disorder can be much higher than is consistent with clinical experience or common sense.[6] Measures of functional impairment have been used as a way of reducing the prevalence estimates to a more manageable level.[18,19] An unsolved problem is how to assess children whose functioning would be impaired if they were not currently in treatment.[2] In practice, rates of treatment are low in the general population[7,19,20] and unlikely to make much difference to global estimates of SED. However, this could be a problem for studies that use clinical samples.

IMPLICATIONS FOR PUBLIC POLICY

The taxonomy of functional impairment has not yet reached the level of sophistication of the taxonomy of psychiatric disorder (E.J.C., D.L.T., and K. Hodges, unpublished reports to the Center for Mental Health Services, 1994). Meanwhile, several federal and state agencies are currently required by law to examine children for both psychiatric disorder and functional impairment, incapacity, or disability, and the result of these evaluations can make a dramatic difference to the resources made available, or denied, to a family for the care of a child. Thus, there is a pressing need for better data on how accurately functional impairment is currently being assessed, and almost certainly a need for better standardized instruments for measuring it more accurately (E.J.C., et al, unpublished report to the Center for Mental Health Services, 1995).

The data presented herein suggest that it is possible to make a fairly detailed assessment of functional impairment even in real-world, nonresearch settings. The Great Smoky Mountains Study was implemented by trained lay interviewers who visited subjects in their homes and used a highly structured protocol. The parts of the interview with a bearing on the diagnosis of SED—psychiatric assessment and evaluation of functioning at home, at school, and in the community—took 1 to 2 hours with parent and child, depending on the number of symptoms and the garrulousness of the informant. This is in the range of time usually allotted for intake assessments in mental health settings and suggests that professionals charged with examining children for SED—social workers, disability examiners, etc—could use standardized assessment methods and instruments routinely if these were available and training programs were developed. A great deal more work is needed, however, to refine the definition and measurement of functioning.

CONCLUSIONS

Our study adds to growing evidence that, as directed by *DSM-III-R*[17] and *DSM-IV*,[1] functioning as well as distress needs to be considered in making a diagnosis and treatment plan. Symptoms and impairment contributed independently to the prediction of need for and use of mental health services. Requiring both a diagnosis and significant impairment for eligibility for treatment or financial aid will undoubtedly reduce the numbers eligible and identify a group of children who are clearly at high need of care. However, only about 1 child in 4 or 5 with SED has recently received any mental health care, so efforts to focus services on the most needy should go hand in hand with efforts to ensure that access to these services is improved.

Accepted for publication February 5, 1996.

This project was supported by grant MH48085 from the National Institute of Mental Health, Bethesda, Md. Additional support was provided through Faculty Scholar awards from the William T. Grant Foundation (Drs Costello and Angold) and a Center grant from the Leon Lowenstein Foundation, New York, NY (Dr Angold).

The field work for this study was supervised by Teresa Sweeney. Ralph Folsom, PhD, of Research Triangle Institute, Research Triangle Park, NC, assisted with the multistage sampling design. We wish to acknowledge with gratitude the help of Superintendents of Schools in the 11-

county area of the study, Jonathan L. Taylor, the Principal Chief of the Eastern Band of the Cherokee Nation, James L. Sanders, MSW, the Director of Social Services on the Qualla Boundary, and Joyce Dugan, the Director of Education there. The cooperation of the entire community of western North Carolina is warmly appreciated.

Reprints: E. Jane Costello, PhD, Developmental Epidemiology Program, Duke University Medical Center, PO Box 3454, Durham, NC 27710.

REFERENCES

1. American Psychiatric Association Committee on Nomenclature and Statistics. *Diagnostic and Statistical Manual of Mental Disorders, Fourth Edition.* Washington, DC: American Psychiatric Association; 1994.
2. Substance Abuse and Mental Health Services Administration (notices). *Federal Register.* May 20, 1993;58:29425.
3. Rutter M, Graham P. Psychiatric disorder in 10- and 11-year-old children. *Proc R Soc Med.* 1966;59:382-387.
4. Zahner GEP, Pawelkiewicz W, DeFrancesco JJ, Adnopoz J. Children's mental health service needs and utilization patterns in an urban community: an epidemiologic assessment. *J Am Acad Child Adolesc Psychiatry.* 1992;31:951-960.
5. Shaffer D, Gould MS, Brasic J, Ambrosini PJ, Fisher PW, Bird HR, Aluwahlia S. A Children's Global Assessment Scale (CGAS). *Arch Gen Psychiatry.* 1983; 40:1228-1231.
6. Shaffer D, Fisher PW, Dulcan M, Davies M, Piacentini J, Schwab-Stone M, Lahey BB, Bourdon K, Jensen P, Bird H, Canino G, Regier D. The NIMH Diagnostic Interview Schedule for Children (DISC 2.3): description, acceptability, prevalences, and performance in the MECA Study. *J Am Acad Child Adolesc Psychiatry.* 1996;35:865-877.
7. Offord DR, Boyle MH, Szatmari P, Rae-Grant NI, Links PS, Cadman DT, Byles JA, Crawford JW, Munroe-Blum H, Byrne C, Thomas H, Woodward CA. Ontario Child Health Study, II: six-month prevalence of disorder and rates of service utilization. *Arch Gen Psychiatry.* 1987;44:832-836.
8. Sanford MN, Offord DR, Boyle MH, Peace A, Racine YA. Ontario Child Health Study: social and school impairments in children aged 6 to 16 years. *J Am Acad Child Adolesc Psychiatry.* 1992;31:60-67.
9. Costello EJ, Angold A, Burns BJ, Stangl DK, Tweed DL, Erkanli A, Worthman CM. The Great Smoky Mountains Study of Youth: goals, design, methods, and the prevalence of *DSM-III-R* disorders. *Arch Gen Psychiatry.* 1996;53:1129-1136.
10. Achenbach TM, Edelbrock C. *Manual for the Child Behavior Checklist and Child Behavior Profile.* Burlington, Vt: University of Vermont; 1983.
11. Angold A, Prendergast M, Cox A, Harrington R, Simonoff E, Rutter M. The Child and Adolescent Psychiatric Assessment (CAPA). *Psychol Med.* 1995;25: 739-753.
12. Farmer EMZ, Angold A, Burns BJ, Costello EJ. Reliability of self-reported service use: test-retest consistency of children's responses to the Child and Adolescent Services Assessment (CASA). *J Child Fam Stud.* 1994;3:307-325.
13. Hodges K, Bickman L, Ring-Kurtz S, Rieter M. Multidimensional measure of level of functioning for children and adolescents. In: Algarian A, Friedman R, eds. *A System of Care for Children's Mental Health: Expanding the Research Base.* Tampa, Fla: Research Training Center for Children's Mental Health; 1991: 149-154.
14. Angold A, Costello EJ. A test-retest reliability study of child-reported psychiatric symptoms and diagnoses using the Child and Adolescent Psychiatric Assessment (CAPA-C). *Psychol Med.* 1995;25:755-762.
15. World Health Organization. *International Classification of Impairments, Disabilities, and Handicaps: A Manual of Classification Relating to the Consequences of Disease.* Geneva, Switzerland: World Health Organization; 1980.
16. Shah BV, Folsom RE, LaVange LM, Wheeless SC, Boyle KE, Williams RL. *SUDAAN Software for the Statistical Analysis of Correlated Data: Statistical Methods and Mathematical Algorithms Used in SUDAAN.* Research Triangle Park, NC: Research Triangle Institute; 1995.
17. American Psychiatric Association Committee on Nomenclature and Statistics. *Diagnostic and Statistical Manual of Mental Disorders, Revised Third Edition.* Washington, DC: American Psychiatric Association; 1987.
18. Bird HR, Canino G, Rubio-Stipec M, Gould MS, Ribera J, Sesman M, Woodbury M, Huertas-Goldman S, Pagan A, Sanchez-Lacay A, Moscoso M. Estimates of the prevalence of childhood maladjustment in a community survey in Puerto Rico: the use of combined measures. *Arch Gen Psychiatry.* 1988;45: 1120-1126.
19. Costello EJ, Costello AJ, Edelbrock C, Burns BJ, Dulcan MK, Brent D, Janiszewski S. Psychiatric disorders in pediatric primary care: prevalence and risk factors. *Arch Gen Psychiatry.* 1988;45:1107-1116.
20. Bird HR, Yager TJ, Staghezza B, Gould MS, Canino G, Rubio-Stipec M. Impairment in the epidemiological measurement of childhood psychopathology in the community. *J Am Acad Child Adolesc Psychiatry.* 1990;29:796-803.

Suicidal Behavior Runs in Families

A Controlled Family Study of Adolescent Suicide Victims

David A. Brent, MD; Jeff Bridge; Barbara A. Johnson, MD; John Connolly, MA

Background: While previous studies have shown an increased rate of suicidal behavior in the relatives of suicide victims, it is unclear if this is attributable merely to increased familial rates of psychiatric disorders. Therefore, we conducted a family study of adolescent suicide victims (suicide probands) and community control probands (controls) to determine if the rates of suicidal behavior were higher in the relatives of adolescent suicide probands even after adjusting for differences in the familial rates of psychiatric disorders.

Method: The relatives of 58 adolescent suicide probands and 55 demographically similar controls underwent assessment for Axis I and II psychiatric disorders, lifetime history of aggression, and history of suicidal behavior (attempts and completions) using a combination of family study and family history approaches.

Results: The rate of suicide attempts was increased in the first-degree relatives of suicide probands compared with the relatives of controls, even after adjusting for differences in rates of proband and familial Axis I and II disorders (odds ratio, 4.3; 95% confidence intervals, 1.1-16.6). On the other hand, the excess rate of suicidal ideation found in the relatives of suicide probands was explained by increased familial rates of psychiatric disorders. Among suicide probands, higher ratings of aggression were associated with higher familial loading for suicide attempts.

Conclusions: Liability to suicidal behavior might be familially transmitted as a trait independent of Axis I and II disorders. The transmitted spectrum of suicidal behavior includes attempts and completions, but not ideation, and the transmission of suicidal behavior and aggression are related.

Arch Gen Psychiatry. 1996;53:1145-1152

THE AGGREGATION of suicide and suicide attempts in the families of suicide victims is well known and has been demonstrated in the relatives of both adolescent[1,2] and adult suicides.[3-5] Adoption and twin studies have also demonstrated a concordance between biological relatives for suicide.[6,7]

The familial clustering of suicidal behavior also extends to the relatives of prepubertal children,[8] adolescents,[9] and adults[10,11] who attempt suicide. Furthermore, those who make the most lethal attempts are most likely to have a positive family history of suicide,[9,10] suggesting a shared familial liability for suicide attempts and completions.

Family history of substance abuse, depression, antisocial and other personality disorders, and assaultive behavior have also been linked to suicidal behavior.[8,12-14] Two reports support the view that the familial transmission of suicide is independent of the transmission of either affective illness[5] or endogenous psychosis.[4,5] However, no published study has examined the familial aggregation of suicidal behavior while controlling for all of these psychopathological conditions. Therefore, we undertook a family study of adolescent suicide victims (suicide probands) and demographically similar community control probands (controls) to test the following hypotheses: (1) The relatives of suicide probands, compared with the relatives of community controls, will show a greater prevalence of suicide and suicidal attempts, even after controlling for an expected increased rate of Axis I disorders. (2) The familial aggregation of suicidal behavior in the relatives of suicide probands will be explained by the familial aggregation of impulsive-aggressive

See Subjects and Methods on next page

From the Western Psychiatric Institute and Clinic, Pittsburgh, Pa.

SUBJECTS AND METHODS

SAMPLE

The sample consists of the first- (mothers, fathers, and siblings) and second-degree relatives (grandparents, uncles, aunts, and half siblings) of adolescent suicide probands and demographically matched adolescent community controls.

Suicide Victims

Fifty-eight adolescent (13-20 years of age) suicide probands were a consecutive series who died within a 28-county region of western Pennsylvania and were assigned a definite verdict of suicide. They represent 78% of all those available during the recruitment period, from July 1989 through May 1994. The suicide probands whose families accepted participation in the study did not differ from refusers with respect to age, gender, race, county of origin, or method of suicide.

Controls

Fifty-eight controls were recruited from an original pool of 173 adolescents obtained by geographic cluster sampling that matched control communities to those of suicide probands with respect to age, gender, median income, population density, and racial composition. Almost all controls (59 of 60, 98%) consented to the interview and of these 93% (55 of 59) of all available controls agreed to participate in the family study. Subsequently, it was found that 3 controls had made serious suicide attempts, and we eliminated these subjects from the control cell, leaving 55 controls. No differences were found between accepters and refusers with respect to age, race, gender, county of origin, family constellation, and socioeconomic status.[15]

Relation of Sample to Other Reports

Forty-three suicide probands and 40 controls have been described previously, but no data on relatives were reported.[16] Family history data have previously been reported on 16 suicide probands and 34 controls, but no family study data have been reported on this sample.[13]

Comparison of Suicide Probands and Controls

As shown in **Table 1**, the 2 groups were similar with respect to age, gender, race, socioeconomic status, and county of origin, but fewer suicide probands than controls lived with both biological parents (*P*=.002). As has been previously reported,[1,2,17] suicide probands showed higher rates than did controls on a broad range of psychiatric disorders (**Table 2**).

Relatives

Our sample consists of the first- and second-degree relatives of the suicide probands and controls: 203 first- and 607 second-degree relatives of 58 suicide probands and 207 first- and 558 second-degree relatives of 55 controls. As shown in **Table 3**, there were no differences between the groups in mean pedigree size, number of direct interviews per family, gender or age distribution of the relatives, or proportion with missing data, with 2 exceptions—the proportion of missing data from the first-degree relatives of suicide probands was greater than that from the relatives of controls (5.0% vs 0.5% [*P*=.005]) and the second-degree relatives of controls were slightly older (*P*=.02).

RECRUITMENT AND INTERVIEW PROCEDURE

Assessment of Suicide Probands and Controls

Approximately 1 to 2 months after the suicide, the families of suicide probands were sent a letter expressing our condolences and inviting family members to participate in the study. This letter was followed up 1 week later by a telephone call from the project clinician responsible for the interview. Families who did not have a telephone were sent an additional postcard to be returned to the clinician that indicated their willingness to participate and how they were to be contacted. On average, the interview took place 5.3 months after the suicide (range, 1.8-15.0 months). For each of the suicide probands, the primary caretaking parent (or parental figure, eg, grandparent or older sibling) served as the main informant. In addition, siblings, friends, other relatives, and professional contacts were interviewed, with a median of 5 informants per subject (range, 1-9). Previous work has indicated that the diagnoses obtained by the psychological autopsy procedure are reliable, valid, and unaffected by state of bereavement of the informant.[18,19] Psychiatric and demographic data were obtained on the controls from the caregiving parent and by self-report.

Interview Procedure With Relatives

On agreeing to participate in the family study, the caregiving parent provided the names, telephone numbers, and addresses of all first- and second-degree relatives and gave permission for an interviewer to contact them.

Diagnostic Procedure

All interviewers were master's level clinicians who had been given extensive training in the administration of semistructured interviews. Best-estimate diagnoses were made by consensus and used all available sources in diagnostic conferences chaired by 2 of us (D.A.B. and B.A.J.).[20] Discrepancies between informants were resolved by reinterview of all informants until consensus could be obtained. Diagnostic assessment and best-estimate conferences were conducted without knowledge of the subject's diagnostic status. Interrater reliability for direct and family history interviews for Axis I and II were high throughout the study (κ values, 0.79-0.95).

Informed consent for all interviews was obtained as approved by the Psychosocial Institutional Review Board of the University of Pittsburgh, Pittsburgh, Pa.

ASSESSMENT

Axis I Psychiatric Disorders

The Schedule for Affective Disorders and Schizophrenia for School-Age Children, Epidemiologic and Present Episode versions (K-SADS)[21,22] were used to assess lifetime and current symptoms and corresponding *DSM-III* diagnoses[23] for all suicide probands, controls, and directly interviewed relatives younger than 18 years. All directly interviewed adult first- and second-degree relatives underwent assessment for the presence of past and current psychiatric disorders by use of the Schedule for Affective Disorders and Schizophrenia, Lifetime Version (SADS-L).[24] The Family History Research Diagnostic Criteria (FH-RDC) method[25] was used to obtain information from those relatives directly interviewed regarding all other first- and second-degree relatives, with diagnostic criteria modified from research diagnostic criteria to *DSM-III* criteria. Because it is known that loss of a family member can increase the risk for subsequent depression,[26,27] we only report disorders in relatives of suicide probands that had a clear onset prior to the suicide.

Axis II Psychiatric Disorders

The Structured Clinical Interview for the *DSM-III-R* Diagnosis of Personality Disorders (SCID-II-R)[28] was used to assess *DSM-III-R*[29] personality disorders in all suicide probands, controls, and directly interviewed relatives older than 13 years. A subset of questions on the interview was modified to make them more appropriate for adolescents. Reliability and validity for this interview have been established previously for adults[29] and for adolescents.[16,30] Based on previous analyses, personality disorder assessment in relatives was restricted to avoidant, antisocial, and borderline personality disorders.[16,31] In addition, questions from the informant version of the SCID-II-R about these personality disorders were added to the FH-RDC interview, allowing us to obtain information about personality disorders on all relatives in the pedigree.

Suicidal Intent

The Beck Suicidal Intent Scale was used to assess suicidal intent among the suicide victims.[32,33] We report on only the first 9 items, relevant to observable behavior, which were administered to the informant(s) for the suicide probands.

Definition of Suicidal Behavior

A suicide attempt was defined as intentional self-harm that is not self-mutilatory in nature. On both the K-SADS and SADS-L, this corresponds to a rating of at least 2 on the medical lethality question of the Suicide Attempt section. Data were also gathered on history of suicidal ideation, which for the purposes of this study refers to suicidal thoughts or threats. All relatives were classified on the basis of their most serious suicidal episode.

Measures of Aggression

The Brown-Goodwin Assessment for Lifetime History of Aggression (BG-LHA), a 12-item interview, was administered to suicide proband and control informants and directly interviewed relatives older than 13 years.[34,35] Internal consistency of the BG-LHA was acceptable (Cronbach α, 0.78). The Assault and Irritability subscales of the Buss-Durkee Hostility Inventory,[36] a self-reported measure of aggressive personality traits, was filled out by the same informants as received the BG-LHA. Internal consistency was adequate for both the Assault and Irritability subscales (Cronbach α, 0.66 and 0.69, respectively). These measures are associated with suicidal behavior and changes in central serotonergic metabolism.[34,35,37] These self-reported questionnaires (filled out by parents) were missing for more suicide probands than controls (33% vs 9% [χ^2=9.45, P=.002]), and for more first-degree relatives of suicide probands than for the relatives of controls (25% vs 9% [χ^2=12.08, P<.001]). We were concerned that these data might not be missing at random. Therefore, we modeled substitution of extreme scores (75th percentile or more) for all missing data with no substantial change in the results. Therefore, data are reported without the substitution.

History of Assaultive Behavior

History of assaultive behavior for suicide probands, controls, and directly interviewed pedigree members was obtained through the assessment of behavioral indicators taken from all available sources (BG-LHA, K-SADS, SADS-L, SCID-II-R, and FH-RDC). For all other relatives, history of assaultive behavior was obtained from the FH-RDC.

DATA ANALYSES

All dependent measures were compared between the relatives of suicide probands and those of the community controls using standard univariate parametric and nonparametric methods. For dichotomous outcomes, the Pearson χ^2 test was used. When any one cell had an expected value of less than 5 or when there was a 0 cell, the Fisher exact test was used. For continuous outcomes, either a 2-sample *t* test or, when the distribution was skewed, the nonparametric equivalent, the Mann-Whitney *U* test, was used.

The rate of suicide attempts and completions for first- and second-degree relatives was compared between groups using either the Pearson χ^2 or Fisher exact test. The age-corrected lifetime rates of attempts and completions between the 2 groups of relatives were compared using Kaplan-Meier analyses.[38] The results using both χ^2 and Kaplan-Meier analyses were similar, so that only the former are reported, although both approaches are displayed in **Table 4**. To determine whether rates of attempts and completions differed between relatives after adjustment on other psychopathological variables (eg, rates of Axis I disorder, assaultive behavior), logistic regression was used. Adjusted hazard ratios were derived from Cox proportional hazards regression models, using the same analytic scheme as was used for the logistic regression analyses.[39]

The familial rate of a disorder was determined by taking the ratio of the number of affected relatives over the total number of relatives (ie, "pooled" data). In addition, we conducted analyses using the family as the unit of analysis, wherein if at least 1 first-degree relative had attempted suicide, that family was considered positive for suicide attempt. Comparisons between groups using the family as the unit of analysis yielded essentially the same results as the pooled data strategy. Therefore, we report only the pooled approach to assessing familial rates. Analyses were computed using the 1990 version of the BMDP software.[40]

Table 1. Demographic Characteristics of Suicide Probands and Community Controls*

Characteristic	Suicide Probands (n=58)	Community Controls (n=55)
Age mean±95% CL, y	17.2±0.5	17.4±0.5
Gender, M:F	51:7	48:7
Race, white:African American	57:1	55:0
Socioeconomic status, %±95% CL†		
I	8.6±7.2	1.8±3.5
II	24.1±11.0	20.0±10.6
III	20.7±10.4	30.9±12.2
IV	32.8±12.1	38.2±12.8
V	13.8±8.9	9.1±7.6
From Allegheny County, %±95% CL	41.4±12.7	38.2±12.8
Lives with both biological parents, %±95% CL	32.8±12.1	65.5±12.6‡

*CL indicates confidence limit.
†Defined in Hollingshead.[15]
‡P<.005.

Table 2. Diagnostic and Clinical Characteristics of Adolescent Suicide Probands and Community Controls*

Diagnosis	Suicide Probands (n=58)	Controls (n=55)
Axis I disorder	77.6±10.7	18.5±10.4†‡
Any affective disorder	36.2±10.0	0.0±0.0†‡
Major depressive disorder	29.3±11.7	0.0±0.0†‡
Dysthymia	12.1±8.4	0.0±0.0§
Substance abuse	36.8±12.5	5.6±6.1†‡
Alcohol	32.8±12.1	5.6±6.1†‖
Other drug	14.3±9.2	0.0±0.0‖
Conduct disorder	38.6±12.6	5.5±6.0†‡
Any anxiety disorder	17.2±9.7	1.9±3.6¶
Any personality disorder	19.0±10.1	0.0±0.0†‖
Cluster A#	1.7±3.3	0.0±0.0
Cluster B**	8.6±7.2	0.0±0.0
Cluster C††	10.5±8.0	0.0±0.0§
Assaultive behavior	28.1±11.7	10.9±8.2§
Brown-Goodwin Lifetime History of Aggression, mean±95% CL	13.2±2.7	4.9±1.6†‡
Buss-Durkee Hostility Inventory, Assault Subscale, mean±95% CL	15.9±0.9	14.5±0.7§
Buss-Durkee Hostility Inventory, Irritability Subscale, mean±95% CL	16.6±0.9	14.4±0.8†‖

*Unless otherwise indicated, data are given as %±95% confidence limit (CL).
†Significant at the alpha <.05 level with Bonferroni correction.
‡P≤.001.
§P<.05.
‖P<.005.
¶P<.01.
#Includes paranoid, schizoid, and schizotypal.
**Includes antisocial, borderline, histrionic, and narcissistic.
††Includes avoidant, passive-aggressive, obsessive-compulsive, and dependent.

(cluster B) personality disorders and tendency to aggressive behavior. (3) The prevalence of suicide and suicidal behavior will be higher among the relatives of suicide probands with high-intent completions, violent completions (ie, firearms, hanging, or jumping), and high levels of aggression.

RESULTS

SUICIDAL BEHAVIOR

The rate of suicide attempts or completions (almost all were attempts [Table 4]) was significantly higher in the first-degree relatives of suicide probands than in the first-degree relatives of controls (11.6% vs 2.4%, χ^2=13.1, *P*<.001; odds ratio [OR], 5.3; 95% confidence interval [CI], 2.0-14.3]). The familial rates of attempts or completions were significantly elevated in mothers (18.2% vs 3.6% [χ^2=5.99, *P*=.01]) and siblings (11.0% vs 2.1% [χ^2=6.12, *P*=.01]), with a nonsignificant trend in the same direction for fathers (5.7% vs 1.8% [χ^2=1.12, *P*=.29]). The rate of suicidal ideation was also higher in relatives of completers than controls (14.7% vs 8.2% [χ^2=4.20, *P*=.04]).

Second-degree relatives of suicide probands were also found to have higher rates of suicide attempts and completions than second-degree relatives of controls (4.9% vs 1.4% [χ^2=10.81; *P*=.001; OR, 3.7; 95% CI, 1.6-8.7]). The rate of suicidal ideation was higher in relatives of suicide probands than those of controls (7.6% vs 4.5% [χ^2=4.63, *P*=.03]).

AXIS I AND II DISORDERS IN RELATIVES

First-degree relatives of suicide probands and controls reported similar rates of most Axis I and II disorders but significant differences between these groups were found for any Axis I disorder (*P*=.03), affective disorder (*P*=.045), dysthymia (*P*=.03), conduct disorder (*P*=.004), and antisocial personality disorder (*P*=.006), largely in keeping with our original hypotheses. Directly interviewed relatives of suicide probands and controls did not differ on any of the 3 measures of impulsive aggression (the BG-LHA or the 2 Buss-Durkee Hostility Inventory subscales), although relatives of suicide probands showed significantly higher lifetime rates of assaultive behavior (*P*=.02).

Among second-degree relatives, higher rates of disorder were also found in families of suicide probands vs controls, with increases in any affective disorder (*P*<.001); substance abuse disorder (*P*=.05); conduct disorder (*P*=.001); anxiety disorder (*P*<.001); antisocial (*P*=.005), avoidant (*P*=.006), and borderline personality disorders (*P*=.03-.005); and assaultive behavior (*P*<.001).

RISK FOR SUICIDAL BEHAVIOR ADJUSTING FOR OTHER PSYCHIATRIC CONDITIONS

First-degree Relatives

A greater risk for attempts and completions persisted in the relatives of suicide probands even after controlling for differences between the relatives with respect to lifetime Axis I psychopathological conditions (ie, affective and conduct disorder [OR, 5.2; 95% CI, 1.7-15.8]). The increased odds of suicidal behavior in the relatives of suicide vs control probands persisted after controlling for differences in rates of Axis I disorders (ie, affective and

Table 3. Demographic Characteristics of Relatives of Suicide Probands and Community Controls*

Characteristic	Suicide Probands (n=58)	Controls (n=55)
Pedigree size, mean± 95% CL, No. of members	14.1±1.2	13.9±1.1
Direct interviews per family, mean±95% CL	5.0±0.8	4.3±0.5
Direct interview, %±95% CL		
Father	53.4±12.8	58.2±13.0
Mother	81.0±10.1	92.7±6.9
Sibling	72.4±9.4	72.2±8.9
First-degree relatives		
No. of relatives	203	207
Gender, M/F	98:105	100:107
Age (mean±95% CL), y	31.8±2.2	31.9±2.1
Father	44.0±2.2	45.9±1.9
Mother	42.1±1.7	43.0±1.5
Sibling	17.2±1.5	17.8±1.0
Missing data, %±95% CL	5.0±3.0	0.5±1.0†
Father	5.2±5.7	0.0±0.0
Mother	5.2±5.7	0.0±0.0
Sibling	4.2±4.5	1.1±2.2
Second-degree relatives		
No. of relatives	607	558
Gender, M/F	304:303	276:282
Age (mean±95% CL), y	49.9±1.4	52.1±1.4‡
Missing data, %±95% CL	7.5±2.1	8.6±2.4

*CL indicates confidence limit.
†P<.01.
‡P<.05.

conduct disorder, Axis II disorder, and assaultive behavior [OR, 4.5; 95% CI, 1.5-14.1]). Inclusion of proband psychiatric disorders and other traits as additional covariates did not substantially change any of these analyses (OR, 4.3; 95% CI, 1.1-16.6). On the other hand, when controlling for these variables, the rate of suicidal ideation was no longer significantly increased in the relatives of suicide probands (OR, 1.6; 95% CI, 0.5-5.1). Parallel analyses, using Cox proportional hazards regression, showed similar results (for suicidal behavior in relatives, OR, 5.3, and 95% CI, 1.4-21.0; for suicidal ideation in relatives, OR, 1.1, and 95% CI, 0.4-3.1).

Second-degree Relatives

Among second-degree relatives, greater risk for attempts and completion in relatives of suicide probands persisted after controlling for familial Axis I covariates (ie, affective, substance abuse, conduct, and anxiety disorders [OR, 2.4; 95% CI, 1.0-5.8). When logistic regression included Axis I and II disorders (avoidant, borderline, and antisocial) and assaultive behavior as covariates, the risk for suicidal behavior in relatives of suicide probands was increased, but the CI included unity (OR, 2.3; 95% CI, 0.9-5.7). The rate of suicidal ideation was not different between the 2 groups when adjusting for the above-noted familial and proband differences (OR, 1.0; 95% CI, 0.4-2.3). Parallel analyses using Cox proportional hazards regression showed similar results (for suicidal behavior in relatives, OR, 2.2, and 95% CI, 0.5-10.9; for suicidal ideation in relatives, OR, 1.3, and 95% CI, 0.6-2.9).

CHARACTERISTICS OF SUICIDE PROBANDS AND FAMILIAL LOADING FOR SUICIDAL BEHAVIOR

There was no relationship between the presence of high suicidal intent or violent method in the suicide probands and familial loading for suicide attempts and completions. Suicide probands who scored above the median on the BG-LHA, compared with those who scored below the median, had much greater familial loading for suicide attempts and completions in first-degree relatives (15.6%±8.1% vs 2.9%±3.9% [χ^2=6.89, *P*<.009]), with a trend in the same direction even after controlling for BG-LHA scores (OR, 4.1; 95% CI, 0.8-21.4) in relatives.

COMMENT

In this family study of adolescent suicide and community control probands, we found increased rates of suicide attempts in relatives of the former compared with relatives of the latter. This increased familial aggregation of suicide attempts in suicide probands persisted, even after controlling for the increased prevalence of Axis I and II disorders in their relatives. Furthermore, familial aggregation of actual suicidal behavior was demonstrated, whereas the excess rate of suicidal ideation in relatives of suicide probands was explained by an increased familial prevalence of psychopathological conditions. While the familial aggregation of suicidal behavior is not completely mediated by the transmission of aggressive behavior, a relationship between familial rates of suicidal behavior and aggression in suicide probands was demonstrated. The implications of these findings will be discussed, after placing them in the context of the limitations of this study.

Most of these limitations are inherent to family studies. In this type of study, family aggregation can be demonstrated, and familial transmission can be inferred, but clear demonstration of familial transmission and its mechanisms require different and more powerful designs. For example, familial aggregation could be due to genetic, environmental, or artifactual causes. The genetic cause of familial aggregation is best demonstrated by adoption or twin studies.[6,7] Family studies are often a precursor to these more powerful designs, because they help to more sharply define the phenotype under investigation. The familial transmission of suicidal behavior can also involve nongenetic mechanisms, such as exposure to family violence, hostility and discord, separation and loss, low parental involvement, or imitation of suicidal behavior in a parent.[41-52] A prospective high-risk design would be best suited to examine the genetic and environmental components of the familial transmission of suicidal behavior. Artifact may also explain the familial aggregation of suicidal behavior, insofar as suicide may affect the report, recall, and actual psychiatric status of relatives.[26,27] However, it has been demonstrated previously that the psychiatric status of parents does not appear to affect their recall or report of psychopathological conditions in suicide victims[18] and that their report appears valid.[19] Furthermore, our estimation of the

Table 4. Lifetime Psychiatric Diagnosis in First- and Second-degree Relatives of Suicide Probands and Community Controls*

Diagnosis in Relatives	Rate, %±95% CL		Morbid Risk±95% CL	
	Suicide Probands (n=58)	Controls (n=55)	Suicide Probands (n=58)	Controls (n=55)
Any Axis I disorder				
First degree	63.6±6.9	52.7±6.9†	0.81±0.08	0.76±0.10
Second degree	48.8±4.2	37.9±4.3‡	0.57±0.06	0.45±0.06§
Any affective disorder				
First degree	34.8±6.8	25.5±6.0†	0.43±0.10	0.32±0.08
Second degree	20.8±3.4	12.9±2.9‡	0.21±0.04	0.13±0.04§
Major depressive disorder				
First degree	24.5±6.1	18.0±5.3	0.29±0.08	0.21±0.06
Second degree	14.7±3.0	10.4±2.7†	0.14±0.04	0.11±0.04
Dysthymia				
First degree	12.7±4.7	6.3±3.3†	0.17±0.08	0.09±0.06†
Second degree	6.3±2.0	2.8±1.4§	0.07±0.02	0.03±0.02†
Mania				
First degree	1.1±1.5	0.5±1.0	0.01±0.02	0.01±0.02
Second degree	0.7±0.7	0.2±0.4	0.006±0.007	0.002±0.005
Hypomania				
First degree	2.1±2.0	1.0±1.4	0.02±0.02	0.01±0.01
Second degree	0.7±0.7	0.2±0.4	0.005±0.006	0.00±0.00
Any anxiety disorder				
First degree	20.8±5.9	18.6±5.3	0.30±0.10	0.32±0.12
Second degree	12.7±2.8	4.9±3.0‡	0.15±0.04	0.07±0.02‡
Alcohol abuse				
First degree	26.5±6.3	21.5±5.6	0.29±0.08	0.31±0.10
Second degree	20.5±3.4	16.9±3.3	0.21±0.04	0.16±0.04
Other drug abuse				
First degree	5.9±3.4	2.4±2.1	0.06±0.04	0.02±0.02†
Second degree	6.2±2.0	2.6±1.4§	0.06±0.02	0.03±0.02†
Conduct disorder				
First degree	16.8±5.4	7.4±3.6‖	0.19±0.08	0.13±0.08
Second degree	8.5±2.4	3.7±1.7‖	0.09±0.04	0.05±0.04†
Any PD¶				
First degree	11.5±4.6	5.1±3.1†	...	...
Second degree	8.6±2.3	2.4±1.3‡	...	...
Antisocial PD¶				
First degree	3.8±2.8	0.0±0.0§		
Second degree	3.3±1.5	0.8±0.8‖	...	...
Avoidant PD¶				
First degree	6.0±3.5	4.6±2.9	...	...
Second degree	4.6±1.8	1.6±1.1§	...	...
Borderline PD¶				
First degree	2.2±2.1	0.5±1.0	...	...
Second degree	1.8±1.1	0.4±0.6†	...	...
Suicide attempt				
First degree	10.6±4.4	2.4±2.1‡	0.14±0.06	0.03±0.02‖
Second degree	4.6±1.8	1.4±1.0‖	0.04±0.02	0.01±0.01§
Suicide completion				
First degree	1.1±1.5	0.0±0.0	0.01±0.02	0.00±0.00
Second degree	0.4±0.5	0.0±0.0	0.004±0.01	0.00±0.00
Suicide ideation				
First degree	14.7±5.0	8.2±3.7†	0.22±0.14	0.09±0.04
Second degree	7.6±2.2	4.5±1.8†	0.07±0.02	0.04±0.02
Assaultive behavior				
First degree	24.5±6.1	15.5±4.9†	0.30±0.08	0.18±0.06†
Second degree	17.2±3.2	7.5±2.3‡	0.15±0.04	0.05±0.02‡
Measures of Aggression#				
Brown-Goodwin Assessment for Lifetime History of Aggression¶				
First degree	5.9±1.1	4.8±0.8	...	...
Second degree	3.8±0.8	4.2±1.2	...	...
Buss-Durkee Hostility Inventory, Assault Subscale¶				
First degree	14.4±0.5	14.0±0.4	...	...
Second degree	13.0±0.5	12.7±0.5	...	...
Buss-Durkee Hostility Inventory, Irritability Subscale¶				
First degree	15.6±0.6	15.3±0.4	...	...
Second degree	14.6±0.5	13.8±0.5	...	...

*Data on mothers, fathers, and siblings are available on request. CL indicates confidence limit; PD, personality disorder.
†P≤.05.
‡P<.001.
§P<.01.
‖P<.005.
¶Morbid risk not applicable.
#Measured as mean±95% CL.

familial morbid risk included only those conditions in relatives of suicide probands that had had their onset prior to death of the suicide victim, so as not to confound preexisting rates of disorder with new-onset conditions precipitated by the stress of the suicide. One further limitation of this particular family study was the relatively low rate of direct interviews for fathers. Although the rate of direct paternal interviews was similar in both groups, we may have underestimated the contribution of familial impulsive aggression on suicidal risk, given that those fathers who were not available for interview may have been more aggressive. However, we did statistically model the substitution of extreme scores of aggression for all missing data without any substantial alteration in the results.

To our knowledge, this study is the first demonstration of the familial aggregation of suicide attempts in the families of suicide victims while controlling for the increased rate of a broad range of Axis I and II psychopathological conditions in relatives. These results strongly suggest that the tendency to suicidal behavior is familially transmitted by a mechanism distinct from the familial transmission of other psychiatric conditions. This finding is consistent with previous reports that the familial aggregation of suicide is distinct from that of either affective illness[5] or endogenous psychoses.[4]

However distinct the familial transmission of liabilities to suicidal behavior and psychopathological conditions are from one another, it appears likely that these 2 sets of liabilities intersect to result in attempted or completed suicide, since the vast majority of those who attempt and complete suicide suffer from at least 1 major psychiatric condition.[1,2,17,45,46,50,53] Conversely, if liability to suicidal behavior alone was sufficient to trigger a suicide attempt or completion, then it would be highly unlikely that such an overwhelming proportion of suicide probands would show evidence of major psychiatric conditions.

What is the spectrum of suicidal behavior that appears to be familially transmitted? Our data suggest that the phenotype for the familial liability to suicidal behavior includes suicide attempts and completions and does not include suicidal ideation. These findings are consistent with those of Pfeffer et al,[8] who reported increased rates of suicide attempts in the relatives of prepubertal suicide attempters, but not in the relatives of suicidal ideators. Similarly, in our study the familial aggregation of attempts persisted after controlling for the increased rate of familial psychopathological conditions in the relatives of suicide probands, whereas the familial aggregation of suicidal ideation was explained by the excess rates of Axis I and II disorders among relatives. The view that suicide attempts and completions represent the expression of a specific liability, whereas ideation is a manifestation of underlying psychopathological condition, is supported by research showing similar changes in serotonergic function in attempted and in completed suicide, but not in suicidal ideation.[37,54-56] In addition, our finding that the relatives of adolescent suicide probands showed a familial excess of suicide attempts supports the view that attempts and completions are part of the same clinical and familial spectrum. The continuity between suicide attempts and completions is also supported by other family studies,[2,9-11] as well as both retrospective[2,17] and prospective studies.[57]

The phenotype of suicidal behavior that is familially transmitted may also include aggressive behavior. Among suicide probands, higher familial loading for suicide attempts was associated with higher ratings of aggression in the probands, even after adjustment for family loading of aggression. Therefore, familial transmission of the liability for suicidal behavior also involves the transmission of liability to aggression. Numerous other studies have reported a relationship between suicidal and aggressive behavior.[1,2,16,17,58,59] Our particular set of findings showing greater family loading for suicide attempts in more aggressive suicide probands is consistent with that of a recent report showing a relationship between a polymorphism of the tyrosine hydroxylase allele and repeated suicide attempts in violent attempters.[60] Since, in our study, familial aggregation for suicidal behavior occurred even after controlling for impulsive aggressive personality disorders, assaultive behavior, and other measures of aggression, familial transmission of suicidal behavior appears to be at least partially independent of the familial transmission of aggression.

These results support further investigations into the familial transmission of suicidal behavior. A high-risk study examining the offspring of attempted suicide victims and a comparison group may be useful in clarifying mechanisms of familial transmission, particularly those mechanisms that may be mediated by nongenetic mechanisms. Genetic investigations using an allele-sharing approach may also be a fruitful avenue of inquiry. Research should focus on clarifying the unique genetic and nongenetic contributions to the familial transmission of suicidal behavior. With a better understanding of familial transmission of suicidal behavior comes the hope of prevention of youthful suicide and suicidal behavior.

Accepted for publication April 1, 1996.

Supported by grants MH43366 and MH44711 from the National Institute of Mental Health, Rockville, Md.

The expert assistance of Patricia Nuss in preparation of the manuscript is gratefully acknowledged. Satish Iyengar, PhD, provided statistical consultation throughout this project, from design through analysis. Mary Jo Auth, Sylvia Bartle, MSW, Robert Brown, Doreen Constantine Richardson, MEd, Sean Curilla, James Matta, MA, Timothy Pitts, MEd, Christine Rather, Mary Wartella, MSW, and Tina White provided interviewing and technical support. Above all, we thank the families for their participation.

Reprints: David A. Brent, MD, University of Pittsburgh School of Medicine, Western Psychiatric Institute and Clinic, 3811 O'Hara St, Pittsburgh, PA 15213.

REFERENCES

1. Shafii M, Carrigan S, Whittinghill JR, Derrick AM. Psychological autopsy of completed suicide in children and adolescents. *Am J Psychiatry.* 1985;142:1061-1064.
2. Shaffer D, Garland A, Gould M, Fisher P, Trautman P. Preventing teenage suicide: a critical review. *J Am Acad Child Adolesc Psychiatry.* 1988;27:675-687.
3. Tsuang MT. Risk of suicide in the relatives of schizophrenics, manics, depressives, and controls. *J Clin Psychiatry.* 1983;44:396-400.

4. Mitterauer B. A contribution to the discussion of the role of the genetic factor in suicide, based on five studies in an epidemiologically defined area (Province of Salzburg, Austria). *Compr Psychiatry.* 1990;31:557-565.
5. Egeland JA, Sussex JN. Suicide and family loading for affective disorders. *JAMA.* 1985;254:915-918.
6. Schulsinger F, Kety SS, Rosenthal D, Wender PH. A family study of suicide. In: Schou M, Stromgren E, eds. *Origin, Prevention and Treatment of Affective Disorders.* Orlando, Fla: Academic Press Inc; 1979:277-287.
7. Tsuang MT. Genetic factors in suicide. *Dis Nerv Syst.* 1977;38:498-501.
8. Pfeffer CR, Normandin L, Tatsuyuki K. Suicidal children grow up: suicidal behavior and psychiatric disorders among relatives. *J Am Acad Child Adolesc Psychiatry.* 1994;33:1087-1097.
9. Garfinkel BD, Froese A, Hood J. Suicide attempts in children and adolescents. *Am J Psychiatry.* 1982;139:1257-1261.
10. Linkowski P, de Maertelaer V, Mendlewicz J. Suicidal behaviour in major depressive illness. *Acta Psychiatr Scand.* 1985;72:233-238.
11. Roy A. Family history of suicide. *Arch Gen Psychiatry.* 1983;40:971-974.
12. Buydens-Branchey L, Branchey MH, Noumair D. Age of alcoholism onset, I: relationship to psychopathology. *Arch Gen Psychiatry.* 1989;46:225-230.
13. Brent DA, Perper JA, Moritz G, Liotus L, Schweers J, Balach L, Roth C. Familial risk factors for adolescent suicide: a case-control study. *Acta Psychiatr Scand.* 1994;89:52-58.
14. Wender PH, Kety SS, Rosenthal D, Schulsinger F, Ortmann J, Lunde I. Psychiatric disorders in the biological and adoptive families of adopted individuals with affective disorders. *Arch Gen Psychiatry.* 1986;43:923-929.
15. Hollingshead A. *Four Factor Index of Social Status.* New Haven, Conn: Yale University Sociology Department; 1975.
16. Brent DA, Johnson BA, Perper J, Connolly J, Bridge J, Bartle S, Rather C. Personality disorder, personality traits, impulsive violence, and completed suicide in adolescents. *J Am Acad Child Adolesc Psychiatry.* 1994;33:1080-1086.
17. Brent DA, Perper JA, Moritz G, Allman C, Roth C, Schweers J, Balach L, Baugher M. Psychiatric risk factors of adolescent suicide: a case control study. *J Am Acad Child Adolesc Psychiatry.* 1993;32:521-529.
18. Brent DA, Perper JA, Kolko DJ, Zelenak JP. The psychological autopsy: methodological considerations for the study of adolescent suicide. *J Am Acad Child Adolesc Psychiatry.* 1988;27:362-366.
19. Brent DA, Perper JA, Moritz G, Allman C, Roth C, Schweers J, Balach L. The validity of diagnoses obtained through the psychological autopsy procedure: use of family history. *Acta Psychiatr Scand.* 1993;87:118-122.
20. Leckman JF, Sholomskas D, Thompson WD, Belanger A, Weissman MM. Best estimate of lifetime psychiatric diagnosis: a methodological study. *Arch Gen Psychiatry.* 1982;39:879-883.
21. Orvaschel H, Puig-Antich J, Chambers W, Tabrizi MA, Johnson R. Retrospective assessment of prepubertal major depression with the Kiddie-SADS-E. *J Am Acad Child Psychiatry.* 1982;21:392-397.
22. Chambers WJ, Puig-Antich J, Hirsch M, Paez P, Ambrosini PJ, Tabrizi MA, Davies M. The assessment of affective disorders in children and adolescents by semistructured interview: test-retest reliability of the Schedule for Affective Disorders and Schizophrenia for School-Age Children, Present Episode Version. *Arch Gen Psychiatry.* 1985;42:696-702.
23. American Psychiatric Association. *Diagnostic and Statistical Manual of Mental Disorders, Third Edition.* Washington, DC: American Psychiatric Association; 1980.
24. Endicott J, Spitzer RL. A diagnostic interview: The Schedule for Affective Disorders and Schizophrenia. *Arch Gen Psychiatry.* 1978;35:837-844.
25. Andreasen NC, Endicott J, Spitzer RL, Winokur G. The family history method using diagnostic criteria: reliability and validity. *Arch Gen Psychiatry.* 1977; 34:1229-1235.
26. Brent DA, Perper JA, Moritz G, Liotus L, Schweers J, Roth C, Balach L, Allman D. Psychiatric impact of the loss of an adolescent sibling to suicide. *J Affect Disord.* 1993;28:249-256.
27. Brent DA, Moritz G, Bridge J, Perper J, Canobbio R. The impact of adolescent suicide on siblings and parents: a longitudinal follow-up. *Suicide Life Threat Behav.* In press.
28. Spitzer RL, Williams JBW, Gibbon M, First MB. *The Structured Clinical Interview for DSM-III-R.* New York, NY: New York State Psychiatric Institute; 1989.
29. American Psychiatric Association. *Diagnostic and Statistical Manual of Mental Disorders, Third Edition, Revised.* Washington, DC: American Psychiatric Association; 1987.
30. Johnson BA, Brent DA, Connolly J, Bridge J, Matta J, Constantine D, Rather C, White T. The familial aggregation of adolescent personality disorders. *J Am Acad Child Adolesc Psychiatry.* 1995;34:789-804.
31. Brent DA, Johnson B, Bartle S, Bridge J, Rather C, Matta J, Connolly J, Constantine D. Personality disorder, tendency to impulsive violence, and suicidal behavior in adolescents. *J Am Acad Child Adolesc Psychiatry.* 1993;32:69-75.
32. Beck AT, Schuyler D, Herman I. Development of Suicidal Intent scales. In: Beck AT, Lettieri DJ, Resnick HLP, eds. *The Prediction of Suicide.* Bowie, Md: Charles Press; 1974:45-55.
33. Pierce DW. The predictive validation of a suicide intent scale: a five year follow-up. *Br J Psychiatry.* 1981;139:391-396.
34. Brown GL, Goodwin FK, Ballenger JC, Goyer PF, Major LF. Aggression in humans correlates with cerebrospinal fluid amine metabolites. *Psychiatry Res.* 1979;1:131-139.
35. Brown GL, Ebert MH, Goyer PF, Jimerson DC, Klein WJ, Bunney WE, Goodwin FK. Aggression, suicide, and serotonin: relationships to CSF amine metabolites. *Am J Psychiatry.* 1982;139:741-746.
36. Buss A, Durkee A. An inventory for assessing different kinds of hostility. *J Consult Clin Psychol.* 1957;21:343-349.
37. Coccaro E, Siever L, Klar HM, Maurer G, Cochrane K, Cooper TB, Mohs RC, Davis KL. Serotonergic studies in patients with affective and personality disorders. *Arch Gen Psychiatry.* 1989;46:587-599.
38. Kaplan EL, Meier P. Nonparametric estimation from incomplete observations. *J Am Stat Assoc.* 1958;53:457-481.
39. Cox DR. Regression models and life-tables. *J R Stat Soc.* 1972;34:187-220.
40. Dixon WJ. *BMDP Statistical Software Manual.* Berkeley: University of California Press; 1990.
41. Asarnow J, Carlson G. Suicide attempts in preadolescent child psychiatry inpatients. *Suicide Life Threat Behav.* 1988;18:129-136.
42. Taylor EA, Stansfeld SA. Children who poison themselves, I: a clinical comparison with psychiatric controls. *Br J Psychiatry.* 1984;145:127-132.
43. Kosky R, Silburn S, Zubrick SR. Are children and adolescents who have suicidal thoughts different from those who attempt suicide? *J Nerv Ment Dis.* 1990;178:38-43.
44. Kienhorst CWM, de Wilde EJ, Van Den Bout J, van Groenou MIB, Diekstra RFW, Wolters WHG. Self-reported suicidal behavior in Dutch secondary education students. *Suicide Life Threat Behav.* 1990;20:101-112.
45. Lewinsohn PM, Rohde P, Seeley JR. Psychosocial risk factors for future adolescent suicide attempts. *J Consult Clin Psychol.* 1994;62:297-305.
46. Garrison CZ, Jackson KL, Addy CL, McKeown RE, Waller JL. Suicidal behaviors in young adolescents. *Am J Epidemiol.* 1991;133:1005-1014.
47. Joffe RT, Offord DR, Boyle MH. Ontario child health study: suicidal behavior in youth age 12-16 years. *Am J Psychiatry.* 1988;145:1420-1423.
48. Kashani JH, Goddard P, Reid JC. Correlates of suicidal ideation in a community sample of children and adolescents. *J Am Acad Child Adolesc Psychiatry.* 1989;28:912-917.
49. Fergusson DM, Lynskey MT. Childhood circumstances, adolescent adjustment, and suicide attempts in a New Zealand birth cohort. *J Am Acad Child Adolesc Psychiatry.* 1995;34:612-622.
50. Reinherz HZ, Giaconia RM, Silverman AB, Friedman A, Pakiz B, Frost AK, Cohen E. Early psychosocial risks for adolescent suicidal ideation and attempts. *J Am Acad Child Adolesc Psychiatry.* 1995;34:599-611.
51. Brent DA, Kolko DJ, Goldstein CE, Allan MJ, Brown RV. Suicidality in affectively disordered adolescent inpatients. *J Am Acad Child Adolesc Psychiatry.* 1990;29:586-593.
52. Harkavy-Friedman JM, Asnis GM, Boeck M, Difiore J. Prevalence of specific suicidal behaviors in a high school sample. *Am J Psychiatry.* 1987;144:1203-1206.
53. Marttunen MD, Aro HM, Henriksson MM, Lonnquist JK. Mental disorders in adolescent suicide: *DSM-III-R* Axis I and II diagnoses in suicide among 13- to 19-year-olds in Finland. *Arch Gen Psychiatry.* 1991;48:834-839.
54. Asberg M, Traskman-Bendz L, Thoren P. 5-HIAA in the cerebrospinal fluid: a biochemical suicide predictor? *Arch Gen Psychiatry.* 1976;33:1193-1197.
55. Mann JJ, McBride PA, Brown RP, Linnoila M, Leon AC, DeMeo M, Mieczkowski T, Myers JE, Stanley M. Relationship between central and peripheral serotonin indexes in depressed and suicidal psychiatric inpatients. *Arch Gen Psychiatry.* 1992;49:442-446.
56. Mann J, Stanley M, McBride A, McEwen BS. Increased serotonin and β-adrenergic receptor binding in the frontal cortices of suicide victims. *Arch Gen Psychiatry.* 1986;43:954-959.
57. Otto U. Suicidal acts by children and adolescents: a follow-up study. *Acta Psychiatr Scand.* 1972;233(suppl):7-91.
58. Virkkunen M, DeJong J, Bartko J, Linnoila M. Psychobiological concomitants of history of suicide attempts among violent offenders and impulsive fire setters. *Arch Gen Psychiatry.* 1989;46:604-606.
59. Pfeffer CR, Newcorn J, Kaplan G, Mizruchi MS, Plutchik R. Suicidal behavior in adolescent psychiatric inpatients. *J Am Acad Child Adolesc Psychiatry.* 1988; 27:357-361.
60. Nielsen DA, Goldman D, Virkkunen M, Tokola R, Rawlings R, Linnoila M. Suicidality and 5-hydroxyindoleacetic acid concentration associated with a tryptophan hydroxylase polymorphism. *Arch Gen Psychiatry.* 1994;51:34-38.

ORIGINAL ARTICLE

Psychosocial Risk Factors of Child and Adolescent Completed Suicide

Madelyn S. Gould, PhD, MPH; Prudence Fisher, MS; Michael Parides, PhD; Michael Flory, PhD; David Shaffer, MD

Background: Few psychosocial risk factors for completed suicide in children and adolescents have been studied systematically. The present study was designed to examine the environmental, social, and familial characteristics of a large representative sample of child and adolescent suicides.

Methods: A case-control, psychological autopsy of 120 of 170 consecutive suicides younger than 20 years and 147 community age-, sex-, and ethnically matched control participants in the greater New York, NY, area.

Results: There was a significant independent impact of the psychosocial factors on increasing suicide risk among children and adolescents, beyond that risk attributable to psychiatric illness. The most notable risks were derived from school problems, a family history of suicidal behavior, poor parent-child communication, and stressful life events. Sex, ethnicity, and age modified the relationships of a few of the psychosocial factors.

Conclusions: Socioenvironmental circumstances add significantly to a teenager's risk of suicide. The overall effect size on increasing suicide risk of the psychosocial factors is comparable with that for diagnostic factors, highlighting the importance of considering socioenvironmental factors when assessing suicide risk.

Arch Gen Psychiatry. 1996;53:1155-1162

Most psychological autopsy studies of children and adolescents have limited their inquiry to psychiatric risk factors. These studies have determined that a majority of those who completed suicide had significant psychiatric problems, including previous suicidal threats and behavior, affective disorder, substance abuse, and conduct disorder.[1-7] Despite the notion that the social environment also impacts on suicidal behavior,[8] there is a relative scarcity of empirical information about the environmental, social, and familial characteristics of adolescent suicide victims. A continuing debate exists over the relative importance of socioenvironmental to psychiatric diagnostic factors in explaining suicidal behavior.[8]

The psychosocial factor that has received the most attention in the psychological autopsy literature is stressful life events. This research generally supports the association of life stressors, such as interpersonal losses and legal or disciplinary problems, with suicide.[9-12] The nature of the stressor has been reported to be related to the underlying psychiatric disorder of the suicide victim,[9,11-13] yet specific stressors, such as legal and disciplinary problems, are still associated with an increased risk of suicide, even after adjusting for psychiatric disorders.[9] Several postmortem studies, relying on record reviews rather than on psychological autopsy interviews,[14-18] have also identified recent stressors in the majority of youth suicides. Only 1[2] of the studies examining stressful life events has included a nonsuicidal comparison group. Without such a comparison group, the specificity of the findings to suicide cannot be determined.

Three psychological autopsy studies with community comparison samples have reported on other environmental, social, and familial risk factors.[2,7,19,20] Two of the studies have been quite small.[7,20] The third, by Brent et al,[2,19] compared 67 adolescent suicide victims in western Pennsylvania with 67 demographically matched community control participants. Significant familial risks included a family history of depression, substance abuse, and parent-

From the Division of Child Psychiatry, Columbia University, College of Physicians and Surgeons/New York State Psychiatric Institute, and the Division of Epidemiology, Columbia University School of Public Health, New York, NY.

See Subjects and Methods on next page

SUBJECTS AND METHODS

A detailed description of the methods of this study has been provided by Shaffer et al.[1] With the exception of social and familial variables that are unique to this article, only a brief description of the sample and methods is given. Several reports describe the robustness of the psychological autopsy method.[1,21,22] The project was approved by the New York State Psychiatric Institute/Columbia University Institutional Review Board, New York.

SAMPLE

Psychological autopsies were conducted on 120 of a consecutive series of 170 suicides completed by persons younger than 20 years within a 2-year period in New York City and 28 surrounding counties in New York State, New Jersey, and Connecticut. The study area represented rural, suburban, and urban areas, with diverse ethnic and socioeconomic characteristics. The percentages of victims who lived in urban, suburban, and rural communities at the time of their death were 28.5%, 57.6%, and 13.9%, respectively. A random comparison sample, stratified on the age, ethnic, and sex distribution of the completed suicide cases, was identified from the study region (N=147 participants from a potential pool of 196 eligible community children and adolescents), using a random-digit dialing procedure. The rural or urban status of the control informants' communities was not significantly different from that of the victims. Participants in both groups did not differ from nonparticipants on demographic variables.[1]

INFORMANTS

Information on completed suicides was obtained from a parent or another adult member of the household in which the victim was living at the time of death, either a sibling or a friend, and between 1 and 3 schoolteachers. Information on community control participants was obtained from the adolescents themselves, a parent or caregiver, and up to 3 schoolteachers. The length of each assessment ranged from 4 to 8 hours. The community control informants were paid $50. The informants were interviewed by 1 of 11 masters- or doctoral-level psychologists or certified social workers. The interval between suicide and assessment ranged from 28 to 976 days (median, 159 days). Fifty-four percent of the sample was assessed within 6 months and 81% within 1 year of the suicide.

ASSESSMENT MEASURES

Demographic Variables

The interview with the informants assessed the household and family constellation during the 3 months before the death (or assessment for the control participants), parental education, occupation, and marital status, and the school or work status of the suicides and control participants.

The 1980 census was used to determine age, sex, and ethnic distributions of the general population aged 19 years and younger in our study area.[23] The Public Use Microdata Sample from the 1980 census provided education and occupation estimates for the reference population of households with children aged 10 through 19 years. The socioeconomic status (SES) for each census household and for each participant family was derived by means of Hollingshead's Four-Factor Index.[24]

Parent-Child Relationships

Six questions addressed the relationship between the subject and his or her parents during the 3 months before death (or assessment). These measured the frequency with which each parent (1) got irritable, (2) nagged, (3) quarreled, or (4) had conversations with him or her; (5) the extent to which the youth confided in the parent; and (6) the parent's satisfaction with the quality of conversations with the adolescent. Identical factor structures emerged in principal-components factor analyses conducted separately for the mothers' and fathers' relationship items. The first scale, "negative interaction," consisted of the frequency of irritability, nagging, and arguments (α=.70 and .72 for mothers' and fathers' relationships, respectively). The second scale, "poor communication," included frequency of conversations, confiding, and sharing, and satisfaction with conversations (α=.46 and .60 for mothers' and fathers' relationships, respectively). The scale scores were dichotomized by means of what we considered to be clinically relevant cutoff points. Only relationships with the *biological* parents were used in the present article. A self-report took precedence when available (85% for mothers and 43% for fathers).

Severe Physical Punishment

Three items assessed the type, frequency, and consequences of punishment the youth received during his or her lifetime. A rating of severe physical punishment was based on frequent (at least once a month) punishment resulting in injuries in the 3 months before death (or assessment); or

child discord. None of the psychological autopsy studies addressed age-, sex-, or ethnicity-specific features.

This report describes the socioenvironmental characteristics, determined by psychological autopsy, of 120 children and adolescents who committed suicide between June 1984 and May 1986 in New York, NY, and its surrounding area. An earlier report described the psychopathological characteristics of the suicide victims.[1] We aimed to identify psychosocial factors that significantly increase the risk of youth suicide and to determine whether these factors yield an incremental suicide risk, beyond that contributed by psychiatric illness. Sex-, ethnicity-, and age-specific effects were examined.

RESULTS

DEMOGRAPHIC CHARACTERISTICS

The demographic characteristics of the suicide victim and community control participants and the general population (1980 census) younger than 20 years in the study areas are presented in **Table 1**. The suicide victims were older (χ^2_2=144.6, *P*<.001), more likely to be boys (χ^2=38.6, *P*<.001), and less likely to be African American (z=2.59, *P*<.01) than the general youth population. Among the suicides, the male-female ratio increased with age, rising from 2.1 to 4.0 in those younger a lifetime history of physical punishment resulting in visible skin lesions 5 or more times or fractures or other internal injuries or punishment resulting in other consequences that led to medical evaluation.

Parental Psychopathologic Characteristics and Family History of Suicidal Behavior

For each parent, a lifetime history (before the suicide) of mood symptoms (depression and dysthymia), psychotic symptoms, alcohol or substance abuse problems, psychiatric treatment, and trouble with the police (other than minor traffic violations or warnings) was ascertained. The symptoms had to meet the duration criterion as specified in *DSM-III* and have resulted in some dysfunction to be scored positive. Only assessments about the *biological* parents were used in the present article. A self-report took precedence when available (78% for mothers and 43% for fathers). Several questions assessed a history of completed or attempted suicide in the first-degree relatives. A positive family history largely reflects suicide attempts, since completed suicides in the families were rare (approximately 1% in each group).

Stressful Life Events

The Coddington Life Event Schedule for Children and Adolescents[25,26] assessed the occurrence of life events during the 3 months before the suicide (or assessment). Composite measures of negative events were derived from 23 of the 50 items, considered undesirable by independent ratings of 3 judges (M.S.G., D.S., and P.F.), and information from direct interview about undesirable events during the month of the death (or assessment). Based on previous psychological autopsy studies,[9] 2 a priori scales were developed to represent legal or disciplinary crises and interpersonal loss. Disciplinary crises included suspension from school, other trouble at school, responsibility for an automobile accident, appearance in juvenile court or other trouble with police, and trouble at work. Interpersonal loss included the death of a relative or friend, disruption of a relationship, and a recent separation. These 2 domains were dichotomized on the basis of the presence of any event within each domain. The few redundant events in the Coddington questionnaire and interview were combined by means of an "either-or" rule.

School or Work Problems

Several questions assessed a history of difficulties in school, including having ever failed a grade, having been suspended within 3 months of death (or assessment), or having dropped out of high school. Work status within 3 months of death (or assessment) was ascertained.

Child and Adolescent Psychiatric Diagnoses

Details about the method of diagnostic assessments were presented by Shaffer et al.[1] Briefly, the symptom-based interview was derived in part from the Schedule for Affective Disorders and Schizophrenia,[27] the Schedule for Affective Disorders and Schizophrenia for Children,[28] and the Present State Examination,[29] supplemented by questions for diagnostic criteria listed in *DSM-III*. The presence of symptoms during the 3 months before death (or assessment) was ascertained. Lifetime assessments were made for some low-frequency events (eg, arrests) and for previous manifestations of suicide-related behavior.

Diagnoses were assigned by computer algorithms, derived from *DSM-III* criteria, by means of a comparable informant base (parents or caretakers only) for suicides and control participants. Superordinate diagnostic categories of mood, disruptive, substance and alcohol, anxiety, and miscellaneous disorders were created because the prevalence of many individual diagnoses was low. The best-estimate clinical diagnoses, incorporating nonblind information from all available informants, were not used in the present analyses because case-control comparisons are not clearly interpretable without a comparable informant base and blinded assessment. Sensitivities for the superordinate diagnoses with the use of best-estimate clinical diagnoses were given in an earlier report.[1]

DATA ANALYSIS

A series of maximum-likelihood logistic regression analyses[30] were performed with the use of each of the psychosocial measures to predict completed suicides. The matching variables of age, sex, and ethnicity were included as covariates in the analyses because the cases and controls were frequency matched rather than individually matched.[31] Socioeconomic status was included as an additional covariate because the community controls had a significantly higher SES than the completed suicides. The analyses tested for interactions with gender, ethnicity, age, and SES. Whether significant ($\alpha<.05$) associations between the psychosocial factors and suicide could be accounted for by their associations with mood, disruptive, and substance and alcohol disorder was examined next. The analyses also examined interactions between diagnostic categories and psychosocial risk factors.

than 15 years to those between 15 and 19 years of age, whereas there were equal proportions of boys and girls at every age among the general population.

The community control participants had a significantly higher SES than the census Public Use Microdata Sample ($\chi^2_4=38.64$, $P<.001$). Therefore, the SES characteristics of the suicide victims and census sample were compared. Only African-American suicide completers, not those who were white or Hispanic, had a significantly higher SES than their general-population counterparts ($\chi^2=11.6$, $P<.05$). Specifically, there was an overrepresentation of the middle class (SES III) and an underrepresentation of the poorest strata (SES IV) among the African-American suicides.

PSYCHOSOCIAL RISKS

Familial Factors

Living Situation. Suicide victims were significantly more likely to come from a nonintact family of origin (48.3%) than were community control participants (33.3%) (odds ratio [OR], 1.9; 95% confidence interval [CI], 1.1-3.3; **Table 2**). Approximately 61% of the victims, in contrast to 76% of community control participants, lived in

Table 1. Demographic Characteristics of Suicides, Community Controls, and General Population Aged 19 Years and Younger

	No. (%)		
	Suicide Victims (n=120)	Community Controls (n=147)	General Population, %*
Age, y			
5-9	1 (0.8)	0 (0)	28.5
10-14	18 (15.0)	23 (15.6)	34.0
15-19	101 (84.2)	124 (84.4)	37.5
Sex			
Female	25 (20.8)	31 (21.1)	49.2
Male	95 (79.2)	116 (78.9)	50.8
Ethnicity			
White	84 (70.0)	111 (75.5)	62.2
African American	13 (10.8)	16 (10.9)	20.3†
Hispanic	18 (15.0)	15 (10.2)	14.6
Other	5 (4.2)	5 (3.4)	2.9
Socioeconomic status‡			
I			
White	14 (16.7)§	27 (24.3)	17.2
African American	1 (7.7)	0 (0)	4.6
Hispanic	0 (0)	1 (6.7)	2.9
II			
White	28 (33.3)	57 (51.4)	32.5
African American	4 (30.8)	6 (37.5)	18.0
Hispanic	3 (16.7)	1 (6.7)	11.1
III			
White	26 (31.0)	17 (15.3)	26.3
African American	7 (53.8)	4 (25.0)	23.9
Hispanic	2 (11.1)	2 (13.3)	16.3
IV			
White	13 (15.5)	10 (9.0)	17.2
African American	1 (7.7)	5 (31.3)	26.8
Hispanic	3 (16.7)	6 (40.0)	28.3
V			
White	3 (3.6)	0 (0)	6.8
African American	0 (0)	1 (6.3)	26.7
Hispanic	10 (55.6)	5 (33.3)	41.4

*See text for description of sources of information.

†African Americans were significantly underrepresented in the suicide group compared with the general population (z=2.59, P<.01).

‡I is the most affluent class, IV the most impoverished.

§The percentage of the ethnic group (within suicides or community controls) who fall in the particular socioeconomic status category. Thus, the percentages are calculated from the division of the cell N by the within-ethnicity/case group N, eg, 14/84=16.7% of white suicides were in socioeconomic status class I.

2-caregiver households (not necessarily the family of origin). Approximately 28% of suicide victims and 20% of control participants were living with a single parent. Of the victims who were not living with any parent (nearly 12%, in contrast to 3% of the control participants), most were living either with another relative (36%) or with a girlfriend or boyfriend or a spouse (36%).

Parent-Child Relationships. Suicide victims had significantly less frequent and less satisfying communication with their mothers (OR, 4.3 [*P*<.01]; 95% CI, 1.6-11.6) and fathers (OR, 4.0 [*P*<.001]; 95% CI, 1.8-9.0). There was no evidence of more negative interactions between victims and their parents, nor a greater history of severe physical punishment.

Table 2. Psychosocial Risks of Suicide, ORs, and CIs*

	No. (%)		
	Suicide Victims (n=120)	Community Controls (n=147)	Adjusted OR (95% CI)†
Parents' marital status			
Nonintact family of origin	58 (48.3)	49 (33.3)	1.9 (1.1-3.3)‡
Parent-child relationships§			
Poor communication with mother	15 (16.1)	10 (7.5)	4.3 (1.6-11.6)‖
Poor communication with father	24 (31.2)	15 (12.8)	4.0 (1.8-9.0)¶
Negative interaction with mother	10 (10.8)	15 (11.5)	0.7 (0.3-1.8)
Negative interaction with father	3 (4.7)	7 (6.3)	0.5 (0.1-2.9)
Severe physical punishment	3 (2.9)	5 (3.6)	1.3 (0.3-6.1)
Parental psychopathology			
Mother			
Mood disorder symptoms	34 (36.6)	30 (21.9)	2.0 (1.1-3.7)‡
Alcohol/substance problems	5 (5.4)	7 (5.1)	1.0 (0.3-3.4)
Trouble with police	2 (2.2)	2 (1.5)	2.6 (0.2-30.9)
Any psychiatric treatment	34 (36.6)	39 (28.5)	1.4 (0.8-2.6)
Father			
Mood disorder symptoms	22 (25.3)	25 (20.5)	1.2 (0.6-2.5)
Alcohol/substance problems	14 (16.1)	16 (13.1)	1.2 (0.5-2.7)
Trouble with police	16 (18.4)	8 (6.6)	4.0 (1.5-10.9)‖
Any psychiatric treatment	18 (20.7)	19 (15.6)	1.5 (0.7-3.3)
Family history of suicidal behavior	20 (17.4)	7 (4.8)	4.6 (1.8-11.7)¶
Stressful life events§			
Disciplinary crises	52 (47.7)	22 (15.5)	5.1 (2.7-9.5)¶
Loss	59 (53.6)	58 (39.7)	1.9 (1.1-3.3)‡
School/work problems			
Failed a grade	25 (25.3)	10 (8.6)	3.3 (1.4-7.7)‖
Suspended from school	16 (16.3)	3 (2.6)	6.1 (1.6-23.4)‖
Dropped out of school#	22 (18.3)	4 (2.7)	5.1 (1.2-20.7)¶
Neither working nor in school#	20 (16.8)	1 (0.7)	44.1 (4.5-432.0)¶**
No college#	37 (94.8)	18 (79.6)	7.8 (2.2-27.3)¶

*OR indicates odds ratio; CI, confidence interval. Numbers of subjects vary for particular variables because of missing data. The pattern of missing data was random. There were no differences in diagnoses, demographic variables, and the other psychosocial factors between those with and those without available data for each specific risk variable, for either cases or controls.

†Controlling for socioeconomic status, sex, ethnicity, and age.

‡P<.05.

§The dichotomously scored factors are presented; the results remained unchanged for their continuously scored counterparts.

‖P<.01.

¶P<.001.

#The analyses are restricted to those who were at risk by nature of their being past high school. The magnitude of the results remained essentially unchanged for total sample.

**The large CI results from small sample sizes. The lower bound of the 95% CI should be used as the conservative estimate of the effect size.

Parental Psychopathologic Characteristics and Family History of Suicidal Behavior. Suicide victims were significantly more likely than control participants to have had a mother with a history of mood disorder symptoms (OR, 2.0 [*P*<.05]; 95% CI, 1.0-3.7), a father with a history of trouble with the police (OR, 4.0 [$P<.01$]; 95% CI, 1.5-10.9), and a family history of suicidal behavior (OR, 4.6 [$P<.001$]; 95% CI, 1.8-11.7).

Nonfamilial Factors

Stressful Life Events. Suicide victims had experienced significantly more negative stressful life events (mean±SD, 4.2±3.0) than community control participants had (1.5±1.8) (t=8.5, $P<.001$). Nearly half of the victims had experienced a recent disciplinary crisis (OR, 5.1 [$P<.001$]; 95% CI, 2.7-9.5) or interpersonal loss (OR, 1.9 [$P<.05$]; 95% CI, 1.1-3.3). The most prevalent disciplinary crisis was suspension from school (Table 2) and appearance in juvenile court (16.1% and 2.6% of suicide victims and control participants, respectively). The majority of the losses represented a breakup with a girlfriend or boyfriend (36% and 16% of suicide victims and control participants, respectively) and a recent separation of the parents (6.2% and 0.9% of suicide victims and control participants, respectively).

School and Work Problems. Difficulties in school, neither working nor being in school, and not going to college posed significant suicide risks. The high percentage of suicide victims (17%) in contrast to control participants (0.7%) who were neither working nor in school at the time of their death (or assessment) was not explained by a disproportionate number of victims residing in residential homes or psychiatric hospitals (only 6% of those victims neither working nor in school).

GENDER INTERACTIONS

Experiencing an interpersonal loss increased the risk of suicide for boys only (OR, 2.6 [$P<.001$]; 95% CI, 1.4-4.8); otherwise, the impact of the psychosocial factors was similar for boys and girls.

ETHNIC INTERACTIONS

Disciplinary crises and failing a grade were the only psychosocial factors that interacted with ethnicity. White and African-American, but not Hispanic, youths were significantly more likely to commit suicide if they had experienced a recent disciplinary crisis (OR, 5.8 [$P<.00$]; 95% CI, 2.8-11.8 for whites; OR, 30.9 [$P<.01$]; 95% CI, 2.8-347.2 for African Americans). Given the extremely large 95% CI for African Americans (because of the small sample size), the lower bound of the CI should be considered the conservative estimate of the effect size. Failing a grade was a risk factor only for white youths (OR, 8.4 [$P<.001$]; 95% CI, 2.6-27.4).

AGE INTERACTIONS

Age modified the impact of only 1 psychosocial factor. Poor communication with the father significantly increased the risk of suicide only for those individuals older than 16 years.

INDEPENDENCE OF CONCURRENT PSYCHOPATHOLOGIC CHARACTERISTICS

The associations between each psychosocial factor and suicide after adjusting for psychiatric disorders in the youths are presented in **Table 3**. Interactions between psychosocial factors and diagnostic categories were also tested in the analyses. Poor communication with the father (for youngsters older than 16 years), the father's history of trouble with the police, a family history of suicidal behavior, disciplinary crises (for whites and African Americans), recent losses (for boys), and school or work problems significantly increased the risk of suicide above the risk contributed by the youth's psychopathology, without exhibiting any significant interactions with psychopathology.

INCREMENTAL EFFECTS ON SUICIDE RISKS

The presence of the significant psychosocial factors has an impact on suicide risk comparable with that of a psychiatric disorder (**Table 4**). The pattern of incremental effects of psychopathology and psychosocial factors is consistent with additive rather than synergistic effects.

COMMENT

Before discussing the novel findings in this study, we will review results consistent with those of earlier psychological autopsy studies. These consistencies emerged despite the use of different methods of ascertainment (eg, parent-only information and nonstandard measures of family history of suicidal behavior and parental psychopathology).

A family history of suicidal behavior greatly increased the risk of completed suicide, as reported in earlier studies.[3,7,17,19,32] This may reflect a genetic factor, rather than a general index of family chaos and psychopathology, since a family history increased suicide risk after controlling for poor parent-child relationships and parental psychopathology (OR, 5.1; 95% CI, 1.8-15.6), similar to the finding by Brent.[33] Our study cannot address whether familial aggregation results from imitation, but other studies[34] do not support this hypothesis. Previous studies have also found high rates of parental psychopathology to be associated with adolescent suicide,[19] consistent with our univariate analyses; however, once we adjusted for the presence of the youth's psychiatric illness, only paternal trouble with police maintained its significant association with youth suicide. Our examination of psychiatric *symptoms* rather than *diagnoses* may account for the inconsistency with earlier studies.

Consistent with other reports, interpersonal losses[2,9,11,13] and disciplinary crises[2,9,11-13,17] increased suicide risk, and the nature of the stressor was related to the underlying psychiatric disorder.[9,11-13] We found a tendency for interpersonal losses to be more common among suicide victims with substance abuse disorders (63% vs 48%, P=.11) and disruptive disorders (66% vs 42%, P=.01); disciplinary crises were more common in victims with disruptive disorders (56% vs 40%, P=.10).

Table 3. Psychosocial Risks of Suicide: ORs and CIs, Association Controlling for Psychiatric Disorders in Youth and Demographic Variables*

	OR (95% CI)		
	Controlling for Disruptive Disorder†	Controlling for Substance Disorder†	Controlling for Mood Disorder†
Nonintact family of origin	1.7 (1.0-3.1)	1.6 (0.9-2.9)	1.9 (1.0-3.6)‡
Parent-child relationships			
Poor communication with mother	4.1 (1.4-11.8)§	3.1 (1.0-9.7)‡	2.2 (0.7-7.4)
Poor communication with father			
Age ≤16 y	NS	NS	NS
Age >16 y	7.2 (2.4-21.8)‖	6.4 (2.1-19.5)‖	6.7 (2.2-21.0)‖
Parental psychopathology			
Mother's mood disorder symptoms	1.6 (0.9-3.0)	1.5 (0.8-2.8)	1.1 (0.6-2.3)
Father's trouble with police	4.2 (1.5-11.5)§	3.6 (1.3-10.1)§	4.2 (1.4-12.1)§
Family history of suicidal behavior	4.4 (1.6-11.6)§	4.7 (1.8-12.7)§	5.1 (1.8-14.5)§
Stressful life events			
Disciplinary crises			
White	5.3 (2.5-11.1)‖	5.3 (2.5-11.3)‖	6.0 (2.6-13.6)‖
African American	30.3 (2.5-360.3)§¶	28.5 (2.5-328.6)§¶	31.4 (2.3-425.6)§¶
Hispanic	NS	NS	NS
Loss			
Girls	NS	NS	NS
Boys	2.3 (1.3-4.4)§	2.2 (1.1-4.1)§	3.4 (1.7-6.8)‖
School/work problems			
Failed a grade			
White	7.5 (2.3-24.9)‖	8.5 (2.5-28.6)‖	7.2 (1.9-26.8)§
African American	NS	NS	NS
Hispanic	NS	NS	NS
Suspended from school	5.4 (1.4-21.1)§	5.3 (1.3-20.7)§	7.0 (1.7-28.5)§
Dropped out of school	5.5 (1.6-18.5)§	5.5 (1.6-18.8)§	6.1 (1.8-21.4)§
Neither working nor in school	22.6 (2.8-183.5)§¶	24.2 (3.0-197.6)§¶	15.3 (1.7-135.6)§¶
No college	7.0 (1.7-28.3)§	11.5 (2.3-59.1)§	9.2 (2.0-43.6)§

**OR indicates odds ratio; CI, confidence interval; NS, not significant.*
†Uses parent/caregiver-only information. Relationships are somewhat attenuated, but the significance remains when best-estimate diagnoses are employed.
‡*P*<.05.
§*P*<.01.
‖*P*<.001.
¶The large CIs result from small sample sizes. The lower bound of the 95% CI should be considered the conservative estimate of the effect size.

NOVEL ASSOCIATIONS

A "failure to communicate" with fathers has not been reported in the psychological autopsy literature but is consistent with the report that fathers' poor relationships with youngsters are more strongly related than those of mothers to suicidal ideation and attempts.[35] It is unlikely that the association of poor father-child communication with suicide reflects merely a silent depressed child or father, since its significance remained after adjusting for the youngster's psychopathology or father's psychiatric symptoms (OR, 7.4; 95% CI, 2.2-24.2 for those older than 16 years).

Youngsters who appear to be "drifting," affiliated with neither a school nor a work institution, were at substantial risk for completing suicide. Shaffer et al[1] noted that many suicides among children younger than 15 years took place after a period of absence from school and that a similar phenomenon had been reported for children who had attempted suicide,[36] suggesting that social isolation associated with absence from school may facilitate suicidal behavior.

African-American suicide victims were from families with a higher SES than that of the general population of African-American youths. Historically, while suicide has been more of a problem among whites, there has been a dramatic rise in the rate among African Americans since 1987.[37] Greater educational and employment opportunities for African Americans may have led to closer identification with the majority white culture, with the unfortunate loss of some traditional protective values among African Americans.[38] The association of SES and suicide within African-American youths is unlikely to have resulted from participation bias, since the SES of the nonparticipant African Americans, approximated by the proportion of the population within their residential zip code who received public assistance,[23] was not significantly different from a comparable macrolevel SES measure derived for participants.

We identified a sex-specific risk not heretofore reported. An interpersonal loss, such as recent romantic breakup, greatly increased the risk of suicide only for boys. "Breaking up" may leave a boy with little social support, since intimacy for boys may tend to be restricted to a single relationship with the opposite sex, whereas teenage girls may establish intimate and confiding relationships with same-sex and opposite-sex peers.[39] Furthermore, it is our clinical impression that the male suicide victims were more

Table 4. Incremental Effects of Psychosocial Factors and Diagnoses on Suicide Risk

Psychosocial Factors*	Psychiatric Diagnosis	Disruptive Disorder		Substance Disorder		Mood Disorder		Any Disruptive, Substance, or Mood Disorder	
		No.	Proportion of Suicides	No.	Proportion of Suicides	No.	Proportion of Suicides	No.	Proportion of Suicides
Absent	Absent	56	0.07	56	0.09	53	0.06	52	0.06
Absent	Present	1	1.00	1	0.00	4	0.50	5	0.40
Present	Absent	144	0.47	161	0.46	143	0.39	111	0.35
Present	Present	42	0.62	25	0.80	43	0.88	75	0.73

Any of the significant psychosocial factors given in Table 3: poor communication with father, father's trouble with police, family history of suicide, disciplinary crises, loss, failed a grade, dropped out of school, neither working nor in school, no college. Suspended from school is not included as a unique psychosocial factor because it was a component item in the measure of disciplinary crises.

likely to develop excessively dependent relationships with members of the opposite sex, making them more vulnerable to overwhelming distress when the relationship was disrupted.

The lack of affiliation with school or work, the loss of a relationship, the inability to confide and share with a father, and being a minority in an upwardly mobile home may have a common aftermath of isolating the youth. This is consistent with the large body of literature on the role of isolation and alienation in suicide.[8,40-43]

ISSUE OF OVERCONTROL

While significant differences in the frequencies of parental psychopathology, parental separation or divorce, and poor mother-child communication existed between the suicide victims and control participants, their impact was no longer significant after controlling for the youths' psychopathology. However, the mother's mood disorder symptoms (or divorce or poor communication) may contribute to the youth's mood disorder, which in turn increases suicide risk. Adolescents whose mothers had mood disorder symptoms were nearly 4 times more likely to have a mood disorder themselves (OR, 3.6; 95% CI, 1.7-7.5). Similarly, having a father who had been in trouble with the police significantly increased the likelihood of a substance disorder in the youth (OR, 4.3; 95% CI, 1.3-13.6). Adjusting for the youth's disorder (a more proximal cause of suicide than the parent's disorder) may remove the link between the parent's disorder and the youth's suicide, resulting in "overcontrol" in the analysis. Therefore, the unadjusted risk estimates (in Table 2) should not be disregarded, since they indicate the factors that may contribute more distally to the suicide and may be excellent ways to identify youths at risk.

LIMITATIONS

Since there is no psychiatric control group, the specificity of the psychosocial factors for suicide risk cannot be determined. By controlling for the youth's psychiatric disorder in the analyses, however, we have accounted for a major source of variation between a psychiatric and community control group and have provided estimates for the unique contribution of the psychosocial factors to suicide, independent of the risks imposed by psychiatric disorder.

We relied on parental-caregiver information to keep the information base comparable for victims and control participants. However, it is generally recognized that there is only modest consistency of reports between adolescents and their parents.[44,45] Although we have obtained only a partial psychosocial history of the youths, the information is recognizable by the parents and could be used for suicide prevention efforts. Furthermore, the relationships remained largely unchanged whether best-estimate diagnoses or parent-only diagnoses were used. Given this consistency, we feel confident that the results are valid.

There was a substantial proportion of missing data in our assessment of father-child (27%) and mother-child (15%) relationships. The primary reason for missing these data (and other psychosocial variables; Table 2) was that several questions that assessed psychosocial domains were added later in the study or changed during the course of the study so that the final set of constructs was not available for the full sample. No systematic bias was evident in the available psychosocial data, since there were no diagnostic, demographic, or psychosocial differences between those with and those without the assessments.

Our reliance on mothers' reports of father-child relationships could reflect the mothers' *perception* of paternal nonavailability, rather than a real problem between father and child. However, when we limited the examination of poor paternal communication to the subsample with fathers' self-reports, its significance remained. The low reliability of the mother-child communication measure may have contributed to its lack of significance.

The limitation of retrospective attribution of significance and denial or forgetting by parents is inherent to all psychological autopsy studies.[21,22] We found no evidence that the time lag between the suicide and the informant interview was correlated with total number of negative events, loss, disciplinary crises, or the youths' severity of psychopathology. Denial does not appear to explain the lack of an association of suicide with severe physical punishment. Of the 5 community-control parents who reported using severe physical punishment, none of their children reported this type of punishment. Additionally, there were no cases in which parents failed to report severe physical punishment reported by the child.

While the absence of underreporting by control parents was reassuring, there is no certainty that the parents of a child who has committed suicide would respond in a similar way.

IMPLICATIONS

The present findings increase our understanding of suicidal behavior as a multidetermined act. The effect size of the psychosocial factors is of a magnitude comparable with that previously reported for psychiatric disorders.[1-3] It is apparent that the psychosocial characteristics of teenagers, as well as their diagnostic profiles, are a necessary component of a suicide risk assessment. The impact of psychosocial factors on suicide is not merely an epiphenomenon of psychiatric illness.

Accepted for publication April 22, 1996.

This work was made possible by William T. Grant Foundation Faculty Scholars Award 84-0954-84, National Institute of Mental Health Research Training Grant T32 MH16434, National Institute of Mental Health Research Grant MH 38198-05A2, and National Institute of Mental Health Center Grant MH 43878-A1 for the Center to Study Youth Depression, Anxiety, and Suicide, Columbia University, New York, NY.

Presented in part at the Fourth Annual Meeting on the Society for Research in Child and Adolescent Psychopathology, Sarasota, Fla, February 7, 1992.

We acknowledge the assistance of the following medical examiners: Catherine Galvin, MD, Robert Goode, MD, Elliot Gross, MD, Charles S. Hirsh, MD, Millard J. Hyland, MD, Leslie Lukash, MD, Sigmund M. Menchel, MD, John M. Zarcone, MD, and Fredierick Zugibe, MD.

Reprints: Madelyn S. Gould, PhD, MPH, 722 W 168th St, New York, NY 10032.

REFERENCES

1. Shaffer D, Gould MS, Fisher P, Trautman P, Moreau D, Kleinman M, Flory M. Psychiatric diagnosis in child and adolescent suicide. *Arch Gen Psychiatry.* 1996;53:339-348.
2. Brent DA, Perper JA, Moritz G, Allan C, Friend A, Roth BS, Schweers J, Balach L, Baugher M. Psychiatric risk factors for adolescent suicide: a case control study. *J Am Acad Child Adolesc Psychiatry.* 1993;32:521-529.
3. Brent DA, Perper JA, Goldstein CE, Kilko DJ, Allan MJ, Allman CJ, Zelenak JP. Risk factors for adolescent suicide: a comparison of adolescent suicide victims with suicidal inpatients. *Arch Gen Psychiatry.* 1988;45:581-588.
4. Marttunen MJ, Aro HM, Henriksson MM, Lonnqvist JK. Mental disorders in adolescent suicide. *Arch Gen Psychiatry.* 1991;48:834-839.
5. Rich CL, Young D, Fowler MD. San Diego Suicide Study, I: young vs old subjects. *Arch Gen Psychiatry.* 1986;45;577-582.
6. Runeson B. Mental disorder in youth suicide: *DSM-III-R* axes I and II. *Acta Psychiatr Scand.* 1989;79:490-497.
7. Shafii M, Carrigan S, Whittinghill JR, Derrick A. Psychological autopsy of completed suicide in children and adolescents. *Am J Psychiatry.* 1985;142:1061-1064.
8. Adams KS. Environment, psychosocial, and psychoanalytic aspects of suicidal behavior. In: Blumenthal SJ, Kupfer DJ, eds. *Suicide Over the Life Cycle.* Washington, DC: American Psychiatric Press; 1990:39-96.
9. Brent DA, Perper JA, Moritz G, Baugher M, Roth C, Balach L, Schweers J. Stressful life events, psychopathology and adolescent suicide: a case control study. *Suicide Life Threat Behav.* 1993;23:179-187.
10. Marttunen MJ, Aro HM, Lonnqvist JK. Precipitant stressors in adolescent suicide. *J Am Acad Child Adolesc Psychiatry.* 1993;32:1178-1183.
11. Rich CL, Fowler RC, Fogarty LA, Young D. San Diego Suicide Study, III: relationships between diagnoses and stressors. *Arch Gen Psychiatry.* 1988;45:589-592.
12. Runeson B. Psychoactive substance use disorder in youth suicide. *Alcohol Alcohol.* 1990;25:561-568.
13. Marttunen MJ, Aro HM, Henrikksson MM, Lonnqvist JK. Psychosocial stressors more common in adolescent suicides with alcohol abuse compared with depressive adolescent suicides. *J Am Acad Child Adolesc Psychiatry.* 1994;33:490-497.
14. Graham C, Burvill PW. A study of coroner's records of suicide in young people, 1986-88 in Western Australia. *Aust N Z J Psychiatry.* 1992;26:30-39.
15. Hoberman HM, Garfinkel BD. Completed suicide in children and adolescents. *J Am Acad Child Adolesc Psychiatry.* 1988;27:689-695.
16. Poteet DJ. Adolescent suicide: a review of 87 cases of completed suicide in Shelby County, Tennessee. *Am J Forensic Med Pathol.* 1987;8:12-17.
17. Shaffer D. Suicide in childhood and early adolescence. *J Child Psychol Psychiatry.* 1974;15:275-291.
18. Thompson TR. Childhood and adolescent suicide in Manitoba. *Can J Psychiatry.* 1987;32:264-269.
19. Brent DA, Perper JA, Moritz G, Liotus L, Schweers J, Balach L, Roth C. Familial risk factors for adolescent suicide: a case-control study. *Acta Psychiatr Scand.* 1994;89:52-58.
20. Dizmang LH, Watson J, May PA, Bopp J. Adolescent suicide at an Indian reservation. *Am J Orthopsychiatry.* 1974;44:43-49.
21. Beskow J, Runeson B, Asgard U. Psychological autopsies: methods and ethics. *Suicide Life Threat Behav.* 1990;20:307-323.
22. Brent DA, Perper JA, Kolko DJ, Zelenak JP. The psychological autopsy: methodological considerations for the study of adolescent suicide. *J Am Acad Child Adolesc Psychiatry.* 1988;27:362-366.
23. *1980 Census of Population, Volume I: Characteristics of the Population, Chapter B. General Population Characteristics.* Washington, DC: US Bureau of the Census; 1980. Part 8, Table 45, p 200, PC80-1-B8; part 32, Table 45, p 405, PC80-1-B32; part 34, Table 45, p 595, PC80-1-B34.
24. Hollingshead AB. *Four Factor Index of Social Status.* New Haven, Conn: Yale University; 1975.
25. Coddington RD. The significance of life events as etiologic factors in the diseases of children, I: a survey of professional workers. *J Psychosom Res.* 1972;16:7-18.
26. Coddington RD. The significance of life events as etiologic factors in the diseases of children, II: a study of a normal population. *J Psychosom Res.* 1972;16:205-213.
27. Endicott J, Spitzer RL. A diagnostic interview: the Schedule for Affective Disorders and Schizophrenia. *Arch Gen Psychiatry.* 1978;35:837-844.
28. Chambers WJ, Puig-Antich J, Hirsch M, Paez P, Ambrosini PJ, Tabrizi MA, Davies M. The assessment of affective disorders in children and adolescents by semi-structured interview: test-retest reliability of the Schedule for Affective Disorders and Schizophrenia for School Age Children, Present Episode Version. *Arch Gen Psychiatry.* 1985;42:696-702.
29. Wing JK, Cooper JE, Sartorius M. *The Measurement and Classification of Psychiatric Symptoms: An Instruction Manual for the Present State Examination and CATEGO Programme.* Cambridge, England: Cambridge University Press; 1974.
30. Hosmer DW, Lemeshow S. *Applied Logic Regression.* New York, NY: John Wiley & Sons Inc; 1989.
31. Kelsey JL, Thompson WD, Evans AS. *Methods in Observational Epidemiology.* New York, NY: Oxford University Press; 1986.
32. Brent DA, Perper JA. Research in adolescent suicide: implications for training, service delivery, and public policy. *Suicide Life Threat Behav.* 1995;25:222-230.
33. Brent DA. Familial factors in suicide and suicidal behavior. *Lifesavers Q Newslett Am Suicide Found.* 1996;8:2-3.
34. Schulsinger F. Biological psychopathology. *Annu Rev Psychol.* 1980;31:583-606.
35. Tousignant M, Bastien MF, Hamel S. Suicidal attempts and ideations among adolescents and young adults: the contribution of the father's and mother's care and of parental separation. *Soc Psychiatry Psychiatr Epidemiol.* 1993;28:256-261.
36. Teicher JD, Jacobs J. Adolescents who attempt suicide. *Am J Psychiatry.* 1966;122:1248-1257.
37. Shaffer D, Gould M, Hicks R. Worsening suicide rate in black teenagers. *Am J Psychiatry.* 1994;151:1810-1812.
38. Shaffer D, Fisher P. The epidemiology of suicide in children and young adolescents. *J Am Acad Child Psychiatry.* 1981;20:545-565.
39. Lagerspetz KMJ, Bjorkqvist K, Peltonen T. Is indirect aggression typical of females? gender differences in aggressiveness in 11- to 12-year-old children. *Aggress Behav.* 1988;14:403-414.
40. Durkheim E. *Suicide: A Study in Sociology.* London, England: Routledge & Kegan Paul; 1952.
41. Maris R. *Pathways to Suicide: A Survey of Self-Destructive Behaviors.* Baltimore, Md: Johns Hopkins University Press; 1981.
42. Maris R. *Social Forces in Urban Suicide.* Homewood, Ill: Dorsey Press; 1969.
43. Trout DL. The role of social isolation in suicide. *Suicide Life Threat Behav.* 1980;10:10-23.
44. Canino G, Bird HR, Rubio-Stipec M, Bravo M. Child psychiatric epidemiology: what we have learned and what we need to learn. *Int J Methods Psychiatr Epidemiol.* 1995;5:1-14.
45. Gould MS, Shaffer D. Epidemiology and child psychiatry. In: Michels R, Cooper AM, Guze SB, Judd LL, Klerman GL, Solnit AJ, Stunkard AJ, eds. *Psychiatry.* Revised edition. New York, NY: JB Lippincott Co; 1991:1-24.

Studies of Ventricular Enlargement

In the September 1995 issue of the ARCHIVES, Elkis et al[1] conclude their meta-analysis of ventricular enlargement in patients with mood disorders with the statement that the statistical power of meta-analysis has allowed them to uncover significant evidence for a greater degree of ventricular enlargement in patients with schizophrenia compared with patients with mood disorders.

However, their emphasis on the small *P* value associated with the finding may be misplaced, as they neglect to discuss in detail the associated importance of their fail-safe N=10 value for their comparison of 11 studies, which were pooled to provide an effect size of 0.2.

It may be worth recalling the importance of the fail-safe N statistic given that Elkis et al actually calculate this value but then fail to fully interpret it. The *fail-safe N* may be defined as the number of new, unpublished or unretrieved, nonsignificant "null-result" studies that, on average, would lower the significance of a meta-analysis to some specified level (eg, to a level that is barely significant or nonsignificant) or alternatively reduce the effect size to a negligible value.[2]

Hence, the statistic indicates the stability of meta-analytic results to the inclusion of additional findings, regardless of their source, unpublished or unretrieved. The need for this calculation arose after realization of a problem that plagued meta-analysis: journals often are filled with the 5% of studies that show type I errors, while the file drawers at the laboratory are filled with the 95% of studies that show nonsignificant results.[2]

The interpretative usefulness of the fail-safe N is analogous in some ways to the confidence interval. In the absence of further information, the best estimate of the true effect size is the mean of the observed values, but the fail-safe N aids in the assessment of the degree of confidence that can be placed in a particular meta-analytic result.

If the fail-safe N is small in comparison with the number of studies in the meta-analysis, then only tenuous conclusions should be drawn, regardless of the magnitude of the effect size or the *P* value. In this context, the 0.2 effect size of Elkis et al was already small. Rosenthal[2] suggests that the ratio of the fail-safe N to the number of studies in the meta-analysis would lead to the calculation of a minimum fail-safe N of 65 for the meta-analysis of Elkis et al. This means that if Elkis et al want to be truly confident about the stability of the result of their meta-analysis concerning the comparison of ventricular enlargement in patients with schizophrenia with patients with mood disorders, a fail-safe N result of at least 65 would be required for their meta-analysis. Because the fail-safe N was only 10 in the meta-analysis by Elkis et al and because this value is so much lower than the necessary value of 65, it would seem that the probable stability of the finding of greater ventricular enlargement in patients with schizophrenia compared with patients with mood disorders will be low in the face of new or undiscovered evidence.

Elkis et al defend their finding against this criticism by drawing attention to the funnel plot they created for their meta-analysis; they note that this plot produces no clear evidence of publication bias, as studies with small N values were published with small positive and negative effect sizes. However, the funnel plot relies on visual inspection, which, particularly when only a few studies are involved, is likely to be a less reliable method for determining the robustness of a finding than relying on the fail-safe N value.[3]

This is because the fail-safe N value of 10 tells us that it would take only 10 unpublished or unretrieved negative or null-result studies to reduce the effect size that Elkis et al found to less than 0.1, which is basically a negligible effect size. The likelihood that 10 such studies already exist, or will soon be part of the literature, cannot be low given that only 11 studies were included in the meta-analysis. Because it is assumed that published studies tend to report greater effect sizes than unpublished studies,[4] the already low average effect size in the meta-analysis by Elkis et al is a cause for some concern.

However, Elkis et al are correct to note that meta-analysis has the power to detect small effects, where large sample sizes are needed to find such effects. However, the neglect of Elkis et al in calculating their fail-safe N value teaches a more sobering lesson. A few studies that are slightly significant, even when their combined *P* value is significant, may well be misleading because only a few unpublished, or yet to be published, studies could change the combined significant result to a nonsignificant result.

Rajendra Persaud, MSc, MPhil, MD, MRCPsych
Croyden Mental Health Services
Warlingham Park Hospital
London, England

1. Elkis H, Friedman L, Wise A, Meltzer H. Meta-analysis of studies of ventricular enlargement and cortical sulcal prominence in mood disorders. *Arch Gen Psychiatry*. 1995;52:735-746.
2. Rosenthal R. The file drawer problem and tolerance for null results. *Psychol Bull*. 1979;86:638-641.
3. Perry A, Persaud R. Misleading meta-analysis. *BMJ*. 1995;310:1604.
4. Shadish WR, Dohery M, Montgomery LM. How many studies are in the file drawer? an estimate from the family/marital psychotherapy literature. *Clin Psychol Rev*. 1989;9:589-603.

In reply

The critique by Persaud of our meta-analysis[1] is based on the following 2 contentions: (1) There is a generally accepted quantitative criterion for the fail-safe N (N_{fs}) and (2) the quantitative criterion of Rosenthal[2]—a criterion that would require us to achieve an N_{fs} equal to 65—is a reasonable criterion to apply to our meta-analysis. In our opinion, both contentions are refutable.

One point that needs to be made before we proceed is that several types of meta-analysis exist. Rosenthal discusses N_{fs} in the context of a "combined significance" meta-analysis, whereas we conducted an "effect size" meta-analysis.[3] (See the book by Hedges and Olkin[3] for a critique of the combined significance approach and a defense of the effect size approach.) Separate formulas for the calculation of N_{fs} are required for these 2 types of meta-analysis. This is not debatable. What is debatable is the method of interpretation of the resulting N_{fs}. Rosenthal suggests a "rough and ready guide" based on the number of studies (ie, k) in the meta-analysis (ie, 5k+10). In our case, with 11 studies in the meta-analysis in question (meta-analysis 3, comparison of the ventricular enlargement between patients with affective disorders and patients with schizophrenia), the resulting criterion is 65. It is the reification of this rough and ready guide that has led Persaud astray.

It is perhaps best to begin with the words Rosenthal uses to introduce his criterion:

> *At the present time no firm guidelines can be given as to what constitutes an unlikely number of unretrieved or unpublished studies. For some areas of research 100 or even 500 unpublished and unretrieved studies may be a plausible state of affairs, whereas for others even 10 or 20 seems unlikely.[2]*

More recently, Iyengar and Greenhouse have noted that Rosenthal's criterion is seldom used:

> *Rosenthal has provided a rough guide to help decide what is an unlikely number of studies in the file drawers, but this guide does not seem to be used, due to its ad hoc nature. Instead, in practice the fail-safe sample size is often used subjectively, relying upon one's knowledge of the field in question to assess the magnitude of the file drawer problem.[4]*

In our meta-analysis,[1] we computed N_{fs} according to the formula provided by Orwin.[5] This formula, which is subsequently detailed, provides for the calculation of N_{fs} in the context of an effect size meta-analysis. In discussing the interpretation of his N_{fs} calculation, Orwin comments on the absence of a statistical model: "A shortcoming of this [Orwin's fail-safe N statistic], as well as Rosenthal's fail-safe N is the absence of a statistical model."[5] Part of the difficulty results from the fact that, by definition, little or nothing is known regarding the hypothesized set of unpublished or unobserved studies. It is for these reasons that the N_{fs} is typically interpreted heuristically and informally. In other words, one makes a judgment about the likelihood that x or more unpublished studies with null effects exist.

A second, very compelling reason to reject the criterion of Rosenthal relates to the relationship between his criterion and effect size. We agree with Persaud that meta-analysis has the power to detect small effect sizes. Apparently, Persaud is unaware that the criterion of Rosenthal is mathematically inconsistent with the detection of a small effect size. Before we proceed to document this mathematical inconsistency, several terms need to be defined:

- Effect size. *The difference between 2 sample means divided by the pooled SD.*
- Small effect size.[6] *0.2.*
- Moderate effect size.[6] *0.5.*
- Large effect size.[6] *0.8.*
- N_{fs}. *Fail-safe N or the number of studies required to reduce the overall effect size to a negligible level.*
- d_c. *A mean effect size that corresponds to the negligible level previously mentioned (in our case, this level was 0.1).*
- d_o. *The mean effect size obtained in a meta-analysis.[5]*
- d_{fs}. *The hypothetical mean effect size of the unpublished studies (usually set to 0.0).*
- k. *The number of studies in the meta-analysis.*

With these symbols defined, 2 formulas need to be established:

(1) 5k+10, which is the formula for the criterion value for N_{fs}, per Rosenthal.

(2) $N_{fs}=k(d_o-d_c)/(d_c-d_{fs})$, which is the equation from Orwin for the computation of N_{fs} in the context of an effect size meta-analysis.

If we set $d_c=0.1$ (a reasonable target negligible effect size) and $d_{fs}=0.0$ (the conventional level), then we can ask the question: Under what circumstances would the application of the N_{fs} formula of Orwin yield an N_{fs} that would exactly satisfy the criterion of Rosenthal? This question can be answered if we set $5k+10=k(d_o-d_c)/(d_c-d_{fs})$; with substitution, $5k+10=k(d_o-0.1)/(0.1)$; and solve for d_o, $d_o=0.6+(1/k)$.

This is the formula we need to document the inconsistency between the criterion of Rosenthal and a meta-analysis with a small composite effect size. With a small k value (number of studies), d_o is greater than 0.6. As k increases, d_o approaches 0.6. In no event can d_o ever be less than 0.6. In other words, for the N_{fs} formula of Orwin to produce an N_{fs} that satisfies the criterion of Rosenthal, the observed effect size must be at least 0.6 (ie, moderate to large). Thus, it is impossible for one to achieve an N_{fs} that meets the criterion of Rosenthal with an effect size less than 0.6.

If we start with a small effect size as a given (ie, $d_o=0.2$), the N_{fs} of Orwin is as follows: $N_{fs}=k(0.2-0.1)/(0.1)$, or $N_{fs}=k$.

In other words, when the effect size is small, N_{fs} equals k, the number of studies in the meta-analysis. In this case, because N_{fs} equals k, N_{fs} can never equal 5k+10. Thus, it is mathematically impossible for a meta-analysis to yield a small effect size and to produce an N_{fs} that meets the criterion of Rosenthal. Therefore, either meta-analyses cannot be used to establish small effect sizes or the criterion of Rosenthal is an inappropriate standard. Since there is no doubt that meta-analysis can be used to establish small effects, the criterion of Rosenthal is an inappropriate standard.

Other grounds support our view that publication bias is not a concern in the interpretation of our meta-analysis 3. Recall that publication bias occurs when researchers only publish statistically significant results, whereas statistically nonsignificant results remain unpublished. If one has strong, a priori evidence that such a bias does not exist in a par-

ticular literature, the entire issue of N_{fs} and its interpretation is irrelevant. In the present case, of the 11 published studies included in our meta-analysis 3, not a single study reported a statistically significant result. In other words, no evidence of publication bias is present in this literature.

There is yet another reason to accept our finding that patients with schizophrenia have slightly larger ventricles than patients with affective disorders. The effect size we report for the difference between patients with affective disorders and control subjects on ventricular enlargement is approximately 0.44. The effect size for the difference between patients with schizophrenia and control subjects reported by Raz and Raz[7] is approximately 0.7. Given these findings, one would expect an effect size between patients with affective disorders and those with schizophrenia to be approximately 0.26. We reported an effect size of 0.21.

Thus, our finding that patients with affective disorders have smaller ventricles than patients with schizophrenia is not likely to be due to publication bias and is entirely consistent with other meta-analytic results. Nevertheless, more primary-level studies are warranted. Furthermore, if primary-level studies are to have sufficient statistical power (0.8) to detect this small effect size, the number of included subjects will have to be much larger (ie, N=310 per group, assuming an effect size of 0.2, 1-tailed test, P<.05) than used in the previous studies (ie, an average of N=45 per group).

Lee Friedman, PhD
John A. Jesberger
Herbert Y. Meltzer, MD
Department of Psychiatry
School of Medicine
Case Western Reserve University
10900 Euclid Ave
Cleveland, OH 44106

Helio Elkis, MD, PhD
São Paulo, Brazil

1. Elkis H, Friedman L, Wise A, Meltzer HY. Meta-analysis of studies of global structural abnormalities in affective disorders and schizophrenia. *Arch Gen Psychiatry*. 1995;52:735-746.
2. Rosenthal R. The 'file drawer problem' and tolerance for null results. *Psychol Bull*. 1979;86:638-641.
3. Hedges LV, Olkin I. *Statistical Methods for Meta-Analysis*. San Diego, Calif: Academic Press Inc; 1985.
4. Iyengar S, Greenhouse JB. Selection models and the file drawer problem. *Stat Sci*. 1988;3:109-135.
5. Orwin RG. A fail-safe N for effect size. *J Educ Stat*. 1983;8:157-159.
6. Cohen J. *Statistical Power Analysis for the Behavioural Sciences*. 2nd ed. Hillsdale, NJ: Lawrence Erlbaum Associates; 1988.
7. Raz S, Raz N. Structural abnormalities in major psychosis: a quantitative review of the evidences from computerized images. *Psychol Bull*. 1990;108:93-108.

The Relationship Between Plasma Haloperidol Concentrations and Clinical Results

The article by Volavka et al[1] in the October 1995 issue of the ARCHIVES supports the existence of an upper limit of haloperidol plasma concentrations of approximately 12 ng/mL for the treatment of patients with acutely exacerbated schizophrenia.

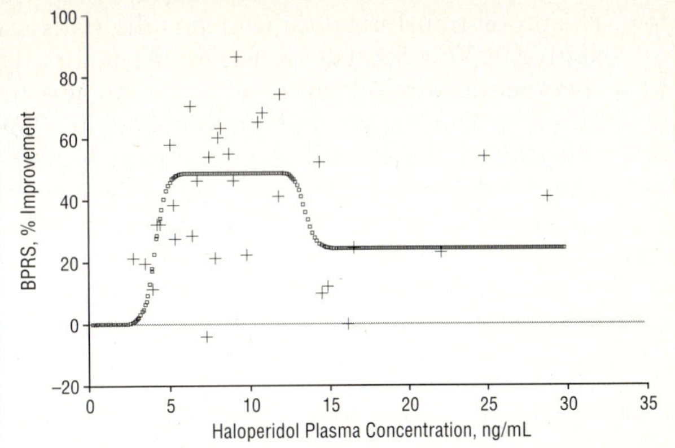

The relationship between the concentrations of haloperidol in the plasma and the change in the Brief Psychiatric Rating Scale (BPRS) total score in 32 patients. A nonlinear regression model was used for the curvilinear relationship (pseudo R^2=.79, P<.01). The optimal range estimated was from 4.6 to 14.4 ng/mL.

Volavka et al[1] do not report a clear lower limit for the antipsychotic activity of plasma concentrations of haloperidol. The authors suggest that a "continuous increase of antipsychotic activity from levels close to 0 to approximately 12 ng/mL" exists.[1] However, the definition of a minimum haloperidol plasma concentration for a meaningful antipsychotic effect may have clinical relevance. The reanalysis of their data using the lower limit found in our study[2] showed that while only 54.8% of the patients with plasma concentrations less than 5.5 ng/mL were considered improved, the value for patients with concentrations greater than that limit was 82.6% (χ^2=4.58, *P*<.05). Other studies have found similar threshold concentrations.[3-5] Furthermore, this is consistent with the finding that an antipsychotic effect occurs when D_2 dopamine-receptor occupancy reaches approximately 65% to 75%.[6,7]

We report the results of a larger sample of our study[2] and compare our design and findings with those of Volavka et al,[1] as we think our comments may be relevant for the interpretation of the results.

In our study, we randomized 32 patients with acutely exacerbated schizophrenia (*DSM-III-R* criteria) to 3 fixed haloperidol dose groups (ie, 10, 20, and 30 mg). The 3 doses were decided on to obtain a range of plasma concentrations. Patients were observed for 3 weeks using a double-blind design; the Brief Psychiatric Rating Scale (BPRS),[8] the Scale for the Assessment of Negative Symptoms, the Scale for the Assessment of Positive Symptoms,[9,10] and the Simpson-Angus Scale for Rating Extrapyramidal Side Effects[11] were used for evaluation. We found an optimal response range close to the one we had obtained previously (ie, 4.6-14.4 ng/mL) (**Figure**). The therapeutic effect of concentrations less than 4.6 ng/mL was small, and improvement decreased at concentrations greater than 14.4 ng/mL. The results of our study differ from the findings of Volavka et al[1] in some aspects.

First, in our study improvement is measured by the total BPRS score, which includes positive and negative symptoms. In the study by Volavka et al,[1] the analysis is independent for the 2 types of symptoms. It would be interesting to know if an analysis using the total BPRS score as the outcome measure would produce different results or support the existence of a therapeutic window. The probit transformation, which is the statistical method used by Volavka et al,[1] is inappropriate for finding a therapeutic window, and we would suggest the model used by Van Putten et al[5] and Palao et al.[2] This model also accounts for a different treatment response for positive and negative symptoms, as we believe the analysis should combine both. Despite these differences, the conclusions agree in the fundamental aspects; when the haloperidol plasma concentration is greater than a certain limit, the antipsychotic treatment may increase negative symptoms while positive symptoms do not improve further. This finding is supported by the results of the crossover in period 3 of the study[1]; the negative symptoms of patients whose conditions do not improve when plasma concentrations are approximately 10 ng/mL decrease when haloperidol plasma concentrations are decreased.

Second, the patients studied by Volavka et al[1] are mostly patients with chronic schizophrenia who have been in the hospital on many occasions. This explains the small magnitude of improvement and the election of only a 20% decrease in the BPRS score as a cutoff point to separate patients who respond to treatment from those who do not respond to the treatment. It can be argued that the small rate of the improvement decreases the possibility of finding notable results. The 20% improvement criterion had been used in studies of patients who were treatment resistant[12] or who had chronic schizophrenia[13] but had not been used for patients with acutely exacerbated schizophrenia. For those patients, a cutoff point of 40%,[14-16] which has a greater clinical significance, has been proposed. For example, in their previous work, Volavka et al[17] used a 50% decrease in the total BPRS score as the cutoff point for a response. In that study,[17] they probably failed to find a clinically meaningful relationship between plasma concentrations of haloperidol and symptomatic improvement because it was based on plasma ranges that were too high. As noted,[2] this also occurred in other previous studies.[18-22]

The existence of an optimal haloperidol plasma concentration range should not be strictly considered. Most authors define it as a range for guidance that is associated with the maximum therapeutic effect for positive and negative symptoms, with minimum side effects.[2-5] The study by Volavka et al[1] does not contradict these conclusions if our considerations are taken into account.

Diego J. Palao, MD
Centre de Salut Mental-Hospital General de Mollet
Cristobal Colon, 1
08100-Mollet
Barcelona
Spain

Alberte Araúxo, MD
Josep M. Haro, MD
Mercé Brunet, MD
Miguel Bernardo, PhD
Barcelona, Spain

1. Volavka J, Cooper T, Czabor P, Meisner M. Plasma haloperidol levels and clinical effects in schizophrenia and schizoaffective disorder. *Arch Gen Psychiatry.* 1995;52:837-845.
2. Palao DJ, Araúxo A, Brunet M, Bernardo M, Haro JM, Ferrer J, González-Monclús E. Haloperidol: therapeutic window in schizophrenia. *J Clin Psychopharmacol.* 1994;14:302-310.
3. Mavroidis ML, Kanter DR, Hirschowitz J, Garver DL. Clinical response and plasma haloperidol levels in schizophrenia. *Psychopharmacology.* 1983;81:354-356.
4. Potkin SG, Shen Y, Zou D, Pardes H, Shu L, Phelps B, Poland R. Does a therapeutic window for plasma haloperidol exist? preliminary chinese data. *Psychopharmacol Bull.* 1985;21:59-61.
5. Van Putten T, Marder SR, Mintz J, Poland RE. Haloperidol plasma levels and clinical response: a therapeutic window relationship. *Am J Psychiatry.* 1992;149:500-505.
6. Farde L, Nordström AL, Wiesel FA, Pauli S, Halldin C, Sedvall G. Positron emission tomographic analysis of central D_1 and D_2 dopamine receptor occupancy in patients treated with classical neuroleptics and clozapine: relation to extrapyramidal side effects. *Arch Gen Psychiatry.* 1992;49:538-544.
7. Nordström AL, Farde L, Wiesel FA, Forslund K, Pauli S, Halldin C, Uppfeldt G. Central D_2-dopamine receptor occupancy in relation to antipsychotic effects: a double-blind PET study of schizophrenic patients. *Biol Psychiatry.* 1993;33:227-235.
8. Overall JE, Gorhamm DR. The brief psychiatric rating scale. *Psychol Rep.* 1962;10:799-812.
9. Andreasen NC, Olsen S. Negative vs positive schizophrenia: definition and validation. *Arch Gen Psychiatry.* 1982;39:789-794.
10. Andreasen NC. Negative symptoms in schizophrenia: definition and reability. *Arch Gen Psychiatry.* 1982;39:784-788.
11. Simpson GM, Angus JWS. A rating scale for extrapyramidal side effects. *Acta Psychiatr Scand.* 1970;212(suppl):11-19.
12. Kane JM, Honigfeld D, Singer J, Meltzer H, the Clozaril Collaborative Study Group. Clozapine for the treatment-resistant schizophrenic. *Arch Gen Psychiatry.* 1988;45:789-796.
13. Marder SR, Meibach RC. Risperidone in the treatment of schizophrenia. *Am J Psychiatry.* 1994;151:825-835.
14. Perry PJ, Pfohl BM, Kelly MW. The relationship of haloperidol concentrations to therapeutic response. *J Clin Psychopharmacol.* 1988;8:38-43.
15. Magliozzi JR, Hollister LE, Arnold KV, Earle GM. Relationship of serum haloperidol levels to clinical response in schizophrenic patients. *Am J Psychiatry.* 1981;138:365-367.
16. Santos JL, Cabranes JA, Almoguera I, Ramos JA, Vazquez C, Angeles F. Clinical implications of determination of plasma haloperidol levels. *Acta Psychiatr Scand.* 1989;79:348-354.
17. Volavka J, Cooper T, Czabor P, Bitter I, Meisner M, Laska E, Gastanaga P, Krakowski M, Chou JCY, Crowner M, Douyon R. Haloperidol blood levels and clinical effects. *Arch Gen Psychiatry.* 1992;49:354-361.
18. Rimon R, Avebuch I, Rozick P, Fijman-Danilovich L, Kara T, Dansberg H, Ebstein RP, Belmader R. Serum and CSF levels of haloperidol by radioimmunoassay and radioreceptor assay during high dose therapy of resistant schizophrenic patients. *Psychopharmacology.* 1981;73:197-199.
19. Bigelow LB, Kirch DG, Braun T, Korpi ER, Wagner RL. Absence of relationship of serum haloperidol concentration and clinical response in chronic schizophrenia: a fixed-dose study. *Psychopharmacol Bull.* 1985;21:66-68.
20. Linkowski P, Hubain P, von Frenckell R, Mendelewick J. Haloperidol plasma levels and clinical response in paranoid schizophrenics. *Eur Arch Psychiatry Neurol Sci.* 1984;234:231-236.
21. Rifkin A, Doddi SR, Karajgi B, Borenstein M, Wachspress M. Dosage of haloperidol for schizophrenia. *Arch Gen Psychiatry.* 1991;48:166-170.
22. Doddi S, Rifkin A, Karajgi B, Cooper T, Borestein M. Blood levels of haloperidol and clinical outcome in schizophrenia. *J Clin Psychopharmacol.* 1994;14:187-195.

In reply

Palao et al believe that a "clear lower limit for the antipsychotic activity of plasma concentrations of haloperidol" exists and that this limit may be found in our data with appropriate analyses. They support this contention by a χ^2 test using our data; our patients with plasma concentrations of haloperidol lower than the alleged lower limit or threshold (ie, 5.5 ng/mL) were less likely to improve than those with plasma concentrations greater than this limit. We computed essentially the same χ^2 statistic and obtained a similar result,[1(p842)] but it did not occur to us that this finding would necessarily imply the existence of a threshold. Why should it? This is a surprising inference.

Palao et al believe that the existence of a threshold is "consistent with the finding that an antipsychotic effect occurs when D_2 dopamine receptor occupancy reaches ap-

proximately 65% to 75%." However, an article that they cite describes 6 patients whose haloperidol plasma concentrations were available; 5 of them reached these occupancy levels at plasma concentrations of haloperidol less than 5.5 ng/mL[2(p539)] (ie, less than the threshold published by Palao et al[3]). Thus, if D_2 dopamine receptor occupancy is important for the antipsychotic effect, the findings of Farde et al[2] are inconsistent with the notion of a 5.5-ng/mL threshold.

Palao et al found a curvilinear relationship between plasma concentrations of haloperidol and the BPRS percentage of improvement (Figure). That curvilinear relationship, they believe, demonstrates the existence of the plasma concentration threshold. Their fitted curve rises continuously from approximately 2 ng/mL to approximately 5 ng/mL of haloperidol in plasma; it flattens out between approximately 5 and 12 ng/mL, and then it turns down and flattens out. But there seem to be only 4 patients with haloperidol plasma concentrations lower than their stated threshold; this number may be too low for a reliable estimate of treatment effectiveness.

Given that most authors agree that raising the plasma concentrations to greater than 12 or 14 ng/mL does not increase the antipsychotic efficacy, and considering the increasing side effects at higher plasma concentrations, the relevant question is as follows: How low can one go with the plasma concentration without losing a notable amount of antipsychotic activity? This question is most directly addressed by limiting the study to the range of plasma concentrations lower than 12 (or 14) ng/mL. The inclusion of higher concentrations will result in a distortion of the relationship that we want to study.

Imagine that all data points greater than 12 ng/mL depicted in the Figure are censored. If that is done, the fitted curve will likely show an increase of antipsychotic activity from concentrations close to 2 to 12 ng/mL. We think that the fitted curve will show no notable discontinuity that would suggest a threshold.

This exercise demonstrates the obvious: the inclusion of patients with high plasma concentrations of haloperidol affects the shape of the fitted curve across the entire spectrum of concentrations. But we have already agreed that concentrations greater than 12 (or 14) ng/mL should be avoided; thus, the part of the curve that fits the points above these concentrations brings little new information.

We believe that neither our data nor the data of Palao et al support the existence of a minimum haloperidol plasma concentration for a meaningful antipsychotic effect. We agree with Palao et al that defining such a concentration may be clinically important. However, determining that concentration based on existing data is impossible.

Jan Volavka, MD, PhD
Thomas B. Cooper, MA
Pal Czobor, PhD
Morris Meisner, PhD
Nathan Kline Institute
140 Old Orangeburg Rd
Orangeburg, NY 10962

1. Volavka J, Cooper TB, Czobor P, Meisner M. Plasma haloperidol levels and clinical effects in schizophrenia and schizoaffective disorder. *Arch Gen Psychiatry.* 1995;52:837-845.
2. Farde L, Nordstrom AL, Wiesel FA, Pauli S, Halldin C, Sedvall G. Positron emission tomographic analysis of central D_1 and D_2 dopamine receptor occupancy in patients treated with classical neuroleptics and clozapine: relation to extrapyramidal side effects. *Arch Gen Psychiatry.* 1992;49:538-544.
3. Palao DJ, Arauxo A, Brunet M, Bernardo M, Haro JM, Ferrer J, Gonzalez-Monclus E. Haloperidol: therapeutic window in schizophrenia. *J Clin Psychopharmacol.* 1994;14:303-310.

ARCHIVES
OF
GENERAL PSYCHIATRY

Index to

Volume 53

January through December 1996

Editor
Jack D. Barchas, MD
New York, NY

Assistant to Editor
Peter M. Marzuk, MD
New York, NY

Editorial Administrator
Angela McGregor
New York, NY

Editorial Board

In this index in alphabetical order are listed names of authors of all articles and letters. Full citation is given under first author only; reference is made from joint authors. Names which begin with a prefix are entered under the prefix. The month is given as a two-letter notation in parentheses.

A

Abel L see Ho AP
Abelson JL, Curtis GC: Hypothalamic-pituitary-adrenal axis activity in panic disorder: 24-hour secretion of corticotropin and cortisol, 323 (Ap)
Abelson JM see Kendler KS
Abram KM see Teplin LA
Adler LE see Freedman R
Aghajanian GK see McDougle CJ
Agosti V see McGrath PJ; Quitkin FM
Akbarian S, Kim JJ, Potkin SG, Hetrick WP, Bunney WE Jr, Jones EG: Maldistribution of interstitial neurons in prefrontal white matter of the brains of schizophrenic patients, 425 (My)
Alaghband-Rad J see Kumra S
Albus KE see Frazier JA; Kumra S
Alexopoulos GS, Meyers BS, Young RC, Kakuma T, Feder M, Einhorn A, Rosendahl E: Recovery in geriatric depression, 305 (Ap)
Alpert NM see Rauch SL
Altaffer F see Dickey B
Alvir JMJ see Chakos MH
Anand A: Schizophrenia and temporal lobe epilepsy (letter) 1062 (No)
Anderson GM see McBride PA
Anderson N see Kushner MG
Andreasen NC see Docherty NM; O'Leary DS
Andreason PJ see Ketter TA
Angold A see Costello EJ
Anton RF, Moak DH, Latham PK: Obsessive-Compulsive Drinking Scale: a new method of assessing outcome in alcoholism treatment studies, 225 (Mr); correction, 576 (Jy)
Araúxo A see Palao DJ
Arndt S see O'Leary DS
Arnsten AFT, Steere JC, Hunt RD: Contribution of α_2-noradrenergic mechanisms to prefrontal cortical cognitive function: potential significance for attention-deficit hyperactivity disorder, 448 (My)
Aro HM see Isometsä ET
Aronson R, Offman HJ, Joffe RT, Naylor CD: Triiodothyronine augmentation in the treatment of refractory depression: a meta-analysis, 842 (Se)
Asher DM see Taller AM
Astrachan BM see Tischler GL
Aylward EH, Harris GJ, Hoehn-Saric R, Barta PE, Machlin SR, Pearlson GD: Normal caudate nucleus in obsessive-compulsive disorder assessed by quantitative neuroimaging, 577 (Jy)
Azeni H see Dickey B

B

Baer L see Breiter HC; Jenike MA
Bailey P see Duval F
Baker JR see Breiter HC
Barchas JD see Beutler LE
Barlow DH, Lehman CL: Advances in the psychosocial treatment of anxiety disorders: implications for national health care, 727 (Au)
Barta PE see Aylward EH
Baxter LR Jr see Schwartz JM
Belliveau JW see Breiter HC
Benjamin B see Zima BT
Berman R see Miller HL
Bernardo M see Palao DJ
Beutler LE, Barchas JD, Marzuk PM: Contribution of psychotherapy and pharmacotherapy research to national mental health care: introduction to the special series, 670 (Au)
Biederman J, Faraone S, Milberger S, Guite J, Mick E, Chen L, Mennin D, Marrs A, Ouellette C, Moore P, Spencer T, Norman D, Wilens T, Kraus I, Perrin J: Prospective 4-year follow-up study of attention-deficit hyperactivity and related disorders, 437 (My)
Blazer DG see Davidson JRT
Block MR see Schulberg HC
Bogert B see Taller AM
Bohman M see Sigvardsson S
Boles Ponto LL see O'Leary DS
Borenstein M see Chakos MH
Breier A see Frazier JA
Breiter HC, Rauch SL, Kwong KK, Baker JR, Weisskoff RM, Kennedy DN, Kendrick AD, Davis TL, Jiang A, Cohen MS, Stern CE, Belliveau JW, Baer L, O'Sullivan RL, Savage CR, Jenike MA, Rosen BR: Functional magnetic resonance imaging of symptom provocation in obsessive-compulsive disorder, 595 (Jy)
Breiter HC see Jenike MA
Brennan P see Raine A
Brennan PA see Hodgins S
Brent DA, Bridge J, Johnson BA, Connolly J: Suicidal behavior runs in families: a controlled family study of adolescent suicide victims, 1145 (De)
Bridge J see Brent DA
Broadhead WE see Olfson M
Brooner RK see Silverman K
Brown AS see Susser E
Brown GL see Fils-Aime M-L
Brunet M see Palao DJ
Buchanan RW see Buckley PF
Buchsbaum MS see Ho AP
Buckley PF, Buchanan RW, Schulz SC, Tamminga CA: Catching up on schizophrenia: the Fifth International Congress on Schizophrenia Research, Warm Springs, Va, April 8-12, 1995, 456 (My)
Bunney WE Jr see Akbarian S; Ho AP
Burns BJ see Costello EJ
Bush T see Katon W
Busquets X see Garcia-Sevilla JA
Buysse DJ see Dew MA

C

Caddell JM see Jordan BK
Camp P see Sherbourne CD
Casey BJ, Cohen JD: Is research in normal and ill children involving radiation exposure ethical? (letter) 1059 (No)
Caspi A, Moffitt TE, Newman DL, Silva PA: Behavioral observations at age 3 years predict adult psychiatric disorders: longitudinal evidence from a birth cohort, 1033 (No)
Castellanos FX, Giedd JN, Marsh WL, Hamburger SD, Vaituzis AC, Dickstein DP, Sarfatti SE, Vauss YC, Snell JW, Lange N, Kaysen D, Krain AL, Ritchie GF, Rajapakse JC, Rapoport JL: Quantitative brain magnetic resonance imaging in attention-deficit hyperactivity disorder, 607 (Jy)
Cavalli-Sforza LL see Hallmayer J
Caviness VS see Jenike MA
Cawthra E see Freedman R
Chakos MH, Alvir JMJ, Woerner MG, Koreen A, Geisler S, Mayerhoff D, Sobel S, Kane JM, Borenstein M, Lieberman JA: Incidence and correlates of tardive dyskinesia in first episode of schizophrenia, 313 (Ap)
Chang G see O'Malley SS
Charney DS see Lam RW; Miller HL
Charuvastra C see Ling W
Chen L see Biederman J
Ciaranello RD see Hallmayer J
Cizadlo T see O'Leary DS
Clarkin JF, Pilkonis PA, Magruder KM: Psychotherapy of depression: implications for reform of the health care system, 717 (Au)
Cloninger CR see Sigvardsson S
Coccaro EF, Kavoussi RJ, Sheline YI, Lish JD, Csernansky JG: Impulsive aggression in personality disorder correlates with tritiated paroxetine binding in the platelet, 531 (Je)
Cohen DJ see Laor N; McDougle CJ
Cohen JD see Casey BJ; Servan-Schreiber D
Cohen MS see Breiter HC
Cohen RM see Zametkin AJ
Cone EJ see Silverman K
Connolly J see Brent DA
Cook EH Jr, Olson K, Pliskin N: Response of organic catatonia to risperidone (letter) 82 (Ja)
Cooper TB see Volavka J
Copeland K see Fletcher JM
Coplan JD see Goetz RR
Cornille TA see Howard KI
Coryell W see Mueller TI
Costello EJ, Angold A, Burns BJ, Erkanli A, Stangl DK, Tweed DL: Great Smoky Mountains Study of Youth: functional impairment and serious emotional disturbance, 1137 (De)
Costello EJ, Angold A, Burns BJ, Stangl DK, Tweed DL, Erkanli A, Worthman CM: Great Smoky Mountains Study of Youth: goals, design, methods, and the prevalence of *DSM-III-R* disorders, 1129 (De)
Coulehan JL see Schulberg HC
Crits-Christoph P see Persons JB
Crits-Christoph P, Siqueland L: Psychosocial treatment for drug abuse: selected review and recommendations for national health care, 749 (Au)
Crocq M-A see Duval F
Csernansky JG see Coccaro EF
Curtis GC see Abelson JL
Czobor P see Volavka J

D

Dahl AA see Wiborg IM
Dahl RE see Goetz RR
Daly E see Murphy DGM
Davidson J see Thase ME
Davidson JRT, Hughes DC, George LK, Blazer DG: Association of sexual assault and attempted suicide within the community, 550 (Je)
Davies M see Kandel DB
Davis CM see Fletcher JM
Davis TL see Breiter HC
DeCarli C see Murphy DGM
Delgado PL see Lam RW; Miller HL
Deliyannides D see Quitkin FM
DeRosa M see Docherty NM
Derrick AM see Shafii M
Dettling M see Heinz A
Devanand DP, Sano M, Tang M-X, Taylor S, Gurland BJ, Wilder D, Stern Y, Mayeux R: Depressed mood and the incidence of Alzheimer's disease in the elderly living in the community, 175 (Fe)
Devanand DP see Sackeim HA
Dew MA, Reynolds CF III, Buysse DJ, Houck PR, Hoch CC, Monk TH, Kupfer DJ: Electroencephalographic sleep profiles during depression: effects of episode duration and other clinical and psychosocial factors in older adults, 148 (Fe)
Dickey B, Normand S-LT, Norton EC, Azeni H, Fisher W, Altaffer F: Managing the care of schizophrenia: lessons from a 4-year Massachusetts Medicaid study, 945 (Oc)
Dickstein DP see Castellanos FX
Diep T-S see Duval F
Dixon MJ see King S
Docherty NM, DeRosa M, Andreasen NC: Communication disturbances in schizophrenia and mania, 358 (Ap)
Donovan SJ see Quitkin FM
Duan N see Zima BT
Dufeu P see Heinz A
Duval F, Mokrani M-C, Crocq M-A, Jautz M, Bailey P, Diep T-S, Macher J-P: Effect of antidepressant medication on morning and evening thyroid function tests during a major depressive episode, 833 (Se)

E

Eaton WW see Magee WJ
Eaves LJ see Kendler KS
Eckardt MJ see Fils-Aime M-L
Eggert M see Virkkunen M
Einhorn A see Alexopoulos GS
Eldadah BA see Taller AM
Elkis H see Friedman L
Endicott J see Mueller TI
Engberg M see Hodgins S
Erkanli A see Costello EJ
Ernst M see Zametkin AJ
Eronen M, Hakola P, Tiihonen J: Mental disorders and homicidal behavior in Finland, 497 (Je)
Escribá PV see Garcia-Sevilla JA

F

Fairbank JA see Jordan BK
Falkai PG see Taller AM
Faraone S see Biederman J
Farber L see Olfson M
Fava M see Thase ME
Feder M see Alexopoulos GS
Fergusson DM, Lynskey MT, Horwood LJ: Comorbidity between depressive disorders and nicotine dependence in a cohort of 16-year-olds, 1043 (No)
Fernald B see Higley JD
Filipek PA see Jenike MA
Fils-Aime M-L, Eckardt MJ, George DT, Brown GL, Mefford I, Linnoila M: Early-onset alcoholics have lower cerebrospinal fluid 5-hydroxyindoleacetic acid levels than late-onset alcoholics, 211 (Mr)
Fischman AJ see Rauch SL
Fisher P see Gould MS; Shaffer D
Fisher W see Dickey B
Fisler RE see Rauch SL
Fiszdon J see Kushner MG

Fletcher JM, Page JB, Francis DJ, Copeland K, Naus MJ, Davis CM, Morris R, Krauskopf D, Satz P: Cognitive correlates of long-term cannabis use in Costa Rican men, 1051 (No)
Flory M see Gould MS; Shaffer D
Foa E see Kushner MG
Forde DR see Stein MB
Francis DJ see Fletcher JM
Frank E see Kupfer DJ
Frank RG, Huskamp HA, McGuire TG, Newhouse JP: Some economics of mental health 'carve-outs', 933 (Oc)
Frazier JA, Giedd JN, Hamburger SD, Albus KE, Kaysen D, Vaituzis AC, Rajapakse JC, Lenane MC, McKenna K, Jacobsen LK, Gordon CT, Breier A, Rapoport JL: Brain anatomic magnetic resonance imaging in childhood-onset schizophrenia, 617 (Jy)
Frazier JA see Kumra S
Freedman R, Adler LE, Myles-Worsley M, Nagamoto HT, Miller C, Kisley M, McRae K, Cawthra E, Waldo M: Inhibitory gating of an evoked response to repeated auditory stimuli in schizophrenic and normal subjects: human recordings, computer simulation, and an animal model, 1114 (De)
Friedman L, Jesberger JA, Meltzer HY, Elkis H: Studies of ventricular enlargement (letter) 1166 (De)
Friedman RA see Kocsis JH

G

Gabrielli WF Jr see Volavka J
Gallagher TJ see Kendler KS
Garcia-Sevilla JA, Escribá PV, Sastre M, Walzer C, Busquets X, Jaquet G, Reis DJ, Guimón J: Immunodetection and quantitation of imidazoline receptor proteins in platelets of patients with major depression and in brains of suicide victims, 803 (Se)
Geisler S see Chakos MH
George DT see Fils-Aime M-L
George LK see Davidson JRT
George MS see Ketter TA
George TP, Spence MW: Alterations of membrane phospholipid metabolism in patients with schizophrenia assessed by phosphorus magnetic resonance spectroscopy (letter) 1065 (No)
Gianoulakis C, Krishnan B, Thavundayil J: Enhanced sensitivity of pituitary β-endorphin to ethanol in subjects at high risk of alcoholism, 250 (Mr); correction, 555 (Je)
Giedd JN see Castellanos FX; Frazier JA
Gill DS see Ketter TA
Gillin JC see Ho AP
Gniwesch L see Kocsis JH
Godec MS see Taller AM
Goetz RR see Johnson JG
Goetz RR, Wolk SI, Coplan JD, Weissman MM, Dahl RE, Ryan ND: Rapid eye movement density among adolescents with major depressive disorder revisited (letter) 1066 (No)
Gold JM, Hermann BP, Weinberger DR: Schizophrenia and temporal lobe epilepsy (letter) 1063 (No)
Goldman D see McGrath PJ; Nielsen DA
Golomb A see Laor N
Goodman AB: Retinoid dysregulation may result in abnormal expression of glutamic acid decarboxylase in schizophrenia (letter) 653 (Jy)
Goodwin DW see Volavka J
Gordis E: Alcohol research: at the cutting edge, 199 (Mr)
Gordon CT see Frazier JA; Kumra S
Gorman JM see Johnson JG; Susser E
Gould MS, Fisher P, Parides M, Flory M, Shaffer D: Psychosocial risk factors of child and adolescent completed suicide, 1155 (De)
Gould MS see Shaffer D
Grady CL see Murphy DGM
Gräf K see Heinz A
Greist JH: Venlafaxine in obsessive-compulsive disorder (letter) 654 (Jy)
Greist JH see Henk HJ
Grewal A see Lam RW
Guimón J see Garcia-Sevilla JA
Guite J see Biederman J
Gurland BJ see Devanand DP

H

Hakola P see Eronen M
Halbreich U see Thase ME
Hallmayer J, Hebert JM, Spiker D, Lotspeich L, McMahon WM, Petersen PB, Nicholas P, Pingree C, Lin AA, Cavalli-Sforza LL, Risch N, Ciaranello RD: Autism and the X chromosome: multipoint sib-pair analysis, 985 (No)
Hamburger SD see Castellanos FX; Frazier JA; Kumra S
Haro JM see Palao DJ
Harris GJ see Aylward EH
Harrison W see Thase ME
Heath AC see Kendler KS; Madden PAF
Hebert JM see Hallmayer J
Heikkinen ME see Isometsä ET
Heinz A, Dufeu P, Kuhn S, Dettling M, Gräf K, Kürten I, Rommelspacher H, Schmidt LG: Psychopathological and behavioral correlates of dopaminergic sensitivity in alcohol-dependent patients, 1123 (De)
Heninger GR see McDougle CJ; Miller HL
Henk HJ, Katzelnick DJ, Kobak KA, Greist JH, Jefferson JW: Medical costs attributed to depression among patients with a history of high medical expenses in a health maintenance organization, 899 (Oc)
Henriksson MM see Isometsä ET
Hermann BP see Gold JM
Herscovitch P see Ketter TA
Hetrick WP see Akbarian S
Hichwa RD see O'Leary DS
Higgins ST see Silverman K
Higley JD, Mehlman PT, Higley SB, Fernald B, Vickers J, Lindell SG, Taub DM, Suomi SJ, Linnoila M: Excessive mortality in young free-ranging male nonhuman primates with low cerebrospinal fluid 5-hydroxyindoleacetic acid concentrations, 537 (Je)
Higley SB see Higley JD
Ho AP, Gillin JC, Buchsbaum MS, Wu JC, Abel L, Bunney WE Jr: Brain glucose metabolism during non-rapid eye movement sleep in major depression: a positron emission tomography study, 645 (Jy)
Hoch CC see Dew MA
Hodgins S, Mednick SA, Brennan PA, Schulsinger F, Engberg M: Mental disorder and crime: evidence from a Danish birth cohort, 489 (Je)
Hoehn-Saric R see Aylward EH
Hoek HW see Susser E
Hofman MA see Purba JS
Hollister JM, Laing P, Mednick SA: Rhesus incompatibility as a risk factor for schizophrenia in male adults, 19 (Ja)
Hoogendijk WJG see Purba JS
Hornbrook MC see McFarland BH
Horwitz B see Murphy DGM
Horwood LJ see Fergusson DM
Houck PR see Dew MA; Schulberg HC
Hoven C see Olfson M
Howard KI, Cornille TA, Lyons JS, Vessey JT, Lueger RJ, Saunders SM: Patterns of mental health service utilization, 696 (Au)
Hughes DC see Davidson JRT
Hunt RD see Arnsten AFT
Hurtig RR see O'Leary DS
Huskamp HA see Frank RG

I

Imber SD see Schulberg HC
Isometsä ET, Heikkinen ME, Henriksson MM, Aro HM, Marttunen MJ, Lönnqvist JK: Parenthood, completed suicide, and mental disorders (letter) 1061 (No)

J

Jackson CA see Sherbourne CD
Jacobsen LK see Frazier JA; Kumra S
Jaffe AJ see O'Malley SS
Jaquet G see Garcia-Sevilla JA
Jautz M see Duval F
Jefferson JW see Henk HJ
Jenike MA, Breiter HC, Baer L, Kennedy DN, Savage CR, Olivares MJ, O'Sullivan RL, Shera DM, Rauch SL, Keuthen N, Rosen BR, Caviness VS, Filipek PA: Cerebral structural abnormalities in obsessive-compulsive disorder: a quantitative morphometric magnetic resonance imaging study, 625 (Jy)
Jenike MA see Breiter HC; Rauch SL
Jensen P see Volavka J
Jesberger JA see Friedman L
Jiang A see Breiter HC
Joffe RT see Aronson R
Johnson BA see Brent DA
Johnson JG, Williams JBW, Goetz RR, Rabkin JG, Remien RH, Lipsitz JD, Gorman JM: Personality disorders predict onset of axis I disorders and impaired functioning among homosexual men with and at risk of HIV infection, 350 (Ap)
Johnson RE see McFarland BH
Jones EG see Akbarian S
Jordan BK, Schlenger WE, Fairbank JA, Caddell JM: Prevalence of psychiatric disorders among incarcerated women: II. convicted felons entering prison, 513 (Je)

K

Kakuma T see Alexopoulos GS
Kandel DB, Davies M: High school students who use crack and other drugs, 71 (Ja)
Kane JM see Chakos MH
Kaplan SH see Meredith LS
Karasu TB see Merriam AE
Kathol R see Olfson M
Katon W, Robinson P, Von Korff M, Lin E, Bush T, Ludman E, Simon G, Walker E: Multifaceted intervention to improve treatment of depression in primary care, 924 (Oc)
Katz R see McGuffin P
Katzelnick DJ see Henk HJ
Katzman GP see Sackeim HA
Kaufman N see Shafii M
Kavoussi RJ see Coccaro EF
Kaysen D see Castellanos FX; Frazier JA
Keller MB see Mueller TI
Kendler KS, Eaves LJ, Walters EE, Neale MC, Heath AC, Kessler RC: Identification and validation of distinct depressive syndromes in a population-based sample of female twins, 391 (My)
Kendler KS, Gallagher TJ, Abelson JM, Kessler RC: Lifetime prevalence, demographic risk factors, and diagnostic validity of nonaffective psychosis as assessed in a US community sample: the National Comorbidity Survey, 1022 (No)
Kendrick AD see Breiter HC
Kennedy DN see Breiter HC; Jenike MA
Kesler ML see O'Leary DS
Kessler RC see Kendler KS; Magee WJ
Ketter TA, Andreason PJ, George MS, Lee C, Gill DS, Parekh PI, Willis MW, Herscovitch P, Post RM: Anterior paralimbic mediation of procaine-induced emotional and psychosensory experiences, 59 (Ja)
Keuthen N see Jenike MA
Key MP see Shafii M
Kim JJ see Akbarian S
King S, Dixon MJ: Influence of expressed emotion, family dynamics, and symptom type on the social adjustment of schizophrenic young adults, 1098 (De)
Kirchner PT see O'Leary DS
Kisley M see Freedman R
Klein DF: Panic attacks: Klein's false suffocation alarm, Taylor and Rachman's data, and Ley's dyspneic-fear theory (letter) 83 (Ja)
Klein DF see Quitkin FM
Kleinman JE see Taller AM
Kleinman M see Shaffer D
Klett CJ see Ling W
Knop J see Volavka J
Kobak KA see Henk HJ
Kocsis JH: Practice guidelines and professional challenges: what psychotherapists need to do, 303 (Ap)
Kocsis JH, Friedman RA, Markowitz JC, Leon AC, Miller NL, Gniwesch L, Parides M: Maintenance therapy for chronic depression: a controlled clinical trial of desipramine, 769 (Se)
Kocsis JH see Thase ME
Koran L see Thase ME
Koreen A see Chakos MH
Krain AL see Castellanos FX
Kraus I see Biederman J
Krauskopf D see Fletcher JM
Krishnan B see Gianoulakis C
Krystal JH see Lam RW; Miller HL
Kuhn S see Heinz A
Kumra S, Frazier JA, Jacobsen LK, McKenna K, Gordon CT, Lenane MC, Hamburger SD, Smith AK, Albus KE, Alaghband-Rad J, Rapoport JL: Childhood-onset schizophrenia: a double-blind clozapine-haloperidol comparison, 1090 (De)
Kupfer DJ, Frank E: Maintenance therapy for chronic depression: a controlled clinical trial of desipramine (commentary) 775 (Se)
Kupfer DJ see Dew MA
Kürten I see Heinz A
Kushner MG, Mackenzie TB, Fiszdon J, Valentiner DP, Foa E, Anderson N, Wangensteen D: Effects of alcohol consumption on laboratory-induced panic and state anxiety, 264 (Mr)
Kwong KK see Breiter HC

L

Labovitz D see Susser E
Laing P see Hollister JM
Lam RW, Zis AP, Grewal A, Delgado PL, Charney DS, Krystal JH: Effects of rapid tryptophan depletion in patients with seasonal affective disorder in remission after light therapy, 41 (Ja)
Lange N see Castellanos FX
Langenbucher JW see McCrady BS
Laor N, Wolmer L, Mayes LC, Golomb A, Silverberg DS, Weizman R, Cohen DJ: Israeli preschoolers under Scud missile attacks: a developmental perspective on risk-modifying factors, 416 (My)
Latham PK see Anton RF
Lave J see Schulberg HC
Lee C see Ketter TA
Lehman CL see Barlow DH
Lenane MC see Frazier JA; Kumra S
Leon AC see Kocsis JH; Mueller TI; Olfson M
Ley R: Panic attacks: Klein's false suffocation alarm, Taylor and Rachman's data, and Ley's dyspneic-fear theory (letter) 83 (Ja)
Lieberman JA see Chakos MH
Lin AA see Hallmayer J
Lin E see Katon W
Lin S see Susser E
Lindell SG see Higley JD

Ling W, Wesson DR, Charuvastra C, Klett CJ: Controlled trial comparing buprenorphine and methadone maintenance in opioid dependence, 401 (My)
Linnoila M see Fils-Aime M-L; Higley JD; Nielsen DA; Virkkunen M
Lipsitz JD see Johnson JG
Lish JD see Coccaro EF
Lönnqvist JK see Isometsä ET
Lotspeich L see Hallmayer J
Luber B see Sackeim HA
Ludman E see Katon W
Lueger RJ see Howard KI
Lundberg GD, Wennberg JE: Quality of care: a call for papers for the annual coordinated theme issues of the AMA journals, 1085 (De)
Lynskey MT see Fergusson DM
Lyons JS see Howard KI

M

Macher J-P see Duval F
Machlin SR see Aylward EH
Mackenzie TB see Kushner MG
MacMillan DR see Shafii M
Madden PAF, Heath AC, Rosenthal NE, Martin NG: Seasonal changes in mood and behavior: the role of genetic factors, 47 (Ja)
Madonia MJ see Schulberg HC
Magee WJ, Eaton WW, Wittchen H-U, McGonagle KA, Kessler RC: Agoraphobia, simple phobia, and social phobia in the National Comorbidity Survey, 159 (Fe)
Magruder KM see Clarkin JF
Mann K see Sass H
Markowitz JC see Kocsis JH
Marrs A see Biederman J
Marsh WL see Castellanos FX
Martin KM see Schwartz JM
Martin NG see Madden PAF
Marttunen MJ see Isometsä ET
Marzuk PM: Violence, crime, and mental illness: how strong a link? 481 (Je)
Marzuk PM see Beutler LE
Mayerhoff D see Chakos MH
Mayes LC see Laor N
Mayeux R see Devanand DP
Mazel RM see Meredith LS
Mazziotta JC: Mapping mental illness: a new era, 574 (Jy)
McBride PA, Anderson GM, Shapiro T: Autism research: bringing together approaches to pull apart the disorder, 980 (No)
McClelland GM see Teplin LA
McCrady BS, Langenbucher JW: Alcohol treatment and health care system reform, 737 (Au)
McDougle CJ, Naylor ST, Cohen DJ, Aghajanian GK, Heninger GR, Price LH: Effects of tryptophan depletion in drug-free adults with autistic disorder, 993 (No)
McDougle CJ, Naylor ST, Cohen DJ, Volkmar FR, Heninger GR, Price LH: Double-blind, placebo-controlled study of fluvoxamine in adults with autistic disorder, 1001 (No)
McFarland BH, Johnson RE, Hornbrook MC: Enrollment duration, service use, and costs of care for severely mentally ill members of a health maintenance organization, 938 (Oc)
McGonagle KA see Magee WJ
McGrath PJ, Nunes EV, Stewart JW, Goldman D, Agosti V, Ocepek-Welikson K, Quitkin FM: Imipramine treatment of alcoholics with primary depression: a placebo-controlled clinical trial, 232 (Mr)
McGrath PJ see Quitkin FM
McGuffin P, Katz R, Watkins S, Rutherford J: Hospital-based twin registry study of the heritability of *DSM-IV* unipolar depression, 129 (Fe); correction, 436 (My)
McGuire TG see Frank RG
McIntosh AR see Murphy DGM
McIntyre JS, Zarin DA, Pincus HA: Role of psychotherapy in the treatment of depression: review of two practice guidelines, 291 (Ap)
McKenna K see Frazier JA; Kumra S
McMahon WM see Hallmayer J
McRae K see Freedman R
Mednick B see Raine A
Mednick SA see Hodgins S; Hollister JM; Raine A; Volavka J
Mefford I see Fils-Aime M-L
Mehlman PT see Higley JD
Meisner M see Volavka J
Meltzer HY see Friedman L
Mennin D see Biederman J
Mentis MJ see Murphy DGM
Meredith LS see Sherbourne CD
Meredith LS, Wells KB, Kaplan SH, Mazel RM: Counseling typically provided for depression: role of clinician specialty and payment system, 905 (Oc)
Merriam AE, Karasu TB: Role of psychotherapy in the treatment of depression: review of two practice guidelines, 301 (Ap)
Meyer RE see O'Malley SS
Meyers BS see Alexopoulos GS
Mick E see Biederman J
Milberger S see Biederman J
Miller C see Freedman R
Miller HL, Delgado PL, Salomon RM, Berman R, Krystal JH, Heninger GR, Charney DS: Clinical and biochemical effects of catecholamine depletion on antidepressant-induced remission of depression, 117 (Fe)
Miller NL see Kocsis JH
Mitchell AJ: Schizophrenia and temporal lobe epilepsy (letter) 1063 (No)
Moak DH see Anton RF
Moeller JR see Sackeim HA
Moffitt TE see Caspi A
Mokrani M-C see Duval F
Monk TH see Dew MA
Montoya ID see Silverman K
Moore P see Biederman J
Moreau D see Shaffer D
Morris R see Fletcher JM
Morton CT: Is research in normal and ill children involving radiation exposure ethical? (letter) 1059 (No)
Mueller TI, Keller MB, Leon AC, Solomon DA, Shea MT, Coryell W, Endicott J: Recovery after 5 years of unremitting major depressive disorder, 794 (Se)
Murphy DGM, DeCarli C, McIntosh AR, Daly E, Mentis MJ, Pietrini P, Szczepanik J, Schapiro MB, Grady CL, Horwitz B, Rapoport SI: Sex differences in human brain morphometry and metabolism: an in vivo quantitative magnetic resonance imaging and positron emission tomography study on the effect of aging, 585 (Jy)
Myles-Worsley M see Freedman R

N

Nagamoto HT see Freedman R
Nahinsky ID see Shafii M
Naus MJ see Fletcher JM
Naylor CD see Aronson R
Naylor ST see McDougle CJ
Neale MC see Kendler KS
Neugebauer R see Susser E
Newhouse JP see Frank RG
Newman DL see Caspi A
Neziroglu FA see Yaryura-Tobias JA
Nicholas P see Hallmayer J
Nielsen DA, Goldman D, Virkkunen M, Tokola R, Rawlings R, Linnoila M: *TPH* replication study: not! (letter) 964 (Oc)
Nobler MS see Sackeim HA
Norman D see Biederman J
Normand S-LT see Dickey B
Norton EC see Dickey B
Nunes E see Quitkin FM
Nunes EV see McGrath PJ

O

Ocepek-Welikson K see McGrath PJ; Quitkin FM
Offman HJ see Aronson R
O'Leary DS, Andreasen NC, Hurtig RR, Kesler ML, Rogers M, Arndt S, Cizadlo T, Watkins GL, Boles Ponto LL, Kirchner PT, Hichwa RD: Auditory attentional deficits in patients with schizophrenia: a positron emission tomography study, 633 (Jy)
Olfson M, Broadhead WE, Weissman MM, Leon AC, Farber L, Hoven C, Kathol R: Subthreshold psychiatric symptoms in a primary care group practice, 880 (Oc)
Olivares MJ see Jenike MA
Olson K see Cook EH Jr
O'Malley SS, Jaffe AJ, Chang G, Rode S, Schottenfeld R, Meyer RE, Rounsaville B: Six-month follow-up of naltrexone and psychotherapy for alcohol dependence, 217 (Mr)
Orlinsky DE see Russell RL
Orr SP see Rauch SL
O'Sullivan RL see Breiter HC; Jenike MA
Ouellette C see Biederman J
Owen RR see Zhang M

P

Page JB see Fletcher JM
Palao DJ, Araúxo A, Haro JM, Brunet M, Bernardo M: Relationship between plasma haloperidol concentrations and clinical results (letter) 1167 (De)
Parekh PI see Ketter TA
Parides M see Gould MS; Kocsis JH
Pearlson GD see Aylward EH
Pediadiatakis N: Occurrence of schizophrenia in monozygotic twins and fractal dendritic development (letter) 85 (Ja)
Penick EC see Volavka J
Perel J see Schulberg HC
Perrin J see Biederman J
Persaud R: Studies of ventricular enlargement (letter) 1165 (De)
Persons JB, Thase ME, Crits-Christoph P: Role of psychotherapy in the treatment of depression: review of two practice guidelines, 283 (Ap)
Petersen PB see Hallmayer J
Petkova E see Quitkin FM
Phelps ME see Schwartz JM
Pietrini P see Murphy DGM
Pilkonis PA see Clarkin JF
Pincus HA see McIntyre JS
Pincus HA, Zarin DA, West JC: Peering into the 'black box': measuring outcomes of managed care, 870 (Oc)
Pingree C see Hallmayer J
Pitman RK see Rauch SL
Pliskin N see Cook EH Jr
Pomeroy KL see Taller AM
Pope SK see Zhang M
Post RM see Ketter TA
Potkin SG see Akbarian S
Preston KL see Silverman K
Price LH see McDougle CJ
Prudic J see Sackeim HA
Purba JS, Hoogendijk WJG, Hofman MA, Swaab DF: Increased number of vasopressin- and oxytocin-expressing neurons in the paraventricular nucleus of the hypothalamus in depression, 137 (Fe)

Q

Quitkin FM, McGrath PJ, Stewart JW, Ocepek-Welikson K, Taylor BP, Nunes E, Deliyannides D, Agosti V, Donovan SJ, Petkova E, Klein DF: Chronological milestones to guide drug change: when should clinicians switch antidepressants? 785 (Se)
Quitkin FM see McGrath PJ

R

Rabkin JG see Johnson JG
Raine A, Brennan P, Mednick B, Mednick SA: High rates of violence, crime, academic problems, and behavioral problems in males with both early neuromotor deficits and unstable family environments, 544 (Je)
Rajapakse JC see Castellanos FX; Frazier JA
Rapoport JL see Castellanos FX; Frazier JA; Kumra S
Rapoport SI see Murphy DGM
Rauch SL see Breiter HC; Jenike MA
Rauch SL, van der Kolk BA, Fisler RE, Alpert NM, Orr SP, Savage CR, Fischman AJ, Jenike MA, Pitman RK: Symptom provocation study of posttraumatic stress disorder using positron emission tomography and script-driven imagery, 380 (My)
Rawlings R see Nielsen DA; Virkkunen M
Reis DJ see Garcia-Sevilla JA
Remien RH see Johnson JG
Reynolds CF III see Dew MA; Thase ME
Risch N see Hallmayer J
Ritchie GF see Castellanos FX
Robinson P see Katon W
Rode S see O'Malley SS
Rodriguez E see Schulberg HC
Rogers M see O'Leary DS
Rommelspacher H see Heinz A
Rosen BR see Breiter HC; Jenike MA
Rosenbaum J see Thase ME
Rosendahl E see Alexopoulos GS
Rosenthal NE see Madden PAF
Rounsaville B see O'Malley SS
Rush AJ: Role of psychotherapy in the treatment of depression: review of two practice guidelines, 298 (Ap)
Russell RL, Orlinsky DE: Psychotherapy research in historical perspective: implications for mental health care policy, 708 (Au)
Rutherford J see McGuffin P
Ryan ND see Goetz RR

S

Sackeim HA, Luber B, Katzman GP, Moeller JR, Prudic J, Devanand DP, Nobler MS: Effects of electroconvulsive therapy on quantitative electroencephalograms: relationship to clinical outcome, 814 (Se)
Salomon RM see Miller HL
Sano M see Devanand DP
Sarfatti SE see Castellanos FX
Sass H, Soyka M, Mann K, Zieglgänsberger W: Relapse prevention by acamprosate: results from a placebo-controlled study on alcohol dependence, 673 (Au); correction, 1097 (De)
Sastre M see Garcia-Sevilla JA
Satz P see Fletcher JM
Saunders SM see Howard KI
Savage CR see Breiter HC; Jenike MA; Rauch SL
Schapiro MB see Murphy DGM
Schlenger WE see Jordan BK
Schmidt LG see Heinz A
Schottenfeld R see O'Malley SS
Schuckit MA, Smith TL: 8-year follow-up of 450 sons of alcoholic and control subjects, 202 (Mr)
Schulberg HC, Block MR, Madonia MJ, Scott CP, Rodriguez E, Imber SD, Perel J, Lave J, Houck PR, Coulehan JL: Treating major depression in primary care practice: eight-month clinical outcomes, 913 (Oc)
Schulsinger F see Hodgins S; Volavka J
Schulz SC see Buckley PF

Schuster CR see Silverman K
Schwartz DJ see Zametkin AJ
Schwartz JM, Stoessel PW, Baxter LR Jr, Martin KM, Phelps ME: Systematic changes in cerebral glucose metabolic rate after successful behavior modification treatment of obsessive-compulsive disorder, 109 (Fe)
Scott CP see Schulberg HC
Servan-Schreiber D, Cohen JD, Steingard S: Schizophrenic deficits in the processing of context: a test of a theoretical model, 1105 (De)
Shaffer D, Gould MS, Fisher P, Trautman P, Moreau D, Kleinman M, Flory M: Psychiatric diagnosis in child and adolescent suicide, 339 (Ap)
Shaffer D see Gould MS
Shafii M, MacMillan DR, Key MP, Derrick AM, Kaufman N, Nahinsky ID: Nocturnal serum melatonin profile in major depression in children and adolescents, 1009 (No)
Shapiro T see McBride PA
Shea MT see Mueller TI
Sheline YI see Coccaro EF
Shera DM see Jenike MA
Sherbourne CD, Wells KB, Meredith LS, Jackson CA, Camp P: Comorbid anxiety disorder and the functioning and well-being of chronically ill patients of general medical providers, 889 (Oc)
Sigvardsson S, Bohman M, Cloninger CR: Replication of the Stockholm Adoption Study of alcoholism: confirmatory cross-fostering analysis, 681 (Au)
Silva PA see Caspi A
Silverberg DS see Laor N
Silverman K, Higgins ST, Brooner RK, Montoya ID, Cone EJ, Schuster CR, Preston KL: Sustained cocaine abstinence in methadone maintenance patients through voucher-based reinforcement therapy, 409 (My)
Simon G see Katon W
Simons AD see Thase ME
Siqueland L see Crits-Christoph P
Smith AK see Kumra S
Smith GR see Zhang M
Smith TL see Schuckit MA
Snell JW see Castellanos FX
Sobel S see Chakos MH
Solomon DA see Mueller TI
Soyka M see Sass H
Spence MW see George TP
Spencer T see Biederman J
Spiker D see Hallmayer J
Stangl DK see Costello EJ
Steere JC see Arnsten AFT
Stein MB, Walker JR, Forde DR: Public-speaking fears in a community sample: prevalence, impact on functioning, and diagnostic classification, 169 (Fe)
Steingard S see Servan-Schreiber D
Stern CE see Breiter HC
Stern Y see Devanand DP
Stevens JR see Taller AM
Stewart JW see McGrath PJ, Quitkin FM
Stoessel PW see Schwartz JM
Suomi SJ see Higley JD
Susser E, Neugebauer R, Hoek HW, Brown AS, Lin S, Labovitz D, Gorman JM: Schizophrenia after prenatal famine: further evidence, 25 (Ja)
Swaab DF see Purba JS
Szczepanik J see Murphy DGM

T

Taller AM, Asher DM, Pomeroy KL, Eldadah BA, Godec MS, Falkai PG, Bogert B, Kleinman JE, Stevens JR, Torrey EF: Search for viral nucleic acid sequences in brain tissues of patients with schizophrenia using nested polymerase chain reaction, 32 (Ja)
Tamminga CA see Buckley PF
Tang M-X see Devanand DP
Taub DM see Higley JD
Taylor BP see Quitkin FM
Taylor S see Devanand DP
Teplin LA, Abram KM, McClelland GM: Prevalence of psychiatric disorders among incarcerated women: I. pretrial jail detainees, 505 (Je); correction, 664 (Au)
Thase ME, Fava M, Halbreich U, Kocsis JH, Koran L, Davidson J, Rosenbaum J, Harrison W: Placebo-controlled, randomized clinical trial comparing sertraline and imipramine for the treatment of dysthymia, 777 (Se)
Thase ME see Persons JB
Thase ME, Simons AD, Reynolds CF III: Abnormal electroencephalographic sleep profiles in major depression: association with response to cognitive behavior therapy, 99 (Fe)
Thavundayil J see Gianoulakis C
Tiihonen J see Eronen M
Tischler GL, Astrachan BM: Funny thing happened on the way to reform, 959 (Oc)
Tokola R see Nielsen DA
Torrey EF see Taller AM
Trautman P see Shaffer D
Tweed DL see Costello EJ

V

Vaillant GE: Long-term follow-up of male alcohol abuse, 243 (Mr)
Vaituzis AC see Castellanos FX; Frazier JA
Valentiner DP see Kushner MG
van der Kolk BA see Rauch SL
Vauss YC see Castellanos FX
Vessey JT see Howard KI
Vickers J see Higley JD
Virkkunen M, Eggert M, Rawlings R, Linnoila M: Prospective follow-up study of alcoholic violent offenders and fire setters, 523 (Je)
Virkkunen M see Nielsen DA
Volavka J, Cooper TB, Czobor P, Meisner M: Relationship between plasma haloperidol concentrations and clinical results (letter) 1168 (De)
Volavka J, Czobor P: Interictal electroencephalographic effects of electroconvulsive therapy: can they elucidate mechanism of action? 826 (Se)
Volavka J, Czobor P, Goodwin DW, Gabrielli WF Jr, Penick EC, Mednick SA, Jensen P, Knop J, Schulsinger F: Electroencephalogram after alcohol administration in high-risk men and the development of alcohol use disorders 10 years later: preliminary findings, 258 (Mr)
Volkmar FR see McDougle CJ
Von Korff M see Katon W

W

Waldo M see Freedman R
Walker E see Katon W
Walker JR see Stein MB
Walters EE see Kendler KS
Walzer C see Garcia-Sevilla JA
Wangensteen D see Kushner MG
Watkins GL see O'Leary DS
Watkins S see McGuffin P
Weinberger DR see Gold JM
Weisskoff RM see Breiter HC
Weissman MM see Goetz RR; Olfson M
Weizman R see Laor N
Wells KB see Meredith LS; Sherbourne CD; Zima BT
Wennberg JE see Lundberg GD
Wesson DR see Ling W
West JC see Pincus HA
Wiborg IM, Dahl AA: Does brief dynamic psychotherapy reduce the relapse rate of panic disorder? 689 (Au)
Wilder D see Devanand DP
Wilens T see Biederman J
Williams JBW see Johnson JG
Willis MW see Ketter TA
Wittchen H-U see Magee WJ
Woerner MG see Chakos MH
Wolk SI see Goetz RR
Wolmer L see Laor N
Worthman CM see Costello EJ
Wu JC see Ho AP
Wyatt RJ: Neurodevelopmental abnormalities and schizophrenia: a family affair, 11 (Ja)

Y

Yaryura-Tobias JA, Neziroglu FA: Venlafaxine in obsessive-compulsive disorder (letter) 653 (Jy)
Young RC see Alexopoulos GS

Z

Zametkin AJ, Schwartz DJ, Ernst M, Cohen RM: Is research in normal and ill children involving radiation exposure ethical? (letter) 1060 (No)
Zarin DA see McIntyre JS; Pincus HA
Zhang M, Owen RR, Pope SK, Smith GR: Cost-effectiveness of clozapine monitoring after the first 6 months, 954 (Oc)
Zieglgänsberger W see Sass H
Zima BT, Wells KB, Benjamin B, Duan N: Mental health problems among homeless mothers: relationship to service use and child mental health problems, 332 (Ap)
Zis AP see Lam RW